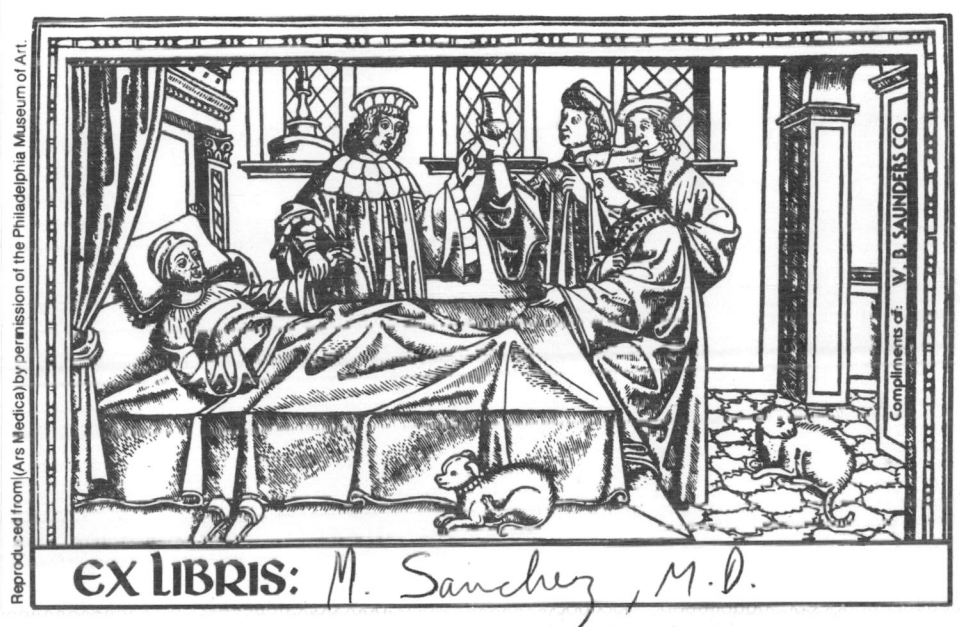

EX LIBRIS: M. Sanchez, M.D.

Harrison's
PRINCIPLES OF INTERNAL MEDICINE

EDITORS OF PREVIOUS EDITIONS

T. R. Harrison, Editor-in-Chief, Editions 1, 2, 3, 4, 5

W. R. Resnik, Editor, Editions 1, 2, 3, 4, 5

M. M. Wintrobe, Editor, Editions 1, 2, 3, 4, 5
      Editor-in-Chief, Editions 6, 7

G. W. Thorn, Editor, Editions 1, 2, 3, 4, 5, 6, 7
      Editor-in-Chief, Edition 8

R. D. Adams, Editor, Editions 2, 3, 4, 5, 6, 7, 8

P. B. Beeson, Editor, Editions 1, 2

I. L. Bennett, Jr., Editor, Editions 3, 4, 5, 6

E. Braunwald, Editor, Editions 6, 7, 8

K. J. Isselbacher, Editor, Editions 6, 7, 8

R. G. Petersdorf, Editor, Editions 6, 7, 8

Harrison's
PRINCIPLES OF INTERNAL MEDICINE

Ninth Edition

Miguel A. Sanchez, M.D.

Editors

KURT J. ISSELBACHER, A.B., M.D.
Mallinckrodt Professor of Medicine, Harvard
Medical School; Physician and Chief,
Gastrointestinal Unit, Massachusetts General
Hospital, Boston

RAYMOND D. ADAMS, B.A., M.A., M.D.,
M.A. (Hon.), D.Sc. (Hon.), M.D. (Hon.)   Bullard
Professor of Neuropathology, Emeritus, Harvard
Medical School; Consultant Neurologist and
Formerly Chief of Neurology Service,
Massachusetts General Hospital; Director, Eunice
K. Shriver Research Center, Boston; Médicin
Adjoint, L'Hôpital Cantonale de Lausanne,
Lausanne

EUGENE BRAUNWALD, A.B., M.D., M.A.
(Hon.)   Hersey Professor of the Theory and
Practice of Physic (Medicine), Harvard Medical
School; Physician-in-Chief, Peter Bent Brigham
Hospital, Boston

ROBERT G. PETERSDORF, A.B., M.D.,
D.Sc. (Hon.)   Professor of Medicine, Harvard
Medical School, Boston; President, Affiliated
Hospitals Center

JEAN D. WILSON, B.A., M.D.   Professor of
Internal Medicine and Director, McDermott Center
for Growth and Development, University of Texas
Health Science Center at Dallas, Dallas

McGRAW-HILL BOOK COMPANY   New York   St. Louis   San Francisco   Auckland   Bogotá
Hamburg   Johannesburg   London   Madrid   Mexico
Montreal   New Delhi   Panama   Paris   São Paulo   Singapore
Sydney   Tokyo   Toronto

Harrison's
Principles of Internal Medicine

1234567890 DODO 7832109

Foreign Editions
FRENCH (Seventh Edition)—Flammarion, © 1975
ITALIAN (Seventh Edition)—Casa Editrice Dr. Francesco Vallardi, © 1976
POLISH (Fifth Edition)—Panstwowy Zakland Wydawnictw Lekarskich, © 1971
PORTUGUESE (Eighth Edition)—Editora Guanabara Koogan, S.A., © 1981 (est.)
SPANISH (Eighth Edition)—La Prensa Medica Mexicana, © 1979
JAPANESE (Eighth Edition)—Hirokawa, © 1978
GREEK (Eighth Edition)—G. Parissianos © 1979

This book was set in Times Roman by Rocappi, Inc.
The editors were J. Dereck Jeffers, Richard S. Laufer, and Timothy Armstrong. The indexer was Philip James; the designer was Merrill Haber; the production supervisor was Jeanne Selzam.
R. R. Donnelley & Sons Company was printer and binder.

Library of Congress Cataloging in Publication Data

Harrison, Tinsley Randolph, date   ed.
   Harrison's Principles of internal medicine.

   Includes bibliographies and index.
   1. Internal medicine.   I. Isselbacher, Kurt J.
II. Title.   III.   Title: Principles of internal medicine.
RC46.H32   1980   616′.026   79-20855
ISBN 0-07-032068-3

        LC CIP DATA (2 vol. ed)
RC46.H32   1980b   616′.026   79-21372
ISBN 0-07-032069-1 (set)

This edition is dedicated to the Editor-in-Chief of this text during its first five editions, Tinsley R. Harrison.

From time to time a personality scintillates across the medical firmament who dazzles all beholders. Tinsley Harrison was such a person. A delightful, vivacious, passionate physician, he stimulated everyone with whom he came in contact, and he placed an indelible stamp on the medical events of his day.

As a thoughtful physician he excelled in the care of the sick, and the words which he penned for the first edition of this book reflect the importance which he attached to his role as a physician:

No greater opportunity or obligation can fall the lot of a human being than to be a physician. In the care of the suffering he needs technical skill, scientific knowledge, and human understanding. He who uses these with courage, humility, and wisdom will provide a unique service for his fellow man and will build an enduring edifice of character within himself. The physician should ask of his destiny no more than this, and he should be content with no less.

These words express the philosophy of the original editors and of all those who have followed. The patient was always in the center of the stage. To put the disease first, to refer to the patient as "a case" would arouse Tinsley's wrath.

Few people of his generation surpassed him as a bedside teacher. He had the remarkable ability to objectify an important clinical finding and to cite all relevant literature without disquieting the patient. Indeed his clinical analysis usually gained the confidence and respect of his patient in a most reassuring manner.

His originality in selecting clinical problems and investigating them by the available physiological methods, especially disorders of the heart and circulation, are familiar to all contemporary scholars. His accounts of his observations and studies were, and continue to be, models of lucid exposition.

To those of us who had the privilege of working with Tinsley on successive editions of this book, he was an unforgettable colleague and friend. It was he and his friend Morris Fischbein, then editor of the *Journal of the American Medical Association*, who saw the need of a textbook suited to the curriculum of American medical schools and resident training programs. It was Ted Philips, then an officer of the Blakiston Publishing Company, who translated Tinsley's ideas into a new type of textbook which soon was to have worldwide influence. Under his superb editorship each edition was a kind of experiment in ways to meet the changing needs of elementary and advanced students of medicine.

In the late summer of 1978, as this edition was being prepared, Tinsley succumbed to a long and distressing illness. It is to the memory of this great physician, whose life and works have so inspired us, that this, the ninth edition of *Harrison's*, is dedicated.

THE EDITORS

ABBREVIATED CONTENTS

CONTENTS

**PART THREE
BIOLOGICAL CONSIDERATIONS IN THE
APPROACH TO CLINICAL MEDICINE**

Section 1 Genetics and human disease

Section 2 Clinical immunology

Diseases of under- and overproduction of
immune globulins 325

Diseases of immune-mediated injury

Section 3 Clinical pharmacology

Section 4 Nutritional disorders

Plates 1 to 8 254

*1-1   Dermatofibroma   1-2   Acrochordon   1-3   Angio-
keratomas   1-4   Café au lait macules   1-5   Acne*

*2-1   Dermatophytosis   2-2   Eczematous dermatitis   2-3
Localized lichenification   2-4   Melasma (chloasma)   2-5
Milia   2-6   Psoriasis*

*3-1   Perleche   3-2   Rosacea   3-3   Seborrheic dermatitis
3-4   Seborrheic keratosis   3-5   Senile angioma ("cherry red
spot")   3-6   Senile lentigo*

*4-1   Senile sebaceous adenoma   4-2   Solar keratosis   4-3
Spider nevus   4-4   Tinea versicolor   4-5   Verruca vulgaris
4-6   Xanthelasma*

*5-1   Necrobiosis lipoidica diabeticorum   5-2   Pretibial myx-
edema   5-3   Pyoderma gangrenosum   5-4   "Palpable" purpura with inflammation occurring in gonococcemia   5-5
Peutz-Jeghers syndrome   5-6   Contact eczematous dermatitis*

*6-1   Lentigo maligna melanoma   6-2   Superficial spreading
melanoma   6-3   Nodular   melanoma   6-4   Superficial
spreading melanoma, superficially invasive*

*7-1   Normal optic nerve and retina   7-2   Glaucomatous optic
disk with secondary atrophy   7-3   Drusen of the optic nerve
head   7-4   Angioid streaks   7-5   Primary optic atrophy
7-6   Early papilledema   7-7   Retentive pigmentosa   7-8
Band keratopathy*

*8-1   Schemic optic neuritis with temporal arteritis   8-2   Cho-
lesterol embolus in retinal arteriole   8-3   Diabetic retinopathy
microaneurysm   8-4   Retinitis proliferans in diabetes mellitus
8-5   Roth spot with subacute bacterial endocarditis   8-6
Central retinal vein thrombosis   8-7   Dislocated lens in Marfan's disease   8-8   Kaiser-Fleisher ring in Wilson's disease*

Plates 9 and 10 285

*9-1   Normal   marrow   9-2   Megaloblastic   marrow   9-3
Erythroid hyperplasia   9-4   Sideroblastic   anemia   9-5
Normal blood smear   9-6   Megaloblastic anemia   9-7
Iron-deficiency anemia   9-8   β thallasemia intermedia   9-9
Myeloid metaplasia   9-10   Uremia   9-11   Liver disease
9-12   Spur-cell anemia   9-13   Hereditary   spherocytosis
9-14   Immunohemolytic anemia   9-15   Traumatic hemolysis
9-16   Sickle-cell anemia*

*10-1   A Normal granulocyte   B Normal monocyte and lym-
phocyte   10-2   A Normal eosinophil   B Normal basophil
10-3   Normal granulocyte precursors in marrow   10-4   Neutrophils with toxic granulation   10-5   Band with Döhle body
10-6   Hypersegmentation   10-7   A Chédiak-Higashi anomaly   B Pelger-Hüet anomaly   10-8   Reactive lymphocytes
(infectious mononucleosis)   10-9   Chronic granulocytic leukemia   10-10   Acute myelogenous leukemia: myeloblast with
Auer rod   10-11   Chronic lymphocytic leukemia   10-12
Acute lymphoblastic leukemia (marrow)   10-13   Hodgkin's
disease: Reed-Sternberg cell in marrow   10-14   Non-Hodgkin's nodular lymphoma (lymph node)   10-15   Multiple myeloma (marrow)*

LIST OF CONTRIBUTORS

RAYMOND D. ADAMS, B.A., M.A., M.D., M.A. (Hon.), D.Sc. (Hon.), M.D. (Hon.)
Bullard Professor of Neuropathology, Emeritus, Harvard Medical School; Consultant Neurologist and Formerly Chief of Neurology Service, Massachusetts General Hospital; Director, Eunice K. Shriver Research Center, Boston; Médicin Adjoint, L'Hôpital Cantonale de Lausanne, Lausanne

JOHN W. ADAMSON, M.D.
Professor of Medicine, University of Washington School of Medicine; Head, Division of Hematology, Veterans Administration Medical Center, Seattle

RAYMOND ALEXANIAN, M.D.
Professor of Medicine, The University of Texas M. D. Anderson Hospital and Tumor Institute, Houston

ELLIOT ALPERT, M.D.
Associate Professor of Medicine, Harvard Medical School; Assistant Physician, Gastrointestinal Unit, Massachusetts General Hospital, Boston

JOSEPH S. ALPERT, M.D.
Professor of Medicine, University of Massachusetts Medical School; Director, Division of Cardiovascular Medicine, University of Massachusetts Medical Center, Worcester

ROBERT J. ANDERSON, M.D.
Associate Professor of Medicine, Division of Renal Diseases, University of Colorado Medical Center, Denver

ARTHUR K. ASBURY, M.D.
Professor of Neurology, University of Pennsylvania School of Medicine; Chairman, Department of Neurology, Hospital of the University of Pennsylvania, Philadelphia

KARL-ERIK ÅSTRÖM, M.D.
Associate Professor of Neuropathology, Harvard Medical School; Associate Neuropathologist, Massachusetts General Hospital, Boston

K. FRANK AUSTEN, M.D.
Theodore B. Bayles Professor of Medicine, Harvard Medical School; Physician-in-Chief, Robert Breck Brigham Hospital, A Division of the Affiliated Hospitals Center, Inc., Boston

ROBERT AUSTRIAN, M.D.
Professor and Chairman, Department of Research Medicine, University of Pennsylvania School of Medicine, Philadelphia

BERNARD M. BABIOR, M.D.
Professor of Medicine, Tufts University School of Medicine; Division of Adult Hematology, New England Medical Center, Boston

JOSEPH H. BATES, M.D.
Chief, Medical Service, Veterans Administration Hospital; Professor of Medicine, University of Arkansas School of Medicine, Little Rock

HARRY N. BEATY, M.D.
Professor and Chairman, Department of Medicine, University of Vermont College of Medicine, Burlington

ARTHUR L. BEAUDET, M.D.
Associate Professor of Pediatrics and Cell Biology, Baylor College of Medicine; Investigator, Howard Hughes Medical Institute, Houston

JOHN E. BENNETT, M.D.
Head, Clinical Mycology Section, LCI, National Institute of Allergy and Infectious Disease, National Institutes of Health, Bethesda

EDWIN L. BIERMAN, M.D.
Professor of Medicine and Head, Division of Metabolism and Endocrinology, Department of Medicine, University of Washington School of Medicine, Seattle

ALAN L. BISNO, M.D.
Professor of Medicine and Chief, Division of Infectious Disease, Department of Medicine, University of Tennessee College of Medicine, Memphis

AREND BOUHUYS, M.D., D.Sc. (Med.), M.A. (Hon.) (deceased)
Professor of Physiology, Physiological Laboratory, University of Utrecht, The Netherlands; Clinical Professor of Environmental Medicine, New York University School of Medicine, New York

ROBERT M. BOYAR, M.D. (deceased)
Associate Professor of Internal Medicine, University of Texas Health Science Center at Dallas, Dallas

WALTER G. BRADLEY, M.D.
Professor of Neurology, Tufts University School of Medicine; Associate Director, Neurology Service, New England Medical Center, Boston

EUGENE BRAUNWALD, A.B., M.D., M.A. (Hon.)
Hersey Professor of the Theory and Practice of Physic (Medicine), Harvard Medical School; Physician-in-Chief, Peter Bent Brigham Hospital, Boston

BARRY M. BRENNER, M.D., M.A. (Hon.)
Samuel A. Levine Professor of Medicine, Harvard Medical School; Physician and Director, Renal Division, Peter Bent Brigham Hospital, Boston

MICHAEL S. BROWN, M.D.
Paul J. Thomas Professor of Genetics, University of Texas Health Science Center at Dallas; Senior Attending Physician, Parkland Memorial Hospital, Dallas

H. FRANKLIN BUNN, M.D.
Professor of Medicine, Harvard Medical School; Director, Hematology Division, Peter Bent Brigham Hospital, Boston

GEORGE P. CANELLOS, M.D.
Associate Professor of Medicine, Harvard Medical School; Chief, Division of Medical Oncology, Sidney Farber Cancer Center; Senior Associate in Medicine, Peter Bent Brigham Hospital, Boston

CHARLES B. CARPENTER, M.D.
Associate Professor of Medicine, Harvard Medical School; Senior Associate in Medicine, Peter Bent Brigham Hospital, Boston

CHARLES C. J. CARPENTER, M.D.
Professor and Chairman, Department of Medicine, Case Western Reserve University School of Medicine; Physician-in-Chief, University Hospitals, Cleveland

WILLIAM A. CAUSEY, M.D.
Associate Professor of Medicine, University of Mississippi School of Medicine; Chief, Medical Service, Veterans Administration Hospital, Jackson

KEITH H. CHIAPPA, M.D.
Instructor in Neurology, Harvard Medical School; Director, EEG Laboratories, Massachusetts General Hospital, Boston

BAYARD CLARKSON, M.D.
Associate Chairman and Chief, Hematology Lymphoma Service, Department of Medicine, Memorial Hospital, Memorial Sloan-Kettering Cancer Center, New York

LEIGHTON E. CLUFF, M.D.
Vice President, The Robert Wood Johnson Foundation, Princeton

FREDRIC L. COE, M.D.
Professor of Medicine and Physiology, Pritzker School of Medicine, University of Chicago; Director, Division of Renal Medicine, Michael Reese Hospital and Medical Center, Chicago

ALAN S. COHEN, M.D.
Chief of Medicine and Director, Thorndike Memorial Laboratory, Boston City University; Conrad Wesselhoeft Professor of Medicine, Boston University School of Medicine, Boston

PETER F. COHN, M.D.
Associate Professor of Medicine, Harvard Medical School; Director, Clinical Cardiology Service, Peter Bent Brigham Hospital, Boston

MAX D. COOPER, M.D.
Professor of Pediatrics and Microbiology, Department of Pediatrics, University of Alabama in Birmingham, The Medical Center, Birmingham

RICHARD A. COOPER, M.D.
Professor of Medicine, University of Pennsylvania School of Medicine; Chief, Hematology-Oncology Section, Hospital of the University of Pennsylvania; Director, University of Pennsylvania Cancer Center, Philadelphia

LAWRENCE COREY, M.D.
Assistant Professor, Laboratory Medicine and Microbiology; Adjunct Assistant Professor, Medicine and Pediatrics, University of Washington School of Medicine; Head, Virology Division, Laboratory Medicine, Childrens Orthopedic Hospital, Seattle

EUGENE P. CRONKITE, M.D.
Chairman, Medical Department, Brookhaven National Laboratory, Associate Universities, Inc., Upton

DAVID C. DALE, M.D.
Professor of Medicine and Associate Chairman, Department of Medicine, University of Washington School of Medicine, Seattle

JAMES E. DALEN, M.D.
Professor and Chairman, Department of Medicine, University of Massachusetts Medical School; Physician-in-Chief, University of Massachusetts Hospital, Worcester

CHANDLER R. DAWSON, M.D.
Professor of Ophthalmology, Francis I. Proctor Foundation for Research in Ophthalmology, University of California, San Francisco; Director, WHO Collaborating Center for Prevention of Blindness and Trachoma, San Francisco

G. ROBERT DELONG, M.D.
Assistant Professor of Neurology, Harvard Medical School; Associate Neurologist and Associate Pediatrician, Massachusetts General Hospital, Boston

VINCENT T. DeVITA, JR., M.D.
Director, Division of Cancer Treatment, National Cancer Institute, National Institutes of Health, Bethesda

JULES L. DIENSTAG, M.D.
Assistant Professor of Medicine, Harvard Medical School; Assistant in Medicine, Gastrointestinal Unit, Massachusetts General Hospital, Boston

JAMES J. DINEEN, M.D.
Assistant Professor of Medicine, Harvard Medical School; Associate Physician, Massachusetts General Hospital, Boston

ROBERT G. DLUHY, M.D.
Associate Professor of Medicine, Harvard Medical School; Senior Associate in Medicine, Peter Bent Brigham Hospital, Boston

KENDALL EMERSON, JR., M.D.
Clinical Professor of Medicine, Emeritus, Harvard Medical School; Physician, Emeritus, Peter Bent Brigham Hospital, Boston

KARL ENGELMAN, M.D., M.A. (Hon.)
Associate Professor of Medicine and Pharmacology, University of Pennsylvania School of Medicine; Chief, Hypertension and Clinical Pharmacology Section, and Director, Clinical Research Center, Hospital of the University of Pennsylvania, Philadelphia

MURRAY J. FAVUS, M.D.
Assistant Professor of Medicine, Pritzker School of Medicine, University of Chicago; Attending Physician, Division of Endocrinology and Metabolism, Michael Reese Hospital and Medical Center, Chicago

ALEXANDER FEFER, M.D.
Professor of Medicine, University of Washington School of Medicine; Head, Division of Oncology, University of Washington Hospital, Seattle

PHILIP J. FIALKOW, M.D.
Professor and Vice-Chairman, Department of Medicine, and Professor of Genetics, University of Washington; Chief, Medical Service, Veterans Administration Medical Center, Seattle

JAMES B. FIELD, M.D.
Rutherford Professor of Medicine and Head, Division of Endocrinology and Metabolism, Baylor College of Medicine; Director, Diabetes Research Laboratory, St. Luke's Episcopal Hospital, Houston

C. MILLER FISHER, M.D.
Professor of Neurology, Harvard Medical School; Neurologist and Neuropathologist, Massachusetts General Hospital, Boston

ALFRED P. FISHMAN, M.D.
William Maul Measey Professor of Medicine, University of Pennsylvania School of Medicine; Director, Cardiovascular-Pulmonary Division, Hospital of the University of Pennsylvania, Philadelphia

THOMAS B. FITZPATRICK, M.D., Ph.D.
Edward Wigglesworth Professor and Chairman, Department of Dermatology, Harvard Medical School; Chief, Dermatology Service, Massachusetts General Hospital, Boston

DANIEL W. FOSTER, M.D.
Professor of Internal Medicine, University of Texas Health Science Center at Dallas, Dallas

PAUL A. FRIEDMAN, M.D.
Assistant Professor of Clinical Pharmacology, Harvard Medical School, Boston

WILLIAM F. FRIEDMAN, M.D.
Professor and Chairman, Department of Pediatrics, Center for the Health Sciences, University of California, Los Angeles; J. H. Nicholson Professor of Pediatric Cardiology, University of California, Los Angeles School of Medicine, Los Angeles

PIERCE GARDNER, M.D.
Professor of Medicine and Pediatrics, Division of Biological Sciences, Department of Medicine, Pritzker School of Medicine, University of Chicago, Chicago

J. BERNARD L. GEE, M.D.
Associate Professor of Medicine, Yale University School of Medicine; Attending Physician, Yale-New Haven Hospital, New Haven

JAMES GERMAN, M.D.
Adjunct Professor, The Rockefeller University; Senior Investigator, The Lindsley F. Kimball Research Institute of the New York Blood Center, New York

ELOISE R. GIBLETT, M.D.
Research Professor of Medicine, University of Washington School of Medicine; Head, Immunogenetics, Puget Sound Blood Center, Seattle

WILLIAM GILL, M.D.
Associate Professor, Department of Surgery (Urology), University of Chicago Hospitals and Clinics, Chicago

BRUCE C. GILLILAND, M.D.
Professor of Medicine and Laboratory Medicine, University of Washington School of Medicine; Medical Director, Providence Hospital, Seattle

RICHARD J. GLASSOCK, M.D.
Professor of Medicine, University of California, Los Angeles School of Medicine; Chief, Division of Nephrology and Hypertension, Harbor-University of California, Los Angeles Medical Center, Los Angeles

GERALD GLICK, M.D.
Senior Consultant, Cardiovascular Institute, Michael Reese Hospital and Medical Center; Clinical Professor of Medicine, Pritzker School of Medicine, University of Chicago, Chicago

ROBERT M. GLICKMAN, M.D.
Associate Professor of Medicine, Columbia University College of Physicians and Surgeons; Chief of Gastroenterology, Presbyterian Hospital, New York

STEPHEN F. GOLDFINGER, M.D.
Associate Professor of Medicine and Associate Dean of Continuing Education, Harvard Medical School; Physician, Gastrointestinal Unit, Massachusetts General Hospital, Boston

PAUL GOLDHABER, D.D.S.
Dean and Professor of Periodontology, Harvard School of Dental Medicine, Boston

JOSEPH L. GOLDSTEIN, M.D.
Paul J. Thomas Professor and Chairman, Department of Molecular Genetics, University of Texas Health Science Center at Dallas; Senior Attending Physician, Parkland Memorial Hospital, Dallas

HARVEY M. GOLOMB, M.D.
Associate Professor of Medicine, Section of Hematology/Oncology, Department of Medicine, Pritzker School of Medicine, University of Chicago, Chicago

ROBERT W. GRAEBNER, M.D.
Assistant Clinical Professor, Department of Neurology, University of Wisconsin, Madison

J. THOMAS GRAYSTON, M.D.
Vice President for Health Affairs, Professor of Epidemiology, School of Public Health and Community Medicine, University of Washington, Seattle

NORTON J. GREENBERGER, M.D.
Professor and Chairman, Department of Medicine, University of Kansas Medical Center, College of Health Sciences, Kansas City

JAMES E. GRIFFIN III, M.D.
Assistant Professor of Internal Medicine, University of Texas Health Science Center at Dallas, Dallas

RICHARD L. GUERRANT, M.D.
Associate Professor of Medicine, Department of Medicine, University of Virginia Medical Center, Charlottesville

JAMES P. HARNISCH, M.D.
Clinical Assistant Professor, Department of Medicine, University of Washington School of Medicine, Seattle

DONALD H. HARTER, M.D.
Charles L. Mix Professor and Chairman, Department of Neurology, The Medical School, Northwestern University, Chicago

HARLEY A. HAYNES, M.D.
Associate Professor of Dermatology, Harvard Medical School; Director, Dermatology Division, Peter Bent Brigham Hospital, Boston

THOMAS R. HENDRIX, M.D.
Professor of Medicine and Chief, Gastroenterology Division, The Johns Hopkins University School of Medicine, Baltimore

JAN V. HIRSCHMANN, M.D.
Assistant Professor of Medicine, University of Washington School of Medicine, Medical Comprehensive Care Unit, Veterans Administration Hospital, Seattle

FRED HOCHBERG, M.D.
Assistant Professor of Neurology, Harvard Medical School; Assistant Neurologist, Massachusetts General Hospital, Boston

PAUL D. HOEPRICH, M.D.
Professor of Medicine and Pathology and Chief, Section of Infectious and Immunologic Diseases, Department of Internal Medicine, University of California-Davis, Sacramento

JOHN H. HOLBROOK, M.D.
Associate Professor of Medicine, Division of General Internal Medicine, Department of Internal Medicine, University of Utah Medical Center, Salt Lake City

MICHAEL F. HOLICK, M.D., Ph.D.
Assistant Professor of Medicine, Harvard Medical School; Clinical Assistant in Medicine, Massachusetts General Hospital, Boston

O. BRYAN HOLLAND, M.D.
Assistant Professor of Internal Medicine, University of Texas Health Science Center at Dallas, Dallas

NORMAN K. HOLLENBERG, M.D.
Professor and Director of Physiologic Research, Department of Radiology, Harvard Medical School; Senior Associate in Medicine, Peter Bent Brigham Hospital, Boston

KING K. HOLMES, M.D.
Professor of Medicine, University of Washington School of Medicine; Head, Infectious Diseases, U.S. Public Health Service Hospital, Seattle

EDWARD W. HOOK, M.D.
Mulholland Professor of Medicine and Chairman, Department of Medicine, University of Virginia Medical Center; Physician-in-Chief, University of Virginia Hospital, Charlottesville

THOMAS H. HOSTETTER, M.D.
Instructor in Medicine, Harvard Medical School; Junior Associate in Medicine, Peter Bent Brigham Hospital, Boston

H. DAVID HUMES, M.D.
Assistant Professor of Medicine, University of Michigan Medical School, Ann Arbor

SIDNEY H. INGBAR, M.D.
William Bosworth Castle Professor of Medicine, Harvard Medical School; Director, Thorndike Laboratory, Beth Israel Hospital, Boston

ROLAND H. INGRAM, JR., M.D.
Associate Professor of Medicine, Harvard Medical School; Physician and Chief, Respiratory Division, Peter Bent Brigham Hospital, Boston

ELI IPP, M.D.
Instructor, Department of Medicine, Pritzker School of Medicine, The University of Chicago, Chicago

KURT J. ISSELBACHER, A.B., M.D.
Mallinckrodt Professor of Medicine, Harvard Medical School; Physician and Chief, Gastrointestinal Unit, Massachusetts General Hospital, Boston

PAUL I. JAGGER, M.D.
Adjunct Professor of Medicine, University of California, San Diego School of Medicine; Codirector, Clinical Research Center, University Hospital, University of California, San Diego Medical Center, San Diego

KHURSHEED N. JEEJEEBHOY, M.B.B.S., Ph.D., F.R.C.P. (Lond.), F.R.C.P. (Edin.), F.R.C.P. (C)
Professor of Medicine, University of Toronto; Head, Gastrointestinal Division, Toronto General Hospital, Toronto

CAROL J. JOHNS, M.D.
Associate Professor of Medicine, The Johns Hopkins University School of Medicine; Physician, The Johns Hopkins Hospital, Baltimore

JOSEPH E. JOHNSON III, M.D.
Professor and Chairman, Department of Medicine, Bowman-Gray School of Medicine, Winston-Salem

BYRON A. KAKULAS, M.D., F.R.A.C.P., M.R.C., Path., F.R.C.P.A.
Professor of Neuropathology, University of Western Australia, Perth; Senior Neuropathologist, Royal Perth Hospital, Perth

SATISH KATHPALIA, M.D.
Instructor in Medicine, Pritzker School of Medicine, University of Chicago; Attending Physician, Division of Renal Medicine, Michael Reese Hospital and Medical Center, Chicago

WILLIAM N. KELLEY, M.D.
Professor and Chairman, Department of Internal Medicine, University of Michigan Medical School, Ann Arbor

WILLIAM M. M. KIRBY, M.D.
Professor of Medicine, Division of Infectious Disease, University of Washington School of Medicine, Seattle

VERNON KNIGHT, M.D.
Professor and Chairman, Department of Microbiology and Immunology, Baylor College of Medicine; Senior Attending Physician, The Methodist Hospital, Houston

RAYMOND S. KOFF, M.D.
Professor of Medicine, Boston University School of Medicine; Chief, Hepatology Section, Boston University Medical Center and Veterans Administration Medical Center, Boston

PETER O. KOHLER, M.D.
Professor and Chairman, Department of Medicine, University of Arkansas for Medical Sciences; Chief, Medical Service, University Hospital, Little Rock

STEPHEN M. KRANE, M.D.
Professor of Medicine, Harvard Medical School; Physician and Chief, Arthritis Unit, Massachusetts General Hospital, Boston

J. THOMAS LaMONT, M.D.
Assistant Professor of Medicine, Harvard Medical School; Associate in Medicine, Division of Gastroenterology, Peter Bent Brigham Hospital, Boston

ALEXANDER R. LAWTON III, M.D.
Professor of Pediatrics and Microbiology, The Medical Center, The University of Alabama in Birmingham, Birmingham

J. MICHAEL LAZARUS, M.D.
Associate Professor of Medicine, Harvard Medical School; Associate in Medicine, Peter Bent Brigham Hospital, Boston

G. RICHARD LEE, M.D.
Professor of Medicine and Dean, University of Utah College of Medicine; University of Utah Hospital, Salt Lake City

A. MARTIN LERNER, M.D.
Professor of Medicine and Head, Division of Infectious Disease, Department of Medicine, Wayne State University School of Medicine; Chief, Hutzel Hospital Medical Unit, Detroit

NORMAN G. LEVINSKY, M.D.
Wade Professor and Chairman, Division of Medicine, Boston University School of Medicine; Physician-in-Chief and Director, Evans Memorial Department of Clinical Research, University Hospital, Boston

BERNARD LOWN, M.D.
Professor of Cardiology, Harvard School of Public Health; Physician, Peter Bent Brigham Hospital, Boston

WALTER C. MacDONALD, M.D.
Professor of Medicine and Head, Division of Gastroenterology, University of British Columbia, Vancouver

JAMES D. MADDEN, M.D.
Clinical Associate Professor of Obstetrics and Gynecology, Health Science Center, University of Texas at Dallas, Dallas

LEONARD L. MADISON, M.D.
Professor, Department of Internal Medicine, University of Texas Health Science Center at Dallas, Dallas

HENRY J. MANKIN, M.D.
Edith M. Ashley Professor of Orthopedic Surgery, Harvard Medical School; Chief, Orthopedic Service, Massachusetts General Hospital, Boston

MART MANNIK, M.D.
Professor of Medicine, Adjunct Professor of Microbiology, and Head, Division of Rheumatology, Department of Medicine, University of Washington School of Medicine, Seattle

ROGER J. MAY, M.D.
Instructor in Medicine, Harvard Medical School; Assistant in Medicine, Gastrointestinal Unit, Massachusetts General Hospital, Boston

JANET W. McARTHUR, M.D.
Professor of Obstetrics and Gynecology, Harvard Medical School; Gynecologist, Massachusetts General Hospital, Boston

E. R. McFADDEN, JR., M.D.
Associate Professor of Medicine, Harvard Medical School; Associate Physician, Peter Bent Brigham Hospital, Boston

J. DENIS McGARRY, Ph.D.
Professor of Internal Medicine and Biochemistry, University of Texas Health Science Center at Dallas, Dallas

JAMES E. McGUIGAN, M.D.
Professor and Chairman, Department of Medicine, University of Florida College of Medicine, Gainesville

RIMA McLEOD, M.D.
Assistant Professor of Medicine, Division of Infectious Disease, Department of Medicine, Michael Reese Hospital and Medical Center, Chicago

JOHN P. MERRILL, M.D.
Professor of Medicine, Harvard Medical School; Director Emeritus, Cardiorenal Section, and Physician, Peter Bent Brigham Hospital, Boston

URS A. MEYER, M.D.
Professor of Clinical Pharmacology, Department of Medicine, University of Zurich Hospital, Zurich

MARTIN C. MIHM, JR., M.D.
Associate Professor of Pathology, Harvard Medical School; Associate Pathologist and Dermatologist, Massachusetts General Hospital, Boston

MYRON MILLER, M.D., F.A.C.P.
Professor of Medicine, State University of New York Upstate Medical Center; Chief, Medical Service, Veterans Administration Medical Center, Syracuse

JAY P. MOHR, M.D.
Professor of Neurology, University of South Alabama; Chief, Neurology Service, South Alabama University Hospital, Mobile

KENNETH M. MOSER, M.D.
Professor of Medicine, University of California, San Diego School of Medicine; Director, Pulmonary Division, University of California, San Diego Medical Center, San Diego

ARNOLD M. MOSES, M.D.
Director of Clinical Research Center and Professor of Medicine, State University of New York Upstate Medical Center; Chief, Endocrinology, Veterans Administration Medical Center, Syracuse

DAVID B. MOSHER, M.D.
Clinical Instructor in Dermatology, Harvard Medical School; Assistant in Dermatology, Massachusetts General Hospital, Boston

JOHN F. MURRAY, M.D.
Professor of Medicine, University of California, San Francisco; Chief, Chest Service, San Francisco General Hospital, San Francisco

ROBERT J. MYERBURG, M.D.
Professor of Medicine and Director, Division of Cardiology, Department of Medicine, University of Miami School of Medicine, Miami

JAMES C. NIEDERMAN, M.D.
Associate Clinical Professor of Epidemiology and Medicine, Department of Epidemiology and Public Health, Yale University School of Medicine, New Haven

HYMIE L. NOSSEL, M.D.
Professor of Medicine, College of Physicians and Surgeons, Columbia University; Attending Physician, Presbyterian Hospital, New York

JOHN A. OATES, M.D.
The Joe and Morris Werthan Professor of Investigative Medicine, Department of Medicine and Pharmacology, Vanderbilt University Hospital, Nashville

JERROLD M. OLEFSKY, M.D.
Professor of Medicine and Head, Division of Endocrinology and Metabolism, University of Colorado Medical Center, Denver

ROBERT A. O'ROURKE, M.D.
Professor of Medicine and Director, Division of Cardiovascular Diseases, University of Texas Health Science Center at San Antonio, San Antonio

JOHN A. PARRISH, M.D.
Associate Professor of Dermatology, Harvard Medical School; Assistant Dermatologist, Massachusetts General Hospital, Boston

MADHUKAR A. PATHAK, M.B., Ph.D.
Senior Associate in Dermatology, Harvard Medical School; Biochemist, Massachusetts General Hospital, Boston

LAWRENCE L. PELLETIER, JR., M.D.
Associate Professor of Internal Medicine, University of North Dakota School of Medicine; Chief, Infectious Diseases Section, Fargo Veterans Administration Hospital, Fargo

PETER L. PERINE, M.D.
Director, Yaws Control Assistance Programs, Research and Development Division, Bureau of Smallpox Eradication, Center for Disease Control, Atlanta

ROBERT G. PETERSDORF, A.B., M.D., D.Sc. (Hon.)
Professor of Medicine, Harvard Medical School, Boston; President, Affiliated Hospitals Center

KIRK L. PETERSON, M.D.
Associate Professor of Medicine, University of California, San Diego School of Medicine; Director, Cardiac Catheterization Laboratory, University of California, San Diego Medical Center, San Diego

JAMES J. PLORDE, M.D.
Professor of Medicine and Laboratory Medicine, University of Washington School of Medicine; Chief, Microbiology Laboratory, Veterans Administration Hospital, Seattle

JOHN W. POPP, JR., M.D.
Clinical Assistant Professor of Medicine, University of South Carolina School of Medicine, Columbia

DAVID C. POSKANZER, M.D., M.P.H.
Associate Professor of Neurology, Harvard Medical School; Associate Neurologist and Epidemiologist, Massachusetts General Hospital, Boston

JOHN T. POTTS, JR., M.D.
Professor of Medicine, Harvard Medical School; Chief, Endocrine Unit, Massachusetts General Hospital, Boston

LAWRIE W. POWELL, M.D.
Professor of Medicine, Department of Medicine, University of Queensland; Physician, Royal Brisbane Hospital, Brisbane

JOEL M. RAPPEPORT, M.D.
Assistant Professor of Medicine, Harvard Medical School; Associate in Medicine, Peter Bent Brigham Hospital, Boston

C. GEORGE RAY, M.D.
Professor of Pathology, Department of Pathology, Microbiology Section, Clinical Laboratories, University of Arizona College of Medicine, Tucson

JEAN J. REBEIZ, M.D.
Assistant Professor of Neurology and Neuropathology, American University of Beirut; Neurologist and Neuropathologist, American University Hospital, Beirut

PETER REICH, M.D.
Associate Professor of Psychiatry, Harvard Medical School; Chief, Psychiatric Services, Affiliated Hospitals Center, Boston

JACK S. REMINGTON, M.D.
Professor of Medicine, Division of Infectious Disease, Department of Medicine, Stanford University School of Medicine; Chief, Division of Allergy, Immunology, and Infectious Disease, Palo Alto Medical Research Foundation, Palo Alto

EDWARD P. RICHARDSON, JR., M.D.
Professor of Neuropathology, Harvard Medical School; Neuropathologist, Massachusetts General Hospital, Boston

ALAN R. RONALD, M.D.
Professor and Head, Department of Medical Microbiology, University of Manitoba, Winnipeg

LEON E. ROSENBERG, M.D.
Professor of Human Genetics, Medicine, and Pediatrics and Chairman, Department of Human Genetics, Yale University School of Medicine; Attending Physician, Yale–New Haven Hospital, New Haven

JOHN ROSS, JR., M.D.
Professor of Medicine, University of California, School of Medicine; Director, Cardiovascular Division, Department of Medicine, University of California, San Diego Medical Center, La Jolla

RICHARD S. ROSS, M.D.
Professor of Medicine (Cardiology) and Dean of the Medical Faculty, The Johns Hopkins University School of Medicine, Baltimore

ARTHUR H. RUBENSTEIN, M.D.
Professor of Medicine, Pritzker School of Medicine, The University of Chicago Medical Center, Chicago

CYRUS E. RUBIN, M.D.
Professor of Medicine, Division of Gastroenterology, University of Washington School of Medicine, Seattle

DANIEL RUDMAN, M.D.
Professor of Medicine and Surgery, Emory University School of Medicine; Director, Clinical Research Facility, Emory University Hospital, Atlanta

FUAD SABRA, M.D., F.A.C.P.
Professor of Neurology and Head, Division of Neurology, Medical School, American University of Beirut; Neurologist, American University Hospital, Beirut

MARIA SALAM-ADAMS, M.D.
Assistant Professor of Neurology, Harvard Medical School; Clinical and Research Fellow in Children's Neurology, Massachusetts General Hospital, Boston

MERLE A. SANDE, M.D.
Professor of Medicine and Vice Chairman, Department of Medicine, University of Virginia Medical Center, Charlottesville

JAY P. SANFORD, M.D.
Dean, Uniformed Services University of the Health Sciences, Bethesda

NICHOLAS A. SAUNDERS, M.B.B.S., F.R.A.C.P., F.R.C.P. (C)
Senior Lecturer, Department of Medicine, University of Newcastle, Newcastle

DENNIS SCHABERG, M.D.
Assistant Professor of Medicine, University of Michigan School of Medicine, Ann Arbor

I. HERBERT SCHEINBERG, M.D.
Professor of Medicine, Albert Einstein College of Medicine; Attending Physician and Head, Division of Genetic Medicine, Hospital of the Albert Einstein College of Medicine, New York

R. NEIL SCHIMKE, M.D., F.A.C.P.
Professor of Medicine and Pediatrics and Chief, Division of Metabolism, Endocrinology, and Genetics, University of Kansas Medical Center, College of Health Sciences, Kansas City

LESLIE J. SCHOENFIELD, M.D.
Professor of Medicine, University of California, Los Angeles; Director, Division of Gastroenterology, Cedars-Sinai Medical Center, Los Angeles

ROBERT W. SCHRIER, M.D.
Professor and Chairman, Department of Medicine, University of Colorado Health Sciences Center, University of Colorado Hospitals, Denver

DAVID A. SHAFRITZ, M.D.
Associate Professor of Medicine and Cell Biology, Albert Einstein College of Medicine, New York

DAVID G. SHAND, Ph.D., M.B.
Professor of Pharmacology and Medicine and Chief, Division of Clinical Pharmacology, Duke University Medical Center, Durham

CHARLES C. SHEPARD, M.D.
Chief, Leprosy and Rickettsia Branch, Center for Disease Control; Adjunct Associate Professor of Microbiology, Emory University School of Medicine, Atlanta

LOUIS M. SHERWOOD, M.D.
Professor of Medicine, Pritzker School of Medicine, University of Chicago, Physician-In-Chief and Chairman, Department of Medicine, Michael Reese Hospital and Medical Center, Chicago

ELIZABETH M. SHORT, M.D.
Assistant Professor of Medicine, Stanford University School of Medicine; Attending Physician, Stanford University Medical Center, Stanford

HARRY L. SHWACHMAN, M.D.
Professor of Pediatrics, Emeritus, Harvard Medical School; Senior Associate in Medicine, Children's Hospital Medical Center, Boston

WILLIAM SILEN, M.D.
Johnson and Johnson Professor of Surgery, Harvard Medical School; Surgeon-in-Chief, Beth Israel Hospital, Boston

FRED E. SILVERSTEIN, M.D.
Associate Professor of Medicine, Division of Gastroenterology, Department of Medicine, University of Washington School of Medicine, Seattle

DAVID W. SMITH, M.D.
Professor and Chairman, Department of Pediatrics, University of Rochester School of Medicine, Rochester

BURTON E. SOBEL, M.D.
Professor of Medicine and Director, Cardiovascular Division, Washington University; Cardiologist-in-Chief, Barnes Hospital, St. Louis

ARTHUR J. SOBER, M.D.
Assistant Professor of Dermatology, Harvard Medical School; Assistant Dermatologist, Massachusetts General Hospital, Boston

EDMUND H. SONNENBLICK, M.D.
Professor of Medicine and Chief, Division of Cardiology, Department of Medicine, Albert Einstein College of Medicine, New York

WESLEY W. SPINK, M.D., D.Sc. (Hon.)
Emeritus Regents' Professor of Medicine and Comparative Medicine, University of Minnesota Health Sciences Center, Minneapolis

WALTER STAMM, M.D.
Assistant Professor of Medicine, Division of Infectious Diseases, University of Washington School of Medicine; Physician, Harborview Medical Center, Seattle

WILLIAM W. STEAD, M.D.
Professor of Medicine, University of Arkansas School of Medicine, Little Rock; Director, Tuberculosis Program, Division of Communicable Diseases, Arkansas Department of Health

DANIEL J. STECHSCHULTE, M.D.
Professor of Medicine, Division of Allergy, Clinical Immunology, and Rheumatology, Department of Medicine, University of Kansas Medical Center, College of Health Sciences, Kansas City

GENE H. STOLLERMAN, M.D.
Professor and Chairman, Department of Medicine, University of Tennessee College of Medicine, Memphis

D. EUGENE STRANDNESS, JR., M.D.
Professor of Surgery, University of Washington School of Medicine, Seattle

DAVID H. P. STREETEN, M.B., D.Phil., F.R.C.P.
Professor of Medicine and Head, Section of Endocrinology, State University of New York Upstate Medical Center, Syracuse

E. DONNALL THOMAS, M.D.
Professor of Medicine and Head, Division of Oncology, University of Washington School of Medicine; Head, Division of Medical Oncology, Fred Hutchinson Cancer Research Center, Seattle

GEORGE W. THORN, M.D., M.A. (Hon.), LL.D (Hon.), D.Sc. (Hon.), M.D. (Hon.), F.R.C.P.
Hersey Professor of the Theory and Practice of Physic, Emeritus, and Samuel A. Levine Professor of Medicine, Emeritus, Harvard Medical School; Physician-In-Chief, Emeritus, Peter Bent Brigham Hospital, Boston

GENNARO M. TISI, M.D.
Associate Professor of Medicine, University of California, San Diego School of Medicine; Chief, Pulmonary Section, Veterans Administration Hospital, San Diego

PHILLIP P. TOSKES, M.D.
Professor of Medicine, University of Florida College of Medicine; Chief, Division of Gastroenterology, Gainesville Veterans Administration Medical Center, Gainesville

MARVIN TURCK, M.D.
Professor of Medicine, University of Washington School of Medicine; Physician-in-Chief, Harborview Medical Center, Seattle

DAVID D. ULMER, M.D.
Professor and Chairman, Department of Medicine, Charles R. Drew Postgraduate Medical School; Physician, Martin Luther King Hospital, Los Angeles

JOHN E. ULTMANN, M.D.
Professor of Medicine, Section of Hematology/Oncology, Department of Medicine; Director, University of Chicago Cancer Research Center; Associate Dean for Research Programs, Biological Sciences Division, Pritzker School of Medicine, University of Chicago, Chicago

ROGER H. UNGER, M.D.
Professor of Internal Medicine, University of Texas Health Science Center at Dallas; Senior Medical Investigator, Dallas Veterans Administration Medical Center, Dallas

HENRI VANDER EECKEN, H.M., M.D.
Professor of Neurology, Faculty of Medicine, University of Ghent; Head of the Department of Neurology, Akademisch Zeikenhuis, Ghent

MAURICE VICTOR, M.D.
Professor of Neurology, Case Western Reserve University School of Medicine; Director, Neurology Service, Cleveland Metropolitan General Hospital, Cleveland

JAMES F. WALLACE, M.D.
Professor of Medicine, University of Washington School of Medicine; Associate Physician-in-Chief, University of Washington Hospital, Seattle

PATRICK C. WALSH, M.D.
Professor and Director, Department of Urology, The Johns Hopkins University School of Medicine; Urologist-in-Chief, James Buchanan Brady Urological Institute, The Johns Hopkins Hospital, Baltimore

JACK R. WANDS, M.D.
Assistant Professor of Medicine, Harvard Medical School; Assistant Physician, Gastrointestinal Unit, Massachusetts General Hospital, Boston

HENRY deF. WEBSTER, M.D.
Head, Section Cellular Neuropathology, National Institute of Neurological Disease and Stroke, National Institutes of Health, Bethesda

LOUIS WEINSTEIN, M.D., Ph.D., Sc.D. (Hon.)
Visiting Professor of Medicine, Harvard Medical School; Physician and Director, Clinical Services, Infectious Diseases Division, Peter Bent Brigham Hospital, Boston

JOHN B. WEST, M.D., Ph.D.
Professor of Medicine, University of California, San Diego School of Medicine; Physician, University Hospital, University of California, San Diego Medical Center, San Diego

GRANT R. WILKINSON, Ph.D.
Professor of Pharmacology, Vanderbilt University School of Medicine, Nashville

GORDON H. WILLIAMS, M.D.
Associate Professor of Medicine, Harvard Medical School; Peter Bent Brigham Hospital, Boston

JEAN D. WILSON, M.D.
Professor of Internal Medicine and Director, McDermott Center for Growth and Development, University of Texas Health Science Center at Dallas, Dallas

MAXWELL M. WINTROBE, B.A., M.D., B.Sc. (Med.), Ph.D., D.Sc. (Hon. Manitoba), D.Sc. (Hon. Utah), M.A.C.P.
Distinguished Professor of Internal Medicine, University of Utah College of Medicine, Salt Lake City

KENNETH A. WOEBER, M.D.
Professor of Medicine, University of California, San Francisco School of Medicine; Chief, Department of Medicine, Mount Zion Hospital and Medical Center, San Francisco

SHELDON M. WOLFF, M.D.
Professor and Chairman, Department of Medicine, Tufts University School of Medicine, Boston

ALASTAIR J. J. WOOD, M.D., M.R.C.P.
Assistant Professor of Medicine and Pharmacology, Vanderbilt University School of Medicine; Attending Physician, Vanderbilt University Hospital, Nashville

THEODORE E. WOODWARD, M.D.
Professor of Medicine and Head, Department of Medicine, University of Maryland School of Medicine, Baltimore

RICHARD J. WURTMAN, M.D.
Professor of Endocrinology and Metabolism and Director, Laboratory of Neuroendocrine Regulation, Massachusetts Institute of Technology; Clinical Associate in Medicine, Massachusetts General Hospital, Boston

SING HEIM YAP, M.D., Ph.D.
Consultant, Division of Gastroenterology and Liver Disease, Department of Medicine, St. Radboud Hospital, University of Nijmegen, Nijmegen

ROBERT R. YOUNG, M.D.
Associate Professor of Neurology, Harvard Medical School; Associate Neurologist and Chief, Clinical Neurophysiology, Massachusetts General Hospital, Boston

PREFACE

Prefaces are always written but they are not frequently read. Hopefully, the readers of this textbook will judge its merits by the substance of its contents and not by the pretexts offered by its editors. Why then a foreword to this ninth edition?

This preface is intended to indicate the ways in which the present edition adheres to the original objectives of this book and at the same time to note some substantive changes which have been made since the last edition.

When the first group of editors met together almost thirty-four years ago, they decided to write a textbook of medicine that would conform to the *clinical method* they had found most useful both as students and as teachers. It was thought that such a book should recapitulate the steps in the process of thinking by which a physician reaches a diagnosis, these being the recording of the patient's symptoms and signs, the consideration of the various disorders that can give rise to them, and the effective utilization of measures which will support and confirm or alter the first impressions and lead ultimately to a firm diagnosis.

The logical first step consistent with this clinical approach is the consideration of the *cardinal manifestations of disease*. Patients present with symptoms, not diagnoses. Consequently, it is basic to good clinical medicine to appreciate the different causes of various manifestations of disease and to understand how they may be produced. This requires an understanding of normal physiology and of the ways in which deviations from the normal lead to disease. For this reason material of fundamental biological importance was incorporated in the first edition and has been regarded as an essential component ever since.

The revolutionary changes in the curricula of many American medical schools, particularly the abbreviation of the standard courses in the sciences basic to clinical medicine and the substitution of shorter "core" courses, has imposed, we believe, additional responsibilities on the modern teacher of clinical medicine and on the modern textbook of medicine. The students who embark on their clinical training now, although far more sophisticated in many ways than their predecessors of even one generation ago, may not possess as much understanding of the mechanisms of symptoms and disease processes as is required to deal intelligently with clinical problems. This book recognizes the challenge to education posed by such curricula. Clinical biochemistry and pathophysiology form an integral part of this book but, insofar as possible, are considered within the clinical setting.

The interpretation of symptoms usually is most effectively achieved by proceeding from the general to the particular. Symptoms often can be grouped as syndromes. Syndromes are the consequence of a variety of etiologic factors or disease mechanisms and, if these can be recognized and understood, measures to restore the normal physiological state can be designed and carried out in a logical, systematic fashion. Furthermore, the method of approaching a diagnosis which is based on an analysis of the symptoms, recognition of the syndrome, and consideration of the various disease mechanisms which may have produced it ensures consideration of the many possible interpretations of the clinical picture which the patient presents. By pursuing such an approach, it is less likely that a disorder which should be considered will be overlooked.

The plan of the book is consistent with this approach. In Part 1, "Introduction to Clinical Medicine," the Editors discuss their general philosophy regarding the approach to the patient. In Part 2, "Cardinal Manifestations of Disease," the mechanisms whereby various symptoms are produced are discussed, an approach to the recognition of the diseases of which these may be manifestations is outlined, and laboratory findings are discussed in relation to the clinical manifestations. Part 3, "Biological Considerations in the Approach to Clinical Medicine," summarizes the important considerations on the following: (1) the genetics of human disease, with discussions of cytogenetics and the prevention and treatment of genetic disorders, including genetic counseling; (2) clinical immunology, which is reviewed in depth; (3) clinical pharmacology and the principles of drug therapy, adverse reactions to drugs, and the clinical pharmacology of the autonomic nervous system; (4) nutritional disorders, with discussions of nutritional requirements, malnutrition and overnutrition (obesity), dietary therapy, and parenteral nutrition; and (5) metabolic disorders, with discussions of derangements of nucleic acid, carbohydrate, and lipid metabolism as well as fluid and electrolyte pathophysiology, including considerations of acidosis and alkalosis. In Part 4, "Disorders Caused by Biological and Environmental Agents," will be found the major discussions of the approach to the diagnosis and treatment of infectious diseases. Chemotherapy of infections and the specific diseases caused by microbial agents are discussed in detail. In addition, disorders of uncertain etiology (such as sarcoidosis and familial Mediterranean fever) and diseases due to environmental hazards such as tobacco smoking, radiation injury, drug overdosage, and alcoholism are considered.

The remainder of the book is concerned with specific disorders and disease entities. In all these sections, the syndromic approach is emphasized insofar as possible. The reader will find at the beginning of most of the sections, either in the introduction or in the first chapter, a discussion of the approach to the patient whose clinical manifestations suggest the type of disease considered in that section.

A deliberate attempt has been made to avoid long bibliographies. The references at the end of the chapters are largely to reviews and monographs. Others refer to a few of the most significant recent articles.

In this ninth edition the editors have attempted to keep pace with the dynamic and ever-changing field of medicine. Since the publication of the last edition only three years ago, new diseases have been discovered (e.g., Legionnaires' disease) and new diagnostic modalities (such as ultrasound, computerized tomography, and endoscopy) have become routine in most medical centers. Consequently, the chapters and sections of this ninth edition have been updated or completely revised as follows.

The section on the *approach to clinical problems* has been extensively updated, especially the chapters on gain and loss in weight and alterations in urinary function. The section dealing with reproductive and sexual functions is completely new, and the dermatology chapters, especially those dealing with skin pigmentation, photosensitivity, and other reactions to light, have been completely revised.

The section on *clinical pharmacology and toxicology* has been revised and updated. The chapter on the clinical pharmacology of the autonomic nervous system is new, and the chapters dealing with the principles of drug therapy and adverse reactions to drugs have been expanded.

The current section on *nutrition,* including the chapters on nutritional problems of the ill patient, anorexia, obesity, and derangements of vitamin metabolism, has been completely revised, and the newest approaches to dietary therapy and parenteral nutrition are discussed.

In the area of *infectious diseases* there are many new chapters, including those on diagnostic procedures, infectious diarrheas and bacterial food poisoning, sexually transmitted infections, immunization practices, Legionnaires' disease, fungus diseases, and urinary tract infections.

In the section on *disorders of the heart,* echocardiography, radionuclide angiography, and other noninvasive methods of cardiac examination have been discussed in greater detail. Major revisions and updating have been carried out in the chapters dealing with the cardiomyopathies, atherosclerosis, and hypertension, with emphasis placed on modern methods of treating the latter two conditions.

The section on *lung diseases* includes new chapters on hypersensitivity pneumonitis and cystic fibrosis in the adult, and the discussions of environmental lung disease and the adult respiratory distress syndrome have been substantially revised. Significant emphasis has been placed on the role of newer diagnostic procedures such as fiberoptic bronchoscopy in the examination of the respiratory system.

The entire *renal section* has been rewritten. The reader will find an up-to-date description of disturbances of renal function and major new chapters on the immunopathogenetic mechanisms of renal injury, glomerulopathies, interstitial diseases of the kidney, and hereditary tubular disorders.

The section on *gastroenterology* includes completely new and up-to-date chapters on peptic ulcer, disorders of the pancreas, and diseases of the gallbladder. The chapters on viral hepatitis (acute and chronic) have also been updated in order to provide the latest information on viral antigens and antibodies and their usefulness in clinical diagnosis of liver diseases. The chapters on intestinal absorption, malabsorption, and inflammatory bowel disease have also been extensively revised.

The sections on *disorders of the hematopoietic system* and *neoplasia* include revisions of the chapters on megaloblastic anemias, bone marrow transplantation, cancer chemotherapy, and Hodgkin's disease. Color plates of disorders of erythrocytes and leukocytes are included in this edition for the first time.

The section on *endocrine and metabolic disorders* has been completely revised. New chapters will be found on the pituitary, hypothalamus, diabetes mellitus, and hypoglycemia. In addition, there are new chapters on disorders of sexual differentiation, diseases of the testes, and disorders of the breast and milk formation.

The section on *disorders of bone and mineral metabolism* has been extensively revised with new illustrations and an updated chapter on vitamin D.

The section dealing with *disorders of the nervous system* includes new and revised chapters on epilepsy and Parkinson's disease. The chapter dealing with cerebrovascular diseases includes an in-depth discussion on the approach to diagnosis and therapy. The section dealing with *diseases of striated muscle* has also been completely revised.

The *Appendix* presents the latest complete set of important laboratory values of clinical importance. Where possible we have also included, for the convenience of the reader, values in *SI units* as well as in conventional units.

With the publication of the eighth edition of this textbook, one of the original editors and the Editor-in-Chief for that edition, Dr. George W. Thorn, retired. We, his colleagues and coeditors, are all indebted to Dr. Thorn, not only for his tremendous contributions to this textbook but also for his major contributions to the field of internal medicine. His distinguished leadership and his creative genius will be sorely missed. His influence will undoubtedly continue to be felt in future editions of this textbook. With this ninth edition we take pleasure in welcoming as a new editor Dr. Jean D. Wilson, an academic colleague who is recognized internationally as an outstanding scholar, teacher, and clinician-scientist.

We also wish to express our appreciation and gratitude to our many associates and colleagues, who as experts in their fields have helped us by providing constructive and valuable criticisms of the chapters in this ninth edition. In addition to the authors and contributors who also reviewed many manuscripts, we wish to thank the following for their many helpful suggestions: David J. Baylink, William J. Bremner, George F. Cahill, George P. Cannelos, Martin C. Carey, Earl Davie, David Donaldson, Thomas D. DuBose, John Ensinck, Z. Myron Falchuk, Donald Farrell, Daniel Federman, Bernard Fields, Clement A. Finch, Stephen Fricker, Ruben Gittes, Charles J. Goodner, Judith G. Hall, Laurence Harker, Holger W. Hoehn, Edward Kass, Juha P. Kokko, Guenter J. Krejs, Robert Labbe, S. Laksminarayan, Lewis Landsberg, Mark Leshin, Lee Levitt, Joseph Martin, James McArthur, George McDonald, Mark McPhee, Donald Miller, Donald E. Moore, Gilbert S. Omenn, C. Alvin Paulsen, James Pennington, Arnold S. Relman, R. Paul Robertson, David S. Rosenthal, David Saunders, Michael Schuffler, C. Donald Scott, Donald Sherrard, Peter Simkin, J. Donald Smiley, R. Graham Smith, George Stamatoyannopoulos, Morton A. Stenchever, Gary E. Striker, Philip D. Swanson, Ira B. Tager, Jerry S. Trier, Shirley Wray, and Joseph E. Zerwekh.

As always, we wish to express our appreciation to our dedicated secretarial coworkers who have been of immeasurable help. We are especially indebted to Mrs. Hilda Gardner, Mrs. Freda Foster, Ms. Patricia Kadlick, Mrs. Mary Jackson, Mrs. Trudy Geissler, Mrs. Cynthia Reid, Mrs. Diane Tasian, and Mrs. Raye Ann Hondroulis.

KURT J. ISSELBACHER
RAYMOND D. ADAMS
EUGENE BRAUNWALD
ROBERT G. PETERSDORF
JEAN D. WILSON

Harrison's
PRINCIPLES OF INTERNAL MEDICINE

VOLUME 1

PART ONE | INTRODUCTION TO CLINICAL MEDICINE

1
THE PRACTICE OF MEDICINE

THE EDITORS

APPROACH TO THE PATIENT

No greater opportunity, responsibility, or obligation is given to an individual than that of serving as a physician. In treating the suffering, there is need for technical skill, scientific knowledge, and human understanding. The person who uses these with courage, with humility, and with wisdom will provide a unique service and will build an enduring edifice of character. The physician should ask of destiny no more than this and be content with no less.

Thirty years ago, the Editors of this book defined what is expected of the physician. Their eloquent words ring as true now as they did then:

Tact, sympathy and understanding are expected of the physician, for the patient is no mere collection of symptoms, signs, disordered functions, damaged organs, and disturbed emotions. He is human, fearful, and hopeful, seeking relief, help and reassurance. To the physician, as to the anthropologist, nothing human is strange or repulsive. The misanthrope may become a smart diagnostician of organic disease, but he can scarcely hope to succeed as a physician. The true physician has a Shakespearean breadth of interest in the wise and the foolish, the proud and the humble, the stoic hero and the whining rogue. He cares for people.

THE ART OF MEDICINE In the practice of medicine the physician employs a discipline which seeks to utilize scientific methods and principles in the solution of its problems, but it is one in which, in the end, both science and art are wedded. The crucial importance of understanding the scientific base of modern medicine is well known; the significance of the art of medicine is not as well appreciated. Thus, to extract from a mass of conflicting physical signs and laboratory data the ones that are of crucial significance, to know in a borderline case when to initiate and when to refrain from a line of investigation or treatment involves judgments based on "assimilated" experience. Skill in accomplishing these necessities of medical art is not usually the outcome of laboratory study alone.

Intuition and maturing wisdom are called upon in developing the more personal relations with patients and the understanding and capacity to peer beneath surface motivations into their behavior. Astute physicians will recognize when the casual mention of an apparently trivial complaint is a device for seeking reassurance regarding a feared disorder such as cancer or heart disease. They will know at once when to probe the more intimate aspects of the patient's life and when to leave them undiscussed, and they will realize when to express a bright and reassuring prognosis and when and how to utter doubt and caution.

Medicine is an art also in the sense that physicians can never be content with the sole aim of endeavoring to clarify the laws of nature; they cannot proceed in their labors with the cool detachment of the scientist whose aim is the winning of the truth, and who, in doing so, conducts a "controlled experiment." It is essential that they maintain objectivity in the study and care of their patients, for this is in the patients' interests; they must use wise judgment and must never forget that their primary and traditional objectives are utilitarian—the prevention and cure of disease and the relief of suffering, whether of body or of mind.

THE PHYSICIAN AND THE PATIENT

An aspect of illness that influences the physician-patient relationship is the real or implied significance of disease in the mind of the patient. Any departure from good health involves a potential threat of physical disintegration or crippling disability, and even the most intelligent and best-informed patients should not be considered immune to forebodings just because they refrain from mentioning them. In fact, most patients are more concerned with the possibility of being rendered dependent by illness than with the disease itself. It is especially important that these fears be borne in mind when dealing with the elderly patient, who is rarely unmindful that "the trap is laid" and death is always near.

The attitude of the patient approaching the doctor must always be tinged, for the most part unconsciously, with distaste and dread; his deepest desire will tend to be comfort and relief rather than cure, and his faith and expectation will be directed towards some magical exhibition of these boons. Do not let yourselves believe that however smoothly concealed by education, by reason, and by confidential frankness these strong elements may be, they are ever in any circumstances altogether absent.

Wilfred Trotter

Illness also constitutes a threat to the individual's status in a social group. Prolonged invalidism during childhood tends inevitably to leave behind an excessive egocentricity, which may become the basis of a lifelong neurosis. In the adult, illness often enforces a return to a posture of dependency, a change usually accompanied by feelings of apprehension and discouragement, sometimes leading to frank anxiety and depression. This explains a number of common psychologic defenses which patients exercise against illness. They may refuse medical aid; or, if they summon the courage to consult a physician, they may minimize or even fail to mention the very symptom about which they are most deeply concerned. Then, too, there are persons whose emotional stability has been tenuous and uncertain, so that the position of dependency imposed by illness comes as a welcome relief from adult responsibility. They appear to enjoy illness and to resent anything that menaces their state of invalidism. Lesser degrees of this tendency are seen among those who consult the physician at the appearance of every new symptom and who are continuously preoccupied with their past illnesses and operations.

During examination in the relatively neutral domain of the hospital ward a patient's emotional life may seem relatively unimportant. Organic lesions have a way of compelling attention to themselves, and further, it may be less exhausting to limit one's focus to the sphere of physical disease. More time,

energy, and experience frequently are necessary to view the patient as an active participant in an enormous moving pageant which includes the personal eccentricities of one's forebears, one's own fears and patterns of reaction, the roles of poverty, insecurity, and perhaps poor vocational and domestic relations. Yet every experienced physician knows that to explain many of the manifestations of illness, it is necessary to view the patient comprehensively as an organism with a vast repository of past experiences, many of which are vaguely remembered, yet have become the foundation of one's current system of meeting daily problems.

THE PHYSICIAN'S RESPONSIBILITIES The physician seeks to respond to and alleviate the patient's complaints, to search out signs of ill health not yet apparent to the patient or abnormalities which may lead to ill health, and to maintain the patient in a state of well-being. To achieve these goals requires a broad orientation. Illness is never limited to one system, nor necessarily to a single disease, and whether the physician is a family practitioner, an internist who provides "primary care," or a subspecialist, the patient must be viewed not as an organ system but as a person.

EXAMINATION OF THE WELL PERSON AND PREVENTION OF DISEASE The intelligent practice of preventive medicine is often considered undramatic; yet few areas of medicine are of greater importance to a single individual or to an entire population. In this aspect of medical practice, the physician deals with individuals or groups who are not overtly ill or whose complaints may be unrelated to the disease process which is to be prevented. The use of the periodic physical examination and the ready availability of multiphasic screening tests allow the physician to detect and to intervene in disease processes early in their course, often before the first symptom becomes manifest.

Physicians who examine well individuals are not "wasting their training." More skill is required to recognize the early signs of ill health than to deal with what is obvious to patients or their families. The discovery and cure of potentially serious disease represent a far greater service to one's patient than ministrations in the course of an incurable condition.

The finding of an elevated arterial blood pressure or an elevated blood sugar, serum uric acid, or cholesterol level in an asymptomatic person or the discussion of milder degrees of nervousness or depression provides an unparalleled opportunity to prevent or retard events of serious consequence. It is not always easy to persuade asymptomatic persons to face situations they had hoped to avoid or to alter their habits or diet in order to follow a therapeutic program throughout the rest of their lives. Nevertheless the value of these efforts is so great that it fully justifies the effort and attention of every physician.

CHANGING PATIENT-PHYSICIAN RELATIONSHIPS The one-to-one patient-physician relationship which traditionally has been the goal of all physicians is changing, primarily because of the changing setting in which medicine is being practiced. In many cases the management of the individual patient requires the active participation of a variety of trained professional personnel—not only physicians, but also nurses, physicians' assistants, dietitians, biochemists, psychologists, and other health care personnel. The patient can benefit greatly from such collaboration, but it is the duty of the physician to guide the patient through an illness. In order to carry out this increasingly difficult task, the physician must have some familiarity with the techniques, skills, and objectives of colleagues in the fields allied to medicine. Their findings must be interpreted not as isolated phenomena, but rather in terms of the total clinical picture. In giving the patient an opportunity to receive all the benefits of the important advances of science, the physician must retain responsibility for the crucial decisions concerning diagnosis and treatment.

An increasing number of patients is being cared for by groups of physicians, clinics, hospitals, and health-maintenance organizations (HMOs) rather than by a single, independent practitioner. There are many potential advantages in the use of such organized medical groups, but there also are hazards, both to the patient and the physician. The identity of the physician who is primarily and continuously responsible for each particular patient must be clearly defined. It is this physician who must have an overview of a patient's problems and who must maintain familiarity with the patient's reaction to illness, to drugs, and to the challenges of daily living. In addition, since a number of physicians may, at any one time, contribute to the care of a particular patient, and since patients as well as physicians are becoming increasingly mobile, accurate and detailed record keeping assumes progressively greater importance. It is imperative that the physician promptly commit all pertinent data obtained from the clinical and laboratory examinations to the patient's permanent medical record. Only in this way can continuity and high quality in the care of the patient be provided.

THE PHYSICIAN AS A PERSON The examining physician is first a human instrument, subject to reactions arising from events in his or her own biography. This background will strongly influence the physician's responses to and understanding of the patient. The student receives much expert coaching in the methods of physical and laboratory diagnosis, and in these areas will most easily develop the skills that permit a comfortable relationship with the patient. The young physician may feel inadequate in dealing with the patient's problems; a sense of insecurity is inevitable. Moreover, the newly acquired role of authority and responsibility may be threatening. Some reactions may be difficult to control: lack of interest in a patient who presents no fascinating problems of organic disease, irritation at the patient's verbosity or lack of clarity and consistency in reciting his or her history, or even disappointment because the patient's illness fails to respond to treatment in the expected manner.

To perceive and understand the problems of the patient, the physician requires not simply instruction but emotional maturity and an interest in and concern for other human beings. The physician must learn to be at ease and to establish rapport with persons of every walk of life, realizing that everyone is born with manifold potentialities determined by their genes and has a personality and character shaped by the emotional climate in which they grow and develop. The physician must relate as much to the person who is ill as to the illness for which he or she seeks relief.

The physician has a special function in society and should be skilled as a psychologist as well as a biologist. With the highly technical knowledge and skills needed to affect the patient's physiologic functions there should also be a feeling of humaneness, a sense of confidence and security based upon the conviction that all will be done that can be done. Such an atmosphere will allow a wholesome personal relationship to develop. The patient must be allowed to feel that his or her unique individuality is recognized and that life's problems are appreciated. This is as important to patients with well-defined organic disease as to those suffering primarily from psychiatric illness.

APPROACH TO DISEASE

HISTORY The written history of an illness should embody all the facts of medical significance in the life of the patient up to

the time that the physician is consulted, but of course, the most recent diseases attract the most attention, for these, obviously, are the reason that a person seeks medical advice. Ideally the narration of symptoms should be in the patient's own words, the principal events being presented in the temporal order in which they occurred. However, few patients possess the necessary powers of observation and talent for lucid, coherent description. Hence, guiding questions from the physician may be required, though one must avoid suggesting answers.

Often a symptom which has concerned a patient has little significance, whereas a seemingly minor complaint may be of importance. Therefore the physician must be constantly alert to the possibility that any event related by the patient, any symptom however trivial or apparently remote, may be the key to the solution of the medical problem. As data are gained from the physical and laboratory examinations, the problems which are presented should be clearly identified.

An informative history is more than an orderly listing of symptoms. Something always is gained by listening to patients and noting the way in which they talk about their symptoms. Inflections of voice, facial expression, and attitude may betray important clues to the meaning of the symptoms to a patient. In listening to the history, the physician discovers not only something about the disease but also something about the patient.

With experience the pitfalls of history taking become apparent. What patients relate for the most part consists of subjective phenomena filtered through minds that vary in their background of past experience. Patients obviously differ widely in their responses to the same stimuli. Their remarks are variably colored by fear of disease, disability, and death, and by concern over the consequences of illness to their families. Additional difficulties are created by language barriers, by failing intellectual powers which deprive the patient of accurate recall, or by disorders of consciousness that make them unaware of their illness. It is not surprising, then, that even the most careful physician may at times despair of collecting factual data and be forced to proceed with evidence that represents little more than an approximation of the truth.

Viewed in another way the symptom marks, in the patient's mind, a departure from normal health; in the physician's mind, it initiates a process of inductive and deductive reasoning that culminates in diagnosis. In pondering the various possible explanations of a given symptom or clinical state, the physician begins a search for other data, elicited by further questioning of the patient and the family, by physical examination, or by laboratory tests. The symptoms alone sometimes will provide the most certain clue, as in angina pectoris or epilepsy, where physical findings and laboratory data collected between attacks may give no evidence of the existence of disease even when it is present with certitude. In most illnesses, however, the history will not be so decisive, though it may narrow the number of diagnostic possibilities and guide the subsequent investigation.

It is in taking the history that the physician's skill, knowledge, and experience are most clearly in evidence. Each symptom is evaluated according to its nature and context; there are times for questioning its credibility and turning to more reliable sources of information, but skepticism must not cause an unusual symptom or manifestation of some new condition to be overlooked. Moreover, there are times when an interrogation must be pressed more deeply in a search for further details and times when the questions must be broader, because "disease often tells its secrets in a casual parenthesis." And finally, the physician knows how to take advantage of the interview in which the history is gathered to obtain the confidence of the patient and allay apprehension and fear, the first steps in therapy.

The family history, all too often obtained in a routine, cursory fashion, is a leading tool of clinical genetics and can provide important evidence regarding the nature of the patient's complaints. Information regarding symptoms like those of the patient which have occurred in blood relatives, or "run in the family," and knowledge of the ethnic origin of the parents and of consanguinity may be exceedingly helpful. The information must be obtained with tact, however, for patients may be embarrassed by such inquiries. The best family history is one which is supported by actual examination of other members of the family. Frequently it is found that some physical deviation from the normal, too subtle to be recognized by a lay person, is quite apparent to the trained observer and that a minor deviation in laboratory data assumes significance when evaluated within a family constellation.

PHYSICAL EXAMINATION Little need be said about the importance of the physical examination, for early in their training physicians learn that physical signs are the objective and verifiable marks of disease. The physical sign represents a solid, indisputable fact. However, its significance is enhanced when it confirms a functional or structural change already evidenced by the patient's history. At other times, the physical sign may stand as the only evidence of disease, especially in those instances in which the history has been inconsistent, confused, or completely lacking.

If full advantage is to be gained from the physical examination, it must be performed methodically and thoroughly. Although attention has usually been directed by the history to the offending organ or part of the body, the examination must extend to all parts of the body. The patient must be scrutinized literally from head to toe in an objective search for abnormalities that may yield information concerning present and possible future illnesses. Unless the examination procedure is systematic, important parts of it may be forgotten, an error against which even the most skilled clinician must guard. The results of the examination, like the details of the history, should be recorded at the time they are elicited, not hours later when they are subject to the distortions of memory. Many inaccuracies stem from the careless practice of writing or dictating notes long after the examination has ended.

Skill in physical diagnosis is acquired with experience, but it is not merely technique that determines success in eliciting signs. The detection of a few scattered petechiae, a faint diastolic murmur, or a small mass in the abdomen is not a question of keener eyes and ears or more sensitive fingers, but of a mind directed to be alert to these findings. Skill in physical diagnosis reflects a way of thinking more than a way of doing.

LABORATORY EXAMINATIONS The marked increase in the number and availability of laboratory diagnostic procedures has inevitably augmented reliance on the knowledge gained from these studies in the solution of clinical problems. It is essential, however, to bear in mind the limitations of such procedures, which by virtue of their impersonal quality and complexity often gain an aura of authority regardless of the fallibility of the individuals or their instruments. More importantly, the accumulation of laboratory data cannot release the physician from the necessity of careful observation and study of the patient. The wise physician understands the merits and limitations of each source of information, whether it be history, physical examination, or laboratory investigation. The physician also must weigh carefully the hazards and the expense involved in every laboratory procedure.

Nowadays, laboratory tests rarely are ordered and reported singly. Rather they are produced as "batteries." A common combination is the M6, which consists of determinations of serum sodium, potassium, carbon dioxide combining power, chloride, blood urea nitrogen, and blood glucose. Even more common is the M12, which reports simultaneously serum calcium, phosphate, proteins, albumin, uric acid, cholesterol, and several enzymes. Some laboratories now perform batteries of 24 and even 40 tests! The various combinations of laboratory tests are often useful. For example, they may provide the clue to such nonspecific symptoms as generalized weakness and increased fatigability by revealing an elevated serum calcium which, in turn, would suggest the diagnosis of hyperparathyroidism.

The thoughtful use of screening tests is not to be confused with indiscriminate laboratory testing; it is based on the fact that a group of laboratory determinations which are known to be frequent harbingers of disease can now be carried out on a single specimen of blood at relatively low cost. Biochemical measurements, together with simple laboratory examinations such as blood count, urinalysis, and sedimentation rate, often provide the major clue to the presence of a pathologic process. This is particularly helpful in identifying organic disease in a patient with evident psychologic or emotional problems. At the same time the physician must learn to evaluate occasional abnormalities among the screening tests that may not necessarily connote significant disease. There is nothing more costly and unproductive than an in-depth work-up following the reporting of an isolated laboratory abnormality in an otherwise well patient.

Discrimination in the ordering of laboratory procedures and judgment in appraising their risk, expense, and possible benefit are important indicators of the effectiveness with which the art and science of medicine have been fused by the individual physician.

THE CLINICAL METHOD AND THE SYNDROMIC APPROACH TO DISEASE The clinical method has as its object the collection of accurate data concerning all the diseases to which human beings are subject, namely, all conditions that "limit life in its powers, enjoyment, and duration." But much more is required in making a diagnosis. Each datum must be interpreted in the light of the known facts of anatomy, physiology, and chemistry. The synthesis of these interpretations yields information concerning the affected organ or body system. Further, from the vantage point afforded by such an anatomic diagnosis the physician may then turn to other data, such as the mode of onset and clinical course of the illness, and to the results of laboratory tests, in order to ascertain the cause of the disease and degree of physiologic impairment.

The clinical method always proceeds in a series of logical steps. The perceptive student will note certain similarities between the clinical method and the scientific method. Each begins with observational data which suggest a series of hypotheses. These are then tested in the light of further observations, some of which are made in the clinic and others in the laboratory. Finally, a conclusion is reached, which in science is called a *theory* and in medicine a *working diagnosis*. The modus operandi of the clinical method, like that of the scientific method, cannot be reduced to a single principle or a type of inductive or deductive reasoning. It involves both analysis and synthesis, the essential parts of cartesian logic. The physician does not start with an open mind any more than does the scientist, but armed with the knowledge of recent cases, the patient's first statement directs one's thinking to certain channels.

It is particularly in the study of more difficult patients that the logical order of the clinical method becomes most important. Here in particular the physician must carefully list each problem indicated by the patient's complaints and physical and laboratory findings and seek answers to each. Anatomic diagnosis regularly precedes etiological diagnosis. The cause and mechanism of a disease can seldom be determined before ascertaining which organ is involved. An intermediate step is syndromic diagnosis. Most physicians attempt consciously or unconsciously to fit a given problem into one of a series of syndromes. The syndrome, in essence, is a group of symptoms and signs of disordered function, related to one another by means of some anatomic, physiologic, or biochemical peculiarity. It embodies a hypothesis concerning the deranged function of an organ, organ system, or tissue. Congestive heart failure, Cushing's disease, and dementia are examples. In congestive heart failure dyspnea, orthopnea, cyanosis, dependent edema, engorged neck veins, pleural effusion, pulmonary rales, and enlarged liver are known to be connected by a single pathophysiologic mechanism—failure of the heart, leading to salt and water retention and high venous pressure. In Cushing's disease the moon faces, hypertension, diabetes, and osteoporosis are the recognized effects of excess corticosteroids acting on many target organs. In dementia deterioration of memory, incoherent thinking, and faulty judgment are related to impairment of the function and destruction of the association areas of the cerebrum.

A syndromic diagnosis does not necessarily identify the precise cause of an illness, but it greatly narrows the number of possibilities and, thus, suggests whatever further clinical and laboratory studies are required. The derangements of each organ system in human beings are reducible to a relatively small number of syndromes. Diagnosis is greatly simplified if a given clinical problem conforms neatly to a well-defined syndrome, because a list of the various diseases that may cause it may be all that is required to make the diagnosis. The search for the cause of an illness that does not conform to a syndrome is much more difficult, for a seemingly infinite number of diseases may then have to be considered. Nevertheless, the principle remains: the clinical method is an orderly intellectual activity which proceeds almost invariably from symptom, to sign, to syndrome, to disease.

THE COMPUTER IN MEDICINE The uses of the computer in managing the economic aspects of medical practice are already well established. However, the role of the computer in clinical medicine is still in an evolutionary stage. It has been used successfully in the clinical laboratory for processing data from automated chemical and microbiological determinations. Several centers have successfully developed computerized medical records for hospital and outpatient use. Automated information systems in pharmacies are becoming sophisticated and are able to assist in prevention of drug-drug interactions and improved monitoring of therapy. Interpretation of electrocardiograms by computer is commonplace. Although these newer developments are noteworthy, computer management of medical data is still in its infancy.

The role of the computer in medical decision making remains elusive but challenging. Considerable progress has been made in using the computer to facilitate differential diagnosis and to evaluate clinical decision-making.

The advantages to the physician who can use computer technology are obvious. Much time and effort can be saved, and more accurate and reliable clinical information can be brought quickly into the hands of the physician.

ACCOUNTABILITY Traditionally, physicians, once licensed to practice medicine, have not had to account for their actions except to their peers. In the past decade, however, there have been increasing demands for physicians to account for the way in which they practice medicine by meeting certain standards prescribed by federal and state governments. Hospitalized patients whose health care is sponsored by the government (Medicare and Medicaid) have been subjected to utilization review. This means that the physician must defend the duration of a patient's hospitalization if it exceeds preset criteria. This concept has been extended in the form of Professional Standard Review Organizations (PSRO) under whose direction norms and standards for the care of patients are developed. The purpose of these regulations is ostensibly to improve the quality of patient care, and, in some instances, this will undoubtedly happen. An equally important reason for implementing these regulations, however, is to contain spiraling health care costs. There is no question but that the insertion of this type of review will be extended to all phases of medical practice and will inevitably alter not only the practice of medicine but the traditional patient-physician relationship.

Physicians also will be expected to give account of their continuing competence by mandatory continuing education, patient record audit, recertification by examination, and relicensure. The American Board of Internal Medicine has administered two voluntary recertification examinations to over 5000 physicians. The American Board of Family Practice is also administering a recertification examination to its recent diplomates.

COST-EFFECTIVENESS IN MEDICAL CARE

As society undertakes greater responsibility for health care, and as the cost of medical care continues to skyrocket, it has become necessary to establish stringent priorities in the expenditure of health dollars. Preventive measures often offer the greatest return per dollar; outstanding examples include vaccination, immunization, reduction in accidents and occupational hazards, and improved environmental control. The cost of "newborn screening" for metabolic diseases is being evaluated. For example, the detection of phenylketonuria by screening of large populations can save many thousands of dollars in hospital costs.

As experience is gained, it will become necessary to weigh the justifiability of performing prohibitively costly operations which provide only a limited life expectancy against the pressing need for more primary care centers for the large segments of population who do not have adequate access to medical services. At the level of the individual patient it has become extremely important to minimize costly hospital admissions as far as possible, if total health care is to be provided at a figure which most can afford. This, of course, implies and depends upon a close cooperative effort between patients, their physicians, third-party carriers, and government, and a constant surveillance of those types of procedures which can be conducted safely and effectively on an ambulatory basis. Equally important in reducing total health care expenditures is the need for individual physicians to monitor carefully both the cost and effectiveness of the drugs they prescribe. In the last analysis the public should depend upon the medical profession for leadership and guidance in matters of health services legislation. It is equally important, however, that consideration of these important socioeconomic aspects of the health care delivery system not be permitted to interfere with the primary humane concern of physicians for the welfare of their patients.

CARE OF THE PATIENT

THE ROLE OF THERAPEUTICS

The care of the patient begins with the development of an interpersonal relationship between the patient and the physician. In the absence of a sense of trust and confidence on the part of the patient, the effectiveness of most therapeutic measures is diminished. In many instances, when there is confidence in the physician reassurance is the best treatment and is all that is needed. Likewise, in those cases which do not lend themselves to easy solutions or for which no effective remedy is available, a feeling on the part of the patient that the physician is doing all that is possible is one of the most important therapeutic measures that the physician can provide.

The discovery of therapeutic agents capable of exerting decisive influence on the course of disease has made it essential that the physician have some understanding not only of the disturbed functions induced by disease, but of the actions of many new drugs, their beneficial effects, and their risks.

Ideally, treatment should strive for the complete restoration of the patient's physical and mental health. When this goal is not attainable, remedies may still be available which will alleviate symptoms and make incurable diseases tolerable to the patient and the family.

IATROGENIC DISORDERS

It is the responsibility of the physician to use the new and powerful therapeutic measures wisely, with due regard for their action, cost, and potential dangers. Every medical procedure, whether diagnostic or therapeutic, has the potentiality of harm, but it would be impossible to afford the patient all the benefits of modern scientific medicine if reasonable steps in diagnosis and therapy were withheld because of possible risks. "Reasonable" implies that the physician has weighed the pros and cons of a procedure and has concluded on rational grounds that it is advisable or essential for the relief of discomfort or the cure or amelioration of disease. When the deleterious effects of the physician's action exceed the advantages that could have been anticipated, one is justified in designating these undesirable effects as iatrogenic. It is necessary only to recall the dangerous or fatal drug reactions that occasionally follow the use of antibiotics given for trivial respiratory infections, the gastric hemorrhage or perforation caused by cortisone administered for mild arthritis, the fatal hepatitis B that may follow needless transfusions of blood or plasma, or the arterial thrombosis or arrhythmia that may complicate coronary angiography.

But the harm that a physician can do to a patient is not limited to the imprudent use of medication. Equally important are ill-considered or unjustified remarks. Since the patient, no matter how apparently placid, approaches the physician with apprehension, anxiety may be enhanced by a too-serious demeanor, a flippant remark, or an unexplained conference concerning the patient's illness. Many persons have developed a cardiac neurosis because the physician expressed a grave prognosis on the basis of a misinterpreted electrocardiogram. Not only the treatment itself but the physician's words and behavior are always capable of causing injury.

The physician must never become so absorbed in the disease as to forget the patient who is its victim. As the science of medicine advances, it is all too easy to become so fascinated by the manifestations of disease that the ailing person's fears and concerns about job and family, the cost of medical care, and the specter of economic insecurity are disregarded. Treatment of a patient consists of more than the dispassionate confrontation of a disease. It embodies also the exercise of warmth, compassion, and understanding. In the now famous words of Peabody,

One of the essential qualities of the clinician is interest in humanity, for the secret of the care of the patient is in caring for the patient.

INFORMED CONSENT

In an era of rapidly advancing technology, patients progressively will require diagnostic and therapeutic procedures that are painful and that pose some risk. These include all surgical procedures, e.g., biopsies of tissues, radiographic maneuvers involving the insertion of catheters, endoscopy, and many others. In most hospitals and clinics, patients undergoing such procedures are required to sign a form consenting to them. More important, however, is the notion that the patient must understand clearly the risk entailed in these procedures; this is the definition of *informed consent*. It is incumbent upon the physician to explain to the patient, in a clearly understandable fashion, the procedures which he or she faces. By doing this conscientiously much of the dread of the unknown that is inherent in hospitalization will be mitigated.

INCURABILITY AND DEATH No problem is more distressing than that presented by the patient with incurable disease, particularly when death is imminent and inevitable. What should the patient and family be told, what measures should be taken to maintain the patient's life, and how is death to be defined?

There is no ironclad rule that the patient must be told "everything," even if he or she is an adult and the head of a family. How much the patient is told will depend upon the patient's own desires and character, the wishes of the family, the state of the patient's affairs, and perhaps religious convictions. First of all the patient must be given an opportunity to speak to the physician and to ask questions. Patients may find it easier to share their feelings about death with their physician who they realize is likely to be more objective and less emotional than their own family members.

One thing is certain: it is not for you to don the black cap and, assuming the judicial function, take hope away from any patient . . . hope that comes to us all.

William Osler

Even when the patient directly inquires, "Doctor, am I dying?" the physician must be circumspect and must attempt to determine whether this is a request for information, a demand for reassurance, or even an expression of hostility. Only further exchanges between the patient and the physician can resolve these questions and guide the physician in what to say and how to say it.

The physician should provide or arrange for emotional, physical, and spiritual support, and must be compassionate, unhurried, and open. Pain should be adequately controlled, human dignity maintained, and isolation from family avoided. The last two, in particular, tend to be overlooked in hospitals, where the intrusion of life-sustaining apparatus can so easily detract from attention to the whole person and instead concentrate on the life-threatening disorder.

The physician must also be prepared to deal with the expiatory attitude of the family when a member becomes gravely or hopelessly ill. The meager resources that may represent the savings of a lifetime may be dissipated in weeks of payment for needlessly expensive rooms, nursing services, and futile therapeutic measures. It is difficult for the physician to oppose these gestures too strenuously, for they serve more to bring consolation to the family than to assuage the distress of the patient, but they need not be encouraged.

Physicians also must be prepared to deal with the feelings of guilt that almost invariably afflict the members of a family when parent or child or spouse has died. They must be assured that everything possible has been done.

Apart from the anguish of facing the terminal phases of disease, to which patient and family react in highly individual ways according to temperament, personal philosophy, and religion, important biologic and medical problems arise as death approaches. At each stage in an illness, the physician must ascertain whether a fatal outcome is inevitable and also whether the surviving patient will suffer a degree of disability that would make life unbearable for the patient and family.

New concepts of death must also be considered. Traditionally, in every society, arrest of heart action has been taken as the only valid medical criterion of death. Lawbooks cite this as the only certain proof that human life has ended. But, as every modern physician knows, the heart may sometimes be restored to action, seemingly miraculously, minutes after it has stopped. On the other hand, other vital organs such as the brain may be destroyed, leaving the individual emotionally and psychologically dead.

When viewed at a cellular level, life is an intricate process of growth and decay in varying proportions at different ages. When decay exceeds growth in organs composed of postmitotic cells such as the musculature and nervous system, where each cell must endure for the lifetime of the individual, death proceeds gradually. This might be termed *cellular death,* and in its most advanced forms organ function may be impaired to a point incompatible with useful life. Of all the organs of humans it is the brain that imparts a meaningful quality to life. Without a functioning cerebrum humans have none of the attributes that distinguish them from other individuals of their own species or from beasts. All awareness of self is permanently effaced; no longer can one think, respond to the physical or social environment, speak, or move. Most thoughtful physicians and many lay people concede that such a state is equivalent to death even though the heart still beats.

Clinical and electrographic criteria are at hand which permit the reliable diagnosis of cerebral death. According to the report of the staff of the Massachusetts General Hospital and the Harvard Committee on Brain Death, one may assume that death has occurred when, as a consequence usually of hypoxia and hypotension, all signs of receptivity and responsivity are in abeyance, including all brainstem and spinal reflexes (pupillary reactions, ocular movement, blinking, swallowing, breathing, tendon and other spinal reflexes), and also, the electroencephalogram is isoelectric. Occasionally, intoxications and metabolic disorders may simulate this state; hence the diagnosis requires expert medical evaluation. Under the aforementioned circumstances, to continue with heroic, highly costly, supportive measures merely for the purpose of preserving cardiac function is in actuality against the best interests of patient, family, and society.

Here, physicians, on contemplating the broad implications of their actions, must either involve themselves in fruitless supportive care or may have to make the difficult decision to abandon their traditional roles of making every effort to preserve life at any cost. If the medical profession, in accord with social sanction, can be brought to redefine life as a state in which cerebral action subserves awareness of environment and the possibility of expressing intellect, emotion, personality, and character, and if it can equate the opposite of this with death, the dilemma can be avoided.

A practice which has been adopted and which has proved most acceptable is as follows:

1 The diagnosis of brain death, based on the above criteria, should be corroborated by another physician, and the clinical examination and EEG should be repeated one or more times over a period of 24 h.
2 The family and nurses should be informed of the irreversibility of brain function but should not be asked or permitted to make the decision whether medical treatment should be discontinued.
3 The physician may withdraw supportive medical measures, assuming that nothing more can be offered and that extraordinary measures to maintain heart function need not be em-

ployed (in agreement with recommendations of Pope Pius XII and others of the clergy).

4 The possibility that such patients may become sources of organs for grafting should not enter into such decisions, although prior to the cessation of heart action the family may be approached by surgeons and asked whether this would be their wish, or the family may suggest that organs be used for this purpose.

It is likely that these criteria will change with the further development of technology to "keep patients alive." In approaching these difficult problems, the physician must combine the art of medicine with its science.

PART TWO | CARDINAL MANIFESTATIONS OF DISEASE: AN APPROACH TO CLINICAL PROBLEMS

2
PROBLEM-ORIENTED MEDICAL RECORD

STEPHEN E. GOLDFINGER
JAMES J. DINEEN

Whatever can be said, can be said clearly.
Whereof one cannot speak, thereof one ought remain silent.

Ludwig Wittgenstein

Medical records, as kept for years, have often failed the purposes of lucid communication, education, and rapid retrieval of stored information. Poorly supported diagnoses, incomplete progress notes, chaotically entered laboratory results, and inadequately expressed plans of management are embarrassingly common findings in records existing at some of the most sophisticated medical institutions. In response to this the problem-oriented medical record (POMR) has been devised to provide a method whereby the medical record will better reflect the health problems of patients and the professional responses to them on the part of physicians, nurses, and other major participants in care.

Central to its formulation is the view that the patient's record must be designed so that it expresses specifically what physicians deal with most frequently—the *problems* of patients. While the ultimate goal of clinical taxonomy is directed toward identification of etiology, pathology, and pathologic physiology, in view of their importance as guides to therapy, it would be both unrealistic and dangerous to require a specific diagnosis for a severely dyspneic patient in the absence of reasonably convincing information concerning the reason for the dyspnea. Until the cause can be established, all diagnostic modalities and therapeutic interventions are oriented to the real and immediate problem *dyspnea*. The same is true of a great variety of symptoms, signs, and laboratory findings which are derived in the process of patient care. A high serum calcium reported in a smooth-muscle antibodies (SMA) screening study, a suspicious pigmented skin lesion, or a sudden unexplained deterioration of intellect are examples of worrisome findings that are most appropriately expressed initially as *problems*. In each instance, a more refined diagnosis in the absence of further data can only represent guesswork; hence, it may be wrong. As data pertaining to each problem become available, the problem may then be expressed at a higher level of understanding, i.e., hyperparathyroidism, malignant melanoma, or subdural hematoma. By offering the physician a system of record keeping compatible with the most frequent focus of attention in the practice of medicine—the problem—an opportunity is provided to reduce distortion and error.

The second and more fundamental aspect of problem orientation is the systematized display of patient care embodied in records. This is best described by considering the elements of medical care and their dynamic interrelationship, as proposed by Weed (Fig. 2-1).

THE DATA BASE All clinical care must start with a data base. A careful and complete history and a physical examination are of fundamental value to the physician. The POMR stresses the importance of this traditional approach to data collection. However, there may be instances when full information is unobtainable as, for example, in the case of an unidentified unconscious patient brought into the emergency room. Management of such a case is nevertheless contingent on data, even though incomplete—primarily the initial physical examination, lumbar puncture, and laboratory results. At the other extreme, one might safely argue that no data base can be absolutely complete on any patient, for a lifetime of psychic and biological events can never be fully recalled, much less transcribed. The POMR brings into focus a defined data base, highlights its deficiencies, and serves as the nucleus for its expansion when desirable. Elements of the data base include:

1 Identifying information (i.e., name, age, sex, race, religion, insurance information, etc.)
2 Patient profile (i.e., occupation, education, marital status, children, hobbies, worries, moods, sleep patterns, habits, etc.)
3 Medical history
  a Chief complaints
  b History of present illnesses
  c Past medical history
  d Review of systems
  e Family history
  f Medications

FIGURE 2-1

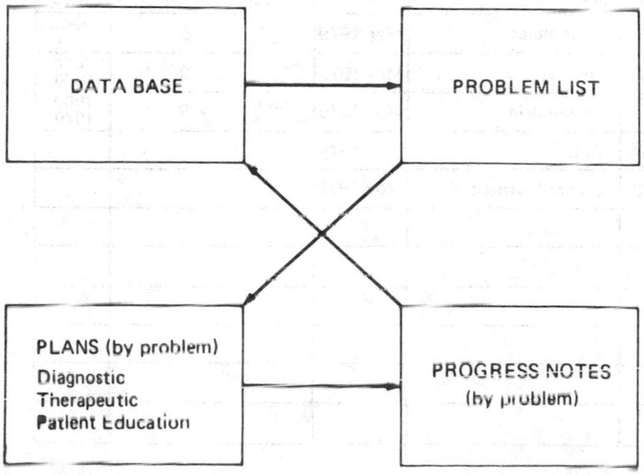

4 Physical examination
5 Laboratory data and physiologic tests (i.e., complete blood count, electrocardiogram, chest x-ray, creatinine, urinalysis, vital capacity, tonometry, etc.)

It is evident that these components do not constitute anything new to conscientious physicians. In using the POMR, they are asked to *define* the data base and to highlight the abnormalities revealed by it as *problems* with which they must deal. Admittedly, an *ideal* data base has not yet been conceived. Such a construct would depend in part on the population served, the resources at hand, and, most importantly, on the relative cost-benefit of various screening studies in regard to prevention of morbidity. Studies of the value of such tests in these terms may lead to the development of a series of risk-related data bases, each applicable to different groups of individuals. Material obtained for each part of the data base is often organized in the record by standardized formats for display. Although some rather sophisticated examples of such data sheets have been designed, it must be emphasized that the ultimate value of a data base depends on the validity of the information that is entered. An inaccurate history, careless examination of the heart, or a faulty piece of laboratory equipment will yield inaccurate data no matter how clearly the results are recorded. Moreover, it should be recognized that the data base must constantly be supplemented by later entries into the record.

THE PROBLEM LIST From the data at hand, a master problem list is formulated. It should include those features in the patient's psychobiological makeup that require continuing attention by the physician and other members of the health team. Thus, the problem list may contain entries relating to social history (e.g., marital discord), risk factors (e.g., familial polyposis of the colon), symptoms (e.g., hemoptysis), physical findings (e.g., splenomegaly), laboratory tests (e.g., anemia), etc. All problems are expressed at a level of highest understanding. For example, if the cause of gastrointestinal bleeding is known to be a duodenal ulcer, the latter becomes the appropriate entry unless severe bleeding in itself constitutes a major health hazard.

FIGURE 2-2

PROBLEM LIST

No.	Active	Date	Inactive	Date
1	Hypertension	1953		
2	Recurrent bronchitis	1958		
3	Penicillin allergy	1958		
4			S/P pyelonephritis	1960
5	Gallstones	Oct 1978	resolved → Cholecystectomy	Mar 1979
6	Arthralgias	Mar 1979	resolved → #9	June 1979
7	Pleurisy	Mar 1979	resolved → #9	June 1979
8	Proteinuria	Apr 1979	resolved → #9	June 1979
9	SLE	Jun 1979		
10	Unemployment	Nov 1979		

The problem list is a *dynamic* entity which is altered as new information and events dictate. All entries are dated, and a separate column permits the recording of resolved and inactive problems (Fig. 2-2).

When kept in this manner, a problem list featured at the beginning of a patient record provides a succinct summary of all important health matters and, moreover, serves as a table of contents for entries within the record which are properly labeled according to problem (see below). Satisfactory problem listing clearly requires periodic revision of this inventory. Also necessary is a sense of proportion, so that a variety of minor, self-limited problems (e.g., colds, sprains, minor gastrointestinal upsets) are excluded from the master problem list, which might otherwise be unduly cluttered with trivial illnesses. When a number of clearly psychosomatic complaints predominate, they may be grouped together as a single entry, e.g., functional symptoms.

PROBLEM-RELATED PLANS Problems regarded as "active" generally require planning for their proper management. The display of these plans, separately listed for each problem, is of critical importance as a reflection of the physician's response to the problems that have been identified. Plans are recorded under three categories:

1 Diagnostic (Dx), i.e., laboratory tests, radiological studies, consultations, continued observation, etc.
2 Therapeutic (Rx), i.e., medications, diet, physiotherapy, corrective surgery, etc.
3 Patient education (Pt ed), i.e., instruction of the patient in various aspects of self-care, education regarding the goal of therapy, the prognosis that has been given, etc.

It is not necessary that all three sections be completed for each problem, inasmuch as planning may at times be concerned with only one or two of them. For example:

1 Diarrhea
 Dx Stool for occult blood, culture, ova, and parasites, microscopic fat, and muscle fibers
   Sigmoidoscopy
   Barium enema if persistent
 Rx Avoid foods that exacerbate
   Propantheline 30 mg tid
 Pt ed Informed that more information is needed to make a diagnosis, will aim for symptomatic therapy for now
2 Pyuria
 Dx BUN
   Repeat urinalysis
   Urine culture
3 Obesity
 Rx 1500 kcal diet
   Weight Watchers
 Pt ed Dangers of obesity cited. *Goal:* 170 lb

PROGRESS NOTES Progress notes are structured on the basis of those problems which have received attention during the office or hospital visit. (Thus, all problems on the list need not be entered.) In a sense, these notes update the course and management of the problem, following the same general schema already described. They are structured in the following manner:

Problem No.
 Subjective (S)   Interval history
       Adherence to program

Problem No.
    Objective (O)   Physical findings
                         Reports of laboratory, x-ray, other tests
    Assessment (A)   Appraisal of progress, interpretation of
                             new findings, etc.
    Plan (P)
        Diagnostic
        Therapeutic
        Patient education
Example:

J   RHD with mitral stenosis
S   2 flight dyspnea, mild fatigue. No orthopnea, hemop-
        tysis, ankle edema. Child has strep throat.
    Medications: chlorothiazide, 500 mg qd.
O   BP 120/70. P 78 regular.
    Neck veins normal, lungs clear.
    Grade iii diastolic rumble, wide opening snap. P_2
        slightly ↑.
    ECG: Early pulmonary mitral; otherwise normal.
A   Stable. Catheterization still not indicated. Risk of
        strep throat present.
P
    Dx   Cardiac fluoroscopy
    Rx   Continue chlorothiazide and penicillin V, 250
            mg bid, 2 weeks
    Pt ed Reinstructed about antibiotic coverage for tooth
            extractions, scheduled for next month. (Will
            contact oral surgeon.)

DATA FLOW SHEETS   At times, the course and management
of a particular problem may be succinctly recorded by using
data flow sheets. Many physicians are familiar with this
method of making brief-interval record entries on patients with
diabetic ketoacidosis or acute gastrointestinal hemorrhage. A
number of other conditions—both acute and chronic—lend
themselves to this manner of sequential description. Data flow
sheets for such problems as hypertension, renal failure, and
respiratory insufficiency serve as excellent adjuncts to effective
patient care within the POMR.

CLINICAL JUDGMENT   This intangible element of patient
care is so crucial that it is cited to emphasize that the style of
recording in itself is no guarantee of excellence. The *content* of
the record—the problems selected from the data base, the nature of the plans evolved, the choice of therapeutic programs—reflects the true quality of the care provided. In this
respect, the initials CJ might appropriately be placed alongside
every arrow in Fig. 2-1 to represent the absolute need for clinical judgment to effectively catalyze the process of sound medical care.

**POTENTIAL BENEFITS OF THE PROBLEM-ORIENTED MEDICAL
RECORD   Allied health personnel**   Several aspects of the
POMR facilitate the team approach to patient care. First, the
requirement that all members of the health team systematically display their thoughts and actions improves communications and potentiates supervision. Second, the existence of a
list of the patient's problems that the health team must manage
reduces errors of omission and treatment out of context. Furthermore, the establishment of a plan for each problem leads
to clearer assignment of specific tasks to each of its members.
Most importantly, the dissection of the health care process into
gathering a data base, formulating problems, and designing a
plan for the management of each problem provides a useful
road map for the intelligent expansion of the role of various
allied health personnel. This breakdown helps physicians as

team leaders to rethink their role in the health care process and
concentrate on the more difficult aspects such as identifying
problems from the data base and organizing approaches to
these problems, while assigning more routine tasks to other
members of the team. Practical experiences in clinical settings
as varied as large hospital clinics and rural offices have suggested the value of the POMR in the team approach to patient
care.

Education and audit   In addition to facilitating patient care, a
good medical record should educate its readers and also be
subject to audit in its own right. By clearly outlining the physician's logic, the POMR reveals the process of patient care in a
manner which can be evaluated. This, in itself, is an educational process. It deemphasizes rote memory and substitutes a
record of the logical steps which are being taken to recognize
the patient's problems and the physician's capacity to act as a
guide in attempting to solve them. Such an endeavor, if begun
early, can set the stage for a lifelong educational process of self
and peer evaluation through effective record audit.

Clinical research   Any record system that clarifies the details
of patient-physician interaction can be a powerful tool in clinical research. A clear data base, an organized system for record
entries, and the use of data flow sheets serve to facilitate rapid
extraction and analysis of clinical information. Efforts to com-
puterize the POMR, if successful, will amass a spectrum of
clinical and epidemiologic data that may prove extremely
valuable in our understanding of illness and the process of
health care.

THE ROLE OF THE POMR IN PATIENT CARE   The POMR is a
system of record keeping which greatly facilitates data retrieval and at the same time highlights the decision-making
role of physicians as they respond to the problems of patients.
It should be evident, nevertheless, that it can only serve the
goal of improved health care when it is used with a sound
intellectual appreciation of disease, based on a full understanding of pathophysiology and a scientific approach to therapy.
The tendency for the POMR to compartmentalize problems
must not preclude creative, synthetic thinking. At some institutions an Initial Assessment entry is placed before the Problem
List to provide an opportunity for the physician to express an
overall perspective and to distinguish the major problems from
others which are less important. Finally, as emphasized in the
preceding chapters, compassion is an element of medical care
that can never be adequately displayed by any record system.
A possible danger of the POMR is that the emotional needs of
patients may receive even less attention from a busy physician
who is intent on writing excellent notes. The patient and not
the record must remain the primary focus of physician care.

REFERENCES

BJORN JC, CROSS HD: *Problem Oriented Practice.* Chicago, Modern
    Hospital Press, McGraw-Hill, 1970
FEINSTEIN AR: The problems of the "problem-oriented medical rec-
    ord." Ann Intern Med 78:751, 1973
GOLDFINGER SE: The problem-oriented record: A critique from a be-
    liever. N Engl J Med 288:606, 1973
HURST W, WALKER HK: *The Problem Oriented System.* New York,
    Medcom Press, 1972
WEED LL: *Medical Records, Medical Education and Patient Care.*
    Cleveland, Case University Press, 1969

section 1 | Pain

3
GENERAL CONSIDERATIONS

RAYMOND D. ADAMS

Pain, it has been said, is one of "Nature's earliest signs of morbidity." Few will deny that it stands preeminent among all the sensory experiences by which humans judge the existence of disease within themselves. There are relatively few maladies that do not have their painful phases, and in many of them pain is a characteristic without which diagnosis must always be in doubt. It seems appropriate, therefore, to begin a section on the cardinal manifestations of disease with a discussion of the more general aspects of pain.

The painful experiences of the sick pose manifold problems for practitioners of medicine, and students should know something of these problems in order to prepare themselves for the task ahead. They must be ready to diagnose disease in patients who have felt only the first rumblings of discomfort, before other symptoms and signs of disease have appeared. To cope effectively with problems of this type requires a sound knowledge of the sensory supply of the viscera and a familiarity with the typical symptoms of many diseases. They will be consulted by some patients who seek treatment for pains that appear to have no obvious structural basis, and further inquiry will disclose that worry, fear, and other troubled emotional states may have aggrandized relatively minor aches and pains. To understand problems of this type requires insight into the psychologic factors which influence behavior and a knowledge of psychiatric disease. Next, they must manage the "difficult pain cases," in which no amount of investigation will bring to light either medical disease or psychiatric illness, and it is here that they will sense the need of a sound and assured clinical approach to the pain problem. Finally, they must care for the patients with intractable pain, often from an established and incurable disease, who demand relief either by drug or by the "less moderate means of surgery." Assessing the possibilities of the latter requires a comprehension of the anatomic pathways of pain.

END ORGANS, AFFERENT TRACTS, AND NUCLEI OF TERMI-NATION OF PAIN PATHWAYS Pain is a sensation which has its own sensory apparatus. The receptors in the skin and deep structures are fine, freely branching nerve endings which form an intricate network throughout the body. A single primary pain neuron with its cell body in the posterior root ganglion subdivides into many small peripheral branches to supply an area of skin of several square millimeters. The cutaneous area of each neuron overlaps with those of other neurons, so that every spot of skin lies within the domain of two to four neurons. These freely branching nerve endings are also found in many of the other specialized sensory receptors in the skin, such as Krause's end bulbs, the ruffinian plumes, and the pacinian corpuscles, which may explain why the extremes of hot, cold, and pressure sensation become painful. Free nerve endings may also serve as receptors for other types of sensa-

tion. They are the only end organ in the cornea, where touch and temperature as well as pain are felt.

The sensory nerve fibers for pain, as they course through somatic and visceral nerves, are mixed with other sensory and motor fibers. All sensory fibers enter the spinal cord through the posterior roots and enter the brainstem through certain of the cranial nerves. The pain fibers are of two sizes, one very small (2 to 4 μm in diameter), called *C fibers* with a slow conducting velocity, the other somewhat larger (6 to 8 μm), called *A-delta fibers,* with more rapid transmission rates. As the posterior root enters the spinal cord, it separates into two divisions, medial and lateral. The medial division, heavily myelinated, synapses either with large secondary sensory neurons in the posterior horn or with anterior horn cells (serving segmental reflexes), or it passes upward in the posterior columns, with some fibers reaching the medulla. The lateral division, of thinly myelinated and nonmyelinated fibers, travels in the tract of Lissauer to reach the substantia gelatinosa, where it synapses with (1) many small neurons whose axons pass into the posterior and anterior horns of the same and adjacent segments of the spinal cord, also effecting reflex connections and (2) large secondary sensory neurons, some of which form the lateral spinothalamic tract and some of which ascend for varying distances near the gray matter as a polysynaptic pathway. The neurons on which the afferent root fibers terminate lie in the first and fifth laminae of the posterior horn, and it is postulated that their reactivity is influenced by large afferent touch fibers or by other inhibitory neurons within the spinal gray matter. Through a mechanism still rather obscure two secondary ascending pathways for pain are activated. One is the lateral spinothalamic tract, the cell bodies of which lie in the posterior horns, with axons crossing through the anterior commissure of the spinal cord within one to two segments of the level of entry. The other is a less well-defined, multineuronal chain which extends upward along the reticular part of the gray matter. The lateral spinothalamic tract, joined in the brainstem by the trigeminothalamic tract, courses through the lateral part of the medulla, pons, and midbrain, giving off many collaterals before terminating in the nucleus ventralis posterolateralis, the posterior nuclear group, and intralaminar thalamic nuclei (Fig. 3-1). The reticular chain of neurons extends cephalad and finally makes connections through the interlaminar nuclei of the thalamus and with the limbic portions of the cerebrum (Bonica).

The secondary spinothalamic and trigeminothalamic tracts synapse with the tertiary sensory neurons of the thalamus whose axons extend to the cortex of the parietal lobe. Physiologists are not agreed as to the cortical terminus for the pain fibers, for electrical stimulation of the cortex in the conscious human being seldom produces a painful sensation, and parietal lobe lesions seldom cause central pain. Presumably their cortical termination is rather diffuse and bilateral in both parietal and frontal regions. Only a few end in the primary somatosensory cortex. The secondary somatosensory cortex receives more fibers than the primary. Most of the pain fibers from the periphery cross to the opposite side of the brain; only a small contingent remains ipsilateral. (See Adams and Victor for more detailed descriptions of pain neurons and tracts.)

Segmental innervation As a means of quick orientation to the anatomy of the peripheral pain pathways it should be remembered that the facial structures and anterior cranium lie in the field of the trigeminal nerves; the back of the head, second cervical; the neck, third cervical; epaulet area, fourth cervical; deltoid area, fifth cervical, radial forearm and thumb, sixth cervical; index finger, seventh cervical; middle finger, eighth cervical; little finger and inner forearm, first thoracic; nipple segment, fifth thoracic; umbilical, tenth thoracic; groin, first lumbar; medial side of knee, third lumbar; great toe, fifth lumbar; little toe, first sacral; back of thigh, second sacral; genitosacral areas, third, fourth, and fifth sacral. The first to fourth thoracic nerve roots are the important sensory pathways for the intrathoracic viscera; the sixth to eighth thoracic, for the upper abdominal organs (Fig. 19-1).

PHYSIOLOGY AND PSYCHOLOGY OF PAIN The stimuli that arouse pain vary for each tissue. Generally the adequate stimuli for skin are those which injure tissue, i.e., pricking, cutting, crushing, burning, and freezing. Interestingly, these same forms of stimulation have little effect when applied to the stomach and intestine. Pain in the gastrointestinal tract is produced instead by local trauma of an engorged or inflamed mucosa, distention or spasm of smooth muscle, and traction on the mesenteric attachment. Pain is induced in skeletal muscles by ischemia (the basis for the condition known as intermittent claudication), as well as by tears of connective tissue sheaths, necrosis, hemorrhage, or the injection of irritating solutions. Prolonged contraction of muscles evokes an aching type of pain. Ischemia, the only proved source of pain in the heart muscle, is responsible for angina pectoris and for the pain of myocardial infarction. Joints are insensitive to pricking, cutting, and cautery, but pain is induced in the synovial membrane by hypertonic saline solution and inflammation. Arteries give rise to pain when pierced with a needle, when induced to pulsate excessively (as in migraine), and in certain diseases of their walls such as exemplified by atherosclerotic thrombosis and arteritis of cranial arteries. Traction and displacement of intracranial vessels and the meningeal structures by which they are supported may cause headache.

In these painful lesions which damage tissues, proteolytic enzymes are released which act on gamma globulins to liberate irritating substances that stimulate nerve endings. Bradykinins, serotonin, acetylcholine, 5-hydroxytryptamine, histamine, prostaglandins, and other similar polypeptides or acid metabolites released by tissue injury have been found to elicit pain when injected intraarterially or applied to the base of a blister. Such substances are viewed as the "mediators" for pain. Strong pressure may also mechanically stimulate free nerve endings.

The sensory experiences resulting from these several modes of stimulation in the skin and in deep skeletomuscular and visceral structures differ in quality. Integumentary stimuli, at the lowest levels of intensity, evoke sensations of touch, pressure, warmth, cold, or tickle. When increased to the point approaching tissue destruction, pain is added, and the resulting experience is thereafter a mixed one. The painful experience itself is one of pricking or burning. The threshold for burning pain from a thermal stimulus is approximately 2000 times the threshold for warmth. This relationship of pain to tissue destruction is the basis of a biologic principle—that pain has a protective, or self-preserving, value to the organism.

A new chapter is being written on the pharmacology of nociception. Salicylates, which are peripherally acting analgesics, exert an inhibitory effect on the synthesis of prostaglandins (potent stimulators of nociceptive endings). Salicylates fail to antagonize other of the putative neurohumors such as bradykinin and histamine. Opiates have a major central analgesic effect. High densities of specific opiate receptors (presumably on the presynaptic terminals of the C and other pain fibers) have been demonstrated in the posterior horns of spinal cord and trigeminal nuclei; others have been demonstrated in the peri-aqueductal gray matter, medial thalamus, infundibulum, amygdaloid nuclei, caudate nuclei, and frontotemporal cortex. Their distribution would appear to account for both the sensory and affective aspects of pain experience. At these receptor sites one expects to find inhibitory and excitatory transmitters. These synaptosomal receptors are blocked by opiates and their antagonists. The identification of these neurotransmitters is incomplete. One type, called the beta endorphin polypeptides, has been isolated from brain tissue; these appear to be the natural CNS transmitters or modulators of opiate action. γ-Aminobutyric acid (GABA) and glycine are potent inhibitory substances. At the cellular level opiates have been shown to inhibit function by causing a decrement in cyclic AMP.

One must ask why the brain contains alkaloid receptors which when blockaded impair the neurologic experience of pain. Guillemin suggests that these receptors were not put there to receive "the poppy" but to recognize and accept some endogenous substance serving the physiology of pain experience, and that because of the configuration of the receptor

FIGURE 3-1

Radiation and sites of reference of cardiac pain (upper) and *gallbladder pain* (lower).

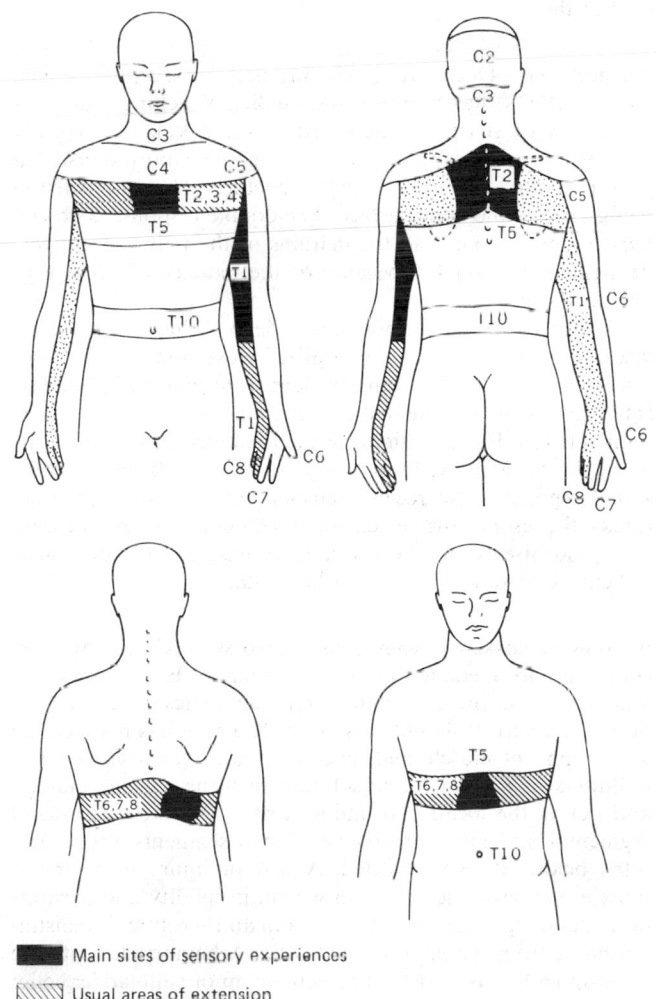

■ Main sites of sensory experiences

▨ Usual areas of extension

▦ Less common areas of extension

binding site both the endogenous substance and opiates are equally effective. Indeed, it has recently been shown that beta endorphins relieve pain and counteract withdrawal symptoms.

The threshold for the perception of pain, i.e., the lowest intensity of stimulus recognized as pain, is approximately the same in all persons. It is lowered by inflammation and raised by local anesthetics (e.g., procaine), lesions of the nervous system, and certain centrally acting analgesic drugs. Distraction and suggestion by turning attention away from the painful part reduce the awareness of and the response to pain. Strong emotion (fear or rage) suppresses pain. Neurotic patients in general have the same pain threshold as normal subjects, but their reaction may be excessive or abnormal. The pain thresholds of frontal lobotomized subjects are also unchanged, but they react briefly if at all to pain. The degree of emotional reaction and the verbalization (complaint) also vary with the personality and character of the patient.

Superficial pain Sensory impulses subserving pricking pain, being transmitted by larger pain fibers, have a more rapid rate of conductivity to the nervous system than burning pain. A hot needle applied to the toe, for example, produces a quick, pricking pain and, only 1 to 2 s later, a burning pain. Together they constitute the "double response" of Lewis. Ischemia of nerve by the application of a tourniquet to a limb abolishes pricking pain before burning pain. Both types of dermal pain are localized with precision (local sign), made possible by the overlap of sensory neurons. Analgesia means the interruption of all pain neurons to an area, and hypalgesia, the interruption of only part of them.

Visceral pain Deep pain (including that of visceral and skeletal structures) has basically the quality of aching, but if intense may be sharp and penetrating (knifelike). Occasionally there is a burning type of pain, as in the heartburn of esophageal irritation and rarely in angina pectoris. The pain is felt as being deep to the body surface. The double response is absent, localization is poor, and the margins of the pain are not well delineated, presumably because of the paucity of nerve endings in viscera.

Actually, the pain originating in deep skeletomuscular and visceral structures cannot be localized closer than two to three sensory segments. For example, pain from myocardial disease is felt to arise within the first to fourth or possibly fifth thoracic segments (see Fig. 3-1, showing theoretic distribution of heart pain). Unfortunately, from the standpoint of diagnosis, these spinal segments also receive sensory fibers from other structures—the esophagus, mediastinal contents, bones, muscles, etc.—and diseases of these structures may cause pain that is difficult to distinguish from cardiac pain.

Deep musculoskeletal pain Since deep skeletal pain and visceral pain are mediated through a common deep sensory system, it is not surprising that their characteristics (type, localization, and referral) should be similar. Kellgren has mapped the topography of muscle and tendinous pain by injecting a few milliliters of normal saline solution into the various muscles and noting the location of induced pain. The ache is usually segmental and may spread one to two segments above (less often below) the site injected. A tear or injury in a lumbar muscle may give rise to a pain which, in quality and localization, including radiation into the groin and scrotum, is indistinguishable from the pain of renal colic. A hemorrhage into the right upper rectus muscle mimics the pain of gallbladder colic; and a lesion in a muscle or ligament deep in the chest wall causes pain referred to the left arm, like that of angina. The

differentiation of these pains must be made on grounds other than location and reference.

Referred pain Deep visceral and somatic pains tend always to be referred superficially to those structures within a given spinal segment that have the most extensive nerve ramifications and therefore the widest cerebral representation (e.g., there are more sensory nerves in the integument than in the viscera, hence the pain in the latter is projected to the body surface). In the case of myocardial pain, sensory impulses entering the first to fourth thoracic nerves activate a pool of sensory neurons, the largest number of which also receive afferents from the skin of the inner side of the arm (T_1 and T_2) and the anterior precordium (T_3 and T_4). More of the sensory neurons from the heart enter the left side of the spinal cord than the right. These anatomic and physiologic data explain why cardiac pain is referred predominantly to the substernal, left precordial, and inner brachial zones.

Aberrant reference of pain occurs not infrequently and is explained in terms of the physiologic status of the spinal pool of sensory neurons. As was stated, a single sensory neuron entering one spinal root presynaptically depolarizes to a varying degree a pool of spinal neurons over four or five spinal segments. Pain then should spread to segments adjacent to the painful lesion, where it also causes cutaneous hyperesthesia and, by activating motor neurons, involuntary muscle contraction. If some preexistent disease in *adjacent* somatic segments has already partially depolarized the spinal pool of sensory neurons, a new painful disease which will further depolarize them causes the pain to spread to them. For example, if gallbladder disease which activated sensory fibers entering at the sixth to eighth thoracic nerve root, or cervical arthritis (at the second to eighth cervical nerve root) were present before a myocardial infarct, the cardiac pain might then be referred to the upper part of the abdomen or neck, respectively. Generally these aberrant referrals occur in segments that are cephalad to the normal segmental distribution of pain because their inhibitory connections are more abundant than those of caudal ones.

Hyperesthesia, hyperalgesia, hyperpathia, involuntary spasms, and other responses It has been customary to use the first two of these terms to designate a lowering of the threshold to touch and pain stimuli and the third for a state of pain with a normal or raised threshold but overreaction. Hyperpathia may even occur with anesthesia, as in *anesthesia dolorosa*. Any real distinction between these states is ephemeral. Probably only with inflammation of the skin is the pain threshold consistently lowered. What is most characteristic of all chronically painful states, and these frequently implicate nerves or central nervous structures, is that the part is unusually sensitive to all stimuli, even those which normally do not evoke pain; and the elicited pain is unnatural, radiant, outlasts the initiating stimulus, and is unusually modifiable by fatigue, emotion, etc. One sees listed here many of the characteristics of causalgia, spinal cord pain, phantom pain, zoster neuralgia, thalamic pain, etc. The explanation currently offered for these states is that at the peripheral as well as the central level the system of pain fibers is no longer in equilibrium with other sensory fibers. A kind of inhibition is exerted on the pain system at all times by the small neurons in the substantia gelatinosa, under the control of other afferent as well as descending pathways. Since the largest afferent peripheral nerve fibers suppress the secondary spinal neurons receiving pain impulses, nerve injury, which tends often to destroy some of the larger fibers, then permits their overresponse. According to Melzack and Wall, the small neurons of the substantia gelatinosa constitute a kind of "gate control system" which modulates input. The activation of large afferent fibers in a peripheral nerve is said to inhibit the gateway cells. While much of the recent physiological evidence has failed to confirm this gateway hypothesis, it has called attention to some type of mechanism that controls the pain threshold and painful states. Some such segmental mechanism must also be under the influence of descending pathways from the cerebrum and from other spinal segments. One might suppose that the activation of some of the sensory fibers controlling "gateway neurons" could be the basis of the effectiveness of *acupuncture;* the psychological mechanism of suggestion may also play a role in acupuncture therapy. There is a wide range of responses to pain to which attention is drawn. Strong, acute pain causes a startle reaction. Intense, persistent pain is usually accompanied by segmental flexion reflexes (e.g., spasm of a segment of the abdominal wall with visceral disease, flexion of knees and hips with peritoneal irritation, extension of neck with meningitis), autonomic responses, postural adjustments, avoidance movements, and vocalization. The obvious biologic function of segmental spasms is to splint the diseased part and to facilitate healing. The altered state of receptivity of the spinal gray matter accounts for stimuli of nonreceptive-type evoking pain, e.g., for subcutaneous pressure being painful.

As pain sensation may be induced by stimulation of the receptors or by irritation of peripheral nerves or roots, it may be abolished by diseases which affect the peripheral or central nervous system, or by a surgical procedure which accomplishes the same result. Pain in a circumscribed region may be terminated by section of the nerve which supplies that region (neurotomy) or by section of the spinal roots (posterior rhizotomy); pain in a limb or one side of the trunk may be abolished by section of the anterolateral spinothalamic tracts (lateral spinal tractotomy in the spinal cord or tractotomy in the lateral medulla or mesencephalon).

Perception of pain   Only upon the arrival of pain impulses at the thalamocortical level of the nervous system is there conscious awareness of the pain stimulus. Clinical study has not informed us of the exact localization of the nervous apparatus for this mental process. It is not entirely abolished by a total hemispherectomy, including the thalamus on one side. It is often said that impulses reaching the thalamus create awareness of the attributes of sensation and that the parietal cortex is necessary for the appreciation of the intensity and localization of the sensation. This seems to be an oversimplification. Probably a close and harmonious relationship between thalamus and cortex must exist in order for a sensory experience to be complete. The traditional separation of sensation (in this instance awareness of pain) and perception (awareness of the nature of the painful stimulus) has been abandoned in favor of the view that sensation, perception, and the various conscious and unconscious responses to a pain stimulus comprise an indivisible process.

Although similar to other sensory or perceptive phenomena in certain respects, such as predictable response to given intensity of stimulus, pain differs in other ways. One of its most remarkable characteristics is the strong feeling tone, or affect, with which it is endowed, nearly always one of unpleasantness. Furthermore, pain does not appear to be subject to negative adaptation. Most stimuli, if applied continuously, soon cease to be effective, whereas pain may persist as long as the stimulus is operative; and, by establishing a central excitatory state, may even outlast the stimulus.

Stereotaxic surgery on the thalamus in cases of intractable pain permits dissection of the anatomy of the pain experience. Lesions in the terminus of the lateral spinothalamic tract in the posterolateral nucleus are said to abolish pain and temperature sensation in the contralateral side of the body while leaving the patient with all the misery or affect of pain. Lesions in the centrum medianum relieve the painful state without altering pain and temperature sensation. Thus, at this level there must also be a balance of inhibitory and facilitatory sensory systems, for one cannot explain intractable pain simply in terms of continuous stimulation of chains of pain neurons.

Psychologic aspects of pain   A discussion of this problem could hardly be complete without some reference to the influence of emotional states or to the importance of racial, cultural, and religious factors on the pain response, especially its overt expressions. It is common knowledge that some individuals, by virtue of training, habit, or phlegmatic character, are relatively stoical, and that others are excessively responsive to pain. And there are rare individuals who are totally incapable of experiencing pain throughout their lifetime, either from a lack of sensory endings or peripheral sensory apparatus, or from some peculiarity of central reception.

Lastly, it is important to keep in mind the devastating effects of chronic pain. As Ambroise Paré remarked, "There is nothing that abateth so much the strength as paine." Continuous pain can be observed to have an adverse effect on the entire nervous system. There are increased irritability, fatigue, troubled sleep, poor appetite, and loss of emotional stability. Courageous individuals are reduced to a whimpering, pitiable state that may arouse only the scorn of a healthy person. They are irrational about illness and may make unreasonable demands on family and physician. The degree of disability exceeds the physical findings. This condition, termed *pain shock,* once established, requires delicate but firm management. Depression (reactive?) is common. Of course, demand for and dependency on narcotic drugs often complicate the picture.

CLINICAL APPROACH TO THE PATIENT WITH PAIN AS THE PREDOMINANT SYMPTOM   One of the first points to keep in mind is that not all pain is the consequence of serious disease. Otherwise healthy individuals have thousands of pains which are part of their daily sensory experience. To mention but a few, there is the momentary, hard pain over an eye, in the temporal region, or in the ear or jaw, which strikes with alarming suddenness; the more persistent ache which arises in some fleshy part, such as the shoulder, neck, thigh, or calf, the darting pain in an arm or leg, the fleeting precordial discomfort that arouses momentarily the thought of heart disease, the breathtaking catch in the side from diaphragmatic cramp, the cluster of abdominal pains with their associated intestinal rumblings, and the brief discomfort upon movement of a joint. These *normal pains,* as they should be called, occur at all ages, tend to be brief, and depart as obscurely as they come. They acquire medical significance only when elicited by an inquiring physician, or when presented as a complaint by a worried patient; and, of course, they must always be distinguished from the *abnormal pains* of disease.

When pain, by its intensity, duration, and the circumstance of its occurrence, appears to be abnormal or constitutes one of the principal symptoms of disease, an attempt should be made to reach a tentative decision as to its cause and the mechanism of its production. This can usually be accomplished by thoroughly questioning and encouraging the patient to relate as accurately as possible the main characteristics of the pain and the circumstances under which it occurs. The physical examination is directed toward a search for evidences of suspected disease and the reproduction of the pain.

Location of pain   When the pain is caused by a superficial lesion, the cause and effect are usually so obvious that no problem is posed. It is the deep lesion, whether involving somatic or visceral structures, that causes trouble, and here exact localization becomes especially important. We have already seen that the pain originating from such tissues is no longer sensed as coming from them, but is instead only roughly segmental, i.e., within the territory of the cord segments innervating the structure. The identification of the segments involved is of value, for it sets the limit on the diagnostic possibilities that must be considered, i.e., they are limited to those structures having a corresponding innervation. Thus an epigastric or subxiphoid pain, or one in the opposite region in the back, obliges one to search for its cause in all those structures innervated by the sixth through eighth thoracic cord segments, i.e., the esophagus, stomach, duodenum, pancreas, biliary tract, the upper retroperitoneal structures, as well as the deep somatic tissues in this region. Also, one must consider the possibility that a lesion in a viscus innervated by spinal segments above or below the sixth through eighth thoracic cord segments may at times be the source of pain that has spread outside its normal boundaries and involved the epigastrium (Fig. 3-1).

Provoking and relieving factors These factors are of greater value than quality of pain in providing important data concerning its mechanism. Pain related to breathing, swallowing, and defecation focuses attention on the respiratory apparatus, the esophagus, and the lower part of the intestinal tract, respectively. A pain coming on a few minutes after the beginning of general bodily movement and relieved almost at once by rest indicates ischemia or a neural mechanism as the probable cause (see Chaps. 9 and 10). Pain occurring several hours after meals and relieved by food or alkali suggests the irritative effect of acid on the raw lining of the stomach or duodenum. Pain that is brought on or relieved by certain movements or postures of parts of the body is usually due to diseased skeletal structures (bones, muscles, ligaments). Pain that is enhanced by cough, sneeze, and strain is usually radicular in origin or arises in ligamentous structures. Pain that is increased or altered by cutaneous stimuli is due to disease in sensory tracts in the peripheral or central nervous system.

Quality and time-intensity characteristics of pain Much reliance is put on the patient's choice of words and account of the intensity of pain. Unfortunately this will depend, in part at least, on the patient's intelligence, vocabulary, and concept of what is taking place. "Crushing" and "squeezing" are commonly employed to describe an anginal pain, and this implication of pressure has some significance since the pain may depend on an associated involuntary contraction of the pectoral muscles. Another patient with the same disease, however, may describe the pain as "exploding" or "burning." Far more important than the adjective used for pain is the information that it is steady and does not fluctuate. Similarly, the pain of peptic ulcer is frequently designated as "gnawing," but again, the deep, steady quality is more important than the word used to denote it. Gallbladder colic and renal colic are misnomers, if by colic is meant a "paroxysmal abdominal pain due to spasm, obstruction, or distention of any of the hollow viscera." *In both these disorders, the pain tends to be steady.* The aching quality of all deep pains is usually characteristic, but there are also several other informative attributes. A true colicky pain, one that is rhythmic and cramping, suggests an obstructive lesion in a hollow viscus. If the patient is a woman who has had children, it is a good idea to ask whether her "cramp" resembles the pains she had during childbirth. A pain that is steady and varies little or not at all from moment to moment means that the stimulus to pain is steady and unwavering, as in angina pectoris and peptic ulcer. Thus, a pain in the anterior midsternal region whose intensity fluctuates appreciably within the space of a minute or two is not due to angina, even

though the history may appear to suggest a relation to exertion. Similarly, a high epigastric pain appearing several hours after a meal and even apparently relieved by food is not caused by an ulcer if the pain fluctuates perceptibly within seconds or a few minutes. The stimulus to ulcer pain does not quickly vary in intensity. A throbbing pain indicates that an arterial pulsation is giving rise to painful stimuli. Sharp, recurrent stabs of pain are caused by disease of nerve roots or sensory ganglions, as exemplified by tic douloureux or tabes, or a single episode may be due to a tear of a muscle or ligament. Once started, in each instance there may be a background of dull, aching pain. Particularly noteworthy here is the abrupt intensification of the dull ache of root pain by cough, sneeze, or strain which momentarily stretches or alters the position of the root.

Mode of onset of pain This factor is also important. A pain reaching its full intensity almost immediately after its appearance suggests a rupture of tissue. The pain of a dissecting aortic aneurysm often develops in this manner. In fact, the suddenness and the severity of the pain, reaching a peak of intensity within seconds or minutes, sometimes provides the first clue in differentiating this type of chest pain from that caused by myocardial infarction. A similarly rapid accession of pain may occur with the rupture of a peptic ulcer.

Duration of pain This is another useful diagnostic attribute. Anginal pain, for example, rarely lasts less than 2 or 3 min or more than 10 to 15 min. Ulcer pain may continue for an hour or more, unless terminated by the ingestion of food or alkali or a tumbler of water.

Severity of pain In any given disease, the severity of pain is subject to wide variation, and patients differ in their tolerance to it. Therefore, one cannot judge the gravity of an illness solely by the patient's report of the intensity of pain. As a rule, pains that completely interrupt work or pleasurable activity, require opiates for relief, enforce bed rest, or awaken the patient from sound sleep are to be taken more seriously than those which have the opposite characteristics.

Time of occurrence An accurate determination must be made of the temporal aspects of the pain. The relationship of ulcer pain to the preceding meal has already been mentioned. Postural aches come after prolonged activity and disappear with rest; arthritic pains are usually most severe during the first movements after prolonged inactivity. The mechanisms for this latter phenomenon are not known, nor do we understand why painful lesions of the bone, such as those caused by metastatic cancer, are likely to be most disturbing during the night. It is possible that the occurrence or aggravation of the latter types of pain is due to enhanced awareness of painful stimuli at a time when the mind is not distracted by other stimuli, or it may be that the pains are now more easily evoked by unconscious movements made during sleep when protective reflexes are in abeyance.

It should be obvious from these remarks that the full significance of a pain is usually not revealed by any one single characteristic. It is only by combining all these data that one can determine its anatomic site and its mechanism. In general, *the most important and revealing clues are obtained from the answers to the questions: What brings on the pain? What relieves it?* Pain is a subjective manifestation, not a state to be observed or measured. The accuracy of our data depends on the skill with which we frame our questions and on the powers of observation and memory of the person answering them.

Finally, the diagnostic value of measures which *reproduce* and *relieve the pain* should be stressed. Not only are they important for diagnosis, but they convince the patient that the physician understands and can control pain and the illness behind it. Climbing several flights of stairs under the physician's supervision may settle the question of the presence or absence of angina pectoris. An injection of procaine into the tender area in the chest wall or some other skeletal structure, with complete disappearance of the pain, may establish its skeletal origin and exclude the possibility of visceral disease. Reproducing the distress sometimes caused by aerophagia merely by distending the esophagus or stomach with air, or reproducing the vague but sometimes alarming sensation of pressure in the chest caused by unconscious hyperventilation by having the patient deliberately hyperventilate are other examples of how the principle of the reproduction of pain may be usefully employed.

A systematic interrogation of the patient will not lead to accurate diagnosis in every instance, but the habit of searching for the identifying characteristics of pain will enable physicians to increase their skill in this difficult field. Furthermore, after becoming familiar with the customary responses to these questions, one becomes more alert to the anxious, the hysterical, or the depressed patient who while complaining of pain seems incapable of describing any of its details, or is unwilling to do so. Instead, there is preoccupation with theories of what is wrong or with the treatments or mistreatments already given.

Obscure and intractable pains Finally, there will always be cases that defy solution, and the physician must develop a systematic clinical approach to them. There are four discernible groups of such pains: (1) the pain of medical and surgical diseases yet undiagnosable; (2) "psychiatric" pains; (3) "neurologic" pains; (4) pains of indeterminate types.

With respect to group 1, neoplasms in retropharyngeal, posterior mediastinal, and retroperitoneal regions and the spine are among the more frequent causes of pain, lasting months before being revealed by the usual methods of diagnosis. In group 2, four psychiatric conditions are associated with pain which may dominate the clinical picture: psychotic depression, hysteria, compensation "neurosis," and constitutional psychopathy; any one of them may be complicated by drug addiction. Since psychiatric illnesses do not preclude another painful disease, the clinical analysis must of necessity rule out the latter while establishing on the basis of history and physical findings the existence and nature of the former. In group 3, neurologic diseases of painful type (causalgia, spinal cord injury, discogenic root disease, and thalamic pain syndrome) are usually diagnosable on the basis of the clinical findings (see Chaps. 19 and 365), but the difficult problems are those in which the neurologic disease is accompanied by depression, malingering, compensation "neurosis," or opiate or other drug addiction. The fourth group includes the cases that are left when the first three are excluded. They defy solution. The physician can proceed only by repeatedly reexamining the patient, explaining the need for continued observation, and enlisting the patient's aid and forbearance during this trying period. Asking the patient to tolerate a certain amount of pain without the use of powerful analgesics is usually effective, particularly when the possibility of drug addiction is explained.

In the relatively rare circumstances when all manner of investigation has failed to throw light on the cause and mechanism of the pain, demands for pain-relieving surgery may become increasingly insistent. The physician may in desperation turn to measures which are more dangerous than the disease. Here the commonest source of error is to operate unnecessarily on the hysterical patient (see Chap. 11), only to discover too late that each operative procedure is followed by a new pain, often at a higher level than the first. Or depressive psychosis may have masqueraded as a painful state and is operated upon

when antidepressant medication, electric shock therapy, or other therapy would have dramatically terminated the illness. Sometimes a half dozen or more operations are unsuccessfully performed on a single patient. The safest rule to follow in these cases is not to use opiates continuously or to recommend operation for the relief of pain unless a reasonable diagnosis has been made. For the pains of metastatic cancer, the thalamic pain of vascular disease of the brain, and other incurable diseases, the relative advantages of the controlled use of opiates versus lateral spinothalamic tractomy or frontal lobotomy must be carefully weighed in each patient. The age of the patient, other diseases, life expectancy, and mental state are all of importance in selecting the treatment procedure. Too often an operation on the spinal cord or brain is chosen in preference to narcotics and the controlled use of drugs. Forgotten is the fact that many patients with cancer were formerly kept relatively comfortable and active by the judicious use of morphine and its analogues and were never subjected to costly operations or deprived of any of those qualities of mind and character which are so treasured by their families.

TREATMENT Superficial pain arising in integumentary structures rarely presents a problem in therapy. Acetylsalicylic acid, 0.30 to 0.60 g, or acetaminophen (Tylenol), 0.30 to 0.60 g, orally every 4 h usually suffices. Acetophenetidin may be added. These two drugs are particularly effective when one element of pain is integumentary. Commercial proprietary preparations of these drugs containing caffeine (e.g., ASA compound, Empirin compound, and aspirin) or amphetamine (e.g., Edrisal) are available in most pharmacies. The caffeine or amphetamine is particularly useful if there is central nervous system depression, and often there is advantage to adding a sedative drug. When this type of pain is not effectively controlled by nonnarcotic analgesics, codeine should be given. Usually the addition of small amounts (8 to 30 mg) of codeine phosphate to the standard dose of acetylsalicylic acid and acetophenetidin is effective. A preparation containing codeine phosphate 8 to 30 mg, acetylsalicylic acid 0.23 g, acetophenetidin 0.16 g, and caffeine 0.032 g is commercially available (Empirin compound with codeine phosphate). Codeine, 20 to 45 mg every 3 h, gives fairly effective analgesia with minimal side effects. Adequate rest and relief of muscle tensions should also be encouraged. The application of moist heat is usually beneficial. Occasionally cold applications are preferred, but with the exception of cooling packs applied to an inflamed, burning skin or to a causalgia, cold is more likely to aggravate than to soothe the painful condition.

Occasionally integumental and deep pains of skeletal structures are of such severity as to require more powerful narcotic analgesics, such as meperidine hydrochloride (Demerol) in doses of 50 to 100 mg orally or intramuscularly, methadone hydrochloride, 5 to 10 mg orally or subcutaneously, or dihydromorphine hydrochloride (Dilaudid), 1 to 2 mg orally and subcutaneously. These drugs are most useful when sedation is not required. When pain is unusually severe and some degree of euphoria is desired, one of the new drugs such as pentazocine hydrochloride (Talwin) should be given in doses of 50 mg orally or subcutaneously every 3 to 4 h. Morphine, although still a valuable drug in doses of 8 to 15 mg, is not used much because of its habit-forming tendency and the frequently associated nausea and vomiting. Since all these narcotic analgesics are, for the most part, detoxified by the liver, they either should not be used or should be given in only half the usual dosage in cases of liver disease, myxedema, adrenal insufficiency, and other states in which·the metabolic rate is reduced. Morphine and related narcotic analgesics tend to cause pruritus and should therefore be used with care in patients with skin irritability. The possibility of initiating addiction in susceptible persons must be carefully evaluated in every instance (cf. Chap. 227).

If the patient exhibits mental tension, insomnia, and restlessness, a sedative drug such as phenobarbital or Amytal Sodium may be given with the analgesic agents. Sedative medications, especially the quick-acting barbiturates, should not be used alone for the control of pain, because they sometimes cause excitement and confusion under these circumstances. If endogenous depression is the underlying illness, it should be managed as outlined in Chap. 25.

Visceral pain originating in the stomach, gallbladder, intestines, or heart is usually very poorly controlled by the nonnarcotic analgesics. The narcotic analgesics are the agents of choice, but of course, they should never be given until the physician is certain that the relief of the pain will not mask the state of the patient. If sedation is not desirable and if constipation is a troublesome problem, the newer synthetic analgesics, such as meperidine in doses of 50 to 100 mg orally or intramuscularly or methadone 5 to 10 mg by mouth or subcutaneously every 4 to 6 h, are recommended. Like morphine, these drugs are habit-forming but less so because they induce milder analgesia, sedation, and euphoria. Patients with severe visceral pain who are also anxious or fearful and unable to relax or sleep should be given morphine sulfate in doses of 8 to 15 mg subcutaneously. The well-known spasmogenic effects of morphine are partially counteracted by atropine sulfate, 0.3 to 0.4 mg. Aminophylline, 0.5 g intravenously, also overcomes much of this undesirable spastic action; a rectal suppository of 0.5 g, although less effective, may be substituted. When pain is due to benign, chronic diseases, every effort should be made to avoid opiate addiction. Here the judicious use of propoxyphene (Darvon), 65 mg every 4 to 6 h; oxycodone hydrochloride (Percodan), 4.5 mg every 6 h, or pentazocine hydrochloride (Talwin), 50 mg every 3 to 4 h, may prove adequate.

Intractable pain due to incurable diseases, such as metastatic carcinoma, is one of the most difficult therapeutic problems. As a rule, one resorts to narcotic drugs because of their strong analgesic action, and habituation is accepted as the lesser of two evils. An alternative is pain-relieving surgery. Section of peripheral nerves, the lateral spinothalamic tracts in the spinal cord (cordotomy) or the lateral part of the medulla, stereotaxic thalamotomy, and lobotomy are relatively safe procedures which have advantages over the continuous use of opiates in selected cases.

REFERENCES

ADAMS RD, VICTOR M: *Principles of Neurology*. New York, McGraw-Hill, 1977, chap 6

BONICA JJ (ed): *Advances in Neurology*. New York, Raven Press, 1974, vol 4

DYKES RW: Nociception. Brain Res 99:229, 1975

GUILLEMIN R: Endorphins, brain peptides that act like opiates. N Engl J Med 296:226, 1977

HARDY JD et al: *Pain Sensations and Reactions*. Baltimore, Williams & Wilkins, 1952

LEWIS T: *Pain*. New York, Macmillan, 1942

MELZACK R, WALL PD: Interaction of fast and slow conducting fiber systems involved in pain and analgesia, in *Pharmacology of Pain*, RKS Lim et al (eds). London, Pergamon, 1968

SNYDER SH, SIMANTOV R: The opiate receptor and opioid peptides. J Neurochem 28:13, 1977

WHITE JC, SWEET WH: *Pain and the Neurosurgeon—A Forty Years Experience*. Springfield, Ill, Charles C Thomas, 1969

4
HEADACHE

RAYMOND D. ADAMS

The term *headache* should encompass all aches and pains located in the head, but in common language its application is restricted to unpleasant sensations in the region of the cranial vault. Facial, pharyngeal, and cervical pain are presented in Table 4-2 and will be described in Chaps. 8 and 376.

Headache, along with fatigue, hunger, and thirst, represents the most frequent human discomforts. Medically speaking, its significance is often abstruse, for it may stand as a symptomatic expression of disease or of some minor tension or fatigue, incident to the affairs of the day. Fortunately, in most instances it reflects the latter, and only exceptionally does it warn of serious disease seated in intracranial structures. But it is this dual significance, benign and potentially malignant, that keeps the physician on the alert. Systematic approach to the headache problem necessitates a broad knowledge of the medical and surgical diseases of which it is a symptom and a clinical methodology which leaves none of the common and treatable causes unexplored.

GENERAL CONSIDERATIONS In the introductory chapter on pain, reference was made to the necessity, when dealing with any painful state, of determining its quality, location, duration and time course, and conditions which produce, exacerbate, or relieve it. When headache is considered in these terms, a certain amount of useful information is obtained by careful history, but perhaps less than one might expect. Unfortunately, physical examination of the head itself is seldom useful.

As to quality of cephalic pain, the patient is rarely helpful in describing it. In fact persistent questioning on that point occasions surprise, for the patient usually assumes that the word *headache* should have conveyed enough information to the examiner about the nature of the discomfort. Most headaches are dull, deeply located, and of aching character, a pain recognizable as of the type that usually arises from structures deep to the skin. Seldom is there reported the superficial burning, smarting, or stinging type of pain localized to the skin. When asked to analogize the sensation to another sensory experience, the patient may make some allusion to tightness, pressure, or bursting feeling, terms which then give clue to a muscular tension or psychologic state.

Queries about the intensity of the pain are seldom of much value since they reflect more the patient's attitude toward the condition and a customary way of reporting things that happen than the true severity. As usual the bluff, hearty person tends to minimize discomfort, whereas the neurotic dramatizes it. Degree of incapacity is a better index. A severe migraine attack seldom allows performance of the day's work. The pain which awakens the patient from sleep at night, or prevents sleep, is also more likely to have a demonstrable organic basis. As a rule, the most intense cranial pains are those which accompany subarachnoid hemorrhage and meningitis, which have grave implications, or migraine and paroxysmal nocturnal orbitotemporal (cluster) headaches, which are benign.

Data regarding *location* of the headache are apt to be more informative. If the source is in deep structures (extracranial, subdermal, or intracranial), as is usually the case, the correspondence with the site of the pain is fairly precise. Inflammation of an extracranial artery causes pain well localized to the site of the vessel. Lesions of paranasal sinuses, teeth, eyes, and upper cervical vertebrae induce less sharply localized pain but one that is still referred in a regional distribution that is fairly constant. Intracranial lesions in the posterior fossa cause pain in the occipital-nuchal region, homolateral if the lesion is one-sided. Supratentorial lesions induce frontotemporal pains, again homolateral to the lesion if it is on one side. But localization can also be very uninformative or misleading. Ear pain, for example, although it may mean disease in the ear, more often is referred from other regions, and eye pain may be referred from parts as remote as the occiput or cervical spine.

Duration and *time-intensity curve* of headaches in both the attack itself and their life profile are most useful. Of course the headache of bacterial meningitis or subarachnoid hemorrhage occurs usually in single attacks over a period of days. Single, brief, momentary (1 to 2 s) pains in the cranium are presently uninterpretable and are significant only because they indicate no serious underlying disease. Migraine of the classic type has its onset in the early morning hours or daytime, reaches its peak of severity in a half hour or so, lasts, unless treated, for several hours up to 1 to 2 days, and is often terminated by sleep. In the life history a frequency of more than a single attack every few weeks is exceptional. A migraine patient having several attacks per week usually proves to have a combination of migraine and tension headaches. In contrast to this is the nightly occurrence (2 to 3 h after onset of sleep) over a period of several weeks to months of the rapidly peaking, nonthrobbing orbital or supraorbital pain of cluster headache, which tends to dissipate within an hour. The headache of intracranial tumor characteristically can occur at any time of day or night, can interrupt sleep, varies in intensity, and lasts a few minutes to hours. The life profile is one of increasing frequency and intensity over a period of months. Tension headache, once commenced, may persist continuously for weeks or months, though waxing and waning from hour to hour.

Headache that bears a more or less constant relationship to certain biologic events and also to physical environmental changes may prove to be informative. Premenstrual headaches most typically relate to premenstrual tension during the period of oliguria and edema formation; they usually vanish after the first day of vaginal bleeding. The headaches of cervical arthritis are most typically intense after a period of inactivity, and the first movements in the morning are both difficult and painful. Hypertensive headaches, like those of cerebral tumor, tend to occur on waking in the morning, but, as with all vascular headaches, excitement and tension may provoke them. Headache from infection of nasal sinuses may appear, with clocklike regularity, upon awakening and in midmorning, and is characteristically worsened by stooping and jarring of the head. Eyestrain headaches naturally follow prolonged use of the eyes, as in reading, peering for a long time against glaring headlights in traffic, or watching the cinema. Atmospheric cold may evoke pain in the so-called "fibrositic" or "nodular" headache or when the underlying condition is arthritic or neuralgic. Anger, excitement, or irritation may initiate common migraine in certain disposed persons; this is more typical of common migraine than of the classic type. Change of position, stooping, straining, cough, and sexual intercourse are each known to produce a special type of headache. Exertional headaches, another well-known type, are usually benign (only 1 in 10 will have an intracranial lesion) and disappear within weeks to months.

PAIN-SENSITIVE STRUCTURES AND MECHANISMS OF HEADACHE Understanding of headache has been greatly augmented by the observations of surgeons during operations. They inform us that the following cranial structures are sensitive to mechanical stimulation: (1) skin, subcutaneous tissue, muscles, arteries, and periosteum of skull; (2) delicate structures of eye, ear, and nasal cavity; (3) intracranial venous sinuses and their tributary veins; (4) parts of the dura at the base of the brain and the arteries within the dura mater and piarachnoid; and (5) the trigeminal, glossopharyngeal, vagus, and first three cervical nerves. The bony skull, much of the piarachnoid and dura, and the parenchyma of the brain lack sensitivity. Interestingly, pain is practically the only sensation produced by stimulation of the listed structures.

The pathways whereby sensory stimuli, whatever their source, are conveyed to the central nervous system are the trigeminal nerves for structures above the tentorium in the anterior and middle fossae of the skull, and the first three cervical nerves for those in the posterior fossa and infradural structures. The ninth and tenth cranial nerves supply part of the posterior fossa and refer the pain to the ear and throat. The tentorium is the border zone between the trigeminal and cervical innervation. The central connections through spinal cord and brainstem to thalamus have already been described in Chap. 3 and will be depicted in Chap. 19.

The pain of intracranial disease is referred, by a mechanism already discussed, to some part of the cranium lying within the areas supplied by the aforementioned nerves (the fifth, ninth, and tenth cranial nerves and the first three cervicals). There may be an associated local tenderness of the scalp at the site of reference. Dental or jaw pain may also have cranial reference. The pain of disease in other parts of the body is not referred to the head, although it may initiate headache by other means.

By analysis of several types of headache, Wolff and his colleagues have demonstrated that most "spontaneous" cranial pains can be traced to the operation of one or more of the following mechanisms:

1 Distention, traction, and dilatation of the intracranial or extracranial arteries
2 Traction or displacement of large intracranial veins or the dural envelope in which they lie
3 Compression, traction, or intrinsic disease of cranial and spinal nerves
4 Voluntary or involuntary spasm and possibly interstitial inflammation and trauma of cranial and cervical muscles
5 Meningeal irritation and raised intracranial pressure

Appenzeller would add to the list hysteria and some "psychogenic" disorders.

More specifically, intracranial mass lesions cause headache only if in a position to deform, displace, or exert traction on vessels and dural structures at the base of the brain, and this may happen long before intracranial pressure rises. In fact, the artificial induction of high intraspinal and intracranial pressure by the subarachnoid or intraventricular injection of sterile saline solution does not result in headache. Some have interpreted this to mean raised intracranial pressure does not cause headache, a conclusion which is called into question by the demonstrable relief of headache by lumbar puncture and lowering the cerebrospinal fluid (CSF) pressure in some patients. Actually, most patients with high intracranial pressure complain of recurrent bioccipital and bifrontal headache, probably due to traction on vessels or dura. As to localization, the pains follow the patterns mentioned above; those lesions deflecting the falx or pressing on superior longitudinal or straight sinuses induce pain behind or above the eye; if the lateral part of the lateral sinus is involved, the pain is felt in the ear. Displacement of tentorium elicits pain felt in the supraorbital region.

Dilatation of the extracranial, temporal, and intracranial arteries with stretching of surrounding sensitive structures is believed to be the mechanism of most of the pain of migraine. Extracranial, temporal, and occipital arteries, when involved in giant cell arteritis (cranial or "temporal" arteritis), a disease which usually afflicts individuals over 50 years of age, give rise to headache of dull aching and throbbing type, at first localized and then more diffuse. Characteristically it is severe and persistent over a period of weeks or months. The offending artery, strangely, is not always tender to pressure, yet section of it, as in biopsy, may relieve the pain (Chap. 67). Evolving atherosclerotic thrombosis of internal carotid, anterior, and middle cerebral arteries is sometimes accompanied by pain in the forehead or temple; with vertebral artery thrombosis the pain is postauricular, and basilar artery thrombosis causes pain to be projected to the occiput and sometimes the forehead.

In *infection or blockage* of *paranasal sinuses,* accompanied usually by pain over the antrum or in the forehead (from the ethmoid and sphenoid sinuses the pain localizes around the eyes on one or both sides or in the vertex or other part of the cranium, especially in disease of the sphenoid sinuses), the mechanism involves changes in pressure and irritation of pain-sensitive sinus walls. Usually it is associated with tenderness of the skin in the same distribution. The pain may have two re-markable properties: (1) When throbbing, it may be abolished by compressing the carotid artery on the same side. (2) It tends to recur and subside at the same hours, i.e., on awakening, with gradual disappearance when the person is upright, and coming again in the late morning hours. The time relations are believed to yield information concerning the mechanism; morning pain is ascribed to the sinuses filling at night, and its relief on arising to emptying after the erect posture has been assumed. Stooping intensifies the pain by pressure change, as do blowing the nose and jarring the head sometimes; and in-halant sympathomimetic drugs such as Neo-Synephrine, which reduce swelling and congestion, tend to relieve the pain. Some believe that the highly sensitive orifice of the sinus is the source, but more probably the pain arises in the sensitive mu-cous membrane of the sinus. However, it may persist after all purulent secretions have disappeared, probably because of mechanism of blockage of the orifice by boggy membranes and a vacuum or suction effect on the sinus wall (*vacuum sinus headaches*). The condition is relieved when aeration is restored. During air flights both earache and sinus headache tend to occur on descent, when the relative pressure in the blocked viscus falls.

Headache of ocular origin, located as a rule in the orbit, forehead, or temple, is of steady, aching type and tends to follow prolonged use of the eyes in close work. Ocular muscle imbalance is believed to be the mechanism. The main faults are hypermetropia and astigmatism (not myopia), which result in sustained contraction of extraocular as well as frontal, tem-poral, and even occipital muscles. Convergence insufficiency is another common disorder. Correction of the refractive error abolishes the headache. Traction on the extraocular muscles during eye surgery, particularly on the iris, will evoke pain. Another mechanism is involved in the raised intraocular pres-sure seen in acute glaucoma or iridocyclitis, which causes steady, aching pain in the region of the eye. When intense, it may radiate throughout the distribution of the ophthalmic di-vision of the trigeminal nerve. As for ocular pain in general, it is important that the eyes should always be refracted, but eye-strain is probably not as frequent as one would expect from the wholesale dispensing of spectacles. The pain of diabetic third nerve palsy, intracranial aneurysm, cavernous sinus thrombo-sis, and Reader's paratrigeminal syndrome may also be re-ferred to the eye.

The mechanism of *headaches accompanying disease of liga-ments, muscles, and apophyseal joints* in the upper part of the spine, which are referred to occiput and nape of neck on the same side, can be in part reproduced by the injection of hyper-tonic saline solution into these structures. Such pains are espe-cially frequent in late life in rheumatoid and hypertrophic ar-thritis and tend also to occur after whiplash injuries to the neck. If the pain is arthritic in origin, the first movements after being still for some hours are both stiff and painful. In fact,

evocation of pain by active and passive motion of the spine should indicate traumatic or other disease of movable parts. The pain of myofibrositis, evidenced by tender nodules near the cranial insertion of cervical and other muscles, is more obscure. There are no pathologic data as to the nature of these vaguely palpable lesions, and it is uncertain whether the pain actually arises in them. They may represent only the deep ten-derness felt in the region of referred pain or the involuntary secondary protective spasm of muscles. Characteristically, the pain is steady (nonthrobbing) and spreads from one to both sides of the head. Exposure to cold or draft may precipitate it. Though severe at times, it seldom prevents sleep. Massage of muscles and heat have unpredictable effects but relieve the pain in some cases.

The *headache of meningeal irritation* (infection or hemor-rhage), which is of acute onset, severe, generalized, deep-seated, constant, especially intense at the base of the skull, and associated with stiffness of neck on bending forward, has been ascribed by some authorities to increased intracranial pressure. Indeed the withdrawal of cerebrospinal fluid may afford some relief. But dilatation and congestion of inflamed meningeal vessels must also be a factor. It seems more probable, there-fore, that the pain is due to the chemical irritation of nerve endings in the meninges.

Lumbar puncture headache, which is characterized by a steady occipital-nuchal pain and also by frontal pain coming on a few minutes after arising from a recumbent position and relieved within a few minutes by lying down, has as its cause a persistent leakage of CSF into the lumbar tissues through the needle site. The CSF pressure is low (often 0 in the lateral decubitus position), and the injection of sterile isotonic saline solution intrathecally relieves it. The headache is usually in-creased by compression of the jugular veins and is unaffected by digital obliteration of one carotid artery. It seems probable that in the upright position a low intraspinal and negative in-tracranial pressure exerts traction on dural attachments and dural sinuses by caudal displacement of the brain. Under-standably, then, headache following cisternal puncture is rare. As soon as the leakage of CSF stops and CSF pressure is gradually restored (usually from a few days up to a week or so), the headache disappears. "Spontaneous" low-pressure headache may follow a sneeze or strain, presumably because of rupture of the spinal arachnoid along a nerve root.

The mechanism of the throbbing or steady headache which accompanies febrile illnesses, located in frontal or occipital re-gions or generalized, is probably vascular. It is much like hista-mine headache in being relieved on one side by carotid artery compression and on both sides by jugular vein compression or the subarachnoid injection of saline solution. It is increased by shaking the head. It seems probable that the meningeal vessels pulsate unduly and stretch pain-sensitive structures around the base of the brain. In certain cases, however, the pain may be lessened by compression of temporal arteries, and in these cases a component of the headache seems to be derived from the walls of extracranial arteries, as in migraine.

The claims of insufferable headaches by the hysteric are undecipherable. The so-called tension headaches of patients with anxiety states and depression are allegedly due to chronic spasm of cranial and cervical muscles. Combinations of the tension and vascular headaches give rise to the "mixed head-aches" of many psychiatric patients.

PRINCIPAL CLINICAL VARIETIES OF HEADACHE Usually there is no difficulty in diagnosing the headache of glaucoma, purulent sinusitis, bacterial meningitis, and brain tumor, and a fuller account of these special headaches will be found where these diseases are described in later sections of the book. It is when headache is chronic, recurrent, and unattended by other important signs of disease that the physician faces one of the most difficult medical problems.

The following types of headache should then be considered.

Migraine The term *migraine* refers to periodic, hemicranial, throbbing headaches which usually begin in childhood, adolescence, or early adult life and recur with diminishing frequency during advancing years.

Two closely related clinical syndromes have been identified. The first is called "neurologic" migraine, the second common. The classic syndrome is ushered in by a disturbance of neurologic function (hemianopsia or central blindness, hemiparesthetic disturbance, slight speech abnormality or aphasia, or hemiparesis) followed in a few minutes by hemicranial headache, nausea, and vomiting, all of which last for hours or as long as a day or two. The other syndrome is characterized by an unheralded onset of hemicranial or generalized headache with or without nausea and vomiting but following the same temporal pattern. Both headache syndromes respond to ergot preparations, if administered early in the attack. Their genetic nature is evidenced by concurrence in several members of the family of the same and successive generations in 60 to 80 percent of cases; but inheritance is somewhat less clear in the common than the classic variety, perhaps because diagnosis is less accurate.

Neurologic migraine presents such a dramatic and at times confusing sequence of events that it merits further description. On awakening in the morning, or at any time of the day, the patient may have a kind of vague premonition of an attack. Then abruptly there is a disturbance of vision consisting usually of bright spots or dazzling zigzag lines which give way within minutes to scotomatous defects; usually they are bilateral and often of homonymous and congruent pattern (corresponding parts of the field of vision of each eye). Soon thereafter, numbness and tingling of lips, face, hand (on one or both sides), slight confusion of thinking, weakness of an arm or leg, mild aphasia, dizziness and uncertainty of gait, drowsiness, or confusion (rarely coma) are added to the clinical picture. Only one or a few of these neurologic phenomena are present in any given patient, and they tend to occur in the same combination in each attack. They last 5 to 15 min or more, and if the weakness or numbness spreads from one part of the body to another or one symptom follows another, it does so slowly in a period of minutes (not in seconds as in a convulsion). Just as inexplicably as they come, they soon begin to recede, and within minutes they are followed by a unilateral throbbing headache, usually on the side of the cerebral disturbance, which slowly increases in intensity. At its peak, in an hour or so, nausea and vomiting may occur. The headache lasts hours or a day or two and is usually the most unpleasant feature of the illness.

Much variation occurs. When this "sick headache," as it is called, is most severe, the patient is forced to lie down and to shun light and noise. Milder forms, especially if partially controlled by medication, do not force withdrawal from accustomed activities. Any one of the three principal components—neurologic derangement, headache, or vomiting—may be absent or occur in different sequence than is described above. Particularly with advancing age there is a tendency for the headache and vomiting to become less severe, finally leaving only the neurologic abnormality. The neurologic symptomatology is also subject to variation. Although visual disturbances are far and away the most common manifestation, they differ in detail from patient to patient; numbness and tingling of the lips and fingers of one hand are probably next in frequency, with transient aphasia or a thickness of speech following in that order. A relatively rare syndrome of vertigo, staggering, drowsiness, and stupor has been delineated by Bickerstaff and called *basilar artery migraine.* Also, he has reported the loss of consciousness at the onset, especially in migrainous young women. Recurrent unilateral headaches associated with extraocular muscle palsies have been called *opthalmoplegic migraine.* A transient third nerve palsy with associated ptosis of one eyelid is the usual picture; rarely, the abducens nerve is affected and lateral movement is impaired. Hemifacial paralysis is another rare variant. Disturbances of the mind may appear—strange excitement, unaccountable irritability or depression, or episodes of mental confusion, which are more common. The headache, though typically hemicranial (the word *migraine* is said to be derived from *megrim,* meaning hemicrania), may be frontal, temporal, or generalized. In children abdominal pain and vomiting, sometimes cyclical, may accompany the headache (abdominal migraine). Another childhood variant is paroxysmal vertigo; this may occur as a prelude to a "sick headache" or without headache (benign paroxysmal vertigo of childhood). The attacks, instead of beginning in childhood and recurring in the usual fashion every few weeks or months with diminishing frequency in middle and late adult years, may begin in adult life or even middle age or suddenly increase in frequency during menopause or when hypertension and vascular disease develop. The neurologic symptoms, instead of being transitory, may leave a permanent deficit (e.g., a homonymous visual field defect) reminiscent of an ischemic stroke or a bleeding vascular malformation. The use of hormones to prevent pregnancy has increased the frequency and severity of migraine and in several reported instances has resulted in a permanent neurologic deficit.

Between attacks the migrainous patient is essentially normal. For a time, when psychosomatic medicine was much in vogue, there was insistence on a migrainous personality characterized by tenseness, rigidity in thinking, meticulousness, and perfectionism. The migrainous attack was said to occur often during the let-down period, after many days of hard work or stress. But further personality analyses have not borne out these ideas, and the temporal relations between headache and the day's activities have not been consistent. Moreover, the fact that the headaches may begin in early childhood, when the personality is relatively amorphous, would argue against this idea.

During an attack, the electroencephalogram reveals a nonspecific slowing of wave frequencies in one-third to one-half of all patients. The cerebral circulation is found by blood flow studies to be slowed early in the attack and speeded up once headache begins.

Migraine is frequent, found in an estimated 5 percent of the general population; women are slightly more susceptible than men, and there is a tendency for the headaches to occur during the period of premenstrual tension and fluid retention. The migrainous attacks usually cease during pregnancy. Reserpine treatment and estrogens and progesterone may increase their frequency. A few patients have linked their attacks to certain articles of diet, such as chocolate, cheese, and wine or other alcoholic beverages. Phenylethylamine, a constituent of such foods and drinks, has been shown to precipitate headaches in migraine patients; tyramine, another constituent, does not. The platelets of migraine patients are deficient in monoamine oxidase, responsible for degrading phenylethylamine. There is no clear relationship, despite many statements to the contrary, between migraine and vascular malformations of the brain and psychoneurosis. The relationship to epilepsy is less clear; convulsions are slightly increased in frequency in migrainous patients and their relatives.

Vasodilatation and excessive pulsation of branches of the external carotid artery have been observed during the headache. Further, as the pulsation decreases, either spontaneously or after the administration of ergotamine, the headache disappears. Vasoconstriction was early postulated as the basis of the neurologic symptoms; it has been confirmed in at least one chance carotid arteriogram and has been inferred from prompt abolition of the visual or neurologic disorder upon administration of nitrites. Thus the vascular theory of migraine has come to be accepted, supported further by surgical observations, that the extracranial arteries can be a source of pain. However, it is quite apparent that the theory does not explain why the intracranial and extracranial arteries should periodically undergo spasm and dilatation in the migrainous individual, nor does it account for the nausea and vomiting (infrequent in all other headaches except those due to tumor) or the tenderness and swelling of the temporal vessels and surrounding tissues.

A hypothesis of current interest postulates that the observed vasospasm and later hyperemic pulsations are induced by a release of amines such as norepinephrine, epinephrine, and serotonin in individuals whose vessels are peculiarly sensitive. These substances are known to be powerful vasoconstrictors. It was found that some migraine patients during their attack excrete increased amounts of the terminal metabolites of the catecholamines, particularly 5-hydroxyindoleacetic acid (5-HIAA) derived from serotonin, and of vanillylmandelic acid (VMA), a product of norepinephrine and epinephrine. A corresponding reduction in serotonin levels in the blood has also been detected. Other observations in line with this are that (1) reserpine, which reduces the level of serotonin in platelets, brain, and other tissues, may provoke migraine; (2) the injection of serotonin gives partial or complete relief of headache, and (3) a serotonin antagonist, methysergide, wholly prevents attacks in many instances. However, it is still difficult to reconcile these data with the finding that a heat-stable polypeptide with some of the properties of bradykinin (one of the plasma kinins) not only can be aspirated from the edematous subcutaneous tissue on the side of the headache but, if reinjected at another site, will cause increased capillary permeability, pain, and lowered skin threshold in the overlying skin. Its algogenic action is potentiated by serotonin. Whether this substance, called *neurokinin*, escapes secondarily during the phase of vasodilatation or initiates the vasodilatation is not known. While this humoral amine theory is incomplete and several of the findings need verification, it nonetheless does promise clarification of the migraine syndrome and possibly other forms of vascular headache. Couch and Hassanein have found an increase in platelet aggregability in migraine patients, especially during an attack of headache, and they suggest that it may be responsible for the stroke that rarely complicates migraine. Clover and his associates have measured a transitory decrease in platelet monoamine oxidase activity during attacks.

DIAGNOSIS Classic migraine should occasion no difficulty in diagnosis if the above facts are kept in mind and if a good history is obtained. That is possible, as a rule, for migraine patients tend to be intelligent.

The real difficulties come from three sources: (1) ignorance of the fact that a progressively unfolding neurologic syndrome may be migrainous in origin; (2) lack of appreciation that the neurologic disorder may occur without headache; (3) lack of awareness that recurrent headaches, which may be an isolated phenomenon, may take many forms, some of which may prove difficult to distinguish from the other common types of headache described in this chapter.

Some of these problems merit further elaboration because of their practical importance, as follows:

The neurologic part of the migraine syndrome may resemble focal epilepsy, the clinical picture of a vascular malformation such as an angioma or aneurysm, or some other vascular disease such as a thrombotic or embolic stroke. Here it is the pace of the neurologic symptoms of migraine more than their character that reliably distinguishes the condition from epilepsy. The clinical profile of the aura of epilepsy is measured in seconds, for it depends on spreading neural excitation, in contrast to the slow progression of migraine, which is based on spreading vascular spasm.

Ophthalmoplegic migraine will always suggest a carotid aneurysm, but in relatively few cases has carotid arteriography revealed such an abnormality. Despite many claims that the question of a vascular malformation should be raised in cases of hemicranial painful attacks occurring invariably on the same side of the head (unlike migraine), in a large series of cases this has only rarely been confirmed by arteriography. Of course, focal epilepsy, protracted headache, stiff neck and bloody cerebrospinal fluid, a persistent neurologic deficit, and cranial bruit would be indicative of a vascular type of headache associated with angioma or aneurysm. Only in the earlier stages, when periodic throbbing headache is the sole symptom, might it be confused with true migraine.

Attacks indistinguishable from epilepsy may also appear in association with the hypertensive and cerebral arteriosclerotic vascular diseases of late life. Here one is aided by late age of onset, more persistent and frequent headaches, and the evidence of vascular disease of heart, lower extremities, and brain.

A special problem relates to paroxysms of throbbing headache, not hemicranial in distribution, not preceded by a neurologic aura, and not accounted for by other known cause. Are they examples of common migraine? Unfortunately, since diagnosis depends on the interpretation of the patient's description of symptoms and since there is as yet no biologically valid confirmatory laboratory test, the controversy as to where migraine begins and ends is of the armchair type. Favoring the diagnosis of migraine are life-long history, childhood onset, positive family history, and response of the headache to ergot derivatives.

A variety of episodic attacks have been described as migraine equivalents: attacks of abdominal pain with nausea, vomiting, and diarrhea; pain localized in the thorax, pelvis, and extremities; bouts of fever; paroxysmal vertigo; transient disturbances in mood (psychic equivalents); recurrent nocturnal orbital (cluster) headache, or migrainous neuralgia. Watson and Steele attribute these associated conditions to a paroxysmal disequilibrium which they find in approximately one-third of migrainous children. The only advantage of considering such attacks as migrainous is that this view protects some patients from unnecessary diagnostic procedures and surgical intervention—but it may also prevent necessary surgery.

From all this discussion the reader should be left with the idea that the migraine syndromes are rather larger and more protean than the rigid stereotyped descriptions we have given would suggest. In these days of complicated diagnostic procedures it is tempting to take x-rays or do computerized tomography (CT scan) of the skull and perform arteriography and electroencephalography on every patient. A conservative approach would lead to temporization, reserving CT scan or EEG for the exceptional case.

Cluster headache This headache is also called *paroxysmal nocturnal cephalalgia, migrainous neuralgia, histamine headache* and Horton's syndrome. It is characterized by a fourfold higher incidence in men than in women, constant, unilateral orbital localization, and onset usually within 2 or 3 h after falling asleep, during the phase of rapid eye movement (REM) sleep (it is infrequent during the waking hours). The pain is intense and steady (nonthrobbing) with lacrimation, blocked nostril, then rhinorrhea, and sometimes flush, miosis, ptosis, and edema of cheek, all lasting approximately an hour or two.

It tends to recur nightly for several weeks or a few months (hence the term *cluster*), followed by complete freedom for years. The pain of a given attack may leave as rapidly as it began. Clusters may recur over the years, being possibly more likely in times of stress, prolonged strain, overwork, and in upsetting emotional experiences. Occasionally alcohol, nitroglycerine, or tyramine-containing foods precipitate an attack. Rarely, the condition may occur in daytime and may not cluster but continue.

The picture is so characteristic that it cannot be confused with any other disease, though to those unfamiliar with it the possibility of a carotid aneurysm, hemangioma, brain tumor, or sinusitis may be suggested. Appropriate roentgenograms and carotid arteriography will always exclude such conditions but usually are unnecessary. In the differential diagnosis orbital, nasociliary, supraorbital, Sluder's sphenopalatine, and neuralgias must also be considered (see Chap. 376).

In the life history profile the clusters of headache may last for weeks. The clusters may be single or recur two, three, or more times, with years of freedom in between, during which such precipitating factors as alcohol are no longer effective. Often the pain involves the same orbit in each cluster. Examples are seen in which the same type of headache may last a year or more or even for a period of 10 to 20 years.

The relationship of the cluster headache to migraine remains conjectural. A portion of the cases have a background of migraine, which led to the earlier postulation of migrainous neuralgia, but the majority do not. The face of the patient with cluster headache turns red (by infrared photography), whereas that of the migraine patient is pale. Some investigators have found a drop in the blood pressure of migraine patients; none occurs in cluster headaches.

Tension headache and various other cranial pains with psychiatric disease The headache is usually bilateral, often with diffuse extension over the top of the cranium. Occipital-nuchal localization is also common. Although the sensation may be described as pain, close questioning may uncover other sensations, viz., fullness, tightness, or pressure (as if the head is surrounded by a band or in a vise), on which waves of aching pain are superimposed. The onset of a given attack is more gradual than in migraine and not infrequently a throbbing "vascular" type of headache is added intermittently to a pressure ache. Tension headache may occur acutely under conditions of emotional excitement or intense worry and lasts for hours or a day or two. More often it persists unremittingly for weeks or months. In fact, this is the only type of headache that exhibits the peculiarity of being absolutely continuous day and night for long periods of time. Although sleep may be possible, whenever the patient awakens, the headache is present; the common analgesic remedies have no beneficial effect unless the pain is intense and of aching type.

As to mechanism, the ascription of it to sustained muscle activity, shown by the electromyogram, is only a partial explanation. The continuous pressing quality of milder cephalic sensations at times when the patient is relaxed hardly seems to be attributable to physiologic stimulation and suggests instead that the condition is maintained by focused attention on the head (occasioned sometimes by worry and fear of intracranial disease). Moreover, it must be remembered that all types of headache in their late stages may give rise to muscle tension, and that this is of an aching rather than a pressure type. In contrast to migraine, in which pain is periodic and lifelong, with tendency to lessen in late adult years, tension headache occurs more often in middle age and usually coincides with anxiety and depression in the trying times of life. Many premenstrual headaches are of this type, and there is an increased incidence of this type of tension headache at menopause.

Psychologic studies of groups of patients with tension headaches have revealed prominent symptoms of depression, anxiety, and to a lesser extent hypochondriasis. Kudrow records that 65 percent of depressed patients have this type of headache and that over 60 percent of his patients with tension headaches were depressed. When psychiatric syndromes are searched for in headache patients, it is evident that the majority of those with anxiety neurosis, hysteria, obsessive-compulsive neurosis, and schizophrenia, in which anxiety is a prominent symptom, exhibit this type of headache. Migraine and traumatic headaches may be complicated by tension headache.

Other odd cephalic pains, e.g., boring pains, "clavus hystericus," may occur in hysteria and raise perplexing problems in diagnosis. Their bizarre character, persistence in the face of every known therapy, absence of other signs of disease, and the presence of the stigmata of the hysterical personality provide the basis for correct diagnosis (see Chap. 11).

Headache of angioma and aneurysm The temporal profile of any given attack shows the onset to be sudden or very acute, with the pain reaching a peak within minutes. Neurologic disturbances such as scintillations, defects in vision, unilateral numbness, weakness, or aphasia may precede or occur after the onset of headache and outlast it. Should hemorrhage occur the headache is often extremely severe and localizes more toward the occiput and neck, lasting many days in association with stiff neck. A cranial or cervical bruit and, of course, blood in the cerebrospinal fluid establish the diagnosis, but it may require verification by arteriography. The claim that vascular malformations may give rise to migraine is probably untenable. Statistical data show migraine to be no more frequent in this group of patients than in the general population. There are however, a few notable exceptions to this statement. Of course, vascular lesions may exist for long periods of time without headache, or the latter may develop many years after other manifestations, such as epilepsy and hemiplegia (see Chap. 365).

Traumatic headaches Severe, chronic, continuous, or intermittent headaches appear as the cardinal symptom of three posttraumatic syndromes, separable in each instance from the headache that immediately follows head injury (i.e., that of scalp laceration and contusion with sanguineous cerebrospinal fluid and increased intracranial pressure). The latter lasts several days or a week or two (see Chap. 366).

Headache of chronic subdural hematoma Headache and dizziness of fluctuating severity, followed by drowsiness, stupor, coma, and hemiparesis, are the usual manifestations of chronic subdural hematoma. The head injury may have been minor and forgotten by patient and family. The headaches are deep-seated, steady, unilateral or generalized, and respond to the usual analgesic drugs. The typical attack profile of the headache and other symptoms is one of increasing frequency and severity over several weeks or months. Diagnosis is now established by CT scan and arteriography (see Chap. 366).

Headache of posttraumatic nervous instability See Chap. 366.

Posttraumatic dysautonomic cephalalgia This term was given by Vijayan and Dreyfus to severe, episodic, throbbing, unilateral headaches accompanied by ipsilateral mydriasis and excessive facial sweating. The condition followed injury to the neck in the region of the carotid sheath. It was postulated that the sympathetic nervous supply of the cranium had been disinhibited, and there was clinical and pharmacologic evidence of sympathetic dysfunction.

Headaches of brain tumor   Headache is the outstanding symptom of cerebral tumor. Unfortunately, the quality of the pain has no specific feature. It tends to be deep-seated, nonthrobbing (or throbbing), and aching or bursting. Attacks last a few minutes to an hour or more and occur once or many times during the day. Activity and frequently change in the position of the head may provoke pain, while rest in bed diminishes its frequency. Nocturnal awakening because of pain, although typical, is by no means diagnostic. Unexpected forceful (projectile) vomiting may punctuate the illness in its later stages. As the tumor grows the pain becomes more frequent and severe; it sometimes is nearly continuous terminally. But there are exceptions: some headaches are mild and tolerable, others as agonizing as that of the headache of bacterial meningitis and subarachnoid hemorrhage. If unilateral, the headache is homolateral to the tumor in 9 out of 10 patients. Supratentorial tumors are felt anterior to the interauricular circumference of the skull; posterior fossa tumors behind this line. Bifrontal and bioccipital headache, coming on after unilateral headache, signifies the development of increased intracranial pressure.

HEADACHES RELATED TO MEDICAL DISORDERS   Experienced physicians are aware of many conditions in which headache figures as a dominant symptom. These include fevers of any cause, carbon monoxide exposure, chronic lung disease with hypercapnia (headaches often nocturnal), hypothyroidism, Cushing's disease, withdrawal of corticosteroid medication, chronic nitrite exposure, occasionally Addison's disease, aldosterone-producing adrenal tumors, use of "the pill" in some instances, acute rises in blood pressure, e.g., from pheochromocytoma, and acute anemia with hemoglobin below 10 g.

With reference to chronic hypertension the relation to headache is less clear. Approximately 50 percent of patients with hypertension complain of headaches. Wolff and colleagues state that except with hypertensive encephalopathy where the intracranial pressure may be increased, the mechanism of the headache is similar to that of migraine, i.e., it is vascular, and in such individuals the headache develops not at a time when the pressure is highest, as in time of stress, but after it has fallen. Perhaps the headache is due to the release of vasodilating prostaglandins. The headaches of renal dialysis tend to increase as the blood pressure falls and sodium and osmolality decrease. Vasoconstricting drugs such as ergotamine often are as effective in hypertensive headaches as in migraine.

An erythromelalgic syndrome (flushing, red hands, numb fingers, blotchy skin) with severe headaches has been described in association with serotonin-secreting tumors, carcinoid tumors, and mastocytosis. In one type reported by Streeter and associates there were high levels of circulating bradykinin.

APPROACH TO THE PATIENT WITH HEADACHE   Obviously very different possibilities are raised by a patient who presents for the first time with severe headache and a patient who has had recurrent headache over a period of years. The chances of uncovering the cause in the first instance are much greater than in the latter, and some of the potential underlying conditions (meningitis, subarachnoid hemorrhage, epidural hematoma, glaucoma, and purulent sinusitis) are more serious. The simple rules to follow are that severe, persistent headache with stiff neck and fever always means meningitis and the same combination without fever, subarachnoid hemorrhage. A lumbar puncture is mandatory. Acute persistent headache over a period of hours or days may occur in systemic infections such as influenza (febrile) or as a manifestation of an acute tension state. The first attack of migraine may present in this way.

In searching for the cause of recurrent headache one should investigate the status of cardiovascular and renal systems by blood pressure and urine examination, eyes by fundoscopic, intraocular pressure, and refraction, the sinuses by transillumination and x-rays, the cranial arteries by palpation (and biopsy?), the cervical spine by effect of passive movement of the head and x-rays, the nervous system by neurologic examination, and psychic function by mental status.

Hypertension is, of course, frequent in the general population and when present is always difficult to prove as a cause of recurrent headaches. Minor elevations of blood pressure may be a result rather than the cause of nervous tension. No doubt severe hypertension with diastolic blood pressures of over 110 mmHg is more regularly associated with headache than is moderate hypertension. If headache is severe and frequent, one should always consider the possibilities of underlying anxiety, tension state, or a common migraine syndrome exacerbated by blood vessel disease. The mechanism of the puzzling hypertensive phenomenon of occipital pain, present on awakening in the morning and wearing off during the day, is uncertain.

The adolescent with daily frontal headaches represents a special type of problem. Often their relationship to eyestrain is unclear, and refraction of the eyes and new eyeglasses do not relieve the condition. Anxiety or tension is probably a factor in such cases, but it is difficult to be certain of a causal relationship. Some of the most persistent and inexplicable headaches, which have led to a survey by a battery of diagnostic procedures for tumor, have proved in the end to be caused by depression.

Equally puzzling is the somber, tense adult whose primary complaint is headache, or the migrainous person who in late life or at menopause begins to have daily headaches. Here it becomes important to assess mental status along the lines suggested in Chaps. 11 and 25, looking for evidences of anxiety, depression, and hypochondriasis. The quality and persistence of the headache are suggestive of the possibility of psychiatric illness. Sometimes a direct question as to the patient's idea of what is the matter may elicit suspicion and fear of brain tumor. Antidepressant drugs given as an empirical test may relieve the headache, thus clarifying the diagnosis.

The most worrisome type of patient is the one who has headache of increasing frequency and severity over a period of months or a year or so. Since an intracranial mass lesion (tumor, abscess, subdural hematoma) is a leading possibility, it becomes necessary to resort to a complete neurologic survey, including careful inspection of optic disk, roentgenograms of skull, electroencephalogram, CT scan, and radioactive isotope.

Every elderly person with severe headache of some few days or weeks duration should be considered as possibly having cranial arteritis. Increased sedimentation rate, fever, and anemia may be conjoined, but only in a minority of cases, unfortunately. The finding of a thickened temporal artery is important, and arterial biopsy and response to corticosteroids establish the diagnosis; treatment with corticosteroids often relieves the pain.

TREATMENT   The most important steps in the treatment of headache are those measures which uncover and remove the underlying disease or functional disturbance.

For the common everyday headache due to fatigue, stuffy atmosphere, or excessive use of alcohol and tobacco, it is simply enough to advise avoidance of the offending activity or agent, and symptomatic therapy in the form of acetylsalicylic acid, 0.6 g (some brand of aspirin such as Anacin), or acetaminophen (Tylenol), 0.6 g, will suffice. Some patients who invariably have headache when constipated and hypochondriacs who not infrequently suffer incapacitating headache, fatigue, and depression whenever bowel elimination does not meet their expectation are not easily helped. Certainly, simple explanation, an anticonstipation regimen, and drugs which counteract depression (see Chap. 11) are preferable to the continuous use of analgesics. Premenstrual headache, if troublesome, can usually be helped by the use of a diuretic compound for the week preceding the menstrual period and a mixture of mild analgesic and tranquilizing medications (acetylsalicylic acid or acetaminophen, 0.6 g, and phenobarbital, 30 mg). If the headaches are severe and incapacitating, they should be treated as common migraine.

Migraine may require no treatment at all, other than an explanation of its nature to the patient and a reassurance that it will do no harm. Some patients know, or allege to know, that certain acts induce attacks, and it is obvious enough that they should be urged to avoid these acts, if possible. In certain instances alcoholic drinks, particularly red wine, are invariably followed by a migraine. Others claim reduction of attacks of headache by an elimination diet, correction of refractive error, or by psychotherapy. However, this is so exceptional that a cause and effect relationship must be doubted in view of the variability of the disease itself.

Treatment of the neurologic aura of migraine is rarely required or possible because of its brevity. If the deficits are lasting, inhalation of an ampul of amyl nitrate should be tried as a preventive measure; it should be used at the first premonition of the attack. The time to initiate treatment of the oncoming headache is during the neurologic disorder. If many of the headaches are mild, the patient may already have learned that 0.6 g acetylsalicylic acid and possibly 5 mg dextroamphetamine sulfate (Dexedrine) will suffice to control the pain. More severe attacks also respond to simple analgesic medication and rest in a quiet, darkened room. Success has been claimed with ergot preparations, and indeed ergotamine tartrate, 0.25 mg by intravenous injection or 1 to 3 mg held under the tongue until dissolved, will interrupt a headache in 80 to 90 percent of cases if given near the onset of the headache. Sometimes the combination of caffeine, 100 mg with 1 mg ergotamine (Cafergot), is preferred. It may be taken in the form of a tablet (two at the onset of headache and a third in half an hour) or as a rectal suppository (2 mg ergotamine and 100 mg caffeine) if vomiting prevents oral administration.

Because of the danger of prolonged vascular spasm in patients who have vascular disease or are pregnant, ergot preparations must be used cautiously, if at all. Even in healthy individuals more than 10 to 15 mg ergotamine per week is risky, for it may in itself produce headache. For the frequent atypical migraine headaches, some of which respond poorly to ergot, one should prescribe a preparation containing 150 mg acetylsalicylic acid, 160 mg acetophenetidin, and dextroamphetamine sulfate, 5 mg, with phenobarbital, 30 mg. This can be repeated once or twice in a severe attack. Once the headache has become intense (after 30 min), ergot is of little help, and one must resort to codeine sulfate, 30 mg, or meperidine (Demerol), 50 mg, as the only means of terminating the pain. If sleep customarily terminates headache, 50 mg of promethazine (Phenergan) orally is helpful; it also relieves vomiting.

In individuals with frequent migrainous attacks (more than one to three times a month), efforts at prevention are worthwhile. Some success has been obtained with preparations of ergot, 0.5 mg, atropine, 0.3 mg, and phenobarbital (Bellergol), 15 mg, two or three times a day for a few weeks. Propranolol (Inderal), 40 mg. tid, has been effective in reducing the frequency and intensity of attacks in approximately one-third of cases. For the most severe forms of the disease, methysergide (Sansert) in a dose of 6 to 8 mg per day given for several weeks or months has proved to be most promising in reducing the frequency of or abolishing attacks. The main contraindication has been retroperitoneal fibrosis; this complication has been reported in several dozen cases when the patient has been treated continuously for more than 4 to 5 months. Discontinu-

ing treatment for 1 month out of every 6 has greatly reduced the incidence of this complication. Recently, claims have been proposed for cloridine hydrochloride (Dixarit), 0.025 to 0.05 mg tid, as a preventative, but it may cause depression in some patients.

All experienced physicians appreciate the importance of helping patients rearrange their schedules so as to control tensions and hard-driving ways of living, so often a feature of many migrainous patients. There is no one way of accomplishing this, but in general, long and costly psychotherapy has not been helpful, or at least one can say there are no substantial data as to its value.

Cluster headaches have proven to be most resistant to treatment. One capsule of Cafergot or 1.0 mg of ergotamine tartrate at bedtime is most widely recommended. However, if the headaches are frequent, severe, and diurnal as well as nocturnal, the intake of ergot may reach dangerous levels. Success has also been claimed for amitryptyline (Elavil), 25 to 100 mg tid, and methysergide, 6 to 8 mg per day, as means of interrupting a cluster. Histamine desensitization, originally proposed by Horton, has been little used in recent years because of inconsistent results. In rare cases of persistent cluster headaches lasting for 10 to 20 years spectacular success has been obtained by indomethacin (Indocin).

Hypertensive headaches respond to agents which lower blood pressure and relieve muscle tension. Chlorothiazide (Diuril), 250 to 500 mg twice a day, and methyldopa (Aldomet), 250 to 500 mg per day, when combined with a small amount of phenobarbital, 15 mg tid, or propranolol (Inderal) 40 mg tid, have given the best results. Meprobamate, 200 mg tid, or chlordiazepoxide hydrochloride (Librium), 5 mg tid, may be administered in place of phenobarbital. For the morning occipital ache a capsule containing sodium nitrite, 30 mg, caffeine sodium benzoate, 0.5 g, and acetophenetidin, 0.6 g, has been useful. A simplified method of treating this kind of headache is to supply the caffeine in a cup of strong black coffee and to give with it acetylsalicylic acid. Blocks under the head of the bed may be helpful.

The muscle tension headaches respond best to massage, relaxation, and a combination of drugs which relieve depression [e.g., amitryptaline (Elavil) or imiprimine (Tofranil)] and anxiety (e.g., phenobarbital, amobarbital, meprobamate, and chlordiazepoxide hydrochloride). Pain-relieving medicine of non-habit-forming type [e.g., acetylsalicylic acid and propoxyphene hydrochloride (Darvon)], should be added when throbbing headache is present. Stronger analgesic medication (codeine or meperidine hydrochloride) should be avoided. Psychotherapy may be helpful in this group of patients.

The headache of the syndrome of posttraumatic nervous instability requires supportive psychotherapy in the form of reassurance and frequent explanation of its benign and transient nature, a program of increasing physical activity, and drugs which allay anxiety and depression. However, the tricyclic antidepressants are generally less effective than in the mixed tension and throbbing headaches of anxious depressions. Tender scars from scalp laceration may be novocainized repeatedly (subcutaneous injection of 5 ml of 1% procaine) with some degree of success. Settlement of litigation as soon as possible works to the patient's advantage.

Heat, massage, salicylates, and indomethacin (Indocin) or phenylbutazone (Butazolidin) usually effect some improvement in those arthritic diseases of the cervical spine which are associated with cervicocranial pain (see Chap. 356).

Corticosteroid therapy is indicated in cranial arteritis to prevent disastrous blindness by occlusion of the ophthalmic

TABLE 4-1
Common types of headache

Type	Site	Age and sex	Clinical characteristics	Diurnal pattern	Life profile	Provoking factors	Associated features	Treatment
Common migraine	Frontotemporal Uni- or bilateral	Children, young to middle-aged adults both sexes	Throbbing and/or dull ache; worse behind one eye or ear Becomes generalized	Upon awakening or later in day Duration: hours to 1-2 days	Irregular interval, weeks to months Tends to disappear in middle age and during pregnancy	Bright light, noise, tension, alcohol Dark room and sleep relieve Scalp sensitive Pressure helps	Nausea in some cases	Ergot preparation at onset Phenergen in established phase Inderal and Bellargol Methysergide (Sansert) for prevention
"Neurologic" migraine	Same as above	Same as above	Same as above	Same as above	Same as above	Same as above	Blindness and scintillating lights Unilateral numbness Disturbed speech Vertigo Confusion	Same as above
Cluster, histamine headache, or migrainous neuralgia	Orbital Temporal Unilateral	Adolescent and adult males (80–90%)	Intense, nonthrobbing pain	Usually nocturnal; occurs one or more hours after falling asleep Rarely diurnal	Nightly for several weeks to months (cluster) Recurrence: years and later	Alcohol in some	Lacrimation, congested eye	Ergot preparation at bedtime Amytryptaline (Elavil) and lithium carbonate for prevention
Tension headaches	Generalized	Adolescents and adults, both sexes	Pressure (nonthrobbing); tightness Aching	Continuous, variable intensity, for weeks and months	One or more periods of months to years	Fatigue and nervous strain	Depression, nervousness, anxiety, insomnia	Antianxiety and antidepressant drugs
Meningeal irritation (meningitis subarachnoid hemorrhage)	Generalized	Any age, both sexes	Intense, steady deep pain, may be worse in neck	Duration: days to a week or more	Single episode	None	Neck stiff on forward bending Kernig and Brudzinski signs	For meningitis or bleeding (see text)
Brain tumor	(See text)	Any age, both sexes	Variable in intensity May awaken patient Steady pain	Lasts minutes to hours; increasing severity	Once in a lifetime: weeks to months	None Sometimes position	Papilledema Vomiting Slow mentation	Corticosteroids Mannitol Glycerol sargicine Treatment of tumor
Temporal arteritis	Unilateral, temporal, or occipital	Over 50 years, either sex	Persistent burning, aching	Continuous or intermittent	Persists for weeks to a few months	Scalp sensitive Tender arteries	Intermittent or permanent loss of sight Rheumatic myalgia Fever	Corticosteroid therapy

SOURCE: *After J Patten, Neurological Differential Diagnosis, London, Harold Starke, Springer-Verlag, 1977.*

TABLE 4-2
Types of facial pain

Types	Site	Clinical characteristics	Aggravating-relieving factors	Diseases	Treatment
Trigeminal neuralgia (tic douloureux)	Second to third division of trigeminal nerve, unilateral	Men:women = 1:3 Over 50 years Paroxysms (10–30 s) of stabbing, burning pain Trigger points, intermittent ache No sensory or motor paralysis	Touching face, chewing, smiling, talking, blowing nose	Idiopathic If in young adults and bilateral, multiple sclerosis Vascular anomaly Tumor of fifth cranial nerve	Carbamazepine (Tegretol) Phenytoin Surgical section of nerve
Atypical facial neuralgia	Unilateral or bilateral	Predominantly female 30–50 years Continuous intolerable pain Mainly maxillary areas	None	Depressive and anxiety states Hysteria Idiopathic	Antidepressant and antianxiety medication
Supraorbital ciliary, infraorbital, sphenopalatine neuralgias	Unilateral in eye, cheek, ear, neck	Persistent, aching pain	Occasional nasal obstruction	Idiopathic Paranasal sinus disease	Decongestant nasal medication ?Nerve section and injection
Postzoster neuralgia	Unilateral Any one of trigeminal divisions	History of zoster Aching, burning pain; jabs of pain Paresthesia, slight sensory loss Dermal scars	Contact, movement	Herpes zoster	Carbamazepine and phenytoin and antidepressants
Costen's syndrome	Unilateral, near temporomandibular joints	Elderly females Severe aching pain, intensified by chewing Tenderness over joints Malocclusion	Chewing, pressure over temporomandibular joint	Loss of teeth, rheumatoid arthritis	Bite correction and surgery
Tolosa-Hunt syndrome	Unilateral, mainly orbital	Intense sharp, aching pain; associated ophthalmoplegias of varying degree Intense sharp, aching pain Pupil inequality, sensory loss	None	?Arteritis and granulomatous lesions	Corticosteroids Nerve section (trigeminal)
Raeder's paratrigeminal syndrome	Unilateral, frontotemporal and maxilla	Intense sharp, aching pain Pupil inequality, sensory loss	None	Tumors, granulomatous lesions, injuries	Depends on type of lesion
Migrainous neuralgia	Orbitofrontal	See cluster headache, Table 4-1	None		Ergot

SOURCE: *After J Patten, Neurological Differential Diagnosis, London, Harold Starke, Springer-Verlag, 1977.*

arteries. The headaches of cranial tumor often respond surprisingly well to large doses of methylprednisolone acetate and like compounds.

In conclusion, it is well to mention the importance of general hygienic measures. Young physicians in particular are apt to seek a specific therapy for each headache syndrome and give little thought to the general health of the patient. We have observed that most of the recurrent and chronic headaches are likely to be more severe and disabling whenever the patient becomes nervous, sick, and tired. A well-rounded diet, adequate rest, a reasonable amount of physical exercise, and a balanced view of the sources of daily anxieties and how to cope with them should be the goal of all therapeutic programs.

REFERENCES

APPENZELLER O: *Pathogenesis and Treatment of Headache.* New York, Spectrum, 1976

CHAPMAN LF: A humoral agent implicated in vascular headache of the migraine type. Arch Neurol 3:223, 1960

CLOVER V et al: Transitory decrease in platelet monoamine oxidase activity during migraine attacks. Lancet 1:391, 1977

COUCH JR, HASSANEIM RS: Platelet aggregability in migraine. Neurology 27:843, 1977

FRIEDMAN AP: *Research and Clinical Studies in Headache.* Baltimore, Williams & Wilkins, 1967

LANCE JW: *The Mechanism and Management of Headache.* London, Butterworth, 1969

LANCE JW, HINTZENBERGER H: The control of cranial arteries by humoral mechanisms and its relation to the migraine syndrome. Headache 7:93, 1967

PARRY CH: *Collections from the Unpublished Medical Writing of the Late Caleb Hillier Parry.* London, Underwood, 1825, vol 1

SICUTERI F: Vasoneuroactive substances and their implication in vascular pain, in A Friedman (ed): *Research and Clinical Studies of Headache.* Baltimore, Williams & Wilkins, 1967, chap 2

SMITH R: *Background of Migraine.* New York, Springer, 1967

STREETER DHP et al: Hyperbradykinism, a new orthostatic syndrome. Lancet 2:1048, 1972

VIJAYAN N, DREYFUS PM: Posttraumatic dysautonomic cephalalgia: Clinical observations and treatment. Arch Neurol 32:649, 1976

VINKEN PJ, BRUYN GW: *Handbook of Clinical Neurology, vol 5: Headache and Cranial Neuralgias.* Amsterdam, North-Holland, 1968

WATSON P, STEELE JC: Paroxysmal dysequilibrium in the migraine syndrome of childhood. Arch Otolaryngol 99:177, 1974

5
CHEST PAIN AND PALPITATION

EUGENE BRAUNWALD

CHEST PAIN

There is little parallelism between the severity of chest pain and the gravity of its cause. Therefore, a frequent problem in patients who complain of chest pain is distinguishing trivial disorders from coronary artery disease and other serious disorders. An incorrect positive diagnosis of a hazardous condition such as angina pectoris is likely to have harmful psychologic and economic consequences, while failure to recognize a serious disorder, such as coronary artery disease or mediastinal tumor, may result in the dangerous delay of much-needed treatment.

The apparently bizarre radiation of pain arising in the thoracic viscera can usually be explained in terms of the known facts concerning nerve supply (Chap. 3). One occasionally sees a patient with extension of pain to a location which cannot be logically explained. In most instances, such a person will be found to have more than one disorder capable of causing pain in the chest. The presence of one condition may affect the radiation of the pain produced by the other disorder. For example, when the pain of angina pectoris extends to the back or abdomen, the patient may be found to have also a significant degree of spinal arthritis or an upper abdominal disorder, such as hiatus hernia, disease of the gallbladder, pancreatitis, or peptic ulcer. The common tendency to assume that the presence of an objective abnormality, such as a hiatus hernia or an electrocardiographic abnormality, necessarily means that an atypical chest pain arises in the stomach or the heart is to be strongly condemned. Such an assumption is justified only if a careful history indicates that the behavior of the pain is entirely compatible with the site of origin suggested by the objective finding.

THE LEFT-ARM MYTH There is a long tradition, widely accepted by physicians and laymen, that pain in the left arm, especially when appearing in conjunction with chest pain, has a unique and ominous significance as being almost certain evidence of the presence of ischemic heart disease. This is a myth that has neither theoretic nor clinical foundation. From a theoretic standpoint, any disorder involving the deep afferent fibers of the left upper thoracic region should be capable of causing pain in the chest, the left arm, or both areas. Hence a pain of trivial significance arising in skeletal tissues innervated by upper (first to fourth) thoracic nerves may produce left-arm-area pain; almost any condition capable of causing pain in the chest may induce radiation to the left arm. Such localization is common not only in patients with coronary disease but also in those with numerous other types of chest pain. Although pain due to myocardial ischemia most frequently is substernal, radiates down the ulnar aspect of the left arm (Chap. 244), and is pressing and constricting in nature, the location, radiation, and quality of pain are of less diagnostic significance than the behavior of the pain, in terms of the conditions which induce it and relieve it.

Most persons also believe that cardiac pain is situated in the region of the left breast, and therefore left inframammary pain is one of the common symptoms that bring the patient to seek medical advice. It differs radically from the pain due to myocardial hypoxia, i.e., angina pectoris, in that it is either momentary, sharp and lancinating, or a long-lasting, dull ache, occasionally accentuated by sharp stabs. Such pain is frequently observed in patients who are tense, easily fatigued, unusually anxious, or psychoneurotic, or who have neurocirculatory asthenia. In contrast to angina pectoris, such precordial pain has no relationship to exertion and may be accompanied by tenderness over the precordium.

PAIN DUE TO OXYGEN DEFICIENCY OF THE MYOCARDIUM
Physiologic considerations of the coronary circulation Pain due to myocardial ischemia occurs when the oxygen supply to the heart is deficient in relation to the oxygen need. The oxygen consumption of this organ is closely related to the physiologic effort made during contraction. It is dependent primarily on three factors: (1) the tension developed by the myocardium, (2) the contractile (inotropic) state of the myocardium, and (3) the heart rate. When these three factors remain constant, or almost so, an elevation of stroke volume produces an efficient type of response because it leads to an increase in the external work of the heart (i.e., in the product of cardiac output and arterial pressure) with little accompanying augmentation of myocardial oxygen requirements. Thus, a rise in flow load causes less increment in myocardial oxygen consumption than does a comparable increase in cardiac work per minute brought about by elevation either of pressure or of heart rate. However, the net effects of these hemodynamic variables depend not on oxygen need alone, but rather on the balance between the demand and the supply of oxygen. The heart is always active, and the coronary venous blood is normally much more desaturated than that draining other areas of the body. Thus the removal of more oxygen from each unit of blood, which is one of the adjustments commonly utilized by exercising skeletal muscle, is already employed in the heart in the basal state. Therefore, the heart must rely on an increase in the coronary blood flow for obtaining additional oxygen.

It follows, from hydrodynamic considerations, that the flow of blood through the coronary arteries is directly proportional to the pressure gradient between the aorta and the ventricular myocardium during systole and the ventricular cavity during diastole, but is proportional to the fourth power of the radius of the coronary arteries. Thus a relatively slight alteration in coronary diameter will produce a large change in coronary flow, provided that other factors remain constant. In the normal heart, coronary blood flow occurs primarily during diastole, when it is unopposed by myocardial constriction of the coronary vessels. Coronary flow is regulated primarily by myocardial oxygen needs, probably through the release of vasodilator metabolites, such as adenosine, and through variations in myocardial P_{O_2}. Although changes in coronary blood flow occur with activation of autonomic nerves to the coronary vessels, these alterations result primarily from the effects of these nervous stimuli on myocardial contraction and therefore on the heart's oxygen consumption. The role of direct neural regulation of the coronary vascular bed is controversial.

The coronary dilatation which normally occurs during exercise and emotion results from the increased myocardial metabolism during these conditions and is impaired in patients with fixed coronary narrowing due to coronary arteriosclerosis. Thus, any condition in which increased heart rate, arterial pressure, or myocardial contractility occurs tends, particularly in the presence of coronary obstruction, to precipitate anginal attacks by increasing myocardial oxygen needs. Bradycardia, when not severe, usually has the opposite effects, and this apparently explains the rarity of angina in patients with complete heart block, even when this disorder is associated with coronary disease.

Causes of myocardial hypoxia By far the most frequent underlying cause is organic narrowing of the coronary arteries secondary to coronary atherosclerosis. Less frequently, narrowing of the coronary orifices due to syphilitic aortitis or to distortion by a dissecting aneurysm may be responsible. There is no evidence that systemic arterial constriction or increased cardiac contractile activity (rise in heart rate or blood pressure, or increase in contractility due to liberation of catecholamines or adrenergic activity) due to emotion can precipitate angina unless there is also structural narrowing of the coronary vessels. While this is usually on an organic basis and secondary to arteriosclerosis, recently it has become clear that coronary artery spasm, with or without accompanying atherosclerosis, can also precipitate angina.

Aside from conditions which narrow the lumen of the coronary arteries, the only other frequent causes of myocardial hypoxia are disorders, such as aortic stenosis and/or regurgitation (Chap. 242), which cause a marked disproportion between the perfusion pressure and the ventricular work. Under such conditions the rise in left ventricular systolic pressure is not, as in hypertensive states, balanced by a corresponding elevation of aortic perfusion pressure. Therefore, an increase in heart rate is especially harmful in patients with aortic stenosis, because it shortens diastole more than systole and thereby decreases the total available perfusion time per minute.

Patients with marked *right ventricular hypertension* may have exertional pain which is, in most respects, identical with that of the common type of angina. It is likely that this discomfort results from relative ischemia of the right ventricle brought about by the increased oxygen needs and by the elevated intramural resistance, with sharp reduction of the normally large systolic pressure gradient which perfuses this chamber. Angina is common in patients with *syphilitic aortitis,* and the relative roles of aortic regurgitation and of coronary ostial narrowing are difficult to assess. The importance of tachycardia, decline in arterial pressure, thyrotoxicosis, or diminution in arterial oxygen content (such as occurs in anemia or arterial hypoxemia) in the production of myocardial hypoxia will be apparent from the above discussion. However, these are precipitating and aggravating factors rather than the underlying cause of angina; as already noted, the latter is, in almost all instances, coronary atherosclerosis.

Effects of myocardial hypoxia The most common of these is anginal pain, which is considered in some detail in Chap. 244. It is usually described as a heavy pressure or squeezing, a sensation of strangling or constriction in the chest, a "burning" or "heavy feeling," or difficulty in breathing, and it occurs particularly on walking, especially after meals, on cold days against a wind or uphill. It is not a stabbing pain. It occurs during exertion, following heavy meals, and with anger, excitement, and other emotional states; it is not precipitated by coughing or respiratory movements. When anginal pain is induced by walking, it forces the patient to stop or to reduce his speed; it is characteristically relieved by rest and nitroglycerin. The exact mechanism of the pain stimulus is still unknown, but it is probably related to an accumulation of metabolites within the heart muscle. Anginal pain occurs most typically in the substernal region, anteriorly across the midthorax; it may radiate to or rarely occur alone in the interscapular region, in the arms, shoulders, and teeth. The more severe the attack, the greater the radiation from the substernal areas to the left arm, especially its ulnar aspect. There is considerable variability in the amount of effort required to bring on anginal pain.

As a rule, myocardial infarction is associated with a pain similar in quality and distribution to that of angina but of greater intensity and longer duration. The pain of myocardial infarction is not relieved by rest or by coronary dilator drugs and may require large doses of narcotics. It may be accompanied by diaphoresis, nausea, and hypotension (Chap. 245).

In addition to chest pain, a second effect of myocardial ischemia consists of electrocardiographic changes (Chaps. 232, 244, and 245). Many patients with angina have normal tracings between attacks, and the record may even remain normal

during the episode of pain. However, often depression of the ST segments appears in leads I, II, aVL, or in those from the left precordium during exertion. The finding of ST-segment depressions of a deep, ischemic type during an attack of pain, with a return to normal after the pain subsides, strongly suggests that the pain is anginal in origin. There is strong experimental evidence that such depressions, as well as the elevations which are usually seen in patients with infarction and are observed in a few patients during anginal attacks, are related to alterations in cellular ionic balance (Chap. 232). The value and limitation of electrocardiographic changes occurring after exercise in the diagnosis of angina pectoris are discussed in Chap. 244.

A third effect of myocardial hypoxia is an alteration in myocardial contraction. It has been shown that the left ventricular end-diastolic and pulmonary vascular pressures may rise during anginal attacks, particularly if they are prolonged. This indicates transient depression of left ventricular function, which is presumably induced by the decreased contractility of the ischemic areas. On auscultation a fourth heart sound is also frequently heard during the anginal episode; paradoxic pulsations may be evident on palpation of the precordium and can be recorded by apex cardiography.

Another characteristic effect of myocardial hypoxia is liability to sudden death (Chap. 32). This may never occur, despite thousands of anginal episodes. However, it may supervene early in the disease and even in the first attack. The usual mechanism is probably ventricular fibrillation, but occasionally in patients with impaired atrioventricular conduction sudden death may be due to ventricular standstill.

PAIN DUE TO IRRITATION OF SEROUS MEMBRANES OR JOINTS Pericarditis The visceral surface of the pericardium is ordinarily insensitive to pain, as is the parietal surface, except in its lower portion, which has a relatively small number of pain fibers carried in the phrenic nerves. The pain associated with pericarditis is believed to be due to inflammation of the adjacent parietal pleura. These observations explain why noninfectious pericarditis (that associated with uremia and with myocardial infarction) and cardiac tamponade with relatively mild inflammation are usually painless or accompanied by mild pain, whereas infectious pericarditis, being nearly always more intense and spreading to the neighboring pleura, is usually associated with pain having some pleuritic features, i.e., it is aggravated by breathing, coughing, etc. Since the central part of the diaphragm receives its sensory supply from the phrenic nerve (which arises from the third to fifth cervical segments of the spinal cord), pain arising from the lower parietal pericardium and central tendon of the diaphragm is felt characteristically at the tip of the shoulder, the adjoining trapezius ridge, and the neck. Involvement of the more lateral part of the diaphragmatic pleura, supplied by branches from the sixth to ninth intercostal nerves, causes pain not only in the anterior part of the chest but also in the upper part of the abdomen or corresponding region of the back, thus sometimes simulating the pain of acute cholecystitis or pancreatitis.

Pericarditis causes three distinct types of pain (Chap. 249):

1 By far the commonest is the pleuritic pain, related to respiratory movements and aggravated by cough or deep inspiration. It is sometimes brought on by swallowing, because the esophagus lies just beyond the posterior portion of the heart. It is often altered by a change of bodily position, becoming sharper and more left-sided. It is frequently referred to the neck or flank and lasts longer than the pain of angina pectoris. This type of pain is due to the pleuritic component of the pleuropericarditis so commonly present in the infectious forms.

2 The next commonest pericardial pain is the steady, crushing substernal pain which mimics that of acute myocardial infarction. The mechanism of this steady substernal pain is not certain, but the pain may arise from marked inflammation of the relatively insensitive inner parietal surface of the pericardium, or from irritated afferent cardiac nerve fibers lying in the periadventitial layers of the superficial coronary arteries.

3 The third type of pain, which is quite uncommon, is synchronous with the heartbeat and is felt at the left border of the heart and left shoulder.

Occasionally two and rarely all three types of pain may be present simultaneously.

The painful syndromes which may follow trauma to or operations on the heart (i.e., the postcardiotomy syndrome) or myocardial infarction are discussed in later chapters (Chaps. 245 and 249). Such pains often but not always arise in the pericardium.

Pleural pain is very common; it generally results from stretching of inflamed parietal pleura and may be identical with that of pericarditis. It occurs in fibrinous pleurisy, as well as when pneumonic processes reach the periphery of the lung. Pneumothorax and tumors involving the pleural space may also irritate the parietal pleura and cause pleural pain; the latter is sharp, knifelike, superficial in quality, and its aggravation by each breath and by coughing readily distinguishes it from the deep, dull, steady unwavering pain of myocardial ischemia.

The pain resulting from *pulmonary embolism* may resemble that of acute myocardial infarction, and in massive embolism it is located substernally. In patients with smaller emboli the pain is located more laterally, is pleuritic in nature, and may be associated with hemoptysis (Chap. 266). Massive pulmonary emboli and other causes of acute pulmonary hypertension may cause severe, persistent substernal pain, presumably due to distention of the pulmonary artery. The pain of mediastinal emphysema (Chap. 269) may be intense and sharp and may radiate from the substernal region to the shoulders; often a distinct crepitus is heard. The pain associated with mediastinitis and mediastinal tumors usually resembles that of pleuritis but is more likely to be maximal in the substernal region, and the associated feeling of constriction or oppression may cause confusion with myocardial infarction. The pain due to *acute dissection of the aorta* or to an expanding aortic aneurysm results from stimulation of the adventitia; it is usually extremely severe, is localized to the center of the chest, lasts for hours, and requires unusually large amounts of analgesics for relief. It often radiates into the back but is not aggravated by changes in position or respiration (Chap. 252).

The *costochondral and chondrosternal articulations* are the commonest sites of anterior chest pain. Objective signs in the form of swelling (Tietze's syndrome), redness, and heat are rare, but sharply localized tenderness is common. The pain may be "neuritic," i.e., darting and lasting for only a few seconds, or a dull ache enduring for hours or days. An associated feeling of tightness due to muscle spasm (see below) is frequent. When the discomfort persists for a few days only, a story of minor trauma or of some unaccustomed physical effort can often be obtained. The variety of this discomfort is common in persons with arthritis of the spine and also in patients with ischemic heart disease, but in many instances no associated disorder is found. It should be emphasized that *pressure on the chondrosternal and costochondral junctions is an essential part of the examination of every patient with chest pain.* A large

percentage of patients with costochondral pain, especially those who also have minor and innocent T-wave alterations (Chap. 232), are erroneously labeled as having coronary disease. The dire consequences of such a mistake have already been emphasized.

Pain secondary to *subacromial bursitis* and *arthritis of the shoulder and spine* may be precipitated by exercise of the local area but not by general exertion. It may be brought about by passive movement of the involved area as well as by coughing.

PAIN DUE TO TISSUE DISRUPTION Rupture or tear of a structure may give rise to pain that sets in abruptly and reaches its peak of intensity almost instantly. Such a story should arouse the suspicion of dissecting aortic aneurysm, pneumothorax, mediastinal emphysema, a cervical disk syndrome, or rupture of the esophagus. However, the patient may be too ill to recall the precise circumstances, or the pain may be atypical and increase gradually in severity. Likewise, other and more benign conditions, such as a slipped costal cartilage or an intercostal muscle cramp, may also produce pain with an abrupt onset.

Dissecting aortic aneurysm usually causes very severe persistent pain located in the anterior chest. It often radiates into the back, and is not intensified by breathing or motion.

CLINICAL ASPECTS OF THE COMMONER CAUSES OF CHEST PAIN Some of the features of pericarditis have already been described, and those of the more serious causes of chest pain such as myocardial ischemia (angina pectoris and infarction), dissecting aneurysm, and disorders of the pleura, esophagus, stomach, duodenum, and pancreas are considered in the appropriate chapters dealing with these problems. Here, we are concerned with the discussion of those causes which are not considered in more detail elsewhere.

Pain arising in the chest wall or upper extremity This may develop as a result of muscle or ligament strains brought on by unaccustomed exercise and felt in the costochondral or chondrosternal junctions or in the chest wall muscles. We mention the upper extremities and especially the left because of the deeply ingrained legend that pain in the left arm has a specific significance in indicting the heart. Other causes are *osteoarthritis* of the dorsal or thoracic spine and *ruptured cervical disks.* Pain in the left upper extremity and precordium may be due to compression of portions of the brachial plexus by a cervical rib or by spasm and shortening of the scalenus anticus muscle secondary to high fixation of the ribs and sternum. Finally, pains in the upper extremity (shoulder-hand syndrome) and in the pectoral muscles may, through unknown mechanisms, occur in patients with ischemic heart disease.

Skeletal pains in the chest wall or shoulder girdles or arms are usually recognized quite easily. Localized tenderness of the affected area is usually present, and the pain is sometimes clearly related to movements involving the painful locus. Thus deep breathing, turning or twisting of the chest, and movements of the shoulder girdle and arm will elicit and duplicate the pain of which the patient complains. The pain may be very brief, lasting only a few seconds, or full and aching and enduring for hours. The duration is, therefore, likely to be either longer or shorter than untreated anginal pain, which usually lasts for only a few minutes.

These skeletal pains often have a sharp or sticking quality. In addition, there is frequently a feeling of tightness, which is probably due to associated spasm of intercostal or pectoral muscles. This may produce the "morning stiffness" seen in so many skeletal disorders. The discomfort is unaffected by nitroglycerin but often is abolished by infiltration of the painful areas with procaine. When chest wall pain is of recent origin and follows trauma, strain, or some unusual activity involving the pectoral muscles, it presents no problem in diagnosis. However, long-standing skeletal pain is frequent in persons who also have angina pectoris. Since both disorders are very common, this association may be coincidental. In other instances, the coronary disease appears to be responsible for the chest wall pain; the exact mechanism is uncertain but probably is similar to that responsible for the well-known shoulder-hand syndrome. This coexistence of the two different types of chest pain in the same patient is a frequent cause of a confusing history, because in the patient's mind the anginal needle may be hidden in the skeletal haystack. Thus every middle-aged or elderly patient who has long-standing anterior chest wall pain merits careful study for the presence of ischemic heart disease.

Detailed questioning may reveal that what was originally thought by the patient to be a single type of discomfort actually comprises two different pains, which, though similar in quality and area, differ in duration and initiating factors. When the history is inconclusive, the exercise electrocardiogram may furnish useful information concerning the existence of myocardial ischemia. In rare instances coronary arteriography may be required. It may be necessary also to learn by direct observation whether exercise alone or postprandial exertion is capable of producing it. Repeated tests may be required, comparing the relative effects of preceding placebos and nitroglycerin on the amount of exertion required to induce the pain. *The confusion created by the presence of innocent skeletal pain impairs the reliability of the history and is probably the commonest cause of errors—both positive and negative—in the diagnosis of angina pectoris.*

Esophageal pain This usually presents as deep thoracic pain; it results from chemical (acid) irritation of the esophageal mucosa or from spasm of the esophageal muscle in the presence of an intraluminal obstruction, and characteristically follows deglutition. Accompanying dysphagia, regurgitation of undigested food, and weight loss direct attention to the esophagus (see Chaps. 34 and 289).

Emotional disorders These are also common causes of chest wall pain. Usually, the discomfort is experienced as a sense of "tightness," sometimes called "aching," and occasionally it may be sufficiently severe as to be designated a pain of considerable magnitude. Since the discomfort has almost always the additional quality of tightness or constriction, and, furthermore, since it is often localized beneath the sternum, although it may be felt in other areas of the anterior part of the chest, it is not surprising that this type of pain is frequently confused with that of myocardial ischemia. Ordinarily, it lasts for a half hour or more and may persist for a day or less with slow fluctuation of intensity. The association with fatigue or emotional strain is usually clear, although this may not be recognized by the patient until called to his attention. The pain probably develops through unconscious and prolonged increase of muscle tone (as in frowning in the face, or as can be quickly produced in the hand by rigidly clenching the fist), often enhanced by an accompanying hyperventilation (by causing a contraction of the chest wall muscles similar to the painful tetany of the extremities). When the hyperventilation and/or the associated adrenergic effect due to anxiety also causes innocent changes in the T waves and ST segments, the confusion with coronary disease is strengthened. However, the long duration of the pain, the lack of any relation to exertion but association rather with fatigue or tension, and the usually periodic occurrence on successive days without any limitation of capacity for exercise usually make the differentiation from ischemic pain quite clear.

As compared with these two causes (the chest wall muscle and ligament strains and the contraction of the pectoral muscles due to reflex influences, fatigue, or tension), the various

other conditions that may cause skeletal discomfort are uncommon and readily recognized after appropriate observation: spinal arthritis, herpes zoster, anterior scalene and hyperabduction syndromes, malignant disease of the ribs, etc.

Other causes of chest pain The several *abdominal disorders* which may at times mimic anginal pain may usually be suspected from the history, which, as in esophageal pain, ordinarily indicates some relationship to swallowing, eating, belching, etc. Pain resulting from gastric or duodenal ulcer (Chap. 290) is epigastric or substernal, commences about 1 to 1½ h after meals, and is usually promptly relieved by antacids or milk. The gastrointestinal roentgenogram is of crucial significance, and roentgenographic examination is also often helpful in differentiating biliary, gastrointestinal, aortic, pulmonary, and skeletal disease pain from angina pectoris. It should be emphasized again that the demonstration of the presence of a coexistent abdominal disorder such as a hiatus hernia does not constitute proof that the chest pain of which the patient complains is due to this. Such disorders are frequently asymptomatic and are not at all uncommon in patients who also have angina pectoris.

Substernal discomfort also frequently occurs in the presence of *tracheobronchitis;* it is described as a burning sensation accentuated by coughing. A variety of *disorders involving the breast,* including inflammatory breast disease, benign and malignant tumors, as well as mastodynia, are common causes of thoracic pain. The localization and superficial swelling and tenderness are of diagnostic importance.

APPROACH TO THE PATIENT WITH PAIN IN THE CHEST Most persons with this complaint will fall into one of two general groups. The first consists of persons with prolonged and often severe pain without obvious initiating factors. Such persons will frequently be gravely ill. The problem is that of differentiating such serious conditions as myocardial infarction, dissecting aneurysm, and pulmonary embolism from each other and from less grave causes. In some such instances, the careful history will provide significant clues, while objective evidence of crucial importance will appear within the subsequent 2 or 3 days. Thus, when the initial examinations are not decisive, a watch-and-wait policy, with repeated electrocardiograms coupled with measurements of serum enzymes, lung scans, and chest roentgenograms, will commonly provide the correct answer.

The second group of patients comprises those who have brief episodes of pain and are otherwise in apparently excellent health. Here, the resting electrocardiogram will rarely supply decisive information, but records taken during or immediately after exercise will often reveal characteristic changes (Chap. 244). However, in many instances it is the study of the subjective phenomenon, i.e., of the pain itself, that will lead to the diagnosis. Of the several methods of investigation which are available for such patients, three are of cardinal importance.

A detailed and *meticulous history* of the behavior of the pain is the most important method. The location, radiation, quality, intensity, and, especially, duration of the episodes are important. Even more so is the story of the aggravating and alleviating factors. Thus a history of sharp aggravation by breathing, coughing, or other respiratory movements will usually point toward the pericardium (because of the associated pleuropericarditis) or mediastinum as the site, although chest wall pain is likewise affected by respiratory motions. Similarly, a pain which regularly appears on rapid walking and vanishes within a few minutes upon standing still suggests the diagnosis of angina pectoris, although here, once again, a similar story will rarely be obtained from patients with skeletal disorders.

When the history is inconclusive, the *study of the patient at the time of the spontaneous episode* will often supply crucial information. Thus the electrocardiogram, which may be normal both at rest and even during or after exercise in the absence of pain, will occasionally demonstrate striking changes when recorded during an anginal episode. Similarly, radiographic study of the esophagus or of the stomach may show no evidence of cardiospasm or of hiatal hernia except when the observation is made during the pain.

The third method of study represents the *attempt to produce and alleviate the pain at will*. This procedure is necessary only when doubt exists following the history or when needed for psychotherapeutic purposes. Thus the demonstration that a localized pain, which can be reproduced by pressure on the chest, is completely relieved by local infiltration with procaine will often be of conclusive importance in convincing the patient that the heart is not the site.

When, as is not rarely the case, the history is atypical, the correct diagnosis of angina pectoris will often depend in large measure on the response to nitroglycerin. Here, a number of pitfalls should be avoided. If the patient has previously had the drug, careful questioning may be necessary to avoid errors. Thus, relief of pain after its sublingual administration does not necessarily prove that there is a cause-and-effect relationship. It is necessary to be certain that the pain vanishes more rapidly (usually within 5 min) and more completely when the drug is used than when it is not employed. A false negative impression concerning the effect of nitroglycerin may be the result of the use of a deteriorated preparation which has been exposed to light. In doubtful instances, repeated exercise tests, with and without preceding administration of nitroglycerin, are necessary. The demonstration that the time required for a given exercise to produce pain is consistently and considerably longer when it is undertaken within a few minutes after a sublingual nitroglycerin pill than after a placebo may, in some instances, represent the sole method for accurate recognition of angina pectoris. A completely negative response to such repeated tests constitutes almost conclusive evidence against angina.

In patients in whom the question of whether there is coronary disease cannot be resolved despite the aforementioned clinical and laboratory tests, including exercise electrocardiography (Chap. 244), cardiac catheterization and coronary arteriography may be required. A useful stress test that can be carried out at the time of catheterization is to elevate the heart rate in stepwise fashion by electrical pacing; the development of ST-segment depressions on the electrocardiogram and the reproduction of the pain support the diagnosis of myocardial ischemia. Coronary arteriography will show severe (more than 75 percent) reduction of the lumen in patients with obstructive coronary artery disease (Chaps. 234 and 244).

PALPITATION

Palpitation is a common, disagreeable subjective phenomenon which may be defined as an awareness of the beating of the heart, an awareness most commonly brought about by a change in the heart's rhythm or rate or by an augmentation of its contractility. Palpitation is not pathognomonic of any particular group of disorders; indeed, often it signifies not a primary physical disorder but rather a psychic disturbance. Even when it occurs as a more or less prominent complaint, the diagnosis of the underlying disease is made largely on the basis of other associated symptoms and data. Nevertheless, palpitation is frequently of considerable importance in the minds of patients, who fear that it may indicate heart disease. Concern is all the more pronounced in patients who know or who have been told that they may have heart disease; to them palpitation may seem to be an omen of impending disaster. Since the resulting anxiety may be associated with increased activity of the autonomic nervous system, with consequent increases of the cardiac rate and rhythm and the vigor of contraction, the patient's awareness of these changes may then lead to a vicious cycle, which may ultimately be responsible for his incapacitation.

Palpitation may be described by the patient in various terms, such as "pounding," "fluttering," "flopping," and "skipping," and in most cases it will be obvious that the complaint is of a sensation of disturbed heartbeat. The wide variability in the sensitivity to alterations in cardiac activity among different individuals must be appreciated. Some patients seem to be unaware of the most serious and chaotic dysrhythmias; others are seriously troubled by an occasional extrasystole. Patients with anxiety states often exhibit a lowered threshold at which disorders of rate and rhythm result in palpitation. Indeed, it is not unusual for palpitation to be the major manifestation of the emotional disorder. The awareness of the heartbeat also tends to be more common at night and during introspective moments, but is less marked during activity. Patients with organic heart disease and chronic disorders of cardiac rate, rhythm, or stroke volume tend to accommodate to these abnormalities and are often less sensitive than normal persons to such events. Persistent tachycardia and/or atrial fibrillation may not be accompanied by continual palpitation, in contrast to a sudden, brief alteration in cardiac rate or rhythm which often causes considerable subjective discomfort. Thus, palpitation is particularly prominent when the precipitating cause for increased heart rate or contractility or arrhythmia is recent, transient, and episodic. Conversely, in emotionally well-adjusted individuals palpitation becomes progressively less disconcerting as the cause (e.g., anemia, frequent extrasystoles, complete atrioventricular block) persists.

PATHOGENESIS OF PALPITATION Under ordinary circumstances the rhythmic heartbeat is imperceptible to the healthy individual of average or placid temperament. Palpitation may be experienced by normal persons who have engaged in strenuous physical effort or have been aroused emotionally or sexually. This type of palpitation is physiologic and represents the normal awareness of an overactive heart—i.e., a heart that is beating at a rapid rate and with an increased contractility. Since palpitation due to overactivity of the heart may occur also in certain pathologic states, e.g., high fever, severe anemia, or thyrotoxicosis, it is commonly assumed that it is the overactivity per se that is responsible for the symptom.

When palpitation is heavy and regular, it is usually caused by an augmented stroke volume, and it should raise the question of aortic or mitral regurgitation, ventricular septal defect, or of a variety of hyperkinetic circulatory states (anemia, arteriovenous fistula, thyrotoxicosis, and the so-called "idiopathic hyperkinetic heart syndrome"). It may also occur immediately after the onset of cardiac slowing, as with the sudden development of heart block, or upon the conversion of sinus rhythm from atrial fibrillation. But unusual movements of the heart within the thorax are also frequently the mechanism of palpitation. Thus, the ectopic beat and/or the compensatory pause may be appreciated, since both are associated with alterations in cardiac motion.

IMPORTANT CAUSES OF PALPITATION See also Chap. 237.

Extrasystoles In most cases the diagnosis will be suggested by the patient's story. The premature contraction and postpremature beat are often described as a "flopping," or the patient may say that he feels as if "the heart turns over." The pause following the premature contraction may be felt as an actual cessation of the heartbeat, in contrast with the complete unawareness of pauses of similar duration when atrial fibrillation with a slow ventricular rate occurs. The first ventricular contraction succeeding the pause may be felt as an unusually vigorous beat and will be described as "pounding" or "thudding."

When extrasystoles are numerous, clinical differentiation from atrial fibrillation can be made by any procedure that will bring about a definite increase in the ventricular rate; at increasingly rapid heart rates, the extrasystoles usually diminish in frequency and then disappear, whereas the ventricular irregularity of atrial fibrillation increases.

Ectopic tachycardias These conditions, which are considered in some detail in Chap. 237, are common and medically important causes of palpitation. Ventricular tachycardia, one of the most serious arrhythmias, rarely is manifested as palpitation; this may be related to the abnormal sequence, and hence impaired coordination and vigor, of ventricular contraction. If the patient is seen between attacks, the diagnosis of ectopic tachycardia and its type will have to depend on the history, but of course the precise diagnosis can be made only when an electrocardiogram and observations on the effect of carotid sinus pressure are made during the episode. The mode of onset and offset gives the most important lead in distinguishing sinus from one of the various forms of ectopic tachycardias; sinus tachycardia commences and ceases over the course of minutes or seconds, but not instantaneously as is characteristic of ectopic rhythms. Monitoring of the electrocardiogram with a portable tape recording system and asking the patient to record the time of onset and cessation of the palpitations are extremely helpful in determining their cause. The technique of ambulatory electrocardiography is discussed in Chap. 237.

Thyrotoxicosis In its fully developed form, thyrotoxicosis will usually be evident and offers little difficulty in the way of diagnosis except in the elderly, in whom so-called "apathetic hyperthyroidism" may be present. Thyrotoxicosis is particularly likely to be overlooked in the presence of myocardial failure (Chap. 335).

Anemia When mild, anemia may cause palpitation during exertion; when severe, palpitation may be present at rest. Palpitation is more prominent the more rapidly the anemia develops. Appropriate studies of the blood will clarify the situation.

Fever Palpitation may be present in acute infections, particularly in the early stages, but here the symptom is merely an insignificant phenomenon in the midst of other obviously more important ones. Palpitation may be a prominent but not usually the principal presenting symptom in an individual suffering from one of the chronic and sometimes more obscure febrile illnesses, such as tuberculosis, chronic brucellosis, subacute infective endocarditis, or acute rheumatic fever with carditis and relatively few or no joint manifestations.

Hypoglycemia Palpitation is often a prominent feature of this condition and appears to be related to release of catecholamines. The diagnosis is confirmed by appropriate blood sugar estimations at the time of symptoms, by reproduction of the symptom following fasting or a 5-h glucose tolerance test, and by prompt relief of all symptoms on the administration of glucose (Chap. 340).

Tumors of the adrenal medulla (pheochromocytomas) Such tumors may give rise to recurrent attacks, including paroxysms

of hypertension and palpitation which are identical with those seen following the injection of epinephrine or norepinephrine. This type of tumor is a rather uncommon cause of palpitation and is mentioned chiefly because cure may be effected by surgical removal (Chap. 337).

Drugs The relationship between the development of palpitation and the use of tobacco, coffee, tea, alcohol, epinephrine, ephedrine, aminophylline, atropine, or thyroid extract is obvious.

Palpitation as a manifestation of the anxiety state Persons who are healthy physically and well adjusted emotionally may have palpitation under certain circumstances. Thus, during or immediately after vigorous physical exertion or during sudden emotional tension, palpitation is common and is usually associated with sinus tachycardia. In poorly conditioned persons without organic heart disease, the sinus tachycardia of exercise may be excessive and associated with palpitation.

In some patients, palpitation may be one of the outstanding manifestations of an episode of acute anxiety. In other persons the palpitation may, with other symptoms, represent prolonged anxiety neurosis or a lifelong disorder characterized by volatile autonomic function. The latter condition has been called *neurocirculatory asthenia*. Whether these illnesses are simply an expression of a chronic, deep-seated anxiety state superimposed on a normal autonomic nervous system or whether they depend on instability of the autonomic nervous system is not clear. At any rate, the clinical significance of the differentiation between the transitory and the enduring forms is that the former is often dissipated by firm reassurance from the physician, whereas the latter is usually resistant even to the most thorough and expert psychiatric care. In the latter case, the patient must be treated with most carefully planned psychologic support and tranquilizing medications. This chronic form of palpitation is known by various names such as *Da Costa's syndrome, soldier's heart, effort syndrome, irritable heart, neurocirculatory asthenia,* and *functional cardiovascular disease.* Aside from palpitation, the chief symptoms are those of an anxiety state.

Physical examination usually reveals the typical findings of the hyperkinetic syndrome. These include a left parasternal lift, a precordial or apical systolic murmur, a wide pulse pressure, rapidly rising pulse, and excessive perspiration. The electrocardiogram may display minor depressions of the ST junction and inversion of T waves and so occasionally lead to a mistaken diagnosis of coronary disease; this is particularly likely to occur when these findings are associated with complaints by the patients of an aching feeling of substernal tightness, commonly present in emotional stress. The presence of any kind of organic disease is one of the commonest causes of the underlying anxiety which frequently precipitates this functional syndrome.

Even when a patient presents undoubted objective evidence of structural cardiac disease, the possibility that a superimposed anxiety responsible for the symptoms when the clinical picture is that which has been described should be considered. Palpitation associated with organic cardiac disease is nearly always accompanied by arrhythmia or by marked tachycardia, whereas the symptom may exist with regular rhythm and with a heart rate of 80 beats per minute or less in patients with the anxiety state. It is noteworthy that an anxiety state, in contrast to heart disease, causes a sighing type of dyspnea. Also pain localized to the region of the apex, either brief and lancinating

TABLE 5-1
Items to be covered in history

Does the palpitation occur:	If so, suspect:
As isolated "jumps" or "skips"?	Extrasystoles
In attacks, known to be of abrupt beginning, with a heart rate of 120 beats per minute or over, or regular or irregular rhythm?	Paroxysmal rapid heart action
Independent of exercise or excitement adequate to account for the symptom?	Atrial fibrillation, atrial flutter, thyrotoxicosis, anemia, febrile states, hypoglycemia, anxiety state
In attacks developing rapidly though not absolutely abruptly, unrelated to exertion or excitement?	Hemorrhage, hypoglycemia, tumor of the adrenal medulla
In conjunction with the taking of drugs?	Tobacco, coffee, tea, alcohol, epinephrine, ephedrine, aminophylline, atropine, thyroid extract, monoamine oxidase inhibitors
On standing?	Postural hypotension
In middle-aged women, in conjunction with flushes and sweats?	Menopausal syndrome
When the rate is known to be normal and the rhythm regular?	Anxiety state

in character or lasting for hours or days and accompanied by hyperesthesia, is due usually to an anxiety state, not to structural cardiac disease. Giddiness due to this syndrome can usually be reproduced by hyperventilation (Chap. 13) or by change from the recumbent to the erect posture.

The *treatment* of the anxiety state with palpitation is difficult and depends on removal of the cause. In many instances a thorough examination of the heart and a statement that it is normal will suffice. Instructions to take more rather than less physical exercise will reinforce these statements. Frequently, the demonstration that the physician can reproduce not only the palpitation but many other symptoms of the anxiety state merely by the subcutaneous injection of 0.5 to 1.0 ml of 1:1000 epinephrine serves to convince the patient that the symptoms are not the result of some mysterious disorder but are rather the effect of a well-understood physiologic mechanism. This is especially true when the initial anxiety has been mainly the result of fear of heart disease. When the anxiety state is a manifestation of chronic anxiety neurosis or depressive psychosis, the symptoms are more likely to persist.

Management of patients with palpitation and the anxiety cardiac syndrome is facilitated by a clear understanding on the physician's part of the mechanisms of the symptoms. The palpitation is probably related to adrenergic stimulation of the heart and to the lower perception threshold. The pain may arise in the intercostal tissues as a result of the pounding of the heart. The hyperventilation with its ensuing train of symptoms (Chap. 13) is analogous to sighing. Explanation of these physiologic mechanisms to the patient and reassurance that they are not indicative of serious disease is one of the most important therapeutic steps.

Table 5-1 summarizes the main points of information to be ascertained in the history in elucidating the significance of palpitation. The recording of the electrocardiogram using a portable tape recorder in an ambulatory subject, and the precise temporal correlation of the cardiac rate and rhythm with the presence of palpitation are extremely useful in the identification or exclusion of a rhythmic disturbance. The effectiveness of antiarrhythmia treatment can also be assessed objectively in this manner, without the necessity of relying only on the patient's subjective symptoms. Beta-adrenergic blockade with propranolol, beginning with 40 mg per day in divided doses, and ranging as high as 240 mg per day, can be extremely effective in patients with palpitation and sinus rhythm or sinus tachycardia. The indications and contraindications for this drug are presented in Chap. 238.

One point merits special emphasis. *As a rule palpitation produces anxiety and fear out of all proportion to its seriousness.* When the cause has been accurately determined and its significance explained to patients, their concern is often ameliorated and may disappear entirely.

REFERENCES

BRAUNWALD E: Control of myocardial oxygen consumption: Physiologic and clinical considerations. Am J Cardiol 27:416, 1971

—— et al: *Mechanisms of Contraction of the Normal and Failing Heart,* 2d ed. Boston, Little, Brown, 1976

BURCH GE et al: Cardiac causalgia. Am Heart J 76:725, 1968

COHN PF: Coronary artery disease, in *Heart Disease,* E Braunwald (ed). Philadelphia, Saunders, 1980, chap 38

DRESSLER W: *Clinical Aids in Cardiac Diagnosis.* New York, Grune & Stratton, 1970

HILLIS DF, BRAUNWALD E: Myocardial ischemia. N Engl J Med 296:971, 1034, 1093, 1977

——, ——: Coronary artery spasm. N Engl J Med 299:695, 1978

HURST JW: Symptoms due to diseases of the heart and blood vessels, in *The Heart,* 4th ed, JW Hurst et al (eds). New York, McGraw-Hill, 1978, p 153

LEVENE DL: *Chest Pain.* Philadelphia, Lea & Febiger, 1977, p 203

WOOD P: The chief symptoms of heart disease, in *Diseases of the Heart and Circulation,* 3d ed. Philadelphia, Lippincott, 1968

6
ABDOMINAL PAIN

WILLIAM SILEN

The correct interpretation of acute abdominal pain is one of the most challenging demands made of any physician. Since proper therapy often requires urgent action, the luxury of the leisurely approach suitable for the study of other conditions is frequently denied. Few other clinical situations demand greater experience and judgment, because the most catastrophic of events may be forecast by the subtlest of symptoms and signs. Nowhere in medicine is a meticulously executed detailed history and physical examination of greater importance. The etiologic classification in Table 6-1, although not complete, forms a useful frame of reference for the evaluation of patients with abdominal pain.

The diagnosis of "acute or surgical abdomen" so often heard in emergency wards is not an acceptable one because of its often misleading and erroneous connotation. The most obvious of "acute abdomens" may not require operative intervention, and the mildest of abdominal pains may herald the onset of an urgently correctable lesion. Any patient with abdominal pain of recent onset requires early and thorough evaluation with specific attempts at accurate diagnosis.

SOME MECHANISMS OF PAIN ORIGINATING IN THE ABDOMEN Inflammation of the parietal peritoneum The pain of parietal peritoneal inflammation is steady and aching in character and is located directly over the inflamed area, its exact reference being possible because it is transmitted by overlapping somatic nerves supplying the parietal peritoneum. The intensity of the pain is dependent upon the type and amount of foreign substance to which the peritoneal surfaces are exposed in a given period of time. For example, the sudden release into the peritoneal cavity of a small quantity of *sterile* acid gastric juice causes much more pain than the same amount of grossly contaminated neutral fecal material. Enzymatically active pancreatic juice incites more pain and inflammation than does the same amount of sterile bile containing no potent enzymes. Blood and urine are often so bland as to go undetected if exposure of the peritoneum has not been sudden and massive. In the case of bacterial contamination, such as in pelvic inflammatory disease, the pain is frequently of low intensity early in the illness until bacterial multiplication has caused the elaboration of irritating substances.

So important is the rate at which the irritating material is applied to the peritoneum that cases of perforated peptic ulcer may be associated with entirely different clinical pictures dependent only upon the rapidity with which the gastric juice enters the peritoneal cavity.

The pain of peritoneal inflammation is invariably accentuated by pressure or changes in tension of the peritoneum, whether produced by palpation or by movement, as in coughing or sneezing. Consequently, the patient with peritonitis lies quietly in bed, preferring to avoid motion, in contrast to the patient with colic, who may writhe incessantly.

Another of the characteristic features of peritoneal irritation is tonic reflex spasm of the abdominal musculature, localized to the involved body segment. The intensity of the tonic muscle spasm accompanying peritoneal inflammation is dependent upon the location of the inflammatory process, the

TABLE 6-1
Some important causes of abdominal pain

I Pain originating in the abdomen
  A Parietal peritoneal inflammation
    1 Bacterial contamination, e.g., perforated appendix, pelvic inflammatory disease
    2 Chemical irritation, e.g., perforated ulcer, pancreatitis, mittelschmerz
  B Mechanical obstruction of hollow viscera
    1 Obstruction of the small or large intestine
    2 Obstruction of the biliary tree
    3 Obstruction of the ureter
  C Vascular disturbances
    1 Embolism or thrombosis
    2 Vascular rupture
    3 Pressure or torsional occlusion
    4 Sickle-cell anemia
  D Abdominal wall
    1 Distortion or traction of mesentery
    2 Trauma or infection of muscles
    3 Distention of visceral surfaces, e.g., hepatic or renal capsules
II Pain referred from extraabdominal sources
  A Thorax—e.g., pneumonia, referred pain from coronary occlusion
  B Spine—e.g., radiculitis from arthritis
  C Genitalia—e.g., torsion of the testicle
III Metabolic causes
  A Exogenous
    1 Black widow spider bite
    2 Lead poisoning and others
  B Endogenous
    1 Uremia
    2 Diabetic coma
    3 Porphyria
    4 Allergic factors (C'1 esterase inhibitor deficiency)
IV Neurogenic causes
  A Organic
    1 Tabes dorsalis
    2 Herpes zoster
    3 Causalgia and others
  B Functional

rate at which it develops, and the integrity of the nervous system. Spasm over a perforated retrocecal appendix or perforated ulcer into the lesser peritoneal sac may be minimal or absent because of the protective effect of overlying viscera. As in pain of peritoneal inflammation, a slowly developing process often greatly attenuates the degree of muscle spasm. Catastrophic abdominal emergencies such as a perforated ulcer have been repeatedly associated with minimal or occasionally no detectable pain or muscle spasm in obtunded, seriously ill, debilitated elderly patients or in psychotic patients.

Obstruction of hollow viscera The pain of obstruction of hollow abdominal viscera is classically described as intermittent, or colicky. Yet the lack of a truly cramping character should not be misleading, because distention of a hollow viscus may produce steady pain with only very occasional exacerbations. Although not nearly as well localized as the pain of parietal peritoneal inflammation, some useful generalities can be made concerning its distribution.

The colicky pain of obstruction of small intestine is usually periumbilical or supraumbilical and is poorly localized. As the intestine becomes progressively dilated with loss of muscular tone, the colicky nature of the pain may become less apparent. With superimposed strangulating obstruction, pain may spread in the lower lumbar region if there is traction on the root of the mesentery. The colicky pain of colonic obstruction is of lesser intensity than that of the small intestine and is often located in the infraumbilical area.

Sudden distention of the biliary tree produces a steady rather than colicky type of pain; hence the term "biliary colic" is misleading. Acute distention of the gallbladder usually causes pain in the right upper quadrant with radiation to the right posterior region of the thorax or to the tip of the right scapula, and distention of the common bile duct is often associated with pain in the epigastrium radiating to the upper part of the lumbar region. Considerable variation is common, however, so that differentiation between these may be impossible. The typical subscapular pain or lumbar radiation is frequently absent. Gradual dilatation of the biliary tree as in carcinoma of the head of the pancreas may cause no pain or only a mild aching sensation in the epigastrium or right upper quadrant. The pain of distention of the pancreatic ducts is similar to that described for distention of the common bile duct but in addition is very frequently accentuated by recumbency and relieved by the upright position.

Obstruction of the urinary bladder results in dull suprapubic pain, usually low in intensity. Restlessness without specific complaint of pain may be the only sign of a distended bladder in an obtunded patient. In contrast, acute obstruction of the intravesicular portion of the ureter is characterized by severe suprapubic and flank pain which radiates to the penis, scrotum, or inner aspect of the upper region of the thigh. Obstruction of the ureteropelvic junction is felt as pain in the costovertebral angle, whereas obstruction of the remainder of the ureter is associated with flank pain, which often extends into the corresponding side of the abdomen.

Vascular disturbances A frequent misconception, despite abundant experience to the contrary, is that pain associated with intraabdominal vascular disturbances is sudden and catastrophic in nature. The pain of embolism or thrombosis of the superior mesenteric artery or that of impending rupture of an abdominal aortic aneurysm certainly may be severe and diffuse. Yet just as frequently, the patient with occlusion of the superior mesenteric artery has only mild continuous diffuse pain for 2 or 3 days before vascular collapse or findings of peritoneal inflammation appear. The early, seemingly insignificant discomfort is caused by hyperperistalsis rather than peritoneal inflammation. Indeed, absence of tenderness and rigidity in the presence of continuous diffuse pain in a patient likely to have vascular disease is quite characteristic of occlusion of the superior mesenteric artery. Abdominal pain with radiation to the sacral region, flank, or genitalia should always signal the possible presence of a rupturing abdominal aortic aneurysm. This pain may persist over a period of several days before rupture and collapse occur.

Abdominal wall Pain arising from the abdominal wall is usually constant and aching. Movement and pressure accentuate the discomfort and muscle spasm. In the case of hematoma of the rectus sheath, now most frequently encountered in association with anticoagulant therapy, a mass may be present in the lower quadrants of the abdomen. Simultaneous involvement of muscles in other parts of the body usually serves to differentiate myositis of the abdominal wall from an intraabdominal process which might cause pain in the same region.

REFERRED PAIN IN ABDOMINAL DISEASES Pain referred to the abdomen from the thorax, spine, or genitalia may prove a vexing problem in differential diagnosis, because diseases of the upper part of the abdominal cavity such as acute cholecystitis, perforated ulcer, or subphrenic abscesses are frequently associated with intrathoracic complications. A most important, yet often forgotten, dictum is that the possibility of intrathoracic disease must be considered in every patient with abdominal pain, especially if the pain is in the upper part of the abdomen. Systematic questioning and examination directed toward detecting the presence or absence of myocardial or pulmonary infarction, pneumonia, pericarditis, or esophageal disease (the intrathoracic diseases which most often masquerade as abdominal emergencies) will often provide sufficient clues to establish the proper diagnosis. Diaphragmatic pleuritis resulting from pneumonia or pulmonary infarction may cause pain in the right upper quadrant and pain in the supraclavicular area, the latter radiation to be sharply distinguished from the referred subscapular pain caused by acute distention of the extrahepatic biliary tree. The ultimate decision as to the origin of abdominal pain may require deliberate and planned observation over a period of several hours, during which time repeated questioning and examination will provide the proper explanation.

Referred pain of thoracic origin is often accompanied by splinting of the involved hemithorax with respiratory lag and decrease in excursion more marked than that seen in the presence of intraabdominal disease. In addition, apparent abdominal muscle spasm caused by referred pain will diminish during the inspiratory phase of respiration, whereas it is persistent throughout both respiratory phases if it is of abdominal origin. Palpation over the area of referred pain in the abdomen also does not usually accentuate the pain and in many instances actually seems to relieve it. The frequent coexistence of thoracic and abdominal disease may be misleading and confusing, so that differentiation might be difficult or impossible. For example, the patient with known biliary tract disease often has epigastric pain during myocardial infarction, or biliary colic may be referred to the precordium or left shoulder in a patient who has suffered previously from angina pectoris. For the explanation of the radiation of pain to a previously diseased area, see Chap. 3.

Referred pain from the spine, which usually involves compression or irritation of nerve roots, is characteristically intensified by certain motions such as cough, sneeze, or strain and is associated with hyperesthesia over the involved dermatomes. Pain referred to the abdomen from the testicles or seminal vesicles is generally accentuated by the slightest pressure on either of these organs. The abdominal discomfort is of dull aching character and is poorly localized.

METABOLIC ABDOMINAL CRISES Pain of metabolic origin may simulate almost any other type of intraabdominal disease. Here several mechanisms may be at work. In certain instances, such as hyperparathyroidism, the metabolic disease itself may produce an intraabdominal process such as pancreatitis. Primary hyperlipemia may also be accompanied by severe pancreatitis, which can lead to unnecessary laparotomy unless recognized. C'l esterase deficiency associated with angioneurotic edema is also often associated with episodes of severe abdominal pain. Whenever the cause of abdominal pain is obscure, a metabolic origin must always be considered. Abdominal pain is also the hallmark of familial Mediterranean fever (Chap. 217).

The problem of differential diagnosis is often not readily resolved. The pain of porphyria and of lead colic usually is difficult to distinguish from that of intestinal obstruction, because severe hyperperistalsis is a prominent feature of both. The pain of uremia or diabetes is nonspecific, and the pain and tenderness frequently shift in location and intensity. Diabetic acidosis may be precipitated by acute appendicitis or intestinal obstruction, so that if prompt resolution of the abdominal pain does not result from correction of the metabolic abnormalities, an underlying organic problem should be suspected. Black widow spider bites produce intense pain and rigidity of the abdominal muscles and of the back, an area infrequently involved in disease of intraabdominal origin.

NEUROGENIC CAUSES Causalgic pain may occur in diseases which injure nerves of sensory type. It has a burning character and is usually limited to the distribution of a given peripheral nerve. Normal stimuli such as touch or change in temperature may be transformed into this type of pain, which is also frequently present in a patient at rest. A helpful finding is the demonstration that cutaneous pain spots are now irregularly spaced, and this may be the only indication of an old nerve lesion underlying causalgic pain. Even though the pain may be precipitated by gentle palpation, rigidity of the abdominal muscles is absent, and the respirations are not disturbed. Distention of the abdomen is uncommon, and the pain has no relationship to the intake of food.

Pain arising from spinal nerves or roots comes and goes suddenly and is of a lancinating type (see Chap. 7). It may be caused by herpes zoster, impingement by arthritis, tumors, herniated nucleus pulposus, diabetes, or syphilis. Again it is not associated with food intake, abdominal distention, or changes in respiration. Severe muscle spasm, as in the gastric crises of tabes dorsalis, is common but is either relieved or is not accentuated by abdominal palpation. The pain is made worse by movement of the spine and is usually confined to a few dermatome segments. Hyperesthesia is very common.

Psychogenic pain conforms to none of the aforementioned patterns of disease. Here the mechanism is hard to define. The most common problem is the hysterical adolescent or young woman who develops abdominal pain; she frequently loses an appendix and other organs because of it. Ovulation or some other natural event that causes brief mild abdominal discomfort may be maximized as an abdominal catastrophe.

Psychogenic pain varies enormously in type and location but usually has no relation to meals. It is often at its onset markedly accentuated during the night. Nausea and vomiting are rarely observed, although occasionally the patient reports these symptoms. Spasm is seldom induced in the abdominal musculature and if present does not persist, especially if the attention of the patient can be distracted. Persistent localized tenderness is rare, and if found, the muscle spasm in the area is inconsistent and often absent. Restriction of the depth of respiration is the most common respiratory abnormality, but this is in the nature of a smothering or choking sensation and is part of an anxiety state (see Chap. 11). It occurs in the absence of thoracic splinting or change in the respiratory rate.

APPROACH TO THE PATIENT WITH ABDOMINAL PAIN There are few abdominal conditions which require such urgent operative intervention that an orderly approach need be abandoned, no matter how ill the patient. Only those patients with exsanguinating hemorrhage must be rushed to the operating room immediately, but in such instances only a few minutes are required to assess the critical nature of the problem. Under these circumstances, all obstacles must be swept aside, adequate access for intravenous fluid replacement obtained, and the operation begun. Many patients of this type have died in the radiology department or the emergency room while awaiting such unnecessary examinations as electrocardiograms or films of the abdomen. *There are no contraindications to operation when massive hemorrhage is present.* Although exceedingly important, this situation fortunately is relatively rare.

Nothing will supplant an orderly painstakingly *detailed history,* which is far more valuable than any laboratory or roentgenologic examination. This kind of history is laborious and time-consuming, making it not especially popular even though a reasonably accurate diagnosis can be made on the basis of the history alone in the majority of cases. The *chronological sequence of events* in the patient's history is often more important than emphasis on the location of pain. If the examiner is sufficiently open-minded and unhurried, asks the proper questions, and listens, the patient will often provide the diagnosis. Careful attention should be paid to the extraabdominal regions which may be responsible for abdominal pain. An accurate menstrual history in a female patient is essential. Narcotics or analgesics should be withheld until a definitive diagnosis or a definitive plan has been formulated, because these agents often make it more difficult to secure and to interpret the history and physical findings.

In the examination, simple critical inspection of the patient, e.g., of facies, position in bed, and respiratory activity, may provide valuable clues. The amount of information to be gleaned is directly proportional to the *gentleness* and thoroughness of the examiner. Once a patient with peritoneal inflammation has been examined in a brusque manner, accurate assessment by the next examiner becomes almost impossible. For example, eliciting rebound tenderness by sudden release of a deeply palpating hand in a patient with suspected peritonitis is cruel and unnecessary. The same information can be obtained by gentle percussion of the abdomen (rebound tenderness on a miniature scale), a maneuver which can be far more precise and localizing. Asking the patient to cough will elicit true rebound tenderness without the need for placing a hand on the abdomen. Furthermore, the brusque demonstration of rebound tenderness will startle and induce protective spasm in a nervous or worried patient in whom true rebound tenderness is not present. A palpable gallbladder will be missed if palpation is so brusque that voluntary muscle spasm becomes superimposed upon involuntary muscular rigidity.

As in history taking, there is no substitute for sufficient time spent in the examination. It is important to remember that abdominal signs may be minimal but nevertheless, if accompanied by consistent symptoms, may be exceptionally meaningful when carefully assessed. Signs may be virtually or actually totally absent in cases of pelvic peritonitis, so that careful *pelvic and rectal examinations are mandatory in every patient with abdominal pain.* The presence of tenderness on pelvic or rectal examination in the absence of other abdominal signs must not

lead the examiner to exclude such important operative indications as perforated appendicitis, diverticulitis, twisted ovarian cyst, and many others.

Much attention has been paid to the presence or absence of peristaltic sounds, their quality, and their frequency. Auscultation of the abdomen is probably one of the least rewarding aspects of the physical examination of a patient with abdominal pain. Severe catastrophes, such as strangulating small-intestinal obstruction or perforated appendicitis, may occur in the presence of normal peristalsis. Conversely, when the proximal part of the intestine above an obstruction becomes markedly distended and edematous, peristaltic sounds may lose the characteristics of borborygmi and become weak or absent even when peritonitis is not present. It is usually the severe chemical peritonitis of sudden onset which is associated with the truly silent abdomen. Assessment of the patient's state of hydration is important. The hematocrit and urinalysis permit an accurate estimate of the severity of dehydration, so that adequate replacement can be carried out.

Laboratory examinations may be of enormous value in the assessment of the patient with abdominal pain, yet with but a few exceptions they rarely establish a diagnosis. Leukocytosis should never be the single deciding factor as to whether or not operation is indicated. A white blood cell count greater than 20,000 per cubic millimeter may be observed with perforation of a viscus, but pancreatitis, acute cholecystitis, pelvic inflammatory disease, and intestinal infarction may be associated with marked leukocytosis. A normal white blood cell count is by no means rare in cases of perforation of abdominal viscera. The diagnosis of anemia may be more helpful than the white blood cell count, especially when combined with the history.

The urinalysis is also of great value in indicating to some degree the state of hydration or to rule out severe renal disease, diabetes, or porphyria. Determination of the blood urea nitrogen, blood sugar, and serum bilirubin levels may also be helpful. The serum amylase determination is overrated, since in carefully controlled series of patients with proved pancreatitis where the determination has been done within the first 72 h, amylase was less than 200 Somogyi units in one-third of the cases, between 200 and 500 in another one-third of the cases, and greater than 500 in one third. Since many diseases other than pancreatitis, e.g., perforated ulcer, strangulating intestinal obstruction, and acute cholecystitis, may be associated with very marked increase in the serum amylase, great care must be exercised in denying an operation to a patient solely on the basis of an elevated serum amylase level. The determination of the amylase-to-creatinine clearance ratio is of much greater accuracy than either serum amylase or lipase determinations in the diagnosis of pancreatitis.

Abdominal paracentesis has proved to be a safe and effective diagnostic maneuver in patients with acute abdominal pain. It is of special value in patients with blunt trauma to the abdomen where evaluation of the abdomen may be difficult because of other multiple injuries to the spine, pelvis, or ribs and where blood in the peritoneal cavity produces only a very mild peritoneal reaction. The gallbladder is the only organ which may continue to seep fluid following accidental perforation, so that the region of this organ must be assiduously avoided. Determination of the pH of the aspirated fluid to ascertain the site of a perforation is misleading, because even highly acid gastric juice is rapidly buffered by peritoneal exudate.

Plain and upright or lateral decubitus roentgenograms of the abdomen may be of the greatest value. They are usually unnecessary in patients with acute appendicitis or strangulated external hernias. However, in cases of intestinal obstruction, perforated ulcer, and a variety of other conditions, films may be diagnostic. During a search for free air, the patient should be kept in the decubitus or upright position for at least 10 min before the appropriate film is taken lest a small pneumoperitoneum be missed. In rare instances, barium or water-soluble medium examination of the upper part of the gastrointestinal tract may demonstrate partial intestinal obstruction which may elude diagnosis by other means. If there is any question of obstruction of the colon, oral administration of barium sulfate should be avoided. On the other hand, barium enema is of inestimable value in cases of colonic obstruction and should be used with greater frequency where the possibility of perforation does not exist.

Sometimes, even under the best of circumstances with all available auxiliary aids and with the greatest of clinical skill, a definitive diagnosis cannot be established at the time of the initial examination. Nevertheless, despite lack of a clear anatomic diagnosis it may be abundantly clear to an experienced and thoughtful physician and surgeon on clinical grounds alone that operation is indicated. Should that decision be questionable, watchful waiting with repeated questioning and examination will often elucidate the true nature of the illness and indicate the proper course of action.

REFERENCES

Bonica JJ: Neurophysiologic and pathologic aspects of acute and chronic pain. Arch Surg 112:750, 1977

Cope Z: *The Early Diagnosis of the Acute Abdomen,* 14th ed. Fairlawn, NJ, Oxford University Press, 1972

Lasser RB et al: The role of intestinal gas in functional abdominal pain. N Engl J Med 293:524, 1975

Leek BF: Abdominal and pelvic visceral receptors. Br Med Bull 33:163, 1977

Staniland JR et al: Clinical presentation of acute abdomen: Study of 600 patients. Br Med J 2:393, 1972

7
PAIN IN THE BACK AND NECK

HENRY J. MANKIN
RAYMOND D. ADAMS

The following remarks concern mainly the lower part of the back, since it is most frequently the site of disabling pain. The lower portions of the spine and pelvis, with their many muscular and tendinous attachments, are relatively inaccessible to palpation and inspection. Although certain physical signs and radiographs are helpful, it is often necessary to depend on the patient's description of a pain (which may not be altogether accurate) and behavior during the execution of certain maneuvers to fully assess the nature of the problem. Seasoned clinicians, for these reasons, come to appreciate the need of a systematic clinical approach the description of which is one of the main purposes of this chapter.

ANATOMY AND PHYSIOLOGY OF THE LOWER PART OF THE BACK

The bony spine is a complex structure, anatomically divisible into two parts. The anterior part consists of a series of cylindrical vertebral bodies articulated by the intervertebral disks and held together by the anterior and posterior longitudinal ligaments. The posterior part consists of more delicate elements that extend from the vertebral body as pedicles and laminae, fused by ligaments to form the vertebral canal. Stout transverse and spinous bony processes project laterally and posteriorly and serve as the attachments of muscles which support and protect the vertebral column. The stability of the spine depends on two types of support: that provided by the bony articulations (principally the posterior elements) and a second type provided by the ligamentous (passive) and muscular (active) supporting structures. The ligamentous structures are quite strong, but because neither they nor the vertebral body-disk complexes have sufficient integral strength to resist the enormous forces acting on the column during even simple movements, voluntary and reflex contractions of the sacrospinalis, abdominal, gluteal, psoas, and hamstring muscles afford most of the stability.

The vertebral and paravertebral structures derive their innervation from the recurrent branches of the spinal nerves. Pain endings and fibers have been demonstrated in the ligaments, muscles, periosteum of bone, outer layers of annulus fibrosus, and synovium of the articular facets. The sensory fibers from these structures and the sacroiliac and lumbosacral joints join to form the sinovertebral nerves which pass via the recurrent branches of the spinal nerves of the first sacral and the fifth to first lumbar vertebrae into the gray matter of the corresponding segments of the spinal cord. Efferent fibers emerge from these segments and extend to the muscles through the same nerves. The sympathetic nerves contribute only to the innervation of blood vessels and appear to play no part in voluntary and reflex movement, though they do contain sensory fibers.

The parts of the back that possess the greatest freedom of movement, and hence are most frequently subject to injury, are the lumbar and cervical. In addition to the voluntary motions required for bending, twisting, and other movements, many actions of the spine are reflex in nature and are the basis of posture.

GENERAL CLINICAL CONSIDERATIONS

TYPES OF LOW BACK PAIN   Of the several symptoms of disease of the spine (pain, stiffness or limitation of movement, and deformity), pain is of foremost importance by virtue of its frequency and its disabling effects. Four types of pain may be differentiated: local, referred, radicular, and that arising from secondary (protective) muscular spasm. One must identify these several types of pain by the patient's description, and here reliance is placed mainly on the character, location, and the conditions which modify them. The mechanism of the several types of pain has already been described in Chap. 3.

Local pain is caused by any pathologic process which impinges upon or irritates sensory endings. Involvement of structures which contain no sensory endings is painless. The central, medullary portion of the vertebral body may be destroyed by tumor, for example, without evocation of pain, whereas cortical fractures, or tears and distortions of the periosteum, synovial membranes, muscles, annulus fibrosus, and ligaments are often exquisitely painful. Although painful states are often accompanied by swelling of the affected tissues, this may not be apparent if a deep structure of the back is the site of disease. Local pain is often described as steady but may be intermittent, varying considerably with position or activity. The pain may be sharp or dull and although often diffuse is always felt in or near the affected part of the spine. Reflex splinting of the spine segments by paravertebral muscles is frequently noted, and certain movements or postures that alter the position of the injured tissues aggravate the pain. Firm pressure or percussion upon superficial structures in the region involved usually evokes tenderness, which is of aid in identifying the site of the abnormality.

Referred pain is of two types, that projected from the spine into regions lying within the area of the lumbar and upper sacral dermatomes and that projected from the pelvic and abdominal viscera to the spine. Pain due to diseases of the upper part of the lumbar spine is usually referred to the anterior aspects of the thighs and legs; that from the lower lumbar and sacral segments is referred to the gluteal regions, posterior thighs, and calves. Pain of this type, although of deep, aching quality and rather diffuse, tends at times to be superficially projected. In general the referred pain parallels in intensity the local pain in the back. In other words, maneuvers which alter local pain have a similar effect on referred pain, though not with such precision and immediacy as in radicular, or "root," pain. Referred pain may be confused with pain from visceral disease, but the latter is usually described as "deep" and tends to radiate from the abdomen through to the back. Also, visceral pain is usually unaffected by movement of the spine, does not improve with recumbency, and may be modified by the activity of the involved viscus.

Radicular, or "root," *pain* has some of the characteristics of referred pain but differs in its greater intensity, distal radiation, circumscription to the territory of a root, and the factors which excite it. The mechanism is distortion, stretching, irritation, or compression of a spinal root, most often central to the intervertebral foramen. Although the pain itself is often dull or aching, various maneuvers which increase the irritation of the root may greatly intensify the pain. Nearly always the radiation of pain is from a central position near the spine to some part of the lower extremity. Cough, sneeze, and strain are characteristically evocative maneuvers; but since they may also jar or move the spine, they may aggravate local pain as well. Any motion which stretches the nerve, e.g., forward bending with the knees extended or "straight-leg raising" in disease of the lower part of the lumbar spine, excites radicular pain; jugular vein compression, which raises intraspinal pressure and may cause a shift in the position of the root, may have a similar effect. The fourth and fifth lumbar and first sacral roots, which form the sciatic nerve, cause pain which extends mainly down the posterior aspects of thigh, the postero- and anterolateral aspects of the leg, and into the foot, in the distribution of this nerve—so called "sciatica." Tingling, paresthesias, and numbness or sensory impairment of the skin, soreness of the skin, and tenderness along the nerve usually accompany radicular pain. Also reflex loss, weakness, atrophy, fascicular twitching, and often stasis edema may occur if motor fibers of the anterior root are involved.

Pain resulting from muscular spasm is usually mentioned in relation to local pain. Muscle spasm may be associated with many disorders of the spine and can produce significant distortions of the normal posture. Chronic tension in muscles may give rise to a dull and sometimes cramping ache. One can in this instance feel the tautness of the sacrospinalis and gluteal muscles and demonstrate by palpation that the pain is localized to them.

Other pains often of undetermined origin are sometimes described by patients with chronic disease of the lower part of the back. In the legs, drawing, pulling, cramping sensations (without involuntary muscle spasm), tearing, throbbing, or jabbing pains, or feelings of burning or coldness are difficult to interpret and, like paresthesias and numbness, should always suggest the possibility of nerve or root disease.

Since it is often difficult to obtain physical or laboratory confirmation of painful disease of the lower region of the spine, it is extremely important to obtain an accurate history. In addition to assessing the character and location of the pain, one should determine the factors which aggravate and relieve it, its

constancy, and its relationship to recumbency and such stereotyped movements and maneuvers as forward bending, cough, sneeze, and strain. Frequently the most important lead comes from the knowledge of the mode of onset and circumstances which initiated the pain. Inasmuch as many painful afflictions of the back are the result of injury incurred during work or in an accident, the possibility of exaggeration or prolongation of pain for purposes of compensation or other personal reasons, or because of hysteria or malingering, must always be kept in mind.

EXAMINATION OF THE LOWER PART OF THE BACK

Much information may be gained by "inspection" of the back, buttocks, and lower extremities in various positions and movements. The normal spine shows a dorsal kyphosis and lumbar lordosis in the saggital plane, which in some individuals may be somewhat exaggerated (swayback). Normally the spine is relatively straight in the coronal plane, although slight curvature is frequent, particularly in females. In spinal disorders, one should observe the spine closely for excessive curvature, list, flattening of the normal lumbar arch, presence of a gibbus (a short, sharp, kyphotic angulation usually indicative of a fracture), pelvic tilt or obliquity, or asymmetry of the paravertebral or gluteal musculature. In severe sciatica, one may observe abnormalities of posture of the affected leg, presumably to reduce tension on the irritated part.

The next step in the examination is observation of the spine, hips, and legs during certain motions. During the procedure it is well to remember that no advantage accrues from trying to find out how much the patient can be hurt. Instead, it is much more important to determine when and under what conditions the pain commences. One looks for limitation of the natural motions of the patient while he or she is disrobing, standing, and reclining. When standing, the motion of forward bending normally produces flattening and reversal of the lumbar lordotic curve and exaggeration of the dorsal curve. With lesions of the lumbosacral region which involve the posterior ligaments, articular facets, or sacrospinalis muscle and with ruptured lumbar disks, protective reflexes prevent stretching of these structures. As a consequence, the sacrospinalis muscles remain taut and limit motion in the lumbar part of the spine. Forward bending then occurs at the hips and at the lumbar-thoracic junction. With disease of the lumbosacral joints and spinal roots, the patient bends in such a way as to avoid tensing the hamstring muscles and putting undue leverage upon the pelvis. In unilateral "sciatica," with its increased curvature toward the side of the lesion, lumbar and lumbosacral motions are splinted, and bending is mainly at the hips; at a certain point the knee on the affected side is flexed to relieve hamstring spasm and tilting of the pelvis and to slacken the lumbosacral roots and sciatic nerve.

It is sometimes of value to record the degree of flexion achieved either by measuring the distance between the fingertips and the floor or by estimating the degree of bending of the spine. Lateral bending is usually less instructive than forward bending. However, in unilateral ligamentous or muscular strain, bending to the opposite side aggravates the pain by stretching the damaged tissues. Moreover, in lateral disk lesions, bending of the spine toward the side from which the trunk lists is restricted. In diseases of the lower part of the spine, flexion while sitting with the hips and knees flexed can normally be performed easily, even to the point of bringing the knees in contact with the chest. The reason is that knee flexion relaxes the tightened hamstring muscles and also relieves stretch of the sciatic nerve.

The study of motions in the supine position yields the same information as study of motions in the standing and sitting positions, with the difference that there is less intradiskal pressure. With lumbosacral lesions and sciatica, passive lumbar flexion causes little pain and is not limited as long as the hamstrings are relaxed and there is no stretching of the sciatic nerve. With lumbosacral and lumbar spine disease (e.g., arthritis), passive flexion of the hips is free, whereas flexion of the lumbar spine may be impeded and painful. Passive straight-leg raising (possible in most normal individuals up to 90° except in those who have unusually tight hamstrings), like forward bending in the standing posture with the legs straight, places the sciatic nerve and its roots under tension, thereby producing pain. It may also cause an anterior rotation of the pelvis around a transverse axis, increasing stress on the lumbosacral joint, and thus causing pain if this segment is arthritic or otherwise impaired. Consequently, in diseases of the lumbosacral joints and lumbosacral roots, this movement is limited on the affected side and to a lesser extent on the opposite side. Lasègue's sign (pain and limitation of movement during elevation of the leg when the knee is extended) is a useful test of this condition. Straight-leg raising of the opposite leg may also cause contralateral pain but of lesser degree and is believed by some to be a sign of a more extensive lesion, such as an extruded disk fragment, rather than a simple prolapse or protrusion. It is important to remember, however, that the evoked

FIGURE 7-1

(1) Costovertebral angle. (2) Spinous process and interspinous ligament. (3) Region of the articular fifth lumbar to the first sacral facet. (4) Dorsum of sacrum. (5) Region of iliac crest. (6) Iliolumbar angle. (7) Spinous processes of fifth lumbar to first sacral vertebrae (tenderness = faulty posture or occasionally spina bifida occulta). (8) Region between posterior superior and posterior inferior spines. Sacroiliac ligaments (tenderness = sacroiliac sprain, often tender with fifth lumbar to first sacral disk.) (9) Sacrococcygeal junction (tenderness = sacrococcygeal injury, i.e., sprain or fracture). (10) Region of sacrosciatic notch (tenderness = fourth to fifth lumbar disk rupture and sacroiliac sprain). (11) Sciatic nerve trunk (tenderness = ruptured lumbar disk or sciatic nerve lesion).

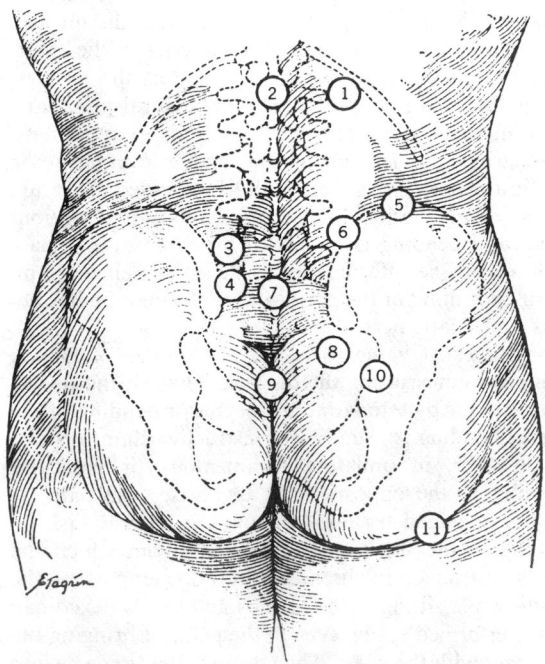

pain is always referred to the diseased side, no matter which leg is flexed.

The motion of hyperextension is best performed with the patient standing or lying prone. If the condition causing back pain is acute, it may be difficult to extend the spine in the standing position. A patient with lumbosacral strain or disk disease can usually extend or hyperextend the spine without aggravation of pain. If there is an active inflammatory process or fracture of the vertebral body or posterior elements, hyperextension may be markedly limited.

Palpation and percussion of the spine are the last steps in the examination. The approach must always be gentle since rough percussion of the designated area of pain may antagonize the patient and only serve to confuse the physician. It is preferable to palpate first those regions which are the least likely to evoke pain. At all times the examiner should know what structures are being palpated (see Fig. 7-1). Localized tenderness is seldom pronounced in disease of the spine because the involved structures are so deep that they rarely give rise to surface tenderness. Mild superficial and poorly localized tenderness signifies only a disease process within the affected segment of the body, i.e., dermatome.

Tenderness over the costovertebral angle often indicates genitourinary disease, adrenal disease (Rogoff's sign), or an injury to the transverse processes of the first or second lumbar vertebra [Fig. 7-1 (1)]. Hypersensitivity on palpation of the transverse processes of the other lumbar vertebrae as well as the overlying sacrospinalis muscles may signify fracture of the transverse process or a strain of muscle attachments. Tenderness of a spinous process or aggravation of pain by the jarring of gentle percussion may be nonspecific but frequently indicates the presence of a disk lesion at the site deep to it, inflammation (as in disk space infection), or pathologic fracture.

In palpation of the spinous processes, it is important to note any deviation in the lateral plane (this may be indicative of fracture or arthritis) or in the anteroposterior plane. A "step-off" forward displacement of the spinous process may be an important clue to a spondylolisthesis, one segment below the displaced level.

Tenderness in the region of the articular facets between the fifth lumbar and first sacral vertebrae is consistent with disease of a lumbosacral disk [Fig. 7-1 (3)]. It is also frequent in rheumatoid arthritis.

Abdominal, rectal, and pelvic examination and assessment of the status of the peripheral vascular system are important parts of the examination of the patient with complaints in the lower back and should not be omitted. They may provide evidence for vascular, visceral, neoplastic, or inflammatory disorders which may extend to the spine or cause pain to be referred to this region.

Finally, a careful neurologic examination should be performed, with special attention given to motor, reflex, and sensory changes (see "Protrusion of Lumbar Intervertebral Disks," below), particularly in the lower extremities.

SPECIAL LABORATORY PROCEDURES Useful laboratory tests, depending on the nature of the problem and the circumstances, include a complete blood count, erythrocyte sedimentation rate (especially helpful in screening for infection or myeloma), measurement of serum calcium, phosphorus, alkaline phosphatase, acid phosphatase (the last mentioned is of importance if one suspects metastatic carcinoma of the prostate), protein electrophoresis, immunoglobulin electrophoresis, tuberculin test, and tests for febrile agglutinins and rheumatoid factor. Roentgenograms of the lumbar part of the spine should be taken in every case of low back pain and sciatica (preferably with the patient standing) in the anteroposterior, lateral, and oblique planes. Special spot views or stereoscopic or laminographic films may provide further information in certain cases. Bone scans are of aid in revealing some fractures and neoplastic and inflammatory lesions. Computerized tomography (CT) scan of the spine and adjacent soft tissues may be particularly helpful in identifying a narrow canal, soft tissue mass, or destructive lesion of the body or posterior elements. Examination of the spinal canal with a contrast medium (air or other contrast myelogram) is often of great value, especially if a spinal cord tumor is suspected or if a patient is thought to have a disk herniation and fails to improve on a conservative regimen. Myelography can be combined with tests of dynamics of the cerebrospinal fluid, and a sample of the fluid should always be removed for cytologic and chemical examination prior to the instillation of the contrast medium (Pantopaque, Myodil, air, or some of the newer contrast media which are resorbed). Injection and removal of Pantopaque require special skill and should not be attempted without previous experience with the procedure. If done properly, the procedure has a very low incidence of significant complications. Injection of contrast medium directly into the intervertebral disk (diskograms) has waxed and waned in popularity over the years but remains controversial. The technique of this procedure is more complicated than that of myelographic examination, and the risk of damage to the disk or nerve roots and the possibility of introduction of infection is not inconsiderable. In the authors' opinion, such a procedure is indicated only under very special circumstances.

PRINCIPAL CONDITIONS WHICH GIVE RISE TO DISABLING PAIN IN THE LOWER PART OF THE BACK

CONGENITAL ANOMALIES OF THE LUMBAR SPINE Anatomic variations of the spine are not at all infrequent, and although rarely of themselves the source of pain and functional derangement, they may predispose an individual to excessive stress because of the altered mechanics or alignment of the spine.

There may be a lack of fusion of the laminae of the neural arch (spina bifida) of one or several of the lumbar vertebrae or of the sacrum. Hypertrichosis or hyperpigmentation in the sacral area may betray the condition, but in most patients the spine defect remains entirely occult until disclosed by x-ray. The anomaly has greater potentiality for pain if accompanied by malformation of vertebral joints. Usually the pain is induced by injury. There are many other congenital anomalies which affect the lower lumbar vertebrae such as asymmetrical facetal joints, abnormalities of the transverse processes, sacralization of the fifth lumbar vertebra (in which L_5 appears to be firmly fixed to the sacrum), or lumbarization of the first sacral vertebra (in which the first sacral resembles a sixth lumbar). Any one of these is occasionally observed in patients with symptoms referable to the low back, but they occur with equal frequency in individuals with no evidence of low back problem. Their role in the genesis of low back derangement is unclear, but in the authors' opinion, they are rarely the cause of specific symptomatology.

Spondylolysis consists of a bony defect, probably congenital, in the pars interarticularis (a segment near the junction of the pedicle with the lamina) of the lower lumbar area. The defect is best visualized on oblique projections. In some individuals the defect is bilateral. Under the circumstance of single or multiple injuries, the vertebral body, pedicle, and superior articular facet move anteriorly, leaving the posterior elements behind. This latter abnormality, known as *spondylolisthesis*, usually results in symptoms. The patient complains of pain in the low back radiating into the thighs, and there is limitation of motion. Often tenderness is elicited near the segment which has "slipped" forward (most often L_5 or occasionally L_4), and

one can feel a "step" on deep palpation of the posterior elements. The pelvis is sometimes rotated and hip flexion limited by hamstring spasm; a variety of neurologic deficits indicative of radiculopathy complete the clinical syndrome. In exceptionally severe cases, the trunk may be shortened and the abdomen protrude, both the result of the forward shift of L_5 on S_1.

TRAUMATIC AFFLICTIONS OF THE LOWER PART OF THE BACK Trauma constitutes the most frequent cause of low back pain.

In severe acute injuries, the examining physician must be careful to avoid further damage. In tests of mobility, all movements must be kept to a minimum until a diagnosis has been made and adequate measures have been instituted for the proper care of the patient. A patient complaining of back pain and inability to move the legs may have a fractured spine. The neck should not be flexed, nor should the patient be allowed to sit up. (See Chap. 375 for further discussion of spinal cord injury.)

Sprains, strains, and derangements The terms lumbosacral *sprain* and *strain* are used loosely by most physicians, and it is probably impossible to distinguish between them. The authors prefer the term *low back derangement* or *strain* for minor, self-limited injuries usually associated with lifting a heavy object, a fall, or a sudden deceleration as may occur in an automobile accident. Occasionally, these syndromes are more chronic in nature, suggesting that postural, muscular, or arthritic factors may play a role. The patients with low back derangement or strain are often acutely discomfited and may assume unusual postures related to spasm of the sacrospinalis muscles. The pain is usually confined to the lower back and is almost invariably relieved by rest. What formerly was regarded as sacroiliac strain or sprain is now known to be due to disk disease in most instances. This is caused by lifting heavy objects with the spine in a position of imperfect mechanical balance, as when lifting and turning at the same time. Sudden, unexpected motion is particularly likely to cause this injury.

The diagnosis of lumbosacral and sacroiliac strains with injury of the various structures of the lower part of the back depends upon the description of the injury, the localization of the pain by the patient, the finding of localized tenderness, and the augmentation of pain when tension is exerted on the involved structures by the appropriate maneuvers. The prompt alleviation of the pain by rest and relaxation indicates the existence of a strain. The rate of recovery depends on the degree of damage, preexisting disk disease, etc. Pain may be immediately relieved by local infiltration of an anesthetic agent, a finding which is also helpful in diagnosis.

Vertebral fractures Most fractures of the lumbar vertebral body are usually the result of flexion injuries and consist of anterior wedging or compression. With more severe trauma the patient may sustain a fracture dislocation, "bursting" fracture, or asymmetrical fracture involving not only the body but the posterior elements. The initiating trauma which causes fractures of the vertebrae is usually a fall from a height (in which case the calcanei may also be fractured) or may result from an automobile accident or other violence. When fractures occur with minimal trauma (or spontaneously), the bone is presumed to have been previously weakened by some pathologic process. Most of the time, particularly in older individuals, the cause of such an event is idiopathic osteoporosis, but there are many other underlying systemic disorders such as osteomalacia, hyperparathyroidism, hyperthyroidism, multiple myeloma, metastatic carcinoma, and a large number of local conditions that may play a role in weakening the vertebral body. Spasm of the lower lumbar muscles, limitation of motion of the lumbar section of the spine, and the roentgenographic appearance of the damaged lumbar portion (with or without neurologic abnormalities) are the basis of clinical diagnosis. The pain is usually immediate, though occasionally it may be delayed in onset for a few days. The patient may develop a mild paralytic ileus or urinary retention during the acute period.

Fractures of the transverse processes are almost always associated with tearing of the paravertebral muscles, principally the psoas. They may cause significant retroperitoneal hemorrhage resulting in a marked depression in hematocrit and, in extensive fractures, hypovolemic shock. Such injuries may be diagnosed by the finding of deep tenderness at the site of the injury, local muscle spasm on one side, and limitation of all movements which stretch the lumbar muscles. Radiologic evidence including body CT scan provides the final confirmation. Fractures of multiple transverse processes, although seemingly trivial, should be the object of considerable concern, and the patient should be carefully watched over the initial period for internal hemorrhage.

Protrusion of lumbar intervetebral disks   This condition is now recognized as the major cause of severe and chronic or recurrent low back and leg pain. It is most likely to occur between the fifth lumbar and first sacral vertebrae, and, with lessening frequency, between the fourth and fifth lumbar, the third and fourth lumbar, the second and third lumbar, and the first and second lumbar vertebrae. Rare in the thoracic portion of the spine, it is next most frequent between the sixth and seventh and fifth and sixth cervical vertebrae. The cause is usually a flexion injury, but in a considerable proportion of cases no trauma is recalled. Degeneration of the posterior longitudinal ligaments and the annulus fibrosus, which occurs in most adults of middle and advanced years, may have taken place silently or have been manifested by mild, recurrent lumbar ache. A sneeze, lurch, or other trivial movement may then cause the nucleus pulposus to prolapse, pushing the frayed and weakened annulus posteriorly. In more severe cases of disk disease, the nucleus may protrude through the annulus or become extruded to lie as a free fragment in the vertebral canal.

The fully developed syndrome of ruptured lumbar intervertebral disk consists of backache, abnormal posture, and limitation of motion of the spine (particularly flexion). Nerve root involvement is indicated by radicular pain, sensory disturbances (paresthesias, hyper- and hyposensitivity in dermatome pattern), coarse twitching and fasciculation, muscle spasms, and impairment of a tendon reflex. Motor abnormalities (weakness and muscle atrophy) may also occur but are usually less prominent than the pain and sensory disorder. Since herniation of the intervertebral lumbar disks most often occurs between the fourth and fifth lumbar vertebrae and the fifth lumbar and first sacral vertebrae with irritation and compression of the fifth lumbar and first sacral roots, respectively, it is important to recognize the clinical characteristics of lesions of these two roots. *Lesions of the fifth lumbar root* produce pain in the region of the hip, groin, posterolateral thigh, lateral calf to the external malleolus, dorsal surface of the foot, and the first or second and third toes. Paresthesias may be in the entire territory or only in the distal parts of these territories. The tenderness is in the lateral gluteal region and near the head of the fibula. Weakness, if present, involves the extensors of the great toe and of the foot. The knee and ankle reflexes are seldom altered, although occasionally, the ankle jerk is moderately depressed. Walking on the heels may be more difficult,

because of weakness of dorsiflexion of the foot, and more uncomfortable than walking on the toes. In *lesions of the first sacral root* the pain is felt in the midgluteal region, posterior part of the thigh, posterior region of the calf to the heel, and the plantar surface of the foot and fourth and fifth toes. Tenderness is most pronounced over the midgluteal region (sacroiliac joint), posterior thigh area, and calf. Rarely it may be referred to the rectum, testicles, or labia. Paresthesias and sensory loss are mainly in the lower leg and outer toes, and weakness, if present, involves the flexor muscles of the foot and toes, abductors of the toes, and hamstring muscles. The ankle reflex is diminished to absent in the majority of cases. Walking on the toes is more difficult, because of weakness of plantar flexors, and more uncomfortable than walking on the heel. With lesions of either root there may be limitation of straight-leg raising during the acute, painful stages.

Degeneration of the intervertebral disk without frank extrusion of a fragment of disk tissue may give rise to low back pain, or the disk may herniate into the adjacent vertebral body, giving rise to a Schmorl's node (seen on x-ray). Such cases often show no signs of nerve root involvement though the back pain may be referred to the thigh and leg.

The rarer *lesions of the fourth and third lumbar roots* give rise to pain in the anterior part of the thigh and knee, with corresponding sensory loss. The knee-jerk is diminished or abolished. An inverted Lasègue sign (pain with hypertension of the limb in relation to the trunk, best elicited with the patient in the prone position) is positive when the third lumbar root is affected.

The lumbar disk syndromes are usually unilateral. Only with massive derangements of the disk or the extrusion of a large, free fragment into the canal do bilateral symptoms and signs occur, and these may sometimes be associated with paralysis of the sphincters. The pain may be mild or severe. All or part of the above syndrome may be present. There may be back pain with little or no leg pain; rarely only leg pain may be experienced. The rupture of multiple lumbar or lumbar and cervical disks is not infrequent, suggesting a diffuse disorder of the connective tissue of the disks, including both the annulus fibrosus and the nucleus pulposus.

When all components of the syndrome are present, the diagnosis is easy; when only one part is present (particularly backache), it may be difficult, especially if there has been a clearly remembered initiating traumatic event. Since similar symptoms may occur without demonstrable disk rupture, other diagnostic procedures are required. Plain roentgenograms usually show no abnormality or at most a narrowing of the intervertebral space, sometimes more on the side of the rupture. Traction spurs, which are indicative of disk degeneration, may be present; in extreme cases, there may be a "vacuum" disk sign, in which a gas-density shadow is present in the intervertebral space, usually on lateral roentgenogram. Frequently however, one must resort to Pantopaque or air myelography, which in most cases will reveal an indentation of the lumbar subarachnoid space or deformity of the root sleeve. Occasionally, with large lesions there is a complete interruption of the flow of contrast material. Conversely, a small ruptured disk may not show any abnormality in the myelogram, especially at the fifth lumbar to first sacral level where there is a large space between the spinal canal and dura. Some clinics use diskograms (opaque material is injected into the disk) to reveal any evidence of extrusion, but the procedure is risky, and the results are difficult to interpret. The electromyogram is helpful in showing denervation of leg muscles (see Chap. 378). The protein level of the cerebrospinal fluid may be elevated in some instances.

Tumor of the spinal canal, epidural or intradural, may produce a syndrome similar to that of ruptured disk (see Chap. 375).

ARTHRITIS Arthritis of the spine is a major cause of backache, cervical pain, and occipital headache.

Osteoarthritis This more frequent type of osteoarthritic spinal disease occurs usually in later life and may involve any part of the spine. It is most prevalent in the cervical and lumbar regions, however, and the exact location determines the localization of the symptoms. Patients often complain of pain centered in the spine, which is increased by motion and is almost invariably associated with complaints of stiffness and limitation of motion. There is a notable absence of systemic symptoms such as fatigue, malaise, and fever, and the pain usually can be relieved by rest. The severity of the symptoms often bears little relation to the radiologic findings; pain may be present when there are minimal findings on an x-ray, and, conversely, marked osteophytic overgrowth with spur formation, ridging, and bridging of vertebrae can be seen in asymptomatic patients in middle and later life. Osteoarthropathic changes in the cervical spine and to a lesser extent in the lumbar spine may by their location compress roots or even the cauda equina or spinal cord, giving rise to the spondylitic form of myelopathy (see Chaps. 375 and 377).

Spondylitic caudal radiculopathy (SCR) is another variant of hypertrophic arthritis. A congenital smallness of the lumbar canal, especially at the L_4 to L_5 level, renders the individual susceptible to either a rupture of an intervertebral disk or arthrosis. The latter condition further narrows the anteroposterior diameter of the canal and leads to compression of lumbosacral roots and even to a block of the spinal canal. The roots are actually caught between the posterior surface of the vertebral body and the ligamentum flavum posterolaterally. Lumbosacral pains are followed by weakening of the lower legs, impairment of ankle and knee reflexes, and numbness and paresthesia in the feet and legs. Extension of the lumbar spine during walking and standing produces or aggravates the neurologic symptoms, and flexion relieves them. The clinical picture and its intermittency correspond to the so-called "intermittent claudication" of the spinal cord. The diagnosis may be suspected on the basis of history and radiographic findings but may be confirmed by myelography or CT scan, both of which will demonstrate the narrowed lumbar canal. Decompression of the spinal canal relieves the symptoms in a considerable proportion of the cases but should be approached with caution since it may lead to instability, necessitating an arthrodesis. SCR is the lumbar equivalent of spondylitic cervical myelopathy (SCM), described below. SCR is a cauda equina syndrome, and its differential diagnosis is discussed in Chap. 375, "Diseases of the Spinal Cord."

Rheumatoid arthritis and ankylosing spondylitis Arthritic disease of the spine takes two distinct forms, ankylosing spondylitis (the more common) and rheumatoid arthritis.

Patients with *ankylosing spondylitis* (also called Marie-Strümpell arthritis) are usually young men who complain of mild to moderate pain, which early in the course of the disease is centered in the back, and on occasion radiates to the back of the thighs. The symptoms may be vague at first (tired back, "catches" up and down the back, sore back) and the diagnosis may be overlooked for a considerable period. Although the pain is often intermittent, the finding of limitation of movement is constant and progressive and over a period of time tends to dominate the picture. Early in the course, this finding is described as "morning stiffness" or increasing stiffness after periods of inactivity, and may be present long before radiologic changes are manifest. Limitation of chest expansion, tenderness over the sternum, and decreased motion and flexion contractures of the hips may also be present early in the course. The radiologic hallmarks of the disease are destruction and subsequent obliteration of the sacroiliac joints, development of

syndesmophytes on the margins of the vertebral bodies, followed by bridging by bone to produce the characteristic "bamboo spine." The entire spine becomes immobilized, often in a flexed position, and usually the pain then subsides. Patterns of restricted movement, indistinguishable from those of ankylosing spondylitis, may accompany Reiter's syndrome, psoriatic arthritis, and inflammatory diseases of the intestine. Patients with these disorders rarely show the joint manifestations of peripheral rheumatoid arthritis, and seldom do they display involvement of the hips or knees. The rheumatoid factor is usually absent, but the sedimentation rate is often rapid, and many of the patients are found to have a HLA-B27 antigen.

Occasionally ankylosing spondylitis is complicated by progressively destructive vertebral lesions. This complication should be suspected whenever the pain returns, after a period of quiescence, or becomes localized. The etiology of these lesions is not known, but they may represent an exaggerated healing response to fracture or excessive production of fibrous inflammatory tissues. Rarely they may result in collapse of a segment of the spine and compression of the spinal cord. Another complication of severe ankylosing spondylitis is bilateral ankylosis of the ribs to the spine, which, coupled with a decrease in the height of axial thoracic structures, causes marked impairment of respiratory function.

Spinal rheumatoid arthritis tends to be localized to the cervical apophyseal joints and atlantoaxial articulation; the pain, stiffness, and limitation of motion are then in the neck and back of the head. Unlike ankylosing spondylitis, rheumatoid arthritis is rarely confined to the spine, and it does not lead to significant degrees of intervertebral bridging. Because of major affection of other joints, the diagnosis is relatively easy to make, but significant involvement of the neck may be overlooked. In the advanced stages of the disease, one or several of the vertebrae may be displaced anteriorly, or a synovitis of the atlantoaxial joint may damage the transverse ligament of the atlas, resulting in forward displacement of the atlas on the axis, i.e., atlantoaxial subluxation. In either instance serious and even life-threatening compression of the spinal cord may occur gradually or suddenly (see Chaps. 356 and 375). Lateral roentgenograms in flexion and extension, performed cautiously, are necessary to visualize dislocation or subluxation.

OTHER DESTRUCTIVE DISEASES **Neoplastic, infectious, and metabolic diseases** Metastatic carcinoma (breast, lung, prostate, thyroid, kidney, gastrointestinal tract), multiple myeloma, Hodgkin's disease, and reticulum cell sarcoma are the malignant tumors which most frequently involve the spine. Since the primary site may be overlooked or asymptomatic the presenting complaint in such patients may be pain in the back. The pain tends to be constant and dull, and is often unrelieved by rest. Indeed, it may be worse at night. Radiographic changes may be absent early in the disease, but when they appear, usually are manifest as destructive lesions in one or several vertebral bodies with little or limited involvement of the disk space, even in the face of a compression fracture. A ^{99m}Tc diphosphonate bone scan is helpful in lighting up "hot spots," indicating areas of increased blood flow and reactive bone formation associated with destructive inflammatory or arthritic lesions.

Infection of the vertebral column is usually the result of pyogenic organisms (staphylococci or coliform bacilli) or tubercule bacilli and is often difficult to distinguish on the basis of clinical findings. Patients complain of pain in the back of subacute or chronic nature that is exacerbated by motion but not materially relieved by rest. There is limitation of motion, tenderness over the spine of the involved segments, and pain with jarring of the spine, such as occurs with walking on the heels. Usually, these patients are afebrile and often do not have a leukocytosis although the erythrocyte sedimentation rate is almost invariably elevated. Radiographs may demonstrate narrowing of a disk space with erosion and destruction of the two adjacent vertebrae. A paravertebral soft tissue mass may be present, indicating an abscess, which may in the case of tuberculosis drain spontaneously, at sites quite remote from the vertebral column. In addition to a bone scan, a gallium scan is somtimes helpful in identifying a soft tissue inflammatory or infectious lesion even when overt bone destruction is not visible in x-rays.

Special mention should be made of the spinal *epidural abscess* (usually staphylococcal), which necessitates urgent surgical treatment. The symptoms are a localized pain, occurring spontaneously, aggravated by percussion and palpation. The patient is febrile and usually has severe radicular complaints, often bilaterial, progressing rapidly to a flaccid paraplegia (see Chap. 368 and 375).

In so-called "metabolic bone diseases" (osteoporosis or osteomalacia) a considerable degree of loss of bone substance may occur without any symptoms whatsoever. Many patients with such conditions do, however, complain of aching in the lumbar or thoracic area. This is most likly to occur following an injury, sometimes of trivial degree, which leads to collapse or wedging of a vertebra. Certain movements greatly enhance the pain, and certain positions relieve it. One or more spinal roots may be involved. Paget's disease of the spine is nearly always painless but may lead to compression of the spinal cord or roots because of encroachment on the canal or foramina by the pagetoid bone. The recognition of these bone disorders is discussed in some detail elsewhere (Chaps. 352 and 353).

In general, patients thought to have neoplastic, infectious, or metabolic disease of the spine should be thoroughly evaluated by means of radiographs, bone scans, myelography, and appropriate laboratory studies (see above).

REFERRED PAIN FROM VISCERAL DISEASE The pain of disease of the plevic, abdominal, or thoracic viscera is often felt in the region of the spine; i.e., it is referred to the more posterior parts of the spinal segment which innervates the diseased organ. Occasionally back pain may be the first and only sign. The general rule is that pelvic diseases are referred to the sacral region, lower abdominal diseases to the lumbar region (centering around the second to fourth lumbar vertebrae), and upper abdominal diseases to the lower thoracic spine (eighth thoracic to the first and second lumbar vertebrae). Characteristically there are no local signs or stiffness of the back, and motion is of full range without augmentation of the pain. However, some positions, e.g., flexion of the lumbar area of the spine in the lateral recumbent position, may be more comfortable than others.

Low thoracic and upper lumbar pain in abdominal disease Peptic ulceration or tumor of the wall of the stomach and of the duodenum most typically induces pain in the epigastrium (see Chaps. 290 and 309); but if the posterior wall is involved, and particularly if there is retroperitoneal extension, the pain may be felt in the region of the spine. The pain may be central in location or more intense on one side, or it may be felt in both locations. If very intense, it may seem to encircle the body. It tends to retain the characteristics of pain from the affected organ; e.g., if due to peptic ulceration, it appears about 2 h after a meal and is relieved by food and antacids.

Diseases of the pancreas (peptic ulceration with extension to the pancreas, cholecystitis with pancreatitis, cyst, or tumor) are apt to cause pain in the back, being more to the right of the

spine if the head of the pancreas is involved and to the left if the body and tail are implicated.

Diseases of retroperitoneal structures, e.g., lymphomas, sarcomas, and carcinomas, may evoke pain in this part of the spine with some tendency toward radiation to the lower part of the abdomen, groins, and anterior thighs. A secondary tumor of the iliopsoas region on one side often produces a unilateral lumbar ache with radiation toward the groin and labia or testicle; there may also be signs of involvement of the upper lumbar spinal roots. An aneurysm of the abdominal aorta may induce pain which is localized to this region of the spine but may be felt higher or lower, depending on the location of the lesion.

The sudden appearance of obscure lumbar pain in a patient receiving anticoagulants should arouse the suspicion of retroperitoneal bleeding.

Lumbar pain with lower abdominal diseases Inflammatory diseases of segments of the colon (colitis, diverticulitis) or tumor of the colon cause pain which may be felt in the lower part of the abdomen between the umbilicus and pubis, in the midlumbar region, or in both places. If very intense, the pain may have a beltlike distribution around the body. A lesion in the transverse colon or first part of the descending colon may be central or left-sided, and its level of reference to the back is to the second to third lumbar vertebrae. If the sigmoid colon is implicated, the pain is lower, in the upper sacral region and anteriorly in the midline suprapubic region or left lower quadrant of the abdomen.

Sacral pain in pelvic (urologic and gynecologic) diseases Although gynecologic disorders may manifest themselves by back pain, the pelvis is seldom the site of a disease which causes obscure low back pain. For the most part the diagnosis of painful pelvic lesions is not difficult, for a thorough palpation of structures by abdominal, vaginal, and rectal examination may be supplemented by methods (sigmoidoscopy, barium enema, pyelography, and culdoscopy) which permit adequate visualization of all these parts.

Menstrual pain itself may be felt in the sacral region. It is rather poorly localized, tends to radiate down the legs, and is of a crampy nature. The most important source of chronic back pain from the pelvic organs, however, is the uterosacral ligaments. Endometriosis or carcinoma of the uterus (body or cervix) may invade these structures, while malposition of the uterus may pull on them. The pain is localized centrally in the sacrum below the lumbosacral joint but may be more on one side. In endometriosis the pain begins during the premenstrual phase and often continues until it merges with menstrual pain. Malposition of the uterus (retroversion, descensus, and prolapse) is thought by some to lead to sacral pain, especially after the patient has been standing for several hours. One may observe the effect of postural influences here as when a fibroma of the uterus pulls on the uterosacral ligaments. Carcinomatous pain due to involvement of nerve plexuses is continuous and becomes progressively more severe; it tends to be more intense at night. The primary lesion may be inconspicuous, being overlooked upon pelvic examination. Papanicolaou smears, pyelogram and CT scan are the most useful diagnostic procedures. X-ray therapy of these tumors may produce sacral pain consequent to swelling and necrosis of tissue. Low back pain with radiation into one or both thighs is a common phenomenon during the last weeks of pregnancy.

Chronic prostatitis, evidenced by prostatic discharge, burning and frequency of urination, and slight reduction in sexual potency, may be attended by a nagging sacral ache; it may be mainly on one side, with radiation into one leg if the seminal vesicle is involved on that side. Carcinoma of the prostate with metastases to the lower part of the spine is another more common cause of sacral or lumbar pain. It may be present without urinary frequency or burning. Spinal nerves may be infiltrated by tumor cells, or the spinal cord itself may be compressed if the epidural space is invaded. The diagnosis is established by rectal examination, roentgenograms of the spine, and measurement of acid phosphatase (particularly the prostatic phosphatase fraction). Lesions of the bladder and testes are usually not accompanied by back pain. When the kidney is the site of disease, the pain is ipsilateral, being felt in the flank or lumbar region.

Visceral derangements of whatever type may intensify the pain of arthritis, and the presence of arthritis may alter the distribution of visceral pain. With disease of the spine in the lumbosacral region, for example, distention of the ampulla of the sigmoid by feces or a bout of colitis may aggravate the arthritic pain. In patients with arthritis of the cervical or thoracic spine the pain of myocardial ischemia may radiate to the back.

OBSCURE TYPES OF LOW BACK PAIN AND THE QUESTION OF PSYCHIATRIC DISEASE The practitioner is frequently consulted by persons who complain of low back pain of obscure origin. Usually the disorder is benign in nature and results from some minor derangement, muscular strain, or diskal prolapse. This is particularly true for those lesions which are of acute onset, aggravated by motion, and relieved by rest. Considerably more difficult are patients with chronic pain, especially those who have had prior back surgery or chronic visceral disease, or those who have severe and progressive pain in which neoplasia or infection is considered.

Even when exhaustive studies have been performed, there remains a group of patients in whom no anatomic or pathologic lesion can be found. These patients generally fall into two categories: those with postural back pain and those with psychiatric illness.

Postural back pain Many slender asthenic individuals and some obese middle-aged individuals have discomfort in the back. Their backs ache much of the time, and the pain interferes with effective work. The physical examination is negative except for slack musculature and poor posture. The pain is diffuse in the mid or low region of the back and characteristically is relieved by bed rest and induced by the maintenance of a particular posture over a period of time. Pain in the neck and between the shoulder blades is a common complaint among thin, tense, active women and seems to be related to taut trapezius muscles.

Psychiatric illness Low back pain may be encountered in compensation hysteria and malingering, in anxiety or neurocirculatory asthenia (formerly called neurasthenia), in depression and hypochondriasis, and in many nervous persons whose symptoms and complaints do not fall within any category of psychiatric illness. It is probably correct to assume that pain in the back in such patients usually signifies diseases of the spine and adjacent structures, and one should always search for a specific cause. However, even when organic factors are found, the pain may be exaggerated, prolonged, or woven into a pattern of invalidism or disability because of coexistent psychologic factors. This is especially true when there is the possibility of secondary gain (notably compensation). Patients seeking compensation for protracted low back pain without obvious structural disease, tend, after a time, to become suspicious, uncooperative, and hostile toward the medical profession or anyone who might question the authenticity of their illness. One notes in them a tendency to describe their pain poorly and to prefer, instead, to discuss the degree of their disability and their mistreatment at the hands of the medical profession. These features and a negative examination of the back should lead one to suspect a psychologic factor. A few patients, usually frank malingerers, adopt the most bizarre attitudes, such as being unable to straighten up or walking with the trunk flexed at almost a right angle (camptocormia) (see Chap. 11).

The depressed and hypochondriac patient represents a troublesome problem, and a common error is to minimize the importance of anxiety and depression or to ascribe them to worry over the illness and its social effects. The more common and minor back ailments, e.g., those due to osteoarthritis and postural ache, are enhanced and rendered intolerable by irritable moodiness and self concern. Such patients are often subjected to surgical procedures which prove ineffective. The disability seems excessive for the degree of spinal malfunction, and misery and despair are the prevailing features of the syndrome. One of the more reliable diagnostic measures is the favorable response to drugs that alleviate the depression (see Chaps. 11 and 25).

PAIN IN THE NECK AND SHOULDER

This topic is discussed to some extent in Chap. 5, and further references are found in Chap. 8.

It is useful to distinguish here three major categories of painful disease—of the spine, brachial plexus (thoracic outlet), and shoulder. Although pain in these three regions of the body may overlap, the patient usually can indicate the site of origin. Pain arising from the cervical spine is felt in the neck and back of the head (though it may be projected to the shoulder and arm), is evoked or enhanced by certain movements or positions of the neck, and is accompanied by tenderness and limitation of motions of the neck. Similarly, pain resulting from abnormalities of the thoracic outlet is experienced in and around the shoulder in the supraclavicular region, or between the shoulders; is induced by the performance of certain tasks and by certain positions; and is associated with tenderness of structures above the clavicle. There may be a palpable abnormality above the clavicle (aneurysms of the subclavian artery, tumor, cervical rib). The combination of circulatory symptoms and signs referable to the lower part of the brachial plexus, manifested in the hand by obliteration of pulse when the patient holds a full breath with the head tilted back or turned (Adson's test), unilateral Raynaud's phenomenon, trophic changes in the fingers, and sensory loss over the ulnar side of the hand with or without interosseous atrophy complete the clinical picture. Roentgenograms showing a cervical rib, deformed thoracic outlet, or superior sulcus tumor of the lung (Pancoast's syndrome) corroborate disease in this location. Electromyography and conduction studies along the plexus from points stimulated above and below the clavicle, and studies of arterial and venous circulation (venograms, noninvasive Doppler techniques) are especially helpful in evaluating this problem.

Pain localized to the shoulder region, often worse at night, associated with tenderness and aggravated by abduction, internal rotation, and extension points toward a lesion of the tendinous structures about the shoulder. Most often these are in the form of a calcific tendonitis or bursitis usually affecting the supraspinatus tendon and the adjacent subdeltoid bursa; occasionally the lesion is more extensive and consists of a rupture of the rotator cuff, in which case the patient may have weakness on abduction and forward flexion. In some such patients there is an adhesive capsulitis, leading to profound limitation of motion, designated as a "frozen shoulder." Shoulder pain may radiate into the arm or hand, but the sensory, motor, and reflex changes which indicate disease of nerve roots, plexus, or peripheral nerves are absent.

Osteoarthritis of the cervical part of the spine may cause pains which radiate into the back of the head, shoulders, and arms on one or both sides of the thorax. Coincident involvement of nerve roots is manifested by paresthesias, sensory loss, weakness, or deep tendon reflex change. Should bony ridges form in the spinal canal (spondylosis) the spinal cord may be compressed (see Chap. 375). A myelogram or CT scan may reveal the degree of encroachment on the spinal canal (narrowing of the canal to less than 11 mm in the anteroposterior diameter) at the level at which the spinal cord is affected. The authors have experienced difficulty in distinguishing spondylosis with or without disk rupture and spinal cord compression from primary neurologic diseases (syringomyelia, amyotrophic lateral sclerosis, or tumor) with an unrelated osteoarthritis of the cervical portion of the spine, particularly at the fifth to sixth and sixth to seventh cervical vertebrae, where the disk spaces are often narrowed in the adult. A combination of nervous tension with osteoarthritis of the cervical part of the spine or a painful injury to ligaments and muscles after an accident in which the neck is forcibly extended and flexed (e.g., whiplash injury to spine) raises extremely vexatious clinical syndromes. If the pain is persistent and limited to the neck, the problem will sometimes prove to have been due to disruption of a disk, but it is often complicated by psychologic factors.

RUPTURED CERVICAL DISKS One of the commonest causes of neck, shoulder, and arm pain is disk herniation in the lower cervical region. As with rupture of the lumbar disks, the complete syndrome includes the disorder of spinal function and evidence of neural involvement. It may develop after trauma either major or minor (sudden hyperextension of the neck, diving, forceful manipulations, etc.). Virtually every patient exhibits an abnormality in range of motion of the neck (limitation and pain). Hyperextension is the movement that most consistently aggravates the pain, although one occasionally sees patients whose principal limitation is in flexion. With laterally situated disk lesions between the fifth and sixth cervical vertebrae, the symptoms and signs are referred to the sixth cervical roots. The full syndrome is characterized by pain felt at the trapezius ridge, tip of the shoulder, anterior upper part of the arm, radial forearm, and often in the thumb; paresthesias and sensory impairment or hypersensitivity in the same regions; tenderness in the area above the spine of the scapula and in the supraclavicular and biceps regions; weakness in flexion of the forearm; diminished to absent biceps and supinator reflexes (triceps retained or exaggerated). When the protruded disk lies between the sixth and seventh cervical vertebrae, the seventh cervical root is involved. Under these circumstances, in the patient with the complete syndrome, the pain is in the region of the shoulder blade, pectoral region and medial axilla, posterolateral upper arm, elbow and dorsal forearm, index and middle fingers, or all the fingers; tenderness is most pronounced over the medial aspect of the shoulder blade opposite the third to fourth thoracic spinous processes, in the supraclavicular area and triceps region; paresthesias and sensory loss are most pronounced in the second and third fingers or tips of all the fingers; weakness is seen in extension of the forearm, in the extension of the wrist, and in the hand grip; the triceps reflex is diminished to absent, and the biceps and supinator reflexes are preserved. Either of these syndromes may be incomplete in that only one of several of the typical findings (e.g., pain) is present. Usually the patient states that cough, sneeze, and downward pressure on the head in the hyperextension position exacerbate pain and traction (even manual) tends to relieve it.

Unlike lumbar disks, the cervical ones, if large and centrally situated, may result in compression of the spinal cord (central disk, all the cord; paracentral disk, part of the cord). The central disk is often nearly painless, and the cord syndrome may simulate a degenerative disease (amyotrophic lateral sclerosis, combined system disease). A common error is to fail to think of a ruptured disk in the cervical region in patients with obscure symptoms in the legs. The diagnosis of ruptured cervical disk should be confirmed by the same laboratory procedures that were mentioned under "Spondylosis," above.

OTHER CONDITIONS Metastases to the cervical spine are fortunately less common than to other parts of the vertebral column. They are frequently painful and the cause of disordered root function. Compression fractures or extension of the tumor posteriorly may lead to rapid development of quadriplegia.

Shoulder injuries (rotator cuff), subacromial or subdeltoid bursitis, the frozen shoulder (periarthritis or capsulitis), tendonitis, and arthritis may develop in patients who are otherwise well, but these conditions are also frequent in hemiplegics or in individuals suffering from coronary heart disease. The pain is often severe and extends toward the neck and down the arm into the hand. The dorsum of the latter may tingle without other signs of nerve involvement. Vasomotor changes also may occur in the hand (shoulder-hand syndrome), and after a time, osteoporosis and atrophy of cutaneous and subcutaneous structures occur (Sudeck's atrophy or Sudeck-Leriche syndrome). These conditions fall more within the province of orthopedics than of medicine and are not discussed here in detail. The physician, however, must know that they can often be prevented by proper exercises (Chap. 253).

The *carpal tunnel syndrome,* with paresthesias and numbness in palmar distribution of the median nerve and aching pain which extends up into the forearm, may be mistaken for disease of the shoulder or neck. Similarly, other less common forms of nerve entrapment may involve the ulnar, radial, or median nerves and lead to a mistaken diagnosis of brachial plexus lesion or cervical syndrome. Electromyography and conduction studies are especially helpful in such conditions (Chap. 377).

MANAGEMENT OF BACK PAIN

Without doubt the preventive aspects of back pain are important. There would be many fewer back problems if adults kept their trunk muscles in optimal condition by regular exercise such as swimming, bicycle riding, walking briskly, running, or calisthenic programs. Morning is the ideal time since the back of the older adult tends to stiffen during the night because of inactivity. This happens regardless of whether a bed board or a stiff mattress is used. Sleeping with back hyperextended and sitting for long times in an overstuffed chair or a badly designed auto seat are particularly risky. It is estimated that pressures between disks are increased 200 percent by changing from a recumbent to a standing position and by 400 percent by sitting slumped in an easy chair. Correct sitting posture lessens this. Long trips in a car or plane without change in position put maximal strain on disk and ligamentous structures in the spine. Lifting from a position of flexed trunk, as in removing a suitcase from the trunk of a car, is dangerous (always lift with the object close to the body). Sudden strenuous activity without conditioning and warm-up also is likely to cause trouble to disks and their ligamentous envelopes (the commonest sources of back pain); certain families seem disposed.

The following diagrams are useful guides in strengthening trunk muscles (Figs. 7-2 to 7-6).

Muscular and ligamentous strains and minor disk prolapses are usually self-limited, responding to simple measures in a relatively short period of time. The basic principle of therapy is rest in a recumbent position for several days to weeks. When weight bearing is resumed, a light lumbosacral support is usu-

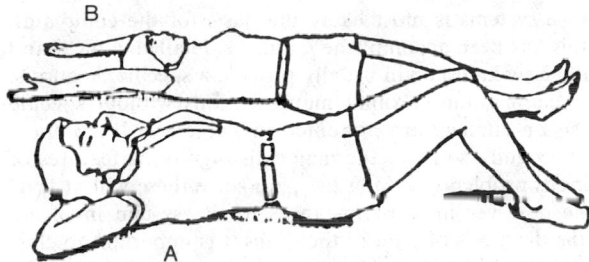

FIGURE 7-2

A. With knees bent, feet flat on floor, and hands clasped behind head, pinch buttocks together, pull in abdomen, and flatten back against floor. At first, hold position for a count of 5, relax for 5, then gradually increase to counts of 20. B. Next do this same exercise with legs extended and arms raised straight overhead. (From U.S. News & World Report. Copyright 1975 U.S. News & World Report).

ally helpful in continuing the immobilization until the patient is restored to full health. Physical measures such as heat, cold, diathermy, or massage are of limited value; of considerably greater importance are active exercises to both reduce the spasm and improve muscle tone. Analgesic medication should be given liberally during the first few days: codeine, 30 mg, and aspirin, 0.6 g, or pentazocine (Talwin), 50 mg, propoxyphene (Darvon), 65 mg, or meperidine (Demerol), 50 mg. Muscle relaxants are often a valuable adjunct, particularly in that such drugs as Valium, 8 to 40 mg in divided doses, and carisoprodol (Soma), 350 mg, twice daily, make bed rest more tolerable. If an inflammatory component is suspected, indomethacin, 75 mg per day (in divided doses), or ibuprofen (Motrin), 400 mg 3 or 4 times daily, may be helpful.

In the treatment of an acute or chronic rupture of a lumbar or cervical disk, complete bed rest is essential, and strong analgesic medication may be required. Traction is of little value in lumbar disk disease, and it is best to permit the patient to find the most comfortable position. Cervical traction with a halter may be of considerable benefit to patients with cervical disk syndrome. It can be administered with the patient in recumbency, or after sufficient improvement to allow ambulation, can be performed intermittently in the erect position using special equipment. During the recumbent phase of treatment of lumbar disk disease, exercises to reduce spasm, muscle relaxants, and anti-inflammatory agents as described above may be

FIGURE 7-3

A. Keeping shoulders flat on floor, draw knees toward chest, clasp hands around knees, and pull knees tightly against chest. B. Next bring forehead up to knees (From U.S. News & World Report. Copyright 1975 U.S. News & World Report.)

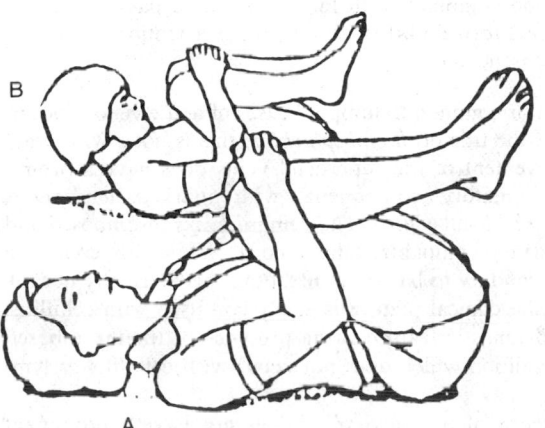

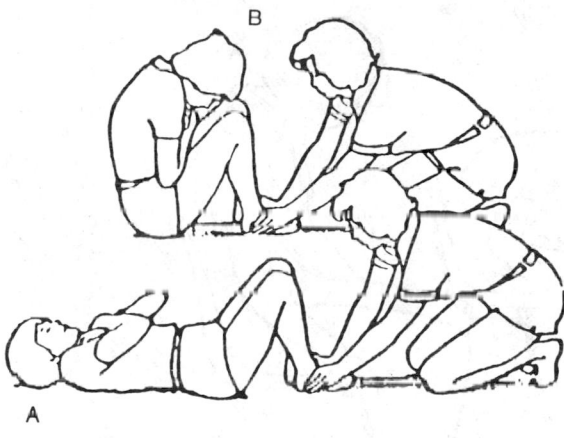

FIGURE 7-4

A. With knees bent, keep feet flat on floor and held or hooked under a heavy piece of furniture to provide leverage. B. Cross arms on chest, raise head and shoulders, and curl up to a sitting position. Keep back round and pull with abdominal muscles. Lower self slowly. (From U.S. News & World Report. Copyright 1975 U.S. News & World Report.)

of considerable value. After 2 to 3 weeks in bed, the patient can be allowed to slowly resume activities, usually with the protection of a brace or light spinal support. Exercise programs designed to increase the strength of the abdominal and gluteal muscles are helpful at this point. The patient may suffer some minor recurrence of the pain but be able to carry on his or her usual activities, and eventually most individuals will recover. If the pain and neurologic findings do not disappear on prolonged, conservative management, or if the patient suffers frequently recurring acute episodes, surgical management may be indicated. This should always be preceded by a myelogram to localize the lesion (and rule out the presence of intra- or extradural tumors). The surgical procedure most often indicated is a hemilaminectomy with excision of the disk involved. Arthrodesis of the involved segments is indicated only in cases in which there is extraordinary instability usually related to an anatomic abnormality (such as spondylolysis) or in the cervical region when an extensive laminectomy has rendered the spine unstable.

Spondylosis of the cervical part of the spine, if painful, is helped by bed rest and traction; if signs of spinal cord involvement are present, a collar to limit movement may halt the progression and even lead to improvement. Decompressive

FIGURE 7-5

A. Bend knees, keeping feet flat on floor and arms straight forward. Raise up and touch head to knees. B. Lower self, then pull knees up tightly against chest and bring forehead up to knees. (From U.S. News & World Report. Copyright 1975 U.S. News & World Report.)

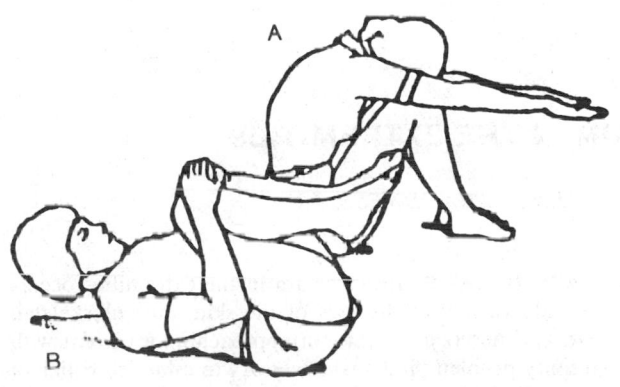

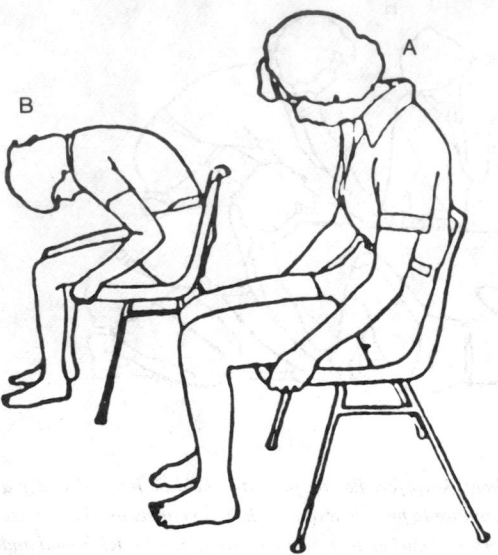

FIGURE 7-6

A. Place hands at edge of chair. B. Bend forward to bring head to knees, pulling in abdomen as you curl forward. Keep weight well back on hips. Release abdominal muscles slowly as you come up. (From U.S. News & World Report. Copyright 1975 U.S. News & World Report.)

laminectomy or anterior fusion is reserved for severe instances of the disease with advancing neurologic symptoms. The shoulder-hand syndrome may benefit from stellate ganglion blocks or ganglionectomy, but the basic treatment is physiotherapy, with or without prednisone, and surgical procedures are used only as measures of last resort.

REFERENCES

ARMSTRONG JR: *Lumbar Disc Lesions,* 3d ed. Baltimore, Williams & Wilkins, 1965

BRADY LP et al: An evaluation of the electromyogram in the diagnosis of lumbar disk lesion. J. Bone Joint Surg 51A:539, 1969

CONVENTRY MB: Anatomy of the intervertebral disk. Clin Orthop 67:9, 1969

EDEIKEN J, PITT MJ: The radiologic diagnoses of disk disease. Orthop Clin N Amer 2:405, 1971

FRIEDENBERG AB, MILLER WT: Degenerative disk disease of the cervical spine. J Bone Joint Surg 45A:1171, 1963

GOLUB B et al: Cervical and lumbar disk disease: A review. Bull Rheum Dis 21:635, 1971

NAYLOR A: The changes in the human intervertebral disk in degeneration and nuclear prolapse. Orthop Clin N Am 2:343, 1971

WATTS C et al: Chymopapain treatment of intervertebral disk disease. J Neurosurg 42:374, 1975

8

PAIN IN THE EXTREMITIES

D. EUGENE STRANDNESS, JR.

APPROACH TO THE PATIENT Pain in the extremities occurs from a wide variety of diseases of the skin, musculoskeletal, vascular, and nervous systems. In approaching a patient with an extremity problem, it is first necessary to establish which of the above systems is most likely the basis for the complaint. Once this has been accomplished, a more detailed clinical and laboratory evaluation will usually provide a specific diagnosis. In this chapter, the cardinal manifestations without specific emphasis on etiology are presented in Table 8-1. It is important to recognize some of the major distinguishing features of the various problems causing the pain since these will at least lead the observer in most instances to the system involved.

In the diagnosis of pain of the limbs it is important to classify the pain and localize the site of involvement. Pain may be classified as superficial, deep, and referred. *Superficial pain* either arising from the skin or spreading from adjacent structures such as joints is well localized and is associated with tenderness and hyperalgesia. *Deep pain* arising from fascia, vessels, periosteum, joints, and supporting structures is often poorly localized and dull, and may be associated with muscular rigidity and deep tenderness. *Referred pain* is usually well localized and similar to pain arising from deep structures (Chap. 3). In persons with acute ischemia of the limbs, with threatened loss of viability, both superficial and deep pain are present.

A thorough examination of the limbs must include inspection for evidence of cutaneous manifestations, palpation for masses and tenderness, and auscultation for arterial bruits. Examination of the peripheral pulses at their accessible sites must always be done. A careful neurologic examination looking for changes in reflexes and sensation is also essential.

In most instances an accurate diagnosis can be made or strongly suspected from the history and physical examination. Special tests such as arteriography, myelography, and nerve conduction studies are often helpful but are primarily reserved for accurate localization of the disease and determination of the extent of involvement.

Acute arterial insufficiency regardless of the cause produces the greatest changes in the *distal* limb. This simple fact, often overlooked, has been a source of confusion to many physicians. It is also important to recognize that the degree of ischemia is a reflection of the available collateral circulation. The dramatic presentation with pain, pallor, and paralysis is rarely missed but lesser symptoms such as transient numbness and a reduction in skin temperature are often overlooked. If there are any questions about the diagnosis, the measurement of the systolic pressure at the ankle and wrist will establish the diagnosis with certainty.

Chronic arterial occlusion produces pain in three circumstances:

1 With exercise (intermittent claudication). The location of the muscle pain depends on the level of occlusion.
2 Pain at rest. As with acute arterial occlusion, the distal limb is most affected, and the condition is recognized by the coexisting dependent rubor, loss of pulses, and improvement in the pain with dependency.
3 Ulceration combined with infection. These patients are often treated for cellulitis without proper attention to the underlying ischemia.

While it is common to lump all cases of acute venous occlusion under the title of *thrombophlebitis,* this is not a wise practice. Involvement of the superficial veins does have a prominent inflammatory component, with marked tenderness, erythema, and local edema. The vein is *always* thrombosed and recognized as a palpable, tender cord. While this condition may be secondary to bacterial infection, this is usually not the case, but the clinical picture is easily confused with cellulitis. The key diagnostic feature is the presence of the thrombosed vein, a condition which does not occur with cellulitis or lymphangitis.

Thrombosis of the deep veins does not have a prominent

inflammatory component and thus is often missed on clinical examination. Tenderness, edema, fever, and prominent superficial veins are so variable that they cannot be relied upon for certainty in establishing the diagnosis. The major point to remember when deep venous thrombosis is suspected is that the diagnosis *must* be established by some independent means, such as noninvasive testing or venography.

Chronic venous disorders of the lower limb are commonly considered in two categories, *varicose veins* and the *postphlebitic syndrome*. Varicose veins, of course, are easily recognized by inspection alone with the patient upright. The most serious sequelae occur secondary to deep vein thrombosis with destruction of the venous valves, which leads to edema, pain in the distal limb, and the stasis skin changes in the vicinity of the medial malleolus. Repeated injury with infection can produce similar skin changes.

PAINFUL SKIN DISEASE The common bacterial and fungous infections may occasionally produce pain, and it can occur in or remote to the involved areas. This is especially true when bacteria have entered the dermis and subcutaneous tissues via the base of the nails or interdigital areas. Depending upon the infecting agent, cellulitis with or without lymphangitis may rapidly ensue and produce local swelling, pain, erythema, and systemic signs of toxicity. If the infection develops in areas such as the pulp of the digits or in plantar or palmar spaces, the pain is severe, throbbing, and may secondarily extend to tendons and joints.

Fungous infections, particularly those of the interdigital areas of the feet, may also become secondarily infected by bacteria, resulting in a spreading cellulitis and lymphangitis. There are also nonbacterial forms of cellulitis. The lymphangitis is diagnosed by the presence of the "red lines" in the involved areas. Pain may also occur in the region of the lymph nodes which drain the infected area and may be the first sign of secondary infection.

Cellulitis, particularly of the lower extremities, may be confused with thrombophlebitis. Differentiating features supporting the diagnosis of cellulitis include: (1) rapidity of onset, (2) prominent cutaneous hyperemia and tenderness, (3) presence of a portal of entry for the infective agent, and (4) the nature of the systemic response (fever, leukocytosis), which is usually much more severe than with thrombophlebitis.

Erythema nodosum (Chap. 49) should be suspected when tender erythematous nodules appear in or under the skin and are associated with fever and joint pains. The articular manifestations often precede the appearance of the nodules. These lesions can be associated with a wide variety of diseases, some of which include tuberculosis, sarcoidosis, coccidioidomycosis, streptococcal infections, and ulcerative colitis. However, in the majority of cases, no underlying disease is found.

MUSCULOSKELETAL PAIN **Bursitis and tendonitis** *Inflammation* of one or more of the bursae may occur as a result of trauma, rheumatoid arthritis, gout, connective tissue disorders, and bacterial infection. The commonly involved bursae are the subdeltoid, olecranon, trochanteric, calcaneal, and prepatellar. When the process is acute, it is characterized by severe local pain and tenderness with marked limitation of activity and mobility. In long-standing cases the symptoms and physical findings are less pronounced. Calcific deposits within the involved bursa develop in some patients and may be seen in an x-ray.

Tenosynovitis of the tendon sheaths of hands or wrists produces pain in restricted regions. Tenosynovitis may arise in association with infection, rheumatoid arthritis, osteoarthritis, or trauma, or occur without explanation. When the sheath of the thumb's abductor longus and extensor brevis tendons at the radial styloid are affected, the condition is called *de Quer-*

vain's disease. The flexor tendons in the palm and finger and the extensor sheaths on the dorsum of the wrist may also be the site of the inflammation. Typically, the pain and tenderness occur in the region of the tendon, and the pain is aggravated by stretching the involved tendons as their muscles contract.

An important variant of tenosynovitis is the *carpal tunnel syndrome,* the symptoms of which may be confused with the thoracic outlet syndrome, cervical disk disease, and local vascular insufficiency. Thickening or swelling of the tendons as they pass through the flexor compartment at the wrist, amyloid deposit with multiple myeloma, or bone enlargement (acromegaly) can exert pressure on the median nerve, causing nocturnal paresthesias and pain in the fingers, wrist, and forearm. As the condition worsens, atrophy of the thenar eminence develops, as well as weakness and sensory loss in the territory of the median nerve. There may be tenderness on pressure over the carpal ligament and electrical tingling in the fingers when the wrist is tapped (Tinel's sign). Nerve conduction may be delayed at the wrist, confirming the diagnosis.

Calcific and *noncalcific tendonitis* is common in the bicipital and supraspinatus tendons, and in the common tendon of origin for the forearm extensors and flexors at the lateral and medial epicondyle of the humerus, respectively (tennis elbow). The diagnosis is suspected by the location of the pain and the painful limitation of motion involved by movement of these tendons.

Painful synovial cysts Cysts of the popliteal space (Baker's cysts) can be an obscure source of pain in the leg. The lesion consists of a cyst in the popliteal fossa, which frequently communicates with the knee joint. While the cause is unknown, such cysts are frequently associated with rheumatoid or osteoarthritis. Trauma may be an inciting factor. Unruptured cysts produce only mild aching in the popliteal space with associated stiffness of the joint. If the cyst ruptures, there is an acute, extensive inflammation of the lower leg with swelling and pain which may be severe. The clinical picture is commonly confused with thrombophlebitis. The diagnosis can easily be made by instilling radiopaque material into the knee joint.

Painful arthritis of extremities Most causes of arthritis can be classified into one of five major groups: (1) infectious, (2) degenerative, (3) posttraumatic, (4) metabolic, and (5) unknown etiology. The synovial membranes and periarticular structures are primarily involved in rheumatoid disease, infectious arthritis, and gout, whereas the cartilage and bone are mainly affected in osteoarthritis and rarer varieties. With acute pyogenic arthritis, gout, and rheumatic fever, the pain is severe even at rest and greatly intensified by even the slightest motion. The local findings of swelling, redness, and heat may be pronounced.

The principal symptom of *osteoarthritis* is pain which is brought on by use and is relieved by rest. Stiffness after sitting and immediately upon rising in the morning is common but seldom persists for more than a few minutes. Some of the more common locations are the terminal phalanges, knees, hips, and spine.

Rheumatoid arthritis most commonly involves the proximal interphalangeal and metacarpophalangeal joints, toes, wrists, ankle, knee, elbow, hip, and shoulder. The onset is often insidious with general fatigue, paresthesias in the extremities, joint pain, and stiffness. The most common symptoms include joint pain at rest which is aggravated by motion. Thickening of the periarticular structures may be marked and accompanied by atrophy of adjacent muscles. Subcutaneous nodules are often

TABLE 8-1
Pain in the extremities

	Chap.	Pain Location	Pain Nature	Pain Duration	Physical findings Inspection	Physical findings Palpation	Physical findings Auscultation	Lab findings
SUDDEN ONSET								
Arterial occlusion (large–medium-sized vessels)	253	Distal limb	Severe	Variable	Pale distal limb	Cool, absent pulses; look for aneurysm	Cardiac arryhmia, murmur, bruits	Positive cardiac findings, ECG abnormal; enzymes; decreased ankle, wrist systolic pressure
Arteriovenous fistula acquired	253	At site of fistula	Mild	Acute phase	Look for site of injury	False aneurysm, palpable thrill	Bruit over fistula	Decrease in systolic pressure distal to fistula
Ruptured synovial cysts	253	Adjacent to ruptured cyst	Severe	Acute phase	Swelling may be marked	Exquisite tenderness in involved area		Positive arthrogram; look for associated rheumatoid arthritis
Nocturnal muscle cramps	383	Muscle group	Severe cramp	Several minutes	Normal	Local tenderness during attack		Not associated with any known disorder
SUDDEN OR GRADUAL ONSET (SEVERAL HOURS)								
Thrombophlebitis (superficial)	253	Involved veins	Severe	Acute phase	Erythema prominent	Severe local tenderness		Elevated WBC count; positive blood culture if septic
Acute venous thrombosis (deep veins)	253	Within involved segments	Mild to moderate	Transient	Usually normal	Edema, degree variable; mild tenderness		Positive noninvasive tests with major venous occlusion; phlebogram diagnostic
Cellulitis		Involved area	Moderate	With inflammation	Marked hyperremia	Local edema, tenderness		Those associated with bacterial infection
Lymphangitis	253	Involved segment	Moderate to severe	Acute phase	"Red streak"	Local edema, tenderness		Those associated with bacterial infection
Arthritis (articular)	355 361	Affected joints	Severe at rest	Acute phase	Joint may be reddened, swollen	Pain increases with motion		Depends on cause
Herniated nucleus pulposus	7	Poorly localized; may radiate	Moderate to severe	Worse with motion	Usually normal	Paravertebral muscle spasm; positive neurologic findings		Narrowing disk space, positive myelogram
Osteomyelitis	360	Affected bone	Severe with motion	Inflammatory phase	Normal to swelling over involved area	Severe pain with motion, palpation		Neutrophilic leukocytosis; elevated sedimentation rate; positive blood cultures; positive x-ray usually evident after second week

TABLE 8-1 (continued)
Pain in the extremities

	Chap.	Pain			Physical findings			Lab findings
		Location	Nature	Duration	Inspection	Palpation	Auscultation	
GRADUAL ONSET (DAYS TO MONTHS)								
Chronic arterial occlusion, moderate	253	Muscle group(s)	Cramp	With exercise	Normal or dependent rubor	Absent pulses	Bruits often present	Decreased ankle systolic pressure; further drop with exercise
Chronic arterial occlusion, severe	253	Distal foot	Severe	Constant	Tissue necrosis; loss of hair; nail changes	Distal limb cool; absent pulses	Bruits often present	Ankle systolic pressure index <0.5
Erythromelalgia	253	Foot; distal leg	Severe burning	During attack only	Foot, distal leg bright red	Increased temperature affected area		Rare cases secondary to myeloproliferative disorders
Sympathetic dystrophy (major)	3	In distribution of injury to nerve	Hyperalgesia; hyperesthesia	Persistent	Normal, late trophic changes	Increased sweating; hyperesthesia		Sympathetic block gives immediate relief?
Causalgia (minor reflex dystrophy)	363	As above	As above		Same as above			May accompany many illnesses, myocardial infarction, neurologic (central and peripheral) infections, severe ischemia
Carpal tunnel syndrome	363	Fingers, wrist, and forearm	Paresthesia burning	Persistent	Possible thenar atrophy			Nerve conduction delayed
Interdigital neuroma		Plantar aspect of foot	Moderate	With pressure or walking	Normal	Pain produced by lateral foot compression		Nothing diagnostic
Bursitis; tendonitis; fibrositis	363	Affected area only	Moderate	Until treated	Normal muscle atrophy, longstanding cases	Local tenderness		Calcium may be seen on x-ray, particularly in cases of bursitis
Rheumatoid arthritis	356	Proximal interphalangeal joints	Moderate	Variable	Periarticular thickening, muscle atrophy	Local tenderness; subcutaneous nodules		Positive rheumatoid factor; antinuclear antibodies; x-ray abnormality
Osteoarthritis	361	Involved joints	Moderate	With exercise	Terminal phalanges may be deformed, enlarged	Minimal tenderness over joints		No specific chemical abnormality; joint space narrow; osteophytes
Erythema nodosum	49	Nodules	Mild	Variable	Reddened subcutaneous nodule	Moderate tenderness with surrounding edema		Usually secondary; extensive workup may be required
Neuritis	377	Along affected nerves	Burning, tearing	Persistent	Usually normal	Areflexia		Nerve conduction delayed

TABLE 8-1 (continued)
Pain in the extremities

		Pain			Physical findings			
	Chap.	Nature	Location	Duration	Inspection	Palpation	Auscultation	Lab findings
GRADUAL ONSET (MONTHS TO YEARS)								
Primary varicose veins	253	Mild	Distal leg	Only with dependency	Dilated superficial veins	Edema if present mild, distal limb		Valvular incompetence confined to superficial veins
Postphlebitic syndrome (secondary to varicose veins)	253	Moderate	Distal leg	Only with dependency	Stasis dermatitis: varicose veins; ulcers often present	Edema, induration in ulcer-bearing zone		Valvular incompetence, superficial and deep veins
Arteriovenous fistula, congenital	253	Mild	Affected limb	With dependency	Prominent venous pattern; increased limb length and girth	Edema variable	Bruits rarely present	Arteriography may show feeding vessels with early venous filling
EPISODIC OR WITH CHANGE OF POSITION								
Thoracic outlet syndromes	253	Moderate	Along distribution of compressed nerve root	Relieved with arm in neutral position	Normal	Decrease in radial pulse in position that produces symptoms, bruit in supraclavicular area		X-ray: cervical rib; osseous abnormality of clavicle, first rib
Vasospastic disorders	253	Mild	Fingers, toes	Transient	Color changes with attack	Pulses usually present	Usually normal	Raynaud's disease, digital circulation normal; secondary form, digital artery occlusions common

found over pressure points. Many of the patients are also subject to cold sensitivity of Raynaud's type. (See Chap. 356.)

Gout, a disease usually of men over 30 years of age, manifests itself often in acute episodes. Most frequently the metatarsophalangeal joint is involved; the affected joint is extremely painful and swells markedly within a few hours, becoming hot and dusky red. The process, particularly in the acute form, may be difficult to distinguish from acute rheumatic fever, gonococcal arthritis, atypical rheumatoid arthritis, traumatic arthritis, cellulitis, suppurative arthritis, and Reiter's syndrome. The presence of tophi and an elevated uric acid clarify the diagnosis. Finding the rodlike crystals of sodium urate in a tophus or synovial fluid establishes the diagnosis with certainty. (See Chap. 92.)

Pyogenic arthritis localizes usually in large joints (hip, knee, and shoulder). Such infections are usually metastatic in origin and remain monoarticular. The cardinal signs of infection, pain, and swelling, and a local increase in temperature with cutaneous hyperemia and fever, usually leave little doubt about the nature of the condition. In suspected cases the joint must be aspirated to identify the organism by Gram's stain and culture. (See Chap. 360.)

Hypertrophic osteoarthropathy, with its characteristic clubbing, periostitis at the ends of long bones, arthritis, and autonomic disorder, causes pain which varies from mild to severe. The pain is deep and aching and along with tenderness is localized to the involved joints and adjacent long bones. This syndrome usually appears in relation to malignancies or suppurative conditions of the lungs, mediastinum, or pleura.

Osteomyelitis   Osteomyelitis may occur following open fractures, open surgical reduction of fractures, or from a distant infective focus. Usually the symptoms commence abruptly with severe pain (aggravated by motion), local swelling, exqui-site tenderness, chills, and fever. There is nearly always a neutrophilic leukocytosis and elevated sedimentation rate, and blood cultures may be positive. X-ray changes may not be evident until the second week or later. The differential diagnosis includes acute pyogenic arthritis, hemarthrosis (particularly in children), cellulitis, and erysipelas. (See Chap. 360.)

Painful disorders of muscle   Disorders of muscles are common causes of severe pain in the limbs. Localized tenderness and pain with motion is most commonly seen after trauma or severe exercise. An acute suppurative myositis is nearly always associated with injury and direct inoculation with bacteria. Clostridial myositis (Chap. 141) must be considered in every case of a deep infection occurring secondary to a puncture wound.

A condition frequently confused with ischemic rest pain is the *nocturnal muscle cramp.* This process of unknown cause occurs in both sexes at all ages but is most often a source of complaints in pregnant women, the middle-aged, and the elderly. Unusually strenuous activity in the daytime increases the liability to cramp at night, especially when the feet are cold. The onset is sudden, usually in one of the muscles of the foot or leg, and it may awaken the patient. The pain subsides with vigorous massage and stretching (Chap. 383) of the part. If frequent and troublesome, 50 mg benadryl taken at bedtime will usually prevent the cramps.

When there is generalized muscle tenderness, weakness, increasing fatigability, and other systemic symptoms, the possibility of polymyositis and dermatomyositis must be considered.

section 2 | Alterations in body temperature

9
DISTURBANCES OF HEAT REGULATION

ROBERT G. PETERSDORF

CONTROL OF BODY TEMPERATURE

INTRODUCTION   In health, the body temperature of human beings is maintained within a narrow range despite extremes in environmental conditions and physical activity. This is also true for most birds and mammals, and such animals are termed *homeothermic,* or warm-blooded. An almost invariable accompaniment of systemic illness is a disturbance in temperature regulation, usually an abnormal elevation, or *fever.* In fact, fever is such a sensitive and reliable indicator of the presence of disease that thermometry is probably the commonest clinical procedure in use. Even in the absence of a frank febrile response, interference with heat regulation by disease is evident. This may take the form of flushing, pallor, sweating, shivering, and abnormal sensations of cold or warmth, or it may consist of erratic fluctuations of body temperature within normal limits when a patient is at bed rest.

HEAT PRODUCTION   The major source of basal heat production is through thyroid thermogenesis and the action of adenosine triphosphatase (ATPase) on the sodium pump of all membranes. The muscles are most important in promoting increased heat production with exercise through increased shivering. Heat production by muscle is of particular importance because the quantity can be varied according to the need. In most circumstances this variation consists of small increases and decreases in the number of nerve impulses to the muscles, causing inapparent tensing or relaxing. When, however, there is a strong stimulus for heat production, muscle activity may increase to the point of shivering, or even to a generalized rigor.

HEAT LOSS   Heat is lost from the body in several ways. Small amounts are used in warming food or drink and in the evaporation of moisture from the respiratory tract. Most heat is lost from the surface of the body, by *convection,* i.e., the transfer of heat to a fluid medium. Heat loss by convection depends on the existence of a temperature gradient between the body surface and the ambient air. A second mechanism for heat loss is *radiation*, which may be defined as an exchange of electromagnetic energy between the body and the radiant environment. *Evaporation* is the third major mechanism for dissipating heat and is particularly important when the ambient temperature exceeds that of the body.

The principal method of regulating heat loss is by varying the volume of blood flowing to the surface of the body. A rich circulation in the skin and subcutaneous tissues carries heat to the surface, where it can escape. In addition, sweating increases heat loss by providing water to be vaporized. The sweat, or eccrine, glands are under the control of the sympathetic nerves which, in this instance, mediate cholinergic stimuli. Heat loss by sweating may be tremendous, and as much as 1 liter per h of sweat may be evaporated. The amount of heat loss through sweating is also dependent upon the humidity in the air. The greater the humidity, the less the ability to lose heat through sweat.

When there is need for conservation of heat, adrenergic autonomic stimuli cause a sharp reduction in the blood flow to the surface. This causes vasoconstriction and transforms the skin and subcutaneous tissue into layers of insulation.

HEAT TRANSFER WITHIN THE BODY This depends upon *conduction*, i.e., the transfer of heat between adjacent organs, and upon *circulatory convection*, which is governed by bulk movement of body fluids and which is responsible for the transfer of heat between the cells and the bloodstream. It is useful, although oversimplified, to visualize the body as a central core at uniform temperatures surrounded by an insulating shell. The role of the shell as a mediator for heat conservation and heat loss is determined in part by its blood supply and by vasoconstriction or vasodilatation. Although insulation is relatively uniform throughout the body, some parts, such as the digits, are particularly susceptible to cold because of the increased surface-to-volume ratio. Moreover, blood that reaches the digits has already been cooled on the way. Insulation may be enhanced by the addition of clothing.

NEURAL CONTROL OF TEMPERATURE The control of body temperature, integrating the various physical and chemical processes for heat production or loss, is a function of cerebral centers located in the hypothalamus. A high-decerebrate animal displays a normal temperature if the hypothalamus is left intact. On the other hand, an animal whose brainstem has been sectioned loses ability to control body temperature, which consequently tends to vary with the environment, a condition referred to as *poikilothermia*. Animal experiments suggest that the preoptic anterior hypothalamus and some centers in the spinal cord have neurons which respond directly to local temperature and act as a sensor for internal temperature. This function is distinct from the integrative function which responds to temperature-sensitive structures all over the body.

Factors affecting neural control of temperature The temperature-regulating system is a negative feedback control system, and possesses three elements essential to such a system: (1) receptors which sense the existing central temperatures; (2) effector mechanisms, consisting of the vasomotor, sudomotor, and metabolic effectors, and (3) integrative structures which determine whether the existing temperature is too high or too low and which activate the appropriate motor response. It is a negative feedback system because a rise in central temperature initiates mechanisms for losing heat while a fall in central temperature activates mechanisms for heat production and heat

conservation. The activation of these effector responses is governed by a central integrative mechanism which may be compared with a thermostat and which responds to a variety of stimuli, such as the sensory impulses engendered in flushing or sweating, behavioral impulses, exercise, endocrine influences, and probably the temperature of the blood circulating through the hypothalamic centers. In a sense all these stimuli reset the thermostat.

A classic example of the endocrine influence on temperature is the effect of menstruation. The mean body temperature of women is higher during the second half of the menstrual cycle than it is between the onset of menstruation and the time of ovulation. The sensations of intense heat followed by diaphoresis that characterize the vasomotor instability experienced by some women at the menopause are undoubtedly the result of endocrine imbalance. The activation of the adrenal medulla in response to cold is another example of the relationship between the endocrine system and the thermoregulatory apparatus.

NORMAL BODY TEMPERATURE It is not practical to designate an exact upper level of normal body temperature because there are small differences among normal persons. There are rare individuals whose temperatures are always elevated slightly above accepted "normal" levels, and there is considerable variation in temperature in a given individual. In general, however, it is safe to regard an oral temperature above 99°F (37.2°C) in a person at bed rest as probable indication of disease. The temperature may be as low as 96.5°F (35.8°C) in healthy persons. Rectal temperature is usually 0.5 to 1.0°F higher than oral temperature. In very hot weather the body temperature may be elevated by 0.5 or even 1.0°F.

There is a distinct diurnal variation in body temperature in healthy human beings. Oral readings of 97°F (36.1°C) are relatively common on arising in the morning. Body temperature rises steadily through the day, reaches a peak of 99°F (37.2°C) or greater between 6 P.M. and 10 P.M., and then drops slowly to reach a minimum at 2 A.M. to 4 A.M. Although it has been postulated that this diurnal variation is dependent upon increasing activity during the day and rest at night, the pattern is not reversed in individuals who work at night and sleep during the day for long periods of time. The febrile patterns of most human diseases also tend to follow this normal diurnal pattern. Fevers tend to be higher, to "spike," in the evening, and many patients with febrile disease have relatively normal temperatures in the early morning hours.

Body temperature is more labile in young children, and transient elevations after relatively slight exertion in warm weather are frequently observed in them.

Severe or prolonged exercise can produce considerable elevation in body temperature. For example, marathon runners often have temperatures between 103.2 and 105.8°F (39 and 41°C). Although this marked increase in temperature with exercise tends to be balanced by compensatory cutaneous vasodilatation, resulting in loss of heat, and hyperventilation, these compensatory mechanisms may fail, leading to hyperpyrexia and, if uncontrolled, to heat stroke. Many of the adverse effects of long-distance running can be prevented by holding races only if the ambient temperature is below 82°F (27.8°C), preferably in the early morning or early evening, and by assuring ample fluid intake both before and during a race.

DISORDERED THERMOREGULATION In exercise, there is a temporary imbalance between heat production and heat loss with prompt reestablishment of normal temperatures at rest due to continuing activation of heat loss mechanisms. In fact, in prolonged exercise, cutaneous vasodilatation in response to an increase in central body temperature stops in order to preserve central temperature. Less adaptation occurs in fever because once a stable body temperature is reached, heat production equals heat loss, but both are greater than in the basal state. Cutaneous blood flow plays a greater role in controlling heat production and heat loss in fever than does sweating. At the beginning of fever, the body temperature as sensed by the thermoreceptors is low and the individual responds physiologically as if he were cold. *Heat production* is increased by shivering, and *heat loss* is decreased by vasoconstriction. These events explain the sensation of cold or chills that characterize the beginning of fever. Conversely, when the cause of fever is removed, the temperature returns to normal, and the individual responds as if he were warm. Cutaneous vasodilatation, sweating, and inhibition of shivering are the compensatory responses.

Deviations of 5°F (approximately 3.5°C) from the normal body temperature do not interfere appreciably with most bodily functions. Convulsions are common at temperatures higher than 106°F (41.1°C) in children, and irreversible brain damage, presumably due to protein denaturation (impairment of normal enzymic functions), is common when temperatures of 108°F (42.2°C) are reached. Fortunately, when hyperthermia reaches dangerous levels, the mechanisms for heat loss are suddenly activated; consequently, oral temperatures above 106°F (41.1°C) are relatively rare in humans. Conversely, when temperatures are lowered to 91°F (32.8°C), loss of consciousness occurs; at 86°F (30°C) poikilothermia sets in, and between 83 and 84°F (28.5°C) slow atrial fibrillation supervenes. Ventricular fibrillation occurs at extremely hypothermic temperatures.

The systemic symptoms accompanying deviations in temperature are poorly understood. For example at temperatures of 102°F (39°C) many patients have malaise, drowsiness, weakness, and generalized aches and pains. Many others, however, feel entirely well. Why some individuals are able to tolerate fever so well while others become markedly ill remains an enigma. Perhaps the inciting stimulus rather than fever per se is the major determinant of systemic complaints.

Diseases of the nervous system   Disease of the regulatory centers in the hypothalamus may affect body temperature. Cases have been observed in which there was destruction of the centers controlling heat-conserving mechanisms, with resulting hypothermia. More commonly, cerebral lesions are manifested by hyperthermia; this may occur with tumors, degenerative diseases, vascular accidents, particularly cerebral hemorrhage, or infections involving the hypothalamus, such as encephalitis. All these may result in loss of neurons and gliosis. Central fever is accompanied by lack of a diurnal variation, absence of sweating, resistance to antipyretic drugs, excessive response to external cooling, and loss of consciousness.

There are several diseases, of which heat stroke is the cardinal example, in which the central mechanisms for cooling suddenly fail and the patient ceases to sweat, despite the fact that his temperature is rising. Some of the highest temperatures ever observed in human beings [112 to 113°F (44.4°C)] have been in cases of heat stroke. A temperature higher than 114°F (45.6°C) is probably not compatible with life.

Increased heat production   Patients with thyrotoxicosis show exaggerated heat production, and their temperature is often 1 to 2°F above the normal range. Dinitrophenol, a drug once used for weight reduction, causes elevation of temperature; this, too, seems to be caused by increased metabolic activity.

Impairment of heat loss   Patients with *congestive heart failure* often have an elevation of body temperature between 0.5 and 1.5°F. Perhaps this elevation is caused by impairment of heat dissipation as a result of diminished cardiac output, decline in cutaneous blood flow (with increasing insulation of the central

temperature core), the insulating effect of edema, and the increased heat production incident to the muscular activity of dyspnea. On the other hand, patients with congestive heart failure are likely to have other causes of fever, such as venous thrombosis, pulmonary embolism and infarction, myocardial infarction, pneumonia, and urinary tract infection. However, since slight fever is so regularly present even in the absence of such complications, the circulatory disturbance may be responsible.

Patients with skin disorders such as *ichthyosis* and *congenital absence of sweat glands* may have fever in a warm environment because of inability to lose heat from the surface of the body. Similarly, individuals taking *drugs which impair sweating*, such as atropine, scopolamine, phenothiazines, monoamine oxidase inhibitors, glutethimide, lysergic acid diethylamide (LSD), amphetamines, and inhalation anesthetics, to mention just some, may have fever in warm weather.

Patients with severe burns tend to be hyperthermic, probably because occlusive dressings interfere with heat loss despite large areas of denuded skin.

PATHOGENESIS OF FEVER

Fever is a consequence of many stimuli, including bacteria and their endotoxins, viruses, yeasts, antigen-antibody reactions, hormonal substances, exemplified by etiocholanolone, drugs, and synthetic polynucleotides like poly I:poly C. These substances, which have been termed collectively *exogenous pyrogens*, are both diverse and complex. It has been postulated that they act through an intermediary substance termed *endogenous pyrogen* (EP). Most of the knowledge concerning EP has come from work in experimental animals.

Endogenous pyrogen is a basic protein of low molecular weight that is derived from leukocytes and macrophages, including Kupffer cells, splenic sinusoidal cells, alveolar macrophages and peritoneal-lining cells. Endogenous pyrogen has not been isolated from lymphocytes, but these cells may react with antigens and, through the action of lymphokines, may stimulate neutrophils and macrophages to release EP.

When stored in cells, such as polymorphonuclear leukocytes, EP is not present in active form. Rather, its release requires synthesis of new messenger ribonucleic acid (RNA) and protein. Because it is present in such small amounts, EP has been difficult to detect in human serum or exudates. However, a radioimmunoassay to detect EP is being developed.

Once released, EP probably acts on the thermosensitive neurons in the preoptic region of the hypothalamus. These neurons control the constancy of body temperature and are the point where fever is initiated.

The action of EP on the hypothalamus is by no means simple. It appears as if there must be a release of 5-hydroxytryptamine (serotonin), a thermogenic amine, to mediate the febrile response. In addition, EP induces synthesis of prostaglandins E_1 and E_2 in the hypothalamus, where they function as central transmitters in the initiation of fever. The action of antipyretics, such as aspirin, has been shown to be the result of their ability to block prostaglandin synthesis. The prostaglandins, in turn, lead to an increase in cyclic AMP, which may be important in the metabolic processes—heat conservation and increased oxygen consumption—that are operative in fever.

All these observations make for a cohesive explanation of the pathogenesis of fever, at least at the level of peripheral tissues, but more studies are needed to elucidate the mechanism of the action of EP in the central nervous system.

DISORDERS ASSOCIATED WITH HIGH TEMPERATURES

CAUSES OF HYPERPYREXIA The incidence of hyperpyrexia, defined as a temperature above 106°F (41.1°C), in adults is not known. In a series of 28 such patients studied at the Massachusetts General Hospital, 11 had infections, 9 had infections plus failure to dissipate heat adequately, such as autonomic dysfunction or occlusive burn dressings, 5 had thermoregulatory failure due to cerebral hemorrhage and heat stroke, and in 3 the cause was not determined. The majority of the hyperpyrexic episodes occurred in summer when the ambient temperature and humidity were high. The mortality was 29 percent and was related primarily to underlying disease; only two deaths were attributed to hyperpyrexia per se. In most patients, the high temperature responded to antipyretic drugs and cooling devices. The good outcome in this series of hospitalized patients was due in part to the early recognition of the high temperature and its intensive treatment.

HEAT SYNDROMES Three clinical syndromes are associated with high environmental temperature: *heat cramps, heat exhaustion,* and *heat pyrexia.* Although each entity may be identified clinically, there is considerable overlap in the changes produced by a high environmental temperature. These alterations are especially prevalent during the first days of a heat wave before effective acclimatization can occur. Prophylaxis by augmenting sodium chloride and fluid intake prior to exposure; by ensuring that susceptible individuals, particularly the elderly or the very young, wear light clothing, take frequent cool baths, and remain in a cool environment; or by restoring a physiologic balance prior to the onset of overt morbidity can help prevent the full-blown syndrome, especially heat pyrexia.

Strenuous physical activity or the presence of an acute or chronic disease may hasten the development of one of the heat syndromes.

Acclimatization The basic mechanism by which humans accommodate to excessive temperatures is unknown. Acclimatization does not increase the threshold for sweating. However, sweating is the most effective natural means of combating heat stress and can occur with little or no change in the core temperature of the body. As long as sweating continues, humans can withstand remarkably high temperatures, provided water and sodium chloride, the most important physiologic constituents of sweat, are replaced. The concentration of sodium chloride varies between that of interstitial fluid and very low concentrations, and the ability to secrete sweat with low sodium chloride content, as well as to increase the quantity of sweat, is a major mechanism for the conservation of salt in hot weather. Dilatation of the peripheral blood vessels in an attempt to dissipate heat is another major way for the body to acclimatize to hot temperatures. Other alterations include a decrease in total circulating blood volume, a decrease in renal blood flow, an increase of antidiuretic hormones (ADH) as well as aldosterone, a decrease in urine sodium, and an increase in respiratory and pulse rates. Ordinarily, acclimatization takes from 4 to 7 days. The hyperaldosteronism may result in severe potassium loss, which may be aggravated by replacement of sodium without concomitant repletion of potassium. Initially there is an increase in cardiac output but as heat stress persists, venous return diminishes and heart failure may occur. If environmental temperatures in excess of the body's temperature persist, heat is retained and hyperpyrexia develops.

Heat cramps Heat cramps, called "miner's cramps" and "stoker's cramps," are the most benign heat syndrome. Cramps are characterized by painful spasms of the voluntary muscles and usually follow strenuous exercise. In general, only individuals in good physical condition develop this syndrome. External temperatures need not exceed the body temperature, and direct exposure to the sun is not necessary. The body temperature is usually not elevated. Muscle cramps usually occur after excessive sweating and may even be precipitated by strenuous exercise in cold environments in untrained persons heavily clothed. Muscles of the extremities bear the brunt of physical activity and hence show the highest incidence of cramps. Physical examination of the patient is normal between the paroxysms. Examination of the blood reveals a concentration of the formed elements and a decreased sodium and chloride concentration. Excretion of these ions in the urine is characteristically low. Treatment consists of sodium chloride; cessation of cramps with replacement of sodium chloride and water is striking and supports the hypothesis that the cause of heat cramps is depletion of these essential electrolytes. Occasionally cramps involve the abdominal musculature, mimicking an intraabdominal emergency. Such patients have had mistaken exploratory surgery performed, often with disastrous results. Replacement of saline prior to surgery would have obviated such operations.

Heat exhaustion Heat prostration, or heat collapse, is probably the most common heat syndrome. It represents a failure of the cardiovascular responses to high external temperatures and is particularly common in elderly individuals who are receiving diuretics. Weakness, vertigo, headache, anorexia, nausea, vomiting, the urge to defecate, and faintness may precede collapse. Heat collapse occurs in both physically active and sedentary individuals. The onset is usually sudden and the duration of collapse brief. During the acute stage, the patient looks ashen-gray. The skin is cold and clammy. The pupils are dilated. The blood pressure may be low and the pulse pressure elevated. Since prostration develops before exposure to heat is prolonged, body temperature is subnormal or normal. The duration of exposure and the extent to which sweat is lost determine the degree of hemoconcentration. Treatment consists of removal of the patient to a cool area and placing him in the recumbent position. Spontaneous recovery then usually takes place. Intravenous administration of saline solution or whole blood is necessary only rarely. Although the pathogenetic mechanism of heat prostration is not primarily a depletion of water and salt, it is likely that maintenance of these electrolytes will prevent heat prostration in individuals exposed to high temperatures.

Heat pyrexia ETIOLOGY Heat hyperpyrexia, heat stroke, or sunstroke is most common in elderly individuals with preexisting chronic disease. Among these are arteriosclerosis and congestive heart failure, particularly when patients receive diuretics. Other predisposing factors include diabetes mellitus, alcoholism, the use of atropinelike drugs, and skin disorders in which it may be difficult to lose heat such as ectodermal dysplasia, congenital absence of the sweat glands, or severe scleroderma. Direct exposure to the sun is not a necessary prerequisite. Heat pyrexia may develop during any period of hot weather, but the incidence in temperate climates increases during prolonged heat waves and at temperatures of 90°F (32.2°C) or higher. High humidity in the range of 60 to 75 percent is a prerequisite to heat stroke. The major pathogenic mechanism of heat stroke is "sweat fatigue," and patients usually stop sweating before the onset of acute symptoms. The cessation of sweating is due to an intrinsic breakdown of the heat regulatory mechanism for reasons not known.

MANIFESTATIONS There may be few premonitory symptoms of heat stroke, and loss of consciousness may be the first sign. Other patients may complain of headache, vertigo, faintness, abdominal distress, confusion, or hyperpnea. Delirium may develop in more severe cases.

Pyrexia and prostration are the significant findings on physical examination. A rectal temperature greater than 106°F (41.1°C) is common and is a grave prognostic sign. Internal body temperatures as high as 112 to 113°F (44.4°C) have been recorded. The skin is hot and dry, and sweating is absent. The pulse rate is increased, and respirations are rapid and weak. The systolic blood pressure may be elevated. The muscles are flaccid, and tendon reflexes may be diminished. Lethargy, stupor, or coma, depending on the severity, is present. Shock is common in fatal cases.

Examination of the blood and urine may show few abnormalities. Leukocytosis is characteristic as are proteinuria, cylinduria, and an elevation in BUN. There is usually a respiratory alkalosis, hypokalemia, and severe hypophosphatemia. The electrocardiogram may show, in addition to tachycardia and sinus arrhythmia, flattening and subsequent inversion of the T wave and depression of the ST segment. Diffuse myocardial necrosis with ECG evidence of myocardial infarction has been reported. Other major laboratory abnormalities include thrombocytopenia; prolonged bleeding, clotting, and prothrombin times; afibrinogenemia and fibrinolysis; and consumptive coagulopathy. All these may be responsible for diffuse bleeding. Liver damage is common; it appears 24 to 36 h after admission and is characterized by clinically apparent jaundice and, often, by abnormalities in hepatocellular enzymes. Renal failure is a common complication of heat stroke.

Patients with heat stroke may die within a few hours after being discovered, or may die of complications such as acute renal failure. However, a number of patients will die several weeks after the acute episode, usually of myocardial infarction, heart failure, renal failure, bronchopneumonia, or complicating bacteremia. In them autopsy may show extensive parenchymal damage to various organs, either from hyperpyrexia per se or from petechial hemorrhages in the brain, heart, kidneys, or liver.

TREATMENT   Heat stroke requires heroic emergency measures. Time is most important. The patient should be placed in a cool place with adequate circulation of fresh air and with most of the clothing removed. Because the pathogenesis of heat stroke involves failure of the heat-regulating mechanism with cessation of sweating, external means of heat dissipation must be employed. The most effective measure is to immerse the patient in an ice-water bath, and there is no effective substitute for this seemingly drastic treatment. An ice-water bath does not induce shock or stimulate significant cutaneous vasoconstriction. The bath should be given with a minimum of delay. The patient should be watched constantly by a nurse or physician and the rectal temperature monitored. The bath may be discontinued when the rectal temperature falls below 101°F (38.3°C), but treatment should be resumed if there is a febrile rebound. Compared with immersion in ice water, other forms of therapy are less effective, but covering the patient with cold wet towels under a fan may be satisfactory if a bath is not available. After the bath the patient should be placed in a cool, well-ventilated room. Massage of the skin aids the acceleration of heat loss and stimulates return of the cool peripheral blood to the overheated brain and viscera. Phenothiazine may be given to reduce shivering. Stimulants such as epinephrine and narcotics are contraindicated. Intravenous fluids should be given with monitoring of the central venous pressure and urinary output. Both dehydration and heart failure must be avoided. Fresh blood should be given in case of bleeding, and clear-cut evidence of disseminated intravascular coagulation calls for heparin (7500 units per hour). Persistent oliguria is an indication for early dialysis.

Malignant hyperthermia   ETIOLOGY   Malignant hyperthermia is an inherited disorder that is characterized by a rapid increase in temperature to 102.2 to 107.6°F (39 to 42°C) in response to inhalational anesthetics such as halothane, methoxyflurane, cyclopropane, and ethyl ether or muscle relaxants, notably succinyl choline. Two forms of the disease exist; in one, where the mechanism of inheritance is autosomal dominant, the individuals are normal between attacks. A second form, which is recessive, occurs in young boys with a number of congenital abnormalities including short stature, undescended testes, lumbar lordosis, thoracic kyphosis, pectus carinatum, webbed neck, winged scapulae, small chin, low-set ears, and an antimongoloid obliquity of the palpebral fissures. The incidence of the autosomal dominant form is 1:50,000 to 1:100,000.

PATHOGENESIS   The triggering anesthetic releases calcium from the membrane of the muscle cell's sarcoplasmic reticulum, which is defective in storing this ion. The result is a sudden increase in myoplasmic calcium. The calcium activates myosin ATPase which converts adenosine triphosphate (ATP) to adenosine diphosphate, phosphate, and heat. There are also inhibition of troponin, uncoupling of oxidative phosphorylation, activation of phosphorylase kinase, and increased glycolysis. Muscular contraction occurs, and it, as well as the chemical events, leads to production of heat.

MANIFESTATIONS   Existence of malignant hyperthermia can be suspected if less relaxation is noted during induction of anesthesia and muscle fasciculations when succinyl choline is given. If the temperature is not monitored, the first signs may be a hot skin and tachycardia or a cardiac arrhythmia. In addition to the high fever, there is muscle rigidity, hypotension, and mottled cyanosis.

Early laboratory abnormalities include respiratory and metabolic acidosis, hyperkalemia and hypermagnesemia, and elevation in blood lactate and pyruvate. Late complications include massive skeletal muscle swelling, pulmonary edema, disseminated intravascular coagulation, and acute renal failure.

PROCAINAMIDE, DANTROLENE SODIUM

TREATMENT   Malignant hyperthermia is a medical emergency. Surgery must be interrupted and the patient cooled with ice. One hundred percent oxygen should be given, along with sodium bicarbonate, to combat the severe metabolic acidosis. A diuresis should be induced with fluids and diuretics to reduce myoglobinemia and hyperkalemia. Specific treatment consists of procainamide 10 mg/kg [0.5 to 1.0 (mg/kg)/min]. An experimental drug, dantrolene sodium, is also effective.

PREVENTION   While the best way to detect this syndrome is to monitor the temperature of all patients under anesthesia, the best way to avert it altogether is to take a thorough family history. Examining patients preoperatively is often not helpful because, between attacks, persons susceptible to malignant hyperthermia may be entirely normal. Some have increased muscle bulk, some have localized areas of muscle weakness, some spontaneous muscle cramps, and a few have generalized muscle weakness. In some of these patients, the creatine phosphokinase (CPK) is elevated, but in many this test is entirely normal. Microscopy of muscle shows marked variation in fiber diameter. In susceptible patients, surgery should be performed under spinal, epidural, or regional anesthesia. If this is not possible, a combination of pentothal and diazepam is probably safest.

DISORDERS ASSOCIATED WITH LOW TEMPERATURES *VOLUME (Replace) when Rewarming*

COLD ACCLIMATIZATION This state of increased resistance to cold injury is the result of exposure to a cold but tolerable environment. Adaptive responses consist of circulatory adjustments protecting the temperatures of exposed portions of the body, metabolic adaptation providing greater heat production to compensate for increased heat loss, and behavioral and neural adaptations minimizing either the actual cold stress or the discomfort resulting from physiologically tolerable hypothermia. In contrast with heat acclimatization, it is not possible to delineate adaptive physiologic changes to cold. Nevertheless, primitive people live at zero temperatures wearing little or no clothing; pain perception is less in persons, such as fishermen, who work periodically with their hands in ice water; and military personnel shiver less during cold exposure after training in the Arctic. Adaptation may take place either by shivering, with production of excess heat, or, as is the case with Australian aborigines, by a drop of internal temperature with only minimal shivering.

Put on Bipass pump? + warm

HYPOTHERMIA Although far less common than is elevation in temperature, hypothermia is of considerable importance because it represents a medical emergency which lends itself to treatment.

Accidental hypothermia This is a well-known complication of exposure and has been reported frequently during the winter months. It usually occurs in elderly individuals after prolonged exposure, not necessarily to excessively low external temperatures. It is attributed not only to exogenous factors such as a cold external environment but also to unknown endogenous factors. The diagnosis of hypothermia has proved elusive largely because *clinical thermometers do not record temperatures below 95°F (35°C). Whenever a patient presents with a temperature below this level, the true temperature should be determined with an incubator thermometer or a thermocouple.* Accidental hypothermia has been found in association with myxedema, pituitary insufficiency, Addison's disease, hypoglycemia, cerebrovascular disease, myocardial infarction, cirrhosis, pancreatitis, and ingestion of drugs or alcohol. For example, it is not uncommon to find a derelict in a railroad yard or under a bridge following an alcoholic debauch with a temperature between 85 and 90°F (28.5 and 32.3°C) or lower. These patients usually appear cold and pale and, when their temperatures are very low, give the appearance of having rigor mortis, so stiff is their musculature. Patients with temperatures less than 80°F (26.7°C) are usually unconscious. The pupils are usually miotic, respirations tend to be shallow and slow, there is bradycardia, and most patients are hypotensive. Generalized edema is often present. Laboratory data tend to show hemoconcentration, mild azotemia, and metabolic acidosis. The acidosis is due in part to hypoxemia in peripheral tissues. At cold temperatures, the hemoglobin dissociation curve is shifted to the left, and there is decreased unloading of oxygen in the peripheral tissues. Some patients have hypoglycemia while others show evidence of diabetes mellitus. Thyroid function tests may give results typical of myxedema. Some patients have elevations in serum amylase, and a few show pancreatitis at autopsy. The electrocardiogram is distorted by muscular tremors and may show bradycardia or slow atrial fibrillation and a characteristic J wave (occurring at the junction of the QRS complex and ST segment). Other arrythmias are common; ventricular fibrillation is usually a terminal event.

TREATMENT Hypothermia is a medical emergency, and therapy should be instituted at once. The following steps are indicated:

1 An airway must be established and maintained, and the patient should be well oxygenated.
2 Blood gases should be monitored; they should be corrected for temperature.
3 Blood volume should be expanded with glucose and saline, low-molecular-weight dextran, or albumin. Maintenance of blood volume is necessary to prevent the infarctions which have been a hallmark in fatal cases and to avert "rewarming shock." *[~ LIKE Post-op Heart]*
4 Because of the tendency to arrythmias, serum potassium should be monitored carefully; a transvenous pacemaker may be indicated.
5 Sodium bicarbonate should be given if pH ≤ 7.25.
6 Although external rewarming with blankets or warm baths may be appropriate in patients with mild hypothermia, patients who are severely hypothermic require reestablishment of core temperature. External rewarming does this poorly because, while it tends to dilate the constricted peripheral blood vessels, it diverts blood from the visceral organs. On the other hand, restoration of the core temperature by hemodialysis, during which the blood is warmed externally, or by peritoneal dialysis, during which the dialysate is warmed to 98.6°F (37°C), is the method of choice. It is particularly important to rewarm the myocardium because, in cases of ventricular fibrillation, defibrillation will not be successful until myocardial temperature is raised to near normal levels.
7 There is a tendency for these patients to develop pneumonia which should be treated promptly with antibiotics.
8 Finally, resuscitative efforts should be vigorous and prolonged despite the poor prognosis which is related primarily to the advanced age and associated debilitating disease of these patients. In younger individuals, some remarkable rescues have been recorded; one young woman was resuscitated even after her temperature had dropped to 69°F (20.6°C).

Hypothermia secondary to acute illness There is a group of patients who develop moderate hypothermia in association with acute diseases including congestive heart failure, uremia, diabetes mellitus, drug overdose, acute respiratory failure, and hypoglycemia. These patients are generally elderly and upon admission to the hospital are found to have temperatures of 92 to 93.9°F (33.3 to 34.4°C). They also have a severe metabolic acidosis, due to increased production of lactic acid, and cardiac arrhythmias. Most of these patients are comatose. This entity differs from accidental hypothermia only in the absence of exposure; these cases have all occurred at normal ambient temperatures. The mechanism appears to be an acute failure of thermoregulation; shivering did not occur in any of these patients. Usually these patients have been rewarmed within a few hours by means of an alcohol-circulating blanket. Upon return to normal temperature, cardiac arrythmias, which were present in most of these patients, responded to treatment, and the sensorium returned to normal. With the exception that core rewarming could be established by external means, other facets of therapy should follow the steps outlined above. In addition, treatment of the underlying disease such as diabetes with insulin, uremia with dialysis, or congestive heart failure with appropriate cardiac drugs and diuretics is essential. The prognosis is good provided the syndrome is recognized early and treatment is instituted at once.

Immersion hypothermia Responses to cold-water immersion may be classified as (1) stimulatory, with deep body temperature normal to 95°F (35°C); (2) depressant, with deep body temperature 95 to 86°F (35 to 30°C); and (3) critical, with deep body temperature 86 to 77°F (30 to 25°C).

The long-distance swimmer is able to maintain a normal body temperature for periods of 15 to 25 h or more in water that may plunge skin temperature to 59°F (15°C) or lower, which is some 28°F below deep body temperature, lending support to the concept of a body core insulated by a body shell. The vasoconstriction operative in cold water greatly reduces heat loss. However, there is great individual variability in heat loss in cold water. The relatively obese swimmer may maintain a normal rectal temperature for 2 h without shivering in 61°F (16°C) water. A lean person under the same conditions, despite violent shivering, may experience a fall in rectal temperature of several degrees and become incapacitated from the rigor. In hypersensitive persons, immersion in cold water may be followed by vascular spasm, vomiting, and syncope.

Other compensatory responses include bradycardia, a slight rise in blood pressure, and an early rise in rectal temperature followed by a fall. At 86°F (30°C), atrial fibrillation is common.

TREATMENT Although rewarming in hot water has been recommended in the treatment of immersion hypothermia, the same objections to sudden diversion of cardiac output to peripheral tissues described above apply. Individuals with this problem should be covered with a light blanket and placed in a room with a moderate ambient temperature. The other measures described for the treatment of accidental hypothermia, including hemodialysis or peritoneal dialysis, should be instituted depending on the clinical picture.

LOCAL COLD INJURIES Mechanisms of freezing injury
These can be divided into phenomena which affect cells and extracellular fluids (direct effects) and those which disrupt the function of organized tissues and the integrity of the circulation (indirect effects).

DIRECT EFFECTS When tissue freezes, ice crystals form and, concomitantly, solutes in the residual liquid become concentrated. The physical dislocation during slow freezing is extreme. Ice crystals many times the size of individual cells form but only in the extracellular spaces. Large ice crystals can develop between cells in soft tissue without producing irreversible injury as long as the percentage of water frozen does not exceed a critical amount. A major source of damage to living cells during freezing and thawing appears to be the strong salt solutions which develop during formation and dissolution of ice; changes in the proportions of lipids and phospholipids in the cell membrane are also of great importance. The discovery of the protective value of such substances as glycerol and dimethylsulfoxide, which enter cells and prevent freezing injury during comparatively slow cooling to low temperatures and rewarming from them, represents a significant advance. This method has been used extensively in banking spermatozoa for subsequent artificial insemination. It has not been possible, however, to protect organs in this manner since the protective substance must be delivered to all cells.

INDIRECT EFFECTS The fulminating vascular reaction and stasis which supervene are associated with production of histamine-like substances which increase the permeability of the capillary bed. Within blood vessels, cellular elements aggregate. Irreversible occlusion of small blood vessels by cell masses has been demonstrated in thawed tissue following

freezing injury. The damaged frozen tissue simulates tissue damage produced by burns.

Manifestations The mildest form of cold injury is called *frostnip* and tends to occur in organs farthest removed from the core of the body such as the earlobes, nose, cheeks, fingers and toes, and hands and feet. It can be prevented by warm clothing and treated with simple rewarming. More consequential, local cold injuries may be divided into freezing (frostbite) and nonfreezing (immersion-foot) injuries. The two types may be observed in the same extremity or in different extremities in the same individual, e.g., trench foot and freezing of the hands but not the feet of shipwreck survivors. The diagnosis of freezing versus nonfreezing injury generally can be made on the basis of history and clinical manifestations.

IMMERSION FOOT This entity is observed in shipwreck survivors or in soldiers (trench foot) whose feet have been wet but not freezing cold for prolonged periods. There is primarily injury to nerve and muscle tissue, but no gross or irreparable pathologic changes occur in blood vessels and skin. The clinical picture reflects primary hypoxic trauma giving rise to three clearly recognizable conditions: (1) *ischemia*, denoted by a pale, pulseless extremity; (2) *hyperemia*, characterized by a bounding pulsatile circulation in red, swollen, painful feet; and (3) the *posthyperemic* or recovery period. The initial cold-induced vasoconstriction, increased blood viscosity, and impaired oxygen transport in the ischemic state are aggravated by such factors as malnutrition, general hypothermia, dehydration, and trauma from relatively fixed, pendant extremities. The problem of rewarming is critical in these patients during the stage of ischemia, when overheating of tissue may lead to gangrene. In the state of hyperemia, the red, swollen feet require judicious cooling. Severe cases may show muscular weakness, atrophy, ulceration, and gangrene of superficial areas. Sensitivity to cold and pain on weight bearing, which may cause discomfort for many years, are sequelae even of milder injuries.

FROSTBITE In contrast with immersion foot, in frostbite the blood vessels may be severely and irreparably injured, the circulation of blood ceases, and the vascular bed of the frozen tissue is occluded by agglutinated cell aggregates and thrombi. The cutaneous injury consists in part of separation of the epidermal-dermal interface. Early, the intravascular clumping is reversible. However, with the passage of time, clumped red blood cells within vessels in injured tissue lose their morphologic identity and take on the appearance of a homogenous, hyalinaceous plug. It has been shown in some, but not all, experimental studies that much of the intravascular aggregation following freezing injury can be reversed and microcirculatory perfusion improved if low-molecular-weight dextran is given intravenously shortly after injury. Frostbitten tissues unfortunately are often neglected and with thawing become macerated; if this is the situation, the method of rewarming is not important. The method of rewarming has been a matter of controversy. It seems most rational to warm the core of the body before treating the local area of frostbite. Following restoration of the core temperature to normal, warming of a frostbitten limb should begin in water at 50 to 59°F (10 to 15°C), which is then increased 9°F (5°C) every 5 min to a maximum of 104°F (40°C).

Most cold injuries do not require warming, and treatment should be conservative and consists of bed rest, elevation of the injured part, tetanus antitoxin, and antibiotics, when indicated; early drainage of blebs and bullae; daily washes with pHisoHex; and early institution of physiotherapy. Alcohol and cigarettes are strongly contraindicated. Surgical amputation and reconstruction is usually not necessary. Regional sympathectomy performed 24 to 48 h after thawing is followed by rapid resolution of edema, earlier demarcation of destroyed tissue, and faster healing. The effect of regional sympathectomy is probably due to ablation of persistent vasospasm and to restoration of cold perception. Intraarterial reserpine has effects similar to sympathectomy, with marked decrease in local vasospasm and decrease in pain and edema.

Some patients with frostbite have residua consisting of excessive sweating, pain, cold feet, numbness, abnormal color, and pain in the joints. The symptoms are generally worse in the winter and following exposure to cold. These patients also often show abnormal nails, discoloration and pigmentation, hyperhydrosis, and, by x-ray, osteoporosis and cystic defects near the joints. These abnormalities tend to be milder in patients who have had sympathetic blockade. Most cold injuries are preventable by graded exposure to cold, as well as appropriate clothing in freezing temperatures.

REFERENCES

Brengelman G: Temperature regulation, in *Physiology and Biophysics*, TC Ruch and HD Patton (eds). Philadelphia, Saunders, 1973

Clowes GHA Jr, O'Donnel TF Jr: Current concepts: Heat stroke. N Engl J Med 291:564, 1974

Dinarello CA, Wolff SM: Pathogenesis of fever in man. N Engl J Med 298:607, 1978

Edelman IS: Thyroid thermogenesis. N Engl J Med 290:1303, 1974

Goulding MR et al: The role of sympathectomy in frostbite, with a review of 68 cases. Surgery 57:774, 1965

Knochel JP et al: The renal, cardiovascular, hematologic and serum electrolyte abnormalities of heat stroke. Am J Med 30:299, 1961

Lask RF et al: Accidental profound hypothermia and barbiturate intoxication: A report of rapid "core" rewarming by peritoneal dialysis. JAMA 201:123, 1966

MacLean D et al: Metabolic aspects of spontaneous recovery in accidental hypothermia and hypothermic myxedema. Q J Med (n.s.) 43(171):371, 1974

O'Donnel TF Jr, Clowes GHA Jr: The circulatory abnormalities of heat stroke. N Engl J Med 287:734, 1972

Penn I, Schwartz SI: Evaluation of low molecular weight dextran in the treatment of frostbite. J Trauma 4:784, 1964

Shibolet S et al: Heat stroke: A review. Aviat Space Environ Med 47:280, 1976

Simon HB: Extreme pyrexia. JAMA 236:2419, 1976

Stephen RC: Malignant hyperthermia. Annu Rev Med 28:153, 1977

Whittle JL, Bates JH: Thermoregulatory failure secondary to acute illness: Complications and treatment. Arch Intern Med 139:418, 1979

Wickstrom P et al: Accidental hypothermia. Am J Surg 131:622, 1976

Wyndham CH: Heat stroke and hyperthermia in marathon runners. Ann NY Acad Sci 301:128, 1977

10
CHILLS AND FEVER

ROBERT G. PETERSDORF

In view of the extensive knowledge of physiologic mechanisms controlling body temperature mentioned in Chap. 9, it is surprising that so little is known about the ways in which disease upsets thermoregulation.

Some bacteria, particularly gram-negative species, produce endotoxins which are pyrogenic, and a few viruses also cause fever when injected into humans or animals. Many microorganisms, however, possess no demonstrable pyrogenic toxin and, of course, fever accompanies diseases which do not involve invasion of the body by any known parasite. Omitting disorders which may involve cerebral thermoregulatory centers directly, such as brain tumors, intracranial hemorrhage or thrombosis, or heat stroke, the following disease states may be accompanied by fever:

1 All *infections*, whether caused by bacteria, rickettsias, viruses, or more complex parasites, cause fever.
2 *Mechanical trauma*, e.g., a crushing injury, frequently gives rise to fever lasting 1 or 2 days. Not infrequently, however, complicating infection sets in.
3 Many *neoplastic diseases* are associated with fever. In most patients, fever in patients with cancer is related to obstruction or infection produced by the tumor. In some solid tumors, however, fever may be due to the tumor per se, particularly following metastasis to the liver. Tumors which are associated with fever include hypernephroma, carcinoma of the pancreas, lung, or bone, and hepatoma. In tumors of the reticuloendothelial system, including Hodgkin's disease, lymphosarcoma, reticulum cell sarcoma, and acute leukemias, fever may be one of the prominent early manifestations.
4 *Hematopoietic disorders*, e.g., acute hemolytic episodes, may be characterized by pyrexia.
5 *Vascular accidents* of any magnitude, e.g., myocardial, pulmonary, and cerebral infarctions, nearly always cause fever.
6 *Diseases due to immune mechanisms* are almost always febrile. These include the collagen diseases, drug fevers, and serum sickness.
7 Certain *acute metabolic disorders*, such as gout, porphyria, hypertriglyceridemia, Fabry's disease, and Addisonian or thyroid crises, sometimes are associated with fever.

ACCOMPANIMENTS OF FEVER **Systemic symptoms** The perception of fever by patients varies enormously. Some persons can tell with considerable accuracy whether their body temperatures are elevated; others, notably patients with tuberculosis, may be wholly unaware of body temperature as high as 103°F (39.4°C). Often, also, patients may pay no attention to fever because of other unpleasant symptoms such as headache and pleuritic pain. Pain in the back, generalized myalgias, and arthralgia without arthritis are common in fever. Whether these symptoms reflect the presence of an infectious agent or are merely a nonspecific accompaniment of pyrexia is not clear.

Chills Abrupt onset of fever with a *chill* or *rigor* is characteristic of some diseases and, in the absence of antipyretic drugs, rare in others. Although repeated rigors are typical of pyogenic infection with bacteremia, a similar pattern of fever may occur in noninfectious diseases such as lymphoma. It is important to differentiate a true chill, which is accompanied by teeth chattering and bed shaking, from the chilly sensation which occurs in almost all fevers, particularly those in viral infections. In some instances, however, a true rigor occurs in viremia. Chills may be evoked or perpetuated by the intermittent administration of aspirin or other antipyretics. These agents may cause a sharp depression in temperature, which is followed by compensatory involuntary muscular contractions, i.e., a chill. This unpleasant side effect of antipyretic drugs can be averted by administering these agents frequently, around the clock, in low doses, rather than by prescribing them only for elevations in temperature above a certain level.

Herpes labialis So-called "fever blisters" result from activation of the herpes simplex virus by elevation in temperature. For reasons which are obscure, fever blisters are common in pneumococcal infections, streptococcosis, malaria, meningococcemia, and rickettsioses but are rare in mycoplasma pneumonia, tuberculosis, brucellosis, smallpox, and typhoid.

Delirium This may result from elevation of body temperature and is particularly common in patients with alcoholism, cerebral arteriosclerosis, or senility.

Convulsions These are not infrequent in febrile children, especially those with a family history of epilepsy, although febrile convulsions do not, in general, reflect serious cerebral disease.

CLINICAL IMPORTANCE OF FEVER The temperature is a simple, objective, and accurate indicator of a physiologic state and is much less subject to external and psychogenic stimuli than the other vital signs, i.e., the pulse, respiratory rate, and blood pressure. For these reasons, determination of the body temperature assists in estimating the severity of an illness, its course and duration, and the effect of therapy, or even in deciding whether a person has an organic illness.

Benefit of fever There are a few infections of humans in which pyrexia appears definitely to be beneficial to the host, such as neurosyphilis and perhaps chronic brucellosis. Certain other diseases, such as uveitis and rheumatoid arthritis, sometimes improve after fever therapy. In experimental animals some pneumococcal and cryptococcal infections have been influenced in favor of the host animal by raising the body temperature. Aged and debilitated patients with infection may have little or no fever, and this is generally interpreted as a bad prognostic sign. In the great majority of infectious diseases, however, there is no reason to believe that pyrexia accelerates phagocytosis, antibody formation, or other defense mechanisms.

Detrimental aspects of fever Fever accelerates all metabolic processes and accentuates weight loss and nitrogen wastage. The work and the rate of the heart are increased. Sweating aggravates loss of salt and water. There may be discomfort due to headache, photophobia, general malaise, or unpleasant sensation of warmth. Fever may precipitate seizures in epileptic patients. The rigors and profuse sweats of hectic fevers are particularly unpleasant for the patient. In elderly individuals with overt or potential cardiac or cerebral vascular disease, fever may be particularly deleterious.

MANAGEMENT OF FEVER Since fever ordinarily does little harm and imposes no great discomfort, antipyretic drugs are rarely necessary and may obfuscate the effect of a specific therapeutic agent or of the natural course of the disease. There are situations, however, in which lowering of the body temperature is of vital importance; e.g., heat stroke, postoperative hyperthermia, delirium due to hyperpyrexia, epileptic seizures, or shock associated with fever and heart failure. Under these circumstances lowering the temperature is indicated. Cooling blankets which can be set at hypothermic temperatures are a highly effective means for external cooling. Alternatively, sponging the body surface with cool saline solution or the application of cool compresses to the skin and forehead may be employed. There is no advantage in sponging with alcohol, which, because of its pungent odor, makes some patients ill. When high internal temperature is combined with cutaneous vasoconstriction, as in heat stroke or postoperative hyperthermia, the cooling measures should be combined with massage of the skin in order to bring blood to the surface, where it may be

cooled. Immediate immersion in a tub of ice water should be considered a lifesaving emergency procedure in patients with heat stroke if the internal body temperature is in excess of 108°F (42.2°C). If cooling blankets are available, they are preferable to immersion in ice in most instances.

If antipyretic drugs, such as aspirin (0.3 to 0.6 g), are employed to bring about a fall in temperature, ill effects such as unpleasant diaphoresis, sometimes associated with an alarming fall in blood pressure and the subsequent return of fever and occasionally accompanied by a chill, may occur. These can be mitigated by enforcing a liberal fluid intake and by administering the drug regularly and frequently at 2- to 3-h intervals. Although adrenal steroids are also potent antipyretics, they must be used with caution because of their tendency to precipitate abrupt falls in temperature accompanied by hypotension. The capacity of these drugs to mask other manifestations of infection also constitutes a relative contraindication to their use.

The discomfort of a rigor can be alleviated in many patients by the intravenous injection of calcium gluconate. This procedure will stop the shivering and chilliness but has no influence on the ultimate height of the fever. Severe disruptive rigors sometimes need to be abolished with morphine sulfate (10 to 15 mg subcutaneously) or with parenteral chlorpromazine.

DIAGNOSTIC CONSIDERATIONS IN FEVER

In many illnesses fever is the most prominent and often the only manifestation of disease. It is not an indication of any particular type of disease; rather it should be considered a reaction to injury comparable with an elevated leukocyte count or a rapid erythrocyte sedimentation rate.

TYPES OF FEVER Fever is classically described as intermittent, remittent, sustained, and relapsing.

Intermittent fever With *intermittent fever* the temperature falls to normal each day. When the variation between the peak and the nadir is very large, the fever is called *hectic* or *septic*. Intermittent fevers are characteristic in pyogenic infections, particularly abscesses, lymphomas, and miliary tuberculosis.

Remittent fever With *remittent fever* the temperature falls each day but does not return to normal. Most fevers are remittent, and this type of febrile response is in no way characteristic.

Sustained fever A *sustained fever* is characterized by persistent elevation without significant diurnal variation. It is exemplified by the fever of untreated typhoid or typhus.

Relapsing fever With *relapsing fever* short febrile periods occur between one or several days of normal temperature. Examples of relapsing fever are seen in the following conditions:

Malaria (Chap. 200) had vanished from the United States almost completely, but for several years Vietnam war veterans constituted an important and sizable reservoir of this infection, as do other persons recently arrived from foreign countries. It is most unusual, however, for malaria to recur after a symptom-free interval of 1 year or more. Febrile bouts recur at 2- or 3-day intervals, or more irregularly in falciparum infections, depending on the maturation cycle of the parasite. The diagnosis depends on demonstration of the parasites in the blood.

Relapsing fever (Chap. 149) occurs in the southwest part of the United States, as far east as Texas, and in many other parts of the world. The recurrences are related to the cyclic development of parasites. Diagnosis is by demonstration of the spirochetal organisms in stained films of the blood.

Rat-bite fever (Chap. 130) is brought about by two agents—*Spirillum minus* and *Streptobacillus moniliformis,* both transmitted by the bite of a rat. Both may cause an illness characterized by periodic exacerbations of fever. The clue to the diagnosis depends on obtaining a history of rat bite 1 to 10 weeks prior to the onset of symptoms. The cause can be established by appropriate laboratory procedures.

Localized *pyogenic infections* in rare instances give rise to periodic bouts of fever separated by afebrile and relatively symptom-free intervals. The so-called "Charcot's intermittent biliary fever," i.e., cholangitis with biliary obstruction due to stones, is an example. *Urinary tract infection,* with episodes of ureteral obstruction due to small stones or inspissated pus, can also cause recurrent fever.

Approximately 5 percent of patients with Hodgkin's disease at some time have so-called "Pel-Ebstein fever"—bouts of fever lasting 3 to 10 days, separated by afebrile and asymptomatic periods of 3 to 10 days. These cycles may be repeated regularly over a period of several months. In rare instances this periodicity of the fever has been sufficiently striking to suggest the correct diagnosis before lymphadenopathy or splenomegaly became evident. However, relapsing fevers indistinguishable from Pel-Ebstein fever usually have causes other than Hodgkin's disease.

EPIDEMIOLOGY OF FEVER The diagnosis of febrile illnesses must take into consideration the context of the epidemiologic setting. For example, an acute 6-day febrile illness in Southeast Asia is probably due to dengue or Chikungunya fever (Chap. 190), malaria (Chap. 200), scrub typhus (Chap. 169), or leptospirosis (Chap. 148); in a college student in the United States it may result from infectious mononucleosis or some other viral infection; and in an octogenarian following prostatectomy it is probably an indication of urinary tract infection, wound infection, pulmonary infarction, or aspiration pneumonia. In children, infections are more likely to be responsible for prolonged fevers than in adults. Likewise, travelers returning from short trips to foreign countries are much more likely to have febrile illnesses indigenous to their home than to the foreign country they have visited.

RARE VERSUS COMMON DISEASES Most of the time fever is a manifestation of a common disease, and fever associated with a pulmonary infiltrate is much more likely to be due to pneumococcal than to pneumocystis pneumonia. Failure to appreciate this cardinal principle has led to many prolonged and futile diagnostic work-ups.

FEBRILE ILLNESSES OF SHORT DURATION Acute febrile illnesses of less than 2 weeks' duration are a common occurrence in medical practice. In many instances they run their course, progressing to complete recovery, and a precise diagnosis is not made. In most instances, however, it is safe to assume that the illness is of infectious origin. Although short febrile illnesses may be noninfectious (e.g., allergic fevers due to drugs, thromboembolic disease, hemolytic crises, or gout), they are decidedly in the minority.

Most undiagnosed acute febrile infectious diseases are probably viral and remain undiagnosed because diagnostic methods are unavailable or cumbersome. It is not practical to carry out tests needed to identify all the known viruses, and, furthermore, there must be a considerable number of still unidentified viruses pathogenic for humans. In bacterial infections, on the other hand, laboratory diagnosis is simpler, and

these infections are often rapidly controlled with chemotherapy.

The following characteristics, though not restricted solely to acute infections, are highly suggestive that infection is present:

1 Abrupt onset
2 High fever, i.e., 102 to 105°F (38.9 to 40.6°C), with or without chills
3 Respiratory symptoms—sore throat, coryza, cough
4 Severe malaise, with muscle or joint pain, photophobia, pain on movement of the eyes, headache
5 Nausea, vomiting, or diarrhea
6 Acute enlargement of lymph nodes or spleen
7 Meningeal signs, with or without spinal fluid pleocytosis
8 Leukocyte count above 12,000 or below 5000 per cubic millimeter
9 Dysuria, frequency, and flank pain

None of the symptoms or signs listed is encountered only in infection. Many of these features could be seen in acute leukemia or disseminated lupus erythematosus. Nevertheless, in a given instance of acute febrile illness with some of or all the manifestations listed, the probabilities strongly favor infection, and the patient may be given reasonable reassurance that he will probably recover in a week or two, regardless of a precise diagnosis.

It is desirable, of course, to establish an accurate diagnosis, and whatever steps are practicable in the circumstances to establish the cause should be taken. Cultures of the throat, blood, urine, or feces should be obtained before institution of antibacterial chemotherapy. Skin and/or serologic tests should be carried out when indicated.

There is a tendency to rely immediately and excessively on the laboratory in ascertaining the cause of fever. In many instances, a thorough history and a complete and, if necessary, repeated physical examination, along with a complete blood count (CBC), urinalysis, and sedimentation rate will provide the answer. Often a little patience, in the form of watchful waiting, before plunging into an expensive and extensive laboratory work-up, will lead to the diagnosis.

PROLONGED FEBRILE ILLNESSES Some of the knottiest problems in the field of internal medicine are found in cases of prolonged fever in which the diagnosis remains obscure for weeks or even months. Eventually, however, the true nature of the illness usually reveals itself, since a disease which causes injury sufficient to evoke temperature elevations to 101°F (38.3°C) or higher for several weeks does not often subside without leaving some clue as to its nature. The elucidation of problems of this sort calls for skillful application of all diagnostic methods—careful history, thorough physical examination, and the carefully considered use of laboratory examinations and roentgenograms.

Fever of unknown origin (FUO) In some patients fever becomes the dominant sign or symptom in a patient's illness, and when its cause escapes detection it is defined as fever of unknown origin (FUO). It is appropriate to use this term only in patients who have elevations in temperature [>101°F (38.3°C)] for a prolonged period (at least 2 to 3 weeks) and in whom the diagnosis cannot be made during at least 1 week of intensive studies. These rigid criteria eliminate from this diagnostic category patients with common bacterial or viral infections, those in whom the diagnosis is obvious, and those whose fever is due to a sequential occurrence of etiologically unrelated diseases. An example is a patient who is febrile following a myocardial infarction, who then develops thrombophlebitis that is associated with fever, and in whom this is followed by multiple pulmonary emboli, also a febrile disease. Much of the confusion in the literature concerning causes of FUO is due to failure to define the criteria employed in classifying patients who have had fever of unknown origin.

DISEASES CAUSING PROLONGED FEVERS

Table 10-1 lists some of the diseases which are responsible for prolonged fever. Some of these disorders must initially be considered to be FUO; in others the diagnosis comes to mind readily.

INFECTION Infections occupy a less prominent position among causes of prolonged fever now than formerly because of the common practice of administering antibiotics to any patient in whom fever persists for more than a few days. Consequently, many infections are at present being eradicated by more or less "blind" therapy without accurate determination of their nature or location. Nevertheless, patients with infections compose approximately 40 percent of any group with FUO. Many times these infections take the form of localized abscesses, osteomyelitis, or bacterial endocarditis; or the organisms are located intracellularly and present as bacteremias.

Tuberculosis (Chap. 143) Tuberculosis remains the most prominent cause of FUO. The diagnosis should be considered strongly in dark-skinned persons. Most of these patients do not have pulmonary tuberculosis but extrapulmonary or miliary disease involving the bones, lymph nodes, genital or urinary organs, peritoneum, or liver. Extrapulmonary or miliary tuberculosis may not be detectable by x-ray until late in the course of the disease. Because many of these patients are debilitated

and have overwhelming disease, the skin test may be negative. A positive skin reaction, on the other hand, does not prove that tuberculosis is causing the illness but requires that the diagnosis be kept in mind until another cause for the fever is found. Occasionally, fungous infections present as FUO, but most often specific organ involvement leads to the diagnosis.

Pyogenic infections UPPER ABDOMINAL INFECTIONS These commonly occur in the right upper quadrant and are related to the gallbladder or liver. Patients with such conditions tend to have mild jaundice, abnormality of liver function, high spiking fevers, and leukocytosis. Bacteremia, often due to enteric pathogens or *Salmonella*, is common. Liver scan is a most useful diagnostic tool, although exploratory laparotomy is often necessary for diagnosis and may achieve cure as well.

LOWER ABDOMINAL INFECTIONS Appendicitis with perforation and abscess formation is a remarkably common cause of prolonged fever, particularly in elderly patients. Persistent right lower quadrant physical signs along with x-ray abnormalities require surgical exploration. Diverticulitis is also common in elderly patients. In younger women, pelvic inflammatory disease may present as FUO.

RENAL INFECTIONS Ordinary pyelonephritis is rarely accompanied by prolonged fever; if pyrexia occurs in these patients, intrarenal or perinephric abscess should be considered. Ureter-

TABLE 10-1
Common disease entities in the United States causing prolonged fever

I Infections
  A Granulomatous infections
    1 Tuberculosis
    2 Deep-seated fungous infections
  B Pyogenic infections
    1 Upper abdominal infections
      a Cholecystitis (stone), empyema of gallbladder
      b Cholangitis
      c Liver abscess
      d Subhepatic abscess
      e Lesser sac abscess
    2 Lower abdominal infections
      a Diverticulitis
      b Appendicitis
    3 Pelvic inflammatory disease
    4 Urinary tract infections
      a Pyelonephritis (rare)
      b Intrarenal abscess
      c Perinephric abscess
      d Ureteral obstruction
      e Prostatic abscess
    5 Sinusitis
  C Bacterial endocarditis (acute and subacute)
  D Bacteremias without overt primary focus
    1 Meningococcemia
    2 Gonococcemia
    3 Vibriosis
    4 Listeriosis
    5 Brucellosis
    6 Coliform bacteremia in patients with cirrhosis
  E Viral, rickettsial, and chlamydial infections
    1 Infectious mononucleosis
    2 Cytomegalovirus
    3 Group B coxsackievirus diseases
    4 Q fever (including endocarditis)
    5 Psittacosis
  F Parasitic diseases
    1 Amebiasis
    2 Malaria
    3 Trichinosis
  G Spirochetal infections
    1 Leptospirosis
    2 Relapsing fever
II Neoplasms
  A Solid (localized)
    1 Kidney

    2 Lung
    3 Pancreas
    4 Liver
    5 Large bowel
    6 Atrial myxoma
  B Metastatic
    1 From gastrointestinal tract
    2 From lung, kidneys, bone
    3 Melanoma
  C Tumors of the reticuloendothelial system
    1 Lymphoma, Hodgkin's disease
    2 Leukemias
    3 Reticulum-cell sarcoma, multiple myeloma (rare)
  D Unclassified
    1 Unclassified lymphatic diseases [immunoblastic lymphadenopathy; lymphamatoid granulomatosis; mucocutaneous lymph node syndrome (children)]
    2 Diffuse sarcoma of bone
III Connective tissue disease
  A Rheumatic fever
  B Systemic lupus erythematosus
  C Rheumatoid arthritis (including Still's disease)
  D Temporal arteritis (polymyalgia rheumatica)
  E Hypersensitivity vasculitis
  F Periarteritis nodosa
  G Wegener's granulomatosis
IV Miscellaneous
  A Drug fever
  B Multiple pulmonary emboli
  C Sarcoidosis
  D Thyroiditis
  E Hemolytic states
  F Cryptic trauma with bleeding into enclosed space
  G Regional enteritis and Whipple's disease
  H Granulomatous hepatitis
  I Dissecting aneurysm (with or without infection)
V Metabolic and inherited diseases
  A Familial Mediterranean fever
  B Hypertriglyceridemia and hypercholesterolemia
  C Fabry's disease
VI Pseudogenic fevers
  A Habitual hyperthermia
  B Factitious fever
VII Periodic fevers (e.g., cyclic neutropenia)
VIII Thermoregulatory disorders
  IX Undiagnosed

al obstruction by either a mass of leukocytes or renal epithelium, as in papillary necrosis, may be accompanied by prolonged fever. Prostatic abscess should be considered in males. These patients may not have dysuria or rectal pain.

RETROPERITONEAL INFECTION Aneurysms that have become filled with organizing clot and debris may become infected. Enteric pathogens (including *Escherichia coli,* bacteroides, and *Salmonella*), have been isolated frequently from patients with such infections. Surgery is mandatory for both diagnosis and therapy. In addition, some patients with dissecting aneurysms have fever without superimposed infections.

Bacterial endocarditis In the classic subacute form of the disease, a heart murmur is nearly always present; therefore, absence of murmur largely eliminates this disease from consideration. The correct diagnosis is likely to be missed in middle-aged or elderly patients, in whom a heart murmur may not be given much weight. For example, an elderly patient with subacute bacterial endocarditis may first come to the physician's attention following the occurrence of a cerebral embolus and may be regarded as having had a hemorrhage or thrombosis because of arteriosclerosis. The best clinical practice is to culture the blood of *every* patient who has fever and a heart murmur. Bacterial endocarditis without cardiac murmurs is seen most frequently in intravenous drug users who develop infection on the tricuspid valve; every such person with fever should be assumed to have endocarditis until proved otherwise. In addition, antibiotics mask subacute bacterial endocarditis (SBE) because they often render the blood culture negative until they have been excreted or metabolized. For this reason, patients suspected of having SBE who have received antimicrobials should have blood cultures taken for several days after administration of the drugs is discontinued.

Bacteremia NEISSERIA Although rare, chronic meningococcemia (Chap. 118) is a well-known cause of prolonged fever. The arthralgia and rash of this disease are sufficiently evanescent to be missed. When this syndrome appears in a young woman, gonococcemia is much more likely (Chap. 119).

SALMONELLA (Chap. 123) Typhoid fever is not often a cause of prolonged fever of obscure origin because cultures of feces and blood will be positive and specific antibodies will be found in the serum. Other *Salmonella* organisms may, however, cause prolonged febrile illness and may present greater diagnostic difficulties. Repeated culture of the blood or bone marrow may yield the cause of this organism. Eventually, the infection may localize in a joint, pleural cavity, or another metastatic focus. Sometimes, salmonella bacteremia occurs spontaneously in patients with cirrhosis, although most often spontaneous bacteremia is due to *E. coli*. Serologic confirmation of a salmonella infection is sometimes helpful.

Brucellosis (Chap. 127) This infection should be considered primarily in farmers, veterinarians, or slaughterhouse workers. Arthralgia and myalgia are common, but arthritis is rare. These patients tend to have normal or depressed leukocyte counts, and their sedimentation rate is often normal. In active febrile disease the blood and bone marrow cultures are frequently positive and specific agglutinins are nearly always present in the serum.

Viral, rickettsial, and chlamydial infections These are rarely the cause of prolonged fevers, but occasionally patients with Epstein-Barr or cytomegalovirus infections may have febrile illnesses, which are often characterized by spontaneous remissions and exacerbations. Cytomegalovirus (with or without *Pneumocystis*) is becoming a progressively more common cause of prolonged fever in immunocompromised hosts. Psittacosis may look much like typhoid fever, and Q-fever endocarditis has been a particularly puzzling and lethal illness that must be treated both with antibiotics and valve replacement.

Parasitic diseases Amebiasis presents as an FUO, primarily in the form of liver abscess. The diagnosis of malaria demands a history of recent exposure.

NEOPLASMS Carcinomas and sarcomas Certain malignant processes are especially likely to cause fever. Notable are sarcomas involving bone or lymphoid tissue, hypernephroma, carcinoma of the pancreas, stomach, or colon, and primary or metastatic cancer of the liver. Occasionally, the clinical picture is strongly suggestive of pyogenic infection, with hectic fever, chills, sweats, and marked leukocytosis; and patients have been subjected to laparotomy with preoperative diagnoses such as empyema of the gallbladder, localized peritonitis, or liver abscess. An elevated alkaline phosphatase level and abnormal retention of Bromsulphalein accompanied by filling defects on a liver scan are important clues to intrahepatic malignancy or other infiltrative hepatic disease.

Hodgkin's disease and lymphomas Fever may be the principal symptom and only objective finding early in the course of Hodgkin's disease, especially when the principal involvement is in the abdominal viscera or retroperitoneal regions. Pel-Ebstein fever is seen in a minority of cases of Hodgkin's disease. The diagnosis of this disorder is usually made by biopsy or occasionally by lymphangiography or staging laparotomy.

Lymphoma-like syndromes Several disease entities have been described which are similar clinically and histologically to lymphoma but which may have a better prognosis, or respond differently to steroids and antitumor agents. Among these entities, all of which may present as FUOs, are immunoblastic lymphadenopathy, lymphadenoid granulomatosis, and, in children, the mucocutaneous lymph node syndrome (Kawasaki's disease). These diseases are discussed more fully in Chap. 55.

Leukemias It is not uncommon for acute leukemia to be mistaken for acute infection at the onset. The acute leukemias are nearly always accompanied by fever, sometimes as high as 105°F (40.6°C). The correct diagnosis is suggested by rapid development of anemia and characteristic changes in peripheral blood and bone marrow. Chronic lymphatic or granulocytic leukemia may be characterized by fever, but such fever is usually due to concomitant infection. Because of the typical changes in circulating leukocytes, fever does not often cause a diagnostic problem. Before it is assumed that fever in a patient with leukemia is due to the blood dyscrasia, infection must be ruled out by appropriate tests and cultures, and often attempts to treat the "most likely" pathogen must be made.

Atrial myxoma Patients with changing heart murmurs, peripheral embolic phenomena, and joint pains are usually suspected of having bacterial endocarditis, rheumatic fever, or occasionally some other connective tissue disease such as lupus erythematosus. In the face of persistence of these symptoms and signs without a positive diagnosis, echocardiography and, if the echocardiogram is positive, angiography should be performed with the possibility that an atrial myxoma may be responsible.

CONNECTIVE TISSUE DISEASE Rheumatic fever Though rheumatic fever is generally easy to detect in children, the diagnosis in adults may be difficult. Attention to unexplained heart murmurs, arrhythmias, pleural and pericardial rubs, arthralgias, and skin rashes should call the diagnosis to mind. These findings, along with an elevated antistreptolysin titer, C-reactive protein, and other acute phase reactants, contribute to the diagnosis. A prompt response to large doses of aspirin is characteristic of rheumatic fever and provides another diagnostic clue.

Systemic lupus erythematosus Fever is a common accompaniment of this disease. Of course, in the presence of arthritis, pleuritis, pericarditis, the classic malar rash, and renal failure, the diagnosis is easy. However, often these findings are absent and fever is the major manifestation. Biopsy of many organs, including the kidney, is generally not helpful; the diagnosis must be made by detecting a high titer of antinuclear or anti deoxyribonucleic (anti-DNA) antibody (Chap. 68).

Rheumatoid arthritis In its classic form, this disease is not difficult to recognize, but in certain patients who initially have FUO arthritis is absent early in the course of the illness; these patients have primarily fever, hepatosplenomegaly, lymphadenopathy, evanescent rashes, anemia, and leukocytosis. Joint changes do not appear until late in the disease. This disease often occurs in young adults, and may be considered the adult counterpart of juvenile rheumatoid disease. The diagnosis is made usually only after prolonged observation, in part because serologic tests for rheumatoid disease are characteristically negative. The prognosis is generally good, and patients respond well to anti-inflammatory drugs.

Temporal arteritis (polymyalgia rheumatica) This is a disease of elderly women who complain of fever, headache, and pain in the muscles and joints. Overt arthritis is unusual. At times, fever is the only symptom, and there are no abnormal physical findings. The sedimentation rate tends to be very rapid, and there may be anemia, leukocytosis, or eosinophilia. Occasionally, the temporal or occipital arteries are inflamed and tender, but usually they are normal. In either instance, the diagnosis must be made by temporal artery biopsy. There may be accompanying visual defects or blindness because of involvement of the retinal artery. This disease responds extremely well to steroids, which may be used as a therapeutic trial.

MISCELLANEOUS CAUSES OF FEVER **Sarcoidosis** Ordinarily fever is not characteristic of sarcoidosis, but it is prominent in a minority of cases, especially those characterized by arthralgia, hilar lymphadenopathy, and cutaneous lesions resembling erythema nodosum, or in those with extensive hepatic lesions. The diagnosis is suggested by lymphoid enlargement, ocular lesions, and hyperglobulinemia and is clinched by biopsy of skin, lymph nodes, muscle, and liver.

Regional enteritis Inflammatory lesions of the large and small intestine rarely present as FUO, but an occasional patient who has only fever, abdominal pain, and subtle changes in bowel habits will be found to have regional enteritis. Likewise, Whipple's disease may make itself known by fever, without arthritis or malabsorption.

Drug fever This is an important cause of cryptic fever; a careful history of drug intake should be taken in every patient with unexplained fever. Fever due to allergy to one of the antibiotics may become superimposed on the fever of the infection for which the drug was given, resulting in a very confused picture. Often fever is due to common drugs, including sulfonamides, arsenicals, iodides, thiouracils, barbiturates, and laxatives, especially those containing phenolphthalein. Any questions of drug fever can be resolved rapidly by discontinuing all medications. The diagnosis can be further substantiated by giving a test dose of the drug after fever has subsided, but this may result in a very unpleasant or even dangerous reaction.

Multiple pulmonary emboli Symptomless thrombosis of deep calf or pelvic veins may cause prolonged febrile illness either because of the thrombophlebitis or as a result of repeated small pulmonary emboli. These emboli may not be manifested by pleuritic pain or hemoptysis, but cough, dyspnea, and vague thoracic discomfort are likely to be present. Careful examination of the legs and repeated examination of the lungs should reveal the diagnosis. Sometimes these patients come to the physician's attention with a nephrotic syndrome due to renal vein thrombosis. Pelvic thrombophlebitis with or without pulmonary emboli is an important cause of FUO in postpartum patients.

Hemolytic episodes Most hemolytic diseases are characterized by bouts of fever, and acute hemolytic crises may give rise to shaking chills and marked elevations of temperature. The difficulty sometimes encountered in differentiating sickle cell disease from acute rheumatic fever is well known. The presence of these hemolytic disorders is suggested by the more rapid development of anemia than occurs in other febrile illnesses and by the usual accompaniment of reticulocytosis and jaundice. Fever is not characteristic of severe anemia due to external blood loss or of the anemia of uremia.

Cryptic trauma Perisplenic and perivesical hematomas, with or without superimposed infection, are among the sites in which accumulated old blood and pus have resulted in prolonged fever. A history of remote trauma is a helpful clue.

Granulomatous hepatitis This disease of unknown etiology is not an uncommon cause of FUO. It is probably a manifestation of hypersensitivity. Liver biopsy shows only nonspecific granulomas. The fever generally subsides spontaneously over a period of weeks or months. Sometimes defervescence can be achieved with steroids, but because the diagnosis of tuberculosis cannot be ruled out completely, patients in whom steroid therapy is given should also be given antituberculous medication.

Habitual hyperthermia Not infrequently, a patient while not appearing acutely ill has been subject to elevation of body temperature above the "normal" range level, i.e., his temperature has been in the range of 99.0 to 100.5°F (37.2 to 38°C). Prolonged low-grade fever may be a manifestation of serious illness, or it may be a matter of no real consequence. Possibly there are some persons whose "normal" temperatures are in this range. However, there is no certain way of identifying such individuals. The possibilities to be considered in such cases vary considerably according to the age groups concerned. A special problem termed *habitual hyperthermia* is encountered in young females. The patient may have temperatures ranging from 99.0 to 100.5°F (37.2 to 38.0°C) regularly or intermittently for years and also usually has a variety of complaints characteristic of psychoneurosis, such as fatigability, insomnia, bowel distress, vague aches, and headache. Prolonged careful study and observation fail to reveal evidence of organic disease. Unfortunately, many of these people go from physician to physician and are subjected to a variety of unpleasant, expensive, and even harmful tests, treatments, and operations. The diagnosis of this syndrome can be made with reasonable certainty after a suitable period of observation and study, and if the patient can be convinced of its validity, a real service will have been rendered.

In a patient past middle age, even low-grade fever should always be regarded as a probable indication of organic disease. The possibilities to be considered in this age group are the same as those discussed earlier under "Prolonged Febrile Illness."

Factitious fever Occasionally, patients will produce purposeful false elevations in temperature. Usually these patients are young women, many of whom are allied health professionals. They fall into two groups—one infects itself with bacteria or other contaminated materials and a second finds a way to cause the thermometer to register higher than the true temperature. If malingering is suspected, all that is necessary to prove it is to repeat the temperature determination immediately after a high reading has been obtained, with someone remaining at the bedside while the thermometer is in place. Other clues to false elevations in the temperature are a dissociation between pulse and temperature, absence of the normal diurnal variation in temperature, and excessively high fevers [greater than 106°F (41.1°C) in adults] and the absence of chills, sweats, or tachycardia. These patients fall into the psychiatric diagnostic category of "borderline syndrome," a state between neurosis and psychosis, in which the prognosis is guarded. Others, mostly young girls, falsify their temperatures to ask for psychiatric help and do well with psychotherapy.

Metabolic causes of fever These include familial Mediterranean fever, hypertriglyceridemia and hypercholesterolemia, Fabry's disease, and, rarely, gout, thyrotoxicosis, and Addison's disease.

Thermoregulatory disorders Rare patients have fever due to an abnormality in their temperature-regulating mechanism. They may be febrile without any other cause or may have exaggerated responses in temperature during the course of other fever-producing diseases. The diagnosis is made by exclusion. Some patients have responded to chlorpromazine.

Cyclic neutropenia See Chap. 56.

DIAGNOSTIC PROCEDURES IN FEVER

With so large a number of possibilities, it is obvious that no single plan can be outlined for the systematic study of every problem in unexplained fever. In any given patient, the history, physical examination, and, most importantly, epidemiologic setting must determine the diagnostic approach. If the features suggest infectious disease, the main dependence will be upon bacteriologic and immunologic methods, whereas when a person in the "cancer age group" has an obscure febrile disorder, the best chance of early diagnosis may lie in x-ray studies, scans, and biopsy.

HISTORY Careful attention to the patient's past history and the chronologic development of symptoms may provide important leads. Places of recent residence, contact with domestic or wild animals and birds, preceding acute infectious diseases such as diarrheal illness or boils, and contact with persons with tuberculosis may provide clues to infection. Localizing symptoms may provide a lead to the affected organ system.

PHYSICAL EXAMINATION Careful search is made for skin lesions and for petechial hemorrhages in the ocular fundi, conjunctivas, nail beds, and skin. The lymph nodes are carefully palpated, with special attention to the supraclavicular, axillary, and epitrochlear areas. The finding of a heart murmur may be important. Detection of an abdominal mass may be the first lead to the diagnosis of neoplastic disease. Palpable enlargement of the spleen suggests infection, leukemia, or lymphoma and points away from a diagnosis of solid tumors. Enlargement of the liver and spleen suggests lymphoma, leukemia, chronic infection, or cirrhosis. A large liver without a palpable spleen points to liver abscess or metastatic cancer. The rectum and the female pelvic organs may reveal masses or abscesses; the testicles may reveal teratoma or tuberculosis.

LABORATORY TESTS Useful examinations include:

1 Cultures of blood, bone marrow (*Brucella* or *Salmonella*), or other body fluids.
2 Serum enzymes, particularly *alkaline phosphatase* and corroborating enzymes such as 5′-nucleotidase and enzymes that measure hepatocellular function, and serum and urinary amylase.
3 Blood smears for abnormal morphology of red or white blood cells or platelets, or for demonstration of parasites.
4 Bone marrow examination for tumor cells, granulomas, lupus erythematosus cells, and abnormal red or white blood cells. Bone marrow biopsy is superior to aspiration for detection of granulomas and tumor cells.
5 Immunologic tests, i.e., antistreptolysin O titers, and other acute-phase reactants, antinuclear and related antibodies, latex fixation tests, and a variety of febrile agglutinins.

ROENTGENOGRAMS The following should be considered:

1 Chest films, which need to be repeated at intervals.
2 Bone x-rays are useful for detecting foci of osteomyelitis or primary or metastatic bone tumors.
3 Intravenous urograms are helpful in finding tumors of the kidney or perinephric or intrarenal abscesses. However, if a renal tumor is suspect on clinical grounds, a negative intravenous pyelogram does not rule out the diagnosis, and renal scan and aortogram should be performed.
4 Abdominal aortography is useful for diagnosing tumors of the kidney, retroperitoneal mass lesions, and, if selective arterial catheterization is performed, tumors of the liver, pancreas, and gut.
5 Intravenous or transhepatic cholangiograms may be helpful in delineating right upper quadrant pathologic changes if the patient is not jaundiced.
6 Visualization of the gallbladder, common bile duct, hepatic ducts, and pancreas may be best accomplished by instilling contrast medium through a flexible endoscope following cannulation of the ampulla of Vater (endoscopic retrograde choledochopancreatography).
7 Echocardiograms should be performed to screen for atrial myxoma; if positive or suggestive, they should be confirmed with angiography.
8 Lymphangiograms are helpful in the diagnosis of abdominal or retroperitoneal lymphomas and may be the only abnormality in these disorders.
9 Upper gastrointestinal x-rays are rarely useful; films of the small intestine may provide clues to Whipple's disease or regional enteritis, and a barium enema may show diverticulitis or tumor.

ULTRASONOGRAPHY This technique has come into vogue to detect abdominal, renal, retroperitoneal, or pelvic mass lesions. Both false-positive and false-negative results are common. Radioactive scanning techniques are usually superior in providing anatomic clues.

RADIOACTIVE SCANS *The liver/spleen scan is the single most useful test in the diagnosis of disease in the right upper quadrant.*

Lung scans may reveal pulmonary emboli, and simultaneous liver and lung scans are useful in delineating subphrenic abscess. Bone scans may detect osseous metastases more readily than x-rays. Renal scans are helpful in the diagnosis of hypernephroma. Gallium scan may be useful in identifying a cryptic focus of infection or infiltration but is rarely the only means for doing so.

There has not been sufficient experience to evaluate the role of total body computerized tomography (CT scan) in the diagnosis of FUO. It is probably most useful in delineating retroperitoneal lesions.

BIOPSIES Often the best means of definitive diagnosis is a biopsy.

1 Bone marrow biopsy may be helpful not only in clarifying the histologic nature of the marrow but also for occasional demonstration of other disease processes such as metastatic carcinoma or granulomas, and for culture.
2 Needle biopsy of the liver is a very helpful procedure and can be done with reasonable safety. It may lead to the diagnosis not only in primary or metastatic disease of the liver, but also may reveal existence of other diseases such as histoplasmosis, schistosomiasis, brucellosis, tuberculosis, sarcoidosis or lymphoma, or granulomatous hepatitis. There has been some controversy about the value of liver biopsy, but it remains very useful when the enzymes indicating infiltrative liver disease are elevated.
3 Lymph node biopsy is helpful in the diagnosis of many diseases, including the lymphomas, metastatic cancer, tuberculosis, and mycotic infections. However, inguinal nodes are notoriously unsatisfactory for biopsy and are too frequently chosen because of their easy accessibility. Axillary, cervical, and supraclavicular nodes are much more likely to yield helpful information, and the node excised need not necessarily be large.
4 Skin and muscle biopsy may be of assistance in the recognition of dermatomyositis, periarteritis nodosa, sarcoidosis, and trichinosis.
5 Lung biopsy may be performed with a needle under direct fluoroscopy or through the bronchoscope. It is of value primarily in solitary mass lesions; diffuse pulmonary disease is rarely diagnosed by needle biopsy; instead, open lung biopsy should be performed.
6 Renal biopsy is rarely helpful, even in connective tissue disease.
7 Pleural and pericardial biopsy with the hook needle technique should be attempted in the presence of effusion.
8 Biopsy of the temporal artery should be considered in elderly women with fever, anemia, hypoalbuminemia, and a rapid sedimentation rate, even though the temporal arteries are not palpable.
9 Biopsy of other accessible masses should not be neglected.

EXPLORATORY LAPAROTOMY Exploratory laparotomy has been advocated as the most definitive diagnostic maneuver in connection with FUO but is valuable only when other investigations including history, physical examination, x-rays, and laboratory data point to the abdomen as a possible source of disease. The clues to intraabdominal disease are often subtle, but they are present nonetheless. Blind exploration of the abdomen simply because the diagnosis is obscure is poor practice. Moreover, often the tissue that is obtained at laparotomy could just as easily have been sampled by external biopsy techniques.

THERAPEUTIC TRIALS It is common practice to give a trial of antibiotic therapy to patients with unidentified febrile disorders. Occasionally, this kind of marksmanship is effective, but in general, "blind" therapy does more harm than good. Undesirable features include drug toxicity, superinfection due to resistant pathogenic bacteria, and interference with accurate diagnosis by cultural methods. Furthermore, a coincidental fall in temperature not due to therapy is likely to be interpreted as response to treatment, with the conclusion that an infectious disease is present. If therapeutic trials are instituted, they should be as specific as possible. Examples are *isoniazid* or *ethambutol* for tuberculosis; *aspirin* for rheumatic fever; *metronidazole* for hepatic amebiasis; *penicillin* and *gentamicin* for enterococcal endocarditis; and *chloramphenicol* for *Salmonella* bacteremia. Shotgun broad-spectrum therapy is contraindicated, because it is unlikely to yield useful information and is more likely to be toxic. Similarly, steroid therapy is often nonspecific. These drugs do have an antipyretic effect and produce euphoria in many persons, but the apparent improvement induced by them tells little about the nature of the underlying disease. Temporal arteritis is an exception to this statement.

PROGNOSIS IN FUO The intelligent application of appropriate diagnostic maneuvers should provide the answer in approximately 90 to 95 percent of patients with prolonged obscure febrile illness. Fortunately, most of the remainder recover spontaneously. Because many of the procedures involved in the diagnosis of FUO are painful, time-consuming, and expensive, it is essential that they be chosen with thoughtfulness and care.

REFERENCES

ADUAN RP et al: Factitious fever and self-induced infection. Ann Intern Med 90:230, 1979

BAKER RR et al: The value of exploratory laparotomy in fever of undetermined etiology. Johns Hopkins Med J 125:159, 1969

BUJAK JS et al: Juvenile rheumatoid arthritis presenting in the adult as fever of unknown origin. Medicine 52:431, 1973

DINARELLO CA, WOLFF SM: Pathogenesis of fever in man. N Engl J Med 298:607, 1978

GHOSE MK et al: Arteritis of the aged (giant cell arteritis) and fever of unexplained origin. Am J Med 60:429, 1976

JACOBY GA, SWARTZ MN: Fever of undetermined origin. N Engl J Med 289:1407, 1973

MITCHELL DP et al: Fever of unknown origin: Assessment of the value of percutaneous liver biopsy. Arch Intern Med 137:1001, 1977

MURRAY HW et al: Fever with dissecting aneurysm of the aorta. Am J Med 61:140, 1976

PETERSDORF RG, BEESON PB: Fever of unexplained origin: Report of 100 cases. Medicine 40:1, 1961

———, WALLACE JF: Fever of unknown origin, in *Diagnostic Approaches to Presenting Syndromes*, JA Barondess (ed). Baltimore, Williams & Wilkins, 1971, p 301

SIMON HB, WOLFF SM: Granulomatous hepatitis and prolonged fever of unknown origin: A study of 13 patients. Medicine 52:1, 1973

VICKERY DM, QUINNELL RK: Fever of unknown origin: An algorithmic approach. JAMA 238:2183, 1977

WOLFF SM et al: Unusual etiologies of fever and their evaluation. Annu Rev Med 26:277, 1975

section 3 | Alterations in nervous function

INTRODUCTION

RAYMOND D. ADAMS

The symptoms and signs of nervous disease are probably the most frequent and complex in all of medicine. To present a lucid exposition of all the many diverse neurologic manifestations is difficult in part because the more complex phenomena may be viewed from either a neurologic or psychologic standpoint. The neurologic physician is inclined to assume that all are manifestations of diseases of the nervous system. The psychiatrically minded physician thinks of many of them in terms of abnormal psychologic reactions. Naturally, our bias is more toward the neurologic for it draws on all the accepted principles of medicine and biologic science. But each extreme can be criticized. The aim, therefore, throughout this section is to avoid entanglement in such theoretical problems, to describe as accurately as possible all the more common expressions of disordered nervous function, and to offer the most generally accepted explanations in terms of anatomy, physiology, biochemistry, and psychology. However, in discussing some of the more abstruse, complex cerebral derangements, a particular effort will be made to present both the neurologic and psychologic conceptions, for the latter have received much attention in recent years.

To provide an initial orientation toward the broad field of neuropsychiatry, it is helpful to think of the subject matter as divisible into two main categories: diseases of the nervous system and disorders based on abnormal psychologic reactions. By *disease* we mean any condition which produces a visible lesion in the nervous system or in which there is actual or presumptive evidence of such. By *abnormal psychologic reaction* we mean a disorder in psychic life and behavior occasioned by abnormal life experiences and maladjustments in social relations. A brain tumor, delirium tremens, and a confusional psychosis would be considered examples of disease; unusually protracted grief, unexplained anxiety, and a character disorder would fall in the category of a reactive psychologic abnormality or one due to the formation of unusual personality traits after repeated psychic traumas and environmental stresses. All diseases of the neuromuscular apparatus, spinal cord, brainstem, and cerebellum and many of those of the cerebrum, fall within the province of neurology, whereas other of the cerebral diseases (especially if they disturb intellect, emotions, and behavior) are of concern to both neurology and psychiatry, and all abnormal psychologic reactions are within the province of psychiatry.

Many nervous disorders are not so easily classified. A psychopathic personality, an anxiety neurosis, or a depression could be considered either as a manifestation of a disease of the brain or an abnormal psychologic reaction. Schizophrenia and manic-depressive psychosis would presently be classified as genetically determined diseases by neurologists and many psychiatrists even though a lesion has never been demonstrated by the conventional techniques of pathology. Other psychiatrists believe psychogenic factors to be important and therefore we have listed these two psychoses as reactive states.

Our objective in the early part of this book is to single out all the common symptoms and signs of diseases of the nervous system as well as the manifestations of certain abnormal psychologic states. In the section on diseases of organ systems, we shall present in one section all the common diseases of the nervous system. The major psychiatric disorders will be subdivided. The neuroses will be presented in Chap. 11 and the two major psychoses, manic-depressive disease and schizophrenia, in Chap. 25.

There are two areas of neuropsychiatry which in a way are even more controversial—the psychosomatic diseases and the sociopathic states. Included under psychosomatic disorders are such conditions as Raynaud's disease, peptic ulcer, ulcerative colitis, bronchial asthma, dysmenorrhea, hypertension, hyperthyroidism, neurodermatitis, rheumatoid arthritis, migraine, and paroxysmal tachycardia. These diseases have been set apart on the basis of three lines of evidence: (1) a large series of observations which have revealed that the malfunctioning organ is excited and possibly deranged by strong emotion and restored to relative normality by tranquility and feelings of security; (2) the discovery in the biographies of such patients of an inordinately high incidence of resentment, hostility, suppressed emotionality, etc.; (3) a demonstrable relationship between onset and exacerbation of the disease and disturbing and frustrating incidents in the patient's life. These psychosomatic diseases differ from the psychoneuroses in that they exhibit different symptoms, are of longer duration, have a known pathologic basis and often a known cause (e.g., allergy in asthma, atopic dermatitis, and hay fever). Finally, the incidence of frank neuroses in this group of diseases is no greater than in the population at large, and neurotics are not more liable to them than normal individuals. For many reasons, not the least of which is that a psychogenic basis has never been proved in any of these diseases, we have chosen to present the relevant facts in the organ systems involved. They are not discussed further in the sections on neurology and psychiatry.

The sociopathies which include those individuals who from childhood exhibit impulsivity, aggressiveness, and various antisocial behaviors (running away, truancy, repeated thefts, alcohol and drug abuse, etc.) involve so many sociologic, educational, economic, and political factors that they fall almost beyond the orbit of medicine. While a medical position is often of value, particularly if there are questions of nervous disease or major psychiatric disorder, there is no clear evidence that medical opinion contributes significantly to the understanding and management of these problems. For these and other reasons such sociopathic states are also eliminated from this section of the book.

NERVOUSNESS, ANXIETY, DEPRESSION, PERSONALITY DISORDERS, AND NEUROSES

RAYMOND D. ADAMS

The majority of patients who enter a physician's office or hospital will admit to being or having been nervous, anxious, or depressed. The stress of contemporary life or the prospect of real or imaginary illness is thought to induce these reactions. If they stand in clear relationship to a stressful event or situation, such as worry over economic reverses or grief over the death of a loved one, such states can be accepted as normal. Only when excessively intense and uncontrollable or when accompanied by obscure derangements of visceral function do they become the basis for medical consultation.

Such problems become more abstruse when similar symptoms occur in persons who are not being subjected to immediately stressful or unhappy experiences, and awareness of such threatening situations, if it exists at all, lies buried in the subconscious mind of the patient. One may assume that it either has been suppressed from consciousness or is part of an elaborate subjective interpretation of which the patient is unaware. The relationship between social stimulus and prevailing anxiety or nervousness, if there is any such association, can then be discovered only by gentle probings by the psychologically sophisticated physician. But once the connection is established and the problem dealt with realistically, the symptoms allegedly become understandable and disappear. One recognizes here all the elements of a *psychoneurotic reaction*. The line of separation between the latter and normal emotional reactions is admittedly ambiguous.

There is still another category of nervousness, anxiety, and depression wherein the emotional states are intense and prolonged, and may occur in cycles, but again without obvious explanation. Such states may overwhelm the individual and cause derangement of all that individual's activities. Delving into the unconscious mind or studying lifelong reaction patterns fails to reveal a plausible psychogenesis. One recognizes here all the elements of a more complete, pervasive *psychotic reaction*. In many such instances a genetic factor appears to operate, and the features of the illness are so stereotyped as to indicate a disease of the parts of the nervous system which control the affective, emotional life. Yet a consistent biochemical change in the blood or brain tissue has not been found, and no lesion has been discerned. Treatment must proceed empirically, along nonpsychologic lines.

The problem confronting every physician is to recognize all these nuances of reaction, personality disorder, and disease, which obviously shade into one another, and to determine to what extent they figure in the medical condition of the patient. Some type of therapeutic maneuver must then be initiated, varying from simple reassurance and realistic management of existing personal difficulties, to suppression of symptoms by drugs. Often, referral to a psychiatrist is necessary for more expert management, including electrotherapy.

In this chapter we shall first consider the cardinal features of these common reactive states and then the personality and character disorders from which they are believed to arise, together with currently accepted views of their origins. The major neuroses of which they may be a part are discussed further on, and the psychoses are discussed in Chap. 25.

NERVOUSNESS By this vague term the lay person usually refers to a state of restlessness, tension, uneasy apprehension, irritability, or hyperexcitability. But it may connote other states, such as thoughts of suicide, fear of killing one's child or spouse, a distressing hallucination, a paranoid idea, or a frankly hysterical outburst. Careful inquiry as to what the patient means when complaining of nervousness is always a necessary first step.

In its most common signification, a period of nervousness may represent no more than a psychic and behavioral state in which an organism is maximally challenged by difficult personal problems, and there are periods in normal life when this is more likely to happen. For example, adolescence rarely passes without its period of turmoil as the person attempts emancipation from parental dominance or adjustment to demands of a scholastic or social nature. The menses are regularly accompanied by increased tension and moodiness, and, of course, the menarche and menopause are other critical periods. Some persons, because of early patterning or character formation, claim to have been nervous in all their social relationships throughout life; one should then suspect a psychoneurosis or unstable character formation or an oncoming psychosis, even though performance within the family unit, at school, and at work were adequate. When nervousness is a recent development, one must consider such conditions as an upheaval in personal affairs, the first attack or exacerbation of a psychoneurosis, an endogenous depression, an endocrine disease (hyperthyroidism, adrenal corticism, or corticosteroid therapy), or withdrawal from a sedative drug (alcohol, barbiturate). Some patients complain of a nervousness that attends or follows the onset of a medical or neurologic disease; and it would then appear to be secondary, occasioned by fear of disability, dependency, or death.

Nervousness, even in its simplest form, is reflected in many important activities of the human organism. There are often a mild somberness of mood and an increased tendency to tears and anger (irritability). Fatigue that bears no proper relationship to activity and rest is frequent, and sleep is often disturbed, as are eating and drinking habits. Headaches may increase in number and intensity. There is a tendency to sweat, tremble, be aware of heart action, feel a bit "queer in the head" or giddy, have an upset stomach, and urinate more often, though these recognized autonomic accompaniments of anxiety are seldom as conspicuous as in anxiety neurosis. Thus, it would appear that nervousness and anxiety constitute a graded series of reactions, the latter in many instances being only a more intense and protracted form of nervousness.

ANXIETY Anxiety is "the fundamental phenomenon and central problem of the neurosis . . . a nodal point, linking up all kinds of most important questions, a riddle of which the solution must cast a flood of light upon our whole mental life" (Freud). From the viewpoint of the social historian, anxiety is said to be "the most prominent mental characteristic of Occidental civilization" (Willoughby). These comments should inform the reader of the broad implications of this reaction.

The more strictly medical meaning of the term *anxiety*, and the one used in this chapter, is a state characterized by a subjective feeling of fear and uneasy anticipation (apprehension), usually with a definite topical content and associated with the physiologic accompaniments of strong emotion, i.e., breathlessness, choking sensation, palpitation, restlessness, increased muscular tension, tightness in the chest, giddiness, trembling, sweating, and flushing. By *topical content* is meant the idea, person, or object about which the person is anxious. The several vasomotor and visceral alterations that underlie the symptoms are mediated through the autonomic nervous system, particularly the sympathetic part of it, and involve also the thyroid and adrenal glands.

Forms of anxiety Anxiety is manifested in acute episodes, each lasting a few minutes and clearly related to a disturbing event in the patient's life; or it may represent an inexplicable protracted state that may last for weeks, months, or years. There may be a succession of acute *attacks,* or *panics* as they are called; the patient is plunged into an inexplicable mental state and fears death, loss of reason or self-control, and insanity, or feels that he or she may commit some horrible crime. The patient is breathless, has a racing heart, chokes, sweats, trembles, and feels gastric distress and anorexia. In a persistent, protracted state the patient experiences lesser and fluctuating degrees of nervousness, restlessness, irritability, fatigue, insomnia, intolerance of physical exertion, and pressure or tension headaches. Discrete anxiety attacks and chronic states of anxiety merge into one another.

Episodic anxiety without disorder of mood (i.e., depression) is usually classified as *anxiety neurosis.* The chronic form with prominent exercise intolerance is called *neurocirculatory asthenia.* Anxiety may, however, be combined with other somatic symptoms in hysteria and may be the restraining factor in *phobic neurosis.* Persistent anxiety with insomnia, lassitude, and fatigue, regardless of mood, should always raise suspicion of a *depressive psychosis,* especially if it begins late in life. Panic attacks are said to occur at the beginning of a schizophrenic illness, but this is rare in our experience. Both anxiety and depression are prominent features of the syndrome of posttraumatic nervous instability (see Chap. 366).

Thus, the differential diagnosis of an anxiety state requires that the physician consider all the major syndromes in psychiatry. Often it is but one component of a far more serious condition, one which may result in suicide or some other antisocial act. Also, without the psychic counterparts of fear and apprehension, the visceral symptoms alone should arouse suspicion of thyrotoxicosis, epilepsy, corticosteroid overdosage, pheochromocytoma, hypoglycemia, or menopause.

DEPRESSION (UNHAPPINESS, GLOOM, AND GRIEF) There are few persons who do not experience periods of discouragement and despair, and these periods become manifestly more frequent in modern society where individual freedom is constrained and one's impulses must be inhibited. As with nervousness and anxiety, depression of mood that is appropriate to a given situation in life is a natural, healthy reaction and seldom is the basis of medical complaint. The patient tends to seek help only when grief or unhappiness becomes uncontrollable. But there are numerous instances in which the patient is miserable, unhappy, and hopeless for reasons which are not apparent. Many of the symptoms are interpreted as ill health, being so similar to those of many disease states as to bring the patient first to the internist. Sometimes another disease is found (such as chronic hepatitis, brucellosis, or postinfluenzal asthenia) or infections in which chronic fatigue is confused with depression, but often an endogenous depression is itself the essential problem. Since the risk of suicide is not inconsiderable, if the illness is mistaken for another or overlooked as a complication, an error in diagnosis may be life-threatening.

Information about depression, like that about all psychiatric syndromes, is gained from three sources: the history obtained from the patient, the history obtained from the family or close friend, and the findings on examination.

From the patient and family it is learned that the patient has been "feeling unwell," "low in spirits," "blue," "glum," "unhappy," or "morbid." There has been a change in emotional reactions of which the patient may not be fully aware. Activities that were formerly pleasurable are no longer so. Often, however, change in mood is less conspicuous than reduction in psychic and physical energy. Fatigue is almost invariable; not uncommonly, it is worse in the morning after a night of restless sleep. The words "loss of pep," "weak," "tired," "no energy to work," "my job seems more trying and difficult" appear in the language of the patient. The outlook is pessimistic. The patient is preoccupied with uncontrollable worry over trivialities. With excessive worry the ability to think with accustomed efficiency is reduced; there is complaint that the mind does not function properly, of being forgetful and unable to concentrate. If the patient is naturally of suspicious nature, paranoid tendencies may assert themselves.

Particularly troublesome in medical diagnosis is the patient's tendency to become hypochondriacal about associated diseases. Indeed, most cases formerly diagnosed as hypochondriasis are now regarded as depression. Pain from whatever cause—a stiff joint, a toothache, fleeting abdominal pains, or other troubles such as constipation, frequency of urination, insomnia, pruritus, burning tongue, weight loss—may become an obsessive focus of complaint. The patient passes from doctor to doctor seeking relief from symptoms that would not trouble the average person, and no amount of reassurance relieves this state of mind. The nervousness and anxiety felt by many of these persons may be obscured by their preoccupation with visceral functions.

When examined, the patient's facial expression is often plaintive, troubled, pained, or anguished. The attitude and manner betray a prevailing mood of depression, discouragement, and despondency. In other words, the affective response, which is the outward expression of feeling, is consistent with the depressed mood. During the interview the patient's eyes may be tearful, or he or she may cry openly. In some there is a kind of immobility of the face that mimics parkinsonism, though others are restless and agitated (pacing the floor, wringing their hands, etc.). Occasionally the patient will smile, but the smile impresses one as more of a social gesture than an expression of feeling.

The stream of speech, from which the ideational content is determined, is slow. At times the patient is mute and speaks neither spontaneously nor in response to questions. Again there may be a long pause between questions and answers. The latter are brief and may be monosyllabic. There is a paucity of ideas. The retardation extends to all topics of conversation and affects movement of limbs as well. The most extreme forms of decreased motor activity, rarely seen in the medical clinic, border on stupor.

Content of speech is found to be abnormal if examined carefully. Conversation is replete with pessimistic thoughts, fears, expressions of unworthiness, inadequacy, inferiority, and sometimes guilt. In severe depressions bizarre ideas, delusions about the body ("blood drying up," "bowels are blocked with cement," "I am half dead") may be expressed.

Etiology and mechanism (see Chap. 25) Like anxiety, depression is a state which may stand as a simple reaction to an environmental circumstance, a form of neurosis or a major psychosis. It is the writer's belief that depression is one of the most commonly overlooked diagnoses in clinical medicine. Part of the trouble is with the word itself, which implies being unhappy about something. The persistent or recurrent endogenous depression or involutional depression should be suspected in all chronic states of ill health, hypochondriasis, multiple complaints involving many organ systems, disability that exceeds manifest signs of a medical disease, neurasthenia, and suicide attempts. Inasmuch as recovery is the rule, the suicide is a tragedy for which the medical profession must often share responsibility.

TABLE 11-1
Personality disorders

Type of disorder	Characteristics
1 Paranoid	Chronic wariness, suspiciousness, litigiousness; lack of insight or humor; tendency to blame others; sense of self-importance and entitlement
2 Cyclothymic	Recurring periods of depression and elation not readily explained by circumstances; severe moodiness
3 Schizoid	Isolation, seclusiveness, secretiveness; discomfort in relationships; often eccentric and lacking in energy; few friends
4 Explosive	Outbursts of rage and aggression not in keeping with usual personality, often in response to minor provocation; sense of loss of control followed by regret
5 Obsessive-compulsive	Chronic worries about standards; excessive concern about self-image; tension in relationships, leading to isolation; inability to relax and excessive inhibitions; predisposition to depression
6 Hysterical	Immaturity, histrionic behavior, sexualization of relationships, low frustration tolerance, and shallow interpersonal ties; dependency
7 Asthenic	Chronic weakness, easy fatigability, sense of vulnerability, poor response to stress, little ambition or aggression
8 Passive-aggressive	Obstructive behavior, stubbornness, intentional errors or omissions; intolerance of authority with struggles over control, often creating difficulties in medical settings; externalization of conflicts and blaming others for untoward events
9 Inadequate	Chronic inability to meet ordinary life demands in the absence of mental retardation; severe dependency on others; tendency to become institutionalized or to become dependent on institutions
10 Antisocial	Unsocialized or antisocial behavior in conflict with society; selfishness, callousness, impulsiveness, lack of loyalty, and little guilt; frustration tolerance is low; tendency to blame others and have a long history of interpersonal and social difficulties and arrests

PERSONALITY DISORDERS When the above nervous states occur repeatedly and without explanation, there is likelihood that they derive from chronic lifelong patterns of maladaptation and peculiarities of character. Psychiatrists speak of such states as *borderline character disorders*, implying that they account for the ways different individuals cope with life.

The origins of these peculiarities of character are obscure. To avoid the dispute as to whether they are conditioned by early life experiences or are the product of genetic factors, the adjective "constitutional" is sometimes used in reference to them. The formal types of neuroses are believed to originate in these personality disorders.

If one examines Table 11-1, the specific personality types clearly shade into particular neuroses, and one wonders if they are not merely milder forms of neurosis, differing from the latter in that they less frequently present as medical problems. Personality disturbances are important to recognize, however, for the perceptive physician must take account of them as well as of the related neuroses in the diagnosis of disease and the management of patients with medical illnesses. Such patients may sabotage a needed diagnostic test or therapy. Actually, it is the physician's knowledge of human nature and skill in the care of these difficult and often exasperating patients that enable him or her to be the leader of a therapeutic team.

NEUROSES When nervousness, anxiety, and depression are persistently or episodically joined with various combinations of irrational fears, obsessive thoughts, compulsions, lassitude and fatigue, insomnia, preoccupation with trivial symptoms, and a number of different somatic disturbances for which no cause can be found, the condition is properly called *neurosis* or *psychoneurosis*.

The neuroses represent a specific group of mental disorders appearing in adolescence and early to middle adulthood in individuals who have already achieved relatively adequate mental function. Since these disorders have no demonstrable organic basis, they are often called "functional," a term that is incorrect, for all functional disorders must have a physical basis. In all instances the neurotic patients are normally alert and correctly oriented, have considerable insight into their troubles, and manifest *"unimpaired reality testing,"* meaning that they do not confuse their subjective experiences and fantasies with external reality, more explicitly that they are not deluded and do not suffer hallucinations. The personality remains organized, and conduct is within socially acceptable limits. Neurotic patients can usually study, work, and function in the family and social circle even though assailed by doubts, loss of self-confidence, and despondency. They know that the troublesome symptoms originate within the mind, but are incapable of overcoming them by force of will, and hence they feel ashamed and inadequate. In these several ways neuroses are to be distinguished from the more pervasive and disorganizing psychoses.

Within this multitude of symptoms certain natural clusterings occur, and these are the basis of the classification in Table 11-2, which has been sanctioned by an international committee of psychiatrists.

In general medicine we have frequently encountered types 1 to 4, whereas type 6 (neurasthenia) and type 8 (hypochondriasis) will usually prove to be manifestations of a depressive state. Type 5 (depressive neurosis) will be difficult to distinguish from the nonpsychotic depression. Type 7 (depersonal-

TABLE 11-2
The neuroses

Type of neurosis	Characteristics
1 Anxiety neurosis	Episodic diffuse anxiety in attacks or waves; somatic complaints such as palpitations, paresthesias, weakness, dizziness; pessimism and irritability
2 Hysterical neurosis:	
a Conversion type	Physical symptoms involving voluntary musculature and sensory system, such as paradoxic paralyses, seizures, sensory deficits, and pain; attitude of indifference
b Dissociative type	Alterations in consciousness and sense of identity, such as fugue states, amnesias, somnambulism; anxiety not evident
3 Phobic neurosis	Intense irrational fears of objects or situations; anxiety attacks may occur with corresponding physical symptoms
4 Obsessive-compulsive neurosis	Persistent or intrusive thoughts, often distressing in content, and uncontrollable minor acts, often to expiate, cleanse, or counteract evil; depression and guilt are prominent; preoccupations with disease may occur
5 Depressive neurosis	Episodic excessive self-criticism, low self-esteem, and lowered vitality, often accompanied by physical complaints
6 Neurasthenic neurosis	Weakness, fatigability, exhaustion, with low self esteem but little self-criticism
7 Depersonalization neurosis	Feelings of unreality and estrangement from self, body, and surroundings; panic may occur
8 Hypochondriacal neurosis	Morbid preoccupations with bodily processes and diseases, accompanied by multiple physical complaints; anxiety and agitation may occur; depression is common

ization neurosis), a relatively rare condition in the author's experience, probably is a form of depression or pseudoneurotic schizophrenia.

For clarity of concept the term neurosis should be reserved for these particular groupings of symptoms and signs, and not loosely applied to individuals who are transiently upset by some circumstance or are emotional or eccentric. Each type may occur in relatively pure form, but often there are overlappings of symptoms. Anxiety, for example, may occur in pure form with a depressive reaction, in hysteria, and with phobic states. These combinations of neuroses are called "mixed neuroses."

The diagnosis of a neurosis depends largely on a thorough history that covers much of the medical biography of the patient. The physical examination seldom yields abnormal findings. Moreover, there is no laboratory test to which one can turn for final confirmation of diagnosis, which is true also of manic-depressive psychosis and schizophrenia. Subjective impressions supersede objective data, reducing accuracy of diagnosis.

Most psychiatrists hold the opinion that the neuroses have their genesis in the early life experiences that mold character and personality; that is, the neurosis stems from a neurotic character (hysterical, hypochondriacal, etc.). Reich and Kelly, who wrote the chapter on neuroses in the eighth edition of this textbook, regard them as psychologic decompensations of a neurotic personality that are basically maladaptive and inappropriate to the level of stress. The form of the neurotic episode is believed to be determined by the personality structure of the patient. But such explanations do not seem relevant to the most frequent of all the neuroses, the anxiety neurosis, which may strike a well-balanced person at any time during life. Furthermore, the stress of urban living conditions seems not to be a factor in the development of neurosis, for surveys of urban and rural populations show approximately the same incidence of neurotic behavior. The lifetime prevalence, regardless of social environment, is approximately 15 percent.

Neuroses vary in severity from mild periods of uneasiness that may not come to medical attention to episodes of severe, incapacitating illnesses that may require hospitalization. Since neuroses are frequent and may masquerade as medical illnesses with which the internist must contend, or complicate certain disease states, the following descriptive data should be fixed in mind.

Anxiety neurosis When anxiety occurs in pure form and is persistent and without explanation as a reaction, whether in an acute self-limiting form or as a chronic state with wavelike intensification of symptoms, it is called anxiety neurosis. The physical manifestations of rapid heart action, smothering, and hyperventilation have already been described. Such patients are seen more frequently by cardiologists than other specialists. Phobias, obsessions, compulsions, and hypochondriacal concerns may appear but are usually transitory and unimportant. Depression of mood is not part of the illness, but herein lies a difficult theoretical problem. Many psychiatrists hold that all persistent anxiety states that do not respond to simple explanation and reassurance are basically *anxious depressions.* The suicide rate in that group is distressingly high, and in not a few instances patients have ended their lives while receiving psychotherapy. The author has known of families afflicted with hereditary endogenous depressions or manic-depressive disease in which one member has developed a typical anxiety neurosis.

Of more general medical importance is the fact that both anxiety and depression can surface in patients hospitalized for a medical illness. The fears that naturally attend a myocardial infarction, a mild stroke, or a tumor may be exaggerated, and the patient may become so agitated as to become unable to listen to explanations or accept reassurance. Unreasonable anger may force the patient to attempt to leave the hospital. Convalescence may be prolonged by "weakness," persistent fatigue, and unwillingness to return to customary activities.

Physiologic and psychologic basis The cause, mechanism, and biologic meaning of anxiety have been the subjects of much speculation, and completely satisfactory explanations are not possible. The psychologist regards anxiety as anticipatory behavior, i.e., a state of uneasiness about something which may happen in the future. William McDougall spoke of it as "an emotional state arising when a continuing strong desire seems likely to miss its goal." The primary emotion, somewhat muted perhaps, is that of fear, and its arousal under conditions not overtly threatening may be explained by conditioning to some recondite component of a formerly threatening stimulus.

The only well-systematized theory is that put forth by the school of psychoanalysis, which looks upon anxiety as a response to a situation that in some manner undermines the security of the individual. The topical content or cause of potential danger lies in the unconscious mind. The postulated danger is internal rather than external; a primitive drive has been aroused that is not compatible with current social practices, and it can be relieved only at risk of harm to the person. In other words, the anxiety protects the individual by preventing the execution of the unacceptable action.

Physicians have searched for evidence of impairments of visceral function without success. The neurocirculatory asthenic is in poor physical condition, has an elevated blood lactate level after exercise, and will not tolerate the work or exercise needed to build up stamina. And even in the resting state lactic acid levels in the blood may be elevated, and infusions containing lactic acid are said to make the symptoms worse. The urinary excretion of epinephrine has been found elevated in some patients; in others, there is an increased urinary excretion of norepinephrine. Aldosterone excretion is raised to two or three times the normal level during intense anxiety. Medical students experiencing fear and anxiety while preparing for an examination also excrete increased amounts of aldosterone. The interpretation of these data (whether as primary or secondary effects) is not certain, but it is becoming increasingly evident that prolonged and diffuse anxiety is a pattern of behavior related to certain biochemical abnormalities of blood, and probably of the brain. A genetic factor seems operative in many cases. Anxiety neurosis and endogenous depressions, which are closely related, tend to run in families.

Easton and Sherman have reviewed the subject of anxiety in relation to adrenergic hyperresponsivity. It has been claimed that in susceptible individuals isoproterenol, when administered by intravenous infusion, induced an anxiety attack. Propranolol (Inderal) gives symptomatic relief. Other investigators have not been able to corroborate these observations and caution against the indiscriminate prescription of propranolol, for it is potentially hazardous in patients with congestive heart failure, atrioventricular block, and asthma (we have found it harmless to most individuals). These observations do, however, emphasize the role of the sympathetic nervous system in anxiety neurosis.

Treatment In the management of acute anxiety states, it is important to explain to patients that they suffer from a real medical illness and not just "nerves," or an imaginary condition. They should be allowed to express their feelings, doubts, and fears. Superficial psychotherapy, involving support, insight, and reeducation proves to be the most practical. Often, as the patient is mobilized and returned to usual activities, the symptoms subside. If the anxiety is persistent and severe, one should be alert to the risk of suicide and be prepared to send the patient to a psychiatric hospital for treatment of depression. If mild, antianxiety drugs such as meprobamate 400 mg tid, chlordiazepoxide 10 to 20 mg tid, diazepam 5 to 10 mg tid, propranolol 40 mg tid, or sodium amytal 100 to 200 mg tid, prescribed in the lowest possible dose, may suffice to bring the symptoms under control.

Hysterical neurosis   Unlike anxiety neurosis, where males and females are equally affected, chronic hysterical neurosis is almost exclusively a female illness. Beginning in late childhood (earliest age around 9 to 10 years), adolescence, or early adulthood, the patient begins to present a variety of inexplicable episodes of illness. Abdominal pains leading to appendectomy or ovariectomy (for cysts), severe and disabling dysmenorrhea, urinary retention requiring catheterization (sometimes followed by permanent injury to bladder), fainting spells and bizarre seizures, recurrent vomiting without weight loss, inexplicable fevers, paraplegias, hemiplegias, ataxias, blindness, deafness, intractable headaches and dizziness, and trancelike states and amnesias (the woman who appears in the emergency ward with lost identity) are some of the principal problems that bring these patients to internists and neurologists. Since these episodes of illness recur over years, one must distinguish between them and all the diseases that are common to this age period. More of these patients are seen on the neurology services of a general hospital than on any other service. By adult years it is not unusual for the patient to have had several unnecessary abdominal operations and many hospitalizations.

Psychiatrists, on the basis of psychoanalytic theory, subdivide the hysterical neurosis into two types, the conversion and the dissociative. All the forms of illness in which there are gross neuromuscular and other somatic derangements are called conversions, with the implication that suppressed anxiety has been converted into the physical symptom. Dissociative states include an alteration of self-awareness resulting in amnesia, fugue states, somnambulism, and split personality. But there are no basic differences between these two forms, and most patients will at some time exhibit both. Strangely, the attitude of the patient is often one of unconcern and apparent indifference to a major physical disability, but typical anxiety symptoms are not infrequent. Most of our patients have been of rather average or low average intelligence. Women working in health care organizations (practical nurses, ward attendants) show a particular susceptibility.

At times, the patient appears to be gaining something by being ill, but this is hard to prove. Nevertheless, it leads to a suspicion of malingering. However, most students of mental illness believe that hysterical symptoms are not under conscious control. And, despite the fact that nurses, ward attendants, and physicians perceive the disability as obviously spurious, the patient seems totally unaware of the unconvincing nature of the symptoms. True malingering usually occurs in immature, sociopathic males who have been in trouble from childhood.

The line between conversion symptoms and malingering is especially vague in a closely related condition called "compensation neurosis" where, following a civilian accident or a frightening experience (an army assignment, a threat of disability) the patient becomes paralyzed or has some other symptom of obscure origin. Such patients differ from the chronic hysterical neurotic in that the potential gain is easily discovered, there is not the history of neurotic illness prior to injury, the patient's lack of insight is less convincing, and males and females are equally susceptible. The author prefers to regard this as a separate illness.

As a rule, a careful physical examination will usually distinguish the hysterical disorders from physical ones, though physicians inexperienced with some of the subtleties of rare medical and neurologic diseases may be misled.

In the management of such patients, prolonged psychotherapy has seldom produced successful results. Often, any suggestion that the illness is psychiatric arouses a hostile reaction, and the patient may refuse to see a psychiatrist. The author has obtained the best results by explaining to the patient and the family that the illness is really a chronic constitutional nervous weakness which is now abating. After all tests for other physical ailments are concluded, the patient is urged to begin walking and resuming normal activities. Sometimes this positive approach can overcome a paralysis within a few minutes, but if it has been present a long time, a vigorous physical program will be needed to restore lost function. Subjective complaints are disregarded, and if the patient continues to emphasize them, reassurance is offered that they will soon recede. Hypnosis, electric stimulation, and dramatic curative methods (Lourdes, acupuncture, etc.) have no advantage. Once rid of the pressing complaint, the patient is best managed by a kindly, understanding physician, sensitive to the nuances of this psychologic disorder, who will analyze each new illness to make sure it is hysterical and not some new intervening disease. Hysterical symptoms should be treated symptomatically, with simple non-habit-forming drugs.

The treatment of compensation neurosis requires a thorough medical survey, reassurance, symptomatic therapy, and early settlement of the compensation claims. The results in the older worker are far from satisfactory.

Phobic and obsessive-compulsive neuroses   These two neuroses, together called psychesthenia by Janet, are relatively rare and need not be described in detail. Individuals with neuroses of this type are rigid and perfectionist; otherwise capable of functioning effectively, they have their lives dominated by a single irrational fear (e.g., of being away from their own home or neighborhood) or by a series of obsessive thoughts or compulsive rituals. Any departure from their restricted mode of life occasions intense anxiety. Overwhelmed by physical symptoms, ashamed and despondent, the patient limps through life with this handicap.

Opinion is divided among psychiatrists as to the efficacy of psychotherapy, including psychoanalysis. Cures have been reported. Several of the author's patients whose phobic state had recently increased to the point where they were disabled, were brought again under partial control by the use of amitryptiline or imipramine. Presumably a depressive state had supervened.

Neurasthenic neurosis   Persistent weakness, fatigability, and exhaustion are common to many mental illnesses, particularly anxiety neurosis and depression. In some instances it seems to be a character type and is lifelong —the asthenic psychopathy of Kahn. This problem will be discussed in Chap. 12.

Hypochondriacal neurosis   Morbid preoccupation with bodily functions and physical symptoms is a frequent condition. Such patients make up a sizeable segment of every medical outpatient clinic. They seem possessed with worries about their bowel functions, tinnitus, arthritic and postzoster pains, old-age vertigo, and many of the other symptoms to which middle-aged and elderly adults are prey. Every minute detail is studied and described, recounted again and again. It is difficult to turn them to any other topic of conversation. Unlike hysteria and anxiety neurosis, one can find no physiologic or somatic derangements.

Most of these patients have a depression, and a few express

frankly delusional ideas about their viscera. Severe hypochondriasis in a young person should always suggest schizophrenia. But there are many individuals who have no other mental illness. They go through life being concerned and worried about disease in themselves and their families. Often, one finds that they have been raised in a family atmosphere of overconcern about health. It has become part of their character.

In hypochondriacal patients, after the proper physical examination procedure and laboratory tests have eliminated serious disease, the physician should tell them that they have a neurosis and need help. Symptomatic therapy, a regulated program of daily activities, frequent visits with an understanding physician for explanation and reeducation, and group psychotherapy are all beneficial. But whenever there is suspicion of despondency and depression, a psychiatric opinion should be sought and antidepressive measures as outlined in Chap. 25 should be initiated.

Depressive neurosis Many patients with any one of the above neuroses may feel trapped, hopeless, and gloomy—a natural reaction to the symptomatology over which they have no control. Unlike the endogenous and involutional depressions, the mood change may be transitory and variable from day to day, and vegetative symptoms such as loss of appetite, weight loss, constipation, loss of libido and impotence do not occur. Many psychiatrists distinguish this neurotic type of depression and the reactive depression from the endogenous or organic types, and they caution that the drugs and electroconvulsive therapy used in the endogenous and organic types are usually unsuccessful in neurotic depressions. The line between the two types is thin, however, and the physician is well advised to let a psychiatric consultant stand responsible for separating them and making sure the patient is not suicidal.

COMMON PROBLEMS IN DIAGNOSIS OF PSYCHIATRIC ILLNESSES THAT PRODUCE PHYSICAL SYMPTOMS The physician's greatest concern is misdiagnosis, and physicians rightly appreciate the difficulty of deciding when mental symptoms appear to accompany, mask, or mimic physical disease. There is often the impression that diagnosis is reduced to inspired guesswork. Shulman, in a discussion of psychogenic illness with physical manifestations, states that the common problems are relatively few and not difficult to recognize. He believes the most frequent source of error to be the too strict application of the law of parsimony, which tries to subsume all symptoms under one diagnosis. At least one-fourth to one-half of all adult medical problems represent a cluster or complex of functional-organic or physical-psychosocial illnesses. Most astute physicians can separate the effects of diseases from the associated psychologic reactions.

Probably the largest and most serious diagnostic error may be committed when there are recurrent symptoms in many organ systems for which no obvious cause can be found. Here one must suspect the *masked depression,* i.e., the form of endogenous illness in which the leading complaint is pain (headache, precordial pain, backache, etc.) or exhaustion, and it is a mistake to consider the despondency a secondary reaction. A safe rule to follow is that whenever an unexplained syndrome is accompanied by complaints in two or three other organ systems, a serious psychiatric illness with anxiety and depression should be suspected. Complications of pharmacologic therapy and chronic liver or pancreatic disease may rarely give rise to a similar picture.

Another perplexing problem is the anxiety state that is misdiagnosed as menopause, thyrotoxicosis, hypoglycemia, pheochromocytoma, carcinoid tumor, left-sided heart failure, or temporal lobe epilepsy. Each of these diseases causes visceral derangements not unlike those of anxiety. But the latter differs descriptively in that there is always a prominent psychic component of fear and apprehension. It is the combination of mental and autonomic symptoms that should always lead to the suspicion of an anxiety state or anxious depression.

And finally there is the problem of misdiagnosing a neurologic disease (e.g., multiple sclerosis) in a patient who has the conversion form of hysteria or a compensation problem. The lifelong history, the context of the illness, and discrepancy between symptoms and signs should direct thinking along the right path.

In all these problems, a good history is the cornerstone of diagnosis, especially if it includes a kind of life chart of key personal events, medical illnesses, and psychologic derangements. The history is more important than the physical examination and laboratory tests. Incongruities between complaints and between symptoms and physical findings and disabilities are the most important leads. It is "the old crock" with a long history of ill health that is most subject to misdiagnosis.

REFERENCES

NICHOLI AM (ed): *The Harvard Guide to Modern Psychiatry.* Cambridge, Mass, Harvard University Press, 1978

SHULMAN R: Psychogenic illness with physical manifestations: A practical approach. Lancet 1:524, 1977

EASTON D, SHERMAN DG: Somatic anxiety attacks and propranolol. Arch Neurol 33:689, 1976

12
LASSITUDE AND ASTHENIA

RAYMOND D. ADAMS

The terms *weakness* and *fatigue* are used by patients to describe a variety of subjective complaints which vary in their import and prognostic significance. The different meanings can usually be fitted into the following classification:

1 Lassitude, fatigue, lack of energy, listlessness, and languor. These terms, though not synonymous, shade into one another. All refer to a weariness and a loss of that sense of well-being typically found in persons healthy of body and mind.
2 Weakness, loss of strength, paresis, paralysis. These may be persistent or episodic.
   a Persistent weakness: This may be (1) restricted to certain muscles or groups of muscles (see Chap. 15) or (2) more or less generalized, i.e., involving the entire musculature (see Chaps. 381 and 382).
   b Episodic, often recurrent: Attacks of weakness may occur in the periodic paralyses. [Many patients confuse "attacks of weakness" with a diminished sense of alertness, lightheadedness, feeling of faintness. These usually turn out to be episodes of partial or threatening syncope, attacks of anxiety or vertigo, or seizures (see Chaps. 11, 14, and 23).]

LASSITUDE AND FATIGUE Of all the symptoms in this group these are among the most frequent and abstruse. More than half of all patients entering a general hospital register direct complaint of fatigability or admit to it when questioned. During the Second World War fatigue was so prominent as to be given a separate place in medical nosology, viz., "combat fatigue," which came to refer to all acute psychiatric illnesses that happened on the battlefield. The common clinical antecedents and accompaniments of fatigue, its significance, and its physiologic and psychologic bases should, therefore, be matters of common medical knowledge.

Patients who complain of weariness and tiredness have a more or less characteristic way of describing their condition. They say that they "are all in," "have lost pep," "have no ambition" or "no interest," are "turned off" or "fed up." They manifest their condition by showing an indifference to the tasks at hand, by talking much about how hard they are working; they are inclined to sit around or lie down, occupying themselves with trivial tasks. On closer analysis one observes that they have a difficulty in initiating activity and also in sustaining it.

This condition is the familiar aftermath of prolonged labor or great physical exertion, and under such circumstances it is accepted as a normal, physiologic reaction. When, however, the same symptoms or similar ones appear in no relation to such antecedents, they are suspected to be the manifestations of disease.

The physician's task begins, then, with an attempt to determine whether the patient is merely suffering from the physical and mental effects of overwork without realizing it. Overworked, overwrought people are everywhere observable in our society. Their actions are both instructive and pathetic. They seem to be impelled by notions of duty and refuse to think of themselves. Or, as is often the case, some personal inadequacy seems to prevent them from deriving pleasure from any activity except their work, in which they indulge themselves as a kind of defense mechanism. Such persons show their fatigue by other symptoms, such as irritability, restlessness, and sleeplessness. Their symptoms and behavior are best understood by referring to psychologic studies of the effect of fatigue on the normal individual.

Effects of fatigue on the normal person According to several authoritative sources, fatigue has both explicit and implicit effects, logically grouped under (1) a series of biochemical and physiologic changes in many organs of the body, (2) an overt disorder in behavior, a reduced output of work, known as *work decrement*, and (3) an expressed dissatisfaction and a subjective feeling of tiredness.

As to the biochemical and physiologic changes, continuous muscular work leads to depletion of muscle glycogen and an accumulation of lactic acid and other metabolites, which in themselves reduce the power of contraction and delay recovery. Extreme degrees of muscle work, in which activity exceeds provision of substrate, results in necrosis of fibers and rise in serum levels of creatine phosphokinase and aldolase even in normal persons. The muscles are slightly swollen and sore for several days. It is said that the injection of blood from a fatigued animal into a rested one will produce overt manifestations of fatigue in the latter. During repeated contractions of muscle, its action is observed to become tremulous, movements are less adept, and the coordination of agonist, antagonist, and synergic muscles is less perfect. The rate of breathing increases, the pulse quickens, the blood pressure rises and pulse pressure widens, and the white blood cell count and metabolic rate are increased. These alterations bear out the hypothesis that fatigue is in part a manifestation of altered metabolism.

The decreased capacity for work or productivity which is a direct consequence of fatigue has been investigated by industrial psychologists. Their findings show clearly the importance of the motivational factor on work output, whether it be in manual or clerical tasks. Individual differences in energy potential appear also to be important, as are differences in physique, intelligence, and temperament.

The subjective feelings of fatigue have been carefully recorded. Aside from feeling weary tired persons are unable to deal effectively with complex problems and tend to be unreasonable, often about trivialities. The number and quality of their associations in psychologic tests are reduced. The ability to deliberate and to reach judgments is impaired; decisions made late at night may appear unsound the next day. The worker after a long, hard day is unable to perform adequately his or her duties as head of a household; the example of the tired businessperson who becomes the proverbial tyrant of the family circle is well known. A disinclination to try and the appearance of ideas of inferiority are other characteristics of the fatigued mind.

Instances of fatigue and lassitude resulting from overwork are not difficult to recognize. Descriptions of patients' daily routines and talks with associates and family will usually suffice. Moreover if they can be persuaded to live at a more reasonable pace and allow time for outside pleasurable activities, their symptoms will promptly subside. A common error in diagnosis, however, is the ascription of fatigue to overwork when actually it is a manifestation of a psychoneurosis or depression.

Fatigue as a manifestation of psychiatric disorder The great majority of patients who enter a hospital because of unexplained chronic fatigue and lassitude have been found to have some type of psychiatric illness. Formerly this state was called *neurasthenia;* but since fatigue rarely exists as an isolated phenomenon, the current practice is to label such cases according to the total clinical picture. The usual associated symptoms are nervousness, irritability, anxiety, depression, insomnia, headaches, difficulty in concentrating, sexual disorders, and loss of bodily appetites. In one series in a general hospital 75 percent of persons admitted because of chronic fatigue and nervousness were diagnosed, finally, as having *anxiety neurosis* and *tension states.* Depression accounted for another 10 percent, and the remainder of the patients had a miscellany of medical and psychiatric illnesses.

Several features are common to the psychiatric group. The fatigue may be worse in the morning. There is an inclination to lie down and rest, but sleep does not come. The fatigue relates more to some activities than to others. Inquiry as to what was happening when the fatigue was first experienced may reveal an unpleasant event, a grief reaction, a surgical operation, or a medical illness. The feeling of fatigue interferes with mental as well as physical activities. The psychic aspects are manifested as difficulty in concentrating on the solution of a problem or in carrying on an involved conversation.

Depressing emotion, as was remarked in the previous chapter, has its characteristic effect on impulse life and energy. Also, it impairs sleep, with a tendency to early-morning waking. Such persons are at their worst in the morning, both in spirit and in energy output. Their tendency is to improve as the day wears on, and they may even feel fairly normal by evening. It is often difficult in them to decide whether the fatigue is a primary manifestation of the depression or is secondary to a lack of interest.

Many physicians question whether all chronically fatigued individuals deviate enough from normal to justify the diagnosis of psychoneurosis or depression. Many people in society, because of circumstances beyond their control, have no purpose in life and much idle time. They are bored with the monotony of their routine. Such circumstances are conducive to fatigue, just as the opposite is also true—that a new enterprise that excites optimism and enthusiasm will dispel fatigue. Other individuals seem normal until some adversity is encountered, arousing worry or fear, and then it becomes apparent that their adjustment is unstable. Such reactions are understandable to anyone who has ever had stage fright or "buck fever" and who remembers the sense of physical weakness, the utter incapacity to act, the intellectual chaos that overwhelms the previously well-ordered mind, and the exhaustion which follows.

Psychologic theories The enervating effect of a strong emotion such as anxiety is well known, and it might be supposed that the simple prolongation of the emotional experience would provide a rational explanation for a chronic fatigue of anxiety. But even if true, however, this explanation does not account for the occurrence of emotion at a time when there is no reason for it.

The dynamic schools of psychiatry, particularly the psychoanalytic, have postulated that chronic fatigue, in the broadest sense, is like the anxiety from which it derives; it is a danger signal that something is wrong—that some attitude or activity has been too intense or too persistent. The fatigue is self-preservative, serving not merely as a protection against physical injury but also as a protection of the individual's self-esteem and confidence in self. As to mechanism, it is claimed that the fatigue is the result of exhaustion of the store of psychic energy required to maintain repression of unacceptable ideas. Others, however, claim to have evidence that fatigue is not a negative symptom, a lack or depletion of energy, but an unconscious desire for inactivity. A reciprocal relationship is said to exist between fatigue and anxiety. Both are protective, but anxiety is the more imperative. It calls for the individual to take some positive action to extricate him- or herself from a predicament, whereas fatigue calls for inactivity. Both operate blindly, however, for the person cannot perceive what it is that must be done or not done. All this happens at the unconscious level.

It is also observed that some persons are low in impulse and energy throughout life, being more so at times of stress. Some psychiatrists believe that they have a constitutional inadequacy. Kahn classifies such individuals as "psychopaths weak in impulse," and points out in his description their inability throughout life to play games vigorously, to compete successfully, to work hard without exhaustion, to withstand or recover quickly from illness, or to assume a dominant role in a social group. The physician caring for them expects greater disability and more prolonged convalescence from every illness.

It is obvious that these several psychologic hypotheses could not all be correct, nor could they be applicable to all situations in which chronic fatigue is the complaint. Undoubtedly there are persons who are underactive and weak because of genetic factors or early life experiences. It is equally clear that psychic and physical energy are closely linked to mood. The more chronic varieties of acquired fatigue, without a basis in medical disease, have in nearly all instances a psychologic basis.

Lassitude and fatigue in chronic infection and in endocrine and other medical diseases Infection is another cause of chronic fatigue, though a much less frequent one. Everyone has at some time or other sensed the abrupt onset of extreme exhaustion, the tired ache in the muscles, an inexplicable listlessness, only to discover later that one is "coming down with the flu." In chronic infections such as hepatitis, tuberculosis, brucellosis, infectious mononucleosis, the infection may not be at once evident. But it should always be suspected when the fatigue is out of proportion to other symptoms such as mood change, nervousness, and anxiety. Often this syndrome will begin with an obvious infection but will persist for several weeks after it should have terminated, and it may then be difficult to decide whether there is still a lingering infection or the infection has been complicated by psychiatric illness during convalescence. In many diseases such as infectious hepatitis, brucellosis, infectious mononucleosis, and a host of other systemic viral infections, long-standing neurotic symptoms appear to have been uncovered. Nevertheless it is difficult to dismiss an obscure secondary metabolic disorder consequent to the infection.

Metabolic and endocrine diseases (see Chaps. 332 and 334) of various types may cause inordinate degrees of lassitude and fatigue. Sometimes there is in addition a true muscular weakness (see Chaps. 13 and 357). In Addison's disease and Simmonds' disease fatigue may dominate the clinical picture. Aldosterone deficiency is another established cause of fatigue (see Chap. 335). In persons with hypothyroidism, with or without frank myxedema, lassitude and sluggishness are frequent complaints. These same symptoms may also be present in patients with hyperthyroidism but are usually less troublesome than nervousness. Uncontrolled diabetes mellitus may be accompanied by excessive fatigability, as are hyperparathyroidism, hypogonadism, and Cushing's disease.

Anemia, when moderate or severe (hematocrit less than 25) should be considered as a possible cause of unexplained lassitude. Mild grades of anemia are usually asymptomatic; lassitude is far too often ascribed to it.

Any type of nutritional deficiency may, when severe, cause lassitude, and in its earlier stages this may be the chief complaint. Weight loss and the history of dietary inadequacy may provide the only other clues to the nature of the illness. Many patients feel weak and tired after a myocardial infarct, but usually there is an accompanying depression.

Among neurologic diseases in which fatigability is a prominent symptom should be mentioned the posttraumatic nervous instability syndrome, Parkinson's disease, and multiple sclerosis. The fatigue of Parkinson's disease may precede the recognition of neurologic signs by months or even years. It is probably a reaction to the increasing disability occasioned by subjective awareness of the akinesia. The majority of patients who recover from a stroke complain of being weak and tired. Hot temperatures worsen the fatigue and other symptoms of the multiple sclerotic patient.

Differential diagnosis If one looks critically at the patients who enter a hospital because of lassitude and fatigability (sometimes incorrectly called weakness), it is clear that the most commonly overlooked diagnoses are psychoneurosis and depression. The correct conclusion can usually be reached by keeping these illnesses in mind as one elicits the principal symptoms of these psychiatric illnesses from patient and family. Difficulty arises when such symptoms are so inconspicuous as not to be appreciated; one comes then to suspect the psychiatric diagnosis only by having eliminated the common medical causes. Observations in the hospital may bear out the existence of a tension state or gloomy mood, as the patient resists attempts to be mobilized. Strong reassurance in combination with a therapeutic trial of 2.5 to 5.0 mg dextroamphetamine morning and noon and 100 to 200 mg sodium amobarbital three times a day may suppress symptoms of which the patient was barely aware and may clarify diagnosis. The danger of mistaking a depression for a neurosis has already been mentioned. Of course, asthenic psychopaths are recognized by their actions as revealed in biographies.

Obscure infections such as pulmonary tuberculosis, brucellosis, subclinical hepatitis, subacute bacterial endocarditis, malaria, hookworm, and parasitic infections should be recognizable, by the characteristic symptoms and signs described elsewhere in the book. An endocrine survey particularly for adrenal insufficiency and thyroid disease, is in order in all obscure cases. There should also be a search for occult tumors. If one has no access to hormone assays, the use of a simple "water excretion test" may prove very helpful in identifying an organic component in a patient's fatigue syndrome, since a wide variety of systemic disorders is associated with a delayed diuresis following the ingestion of water. It is thought that the "sick cell" with impaired permeability of cell membrane "traps" water and then releases it slowly. The test consists in the administration of 500 ml water at 8:00, 8:15, and 8:30 A.M. for a total intake of 1500 ml with the patient fasting and lying in a horizontal position. Smoking is not permitted. The water should be room temperature, *not cold.* Urine volume is measured hourly for 3 to 4 h. A normal response will usually include a diuresis of 400 to 600 ml in the first, second, and third hours, with a total volume of at least 80 percent in 3 to 4 h (1200 ml). An impaired response in the horizontal position suggests *organic disease.* It should be remembered that chronic intoxications with barbiturates, alcohol, or bromides, some of which are given to suppress nervousness, may contribute to fatigability.

Finally, when onset of fatigue is rapid and recent, the cause is likely to be an infection, a disturbance in fluid balance, or rapidly developing circulatory failure of either peripheral or cardiac origin.

GENERALIZED WEAKNESS AND ASTHENIA As can be judged from the foregoing remarks, weakness must be distinguished from lassitude and fatigue. The demonstration of reduced muscular power sets the case analysis along rather different lines, for it raises consideration more particularly of diseases of the nervous system or of the musculature.

True neural or myopathic weakness is probably never due to psychologic factors, though the hysteric or malingering patient may claim weakness. Usually this can be detected by the criteria outlined in Chap. 11. In anemia, chronic infection, malignancy, and nutritional depletion (except when polyneuropathy is present), the thin muscles are always stronger during tests of peak contraction than one would expect, though of course strength falls short of that of a healthy individual (see Chap. 378 for description of tests of peak power and endurance of muscles).

The proper ascertainment of muscular weakness depends on two lines of inquiry: (1) a history of reduced efficiency; and (2) demonstrable failure in ability to contract the muscles forcefully one or more times. If one proceeds to test each of the major groups of muscles from head to foot, comparing the patient's performance with one's idea of normalcy for man or woman, one may ascertain whether all or certain groups fall below standard. Quantitative and qualitative changes (myasthenia, inverse myasthenia, myotonia, paramyotonia, pathologic cramping) may also be detected by the methods outlined in Chap. 378. The topography of weakness and associated neurologic findings permit distinction between the various types of spinal, peripheral nerve, and myopathic pareses. Rare diseases, difficult to diagnose, that cause inexplicable muscle weakness are masked hyperthyroidism, hyperparathyroidism, ossifying hemangiomas with hypophosphatemia, some of the kalemic periodic paralyses, and hyperinsulinism.

REFERENCES

ADAMS RD: *Pathology of Muscle Diseases,* 3d ed. New York, Harper & Row, 1976

MAYER-GROSS W et al: *Clinical Psychiatry,* 3d ed. Baltimore, Williams & Wilkins, 1969

WALTON JN (ed): *Disease of Voluntary Muscle,* 3d ed. London, Churchill, 1975

13
FAINTNESS, SYNCOPE, AND EPISODIC WEAKNESS

RAYMOND D. ADAMS
EUGENE BRAUNWALD

Episodic faintness, lightheadedness or giddiness, and reduced alertness are frequently difficult to distinguish, tending to shade into one another. And the difference between faintness and frank syncope is only quantitative. Types of episodic weakness, such as myasthenia gravis, cataplexy, and familial periodic paralysis, which cause striking reduction of muscular strength but no impairment of consciousness, should be set apart (see Chaps. 381 and 382); epilepsy, which is also associated with episodic unconsciousness, differs from syncope in most other respects and is discussed in Chap. 23.

CARDINAL FEATURES

Syncope comprises a generalized weakness of muscles, with inability to stand upright, and a loss of consciousness. The term *faintness*, in contrast, refers to lack of strength, with sensation of impending loss of consciousness. At the beginning of a syncopal attack the patient is nearly always in the upright position, either sitting or standing [the Stokes-Adams attack (see Chap. 237) is exceptional in this respect]. Usually an individual is warned of the impending faint by a sense of "feeling bad." The patient is assailed by giddiness, the floor seems to move, and surrounding objects begin to sway. The senses become confused; the patient yawns or gapes, there are spots before the eyes, vision may dim, and the ears may ring. Nausea and sometimes vomiting accompany these symptoms. There is a striking pallor or ashen grey color of the face, and very often the face and body are bathed in cold perspiration. The deliberate onset may often allow the patient time for protection against injury; a hurtful fall is exceptional. If the patient can lie down promptly, the attack may be averted without complete loss of consciousness.

The depth and duration of unconsciousness vary. Sometimes the patient is not completely oblivious of the surroundings, or there may be profound coma with complete lack of awareness and of capacity to respond. The patient may remain in this state for seconds to minutes or even as long as half an hour. Usually the patient lies motionless with skeletal muscles relaxed, but a few clonic jerks of the limbs and face may occur shortly after the beginning of the unconsciousness. Generalized tonic-clonic convulsions are never a part of syncope. Sphincter control is usually maintained. The pulse is feeble or cannot be felt; the blood pressure may be low and breathing almost imperceptible. Once the patient is in a horizontal position, perhaps from having fallen, gravitation no longer hinders the flow of blood to the brain. The strength of the pulse then improves, color begins to return to the face, breathing becomes quicker and deeper, and consciousness is regained. There is from this moment onward a correct perception of the environment. The patient is, nevertheless, keenly aware of physical weakness, and rising too soon may precipitate another faint. Headache and drowsiness, which, with mental confusion, are the usual sequelae of a convulsion, do not follow a syncopal attack.

ETIOLOGY

The list of causes in Table 13-1 is based on established or assumed physiologic mechanisms. The commoner types of faint are reducible to a few simple mechanisms. Syncope results essentially from a sudden impairment of brain metabolism usually brought about by a hypotensive reduction of cerebral blood flow.

Nature has provided humans with several mechanisms by which circulation adjusts to the upright posture. Approximately three-fourths of the systemic blood volume is contained in the venous bed, and any interference with venous return may lead to a reduction in cardiac output. Cerebral blood flow may still be maintained, as long as systemic arterial vasoconstriction occurs; but when this adjustment fails, serious hypotension with resultant cerebral underperfusion to less than half of normal results in syncope. Normally, the pooling of blood in the lower parts of the body is prevented by (1) pressor reflexes which induce constriction of peripheral arterioles and venules; (2) reflex acceleration of the heart by means of aortic and carotid reflexes; and (3) improvement of venous return to the heart by activity of the muscles of the limbs and by increased rate of respiration. Placing a normal person on a tilt table to relax the muscles and tilting upright slightly diminishes cardiac output, and allows the blood to accumulate in the legs to a

TABLE 13-1
Causes of recurrent weakness, faintness, and disturbances of consciousness

I Circulatory (deficient quantity of blood to the brain)
  A Inadequate vasoconstrictor mechanisms
    1 Vasovagal (vasodepressor)
    2 Postural hypotension
    3 Primary autonomic insufficiency
    4 Sympathectomy (pharmacologic or surgical)
    5 Diseases of central and peripheral nervous systems, including autonomic nerves (Chap. 377)
    6 Carotid sinus syncope (see also Bradyarrhythmias, below)
  B Hypovolemia
  C Mechanical reduction of venous return
    1 Valsalva maneuver
    2 Cough
    3 Micturition
    4 Atrial myxoma, ball valve thrombus
  D Reduced cardiac output
    1 Obstruction to left ventricular outflow: aortic stenosis, hypertrophic subaortic stenosis
    2 Obstruction to pulmonary flow: pulmonic stenosis, primary pulmonary hypertension, pulmonary embolism
    3 Myocardial: massive myocardial infarction with pump failure
    4 Pericardial: cardiac tamponade
  E Arrhythmias (Chap. 237)
    1 Bradyarrhythmias
      a Atrioventricular (AV) block (11° and 111°), with Stokes-Adams attacks
      b Ventricular asystole
      c Sinus bradycardia, sinoatrial block, sinus arrest
      d Carotid sinus syncope (see also Inadequate Vasoconstrictor Mechanisms, above)
      e Glossopharyngeal neuralgia (and other painful states)
    2 Tachyarrhythmias
      a Episodic ventricular fibrillation with or without associated bradyarrhythmias
      b Ventricular tachycardia
      c Supraventricular tachycardia without AV block
II Other causes of weakness and episodic disturbances of consciousness
  A Altered state of blood to the brain
    1 Hypoxia
    2 Anemia
    3 Diminished carbon dioxide due to hyperventilation (faintness common, syncope seldom occurs)
    4 Hypoglycemia (episodic weakness common, faintness occasional, syncope rare)
  B Cerebral
    1 Cerebrovascular disturbances (cerebral ischemic attacks, see Chap. 365)
      a Extracranial vascular insufficiency (basilar-vertebral, carotid)
      b Diffuse spasm of cerebral arterioles (hypertensive encephalopathy)
    2 Emotional disturbances, anxiety attacks, and hysterical seizures (see Chaps. 11 and 25)

slight degree. This may then be followed by a slight transitory fall in systolic arterial pressure and, in patients with defective vasomotor reflexes, may be a means of reproducing faints.

TYPES OF SYNCOPE

VASOVAGAL (VASODEPRESSOR) SYNCOPE This is the common faint that may be experienced by normal persons; it is frequently recurrent and tends to take place during emotional stress (especially in a warm, crowded room), after an injurious, shocking accident, and during pain. Mild blood loss, poor physical condition, prolonged bed rest, anemia, fever, organic heart disease, and fasting are other factors which increase the possibility of fainting in susceptible individuals. A short premonitory phase is characterized by nausea, perspiration, yawning, epigastric distress, hyperpnea, tachypnea, weakness, confusion, tachycardia, and pupillary dilatation. Physiologically, there is first a marked fall in arterial pressure and systemic vascular resistance which is most notable in the skeletal muscular beds. Cardiac output may be within normal limits, but it fails to exhibit the expected increase which normally occurs with hypotension. It declines when vagal activity leads to marked bradycardia, replacing tachycardia, resulting in further lowering of arterial pressure and reduction of cerebral perfusion. Assumption of the supine posture with elevation of the legs and removal of the offending stimulus will rapidly restore consciousness.

POSTURAL HYPOTENSION WITH SYNCOPE This type of syncope affects persons who have a chronic defect in or variable instability of vasomotor reflexes. Though the character of the syncopal attack differs little from that of the vasovagal or vasodepressor type, the effect of posture is its cardinal feature; sudden arising from a recumbent position or standing still are the circumstances under which it is most likely to happen.

Postural syncope tends to occur under the following conditions: (1) in otherwise normal persons who for some unknown reason have defective postural reflexes (this may be familial); (2) rarely, as part of a syndrome named *primary autonomic insufficiency,* which includes chronic orthostatic hypotension either in pure form or in association with symptoms of peripheral preganglionic autonomic and cerebellar or extrapyramidal disorder; (3) after physical deconditioning, e.g., after prolonged illness with recumbency, especially in elderly individuals with flabby muscles; (4) after a sympathectomy that has abolished vasopressor reflexes; (5) in diabetic, alcoholic, and other neuropathies, tabes dorsalis, syringomyelia, subacute combined sclerosis, and diseases of the nervous system which cause muscular atrophy and paralysis of vasopressor reflexes; (6) in patients receiving antihypertensive and vasodilator drugs as well as those who may be hypovolemic because of diuretics, excessive sweating or adrenal insufficiency.

In the otherwise normal individuals who faint if tilted on a table, it has been found that at first the blood pressure diminishes slightly and then stabilizes at a lower level. Shortly thereafter the compensatory reflexes suddenly fail, and the arterial pressure falls precipitously. This reaction also may be observed in some of the conditions listed above. In others, e.g., after pharmacologic sympathectomy, in diseases of the sympathetic nervous system, and in the unusual condition known as chronic orthostatic hypotension, the arterial pressure never stabilizes after tilting but falls steadily to a level at which cerebral circulation cannot be maintained.

ORTHOSTATIC HYPOTENSION Here a critical fall in blood pressure on assumption of upright posture is due to a loss of vasoconstrictor reflexes in resistance and capacitance vessels of the lower extremities. Peripheral (postganglionic) or central (preganglionic) neurons may be defective.

The most common form of neurogenic orthostatic hypotension is that which accompanies diseases of the peripheral nervous system. Diabetic polyneuropathy, beriberi, amyloid polyneuropathy, and the Adie syndrome are examples. Usually the orthostatic hypotension is associated with disturbances in sweating, impotence, and sphincter difficulties. Presumably the lesion involves postganglionic, nonmedullated fibers in peripheral nerves (see Chap. 377).

There are other forms of severe orthostatic hypotension which occur in the absence of all signs of sensory-motor nerve involvement. These are called *primary autonomic insufficiencies* or *dysautonomias*. At least three syndromes have been delineated.

1 *Acute or subacute dysautonomia.* In this disease an otherwise healthy adult or child is afflicted over a period of a few days or weeks with a partial or complete paralysis of the parasympathetic and sympathetic nervous systems. Pupillary reflexes are lost, as are lacrimation, salivation, and sweating; and there is impotence, paresis of bladder and bowel musculature, and orthostatic hypotension. The CSF protein is increased. Sensory and motor nerve fibers are demonstrably intact, but nonmedullated autonomic ones have degenerated. Recovery occurs within a few months, possibly hastened by prednisone therapy. The disease is believed to represent a variant of acute idiopathic polyneuritis, akin to Landry-Guillain-Barré syndrome (Young et al.).

2 *Chronic postganglionic autonomic insufficiency.* This is a disease of middle-aged and elderly individuals who gradually become troubled by chronic orthostatic hypotension, sometimes in conjunction with anyhydrosis, impotence, and sphincter disturbances. Upon standing for 5 to 10 min the blood pressure decreases at least 35 torr and the pulse pressure narrows, both without increase in pulse rate, pallor, or nausea. Men are more often affected than women. The condition is relatively benign and seemingly irreversible.

3 *Chronic preganglionic autonomic insufficiency.* In this condition orthostatic hypotension with variable anyhydrosis, impotence, and sphincter disturbances is combined with any one of three or more disorders of the central nervous system. These include (*a*) tremor, extrapyramidal rigidity, and akinesia (Shy-Drager syndrome); (*b*) progressive cerebellar degeneration, some instances of which are familial; and (*c*) a more variable extrapyramidal and cerebellar disorder (strionigral degeneration). These syndromes lead to disability and often death within a few years.

The differentiation of the chronic peripheral postganglionic and central preganglionic insufficiency is based on pathologic and pharmacologic evidence. In the postganglionic type, neurons of the sympathetic ganglia degenerate, whereas in the central type, the lateral horn cells of the spinal cord degenerate. In the postganglionic peripheral type, the resting levels of norepinephrine are subnormal because of failure of release from postganglionic endings, and there is hypersensitivity to injected norepinephrine. In the central type, the resting levels of norepinephrine are normal. On standing, unlike the normal individual, there is little if any rise in norepinephrine levels in either type. And in both types, the levels of plasma dopamine β-hydroxylase (the enzyme that converts dopamine to norepinephrine) are subnormal (Ziegler et al.).

This distinction of types has therapeutic significance. In the peripheral postganglionic type, the most effective treatment of the orthostatic hypotension is a 9α-fluorohydrocortisone (oral dose 0.5 to 2.0 mg per day) and salt loading to increase blood volume, supplemented by mechanical devices to prevent pooling of blood in the legs and lower trunk (g suit). For the central preganglionic type, there has been greater success with use of a sympathomimetic amine such as tyramine (which releases norepinephrine from intact postganglionic endings) supplemented by a monoamine oxidase inhibitor (to prevent destruction of the amine), and possibly propranolol (Inderal).

Micturition syncope, a condition usually seen in the elderly during or after urination, particularly after arising from the recumbent position, is probably a special type of postural syncope. It has been suggested that release of intravesicular pressure causes sudden vasodilatation, augmented by standing and that vagally mediated bradycardia is a contributory factor (Johnson and Spaulding).

SYNCOPE OF CARDIAC ORIGIN (CARDIAC SYNCOPE) Cardiac syncope results from a sudden reduction in cardiac output, caused most commonly by a cardiac arrhythmia. In normal individuals slow ventricular rates, but above 35 to 40 beats per minute, and fast ones not exceeding 180 beats per minute do not reduce cerebral blood flow, especially if the person is in the supine position, but changes in pulse rate outside these limits may impair cerebral circulation and functions. The upright posture, cerebrovascular disease, anemia, and coronary, myocardial, or valvular disease all reduce the tolerance to alterations in rate.

Complete atrioventricular block is the commonest arrhythmia that leads to fainting, and syncopal episodes associated with this arrhythmia are known as the Stocks-Adams-Morgagni syndrome. The etiology of disturbances in atrioventricular conduction is considered elsewhere (Chap. 237), but in patients with these attacks the block may be persistent or intermittent; it is often preceded or followed by disturbed conduction in one or two of the three fascicles through which the ventricles are normally activated, by second degree atrioventricular block (Mobitz type II), or bifascicular or trifascicular block. When the block is complete and the pacemaker below the block fails to function, syncope occurs. A brief bout of ventricular tachycardia or fibrillation may also be responsible for the syncopal episode. Recurrent syncope due to ventricular fibrillation, characterized by a prolonged QT interval (sometimes associated with congenital deafness), has been reported; this condition may be familial or sporadic.

Stokes-Adams attacks occur usually without more than a momentary sense of weakness, the patient suddenly losing consciousness. After cardiac standstill of more than several seconds, the patient turns pale, falls unconscious, and, as in other types of fainting, may exhibit a few clonic jerks. With longer periods of asystole, the ashen gray pallor gives way to cyanosis, stertorous breathing, fixed pupils, incontinence, and bilateral Babinski signs. Prolonged confusion and neurologic signs due to cerebral ischemia may occur in some patients, and permanent impairment of mental function may also occur, although focal neurologic signs are rare. Cardiac faints of this type may recur several times a day. Occasionally the heart block is transitory, and the electrocardiogram taken later may not show any arrhythmia.

Less commonly, a decreased rate of discharge of the sinoatrial node leads to syncope. Recurrent attacks of tachyarrhythmias—including atrial flutter and paroxysmal atrial and ventricular tachycardia with normal AV conduction—may also suddenly reduce cardiac output to a degree sufficient to cause syncope.

In another form of cardiac syncope the heart block is reflexive and is due to irritation of the vagus nerves. Examples of this phenomenon have been observed in patients with esophageal diverticula, mediastinal tumors, gallbladder disease, carotid sinus disease, glossopharyngeal neuralgia, and pleural and pulmonary irritation. However, in these conditions reflex bradycardia is more commonly of the sinoatrial than the atrioventricular type.

Cardiac syncope may also result from *acute massive myocardial infarction*, particularly when associated with cardiogenic shock. *Aortic stenosis* often sets the stage for exertional syncope, most commonly by limiting cardiac output in the face of peripheral vasodilatation, but sometimes during exertion, with resultant myocardial and cerebral ischemia and occasionally arrhythmias. *Idiopathic hypertrophic subaortic stenosis* may also lead to exertional syncope, because of intensified obstruction and/or ventricular arrhythmias (Chap. 237). In *primary pulmonary hypertension* a relatively fixed cardiac output and bouts of acute right ventricular failure may be associated with syncope (Chap. 265). However, vagal reflexes may be involved in this condition as well as in the syncope that occurs with *pulmonary embolism*. Ball valve thrombus in the left atrium, left atrial myxoma, or thrombosis or malfunction of a prosthetic valve may produce sudden mechanical obstruction of the circulation and syncope. *Tetralogy of Fallot* is the congenital cardiac malformation most commonly responsible for syncope. In this condition systemic vasodilatation, perhaps associated with infundibular spasm, greatly increases the right-to-left shunt and produces arterial hypoxia, which leads to syncope (Chap. 240).

CAROTID SINUS SYNCOPE The carotid sinus is normally sensitive to stretch and gives rise to sensory impulses carried via the nerve of Hering, a branch of the glossopharyngeal nerve, to the medulla oblongata. Massage of one or both of the carotid sinuses, particularly in elderly persons, causes (1) a reflex cardiac slowing (sinus bradycardia, sinus arrest, or even atrioventricular block), the so-called vagal type of response, (2) a fall of arterial pressure without cardiac slowing, the so-called "depressor" type of response, and (3) an interference with the circulation of the ipsilateral cerebral hemisphere, the so-called "central" type. Two or three types of carotid sinus response may coexist.

Syncope due to carotid sinus sensitivity may be initiated by turning of the head to one side, by a tight collar, or, as in a few reported cases, by shaving over the region of the sinus. But the absence of such stimuli is of no aid in diagnosis, since spontaneous attacks may occur. The attack nearly always begins when the patient is in an upright position, usually when standing. The period of unconsciousness seldom lasts longer than a few minutes. The sensorium is immediately clear when consciousness is regained. The majority of the reported cases have been in men. In a patient displaying faintness on compression of one carotid sinus, it is important to distinguish between the benign disorder (hypersensitivity of one carotid sinus) and a much more serious condition—atheromatous narrowing of the opposite carotid or of the basilar artery (see Chap. 365).

Other forms of vasovagal syncope have been described. Exceptionally intense pain of visceral origin may inhibit cardiac action through vagal stimulation, e.g., cardiac standstill during an attack of gallbladder colic, a lesion of the esophagus or mediastinum, bronchoscopy, pleural or peritoneal taps, intense vertigo from labyrinthine or vestibular disease, and needling of body cavities.

VAGAL AND GLOSSOPHARYNGEAL NEURALGIA Occasionally this induces a reflex type of fainting. Again the sequence is always pain, then syncope; in this instance the pain is localized to the base of the tongue, pharynx or larynx, tonsillar area, and ear. It may be triggered by pressure at these sites. Section of the appropriate branches of the ninth or tenth cranial nerve relieves the condition. The cardiovascular effects are attribut-

able to excitation of the dorsal motor nucleus of the vagus via collateral fibers from the nucleus of the tractus solitarius.

TUSSIVE SYNCOPE (LARYNGEAL VERTIGO) This is a rare condition that results from a paroxysm of coughing, usually in men with chronic bronchitis. After hard coughing the patient suddenly becomes weak and loses consciousness momentarily. The intrathoracic pressure becomes elevated and interferes with the venous return to the heart, as does the Valsalva maneuver (exhaling against a closed glottis). Episodes of faintness and lightheadedness are not infrequent in pertussis and chronic laryngitis.

SYNCOPE ASSOCIATED WITH CEREBROVASCULAR DISEASE This is usually caused by partial or complete occlusion of the large arteries in the neck. Physical activity may then critically reduce blood flow to the upper part of the brainstem, causing abrupt loss of consciousness (see Chap. 365).

PATHOPHYSIOLOGY OF SYNCOPE

In the final analysis the loss of consciousness in these different types of syncope is caused by a change in the nervous elements in those parts of the brain which subserve consciousness. Syncope resembles epilepsy in this respect; yet there is an important difference. In epilepsy, whether major or minor, the arrest in mental function is almost instantaneous, and, as revealed by the electroencephalogram, it is accompanied by a paroxysm of activity in certain groups of cerebral neurons. Syncope, on the other hand, is not so sudden. The difference relates to the essential pathophysiology—a sudden spread of an electric discharge in epilepsy, and the more gradual failure of the cerebral circulation in syncope.

During syncopal attacks, there are demonstrable reductions in cerebral blood flow, cerebral oxygen utilization, and cerebral vascular resistance. The electroencephalogram reveals high-voltage slow waves, two to five per second, coincident with the loss of consciousness. If the ischemia lasts only a few minutes, there are no lasting effects on the brain. If it persists for a longer time, it may result in necrosis of the border zones between the major cerebral and cerebellar arteries.

DIFFERENTIAL DIAGNOSIS OF CONDITIONS INVOLVING EPISODIC WEAKNESS AND FAINTNESS BUT NOT SYNCOPE

ANXIETY ATTACKS AND THE HYPERVENTILATION SYNDROME These are discussed in detail in Chaps. 11 and 25. The giddiness of anxiety is frequently interpreted as a feeling of faintness without actual loss of consciousness. Such symptoms are not accompanied by facial pallor and are not relieved by recumbency. The diagnosis is made on the basis of the associated symptoms, and part of the attack can be reproduced by hyperventilation. Two of the mechanisms known to be involved in the attacks are reduction in carbon dioxide as the result of hyperventilation and the release of epinephrine. Hyperventilation results in hypocapnia, alkalosis, increased cerebrovascular resistance, and decreased cerebral blood flow.

HYPOGLYCEMIA When severe, hypoglycemia is usually traceable to a serious disease, such as a tumor of the islets of Langerhans or advanced adrenal, pituitary, or hepatic disease, or to excessive administration of insulin. The clinical picture is one of confusion or even a loss of consciousness. When mild, as is usually the case, hypoglycemia is the reactive type (Chap. 339), occurring 2 to 5 h after eating, and is not usually associated with a disturbance of consciousness. The diagnosis depends on the history, the documentation of reduced blood sugar during an attack, and the reproduction by an injection of insulin of a symptom complex exactly similar to that occurring in the spontaneous attacks.

ACUTE HEMORRHAGE Acute blood loss, usually within the gastrointestinal tract, is an occasional cause of syncope. In the absence of pain and hematemesis the cause of the weakness, faintness, or even unconsciousness may remain obscure until the passage of a black stool.

CEREBRAL ISCHEMIC ATTACKS These occur in some patients with arteriosclerotic narrowings or occlusion of the major arteries of the brain. The main symptoms vary from patient to patient and include dim vision, hemiparesis, numbness of one side of the body, dizziness, and thick speech, and to these may be added an impairment of consciousness. In any one patient all attacks are of identical type and indicate a temporary deficit of the function in a certain region of the brain due to inadequate circulation.

HYSTERICAL FAINTING Hysterical fainting is rather frequent and usually occurs under dramatic circumstances (Chap. 11). The attack is unattended by any outward display of anxiety. The evident lack of change in pulse and blood pressure or color of the skin and mucous membranes distinguishes it from the vasodepressor faint. The diagnosis is based on the bizarre nature of the attack in a person who exhibits the general personality and behavioral characteristics of hysteria.

DIFFERENTIAL DIAGNOSIS OF SEIZURE AND SYNCOPE

Most typical varieties of syncope must be distinguished from other disturbances of cerebral function, the most frequent of which is akinetic or some other form of epilepsy (see Chap. 23). The epileptic attack may occur day or night, regardless of the position of the patient; syncope rarely appears when the patient is recumbent, the only common exception being the Stokes-Adams attack. The patient's color does not usually change in epilepsy; pallor is an early and invariable finding in all types of syncope, except chronic orthostatic hypotension and hysteria, and it precedes unconsciousness. Epilepsy is more sudden in onset, and if an aura is present, it rarely lasts longer than a few seconds before consciousness is abolished. The onset of syncope is usually more deliberate and without aura. Injury from falling is frequent in epilepsy and rare in syncope, for the reason that only in epilepsy are protective reflexes instantaneously abolished. Tonic-convulsive movements with upturning eyes are a feature of epilepsy and not syncope. The period of unconsciousness tends to be longer in epilepsy than in syncope. Urinary incontinence is frequent in epilepsy and rare in syncope, but since it may be observed occasionally in syncope, it cannot be used as a means of excluding epilepsy. The return of consciousness is prompt in syncope, slow in epilepsy. Mental confusion, headache, and drowsiness are common sequelae in epilepsy; physical weakness with clear sensorium characterizes the postsyncopal state. Repeated spells of unconsciousness in a young person at a rate of several per day or month are more suggestive of epilepsy than of syncope. No one of these points will absolutely differentiate epilepsy from syncope, but taken as a group and supplemented by electroencephalograms, they provide a means of distinguishing the two conditions.

DIFFERENT TYPES OF SYNCOPE Differentiation of the several conditions that diminish cerebral blood flow is discussed in greater detail in Chap. 30.

When faintness is related to reduced cerebral blood flow

resulting directly from a disorder of cardiac function, there is likely to be a combination of pallor and cyanosis. When, on the other hand, the peripheral circulation is at fault, pallor is usually striking but is not accompanied by cyanosis or respiratory disturbances. When the primary disturbance lies in the cerebral circulation, the face is likely to be florid and the breathing slow and stertorous. During the attack a heart rate faster than 150 beats per minute indicates an ectopic cardiac rhythm, while a striking bradycardia (rate of less than 40 beats per minute) suggests complete heart block. In a patient with faintness or syncope attended by bradycardia, one has to distinguish between the neurogenic reflex and the cardiogenic (Stokes-Adams) types. The electrocardiogram is decisive, but even without it, the Stokes-Adams seizures can be recognized clinically by their longer duration, by the greater constancy of the slow heart rate, by the presence of audible sounds synchronous with atrial contraction, by atrial contraction (A) waves in the jugular venous pulse, and by marked variation in intensity of the first sound, despite the regular rhythm (Chap. 237).

It is of primary importance to know the circumstances and the precipitating and alleviating factors in a given episode of weakness or fainting.

TYPE OF ONSET When the attack begins over the period of a few seconds, carotid sinus syncope, postural hypotension, sudden atrioventricular block, ventricular standstill, or fibrillation is likely. When the symptoms develop gradually during a period of several minutes, hyperventilation or hypoglycemia should be considered. Onset of syncope during or immediately after exertion suggests aortic stenosis or idiopathic hypertrophic subaortic stenosis and, in elderly subjects, postural hypotension. Exertional syncope is seen occasionally in persons with aortic insufficiency and with severe occlusive disease of cerebral arteries. In patients with ventricular standstill or ventricular fibrillation, loss of consciousness occurs several seconds later, followed rapidly by cessation of electroencephalographic activity and then often by brief clonic contractions.

POSITION AT ONSET OF ATTACK Epilepsy and syncopal attacks due to hypoglycemia, hyperventilation, or heart block are likely to be independent of posture. Faintness associated with a decline in blood pressure (including carotid sinus attacks) and with ectopic tachycardia usually occurs only in the sitting or standing position, whereas faintness resulting from orthostatic hypotension is apt to set in shortly after change from the recumbent to the standing position.

ASSOCIATED SYMPTOMS Palpitation is likely to be present when the attack is due to anxiety or hyperventilation, to ectopic tachycardia, or to hypoglycemia. Numbness and tingling in the hands and face are frequent accompaniments of hyperventilation. Genuine convulsions during the attack, although characteristic of epilepsy, may occasionally occur with heart block, ventricular standstill, or fibrillation.

DURATION OF ATTACK When the duration is very brief, i.e., a few seconds to a few minutes, carotid sinus syncope or one of the several forms of postural hypotension is most likely. A duration of more than a few minutes but less than an hour suggests hypoglycemia or hyperventilation.

SPECIAL METHODS OF EXAMINATION

In many patients who complain of recurrent weakness or syncope but do not have a spontaneous attack while under observation of the physician, an attempt to reproduce attacks is of great assistance in diagnosis.

When hyperventilation is accompanied by faintness, the pattern of symptoms can be reproduced readily by having the subject breathe rapidly and deeply for 2 to 3 min. This test is often of therapeutic value also, because the underlying anxiety tends to be lessened when the patient learns that the symptoms can be produced and alleviated at will simply by controlling breathing.

Among other conditions in which the diagnosis is commonly clarified by reproducing the attacks are carotid sinus hypersensitivity (massage of one or the other carotid sinus), orthostatic hypotension and orthostatic tachycardia (observations of pulse rate, blood pressure, and symptoms in the recumbent and standing positions), and tussive syncope (by inducing the Valsalva maneuver). In all these instances the crucial point is not whether symptoms are produced (the procedures mentioned frequently induce symptoms in healthy persons) but whether the exact pattern of symptoms that occurs in the spontaneous attacks is reproduced in all the artificial ones. Careful, continuous monitoring of the electrocardiogram in the hospital or the recording of the electrocardiogram over 1 or 2 days using a portable lightweight tape recorder in an ambulatory patient may be extremely useful in identifying an arrhythmia responsible for the syncopal episode. Monitoring is most helpful if it shows that the syncopal episode is characterized by a bout of cardiac standstill, extreme bradycardia, or tachyarrhythmia.

The electroencephalogram may be helpful in differentiating syncope from epilepsy. In the interval between epileptic seizures it may show some degree of abnormality in 40 to 80 percent of cases. In the interval between syncopal attacks it should be normal.

TREATMENT

Fainting in most instances is relatively benign. In dealing with patients who have fainted, the physician should think first of those causes of fainting that consitute a therapeutic emergency. Among them are massive internal hemorrhage and myocardial infarction, which may be painless, and cardiac arrhythmias. In elderly persons a sudden faint, without obvious cause, should arouse the suspicion of complete heart block, even though all findings are negative when they are seen by a physician.

Patients seen during the preliminary stages of fainting or after they have lost consciousness should be placed in a position which permits maximal cerebral blood flow, i.e., with head lowered between the knees, if sitting, or in the supine position. All tight clothing and other constrictions should be loosened and the head turned so that the tongue does not fall back into the throat, blocking the airway. Peripheral irritation, such as sprinkling or dashing cold water on the face and neck or the application of cold moist towels, is helpful. If the temperature is subnormal, the body should be covered with a warm blanket. If available, aromatic spirit of ammonia may be given cautiously by inhalation. Since emesis is frequent, one should be prepared for a possible aspiration. Nothing should be given by mouth until the patient has regained consciousness. Then one-half a teaspoon of aromatic spirit of ammonia in one-half a glass of cold water, or a sip of brandy or whiskey, may be given. Patients should not be permitted to rise until the sense of physical weakness has passed, and they should be watched carefully for a few minutes after rising.

The *prevention* of fainting depends on the mechanisms in-

volved. In the usual vasovagal faint of adolescents, which tends to occur in periods of emotional excitement, fatigue, hunger, etc., it is enough to advise the patient to avoid such circumstances. In postural hypotension, patients should be cautioned against arising suddenly from bed. Instead, they should first exercise their legs for a few seconds, then sit on the edge of the bed and make sure they are not lightheaded or dizzy before starting to walk. Sleeping with the headposts of the bed elevated on wooden blocks 8 to 12 in high and wearing snug elastic abdominal binder and elastic stockings are often helpful. Drugs of the ephedrine group may be useful if they do not cause insomnia. If there are no contraindications, a high intake of sodium chloride, which expands the extracellular fluid volume, may be beneficial.

In the syndrome of chronic orthostatic hypotension, special corticosteroid preparations (Florinef acetate tables, 1 to 2 mg per day in divided doses) have given relief in some cases. Binding of the legs (g suit) and sleeping with head and shoulders elevated are helpful.

The treatment of carotid sinus syncope involves first of all instructing the patient in measures that minimize the hazards of a fall (see below). Loose collars should be worn, and the patient should learn to turn the whole body, rather than the head alone, when looking to one side. Atropine or the ephedrine group of drugs should be used, respectively, in patients with pronounced bradycardia or hypotension during attacks. If atropine is not successful, a demand pacemaker should be inserted into the right ventricle. Radiation or surgical denervation of the carotid sinus has apparently yielded favorable results in some patients, but it is rarely necessary. Once it has been concluded that the attacks are due to a narrowing of major cerebral arteries, some of the surgical measures discussed in Chap. 365 must be considered.

The treatment of the various cardiac arrhythmias which may induce syncope is discussed in Chap. 237. The treatment of hypoglycemia will be found in Chap. 339 and of the hyperventilation syndrome and hysterical fainting in Chaps. 11 and 12, respectively.

The chief hazard of a faint in most elderly persons is not the underlying disease but rather fracture or other trauma due to the fall. Therefore, patients subject to recurrent syncope should cover the bathroom floor and bathtub with rubber mats and should have as much of their home carpeted as is feasible. Especially important is the floor space between the bed and the bathroom, because faints are common in elderly persons when walking from bed to toilet. Outdoor walking should be on soft ground rather than hard surfaces, and the patient should avoid standing still, which is more likely than walking to induce an attack.

REFERENCES

HICKLER R: Fainting, in *Signs and Symptoms,* 6th ed, RS Blacklow (ed). Philadelphia, Lippincott, 1977, chap 33

JOHNSON RH, SPAULDING JMK: *Disorders of the Autonomic Nervous System.* Philadelphia, Davis, 1974

LEE JE et al: Episodic unconsciousness, in *Diagnostic Approaches to Presenting Syndromes,* JA Barondess (ed). Baltimore, Williams & Wilkins, 1971, pp 133–167

WEISSLER AM, WARREN JV: Syncope and shock, in *The Heart,* 4th ed, JW Hurst (ed). New York, McGraw-Hill, 1978, p 705

WRIGHT KE JR., MCINTOSH MD: Syncope: Review of pathophysiological mechanisms. Prog Cardiovasc Dis 13:580, 1971

YOUNG RR et al: Pure pandysautonomia with recovery. Trans Am Neurol Assoc 94:355, 1969

ZIEGLER MG et al: The sympathetic nervous system defect in primary orthostatic hypotension. New Engl J Med 296:293, 1977

DIZZINESS AND VERTIGO

MAURICE VICTOR
RAYMOND D. ADAMS

Dizziness and other sensations of unbalance occur in a wide variety of diseases. In many instances the clue to an important medical disorder is afforded by the correct analysis of the complaint.

The term *dizziness* covers a number of different sensory experiences—true vertigo, which refers to a feeling of whirling or rotation, as well as nonrotatory swaying, weakness, faintness, and lightheadedness. Blurring of vision, feelings of unreality, syncope, and even petit mal may be incorrectly called dizzy spells; hence a close questioning as to how the patient is using the term becomes a necessary first step in clinical study. A distinction is sometimes drawn between subjective vertigo, meaning a sense of turning one's body, and objective vertigo, an illusion of movement of objects in the environment, but its validity is doubtful.

In this chapter the term *vertigo* is used to refer to all subjective and objective illusions of rotation. *Giddiness* refers to a swaying type of dizziness. *Equilibrium,* the state of equipoise whereby the posture of the body is maintained against the forces of gravity, is deranged in vertigo but is also affected by other disorders as well, e.g., loss of joint or muscle sense (sensory ataxia), cerebellar disease (cerebellar ataxia), and motor abnormalities (spasticity and rigidity, myotonia, and the pseudomyotonia of hypothyroidism).

ANATOMIC, PHYSIOLOGIC, AND PSYCHOLOGIC CONSIDERATIONS Several mechanisms maintain balanced posture and awareness of the body's positions in relation to its surroundings. The most important of these are:

1 Impulses from the retinas of the eyes which are coordinated by ocular motor mechanisms to supply information about the position and movement of the body and its surroundings.
2 Impulses from the labyrinths of the inner ears—specialized spatial proprioceptors whose primary function is to register changes in the direction of motion (either acceleration or deceleration) and position of the body. [*Note:* The semicircular canals respond to movement and angular momentum, whereas the otoliths (sense organs of the utricle and saccule) are mainly concerned with orienting the organism with reference to gravitational force.]
3 Impulses from the proprioceptors of joints and muscles—essential to all reflex, postural, and volitional movements. Those of the neck are of special importance in relating the position of the head to that of the rest of the body.

The cerebellum and certain ganglionic centers in the brainstem (particularly the vestibular nuclei, oculomotor nuclei, and red nuclei) and in the basal ganglia are the important coordinators of these sensory data and provide for postural adjustment, upright stance, and locomotion.

Important psychophysiologic mechanisms are also involved in the maintenance of equilibrium and the proper relationship of our bodies to the external world. Early in life we come to coordinate the parts of our body in relation to one another and to perceive that portion of space occupied by our bodies. The construct of these integrated sensory data has been designated by Russell Brain as the *body schema.* The space around our body is said to be represented by another set of data, the *environmental schema.* These two schemata are dynamic and interdependent, since both are simultaneously changed in every activity. For example, we learn to see objects as being stationary when we are moving. Thus, the motion of ourselves and of objects in space is always relative. At times, when sensory information is incomplete, we mistake movement of our surroundings for those of our own body, as in the illusion caused by motion of a neighboring train. A disturbance in the awareness of one's own body schema is postulated by some psychiatrists as the basis of neurotic disorientation and psychotic feelings of unreality.

CLINICAL CHARACTERISTICS OF VERTIGO AND GIDDINESS
The clinical recognition of *vertigo* proves to be relatively easy when the patient states that objects in the environment turned or moved in one direction or that the head and body whirled. Often, however, the patient is not so explicit. The feeling may be described as oscillation, or of veering, of being pulled to one side or to the ground, as though drawn by a magnet (impulsion). Again, the floor or walls may seem to tilt, sink, or rise up. The feeling of impulsion is particularly characteristic of vertigo.

All but the mildest forms of vertigo are accompanied by perspiration, pallor, nausea, and vomiting. The nystagmus which is invariably present causes objects in the field of vision to move rhythmically in one direction. As a rule the patient can walk only with difficulty or not at all, should the vertigo be intense. A sudden attack may even catapult the patient to the ground, and only when down is vertigo experienced. Forced to lie down the patient realizes that one position, usually on one side with eyes closed, reduces the vertigo and nausea, and that the slightest motion of the head aggravates them. One form of vertigo, the benign positional vertigo of Bárány, occurs only for a few seconds after lying down and sitting up. If the vertigo is less severe, the patient can walk unsteadily but may veer to one side. The ataxia of gait with vertigo (vertiginous ataxia) is recognized always as being a "dizziness in the head," not a trouble in the control of the legs and trunk. It is noteworthy that in these circumstances the coordination of the individual movements of the limbs is not impaired—a point of difference from cerebellar disease. There may be headache, especially in the region of the offending ear. Loss of consciousness as part of a vertiginous attack nearly always signifies another type of disorder (seizure or faint).

Giddiness and other types of pseudovertigo are usually described as feelings of swaying, lightheadedness, a swimming sensation, and, more rarely, as though walking on air, "queer in the head," uncertain, about to fall or "pass out." These sensory experiences are particularly common in psychiatric illnesses featured by anxiety attacks. They may be reproduced by hyperventilation, and then it is appreciated that panic and apprehensiveness, palpitation, breathlessness, trembling, and sweating are concurrent.

Other pseudovertiginous symptoms are less definite. In severe anemic states weakness and languor may be attended by a lightheadedness related to postural change and exertion. In the emphysematous patient physical effort may be associated with weakness and peculiar cephalic sensations, and coughing may lead to giddiness and even fainting (tussive syncope) because of impaired return of venous blood to the heart. The dizziness that so often accompanies hypertension is more difficult to evaluate. Sometimes it is an expression of anxiety, or it may be due to an unstable adjustment of cerebral blood flow. *Postural dizziness* is another example of unstable vasomotor reflexes preventing a constancy of cerebral circulation and is notably frequent in persons recently bedfast, in the weak and ill, and the elderly. Abrupt arising from a recumbent or sitting position is followed immediately by a swaying type of dizziness, dimming of vision, and spots before the eyes which last a few seconds. The patient is forced to stand still and hold onto a nearby object until steady. A syncopal attack may occur at this time (see Chap. 13).

In practice it is not difficult to separate these types of pseudovertigo from true vertigo, for there is none of the feeling of rotation or impulsion so characteristic of the latter. Lacking also are the other ancillary symptoms of true vertigo, namely, nausea, vomiting, tinnitus and deafness, nystagmus, and staggering.

NEUROLOGIC AND OTOLOGIC CAUSES OF VERTIGO Vertigo may constitute the aura of an epileptic seizure, but this event is rare. The lesion is then on the posterolateral aspects of the temporal lobe near the sylvian fissure. A sensation of movement, either of the body away from the side of the lesion or of the environment in the opposite direction, lasts for a few seconds before being submerged in other seizure activity. Vertiginous sensations may rarely serve as a stimulus for *reflex epilepsy* (see Chap. 23), and the test for this form of vertigo provokes the seizure.

Oculomotor disorders are a source of a spatial disorientation simulating dizziness. This is maximal when the patient looks in the direction of action of the paralyzed muscle; it is attributable to the receipt of two conflicting visual images. In fact some normal individuals even experience dizziness for a time when adjusting to bifocal glasses or when looking down from a height.

Whether lesions of the cerebellum can produce vertigo seems to depend on the part of it involved. Large destructive processes in the cerebellar hemispheres and vermis may cause no vertigo whatsoever, unless they extend to central vestibulocerebellar connections. However, Duncan, Parker, and Fisher report definite vertigo in verified lesions of the posterior-inferior part of the hemisphere due to occlusion limited to the cerebellar branch of the inferior cerebellar artery.

Labyrinthine (aural) lesions are the usual causes of paroxysmal vertigo. In the classic variety, that of Ménière's disease, the onset is abrupt, the vertigo is clearly of the rotary type, and it lasts a few minutes to hours. Concomitant tinnitus, fullness in the ear, high-tone deafness with auditory recruitment (see Chaps. 18 and 376), nystagmus, nausea, vomiting, and staggering constitute the full syndrome. The patient preferentially lies with the faulty ear uppermost and is disinclined to look toward the normal side because of exaggeration of the nystagmus and dizziness. The nystagmus is fine, rotatory, and most pronounced when the eyes are turned away from the offending ear. Vertiginous attacks of this type may recur and give rise to mild, chronic states of disequilibrium which may persist for days. Seldom does the vertigo last, however, for central mechanisms compensate for permanent deficits of one labyrinth. Chronic vertigo may be complicated by the giddiness of a secondary anxiety state. *Vestibular neuronitis* is a term that refers to severe vertigo, often of several days' duration, without tinnitus or deafness. Its pathologic basis is uncertain. Episodic vertigo occurs in the syndrome known as *Bárány's benign positional vertigo* and the more malignant positional vertigo of posterior fossa tumors and other lesions, and lasts only a few seconds (Chap. 376).

Vertigo of acoustic nerve origin, the commonest cause of which is an acoustic neuroma, tends usually to be mild and intermittent (lasting weeks or months). Seldom does it come in discrete attacks separated by free intervals. Vertigo has rarely been observed as the initial symptom with eighth nerve tumors, but the usual sequence is deafness of high-frequency type (without recruitment), followed some time later by a sense of imbalance and impaired caloric responses, then cranial nerve palsies (involving the eighth, fifth, and tenth nerves), ipsilateral ataxia of limbs, and headache, the other common signs of a cerebellopontine angle tumor (see Chap. 367).

A number of ototoxic drugs may result in labyrinthine and auditory symptoms, sometimes permanent (see Chap. 376).

Vertigo of brainstem origin implicates vestibular nuclei and their connections. In these cases auditory function is nearly always spared, since the vestibular and cochlear fibers separate upon entering the medulla and pons. The nystagmus which accompanies such central lesions tends to be coarse, protracted, and variable; it is more marked on lateral gaze to one side than the other. There may also be a nonrotary vertical component. The central localization is evidenced further by the attendant signs of involvement of other structures within the brainstem (cranial nerves, sensory and motor tracts, etc.) Mode of onset, duration, and other features of the clinical picture depend upon the nature of the causative disease, usually vascular (basilar artery, vertebral artery, or labyrinthine artery occlusion), traumatic, neoplastic, or demyelinative.

Electronystagmography is often helpful in the diagnosis of central vertigo. It will reveal vertical nystagmus with eyes closed, types I and II positional nystagmus, perverted nystagmus on caloric stimulation, and ocular deviations with eyes closed.

APPROACH TO THE PATIENT WITH DIZZINESS As already stated, a careful history and physical examination of the dizzy patient usually afford a basis for separating true vertigo from the swaying dizziness of the hyperventilating, anxious patient and from the other types of pseudovertigo (such as partial syncope and feelings of unreality). If the patient is unobservant or imprecise in descriptions, a helpful tactic is to provoke a number of dissimilar sensations by rotating the patient, irrigating the ears with warm or cold water, by asking the patient to stoop for a minute and straighten up, by hyperventilating for 3 min, and by measuring the blood pressure as the patient changes from a recumbent to a standing position and remains upright for 3 to 4 min. Should the patient be unable to distinguish among these several types of induced sensation or to ascertain the similarity of one of the types to his or her own condition, the history is probably too inaccurate for purposes of diagnosis.

When vertigo is mild or difficult for the patient to describe, small items of the history, such as disinclination to walk during an attack, tendency to list to one side, aggravation by riding in a vehicle, preference for one position, are helpful. They distinguish vertigo from giddiness.

In some patients an attack of vertigo is so abrupt and violent that they are virtually flung to the ground, sometimes with a serious injury. These attacks have been called by the quaint term "otolithic crises of Tumarken," but without proof of involvement of the utricle or saccule. The diagnosis is usually substantiated by the presence of vertigo, nausea, and vomiting while on the ground, distinguishing it from a seizure, faint, or cataplexy. Probably it differs from other forms of labyrinthine vertigo only in its severity.

In the differentiation of types of labyrinthine and vestibular nerve disease, inspection of eardrums, x-rays of mastoids, middle ears, and inner ears, and auditory and caloric tests are useful, especially in excluding labyrinthitis. In caloric testing, the patient's head is tilted forward 30° from the horizontal (bringing the horizontal semicircular canal into a vertical plane), which is the position of maximal sensitivity to thermal stimuli. The external auditory meati are irrigated in turn for 40 s with water at 30 and 44°C (7°C below and above body temperature). Cold water induces nystagmus to the opposite side (direction of the fast phase), and warm water to the same side.

The nystagmus begins in 20 s and should persist 90 to 120 s. Comparison of the two ears reveals which one is paretic or hypersensitive. Special rotational chairs and electronystagmography are other more refined means of assessing disordered labyrinthine function. The diagnosis of benign positional vertigo is settled at the bedside by reproducing a brief vertigo and nystagmus (lasting up to a minute) by moving the patient from the sitting position to recumbency with head to one side in one trial and to the other in the second. Going from a recumbent to a sitting position reverses the direction of vertigo and nystagmus. This specific pattern and its reversibility are not observed in the more malignant positional vertigo of posterior fossa tumors and other lesions. The application of some of the maneuvers designed to elicit weakness and syncope (see Chap. 13) will distinguish these forms of pseudovertigo.

The association of vertigo with auditory signs and symptoms always signifies a disease process of end organ or eighth nerve. Labyrinthine and auditory tests and the presence or absence of neurologic signs of structures adjacent to the eighth cranial nerve nuclei are useful in their differentiation.

Pure vertigo as a manifestation of disease of the brainstem is rare, and the rule we have found trustworthy is that unless other symptoms and signs appear within 1 to 2 weeks, one can nearly always postulate an aural origin and exclude vascular disease of the brainstem. This is also true of multiple sclerosis, which may be the explanation of a persistent vertigo in some adolescents or young adults.

REFERENCES

ADAMS RD, VICTOR M: *Principles of Neurology.* New York, McGraw-Hill, 1977

ALTMANN F: Diagnostic significance of vertigo, in *The Vestibular System and Its Diseases,* RJ Wolfson (ed). Philadelphia, University of Pennsylvania Press, 1966, p 353

DIX MR: Modern tests of vestibular function, with special reference to their value in clinical practice. Br Med J 3:317, 1969

DUNCAN GW et al: Acute cerebellar infarction in the PICA territory. Arch Neurol 32:364, 1975

FISHER CM: Vertigo in cerebrovascular disease. Arch Otolaryngol 85:529, 1967

SPECTOR M: *Dizziness and Vertigo.* New York, Grune & Stratton, 1967

15
MOTOR PARALYSIS

RAYMOND D. ADAMS

Impairments of motor function may be subdivided into (1) paralysis due to affection of lower motor neurons, (2) paralysis due to disorder of upper motor (corticospinal and corticobrainstem) neurons, (3) abnormalities of coordination (ataxia) due to lesions in the cerebellum, (4) abnormalities of movement and posture due to disease of the extrapyramidal motor system, and (5) apraxic or nonparalytic disturbances of purposive movement due to involvement of the cerebrum. The first two types of motor disorder and the cerebral disorders of movement are discussed briefly in the following pages; purely muscular weakness and paralysis will be discussed in Chap. 378; cerebellar ataxia and extrapyramidal motor abnormalities are considered in Chap. 16.

DEFINITIONS When applied to voluntary muscles, *paralysis* means loss of contraction due to interruption of one of the motor pathways from the cerebrum to the muscle fiber. Lesser degrees of paralysis are sometimes spoken of as *paresis,* but in everyday medical parlance motor paralysis usually stands for either partial or complete loss of function. The word *plegia* comes from the Greek word meaning stroke; and the word *palsy,* from an old French word, has the same meaning as paralysis. It is preferable to use *paresis* for slight and paralysis or plegia for severe loss of motor function.

PARALYSIS DUE TO DISEASE OF THE LOWER MOTOR NEURONS Each motor nerve cell, through the extensive arborization of the terminal part of its fiber, comes into contact with 100 to 200 or more muscle fibers; altogether they constitute "the motor unit." All the variations in force, range, and type of movement are determined by differences in the number and size of motor units called into activity and the frequency of their action. Feeble movements recruit few units, stronger ones many more units of increasing size. Histochemical methods show that motor units involved in slow, tonic contractions (type I) have muscle fibers rich in oxidative enzymes and mitochondria, and those involved in fast, phasic contractions (type II), more phosphorylase. When a motor neuron becomes diseased, as in progressive muscular atrophy, it may manifest increased irritability, and all the muscle fibers that it controls may discharge sporadically, in isolation from other units. The result of the contraction of one or several such units is a visible twitch, or *fasciculation,* which can be seen and recorded in the electromyogram as a large diphasic or multiphasic action potential. If the motor neuron is destroyed, all the muscle fibers to which it is attached undergo a profound atrophy, namely, denervation atrophy. For some unknown reason the individual denervated muscle fibers now begin to be hypersensitive and to contract spontaneously, though they can no longer do so in response to a nerve impulse as a part of the motor unit. This isolated activity of individual muscle fibers is called *fibrillation* and is so fine that it cannot be seen through the intact skin and can be recorded only as a repetitive short-duration spike potential in the electromyogram. The motor nerve fibers of each anterior root intermingle with adjacent roots as they join to form plexuses, and although the innervation of the muscles is roughly according to segments of the spinal cord, each large muscle comes to be supplied by two or more roots. In contrast, a single peripheral nerve usually provides the complete motor innervation of a muscle or group of muscles. For this reason the distribution of paralysis due to disease of the anterior horn cells or anterior roots differs from that which follows a lesion of a peripheral nerve.

All motor activity, even the most elementary reflex type, requires the cooperation of several muscles. The analysis of a relatively simple movement, such as clenching the fist, affords some idea of the complexity of the underlying neural arrangements. In this act the primary movement is a contraction of the flexor muscles of the fingers, the flexor digitorum sublimis and profundus, the flexor pollicis longus and brevis, and the abductor pollicis brevis. These muscles act as *agonists,* or *prime movers,* in this act. In order for flexion to be smooth and forceful, the extensor muscles (antagonists) must relax at the same rate at which the flexors contract. The muscles which flex the fingers also flex the wrist; and since it is desired that only the fingers flex, the muscles which extend the wrist must be brought into play to prevent its flexion. The action of the wrist extensors is *synergic,* and these muscles are called synergists in this particular act. Lastly the wrist, elbow, and shoulder must be stabilized by appropriate flexor and extensor muscles, which serve as *fixators.* The coordination of agonists, antagonists, synergists, and fixators involves reciprocal innervation and is managed entirely by segmental spinal reflexes under the guidance of proprioceptive sensory stimuli. Only the agonist movement in a voluntary act is believed to be initiated at a cortical level.

In addition, there are many basic motor activities, such as the maintenance of certain postures and stepping movements, which do not involve reciprocal innervation. For these activities agonists and antagonists contract simultaneously. The alternating movements of spinal stepping represent an even more elaborate type of coordination. Also in the support of the body in an upright posture, when the limb must be as rigid as a pillar, and in shivering the agonists and antagonists must act together. In general, the more delicate the movement, the more precise the coordination between agonist and antagonist muscles.

If all or practically all peripheral motor nerves supplying a muscle are destroyed, all voluntary, postural, and reflex movements are abolished. The muscle becomes soft and yields excessively to passive stretching, a condition known as flaccidity. Muscle tone—the slight resistance that normal relaxed muscle offers to passive movement—is reduced (hypotonia or atonia). The denervated muscles undergo extreme atrophy, usually being reduced to 20 to 30 percent of their original bulk within 3 months. The reaction of the muscle to sudden stretch, as by tapping its tendon, is lost. And, finally, it may be demonstrated that the muscle will no longer respond to electric stimuli of short duration, i.e., faradic stimuli, but still responds to currents of long duration, i.e., to galvanic stimuli. This alteration of electric response is known as *Erb's reaction of degeneration.* If only a part of the motor units in the muscles is affected, partial paralysis will ensue. Quantitative testing by determination of strength-duration curves is a means of showing partial denervation, and electromyographic evidence of fibrillations may also be obtained.

The tonus of muscle and the tendon reflexes are known to depend on the muscle spindles and the afferent fibers to which they give origin and on the small anterior horn cells whose axons terminate on the small muscle fibers within the spindles. These small spinal motor neurons are called *gamma neurons,* in contrast to the large *alpha neurons.* Two different gamma neurons are now recognized, one, connected with nuclear bag spindle muscle fibers for phasic actions; the other, with nuclear chain spindle fibers for tonic actions. A tap on a tendon, by stretching the spindle muscle fibers, activates afferent neurons which transmit impulses to alpha motor neurons. The result is the familiar brief muscle contraction or tendon reflex. The spindle muscle fibers are then relaxed (unloaded), which terminates the reflex. Thus the setting of the spindle fibers and the state of excitability of the gamma neurons (normally inhibited by the corticospinal fibers and other supranuclear neurons) determine the level of activity of the tendon reflexes and the responsiveness of muscle to stretch. Other mechanisms of an inhibitory nature, involving Golgi tendon organs, are brought into play in more powerful stretching of muscle.

Lower motor neuron paralysis is the direct result of physiologic arrest or destruction of anterior horn cells or their axons in anterior roots and nerves. The signs and symptoms vary according to the location of the lesion. Probably the most important question for clinical purposes is whether sensory changes coexist. The combination of flaccid, areflexic paralysis and sensory changes usually indicates involvement of mixed motor and sensory nerves or affection of both anterior and posterior roots. If sensory changes are absent, the lesion must be situated in the gray matter of the spinal cord, in the anterior roots, in a purely motor branch of a peripheral nerve, or in motor axons alone. The distinction between nuclear (spinal) and anterior root (radicular) lesions may at times be impossible to make. Retention of reflexes and spasticity in muscles

weakened by a spinal lesion point to a lesion of the corticospinal tracts and integrity of the segments below the level of the lesion.

PARALYSIS DUE TO DISEASE OF THE CORTICOSPINAL AND CORTICO-BRAINSTEM NEURONS It was formerly believed that the corticospinal tract originated from the large motor cell of Betz in the fifth layer of the precentral convolution. However, there are only about 25,000 to 30,000 Betz cells, whereas the corticospinal tract at the level of the medulla contains approximately 1 million axons. This tract must, therefore, contain many fibers that arise not from the giant Betz cells of the motor cortex (area 4 of Brodmann) but rather from the smaller Betz cells of area 4, the cells of the adjacent precentral cortex (area 6), as well as those of the secondary motor cortex in the superior frontal convolution and postcentral cortex (areas 1, 2, 3, 5, 7). The most critical degeneration studies of van Crevel have shown that when areas 4, 6, 1, 2, 3, 5, and 7 are removed in the cat, if one waits several months, all of the pyramidal fibers will be found to have degenerated. The corticospinal tract is the only long-fiber connection between the cerebrum and the spinal cord. At the level of the internal capsule these corticospinal fibers are intermingled with many others destined to end in the globus pallidus, substantia nigra, red nucleus, and reticular substance and with others ascending from the thalamus. The fibers to the cranial nerve nuclei become separated at about the level of the midbrain and cross the midline to the contralateral cranial nerve nuclei (Fig. 15-1). These fibers form the corticomesencephalic, corticopontine, and corticobulbar tracts, and since they have functions similar to those of the corticospinal tract, they may be included in the pyramidal system of motor neurons. The decussation of the corticospinal tract at the lower end of the medulla is variable in different persons. Most of the crossing fibers come to occupy a position in the posterolateral part of the lateral funiculus; a few cross to form an anterior fasciculus. A small number of fibers, 10 to 20 percent, do not cross but descend ipsilaterally as the uncrossed

FIGURE 15-1

Diagram of the corticospinal and corticobulbar tracts. Lesion at A produces ipsilateral oculomotor palsy and contralateral paralysis involving face, arm, and leg. Lesion at B causes ipsilateral facial paralysis of peripheral type and contralateral paralysis of arm and leg. Lesion at b results in ipsilateral facial weakness of upper motor neuron of central type and contralateral paralysis of arm and leg. (Courtesy of Bergmann and Staehln, Krankheiten des Nervensystems, Berlin, Springer-Verlag, 1939.)

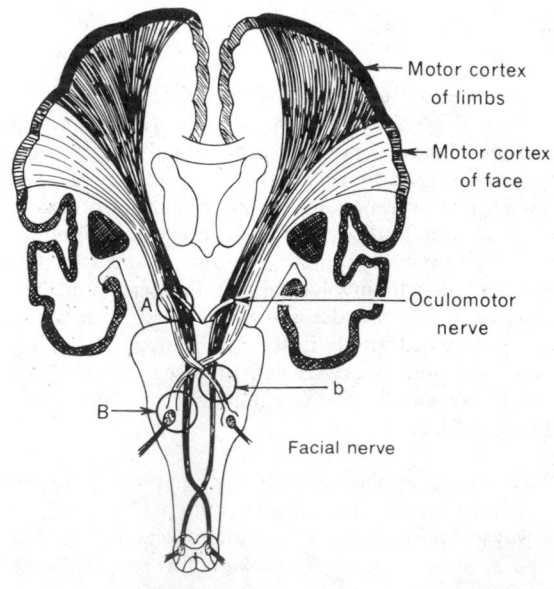

Motor cortex of limbs

Motor cortex of face

Oculomotor nerve

b

Facial nerve

corticospinal tract. Exceptionally, all of them cross; rarely, none. The termination of the corticospinal tract is in relation to nerve cells in the intermediate zone of gray matter, and not more than 10 to 15 percent establish direct synaptic connection with anterior horn cells. These facts, derived from degeneration studies, must of necessity modify current views of the anatomy of the corticospinal tract and suggest new interpretations.

The motor area of the cerebral cortex is difficult to define. It includes that part of the precentral convolution which contains Betz cells (area 4), but, as already mentioned, it probably extends anteriorly into area 6 and the secondary motor area of the superior frontal convolution and posteriorly into the anterior parietal lobe, where it overlaps the sensory areas. Physiologically it is defined as the region of electrically excitable cortex from which isolated movements can be evoked by stimuli of minimal intensity. The muscle groups of the contralateral face, arm, trunk, and leg are represented in the motor cortex, those of the face being at the lower end of the precentral convolution and those of the leg in the paracentral lobule on the medial surface of the cerebral hemisphere. The parts of the body capable of the most delicate movements have, in general, the largest cortical representation. Very strong stimuli elicit movements from a wide area of premotor frontal and parietal cortex, and the same movements may be obtained from several points. From this it may be assumed that one of the functions of the motor cortex is to synthesize simple movements into an infinite variety of finely graded, highly differentiated patterns.

Corticospinal motor neuron paralysis may be due to lesions in the cerebral cortex, subcortical white matter, internal capsule, brainstem, or spinal cord. Usually much more is involved than the corticospinal, or pyramidal, tract. There has been a dispute as to the effects of a pure lesion of the corticospinal system. A lesion which severs the corticospinal system at midbrain level is said to cause only hemiparesis. However, in the 11 proven cases of destruction of the pyramid in the medulla, a flaccid then spastic hemiplegia was observed. In part, difference in the degree of dysfunction is a function of completeness of the corticospinal lesions (Trelles et al.). The distribution of the paralysis varies with the locale of the lesion, but there are certain common features. Paralysis due to a lesion of these supranuclear motor neurons always involves a group of muscles, never individual muscles. If any volitional movement is possible, the maximum effort is attained more slowly than in the normal limb, and there is a lesser degree of multiple motor unit recruitment and frequency of single-unit discharge. The paralysis never involves all the muscles on one side of the body, even in the hemiplegia resulting from a complete lesion of the internal capsule. Movements that are invariably bilateral, such as those of the eyes, jaw, pharynx, larynx, neck, thorax, and abdomen, are little if at all affected. The hand and arm muscles suffer most severely, the leg muscles next, and of the cranial musculature only the muscles of the lower part of the face and tongue are involved to any significant degree. Clinical observation informs us that the cortical control of all movements is to some extent bilateral. Examples that prove this are hemiplegias that worsen when the other corticospinal tract is interrupted by disease. Corticospinal motor paralysis is rarely complete for any long period of time; in this respect it differs from the total and absolute paralysis due to a complete destruction or interruption of anterior horn cells and their axons. The paralyzed arm may suddenly move during yawning and stretching, and various spinal reflexes can be elicited at all times.

Acute disorders of the corticospinal motor system, at lower levels such as the cervical cord, may not only cause a paralysis of voluntary movement but may also abolish temporarily the spinal reflexes subserved by segments below the lesion. This condition is known as *spinal shock*. After a few days to weeks the shock disappears and gives way to a phenomenon known as *spasticity*. The latter is a feature of all acute and chronic lesions of the pyramidal system at cerebral, capsular, midbrain, and pontine levels. In cerebral and brainstem lesions it does not usually appear immediately, and in exceptional cases the paralyzed limbs remain flaccid but with reflexes. Spasticity is related to the excessive activity of the released or disinhibited spinal motor neurons. The tendon reflexes are hyperactive, and clonus may appear. The posture of the arm and leg inform us that certain spinal neurons are more active than others. The arm, for example, is maintained in a pronated, flexed position and the leg in an adducted, extended position. Any attempts to extend the arm or flex the leg passively will encounter, after a brief free interval, a resistance which quickly yields (clasp-knife phenomenon). When the limb is left in the new position, the resistance reappears (lengthening and shortening reactions). Actually the clasp-knife type of spasticity is infrequent. It is more usual for corticospinal lesions to produce a sustained resistance to movement, as pointed out by Colne. But the tendon reflexes are hyperactive and the muscles weakened. The nocifensive spinal flexion reflexes, of which Babinski's sign is a part, are also released, and the cutaneomuscular abdominal and cremasteric reflexes abolished. The flexion reflexes are not actually a component of spasticity. In the hemiplegic patient they are less prominent than in the spinal paraplegic or quadriplegic patient. With cerebral lesions exaggerated stretch and cutaneous cranial reflexes can also be elicited in cranial as well as limb and trunk muscles, and when the corticospinal disorder is bilateral, there is pseudobulbar paralysis (dysarthria, dysphonia, and dysphagia with bifacial paralysis). Prolonged flexor and extensor spasms may occur with lesions of the spinal cord; they are due to a release of tonic myotatic reflexes.

Spasticity may be present when the limbs are not paralyzed but only paretic, and it then produces interesting effects on voluntary movements. As the patient flexes and then extends the forearm, for example, the contraction of the biceps and brachioradiales persists during extension. It would appear that there is not only a diminution of anterior horn cell activation (the negative effect), but also a deficit in the "dynamic range and degree of reciprocal motor neuron control" (Sohrman and Norton). Moreover attempts by the patient to move the hemiplegic limbs voluntarily may result in a variety of associated movements. When asked to rotate one arm, the quadriparetic patient makes the same movement in the other (mirror movement). Flexion of the arms results in involuntary pronation; flexion of the leg causes the foot to dorsiflex and invert automatically (Strumpell's tibialis sign) and the thigh to flex on the trunk. Flexion of one leg is associated with involuntary extension of the other.

Table 15-1 shows the main differences between corticospinal and lower motor neuron syndrome.

Not all hemiplegias of cerebral origin are spastic.

APRAXIC OR NONPARALYTIC DISORDERS OF MOTOR FUNCTION Aside from upper and lower motor neuron paralysis with cerebral lesions, there may be loss of purposive movement without paralysis. This is called *apraxia* and may be explained as follows. Many simple actions are acquired by learning or practice. These depend on the formation of movement patterns, particularly those which involve the use of tools and instruments as well as gestures. Once established, they are remembered and may be reproduced under the proper circumstances. Any purposive act may be conceived as occurring in several stages. First, the idea of an act must be aroused in the mind of the subject by an appropriate stimulus situation, perhaps by a spoken command to do something. This idea is then translated into action by excitation of patterns of premotor or motor cortical neurons in proper sequence, which are transmitted to lower centers by the corticospinal tracts. These initiate particular movements of individual muscle groups but also modify or suppress the subcortical mechanisms that control the basic attitudes and postures of the body. In right-handed and most left-handed persons the neural mechanisms for the formulation of an idea of an act (motor schema or image) in response to a spoken command or a verbal stimulus and its reproduction are believed to be centered in the posterior and inferior parts of the left parietal lobe; these areas, near the language mechanism, are connected with the left premotor regions for the control of the right hand and thence with the motor areas of the right cerebral hemisphere through the corpus callosum for the control of the left side.

A failure to execute certain acts in the correct context while retaining the ability to carry out the individual movements upon which such acts depend is the main feature of *apraxia*. The most adequate clinical test of motor deficits of this type is to observe a series of self-initiated actions such as using a comb, a razor, a toothbrush, or a common tool, or gesturing, e.g., waving goodbye, saluting, shaking the fist as though angry, or blowing a kiss. These actions may be called forth by a command or a request to imitate the examiner. Of course, failure to follow a spoken or written request may be due to an aphasia that prevents understanding of what is asked, or an agnosia may prevent recognition of the tool or object to be used. But when these difficulties are excluded, there remains a peculiar motor deficit in which the patient appears to understand but has lost the memory of how to perform a given act, especially if it is called for in an unnatural setting. The patient may have the idea of what to do, but cannot translate the idea of the sequence of movements into a precise, well-executed act. This is sometimes called *ideomotor apraxia*. The failure may be evident both after a spoken command and in requests to imitate the gestures of the examiner. Sometimes these two conditions may be dissociated; the patient, while not aphasic, cannot execute a spoken command but can still imitate the act if it is called forth by gesture. Also if merely given the tool the patient may use it properly in an automatic fashion.

Apraxia may be limited to one group of muscles, such as tongue or lips, as in Broca's aphasia (Chap. 24), or the loss of commanded actions of the left arm and leg in right-sided hemiplegics (sympathetic apraxia). (See Chap. 25.)

If this motor disorder can be singled out, it reflects a specific loss of certain learned patterns of movement (a "specific amnesia," so to speak, analogous to the amnesia of words in aphasia). The added element of mental confusion tends often to obscure the disorder.

DIFFERENTIAL DIAGNOSIS OF PARALYSIS The diagnostic consideration of paralysis may be simplified by the following subdivisions, which relate to the location and distribution of weakness.

Monoplegia The examination of patients who complain of weakness of one extremity often discloses an unnoticed weakness in another limb, and the condition is actually hemiplegia or paraplegia. Or instead of weakness of all the muscles in a limb, only isolated groups are found to be affected. Ataxia, sensory disturbances, or pain in an extremity will often be interpreted by the patient as weakness, as will the mechanical limitation resulting from arthritis or the rigidity of parkinsonism.

In general, the presence or absence of atrophy of muscles in a monoplegic limb can be of diagnostic help.

PARALYSIS WITH LITTLE OR NO ATROPHY Long-continued disuse of a limb may lead to atrophy, but this is usually not so marked as in diseases that denervate muscles; the tendon reflexes are normal, and the response of the muscles to electric stimulation and the electromyogram are unaltered.

The most frequent cause of monoplegia without muscular wasting is a lesion of the cerebral cortex. Only occasionally does it occur in diseases which interrupt the corticospinal tract at the level of the internal capsule, brainstem, or spinal cord. A vascular lesion (thrombosis or embolus) is the commonest cause, and, of course, a tumor or abscess may have the same effect. Multiple sclerosis and spinal cord tumor, early in their course, may cause weakness of one extremity, usually the leg. Weakness due to damage to the corticospinal system is usually accompanied by spasticity, increased reflexes, and an extensor plantar reflex (Babinski's sign), and the electric reactions and electromyogram are normal. However, acute diseases that destroy the motor tracts in the spinal cord may at first (for several days) reduce the tendon reflexes and cause hypotonia (*spinal shock*). This does not occur in partial or slowly evolving lesions and occurs only to minimal degree, if at all, in lesions of brainstem and cerebrum. In acute diseases affecting the lower motor neurons the tendon reflexes are always reduced or abolished, but atrophy may not appear for several weeks. Hence one must take into account the mode of onset and the duration of the disease in evaluating the tendon reflexes, muscle tone, and degree of atrophy before reaching an anatomic diagnosis.

PARALYSIS WITH MUSCULAR ATROPHY This is more frequent than paralysis without muscular atrophy. In addition to the paralysis and reduced or abolished tendon reflexes, there may be visible fasciculations. If completely paralyzed, the muscles exhibit an electric reaction of degeneration, and the electromyogram shows reduced numbers of motor units (often of large size), fasciculations at rest, and fibrillations. The lesion may be in the spinal cord, spinal roots, or peripheral nerves. Its location can usually be decided by the distribution of the palsied muscles (whether the pattern is one of nerve, spinal root, or spinal cord involvement), by the associated neurologic symptoms and signs, and by special tests (cerebrospinal fluid examination, roentgenogram of spine, and myelogram).

Brachial atrophic monoplegia is relatively rare, and when present, it should suggest in an infant a brachial plexus trauma, in a child poliomyelitis, in an adult poliomyelitis, sy-

TABLE 15-1
Differences between paralysis of corticospinal and lower motor neurons

Upper, corticospinal motor paralysis	Lower, spinomuscular, or nuclear-infranuclear paralysis
Muscle groups affected diffusely, never individual muscles	Individual muscles may be affected
Atrophy slight and due to disuse	Atrophy pronounced, 70 to 80 percent of total bulk
Spasticity with hyperactivity of the tendon reflexes	Flaccidity and hypotonia of affected muscles with loss of tendon reflexes
Extensor plantar reflex, Babinski's sign	Plantar reflex, if present, is of normal flexor type
Fascicular twitches not produced	Fascicular twitches may be present
Normal reactions to galvanic and faradic current	Loss of faradic reaction, retention of galvanic action (reaction of degeneration)

ringomyelia, amyotrophic lateral sclerosis, or other brachial plexus lesions. Crural monoplegia is more frequent and may be caused by any lesion of thoracic or lumbar cord, i.e., trauma, tumor, myelitis, multiple sclerosis, etc. Multiple sclerosis almost never causes atrophy, and ruptured intervertebral disk and the many varieties of neuritis rarely paralyze all or most of the muscles of a limb. Muscle dystrophy may begin in one limb, but by the time the patient is seen the typical more or less symmetric pattern of proximal limb and trunk involvement is evident. A unilateral retroperitoneal tumor may paralyze the leg by implicating the lumbosacral plexus.

Hemiplegia Loss of strength in arm, leg, and sometimes face on one side of the body is the most frequent distribution of paralysis in humans. With rare exceptions (a few unusual cases of poliomyelitis or motor system disease) this pattern of paralysis is due to involvement of the corticospinal tract.

LOCATION OF LESION-PRODUCING HEMIPLEGIA   The site or level of the lesion can usually be deduced from the associated neurologic findings. Diseases localized in the cerebral cortex, cerebral white matter (corona radiata), and internal capsule usually evoke weakness or paralysis of the face, arm, and leg on the opposite side. The occurrence of convulsive seizures or the presence of a defect in speech (aphasia), a cortical type of sensory loss (astereognosis, loss of two-point discrimination, etc.), anosognosia, or defects in the visual fields suggest a cortical or subcortical location. A pure, isolated hemiplegia affecting simultaneously the face, arm, and leg indicates a lesion in the posterior limb of the internal capsule, often a vascular lacuna.

Damage to the corticospinal and cortico-brainstem tracts in the upper portion of the brainstem (see Fig. 15-1) may cause paralysis of the face, arm, and leg on the opposite side. The lesion in such cases is localized by the presence of a paralysis of the muscles supplied by the oculomotor nerve on the same side as the lesion (Weber's syndrome) or other neurologic findings. With low pontine lesions a unilateral abducens or facial palsy is combined with a contralateral weakness or paralysis of the arm and leg (Millard-Gubler syndrome). Lesions of the lowermost part of the brainstem, i.e., in the medulla, affect the tongue and sometimes the pharynx and larynx on one side and arm and leg on the other side. These "crossed paralyses," so common in brainstem diseases, are described in Chap. 376. Ataxic hemiplegia with or without dysarthria also indicates lesion in the contralateral basis pons. Here Fisher has traced the involvement to the uncrossed corticospinal, corticobulbar, and corticopontocerebellar tracts.

Rarely, a homolateral hemiplegia (sparing cranial muscles) may be caused by a lesion in the lateral column of the cervical spinal cord. At this level, however, the pathologic process often induces bilateral signs, with resulting quadriparesis or quadriplegia. Homolateral paralysis, if combined with a loss of vibratory and position sense on the same side and a contralateral loss of pain and temperature (Brown-Séquard syndrome), signifies disease of the spinal cord on one side (Chaps. 19 and 375).

Muscle atrophy of minor degree often follows lesions of the corticospinal system but never reaches the proportions seen in diseases of the lower motor neurons. The atrophy is due to disuse. When the motor cortex and adjacent parts of the parietal lobe are damaged in infancy or childhood, the normal development of the muscles and the skeletal system in the affected limbs is retarded. The palsied limbs and even the trunk on one side are small. This does not occur if the paralysis begins after the greater part of skeletal growth is attained (after puberty). In the hemiplegia due to spinal cord injury, muscles at the level of the lesion may undergo atrophy if there is associated damage to anterior horn cells or ventral roots.

CAUSES OF HEMIPLEGIA   In this condition vascular diseases of the cerebrum and brainstem exceed all others in frequency. Trauma (brain contusion, epidural and subdural hemorrhage) ranks second, and other diseases such as brain tumor, brain abscess and encephalitis, demyelinative diseases, complications of meningitis, tuberculosis, and syphilis are of decreasing order of importance.

Paraplegia Paralysis of both lower extremities may occur in diseases of the spinal cord and the spinal roots or of the peripheral nerves. If the onset is acute, it may be difficult to distinguish spinal from neural paralysis, for in any acute myelopathy spinal shock may result in abolition of reflexes and flaccidity. As a rule in acute spinal cord diseases with involvement of corticospinal tracts, the paralysis affects all muscles below a given level; and often, if the white matter is extensively damaged, sensory loss below a particular level (loss of pain and temperature sense with lateral spinothalamic tracts and loss of vibratory and position sense with posterior columns) is conjoined. Also, in bilateral disease of the spinal cord, the bladder and bowel sphincters are paralyzed. Alterations of cerebrospinal fluid (dynamic block, increase in protein or cells) are frequent. In peripheral nerve diseases both sensory loss and motor loss tend to involve the distal muscles of the legs more than the proximal ones (an exception is acute idiopathic polyneuritis), and the sphincters are spared or only briefly deranged in function. Sensory loss, if present, is more likely to consist of distal impairment of touch, vibration, and position sense, with pain and temperature sense spared in many instances. The cerebrospinal fluid protein level may be normal or elevated.

Acute paraplegia beginning at any age is relatively infrequent. Fracture dislocation of the spine with traumatic necrosis of the spinal cord, spontaneous hematomyelia with bleeding from a vascular malformation (angioma, telangiectasis), thrombosis of a spinal artery with infarction (myelomalacia), and dissecting aortic aneurysm or atherosclerotic occlusion of nutrient spinal arteries arising from the aorta with resulting infarction (myelomalacia) are the commonest varieties of sudden paraplegia (or quadriplegia, if the cervical cord is involved). Postinfectious or postvaccinal myelitis, acute demyelinative myelitis (Devic's disease if the optic nerves are affected), necrotizing myelitis, and epidural abscess or hemorrhage with spinal cord compression tend to develop somewhat more slowly, over a period of hours or days, or they may have an acute onset. Poliomyelitis, a purely motor disorder with meningitis, must be distinguished from the other acute myelopathies.

In adult life multiple sclerosis, subacute combined degeneration, spinal cord tumor, ruptured cervical disk and cervical spondylosis, syphilitic meningomyelitis, chronic epidural infections (fungous and other granulomatous diseases), Erb's spastic paraplegia and motor system disease, familial spastic paraplegia, and syringomyelia represent the most frequently encountered forms of spinal paraplegia. (See Chap. 375 for discussion of these spinal cord diseases). The several varieties of polyneuritis and polymyositis must be considered in their differential diagnosis, for they, too, may cause paraparesis. Friedreich's ataxia and familial paraplegia, progressive muscular dystrophy, and the chronic varieties of polyneuritis tend to appear during late childhood and adolescence and are slowly progressive.

Quadriplegia All that has been written about the common causes of paraplegia applies to quadriplegia. The lesion is usually in the cervical rather than the thoracic or lumbar segments of the spinal cord. If it is situated in the low cervical segments and involves the anterior half of the spinal cord, as in occlusion of the anterior spinal artery, the arm paralysis may be flaccid and areflexic and the leg paralysis spastic (anterior spinal syndrome). There are only a few points of difference between the common paraplegic and quadriplegic syndromes. Repeated cerebral vascular accidents may lead to bilateral hemiplegia, usually accompanied by pseudobulbar palsy.

Isolated paralysis Paralysis of isolated muscle groups usually indicates a lesion of one or more peripheral nerves. The diagnosis of a lesion of an individual peripheral nerve is made on the presence of weakness or paralysis of the muscle or group of muscles and impairment or loss of sensation in the distribution of the nerve in question (Chap. 337). Complete transection or severe injury to a peripheral nerve is usually followed by atrophy of the muscles it innervates and by loss of their tendon reflexes. Trophic changes in the skin, nails, and subcutaneous tissue may also occur. It is of considerable importance to decide whether the lesion is a temporary one of conduction only (neuropraxia) or whether there has been a pathologic dissolution of continuity, requiring nerve regeneration for recovery. Electromyography may be of value here.

EXAMINATION SCHEME FOR MOTOR PARALYSIS AND APRAXIA The first step is to inspect the paralyzed limb, taking note first of its posture and of the presence or absence of muscle atrophy, hypertrophy, and fascicular twitchings. The patient is then called upon to move each muscle group, and the power and facility of movement are graded and recorded. The range of passive movement is then determined by moving all the joints. This provides information concerning alterations of muscle tone, i.e., hypotonia, spasticity, and rigidity. Dislocations, diseased joints, and ankyloses may also be revealed by these same maneuvers. Muscle bulk is then inspected. Slight atrophy may be due to disuse from any cause, i.e., pain, fixation as the result of a cast, or any type of paralysis. Pronounced atrophy usually occurs only with denervation of several weeks' or months' standing.

The tendon reflexes are then tested. The usual routine is to try to elicit the jaw jerk (increased in pseudobulbar palsy) and the supinator, biceps, triceps, quadriceps, and Achilles tendon reflexes. Two cutaneous reflexes are then tested, the abdominal and plantar reflexes.

If there is no evidence of upper or lower motor neuron disease, but certain acts are nonetheless imperfectly performed, one should look for a disorder of postural sensibility or of cerebellar coordination or rigidity with abnormality of posture and movement due to disease of the basal ganglions (Chap. 16). In the absence of these disorders, the possibility of an apraxic disorder may be investigated by watching the patient's own movements and those called forth by specific command and gesture.

Hysterical paralysis may pose problems. Usually it is easily distinguished from chronic lower motor neuron disease by absence of areflexia and severe atrophy. Diagnostic difficulty arises only in certain acute cases of upper motor neuron disease that lack all the usual changes in reflexes and muscle tone. In hysterical paralysis one arm or one leg or all one side of the body may be affected. The hysterical gait is sometimes diagnostic (Chap. 17). Often there is loss of all forms of sensation (touch, pain, smell, vision, and hearing) in the paralyzed side, a group of sensory changes that is never seen in organic brain disease. The patient should be asked to move the affected limbs; the movement is seen to be slow and jerky, often with contraction of both agonist and antagonist muscles simultaneously or intermittently. Hoover's sign and Babinski's combined leg flexion test are helpful in distinguishing hysterical from organic hemiplegia. To elicit Hoover's sign, the patient, lying on the back, is asked to raise one leg from the bed against resistance; in a normal individual the back of the heel of the contralateral leg is pressed firmly down, and the same is true when the patient with organic hemiplegia attempts to lift the paralyzed leg. The hysteric will contract the good leg more strongly under these circumstances than as a primary willed action. To carry out Babinski's combined leg flexion test, a patient with an organic hemiplegia is asked to sit up without using the arms; in doing this, the paralyzed or weak leg flexes at the hip, and the heel is lifted from the bed while the heel of the sound leg is pressed into the bed. This sign is absent in hysterical hemiplegia.

MUSCULAR PARALYSIS AND SPASM UNATTENDED BY VISIBLE CHANGE IN NERVE OR MUSCLE A group of diseases appears to have no basis in visible structural change in motor nerve cells, nerve fibers, motor end plates, and muscular fibers. This group is composed of myasthenia gravis, myotonia congenita (Thomsen's disease), familial periodic paralysis, disorders of potassium, sodium, calcium, and magnesium metabolism, tetany, tetanus, botulinus poisoning, black widow spider bite, and the thyroid myopathies. In these diseases, each of which possesses a fairly distinctive clinical picture, the abnormality is purely biochemical, and even if the patient survives for a long time, no visible microscopic changes develop. An understanding of these diseases requires knowledge of the processes involved in nerve and muscle excitation and the contraction of muscle. They are discussed in Chaps. 378 and 383.

REFERENCES

Brodal A: *Neurological Anatomy in Relation to Clinical Medicine.* New York, Oxford, 1969

Calne DB: Drug treatment of spasticity and rigidity, in *Modern Trends in Neurology,* 6th ed, D Williams (ed). London, Butterworths, 1975

Fisher CM: Ataxic hemiparesis—a pathological study. Arch Neurol 35:126, 1978

Sohrman SA, Norton BJ: The relationship of voluntary movement to spasticity in the upper motor neuron syndrome. Ann Neurol 2:460, 1977

Trelles JO et al: Spasticity in hemiplegia due to lesion of anterior pyramid. Rev Neurol 129:105, 1973

16
TREMOR, CHOREA, ATHETOSIS, ATAXIA, AND OTHER ABNORMALITIES OF MOVEMENT AND POSTURE

RAYMOND D. ADAMS

In this chapter are discussed the automatic, static, and less modifiable postural activities of the human nervous system. These are believed, on good evidence, to be an expression of the function of the *older motor system,* meaning the motor structures in the basal ganglia and brainstem.

In health, the activities of the motor systems of basal ganglia and cerebellum are blended and modulate the corticospinal and cortico-brainstem-spinal systems. The static postural activities of the former are indispensable to the voluntary or willed movements of the latter.

This close association of the corticospinal (formerly pyramidal) and extrapyramidal systems is shown by human disease. Lesions of the corticospinal tracts result not only in paralysis of volitional movements of the contralateral half of the body but in the appearance of a fixed posture or attitude in which the arm is maintained in flexion and the leg in extension (predilection type of Wernicke-Mann or hemiplegic dystonia of Denny-Brown). Similarly, decerebration from a lesion in the upper pons or midbrain releases another posture in which all four extremities are extended and the cervical and thoracolumbar spine is dorsiflexed. In these released action patterns one has evidence of extrapyramidal postural and righting reflexes which are mediated through bulbospinal and other brainstem-spinal systems.

The student may be dismayed to read in current articles trenchant criticism of the validity of the concept of the corticospinal tract and the division of the motor system into corticospinal and extrapyramidal. Extremists claim the corticospinal tract may be severed in animals and even in humans without lasting motor deficits. But it must be remembered that this tract is so puny in most mammals, even in small monkeys, that it can hardly be compared with that of humans, and there has yet to be a pathologically proved example in humans of complete interruption of this tract with preserved voluntary motor function.

If an oversimplification may be permitted for clarity of exposition, the extrapyramidal motor system may be subdivided into two parts: (1) the striatopallidonigral and (2) the cerebellar. Disease in either of these parts will result in disturbances of movement and posture without significant paralysis. These two major systems and the symptoms that result when they are diseased are reviewed on the following pages.

BASAL GANGLIA: PATHOLOGIC ANATOMY

As an anatomic entity the basal ganglia have no precise definition. The list of basal structures originally thought to have some part in motor function, such as the caudate and lenticular nuclei, has been greatly expanded by physiologists to include the field of Forel and zona incerta, subthalamic nucleus of Luys, substantia nigra, red nucleus, dentate nucleus of cerebellum, and the reticular formation of the brainstem.

For the convenience of the reader, a diagram (Fig. 16-1) is included to show the principal structures and their connections. Attention is drawn to the wide range of corticostriate connections; the caudate nucleus and putamen (striatal) connections with the outer and inner segments of the globus pallidus; the direct striatonigral and nigrostriatal circuit; the globus

pallidus–ventrolateral thalamus (ansa and striatal lemnisci) pathway; the striatothalamic and thalamostriatal circuit; and the connection between outer pallidum and subthalamic nucleus. The details of these relationships are well presented in Carpenter's neuroanatomy monograph, but unfortunately a fine map of the connections of the individual cell types, their chemical transmitters, and their philosophy in the workings of the motor system have yet to be established.

The principal new anatomic datum to emerge in recent years is the central physiologic role of the ventrolateral (and anterior) nucleus of the thalamus. It is a vital link in an ascending fiber system from the lenticular nucleus and cerebellum to the motor cortex. Indeed, it would seem that most of the basal ganglionic and cerebellar influence on the motor system is funneled through the ventral plane of thalamic nuclei, thus effecting a number of corticocortical circuits. Descending pathways to the spinal cord are disputed; probably there are polysynaptic descending fibers through the reticular formation of the pons and medulla to the motor neurons of the spinal cord. It is noteworthy that these ascending thalamocortical fibers pass through the internal capsule and cerebral white matter; hence lesions in these parts may simultaneously affect both corticospinal and extrapyramidal systems.

NEUROPHARMACOLOGY

In recent years it has been discovered that the neurons of these several striatopallidothalamic, striatonigral, striatothalamic, and pallidosubthalamic circuits are activated by chemical transmitters. Acetylcholine (ACh), norepinephrine (NE), 5-hydroxytryptamine (5-HT), dopamine (DA), and the inhibitory transmitter γ-aminobutyric acid (GABA) have been localized to certain neurons of the basal nuclei and hypothalamus.

Particular neurotransmitters appear to figure prominently in extrapyramidal diseases. In Parkinson's disease, which is manifested by a combination of akinesia, tremor, rigidity, and flexed posture, the DA content of the striatum is depleted, presumably due to a loss of neurons in the substantia nigra and degeneration of the nigrostriatal tract to which they give rise. This loss of DA is believed to upset the normal balance between DA and ACh. Restoration of this equilibrium, by giving L-dopa and anticholinergic medication (belladonna alkaloids) has been shown to suppress this neurologic disorder (see Fig.

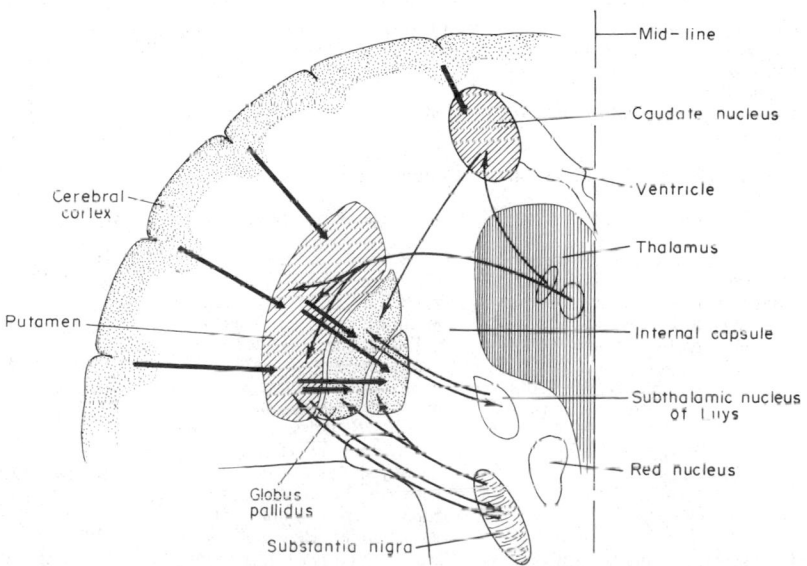

337-1 for diagram of metabolic pathways of DA). Reserpine and tetrabenzine, which cause a more or less typical parkinsonian syndrome, also reduce the content of DA in this part of the brain (and also its NA and 5-HT).

Another point of interest is the observation that an excess of L-dopa in the patient with Parkinson's disease, probably by the stimulation of receptors in the striatum, induces a wide variety of abnormal movements. This seems to be dose-related. The most frequent of these is craniofacial athetosis, but a more generalized choreoathetosis, facial and cervical spasms, tremors and myoclonic jerks (see below) may also occur. Presumably certain striatal neurons, not the ones causing the Parkinson's syndrome, have been rendered hypersensitive, for L-dopa appears not to have this effect on normal individuals. Moreover, drugs of the phenathiazine and butyrophenone groups (Chap. 229), for reasons that are unclear, are capable of evoking acute dystonic reactions, akathesia (motor restlessness, repetitive tapping and fiddling with hands and feet, and facial mannerisms) and tardive dyskinesias. In Huntington's chorea, L-dopa worsens the chorea. Physostigmine enhances the activity of the cholinergic transmitters by blocking cholinesterase and is said to lessen it. This may be explained by the reduction in acetylcholine transferase, the enzyme necessary for acetylcholine formation, in the caudate nuclei in this disease. GABA is also reduced.

While these findings cannot be integrated into a coherent theory of central neurotransmitters, they nonetheless offer prospects of a new pathophysiology of extrapyramidal chemical phenomena and of basal ganglionic diseases. (Further information concerning the biochemistry of norepinephrine and serotonin may be found in Chaps. 91 and 373.)

Some of the most significant facts about clinicopathologic relationships in humans are indicated in Table 16-1, which presents clinicopathologic correlations accepted by many neurologists; however, there is still much uncertainty as to finer details.

The symptoms that lend themselves best to clinical analysis are akinesia, rigidity, chorea, athetosis, dystonia, myoclonus, and tremor.

TABLE 16-1
Clinicopathologic correlations

Symptoms	Principal location of morbid anatomy
Unilateral plastic rigidity with static tremor and regular slowness of movement (Parkinson's syndrome)	Contralateral substantia nigra plus (?) other structures
Unilateral hemiballismus and hemichorea	Contralateral subthalamic nucleus of Luys, prerubral area, and Forel's fields
Chronic chorea of Huntington's type	Caudate nucleus, putamen
Athetosis and dystonia	Contralateral putamen or thalamus
Cerebellar ataxia, i.e., intention tremor; irregular slowness in starting and stopping alternating voluntary movements; hypotonia; rebound phenomenon	Homolateral cerebellar hemisphere or middle and inferior cerebellar peduncles, superior brachium conjunctivum (ipsilateral if below the decussation, contralateral if above)
Decerebrate rigidity, i.e., opisthotonos, extension of arms and legs	Lesion usually bilateral in tegmentum, involving upper brainstem, particularly red nucleus or structures between red nucleus and vestibular nuclei
Palatal and facial myoclonus (rhythmic)	Lesion in the central tegmental tract, inferior olivary nucleus, and olivodentate connections
Diffuse myoclonus	Cerebellar cortex (?), thalami (?)

AKINESIA

When extrapyramidal disease is analyzed along classic neurologic lines into primary functional deficits and secondary release effects, akinesia stands as the principal negative or deficit symptom. By the term *akinesia* one refers to the disinclination of the patient to use an affected part of the body, to engage it freely in all the natural actions of the body. In contrast to paralysis, the negative symptom of corticospinal lesions, strength is relatively undiminished in the part, and it can be used effectively in the desired movement under conditions of maximal motivation. In this respect, too, it is unlike apraxia, where movements are lost because of a lesion which erases the memory of the motor schema that forms a sequence of movements for intended action. Parkinsonian patients exhibit the phenomenon of akinesia most clearly in their extreme underactivity. They sit motionless for long times. In looking to the side they move the eyes, not the head. In arising from a chair they fail to make all the little adjustments needed (putting feet back, putting hands on arms of chair, etc.). They neglect the affected arm. Yet they are not weak (paretic) or apraxic. Formerly, akinesia was attributed to rigidity, which could reasonably hamper all movements, but now that stereotaxic surgery has been shown to abolish both tremor and rigidity, it becomes clear that the motor deficit, or akinesia, is still there. Strictly interpreted, it would appear that apart from their contribution to the maintenance of postures, the basal ganglia must provide something essential to the performance of the large variety of semiautomatic actions that make up the full repertoire of natural human motility.

ALTERATIONS OF MUSCLE TONE (SPASTICITY, RIGIDITY, HYPOTONIA)

It has been pointed out that muscle tone (the small resistance to muscle stretch offered by healthy muscle) is enhanced in the many conditions that cause a paralysis of voluntary movement by interrupting the corticospinal tract. The special distribution of the increased tone (i.e., greater in antigravity muscles—leg extensors and arm flexors in humans), the sudden augmentation of tone with gradual yielding upon quick movement (the lengthening reaction or clasp-knife phenomenon), the absence of resistance upon slow movement and its disappearance in relaxed muscle with "electromyographic silence when relaxed," and exaggerated tendon (phasic myotatic) reflexes are the identifying characteristics of spasticity. This type of hypertonus is believed to be due in some instances to hyperactivity of the small gamma motor neurons, resulting in increase in the sensitivity of the spindle muscle fibers to stretch. In other instances especially when a voluntary movement evokes a persistent, diffuse resistance to active and passive movement (tonic myotatic reflex activity), it seems clearly related to excessive activity (or disinhibition) of the larger alpha motor neurons. The "gamma spasticity" is abolished by procaine injection of the motor nerve, which paralyzes the small gamma motor and sensory fibers, leaving the larger ones intact, without weakening the willed contractions of the muscle; the "alpha spasticity" is not affected by procaine.

In the state known as *rigidity* the muscles are continuously or intermittently firm, tense, and prominent; and the resistance to passive movement is intense and even, like that noted in bending a lead pipe or in stretching a strand of toffee. Although rigidity is present in all muscle groups, both flexor and extensor, on the whole it tends to be more prominent in those which maintain a flexed posture, i.e., the flexor muscles of trunk and limbs. It appears to be somewhat greater in the large muscle groups, but this may be merely a question of muscle mass. Certainly the smaller muscles of the face and tongue and even those of the larynx are often affected. Nevertheless, like "gamma spasticity," this rigidity is said to be abolished by procaine, and Foerster earlier demonstrated that it is eradicated by posterior root section. In the electromyographic tracing, motor unit activity tends to be more continuous than in spasticity, persisting even after relaxation (Table 16-2).

A special type of rigidity is the *cogwheel phenomenon.* When the hypertonic muscle is passively stretched, the resistance may be rhythmically jerky, as though the resistance of the limb were controlled by a ratchet. A number of different explanations of this phenomenon have been suggested. Wilson postulated that it might be due to a minor form of the lengthening-shortening reaction, but a more likely explanation is an associated static tremor that is masked by rigidity during an attitude of repose but emerges faintly during manipulation.

Rigidity is prominent in extrapyramidal diseases such as paralysis agitans, postencephalitic Parkinson's syndrome, and dystonia musculorum deformans.

The *tension hypertonus of athetosis* differs from both spasticity and rigidity. Strictly speaking, it takes two forms, one which occurs during the involuntary athetotic movement, and another which appears in the absence of any involuntary motion. Clinically these forms of hypertonus are variable from one moment to the next and are paradoxic in that they sometimes disappear during a rapid passive movement or when the limb is passively shaken. The tendon reflexes may be normal or brisk. The lengthening and shortening reactions are absent. This form of variable hypertonus is found in double athetosis and choreoathetosis and in some cases of dystonia musculorum deformans. Usually in Sydenham's and Huntington's chorea a state of hypotonia prevails, sometimes as strikingly as in sensory polyneuropathies and lower motor neuron paralyses.

INVOLUNTARY MOVEMENTS

CHOREA Derived from the Greek word meaning "dance," *chorea* refers to widespread arrhythmic movements of a forcible, rapid, jerky type. These movements are involuntary and are noted for their irregularity, variability, relative speed, and relatively brief duration. They may be simple or quite elaborate and of variable distribution. In some respects they resemble a voluntary movement in their complexity, yet they are never combined into a coordinated act. The patient may, how-

TABLE 16-2
Nontremorous extrapyramidal movement disorders

Type	Physiologic characteristics	Pathologic anatomy	Common diseases	Treatment
Plastic rigidity, static tremor, slowness of movement (Parkinson's syndrome)	Present during rest and activity Worsened by excitement No change in tendon or cutaneous reflexes unilateral or bilateral See Table 16-3	Substantia nigra- and nigrostriatal pathway Contralateral if one-sided	Paralysis agitans (Parkinson's disease) Postencephalitic parkinsonism Wilson's disease Hallevorden-Spatz disease Phenothiazine effect	Anticholinesterase drugs L-Dopa Amantadine Stereotaxic thalamic surgery
Chorea and choreoathetosis: Generalized	Moderately fast, arrhythmic, usually with hypotonia but without change in reflexes or ataxia	Striatum, caudate nucleus, and putamen	Rheumatic (Sydenham's chorea) Huntington's chorea Senile chorea Tardive dyskinesia Rarely thyrotoxicosis, "the pill," lupus erythematosus, polycythemia vera, hypernatremia Sydenham's chorea	Prednisone Haloperidine Diazepam
Unilateral or localized	Same	Contralateral striatum	Infarct or hemorrhage in thalamus or striatum (contralateral)	Rest, quiet, sedatives Stereotaxic thalamic surgery
Athetosis and dystonia: Generalized	Present at rest, worse on willed movement Aggravated by excitement Reflexes normal or abnormal	Anterior thalamus or ventricular nuclei with intact pyramidal tracts	Cerebral palsy Wilson's disease Rigid form of Huntington's chorea Overdose of L-dopa Postanoxic sequela Other degenerative diseases Dystonia musculorum deformans	Stereotaxic thalamic surgery
Unilateral (restricted dystonias, see text)	Same	Same	Posthemiplegic states	As above Surgical denervation of affected muscles
Hemiballismus	Arrhythmic; large excursion; usually unilateral; no weakness or pyramidal signs	Contralateral subthalamic nucleus	Vascular lesions (hemorrhage or infarct) Posttraumatic (rare)	Surgical section of cerebral peduncles Stereotaxic thalamic surgery Diazepam and other sedatives
Myoclonus: Arrhythmic	Movements quicker than chorea Associated ataxia (often) or dementia and seizures	Cerebellum, ?cortex, ?dentate nuclei, ?thalamus	Postanoxic Lipidoses Jakob-Creutzfeld disease Subacute sclerosing encephalitis Familial myoclonic epilepsy and other degenerative diseases	5-Hydroxytryptophane Anticonvulsant and sedative medications
Rhythmic (restricted, palatal myoclonus)	Continuous, awake and asleep; other brainstem signs	Central segmental tracts of pons, medulla, and inferior olivary nuclei	Vascular lesions, gliomas	None known

ever, incorporate them into a deliberate movement, as if to make them less noticeable. When superimposed on voluntary movements, these may take on a grotesque and exaggerated character. Grimacing and peculiar respiratory sounds may be other expressions of the movement disorder. Usually the movements are discrete, but if very numerous, they may flow into one another; the resultant picture then resembles athetosis. They may be limited to a limb or one side of the body (hemichorea), or they may involve all parts of the body. Normal volitional movements are, of course, possible, for there is no paralysis, but they too may be excessively quick and poorly sustained. The limbs are often unusually slack, or hypotonic. A choreic movement may be superimposed on a tendon reflex, giving rise to the "hung-up reflex." The tendon reflexes tend to be pendular because of the associated hypotonia; when the knee jerk is elicited with the patient sitting, the leg swings back and forth four or five times, like a pendulum, rather than one or two times as in a normal person. (See Table 16-2 for list of common pathologies.)

A special variety of chorea (sometimes choreoathetosis or dystonia) is clearly paroxysmal and sometimes familial (dominant inheritance). Paroxysms lasting minutes to hours appear during childhood or adolescence and continue throughout life. In one special subtype the chorea is kinesogenic, meaning that it is initiated by a sudden voluntary movement. Alcohol, hypernatremia, and diphenylhydantoin (especially in patients who have had Sydenham's chorea in childhood) are other factors in paroxysmal chorea. Lance has discussed this in terms of a dopaminergic "sensitivity." In some cases anticonvulsive drugs (clonazepam, phenobarbital) have prevented attacks and in others L-dopa has been effective.

ATHETOSIS This term is from a Greek word meaning "unfixed" or "changeable." The condition is characterized by an inability to sustain the fingers and toes, tongue, or any other group of muscles in one position. The maintained posture is interrupted by continuous, slow, sinuous, purposeless movements. These are most pronounced in the digits and the hands but often involve the tongue, throat, and face. One can detect as basic patterns of movement an extension and pronation and flexion and supination of the arm, and alternating flexion and extension of the fingers. They may be unilateral, especially in children who have suffered a hemiplegia at some previous date (posthemiplegic athetosis). The movements are slower than those of chorea, but in many cases gradations between the two (choreoathetosis) are seen. Most athetotic patients exhibit variable degrees of motor deficit due in some instances to associated corticospinal tract disease. Discrete individual movements of the tongue, lips, and hand are often impossible, and attempts to perform such voluntary movements result in a contraction of all the muscles in the limb and other parts of the body (*intention spasm*). Variable degrees of rigidity are generally associated, and these may account for the slower quality of athetosis, in contrast to chorea. It must be admitted, however, that in some cases it is almost impossible to distinguish between chorea and athetosis.

TORSION SPASM OR DYSTONIA Torsion spasm is closely allied to athetosis, differing only in that the larger axial muscles (those of the trunk and limb girdles) rather than appendicular muscles are involved. It results in bizarre, grotesque movements and positions of the body. The word *dystonia* has been given to these movements but, unfortunately, is also applied to any fixed posture which may be the end result of a disease of the motor system. Thus Denny-Brown speaks of hemiplegic dystonia, the flexion dystonia of parkinsonism, and extensor dystonia with retraction of the head and arching or twisting of the back. If the latter meaning is given, it would be better to speak of athetosis of the trunk as torsion spasms or phasic dystonia, in contrast to fixed dystonia. The former, like athetosis, may show remarkable fluctuations; sometimes the whole musculature of the body may be thrown into spasm by an effort to move an arm or to speak. If mild, the torsion spasm may be limited to the lumbar or cervical muscles or those of one limb and may cease when the body is at rest (see below).

Torsion spasm may be seen in the condition of double athetosis after hypoxic damage to the brain, in kernicterus, in chronic manganese intoxication, and, rarely, in Wilson's hepatolenticular degeneration. It is most characteristic of the syndrome designated *dystonia musculorum deformans* but also occurs in other conditions such as the postphenothiazine dyskinesias and Hallevorden-Spatz disease (Chap. 373).

Chorea, athetosis, and torsion spasm are all closely related. The movements are elaborate and depend for their expression on cortical mechanisms. Paralytic lesions involving the corticospinal tract abolish these involuntary movements. The hypotonia in chorea and some cases of athetosis, the pendular reflexes, and some degree of interference with natural movements are also reminiscent of the syndrome that follows disease of the cerebellum. Lacking, however, are intention tremor and true incoordination or ataxia.

MYOCLONUS This term refers to several different motor disorders, some localized, others diffuse. As in chorea, the myoclonic movement is involuntary and arrhythmic, but it is much faster than chorea, being concluded in a few hundred milliseconds or less. Variations in degree are noteworthy; it may consist of no more than a flick of a single muscle or part of a muscle, but the larger movements always betray its nature, involving as they do a group of muscles. Thus myoclonus may be distinguished from fasciculation. Sensory relationships are another prominent attribute. Flickering light, a series of loud sounds, or abrupt contact with some part of the body in some instances may regularly initiate a jerk, sometimes as a direct sensorimotor effect, again through the mechanism of startle. One special variety is evoked by willed movement, presumably through a proprioceptive mechanism. Hence, one may speak of action or intention myoclonus, auditory or visual myoclonus. A series of intense stimuli may recruit a series of myoclonic jerks that progress to a full-blown seizure, as happens often in the familial myoclinic epilepsy syndrome of Unverricht-Lundborg. The pathologic disturbance in the latter is usually a lipid storage disease or an amyloid Lafora body inclusion disease (Chap. 373). See Table 16-2 for list of common causes.

The term *myoclonus* unfortunately has also been assigned to a rather different motor phenomenon—that of repetitious, rhythmic clonus of some part of the "branchial cleft" or craniocervical musculature. Examples are "nystagmus of the palate" (rhythmic contractions at the rate of 10 to 50 or more per minute of the soft palate) and rhythmic contractions of the pharyngeal muscles, vocal cords, facial muscles, and diaphragm. The lesions producing this state, which we would prefer to designate as a form of continuous *bulbar, facial,* or *diaphragmatic clonus,* have been situated in all instances in the central tegmental tract, inferior olivary nucleus, or olivocerebellar tract. The causative lesions have been infarcts, tumors, and encephalitic processes.

The main fault with our concept of myoclonus is that it covers too many motor disorders. When movements are grouped according to their brevity or involuntary nature, one must include the normal dormescent start or jerk of a limb as one falls asleep, and the motor components of a natural startle reaction. The obligatory Moro response also falls within the group, as well as the form of epilepsy known as infantile or salaam spasms and the falling spells of the petit mal triad. Metrazol injections cause myoclonus of the limbs, which has been shown to depend on a lower brainstem (medullary reticular) mechanism. Another problem arises on the clinical side in distinguishing diffuse myoclonus from other abrupt involuntary movements such as tremors, chorea, and restricted forms of epilepsy (epilepsia partialis continua). Speed of movement, lack of rhythmicity, and relationships to sensory stimulation prove to be the most reliable identifying features of the larger group of myoclonic disorders. There is an advantage in separating the arrhythmic diffuse form from the rhythmic restricted form in that each stands as a diagnostic attribute of a separate category of nervous diseases.

TREMOR This consists of a more or less regular rhythmic oscillation of a part of the body around a fixed point. The rate varies from three to eight oscillations per second; in a particular person the rate is fairly constant in all affected parts, regardless of the size of the muscle or of the part of the body. Tremors usually involve the distal part of the limbs, the head, tongue, or jaw, and rarely the trunk.

There are many different types of tremor, and only a few are recognized as bearing any meaningful relationship to disease of the extrapyramidal motor system; but since tremors have not been discussed elsewhere, all the different types will be considered here.

Tremors may be subdivided according to their distribution, amplitude, regularity, and relationship to volitional movement. The tremors described in the following paragraphs should be familiar to every physician (Table 16-3).

Static (parkinsonian) tremor This is a coarse, rhythmic tremor, with an average rate of four to five beats per second,

most often localized in one or both hands, and, occasionally, in the jaw or tongue. Its most characteristic feature is that it occurs when the limb is in an attitude of repose, and willed movement at least temporarily suppresses it. If the tremulous limb is completely relaxed, the tremor usually disappears, but the average patient rarely achieves this state. In some cases the tremor is constant; in others it varies from time to time and with the progress of the disease extends from one group of muscles to another. In paralysis agitans the tremor tends to be rather gentle and more or less limited to the distal muscles, whereas in postencephalitic parkinsonism and hepatolenticular degeneration it often has a wider range and involves proximal muscles. In many cases there is a variable degree of rigidity of a plastic type in the tremulous limb or elsewhere. The tremor interferes with voluntary movements surprisingly little; it is not uncommon to see a patient who has been trembling violently raise a full glass of water to the lips and drain the contents without spilling a drop. The handwriting of these patients is often small and cramped (micrographia). The gait may be of festinating type (see Chap. 17). It is the combination of static tremor, slowness of movement, rigidity, and flexed postures without true paralysis that constitutes Parkinson's syndrome (also called *amyostatic* syndrome).

The exact pathologic anatomy of static tremor is unknown. In paralysis agitans and postencephalitic Parkinson's syndrome, the visible lesions are predominantly in the substantia nigra. In hepatocerebral degeneration, where this syndrome is

TABLE 16-3
Tremors

Types	Physiologic characteristics	Anatomic pathology	Common diseases	Treatment
Fast frequency (7–10 per second), slightly arrhythmic action tremor	Generalized (usually) Present during activity; increased in precise movement and excitement; ceases during full relaxation Increased by epinephrine	Unknown ?Peripheral or spinal	One of hereditary types Hyperthyroidism Intense fright Corticosteroid and lithium therapy Pheochromocytoma and carcinoid Alcoholic withdrawal	Reduced by propranolol (Inderal) and beta-blocking agents Reduced by alcohol Sometimes helped by diazepam
Medium frequency (5–7 per second), rhythmic action tremor	Same as above except for rhythmic alternations of agonists and antagonists	Unknown ?Central (spinal or higher centers)	One of hereditary types General paresis (syphilis) Rare in other diseases Some cases of corticosteroid therapy	Variably reduced by Inderal and alcohol Reduced by diazepam
Ataxic intention tremor (4–6 per second)	Present in terminal phase of projected (willed) movement; absent during relaxation May be unilateral Associated with cerebellar ataxia	Cerebellum—especially dentatothalamic tracts (superior cerebellar peduncle and brachium conjunctivum)	Multiple sclerosis Cerebellar and brainstem tumors Vascular lesions	None Drugs ineffective
Combined rest and intention tremor (4–6 per second, erroneously called "rubral tremor")	Wide range and rhythmic; worse during willed movement, but present at rest Associated with cerebellar ataxia and/or parkinsonism May be unilateral	Tegmentum of midbrain and subthalamus ?Brachium conjunctivum	Multiple sclerosis Wilson's disease Vascular lesions and traumatism	Stereotaxic surgery of ventromedial nucleus may help Drugs ineffective
Tremor at rest (4–5 per second, static tremor or "parkinsonian tremor")	Rhythmic alternation of agonist antagonist muscles Present in attitude of repose; temporarily abolished by willed movement May be combined with fast-frequency tremor Usually associated with rigidity and slowness of movement	Lesions in substantia nigra and nigrolenticular pathway	Paralysis agitans (Parkinson's disease) Postencephalitic parkinsonism Wilson's disease Senile syndromes Postphenothiazine (tardive) dyskinesia	Reduced by anticholinergic drugs and L-dopa Reduced by stereotaxic surgery (ventral thalamus and pallidum)

mixed with cerebellar ataxia, the lesions are more diffuse. A similar tremor, without rigidity, slowness of movement, flexed postures, or masked facies, is seen in senile persons. Unlike Parkinson's disease, it does not progress to motor disability and does not respond to antiparkinson drugs.

Action tremor   This term refers to a tremor present when the limbs are actively maintained in a certain position, as when outstretched, and throughout voluntary movement. It may increase slightly as the action of the limbs becomes more precise, but it never approaches the degree of augmentation in fine movement seen in intention tremor. It is easily made to disappear when the limbs are relaxed. Probably some of the *action tremors* are but an exaggeration of normal or physiologic tremor, which ranges from six to eight per second, being slower in childhood and old age. In adults the tremor is of small excursion, has a frequency of seven to eight per second, and is somewhat irregular. The tremor involves the outstretched hand, head, and, less often, the lips and tongue, and it interferes little with voluntary movements such as handwriting and speech. This type of tremor is seen in numerous medical, neurologic, and psychiatric diseases and is therefore more difficult to interpret than static tremor. There are somewhat slower frequencies of action tremor, and instead of rather irregular potentials in both agonist and antagonist muscles (as in the aforementioned type), their activity alternates. Either form, when occurring as the only neurologic abnormality in several members of a family, is known as *familial* or *hereditary tremor*. Familial tremor may begin in childhood, but usually comes on later and persists throughout adult life. Being worse when the patient is under observation, it becomes a source of embarrassment because it suggests to the onlooker that the patient is nervous. A curious fact about familial tremors is that one or two drinks of an alcoholic beverage may abolish them, and they may become worse after the effects of the alcohol have worn off. Similar fast-frequency action tremors are seen in delirious states, such as delirium tremens, in chronic alcoholism as an isolated symptom (the morning shakes), and in general paresis. An action tremor, usually more rapid than the above, is also characteristic of hyperthyroidism and other toxic states, and a similar tremor is frequently observed in patients suffering intense anxiety. In fact it can be reproduced by injections of epinephrine. Severe action tremor may also accompany certain diseases of the basal ganglia, including parkinsonism. Some of the fast-frequency action tremors are suppressed by beta-adrenergic blocking agents such as propranolol (Inderal, 40 mg tid).

Intention tremor   The word *intention* is ambiguous in this context because the tremor itself is not intentional. The term means, instead, that the tremor requires for its full expression the performance of an exacting, precise, willed movement. The term *ataxic tremor* has been suggested because it is always combined with and adds to cerebellar ataxia. The tremor is absent when the limbs are inactive and during the first part of a voluntary movement, but as the action continues and greater precision is demanded (e.g., in touching a target such as the patient's nose or the examiner's finger), a jerky, more or less rhythmic interruption of forward progression, with side-to-side oscillation, appears. It continues for a fraction of a second or so after the act is completed. The tremor may seriously interfere with the patient's performance of skilled acts. Sometimes the head is involved (titubation). This type of tremor invariably indicates disease of the cerebellum and of its connections. When the disease is very severe, every movement, even the lifting of a limb, results in a wide-ranging tremor of such violence as to throw the patient off balance. This latter state is

occasionally seen in multiple sclerosis, Wilson's disease, and vascular, traumatic, and other lesions of the tegmentum of the midbrain and subthalamus but not of the cerebellum.

OTHER INVOLUNTARY MOVEMENTS   There are other abnormalities of movement, about which only a few words can be said. They vary from simple irritative phenomena to complex psychologically related disorders, such as compulsions, mannerisms, etc.

The first group are the isolated or restricted dystonias (dyskinesias) of adult life. These include idiopathic spasmodic torticollis, oromandibular dystonia, blepharospasm, spastic dysphonia, and dystonic writer's cramp.

Spasmodic torticollis   This is an intermittent or continuous spasm of sternomastoid, trapezius, and other neck muscles, usually more pronounced on one side, with turning or tipping of the head. It is involuntary and cannot be inhibited and thereby differs from habit spasm or tic. This condition should be considered a form of dystonia. It is worse when the patient sits, stands, or walks, and usually contactual stimulation of the chin or of the back of the head partially alleviates the muscle imbalance.

Women are affected twice as often as men and the average age of onset is 40 years. Rarely is it seen in early adult life or adolescence. Extranuchal dystonia, tremor, and facial masking are seen in some cases.

Various modes of therapy have been tried with inconsistent results. L-Dopa (1 g per day) or carbidopa, carbamazepine (Tegretol, 200 to 1200 mg per day), haloperidal (2 to 12 mg per day) and biofeedback therapy have each been beneficial in certain cases. Psychiatric treatment is ineffectual. In severe cases muscle sectioning, neurectomy, or section of the anterior cervical roots has given favorable results.

Other craniocervical spasms   Blepharoclonus (inability to keep the eyes open), lingual spasms, "spastic" dysphonia, facial spasms, cervicothoracic spasms, and writer's cramp are all special varieties of involuntary movement, appearing usually in late middle life and the senium. Such facial, cervical, and thoracic spasms have occurred with striking frequency during phenothiazine medication, but they also appear de novo. Marsden refers to them as restricted dystonias. Nonprogressivity, unresponsiveness to psychotherapy, and uncertain amelioration by all pharmacologic agents characterize most of them. Exceptionally, when these disorders are induced by drugs of the phenothiazine class, they persist after discontinuance of the drug (tardive or postphenothiazine dyskinesias). Once started they tend to persist indefinitely, and the only therapy of value has been surgical denervation of the affected muscles (C_1 to C_3 and unilateral C_4 roots) in spasmodic torticollis.

Tics and habit spasms   Many persons throughout life are given to habitual movements, such as sniffing, clearing the throat, protruding the chin, or blinking, whenever they become tense. The patient admits that the movements are voluntary and that he or she feels compelled to make them in order to relieve tension; they can be inhibited for a time by an effort of will but reappear when attention is diverted. Children between five and ten years of age are especially likely to have habit spasms. The movements are often purposive coordinated acts which normally serve the organism; it is only their incessant repetition when uncalled for that constitutes a habit. In certain cases they become so ingrained that the person is unaware of them and unable to control them. Stereotypy purposelessness, and repetitiveness at irregular intervals are their main identifying features. Multiple convulsive tics with coprolalia (compulsive utterance of vile words; *Gilles de la Tourette's disease*) constitute a more severe and often unremitting form of the same condition. In children with transitory habit spasms it is best to ignore the habit spasm and at the same time to arrange for more rest and calmer environment. In adults, relief of nervous tension by tranquilizing drugs (chlorpromazine, 25 to 75 mg tid) and psychotherapy is helpful, but the disposition to tic formation persists. In the chronic tic or Tourette's syndrome large doses of haloperidol (10 to 20 mg per day orally) have been beneficial in some cases.

Mentally backward children and adults often display, when idle, a wide variety of rhythmic body-rocking, head-bobbing, arm-and-finger movements. These are of the nature of mannerisms and have no known basal ganglion pathology.

It would be a mistake to assume that each of the above disorders of movement occurs separately in specific relationships to certain diseases. This may happen, as in paralysis agitans; but there is sometimes much overlap in the degenerative diseases and birth injuries.

EXTRAPYRAMIDAL MOTOR DISTURBANCES DUE PRIMARILY TO DISEASES OF THE CEREBELLUM

Isolated lesions in the midline flocculonodular lobe result in grave disturbances of equilibrium. Often the symptoms are exhibited only when the patient attempts to stand and walk. Then sways, staggers, titubates, and reels occur (see "Disturbance of Movement and Posture," below). There may be no disturbance in coordination and no intention tremor of the limbs. A midline tumor of the cerebellum such as medulloblastoma, hemorrhage, or other lesion usually produces this syndrome.

Extensive lesions of one cerebellar hemisphere, especially the anterior lobe, cause disturbances in coordination of volitional movements of the ipsilateral arm and leg. This is known as *ataxia*. The movements are characterized by an inappropriate range, rate, and strength of each of the various components of a motor act and by an improper combination of those components. Electromyographic analysis has shown that ataxia is manifested as a decomposition of movement consisting of abnormal duration and timing of bursts of contraction and relaxation of agonists and antagonists of a joint, usually a large one. This incoordination is also called *asynergia*. The defects are particularly noticeable in acts that require rapid alternation of movements. Irregular slowness in acceleration and deceleration, which is almost invariably present, impedes the performance (dysdiadochokinesis). The direction of projected (purposive) movement is frequently inaccurate. Owing to delay in arresting a movement, the patient may overshoot the mark. The antagonist muscles do not come into play at the proper time, possibly because of the hypotonia that is almost always present. This may be demonstrated by having the patient flex the arm against a resistance that is suddenly released. The patient with cerebellar disease will sometimes strike the face because of failure to check the flexion movement. In movements requiring accurate direction, as the limb approaches its destination it may stop short and then advance by a more or less rhythmic series of jerks and oscillations (intention tremor). In addition to hypotonia, there may be, in acute cerebellar lesions, some slight weakness.

A similar ataxia, asynergia, and dysmetria, usually with hypotonia and only a little intention tremor, may accompany lesions of the lateral and inferior parts of the cerebellar hemisphere. Bilateral lesions of the cerebellar hemispheres and midline flocculonodular lobe lead to such a severe disturbance in all movements that the patient may be unable to stand or walk or use the limbs effectively. In addition, there are ocular and speech disturbances, namely, nystagmus, dysmetria and skew deviation of the eyes, and dysarthria. Lesions of the cerebellar peduncles have the same effect as extensive hemispheral le-

sions. This syndrome, due to involvement of one cerebellar hemisphere, may be observed in a tumor or abscess or in vascular lesions of the brainstem and cerebellar peduncles. The ataxia tends to be bilateral and symmetric in primary atrophy or degeneration of the cerebellum.

There have been numerous attempts to explain in physiologic terms the hypotonia, mild degrees of weakness and fatigability, and abnormalities in the rate and regularity of projected movement that accompany cerebellar lesions in humans. It has been found that depression of fusimotor (spindle) efferent activity in the spinal cord leads to decreased spindle afferent discharge and lessened tonic facilitation of alpha motor neuron activity. The cerebellar facilitation that is lost with acute lesions is normally mediated through two systems of fibers—the fastigioreticulospinal and the dentatorubrothalamocortical. The latter, acting specifically on cortical areas 4 and 6, is the more important in humans. Although the corticospinal tract is probably essential for expression of cerebellar deficits in humans, in the primate any pathway subserving specifically projected movements into environment may support tremor and other parts of the syndrome. Tremor, ataxia, and hypotonia seem to be separable, independent entities, but all are believed related to the disturbed fusimotor activity.

A kind of pseudoataxia, especially of gait, may be caused by the improper timing of the components of complex actions, e.g., with defects in postural sense (sensory ataxia) and with slow relaxation of muscles in hypothyroidism (myxedema with ataxia).

SOME GENERAL FEATURES OF ALL EXTRAPYRAMIDAL MOTOR DISTURBANCES

From the above discussion of many special types of motor disorder the reader must not think that they always appear in pure form. Various combinations occur in diseases. For example, Wilson's disease usually presents with a Parkinson-like picture of tremor, rigidity, slowness of movement, and flexion dystonia of trunk, but exceptionally there is athetosis, tonic innervation (inability to relax a voluntary movement), phasic dystonia, and intention tremor. Hallervorden-Spatz disease may take the form of universal rigidity and flexion dystonia or choreoathetosis. Occasionally the degeneration of Huntington's chorea leads to rigidity rather than choreoathetosis. Corticospinal and various of these extrapyramidal disorders may be associated in patients with cerebral diplegia. Nonetheless certain combinations tend to occur with greater or lesser frequency in certain diseases, as discussed in Chaps. 373 and 374.

In broad terms all the extrapyramidal disorders should be viewed in terms of the primary deficit (negative symptom) and of the new phenomena (movements, abnormal postures, tremors, etc.) which have appeared. These latter positive symptoms are presently ascribed to release from or disequilibrium of undamaged motor parts of the nervous system. The clearest negative effect is usually evidenced as an akinesia, or disinclination to use the affected muscles. The difficulty in rapid alternating sequences of movement stands as another negative effect in diseases of both the basal ganglia and the cerebellum. In fact this latter symptom, presenting as a clumsiness, may be the only fault manifest in certain congenitally maladroit children. Stress and nervous tension characteristically worsen both the motor deficiency and the abnormal movements in all these extrapyramidal syndromes, just as relaxation helps the motor performance. All the movement disorders are abolished in sleep.

One of the most remarkable discoveries of recent years, to

be credited largely to the pioneering efforts of neurosurgeons (Cooper), has been the abolition of tremors, rigidity, and involuntary movements of the limbs by a surgical lesion in the medial segment of the globus pallidus or the ventrolateral nucleus of the thalamus. The effects are contralateral. Usually the lesion has been made first by the injection of procaine (Novocain) and then by use of alcohol, cooling and freezing (Cooper), or electrocoagulation. The operation has been successful in temporarily alleviating tremor or rigidity (or both) on one side. The procedure is successful in approximately 80 percent of cases of paralysis agitans, and the postural abnormality in dystonia musculorum deformans and double athetosis has responded somewhat less consistently. The operations have been perfected to the point at which the mortality rate is less than 1 percent, and the risk of hemiplegia or some other sequel is less than 10 percent. Of course, as the disease progresses, the beneficial effects are lost. The therapeutic procedure indicates that the pallidum and ventrolateral nucleus, probably through their connections with the cerebral cortex (motor cortex and its corticospinal pathway), are essential for the expression of these extrapyramidal syndromes. The indications for these surgical procedures are discussed in Chap. 373.

DISTURBANCE OF MOVEMENT AND POSTURE: EXAMINATION AND DIFFERENTIAL DIAGNOSIS

In Chap. 15 the methods of examining the motor system are described at some length, so only a few additional remarks concerning extrapyramidal disorders need be made here. These abnormalities are best demonstrated by seeing the patient in action. Patients who complain of a limp after walking a distance or of difficulty in climbing stairs should be observed under these conditions. Tests of rate, regularity, and coordination of voluntary movement must be sufficiently varied and demanding of the patient's motor coordination to bring out the defect. The physician must cultivate the habit of accurately observing and describing abnormalities of movement and must not be content merely to give the condition a name or to force it into some category such as chorea, tic, or myoclonus. The main postures of the body in all common acts should be noted. Aside from the assessment of muscle power and of gait, the usual test applied to the upper limb is to ask the patient to touch the examiner's fingertip and then the tip of his or her own nose repeatedly (*finger-to-nose test*). To test the leg, the patient is asked to place a heel on one knee and then to run it down the shin and back to the knee (*heel-to-knee-to-shin test*). Finer movements of the hand may be tested by having the patient successively touch each finger to the thumb, pat a thigh rapidly, or use tools or handle objects. Rapidly alternating movements such as repeatedly touching the index finger with the thumb, pronation and supination of wrist, or opening and closing the hands are valuable tests.

The fully developed extrapyramidal motor syndromes can be recognized without difficulty once the physician has become familiar with the typical pictures. The mental picture of Parkinson's syndrome, with its slowness of movement, poverty of facial expression, and static tremor and rigidity should be fixed in mind. Similarly, the gross distortions and postural abnormalities of dystonia, whether widespread in trunk muscles or involving only neck muscles, as in spasmodic torticollis, once seen should thereafter be familiar. Athetosis, with its instability of postures and ceaseless movements of fingers and hands; intention spasm, chorea, with its more rapid and complicated movements; and the abrupt movements of myoclonus that flit over the body are other standard syndromes. Characteristic of all is a mild defect in the voluntary use of the affected parts.

The clinical differences between corticospinal and extrapyramidal disorders are summarized in Table 16-2.

Early or mild forms of these conditions, like all medical diseases, may offer special difficulties in diagnosis. Cases of paralysis agitans, seen before the appearance of tremor, are often overlooked. The patient may complain of being nervous and restless or may have experienced an indescribable stiffness and aching in certain parts of the body. Because of the absence of weakness or of reflex changes, the case may be considered psychogenic or rheumatic. It is well to remember that Parkinson's syndrome often begins in a hemiplegic distribution, and for this reason the illness may be misdiagnosed as cerebral thrombosis. A slight masking of the face, a suggestion of a limp, blepharoclonus (uninhibited blinking of eyes when the bridge of the nose is tapped), a mild rigidity, failure of an arm to swing naturally in walking, or loss of certain movements of cooperation will help in diagnosis at this time. Every case presenting the syndrome of Parkinson or other abnormality of movement and posture in adolescence or early adult life should be surveyed for hepatolenticular degeneration by tests of liver function and slit-lamp examination for corneal pigmentation (Kayser-Fleischer ring); if facilities are available, urinary amino-nitrogen excretion and copper excretion should be determined.

Mild or early chorea is often mistaken for simple nervousness. If one sits for a time and watches the patient, the diagnosis will often become evident. There are cases, nonetheless, in which it is impossible to distinguish simple nervousness from early Sydenham's chorea, especially in children, and there is no laboratory test upon which one can depend. The first postural manifestation of dystonia may suggest hysteria, and it is only later, when the fixity of the postural abnormality, the lack of the usual psychologic picture of hysteria, and the relentlessly progressive character of the illness become evident, that accurate diagnosis is reached. Another common error is to assume that a bedfast patient who has complained of dizziness, staggering, and headaches and exhibits no other neurologic abnormality is suffering from hysteria. The flocculonodular cerebellar syndrome is demonstrable only when the patient attempts to stand and walk.

The uncertainty of balance and short-stepped gait (*marche à petit pas*) in the elderly is often incorrectly attributed to loss of confidence and fear of falling.

REFERENCES

CARPENTER M: Anatomy of the basal ganglia and related nuclei: A review, in *Advances in Neurology,* vol 14: *Dystonia,* D Williams (ed). London, Butterworths, 1975

COOPER IS: *Involuntary Movement Disorders.* New York, Hoeber, 1969

CUMINGS JN: Biochemistry of the basal ganglia, in *Handbook of Clinical Neurology,* vol 6, PJ Vinken, GW Bruyn (eds). Amsterdam, North-Holland, 1968, p 116

DENNY-BROWN D: Clinical symptomatology of disease of the basal ganglia, in *Handbook of Clinical Neurology,* vol 6, PJ Vinken, GW Bruyn (eds). Amsterdam, North-Holland, 1968, p 133

LANCE JW: Familial paroxysmal dystonic choreoathetosis and its differentiation from related syndromes. Ann Neurol 2:285, 1977

MARSDEN CD: The neuropharmacology of abnormal involuntary movement disorders (the dyskinesias), in *Modern Trends in Neurology,* D Williams (ed). London, Butterworths, 1975

DISTURBANCES OF EQUILIBRIUM AND OF GAIT

MAURICE VICTOR
RAYMOND D. ADAMS

All that has been said previously in Chap. 14, "Dizziness and Vertigo," refers in large measure to the patient's awareness of a disorientation in space; however, there are forms of neurologic abnormality with a prominent disequilibrium of the body but no dizziness whatsoever. Since these are manifested most clearly as an impairment of upright stance and locomotion, their evaluation depends on a knowledge of the nervous mechanisms underlying these peculiarly human functions.

Since normal body posture and locomotion require visual information, labyrinthine function, and proprioception, it is of interest to note the effect of deficits in these senses on normal function. Blind persons or persons with sight who are blindfolded may walk very well. They move cautiously, to avoid collision with objects, and on smooth pavement shorten their step slightly; with the shortening there is less rocking of the body, and they seem unnaturally stiff. A person deprived of labyrinthine function shows a slight unsteadiness in walking and an inability to descend stairs without holding onto a banister. Running is also difficult. Characteristically, there is great difficulty in focusing on a stationary object when the individual is moving, so that he or she cannot drive a car. Proof of dependence on visual cues comes from blindfolded performance, when unsteadiness and staggering increase to some extent, but usually not to the point of falling. A loss of proprioception, as in a complete lesion in the posterior columns of the spinal cord in the high cervical region, abolishes for a long time the capacity for independent locomotion. After years of training, the patients will still have difficulty in starting to walk and in propelling themselves forward. As Purdon Martin has illustrated, they hold the hands in front of the body, bend body and head forward, walk with a wide base with irregular uneven steps but do rock the body. If they lose balance, they show no reaction to the altered posture. If they fall, they cannot arise without help, and they cannot get up from a chair. They are unable to crawl or to get into an all-fours posture. When standing, if blindfolded, they immediately fall. Thus the postural reactions are demonstrably more dependent on proprioceptive than on visual or labyrinthine information.

CLINICAL APPROACH TO GAIT DISORDERS When confronted with a disorder of gait, the examiner must observe the patient's natural stance and the attitude and dominant positions of the legs, trunk, and arms. Questions about coexistent vertigo and giddiness should be asked. If present, one proceeds as outlined above. It is good practice to watch while patients walk into the examining room, because they are apt to walk more naturally then than during special tests. They should be asked to stand with the feet together, head erect, with eyes first open and then closed. Swaying due to nervousness may be overcome by diverting the patient's attention as in asking the patient to touch the tip of the nose with the finger of first one hand and then the other. Next the patient should be asked to walk forward and backward, with the eyes first open and then closed. Any tendency to reel to one side, as in cerebellar disease, can be checked by having the patient walk around a chair. When the affected side is toward the chair, the patient tends to walk into it; when it is away from the chair, the patient veers outward in ever-widening circles. More delicate tests of gait are walking a straight line heel to toe or having the patient arise quickly from a chair, walk briskly, and then stop or turn suddenly. If all these tests are successfully executed, it may be assumed that any difficulty in locomotion is not due to disease of the proprioceptive mechanisms or cerebellum. Detailed neurologic examination is then necessary in order to determine which of the many other possible diseases is responsible for the patient's disorder of gait.

The following abnormal gaits are so distinctive that with a little practice they can be recognized at a glance.

Cerebellar gait The main features of this gait are *wide base* (separation of legs), *unsteadiness, irregularity,* and *lateral reeling.* Steps are uncertain, some are shorter and others longer than intended, and the patient may lurch to one side or the other. The unsteadiness is more prominent on quickly arising from a chair and walking, on stopping suddenly while walking, or on turning abruptly. If the ataxia is severe, the patient cannot stand without assistance. If it is lesser in degree, standing with feet together and head erect, with eyes either open or closed, may be difficult. In its mildest form the ataxia is best demonstrated by having the patient walk a line heel to toe. After two or three steps there is loss of balance and the patient must place one foot to the side to avoid falling. Romberg's sign, i.e., marked swaying or falling with the eyes closed but not with the eyes open, is not a feature of cerebellar disease. Compensation may be effected by shortening the step and shuffling, i.e., keeping both feet simultaneously on the ground. The defect in the cerebellar gait is not in antigravity support, steppage, or propulsion but in the coordination of proprioceptive, labyrinthine, and visual information in reflex coordination of movements. The abnormality of gait may or may not be accompanied by other signs of cerebellar incoordination and intention tremor of the arms and legs. The presence of the latter signs depends on involvement of the superior midline structures as distinct from cerebellar hemispheres; if the lesion is unilateral, the signs are always on the same side.

Cerebellar gait is in some instances the major symptom in multiple sclerosis, cerebellar tumors, particularly medulloblastoma of the cerebellar vermis, paraneoplastic diseases, and the cerebellar degenerations. In certain forms of cerebellar degeneration (e.g., the type associated with chronic alcoholism) the disease process reaches a plateau and then remains stable for many years, and the gait disorder, in these circumstances, becomes altered to some extent. The base is wide and the steps are still short, but more regular; the trunk is inclined slightly forward, the arms are held away from the sides, and the gait assumes a somewhat rhythmic quality. In this way the patient can walk for long distances but lacks the capacity to make the necessary postural adjustments in response to sudden changes in position.

A slowness in muscle relaxation as in myxedema may also lead to a kind of gait disorder that simulates a cerebellar defect.

Gait of sensory ataxia This gait is due to an impairment of proprioception resulting from interruption of afferent nerve fibers in the peripheral nerves, posterior roots, posterior columns of the spinal cords, or medial lemnisci; it may also be produced occasionally by a lesion of both parietal lobes. Whatever the location of the lesion, the patient is deprived of knowledge of the position of the limbs. The principal features of the resulting gait disorder are *uncertainty, irregularity,* and the *stamp* of the feet. Hunt characterized this type of gait very well when he said that the ataxic patient is recognized by "his stamp and stick." More explicitly, there are varying degrees of difficulty in standing and walking, and in advanced cases a complete failure of locomotion, even though muscular power is retained. The legs are kept far apart to correct the instability, and the patient carefully watches the ground and the feet. As the patient steps out, the legs are flung abruptly forward and outward, often lifted higher than necessary. The steps are of variable length, and many are attended by an audible stamp as the foot is banged down on the floor. The body is held in a slightly flexed posture, and the weight may be supported on the cane that the severely ataxic patient usually carries. The incoordination is greatly exaggerated when the patient is deprived of visual cues, as in walking in the dark. Most patients, when asked to stand with feet together and eyes closed, show greatly increased swaying or actual falling (Romberg's sign). It has been said that a lame person whose shoes are not worn in any one place is probably suffering from sensory ataxia. There is invariably a loss of vibratory and position sense in the feet and legs. A disordered gait of this type is observed in tabes dorsalis, Friedreich's ataxia, subacute combined degeneration, syphilitic meningomyelitis, chronic polyneuritis, and those cases of multiple sclerosis in which posterior column disease predominates.

Hemiplegic and paraplegic (spastic) gait   In hemiplegia the leg is held stiffly and does not flex freely and gracefully at the knee and hip. It tends to rotate outward and describes a semicircle, first away from and then toward the trunk (circumduction). The foot scrapes along the floor, and the toe and outer side of the sole of the shoe are worn. One can diagnose the hemiplegic gait by hearing the slow rhythmic scuff of the foot along the floor. The other muscles of the body on the affected side are weak and stiff to a variable degree, particularly the arm, which is carried in a flexed position and does not swing naturally. This type of gait disorder is most frequently associated with vascular disease of the brain.

The spastic paraplegic gait is entirely different from the gait of sensory ataxia, though the two may be combined. Each leg is advanced slowly and stiffly with restricted motion at the knee and hip. The patient looks as though wading in water. The legs are extended or slightly bent at the knees and may be strongly adducted at the hips, tending almost to cross ("scissors" gait). The steps are regular and short. Movements of the legs are slow, and the patient may be able to advance only with great effort. An easy way to remember the main features of the hemiplegic and paraplegic gait is by the letter S, which begins each of its descriptive adjectives—spastic, slow, scuffing. The defect is in the stepping mechanism and in propulsion, not in support or equilibrium. Cerebral spastic diplegia, multiple sclerosis, syringomyelia, spinal syphilis, combined system disease, spinal cord compression, and familial spinal spastic ataxia are the common causes of spastic paraparesis.

Festinating gait   The term *festinating* comes from the Latin *festinare,* to hasten, and appropriately describes the involuntary increase or hastening of the gait that characterizes both paralysis agitans and postencephalitic Parkinson's syndrome (see Chap. 373). *Rigidity* and *shuffling,* in addition to *festination,* are the cardinal features of this gait. When they are joined to the typical tremors, rigidity, and slowness of movement, there can be little doubt as to the diagnosis.

The general attitude of the patient is one of flexion; rigidity and immobility of the body are other conspicuous features. There is a paucity of the automatic movements made in sitting, standing, and walking; the head does not turn in looking to one side, the arms are seldom folded, and the legs are rarely crossed. The arms are held stiffly as though in preparation for writing, and the facial expression is unblinking and masklike.

This slight, generalized stiffening is common in psychiatric patients treated with phenothiazine drugs.

In walking, the trunk is bent forward and the arms are carried ahead of the body and do not swing. The legs are stiff and bent at the knees and hips. The steps are short, and the feet barely clear the ground as the patient shuffles along. Once forward or backward locomotion is started, the upper part of the body advances ahead of the lower part, as though the patient were chasing the center of gravity. Steps become more and more rapid, and the patient may fall if not assisted. This is the festination, and it may occur when the patient is walking forward or backward, taking the form of either propulsion or retropulsion. The defect is in rocking the body from side to side so as to clear the floor and in moving the legs quickly enough to catch the center of gravity in forward propulsion. Other unusual gaits are sometimes observed in postencephalitic patients. For example, they may be unable to take the first step forward because they cannot lift one foot, or they may be unable to step forward until they hop or take one step backward; walking may be initiated by a series of short steps that give way to a more normal gait; occasionally such a patient may run better than walk or walk backwards better than forward. Choreoathetotic movements may be added to the festinating gait in the L-dopa-treated patient with Parkinson's disease.

Athetotic, dystonic, and choreic gaits   Diseases that are characterized by involuntary movements and abnormal postures seriously affect gait. In fact, a disturbance of gait may be the initial and dominant manifestation of these diseases, and the testing of gait often serves to provoke abnormalities of movement and posture that are otherwise not conspicuous. The *athetotic* patient often assumes the most grotesque postures. One arm may be held aloft and the other one behind the body with wrist and fingers alternately undergoing slow flexion, extension, and rotation. The head may be inclined in one direction, the lips alternately retract and then purse as part of a grimace, and the tongue intermittently protrudes from the mouth. The legs advance slowly and awkwardly, the result of superimposed involuntary movements and postures. Sometimes the foot is plantar-flexed at the ankle, and the weight is carried on the toes; or it may be dorsiflexed or inverted or flung to one side. This type of gait is typical of congenital athetosis and Huntington's chorea.

In *dystonia musculorum deformans* the first symptom may be a limp due to inversion or plantar flexion of the foot or a distortion of the pelvis. The patient stands with one leg rigidly extended or one shoulder elevated. The trunk may be in a position of exaggerated lordosis, and the hips are partly flexed, with a tilting forward of the pelvis. Because of the muscle spasms that deform the body in this manner, the patient may have to walk with knees flexed. The gait may seem normal as the first steps are taken, but as the patient walks, one or both legs become flexed, giving rise to the "dromedary gait." In the more advanced stages walking becomes impossible, owing to torsion of the trunk or the continuous flexion of one leg.

In *Sydenham's chorea* the gait is often bizarre (see Chap. 373). As the patient stands or walks, there is a continuous play of irregular "choreic" movements affecting the face, neck, hands, and, in the advanced stages, the large proximal joints and trunk. The positions of the trunk and upper parts of the body vary with each step. There are jerks of the head, grimacing, squirming, twisting movements of the trunk and limbs, and peculiar respiratory noises.

Drop-foot, steppage, or equine gait   This is caused by paralysis of the pretibial and peroneal muscles. The legs must be lifted abnormally high in order for the feet to clear the ground. There is a slapping noise as the foot strikes the floor. The anterior and lateral borders of the sole of the shoe become worn. The steps are regular and even; otherwise, walking is not remarkable. Foot drop may be unilateral or bilateral and occurs in diseases that affect the peripheral nerves of the legs or motor neurons in the spinal cord, such as poliomyelitis, progressive muscular atrophy, and Charcot-Marie-Tooth disease (peroneal muscular atrophy). It may also be observed in patients with peripheral types of muscular dystrophy. The most common cause of unilateral foot drop is compression of the anterior tibial nerve, where it crosses the head of the fibula (see Chap. 377).

Waddling gait   This gait is characteristic of progressive muscular dystrophy. The attitude of the body may be straight, but more often the lumbar lordosis is accentuated. The steps are regular but a little uncertain. With each step there is an exaggerated elevation of one hip and depression of the other; once the weight is on the hip it yields to an abnormal degree, so that the upper trunk then inclines to that side. This alternation of lateral trunk movements results in the rolling gait, or *waddle*, a term suggested by Oppenheim. The gluteal musculature is weak and inefficient, although leg muscles may appear well developed. Muscular contractures leading to an equinovarus position of the foot may complicate childhood cases, so that the waddle is combined with circumduction of the legs and "walking on the toes."

Staggering or drunken gait   This is characteristic of alcoholic and barbiturate intoxication. The drunken patient totters, reels, tips forward and then backward, threatening each moment to lose balance and fall. Control over trunk and legs is greatly impaired. The steps are irregular and uncertain. The patient appears stupefied and indifferent to the quality of performance, but under certain circumstances can momentarily correct the defect.

The frequently used adjectives *drunken* and *reeling* do not describe aptly the gait of cerebellar disease, except, perhaps, the most acute and severe cases. The intoxicated patient reels in many different directions, unlike the patient with cerebellar disease, and no effort is made to correct the staggering by watching the legs or the ground, as in cerebellar or sensory ataxia. In the drunken patient, despite a wide diversity of excursions of all parts of the body, balance may be exquisitely maintained. In contrast, patients with cerebellar disease have great difficulty in maintaining balance if they sway or lurch too far to one side.

Hysterical gait   This may take one of several forms— monoplegic, paraplegic, or hemiplegic. The monoplegic or hemiplegic patient does not lift the foot from the floor while walking; instead, it is dragged as a useless member or pushed ahead as though it were a skate. The characteristic circumduction is absent in hysterical hemiplegia, and the typical hemiplegic posture, hyperactive tendon reflexes, and Babinski sign are missing. The hysterical paraplegic cannot very well drag both legs, and usually depends on a crutch or remains helpless in bed; the muscles may be rigid with pseudocontractures or flaccid. The gait may be quite dramatic. Some patients look as though they were walking on stilts, and others lurch wildly in all directions, actually demonstrating by their gyrations a remarkable ability to make rapid postural adjustments.

Astasia-abasia, in which the patient, though unable to either stand or walk, retains normal use of the legs while in bed, is nearly always hysterical. When such patients are placed on their feet, they take a few normal steps and then become unable to advance the feet; they lurch widly and crumple to the floor if not assisted.

Frontal lobe ataxia   Equilibrium and the capacity to stand and walk may be severely disturbed by diseases that affect the frontal lobes, particularly their medial parts. Although this disorder of gait is sometimes spoken of as an ataxia or as an *apraxia*, since the difficulty in walking cannot be accounted for by weakness or loss of sensation, it is probably neither. It most likely represents a loss of integration at the cortical and basal ganglionic level of the essential elements of stance and locomotion which were acquired in infancy and are often lost in senility.

These patients assume a posture of slight flexion, with the feet placed farther apart than normal. They advance slowly, with small, shuffling, hesitant steps. At times they halt, unable to advance without great effort, although they do much better with a little assistance. Turning is accomplished by a series of tiny, uncertain steps which are made with one foot, the other being planted on the floor as a pivot. The initiation of walking becomes progressively more difficult, and in advanced cases patients may be unable to take a step, as though the feet were glued to the floor. Finally they become unable to stand or even to sit, and without support fall backward or to one side.

Some patients are able to make complex movements with their legs, such as drawing imaginary figures, at a time when their gait is seriously impaired. Eventually, however, all movements of the legs become slow and awkward, and the limbs, when passively moved, offer variable resistance (gegenhalten). An inability to turn and sit in a chair or to lie down on a bed is highly characteristic, and may eventually become complete. These motor disabilities are usually associated with dementia, but there need be no parallelism in their evolution. Grasping, groping, hyperactive tendon reflexes, and Babinski signs may or may not be present. The end result in many cases is a "cerebral paraplegia in flexion" (Yakovlev), in which the patient lies curled up in bed, immobile and mute, the limbs fixed by contractures in an attitude of flexion.

Senile gait   Elderly persons often complain of difficulty in walking, and examination may disclose no abnormality other than the slightly flexed posture of the senile and short uncertain steps, *marche à petit pas*. Speed, balance, and all the graceful, adaptive movements are lost. The exact nature of this gait disorder is not understood. Probably it is a combination frontal lobe and basal ganglionic defect. It should be noted, however, that a short-stepped, cautious gait lacks specificity, being a general defensive reaction to all forms of defective locomotion.

REFERENCES

ADAMS RD, VICTOR M: *Principles of Neurology*. New York, McGraw-Hill, 1977
DIX MR: Modern tests of vestibular function, with special reference to their value in clinical practice. Br Med J 3:317, 1969

18
COMMON DISTURBANCES OF VISION, OCULAR MOVEMENT, AND HEARING

MAURICE VICTOR
RAYMOND D. ADAMS

Diseases of the eyes and ears, by virtue of their frequency, unusual nature, and serious consequences, make up separate medical specialties and, therefore, fall outside the field of internal medicine. Yet disturbances of visual and auditory function may be the initial or leading manifestations of many systemic diseases. Of more general interest is the fact that these two senses represent the most finely developed parts of the entire afferent apparatus of the nervous system; hence the study of their disorders may yield important information about neurologic diseases.

THE EYE AND DISORDERS OF VISION

The eye, with its diverse epithelial, vascular, collagenous, neural, and pigmentary components, is a medical microcosm, susceptible to manifold diseases. Moreover, its transparency makes it accessible to direct inspection by the ophthalmoscope, an instrument found in the consulting room of every physician, and affords an opportunity to observe many of the specific lesions of medical diseases.

Since the eye is the organ of vision, it is obvious that impairment of visual acuity of varying degree should stand as the most frequent symptom of eye disease. Strabismus and diplopia, ocular pain, irritation, redness and photophobia, inability to read or recognize objects and people, and drooping or closure of the eyelids are also important. The impairment of eyesight may be unilateral or bilateral, sudden or gradual, episodic or enduring. The common causes vary with age. In late childhood and adolescence increasing difficulty in focusing the eyes and in seeing clearly usually can be traced to *myopia*, though an optic nerve disorder or suprasellar tumor must be excluded. In middle age *presbyopia* is almost invariable and requires refraction and eyeglasses. Still later in life *cataracts, glaucoma,* and *retinal hemorrhages* and *detachments* are the most frequent causes of visual disturbance. Episodic blindness in early life is usually due to migraine; later, amaurosis fugax is caused by stenosis of the carotid artery or cranial arteritis. Cerebrovascular disease deranges vision with increasing frequency in late life.

Thus failing eyesight may be due to an abnormality of the refractive media of the eye or to a lesion of the retina or optic nerve or the parts of the brain with which they are connected. In approaching this problem one begins always by inquiring as to precisely what patients mean when they say they cannot see properly, for they may be referring to symptoms as varied as excessive tearing, diplopia, partial syncope, or even giddiness or dizziness. Fortunately these statements can be checked by the measurement of visual acuity, a technique which is the single most important part of the ocular examination. If visual acuity is less than 20/20 and cannot be improved by refraction and if the media of the eye are transparent, there is some sensory defect, the nature of which must be ascertained.

In the measurement of visual acuity the *Snellen chart,* which contains rows of letters of diminishing size (those of each row subtending 5 min of an arc when held at various distances from the eye), is utilized. The letters at the top of the chart subtend 5 min of an arc at a distance of 200 ft; those at the bottom subtend an arc of 5 min at 20 ft. Thus if the patient can see only the top letters at 20 ft, rather than 200 ft, vision is 20/200; if those letters at the bottom are seen at this distance, the acuity is 20/20. The patient with a corrected refractive error should wear eyeglasses for the test; if the visual acuity is then less than 20/20, either the refractive error has not been properly corrected or there is some other reason for it. The former possibility can be ruled out if the patient sees clearly while looking through a pinhole of 2 to 3 mm in a cardboard with the glasses still on. The pinhole permits a narrow shaft of light to fall on the fovea without being refracted.

Light entering the eye is focused on the outer layer of the retina (the rods and cones). Consequently the media (tissues and fluids) through which the light passes must be transparent. These media are the cornea, the aqueous humor of the anterior chamber, the lens, the vitreous humor of the vitreous cavity, and the retina itself. The clarity of these media can be determined ophthalmoscopically, but this examination requires that the pupil be dilated to at least 6 mm in diameter. This is best accomplished by instilling a few drops of 10% phenylephrine (Neo-Synephrine) in each eye after the visual acuity is measured, the pupillary response recorded, and the intraocular pressure estimated. *An attack of angle-closure glaucoma may be precipitated by pupillary dilatation, but this happens rarely;* this complication should be treated by the intravenous administration of mannitol (50 g of a 20% solution) and oral administration of the carbonic anhydrase inhibitor, acetazolamide (Diamox, 250 mg qid), followed by the topical instillation of 4% pilocarpine. The cycloplegic action of phenylephrine lasts only an hour or two. Looking through a +6 ophthalmoscopic lens from a distance of 15 to 20 cm permits the visualization of any opacity in refractive media against the diffuse bright red of reflected light from the retina. By adjusting the lens of the ophthalmoscope from high + to 0 or −, one can "depth-focus" from the cornea to the retina. Clarity of all media means that reduced vision uncorrected by glasses must be due to a lesion in the macula, optic nerve, or structures further back in the visual system.

More specifically, the alterations in the refractile media that affect vision have certain medical implications, as follows.

CORNEAS In hypercalcemia secondary to sarcoid (Chap. 216), hyperparathyroidism (Chap. 350), and vitamin D intoxication (Chap. 351), calcium phosphates and carbonates precipitate, primarily beneath the corneal epithelium in a plane corresponding to the interpalpebral tissue—so-called *band keratopathy* (see Plate 7-8); cystine crystals are deposited in cystinosis (Chap. 90), cholesterol esters in hypercholesterolemia (*arcus senilis*) (Chap. 100), chloroquine crystals in treatment of discoid lupus by this drug, and copper in hepatolenticular degeneration [Kayser-Fleischer ring (Plate 8-8 and Chap. 95)]. Opacification of the cornea (keratitis) may also occur after herpes simplex and herpes zoster infections (Chaps. 193 and 185); or it may be combined with uveitis and iritis in Behçet's disease, Reiter's disease (Chap. 358), Stevens-Johnson disease (Chap. 67), and idiopathic infections, Keratitis may be a manifestation also of congenital syphilis (Chap. 146) and of more innocent states such as drying and injury of eyes during coma.

AQUEOUS HUMOR The common problem is one of high pressure due to impediment of the outflow of the aqueous fluid. This is termed *glaucoma*. In 90 percent of cases (of the wide-angle type) the cause is unknown; in 5 percent the angle between pupil and lateral cornea is narrow and blocked when the pupil is dilated; and in the remaining 5 percent the condition is secondary to some disease process that blocks outflow channels (inflammatory debris of uveitis, or red blood cells from hemorrhage in the anterior chamber, i.e., hyphema). Glaucoma occurs in 2 percent of all patients over the age of 40; it may be asymptomatic and go unrecognized for years before it progresses to rapid loss of vision. Therefore, the intraocular pressure should be measured routinely, using a Schiotz tonometer. This is a simple procedure which should be practiced by every physician. With the patient supine, a drop of local anesthetic is put into each eye and the tonometer is then placed on the cornea so that the instrument is perfectly vertical. When the tonometer is pressed against the eye, the scale is read and the units are converted into millimeters of mercury from the chart in the tonometer case. The normal pressure is about 15 mmHg. Pressures of 20 to 30 mmHg may damage the optic nerve, leading first to a nasal quadrant defect and finally to blindness. With the ophthalmoscope one can see also that the optic disk is excavated and, in some instances, atrophic (Plate 7-2).

THE LENS Opacities form in diabetes mellitus (Chap. 337) and galactosemia ("sugar cataracts") from sustained high levels of blood glucose and galactose, which are changed to sorbitol or dulcitol (the accumulation of which leads to a high osmotic gradient within the lens fibers); in hypoparathyroidism (Chap. 350), which by lowering the concentration of calcium in the aqueous humor opacifies newly forming lens fibers; after prolonged high doses of chlorpromazine and corticosteroid therapy, which are believed to result in lenticular opacities; and in myotonic dystrophy (Chap. 380), which is associated with a special type of cataract. Weakening of the zonular ligaments of the lens allows a dislocation (iridodenesis) in both Marfan's syndrome and homocystinuria (Plate 8-7 and Chap. 58).

VITREOUS HUMOR Hemorrhage may occur from rupture of a retinal vessel, causing a shower of black or red dots. It is also seen in diabetes mellitus, where it may occur following rupture of newly formed retinal vessels, i.e., *retinitis proliferans,* or after a retinal tear which may progress to retinal detachment. The vitreous humor may also be affected by deposition of calcium soaps (seen as small white opacities with the ophthalmoscope)—so-called "asteroid hyalosis" of diabetes mellitus.

RETINA AND OPTIC NERVE The search for neurologic explanations of reduced vision begins with an ophthalmoscopic examination of the retina. This thin (0.4 mm) sheet of transparent tissue and the optic nerve head into which the visual information is channeled are the only parts of the central nervous system that can be inspected during life.

Light entering the eye passes through the full thickness of the retina to reach the receptor layer of rods and cones. Impulses arising in these photoreceptors are transmitted via secondary neurons, the bipolar cells, to the innermost ganglion cell layer, the axons of which in turn travel through the optic nerve head, optic nerve, chiasm, and optic tracts to the lateral geniculate bodies. These retinal neurons normally acquire a myelin sheath only after piercing the lamina cribrosa. The macular region, which lies two disk diameters or 3 mm lateral to the optic disk, is the most sensitive part of the retina. The vascular supply comes from the ophthalmic branch of the internal carotid artery, which in turn gives origin to the central retinal artery. The latter, upon issuing from the optic disk, divides into four arterioles, which supply the four quadrants of the retina (Plate 7-1). The ganglion cells and bipolar cells receive their blood supply from these arterioles and their capillaries, whereas photoreceptor elements receive nourishment from the underlying choroidal vascular bed.

These small vessels react in disease states like vessels of corresponding size in the brain. Since the walls of the retinal arterioles are transparent to the ophthalmoscope, what is seen is a column of blood. In arteriosclerosis (usually coexistent with hypertension), the lumens of the vessels are narrowed because of fibrous tissue replacement of the media and thickening of the basement membrane. The light reflection from the vessel then has a different refractive index than the adjacent retinal tissue. Tortuosity of vessels, arteriole-venous compressions, and narrowed segments are other signs of hypertension and arteriolosclerosis. In malignant hypertension there are, in addition, cotton-wool exudates, splinter hemorrhages, and papilledema, changes that may also be present in the intracranial arterioles. Atheromatous deposits, which form in larger arteries, are observed in the retina only with extreme degrees of hyperlipemia because of the small size of the vessels. Occasionally atheromatous and other emboli from the carotid and aorta

may lodge in them. Capillary-venular aneurysms may develop, most often in diabetes mellitus (Plate 8-3). Since the central retinal vein and artery share a common adventitial sheath, atheromatous plaques in the artery may result in thrombosis of the vein. Round or oval hemorrhages always lie in the outer plexiform layer and linear or flame-shaped ones in the superficial layer of the retina, as occurs in conditions with extremely high intracranial pressure, such as ruptured intracranial saccular aneurysm and hemangioma; occasionally brain hemorrhage or cranial trauma permits blood to cover the retina and extend beneath the vitreous humor (subhyaloid hemorrhage).

The systemic coagulopathies of thrombotic thrombocytopenia and disseminated intravascular coagulopathy may cause clotting, preferentially in the submacular choriocapillaries. Sometimes this is associated with choroidal hemorrhage and detachment of the retina. The patient will complain of blurred vision because of a scotoma.

Aside from visible vascular lesions, other more specific alterations of the retina may impair vision. The most important of these are tears and separations and detachments and degenerations.

1 *Degeneration of the outer receptor layer and subjacent pigment epithelium* occurs as a hereditary trait in *retinitis pigmentosa* (Plate 7-7), and also in Laurence-Moon-Biedl syndrome, progressive ophthalmoplegia, Bassen-Kornzweig disease (Chap. 100), Refsum's disease (Chap. 377), Batten-Mayou juvenile lipid storage disease, and idiopathic senile macular degeneration (Chaps. 100 and 373).
2 *Degeneration in Bruch's membrane* (which supports the layer of pigment epithelium next to the rods and cones) and its repair by fibrosis give rise to angioid streaks (Plate 7-4) typical of pseudoxanthoma elasticum (Chap. 363), Paget's disease (Chap. 353), hyperphosphatemia, and acromegaly.
3 *Deposits of phenothiazine conjugate with the melanin* of the pigment layer result in degeneration of the outer retinal layers. When these drugs are used, the doses should be kept low and the central visual fields tested with small colored test objects.

Sarcoidosis, toxoplasmosis, and *histoplasmosis* involve both the retina and the choroid. The latter is the site of noninfective inflammatory reactions, often in association with iridocyclitis.

The optic nerves, chiasm, and tracts which constitute the third visual neuron can be inspected only in part, from the foveal or macular region to the optic disk. The latter reflects raised intracranial pressure (papilledema or choked disk), papillitis (disease of the optic nerve close to the disk), optic nerve atrophy, and glaucoma (Plates 7-2, 7-5, and 7-6).

Central visual disturbances (caused by defects in the retina, optic nerves and tracts, lateral geniculate bodies, geniculocalcarine path, and striate cortex of occipital lobes) are evidenced by changes in the visual fields. In good light, if one of the patient's eyes is covered and the other aligned with the corresponding eye of the examiner and a cotton pledget or white disk on a stick is brought from the outside toward the center, the periphery of the patient's visual field can be compared with that of the examiner. The types of visual field defect resulting from lesions in different parts of the visual pathways are shown in Fig. 18-1. A prechiasmal lesion causes either a scotoma (an island of impaired vision within the visual field) or a cut in the peripheral part of the visual field. A small scotoma in the macular part of the visual field may seriously impair visual acuity in the early stages of macular disease, giving rise to a central scotoma; patients may complain of distortion of vision, particularly for straight lines (metamorphopsia). One may test for this at the bedside by asking the patient to look at the center of a checkerboard or a jigsaw puzzle. The straight lines in the center appear curved or kinked. Metamorphopsia is diagnostic of retinal disease and aids in the distinction between a macular lesion and one in the optic nerve or occipital lobe. Demyelinative, toxic (methyl alcohol, quinine, and certain of the phenothiazine tranquilizing drugs), nutritional (so-called "tobaccoalcohol" amblyopia), and vascular diseases are the usual causes of scotomas. The toxic states are characterized by symmetric bilateral scotomas, and the nutritional disorders by more or less symmetric central scotomas (involving the fixation point) or centrocecal scotomas (involving both the fixation point and the blind spot). These latter scotomas are predominantly in the distribution of the papillomacular bundle, but their presence does not establish whether the primary effect is on the nerve fibers or the ganglion cells. Demyelinative diseases are characterized by unilateral or asymmetric bilateral scotomas. If the lesion is near the optic disk, there may be swelling of the optic nerve head, i.e., *papillitis*, which can usually be distinguished from papilledema by the marked impairment of vision it produces. Vascular lesions as a rule give rise to unilateral scotomas. The lesions take the form of retinal hemorrhages, hard exudates, or occluded vessels which cause infarction of the retina. The common cotton-wool patches are in reality small retinal infarcts. Large zones of retinal infarction may follow occlusion of a branch of the central retinal artery (Plates 8-1, 8-2, 8-4, and 8-5).

FIGURE 18-1

Diagram showing the effects on the fields of vision produced by lesions at various points along the optic pathway. A. Complete blindness in left eye. B. Bitemporal hemianopsia. C. Nasal hemianopsia of left eye. D. Right homonymous hemianopsia. E and F. Right upper and lower quadrant hemianopsia. G. Right homonymous hemianopsia with preservation of central vision. (From Homans, A Textbook of Surgery, Springfield, Ill, Charles C Thomas, 1945.)

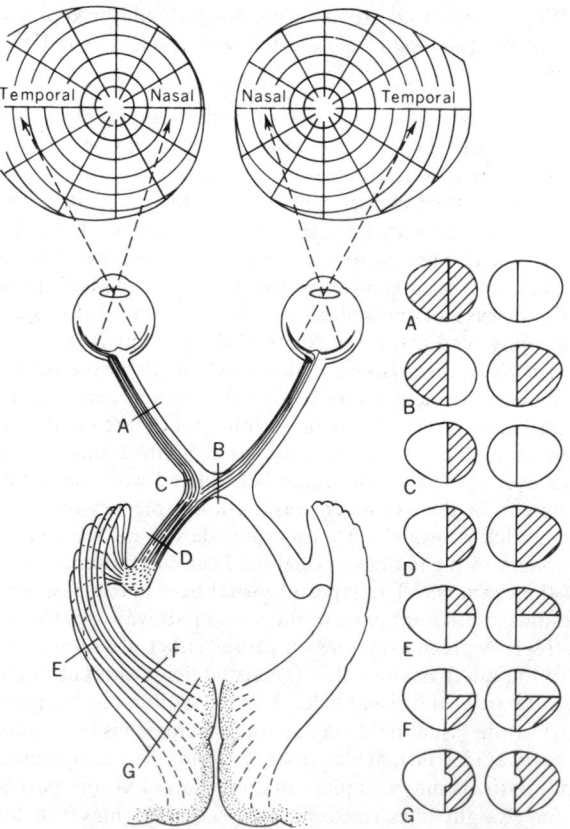

Ischemic optic neuropathy is another well-recognized entity. The onset is abrupt, usually in an elderly person. It may be painful. Vision may be abolished completely, or there may be an altitudinal or segmental defect in one eye. Examination of the fundus may show no abnormality, but later the optic disk may become pale; rarely there is congestion, hemorrhage, and swelling of the disk. The pathologic basis of this disturbance is thrombosis or embolism of the posterior ciliary artery. If preceded by headache, pain on chewing, and arthralgia, the diagnosis is usually temporal arteritis. Both eyes may be affected simultaneously or in succession. Prognosis for recovery of vision is poor. Fluorescein retinography (see below) is a valuable method for revealing retinal vascular abnormalities.

Another common defect encountered on visual field examination is concentric constriction. This may be due to papilledema, in which case it is usually accompanied by an enlargement of the blind spot. A concentric constriction of the visual field, at first unilateral and later bilateral, and pallor of the optic disks (optic atrophy) should suggest chronic syphilitic meningo-optic neuritis. Glaucoma is another cause of this type of field defect. Tubular vision, i.e., constriction of the visual field to the same degree regardless of the distance of the visual test stimulus from the eye, is a sign of hysteria. In organic disease, for example, chorioretinitis, the area of the constricted visual field naturally enlarges as the distance between the patient and the stimulus increases.

With most diseases of the optic nerve, the nerve will eventually become pale (optic atrophy). This may require several weeks or months to occur, as illustrated by the delay between the sudden blindness of a traumatic severance of one optic nerve and the pallor. If the optic nerve degenerates [e.g., in multiple sclerosis, Leber's hereditary optic atrophy (Chap. 373), or syphilitic optic atrophy], the disk becomes chalkwhite, with sharp, clean margins. If the atrophy is secondary to papillitis or papilledema, the margins are obscure and irregular, with pigment deposits in the adjacent retina.

Hemianopsia means blindness in one-half of the visual field. *Bitemporal hemianopsia* indicates a lesion of the decussating nasal retinal fibers of the optic chiasm and is due usually to tumor of the pituitary gland or of the infundibulum or third ventricle, to meningioma of the diaphragm of the sella, or occasionally to a large suprasellar aneurysm of the circle of Willis. *Homonymous hemianopsia* (a loss of vision in corresponding halves of the visual fields) signifies a lesion of the visual pathway behind the chiasm and, if *complete*, gives no more information than that. *Incomplete homonymous hemianopsia* has more localizing value: if the field defects in the two eyes are identical (*congruous*), the lesion is likely to be in the calcarine cortex; if *incongruous*, the visual fibers in the parietal or temporal lobe are more likely to be implicated. Since the fibers from the peripheral lower quadrants of the retina extend for a variable distance into the temporal lobe, lesions of this lobe may be accompanied by a homonymous upper quadrantic field defect. Parietal lobe lesions may affect the lower quadrants more than the upper.

If the entire optic tract or calcarine cortex on one side is destroyed, there is complete homonymous hemianopsia, including that part of the field supplied by the macula. Incomplete lesions of the optic tract and radiation usually spare central (macular) vision. Apparent macular sparing is frequently due to imperfect fixation of gaze. A lesion of the tip of one occipital lobe produces central homonymous hemianopsia because half the macular fibers of both eyes terminate there. Lesions of both occipital poles (as in embolization of the posterior cerebral arteries) result in bilateral central scotomas; if all the calcarine cortex on both sides is completely destroyed, there is "cortical" blindness. Altitudinal or horizontal hemianopsias are more often due to lesions of the occipital lobes below or above the calcarine sulcus than to lesions of the optic chiasm.

In addition to blindness, i.e., "visual anesthesia," there is another category of visual impairment, which consists of a defect of visual perception, i.e., *visual agnosia*. These patients can see but cannot recognize objects unless they hear, smell, taste, or palpate them. The failure of visual recognition of words alone is called *alexia*. The ability to recognize visually presented objects and words depends upon the integrity not only of the visual pathways and primary areas of the cerebral cortex but also of those secondary and tertiary visual cortical areas which lie just anterior to them and the angular gyrus of the dominant hemisphere. Visual-object agnosia and alexia result from lesions of these latter areas or from a lesion of the left calcarine cortex combined with one which interrupts the fibers crossing from the right occipital lobe. These subjects are discussed further in Chaps. 19 and 25.

Other disturbances of vision include various types of distortion in which the perceived objects appear too small (micropsia), too large (macropsia), or askew. If this disturbance is in only one eye, a local retinal lesion should be suspected. When bilateral, such phenomena suggest disease of the temporal lobes, in which case the visual disturbances tend to occur in attacks and are accompanied by complex visual hallucinations and other manifestations of temporal lobe seizures (Chap. 23).

The optic nerves also contain the afferent fibers for the pupillary reflexes. These fibers leave the optic tract and terminate in the pretectal region of the midbrain. A lesion of the optic nerve or tracts may abolish the pupillary light reflex; the pupil is dilated and unreactive. Cerebral lesions, on the other hand, leave the pupillary light reflex unaltered. The lack of direct reflex in the blind eye and of consensual reflex in the sound one means that the afferent limb of the reflex arc (optic nerve) is the site of the lesion. A lack of direct light reflex with retention of the consensual reflex places the lesion in the efferent limb of the reflex (the homolateral oculomotor nucleus or nerve). Loss of light reflex without visual impairment or ocular palsy (Argyll Robertson pupillary phenomenon) is thought to be due to a lesion in the superior colliculi or periaqueductal region (see "Alterations of Pupils," below).

Amaurosis refers to blindness from any cause. *Amblyopia* refers to an impairment or loss of vision which is not due to an error of refraction or to other disease of the eye. *Nyctalopia* means poor twilight or night vision and is associated with either vitamin A deficiency or pigmentary degenerations of the retina.

Papilledema (choked disk) refers to venous congestion and edema and elevation of disk margins. The depression of the optic disk is obliterated. The elevation ranges from 1 to 4 mm and when extreme may be surrounded by hemorrhages. Visual acuity is little affected until late, except for constriction of visual fields and enlargement of blind spots, which is in contrast to papillitis where visual loss occurs early. The cause is raised intracranial pressure (tumors, abscesses, hemorrhages) which is transmitted to the subarachnoid space around optic nerves. This leads, after some days, to obstruction of venous outflow from the retinas, usually more so on the side of the lesion (see Plates 7-3 and 8-6).

Minor degrees of disk swelling are difficult to distinguish from the disk of the normal hyperopic eye. Lack of vein pulsation suggests increased pressure. Fluorescein retinography reveals early papilledema by the leakage of the dye into the disk and surrounding retina. Myelination of optic nerve fibers and drusen must not be confused with papilledema.

In the analysis of retinal, optic nerve and tract, and geniculocalcarine lesions, two other techniques are especially valuable—the electroretinogram (ERG) and the patterned stimulus visual-evoked responses (VER) to light flash. The human ERG is a mass response that is reduced only in diseases of the retina.

The VER provides evidence of the speed of visual impulse conduction between the retina and occipital lobe. With diseases of the optic nerve, even with normal visual acuity and a normal appearance of the retina, it may be abnormal.

DIPLOPIA, STRABISMUS, AND DISORDERS OF THE THIRD, FOURTH, AND SIXTH NERVES *Strabismus* (squint) refers to a muscle imbalance that results in improper alignment of the two eyes. It may be due to paralysis of an eye muscle or the ocular deviation resulting from the unrestrained activity of the opposing muscle; or it may be due to inequality of tone in the muscles that yoke the two eyes together in a central position. The former is called *paralytic strabismus* and is primarily a neurologic problem; the latter is *nonparalytic strabismus* (referred to as comitant strabismus if the angle between the visual axes is the same in all fields of gaze) and is an ophthalmologic problem. Once binocular fusion is established, any type of ocular muscle imbalance causes diplopia, for the reason that images then fall on disparate or noncorresponding parts of the two retinas. After a time, however, the patient learns to suppress the image of one eye. This almost invariably happens early in comitant strabismus of congenital nature, and the person may then have a diminished visual acuity in that eye (*amblyopia ex anopsia*). The vision may remain normal in both eyes when the eyes are used alternately for fixation; this is *alternating strabismus*.

The oculomotor, trochlear, and abducens nerves innervate the extrinsic musculature of the eye. A knowledge of their origin and anatomic relationships is essential to an understanding of the various paralytic ocular syndromes. The oculomotor nucleus consists of several groups of nerve cells ventral to the aqueduct of Sylvius, at the level of the superior colliculi. All nuclear neurons send fibers to the ipsilateral eye except those innervating the superior rectus muscle, which are contralateral like those of the trochlear nucleus. The nerve cells that innervate the iris and ciliary body are situated dorsally in the so-called "Edinger-Westphal nucleus." Ventral to this nucleus are the cells for the levator of the lid, superior and inferior recti, inferior oblique, and medial rectus muscles, in this dorso-ventral order. Convergence is under the control of an unpaired medial group of cells. The cells of origin of the trochlear nerves are just inferior to those of the oculomotor nerves. The sixth nerve arises at a considerably lower level, from a paired group of cells in the floor of the fourth ventricle at the level of the lower pons. The intrapontine portion of the facial nerve loops around the sixth nerve nucleus before it turns anterolaterally to make its exit; a lesion in this locality usually causes a homolateral paralysis of both the lateral rectus and facial muscles.

All three nerves, after leaving the brainstem, course anteriorly and pass through the cavernous sinus, where they come into close proximity with the ophthalmic division of the fifth nerve, and together they enter the orbit through the superior orbital fissure. The oculomotor nerve supplies all the extrinsic ocular muscles except two—the superior oblique and the external rectus—which are innervated by the trochlear and the abducens nerves, respectively. The levator palpebrae muscle is also supplied by the oculomotor nerve, the involuntary part being under the control of autonomic fibers. Parasympathetic fibers of the oculomotor nerve supply the sphincter pupillae and the ciliary muscles (muscles of accommodation).

Although all the extraocular muscles probably participate in every movement of the eyes, particular muscles move the eyes in certain fields. The lateral rectus deviates the eye outward; the medial rectus, inward. The function of the vertical recti and the oblique muscles varies according to the position of the eye. When the eye is turned outward, the elevators and depressors of the eye are the superior and inferior recti; when the eye is turned inward, they are the inferior and superior oblique muscles, respectively. In contrast, torsion of the eyeball is effected by the oblique muscles when the eye is turned outward.

Accurate binocular vision is achieved by the associated action of the ocular muscles, which allows a visual stimulus to fall on exactly corresponding parts of the two retinas. Conjugate movement of the eyes is controlled by centers in the cerebral cortex and brainstem. Area 8 in the frontal lobe is the center for voluntary conjugate movements of the eyes to the opposite side. In addition, there is a center in the occipital lobe concerned with contralateral following movements. Fibers from these centers pass to the opposite sides of the brainstem, where they connect with lower centers for conjugate movements: those for right lateral gaze are thought to be in the proximity of the right abducens nucleus; those for left lateral gaze are near the left abducens. Simultaneous innervation of one internal rectus and the other external rectus during lateral gaze is mediated through the medial longitudinal fasciculus which connects one abducens nucleus with the opposite oculomotor nucleus. The arrangements of nerve cells and fibers for vertical gaze and convergence are situated in the pretectal areas and paramedian zones of the midbrain tegmentum.

The coordination of eye movement by those cerebral and brainstem structures involves the interaction of five physiologic systems: those for voluntary, saccadic, pursuit, vergence, and vestibular and fixation. The clinical importance of this subdivision relates to the fact that each system may be affected independently by disease (Bach-y-Rita and Collins).

OCULAR MUSCLE AND GAZE PALSIES   There are three types of paralysis of extraocular muscles: (1) paralysis of isolated ocular muscles, (2) paralysis of conjugate movements (gaze), and (3) syndromes of mixed gaze and ocular muscle paralysis.

Characteristic clinical disturbances result from single lesions of the third, fourth, or sixth cranial nerves. A complete third nerve lesion causes ptosis (since the levator palpebrae is supplied mainly by the third nerve), an inability to turn the eye upward, downward, or inward; a divergent strabismus due to unopposed action of the lateral rectus muscle; a dilated nonreactive pupil (iridoplegia); and paralysis of accommodation (cycloplegia). When only the muscles of the iris and ciliary body are paralyzed, the condition is termed *internal ophthalmoplegia*. Fourth nerve lesions result in an extorsion of the eye and a weakness of downward gaze most marked when the eye is

turned inward, so that patients commonly complain of special difficulty in going downstairs. Head tilting, to the opposite shoulder, is especially characteristic of a fourth nerve lesion. Such patients may also have difficulty in reading with their bifocal glasses. When the difficulty is bilateral, there is often a V-pattern isotropia that is most marked on looking down and minimal on looking up. The patient compensates for this by keeping the chin down to minimize the diplopia. This maneuver puts the eye in a position where the superior oblique is relaxed, thereby facilitating binocular vision. Lesions of the sixth nerve result in paralysis of abduction and a convergent strabismus, owing to the unopposed action of the internal rectus muscles. With incomplete sixth nerve palsies, turning the head toward the side of the paretic muscle may overcome diplopia by relaxing the affected lateral rectus muscle. (The foregoing signs may occur with various degrees of completeness, depending on the severity and site of the lesion or lesions.)

Ocular palsies may be central, i.e., due to a lesion of the nucleus or the intramedullary portion of the cranial nerve, or peripheral. Opthalmoplegia due to a lesion in the brainstem is usually accompanied by involvement of other cranial nerves or long tracts. Peripheral lesions, which may or may not be solitary, have a great variety of causes; the most common are *aneurysm of the circle of Willis,* tumors of the base of the brain, carcinomatosis of the meninges, herpes zoster, *syphilitic* and other chronic forms of *meningitis*. A practical rule is that any nontraumatic oculomotor palsy with a dilated, unreactive pupil will usually be traced to a tumor or aneurysm. The third nerve palsy that occurs with diabetes is most often due to infarction of the third nerve, and the prognosis for recovery in such cases, as with other nonprogressive diseases of the peripheral nerve, is usually excellent. The points of difference between lesions within and outside the brainstem are tabulated in Table 18-1, and the various intramedullary and extramedullary cranial nerve syndromes are described in Tables 376-1 and 376-2. See also the diagrams in Chap. 365.

Paralysis of conjugate movement (gaze)   The term *conjugate gaze,* or *conjugate movement,* refers to the simultaneous movement of the two eyes in the same direction. An acute lesion, such as an infarct, in one frontal lobe may cause paralysis of contralateral gaze, and the eyes will turn toward the side of the lesion. The ocular disorder in this circumstance is temporary (several days' duration). In bilateral frontal lesions the patient may be unable to turn the eyes voluntarily in any direction—up, down, or to the side—but retains fixation and following movements, which are believed to be occipital lobe functions. Gaze paralysis of cerebral origin is not attended by strabismus or diplopia. The usual causes are vascular occlusion with infarction, hemorrhage, and abscess or tumor of the frontal lobe. With certain extrapyramidal disorders, e.g., postencephalitic parkinsonism, Huntington's chorea, and progressive supranuclear palsy, ocular movements may be limited in all directions, especially upward. Lesions of the superior colliculi and tegmentum, near the posterior commissure, interfere with voluntary upward gaze, and often movements of convergence as well as the pupillary light reflex are abolished (Parinaud's syndrome). There also exists a pontine center for conjugate lateral gaze, probably in the vicinity of the abducens nucleus. A lesion here causes ipsilateral gaze palsy, with the eyes turning to the opposite side. Vertical and lateral gaze palsies are combined in Steele-Richardson disease. The palsy is persistent, unlike that of cerebral lesions, and is frequently accompanied by other signs of midbrain disease. Fully developed forms of gaze paralysis are readily discerned, but lesser degrees may be overlooked unless one pays special attention to the predominant position of the eyes at rest and the ability to sustain conjugate movement.

Ocular apraxia is another special gaze disorder. Normally,

TABLE 18-1
Comparison of lesions within and outside the brainstem

Effect	Lesions within the brainstem	Lesions external to the brainstem
Involvement of multiple contiguous nerves	±	+
Involvement of sensorimotor tracts	+, often "alternating" or crossed sensory motor palsies	±
Disturbance of consciousness	+	0 (+ late)
Evidence of other segmental disturbances of the brainstem such as decerebrate rigidity, tonic neck reflexes, pseudobulbar palsy	+	0 (+ late)
X-ray evidence of erosion of cranial bones or enlargement of foramens	0	+

on looking to the side, the eyes and head turn together, but in this condition the head turns and the eyes actually go in the opposite direction. The head is flung too far, in order not to lose sight of the target, and then the eyes "catch up." This may be a solitary congenital abnormality (Cogan), the anatomy of which is unknown, or it may be acquired as in ataxia telangiectasia (see Chap. 374).

In skew deviation, a poorly understood disorder of gaze, the eyes diverge, one looking down, the other up. The deviation is constant in all fields of gaze. It may occur with any lesion of the posterior fossa but particularly with one in the brainstem. The lesion is on the side of the lower eye.

Mixed gaze and ocular paralyses These are always a sign of intrapontine or mesencephalic disease. A lesion of the lower pons in or near the sixth nerve nucleus causes a homolateral paralysis of the lateral rectus muscle and a failure of adduction of the opposite eye, i.e., a combined paralysis of the sixth nerve and of conjugate lateral gaze. Lesions of the medial longitudinal fasciculi interfere with lateral conjugate gaze in another way. When the patient looks to the right, the left eye fails to adduct; when looking to the left, the right eye fails to adduct. The abducting eye may show nystagmus. This condition is referred to as *internuclear ophthalmoplegia* and should always be suspected when only adduction of the eyes is affected. It may be unilateral or bilateral. If unilateral, the lesion is always on the side of the weak adducting eye. If the lesion is in higher (midbrain) part of the medial longitudinal fasciculus, convergence may be lost, occurring with paralysis of the medial recti on attempted lateral gaze (anterior internuclear ophthalmoplegia); if the lesion is in the lower (pontine) part, convergence is normal, but there may be some degree of associated limitation of conjugate lateral gaze or sixth nerve palsy (posterior internuclear opthalmoplegia).

NYSTAGMUS AND OTHER INVOLUNTARY EYE MOVEMENTS
Nystagmus refers to involuntary rhythmic movements of the eyes. It is usually subdivided into two types, oscillating (pendular) and rhythmic (jerk). Although practical, this classification is an oversimplification. In jerk nystagmus, the movements are distinctly faster in one direction than the other; in pendular nystagmus, the oscillations are roughly equal in rate for the two directions, although on conjugate lateral gaze the pendular type may resemble the jerk type, with the fast component to the side of the gaze.

In testing for nystagmus, the eyes should first be examined in the central position and then during upward, downward, and lateral movements. If nystagmus is monocular, each eye should be tested separately, with the other one covered. Labyrinthine nystagmus is most obvious when visual fixation is prevented by shielding the eyes; and brainstem nystagmus and cerebellar nystagmus are brought out best by having the patient fixate on a finger. Labyrinthine nystagmus may vary with the position of the head; hence, these various tests should be performed with the head in several different positions. In particular, the postural nystagmus of Bárány is evoked by hyperextension of the neck, with the patient supine. A series of moving visual stimuli also evoke nystagmus. This optokinetic nystagmus should be tested by asking the patient to look at a rotating cylinder on which several stripes have been painted or at a striped cloth moved across the field of vision.

A few irregular jerks are observed in many normal individuals when the eyes are turned far to the side. These so-called "nystagmoid movements" are probably similar to the tremulousness of a muscle that is contracted maximally. Occasionally a fine rhythmic nystagmus may be found in extreme lateral gaze, but if it is bilateral and disappears as the eyes move a few degrees toward the midline, it usually has no clinical significance.

Pendular nystagmus is found in a variety of conditions in which central vision is lost early in life, such as albinism and in various other diseases of the retina and refractive media. Occasionally it is observed in patients with multiple sclerosis and as a congenital abnormality, even without poor vision. The syndrome of miners' nystagmus, formerly a common cause of industrial disability, occurs after many years of work in comparative darkness. The oscillations of the eyes are very rapid, increase on upward gaze, and are often associated with vertigo, head tremor, and intolerance of light.

Jerk nystagmus is the commoner type. It may be lateral or vertical, particularly on ocular movement in these planes, or it may be rotary. By custom, the direction of the nystagmus is named according to the direction of the fast component. There are several varieties of jerk nystagmus. When one is watching a moving object—e.g., the passing landscape from a train window or a rotating drum with vertical stripes— rhythmic jerk nystagmus, *optokinetic nystagmus,* normally appears. The slow phase is a result of visual fixation; the quick phase is compensatory. With unilateral cerebral lesions, particularly in the parietooccipital region, optokinetic nystagmus is lost when the moving stimulus, e.g., the drum, moves toward the side of the lesion.

Aside from optokinetic nystagmus, lateral and vertical nystagmus are most frequently due to barbiturate intoxication. Jerk nystagmus may signify disease of the labyrinthine-vestibular apparatus. Labyrinthine stimulation or irritation by cold water in the external auditory meatus produces a nystagmus with the fast phase to the opposite side. The slow component reflects the effect of impulses derived from the semicircular canals, and the fast component is a corrective movement. Vestibular-labyrinthine nystagmus may be horizontal, vertical, or, most characteristically, rotary. Vertigo, nausea, vomiting, and staggering are the usual accompaniments (Chap. 14). Brainstem lesions often cause a coarse unidirectional nystagmus, which may be horizontal or vertical; the latter is brought out usually on upward gaze and rarely on downward gaze. The presence of vertical nystagmus is pathognomic of disease in the tegmentum of the brainstem and possibly of cerebellar connections. Vertigo is inconstant, and signs of disease of other nuclear structures and tracts in the brainstem are frequent. Upward jerk nystagmus of this type is frequent in demyelinative or vascular disease, in tumors, and in Wernicke's disease and syringobulbia. Vertical downward nystagmus is most often associated with lesions at the cervicomedullary junction, such as meningeal cysts, meningiomas, and the Arnold-Chiari malformation. Cerebellopontine angle tumors cause a coarse bilateral horizontal nystagmus, coarser to the side of the lesion. We have also observed nystagmus with a single lesion of the inferior cerebellar hemisphere. Periodic alternating nystagmus (horizontal nystagmus on straight-ahead gaze in one direction for 1 or 2 min and then reversing direction) has been observed with lesions of the fastigial nuclei and flocculonodular lobe of the cerebellum. The nystagmus that occurs only in the abducting eye and is said to be a pathognomonic sign of multiple sclerosis probably represents an incompletely developed form of internuclear opthalmoplegia.

Convergence nystagmus is a rhythmic oscillation in which a quick movement of adduction is followed by a slow abduction of the eyes in respect to each other. It is usually accompanied by other types of nystagmus and by one or more features of Parinaud's syndrome. Occasionally there is also a rhythmic retraction movement of the eyes (*nystagmus retractorius*) or eyelids, or a maintained spasm of convergence, best brought out on attemped elevation of the eyes to command. These unusual phenomena all point to a lesion of the upper midbrain tegmentum and are usually manifestations of vascular disease or of pinealoma. *Seesaw nystagmus*—one eye moving up, the other down—is occasionally observed in conjunction with bitemporal hemianopia. Its mechanism is unknown. In children it occurs with gliomas of the optic chiasm; in adolescents and adults it is most frequent with craniopharyngiomas and pituitary adenomas.

Oscillopsia refers to illusory movement of the environment, in which objects seem to move back and forth, to jerk, or to wiggle. It may or may not occur with turning of the eyes and consequent displacement of the image on the retina. Such movement of all objects in the environment appears with coarse central nystagmus or opsoclonus. Movement or distortion of position of single visualized objects may be part of a metamorphopsia from cerebral lesions.

Opsoclonus is the term applied to either sustained, irregular, conjugate "dancing" movements of the eyes in a horizontal, rotary, and vertical direction or a fast-frequency flutter. The neurologic basis for these movements is not clear, but in most cases they are associated with signs of cerebellar disease, a viral infection, or occult neuroblastoma. In some viral infections causing stupor or coma, the eye movements are constant and chaotic. Slow downward movement of both eyes with a fast upward movement (called "ocular bobbing" by Fisher) is characteristic of pontine lesions such as hypertensive hemorrhage.

Ocular dysmetria consists of an overshoot of the eyes on attempted fixation, followed by several cycles of oscillations of diminishing amplitude until precise fixation is attained. The overshoot may occur on eccentric fixation or on refixation in the primary position of gaze. This sign occurs in disease of the cerebellum or its pathways and is analogous to cerebellar dysmetria of the limbs.

ALTERATIONS OF PUPILS Pupil size is determined by the balance of innervation between the dilator and constrictor fibers. The pupillodilator fibers arise in the posterior part of the hypothalamus and descend in the lateral tegmentum of the midbrain, pons, medulla, and cervical spinal cord to the eighth cervical and first thoracic segments, where they synapse with the lateral horn cells. These give rise to preganglionic fibers that synapse in the superior cervical ganglion; the postganglionic fibers course along the internal carotid artery and traverse the cavernous sinus to join the first division of the trigeminal nerve, finally reaching the eyes as the long ciliary nerves. The pupilloconstrictor fibers arise in the nucleus of Edinger-Westphal, join the oculomotor nerve, and synapse in the ciliary ganglion with the postganglionic neurons that innervate the iris and ciliary body.

The pupils are usually equal in size, though if the eyes are turned to one side, the pupil of the abducting eye dilates slightly. Pupil size varies with light intensity; as one pupil constricts under a bright light (direct reflex), the other unexposed pupil does likewise (consensual reflex). Pupillary constriction is also part of the act of convergence and accommodation for near objects.

Interruption of the sympathetic fibers either centrally, between the hypothalamus and their point of exit from the spinal cord (first thoracic segment), or peripherally (superior or cervical ganglion in the neck or along the carotid artery) results in miosis and ptosis (because of paralysis of Müller's muscle), with loss of sweating of the face, and occasionally enophthalmos (Bernard-Horner syndrome). Stimulation or irritation of the pupillodilator fibers has the opposite effect, i.e., lid retraction, slight proptosis, and dilatation of the pupil. The ciliospinal pupillary reflex, evoked by pinching the neck, is effected

through these efferent sympathetic fibers. Abnormal dilatation of the pupils (mydriasis), often with loss of pupillary light reflexes, may result from midbrain lesions and is a frequent finding in cases of deep coma. Extreme constriction of the pupils (miosis) is commonly observed with pontine lesions, presumably because of bilateral interruption of the pupillodilator fibers.

The functional integrity of the sympathetic and parasympathetic nerve endings in the iris may be determined by the use of certain drugs. Atropine and homatropine dilate the pupils by paralyzing the parasympathetic nerve endings; physostigmine and pilocarpine constrict them, the former by inhibiting cholinesterase activity at the neuromuscular junction, and the latter by direct stimulation of the sphincter muscle of the iris. Cocaine dilates the pupils by preventing the reuptake of norepinephrine into the nerve endings. Morphine acts centrally to constrict the pupils.

In chronic syphilitic meningitis and other forms of late syphilis, particularly tabes dorsalis, the pupils are usually small, irregular, and unequal; they do not dilate properly in response to mydriatic drugs and fail to react to light, although they do constrict on accommodation. In some cases there is an associated atrophy of the iris. This is known as the *Argyll Robertson pupil*. The exact locality of the lesion is not certain; it is generally believed to be in the tectum of the midbrain proximal to the oculomotor nuclei, where the descending pupillodilator fibers are in close proximity to the light-reflex fibers. A dissociation of the light reflex from the accommodation-convergence reaction is sometimes observed with other midbrain lesions, e.g., pinealoma, multiple sclerosis, and diabetes mellitus; in these diseases miosis, irregularity of pupils, and failure to respond to a mydriatic are not constantly present. However, in the usual Argyll Robertson pupillary abnormality of tabes and of diabetic and amyloid polyneuropathy the lesion is probably peripheral, in the oculomotor nerve or ciliary ganglion. Another interesting pupillary abnormality is the myotonic reaction, sometimes referred to as *Adie's pupil*. The patient may complain of blurring of vision or may have suddenly noticed that one pupil is larger than the other. The reaction to light and convergence are absent if tested in the customary manner, although the size of the pupil will change slowly on prolonged stimulation. Once contracted or dilated, the pupils remain in that state for some minutes. The affected pupil reacts promptly to the usual mydriatic and miotic drugs but is usually sensitive to a $1/16\%$ solution of pilocarpine or a 2.5% solution of methacholine (Mecholyl), a strength that will not affect a normal pupil. The myotonic pupil usually appears during the third or fourth decade of life; it may be associated with absence of knee or ankle jerks and hence be mistaken for tabes dorsalis.

Ocular movement, pupillary contraction, and visual acuity may be affected by diseases which alter the contents of the orbit. Usually this is accompanied by bilateral exophthalmos, as in thyroid or pituitary disease (Chap. 334). Unilateral exophthalmos may occur with orbital tumors (dermoids, adenoma of lacrimal gland, optic nerve glioma, neurofibroma, metastatic carcinoma, meningioma) or granuloma, or cavernous sinus thrombosis (Chap. 368). Sometimes thyroid disease will have an asymmetric effect with more exophthalmos and/or limitation of motion on one side than the other. Progressive paralysis of the eyelids, which may obstruct vision, occurs separately or as part of an external paralysis, as in ocular dystrophy or in oculopharyngeal dystrophy.

DISTURBANCES OF HEARING

Tinnitus and *deafness* are frequent symptoms and always indicate disease of the ear or of the auditory nerve and its central connections.

Tinnitus, or ringing in the ears, is a purely subjective phenomenon and may also be reported as a buzzing, whistling, hissing, or roaring sound. It is a very common symptom in adults. Low-frequency vibratory clicks, pops, roarings, etc., are invariably due to diseases of the middle ear and eustachian tube. High-pitched tonal, nonvibratory tinnitus means disease of the cochlea and eighth nerve. Severe and prolonged tinnitus in the presence of normal hearing is very rare. If tinnitus is localized to one ear and is described as having a low-pitched tonal character, such as ringing or a bell-like tone, and particularly if there is reduced hearing with the recruitment phenomenon (see below), it is probably cochlear in origin. Clicking sounds are caused by intermittent contraction of the tensor tympani. A pulsating tinnitus synchronous with the pulse may be related to an intracranial vascular malformation; however, this symptom must be carefully judged, since introspective persons often report hearing their pulse when lying with one ear on a pillow. Certain drugs such as salicylates and quinine produce tinnitus and transient deafness. Nervous persons are less tolerant of tinnitus than more stable ones; depressed or anxious patients may demand relief from tinnitus that has existed for years.

Examination of hearing should always begin with inspection of the external auditory canal and the tympanic membrane. A ticking watch or whispered words are suitable means of testing hearing at the bedside, the opposite ear being closed by the finger. If there is any suspicion of deafness or a complaint of tinnitus or vertigo, or if the patient is a child with a speech defect, then hearing must be tested further. This can be done with the use of tuning forks of different frequencies, but the most accurate results are obtained by the use of an electric audiometer and the construction of an audiogram which reveals the entire range of hearing at a glance.

Deafness is frequent. In the United States it is estimated that there are more than 6 million persons with hearing loss; in one-third to one-half of these persons the loss is hereditary. Deafness is of two types: (1) nerve deafness (also called perceptive or sensorineural), due to disease of the cochlea or of the cochlear division of the eighth cranial nerve, and (2) conductive deafness, due to disease of the middle ear, such as otosclerosis or chronic otitis, or to occlusion of the external auditory canal or eustachian tube. In differentiating these two types, the tuning fork tests are of value. When a tuning fork vibrating at 256 Hz is held about one inch from the ear (the test for air conduction), sound waves can be appreciated only as they are transmitted through the middle ear and are reduced with disease in this location. When the fork is applied to the skull (test for bone conduction), the sound waves are conveyed directly to the cochlea, without the intervention of the middle ear apparatus, and are therefore not reduced or lost. Normally air conduction is better than bone conduction. These principles form the basis for several tests of auditory function.

In *Weber's test,* the vibrating fork is applied to the forehead in the midline. In middle ear deafness the sound is localized in the affected ear; in nerve deafness, in the normal ear. In *Rinné's test,* the vibrating fork is applied to the mastoid process, the other ear being closed by the observer's finger. At the moment the sound ceases, the fork is held at the auditory meatus. In middle ear deafness the sound cannot be heard by air conduction after bone conduction has ceased (abnormal or negative Rinné's test). In nerve deafness the reverse is true (normal or positive Rinné's test), although both air and bone conduction may be quantitatively decreased. In *Schwabach's test,* the patient's bone conduction is compared with that of a normal observer. In general, high-pitched tones are lost in nerve deafness and low-pitched ones in middle ear deafness, but there are frequent exceptions to this rule.

The following audiologic tests, taken together, help distinguish between cochlear and retrocochlear (nerve) lesions:

1 *Auditory recruitment:* the difference in hearing between the two ears is estimated, and the loudness of the stimulus delivered to each ear is then increased by regular increments. In nonrecruiting deafness (characteristic of nerve trunk lesion) the original difference in hearing persists in all comparisons of loudness above threshold. In recruiting deafness (as occurs in Ménière's disease) the more defective ear gains in loudness and finally is equal to the better one.

2 *Speech discrimination:* retrocochlear lesions are indicated by a failure to recognize more than 30 percent of phonetically balanced monosyllabic words (e.g., *thin and sin*) at suprathreshold levels.

3 *Short-increment sensitivity index* (SISI), in which the patient responds to a series of twenty 1-decibel (dB) increments in amplitude superimposed on a steady tone of the same frequency presented at a sensation level of 20 dB. The patient's score is the percentage of these 20-dB increments which he or she is able to detect at a given frequency. Low SISI scores, below 60 percent, point to an end-organ lesion.

4 *Threshold sensitivity* recorded via *Békésy audiometry* for both continuous and interrupted tonal stimuli. Four types of tracing may be obtained; the type II tracing is obtained in patients with end-organ lesions, and type III or IV, usually the former, characterizes retrocochlear lesions.

5 *Threshold tone decay:* this test quantifies auditory adaptation and requires only a conventional pure tone audiometer. Retrocochlear lesions yield greater amounts of decay than cochlear ones.

The common causes of middle ear deafness are otitis media, otosclerosis, and rupture of the eardrum. Nerve deafness has many causes. The internal ear may be aplastic from birth (hereditary deaf-mutism), or it may be damaged by rubella in the pregnant mother. Acute purulent meningitis or chronic infection spreading from the middle ear may cause nerve deafness in childhood. The auditory nerve may be involved by tumors of the cerebellopontine angle or by syphilis. Deafness may also result from a demyelinative plaque in the brainstem. A large series of genetically determined syndromes which feature a neural type of deafness, some congenital, others progressive, has come to light (see article by Konigsmark). The most interesting of these are dominant progressive nerve deafness, dominant unilateral deafness, dominant low-frequency hearing loss, recessive congenital deafness, sex-linked congenital neural deafness, several types of deafness (neural and conductive) with malformations of external ears, face, and neck (Treacher-Collins disease and Engelmann's diaphyscal dysplasia); hereditary deafness with goiter (Pendred's disease); hereditary heart disease with deafness; hereditary deafness with various combinations of mental retardation, retinitis pigmentosa, and polyneuropathy (as in Hallgren's disease, Alstrom's disease, Refsum's disease); hereditatry deafness with skin abnormalities such as albinism, lentigines, piebaldness, white forelock (Waardenburg's disease), onchydystrophy and pegged teeth, atopic dermatitis, and anhydrosis.

Of the types of progressive conduction deafness, hereditary otosclerosis is the most frequent (cause of 50 percent of deafness in adulthood). Hysterical deafness may be difficult to distinguish from organic disease. In the case of bilateral deafness, the distinction can be made by observing a blink (cochleoorbicular reflex) or an alteration in skin sweating (psychogalvanic skin reflex) in response to a loud sound. Unilateral hysterical deafness may be detected by an audiometer, with both ears connected, or by whispering into the bell of a stethoscope attached to the patient's ears, closing first one tube and then the other without the patient's knowledge.

In otosclerosis and hereditary sensorineural deafness, vestibular function is usually retained (caloric responses are normal).

REFERENCES

ASHWORTH B: Neuro-ophthalmology, in *Recent Advances in Clinical Neurology,* WB Mathews (ed). Edinburgh, Churchill-Livingstone, 1975

BACH-Y-RITA P, COLLINS CC: *The Control of Eye Movements.* New York, Academic, 1971

BENDER MB: Neurophthalmology, in *Clinical Neurology,* AB Baker (ed). New York, Hoeber-Harper, 1962, vol 1, chap 4

COGAN DG: *Neurology of the Ocular Muscles,* 2d ed. Springfield, Ill, Charles C Thomas, 1956

GLASER JM: *Neuro-ophthalmology.* New York, Harper & Row, 1978

KONIGSMARK BW: Medical progress. Hereditary deafness in man. N Engl J Med 281:713, 774, 827, 1969

TILLMAN TW: Special hearing tests in otoneurologic diagnosis. Arch Otolaryngol 89:25 1969

19
DISORDERS OF SENSATION

MAURICE VICTOR
RAYMOND D. ADAMS

Loss or perversion of somatic sensation not infrequently is the principal manifestation of disease of the nervous system. The reason for this is clear enough, since the major anatomic pathways of the sensory system are distinct from those of the motor system and may be selectively disturbed by disease. An understanding of these sensory disorders may provide important leads to neurologic diagnosis.

GENERAL CONSIDERATIONS Unfortunately, space does not permit here a more detailed review of the anatomy of the sensory system or of its physiology. The interested reader may turn to the references at the end of the chapter. The cutaneous distribution of sensory spinal roots may be observed in Fig. 19-1 (see also Chap. 3).

Disorders of the somatic sensory apparatus pose special problems for these patients. They are confronted with derangements of sensation which may be unlike anything they have previously experienced, and they have few words in their vocabulary to describe what they feel. They may say that a limb feels "numb" and "dead" when in fact they mean it is weak. Observant individuals may occasionally discover a loss of sensation, for example, inability to feel discomfort on touching an object hot enough to blister the skin or unawareness of articles of clothing and other objects in contact with the skin. But more often disease has induced a new and unnatural series of sensory experiences. If nerves, spinal roots, or spinal tracts are only partially interrupted, a touch may arouse tingling or pricking, meaning presumably that at least some of the remaining touch and pain fibers are functional but are acting abnormally. Tightness and drawing and pulling sensations, a feeling of a band or girdle around the limb or trunk, are common with partial involvement of pressure fibers. Similarly, burning and pain (causalgia) may represent overactivity of surviving thermal and pain fibers. The responsible lesion may be in the peripheral nerve, the lateral spinothalamic tract in the spinal cord or brainstem, or the thalamus. Also, hyperesthesia and hyperpathia are frequent. These abnormal sensations are called *paresthesias,* or *dysesthesias,* if they are unpleasant; and their character and distribution inform us of the anatomy of the lesion involving the sensory system.

EXAMINATION OF SENSATION The examination of sensation is the most difficult part of the neurologic examination. For one thing, test procedures are relatively crude and inadequate. And, embarrassingly often, no objective sensory loss can be demonstrated despite symptoms that clearly indicate the presence of such a deficit. Also, a response to a sensory stimulus is difficult to evaluate objectively, since the examiner's conclusions depend on the patient's interpretations of sensory experiences. This presupposes a general responsiveness, alertness, and a desire to cooperate, as well as intelligence and a certain level of education. Hypersuggestibility and fatigue may interfere with the obtaining of accurate test data.

The detail in which sensation is tested will be determined by the clinical situation. If the patient has no sensory complaints, it is sufficient to examine vibration and position sense in the fingers and toes, to test the appreciation of pain over the face, trunk, and extremities, and to determine whether the sensory findings are the same in symmetric parts of the body. A rough survey of this sort may detect sensory defects of which the patient is unaware. On the other hand, more thorough testing is in order if the patient has complaints referable to the sensory system or if there is localized atrophy or weakness, ataxia, trophic changes of joints, or painless ulcers.

A few other general principles should be mentioned. One should not press the sensory examination in the presence of fatigue, for an inattentive patient is a poor witness. The exam-

FIGURE 19-1

Distribution of the sensory spinal roots on the surface of the body. (From G Holmes, Introduction to Clinical Neurology, 2d ed, Baltimore, Williams & Wilkins, 1952.)

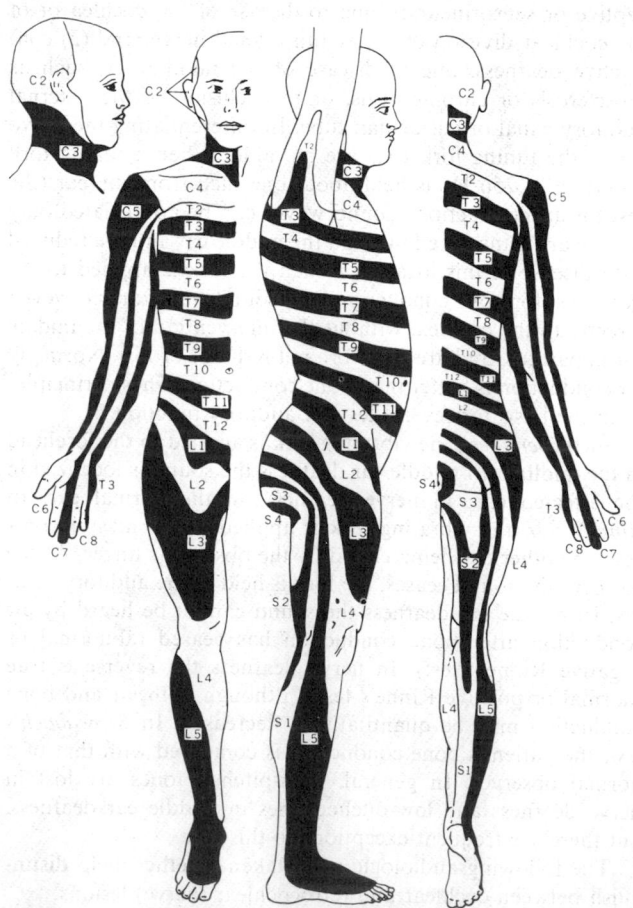

iner must also avoid suggesting symptoms to the patient. After having explained in the simplest terms what is required, as few questions and remarks should be interposed as possible. Consequently, patients must not be asked, "Do you feel that?" each time they are touched; they should simply be told to say "yes" or "sharp" every time they have been touched or feel pain. The patient should not be permitted to see the part under examination. For short tests it is sufficient to close the eyes; during more detailed testing it is preferable to screen the eyes from the part being examined. Quantitative methods are available, utilizing graded sensory stimuli (Dyck et al.). Finally, the findings of the sensory examination should be accurately recorded on a chart.

Sensation is frequently classified as *superficial* (cutaneous, exteroceptive) and *deep* (proprioceptive); the former comprises the modalities of light touch, pain, and temperature; the latter includes the sense of position, passive motion, vibration, and deep pain.

Sense of touch This is usually tested with a wisp of cotton. The patient is first made acquainted with the nature of the stimulus by applying it to a normal part of the body and is then asked to say "yes" each time various other parts are touched. A patient simulating sensory loss may say "no" in response to a tactile stimulus. Cornified areas of skin, such as the soles and palms, will require a heavier stimulus than normal, and the hair-clad parts a lighter one because of the numerous nerve endings around the hair follicles. The patient is more sensitive to a moving contactual stimulus of any kind than a stationary one. The gentle movement of the examiner's or preferably the patient's finger tip over the skin is a useful method of mapping out an area of tactile loss.

Sense of pain This is most efficiently estimated by pinprick, although it may be evoked by a great diversity of noxious stimuli. The patient must understand that he or she is to report the degree of sharpness of the pin, not simply the feeling of contact or pressure of the point or even a special sensation due to penetration of the skin. If the pinpricks are applied rapidly, their effects may be summated and excessive pain may result; therefore, they should be delivered not too rapidly, about one per second, and not over the same spot.

If an area of diminished or absent touch or pain sensation is encountered, its boundaries should be demarcated to determine whether it has a segmental or peripheral nerve distribution or whether sensation is lost below a certain level. Such areas are best delineated by proceeding from the region of impaired sensation toward the normal, and the changes may be confirmed by dragging a pin lightly over the skin.

Deep pressure sense One can estimate this sense simply by pinching gently or pressing deeply on the tendons and muscles. Pain can often be elicited by heavy pressure even when superficial sensation is diminished; conversely, in some diseases, such as tabetic neurosyphilis, the loss of deep pressure sense may be more prominent.

Thermal sense The following procedure for testing thermal sensation is suggested. The areas of skin to be tested should be exposed for some time before the examination. The test objects should be large, preferably Erlenmeyer flasks containing hot and cold water. Thermometers which extend into the water through the flask stoppers indicate the temperature of the water at the moment of testing. At first, extreme degrees of heat and cold (e.g., 10 and 45°C) may be employed to delineate roughly an area of thermal sensory disturbance; the patient will report that the flask feels "less hot" or "less cold" over such an area than over a normal part. If areas of impaired sensation are found, the borders may be accurately determined

by moving the flask along the skin from the insensitive to the normal region. The qualitative change should then be quantitated as far as possible by estimating the *differences in temperature* which the patient is able to recognize. The patient is asked to report whether one stimulus is *warmer or colder* than another not whether a given stimulus is warm or cold, since the cooler of the two may be interpreted as warm. The range of temperature difference between the two flasks is gradually narrowed by mixing their contents. A normal person is capable of detecting a difference of 1°C when the temperature of the flasks is in the range of 28 to 32°C. In the warm range one should readily recognize differences between 35 and 40°C, and in the cold range, between 10 and 20°C. In many normal older persons and in others with poor peripheral circulation (especially in cold weather), the responses may be modified.

The sensation of heat or cold depends not only on the temperature of the stimulus but also on the duration of the stimulus and the area over which it is applied. This principle may be employed to detect slight degrees of sensory impairment; the patient may be able to distinguish small differences in temperature when the bottom of the flask is applied for 3 s but unable to do so if only the side of the flask is applied for 1 s. Throughout the test procedure, especially when small temperature differences are involved, the area of sensory disturbance should be continually checked against perception in normal parts.

Postural sense and the appreciation of passive movement These modalities are usually lost together, although in any particular case one may be disproportionately affected.

Abnormalities of postural sensation may be revealed in several ways. When the patient extends the arms forward and closes the eyes, the affected arm will wander from its original position; if the fingers are spread apart, they may undergo a series of slow-changing postures ("piano-playing" movements, or *pseudoathetosis*). In attempting to touch the tip of the nose with the index finger, the patient may miss the target repeatedly.

The lack of position sense in the legs may be demonstrated by displacing the limb from its original position and asking the patient to point to the large toe. If postural sensation is defective in both legs, the patient will be unable to maintain balance with feet together and eyes closed (Romberg's sign). This sign should be interpreted with caution. Even a normal person in the Romberg position will sway slightly more with the eyes closed than open. A patient with lack of balance due to motor disorders or cerebellar disease will also sway more if visual cues are removed. Only if there is a marked discrepancy between the state of balance with eyes open and closed can one confidently state that the patient shows Romberg's sign, i.e., loss of joint-position sense. Mild degrees of unsteadiness in nervous or suggestible patients may be overcome by diverting their attention, e.g., by having them alternately touch the index finger of each hand to their nose while standing with their eyes closed.

The appreciation of passive movement is first tested in the fingers and toes, and the defect, when present, is reflected maximally in these parts. It is important to grasp the digit firmly at the sides opposite the plane of movement; otherwise the pressure applied by the examiner in displacing the digit may allow the patient to identify the direction of movement. This applies to the testing of the more proximal segments of the limb as well. The patient should be instructed to report each movement as "up" or "down" in relation to the previous stationary position. It is useful to demonstrate the test with a large and easily identified movement, but once the idea is clear to the patient, the smallest detectable changes in position should be tested. The range of movement normally appreciated in the digits is said to be as little as 1°. Clinically, however, defective appreciation of passive movement is judged by comparison with a normal limb or, if bilaterally defective, on the basis of what the examiner has through experience learned to regard as normal. Slight impairment may be disclosed by a slow response or, if the digit is displaced very slowly, by a relative unawareness that movements have occurred; or after the digit has been displaced in the same direction several times, the patient may misjudge the first movement in the opposite direction; or after the examiner has moved the toe, the patient may make a number of small voluntary movements of the toe, in an apparent attempt to determine its position or the direction of the movement.

The sense of vibration This is a composite sensation comprising touch and rapid alterations of deep pressure sense, the end organ of which is the pacinian corpuscle. Its conduction depends on both cutaneous and deep afferent fibers which ascend in the dorsal columns of the cord. It is therefore rarely affected by lesions of single nerves but will be disturbed in cases of polyneuritis and disease of the dorsal columns, medial lemniscus, and thalamus. For this reason, vibration and position sense are usually lost together, although one of them (usually vibration sense) may be affected disproportionately. With advancing age, vibration sense may be diminished at the toes and ankles.

Vibration sense is tested by placing a tuning fork with a low rate (and long duration) of vibration (128 Hz) over the bony prominences. The examiner must make sure that the patient responds to the vibration, not simply to the pressure of the fork. Although there are mechanical devices to quantitate vibration sense, it is sufficient for clinical purposes to compare the point tested with a normal part of the patient or the examiner. Thus, if the fork is allowed to run down until vibration is no longer appreciated but is still felt at an analogous point on the opposite limb, and if this finding is consistent, one can be certain of a significant impairment of vibration sense. In a similar way, the appreciation of vibration at the tibial tuberosity after it has disappeared in the ankle, or at the iliac portion of the spine after it has disappeared at the tibial tuberosity, is an indication of a peripheral nerve lesion. The level of vibration-sense loss due to spinal cord lesions may be estimated by placing the fork over successive vertebral spines.

DISCRIMINATIVE SENSORY FUNCTIONS Damage to the sensory cortex or to the sensory projections from thalamus to cortex results in a special type of disturbance that affects mainly the patient's ability to make sensory discriminations. Lesions in these structures may disturb postural sense but leave the so-called "primary modalities" (touch, pain, temperature, and vibration sense) relatively little affected. In such a situation, or if a cerebral lesion is suspected on other grounds, discriminative function should be tested further in the following ways:

Two-point discrimination The ability to distinguish two points from one is tested by using a compass, the points of which should be blunt and applied simultaneously and painlessly. The distance at which such a stimulus can be recognized as double varies greatly; 1 mm at the tip of the tongue, 2 to 3 mm on the lips, 3 to 5 mm on the dorsa of the hands and feet, and 4 to 7 cm on the body surface. It is characteristic of the patient with a lesion of the sensory cortex to mistake two points for one, although occasionally the opposite occurs.

Cutaneous localization and number writing The ability to localize cutaneous stimuli is tested by touching various parts of

the patient's body and asking the patient to point to the part touched or the corresponding part on the examiner's limb. Recognition of numbers or letters (these should be larger than 4 cm) or of the direction of lines drawn on the skin also depends on localization of tactile stimuli.

Appreciation of texture, size, and shape Appreciation of texture depends mainly on cutaneous impressions, but the recognition of shape and size of objects is based on impressions from deeper receptors as well. The lack of recognition of shape and form, therefore, though frequently found with cortical lesions, may also be present with lesions of the spinal cord and brainstem because of interruption of tracts transmitting postural and tactile sensation. The latter type of sensory defect, called stereoanesthesia, should be distinguished from astereognosis, which connotes an inability to identify an object by palpation, the primary sense data (touch, pain, temperature, and vibration) being intact. In practice, a pure astereognosis is rarely encountered, and the term is employed where the impairment of superficial and vibratory sensation in the hands is of insufficient severity to account for the defect. Defined in this way, astereognosis may be the product of a lesion in *either* hemisphere, in the postcentral gyrus or the thalamoparietal projections. Astereognosis may be confused with *tactile agnosia.* The latter disorder is due to a lesion lying posterior to the postcentral gyrus of the *dominant* parietal lobe, and causes an inability to recognize an object by touch or handling in one or both hands. In contrast, the patient with astereognosis may not appreciate the size, form, consistency, and weight of an object placed in the hand, and therefore cannot identify it.

Extinction of sensory stimuli and sensory inattention In response to bilateral simultaneous testing of symmetric parts, the patient may acknowledge only the stimulus on the sound side or may improperly localize the stimulus on the affected side, whereas stimuli applied to each side separately are properly appreciated. This phenomenon of extinction, or cortical inattention, is characteristic of parietal lobe lesions, the symptoms of which are considered in Chap. 25.

A few other terms require definition, since they may be encountered in descriptions of sensation. *Anesthesia* refers to a loss of all forms of sensation, and *hypesthesia* to a diminution of all sensation. Loss or impairment of specific cutaneous sensations is indicated by an appropriate prefix or suffix, e.g., thermoanesthesia or thermohypesthesia, analgesia (loss of pain) or hypalgesia, tactile anesthesia (loss of sense of touch), and pallanesthesia (loss of vibratory sense). The term *hyperesthesia* requires special mention; although it implies a heightened receptiveness of the nervous system, careful testing will usually demonstrate an underlying sensory defect, i.e., an elevated threshold to tactile, painful, or thermal stimuli; once the stimulus is perceived, however, it may have a severely painful or unpleasant quality (hyperpathia).

SYNDROMES OF SENSORY ABNORMALITY **Sensory changes due to single nerve involvement** Sensory changes may be due to interruption of a single peripheral nerve. These changes will vary with the composition of the nerve involved, depending on whether it is predominantly muscular, cutaneous, or mixed. In lesions of cutaneous nerves, the area of tactile anesthesia is more extensive than the one for pain, because of greater overlapping of pain fibers. Also, because of overlap from adjacent nerves, the area of sensory loss following division of a cutaneous nerve is always less than its anatomic distribution. If a large area of skin is involved, the sensory defect characteristically consists of a central portion, in which all forms of cutaneous sensation are lost, surrounded by a zone of partial loss, which becomes less marked as one proceeds from the center to the periphery. The senses of deep pressure and passive movement are intact because they are carried by special nerve fibers from subcutaneous structures and joints. Along the margin of the hypesthetic zone the skin becomes excessively sensitive. According to Weddell, this is because of collateral regeneration from surrounding healthy nerves into the denervated region (see Chap. 3).

Particular types of lesions differentially affect the fibers in a sensory nerve. Compression paralyzes large touch and pressure fibers more than the small pain, thermal, and autonomic motor fibers; procaine and cocaine have opposite effects.

In lesions involving the brachial and lumbosacral plexuses, the sensory disturbance is no longer confined to the territory of a single nerve and is almost invariably accompanied by muscle weakness and reflex change.

Sensory changes due to multiple nerve involvement (polyneuropathy) In most instances of polyneuropathy the sensory changes are accompanied by varying degrees of motor and reflex loss. Usually the sensory impairment is symmetric, with notable exceptions in some instances of diabetic and periarteritic neuropathy. Since the longest and largest fibers tend to be the most affected, the sensory loss is most severe over the feet and legs and less severe over the hands. The abdomen, thorax, and face are spared except in the most severe cases. The sensory loss usually involves all the modalities, and although it is manifestly difficult to equate the impairment of pain, touch, temperature, vibration, and position sense, one of these may seemingly be impaired out of proportion to the others. One cannot accurately predict from the patient's symptoms which mode of sensation will be disproportionately affected. The term *glove-and-stocking anesthesia* is frequently employed to describe the sensory loss of polyneuropathy and draws attention to the predominantly distal pattern of involvement. It is an inaccurate term insofar as the border between normal and impaired sensation is not so sharp; the sensory loss shades off gradually. In hysteria, by contrast, the border between normal and absent sensation is usually sharp. (See Chap. 377 for description of special varieties of sensory changes in polyneuropathies.)

Sensory changes due to involvement of single or multiple spinal nerve roots Because of considerable overlap from adjacent roots, division of a single sensory root does not produce complete loss of sensation in any area of skin. Compression of a single sensory cervical or lumbar root (e.g., in herniated intervertebral disks) causes varying degrees of impairment of cutaneous sensation in a segmental pattern, however. When two or more roots have been completely divided, a zone of sensory loss can be found in which reduction of pain perception is greater in extent than touch. Surrounding the area of complete loss is a narrow zone of partial loss, in which a raised threshold accompanied by overreaction (*hyperpathia*) may or may not be demonstrated. The presence of muscle paralysis, atrophy, and reflex loss indicates involvement of ventral roots as well.

Tabetic syndrome This, too, is a radicular syndrome, resulting from damage to the large proprioceptive and other fibers of the posterior lumbosacral roots. It is usually caused by neurosyphilis, less often by diabetes mellitus, meningeal tumors, etc. Numbness or paresthesias and lightning pains are frequent complaints, and areflexia, atonicity of the bladder, abnormalities of gait (Chap. 17), and hypotonia without muscle weakness are found on examination. The sensory loss may consist only of loss of vibration and position sense in the lower extremities, but in severe cases, loss or impairment of superficial or deep pain sense or of touch may be added. The feet and legs are most affected, much less often the arms and trunk.

Complete spinal sensory syndromes In a complete transverse lesion of the spinal cord, all forms of sensation are abolished below a level that corresponds to the lesion. There may be a narrow zone of "hyperesthesia" at the upper margin of the anesthetic zone. During the evolution of such a lesion there may be a discrepancy between the level of the lesion and that of the sensory loss, the latter ascending as the lesion progresses. This can be understood if one conceives of a lesion evolving from the periphery to the center of the cord, affecting first the outermost fibers carrying pain and temperature sensation from the legs. Conversely, a lesion advancing from the center of the cord may affect these modalities in the reverse order. (See Chap. 375 for more complete discussion.)

Partial spinal sensory syndromes (hemisection of the spinal cord, Brown-Séquard syndrome) In rare instances disease is confined to one side of the spinal cord; pain and heat sensation are affected on the opposite side, and proprioceptive sensation is affected on the same side as the lesion. The loss of pain and temperature sensation begins two or three segments below the lesion. An associated motor paralysis on the side of the lesion completes the syndrome. Tactile sensation is not involved, since the fibers from one side of the body are distributed in tracts on both sides of the cord.

Lesions of the central gray matter (syringomyelic syndrome) Since fibers conducting pain and temperature cross the cord in the anterior commissure, a lesion in this location will characteristically abolish these modalities on one or both sides but will spare tactile sensation. The commonest cause of such a lesion is syringomyelia, less often tumor and hemorrhage. This type of dissociated sensory loss usually occurs in a segmental distribution (the sensation is normal above and below the affected segment), and since the lesion frequently involves other parts of the gray matter, varying degrees of segmental amyotrophy and reflex loss may be added. If the lesion has spread to the white matter, signs of involvement of corticospinal and spinothalamic tracts and posterior columns will be present as well.

Posterior column syndrome There is loss of vibratory and position sense below the lesion, but the senses of pain, temperature, and touch are affected relatively little or not at all. This condition may be difficult to distinguish from an affection of large fibers in sensory roots (tabetic syndrome). In some diseases vibratory sensation may be involved predominantly, whereas in others position sense is more affected. An interruption of proprioceptive fibers may interfere with discriminative sensory function, such as two-point discrimination and recognition of size, shape, and weight; and impairment of these functions may occur with posterior column disease alone. Paresthesias in the form of tingling and "pins-and-needles" sensations or girdle sensations are a common complaint with diseases of posterior columns, and pain stimuli may also produce unpleasant sensations.

The "anterior spinal artery syndrome" With occlusion of the anterior spinal artery or other destructive lesions that predominantly affect the ventral portion of the cord, there is a relative or absolute sparing of the posterior column functions and only a loss of pain and temperature sensation below the level of the lesion. Since the corticospinal tracts and the ventral gray matter also fall within the area of distribution of the anterior spinal artery, paralysis of motor function forms a prominent part of this syndrome.

Disturbances of sensation due to lesions of the brainstem A characteristic feature of lesions of the medulla and lower pons is crossed sensory disturbance, i.e., loss of pain and temperature sensation of one side of the face and of the opposite side of the body. This is accounted for by involvement of the trigeminal tract or nucleus and the lateral spinothalamic tract on one side of the brainstem. This is nearly always due to a lateral medullary infarction (Wallenburg's syndrome). In the upper pons and midbrain, where the spinothalamic tracts and the medial lemniscus become confluent, an appropriately placed lesion may cause a loss of all superficial and deep sensation over the contralateral side of the body. Cranial nerve palsies, cerebellar ataxia, or motor paralysis are often associated (see Chap. 376).

Sensory loss due to a lesion of the thalamus (syndrome of Dejerine-Roussy) Involvement of the nucleus ventralis posterolateralis of the thalamus, usually due to a vascular lesion or tumor, causes loss or diminution of all forms of sensation on the opposite side of the body. Position sense is affected more frequently than any other sensory function, and deep sensory loss is usually, but not always, more profound than cutaneous loss. Sooner or later, often as sensation improves, spontaneous pain or discomfort ("thalamic pain"), sometimes of the most torturing and disabling type, appears on the affected side of the body; and any form of stimulus may acquire a diffuse, unpleasant, lingering quality. Emotional disturbance also aggravates the painful state. The thalamic pain syndrome may occasionally accompany lesions of the white matter of the parietal lobe (Chap. 25).

Sensory loss due to lesions in the parietal lobe There is a unique disturbance mainly of discriminative sensory functions on the opposite side of the body, particularly the face, arm, and leg. Loss of position sense, impaired ability to localize touch and pain stimuli, elevation of two-point threshold, a general inattentiveness to sensory stimuli on one side of the body, and astereognosis (if the lesion is in the dominant hemisphere) are the most prominent findings. With cortical lesions, the patient's reports are variable; one examination may disclose no sensory abnormalities, whereas another does. This type of response is often attributed to hysteria. As to the anatomic localization of lesions that impair tactile discrimination, they have been found consistently in the postcentral gyrus of the contralateral parietal lobe (Roland). Other features of parietal lobe symptomatology and the differences between dominant and nondominant parietal lobe syndromes are considered in Chap. 25. More frequent with lesions of the parietal lobe is a global reduction of all forms of somatic sensation on the opposite side of the body.

Sensory loss due to suggestion and hysteria Hysterical patients almost never complain spontaneously of cutaneous sensory loss, although they may use the term *numbness* to indicate a paralysis of a limb. Complete hemianesthesia, often with reduced hearing, sight, smell, and taste, as well as impaired vibration sense over only half the skull, is a common finding in hysteria. Anesthesia of one entire limb or a sharply defined sensory loss over part of a limb, not conforming to the distribution of root or cutaneous nerve, is also frequently observed. Postural sensation is rarely affected. The diagnosis of hysterical hemianesthesia is best made by eliciting the other relevant symptoms of hysteria or, if this is not possible, by noting the discrepancies between this type of sensory loss and that which occurs as part of the usual sensory syndromes.

REFERENCES

BRODAL A: The somatic afferent pathways, in *Neurological Anatomy.* New York, Oxford, 1969, chap 2

DYCK PJ et al: Clinical vs. quantitative evaluation of cutaneous sensation. Arch Neurol 33:651, 1976

MAYO CLINIC: *Clinical Examinations in Neurology,* 3d ed. Philadelphia, Saunders, 1972

MOUNTCASTLE VB: Central nervous mechanisms in sensation, in *Medical Physiology,* 12th ed, VB Mountcastle (ed). St. Louis, Mosby, 1968, vol 2, chaps 61–63

ROLAND PE: Astereognosis: Tactile discrimination after localized hemispheric lesions in man. Arch Neurol 33:543, 1976

20
COMA AND RELATED DISTURBANCES OF CONSCIOUSNESS

RAYMOND D. ADAMS

The practitioner of medicine is frequently called upon to treat patients whose principal abnormality is an impairment of consciousness, which varies from inattentiveness and simple confusion to coma. In large municipal hospitals it is estimated that as many as 3 percent of total admissions to the emergency ward are due to diseases that have caused coma; although this figure seems high, it serves to emphasize the importance of this class of neurologic diseases and the necessity for every student of medicine to acquire a theoretic as well as practical knowledge of them.

The terms *consciousness, confusion, stupor, unconsciousness,* and *coma* have been endowed with so many meanings that it is almost impossible to avoid ambiguity in their usage. They are not strictly medical terms, but literary, philosophic, and psychologic ones as well. The word *consciousness* is the most difficult of all. William James once remarked that everyone knew what consciousness was until attempting to define it. To the psychologist consciousness denotes a state of awareness of one's self and one's environment. Knowledge of one's self, of course, includes all "feelings, attitudes and emotions, impulses, volitions, and the active or striving aspects of conduct"—in short, an awareness of all one's own mental functioning, particularly of the cognitive processes. These can be judged only by the patient's verbal account of introspections and, indirectly, by actions. Physicians, being practical persons for the most part, have learned to place greater confidence in their observations of the patient's general behavior and reactions to overt stimuli than in what the patient says. For this reason when they employ the term *consciousness,* they usually do so in its commonest and simplest signification, namely, a state of awareness of the environment. This narrow definition has another advantage in that the word *unconsciousness* is its exact opposite—a state of unawareness of environment or a suspension of those mental activities by which humans are made aware of their environment. To add to the ambiguity, psychoanalysts have given the word *unconscious* a still different meaning; for them it stands for the repository of impulses and memories of previous experiences that cannot immediately be recalled to the conscious mind.

Description of states of normal and impaired consciousness The following definitions, though admittedly unacceptable to most psychologists, are of service to medicine, and they will provide the students with a convenient terminology for describing the mental states of their patients.

Normal consciousness This is the condition of the normal person when fully awake, who is responsive to psychologic stimuli and "indicates by his behavior and speech that he has the same awareness of himself and his environment as ourselves." This normal state may fluctuate during the course of the day from keen alertness or deep concentration with a marked constriction of the field of attention to general inattentiveness and drowsiness.

Sleep Sleep is a state of physical and mental inactivity from which the patient may be aroused to normal consciousness. A person in sleep gives little evidence of being aware of self or environment and in this respect is unconscious. Yet such a person differs from a comatose patient in that the former may still respond to unaccustomed stimuli and at times is capable of some mental activity in the form of dreams, which leave their traces in memory. Also, he or she is arousable.

Inattention, confusional, and cloudy states of consciousness In these conditions the patient does not take into account all elements of the immediate environment. As in delirium, there is always an element of sensorial clouding or imperceptiveness and distractibility of attention. The term *confusion* lacks precision, for often it is meant to denote an inability to think with customary speed and coherence. Here the difficulty is in defining *thinking,* a term which invariably refers to problem solving and coherence of ideas about a subject.

An inattentive, severely confused person is usually unable to do more than carry out a few simple commands. Few if any thought processes are in operation. The capacity for speech may be limited to a few words or phrases, or the patient may be voluble. These patients are unaware of much that goes on around them and do not grasp the immediate situation. Moderately confused persons can carry on simple conversations for short periods of time, but their thinking is slow and incoherent, and they are unable to stay on one topic. They are distractible and at the mercy of every stimulus. Usually they are disoriented in time and place. In mild degrees of confusion, the disorder may be so slight that it is overlooked unless the examiner is scrutinizing the patient's behavior and conversation. The patient may even be roughly oriented as to time and place and able to speak freely on almost any subject. Only occasional irrelevant remarks betray an incoherence of thinking. Patients with mild or moderately severe confusion may be subjected to psychologic testing. The degree of confusion often varies from one time of day to another and tends to be least pronounced in the early morning. Severe confusion or stupor may resemble semicoma during periods when the patient is drowsy or asleep. Many events that happen to the confused patient leave no apparent trace in the memory; in fact, capacity to recall later the events that transpired in any given period is one of the most delicate tests of mental clarity. However, careful analysis will show the defect to be one of inadequate registration and fixation of items rather than a fault in retentive memory.

Some neurologists regard *delirium* as a state of confusion with excitement and hyperactivity, and in some medical writings the terms *delirium* and *confused-cloudy states* are used interchangeably. It is undoubtedly true that the delirious patient is nearly always confused. However, the inability to sleep, vivid hallucinations, the relative inaccessibility of the patient to other events than those to which he or she is reacting at any one moment, extreme agitation and tremulousness, and the tendency to convulse, all of which characterize delirious states, suggest a cerebral disorder of a somewhat different type. The clearest evidence of the relationship of inattention, confusion, stupor, and coma is that the patient may pass through all these states while becoming comatose or emerging from coma. The

author has not observed any such relationship between coma and delirium. These distinctions are drawn with greater clarity in Chap. 25.

At times a patient with certain types of aphasia, especially jargon aphasia, may create the impression of confusion, but close observation will reveal that the disorder is confined to the sphere of language and that behavior is otherwise natural.

Stupor In stupor mental and physical activity are reduced to a minimum. Although inaccessible to many stimuli, the patient opens the eyes, looks at the examiner, and does not appear to be unconscious. Response to spoken commands is either absent or slow and monosyllabic. As a rule tendon or plantar reflexes are not altered. On the other hand, tremulousness of movement, coarse twitching of muscles, restless or stereotyped motor activity, and grasping and sucking reflexes are not infrequent, depending on the way in which disease affects the nervous system. In psychiatry the term *stupor* means a state in which impressions of the external world are normally received but activity is suspended or marked by negativism, e.g., catatonic stupor of schizophrenia and mania.

Coma The patient who appears to be asleep and is at the same time incapable of sensing (unreceptive) and responding adequately to either external stimuli or inner needs (unresponsive) is in a state of coma. Coma may vary in degree, and in its deepest stages no reaction of any kind is obtainable. Corneal, pupillary, pharyngeal, tendon, and plantar reflexes are all absent, and there may or may not be extensor rigidity of the limbs and opisthotonos, signs which, as Sherrington showed, indicate decerebration. Respirations are often slow or rapid and may be periodic, i.e., Cheyne-Stokes breathing. With lesser degrees of coma, pupillary reflexes and ocular movements and other brainstem reflexes are preserved; in still lighter stages, referred to as *semicoma,* most of the above reflexes can be elicited, and the plantar reflexes may be either flexor or extensor (Babinski's sign). Moreover, pricking or pinching the skin, shaking and shouting at the patient, or an uncomfortable distention of the bladder may cause the patient to stir or moan and respirations to quicken. Coma differs from akinetic mutism (a state in which a patient is awake but lacking in impulse to speech and action) and the "locked-in" syndromes (a global paralysis of limbs and cranial musculature) in which the patient is still receptive but unresponsive.

ELECTROENCEPHALOGRAM AND DISTURBANCES OF CONSCIOUSNESS One of the most delicate confirmations of the fact that these states of altered consciousness are expressions of neurophysiologic changes is the electroencephalogram. In the normal waking state the electric potentials of the cortical neurons are integrated into regular waves of two frequency ranges, from 8 to 15 per second (alpha rhythm) and from 16 to 25 per second (beta rhythm). These waveforms are established by the time one reaches adolescence, but certain individual differences in general pattern and dominance of alpha waves are maintained throughout adult life. With sleep these cortical potentials slow down, and amplitude (voltage) of the individual waves increases. At one stage in light sleep characteristic bursts of 14 to 16 waves per second appear, the so-called "sleep spindles," and in deep [nonrapid eye movement (NREM)] sleep all the waves of normal frequency and amplitude are replaced by slow ones of high voltage (1¼ to 3 per second). In rapid eye movement (REM) sleep the brain waves return to normal (see Chap. 22). Similarly, some alteration in brain waves occur in all disturbances of consciousness except the milder degrees of confusion. This alteration usually consists of a disorganization of the electroencephalographic pattern, which shows random, slow waves of high voltage in stages of confusion; more regular, slow, 2- to 3-per-second waves of high voltage in stupor and semicoma; and slow waves or even suppression of all organized electric activity (isoelectric state) in the deep coma of hypoxia and ischemia, the so-called "brain-death syndrome." The electroencephalograms of deep sleep and of light coma resemble each other. However, not all diseases that cause confusion and coma have the same effect on the electroencephalogram. Some, such as barbiturate intoxication, may cause an increase in frequency and amplitude of the brain waves. In epilepsy the disturbance of consciousness is usually attended by paroxysms of "spikes" (fast waves of high amplitude) or by the characteristic alternating slow waves and spikes of petit mal. Other diseases, such as hepatic coma, characteristicially cause a slowing in frequency and an increasing amplitude of "brain waves" and special triphasic waves. Whether all metabolic diseases of the brain induce similar changes in the electroencephalogram has not been determined. Probably there are differences among them, some of which may be significant (see Chap. 371).

MORBID ANATOMY AND PHYSIOLOGY OF COMA In recent times there has been some clarification and amplification of earlier neuropathologic observations that the smallest lesions associated with protracted coma are always to be found in the midbrain and thalamus. The essence of more recent neurophysiologic studies, to be found in the writings of Bremer, of Morison and Dempsey, and of Moruzzi and Magoun, is that a systematic series of destructive lesions of spinal cord, medulla, pons, and cerebellum has no effect on the state of consciousness until the level of midbrain and diencephalon (thalamus) is reached. High brainstem transections invariably induce states of prolonged unresponsiveness, whereas stimulation of the upper brainstem reticular formation causes a drowsy or sleeping animal to become suddenly alert and its EEG to change correspondingly. As anesthetic agents abolish consciousness, they are found to suppress the activity of the upper reticular activating system, without interfering, at least at certain levels, with the transmission of specific sensory impulses en route to parietal lobe cortex.

Anatomic studies show the reticular activating system of the upper brainstem to receive collaterals from the specific sensory pathways and to project, not just to the sensory cortex of the parietal lobe, as do the thalamic relay nuclei for somatic sensation, but to the whole of the cerebral cortex. The latter has corticofugal connections which feed back nerve impulses to the reticular formation. Sensory stimulation, it would seem, then, has the double effect of conveying to the brain information about the outside world and also of providing some of the energy for activating those parts of the nervous system on which consciousness depends.

These new data are in line with the older ideas of Herbert Spencer and Hughlings Jackson—that the diencephalon and cerebral cortex always function together as a unit and represent the highest levels of integrative nervous activity, called by Penfield *centrencephalic*. Though anatomic details have yet to be worked out and the precise physiology of the reticular activating system leaves much to be desired, being more complicated than this simple formulation woud suggest, nevertheless, as a working idea it will make some of the following neuropathologic observations more comprehensible.

The study of a large series of human cases in which coma has preceded death by several days will bring to light two major types of lesion. In the first group a macroscopically visible lesion such as a tumor, abscess, intracerebral, subarachnoid, subdural, or epidural hemorrhage, massive infarct, or meningitis is demonstrable; usually the lesion involves a portion only of the cortex and white matter, leaving much of the cerebrum intact. Rarely, it is located in the thalamus or midbrain, which would make the coma understandable. In the mass-type lesions the coma will always be related to a *temporal lobe–tentorial herniation* with compression, ischemia, and secondary hemorrhage in the midbrain and lower thalamus or with downward displacement of the brainstem (see Chap. 367). A detailed clinical record will show the coma to have coincided with these secondary displacements and herniations. Exceptionally, widespread bilateral damage to the cortex and subcortical white matter will be found—the result of bilateral infarcts or hemorrhages, viral encephalitis, hypoxia, or ischemia—without thalamic or midbrain lesions. In the second group (and this is larger than the first) no visible lesion is seen by the naked eye, and often no abnormality is divulged by any technique of pathology. The lesion here is caused by a metabolic or toxic state which may be impossible to detect morphologically. In some instances the grossly normal brain will reveal a demonstrable cellular change under the light microscope which may be characteristic, e.g., hepatic coma. Usually, in these latter instances the microscopic lesions are too diffuse for clinicoanatomic correlation. Thus, pathologic changes are compatible with physiologic deductions—that the state of prolonged coma correlates with lesions of all parts of the cortical-diencephalic systems of neurons, but it is only in the upper brainstem that they may be small and discrete.

MECHANISMS WHEREBY CONSCIOUSNESS IS DISTURBED IN DISEASE Knowledge of diseases of the nervous system is so limited that is is not possible to identify all the different mechanisms by means of which consciousness is disturbed. Already several different ways in which the mesencephalic-diencephalic-cortical systems are deranged have been identified; there are probably many others.

In a number of disease processes there is evidence of direct interference with the metabolic activities of the nerve cells in the cerebral cortex and central thalamic nuclei of the brain and depletion of putative transmitters (serotonin, dopamine, acetylcholine, norepinephrine, γ-aminobutyric acid, choline, and glutamic acid). Hypoxia, hypoglycemia, hyper- and hypo-osmolar states, acidosis, alkalosis, hyper- and hypokalemia, hyperammonemia, and deficiencies of thiamine, nicotinic acid, vitamin B_{12}, pantothenic acid, and pyridoxine are well-known examples (see Chap. 371). Relevant points for our discussion are that cerebral metabolism or blood flow is reduced in all the metabolic disorders leading to coma. Oxygen values below 2 ml per 100 g brain tissue per minute are incompatible with an alert state. In hypoglycemia the cerebral blood flow is normal or above normal, whereas the cerebral metabolic rate is diminished, owing to deficiency of substrate. In thiamine and vitamin B_{12} deficiency the cerebral blood flow is normal or slightly diminished, and the cerebral metabolic rate is diminished, presumably because of insufficiency of coenzymes. Extremes of body temperature, either hyperthermia (temperature over 41°C) or hypothermia (temperature below 35°C), probably induce coma by exerting a nospecific effect on the metabolic activity of neurons.

Diabetic acidosis, uremia, hepatic coma, and the coma of systemic infections are examples of endogenous intoxications. The identity of the toxic agents is not entirely known. In diabetes acetone bodies (acetoacetic acid, β-hydroxybutyric acid, and acetone) are present in high concentration or in the nonketotic form a lactic acidosis, and in uremia there is probably accumulation of dialyzable toxins, perhaps phenolic derivatives of the aromatic amino acids. In both conditions "dehydration" and serum acidosis (pH < 7.3, $P_{CO_2} < 35$ mmHg, $[HCO_3^-] < 10$ meq per liter) may also be significant. In many cases of hepatic coma, elevation of blood NH3 to levels five to six times normal has been found. Lactic acidemia and other organic acids may affect the brain by lowering its pH. The mode of action of bacterial toxins is unknown. In all these conditions the cerebral metabolic rate tends to be reduced, whereas cerebral blood flow remains normal. Extreme hypoglycemia (blood glucose concentration <10 to 15 mg per 100 ml) critically reduces substrate for cerebral function, and hyperglycemia (500 mg per 100 ml) affects cerebral function by causing hyperosmolality. In water intoxication hypoosmolality the membrane excitability of nerve cells is altered by hyponatremia and changes in intracellular K levels. In respiratory acidosis (serum [HCO3] > 20 meq per liter, P_{CO_2} > 45 mmHg, pH<7.30) from depressant drug poisoning or chronic pulmonary disease, coma is caused by a combination of hypercapnia and hypoxia. In respiratory alkalosis and metabolic alkalosis (pH>7.45) from cardiopulmonary disease, central neurogenic hyperventilation, alkali ingestion, etc., cerebral function is disturbed because of altered neuronal membrane activity.

Drugs such as barbiturates, bromides, diphenylhydantoin (Dilantin), alcohol, glutethimide, and phenothiazines induce coma by their direct suppressive effect on the neurons of the cerebrum and diencephalon. Others such as methyl alcohol, paraldehyde, and ethylene glycol result in metabolic acidosis. Many additional pharmacologic agents have no direct action on the nervous system but may lead to coma through the mechanism of circulatory collapse and inadequate cerebral blood flow. In toxic and metabolic diseases, although the patient usually approaches coma through stages of drowsiness, confusion, and stupor, and the reverse sequence occurs while emerging from it, each disease has its special effects, manifesting itself by a characteristic clinical picture. This means that the mechanism and topography of the lesion will be different.

A critical fall in blood pressure, usually to a systolic level below 70 mmHg, affects neural structures by causing a critical decrease in oxygenation, which reduces cerebral blood flow by half, and secondarily, a diminution in cerebral metabolic rate. If decline in blood pressure is episodic, the corresponding clinical picture is one of physical weakness usually preceding and following the loss of consciousness, i.e., syncope, the whole process being acute and promptly reversible. Cardiac arrest completely interrupts cerebral circulation and abolishes consciousness in 5 to 10 s.

The sudden, violent, and excessive discharge of *epilepsy* is another mechanism. Usually a Jacksonian convulsion has little effect on consciousness until it spreads from one side of the body to the other. Coma immediately ensues, presumably because the spreading of the seizure discharge to central neuronal structures paralyzes their function. Other types of seizure in which consciousness is interrupted from the very beginning are believed to originate in the diencephalon.

Concussion exemplifies still another special pathophysiologic mechanism. In "blunt" head injury it has been shown that there is an enormous increase in intracranial pressure of the order of 200 to 700 lb/in², lasting a few thousandths of a second. Either the vibration set up in the skull and transmitted to the brain or this sudden high intracranial pressure is believed to be the basis of the abrupt paralysis of the nervous system that follows head injury. A separate rotatory motion of the brain within the skull is another more likely possibility. Raising the intraventricular pressure to a level approaching diastolic blood pressure has abolished all vital functions in the experimental animal.

As was pointed out above, large, destructive, supratentorial, space-consuming lesions of the brain, such as hemorrhage, tumor, or abscess, interfere with consciousness in two ways. One is by direct destruction of the midbrain and diencephalon; the other, far more frequent, is by producing herniation of the

medial part of the temporal lobe through the opening of the tentorium and crushing the upper brain against the opposite free edge of the tentorium or lateral and downward displacement of brainstem. Here the mechanism is again mechanical, and probably circulatory as well.

CLINICAL APPROACH TO THE COMATOSE PATIENT   Coma is not an independent disease entity but is always a symptomatic expression of disease. Sometimes the underlying disease is perfectly obvious, as when a healthy individual is struck on the head and rendered unconscious. All too often, however, the patient is brought to the hospital in a state of coma, and little or no information is immediately available. The physician must then subject the clinical problem to careful scrutiny from many directions. To do this efficiently requires a broad knowledge of disease and a systematic approach that leaves none of the common and treatable causes of coma unexplored.

It should be pointed out that when the comatose patient is seen for the first time, simple therapeutic measures take precedence over diagnostic procedures. In a quick survey one makes sure that the comatose patient has a clear airway and is not in shock (circulatory collapse) or, if trauma has occurred, that the patient is not bleeding from a wound. In patients who have suffered a head injury there may be a fracture of the cervical vertebrae, and therefore one must be cautious about moving the head and neck lest the spinal cord be inadvertently crushed. There must be an immediate inquiry as to the previous health of the patient: whether he or she had suffered a head injury or had been seen in a convulsion, and the circumstances in which the patient was found. The persons who accompany the comatose patient to the hospital should not be permitted to leave until they have been questioned.

Diagnosis   The temperature, pulse, respiratory rate and pattern, and blood pressure are of aid in diagnosis. Fever suggests a severe systemic infection such as pneumonia, bacterial meningitis, or a brain lesion that has disturbed the temperature-regulating centers. An excessively high body temperature, 41 to 44°C, associated with dry skin should arouse the suspicion of heat stroke. Hypothermia is frequently observed in alcoholic or barbiturate intoxication, extracellular fluid deficit, peripheral circulatory failure, or myxedema. Slow breathing points to morphine, barbiturate intoxication, central alveolar hypoventilation, metabolic alkalosis, or hypothyroidism, whereas deep, rapid breathing suggests pneumonia but may occur in diabetic or uremic acidosis or exogenous organic acid intoxication (Kussmaul's respiration) or with intracranial diseases, as in central neurogenic hyperpnea. The rapid breathing of pneumonia is often accompanied by an expiratory grunt, cyanosis, and fever. Diseases that elevate the intracranial pressure or damage the brain, especially the brainstem or cerebrum, often cause slow, irregular, or periodic (Cheyne-Stokes) breathing. The pulse rate is less helpful, but if exceptionally slow, it should suggest heart block, or if combined with periodic breathing and hypertension, an increase in intracranial pressure. A tachycardia of 140 heartbeats per minute or above calls attention to the possibility of an ectopic cardiac rhythm with insufficiency of cerebral circulation. Marked hypertension occurs in patients with cerebral hemorrhage and hypertensive encephalopathy and, at times, in those with increased intracranial pressure, whereas hypotension is the usual finding in the coma of alcohol or barbiturate intoxication, or internal hemorrhage, myocardial infarction, gram-negative bacillary septicemia, and Addison's disease.

Inspection of the skin may also yield valuable information.

Cyanosis of the lips and nail beds means inadequate oxygenation. Cherry-red coloration indicates carbon monoxide poisoning. Multiple bruises, and in particular a bruise or boggy area in the scalp, favor cranial trauma. Bleeding from an ear or the nose or orbital hemorrhage also raises the possibility of trauma. Puffiness and hyperemia of face and conjunctivas and telangiectasia are the usual stigmas of alcoholism; marked pallor suggests internal hemorrhage. The presence of a maculo-hemmorrhagic rash indicates the possibility of meningococcal infection, staphylococcus endocarditis, typhus, or Rocky Mountain spotted fever. Pellagra may be diagnosed from the typical skin lesions on face and hands. The myxedematous appearance of the face is indicative of hypothyroid stupor or coma. In pituitary hypoadrenalism the skin is sallow. Excessive sweating suggests hypoglycemia or shock, and dry skin diabetic acidosis and uremia. Skin turgor is reduced in dehydration. Hemorrhagic blisters will have formed over pressure points if the patient has been motionless for a time.

The odor of the breath may provide clues to the nature of a disease causing coma. The odor of alcohol is easily recognized (except for vodka, which is odorless). The spoiled-fruit odor of diabetic coma, the uriniferous odor of uremia, and the musty fetor of hepatic coma are distinctive enough to be identified by physicians who possess a keen sense of smell.

The next step in the physical examination should give special attention to the status of the nervous system. Although the examination is limited in many ways, careful observation of the stuporous or comatose patient may yield considerable information concerning the function of different parts of the nervous system. One of the most helpful procedures is to sit at the bedside for 5 to 10 min and observe what the patient does. The predominant postures of the body, the position of the head and eyes, the rate, depth, and rhythm of respiration, and the pulse should be noted. The state of responsiveness should then be estimated by noting both the reaction when the patient's name is called and the capacity to execute a simple command or to respond to painful stimuli. The most effective painful stimuli are supraorbital pressure, sternal pressure, or pinching the side of the neck or inner parts of the upper arms or thighs. By grading these stimuli, one may titrate the response, so to speak, and evaluate both the degree of coma and changes from hour to hour in the course of the disease. Vocalization may persist in stupor and light coma and is the first response to be lost. Deft avoidance movements of parts stimulated, and grimacing are preserved in light coma and substantiate the integrity of corticomedullary and corticospinal tracts.

Usually it is possible to determine whether the coma is accompanied by meningeal irritation or focal disease in the cerebrum or brainstem. With meningeal irritation from either bacterial meningitis or subarachnoid hemorrhage, there is resistance to active and passive flexion of the neck but not to extension, turning, or tipping the head. Resistance to movement of the neck in all directions indicates disease of the cervical spine or is part of generalized rigidity. In infants, bulging of the anterior fontanel is at times a more reliable sign of meningeal irritation than stiff neck. A temporal lobe or cerebellar pressure cone or decerebrate rigidity may also limit passive flexion of the neck and may be confused with meningeal irritation.

Evidence of disease of a cerebral hemisphere, diencephalon, midbrain, pons, or medulla can be obtained even though the patient is comatose by noting the residual movement, prevailing postures of the body, respiratory rhythm and frequency, and status of cranial nerves. This is of more than passing importance, because severe and persistent derangements of these functions are frequent with mass lesions of the brain and rare in metabolic disorders (except in terminal stages). A hemiplegia, in most instances, reflects a contralateral hemispheral lesion and is revealed by lack of restless movements, grasp reflex, and avoidance movements. The paralyzed limbs are slack and remain in uncomfortable positions. If lifted from the bed, they "fall flail." The cheek puffs out in expiration on the paralyzed side, and the eyes are often turned away from the paralysis (toward the lesion). Painful stimuli may provoke a moan or grimace on one side and not the other, reflecting a hemianesthesia. A homonymous hemianopia in a stuporous patient is revealed by attraction of eyes to visual stimuli presented on one side and not the other or lack of blink in reaction to threat on one side.

Of the various tests of brainstem function those which have been most useful are pattern of breathing, pupillary size and reactivity, and ocular movement and oculovestibular reflexes. As to patterns of abnormal breathing in progressive lesions which reduce the state of consciousness from confusion and inattention to stupor and coma, the earliest abnormality with cerebral lesions is the appearance of posthyperventilation apnea (period of apnea after 5 to 10 deep breaths). Its presence indicates bifrontal disease, wherein lies the mechanism, according to Plum, for activating rhythmic breathing when CO_2 is reduced. In coma due to massive cerebral lesions the rate of respiration increases slightly, and as it progresses an irregularity appears which gives way to the waxing-waning Cheyne-Stokes respiration (CSR). This means that the centers in the brainstem, now isolated from the cerebrum, are rendered more sensitive than usual to CO_2 (hyperventilation drive); and by intermittently reducing plasma CO_2 to low levels, a temporary apnea follows. With midbrain–upper pontine lesions a state of central neurogenic hyperpnea (CNH), rather like Kussmaul breathing, supervenes. Here respirations are increased in rate (up to 100 per minute) and in depth, to the extent that respiratory alkalosis may result. The reflex mechanisms for respiratory control in the lower brainstem have in this instance been released, and the threshold of respiratory activation is low. This respiratory drive continues despite low arterial CO_2 tensions and elevated pH. Oxygen therapy (unlike the hyperventilation of pneumonia, pulmonary congestion, etc.) does not modify the pattern. Low pontine-level lesions sometimes cause apneustic breathing (where there is a pause of 2 to 3 s after full inspiration) or other abnormal patterns, such as short cycle clusters [three to four respirations without a waxing or waning followed by a pause (Biot respirations)]; or respiration alternans, in which a few breaths are omitted from time to time. With lesions of the medulla the rhythm of breathing is chaotic, being irregularly interrupted, the breath varying in rate and depth. This has been called "ataxic breathing," not a very appropriate term. The latter progresses to apnea, as may also CSR or CNH; in fact, respiratory arrest is the mode of death of most patients with serious central nervous system disease. As Plum and Fisher both point out, when certain supratentorial brain lesions progress to the point where the temporal lobe and cerebellum herniate, one may observe a succession of respiratory patterns (CSR–CNH–Biot breathing to ataxic breathing), indicating extension of the functional disorder from upper to lower brainstem.

With midbrain lesions the pupils dilate to 4 or 5 mm and become unreactive to light; with severe destruction of the tissue at this level (anoxic pannecrosis), they will finally dilate widely to 8 to 9 mm and not respond. Pontine and midbrain tegmental lesions cause miotic pupils with only slight reaction to strong light. Thus, normal-sized pupils and the preservation of pupillary light reflexes indicate integrity of the pupillary dilatation and constrictive mechanisms in the midbrain. Ciliospinal pupillary dilatation is also lost in brainstem lesions (see Chap. 18). Unilateral Horner's syndrome (miosis, ptosis, exophthalmos, and reduced sweating) may be observed homolateral to a predominantly one-sided lower brainstem lesion, usually medullary. The pupillary reactions are of great importance, because drug intoxications and metabolic disorders which cause coma leave the pupils unaffected. Exceptions are glutethimide (Doriden) and deep ether anesthesia, which cause the pupils to be of medium size or slightly enlarged and unreactive for several hours; opiates (heroin and morphine), which cause pinpoint pupils with light reflex so small that it can be seen only with a magnifying glass, and atropine poisoning, in which the pupils are widely dilated and fixed.

Ocular movements are altered in a variety of ways. In light coma from metabolic abnormalities the eyes rove from side to side in random fashion like the slow eye movements of light sleep. They disappear as brainstem function becomes depressed. Oculocephalic reflexes (doll's eye movements), elicited by briskly turning or tilting the head, with eyes moving conjugately in the opposite direction, are easily elicited. They are not present in the normal person, and if they are elicitable, evidence is obtained of release from cerebral control and integrity of the tegmental structures of the midbrain and pons, which integrate ocular movements, and of the third, fourth, and sixth cranial nerves. Irrigation of each ear with 30 to 100 ml ice water (or just cold water if the patient is not completely comatose) will normally cause nystagmus away from the stimulated side (see Chap. 18). In comatose patients in whom the fast corrective "cortical" phase of nystagmus is lost, the eyes are deflected to the side irrigated with cold water or away from the side irrigated with hot water. The position is held for 2 to 3 min. These vestibuloocular reflexes are also lost in brainstem lesions. If only one eye abducts and the other fails to adduct in the lateral conjugate movement, there is indication of interruption of the medial longitudinal fasciculus (on the side of adductor paralysis). Irrigating both ears with ice water with the head extended to 60° will sometimes induce vertical conjugate movements. An abducens palsy (sixth nerve) is reflected by a turning in of the eye because of unopposed action of the abducens muscle. The eyes may be held conjugately to one side at all times in a coma—away from the side of the paralysis with large cerebral lesions (looking at the lesion) and toward the side of the paralysis with unilateral pontine lesions (looking away from the lesion). And during a one-sided seizure, the eyes jerk toward the convulsing side of the face, arm, and leg (opposite the irritative focus). The eyes may be turned down and inward (looking at the nose) in thalamic and upper midbrain lesion (Parinaud's syndrome, see Chap. 18). Retraction and convergence nystagmus and ocular bobbing [brisk downward movements of both eyes with slow elevation to the original position (2 or 3 times a minute)] occur with lesions in the midbrain tegmentum and lower pons, respectively. The major brainstem structural lesions, including temporal lobe herniation, abolish most, if not all, conjugate ocular movements when producing coma, whereas metabolic disorders do not. Barbiturates and diphenylhydantoin (Dilantin) are the only common intoxicating drugs which affect ocular movements, but they leave pupillary reactions intact.

As to the meaning of the forced postures and movements in the comatose patient, it may be said that restless, grasping, picking movements of one arm or arm and leg or all four extremities signify that the corticospinal tract(s) is intact; variable resistance to passive movement (paratonic rigidity) and strong grasping or complex avoidance movements have the same signification, and if they are bilateral, the coma usually is not deep. Focal seizures require an intact corticospinal motor system and are seldom seen in the paralyzed side with massive destruction of a cerebral hemisphere. Often these elaborate forms of semivoluntary movement are present on the "good side" in patients with extensive disease in one hemisphere and probably represent some type of disequilibrium of cortical and subcortical movement patterns. Definite choreic, athetotic, or even hemiballismic movements indicate disorder of the subthalamic and basal ganglionic structures, just as they do in the alert patient. *Decerebrate rigidity,* with jaw clenched, neck retracted, arms and legs stiffly extended and internally rotated, appears in the condition of diencephalic-midbrain compression by temporal lobe pressure cone, with hemorrhages and infarction of the upper pons and midbrain and with certain metabolic disorders such as hypoglycemia and hypoxia. Occasionally the mechanism of the decerebrate posture is unclear, as with certain bilateral subacute encephalitic, demyelinative, and infarctive cerebral lesions. In some instances the lesions are clearly in the cerebral white matter or basal ganglia. *Decorticate rigidity,* with arm or arms in flexion and adduction and leg(s) extended, signifies higher lesions in cerebral white matter, internal capsules, and thalamus. *Diagonal postures,* opposite arms and legs flexed and extended, probably mean supratentorial lesions; extended arms and flexed legs are probably fragments of decerebrate postures and point to midpontine lesions. *Abolition of all postures and movements* indicates acute bilateral corticospinal interruption and low pontine-medullary lesions involving reticular facilitatory (extrapyramidal) mechanisms. The coma is usually profound.

Lower brainstem reflexes are seldom helpful in the analysis of coma. Only in the most profound metabolic comas and intoxications and in the hypoxemic pannecrosis of the entire brain (brain-death syndromes) are blinking, coughing, swallowing, and spontaneous respirations all abolished. Further, the tendon and plantar reflexes give little indication of what is happening. Tendon reflexes may be preserved until late and may be normal or slightly reduced on the hemiplegic side. The plantar reflexes may be absent or extensor. Only in deep coma or in states of decerebrate rigidity will a cerebral hemiplegia not be detected by flaccidity and motionless arm and leg.

A history of headache before or at the onset of coma, recurrent vomiting, and papilledema afford the best clues to increased intracranial pressure. The lesion is most safely evidenced by computerized tomography (CT scan); however, if there is a question of subarachnoid hemorrhage or meningitis, a lumbar puncture will help. It is usually safe unless there is a herniation of the temporal lobe through the tentorium or of the cerebellum through the foramen magnum. In the latter instance the cerebrospinal fluid pressure may not reflect intracranial pressure. Papilledema may develop within 12 to 24 h in brain trauma and brain hemorrhage but, if pronounced, usually signifies a lesion of longer duration such as a brain tumor or abscess. Multiple retinal or large subhyaloid hemorrhages are usually associated with ruptured saccular aneurysm or hemorrhage from an angioma. Papilledema, with widespread retinal exudates, hemorrhages, and arteriolar changes, is an almost invariable accompaniment of hypertensive encephalopathy. See Chap. 18 for further discussion of retinal changes.

Laboratory procedures Unless the diagnosis is established at once by history and physical examination, it is necessary to carry out a number of laboratory procedures. If poisoning is suspected, the gastric contents must be aspirated and saved for later chemical analysis. A catheter is passed into the urinary bladder, and a specimen of urine is obtained for determination of specific gravity, sugar, acetone, and albumin content. Urine of low specific gravity and high protein content is nearly always found in uremia, but proteinuria may also occur for 2 or 3 days after a subarachnoid hemorrhage or with fever. Urine of high specific gravity, glycosuria, and acetonuria are almost invariable in diabetic coma; but glycosuria and hyperglycemia may result from a massive cerebral lesion. If diphenylhydantoin, bromide, or barbiturate or other intoxication is suspected, it can be verified by special tests for these substances in the blood. A blood count is made, and in malarial districts a blood smear is examined for malarial parasites. Neutrophilic leukocytosis occurs in bacterial infections and also with brain hemorrhage and softening. A blood sample should be examined for glucose, BUN, P_{CO_2}, P_{O_2}, pH, NH_3, Na, K, Cl, and Ca. The cerebrospinal fluid must be drawn if there are no lateralizing signs (CT scan if there are), and the pressure, presence of blood, white cell count, and results of Pandy's test should be recorded. Bloody cerebrospinal fluid (CSF) occurs in cerebral contusion, subarachnoid hemorrhage, brain hemorrhage, and occasionally with hemorrhagic infarcts due to arterial embolism and thrombophlebitis. If there is pleocytosis, a stained smear of the sediment should be searched for bacteria, and a rough quantitative sugar determination should be done. The standard cerebrospinal fluid formula in bacterial meningitis is elevated pressure, high white cell count (5000 to 20,000 per cubic millimeter), elevated protein level, and subnormal sugar values, but exceptionally bacteria may be seen with relatively low white cell counts. The fluid should be saved for quantitative tests for sugar and protein, and a bacterial culture and Wassermann reaction should be performed. If it is suspected that the pressure is elevated, a No. 22 needle should be used. A very high pressure must be slowly reduced by removal of 10 to 15 ml over a period of 15 to 20 min, and urea, mannitol, or other hypertonic solutions should be given to reduce brain swelling over a longer period of time. Jugular compression tests are obviously contraindicated. X-rays of the skull and CT scan should be obtained immediately if there is clinical evidence of mass lesion (one-sided neurological signs with or without papilledema), preferably between the emergency ward and the hospital room. Tests to be done later are: liver function tests, blood and CSF culture, full electrolyte evaluation, and EEG.

CLASSIFICATION OF COMA AND DIFFERENTIAL DIAGNOSIS
The demonstration of focal brain disease or meningeal irritation with cerebrospinal fluid abnormality helps in differential diagnosis. The disease that frequently cause coma may be conveniently divided into three classes, as follows:

I Diseases that cause no focal or lateralizing neurologic signs or alteration of the cellular content of the cerebrospinal fluid
  A Intoxications (alcohol, barbiturates, opiates, etc.) (Chaps. 226 to 227)
  B Metabolic disturbances (diabetic acidosis, uremia, Addisonian crises, hepatic coma, hypoglycemia, hypoxia) (Chap. 371)
  C Severe systemic infections (pneumonia, typhoid fever, malaria, Waterhouse-Friderichsen syndrome) (Chaps. 115 and 118)
  D Circulatory collapse (shock) from any cause, and cardiac decompensation in the aged (Chaps. 30 and 109)
  E Epilepsy (Chap. 23)
  F Hypertensive encephalopathy and eclampsia (Chap. 365)
  G Hyperthermia or hypothermia (Chap. 9)
  H Concussion (Chap. 366)
II Diseases that cause meningeal irritation, with either blood or an excess of white cells in the cerebrospinal fluid, usually without focal or lateralizing signs
  A Subarachnoid hemorrhage from ruptured aneurysm, occasionally trauma (Chap. 365)
  B Acute bacterial meningitis (Chap. 368)
  C Some forms of virus encephalitis (Chap. 369)
  D Acute hemorrhagic leukoencephalitis (Chap. 370)

III Diseases causing focal or lateralizing neurologic signs, with or without changes in cerebrospinal fluid
  A Brain hemorrhage (Chap. 365)
  B Brain softening due to thrombosis or embolism (Chap. 365)
  C Brain abscess (Chap. 368)
  D Epidural and subdural hemorrhage and brain contusion (Chap. 366)
  E Brain tumor (Chap. 367)
  F Miscellaneous, i.e., thrombophlebitis, some forms of virus encephalomyelitis (Chap. 369)

With the clinical laboratory tests outlined above clearly in mind, one can usually ascertain whether a patient with coma falls in one of these three classes. Concerning the group of comas without focal, lateralizing, or meningeal signs, which includes most of the secondary metabolic diseases of the brain, intoxications (both exogenous and endogenous), concussion, and postseizure states, it should be point out that a previous neurologic disease may have left residues which confuse the clinical picture. An earlier hemiparesis from vascular disease or trauma may reveal itself in an alcoholic or hepatic coma, uremia, or hyperglycemic encephalopathy. Also, in hypertensive encephalopathy transitory focal signs may sometimes be present. And occasionally, for no understandable reason, one leg may seem to move less or one plantar reflex be extensor in a metabolic coma. In actuality, the diagnosis of postepileptic coma or concussion depends on observation of the precipitating event or indirect evidence thereof; usually the diagnosis is not too long obscure, for another fit may occur and recovery of consciousness, once the seizures cease, is usually prompt. The final determination of the exact toxic or metabolic disorder requires a variety of clinical and laboratory tests, which are described in other parts of the book.

With respect to the comas of group II, the signs of meningeal irritation (head retraction, stiffness of neck on forward bending, Kernig and Brudzinski leg flexion signs) can usually be elicited in both bacterial meningitis and subarachnoid hemorrhage. However, if the coma becomes deep, stiff neck may disappear or be absent from the beginning. In such cases diagnosis is established by CSF examination. In the coma of bacterial meningitis, unless it is associated with brain swelling and cerebellar herniation, the CSF pressure is not exceptionally high (usually less than 400 mmHg); if the pressure is high, as death approaches there are signs of compression of the medulla, with fixed, dilated pupils, arrest of respiration, and fall in arterial blood pressure. Patients in coma from ruptured aneurysms also have high CSF pressure and often a massive hemispheral and ventricular extension of the hemorrhage.

In patients with group III type of coma it is the inequality of sensorimotor disturbances in the two arms and legs and the aforementioned changes in respiratory pattern, pupillary and ocular reflexes, and the remaining postural states that provide clues to serious structural lesions in the cerebrum and segmental brainstem apparatus. As the latter become prominent, they may obscure earlier signs of cerebral disease. It is noteworthy that bilateral cerebral infarction or hemorrhage or traumatic necrosis and hemorrhage may resemble the comatose state of metabolic and toxic disease, since brainstem mechanisms may be preserved; contrariwise, hepatic, hypoglycemic, and hypoxic coma will sometimes look like the coma of brainstem lesion by causing decerebrate postures. Usually, however, the CSF pressure is elevated and the fluid sanguineous in massive cerebral hemorrhage. Unilateral infarction due to anterior, middle, or posterior cerebral artery occlusion seldom produces more than a stupor or light coma; if infarction is bilateral, however, coma may be profound. Evidence of brainstem displacement and temporal lobe herniation is manifested by increased or altered ventilation (CSR, CNH), bilateral Babinski signs, dilated pupil and drooped eyelid on the side of the lesion, decerebrate postures, later dilated pupils, and loss of full ocular movements. The coma itself gives no clue to the nature of the original mass lesion. The terminal pattern of a descending gradient of diencephalic, mesencephalic, pontomedullary paralysis of nervous system is identical in all. Differential diagnosis must depend on the other data.

An error which must be cautioned against is the diagnosis of irreversible coma (brain-death syndrome) on the basis of complete abolition of all brainstem and cerebral activity and isolectric (flat) EEG if there is hypothermia or evidence of intoxication. Only with hypoxia and cerebral ischemia can this diagnosis be made securely.

Diagnosis has as its prime purpose the direction of therapy, and it matters little to the patient if we diagnose a disease for which we have no treatment. The treatable forms of coma are drug intoxications, toxemia from systemic infections, epidural and subdural hematoma, brain abscess, bacterial and tuberculous meningitis, diabetic acidosis, and hypoglycemia.

RELATIVE INCIDENCE OF DISEASES THAT CAUSE COMA

There have been only a few attempts to determine the relative incidence of diseases that lead to coma. A report from the Boston City Hospital (Solomon and Aring) included the largest series of clinical cases but was heavily skewed by the large local problem of chronic alcoholics, which made up 60 percent of all admissions in coma. Trauma (13 percent), cerebral vascular disease (10 percent), poisonings (3 percent), epilepsy (2.4 percent), diabetes, bacterial meningitis, pneumonia, uremia, and eclampsia followed in that order. In a series of 386 cases of coma of uncertain cause Plum and Posner observed that approximately 40 percent turned out to be metabolic; 25 percent, drug intoxications; and the remainder, neurologic disease of supra- or infratentorial structures.

Of course, figures like these do not provide information concerning coma caused by multiple factors. For example, a patient with a cerebral vascular lesion, old or recent, and diabetes mellitus may lapse into coma during an insulin reaction at a time when there is still sugar in the urine. Only by appreciating the interplay of these several common factors is one likely to reach the correct diagnosis.

The differential diagnosis of diseases that cause focal or lateralizing signs and meningitis is taken up under the dicussions of traumatic, neoplastic, vascular, and infective diseases of the brain.

CARE OF THE COMATOSE PATIENT

Impaired states of consciousness, regardless of their cause, are often fatal because they not only represent an advanced stage of many diseases but also add their own characteristic burden to the primary disease. The main objective of therapy is, of course, to find the cause of the coma, by utilization of procedures already outlined, and to remove it. Often, however, the disease process is one for which there is no specific therapy; or, as in hypoxia or hypoglycemia, the disease process may already have expended itself before the patient comes to the attention of the physician. Again, the problem may be infinitely complex, for the disturbance may be attributable not to a single cause but to several possible factors acting in unison, no one of which could account for the total clinical picture. In lieu of direct therapy, supportive measures must be used, and, indeed, it may be said that the patient's chances of surviving the original disease often depend in large measure on their effectiveness.

The physician must give attention to every vital function in the insensate patient. A brief outline of the more important procedures follows. In order for them to be carried out successfully, a well-coordinated team of nurses under constant guidance of a physician is needed.

1 If the patient is in shock, this takes precedence over all other abnormalities. The treatment of shock is discussed in Chap. 30.

2 Shallow and irregular respirations and cyanosis require the establishment of a clear airway and oxygen. The patient should be placed in a lateral position so that secretions and vomitus do not enter the tracheobronchial tree. Pharyngeal reflexes are usually suppressed, and therefore an endotracheal tube can be inserted without difficulty. Stagnant secretions should be removed with a suction apparatus as soon as they accumulate, since they will lead to atelectasis and bronchopneumonia. Oxygen can be administered by mask in a 100% concentration for 6 to 12 h, alternating with 50% concentration for 4 h. The depth of respiration can be increased by the use of 5 to 10% carbon dioxide for periods of 3 to 5 min every hour. Atropine should not be given; edema of the lungs and fluid in the tracheobronchial passages are not glandular secretions. Furthermore, atropine thickens the fluid and also may disturb temperature regulation of the body. Aminophylline is helpful in controlling Cheyne-Stokes breathing. Respiratory paralysis dictates the use of endotracheal intubation and a positive pressure respirator, but in the author's experience neither has been effective in comatose states in which there is disorganization of respiratory centers.

3 The temperature-regulating mechanisms may be disturbed, and extreme hypothermia, hyperthermia, or an unrecognized poikilothermia may occur. In hyperthermia, removal of blankets and use of alcohol sponges and cooling solutions are indicated. An optimal temperature is 1 to 2°C below the normal level.

4 The bladder should not be permitted to become distended. If the patient does not void, a retention catheter should be inserted. If more than 500 ml urine is found in the bladder, decompression must be carried out slowly over a period of hours. Urine excretion should be kept between 500 and 1000 ml per day. The patient should not be permitted to lie in a wet or soiled bed.

5 Diseases of the central nervous system may upset the control of water, glucose, and salt. The unconscious patient can no longer adjust the intake of food and fluids by hunger and thirst. Salt-losing and salt-retaining syndromes have both been described with brain disease. Water intoxication and severe hyponatremia may of themselves prove fatal. The maintenance of water and electrolytes is discussed in Chap. 84. If coma is prolonged, the insertion of a stomach tube will ease the problem of feeding the patient and maintaining fluid and electrolyte balance.

6 Aspiration pneumonitis should be avoided by prevention of vomiting (stomach tube), position, and restriction of oral fluids. Should it occur, corticosteroid therapy is beneficial. The legs should be examined each day for signs of thrombophlebitis.

7 If the patient is capable of moving, suitable restraints should be used to prevent a possible fall out of bed.

8 Convulsions should be controlled by measures outlined in Chap. 23. However, anticonvulsant medication should be used cautiously. An occasional seizure is less harmful than is deep coma from excessive medication.

REFERENCES

FISHER CM: Neurological examination of the comatose patient. Acta Neurol Scand 45(suppl 36):5, 1969

PLUM F, POSNER J: *Diagnosis of Stupor and Coma*, 2d ed. Philadelphia, Davis, 1975

21

DELIRIUM AND OTHER ACUTE CONFUSIONAL STATES

RAYMOND D. ADAMS
MAURICE VICTOR

All physicians sooner or later discover through clinical experience the need for special competence in assessing the mental faculties of their patients. They must be able to observe with detachment and complete objectivity their character, intelligence, mood, memory, judgment, and other attributes of personality, in much the same fashion as they observe the nutritional state and the color of the mucous membranes. The systematic examination of these affective and cognitive functions permits the physician to reach certain conclusions regarding patients' mental status, and these are also of value in understanding the patient and the illness. Without data obtained from the study of mental status, errors will be made in evaluating the reliability of the patients' histories, in diagnosing the neurologic or psychiatric diseases from which they suffer, and in conducting any proposed therapeutic program.

DEFINITION OF TERMS

The definition of normal and abnormal states of mind is difficult because the terms used to describe these states have been given so many different meanings in both medical and non-medical writings. Compounding the difficulty is the fact that the pathophysiology of the confusional states, delirium and dementia, is not fully understood, and the definitions depend on their clinical relationships, with all the lack of precision which this entails. The following nomenclature, though tentative, is useful, and is employed throughout this textbook.

Confusion is a general term denoting an incapacity of the patient to think with customary speed and clarity. This abnormality may depend on any one of several factors. In delirium, for example, inattention and the intrusion of illusory and hallucinatory experiences are mainly responsible. At certain stages in the evolution or devolution of stupor and coma, as indicated in Chap. 20, confusion is aligned with a disorder of conscious awareness and perception. In patients with dementia, confusion is related to a derangement of intellectual function, i.e., an inability to learn, remember, calculate, make appropriate deductions from given premises, reason abstractly, etc.

The term *delirium* is used here to denote a special type of confusional state, acute in onset and transient in nature, and characterized by gross disorientation in the presence of alertness and vigilance, disorder of perception in which illusions and vivid hallucinations are prominent, and overactivity of psychomotor and autonomic nervous functions. Implicit in the definition are certain nonmedical connotations of the term—intense agitation, frenzied excitement, and creations of the imagination. Most stuporous and some demented patients, in contrast to those with delirium, show a *reduced* state of alertness and attentiveness, *decreased* psychomotor activity, and a *relatively slight* tendency to hallucinate. For these reasons, and also because of the particular clinical settings in which they occur, it seems worthwhile to set the delirious states apart from those of depressed consciousness on the one hand and of dementia and amnesia on the other. Such a concept is far from new. To a greater or lesser extent, the terms exogenous reaction type, symptomatic psychosis, toxic psychosis, infective-exhaustive psychosis, and drug, traumatic, or fever delirium all have reference to the syndrome of delirium. All these terms convey the idea of an acute and transient (reversible) confusional state, occurring in a particular clinical setting and carrying a serious prognosis, by virtue of adding its burden to an already serious medical illness.

It should be pointed out that not all neuropsychiatrists agree with our distinction between *confusion* and delirium. There are some, such as Engel and Romano, and Lipowski, who use the term delirium in reference to both conditions. Our insistance on their separation is based on their different clinical manifestations and the clinical settings in which they occur.

The term *amnesia* refers to a loss of past memories coupled with an inability to form new memories, i.e., to learn. It presupposes an alert state of mind, an ability to grasp the problem, to use language normally, and to maintain adequate motivation. The failure is mainly one of retention, recall, and reproduction, and it should be distinguished from the loss of memory that accompanies states of drowsiness and acute confusion, in which information seems never to have been adequately registered in the first place or assimilated.

Dementia means loss of reason or, more particularly, a deterioration of all intellectual or cognitive functions, without clouding of consciousness or disturbance of perception. Implied in the word is the idea of a gradual enfeeblement of mental powers in a person who formerly possessed a normal mind and in most instances irreversibility. *Amentia*, by contrast, indicates a congenital feeblemindedness.

OBSERVABLE BEHAVIOR AND ITS RELATION TO CONFUSION, DELIRIUM, AMNESIA, AND DEMENTIA

The components of mentation and behavior that lend themselves to bedside examination are (1) the processes of sensation and perception; (2) the capacity for memorizing; (3) the ability to think, reason, and form logical conclusions; (4) temperament, mood, and emotion; (5) initiative, impulse, and drive; (6) insight. Of these (1) is sensorial, (2) and (3) may be considered cognitive, (4) affective, and (5) conative or volitional. Insight includes all introspective observations made by patients concerning their own normal or disordered functioning. Each component of behavior and intellection has its objective side, expressed in the manifest effects of certain stimulus conditions on patients and their behavioral responses, and its subjective side, expressed in what patients say they think and feel in relation to the stimuli.

DISTURBANCES OF PERCEPTION Perception, i.e., the processes utilized in acquiring through the senses a knowledge of the "world about" or of one's own body, involves many things aside from the simple sensory phenomenon of being aware of the attributes of a stimulus. It includes the selective focusing and maintaining of attention, elimination of all extraneous stimuli, and recognition of the stimulus by knowing its relationship to personal remembered experience. The perception of an object undergoes predictable types of derangement in disease. Most often one finds a reduction in the number of perceptions in a given unit of time and failure to synthesize them properly and relate them to the ongoing activities of the mind. There may be inattention or fluctuations of attention, distraction (pertinent and irrelevant stimuli now having equal value), and inability to persist in an assigned task. Qualitative changes also appear, mainly in the form of sensory distortions and misinterpretation and misidentification of objects and persons (illusions). These changes, at least in part, form the basis of hallucinatory experience in which the patient reports and reacts to stimuli not present in the environment. There is also an inability to perceive simultaneously all elements of a large complex of stimuli, which is referred to by some as a "failure of subjective reorganization." These major disturbances in the perceptual sphere, sometimes called "clouding of the sensorium," occur most often in acute confusional states and deliria, but quantitative deficiency may also become evident in the advanced stages of amentia and dementia.

DISTURBANCES OF MEMORY Memory, i.e., the retention of learned experiences, is involved in all mental activities. It may be arbitrarily subdivided into several parts, namely, (1) registration, which includes all that was mentioned under perception; (2) mnemonic integration and retention; (3) recall; and (4) reproduction. In disturbances of perception and attention there may be a complete failure of learning and consequently of memory for the reason that the material to be learned was never registered and assimilated. In Korsakoff's amnesic syndrome, newly presented material appears to be temporarily registered but cannot be retained for more than a few minutes, and there is always an associated defect in the recall and reproduction of memories formed some days, weeks, or months before the onset of the illness (retrograde amnesia). Dislocation of events in time and the fabrication of stories, *confabulation*, constitutes a third, but not invariable feature of the syndrome. Sound retention with failure of recall is at times a normal state; when it is severe and extends to all events of past life, it is usually due to hysteria or malingering. Proof that the processes of registration and retention are intact under these circumstances comes from hypnosis and suggestion, and questioning under amytal or pentothal narcosis, whereby the lost items are fully recalled and reproduced. In Korsakoff's amnesic state the patient fails on all tests of learning and recent memory, and behavior accords with the deficiencies of information. Since some aspect of memory is involved to some extent in all mental processes, it becomes the most testable component of mentation and behavior.

DISTURBANCES OF THINKING Thinking, which is central to so many important intellectual activities, remains one of the most elusive of all mental operations. If by thinking we mean selective ordering of symbols for problem solving and capacity to reason and form sound judgments (the usual definition), obviously the working units of most complex experiences of this type are words and numbers. The activity of substituting word and number symbols for the objects for which they stand (symbolization) is a fundamental part of the process. These symbols are formed into ideas or concepts, and the arrangement of new and remembered ideas into certain orders or relationships, according to the rules of logic, constitutes another intricate part of thought. One test is problem solving—the capacity to formulate a problem into several hypotheses, to analyze critically the evidence for and against each hypothesis, and to make a correct choice. In a general way one may examine thinking for speed and efficiency, ideational content, coherence and logical relationships of ideas, quantity and quality of associations to a given idea, and the propriety of the feeling and behavior engendered by an idea.

Information concerning the thought processes and associative functions is best obtained by analyzing the patient's spontaneous verbal productions and by engaging him or her in conversation. If the patient is taciturn or mute, one may then have to depend on the responses to direct questions or upon written material, i.e., letters, etc. One notes the prevailing trends of the patient's thoughts; whether the ideas are reasonable, precise, and coherent or vague, circumstantial, tangential, and irrelevant; and whether the thought processes are shallow and fragmented. Disorders of thought are frequent in confusional states and in degenerative and other types of cerebral disease. The organization of thought may be disrupted with fragmentation, repetition, and perseveration. This is spoken of as *incoherence* and characterizes many acute confusional and delirious states. The patient may be excessively critical, rationalizing, and hairsplitting; this is a type of thinking often manifest in depressive psychoses. Derangements of thinking may also take the form of a flight of ideas. The patient moves nimbly from one idea to another, and associations are numerous and loosely linked. This is a common feature of hypomanic or manic states. The opposite condition, poverty of ideas, is characteristic both of depression, where it is combined with gloomy thoughts, and of dementing disorder, where it is part of a general reduction in intellectual activity. Thinking may be distorted in such a way that the patient fails to check his or her ideas against reality. When a false belief is maintained in spite of normally convincing contradictory evidence, the patient is said to have a *delusion*. Delusions are common to many illnesses, particularly manic-depressive and schizophrenic states. Ideas may seem to the patient to have been implanted in the mind by some outside agency such as radio, television, or atomic energy. These reflect the passivity feelings characteristic of schizophrenic psychoses. Other distortions of thinking, such as gaps or condensations of logical associations are also typical of schizophrenia, of which they constitute a diagnostic feature.

DISTURBANCES OF EMOTION, MOOD, AND AFFECT The emotional life of the patient is expressed in a variety of ways. In the first place, rather marked individual differences in basic temperament are to be observed in the normal population; some persons are throughout their life cheerful, gregarious, optimistic, and free from worry, whereas others are just the opposite. The unusually volatile, cyclothymic person is believed to be liable to manic-depressive psychosis, and the suspicious, withdrawn, introverted person to schizophrenia and paranoia. Strong, persistent emotional states such as fear and anxiety may occur as reactions to life situations and may be accompanied by derangements of visceral function. If excessive and disproportionate to the stimulus and persistent, they are usually manifestations of an anxiety neurosis, depression, or autism and schizophrenia. Variations in the degree of responsiveness to emotional stimuli are also frequent and, when excessive and persistent, assume importance. In depression all stimuli tend to enhance the somber mood of unhappiness. Emotional response that is excessively labile, variable from moment to moment, and poorly controlled or uninhibited is a condition common to many diseases of the cerebrum, particularly those involving the corticopontine and corticobulbar pathways. It constitutes a part of the syndrome of pseudobulbar palsy. All emotional expression may be lacking, as in apathetic states or severe depressions, or the patient may be a victim of every trivial problem in daily life; i.e., cannot control worries. Finally, the emotional response may be inappropriate to the stimulus, e.g., a depressing or morbid thought may seem amusing and be attended by a smile or arouse no emotional reaction, as in schizophrenia.

Since there are relatively few overt manifestations of temperament, mood, and other emotional experiences described above, the physician must evaluate these states by the appearance of the patient and by verbalized accounts of feelings. For these purposes it is convenient to divide emotionality into mood and feeling or affect. By *mood* is meant the prevailing emotional state of the individual without reference to the stimuli immediately impinging upon him or her. It may be pleasant and cheerful or melancholic. The language, e.g., the adjectives used, and the facial expressions, attitudes, postures, and speed of movement most reliably betray the patient's mood. By contrast, *feelings* (or *affect*) are said to be emotional experiences evoked by particular stimuli.

DISTURBANCES IN IMPULSE Impulse, that basic biologic urge, driving force, or purpose, by which every organism is directed to reach its full potentialities, appears to be another extremely important and observable, though somewhat neglected, dimension of behavior. Again, one notes wide normal variations from one person to another in strength of impulse to action and thought, and these individual differences are present throughout life. One of the most conspicuous pathologic deviations is an apparent constitutional weakness in impulse in certain neurotic persons. Moreover, with many types of cerebral disease (particularly those which involve the posterior orbital parts of the frontal lobes, medial forebrain tracts, and lateral hypothalamus), a reduction in impulse is coupled with an indifference or lack of concern about the consequences of actions. In such cases all other measurable aspects of psychic function may be normal. Extreme degrees of lack of impulse, or *abulia,* may take the form of mutism and immobility, a state sometimes called *akinetic mutism.* Psychomotor retardation is a lesser degree of the same state and is a feature of both cerebral disease and depression. In the latter instance mood alteration and extreme fatigability are conjoined.

LOSS OF INSIGHT Insight, the state of being fully aware of the nature and degree of one's deficits, becomes manifestly impaired or abolished in relation to all types of cerebral disease that cause complex disorders of behavior. Rarely does the patient with any of these disorders seek advice or help for the illness. Instead, the family usually brings the individual to the physician. Thus, it appears that the diseases which produce many of the high-order or complex mental abnormalities not only evoke observable changes in mentation and behavior but also alter or reduce the patient's capacity for self-observation.

DELIRIUM

CLINICAL FEATURES These are most perfectly depicted in the alcoholic patient. The symptoms usually develop over a period of 2 or 3 days. The first indications of the approaching attack are difficulty in concentrating, restless irritability, tremulousness, insomnia, and poor appetite. One or several generalized convulsions are the initial major symptom in almost 30 percent of the cases. The patient's rest becomes troubled by unpleasant and terrifying dreams. There may be momentary disorientation or an occasional inappropriate remark.

These initial symptoms rapidly give way to a clinical picture that, in severe cases, is one of the most colorful and dramatic in medicine. The state of consciousness becomes altered ("clouded"); it is clouded in that the patient is inattentive and unable to perceive all elements of the situation. There may be incessant talking, and the patient may be incoherent and look distressed and perplexed; his or her expression is in keeping with vague notions of being annoyed or pursued by some threatening person. From the patient's manner and from the content of his or her speech it is evident that the patient misinterprets the meaning of ordinary objects and ambient sounds and has vivid visual, auditory, and tactile hallucinations, often of a most unpleasant type. At first the patient can be brought momentarily into touch with reality and may in fact answer questions correctly; but almost at once there is a relapse into the preoccupied, confused state; the patient gives wrong answers, is unable to think coherently, and is incapable of proper self-orientation. Before long the patient is unable to shake off the hallucinations even for a second and does not recognize family or physician. Tremor and restless movements are usually present and may be violent. Sleep is impossible or occurs only in brief naps. The countenance is flushed, the pupils are dilated, and the conjunctivas are injected; the pulse is rapid,

and the temperature may be raised. There is much sweating, and the urine is scanty and of high specific gravity. The signs of overactivity of the autonomic nervous system, more than any other, distinguish delirium from all other confusional states.

The symptoms abate, either suddenly or gradually, after 2 or 3 days, although in exceptional cases they may persist for several weeks. The most certain indication of the end of the attack is the occurrence of sound sleep and of lucid intervals of increasing length. Recovery is usually complete.

Delirium is subject to all degrees of variability, not only from patient to patient but in the same patient from day to day and hour to hour. The entire syndrome may be observed in one patient and only one or two components in another. In its mildest form, as so often occurs in febrile diseases, it consists of an occasional wandering of the mind and incoherence of verbal expression, interrupted by periods of lucidity. This form, lacking motor and autonomic overactivity, is sometimes referred to as a *quiet delirium* (or *hypokinetic delirium*) and is difficult to distinguish from other confusional states. The most severe form, best exemplified by delirium tremens, may progress to a "muttering stupor" and in about 10 percent of patients ends fatally.

MORBID ANATOMY AND PATHOPHYSIOLOGY The brains of patients who have died in delirium tremens usually show no pathologic changes of significance. A number of diseases, however, may cause delirium and also give rise to focal lesions in the brain, such as focal embolic encephalitis, viral encephalitis, Wernicke's disease, or trauma. The topography of these lesions is of particular interest. They tend to be localized in the midbrain and subthalamus and in the temporal lobes, where they involve the reticular activating and limbic systems.

Penfield's studies of the human cortex during surgical exploration clearly indicate the importance of the temporal lobe in producing visual, auditory, and olfactory hallucinations. With subthalamic and midbrain lesions there may be visual hallucinations that are not unpleasant, animated, and accompanied by good insight (the peduncular hallucinosis of Lhermitte).

The electroencephalogram in delirium may show nonfocal slow activity in the 5- to 7-per-second range, a state that rapidly returns to normal as the delirium clears. In other cases only low voltage, fast activity in the fast beta frequency range is seen, and in milder degrees of delirium there is usually no abnormality at all.

An analysis of the several conditions conducive to delirium suggests at least three different physiologic mechanisms. The withdrawal of alcohol, barbiturates, or other sedative hypnotic drugs, following a period of chronic intoxication is the most common cause of delirium (Chaps. 226 and 228). These drugs are known to have a strong depressant effect on certain areas of the central nervous system; presumably the release and overactivity of these parts, after withdrawal of the drug, are the basis of delirium. In the case of bacterial infections and poisoning by certain drugs, such as atropine and scopolamine, the delirious state probably results from the direct action of the toxin or chemical agent on these same parts of the brain. Thirdly, destructive lesions, such as acute inclusion body encephalitis of the temporal lobes, may cause delirium by disturbing the function of certain areas, particularly the inferotemporal portions of the temporal lobes.

ACUTE CONFUSIONAL STATES ASSOCIATED WITH REDUCED MENTAL ALERTNESS AND RESPONSIVENESS

In the most typical examples, all mental functions are reduced to some degree, but alertness, attentiveness, and the ability to grasp all elements of the immediate situation suffer most. In the mildest form the patient may pass for normal, and only failure to recollect and reproduce happenings of the past few hours or days reveals the inadequacy of mental function. The more obviously confused patient spends much time in idleness, and what is done may be inappropriate and annoying to others. Only the more automatic acts and verbal responses are properly performed, but these may permit the examiner to obtain from the patient a number of relevant and accurate replies to questions about age, occupation, and residence. Reactions are slow and indecisive, and it is difficult for the patient to sustain a conversation. There may be dozing during the interview and the patient may sleep more hours each day than is natural or the same number at more irregular intervals. Responses tend to be rather abrupt, brief, and mechanical. Disturbances of perception are frequent, and voices, common objects, and the actions of other persons are frequently misinterpreted. Often one cannot discern whether the patient hears voices and sees things that do not exist, i.e., whether the person is hallucinating, or merely misinterpreting stimuli in the environment. Inadequate perception and forgetfulness result in a constant state of bewilderment. Failing to recognize the surroundings and having lost all sense of time, the patient repeats the same question and makes the same remarks over and over again. Irritability may or may not be present. Some patients are extremely suspicious, demanding, and aggressive; in fact, a paranoid trend may be the most pronounced and troublesome feature of the illness.

As the confusion deepens, conversation becomes more difficult, and at a certain stage the patient no longer notices or responds to much of what is occurring. Replies to questions may be with a single word or a short phrase spoken in a soft tremulous voice or whisper. The patient may be mute. In its most advanced stages confusion gives way to stupor and finally to coma. As the patient improves, there may again be a stage of stupor and confusion, occurring in the reverse order. All this informs us that at least one category of confusion is but a manifestation of the same disease processes that in their severest form cause coma.

In the most typical cases, this type of confusional state is readily distinguished from delirium; in others with more than the usual degree of irritability and restlessness, one cannot fail to notice the resemblance to delirium. Similarly, certain cases of delirium, in which tremor, vivid hallucinations, vigilant excited attitude, and insomnia, are relatively inconspicuous, are difficult to distinguish from other acute confusional states. The same diagnostic difficulty arises when a delirium is complicated by an illness that superimposes stupor (e.g., delirium tremens with pneumonia or meningitis).

When clouding of consciousness is minimal and the confusion is of insidious onset and several weeks duration, it may mimic dementia. Lipowski has called it "reversible dementia," claiming it to be an intermediate state between delirium and dementia and still potentially reversible. We would classify it as a protracted confusional state.

SENILE DEMENTIA AND OTHER CEREBRAL DISEASES COMPLICATED BY MEDICAL OR SURGICAL ILLNESS (BECLOUDED DEMENTIA)

Many elderly patients who enter the hospital with medical or surgical illness are mentally confused. Presumably the liability to this state is determined by preexisting brain disease, in this instance senile dementia, which may or may not have been obvious to the family before the onset of the complicating illness. Other cerebral diseases (vascular, neoplastic, demyelinative) may have the same effect of increasing the patient's liability to confusion.

All the clinical features of hypokinetic delirium or of acute confusion may be present. The severity may vary greatly. The confusion may be reflected only in the patient's inability to relate sequentially the history of the illness, or it may be so severe that the patient is virtually *non compos mentis*.

Although almost any complicating illness may bring out the confusion, it is particularly frequent with infectious disease; with posttraumatic and postoperative states, notably after concussive brain injuries; with the removal of cataracts (in which case the confusion is probably related to being temporarily deprived of vision); and with congestive heart failure, chronic respiratory disease, and severe anemia, especially pernicious anemia. Often it is difficult to determine which of several possible factors is responsible for the confusion in this heterogeneous group of illnesses, and there may be more than one. A cardiac patient with a confusional psychosis may be febrile, have marginally reduced cerebral blood flow, be intoxicated by one or more drugs, and be in electrolyte imbalance.

When these patients recover from a medical or surgical illness, they usually return to their premorbid state, though their shortcomings, now drawn to the attention of the family and physician, may be more obvious than before.

CLASSIFICATION AND DIAGNOSIS (See Table 21-1)

The first step in *diagnosis* is to recognize that the patient is confused. This is obvious in most cases, but, as pointed out above, the mildest form of confusion, particularly when some other acute alteration of personality is prominent, may be overlooked. In these mild forms a careful analysis of the thought patterns as the patient gives the history of the illness and the details of personal life will usually reveal an incoherence. Digit span and serial subtraction of 3s and 7s from 100 are useful bedside tests of the patient's capacity for sustained mental activity. Memory of recent events is one of the most delicate tests of adequate mental function and may be accomplished by having the patient relate all the details of entry into the hospital, laboratory tests, etc.

A certain proportion of psychoses of the schizophrenic or manic-depressive type first become manifest during an acute medical illness or following an operation or parturition. A causal relationship between the two is usually sought but cannot be established. Usually the psychosis began long before but was not recognized. The diagnostic studies of the psychiatric illness must proceed along the lines suggested below. Close observation will usually reveal a clear sensorium and relatively intact memory, which permits differentiation from the acute confusional states.

Once it is established that the patient is confused, the differential diagnosis must be made among delirium, acute confusional states associated with psychomotor underactivity, and a beclouded dementia. This can be done usually by careful attention to the patient's degree of alertness and wakefulness, capacity to solve new problems, memory, accuracy of perception, and hallucinations. The distinction between confusional states and dementia may be difficult at times.

CARE OF THE DELIRIOUS AND CONFUSED PATIENT

The physician must be secure in the ability to manage the delirious and confused patient because such illnesses are observed almost daily on the medical and surgical wards of a general hospital. Occurring as they do during an infective fever, in the course of another illness such as cardiac failure, or following an injury, operation, or withdrawal from alcohol, they never fail to create grave problems. The physician's program of treatment may constantly be threatened by the patient's agitation, sleeplessness, and uncooperative attitude. The nursing personnel are often sorely taxed by the necessity of providing a satisfactory environment for the convalescence of the patient and, at the same time, maintaining a tranquil atmosphere for the other patients. And the family is appalled by the sudden specter of insanity and all that it entails.

The primary therapeutic effort is directed to the control of the underlying medical disease. Other important objectives are to quiet the patient and protect him or her against injury. A private nurse, an attendant, or a member of the family should be with the patient at all times, if this can be arranged. Depending on how active and vigorous the patient is, a locked room, screened windows that cannot be opened by the patient, and a low bed or mattress on the floor should be arranged. It is often better for the patient to be allowed to walk about the room rather than be tied into bed, which may excite or frighten him or her into struggling to the point of complete exhaustion and collapse. If less active, the patient can usually be kept in bed by leather wrist restraints, a restraining sheet, or a net thrown over the bed. Unless it is contraindicated by the primary disease, the patient should be permitted to sit up or walk about the room part of the day.

TABLE 21-1
Classification of delirium and acute confusional states

I Delirium
  A In a medical or surgical illness (no focal or lateralizing neurologic signs; cerebrospinal fluid usually clear)
    1 Typhoid fever
    2 Pneumonia
    3 Septicemia, particularly erysipelas and other streptococcal infections
    4 Rheumatic fever
    5 Thyrotoxicosis and ACTH intoxication (rare)
    6 Postoperative and posttraumatic states
  B In neurologic disease that causes focal or lateralizing signs or changes in the cerebrospinal fluid
    1 Vascular, neoplastic, or other diseases, particularly those involving the temporal lobes and upper part of the brainstem
    2 Cerebral contusion and laceration (traumatic delirium)
    3 Acute bacterial and tuberculous meningitis
    4 Subarachnoid hemorrhage
    5 Viral encephalitis
  C The abstinence states, exogenous intoxications, and postconvulsive states; signs of other medical, surgical, and neurologic illnesses absent or coincidental
    1 Withdrawal of alcohol (delirium tremens), barbiturates, and nonbarbiturate sedative drugs, following chronic intoxication (Chaps. 226 and 228)
    2 Drug intoxications: camphor, caffeine, ergot, bromides, scopolamine, atropine, amphetamine
    3 Postconvulsive delirium
II Acute confusional states associated with psychomotor underactivity
  A Associated with a medical or surgical disease (no focal lateralizing neurologic signs; cerebrospinal fluid clear)
    1 Metabolic disorders: hepatic stupor, uremia, hypoxia, hypercapnea, hypoglycemia, porphyria
    2 Infective fevers
    3 Congestive heart failure
    4 Postoperative and posttraumatic psychoses
  B Associated with drug intoxication (no focal or lateralizing signs; cerebrospinal fluid clear): opiates, barbiturates, bromides, Artane, etc.
  C Associated with diseases of the nervous system (the focal or lateralizing neurologic signs and cerebrospinal fluid changes of these conditions are commoner than in delirium)
    1 Cerebral vascular disease, tumor, abscess
    2 Subdural hematoma
    3 Meningitis
    4 Encephalitis
  D Beclouded dementia, i.e., senile or other brain disease in combination with infective fevers, drug reactions, heart failure, or other medical or surgical disease

All drugs that could possibly be responsible for delirium—particularly opiates, barbiturates, bromides, atropine, hyoscine, cortisone, adrenocorticotropic hormone (ACTH), and salicylates in large doses—should be discontinued (unless withdrawal effects are believed to underlie the illness). Paraldehyde and choral hydrate are trustworthy sedatives under these circumstances. Paraldehyde, which is preferred, may be given orally or rectally in doses of 10 to 12 ml. For oral administration, mixing it with fruit juices makes it more palatable. Chlorpromazine, chlordiazepoxide, and diazepam are often extremely effective if given in full doses, and should be continued until natural sleep is restored. One must be cautious in attempting to suppress agitation completely. To accomplish this may require very large doses of drugs, and vital functions may then be dangerously impaired. The purpose of sedation is to ensure rest and sleep so that the patient does not become exhausted.

Confusional states related to antidepressant drugs, e.g., amitriptyline, are said to be reversed by a 2-mg dose of physostigmine.

A fluid intake and output chart should be kept, and any fluid and electrolyte deficit should be corrected. The pulse and blood pressure should be recorded at intervals of 2 h in anticipation of circulatory collapse. Transfusions of whole blood and vasopressor drugs may be lifesaving.

Finally, the physician should be aware of many small therapeutic measures that may allay fear and suspicion and reduce the tendency to hallucinations. The room should be kept dimly lighted at night, and if possible the patient should not be moved from one room to another. Every procedure should be explained in detail, even such simple ones as the taking of blood pressure or temperature. The presence of a member of the family may enable the patient to maintain contact with reality.

Most delirious patients tend to recover if they are placed in good hygienic surroundings and competently nursed. The family should be reassured on this point and must also understand that the abnormal behavior and irrational actions of the patient are not willful but rather are symptomatic of a brain disease. Once recovered, the patient will be at least partly amnesic for the period of the delirium or confusion, a gap which must be filled by information provided by physician and family.

REFERENCES

ADAMS RD, VICTOR M: *Principles of Neurology*. New York, McGraw-Hill, 1977

BENSON FD, BLUMER D: *Psychiatric Aspects of Neurologic Disease*. New York, Grune & Stratton, 1975, chap 2

LIPOWSKI ZJ: Delirium, clouding of consciousness and confusion. J Nerv Ment Dis 145:227, 1967

22
SLEEP AND ITS ABNORMALITIES

RAYMOND D. ADAMS

NORMAL SLEEP The pattern of sleeping varies in the different epochs of life. A nocturnal predominance begins to appear after the first few weeks of postnatal life, resulting in the biphasic pattern of sleeping and waking which persists throughout adolescence and adult years, unless altered by disease. Not until old age does it break down progressively. Night awakenings then increase in frequency, and the daytime waking period becomes interrupted frequently by paroxysmal bursts of sleep lasting 1 to 10 s (microsleep) and by longer naps. Throughout most of life females are said to need about an hour more sleep than males.

Physiologic mechanisms By means of electroencephalographic analysis five stages of sleep, associated with two alternating physiologic mechanisms, have been defined. Relaxed wakefulness is found to be accompanied by sinusoidal alpha waves of 8 to 12 cycles per second (cps) and low-voltage fast activity of mixed frequency in the EEG; there are the usual associated blinks, eye and limb movements, and moderate tone in all the skeletal muscles. As a person falls asleep and the muscles relax, the eyelids droop, the eyes begin to roll from side to side, and the EEG pattern changes to one of progressively lower voltage and mixed frequency. This is called stage I sleep. As sleep deepens into stage II, bursts of 12- to 14-cps waves (sleep spindles) and high-amplitude, sharp, slow-wave (k) complexes appear. By now eye movements have ceased, but muscle tone is maintained. The deep sleep of stages III and IV is featured by an increasing proportion of high-voltage, slow-wave activity in the EEG. In stage V, rapid eye movements return and muscle tension increases in the jaw, whereas the neck, trunk, and limb muscles, after a few quivering, tremulous, or myoclonic movements, become completely slack. The first four stages are called *nonrapid eye movement sleep* (NREMS); the last stage is variously designated as *rapid eye movement sleep* (REMS), *paradoxic sleep* (PS), or *activated sleep* (AS).

In a typical night the normal drowsy adult passes successively through stages I, II, III, and IV of NREMS. After about 70 min, mostly spent in stages III and IV, the first REMS period occurs, usually heralded by an increase in body movements and a shift in the EEG pattern from stage IV to II. This NREMS-REMS cycle (activity-rest cycle of Kleitman) is repeated at about the same interval four to six times during the night, depending on the length of sleep. The first REMS cycle may be brief, and the later cycles include less stage IV NREMS.

There is some evidence that the two alternating physiologic sleep mechanisms for NREMS and REMS lie in the brainstem and are influenced by biogenic amines, particularly 5-hydroxytryptamine (serotonin) and norepinephrine. The serotoninergic neurons are known to be located in the medial tegmentum of the medulla, pons, and lower midbrain and to project upward to the hypothalamus and thalamus and to the orbital frontal and medial temporal (limbic) cortex. Activation of serotoninergic neurons, presumably by factor S (see below), suppresses the higher reticular formation subserving consciousness and causes hypersomnia with increase in NREMS and REMS; their destruction or pharmacologic suppression by serotonin antagonists results in insomnia, with disappearance of both NREMS and REMS. Another group of neurons, presumably responsive to dopamine and norepinephrine, lies in the lateral tegmentum of the pons, the locus ceruleus, substantia nigra, and hypothalamus and are necessary for REMS. Their activation increases REMS and their destruction or suppression by norepinephrine antagonists reduces or abolishes it. However, REMS is primed by NREMS serotoninergic neurons, and the two types of sleep are always closely related. Only under conditions of narcolepsy, cataplexy, and sleep paralysis (see below) is REMS separated from NREMS. Monoamine oxidase inhibitors selectively diminish or abolish REMS. Thus, normal sleep involves both a serotoninergic mechanism and a catecholaminergic or adrenergic mechanism.

The details of the neuropharmacology of sleep have not yet been fully ascertained. In some mysterious way, a product(s) of fatigue or some obscure hypnotoxin activates the serotoninergic neurons subserving NREMS and at the same time suppresses the effects of afferent stimulation of the upper reticular

formation. It is not known how neuronal systems of REMS are suppressed for a time during NREMS and periodically become active and interrupt it. The plasma of drowsy or sleeping animals has been shown by Monnier to contain factor delta, a substance with properties that induce somnolence and increase NREMS in alert animals. More recently Pappenheimer and his associates have isolated a factor S from the cerebrospinal fluid and brain of animals deprived of sleep. When injected into rats and rabbits, it induces slow-wave sleep lasting 4 to 6 h. Its molecular weight is about 350, and it is destroyed by pronase, indicating the presence of peptides. Probably it is similar if not identical to the sleep-promoting factor isolated by Nagasaki.

EFFECTS OF SLEEP LOSS Of all the conditions that make for human efficiency and sense of well-being, sleep is one of the most important. Deprived of sleep, experimental animals will die within a few days, no matter how well they are fed, watered, and housed; under similar circumstances human beings suffer a variety of unpleasant symptoms that must be separated from the diseases that cause insomnia.

Human beings deprived of sleep (NREM and REM) for periods of 60 to 200 h experience increasing fatigue and irritability and find it difficult to concentrate, to perceive accurately, and to maintain their orientation. Illusions and hallucinations intrude into consciousness, primarily in the visual and tactile sensory fields, becoming more intense as the period of sleeplessness is prolonged. Performance of motor tasks deteriorates. If the tests are of short duration and of slow pace, the subject can keep up, but cannot if speed and perseverance are demanded. Incentive to work weakens, and sustained action is interrupted by lapses of attention. Neurologic signs include mild and fleeting nystagmus, a slight tremor of the hands, ptosis of eyelids, expressionless face, and thickness of speech, with mispronunciation and incorrect choice of words. A decrement of alpha waves appears in the EEG, and closing of the eyes no longer generates alpha activity. The concentration of 17-hydroxycorticosteroids increases in the blood, and catecholamine output rises.

Recovery after prolonged sleep deprivation shows that the amount of sleep required to recuperate is never equal to the amount lost. At first, the subject rapidly falls into stage IV of NREMS, often with "supernormal" slow waves in the EEG and remains there, at the expense of stage II sleep; stage IV is interrupted from time to time by REM which remains in the usual proportion. But by the second night, REMS rebounds and exceeds that of the predeprivation period. Stage IV NREMS seems, then, to be the most valuable stage in restoring the flagging functions of the nervous system.

The effects of partial and differential deprivation are somewhat different. If prevented night after night from having REMS, subjects show a greater tendency to become hyperactive and emotionally labile, and less able to control their impulses, a state which corresponds to the heightened activity, excessive appetite, and oversexuality of REMS-deprived animals. Differential deprivation of NREMS (stages III and IV) leads, instead, to hyporesponsiveness.

Of course, since the need for sleep is known to vary from person to person in everyday life, it is difficult to decide what is partial sleep deprivation. Some individuals function perfectly on as little as 3 or 4 h per night, and others, who sleep long hours, claim not to obtain the maximum benefit from it.

DERANGEMENTS OF SLEEP **Insomnia** This word signifies want of sleep, and is used popularly to indicate any impairment in its duration, depth, or restorative properties. Quantitative precision as to what constitutes insomnia is impossible because of the uncertainty as to the natural requirement of sleep and also its role in the economy of the human body.

Two classes of insomniacs may be defined: one in which there appears to be a primary disturbance of the normal sleep mechanism, the other in which sleep impairment is secondary to another disease or condition. The latter is encountered frequently in medical practice and may usually be ascribed to pain or some other annoying sensation, or to nervousness, anxiety, and worry.

The term *primary insomnia* should be reserved for those persons who throughout their lives have never enjoyed restful slumber, and in whom none of the usual symptoms of neurosis, depression, or other psychiatric or medical diseases can be elicited. Unlike the rare individuals who seem to thrive on 3 to 4 h sleep a night, they suffer the effects of partial sleep deprivation and resort to drugs and various techniques to induce or maintain sleep. Their life comes so obviously to revolve around sleep that they have been called "sleep pedants" or "sleep hypochondriacs." They sleep for shorter periods than normal persons, awaken more often, spend less time in REMS and more in stage II NREMS, move more often, have more rapid pulse, peripheral vasoconstriction, and higher body temperature, and show a heightened physiologic arousal. Thus their sleep is both quantitatively and qualitatively different from that of "good sleepers."

While there is no doubt that the victims of insomnia, regardless of the cause of their wakefulness, are likely to exaggerate the amount of sleep lost, *primary insomnia* should be recognized as an entity and not passed off as a neurotic quirk.

Of the sensory disorders conducive to abnormal wakefulness, pain in the spine with or without nerve root involvement stands out, as does abdominal discomfort from peptic ulcer and carcinoma. Tired, aching, restless legs, an obscure benign state known as the "restless leg syndrome" (anxietas tibialis), may regularly delay the onset of sleep. Excessive fatigue may give rise to many abnormal muscular sensations of similar nature. Acroparesthesias, peculiar nocturnal tingling and numbness of palms and fingers due to tight carpal ligaments (carpal tunnel syndrome), may awaken the patient at night, as does cluster or histamine headache, which nearly always occurs 2 to 3 h after falling asleep.

Severe insomnia is a frequent complaint of patients suffering from psychiatric disease (more than 85 percent of a group of insomniacs in one series). Its simplest form occurs in a reactive nervous state in which domestic and business worries keep the patient's mind in a turmoil. Also, vigorous mental activity late at night or excitement which leaves the muscles tense counteracts drowsiness and sleep. Under these circumstances there is difficulty in falling asleep and a tendency to sleep late in the morning.

Sleeplessness is also commonly recorded in the histories of patients suffering from psychoneuroses and psychoses. Illnesses in which anxiety and fear are prominent symptoms usually result in difficulty in falling asleep and light, fitful, or intermittent sleep. Also, disturbing dreams are frequent and may awaken the patient; exceptionally, the patient may even try to stay awake in order to avoid them. The diurnal-nocturnal timing of sleep is altered, but quality and quantity are little if at all changed. In contrast, the depressive illnesses, particularly the manic-depressive or involutional type, cause either light sleep in the early part of the night or early morning waking and inability to return to sleep. Quantity of sleep is reduced, and nocturnal mobility is increased. The REMS, although not reduced, comes earlier in the night; this is termed the *increased pressure of REMS*. If anxiety is combined with depression,

both the above patterns are observed. In states of mania, sleep diminishes and REMS may be abolished. The sleep rhythm may be totally deranged in acute confusional states and delirium, and REMS increases. In the latter the patient may only doze for short periods, both day and night. The total amount and depth of sleep in a 24-h period are reduced. Frightening hallucinations may prevent sleep. The senile and arteriosclerotic patient tends to catnap during the day and then refuses to go to bed at night. The nocturnal sleep is intermittent; its total amount may be either increased or decreased.

Disturbances in the transitional period of sleep As sleep comes on, certain nervous centers may be excited to a burst of insubordinate activity. The result is a sudden start that arouses the incipient sleeper. It may involve one or both legs or the trunk, less often the arms. If the start occurs repeatedly during the process of falling asleep and is a nightly event, it may become a matter of great concern to the patient.

Sensory centers may be disturbed in a similar way, either as an isolated phenomenon or in association with phenomena that induce motion. The patient may drop off to sleep but be aroused by a sensation that darts through the body. Or a sudden clang or crashing sound disturbs commencing sleep. Sometimes there is a sudden flash of light or a sensation of being lifted and dashed to earth or of being turned. These symptoms are probably similar sensory paroxysms involving the labyrinthine mechanism.

Sleep palsies and acroparesthesias Curious and at times distressing paresthetic disturbances develop during sleep. Everyone is familiar with the phenomenon of an arm or leg "falling asleep." The immobility of the limbs and the maintenance of uncomfortable postures without being aware of them permit pressure to be applied to exposed nerves. The ulnar, radial, and peroneal nerves are quite superficial in places; pressure of the nerve against an underlying bone may interfere with intraneural circulation of the compressed segment. If such pressure is continued for half an hour or longer, a sensory and motor paralysis sometimes referred to as *sleep palsy* may develop. This condition usually lasts only a few minutes or hours, but if the compression is prolonged, the nerve may be severely damaged so that functional recovery awaits remyelination or regeneration. Unusually deep sleep, as in alcoholic intoxication, renders the patient especially liable to sleep palsies merely because the patient does not heed the discomfort of an unnatural posture.

Acroparesthesias are frequent in adult women and are not unknown to men. The patient complains of being awakened by an intense numbness, tingling, prickling, a feeling of "pins and needles" in the fingers and hands after being asleep for a few hours. There are also aching, burning pains or tightness and other unpleasant sensations. At first there is a suspicion of having slept on the arm, but the usual bilaterality and the occurrence regardless of the position of the arms dispel this notion. Usually the paresthesias are in the distribution of the median nerves. Vigorous rubbing of the hands restores normal sensation, and the paresthesias subside within a few minutes, only to return later upon first awakening in the morning. The condition seldom occurs during the daytime unless the patient is lying down or sitting with the arms and hands in one position. When acroparesthesias are frequent, the hands may at all times feel swollen, stiff, clumsy, slightly numb, and sometimes distressingly painful. More severe degrees of this condition merge with the compression syndrome of the median nerve (carpal tunnel syndrome) described in Chaps. 19 and 377.

Nightmares and night terrors (pavor nocturnus) Awakening in a state of terror has happened to nearly everyone. Children are especially susceptible. Fever disposes to it, as may many other conditions, such as indigestion. Bad dreams, stimulated directly by the reading of blood-curdling stories or seeing exciting television programs before bedtime, may be followed by a nightmare. Nightmares differ from night terrors only in the greater intensity of the anxiety and extreme degree of autonomic discharges in the latter. In addition there is more vocalization and motor activity, even to the point of running as if pursued. Then night terror and somnambulism are combined. Gastaut and his associates, who have compared nightmares and night terrors, found the latter to occur in stage IV NREMS often within a half hour of falling asleep. The patient suddenly develops an arousal response (imperfect) with return of alpha rhythm in the EEG and a pattern of extreme motility. Vocalizations, walking, screams, tachycardia (130 to 170 beats per min) and increase in respiratory rate, all lasting a few minutes, may occur.

Such phenomena are of little significance as isolated events in childhood. Indeed, few children have escaped the more frequent experience of nightmare. Only if persistent and frequent do they become matters of pressing medical complaint. Of greater importance is the differentiation of both the nightmare and night terror from nocturnal epilepsy, which also may have a tendency to occur only during a specific stage of sleep. Pharmacologic agents which interfere with the metabolism of either serotonin or norepinephrine offer a possible therapeutic approach to both nightmares and night terrors.

Somnambulism and sleep automatism Examples of sleepwalking occasionally come to the attention of the practicing physician. This condition likewise occurs more often in children than in adults. After being asleep for a time, the patient arises from bed, walks about the house, and may turn on a light or perform some other familiar act. There is no outward sign of emotion; the eyes are open, and the sleeper is guided by vision, thus avoiding familiar objects. The sight of an unfamiliar object may awaken the sleeper. If spoken to, there is no response; if told to return to bed, the sleeper may do so but more often must be led back to it. Sometimes strange phrases or sentences are muttered over and over. The following morning there is usually no memory of the episode. Talking in one's sleep is probably a minor variant.

Nocturnal epilepsy Paroxysmal abnormalities of the brain waves of the type seen in epilepsy tend to occur in epileptic patients during or shortly after the onset of sleep. Not infrequently an individual subject to grand mal attacks will have them only at night during sleep.

Nocturnal jerks of the legs, also called *nocturnal myoclonus*, are another troublesome symptom because they interfere with sleep night after night. This condition differs from the restless leg syndrome in that involuntary movements occur. Only recently has it been classified as a myoclonic form of epilepsy. It is unaccompanied by all other epileptic manifestations. Anticonvulsant drugs are said to control it, though in two cases the author has had better success with an occasional dose of purified opium alkaloids (Pantopon). Obviously an opiate cannot be prescribed for its control.

THE HYPERSOMNIAS *Prolonged states of sleep* are characteristic of patients suffering from encephalitis lethargica (Chap. 369), trypanosomiasis, and a variety of other diseases localized to the floor and walls of the third ventricle. Small tumors in the posterior hypothalamus and midbrain have been associated with arterial hypotension, diabetes insipidus, and somnolence lasting many weeks. Such patients can be aroused, but if left alone, immediately fall asleep. Tumors of the brain, in general, show a tendency to cause drowsiness and increase in time spent in sleep, but those of the diencephalon more so than any others (e.g., more so than those of the posterior fossa). Traumatic brain lesions and other diseases have been found to produce similar clinical pictures. Myxedema, if severe, may cause hypersomnia.

There are two special varieties of hypersomnia, the Kleine-Levin and Pickwickian syndromes. The Kleine-Levin syndrome consists of periodic hypersomnolence lasting for periods of 2 to 3 weeks and hyperphagia (bulimia). The attacks occur two or three times a year. Onset is usually during adolescence with a striking male predominance. The pathogenesis is obscure. The Pickwickian syndrome of obesity, dyspnea, hypercapnea, and drowsiness are discussed in Chap. 371. This condition may be accompanied by a distressing *sleep apnea*.

NARCOLEPSY AND CATAPLEXY The essential characteristic of narcolepsy is uncontrollable sleepiness. Many times a day the individual is assailed by an uncontrollable desire to sleep. The eyes close, muscles relax, breathing slows, and the person appears to be dozing. A noise or a touch is enough to awaken these individuals, and they may feel refreshed momentarily. As a rule the condition begins in adolescence or early adult life. The periods of sleep may occur at any time of day, especially when the patient is physically inactive. The impulse to sleep is so insistent that the victim may be unable to sit through a single class in school or a meeting without at once falling asleep. A given period of sleep usually lasts up to 15 min, seldom as long as an hour unless lying down. At the onset there may be blurring of vision, diplopia, and ptosis which may raise the question of an ophthalmologic disorder. The condition is often associated with cataplexy (70 percent of cases), sleep paralysis (50 percent), and hypnagogic hallucination (25 percent).

Cataplexy consists of the sudden loss of muscle tone provoked by exaggerated emotion such as excessive laughter or anger. Approximately 70 percent of patients with narcolepsy, if questioned carefully, will admit to having cataplexy. Reference here is made to the curious circumstance that hearty laughter, sadness, or anger will cause the patient's head to fall forward, the jaw to drop open, the knees to buckle, even with falling to the ground, and all with preservation of consciousness. The attack lasts only a minute or two.

The other components of the narcoleptic tetrad are sleep paralysis and hypnagogic hallucinations. In sleep paralysis individuals, while falling asleep or awakening, become conscious of an inability to move or speak. They have the helpless feeling that a word from someone or a touch would break the spell. Recovery occurs in a minute or two. Vivid hallucinations may also occur in this period or separately in a brief nap.

Narcolepsy and cataplexy usually begin in adolescence or early adult life and, once started, continue throughout the adult period, possibly being less frequent in old age. Males are affected more than females, and there is suggestion of a genetic factor. The attack of narcolepsy resembles REMS, as is also true of cataplexy, sleep paralysis, and the hallucinations. The night sleep pattern may also begin with REMS. The EEG is usually normal. No complete pathologic studies are available. There are no other neurologic abnormalities. The condition must be distinguished from the somnolence of obesity, hypothyroidism, heart failure, and excessive use of drugs and alcohol. In these latter cataplexy is always absent.

OTHER CAUSES OF EXCESSIVE DAYTIME DROWSINESS Diurnal hypersomnia of nonnarcoleptic type is another common complaint. Idleness and imposed inactivity due to medical disease increase the amount of daytime sleep, especially in certain parts of the day—after breakfast, after lunch, around dinner time. In part it may be occasioned by poor nocturnal sleep or drugs. Certain medical conditions such as cardiac decompensation, pulmonary disease with hypercapnea, hypothyroidism, and brain tumor cause diurnal drowsiness.

In an analysis of more than 200 cases of diurnal hypersomnia, Guilleminault and Dement found more than half had narcolepsy and the rest heavy snoring with "upper airway sleep apnea," narcolepsy with sleep apnea, drug dependency, or other disorders.

SLEEP IN RELATION TO MEDICAL DISEASES Patients with a variety of nocturnal medical complaints have been found to undergo other important physiologic changes in relation to certain phases of sleep. Anginal attacks at night appear usually with REMS and peptic ulcer pain increases during REMS when production of hydrochloric acid increases. On the other hand, attacks of bronchial asthma during the night may appear in any phase of sleep.

TREATMENT OF SLEEP DISORDERS Insomnia In general, there are three varieties of wakefulness. For best management, treatment should be based on the type exhibited by the patient. One type, infrequently observed in younger patients, is the inability to fall asleep. Individuals affected by this type have become more and more tense during the day and are unable to relax. This type of insomnia usually lasts from 1 to 3 h, and then the individual sinks into an exhausted, deep sleep which continues through the night. For these patients any fairly quick-acting, rapidly destroyed hypnotic such as secobarbital (Seconal), 0.1 g, flurazepam (Dalmane), 30 to 60 mg, chloral hydrate (Noctec), 500 to 1000 mg, glutethimide (Doriden), 500 mg, or methaqualone (Sopor), 150 to 300 mg, given 15 to 30 min before going to bed is useful in inducing and maintaining sleep. After a week or two, however, their effect wanes. Kales and Kales found only flurazepam to retain its power of reducing sleep latency and awake time after sleep onset.

The second type of insomnia is exhibited by patients who are able to go to sleep but who awaken in 2 or 3 h and lose sleep in the middle of the night. They awaken during the period when sleep normally lightens, and some are alternately awake and asleep all the rest of the night. Often these are sick persons with a debilitating or painful illness which generates more pain and restlessness as muscles relax and leave painful areas unsplinted. In others, fever, sweats, dyspnea, or other distressful symptoms develop and demand attention. Frequently, these patients secure relief from pentobarbital (Nembutal), 0.1 g, or flurazepam (Dalmane), 30 to 60 mg, given at bedtime. For cardiac patients who have Cheyne-Stokes respiration or moderate orthopnea, a rectal suppository of aminophylline, 0.5 g given at bedtime, will frequently relieve the respiratory distress and promote sleep. When pain is a factor in insomnia, acetylsalicylic acid, 0.3 to 0.6 g, should be given with the sedative. Occasionally, codeine phosphate, 30 mg, meperidine (Demerol), 50 mg, or morphine sulfate, 10 to 15 mg, may be required when pain is severe.

The third type of insomnia is seen in patients who go to sleep promptly and sleep well most of the night, only to awaken too early in the morning. Most of these individuals are older persons who turn night into day. They go to bed and get up earlier and earlier so that soon they are sleeping during the day and are alert during the night. Into this category also fall those individuals who are under great tension, worry, or anxiety or are overworked and exhausted. These people sink into bed and sleep through sheer exhaustion, but around 4 or 5 A.M. they awaken with their worries and are unable to get back to sleep. Most of these patients are benefited by barbital, 0.3 g,

given with fruit juice or milk at bedtime. For debilitated patients the compressed tablets of insoluble material should be crushed to ensure proper absorption, or sodium barbital should be substituted. Chloral hydrate, 500 mg given with fruit juice at bedtime, is also effective and may be substituted for barbital.

Patients with serious mental agitation, delirium, or excitement who require prompt, easily controlled, relatively safe sedation should receive whiskey, 30 to 60 ml by mouth, or paraldehyde, 15 to 30 ml by mouth in iced fruit juice, or the same dose of the latter by rectum but diluted with 200 ml physiologic saline or 120 ml olive oil. For frankly delirious patients 25 to 50 mg chlorpromazine tid or a similar psychotropic drug has been a most helpful medication. Generally, it is wise to avoid barbiturates with highly agitated patients, since occasionally they may precipitate serious mental confusion, excitement, or even manic tendencies. Chloral hydrate, 1 to 2 g by mouth, is also useful in the management of these individuals and frequently proves more satisfactory than the barbiturates.

A word of caution about oversedation is wise in any discussion of sedative drugs. All too frequently they are abused in that they are given when not needed, the dosage is too great, or the wrong preparation is chosen. These drugs are a common source of constipation, lead to fatigue and lack of energy and strength, and interfere with the patient's recovery from illness.

When large dosages of quicker-acting barbiturates, 0.4 to 0.6 g daily, or other of the soporific drugs are given for more than a few weeks, there is real danger of habituation, which, once developed, is pernicious in character. Withdrawal, unless accomplished skillfully and in graded steps, may cause serious mental disturbance or precipitate convulsions. The chronic insomniac who has no other symptoms should not be permitted to use sedative drugs as a crutch on which to limp through life. The solution to the problem is rarely to be found in medication. One should search out and correct the underlying difficulty, using medication only as a temporary helpful tool. A good book, pleasure in staying awake, and belief that the human organism will always get as much sleep as needed are helpful.

Since psychologic factors have not been demonstrated in such cases, a conservative program of medical management and pharmacologic treatment is indicated. Diazepam (Valium), which suppresses stage IV NREMS, is helpful in controlling night terrors, and if their differentiation from nocturnal epilepsy is impossible, a trial on diphenylhydantoin (Dilantin) and phenobarbital is indicated. (See Chap. 23 for further information concerning anticonvulsant medication.)

Narcolepsy and cataplexy For narcolepsy and cataplexy there is no therapy which will control all the symptoms. The narcoleptic responds best to (1) strategically placed naps (during lunch hour, before or after dinner, etc.) and (2) the use of analeptic drugs, such as amphetamine sulfate (Benzedrine), methylphenidate (Ritalin), or pipradrol (Meratran). The time of medication should be adjusted to the study or work habits of the patient. The usual dose of amphetamine varies from 5 to 10 mg given three to five times a day. This is ordinarily well tolerated and does not cause wakefulness at night. The dose of Ritalin is 10 to 20 mg thrice daily, and of Metratran, 2.5 to 5.0 mg 2 or 3 times daily. These have rather little effect on cataplexy but are partially effective in the Kleine-Levin syndrome. Fortunately the latter is less frequent, and some psychiatrists have claimed that it can be controlled by avoidance of emotionally charged situations. The newest addition to the pharmacology of cataplexy is imipramine (Tofranil), which, in doses of 25 mg three to four times a day, markedly reduces attacks, presumably by abolishing REMS.

REFERENCES

ADAMS RD, VICTOR M: *Principles of Neurology.* New York, McGraw-Hill, 1977

GUILLEMINAULT C, DEMENT W: Two hundred thirty-five cases of excessive daytime sleepiness: Diagnosis and tentative classification. J Chronic Dis 29:733, 1976

KALES A, KALES JD: Recent findings in the diagnosis and treatment of disturbed sleep. N Engl J Med 290:487, 1974

PAPPENHEIMER JR, SETCHELL BP: The measurement of cerebral blood flow in the rabbit and sheep. J Physiol (Lond) 226:48P, 1972

23
THE CONVULSIVE STATE AND IDIOPATHIC EPILEPSY

MARIA SALAM-ADAMS
RAYMOND D. ADAMS

The magnitude of the problem of convulsion as a leading manifestation of a medical or neurologic disease can hardly be overstated. The statistics of Hauser and Kurland show that at least 1 million persons in the United States are subject to recurrent seizures and that at least ten times that number consult a physician or go to a hospital at some time in their lives because of a seizure.

A solitary or brief outburst of convulsions may occur during the course of many medical illnesses; its significance derives from the fact that it indicates involvement of the nervous system and by its very nature, if repeated every few minutes, as in status epilepticus, may threaten life. Recurrent convulsions over long periods of life, most of the episodes being more or less identical in type, represent a different sort of problem. On the one hand they may be a manifestation of an ongoing primary neurologic disease that demands diagnosis and therapy, as in brain tumor. On the other hand, they may call attention to a long-standing, occult, episodic, corticothalamic derangement that began some time in the distant past and remains in some instances as a fibroglial scar. Not infrequently the original disease was unnoticed; perhaps it occurred in utero, at birth, or during childhood in parts of the brain that were too immature to test; or it may have affected a silent area of the mature brain. Patients with such old lesions, who make up the majority of those with recurrent seizures, are necessarily classified as having "idiopathic epilepsy," because it is impossible to obtain data regarding the original disease. The seizure may be the only sign of the brain abnormality.

The convulsive disorder is the expression of a sudden, excessive, disorderly discharge of neurons in either a structurally normal or diseased cortex. The discharge results in an almost instantaneous disturbance of sensation, loss of consciousness, convulsive movement, or some combination thereof. A terminologic embarrassment arises from the diversity of the clinical manifestations. It seems improper to call a condition a "convulsion" when only an alteration of sensation or of consciousness takes place. The word "seizure" is preferable, as a generic term, and also lends itself to qualification. Motor or convulsive seizure is not, therefore, tautologic, and one may also speak of sensory seizure.

COMMON TYPES OF CONVULSIVE DISORDER The generalized convulsion ranks as the most frequent type, being both a common expression of a number of ongoing diseases and the lasting mark of some obscure disease in the past. As in petit mal, another special type of spell noted for its brevity, the cause of the lesion and its location are unknown. Presumably the generalized seizure involves the entire cerebral cortex and diencephalon. Various other patterns of seizure, such as the psychomotor, which is associated with disease of the temporal lobe, usually have a demonstrable cortical focus, either actively progressing or stationary.

When the idiopathic recurrent types of convulsive disorder are analyzed as a group, as in the survey of nearly 2000 patients by Lennox, it was found that 51 percent had generalized convulsions; 8 percent, petit mal; and the remaining 41 percent, focal and mixed types, of which psychomotor was the most frequent.

Generalized convulsion (other than grand mal) Certain intercurrent medical diseases manifest themselves at one stage by a seizure or a series of seizures beginning as immediate loss of consciousness, with stiffening, then clonic rhythmic jerking of the limbs or only with the latter. The focality of the initiating lesion may be indicated by tonic or clonic spasm of the muscles of only one part of the body or a turning of eyes and head to one side. Consciousness tends to be reinstated soon after the cessation of the generalized motor activity. A single myoclonic jerk or multiple ones may be a prelude to the major seizure or may follow it or be interspersed between seizures. In some instances, especially in metabolic disorders of the brain, the focal motor seizures may appear first on one side of the body, then on the other, progressing to a generalized seizure.

Generalized convulsion (grand mal) The recurrent generalized seizure of grand mal type is more elaborate and demonstrates more clearly the effect of the epileptic discharge on the physiology of the nervous system. It begins with a sudden loss of consciousness, a cry, a fall to the ground, tonic then clonic movements of muscles of cranium and limbs, sometimes sphincteric incontinence, and other autonomic disorders. The motor activity soon terminates, leaving the patient in a state of coma, which lasts for many minutes or even as long as a half-hour. As the coma recedes, mental confusion, drowsiness, and headache become evident.

Petit mal (minor epilepsy, l'absence) This type of seizure, occurring most frequently between the fourth year of life and adolescence, comes without warning and is notable for its brevity and minimal motor accompaniment. It consists essentially of a brief loss of consciousness, lasting a few seconds. A few 3-per-second blinks or jerks of eyelids and sometimes arms may be conjoined. Petit mal may be more variable (atypical) with 2-per-second motor and EEG pattern and then is more likely to be combined with sudden falling episodes or single, brief, generalized myoclonic contractions of limbs or other types of seizures (laughing or "gelastic" spells, unilateral tonic or clonic spasms). These mixed types are especially difficult to control.

COMMON FOCAL SEIZURE PATTERNS **Psychomotor epilepsy** Certainly this is the most frequent and interesting type of focal seizure pattern. The aura, if it occurs, often takes the form of a complex hallucination or perceptual illusion. There may be an unpleasant smell or taste, or the revival of a complicated visual scene involving people, dwellings, etc., usually taken from past experiences and resembling a dream. There may be recurrence of a certain thought. Furthermore, the patient's perception of what is seen and heard and relationship to the outside world are altered. Objects appear to be far away or unreal (*jamais vu*); or strange objects or persons may seem familiar (*déjà vu phenomenon*). Hughlings Jackson applied the term *dreamy state* to these psychic disturbances. In the seizure patients behave as though partially conscious. They may get up and walk about, unbutton or remove clothes, attempt to speak, or even continue such habitual acts as driving a car. If asked a specific question or given a command, it is evident that they are out of contact with the examiner and do not understand. When restrained, they may resist with great energy and at times may be violent. This type of behavior is said to be *automatic*, presumably because the patient behaves like an automaton. Convulsive movements, when present, are likely to consist of chewing, smacking and licking of the lips, and, less often, tonic spasms of the limbs or turning of the head and eyes to one side.

In any given case one or several of these phenomena may be observed. In the series studied by Lennox and Lennox, which numbered 414 cases, 43 percent of patients displayed some of these motor or psychomotor phenomena; 32 percent, the automatic state; and 25 percent, the psychic changes. Some psychomotor seizures are very brief, lasting only for seconds, and others continue for hours. This calls to mind that the duration of the seizure is an unsatisfactory criterion for classification.

LOCALIZED MOTOR SEIZURES A lesion in one or the other frontal lobe may give rise to a generalized or major convulsive seizure of the type described above, without an introductory aura. In some cases there is a turning movement of the head and eyes to one side, simultaneously with loss of consciousness. It has been postulated that in both types of seizure, the one with and the one without contraversive movements, the discharge from the frontal lobe spreads rapidly into an integrating center such as the thalamus, with immediate loss of consciousness.

The *Jacksonian motor seizure* begins usually with a tonic contraction or a clonic rhythmic twitching of the fingers of one hand, the face on one side, or one foot. The twitching may occur in bursts, or paroxysms. The disorder then spreads, or marches, from the part first affected to other muscles on the same side of the body—from the face to the neck, hand, forearm, arm, trunk, and leg; if the first movement is in the foot, the order is reversed. A high incidence of onset in the lips, fingers, and toes probably is related to the greater cortical representation of these parts of the body. The disease process or focus of excitation is usually the rolandic cortex, area 4 (Fig. 25-1) on the opposite side; in a few cases it has been found in the postrolandic convolution. Lesions confined to the premotor cortex (area 6) are said to induce tonic contractions of an arm, face, neck, or all of one side of the body. Perspiration and piloerection, sometimes only of the parts of the body involved in a focal motor seizure, suggest that these autonomic functions have cortical representation in the rolandic area.

Another type of focal motor epilepsy consists of rhythmic clonic movements of one group of muscles, usually in the face, arm, or leg. These may continue for a variable period of time, from minutes to weeks or months (epilepsia, partialis continua). The seizure does not occur in bursts or paroxysms and usually does not "march" to other parts of the body. Its localizing value has not been settled. Some patients have a lesion in the opposite sensorimotor areas of the cerebral cortex.

SOMATIC, VISUAL, AND OTHER SENSORY SEIZURES Somatic sensory seizures, either focal or marching to other parts of the body on one side, nearly always indicate a parietal lobe lesion. The usual *sensory disorder* is described as a numbness, a tingling, or a "pins-and-needles" feeling. Other variations are sensations of crawling (formication), buzzing, electricity, or vibration. Pain and thermal sensations are infrequent. The onset is in the lips, fingers, and toes in the majority of cases, and the spread to adjacent parts of the body follows a pattern determined by sensory arrangements in the postcentral (postrolandic) convolution of the parietal lobe. In the series of Kristiansen and Penfield the seizure focus was found in the postcentral convolution in 24 of 55 cases; it was central (both pre- and postrolandic) in 18, and precentral in 7 cases. If localized in the cranial muscles, the focus is in the lowest part of the convolution, near the sylvian fissure; if in the foot or leg, the upper part near the superior sagittal sinus is involved.

Lesions in or near the striate cortex of the occipital lobe usually produce a sensation of lights, of darkness, or of color. The patient may tell of seeing stars or moving lights in the visual field on the side opposite the lesion. Sometimes they appear to be straight ahead of the patient. Often, if they occur on only one side of the visual field, the patient believes only one eye to be affected, the one opposite the lesion, probably because the average person is unaware that there are two corresponding visual fields. It is curious that a seizure arising in one occipital lobe may cause momentary blindness in both eyes. It has been noted that seizures arising in the lateral surface of the occipital lobes (Brodmann's areas 18 and 19) are more likely to cause twinkling or pulsating lights. Complex visual hallucinations are usually due to a focus more anterior in the visual association areas at the junction of occipital, parietal, and the posterior part of the temporal lobe, and they may be associated with auditory hallucinations. Often the visual images, either those of the hallucination or of objects seen, are distorted or seem too small (*micropsia*) or unnaturally arranged.

Auditory hallucinations are rather infrequent as an initial manifestation of a seizure. Occasionally a patient with a focus in the superior temporal convolution on one side will report a buzzing or a roaring in the ears. A human voice sometimes repeating recognizable words has been reported a few times by patients with lesions in the more posterior part of the dominant temporal lobe.

Vertiginous sensations of a type suggesting vestibular stimulation may be the first symptom of a seizure. The lesion is usually localized in the superior posterior temporal region or at the junction between the parietal and temporal lobes. Occasionally, with a temporal focus, vertigo is followed by an auditory sensation.

Olfactory hallucinations are often associated with disease of the inferior and medial parts of the temporal lobe, usually in the region of the hippocampal convolution or the uncus (hence the term *uncinate seizures*, after Jackson). Usually the smell is exteriorized, i.e., projected to someplace in the environment, and is of a disagreeable nature. Gustatory hallucinations have also been recorded in proved cases of temporal lobe disease. Sensations of thirst and salivation may be associated. Seizures arising in and stimulation of the upper surface of the temporal lobe in the depths of the sylvian fissure during neurosurgical operations have produced peculiar sensations of taste.

Visceral sensations arising in the thorax, epigastrium, and abdomen are among the most frequent of the auras. They are described as a vague, indefinable feeling, a sinking sensation in the pit of the stomach, and a weakness in the epigastrium or substernal area that rises to the throat and head. The seizure discharge may be localized to the upper bank of the sylvian fissure or in the upper intermediate or medial frontal areas near the cingulate gyrus. Palpitation and acceleration of pulse at the beginning of the attack have also been related to a temporal lobe focus.

PSYCHIC PHENOMENA A close relationship between psychic changes and temporal lobe foci has been established. Disease of either temporal lobe may be accompanied by seizures that have many of the characteristics of psychomotor epilepsy. In addition, complex visual and auditory hallucinations with feelings of unreality, and partial or complete interruption of consciousness, may be observed more often in the dominant than the nondominant temporal lobe. Compulsive thought or action may recur in a fixed pattern during each seizure. Automatic behavior or even frank psychoses resembling confusional states or schizophrenia, and lasting for hours or days, may be induced by seizure discharges or electrical stimulation of the temporal lobe.

The various motor, sensory, or psychic phenomena may be combined in many different sequences. These presumably indicate the spread of a seizure discharge from one cortical area to another. A flash of light followed by tingling of one side of the body suggests that the epileptic discharge began in the occipital lobe and extended to the somatic sensory areas in the parietal lobe. A smell of something burning, followed by chewing and smacking movements, and then loss of speech would be interpreted as a spread of the seizure discharge from the region of the uncus to the upper parts of the temporal and the inferior frontal lobes. A focal motor seizure followed by a tonic contraction of one side of the body and then by turning of the head and eyes contralaterally would indicate a successive involvement of the motor, premotor, and contraversive cortical field for head and eyes. Little is known about the factors that facilitate or inhibit the spread of seizure discharges from one part of the brain to another.

EVOCATION OF SEIZURES (REFLEX EPILEPSY) Seizures can sometimes be evoked in susceptible persons by a physiologic or psychologic stimulus. Approximately 1 in every 15 patients will have remarked that their seizures occur under special circumstances, such as being exposed to flickering light, passing from darkness to light or the reverse, being startled by a loud noise, hearing a series of monotonous sounds or music, touching, rubbing, or hurting a particular part of the body, making certain movements (e.g., eating, reading, carrying out some complex mental task), or being subjected to fright or other strong emotion. The evoked seizure may be focal (beginning often in the part of the body that has been stimulated) or generalized. In a few instances this reflex epilepsy, as it is called, has been due to a focal cerebral disease, such as a tumor, but more often its cause cannot be ascertained. A special type of reflex myoclonic epilepsy with a strong tendency to familial incidence can be elicited by photic stimulation (photic epilepsy). Another point of interest in these cases of evoked seizure has been the phenomenon of willfully averting the seizure by undertaking some mental task, e.g., thinking about some distracting subject or counting, or by initiating some physical activity.

PATHOPHYSIOLOGY OF THE CONVULSION Reflex epilepsy suggests that epilepsy is a natural state, a physiologic event resulting from excitation and subsequent inhibition of a damaged part of the cerebrum. Eventually the physiologic event that initiates the seizure is a high-voltage discharge of an assemblage of cortical neurons. There need not be a visible lesion for, under the proper circumstances, it can be initiated in entirely normal cerebral cortex, as when the cortex is functionally altered by low-intensity electric stimulation that does not in itself produce seizures but leaves an epileptic focus (kindling effect of Goddard), or is activated by a drug or injured by hypoxia. But it is the visible focal lesion that has been the most thoroughly investigated. Some of the electric properties of the cortical focus suggest that its neurons have been deafferented. Deafferented neurons are known to be hypersensitive; they remain chronically in a state of partial depolarization, and the cytoplasmic membranes have an increased permeability which renders them susceptible to activation by hyperthermia, hypoxia, hypoglycemia, and hyponatremia, as well as by repeated sensory (e.g., photic) stimulation and during certain phases of sleep (when hypersynchrony of neurons is known to occur). Another hypothesis is that the lesion of the cortex has

resulted in the removal of a normal diencephalic inhibitory effect. An excellent review of these and other pathophysiologic mechanisms is to be found in the monograph of Jasper et al.

The biochemical studies of the involved clone of neurons of a seizure focus have suggested some interesting possibilities. Epileptic foci are known to be sensitive to the facilitatory transmitter substance acetylcholine and to be slower in binding and removing it than normal cerebral cortex; a deficiency of γ-aminobutyric acid (GABA), the inhibitory transmitter, a disturbance of cytochrome oxidase with decrease in ATP production, a reduction in the Krebs cycle function with a shift to GABA-succinate shunt, and disturbance in local regulation of extracellular K, Na, Ca, Mg are other hypotheses. An interesting proposal is that astrocytes adjacent to neurons and presynaptic terminals have altered relationships in cortical scars and are no longer able to modulate fluxes of extracellular potassium.

Once the intensity of the seizure discharge exceeds a certain point, it spreads to adjacent cortical and to thalamic and brainstem nuclei. It is then that the first clinical manifestation of the convulsion begins. Presumably the excitatory activity is fed back from the thalamus to the original focus and to other parts of the forebrain, giving rise to the characteristic high-frequency discharge in the EEG, and there is propagation downward to spinal neurons via corticospinal and reticulospinal pathways. Shortly thereafter a diencephalocortical inhibition begins and intermittently interrupts the focal and generalized seizure discharge, changing it from the persistent discharge of the tonic phase to the intermittent bursts of the clonic phase. These become less and less frequent and finally cease altogether, leaving in their wake strong inhibition or paralysis of the neurons of the epileptic focus. This latter is the presumed basis of *Todd's postepileptic paralysis* which is accompanied by diffuse slow waves in the EEG in all parts of the cerebrum. In petit mal it is thought that the high-voltage spike-slow-wave discharge originates in the thalamus, and this may also be true of some cases of grand mal, in both of which consciousness is at once abolished. On the other hand, atypical petit mal and possibly the typical type as well can be induced by a mesial frontal lesion. Temporal lobe seizures are known to arise in foci in the medial temporal lobe, amygdaloid nuclei, and hippocampus. Electric stimulation in these areas reproduces a partial loss of conscious contact with environment, feelings of depersonalization, and automatic behavior.

A discovery of no little importance is that a seizure focus, if active for a time, may establish via commissural and corticocortical connections, a secondary focus in the corresponding area of cortex in the opposite hemisphere (mirror focus) or in adjacent regions. The nature of this development is not fully understood, but probably it is similar to the kindling effect. This becomes a source of confusion in trying to identify electrographically the side of the primary lesion.

Severe seizures may disturb the chemistry of the brain by causing hypoxia, acidosis with rise in P_{CO_2}, and an accumulation of lactic acid. Some of these effects are secondary to respiratory spasm, blockage of airway, and excessive muscular activity at a time when the metabolic activity of the involved cerebral tissue is maximal. These biochemical changes give rise to secondary cerebral lesions. The latter are especially frequent in the temporal lobes and cerebellum and may themselves later become epileptic foci. Ohmsted and others explain the rising frequency of temporal lobe foci in the epileptic individual in this way. A violent epileptic discharge of the brain may cause respiratory arrest or cardiac standstill, with death ensuing immediately or if there is survival, a severe hypoxic (postepileptic) encephalopathy.

The electroencephalogram provides a delicate proof of Hughlings Jackson's theory of epilepsy—that it is an excessive, disorderly discharge of cortical neurons. At the onset of the focal seizure this is registered in or near the focus as a series of spikes or sharp waves interrupting the normal alpha and beta waves. The clinical spread of the seizure has its electroencephalographic equivalent in the extension of the abnormal electrical waves; with generalization of the seizure (grand mal), the entire electroencephalographic recording surface of the brain exhibits spikes of high voltage. Petit mal is accompanied by a characteristic 3-per-second wave-spike complex occurring simultaneously in all cortical leads and presumably taking origin from a diencephalic focus. At first there was thought to be a characteristic electroencephalographic picture for psychomotor epilepsy, but further studies have not confirmed this. The postseizure state, sometimes called *postconvulsive paralysis of cerebral function*, also has its electroencephalographic correlate in random generalized slow waves. With recovery of normal mentation the electroencephalogram returns to normal. If the electroencephalographic tracing is obtained during the interval between seizures, it is abnormal to some degree in approximately 40 percent of fully conscious and 75 percent of sleeping patients.

The epileptic lesion Of the innumerable diseases that are epileptogenic it has not been possible to distinguish the component of the lesion that is responsible for the seizures from one that is not. In other words one cannot say from microscopic examination whether any given lesion was epileptic. Gliosis, fibrosis, vascularization, meningocerebral cicatrix have all been incriminated, but they occur as well in nonepileptic foci. Partial disconnection of groups of cortical neurons from those of neighboring cortex, of the other cerebral hemisphere, and of the thalamus seems likely to have occurred. Or certain systems of inhibiting neurons may have been destroyed. Once a gliotic focus of whatever cause, bordered by groups of discharging neurons, becomes epileptogenic, it may remain so throughout the lifetime of the patient. Of course, none of these remarks apply to the "kindled focus" in which the structurally normal cortical neurons are capable of giving rise to seizures for a year or more.

DISEASES CAUSING SYMPTOMATIC SEIZURES Among the medical diseases which may be complicated by a burst of seizures, the following are the most frequent.

Generalized convulsions mixed in some instances with unilateral muscular contractions of clonic type appear prominently during an abstinence or withdrawal period in patients addicted to *alcohol* or *barbiturates*. Suspicion of this mechanism is raised by the telltale marks of alcoholic excesses or the history of a prolonged nervousness requiring sedation. Also disturbances of sleep, disorientation, illusions, and visual hallucinations often precede and follow the convulsive phase of the illness. The convulsive period lasts several days and is accompanied and followed for several more by a confusional state.

Bacterial meningitis is another type of illness with a strong convulsive tendency, more pronounced in children than in adults. Fever and stiff neck usually provide the clue, and lumbar puncture yields the salient laboratory data.

Uremia is another condition with a prominent convulsive aspect. Of interest is the sequence of events in complete anuria. This condition is tolerated for 2 to 3 days without neurologic signs, and then there is a rapid onset of twitching, trembling, myoclonic jerks, and generalized motor seizures. Tetany may

be added (see Chap. 275). The motor display, one of the most dramatic in medicine, lasts several days until the patient sinks into terminal coma or recovers. When this syndrome accompanies lupus erythematosus, delirium tremens, idiopathic epilepsy, or generalized neoplasia, one can nearly always be sure that it has a basis in renal failure.

Cardiac arrest, suffocation or respiratory failure, NO_2 anesthesia, CO poisoning—the common causes of hypoxic encephalopathy—usually induce a diffuse myoclonic jerking of all the musculature and generalized seizures as soon as cardiac function is resumed. The convulsive phase of this condition may last only a few days, in association with coma, stupor, or confusion; or it may persist indefinitely as an intensive myoclonic-convulsive state.

Other acute illnesses complicated by generalized and multifocal motor seizures are hyponatremia and water intoxication, thyrotoxic storm, hypertensive encephalopathy, porphyria, hypoglycemia, pyridoxine deficiency, argininosuccinic aciduria, and phenylketonuria. Picrotoxin and pentylenetetrazol (Metrazol) are two of the most highly convulsant drugs in use, and lead and arsenic the most frequent convulsive metallic intoxicants.

Generalized seizures with or without twitching may occur in the terminal phases of many other illnesses, such as gram-negative septicemias with shock, liver coma, and intractable congestive heart failure.

There are several primary diseases of the brain which are announced by an acute convulsive state. Myoclonic jerking and seizures appear early in acute inclusion-body encephalitis and other forms of viral, treponemal, and parasitic encephalitis, subacute sclerosing encephalitis, as well as in lipid storage diseases, Jakob-Creutzfeldt disease, and diffuse gliomatosis of the brain.

It seems strange that difficult problems of a convulsive nature seldom occur in patients suffering from cerebrovascular disease. Seizures hardly ever occur in limbs paralyzed by cerebral infarction and hemorrhages, and limbs that are involved in seizures in a comatose patient will later prove to have retained their normal power. However, old cortical infarcts, usually of embolic origin or due to an old subcortical hemorrhage, become epileptogenic in approximately 20 percent of cases. The rupture of an aneurysm is occasionally marked by one or two generalized convulsions. Thrombotic occlusions of cerebral arteries are almost never convulsive in the opening phases of the stroke. The rare thrombophlebitis with cortical ischemia and infarction is probably the most highly convulsive vascular lesion. Tumor, on the other hand, is a frequent cause of focal or generalized seizures, the latter present in more than 30 percent of cases if located in the central parts of the cerebrum. Nearly 40 percent of cerebral abscesses have in their wake recurrent convulsions. Cerebral traumatism is the other common convulsive disease. Thirty to forty percent of all penetrating and contusing cerebral injuries will be followed by focal epilepsy. (See Chaps. 366 to 368.)

IDIOPATHIC EPILEPSY Idiopathic epilepsy tends to express itself with maximal frequency at two periods in life, between the ages of 2 and 5 years and around puberty. More often than not the first seizure is generalized, though a series of petit mal, "staring spells," may precede its appearance. Up to this moment development may have been normal, and a neurologic examination is likely to disclose no other abnormality. In a smaller proportion other types of seizures (neonatal, infantile spasms, severe febrile seizures, etc.) have occurred earlier in life. Although the seizures may be either of generalized motor type (51 percent of cases) or petit mal (8 percent) in the beginning, as the years pass and the seizures continue, approximately 40 percent of patients will have both these types or psychomotor seizures.

The severity of the convulsive state varies from a single attack every several years to many per day. If the generalized seizures are at all frequent, they pose a constant threat of injury and social embarrassment, often preventing the further education of the child or the gainful occupation of the adult, and they may interfere with the development of a stable, mature personality. Of the milder form of disorder, however, sufficient medical control may be achieved so that there is no interference with normal life activities. In enlightened communities no longer is an intelligent epileptic ostracized by teachers or employers, and virtually all patients without other neurologic abnormalities can find their place in society. If there is evidence of mental retardation, character changes, hemiparesis, etc., as not infrequently happens, the other problems may be as important as the idiopathic epilepsy.

The common diagnostic procedures performed in the interval between seizures are usually uninformative, i.e., the cerebrospinal fluid is normal, x-rays of skull are normal, pneumoencephalogram and arteriograms, where they have been done, are negative. Only the electroencephalogram will demonstrate an abnormality in 40 to 75 percent of cases, either a generalized paroxysmal 3-per-second spike-slow-wave complex (dartdome), sharp waves, or some other less specific alterations.

Without doubt the appearance of a convulsion poses a serious problem for the patient, family, and physician. There is first of all the possibility of its being the initial manifestation of a neurologic disease which will take the life of the patient (e.g., infiltrating glioma). But even if the convulsion is due to a stationary, healed lesion, life expectancy is slightly reduced owing to the danger of injury or, rarely, unexplained death. If seizures are frequent or difficult to control, mentation may be altered; the patient is dull, vague, querulous, often hyperreligious, and illogically argumentative. If seizures are infrequent and the EEG relatively normal between attacks, prognoses for successful schooling, occupational adjustment, and marriage are excellent. Mental deterioration, fortunately, occurs rarely, contrary to lay opinion, and when it becomes evident over a few weeks, months, or years one must suspect (1) wrong initial diagnosis (not idiopathic epilepsy but seizures due to some definable cerebral disease), (2) drug intoxication from anticonvulsant medication, (3) recurrent subclinical seizures, (4) hypoxic-hypotensive crisis during a bout of prolonged seizures, (5) subdural hematoma resulting from head injury.

APPROACH TO THE CLINICAL PROBLEM OF RECURRENT SEIZURES A history of recurrent attacks of loss of consciousness or awareness associated with abnormal movements or confusion is usually sufficient to establish a diagnosis of epilepsy. With such patients a thorough history, a complete physical and neurologic examination, testing of the visual fields, and laboratory studies, including computerized tomography (CT scan) of the skull and an electroencephalogram, should be done. The results of these essential procedures will determine to which of the categories in the above classification the case belongs or whether one is justified in making the diagnosis of idiopathic epilepsy.

If a patient not known to have been epileptic has an acute illness with frequent generalized or one-sided seizures, a search must be conducted for clinical and laboratory signs of infection, metabolic and endocrine diseases, and intoxications.

If convulsions have occurred in the past, an inquiry as to epilepsy in the family history and occurrence of head trauma or cerebral infections in the past must be made; careful description of the seizure itself, including prodromata, aura, manifestations during the seizure and the postictal period, must be obtained. Seizures in other members of the family favor slightly the diagnosis of *idiopathic epilepsy*. Signs of pulmonary or ear infection or of congenital heart disease with a right-to-left shunt should suggest, in a patient with recently

acquired seizures, the possibility of a *brain abscess*. The presence of a heart murmur and fever or of atrial fibrillation favors embolism. Head trauma of a serious nature, followed by seizures after an interval of several weeks to 2 years, indicates that an injury may have given rise to convulsions. A regularly recurring aura, especially of a focal nature, may indicate a localized lesion in the brain. Similarly, a focal convulsive movement at the onset of the seizure probably indicates a localized cerebral lesion. A transient monoplegia or hemiplegia or aphasia or hemisensory loss (Todd's paralysis) in the postictal period also has considerable significance in localizing a lesion. In fact, its presence may provide the best clue to a focal brain lesion. A history of other neurologic symptoms such as headache, localized paralysis, or mental changes often indicates the need for special diagnostic studies.

A general physical examination may provide clues to the legion of conditions associated with epilepsy. Protuberances over the skull may suggest an underlying pathologic condition. Vascular nevi over the body, especially over the face and in the retina, may be associated with vascular abnormalities within the skull. Small tumors, often pedunculated, distributed over the body surface bring to mind the diagnosis of von Recklinghausen's disease and, when associated with seizures, may indicate an intracranial glioma or neurofibroma. White spots over the trunk and limbs and sebaceous adenomas of the face point to the diagnosis of tuberous sclerosis. Smallness of an arm or leg indicates a lesion acquired at an early age. Cranial nerve disturbances are also helpful in diagnosis; thus, a sixth-nerve paralysis is often associated with increased intracranial pressure. Localized weakness, differences in reflexes, or the presence of abnormal reflexes, such as Babinski's response, all have localizing value.

The question of what laboratory procedures should be done in cases of epilepsy can be answered only on the basis of the clinical findings. With recent onset of generalized convulsions simple blood chemistry tests are among the first measures to be carried out. The determination of blood glucose helps orient the examiner in instances of hypoglycemia and hyperglycemia; the calcium level provides the main clue to hypocalcemia, the blood urea nitrogen (BUN) to kidney disease, and sodium and potassium levels to multiple metabolic disturbances, including dilutional hyponatremia. X-rays of the skull, and more particularly a CT scan, if available, should be taken in all cases. Significant findings related to increased intracranial pressure include erosion of the clinoid processes and, in infants and children, separation of the sutures. Hyperostoses, erosions of the skull, abnormal vascular markings, and intracranial calcifications are other findings of importance that may appear in skull x-rays. In the CT scan one looks for defects in cerebral tissue, ventricular distortion, and areas of enhancement (with contrast techniques). Because of the frequency of cerebral metastases from primary carcinoma of the lung, chest x-rays should be made in all patients suspected of having intracranial neoplasm.

Lumbar puncture can be of considerable value in elucidating the causes of epilepsy. If the history, neurologic examination, or skull x-rays show any abnormality, especially if a focal lesion in the brain is suggested, then a lumbar puncture is mandatory (unless there are signs of high intracranial pressure). Of special importance are determination of the pressure, cell count, total protein, and serologic tests. An abnormal cell count usually indicates an infectious process. An elevation only of total protein (greater than 100 mg per 100 ml) favors the diagnosis of a tumor. If the pressure is normal but other symptoms or signs point to a recently acquired, localized brain lesion, an arteriogram, radionuclide scans, or pneumoencephalogram may be needed to supplement the findings on CT scan. The visualization of the cerebral hemisphere by these procedures may be of particular help to the neurosurgeon in localizing the lesion and in planning a surgical approach to it.

The electroencephalogram, although now routinely employed in the definitive diagnosis of cases with epilepsy, is not absolutely conclusive, since it may be normal in some patients, particularly if the seizures are relatively infrequent, or abnormal in diseases that do not cause epilepsy. The test is of particular value in diagnosing petit mal, for here clinical or subclinical attacks are apt to be frequent enough to register during the electroencephalographic test. Abnormal electric waves may manifest themselves in other types of epilepsy as well, and the electroencephalogram may be abnormal during the interseizure period, demonstrating either focal or generalized abnormalities of cortical activity. Activation of the electroencephalogram by photic stimulation and drug-induced sleep is now standard procedure in many laboratories (see Chap. 364).

The type of clinical study in any given case is dictated to some extent by the age of the patient and the length of time the patient has been having seizures. Up until early adulthood most patients turn out to have idiopathic epilepsy. With increasing age, the incidence of idiopathic epilepsy becomes less and that of symptomatic epilepsy increases. Thus the appearance of convulsions for the first time in early or middle adult life should be presumptive evidence of brain tumor until every effort has been made to rule it out (see Table 23-1). If seizures have been occurring for 15 to 20 years or more, the likelihood of tumor or other progressive neurologic disease is so remote that most diagnostic tests are not worthwhile.

DIFFERENTIAL DIAGNOSIS The clinical differences between a seizure and a syncopal attack are presented in Chap. 13 and need not be repeated here. It must be emphasized once again that there is no single criterion for distinguishing between them. The author has erred in calling akinetic seizures simple faints and in mistaking cardiac or carotid sinus faints for seizures. Petit mal may be difficult to identify because of the brevity of attacks. One helpful maneuver is to have the patient count for 5 to 10 min. If having petit mal, the patient will blink or stare, pause in counting, or skip one or two numbers. Hyperventilation is a useful way of evoking this type of seizure. Psychomotor seizures are the most difficult of all to diagnose. These attacks are so variable in character and so likely to induce minor disturbances in conduct rather than obvious interruptions of consciousness that they may be misdiagnosed as temper tantrums, hysteria, psychopathic behavior, or acute psychosis.

A special problem in diagnosis is offered by states of mental dullness and confusion. Epileptic patients as seen in hospital and office practice usually show no mental deterioration, regardless of the type of seizure. Therefore, the appearance of dementia, confusion, or some other derangement of mental function should suggest the possibility of recurrent subclinical seizures not controlled by medication, drug intoxication, postseizure psychosis, or a brain disease that has caused both dementia and seizures. To distinguish these clinical states may require careful observation, along the lines suggested in Chap. 21, and electroencephalography (Chap. 364).

TREATMENT AND MANAGEMENT OF THE CONVULSING AND EPILEPTIC PATIENT   Status epilepticus   Rarely does a single seizure terminate life, although instances do occur presumably from a cardiac arrhythmia, suffocation, or aspiration. Recovery from a single seizure is usually prompt and requires no special treatment.

It is necessary to protect the convulsing patient from injury and to make sure that there is a clear airway. A soft object that cannot be swallowed may be placed between the teeth to protect the tongue, but once the jaws are set in a tonic spasm, one should not try to force them open because of the risk of breaking teeth.

Once the seizures are under control, further anticonvulsant therapy depends on the nature of the disease. If a causative lesion is eliminated by medication, e.g., meningitis, no further therapy is needed. When seizures are associated with a surgically removable lesion of the brain, such as a tumor or abscess, its excision may eradicate the discharging focus. This is unpredictable, however, for convulsive seizures are relieved in only about 50 percent of cases of meningioma and an even smaller percentage of cases of glioma or abscess of the cerebrum.

A series of seizures without restoration of consciousness between (status epilepticus) is more dangerous and demands admission to a hospital and prompt pharmacotherapy. Often the patient is already receiving a maintenance dose of anticonvulsant medication, but if not, intravenous therapy should be initiated at once. Diphenylhydantoin (Dilantin) in a loading dose of 1000 mg (in single or divided doses) should be given, supplemented by diazepam (5 mg) or sodium phenobarbitol (100 mg). Intravenous injection of diazepam (Valium) should be made slowly over the period of a minute into a large vein and repeated every 2 to 4 h if necessary. Rapid injection may cause apnea or cardiac arrest. The alternative, sodium phenobarbital, may also be given intravenously, in a dose of 200 mg, to be repeated if necessary every 4 h. For *focal* status epilepticus paraldehyde, 1 to 3 ml given slowly by intravenous route or 5 to 10 ml intramuscularly (avoiding nerves), is sometimes useful. Once the cycle of status epilepticus is broken, one may rely on the standard oral anticonvulsant medications. If the seizures are not responsive to the above doses of Valium or sodium phenobarbital, it is better for the patient to have a few seizures than to be rendered comatose by increasing doses of medication.

The type of disease causing the seizures and its treatment is another important consideration. Antibiotic medication usually arrests the seizure tendency in bacterial meningitis. NaCl in a 3% solution usually terminates the seizures in hyponatremia, and 5% glucose solution has a similar effect in hypoglycemic seizures. $MgSO_4$ and calcium gluconate often help in uremic seizures. Abstinence seizures cease usually within a few days and are rarely severe and frequent. In all these conditions or in idiopathic epilepsy if status epilepticus occurs, occasional seizures are of less serious consequence than a deepening drug-induced coma from excessive doses of anticonvulsant medication.

Recurrent seizures including idiopathic epilepsy   Of course success in the management of patients with epilepsy depends in large measure on the deployment of drugs for the prevention

TABLE 23-1
Causes of recurrent convulsion in different age groups

Age of onset, years	Probable cause
Infancy, 0–2	Congenital maldevelopment, birth injury, metabolic disorder (hypocalcemia, hypoglycemia), vitamin B_6 deficiency, phenylketonuria
Childhood, 2–10	Birth injury, trauma, infections, thrombosis of cerebral arteries or veins, beginning of idiopathic epilepsy
Adolescence, 10–18	Idiopathic epilepsy, trauma, congenital defects
Early adulthood, 18–35	Trauma, neoplasm, idiopathic epilepsy, alcoholism, drug addiction
Middle age, 35–60	Neoplasm, trauma, vascular disease, alcoholism, drug addiction
Late life, over 60	Vascular disease, degeneration, tumor

of seizures. If managed well with anticonvulsants, fully 75 percent of patients may have their seizures controlled or reduced in frequency.

The drugs in common use for this purpose are the barbiturates, hydantoins, and oxazoladinediones, and to a lesser extent acetylureas and benzodiazepams. The available products which have received a thorough clinical trial and their daily dosages are listed in Table 23-2.

Certain drugs are more effective in one type of seizure than in another, and it is necessary to use the proper drugs in the optimum dosages for the different types of seizures. If satisfactory results are not obtained with one of the drugs, the others should be tried, but frequent shifting of drugs is not advisable, and each should be given in adequate trial before another is substituted. In some patients a combination of two or more drugs will produce better results than one alone.

Intelligent administration of drugs depends on having the patients chart daily their medication and the number, time, and circumstances of their seizures. Ideally such a baseline should be established before medication is begun, since each patient tends to have an individual pattern of seizures, but often this is impractical. Changes in medication should be made only when a given program is shown to be inadequate. Frequent measurements of blood levels of diphenylhydantoin, barbiturate and other drugs are useful. For Dilantin the therapeutic level is 10 to 15 μg/ml, and one-half of patients have side effects at 30 or more μg/ml. These consist of ataxia, slurred speech, staggering, nystagmus, diplopia, mental dullness, forgetfulness, and confusion. Stupor or coma may occur when the level exceeds 50 μg/ml. Clinical and electroencephalographic improvement are not usually obtained if the level is below 10 μg/ml. The therapeutic level for phenobarbital is probably about 10 to 15 μg/ml, though the range varies with the type of barbiturate used. Side effects appear in patients on long-term treatment with phenobarbital levels above 30 μg/ml.

When changing medication, the dosage of the new drug should be gradually increased to an optimum level at the same time as the dosage of the old drug is gradually decreased. The sudden withdrawal of a drug may lead to status epilepticus, even though a new drug is substituted. Once an anticonvulsant or a combination of anticonvulsants is found to be effective, its use should be maintained for a period of years.

The therapeutic dose for any patient must be determined to some extent by trial and error. Not uncommonly a drug is discarded as being ineffective, when a slightly increased dosage would have led to a complete disappearance of the seizures. It is, however, inadvisable to administer a drug to the point where the patient is so dull and stupid as to be more incapacitated by the toxic effects than by the seizures. There is no evidence to prove that the prolonged administration of anticonvulsant medication is a factor in the development of the mental deterioration that occurs in a small percentage of the patients with convulsive seizures. It is not uncommon to note an improvement in the mental faculties of some patients following control of the seizures by the use of anticonvulsant drugs.

An antifolate effect on blood serum and a reduction of protein-bound iodine (without lowering of the BMR) have been reported. Some of the anticonvulsant drugs [primidone (Mysoline) or Dilantin] cause hirsutism, gum hypertrophy (Dilantin), and coarsening of the features of a growing child. Mild polyneuropathy (abolition of reflexes in legs and numb feet) has also been reported. Some adult males complain of reduced sexual potency and both Dilantin and carbamazepine (Tegretol) have been shown to decrease 17-corticosteroids (Luhdorf et al.). When this happens, the drug should be changed.

TABLE 23-2
Anticonvulsant medications*,†

Generic name	Trade name	Total daily dose per kg body wt and usual adult dose	Principal therapeutic purposes	Serum half-life, h	Effective blood level, μg per 100 ml	Toxic level, μg per 100 ml
Phenobarbital	Luminal	1–5 mg; 60–200 mg	Major seizures; partial seizures; psychomotor seizures; and petit mal	96 ± 12	15	40
Diphenylhydantoin	Dilantin	4–7 mg; 200–500 mg	Major seizures; psychomotor seizures; partial epilepsy	24 ± 12	10	20
Primidone	Mysoline	10–25 mg; 750–1500 mg	Major seizures; psychomotor seizures; partial epilepsy	12 ± 6	5	12
Ethosuximide	Zarontin	20–30 mg; 1000–1500 mg	Petit mal	30 ± 6	40	100
Trimethadione	Tridione	10–25 mg; 500–1250 mg	Petit mal			
Paramethadione	Paradione	10–25 mg; 500–1250 mg	Petit mal			
Mephenytoin	Mesantoin	7–12 mg; 300–600 mg	Major seizures; psychomotor seizures; focal epilepsy			
Mephobarbital	Mebaral	2.5–10 mg; 200–500 mg	Same as phenobarbital; myoclonic epilepsy			
Methsuximide	Celontin	10–20 mg; 500–1000 mg	Petit mal			
Phensuximide	Milontin	10–20 mg; 500–1250 mg	Petit mal			
Acetazolamide	Diamox	5–15 mg; 250–750 mg	Petit mal; infantile spasms; major seizures			
Diazepam	Valium	0.15–2 mg; 15–30 mg	Petit mal; major seizures; status epilepticus			
Nitrazepam	Mogadon	0.15–2 mg; 10–100 mg	Infantile spasms; myoclonic epilepsy			
Ethotoin	Peganone	10–20 mg; 500–1000 mg	Major seizures; focal seizures			
ACTH		40–60 units per day	Infantile spasms			
Carbamazepine	Tegretol	10–20 mg; 1000–1200 mg	Tonic-clonic seizures; complex partial seizures	12 ± 3	4	8
Clonazepam	Rivotril	1–12 mg per day	Atypical petit mal			
Sodium valproate		400 mg qid	Intractable epilepsy of all types, especially atypical petit mal			

* Children usually need larger doses than adults, if dose is calculated according to body weight. Excessive drowsiness can often be diminished by dextroamphetamine (Dexedrine), methamphetamine (Desoxyn), or methylphenidate (Ritalin).
† This table lists only drugs in common use; for a complete list and discussion consult JK Penry (ed), Epilepsy: Eighth International Symposium, New York, Raven Press, 1977.

Indications for use of specific drugs GRAND MAL SEIZURES For those patients with infrequent grand mal seizures (from one to four per year), phenobarbital can be tried first because of its high therapeutic index and its relatively low toxicity. When the seizures are more frequent, Dilantin is the drug of choice. A combination of Dilantin (0.3 to 0.4 g) and phenobarbital (0.1 to 0.2 g) is more often effective than either of the drugs used alone. When these drugs are used in combination, a full therapeutic dose of each drug must be given. Occasionally, mephenytoin (Mesantoin) or a combination of this drug with the Dilantin or Mysoline will succeed where Dilantin alone has failed. In the more difficult cases carbamazepine, 400 mg tid, clonazepam, 2 mg tid, and sodium valproate, 400 mg qid, have controlled the seizures, though the carbamazepine is more effective in minor seizures.

The toxic effects of phenobarbital, which are drowsiness and mental dullness, nystagmus, and staggering, should be used as indications of excess dosage. Only skin eruption is a contraindication to its further use; otherwise these symptoms can be controlled by reducing the dose. Dilantin almost always leads to hypertrophy of gums, and, as was stated above, ataxia, stupor, or coma if given in excess dosages. If skin rashes and other hypersensitivity phenomena (polyarteritis) occur, discontinuation of the medication is necessary. Reduction of dose controls the other symptoms. The most important side effects of clonazepam and sodium valproate are drowsiness and lassitude. Nausea, vomiting, and diarrhea occur in approximately 10 percent of patients receiving clonazepam.

PSYCHOMOTOR ATTACKS Drugs effective in the treatment of grand mal seizures are effective in the treatment of patients with psychomotor attacks. Dilantin, 300 to 400 mg per day, and Mysoline, 750 to 1000 mg per day, have given the best results. The results on the whole are not as good as in grand mal epilepsy. Carbamazepine has had a notable success in many patients with this type of seizure. One should begin with a low dosage (100 mg bid or tid) and increase to 1200 mg per day.

PETIT MAL ATTACKS As a rule, drugs effective in the treatment of grand mal and psychomotor seizures are relatively ineffective in the treatment of patients with petit mal attacks. Ethosuximide (Zarontin), 750 to 1500 mg per day, has been most successful and has the advantage over trimethadione (Tridione), paramethadione (Paradione), and phensuximide (Milontin) in producing fewer side effects. It is wise to begin with a single dose of 250 mg per day and increase it every week until therapeutic effect is achieved. Toxic symptoms to Tridione and Paradione are skin eruptions and photophobia. Aplastic anemia has been reported; hence monthly blood counts during the first year are indicated. Methsuximide (Celontin; adult dose 0.3 g three or four times a day) and acetazolamide (Diamox; adult dose 0.25 to 0.75 g per day) have been useful in controlling difficult cases of petit mal and massive myoclonus in children. Atypical varieties of petit mal (2-per-second wave and spike EEG paroxysms) in association with myoclonus and akinetic falling spells or brief focal tonic or clonic seizures may be exceedingly resistant to medication. Methsuximide (Celontin) and acetazolamide (Diamox) or carbamazepine (Tegretol; adult dose 1.0 to 1.2 g per day) have had some success. Clonazepam, recently introduced (1.0 to 4.0 mg tid) and particularly sodium valproate (400 mg qid), are reported to have controlled atypical petit mal better than Zarontin.

MINOR SEIZURES AND FOCAL ATTACKS The same drugs effective in the treatment of grand mal and psychomotor seizures are effective against minor seizures and focal attacks. Minor seizures, which appear in patients whose grand mal attacks have been controlled, can occasionally be checked by simply increasing the dose of the drug or drugs that the patient is already taking. If the minor attacks are very infrequent and nonincapacitating, no great effort need be made to treat them.

PETIT MAL PLUS OTHER TYPES When patients are subject to petit mal seizures as well as grand mal or psychomotor seizures, they should receive Zarontin plus diphenylhydantoin sodium, phenobarbital, or sodium valproate.

MYOCLONIC EPILEPSY Mephobarbital (Mebaral), 0.2 to 0.5 g, and phenobarbital, 0.1 to 0.2 g, have been the most effective agents in this type of seizure, but in intractable cases clonazepam and sodium valproate should be tried. In the treatment of massive myoclonus in infants, ACTH or a combination of nitrazepam (Mogadon) and Diamox have been most effective.

Other treatments and management Surgery has been advocated for the removal of cortical scars secondary to cerebral trauma, of vascular lesions, and birth injuries on the assumption that such scars are surrounded by irritable foci which act as a trigger mechanism for the seizures. Reduction in the frequency of seizures has been reported as a sequel to these operations by a number of neurosurgeons. This treatment should be limited to the group of patients with focal attacks which do not respond to medical therapy. In addition, such lesions should be excised only by neurosurgeons who have facilities for the adequate localization of the lesion. Further medical treatment will still be required for most of these patients after operation.

The anterior tip of the temporal lobe and the amygdaloid nuclei have been removed or destroyed by stereotaxis in patients with psychomotor seizures who have failed to respond to medical therapy and in whom it was possible to demonstrate a temporal lobe focus by electroencephalography. Favorable results have been reported with this procedure by some neurosurgeons, but experience is too limited to evaluate its efficacy. The same may be said of implantation of cerebellar stimulators and section of the corpus callosum to prevent spread of seizure.

Biofeedback in which the patient is warned of the abnormal brainwaves and is trained to control them has attracted attention in the lay press, but the studies are so poorly controlled and so limited that no conclusions can be drawn.

Since epilepsy is a long-term medical problem, general hygienic measures are important, for they tend to stabilize the neurophysiologic state of the cerebrum. They should include regular hours of sleep, balanced diet, daily exercise, avoidance of constipation, and abstinence from alcohol. With proper safeguards even the more dangerous sports such as swimming and football may be permitted. The uncontrolled epileptic obviously should not be allowed to drive a car, operate unguarded machines, climb to heights, and so forth. Patients whose seizures are under medical control are no more dangerous on the highways than the average nonepileptic citizen.

Psychotherapy will help prevent or overcome feelings of inferiority and self-consciousness or shame. Both the patient and family will benefit from such therapy, and proper attitudes may be established. Oversolicitude and overprotection are to be discouraged. It is important for the patient live as normal a life as possible.

Every effort should be made to keep children in school, and adults should stay at work. Many communities have a branch of the American Committee against Epilepsy or a vocational rehabilitation center, and advantage should be taken of such facilities. Patients should participate in available recreational activities such as movies, dancing, and parties.

Not infrequently the convulsive disorder is but one manifestation of a widespread static cerebral disease that in itself interferes with education and work. Then realistic planning for activities that lie within the patient's scope is desirable.

As with all medications there are side effects. Toxic levels may cause confusion, stupor, or coma. Diphenylhydantoin may induce cerebellar ataxia, nystagmus, ocular palsies, asterixes, chorea, or choreoathetosis; chronic overdose may leave in its wake a permanent cerebellar ataxia due presumably to degeneration of Purkinje cells. Chronic usage of barbiturates leads to addiction and withdrawal effects (see Chap. 228).

REFERENCES

Adams RD, Victor M: *Principles of Neurology.* New York, McGraw-Hill, 1977

Glazer GH: Epilepsy, in *Recent Advances in Clinical Neurology*, WB Mathews (ed). Edinburgh, Churchill Livingstone, 1975, pp 23–68

Hauser WA, Kurland LT: The epidemiology of epilepsy in Rochester, Minnesota. Epilepsia 16:1, 1975

Jasper HH et al (eds): *Basic Mechanisms of the Epilepsies.* Boston, Little, Brown, 1969

Lennox W, Lennox M: *Epilepsy and Related Disorders.* Boston, Little, Brown, 1960

Lühdorf K et al: Epilepsy, in *Eighth International Symposium*, JF Penry (ed). New York, Raven Press, 1977, pp 209–214

Schmidt RP, Wilder BJ: *Contemporary Neurology Series*, vol 5: *Epilepsy*, F Plum, FH McDowell (eds). Philadelphia, Davis, 1968

24
AFFECTIONS OF SPEECH

JAY P. MOHR
RAYMOND D. ADAMS

Language and speech are of fundamental significance to humanity both in social intercourse and private intellectual life. When disordered as a consequence of disease of the brain, the loss exceeds in gravity even blindness, deafness, and paralysis.

GENERAL CONSIDERATIONS

The terms *speech* and *language* refer to some of the most complex and poorly understood integrating activities of the cerebrum. The terms are not synonymous.

Speech involves the execution of acquired skills by which vocal, manual, auditory, and visual systems are utilized to permit the conveyance of communicative efforts. These skills include: pronunciation of words, variations in stress, intonation, and melody; the production of graphic marks in the accepted spatial orientation; the discrimination of spoken speech and its classification as to speaker; the discrimination of handwritten or printed speech, the visual search patterns involved in scanning a text; and the use of other, less specifiable behaviors. Deficiencies in these skills impede interpersonal communication apart from any separate impairment in language usage; when intact, these skills do not suffice for any but elemental communication, such as that between two individuals who speak languages unfamiliar to each other.

Language has a wider connotation and refers to the selection and serial ordering of individual words according to accepted rules that permit a person using the speech modalities to modify the behavior of another and to externalize that poorly understood cerebral activity referred to as *thinking*. A disturbance of language usage, usually accompanied by a disturbance in speech from cerebral dysfunction, is referred to as *aphasia*, or more properly as *dysphasia* (see below).

CEREBRAL DOMINANCE AND ITS RELATIONSHIP TO SPEECH AND HANDEDNESS

The functional supremacy of one cerebral hemisphere is crucial to language function. There are three ways of determining that the left side of the brain is dominant: (1) the loss of speech when disease occurs in certain parts of the left hemisphere and its preservation in diseases involving corresponding parts of the right hemisphere; (2) the greater facility in the use of the right hand, foot, and eye; (3) the arrest of speech immediately after the injection of amobarbital (Amytal sodium) or some other drug in the left internal carotid artery. Only (2) and (3) are of use in deciding the cerebral dominance of a living, healthy patient. Unfortunately the Amytal sodium, or Wada, test does not reproduce the syndrome of major hemisphere inactivation. There is only mutism, followed by a brief period of groping for names. Presumably it gives information about the localization of motor output areas rather than of sensory ones.

Of the general population approximately 90 to 95 percent are right-handed; the remainder prefer the left hand. A person who chooses the right hand for intricate, complex acts and is more skillful with it is said to be right-handed. The preference is more complete in some persons than in others. Most individuals are neither right-handed nor completely left-handed but favor one hand for more complicated tasks.

The reason for hand preference is still controversial. There is strong evidence of a hereditary factor, but the mode of inheritance is uncertain. Learning is also a factor; many children are shifted at an early age from left to right (shifted sinistrals) because it is a handicap to be left-handed in a right-handed world. Many right-handed persons sight with the right eye, and it has been said that eye preference determines hand preference.

Anatomic differences between the dominant and the minor cerebral hemispheres have recently attracted attention. The left planum temporale, part of Wernicke's language zone, in the left hemisphere, is larger, and other evidence of asymmetries elsewhere are being uncovered; it is suggested that they are related to functional hemispheral differences.

Left-handedness may result from disease of the left cerebral hemisphere in early life; this fact probably accounts for its higher incidence among the feebleminded and brain-injured. Presumably the neural mechanisms for language then become centered in the right cerebral hemisphere. Handedness and cerebral dominance may fail to develop in some individuals; this is particularly true in certain families.

In studies of groups of left-handed individuals who suffer cerebral derangements of speech, it has been noted that approximately 75 percent have had lesions in the left cerebral hemisphere. Further, in those extremely rare cases of aphasia due to right cerebral lesions, the patient is nearly always left-handed, and the speech disorder tends to be less severe and enduring. The latter may take the form of an expressive disturbance, with prominent faults in calculation, implicit unawareness of the neurologic deficits (anosognosia), and visuoconstructive troubles.

The functional capacities of the minor hemisphere in speech are not fully understood despite careful anatomic studies. An additional problem in assessment is the uncertainty as to whether any residual function after lesions of the major hemisphere is due to recovery of parts of its language zones or to the activity solely of the minor hemisphere. The following functions are not disturbed in lesions of the left hemisphere: motor responses of mimicry, social anticipation (smiling, hand-shaking, modesty reactions) and self-care (washing and feeding), avoidance behavior to noxious stimuli, and capability of training in performances of cross-matching visually presented simple words with pictures.

TYPES OF LANGUAGE DISORDERS ENCOUNTERED IN MEDICAL PRACTICE

These may be divided into four categories:

1 *Cerebral disturbances* in which there is a loss more or less exclusively of the production and/or comprehension of spoken and/or written speech and language. Such a condition is called *aphasia,* or, in milder degrees, *dysphasia.*
2 *Defects in articulation* with intact mental functions and normal comprehension and memory of words. These are pure motor disorders of the muscles of articulation and may be due to flaccid or spastic paralysis, rigidity, repetitive spasms (stuttering), or ataxia. The terms *anarthria* and *dysarthria* have been applied to some of these conditions.
3 *Loss of voice* due to a disease of the larynx or its innervation, with resultant *aphonia* or *dysphonia.*
4 *Disturbances of speech* that occur with diseases affecting the higher nervous integrations, namely delirium and dementia (see Chaps. 21 and 25). Speech is seldom lost in these conditions but is instead merely deranged as part of a general impairment of all elements of language.

APHASIA OR DYSPHASIA In the scientific study of aphasia one faces formidable problems since there are no experimental models; this prevents the easy testing of hypotheses of speech and language function. The only reliable source materials are humans with cerebral disease, and the study of such cases is hampered by a number of uncontrollable variables such as the difficulty in delineating the basic functional deficit and the changes in symptomatology at different periods in the timecourse of the disease. The anatomic site of the lesion is often imprecisely characterized which makes for difficulty in clinicoanatomic and clinicopathologic correlation. And, finally, of theoretical importance is the problem of ascribing normal function to a part of the cerebrum by a study of the abnormal diseased brain.

As a general orientation, most of the lesions that lead to aphasia are known to be located in the perisylvian or *opercular* regions (frontal, temporal, and parietal) that cover the insula of the dominant cerebral hemisphere, i.e., the left in right-handed individuals.

The clinical deficit is most easily demonstrated in the acute phase. The changes that occur with time make estimation of lesion site and size more difficult later on, especially with the smaller lesions. Lesions one or more centimeters in diameter are often found at autopsy in cases whose clinical deficit was evanescent and had faded to functional insignificance within weeks or months. Diseases affecting the cerebral surface gray matter produce a more significant deficit than those more confined to the white matter; tumors, for example, confined as they are largely to the white matter, may reach discouragingly large size before speech or language deficit is evident. The site is more significant than the size of the lesion, for the former determines the qualitative features of the deficit, but the size determines the quantitative features and, in the larger lesions, appears to produce additional qualitative features not present in the smaller lesions. In particular, deficits in speech function are more evident in smaller lesions, while deficits in language as well as speech functions occur in the larger lesions.

The importance of site of lesion is well illustrated by a study of the types of aphasia observed in diseases affecting the sylvian territory. Those that lie anteriorly produce deficits in the acts of speaking. These disorders include mutism, impaired articulation, disordered transitions from syllable to syllable, and defective stress, intonation, and melody. Those located more posteriorly produce malpositioning of the oral cavity and some anticipatory errors out of sequence that result in gross mispronunciations of the intended syllables and words, more evident when the expected utterance is lengthy. Lesions grouped around the posterior sylvian fissure including the superior temporal lobe and its auditory gyri are manifested by disordered discrimination of spoken words, resulting in poor repetition of speech sounds and faulty understanding of spoken language.

Language deficits are well understood and less well correlated with anatomic pathology. Many formulations of aphasia envision only one "true" language deficit, the detection of which by any method of testing suffices to label the patient as aphasic. But those formulations based more on pathoanatomic correlations are leaning more toward separation of two large categories of disorder. That disorder reflecting large lesions involving the bulk of the frontal operculum and insula shows *agrammatism,* which features sharply contracted sentence structure, lacking most small grammatic words, often with faulty use of grammar in the words remaining, the surviving words serving mainly a predicative or substantive function. Large posterior sylvian lesions show almost the opposite, with substantive elements missing or substituted by errors in which the desired response is only approximated (paraphasias). These latter may consist of faulty pronunciations (literal paraphasias) or faulty word selections (verbal paraphasias). Disturbances in understanding language through auditory and visual speech forms reflect both types of major paraphasias.

Lesions in other parts of the cerebrum either cause no disturbance of human communicative skills or alter them only secondarily. An example of the latter is the lesion of the frontal lobes, especially the medial and orbital parts which impairs all motor activities, and often results in abulia, verging on akinetic mutism. The speech is laconic with long pauses between utterances, and there is an inability to sustain monologue and narrative. Extensive occipital lesions impair reading and reduce the utilization of all visual, lexic stimuli. Thalamic and deep cerebral lesions impair alertness and cause fluctuant states of inattention and disorientation, thereby inducing fragmentation of words (neologisms) and phrases, and protracted uncontrollable talking (logorrhea). Strong stimulation which momentarily stabilizes behavior and speech informs us of the essential integrity of language mechanisms.

In the initial formulations of cerebral function in the last century, it was easily concluded that lesions of the frontal (motor) regions produced syndromes independent from those of the posterior (sensory) regions, that the dysphasias could be classified as motor (Broca's) or sensory (Wernicke's), and could be further specified as subcortical, cortical, or transcortical in type. Subcortical lesions were envisioned to cut off the main efferent or afferent projections of the cortical "center." Cortical lesions involved the "centers" themselves. Transcortical lesions isolated the "centers" from one another, i.e., a kind of "conduction" aphasia, or from other regions of the brain. In modern times, the difficulties in attempting to understand the disorders of language that usually accompany the disorders of speech in focal brain disease, the improvements in techniques to document the extent of the lesion, and data available in longitudinal studies have led to a greater awareness of the complexity of these relationships.

TYPES OF APHASIA The examination of patients with disturbances of speech and language discloses a number of different abnormalities. Attempts have been made to classify them in terms of their predominant form, their presumed physiologic or psychologic bases, or the anatomy of the underlying diseases. No one of the many schemes has been accepted, and the leading students of language have railed against the premature acceptance of incomplete simplistic theories of language.

The most readily recognized type of aphasia is one that is complete or global, in which all modes of expression (spoken word, written word, and gesture) as well as the capacity for reading and understanding of spoken words are abolished. If more or less permanent, large perisylvian lesions of the left cerebral hemisphere are demonstrable, they usually reflect involvement of both divisions of the left middle cerebral artery. A second major type involves the motor, verbal, and executive side of the language and is named *Broca's aphasia*. The lesion is large, involving the bulk of the anterosuperior sylvian operculum and insula, in the territory of supply of the upper division of the left middle cerebral artery. A third major type involves the receptive, sensory, and central aspects of language and is named *Wernicke's aphasia*. The syndrome is ascribed to a large lesion involving the left posterior temporal and parietal regions, in the territory of supply of the lower, posterior division of the left middle cerebral artery. There are in addition a number of so-called "dissociative" aphasias such as "conduction" aphasia, "pure" word deafness, "pure" word blindness, "amnestic" aphasia, and "pure" agraphia, each attributed to smaller lesions within the speech areas or in their afferent and efferent connections. Scrutiny of these syndromes has shown that their anatomy is poorly established, and ideas about them are more in tune with theory of language than observed fact.

The practical student might question the purpose of these classifications. There are several. Many of these syndromes have fairly specific anatomic localizing value and are of clinical assistance to the physician in cases having surgical implications. In addition, the different prognoses attached to several syndromes are helpful in management and in the use of different corrective measures in therapy. And, finally, such data might become the basis of a unified theory of language.

Complete (global) aphasia This syndrome is due to a lesion that destroys a large part of the speech areas of the major cerebral hemisphere. As such, it represents the maximal aphasic deficit possible and shows the least improvement of all aphasic syndromes. Since the middle cerebral artery nourishes all the speech areas, nearly all aphasic syndromes due to vascular occlusion are caused by involvement of this artery or its branches. In complete aphasia, occlusion of the left internal carotid or the middle cerebral artery at its origin is usually responsible. Less often, the syndrome may be caused by a large hemorrhage, tumor, other lesions, or even temporarily as a postictal effect of grand mal epilepsy.

Most patients with total aphasia can say at most a few words; they cannot read or write, and they understand only a few words and phrases of the speech of others. Related signs include right hemiplegia, hemianesthesia, and homonymous hemianopia. The state of consciousness may vary from full alertness to semicoma. The alert patient may participate in common gestures of greeting, may show modesty and avoidance reactions, and is able to engage in self-help activities. With the passage of time some degree of understanding of spoken speech may be evident, and a few spoken words may emerge. Early appearance of clearly vocalized stereotyped words, such as "hi," are often falsely encouraging signs and may reflect the uninhibited function of the right hemisphere. Rapid improvement frequently occurs when the main cause is edema, postconvulsive paralysis, or transient metabolic derangements such as infection, or hyponatremia, which worsen old aphasic lesions. Although speech loss from a disintegrating embolus of the left middle artery may be transient, some part of the deficit may persist, being easily demonstrated by presenting the patient with complex words or double negatives in sentences.

Broca's aphasia (major motor aphasia) This term is used to designate a complex syndrome, predominantly a failure of motor aspects of speaking and writing, with an accompanying *agrammatism* and a variable impairment in language comprehension. Although commonly thought due to a circumscribed lesion in the inferior frontal convolution (Broca's area), this major syndrome is usually the result of a larger lesion, involving cortical and subcortical structures along the frontal and superior sylvian fissure including the insula, in the territory of supply of the upper division of the left middle cerebral artery.

The large extent of the lesion, and involvement of the sensorimotor rolandic region, account for the more or less dense right hemiparetic and hemisensory syndrome that almost invariably accompanies the aphasia and usually persists. Initially, a transient right hemianopia and an ipsilateral deviation of the eyes are observed.

In the acute phase of the syndrome, the entire language mechanism appears inactivated, and the helplessly mute, noncommunicative, and uncomprehending patient presents the syndrome of *total aphasia*, indistinguishable by present methods from the previously described form of total aphasia coming from infarction of the whole left middle cerebral artery territory. Within weeks to years, the disorder of comprehension abates somewhat but remains forever easily detected by formal testing. This improvement in comprehension exceeds that in speaking and writing, where deficits are sufficient to stamp the syndrome traditionally as *motor aphasia*.

In the chronic stage of the syndrome, the patient will have severe difficulties in speaking aloud. The lower part of the face on the right side is weak and sags, and the tongue also deviates to the weak side, usually accompanied by weakness of the right arm and leg. For a time, despite satisfactory comprehension of spoken words and ability to read simple commands, an apraxia of the linguooropharyngeal apparatus is manifested in faulty efforts to smack the lips and to make other purposeful or commanded movements. In these circumstances imitation of the examiner's actions are better performed than execution of acts on command. Self-initiated actions, by contrast, are often normal. The patient who speaks at all may repeat a few remaining words over and over, as if compelled to do so. Certain stereotyped phrases such as "hi," "good morning," "how are you" seem to be more easily emitted, as are the words of popular songs when sung. When angered or excited, the patient may curse. Thus, it is evident that although "speechless" the person is not "wordless." The patient's efforts and facial expressions suggest an awareness of his or her own ineptitudes and mistakes. Repeated failures cause exasperation and despair.

As improvement occurs and in the milder forms of motor aphasia, the patient is able to speak aloud to some degree. Words are enunciated slowly and laboriously. Articulation and the melody of speech (prosody) are impaired. This dysfluency takes the form of improper accent or stress on certain syllables, incorrect phrasing of words in a series, pacing of the speed of word sequences, and even a stammering stuttering quality to the uttered phrases. Speech is sparse and consists mainly of nouns, transitive verbs, and important adjectives; many of the small words (articles, prepositions, conjunctions) are omitted, giving the speech an agrammatic and telegraphic character. The substantive content allows the patient to communicate to some extent despite the gross mechanical and language difficulties. Once fully established, these speech impediments persist and improve only slightly despite years of speech therapy.

Most patients with Broca's aphasia have a correspondingly severe impairment in writing. Should their right hand be paralyzed, they cannot print with their left one; if manual mobility is spared, they fail as completely in writing out their commands or replies to questions as in speaking them. Writing from dictation is severely impaired, though letters and words can still be copied. On careful testing, communication by writing can be shown superior to that of speaking, suggesting a certain independence between these two acts as vehicles of language.

The lesion of Broca's aphasia is most often an infarction of frontal, anterior parietal, and anterior insular parts of the cerebrum due to embolic occlusion of the upper division of the left middle cerebral artery. Major putaminal hypertensive hemorrhage is also a common cause. A huge frontal lobe tumor or abscess is occasionally responsible; metastatic lesions, subdural hematoma, and encephalitis only rarely cause the syndrome.

Minor motor aphasia Sharp focal lesions along the anterior and superior sylvian operculum and insula produce remarkably circumscribed effects on the mechanical elaboration of speech which can be observed alone or in combinations, depending on the site and extent of the lesion. However, *none of these focal lesions produces significant or lasting deficits in language usage;* the experienced listener can easily detect the error patterns in speech and, through them, discern the communicative efforts of the sufferer, who is acutely aware of and discouraged by the deficit. The effects on speech of focal opercular lesions take several forms. *Broca's area infarction* involves the lower premotor cortex adjacent to the motor cortex for the oropharynx, larynx, and respiratory apparatus; the infarct interrupts skilled movements of these muscle groups, and the resultant dyspraxia in speech takes the form of impaired transitions between syllables and words, and disruption of the melodic intonation of phrases (dysprosody). Involvement of this region appears insufficient to produce the major syndrome referred to as Broca's aphasia. *Rolandic infarction* involves the sensorimotor cortex itself; poor articulation, lowered volume and pitch of speech, and a nasal quality to the voice reveal the pareses of the involved musculature. *Postcentral, anterior parietal infarction* appears to be associated with errors in the positioning of the oral cavity for individual sounds, syllables, and whole words; the acoustic features of the utterance are often distorted by these malpositions of the oral cavity and strike the listener's ear as literal paraphasias. Since they are easily produced in tests of repeating and reading aloud and occur in conversation, the patient could be labeled as having "conduction" aphasia. The important point with all these minor motor aphasias is that at first they may resemble major motor aphasia except for the satisfactory understanding of spoken and written words. The prognosis for nearly full recovery is excellent.

Most lesions sufficiently focal as to produce such circumscribed deficits are embolic in nature. The sequential branching of the upper division of the middle cerebral artery provides a series of separate sites for emboli to lodge. Deeper, larger lesions, or larger emboli involving the stem of the upper division, encompass several deficit types in a single patient, making these individual distinctions less clear, and blend with the major syndromes of Broca's aphasia. Facial, lingual, and sometimes brachial paresis and ideomotor dyspraxia of the face and *left,* nondominant limbs commonly accompany the speech disorder. Most of these syndromes fade in clinical significance within weeks or months.

Wernicke's aphasia (major central or sensory aphasia) This term encompasses a wide range of syndromes reflecting lesions from the posterior perisylvian structures to the posterior parietooccipital regions supplied by the lower division of the middle cerebral artery. There is disruption of the whole array of language behavior. When more restricted to the temporal lobe, the main disturbance is most evident in language tasks involving words heard; when more parietooccipital, in words seen.

In brief, spoken and written efforts at communication as well as in auditory and visual comprehension are affected, a combination which justifies the term *central aphasia.* The older term, *sensory aphasia,* was formerly used to accentuate the contrast from motor (Broca's) aphasia; instead of the difficult articulation, faulty transitions, dysmelodic speaking, and disproportionate condensation of grammatical forms that characterize Broca's aphasia, the speech of Wernicke's aphasia is fluent. Hence the name "fluent aphasia." We prefer the eponym, *Wernicke's aphasia,* for it serves to encompass all the syndromes while avoiding the many sharp controversies that still surround unsuccessful attempts to characterize these aphasias by a single functional term.

In severe cases, the patient utters a series of incomprehensible syllables, makes illegible marks on a page in attempts at writing, cannot be made to repeat aloud or copy at sight correctly, and treats the examiner's attempts at written and verbal communication as if they were in a wholly unfamiliar foreign language. In less severe cases, the patient can be made to repeat aloud and copy, but in so doing frequently echoes the words heard with faulty pronunciation, or copies the words seen in a slavish manner, imitating even the examiner's handwriting style. It is as though the test words were unfamiliar. Clearly the disturbance in language does not simply reflect a disturbance in hearing or in vision. In the mildest cases, the deficits are reflected in errors in word comprehension and usage that show some approximation to the desired response, the words often belonging to the same functional class (i.e., "cow" for "pig," but not "cow" for "yellow"); errors in word structure, with improper tenses, prefixes, suffixes (i.e., "beautifuling"); and other errors that resemble performances by normal people unfamiliar with the language in question. Some such patients pass for normal in casual conversation. Their speech resembles the performance of people tired or distracted, and their abnormality is detected only on tests of complex language function. This state is often the residual of a more severe initial deficit.

As a rule, the syndrome is due to an embolic occlusion of the lower division of the left middle cerebral artery. A "slit hemorrhage" in the subcortex of the temporoparietal region or involvement of the temporal isthmus and adjacent white matter by tumor, abscess, or extension of a small putaminal or thalamic hemorrhage may have similar effects. The posterior sylvian region, comprising posterosuperior temporal, opercular supramarginal, and posterior insular gyri, appears to encompass a variety of language functions, since seemingly minor changes in size and locale of the lesion are associated with important variations in the elements of Wernicke's aphasia detailed below.

Minor central aphasia syndromes In time the patient with Wernicke's aphasia improves, and in so doing a number of lesser syndromes appear. These latter, however, may be present in comparatively pure form from the beginning, when only small restricted lesions involve some part of the territory of the lower division of the middle cerebral artery. Depending on the exact locale of lesion, language behavior dependent on auditory function (hearing spoken words, echoing sounds and speech, relating the spoken to the written word, and finally repeating and writing it) may be deranged partially or in its entirety. The same is true of language behavior dependent upon visual function, when the left posterior parietal lobe is involved.

These partial syndromes have been traditionally labeled as conduction aphasia, pure word deafness, and pure word blindness.

Attempts to correlate complete and partial posterior sylvian syndromes with arteriographic findings during life frequently fail. Since most partial vascular aphasias are due to cerebral embolism, the latter may have lodged in the artery long enough to cause infarction and then disintegrate. The arteriogram done after this happens is normal. Or a fragment of the disintegrating embolus may drift distally and permanently block only a more distal branch, sometimes permitting part of the ischemic tissue to recover. Computerized tomography (CT scan) has proved a helpful addition to attempts to delineate the areas involved.

Dissociative speech syndromes These disorders are characterized by an interruption of afferent nervous impulses to the language mechanism or efferent ones from these centers to other motor structures. This concept is an interesting one and has had the heuristic value of indicating certain lines of anatomicophysiologic separation of language functions. However, the anatomy of several of the following conditions is far from proved, and the theories that derive from such data as are available lead one to a naïve conception of the language mechanisms in terms of a kind of telephonic circuitry. With these reservations we present the following syndromes.

CONDUCTION APHASIA: SEPARATION OF WERNICKE'S AND BROCA'S LANGUAGE AREAS   Here the principal abnormality resembles Wernicke's aphasia in certain respects. There is the same paraphasia in self-initiated speech, in repeating what is heard, and in reading aloud. In contrast, no difficulty is shown in comprehending words that are heard or seen. Nor is any element of dysarthria or dysprosody detected. The patient is alert and aware of the deficit. One of the best ways of eliciting the defect is to have the patient repeat nonsense syllables. The mistakes are then manifestly of a type observed in literal paraphasia, i.e., close similarity but detectably different sounds occasioned by improper positioning of the oropharyngeal apparatus. The disorder in repeating from dictation becomes more apparent when the rate of presentation of auditory material is increased and as the uttered words become more polysyllabic. Since nouns are the longest words in the sentence, one may gain an impression that they are specifically affected.

The lesion in autopsied cases is located in the cortex and subcortical white matter in the upper bank of the sylvian fissure, involving the supramarginal gyrus of the inferior parietal lobule and occasionally the posterior part of the superior temporal region. Presumably fiber systems in the insula are interrupted. The usual cause is an embolus in the ascending parietal or posterior temporal branch of the middle cerebral artery. Deeper, larger lesions in position to interrupt the arcuate fasciculus connecting the temporal and frontal lobes usually involve other pathways as well, giving rise to a more extensive speech deficit (central, Wernicke's aphasia, or amnestic aphasia). However, these latter types of aphasia, as they regress, may resolve into conduction aphasia. More anterior insular lesions usually include some degree of Broca's aphasia.

"PURE" WORD DEAFNESS   This syndrome could be considered the auditory form of Wernicke's aphasia, in which the most obvious findings are an impaired auditory comprehension and inability to repeat what is said or to write to dictation. Spoken language is far better performed but is rarely normal, and occasionally the patient is initially diagnosed as having Wer-

nicke's aphasia. By audiometric testing no hearing defect is found, or minor abnormalities appear which may well reveal the underlying deficit in individual cases. Ordinary sounds can be distinguished. The patient is forced to depend heavily on visual cues in understanding the remarks of others and frequently uses these cues well enough to obviate much of the difficulty. But tests which prevent the use of visual cues readily uncover the deficit. Comprehension of visually presented material, for example, printed matter such as newspapers, is far better than auditory comprehension; it occasionally approaches normal, and justifies use of the traditional term, *pure word deafness.*

In most recorded autopsy studies the lesion has been embolic, bilateral in the superior temporal gyrus, and in position to damage the primary auditory cortex in the transverse gyrus of Heschl and its relations to the association areas of the superior, posterior part of the temporal lobe. The few unilateral lesions are localized in this part of the major (dominant) temporal lobe and encroach on those regions whose involvement precipitates the larger syndrome of Wernicke's aphasia.

DYSLEXIA WITH DYSGRAPHIA   This syndrome features a language disturbance most evident in reading and writing. The errors take a form typical of those encountered in the larger syndrome of Wernicke's aphasia. Yet auditory comprehension is so much superior to visual comprehension that the syndrome could be considered the visual form of Wernicke's aphasia. Since conversational testing frequently is the extent of many casual clinical evaluations of such patients, satisfactory auditory comprehension, ability to repeat aloud, and mild paraphasic errors in spontaneous speech frequently lead to a diagnosis of very mild Wernicke's aphasia. Detailed testing of reading aloud and for comprehension, and tests of spontaneous writing and writing in response to dictated and visually presented material, will reveal a far greater disturbance on these tasks and expose the syndrome. This type of aphasia is often the late sequel of the larger syndrome of Wernicke's aphasia.

The parietooccipital region is the anatomic site of this deficit. A lesion here is unusual in embolism, which more often affects structures more proximal in the territory of the lower division of the middle cerebral artery. Tumors, abscess, and the like disrupt other structures as well, and this syndrome is often a less conspicuous part of a larger clinical picture. Systemic hypotension and hypoxia may leave as a residual abnormality dyslexia with dysgraphia; but more often they have produced a more severe defect described below under "Isolation of speech areas."

"PURE" WORD BLINDNESS   In this state literate persons lose their ability to read and often to name colors. They can no longer name or point on dictated command to visual letter stimuli or the words of which they are composed. However, understanding spoken language, repetition of what is heard, writing to dictation, and conversation are all intact. Often the patient is unaware of the difficulty and registers no complaint; it is discovered almost by accident. In lesser degrees of the affection, reading aloud is possible, but the patient manages only a single letter at a time (this may be seen in otherwise normal patients who have bilateral hemianopia with only central vision remaining); commonly letter or name responses that seem to have little connection with the presented ones are expressed. The response may be corrected and the defect obscured if other visual cues are available, such as the bottle on which the words Coca-Cola appear. The naming of common colors presented singly and of objects is also impaired. When the dominant hemisphere is involved, as it usually is in such cases, there may be a right homonymous hemianopia, an amnestic defect (see Chap. 25), and a hemisensory defect on the right due to involvement of the left occipital lobe, the left fornix and its decussation, and the left thalamus, respectively, a combination which nearly always signifies thrombosis or embolism of the left posterior cerebral artery.

The autopsy of such lesions has usually demonstrated a lesion that destroys the left visual striate cortex (area 17) and visual association areas (18 and 19), as well as the connections of the right visual cortex and association areas with the temporoparietal region. This latter "disconnection" usually is due to interruption of the fibers passing through the posterior part (splenium) of the corpus callosum, which connect the visual association areas of the two hemispheres. A lesion deep in the left parietooccipital region may also prevent visual information from both occipital lobes reaching the left angular gyrus. In this case the right homonymous hemianopia may be absent. With purely left cerebral lesions, aside from vascular lesions there may be a primary or secondary tumor, or, rarely, multifocal leukoencephalopathy may be the underlying disease.

ISOLATION OF SPEECH AREAS Following prolonged hypotension or carbon monoxide poisoning, widespread cerebral ischemia affects the vascular anatomic border zones linking the major cerebral arteries and their distal branches on the cerebral surfaces, and spreads centripetally into their adjacent territories. The central fields of supply of these arteries are spared. In the middle cerebral artery territory, this sparing leaves largely intact the sylvian region and its speech areas. With much of the rest of the brain out of action in patients who have survived such hypoxic-hypotensive accidents, the speech mechanism is preserved and can be activated by spoken words. There is parrot-like repetition of words and sounds (echolalia) and similar findings which indicate that the auditory-vocal loop remains functional. Scant evidence of comprehension or self-initiated conversation has been observed, findings that are thought to reflect the widespread injury outside the speech regions. The syndrome is of great theoretic interest, and may prove common in cases surviving cardiac arrest.

Amnestic-dysnomic aphasia This may be a relatively early or an isolated manifestation of disease of the nervous system. The patient loses only the ability to produce names on demand, including nouns, adjectives, and other descriptive parts of speech. There are typical pauses in speech, groping for words, and substitution of another word or phrase that conveys the meaning (circumlocution). When shown a series of common objects, the patient may tell of their use instead of giving their names. The difficulty applies not only to objects seen but to the names of things heard or felt. By contrast, other verbal tasks, including recall of the names for letters, digits, reading, writing, spelling, etc., are almost invariably preserved. That the deficit is principally one of naming is shown by the patient's correct use of the object and, usually, by an ability to point to the correct object on hearing or seeing the name. There is a tendency among patients to attribute their failure to forgetfulness, or to give some other lame excuse for the disability, suggesting that they are not completely aware of the nature of their difficulty.

The causative lesion is usually deep in the temporal lobe, in position, probably, to interrupt connections of sensory speech areas with the hippocampal-parahippocampal regions concerned with learning and memory. Mass lesions, such as a tu-

mor or an otogenic abscess, are the most frequent, and as they enlarge, an upper contralateral quadrantic visual field defect or Wernicke's aphasia is added. Occasionally, dysnomia appears with diseases which occlude the temporal branches of the posterior cerebral artery. Alzheimer's disease and senile dementia may begin with a dysnomic or amnestic type of aphasia. By the time the patient's difficulty is fully recognized, other disorders of speech and indifference, apathy, and abulia are conjoined. This deficit may also be discovered in testing patients with a confusional state caused by metabolic, infectious, intoxicative, or other acute medical illnesses, but then it has no certain localizing value.

DISORDERS OF ARTICULATION AND PHONATION In simple dysarthria there is no abnormality of the cortical centers. Dysarthric patients are able to understand perfectly what they hear, and if literate, read and have no difficulty in writing, even though they are unable to utter a single intelligible word. This is the strict meaning of being inarticulate.

The act of speaking is a highly coordinated sequence of contractions of the larynx, pharynx, palate, tongue, lips, and respiratory musculature. These are innervated by the hypoglossal, vagal, facial, and phrenic nerves. The nuclei of these nerves are controlled through the corticobulbar tracts by both motor cortices. As with all movements, there are also extrapyramidal influences from the cerebellum and basal ganglia. A current of air is produced by expiration, and the force of it is finely regulated by the activity of the various muscles engaged in speech. *Phonation,* or the production of vocal sounds, is a function of the larynx. Changes in the size and shape of the glottis and in the length and tension of the vocal cords are controlled by the action of the laryngeal muscles. Vibrations are set up and transmitted to the column of air passing over the vocal cords. Sounds thus formed are modified as they pass through the nasopharynx and mouth, which act as resonators. Articulation consists of contractions of the tongue, lips, pharynx, and palate, which interrupt or alter the vocal sounds. Vowels are of laryngeal origin, as are some consonants, but the latter are formed for the most part during articulation. For instance, the consonants *m, b,* and *p* are labial, *l* and *t* are lingual, and *nk* and *ng* are nasoguttural.

Defective articulation and phonation are recognized at once by listening to patients during ordinary conversation or while they are reading aloud from a newspaper or book. Test phrases or attempts at rapid repetition of lingual, labial, and guttural consonants (e.g., la-la-la-la or me-me-me-me) bring out the particular abnormality. Disorders of phonation call for a precise analysis of the voice and its apparatus. The movements of the vocal cords should be inspected with the aid of a hand mirror, or, even better, a laryngoscope, and those of the tongue, palate, and pharynx by direct observation.

Defects in articulation may be subdivided into several types; paretic dysarthria, spastic and rigid dysarthria, choreic, myoclonic, and ataxic dysarthria.

Paretic dysarthria This is due to a neural or bulbar (medullary) weakness or paralysis of the articulatory muscles (lower motor neuron paralysis). In the latter condition the shriveled tongue lies inert on the floor of the mouth, and the lips are relaxed and tremulous. Saliva constantly collects in the mouth because of dysphagia, and spills over the lips causing drooling. Speech becomes less and less distinct. There is a special difficulty in the correct utterance of vibratives, such as r; as the paralysis becomes more complete, lingual and labial consonants are finally not pronounced at all. Degrees of this abnormality are observed in myasthenia gravis. Bilateral paralysis of the palate may occur with diphtheria, poliomyelitis, and progressive bulbar palsy. Bilateral paralysis of the lips, as in the facial diplegia of idiopathic polyneuritis, interferes with enunciation of labial consonants; *p* and *b* are slurred and sound more like *f* and *v*.

Spastic and rigid dysarthria These are more frequent than the paralytic variety. Diseases that involve the corticobulbar tracts, usually vascular disease or motor system disease, result in the syndrome of pseudobulbar palsy. The patient may have had a minor stroke some time in the past affecting the corticobulbar fibers on one side; but since the bulbar muscles are probably represented in both motor cortices, there is no impairment in speech or swallowing from a unilateral lesion. Should another stroke then occur, involving the other corticobulbar tract and possibly the corticospinal tract at the pontine, midbrain, or capsular level, the patient immediately becomes anarthric or dysarthric and dysphagic. Often the muscles of facial expression on both sides are weakened as well. Unlike bulbar paralysis due to lower motor neuron involvement, this condition entails no atrophy or fasciculation of the paralyzed muscles; the jaw jerk and other facial reflexes soon become exaggerated; the palatal reflexes are retained; emotional control is poor (pathologic laughter and crying); and sometimes breathing becomes periodic (Cheyne-Stokes). When the frontal operculum alone is involved, the speech deficit may be a pure dysarthria but usually without the impairment in emotional control. In the beginning, the patient may be totally anarthric and aphonic, but as improvement occurs or in mild degrees of the same condition, speech is notably slow, thick, and indistinct, much like that of partial bulbar paralysis.

In paralysis agitans, or postencephalitic Parkinson's syndrome, one observes an extrapyramidal disturbance of articulation. The patient speaks hastily and articulates poorly, slurring over many syllables and trailing off the end of sentences. The words are pronounced hastily. The voice is low-pitched, monotonous, and lacks inflection; voice volume diminishes. In advanced cases speech is almost unintelligible; only whispering is possible. It may happen that the patient finds it impossible to talk while walking but can speak if sitting or lying down.

Pyramidal and extrapyramidal disturbances of speech may be combined in generalized cerebral diseases such as general paresis, in which slurred speech is one of the cardinal signs.

In many cases of capsular hemiplegia or partially recovered Broca's aphasia the patient is left with a dysarthria that may be difficult to distinguish from a pure articulatory defect. Careful testing of other language functions, especially writing, will reveal the aphasic quality.

Choreic and myoclonic dysarthria In chorea and myoclonus, speech may also be affected in a highly characteristic way. Unlike the defect of pseudobulbar palsy or paralysis agitans, chorea and myoclonus abruptly interrupt the pronunciation of words by the abnormal movements. The idea is best conveyed by the phrase "hiccup speech," in that the breaks are as unexpected as in singultus. Grimacing and other characteristic motor signs must be depended upon for diagnosis.

Ataxic dysarthria This is characteristic of acute and chronic cerebellar lesions. It may be observed in multiple sclerosis, Friedreich's ataxia, cerebellar atrophy, and heat stroke. The principal speech abnormality is slowness; imprecise enunciation, monotony, and unnatural, irregular separation of the syllables of words (scanning) are other features. Coordination of speech and respiration are poor. There may not be enough breath to utter certain words, and others may be ejaculated explosively. *Scanning dysarthria* is distinctive, but in some cases, especially if there is a possibility of spastic weakness of the tongue from corticobulbar tract involvement, it is impossible to predict the anatomy of disease from analysis of speech alone. Myoclonic jerks involving the speech musculature may be superimposed on cerebellar ataxia in a number of diseases.

APHONIA AND DYSPHONIA Finally, a few points should be made concerning the group of speech disorders involving disturbances of voice.

Paresis of the respiratory movements, as in poliomyelitis and acute infectious polyneuritis, may affect voice because insufficient air is provided for phonation and speech. Also, disturbances in the rhythm of respiration may interfere with the fluency of speech. This is particularly noticeable in so-called "extrapyramidal diseases," where one may observe that the patient does not allow sufficient air during expiration to complete a phrase. In the latter conditions reduced volume of speech due to limited excursion of the breathing muscles is another common feature; the patient is unable to speak above a whisper or to shout. Whispering speech is also a feature of stupor, but strong stimulation may make the voice audible.

Paresis of both vocal cords causes complete aphonia. There is no voice, and the patient can speak only in whispers. Since the vocal cords normally separate during inspiration, their failure to do so when paralyzed may result in an inspiratory stridor. If one vocal cord is paralyzed, the voice becomes hoarse, low-pitched, and rasping. Involvement of one of the tenth cranial nerves by tumor, for example, may also cause a certain nasality of voice because the posterior nares do not close during phonation. Certain consonants such as *b*, *p*, *n*, and *k* are followed by escape of air into the nasal passages. The abnormality is sometimes less pronounced in recumbency and increases when the head is thrown forward. Hoarseness may also be due to structural changes in the vocal cords caused by cigarette smoking, chronic inflammation, polyps, etc.

Another curious condition about which little is known is *spastic dysphonia*. The authors have seen many patients, middle-aged or elderly men and women, otherwise healthy, who gradually lose the ability to speak quietly and fluently. Any effort to speak results in contraction of all the speech musculature so the patient's voice is strained and phonation is labored. This is apparently a neurologic disorder similar to writer's cramp, i.e., a kind of restricted dystonia. The patients are not neurotic, and psychotherapy and speech therapy have been ineffective. This condition differs from the stridor caused by spasm of the laryngeal muscles in tetany. It is nonprogressive but in some instances is combined with other of the restricted extrapyramidal disorders such as blepharospasm and spasmodic torticollis.

CLINICAL APPROACH TO LANGUAGE DISORDERS Aphasia In investigating a case of aphasia, it is first necessary to inquire into the patient's native language, handedness, and previous education. Many naturally left-handed children are trained to use their right hand for writing; therefore, in determining this point we must ask which hand is used for throwing a ball, threading a needle, or using a spoon and common tools such as a hammer, saw, or bread knife. It is important before the beginning of the examination to determine whether the patient is alert and can be made to participate reliably in testing, as accurate assessment of language depends on these factors. One should quickly ascertain whether the patient has other signs of a gross cerebral lesion such as hemiplegia, facial weakness, homonymous hemianopia, or cortical sensory loss. When hemiplegia, hemianesthesia, and homonymous hemianopia coexist, the aphasic disorder is usually complete or global. Such a constellation of major neurologic signs is seldom associated with the less complete forms of language disorder, the posterior sylvian syndromes, or one of the dissociative syndromes. Dyspraxia of limbs and speech musculature, in response to spoken commands or to visual mimicry, is generally associated with Broca's aphasia and sometimes with Wernicke's aphasia. Bilateral or unilateral homonymous hemianopia without motor weakness tends often to be linked to "pure" word blindness (alexia or dyslexia) or to amnestic-dysnomic aphasia. Bilateral hemiplegias due to extensive frontal lesions are accompanied not infrequently by "pure" word muteness. The special types of aphasia—alexia, "pure" word deafness, etc.—are often associated with evidence of embolism to other parts of the brain or other organs.

Conversational testing permits quick assessment of the motor aspects of speech (praxis and prosody) and apparent language formulation and auditory comprehension.

Disabilities in the purely motor aspects of speech suggest a motor aphasia, and this possibility can be pursued further by tests of repeating from dictation and by special tests of praxis of the oropharyngeal and respiratory apparatus. Disabilities in language formulation in the form of literal paraphasias with impaired comprehension are indicative of Wernicke's aphasia. Impaired comprehension but perfectly normal formulated speech suggest the rare syndrome of pure word deafness. Disorders confined to naming, generally without paraphasias, when other language functions (reading, writing, spelling, etc.) are found adequate, are diagnostic of amnestic dysnomia.

When conversation shows virtually no disabilities, other tests may still be revealing. Reading aloud single letters, words, and text may reveal the dissociative syndrome of pure word blindness, while tests of writing in this syndrome will show little abnormality. Literal and verbal paraphasic errors may appear in milder cases of Wernicke's aphasia as the patient reads aloud from text or from words in the examiner's handwriting. Similar errors appear even more frequently when the patient is asked to explain the text, read aloud, or give explanations in writing. Should such tests still be unrevealing of deficits, the examiner may find it useful to increase the complexity of the tests. If the patient then succeeds, one may be sure that there is no disorder of adequacy of reception. Adequacy of response channels is next determined by presenting the patient with tasks that permit a response physically identical with the test stimulus. Copying visual stimuli and repeating aloud from auditory stimuli are examples of this kind of testing. Inadequacy of receptive or response channels will then preclude further analysis of the deficit involving that channel in more complex types of tests, except in the unlikely instance that the more complex test is better performed. If reception and response channels are found adequate in these initial tests, they may then be used in tests requiring all types of language function, such as writing from dictation, vocal naming of visual stimuli, matching physically dissimilar stimuli having a name in common (i.e., the word "cow" and a picture of a cow). By utilizing the same test material used in the earlier tests, direct comparison of performances in spoken naming, written naming, and matching can be compared from visual, auditory, and palpated stimuli. A performance profile can be constructed separately for each type of stimulus material tested (i.e., objects, pictures, words, letters, numbers, colors, etc.). The resultant profile can then be used to determine whether the main deficits fall across one or more input or response channels. These data then provide a baseline against which later changes may be compared.

Articulatory-phonation disorders Disturbances of articulation point to involvement of a different set of neural structures, such as the motor cortices, the corticobulbar pathways, the seventh, ninth, and tenth nuclei, the brainstem, and extrapyramidal nuclei and tracts. Often it is necessary to use other neurologic findings to decide which of these are implicated in any given case. The important distinction between the pseudobulbar or supranuclear palsies and the bulbar palsies is grasped only with difficulty by the average student. The information obtained by localizing these two major types of dysarthria is extremely helpful in differential diagnosis.

Dysphonia should lead to an investigation of laryngeal disease, either primary or secondary to an abnormality of innervation. Inspection of vocal cords is a necessary step in the clinical study.

TREATMENT The sudden loss of speech would be expected to cause great apprehension, but except for almost pure motor defects, most patients show remarkably little concern. It appears that the very lesion that deprives them of speech also causes a partial loss of insight into their own disability. This reaches almost a ludicrous extreme in some cases of Wernicke's aphasia, in which patients become indignant when others cannot understand their jargon. Nonetheless, as improvement occurs, many patients do become discouraged. Reassurance and a positive program of speech rehabilitation are the best ways of helping the patient at this stage.

Most aphasic difficulties are due to vascular disease of the brain, and nearly always this is accompanied by some degree of spontaneous improvement in the days, weeks, and months that follow the stroke. Sometimes recovery is complete within hours or days; at times not more than a few words are regained after a year or two of assiduous speech training. Nevertheless, it is the opinion of many experts in the field that speech training is worthwhile.

One must decide for each patient whether speech training is needed and when it should be started. As a rule, therapy is not advisable in the first few days of an aphasic illness, because one does not know how lasting it will be. Also, if the patient suffers a severe global aphasia and can neither speak nor understand spoken and written words, the speech therapist is helpless. Under such circumstances, one does well to wait a few weeks until some one of the language functions has begun to return. Then the physician may begin to encourage and help the patient to use the function to a maximal degree. In milder aphasic disorders the patient may be sent to the speech therapist as soon as the illness has stabilized.

The methods of speech training are specialized, and it is advisable to call in a person who has been trained in this field.

There is no special treatment for the dysarthric disturbance of speech.

PROGNOSIS The outcome of aphasia depends on the nature of the underlying disease and the magnitude of the lesion within the speech areas. Global aphasias lasting more than a week or two usually have a bad outcome. Seldom is there enough recovery of communicative speech to permit resumption of occupation or profession. Partial aphasias frequently improve, sometimes to a gratifying degree, if of vascular or encephalitic origin. Aphasias due to embolism, whether global or restricted, may disappear in hours to days, like all cerebral embolic deficits, or persist.

REFERENCES

BRAIN R: Aphasia, apraxia, agnosia, in *Neurology*, 2d ed, SAK Wilson, N Bruce (eds). Baltimore, William & Wilkins, 1955, vol 3, chap 83

GESCHWIND N: Disconnection syndromes in animals and man. Brain 88:237, 585, 1965

MOHR JP: Broca's area and Broca's aphasia, in *Studies in Neurolinguistics*, H Whitaker (ed). New York, Academic, 1975, chap 6

———, SIDMAN M: Aphasia: Behavioral aspects, in *American Handbook of Psychiatry*, vol 4, M Reiser (ed). New York, Basic Books, 1975, pp 279–298

NIELSEN JM: *Agnosia, Apraxia, Aphasia: Their Value in Cerebral Localization*, 2d ed. New York, Hafner, 1962

DERANGEMENTS OF INTELLECT, MOOD, AND BEHAVIOR, INCLUDING SCHIZOPHRENIA AND MANIC-DEPRESSIVE STATES

RAYMOND D. ADAMS
MAURICE VICTOR

Increasingly, as mental, emotional, and behavioral disorders are recognized as manifestations of diseases of the brain, the internist is consulted because an otherwise healthy person begins to lose the capacity to function effectively as a student, a worker, or head of a family. This may have several meanings—the beginning of a brain tumor, the formation of chronic subdural hematoma, the development of chronic drug intoxication, chronic meningoencephalitis (syphilis), degenerative cerebral disease, or a schizophrenic psychosis. In former times, when there was little that could be done about any of these clinical states, no great premium was attached to diagnosis, but modern medicine now offers the means of treating several of these conditions and in some instances of restoring the patient to normal health and effectiveness. Early recognition of the underlying pathologic process improves the chances of recovery.

In this chapter we consider first the global deterioration of mental functions subsumed under the term dementia and then certain special impairments such as Korsakoff's amnesic state, schizophrenia, and manic-depressive psychosis. The last part of the chapter will be devoted to the clinical manifestations of focal cerebral diseases, exclusive of aphasia and convulsions.

THE CLINICAL SYNDROME OF DEMENTIA

The term *dementia* usually denotes a clinical state composed of failing memory and loss of other intellectual functions due to chronic progressive degenerative disease of the brain. It may or may not be associated with signs of disease in one or more of the motor, sensory, or language areas of the cerebrum. The chronicity of the process is ordinarily emphasized, but the illogic of setting apart any one constellation of cerebral symptoms on the basis of their speed of onset, rate of evolution, or duration is obvious. We would insist that the state of dementia is a generic syndrome of multiple causation and mechanism, and that a diffuse degeneration of neurons is only one of the types.

Clinical findings The earliest signs of dementia may be so subtle as to escape the notice of even the most discerning physician. Often an observant relative of the patient or an employer is the first to become aware of certain lack of initiative, irritability, loss of interest, and inability to perform up to the usual standard. Later there is distractibility of attention, inability to think with accustomed clarity, reduced general comprehension, perseveration in speech, action, and thought, and defective memory, especially for recent events. Frequently a change in mood becomes apparent, deviating more often toward depression than elation. The direction of this deviation is said to depend on the previous personality of the patient rather than upon the character of the disease. Excessive lability of mood may be observed, i.e., easy fluctuation from laughter to tears on slight provocation. Lapses in social graces and conduct occur, and judgment becomes impaired, early in some cases and late in others. Paranoid ideas and delusions may develop. As a rule, the patient has little or no realization of these changes in behavior and lacks insight into their meaning.

As the condition progresses, there is loss of almost all intellectual faculties. Dysarthria, aphasia, and sphincteric incontinence, reduced responsivity, and finally mutism may be added to the clinical picture. In a late stage a secondary physical deterioration also takes place. Food intake, which may be increased in the beginning of the illness, is in the end usually limited, with resulting emaciation. Any febrile illness or metabolic upset induces a marked increase in confusion and even stupor or coma, indicating the precarious state of cerebral compensation. Finally, the patient remains in bed most of the time and dies of pneumonia or some other intercurrent infection. This whole process may evolve over a period of months or years, usually the latter.

Many of the alterations of behavior are the direct result of disease of the nervous system; expressed in another way, the symptoms are the primary manifestations of neurologic disease. Others are secondary; i.e., they are reactions to the catastrophe of losing one's mind. For example, the dement is said to seek solitude to hide the affliction and may thus appear asocial or apathetic. Again, excessive orderliness may be an attempt to compensate for failing memory; apprehension, gloom, or irritability may reflect general dissatisfaction with a necessarily restricted life. It would appear that even in a state of fairly advanced deterioration the patient is still capable of reacting to the illness and to the persons who care for him or her.

Degenerative diseases may terminate in virtually complete decortication. The patient is unaware of what is happening but lies with eyes open. He or she no longer responds to spoken commands or speaks. There is no interest in food or drink, though they are swallowed if placed in the mouth. The facial and limb muscles are stiff with increased tendon reflexes and Babinski signs. Grasping and sucking are prominent. The sphincters are incontinent.

Morbid anatomy and pathologic physiology of dementia Dementia is related usually to obvious structural disease of the cerebrum and the diencephalon. In some, such as the Alzheimer-senile dementia complex and Pick's disease, the main process appears to be a degeneration and loss of nerve cells in the association areas, with secondary changes in the cerebral white matter. A degeneration of neurons confined to the thalamus may also cause dementia. In others, such as Huntington's chorea and certain of the cerebral-basal ganglionic degenerations, loss of neurons in the cerebral cortex is accompanied by a similar degeneration of neurons in the putamen and caudate nuclei and cerebellum. Arteriosclerotic vascular disease may result in multiple foci of infarction throughout the thalami, basal ganglia, brainstem, and cerebrum. Cerebral involvement may include the motor, sensory, or visual projection areas as well as the association areas. Severe trauma may cause contusions of cerebral convolutions and white matter as well as necroses and hemorrhages in the midbrain, lesions which are responsible for protracted stupor, coma, or dementia. Most diseases that produce dementia are quite extensive, and the frontal lobes are affected more often than other parts of the cerebrum.

Mechanisms other than the destruction of brain tissue may be operative in some cases. Chronic increased intracranial pressure or chronic hydrocephalus (with large ventricles the pressure may not exceed 180 mmHg), regardless of cause, is often associated with a general impairment of mental function. Compression of cerebral white matter is the main factor. The compression of one or both of the cerebral hemispheres by chronic subdural hematomas may cause a widespread disturbance of cortical function. A diffuse inflammatory process is at least in part the basis for dementia in syphilis and in certain virus infections such as "inclusion body encephalitis"; presumably there is loss of some neurons as well as inflammatory derangement of the function of other neurons. Lastly, several of the toxic and metabolic diseases discussed in Chap. 371 may interfere with nervous function over a period of time and create a clinical picture similar to, if not identical with, that of dementia. One must suppose that the altered biochemical environment has affected the excitability of the neurons.

Bedside classification of dementia

I Diseases in which dementia is usually the only evidence of neurologic or medical disease
  A Alzheimer's disease and senile dementia
  B Pick's disease

II Diseases in which dementia is associated with other neurologic signs but not with other obvious medical disease
  A Invariably associated with other neurologic signs
    1 Huntington's chorea (choreoathetosis)
    2 Schilder's disease, metachromatic leukodystrophy, and related demyelinative diseases (spastic weakness, pseudobulbar palsy, blindness, deafness)
    3 Lipofuscinosis and other lipid-storage diseases (myoclonic seizures, blindness, spasticity, cerebellar ataxia)
    4 Myoclonic epilepsy (diffuse myoclonus, generalized seizures, cerebellar ataxia)
    5 Jakob-Creutzfeldt disease (diffuse myoclonus and cerebellar ataxia)
    6 Cerebrocerebellar degeneration (cerebellar ataxia of olivopontocerebellar type and others)
    7 Cerebral-basal ganglionic degenerations (apraxia-rigidity)
    8 Dementia with spastic paraplegia
    9 Basal ganglia calcification (idiopathic and hypoparathyroidism)
    10 Hallervorden-Spatz disease
    11 Dementia with Parkinson's disease
  B Often associated with other neurologic signs
    1 Cerebral arteriosclerosis
    2 Brain tumor
    3 Brain trauma, such as cerebral contusion, midbrain hemorrhage, chronic subdural hematoma
    4 Marchiafava-Bignami disease (often with apraxia and other frontal lobe signs)
    5 Low-pressure hydrocephalus (always with ataxia of gait and often with sphincteric incontinence)

III Diseases in which dementia is usually associated with clinical and laboratory signs of other medical disease
  A Hypothyroidism
  B Cushing's disease
  C Nutritional deficiency states such as pellagra, the Wernicke-Korsakoff syndrome, and subacute combined degeneration of spinal cord and brain (vitamin B_{12} deficiency)
  D Neurosyphilis: general paresis and meningovascular syphilis
  E Hepatolenticular degeneration, familial and acquired
  F Bromidism, chronic barbiturate intoxication

The degenerative diseases that cause dementia are discussed in Chap. 373. The special features of the dementia that accompanies arteriosclerotic, senile, syphilitic, traumatic, nutritional, and degenerative diseases are discussed in the appropriate chapters.

Differential diagnosis The first task in dealing with this class of patients is to make sure that the central problem is one of general deterioration of intellect and personality change. It may be necessary to examine the patient several times before one is confident of the clinical findings.

An easy mistake is to assume that mental function is normal if there is complaint only of nervousness, fatigue, insomnia, or vague somatic symptoms, and to label such patients as psychoneurotic. *This will be avoided if one keeps in mind that psychoneuroses rarely begin in middle or late adult life.* A practical rule is to assume that all mental illnesses beginning during this period are due either to structural disease of the brain or to a depressive psychosis.

A mild dysphasia must not be mistaken for dementia. Aphasic patients appear uncertain of themselves, and their speech may be incoherent. Furthermore, they may be anxious and depressed over this ineptitude. Careful attention to the language performance of these patients will lead to the correct diagnosis in most instances. Further observation will disclose that their behavior, except that which is related to the language disorder, is within normal limits.

Depressed patients present another type of problem. They may remark that their mental function is poor or that they are forgetful and cannot concentrate. Scrutiny of these remarks will show, however, that they actually remember the details of their illness and that no qualitative change in mental ability has taken place. The difficulty is either a lack of energy and interest or an anxiety that prevents the focusing of attention on anything except their own problems. Even during mental tests their performance may be impaired by their emotions in much the same way as the performance of worried students is impaired during examinations. This condition of emotional blocking is called *experiential confusion.* When patients are calmed by reassurance and given more time in the performance of tests, mental function improves, indicating that intellectual deterioration has not occurred. Hypomanic patients fail in tests of intellectual function because of restlessness and distractibility. It is helpful to remember that demented patients, except in the early phases of their illness, rarely have sufficient insight to complain of mental deterioration and those who admit to poor memory seldom realize the degree of their disability. The physician must never rely on patients' statements of the efficiency of mental function and must always evaluate a poor performance on tests in the light of the emotional state and motivation at the time the test is given.

The neurologic syndromes associated with metabolic or endocrine disorders, i.e., ACTH therapy, hyperthyroidism, Cushing's disease, Addison's disease, or the postpartum state may be difficult to separate from that of dementia because of the wide variety of clinical pictures by which they manifest themselves. Some such patients appear to be suffering from a dementia, others from an acute confusional psychosis; or if mood change or negativism predominates, a manic-depressive psychosis or schizophrenia is suggested. In these conditions some degree of clouding of sensorium and impairment of intellectual function can usually be recognized, and these findings alone should be enough to exclude schizophrenia and manic-depressive psychosis. It is well to remember that acute onset of mental symptoms always suggests confusional psychosis or delirium. Inasmuch as many of these conditions are completely reversible, they must be distinguished from the dementia of degenerative diseases (see Chap. 21).

Once it is decided that the patient suffers from a dementing disease, the next step is to determine by careful physical examination whether there are other neurologic signs or indications of a particular medical disease. This enables the physician to place the case in one of the three categories in the bedside classification. X-rays of the skull, electroencephalogram, lumbar puncture, and computerized tomography (CT) scans should be carried out in most cases. Usually these procedures necessitate admission to a hospital. The final step is to determine by the total clinical picture which disease within any one category the patient has.

SPECIAL TYPES OF INTELLECTUAL IMPAIRMENT

KORSAKOFF'S PSYCHOSIS (AMNESIC CONFABULATORY PSYCHOSIS) Clinical findings These terms are used interchangeably to designate a unique but common disorder of cognitive function, in which memory is deranged out of all proportion to other components of mentation and behavior. It possesses two salient features which may vary in severity but are always conjoined: (1) an impaired ability to recall events and other information that has been recorded in the mind before the onset of the illness (retrograde amnesia); and (2) an impaired ability to acquire new information, i.e., to learn or to form new memories (anterograde amnesia). Other cognitive functions (particularly the capacity for concentration, spatial organization, visual and verbal abstraction), which depend little or not at all on memory, may also be impaired but to a relatively minor degree. The patient tends to be lacking in initiative and spontaneity. *Confabulation*, meaning false or fabricated accounts of recent events, is present in most cases, especially in the acute phase of the illness.

The definition of Korsakoff's psychosis demands also that certain aspects of behavior and mental function be intact. The patient should be alert, attentive, responsive, and capable of understanding the written and spoken word, of making appropriate deductions from given premises, and of solving such problems as can be concluded within the his or her forward memory span. These "negative" features are of particular importance because they help to distinguish Korsakoff's psychosis from a number of other disorders in which the basic defect is not necessarily in retentive memory but in some other psychologic mechanism, e.g., in attention and perception (as in the delirious, confused, or stuporous patient), in recall (as in the hysterical patient), or in volition (as in the patient with frontal lobe disease).

Pathologic anatomy The anatomic structures of particular importance in memory function are the diencephalon (specifically the medial portions of the medial dorsal nuclei of the thalamus) and the inferomedial portions of the temporal lobes, particularly the hippocampal formations and underlying white matter. Bilaterally placed lesions in either of these regions derange memory and learning out of all proportion to other cognitive functions, and even unilateral lesions in the dominant hemispheres produce a lesser degree of the same effect. It would appear that the aforementioned anatomic structures are involved in all forms of learning and integration of newly formed memories and that they form a tenuous but vital link between the high brainstem reticular formation (the integrity of which is necessary to maintain an alert state of mind, a prerequisite for any learning) and the cerebral cortex, which is the locus for special memories such as words, geometric figures, and numbers.

Classification of diseases characterized by an amnesic syndrome

I Amnesic syndrome of sudden onset—usually with gradual but incomplete recovery
  A Bilateral hippocampal infarction due to atherosclerotic-thrombotic or embolic occlusion of the posterior cerebral arteries or their inferior temporal branches
  B Trauma to the diencephalic or inferomedial temporal regions

  C Spontaneous subarachnoid hemorrhage
  D Carbon monoxide poisoning and other hypoxic states (rare)
II Amnesia of sudden onset and brief duration with full recovery
  A Temporal lobe seizures
  B Postconcussive states
  C "Transient global amnesia"
III Amnesic syndrome of subacute onset with varying degrees of recovery, usually leaving permanent residue
  A Wernicke-Korsakoff disease
  B Inclusion body (herpes simplex) encephalitis
  C Tuberculous and other forms of meningitis characterized by a granulomatous exudate at the base of the brain
IV Slowly progressive amnesic states
  A Tumors involving the walls of the third ventricle and temporal lobes
  B Alzheimer's disease and other degenerative disorders (early stage only)

The differentiation of the diseases that give rise to the amnesic syndrome proceeds along the lines indicated in Chaps. 265, 366, 369, 372, and 373.

THE DELUSIONAL-HALLUCINATORY (SCHIZOPHRENIFORM) SYNDROME AND RELATED MENTAL STATES (PSYCHOSES)

From the neurologist's standpoint this syndrome is basically a subtle disorder in attention and thinking associated with hallucinatory experiences, delusions, and an inability to distinguish subjective experience from reality. Conjoined often are disturbances in affect, verbal expression, motor activity, and social behavior.

Originally Kraepelin, one of the pioneers in German psychiatry, referred to this syndrome as *dementia praecox,* but it soon became evident that it bore little resemblance to the general intellectual deterioration described above under dementia. Indeed, memory function, lost early in the latter syndrome, is usually preserved except in the most advanced stages. Even then the sensorium tends to remain clear, and language functions, arithmetic ability, and all gnosic and praxic activities of the brain are preserved. Bleuler decided that the term schizophrenia, meaning a splitting of the mind (or dissociation of content of thought and affect) was more appropriate. He emphasized disturbances in the association of ideas, an inclination to withdraw from reality, and a preference for rumination and fantasy (autism) as the fundamental derangements.

Discerning analyses of abnormal mentation, mood, and behavior inform us that this more or less unique syndrome, readily recognizable in its most typical form, has multiple causes. While characteristic of a genetic disease known to the medical world as *schizophrenia*, the syndrome may also be the clinical expression of manic-depressive psychosis, alcoholic auditory hallucinosis, *amphetamine psychosis, temporal lobe epilepsy,* some of the *puerperal* and *endocrine psychoses*, and rarely a focal cerebral disease of other type.

Clinical aspects of the syndrome This clinical state is the most abstruse of any in the realm of neuropsychiatry. Thinking and behavioral abnormalities are both present. In some instances they may be so obvious that diagnosis offers no difficulty whatsoever, but in many others the symptoms may be subtle, vague, and difficult to elicit. The clinician must always depend for diagnosis on the verbal expressions and actions of the patient. If the patient is mute, taciturn, incapable of freely expressing his or her thoughts, or reluctant to talk because of hostility and suspicion toward the examiner, the primary disorder of thought may not be discovered or may be only inferred from his or her actions. A detailed account of the patient's speech and behavior by an observant member of the family then is particularly helpful.

The most striking feature of the syndrome is a curious alteration of awareness of what is going on. Such patients are seemingly preoccupied with their own thoughts so that their responses to questions are neither constant nor prompt. In their replies to questions and spontaneous remarks, one finds that orientation to time, place, and person is intact, and usually the names of doctors, nurses, medications, etc., can be given accurately. In other words, the general aspects of formal intelligence are preserved. However, during the most intense phases of the syndrome, in which mental disorganization is profound, there may be inattentiveness to ambient surroundings.

The thoughts of these patients are often interrupted by hallucinations (usually auditory) and unreal dreamlike experiences. Sometimes the hallucinations consist of voices coming from outside the body, but often no clear distinction is drawn between a hallucination and an idea that has been planted in the mind. In the struggle to retain sanity, patients try vainly to separate their own thoughts and perceptual experiences from those of others who are ostensibly trying to control them. Communication of this melange of confusing experiences is difficult. Even when obviously preoccupied with voices, the patients may be reluctant or unable to admit that they are hallucinating.

The patients may feel that their thoughts are being read by others or that they are under outside control. When extraneous ideas are forced upon them they may feel powerless, as though they are passive recipients of the ideas of others (passivity feelings). They may believe these ideas have been transmitted to them by wireless electronic devices, laser beams, or whatever is culturally in vogue. Sometimes they may believe that their own thoughts are made known to others by similar devices. Trying to cope with this confusion of strange and disturbing ideas, patients become so self-absorbed that simple questions may evoke no reply or only one that seems tangential, inappropriate, and incomplete.

Psychologists have attempted for decades to categorize this thought disorder and to educe its essential character. They have remarked on the apparent "disregard for the logical limits of time and space," the "confusion of parts for wholes," "the lumping and condensation of separate items," the acceptance of "the identity of opposites," and the inability to think abstractly. None of these attributes appear to be inclusively descriptive.

Associated with this thought disorder are delusions. These are expressed at some time in the majority of cases. Patients may come to believe they have a disease, that their lives are in danger, that they have been singled out or are threatened for some obscure reason, or that they have suddenly gained remarkable insight into world events. The delusions, based as they are on accusatory or controlling hallucinatory and imagined experiences, cannot be eradicated by logical argument. Such thoughts may be acted upon and occasionally lead to suicide or homicide.

This disorder of thought may vary in intensity from time to time. If it is severe and persistent, patients appear overwhelmed; they may lie mute and frozen in a state of suspended activity (catatonia), or they may be found wandering aimlessly, perplexed, and fearful or excited. The mental state then may resemble a confusion or delirium but without the characteristic clouding of consciousness. If the thought disorder is mild, there are periods when patients appear relatively normal and only withdrawal, disregard of social customs, and preoccupations prevent adequate school or work performance. However, at any time the thought disorder may break through, and seemingly well persons may for no obvious reason once again become vague, preoccupied, and deluded.

The typical and allegedly characteristic affect of the delusional-hallucinatory syndrome is difficult to interpret. Often it seems to be a reflection of the patients' mental state and content of thought. When they are preoccupied, they appear to be detached and indifferent to surroundings. Irritability and undue sensitivity are prominent in some patients and are expressed as resentment toward the therapist and sometimes as unreasonable hostility. If voices and ideas threaten, they first excite patients, but later, if the threats continue, patients become more or less inured to them. While some of the emotional reactions seem inappropriate to the immediate situation, it is usually discovered that they are not inappropriate to the patients' thoughts and mental preoccupations. If one can probe the content of thought, one may then find that the emotions are not at all incongruous, but in some instances the incongruity of thought and feeling is obvious and impossible to understand.

In summary, it is the combination of a subtle *alteration of clear awareness and the intrusion of hallucinatory and dreamlike experiences,* occurring all during the waking hours and making separation of fantasy and reality impossible, and *the delusional systems of ideas* that identifies this psychotic syndrome. Semiologically it falls between delirium on one side and a vague personality and character disorder on the other.

Schizophrenia This is a hereditary lifelong disease of the nervous system which begins in early life, pursues a recurrent course without full remissions, and is characterized by the above syndrome or some variant thereof.

The disease is frequent and worldwide. Prevalence rates are in the order of 0.2 to 0.5 percent, and life expectancy rates (chance of manifesting schizophrenic symptoms sometime during life) are at least 1.0 percent. New cases each year number about 0.05 to 0.1 percent of the total population. World prevalence is 10 to 20 million cases. Males and females are equally affected. Family studies show that the closer a person is related to a schizophrenic, the greater the risk of the disease for that person. If both parents have schizophrenia, the risk to a child is approximately 50 percent; this holds whether the child is raised with the biologic parents or in a foster home. A monozygotic twin has three to four times the risk of a dizygotic twin or sibling. However, the hereditary pattern does not conform to any known mendelian type, and the importance of environmental stress, which is emphasized by many psychiatrists, is difficult to evaluate.

CLINICAL FINDINGS The onset of the clinical manifestations occurs usually during adolescence or early adult life, but in approximately half the cases the psychotic episode occurs in an individual who throughout childhood is known to have been eccentric, timid, aloof, or socially maladjusted in some way. In some instances the onset is acute and at a time of stress, and the disease is so disturbing to the patient and family as to require hospitalization. The symptoms subside within a few weeks or months, especially under the influence of medication. Equally as frequent is a gradual onset with drift into an inactive, withdrawn, delusional state where the beginning of the illness is impossible to date. Even after recovery from an acute episode, patients tend not to be normal and are unable to function up to their previous intellectual level. These patients tend to be vague, poorly motivated, worried, and concerned about matters of little importance to a healthy mind. Relapse is frequent throughout the remainder of their lives.

The psychosis may vary in its outward manifestations.

Some patients are strikingly paranoid, others catatonic or remarkably disorganized and silly in their delusional behavior (hebephrenia); or the illness may resemble a severe and persistent neurosis (pseudoneurotic) or a pervasive character disorder. One may question whether these are variations of a single disease or several diseases, closely related in their clinical expression (cf., *Harvard Guide in Modern Psychiatry*).

In this disease complete recovery after an acute episode of the schizophrenic syndrome is said to occur in approximately 30 percent of cases, but this is disputed. Probably many of the complete recoveries are in patients who have the delusional-hallucinatory syndrome but not schizophrenic disease. For example, an acute hypomania or mixed manic-depressive state in an adolescent, as will be pointed out below, may be virtually indistinguishable from the psychosis of schizophrenia.

According to Robins and Guze the diagnosis of schizophrenia becomes reliable only when, over a period of at least 6 months, a patient exhibits the delusional-hallucinatory syndrome (with clear consciousness and orientation), along with a type of "verbal production that makes communication difficult because of lack of logical or understandable organization." Usually the individual is unmarried and has had poor premorbid social adjustment and work history, and a family history of schizophrenia. The onset of illness before the age of 40 years and the absence of drug or alcohol abuse and of manic and depressive symptoms increase the probability of accuracy of this diagnosis to over 90 percent.

ETIOLOGY AND PATHOGENESIS   Theories are legion, but a textbook of medicine is hardly the place to discuss them. Many psychiatrists are committed to a psychogenic etiology, but this remains entirely unproved. In recent years attention has been focused largely on biological factors, particularly chemical derangement of certain structures in the limbic portions of the brain (nucleus accumbens, bed nucleus of stria terminalis, ventral septum, and mammillary bodies). In several cases of chronic paranoid schizophrenia the norepinephrine levels in these regions have been significantly increased (McCullough et al.). This finding, if verified, would incriminate a disorder in neurotransmitter dynamics as the chemical pathology of this hereditary disease.

The morphologic substratum of this disease has eluded all neuropathologic techniques. The possible ways in which a genetic factor can be translated into disordered function of certain parts of the brain without visibly altering neuronal structure has been reviewed by Kety. He finds all current biochemical hypotheses to be unsubstantiated.

TREATMENT   The treatment of schizophrenia is relatively unsatisfactory and is usually left to the psychiatrist. Chlorpromazine (Thorazine) in a dose usually of 200 to 300 mg per day (range 200 to 2000 mg per day) is the most widely used medication for acute psychotic episodes. However, it carries the risk of extrapyramidal side effects, some of which are permanent (tardive dyskinesia), even when treatment is combined with antiparkinson drugs. There are now many new drugs, some of which are modifications of the original phenothiazines, including the piperazine derivatives, which are higher in their per milligram potency [e.g., fluphenazine (Prolixin), trifluoperazine (Stelazine), and perphenazine (Trilafon)]. Other drugs in common use are chlorprothixene (Taractan), butyrophenone (Haldol), and loxapine (Loxitene). These medications do not merely tranquilize, but suppress hallucinations and delusions and improve the organization of thought. Electroconvulsive therapy (ECT) is sometimes used for stuporous or agitated patients, but its general efficacy is questionable. The value of psychotherapy is unproved, and most psychiatrists agree with Baldessarini, who stated that it has little to offer "as a primary mode of treatment." A few psychoanalysts claim to have suc-

cessfully treated schizophrenia. Active supportive medical and psychotherapy directed to helping the patient maintain a grasp on reality and to readjust to home and work situations are clearly indicated. In combination with drug therapy, a large proportion of schizophrenic patients are now able to leave psychiatric hospitals and return to a sheltered existence in the community.

Psychotic form of manic-depressive disease   Descriptions of manic-depressive disease and dementia praecox, from the earliest ones by Kraepelin, cannot fail to impress the readers with the similarities between these disease states. Contemporary psychiatrists attest to the difficulty in distinguishing some cases of these two diseases by positing a category of *schizoaffective* or *schizothymic* states in which are combined attributes of both. Pope and Lipinski, after a review of the literature and a 4-year personal experience with admissions to the McLean Hospital, and Robins and Guze and their associates, observe that the full delusional-hallucinatory psychotic syndrome of schizophrenia occurs frequently in manic-depressive disease. They insist that this syndrome when viewed in "cross section" is not diagnostic of either schizophrenia or manic-depressive disease; i.e., it is nonspecific. If it occurs acutely in association with a prominent affective or mood disorder in a previously well-adjusted individual, especially if it is preceded by euphoria, hyperactivity, flight of ideas, pressure of speech, grandiosity, hostility and sleeplessness (the usual symptoms and signs of mania), the diagnosis will usually turn out to be manic-depressive disease. The hypomanic patient often will have a family history of manic-depressive disease, and over 70 percent will respond to lithium therapy and make a full recovery within a few months. Schizophrenia differs in the lack of manic-depressive disease in the family, lack of affective symptoms and an emotional state incongruent with thought content, a more gradual onset, incomplete recovery, and little or no response to lithium. Depressive states of nonpsychotic type are more fully discussed below.

Alcoholic auditory hallucinosis   This disease begins as a withdrawal or abstinence syndrome in the chronic alcoholic. Usually it subsides in 1 to 2 weeks, but in some the hallucinosis persists indefinitely. The illness comes in time to resemble schizophrenia (see Chap. 226). Affected individuals do not have a premorbid schizoid personality and have no family history of schizophrenia. Such cases reinforce the authors' argument that a slightly altered consciousness, delusions, and hallucinatory experiences stand as the primary abnormalities in the schizophrenic syndrome and are not of themselves diagnostic of the disease schizophrenia.

Schizophrenic psychosis in patients with temporal lobe epilepsy   Quite apart from the psychomotor seizures, which in themselves induce curious behavioral abnormalities, such patients may develop an acute psychosis with prominent thought disorder, hallucinations and delusions, ideas of reference, remoteness, and a disorganization of activity and social relations that simulates schizophrenia. The psychosis appears not to be due to continuous subclinical firing of a seizure focus, for the EEG contains no paroxysmal discharge. The patients respond to antipsychotic drugs and recover within a few weeks.

Amphetamine psychosis   High dosage and prolonged usage of amphetamines can induce a typical paranoid psychosis with characteristic autistic thought disorder, delusions, and hallucinations. Once started it may continue for several weeks and is

152

said to respond to antipsychotic drugs. A similar syndrome is occasionally observed in a metabolic disease, and after marijuana and lysergic acid overdosage. The authors have had little experience with these states and cannot document the similarity of such syndromes to the one under consideration.

Puerperal psychosis Brief psychologic disturbances are not infrequent in the puerperium. The most typical reaction is a depression which may last for days, weeks, or months, and may recur after the next pregnancy. There is another type of psychosis featured by variable degrees of confusion and autistic thought disorder. The deluded mother may claim the baby not to be her own, and there are tragic instances where she has killed the infant. Recovery occurs over many weeks or months, and opinion is divided as to whether this is a confusional psychosis or delirium or is a delusional-hallucinatory psychosis of either schizophrenic or manic type.

Endocrine psychosis In patients receiving high-dose corticosteroid or ACTH therapy and occasionally in a person suffering from hyperthyroidism, there may occur poor sleep, hallucinations, delusions, disordered thought, and frenzied excitement in varying combinations. Discontinuation of the steroid or treatment of the thyrotoxicosis usually restores the patient to normalcy within a few weeks. Here once again is an example of an illness that overlaps the acute confusional and delirious state where there is clouding of consciousness on the one hand and the more protracted delusional-hallucinatory syndrome with relatively clear consciousness on the other.

Differential diagnosis At times a schizophrenic illness that never explodes into an overt psychosis but leads to persistent inability to function in school, at work, or as a member of a family unit may be difficult to distinguish from one in which there is adolescent turmoil, maladjustment, preoccupation with philosophical ideas and Eastern religions, and involvement in the activist affairs of the counterculture. Abuse of drugs adds to the problem. Suspiciousness, dramatic behavior, unreasonable attitudes, and indifference to conventional practices are common to both conditions. Only by identification of the basic cognitive disorders of the schizophrenic syndrome with the added stipulation that it persist for many months will the diagnosis of schizophrenia be established, and this may require a period of observation in the neutral environment of a hospital. It is said that some social derelicts, vagrants, chronic drug abusers, and sociopathic individuals are actually suffering from simple schizophrenia.

The elderly patient who becomes paranoid while still mentally intact and who is not depressed presents another difficult clinical problem. Such cases need to be studied over a period of time before one can eliminate the possibility of a dementing illness or a depressive psychosis. Only if the latter are excluded is one justified in the conclusion that they have the rare and special psychiatric illness known as pure *paranoia*.

SYNDROMES OF EMOTIONAL (AFFECT AND MOOD) DISTURBANCE
The term *emotion* is used in medical practice in so many ways that it virtually loses all meaning. It refers indiscriminately to the nervous, the neurotic, the unhappy and maladjusted, and to the patient with obscure medical disease. The neurologist assigns to it a more precise definition—a complex state of the organism comprised of a mental component of fear, anger, love, or hate in association with certain visceral changes that are mainly under the control of the autonomic nervous system and lead to a certain pattern of motor expression. Intense emotion may disturb rational thought, and the

resulting behavior, while apparently degraded and stereotyped, is nonetheless protective of the organism. Mild emotion may take the form of anxiety, depression, or elation with only the most subtle visceral accompaniments and somatic manifestations.

Human emotion upon strict analysis consists of a stimulus, the accurate perception of which requires the memory of specific associations drawn from previous experience. The psychic state aroused by the perception includes a *feeling* or *affect* known only to the experiencing individual and manifested through verbal expressions and behavior. Thus, on the one side, an emotion includes the same perceptive-cognitive processes as does any induced sensory experience, but it differs with respect to its affective component with the associated visceral reactions and with respect to certain specific patterns of behavior.

Cannon and Bard and their associates studied the ways in which the two parts of the autonomic nervous system participate in the emotional state—the parasympathetic mediating trophotropic, restorative, and reproductive functions, viz., the general homeostatic functions; and the sympathetic (including the adrenal glands) mediating self-protective or ergotropic functions. Hess and Bard localized the central control mechanisms in the hypothalamus which are ideally situated to send impulses via descending tracts to the parasympathetic and sympathetic segmental apparatus and via releasing factors to the pituitary-adrenal-thyroid system. This entire complex of emotional activities, including visceral, glandular, and motor reactions, could be elicited from decerebrate animals as long as the hypothalamus remained intact. Papez postulated that the limbic parts of medial temporal and orbital-frontal lobes, which have rich connections with the hypothalamus, could sustain and modulate the long-acting emotional states.

Clinical observations The affective and emotional apparatus is known to be disordered in a number of ways by diseases of the brain. There may be an unnatural *apathy* and *placidity*, wherein the usual stimuli of fear, anger, love, and anxious concern have little or no effect on the patient. Bilateral temporal lesions may result in this condition, along with a remarkable failure of visual recognition, a tendency to examine every object by touch or oral exploration, and either hyper- or hyposexuality. This entire complex is known as the *Kluver-Bucy syndrome*. The right parietal (nondominant) lobe seemed very important in emotional experience, and large lesions here result in an unusual blunting of all emotional reactions. In contrast, a focal lesion in the dominant temporoparietal region rarely may plunge the patient into a state of frenzied excitement, rage, and fear; every stimulus, even innocuous ones, excite the individual, who may lash out blindly at everyone who approaches. One may imagine that the dominant cerebral lesion has disinhibited the intact right parietal lobe. Inferior bifrontal lesions may cause either apathy along with abulia or, rarely, excitement and aggressive behavior, depending on their anatomy. Complete disinhibition of the facial-respiratory apparatus for laughter and crying (syndrome of forced or pathologic laughter and crying) is a frequent accompaniment of pseudobulbar palsy. Here it is the apparatus for emotional expression and not the mental state that is out of control. Lesser degrees of this, in the forms of emotional lability, occur in many cerebral diseases.

The emotional disorders that are the most subtle and difficult to comprehend are *acute* and *chronic anxiety, depression,* and *mania*. They stand as separate syndromes that may appear as the dominant features of certain mental disturbances. They bear no clear relationship to the circumstances which may have occurred in the patient's life. In some instances the prevailing emotional state, on close examination, has been induced by a hallucination or delusion. In a delirium or the schizophreniform syndrome, for example, voices which threaten the patient's life naturally excite fear. In other mental illnesses, the patient experiences an overwhelming anxiety or depression. Unlike the normal person, in whom anxiety, depression, and elation are the natural reactions to life situations such as loss of livelihood or grief over the death of a loved one, or the winning of a coveted treasure, these patients have no conscious awareness of any provocative stimulus. In this sense their emotional state is endogenous. Manic-depressive psychosis, involutional melancholia, and anxiety neurosis (actually a form of depression in most instances) are the most familiar examples, and in the opinion of most neurologists and many psychiatrists they represent diseases of the brain.

Manic-depressive disease   Manic-depressive psychosis is a disease characterized by a cyclic disorder of mood. There may be episodes of depression or of mania, appearing once or many times during the lifetime of the patient. Depression is more frequent than mania, and some patients have only depressions. Thus, the mood disorder may be subdivided into monopolar or bipolar type; but in some individuals, there may be both features within a given episode, i.e., mixed manic-depressive.

The disease was given its name by Kraepelin in 1896, and he fully delineated its most distinctive features. Unlike schizophrenia, which usually leaves the patient permanently disabled, between attacks of manic-depressive disease the patient is usually entirely normal.

The incidence of this disease is difficult to determine because of inaccuracy of diagnosis. As pointed out above, many young adults who are said to have recovered from schizophrenia actually have had a manic psychosis. In the author's clinical experience manic-depressive disease is several times more frequent than schizophrenia, at least on the wards of a general hospital. The worldwide incidence is 3 to 4 per 1000 population. In certain countries as many as 5 percent of males and 8 to 9 percent of females will have symptoms of this disease sometime in their lifetime.

The onset is most frequent in middle adult life, but typical episodes may be seen in children, adolescents, and young adults. In fact, it is the most frequent cause of admission of adolescents and young adults to a psychiatric hospital. Any one episode may last months or years, being shortened by therapy.

CLINICAL PICTURE   The fully developed depression may evolve within a few days or develop more slowly. The symptoms and signs have already been described in Chap. 11. It need only be restated that the patient, without obvious cause, begins to feel helpless, discouraged, and despondent. Life seems worthless and without purpose, and there is self-blame for the condition. Energy for both mental and physical activity is reduced; the powers of concentration and capacity to maintain interest in the ordinary tasks of the day are lowered, and the least effort is exhausting. It becomes impossible to cope with everyday worries and concerns. Indecisiveness, pain, and many of the bodily effects of frank anxiety are other prominent symptoms. Thoughts of suicide assert themselves. As the depression worsens the patient talks less and finally becomes motionless and mute. Delusions of a somatic or paranoid type often appear and are a source of distress. Finally there is indifference even to nutritional needs; anorexia, weight loss, constipation, insomnia, and loss of libido are the most prominent vegetative effects and will last until the patient begins to emerge from the depression.

In the manic phase the symptoms are the opposite to those of depression. The patient becomes more energetic and is full of enthusiasm and the joy and zest for life. New schemes are embarked upon with great drive and confidence but are seldom carried to completion. New ideas flood the mind, and

there is a great pressure of speech. Judgment is poor, and irritability may become apparent even to the point of hostility if the patient is thwarted or criticized. The euphoria and expansiveness may increase and give way to delusions of grandeur, supernatural power, and self-importance. As in depressive psychosis, paranoid and somatic delusions may appear along with hallucinations. In a more advanced phase of the disease, the patient may have ideas of reference, look disheveled, and neglect personal hygiene. In a *delirious mania*, as was pointed out above, behavior is totally disorganized; the patient is disoriented, hallucinates, and may lapse into catatonia. This extreme form is rare. *Hypomania* refers to the milder degrees of mania.

First attacks of either mania or depression usually last an average of 6 months, but treatment may reduce this by half. Over 90 percent of patients recover from their first attack. Episodes tend to be longer in old age.

ETIOLOGY AND PATHOGENESIS   The hereditary factor is the most important biologic attribute of the disease. If one parent has the disease, there is at least one chance in five that one of the children will have it. Not infrequently it can be traced through three or four generations, involving as many as a dozen individuals. If one of identical twins has the disease, the chances are over three out of four that the other will have it, whereas the coincidence in dizygotic twins is about 20 percent.

The discoveries that reserpine may cause depression, that iproniazid may cause elation, and that certain tricyclic drugs and monoamine oxidase inhibitors may relieve depression has aroused great interest in the role of biogenic amines (norepinephrine, serotonin, dopamine) in the causation of hereditary manic-depressive disease. This subject has been reviewed by Maas, who points out that one group of depressive patients (bipolar type) have a consistently low urinary excretion of 3-methoxy-4-hydroxyphenethyleneglycol, one of the major metabolites of brain norepinephrine. This group, interestingly, responds well to imiprimine (Tofranil), desipramine, and dextroamphetamine. A central adrenergic disorder is postulated. In another group excretion of this metabolite is normal or increased, and there is little or no response to these drugs. Instead, amitriptyline (Elavil), which acts on serotonin metabolism, is more effective. These studies of biogenic amine metabolism suggest a biochemical heterogeneity of depressive illness, a concept which is also in line with clinical data.

Psychoanalytic theory postulates a personality type that is prone to depressive illness and attempts to discover a psychogenesis, but there is no convincing proof of this hypothesis. Further, psychotherapy has been of no apparent value in terminating an episode of either depression or mania or in preventing another episode.

Involutional melancholia   This form of depression, probably a variant of manic-depressive disease, differs from that disease in several ways: later age of onset (more or less), more prominent anxiety and agitation, higher incidence in women, absence of manic phase, possibly greater frequency of obscure pains, and hypochondriasis.

DIFFERENTIAL DIAGNOSIS   Endogenous depression and involutional melancholia, conditions that are closely related if not identical, are among the most frequently misdiagnosed of all diseases. Chronic pains of obscure type (headache, atypical facial pain, backache, uncomfortable and fatigable muscles, pseudoangina pectoris at rest (without ECG change) in the middle-aged and elderly usually turn out to be "masked depressions." Hypochondriasis of persistent type is so frequently a manifestation of depression that it no longer stands as a separate nosologic entity in psychiatry. Chronic anxiety symptoms (giddiness and dizziness, rapid heart action, smothering, trembling, and uneasy apprehension) of longer than a month's duration and unresponsive to reassurance are virtually always due to depression, especially in the middle-aged and elderly. Paranoid and somatic delusions should be regarded as having a depressive origin until proved otherwise. At any age an acute episode of hallucinations and disorganization of thought and delusions in a person whose consciousness is unclouded and who has been previously well-adjusted and is not abusing alcohol or drugs is more likely to be manic-depressive disease than schizophrenia. Persistent weakness and fatigability in association with multiple complaints in various organ systems, often mistakenly attributed to chronic infection (brucella, viral hepatitis, postinfluenzal asthenia), mild anemia, hypothyroidism, and adrenal insufficiency, frequently prove to be due to a depressive illness. Thoughts of or frank attempts at suicide are always to be judged as expressions of a depression, though schizophrenics may also commit suicide and hysterics may make dramatic but not serious attempts. Persistent depression should not be passed off as a natural reaction to some circumstance in life unless the relationship is convincing.

Treatment For the depressed phase of manic-depressive psychosis and for involutional melancholia the plan of therapy embraces five points.

1 *Enlisting the help of a psychiatrist.* The untrained physician would be rash to attempt the management of these patients without psychiatric assistance.
2 *The prevention of suicide.* This involves the question of hospitalization. If there is any doubt about the patient's intention of suicide, it is better to hospitalize the individual than to take a chance. In manic-depressive illness, attacks of depression or elation are remarkably similar in the same individual. Thus one can predict the course and content of the present spell on the basis of the last. If suicide attempts were made then, the chance is they will be made again.
3 *Antidepressant medication.* There are two categories of antidepressants, the tricyclic compounds and the monoamine oxidase (MAO) inhibitors. Representing the former are imipramine (Tofranil) and amitriptyline (Elavil), and the latter, phenelzine (Nardil) and tranylcypromine (Parnate). In the treatment of depression, most psychiatrists start with the tricyclic antidepressants because they are far safer. With imipramine and amitriptyline, doses range from 100 to 200 mg each day. The starting dose is usually 100 mg per day, which is then raised in stepwise fashion as needed. The therapeutic effect of tricyclic medication is often not evident for 2 or 3 weeks after treatment has been initiated, so that it would be premature to stop the drug before that time. Common side effects are orthostatic hypotension, dry mouth, constipation, tachycardia, and urinary retention. Because of their effect on the cardiovascular system, the tricyclic compounds should not be given to patients who have coronary heart disease. If these are not effective, they are discontinued for 2 weeks and administration of an MAO inhibitor is started. Phenelzine is regarded as the least likely of the MAO inhibitors to produce serious side effects. The usual starting dose is 15 mg tid, which is gradually increased as needed to a maximum of 45 mg tid. The most serious side effect of this class of antidepressants is hypertensive crisis. As a consequence, all MAO inhibitors should be dispensed with extreme caution in patients with a history of cardio- or cerebrovascular disease. Patients taking MAO inhibitors should avoid foods with high tyramine content. The latter is

a pressor amine that is normally inactivated by MAO, and ingestion under such circumstances may result in a hypertensive crisis. Proscribed foods (aged cheese, pickled herring, chicken liver, etc.) are always listed on the manufacturer's information insert.

Since patients are usually responsive to one or the other but not to both, it is important to find out whether tricyclics or MAO inhibitors have been more helpful in the past. This will guide one in current management. Interestingly enough, it has been found that members of the same family are apt to have a similar response to the same antidepressant. Thus, if a patient's mother was helped by an MAO inhibitor, then her children would probably react well to drugs in this category.

4 *Lithium carbonate.* Lithium carbonate has been used since 1949. It is the drug of choice in treating the manic phase of manic-depressive illness. Because it takes a few days to weeks to act effectively against mania, the patient should be hospitalized and sedated with chlorpromazine or haloperidol until the lithium has taken effect. Lithium carbonate has been found to be an effective prophylactic against further attacks of mania and possibly depression. Since it is not a specific antidepressant, the depression must be controlled by either an antidepressant or electroconvulsive therapy before lithium can be started. The blood level of lithium must be followed closely, both to ensure that a therapeutic dose is being given and to guard against toxicity.
5 *Electroconvulsive therapy (ECT).* Electroconvulsive therapy is an effective treatment for the depressed phase of manic-depressive psychosis and involutional melancholia and can also be used to interrupt manic excitements. The last disorder often requires only two or three treatments. The technique is quite simple. The patient is premedicated with a muscle relaxant (Anectine) and then anesthetized by an intravenous injection of a short-acting barbiturate (Brevital). An electrode is then placed over each temple, and an alternating current of about 400 mA and 70 to 120 V is passed between them for $\frac{1}{10}$ to $\frac{1}{2}$ s. The Anectine prevents strong and sometimes injurious muscle spasm. The patient is awake within 5 to 10 min and is up and about in $\frac{1}{2}$ h. Convulsions can also be induced chemically by injecting Metrazol or by inhaling the gas Indoklon. The mechanism by which convulsive therapy works is not known. In treating depression, ECT is usually given every other day for 14 to 20 treatments. The only absolute contraindication is the presence of an intracranial mass such as a neoplasm or hematoma. Its one major drawback is a transient impairment of recent memory for the period of treatment and the days which follow, the degree of impairment being related to the number of treatments given. Placing both electrodes on the nondominant side (unilateral ECT) produces less memory disturbance but is thought to be less effective against the depression.

In manic-depressive illness the best program of management relies on a physician who is willing to follow the patient's course over a long period of time and who is known to the family. Although the prognosis for any individual attack is relatively good, it is wise to arrange for a plan of action which is set in operation as soon as the first symptoms of a recurrence become manifest. A physician who works in conjunction with the family and who has ready access to a psychiatrist would be helpful in arranging for the early treatment of each recurrence.

The manic phase of manic-depressive psychosis also usually requires hospitalization to prevent patients from impulsive and often aggressive behavior which might jeopardize their career or standing in the community. Judgment is so poor in mania that patients may gamble away fortunes or make reckless investments. Chlorpromazine (Thorazine) or haloperidol (Haldol) can be used to control the mania while lithium carbonate is started. If tranquilizers are ineffective in slowing hyperactivity, ECT can be used.

SYNDROMES CAUSED BY DISEASES OF SPECIAL PARTS OF THE CEREBRUM

FRONTAL LOBES In Fig. 25-1, it is seen that the frontal lobes lie anterior to the central, or rolandic, sulcus and superior to the sylvian fissure. They consist of several functionally different parts, which are conventionally designated in the neurologic literature by numbers (according to a scheme devised by Brodmann) and by letters (according to a scheme of von Economo and Koskinas).

The posterior parts, areas 4 and 6 of Brodmann, are specifically related to motor function. Voluntary movement in humans depends on the integrity of these areas, and lesions in them produce spastic paralysis of the contralateral face, arm, and leg. This is discussed in Chap. 15. Lesions limited more or less to the premotor areas (area 6) are accompanied by prominent grasp and sucking reflexes. Lesions in area 8 of Brodmann interfere with the mechanism concerned with turning the head and eyes contralaterally. Lesions in area 44 (Broca's area) of the dominant cerebral hemisphere, usually the left one, have often resulted in at least a temporary loss of verbal expression. Lesions in the medial limbic or piriform cortex (areas 23 and 24), wherein are bilaterally organized the mechanisms controlling respiration, circulation, and micturition, have relatively unclear clinical effects.

The remaining parts of the frontal lobes (areas 9 to 13 of Brodmann), sometimes called the *prefrontal areas*, have less specific and measurable functions. In contrast to the motor areas of the frontal lobes and other areas of the brain, stimulation of the prefrontal areas in humans has yielded a paucity of findings. Many patients with gunshot wounds of these areas have shown only mild and inconsistent abnormalities of behavior. Nevertheless, the following groups of symptoms have been observed in patients with large lesions of one or both of the frontal lobes or of the central white matter and the anterior part of the corpus callosum by which they are joined:

1 Lack of initiative and spontaneity in conjunction with diminished speech and motor inactivity (apathetic-akinetic-abulic state). Necessary daily activities are neglected. Interpersonal social reactions are reduced and shallow.
2 Change of personality, usually expressed as lack of concern over the consequences of any action, which may take the form of a childish excitement, an inappropriate joking and punning, or an instability and superficiality of emotion, or irritability. This puerility and euphoria may at times assume a pseudopsychopathic form.
3 Slight impairment of intelligence, usually described as lack of concentration, vacillation of attention, inability to carry out planned activity, difficulty in changing from one activity to another, or slight loss of recent memory. According to Luria, who views the frontal lobe as a regulating mechanism of the organism's activities, planned action is deficient with respect to steady control and goal orientation.
4 Motor abnormalities such as decomposition of gait and upright stance, wide base, flexed posture, and small shuffling steps, culminating in an inability to stand (truncal ataxia of Bruns), abnormal postures, reflex grasping or sucking, and incontinence of sphincters.

Some differences have been noted between the dominant (left) and right frontal lobes. In psychologic tests left frontal lesions impair verbal fluency and right frontal the learning of visual spatial patterns (see Hecaen and Albert for further details).

TEMPORAL LOBES The boundaries of the temporal lobes may be seen in Fig. 25-1. The sylvian fissure separates the superior surface of each temporal lobe from the frontal and anterior parts of the parietal lobes. There is no definite anatomic boundary between the temporal and occipital lobes or between posterior temporal and parietal lobes. The temporal lobe includes the superior, middle, and inferior temporal, fusiform, and hippocampal convolutions and the transverse convolutions of Heschl, which are the auditory receptive area present on the superior surface within the sylvian fissure. The hippocampal convolution was once believed to be related indirectly to the olfactory bulb, but now it is known that lesions here do not cause anosmia. The lower fibers of the geniculocalcarine pathway (from the inferior retina) swing in a wide arc over the temporal horn of the ventricle into the white matter of the temporal lobe en route to the occipital lobes, and lesions that interrupt them characteristically produce a contralateral homonymous upper quadrant defect of visual fields. Hearing, also localized in the temporal lobes, is bilaterally represented, which accounts for the fact that unless both temporal lobes are affected, there is little or no demonstrable loss of hearing. Loss of equilibrium has not been observed with temporal lobe lesions. Extensive disease in the superior and middle convolutions of the left temporal lobe in right-handed individuals results in Wernicke's aphasia. This syndrome, discussed in Chap. 24, consists of jargon aphasia and inability to read, to write, or to understand the meaning of spoken words.

FIGURE 25-1

Diagram to show cortical areas, numbered according to the scheme of Brodmann. The speech areas are in black, the three main ones of which are 39, 41, and 45. The zone marked by vertical stripes in the superior frontal convolution is the secondary motor area which, like Broca's area 45, if stimulated, causes vocal arrest. (After Handbuch der Inneren Medizin, Berlin, Springer-Verlag, 1939.)

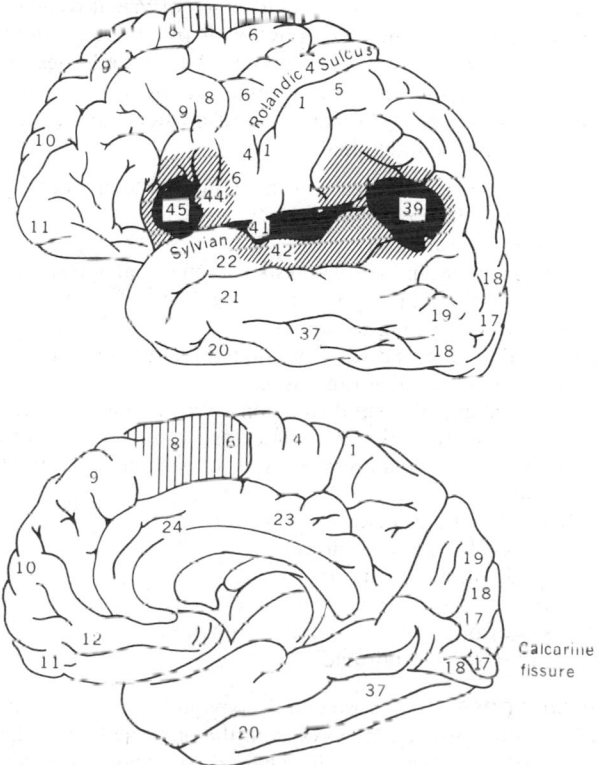

Between the auditory and olfactory projection areas there is a large expanse of temporal lobe which has no assignable function. This is the temporal association area. Dysnomia has been the most frequent symptom in lesions of the dominant hemisphere. The most careful psychologic studies have shown a difference between cases involving loss of the dominant and nondominant temporal lobe. With lesions of the dominant side there is impairment in learning auditorially presented material; with nondominant lesions there is a similar failure in tests with visually presented material. In addition, about 20 percent of both right and left lobectomy patients have shown a syndrome similar to that described for the prefrontal parts of the brain; but more significant is the fact that the other cases exhibited little or no alteration of personality. The study of cases of uncinate epilepsy, with the characteristic dreamy state, olfactory or gustatory hallucinations, and masticatory movements, suggests that all these functions are organized through the temporal lobes. Similarly, stimulation of the posterior parts of the temporal lobes of fully conscious epileptic patients during surgical procedures has brought to light the interesting fact that complex memories and visual and auditory images, some with strong emotional content, can be aroused. Studies of the effect of stimulation of the amygdaloid nucleus, which is in the anterior and medial part of the temporal lobe, have shed additional light on this subject. Symptoms not unlike some of those of schizophrenic and manic patients may be evoked. Complex emotional experiences that have occurred previously may be revived. There are remarkable autonomic effects: blood pressure rises, pulse increases, respirations increase in frequency and depth, and the patient looks frightened. In temporal lobe epilepsy, recently reviewed by Geschwind, there may be an intensification of the patient's emotional reactions, an intense concern about moral and religious issues, a tendency to write excessively, and sometimes aggressiveness. Ablation of the amygdaloid nuclei has eliminated uncontrollable rage reactions in psychotic patients. Hippocampal and adjacent convolutions have been excised bilaterally, with a disastrous loss of ability to learn or to establish new memories (Korsakoff's psychosis). Bilateral destruction of the temporal lobes in both humans and monkeys results in placidity, loss of visual recognition, tendency to examine objects by touch and mouthing, and hypersexuality (Kluver-Bucy syndrome). All this indicates an important role of the temporal lobes in auditory and visual perception and imagery, in learning and memory, and in the emotional life of the individual.

I Effects of unilateral disease of the dominant temporal lobe
  A Homonymous quadrantanopia
  B Wernicke's aphasia
  C Impairment in verbal tests of material presented through the auditory sense
  D Dysnomia or amnesic aphasia
II Effects of unilateral disease of nondominant temporal lobe
  A Homonymous quadrantanopia
  B Impairment of mental function with inability to judge spatial relationships in some cases
  C Impairment in nonverbal tests of visually presented material
III Effects of bilateral disease
  A Korsakoff's amnesic defect
  B Apathy and placidity
  C Loss of sexual capacity
  D Loss of other of the unilateral functions
  E Kluver-Bucy syndrome

PARIETAL LOBES The postcentral convolution is the terminus of somatic sensory pathways from the opposite half of the body. However, destructive lesions here do not abolish cutaneous sensation but instead cause mainly a defect in sensory discrimination with variable impairment of primary sensation. In other words, the perception of painful, tactile, thermal, and vibratory stimuli is more or less normal, whereas stereognosis, sense of position, distinction between single and double contacts (two-point threshold), and the localization of sensory stimuli are impaired or lost. There is also the phenomenon of extinction; i.e., if both sides of the body are touched simultaneously, only the stimulus on the normal side is perceived. This type of sensory disturbance, sometimes called *cortical sensory defect,* is discussed in Chap. 19. Extensive lesions deep in the white matter of the parietal lobes produce an impairment of all forms of sensation contralaterally as well as a contralateral homonymous hemianopia, often incongruous and greater in the inferior quadrants. Lesions in the angular gyrus of the dominant hemisphere result in an inability to read.

More recent investigations have centered on the function of the parietal lobes in the perception of one's position in space and of the relationship of the various parts of the body to one another. Since the time of Babinski it has been known that patients with a large lesion of the minor parietal lobe are often unaware of their hemiplegia and hemianesthesia. Babinski called this condition *anosognosia.* Related psychologic disorders are lack of recognition of the left arm and leg, neglect of the left side of the body (as in dressing) and of external space on the left side, and constructional apraxia (an inability to perform the movements of constructing simple figures). All these disorders of parietal lobe function may occur with left-sided lesions as well but are observed only infrequently, since aphasic difficulties with lesions of the left hemisphere make it difficult to adequately test these functions.

Another frequent constellation of symptoms, usually referred to as *Gerstmann's syndrome,* occurs only with lesions of the dominant parietal lobe. This consists of inability to write (agraphia), inability to calculate (acalculia), failure to distinguish right from left, and loss of recognition of various fingers and toes. This is a true *agnosia,* since it represents a defect in the formulation and use of symbolic concepts, including the significance of numbers and letters and the names of parts of the body. An ideomotor apraxia may or may not be associated. *Apraxia and agnosia* are discussed in Chaps. 15 and 19.

The effects of disease of the parietal lobes may be organized into three major categories:

I Effects of unilateral disease of the parietal lobe, right or left
  A Cortical sensory syndrome and sensory extinction (or total hemianesthesia with large acute lesions of white matter)
  B Mild hemiparesis, unilateral muscular atrophy in children
  C Homonymous hemianopia or visual inattention, and sometimes anosognosia, neglect of one-half of the body and of extrapersonal space
  D Abolition of opticokinetic nystagmus to one side
II Effects of unilateral disease of the dominant parietal lobe (left hemisphere in right-handed patients), additional phenomena
  A Disorders of language (especially alexia)
  B Gerstmann's syndrome
  C Bimanual astereognosis (tactile agnosia)
  D Bilateral apraxia of the ideomotor type
III Effects of nondominant parietal lobe (additional phenomena)
  A Dressing apraxia
  B Constructional apraxia
  C Misidentification of left arm and leg
  D Bland mood, indifference to illness, or neurologic defects

In all these lesions, if the disease is sufficiently extensive, there may be a reduction in the capacity to think clearly, inattentiveness, and impaired memory.

OCCIPITAL LOBES The occipital lobes are the terminus of the geniculocalcarine pathways and are essential for visual sensation and perception. Lesions in one occipital lobe result in homonymous defects in the contralateral visual fields. Most often the defect takes the form of loss of vision in part or all of the homonymous fields. Occasionally patients complain of changes in the form and contour of visually perceived objects (metamorphopsia), as well as illusory displacement of images from one side of the visual field to another (visual allesthesia), or of abnormal persistence of the visual image after the object has been removed (palinopsia). Bilateral lesions cause "cortical" blindness, a state of blindness without change in optic fundi or pupillary reflexes. Visual illusions, hallucinations, and metamorphopsias (distortion of form, size, movement, and color) may also occur.

Lesions in Brodmann's areas 18 and 19 of the dominant hemisphere (Fig. 25-1) cause a loss of visual recognition with retention of some degree of visual acuity, a state termed *visual agnosia.* In the classic form of this blindness individuals with intact mental powers are unable to recognize objects, even though by tests of visual acuity and perimetry they appear to see sufficiently well to do so; they are able to recognize objects by tactile or other extravisual sense. In these terms, *alexia,* or inability to read, represents a visual verbal agnosia or "word blindness." Patients can see letters and words but cannot recognize their meaning, although they can still recognize them through tactile or auditory senses. Other types of agnosia for recognition of faces (prosopagnosia), for a complex of objects the elements of which are perceived but not the whole (simultanagnosia), color agnosia, and Balint's syndrome (inability to look at and grasp an object and inattention) are observed with unilateral and bilateral occipital lesions (see Adams and Victor).

CORPUS CALLOSUM AND THE DISCONNECTION SYNDROMES Considerable attention has been devoted to the study of each of the two cerebral hemispheres in isolation. This is possible only when the corpus callosum which forms a bridge between the two hemispheres is congenitally defective, surgically sectioned (for epilepsy), or destroyed by infarction or tumors. From these studies emerges the well-known fact that the left hemisphere is dominant in all language functions and auditory perception and the right hemisphere is superior in spatial and visual perception. Partial lesions of the corpus callosum or of the long tracts in the cerebral white matter are found to be associated with a number of interesting syndromes (commissural and intrahemispheric) which will be described below. (See reference to disconnection syndromes by Dimond.)

When the entire corpus callosum is missing because of a congenital defect or destroyed by a surgical procedure or anterior cerebral artery occlusion (anterior four-fifths), the speech and perceptual areas of the left hemisphere are isolated from those of the right hemisphere. These patients, if blindfolded, are unable to match an object held in one hand with that in the other hand. Further, they cannot match an object seen in the right half of the visual field with one in the left half. If given verbal commands to execute, they perform correctly with the right hand but not with the left. Without vision, objects placed in the right hand are named correctly, but not those in the left. In lesions confined to the posterior fifth of the corpus callosum (splenium), only the visual part of the disconnection syndrome occurs. Occlusion of the left posterior cerebral artery provides the best examples of the latter. Since infarction of the left occipital lobe causes a right homonymous hemianopia, thereafter all visual information needed for activating the speech areas of

the left hemisphere must come from the right occipital lobe and cross the splenium of the corpus callosum. If there is a lesion in the corpus callosum the patient cannot read or name colors because the visual information cannot reach the left angular gyrus. There is no difficulty in copying words (though the patient cannot read what has been written); apparently the visual information for activating the left motor area crosses the corpus callosum more anteriorly. Matching of colors without naming them is done without error.

A disconnection in the anterior third of the corpus callosum, where fiber systems between right and left motor areas pass, results only in failure of the left hand to obey commands, the right one performing perfectly (left-sided apraxia). The left one can still imitate the examiner's movements.

Of intrahemispheric disconnections, those listed below are the most important:

1 Conduction (also called "central") aphasia. The patient has fluent but paraphasic speech and writing with nearly perfect comprehension of spoken or written language. Repetition is severely affected. The lesion is presumably in the arcuate fasciculus, which connects Wernicke's area with Broca's area.
2 Sympathetic apraxia in Broca's aphasia. A lesion in the subcortical white matter, underlying Broca's area, by destroying the origin of the fibers that connect the left and right motor association cortices causes an apraxia of command movements of the left hand.
3 Pure word deafness. Although the patient is able to hear and to identify nonverbal sounds, there is loss of ability to comprehend spoken language. The patient's speech remains normal. This defect has been attributed to a subcortical lesion sparing Wernicke's area.
4 Alexia and inability to name colors without agraphia. This is due to a lesion in the left occipital lobe and splenium of corpus callosum.

OTHER BEHAVIORAL DISORDERS ASSOCIATED WITH CEREBRAL DISEASE

When one attempts to categorize all the patients with relatively acute or subacute disorders of mentation and behavior under the section headings above, there are still a considerable number that remain difficult to classify. They present themselves as an almost infinite variety of syndromes in which the following abnormalities of function may occur: reduced or increased levels of speech, thought, and action; disorientation as to time and place; idleness and lack of interest; loss of spontaneity and sense of humor; muteness and hypokinesia, resistiveness and negativism; hostility, lack of observance of social customs, use of abusive and vulgar language; inexplicable fright, euphoria, and lack of proper concern; complaint of visual distortion, of excess sensitivity to sounds; distortions of smell and taste; inability to find the names of objects, to follow a conversation, to think coherently; sexual indiscretion, lack of modesty, and other signs of disinhibition; seizures; disturbances of sleep. Obviously these many symptoms do not all have the same basic significance, and the majority possess only relative localizing value. They may be associated with definite hemiparesis, hemihypesthesia, frank aphasia, or homonymous hemianopia, but even without these lateralizing signs they point to the existence of cerebral disease.

Syndromes comprising these elements may be observed in subacute sclerosing panencephalitis, listeriosis with meningoencephalitis, Behçet's meningoencephalitis, adult toxoplasmosis, infectious mononucleosis, acute or subacute demyelinative diseases (acute or subacute recurrent multiple sclerosis), granulomatous and other forms of angiitis, gliomatosis cerebri, carcinomatosis with encephalopathy of multifocal type, multiple tumor metastases, acute and subacute bacterial endocarditis, and thrombopenia with multiple-platelet thromboses in small vessels (Moschkowitz's disease). A fuller account of some of the cerebral symptoms enumerated above is found in chapters dealing with these diseases.

APPROACH TO THE PATIENT

The physician presented with a patient suffering from delirium, confusional states, dementia and psychoses of manic-depressive or schizophrenic type must adopt an examination technique designed to expose fully the intellectual defect. Abnormalities of posture, movement, sensation, and reflexes cannot be relied upon for the full demonstration of the neurologic deficit, for it must be remembered that the association and limbic areas of the brain may be severely damaged without demonstrable neurologic signs of this type.

Three sources of data are required for the recognition and differential diagnosis of these mental disorders:

1 A reliable history of the illness
2 Findings on mental examination, i.e., so-called "mental status," as well as on the rest of the neurologic examination
3 Special laboratory procedures, lumbar puncture, x-rays of the skull, electroencephalogram, CT and radionuclide scanning of the brain, and sometimes pneumoencephalogram

The history should always be supplemented by information obtained from a person other than the patient. Through lack of insight, patients are often unaware of their illness; indeed, they may be ignorant even of their chief complaint. Special inquiry should be made about the patient's general behavior, social adjustment, capacity for work, personal habits, etc., and family history.

This examination of the mental status must be systematic. At a minimum it should provide answers to the questions listed below.

I Insight (patients' replies to questions about their chief symptoms): What is your difficulty? Are you ill? When did your illness begin?
II Orientation (knowledge of personal identity and present situation): What is your name? What is your occupation? Where do you live? Are you married? Where are you now?
  A Place: What is the name of the place where you are now? How did you get here? What floor is it on? Where is the bathroom? What are you doing now?
  B Time: What is the date today? What time of day is it? What meals have you had? When was the last holiday?
III Memory:
  A Remote: Tell me the names of your children and their birth dates. When were you married? What was your mother's maiden name? What was the name of your first school teacher? What jobs have you held?
  B Recent past: Tell me about your recent illness (compare with previous statements). What did you have for breakfast today? What is my name or the nurse's name? When did you see me for the first time? What tests were done yesterday? What were the headlines in the newspaper today? Give patients a simple story, oral or written, and ask him to recall it after 3 to 5 min.
  C Immediate recall (short-term memory): Repeat these numbers after me (give a series of 3, 4, 5, 6, 7, and then 8 digits at the speed of one per second). Now when I give a series of numbers, repeat them in reverse order.
  D Visual span: Show patients a picture of several objects, ask them to name what they have seen and note any inaccuracies.
IV General information: Ask about names of presidents, well-known historic dates, the names of large rivers or cities, etc.
V Capacity for sustained mental activity:
  A Calculation: Test ability to add, substract, multiply, and divide. Serial subtraction of 7s or 3s from 100 is a good test of calculation as well as of concentration.
  B Abstract thinking: See if patients can detect similarities and differences between classes of objects, or explain a proverb or a fable.
VI General behavior: Attitudes, general bearing, attentiveness, manner of dress, etc.
  A Content of thought: What ideas occupy the thoughts of patients? Do they believe that their thoughts and actions are controlled or are being broadcast to others? Are there hallucinations and/or delusions? Is there a press of speech or lack of speech?
  B Mood: Do patients appear gay or sad? How do they feel? Are they nervous and worried or apprehensive? What feeling is revealed through speech, attitude, facial expression?
VII Special tests of localized cerebral functions: grasping, sucking, aphasia battery, praxis with both hands, cortical sensory function, drawing of clock face, map of United States or Europe, floor plan of patient's house, etc.

In order to enlist the full cooperation of patients, physicians must prepare them for questions of this type. Otherwise, their first reaction will be one of embarrassment or anger because of the implication that their mind is not sound. It should be pointed out to patients that some individuals are rather forgetful and that it is necessary to ask specific questions in order to form some impression about their degree of nervousness when being examined. Reassurance that these are not tests of intelligence or of sanity is helpful. A more formal and reliable method of examining the mental capacity of adults is the Wechsler-Bellevue test.

Correct diagnosis of treatable forms of mental disease (e.g., general paresis, subdural hematoma, brain tumor, bromide or other chronic drug intoxication, normal-pressure hydrocephalus, pellagra and other deficiency states, and hypothyroidism) is of greater practical importance than the diagnosis of the untreatable ones.

The separation of the Korsakoff amnesic syndrome and dementia depends on the relative integrity of all cognitive functions except retentive memory. The two major so-called "functional psychoses," schizophrenia and manic-depressive disease, are distinguished from the amnesic state and dementia on the basis of the retention of an alert state of mind, retention of all cognitive functions including retentive memory, and the identification of disordered thinking with prominent hallucinations, delusions, and/or alteration of mood. The separation of these two latter types of mental illness, both of which are chronic, is based on the presence or absence of premorbid psychic peculiarity, age of patient, mode of onset, duration of illness, recovery, recurrence, etc. If of recent onset while using drugs and alcohol, or associated with temporal lobe seizures or an endocrine disease, a period of observation may be required before the diagnosis can be settled.

MANAGEMENT OF THE PATIENT

These major mental derangements and psychoses are clinical states of the most serious nature, and usually it is worthwhile to admit the patient to the hospital for a period of observation. The physician then has an opportunity to see the patient several times in a neutral and fairly constant hospital environment, and certain special procedures such as x-rays of the skull, lumbar puncture, analysis of blood for drugs, basal metabolic rate, an electroencephalogram, CT scan, and sometimes a pneumoencephalogram can be carried out at this time. The management of the demented patient in the hospital may be relatively simple if the person is quiet and cooperative. If the disorder of mental function is severe, i.e., the patient is psychotic, a nurse, attendant, or member of the family must stay with the patient at all times. Provision must be made for adequate food and fluid intake and control of infection, using the same measures outlined for the delirious patient (see Chap. 21).

Once it is established that the patient has an untreatable dementing, amnesic, schizophrenic, or manic-depressive brain disease, a responsible member of the family should be apprised of the medical facts. The patient should be told that he or she has a nervous condition for which rest and treatment has been prescribed. Nothing is accomplished by telling the individual more. The family should be given diagnosis and prognosis if the diagnosis is sufficiently certain for this to be done. If the psychic or mood abnormalities are slight and circumstances are suitable, the patient should remain at home, continue appropriate activities, and receive appropriate medication. If he or she is depressed and suicidal, the patient should remain in a psychiatric hospital. The individual should be spared responsibility and guarded against injury that might result from imprudent action. If the patient becomes demented while still at work, plans for occupational retirement should be carried out. In more advanced stages of disease, mental and physical enfeeblement become pronounced and institutional care should be advised. Seizures should be treated symptomatically. Nerve tonics, vitamins, and hormones are of no value in checking the course of dementia or in regenerating decayed tissue. They may, however, offer some support to the patient and family.

Sometimes, stimulants in the form of dextroamphetamine, caffeine, and nicotinic acid cause transitory improvement in mental function. Undesirable restlessness, nocturnal wandering, belligerency, or anxiety may be reduced by some of the "minor" tranquilizing drugs (see Chap. 227).

REFERENCES

ADAMS RD, VICTOR M: *Principles of Neurology* New York, McGraw-Hill, 1977

ARMAND MN (ed): *Harvard Guide to Modern Psychiatry.* Cambridge, Mass, Harvard University Press, 1978

BENSON L, BLUMER D: *Psychiatric Aspects of Neurologic Disease.* New York, Grune & Stratton, 1975

DIMOND SJ: The disconnection syndrome, in *Modern Trends in Neurology*, E Williams (ed) London, Butterworths, 1975

GESCHWIND N: Temporal lobe epilepsy. Arch Neurol 34:454, 1977

HECAEN H, ALBERT ML: Disorders of mental functioning related to frontal lobe, in *Modern Trends of Neurology*, E Williams (ed). London, Butterworths, 1975

HOREL JA: The neuroanatomy of amnesia. A critique of the hippocampal memory hypothesis. Brain 101:403, 1978.

LURIA AR: *Higher Cortical Functions in Man.* New York, Basic Books, 1966

MAAS JW: The clinical and biochemical heterogeneity of the depressive disorders. Ann Intern Med 88:556, 1978

McCULLOUGH E et al: Norepinephrine in chronic paranoid schizophrenia: Above-normal levels in limbic forebrain. Science 200:456, 1978

POPE HG, LIPINSKI JF: Diagnosis in schizophrenia and depressive illness. Arch Gen Psychiatry (in press)

ROBINS E et al: Diagnostic criteria for use in psychiatric research. Arch Gen Psychiatry 26:57, 1972

section 4 | Alterations in circulatory and respiratory function

26
COUGH AND HEMOPTYSIS

GENNARO M. TISI
EUGENE BRAUNWALD

COUGH

Cough, one of the most frequent cardiorespiratory symptoms, is an explosive expiration which provides a means of clearing the tracheobronchial tree of secretions and foreign bodies.

MECHANISM Coughing may be initiated either voluntarily or reflexly. As a defensive reflex it has both afferent and efferent pathways. The *afferent limb* includes cough receptors within the sensory distribution of the trigeminal, glossopharyngeal, superior laryngeal, and vagus nerves. The *efferent limb* includes the recurrent laryngeal nerve (which causes glottic closure) and the spinal nerves (which cause contraction of the thoracic and abdominal musculature). The *sequence of a cough* includes an appropriate stimulus which initiates a deep inspiration. This is followed by glottic closure, relaxation of the diaphragm, and muscle contraction against a closed glottis so as to produce maximally positive intrathoracic and intraairway pressures. These positive intrathoracic pressures result in a narrowing of the trachea, produced by an infolding of its more compliant posterior membrane. Once the glottis opens, the combination of a large pressure differential between the airways and the atmosphere coupled with this tracheal narrowing produces flow rates through the trachea close to the speed of sound. The shearing forces which are developed aid in the elimination of mucus and foreign materials. A tracheostomy short-circuits glottic closure and therefore decreases the effectiveness of the cough mechanism.

ETIOLOGY Cough is produced by inflammatory, mechanical, chemical, and thermal stimulation of the cough receptors. *Inflammatory* stimuli are initiated by edema and hyperemia of the respiratory mucous membranes, and by irritation from exudative processes. Such stimuli may arise either in the airways (as in laryngitis, tracheitis, bronchitis, and bronchiolitis) or in the alveoli (as in pneumonitis and lung abscess). *Mechanical* stimuli are produced by inhalation of particulate matter, such as dust particles, and by compression of the air passages and pressure or tension upon these structures. Lesions associated with airway compression may be either extramural or intramural in type. The former include aortic aneurysms, granulomas, pulmonary neoplasms, and mediastinal tumors; intramural lesions include bronchogenic carcinoma, bronchial adenoma, foreign bodies, granulomatous endobronchial involvement, and contraction of airway smooth muscle (bronchial asthma). Pressure or tension upon the air passages is usually produced by lesions associated with a decrease in pulmonary compliance. Examples of specific causes include acute and chronic interstitial fibrosis (Chap. 264), pulmonary edema, and atelectasis. *Chemical* stimuli may result from inhalation of irritant gases, including cigarette smoke and chemical fumes. Finally, *thermal* stimuli may be produced by inhalation of either very hot or cold air.

DIAGNOSTIC EVALUATION When one is considering the above list of causes, answers to the following general questions will significantly narrow the diagnostic possibilities: Is the cough acute or chronic? Is it productive of sputum or nonproductive? A chronic productive cough may be caused by diseases such as chronic bronchitis, pulmonary tuberculosis, and pulmonary neoplasms. Are the findings on physical examination of the chest normal or abnormal? Is the chest roentgenogram normal or abnormal?

Features of the history, physical examination, chest roentgenogram, screening pulmonary function studies (static lung volumes and dynamic flow rates), and sputum examination may indicate a specific cause. The *history* may indicate specific diagnoses. Acute episodes of cough may be associated with such viral infections as acute tracheobronchitis or pneumonitis or with bacterial bronchopneumonia. Cough associated with an acute febrile episode and associated with hoarseness is usually produced by viral laryngotracheobronchitis. The character of the cough may suggest the anatomic site of involvement: the patient with a "barking" type of cough may have epiglottal involvement, while the cough associated with tracheal or major airway involvement is often loud and "brassy." Cough associated with generalized wheezing may be produced by acute bronchospasm. The time of occurrence of a cough may indicate a specific cause: a cough which occurs selectively at night suggests congestive heart failure; one related to meals suggests a tracheoesophageal fistula, a hiatal hernia, or an esophageal diverticulum; a cough precipitated by a change in position suggests a lung abscess or a localized area of bronchiectasis. The description of sputum or secretions produced in conjunction with the cough may also be helpful: putrid sputum suggests a lung abscess; bloody sputum, bleeding (see "Hemoptysis," below); frothy and pink-tinged sputum, pulmonary edema; mucoid and massive sputum, alveolar cell carcinoma; purulent and/or large amounts of sputum, lung abscess and bronchiectasis.

On *physical examination* the character of the auscultatory findings may suggest the site of disease: inspiratory stridor and wheezing may be present in laryngeal disease; inspiratory and expiratory rhonchi favor tracheal and major airway involvement; coarse subcrepitant inspiratory rales may indicate interstitial fibrosis and/or edema; fine crepitant rales may indicate

a process such as pneumonitis or pulmonary edema, which fills the alveoli with fluid. The *chest roentgenogram* may reveal the cause of the cough; it may show an intrapulmonary mass lesion which may be either central or peripheral (Chap. 268), an alveolar filling process which may be pneumonic or nonpneumonic, an area of honeycombing and cyst formation which may indicate an area of localized bronchiectasis, or bilateral hilar adenopathy which may indicate sarcoidosis or a lymphoma.

Screening pulmonary function studies may also indicate specific diagnoses. Significant expiratory obstruction to airflow (as determined from a forced expiratory flow maneuver), coupled with a history of cough and significant sputum production, suggests that irrespective of other lesions the patient has significant bronchitis. Decreased lung volume (as determined from the static lung volumes) indicates that a restrictive type of lung disease is present—reduction of lung volumes produced by thoracic, pleural, alveolar, or interstitial disease. Finally, a careful *sputum examination* may be more enlightening than a patient's description of the character of the sputum. Examination shows whether the sputum is thin or viscid, purulent or not, foul-smelling or not, blood tinged or not, scant or copious. Gram stain and culture of the deep-cough specimen may reveal a specific bacterial, fungal, or mycoplasmal causation, while sputum cytology may result in a positive diagnosis of a pulmonary neoplasm.

Two features of cough should be highlighted: (1) A cough is often so common in the cigarette smoker as to be ignored or minimized. *Any changes in the nature and character of a chronic cigarette cough should initiate immediate diagnostic evaluation, with particular attention directed to detection of bronchogenic carcinoma.* (2) Female patients are inclined to swallow sputum and not to expectorate as male patients do. This tendency may lead to the incorrect conclusion that a cough in a female patient is irritative and nonproductive.

COMPLICATIONS Three complications may be produced by the coughing mechanism: paroxysms of coughing may precipitate syncope (cough syncope, Chap. 13), and strenuous coughing may produce rupture of an emphysematous bleb and rib fractures. A potential mechanism for cough syncope includes the development of markedly positive intrathoracic and alveolar pressures which decrease venous return, producing a decrease in cardiac output and resultant syncope. Although cough fractures of the ribs may occur in otherwise normal patients, their occurrence should at least raise the possibility of pathologic fractures, which are seen in multiple myeloma, osteoporosis, and osteolytic metastases.

THERAPY Specific treatment of cough depends upon the underlying cause. An irritative, nonproductive cough may be suppressed by an antitussive agent, such as codeine or dextromethorphan, 15 mg qid. These drugs are particularly useful in interrupting prolonged, self-perpetuating paroxysms. However, a cough productive of significant quantities of sputum should not be suppressed, since retention of sputum in the tracheobronchial tree may interfere with alveolar aeration and impair the ability of the lung to resist infection. When secretions are tenacious and thick, adequate hydration, expectorants (such as potassium iodide), and humidification of the air with an ultrasonic nebulizer may be helpful.

HEMOPTYSIS

For purposes of definition hemoptysis includes both blood-streaked sputum and gross hemoptysis. It is apparent that any patient with gross hemoptysis should be given appropriate diagnostic tests so that a specific cause may be found. The patient with blood-streaked sputum should also be studied unless one can be certain that this type of hemoptysis is due to a benign condition. A major pitfall in dealing with hemoptysis is to ascribe recurrent episodes of hemoptysis to a previously established diagnosis, such as chronic bronchiectasis or bronchitis. Such an approach may result in missing a serious but potentially treatable lesion. The safest approach to a recurrent episode of hemoptysis is to treat it as if it were the initial episode and proceed with a complete diagnostic evaluation.

ETIOLOGY AND INCIDENCE   Prior to embarking upon an extensive diagnostic workup of hemoptysis, it is essential to determine that the blood is in fact coming from the respiratory tract, not from the nasopharynx or gastrointestinal tract. Once this point is established, the diagnostic tests for hemoptysis may proceed. Although there are numerous single case reports of diseases which have been associated with hemoptysis, Table 26-1 presents the more common disorders.

The incidence of the diagnoses listed in Table 26-1 depends upon the nature of the series reported and whether one includes both gross bleeding and blood streaking of the sputum. If both types of bleeding are included, then the major causes (approximately 60 to 70 percent) are chronic bronchitis and bronchiectasis. If the definition is restricted to gross bleeding (greater than several tablespoons) then the incidence depends upon the type of series reported. Surgical series favor the incidence of mass lesions and operable lesions (carcinoma, 20 percent; localized, segmental, or lobar bronchiectasis, 30 percent). Those from centers with a large tuberculosis population favor this condition (incidence varying between 2 and 40 percent). Combined medical-surgical series include a wider representation of those lesions which present with hemoptysis (carcinoma, 20 percent; bronchiectasis, 30 percent; bronchitis, 15 percent; other inflammatory lesions including tuberculosis, 10 to 20 percent; other lesions including the vascular, traumatic, and hemorrhagic etiologies listed in Table 26-1, 10 percent). Despite the most extensive of evaluations, 5 to 15 percent of cases entailing gross hemoptysis remain undiagnosed.

Two points should be highlighted with reference to diseases associated with hemoptysis: (1) *hemoptysis is rare in metastatic carcinoma to the lung*; (2) *although hemoptysis may occur at some time during the course of a viral or pneumococcal pneumonia, it is usually scanty and its occurrence should always raise the question of a more serious underlying process.*

DIAGNOSIS   The *history* may suggest specific diagnoses: recurrent, chronic hemoptysis in a young, otherwise asymptomatic female favors the diagnosis of a bronchial adenoma; recurrent hemoptysis with chronic, marked sputum production associated with ring shadows, tram lines (abnormal air bronchograms), and cyst formation on the roentgenogram suggests a diagnosis of bronchiectasis; putrid sputum production suggests a lung abscess; weight loss and anorexia in a male smoker over the age of 40 raises the possibility of a bronchogenic carcinoma; a recent history of blunt trauma to the chest suggests a lung contusion; and acute pleuritic chest pain raises the possibility of pulmonary embolism with infarction or some other pleurally based lesion (lung abscess, coccidiomycosis cavity, and vasculitis). Several findings on the *physical examination* may also suggest a specific diagnosis: a pleural friction rub suggests those diagnoses just mentioned in connection with pleuritic pain; the findings of pulmonary hypertension raise the diagnostic possibilities of primary pulmonary hypertension, mitral stenosis, recurrent or chronic thromboembolism, and Eisenmenger's syndrome; a localized wheeze over a major lobar airway suggests an intramural lesion such as a bronchogenic carcinoma or a foreign body; systemic arteriovenous communications or the presence of a murmur over the lung fields suggest the diagnosis of Osler-Weber-Rendu disease with pulmonary atrioventricular malformation; evidence of signifi-

cant expiratory obstruction to airflow coupled with sputum production suggests that whatever other lesion may be present, the patient has significant bronchitis. Finally, the *chest roentgenogram* is critical to diagnosis. The presence of ring shadows favors a diagnosis of bronchiectasis; an air-fluid level, the diagnosis of a lung abscess; and a mass lesion, the diagnosis of a central or peripheral pulmonary neoplasm. A mass lesion which may cause hemoptysis should be distinguished from an area of blood pneumonitis caused by aspiration of blood into contiguous areas.

One of the most demanding diagnostic problems is the identification of the side of bleeding in a patient with normal findings on physical examination and a normal roentgenogram of the chest. A patient with hemoptysis tends to keep the bleeding side dependent. Otherwise, gravitational drainage would cause aspiration into the noninvolved dependent lung. The patient may also be able to give a history of a burning or deep pain which may localize the side of bleeding; bronchoscopy may then be useful. This procedure generally is most helpful when the bleeding is scant, and of least help when the bleeding is massive, since blood may be aspirated into contiguous airways.

Following the history and physical examination, the diagnostic approach to a patient with hemoptysis includes whatever specialized studies and procedures are required to make a specific diagnosis. The first step is to obtain a roentgenogram. Usually bronchoscopy is the procedure employed next. The recent introduction of fiberoptic bronchoscopy (Chap. 256) has improved visualization of the upper lobes and included within the range of visualization airways as small as several millimeters in diameter. This endoscopic technique may provide definitive visual, biopsy, or cytologic information. Since direct visualization of more peripheral portions of the airway system is now possible, the indications for bronchography in the evaluation of hemoptysis are being modified. The principal indications for bronchography in such patients are (1) to establish the presence of localized bronchiectasis (including a sequestered lobe) and (2) to rule out the presence of more generalized bronchiectasis in a patient with localized disease who is regarded as a surgical candidate because of either repetitive hemoptysis or recurrent infections. The majority of patients with bronchiectasis have a normal chest roentgenogram. If bronchoscopy in such patients is also negative, bronchography is the only means of establishing an anatomic diagnosis of bronchiectasis. If the chest roentgenogram is abnormal, revealing

TABLE 26-1
Causes of hemoptysis

I Inflammatory
  A Bronchitis
  B Bronchiectasis
  C Tuberculosis
  D Lung abscess
  E Pneumonia, particularly *Klebsiella*
II Neoplastic
  A Lung cancer: squamous cell, adenocarcinoma, oat cell
  B Bronchial adenoma
III Other
  A Pulmonary thromboembolism
  B Left ventricular failure
  C Mitral stenosis
  D Traumatic, including foreign body and lung contusion
  E Primary pulmonary hypertension; arteriovenous malformation; Eisenmenger's syndrome; pulmonary vasculitis including Wegener's granulomatosis and Goodpasture's syndrome; idiopathic pulmonary hemosiderosis; and amyloid
  F Hemorrhagic diathesis including anticoagulant therapy

either ring shadows or tram lines, a diagnosis of bronchiectasis may be made without the need for bronchography.

THERAPY Since hemoptysis is such an alarming symptom, there is a tendency to overtreat the patient. Usually hemoptysis is scant and will stop spontaneously without specific therapy. If the hemoptysis is substantial, the mainstays of therapy include keeping the patient calm, instituting complete bed rest, excluding unnecessary diagnostic procedures until the hemoptysis has begun to subside, and suppressing cough if it is present and an aggravating feature of the hemoptysis. The emergency care of such a patient demands that intubation and suctioning equipment be at the bedside. In patients in danger of asphyxiation by flooding of the lung contralateral to the site of hemorrhage, intubation by a technique which isolates the hemorrhaging lung and prevents contralateral aspiration of blood should be carried out. This can be accomplished by strategic location of a balloon catheter whose introduction into the bronchus in question is facilitated by direct visualization through a fiberoptic bronchoscope.

The management of potentially lethal massive hemoptysis remains controversial. The choice between a medical approach and surgical intervention hinges on the words *potentially lethal.* Massive hemoptysis, usually defined as greater than 1000 ml in 24 h, is an alarming clinical situation in which asphyxiation due to aspiration of blood represents the principal threat to life. The choice between surgical and medical management relates most often to the anatomic basis for the massive hemoptysis. In patients with cavitary tuberculosis, anaerobic lung abscess, and lung cancer, the risk of mortality is far greater than when the cause for the hemoptysis is bronchitis or bronchiectasis. Operation may occasionally be necessary in the former, but virtually never in the latter group. In either case the initial management should include the conservative measures suggested above. With such management, spontaneous cessation of bleeding usually occurs. Surgical intervention should be considered in that small group of patients with a definable lesion or chest roentgenogram (i.e., cavitary disease, lung abscess, lung cancer) who have evidence of uncontrollable respiratory or hemodynamic compromise. If a patient is a surgical candidate, bronchoscopy should be performed to identify the specific site of bleeding. Otherwise bronchoscopy should be deferred for several days because of the tendency of this procedure to aggravate cough and thereby perpetuate the hemoptysis. Bronchial arterial catheterization and embolization are new modalities of treatment currently under evaluation for the nonsurgical control of massive hemoptysis, especially in patients with nonresectable lung cancer.

REFERENCES

BATES DV et al: *Respiratory Function in Disease.* Philadelphia, Saunders, 1971, p 584ff

COMMITTEE ON ETIOLOGY OF CHRONIC BRONCHITIS, MEDICAL RESEARCH COUNCIL: Definition and classification of chronic bronchitis. Lancet 1:775, 1965

COMMITTEE ON THERAPY, AMERICAN THORACIC SOCIETY: The management of hemoptysis. Am Rev Resp Dis 93:471, 1966

KARY RC, SMITH JR: Medical history and physical examination in the assessment of pulmonary disease, in *Textbook of Pulmonary Diseases*, 2d ed, GL Baum (ed). Boston, Little, Brown, 1974, p 3

LOUDON RG, SHAW GB: Mechanics of cough in normal subjects and in patients with obstructive respiratory disease. Am Rev Resp Dis 96:666, 1967

PIERCE J: Cough and hemoptysis, in *Signs and Symptoms*, 6th ed, RS Blacklow (ed). Philadelphia, Lippincott, 1979, chaps 17, 18

WOLFE JD, SIMMONS DH: Hemoptysis: Diagnosis and management (medical progress). West J Med 127:383, 1977.

27
DYSPNEA AND PULMONARY EDEMA

ROLAND H. INGRAM, JR.
EUGENE BRAUNWALD

DYSPNEA

INTRODUCTION For an average 70-kg adult at rest the normal breathing pattern consists of an average frequency of 14 breaths per minute and has a mean tidal volume of 600 ml. It is not surprising that a normal, resting person is unaware of the act of breathing since it originates in the more vegetative portions of the central nervous system and is modulated by both lower central and peripheral vagal pathways. The breathing pattern is changed by a series of higher central and peripheral control mechanisms which can increase ventilation in excess of metabolic demands in conditions such as anxiety and fear, and can increase ventilation appropriate to increased metabolic demands during physical activity. Although a person may become conscious of breathing during mild to moderate exertion, no discomfort is experienced. However, during and following exhausting exertion an individual may become unpleasantly aware of breathing, yet feel reasonably assured that the sensation will be transitory and is appropriate to the level of exercise. Therefore, as a cardinal symptom of diseases affecting the cardiorespiratory system, dyspnea is defined as an *abnormally uncomfortable awareness of breathing.*

Although dyspnea is not painful in the usual sense of the word, it is, like pain, involved with both the perception of a sensation and the reaction to that perception. Thus, since it is a symptom, dyspnea is present whenever a patient experiences it. Patients experience a number of uncomfortable sensations related to breathing and use an even larger number of verbal expressions to describe these sensations, such as "cannot get enough air," "air does not go all the way down," "smothering feeling in the chest," "tightness in the chest," "fatigue in the chest," and a "choking sensation." It may be necessary, therefore, to review meticulously the patient's history in order to ascertain whether the more abstruse descriptions do, in fact, represent dyspnea. Once it is established that a patient does have dyspnea, it is of paramount importance to define the circumstances in which it occurs and to assess associated symptoms. There are situations in which breathing appears labored but in which dyspnea does not occur. For example, the hyperventilation in association with metabolic acidemia is rarely accompanied by dyspnea. On the other hand, patients with apparently normal breathing patterns may complain of shortness of breath.

QUANTITATION OF DYSPNEA The gradation of dyspnea may usefully be based upon the amount of physical exertion required to produce the sensation. In actual practice the major functional classifications of patients with heart or lung disease are based largely on dyspnea in relation to degree of exertion. However, in assessing the severity of dyspnea, it is important to obtain a clear understanding of the patient's general physical condition, work history, and recreational habits. For example, the development of dyspnea in a trained runner upon running 2 mi may signify a more serious disturbance than a similar degree of breathlessness on running a fraction of this distance in a sedentary person. It is also important to note that some patients with lung or heart disease may have such reduced capabilities due to other disease that exertional dyspnea is precluded despite serious impairment of pulmonary or cardiac function; in contrast, others who decrease their physical activities gradually may avoid dyspnea because they do not stress themselves.

Some patterns of dyspnea are not directly related to physical exertion. Sudden and unexpected dyspneic episodes at rest can be associated with pulmonary emboli, spontaneous pneumothorax, or anxiety. Nocturnal episodes of severe paroxysmal dyspnea and diaphoresis are characteristic of congestive heart failure in association with hypertensive cardiovascular disease. Dyspnea upon assuming the supine posture, *orthopnea* (see below), thought to be mainly characteristic of congestive heart failure, may also occur in some patients with asthma and chronic obstruction of the airways and is a regular finding in the rare occurrence of bilateral diaphragmatic paralysis. The term *trepopnea* is used to describe the unusual circumstance in which dyspnea occurs only in the left or right lateral decubitus position, most often in patients with heart disease, while *platypnea* is dyspnea which occurs only in the upright position. Both of these patterns remain to be fully explained but may be related to positional alterations in ventilation-perfusion relations.

MECHANISMS OF DYSPNEA Physicians usually relate the symptom of dyspnea to a process such as obstruction of the airways or congestive heart failure and generally proceed with further diagnostic and/or therapeutic attempts, having satisfied themselves that they understand the mechanism of the dyspnea. In fact, elucidation of the *actual* mechanism(s) of dyspnea has eluded clinical investigators.

It is well known that dyspnea occurs whenever the work of breathing is excessive. Increased force generation is required of the respiratory muscles to produce a given volume change if the chest wall or lungs are less compliant or if resistance to airflow is increased. Although it is true that an individual is more apt to become dyspneic when the work of breathing is increased, the work theory does not account for the perceptual difference between a deep breath with a normal mechanical load and a normal-sized breath with an increased mechanical load. The work might be the same with both breaths, but the normal one with the increased load will be associated with discomfort. In fact, with respiratory loading, such as adding a resistance at the mouth, there is an increase in respiratory center output, as gauged by newer indices, that is disproportionate to the increase in work of breathing. Hence, a more appealing theory is one that links inappropriate length to tension in the respiratory muscles. Campbell has proposed that a sense of discomfort arises when there is misalignment of the nerve spindles, which are sensing tension, in relation to muscle length. This misalignment would lead to the sensation that a person is getting an insufficient breath for the tension generated by the respiratory muscles. Such a theory is difficult to test and, if tested and proved in some circumstances, would still not explain why patients who are completely paralyzed, either by cord transections or neuromuscular blockade, experience dyspnea although aided by a mechanical ventilator. It is probable, in these circumstances, that signals from the lungs and/or airways travel via the vagus nerve to the central nervous system to account for the sensation.

In all likelihood a number of different mechanisms operate to different degrees in the various clinical situations in which dyspnea occurs. Perhaps, in some circumstances, dyspnea is evoked by stimulation of receptors in the upper respiratory tract; in others it may originate from receptors in the lungs, airways, respiratory muscles, or some combination of those structures. In general, there is a reasonably good correlation between the severity of dyspnea and the disturbances of pulmonary or cardiac function which are responsible.

DIFFERENTIAL DIAGNOSIS Obstructive disease of airways (see also Chaps. 257 and 263) Obstruction to airflow can be present anywhere from the extrathoracic airways out to the small airways in the periphery of the lung. Large extrathoracic airway obstruction can occur acutely, as with aspiration of food or a foreign body or with angioneurotic edema of the glottis. Circumstantial evidence or testimony from witnesses should cause the physician to suspect aspiration, and an allergic history together with a few scattered hives should raise the possibility of glottic edema. The acute form of upper airway obstruction is a medical emergency. More chronic forms can occur with tumors or with fibrotic stenosis following tracheostomy or prolonged endotracheal intubation. Whether acute or chronic, the cardinal symptom is dyspnea, and the characteristic signs are stridor and retraction of the supraclavicular fossae with inspiration.

Obstruction of intrathoracic airways can occur acutely and intermittently or can be present chronically with worsening during respiratory infections. Acute intermittent obstruction with wheezing is typical of *asthma*. Chronic cough with expectoration is typical of *chronic bronchitis* and *bronchiectasis*. Most often there is a prolongation of expiration and coarse rhonchi which are generalized in chronic bronchitis and may be localized in the case of bronchiectasis. Intercurrent infection results in worsening of the cough, increased expectoration of purulent sputum, and more severe dyspnea. During such episodes the patient may complain of nocturnal paroxysms of dyspnea with wheezing relieved by cough and expectoration of sputum.

Many years of exertional dyspnea progressing to dyspnea at rest characterize the patient with predominant *emphysema*, a condition which is defined as dilatation of the terminal air sacs with disruption of alveolar septa. Although a parenchymal disease by definition, emphysema is invariably accompanied by obstruction of airways. The signs are prominent usage of accessory muscles which lift the anterior thorax, retraction of the lower intercostal spaces with inspiration, distant breath sounds with a hyperresonant percussion note, and end-expiratory wheezes.

With severe chronic bronchitis and/or emphysema, the signs of cor pulmonale may either appear or increase during a respiratory infection. Spirometry and measurements of lung volumes and arterial blood gases (Chap. 255) not only are helpful in establishing a diagnosis but also serve to assess the severity of the process in guiding therapy.

Diffuse parenchymal lung diseases (see also Chap. 264) This category includes a large number of diseases ranging from acute pneumonia to chronic disorders such as sarcoidosis and the various forms of *pneumoconiosis*. History, physical findings, and radiographic abnormalities often provide clues to the diagnosis. The patients are often tachypneic with arterial P_{CO_2} and P_{O_2} values below normal. Exertion often further reduces the arterial P_{O_2}. Lung volumes are decreased and the lungs are stiffer, i.e., less compliant.

Pulmonary vascular occlusive diseases (see also Chap. 266) Whether due to repeated emboli or intrinsic vascular disease, right ventricular hypertrophy or signs of right ventricular failure in the absence of obvious parenchymal lung disease should suggest the possibility of pulmonary vascular occlusive disease. Repeated episodes of dyspnea at rest often occur with repeated emboli. A source for emboli, such as phlebitis of a lower extremity or the pelvis, is quite helpful in leading the physician to suspect the diagnosis. Arterial blood gases are almost invariably abnormal, but lung volumes are frequently normal or only minimally abnormal.

Diseases of the chest wall or respiratory muscles (see also Chap. 270) The physical examination establishes the presence of a chest wall disease such as severe kyphoscoliosis, pectus excavatum, or spondylitis. Although all three of these deformities may be associated with dyspnea, only severe kyphoscoliosis regularly interferes with ventilation sufficiently to produce chronic cor pulmonale and respiratory failure.

Both weakness and paralysis of respiratory muscles can lead to respiratory failure, but most often the signs and symptoms of the neurologic or muscular disorder are more prominently manifested in other systems. A reduction in total lung capacity and vital capacity along with an increased residual volume in the absence of apparent heart or lung disease suggests the diagnosis. Such a pattern can be explained by muscle weakness, which can be confirmed by measuring maximal voluntary static pressures.

Anxiety neurosis Dyspnea experienced by someone with an anxiety neurosis is a difficult symptom to evaluate. The signs and symptoms of acute and chronic hyperventilation do not serve to distinguish between anxiety neurosis and other processes, such as recurrent pulmonary emboli. A rather extensive series of pulmonary and cardiac function tests, carried out both at rest and during exercise, may be needed to be certain that anxiety is, in fact, the cause of the dyspnea. Certain clues are helpful in leading one to suspect a psychogenic origin. Frequent sighing respirations and a bizarre, irregular breathing pattern are helpful. Often the breathing pattern returns to normal during sleep.

Heart disease In patients with cardiac disease exertional dyspnea occurs most commonly as a consequence of an elevated pulmonary capillary pressure; aside from uncommon causes such as obstructive disease of the pulmonary veins (Chap. 240), pulmonary capillary hypertension is a consequence of left atrial hypertension, which in turn may be due to left ventricular dysfunction (Chaps. 235 and 236), reduced left ventricular compliance, and mitral stenosis. The elevation of hydrostatic pressure in the pulmonary vascular bed tends to upset the Starling equilibrium (see "Pulmonary Edema" below) with resulting transudation of fluid into the interstitial space, reducing the compliance of the lungs. A diminution in compliance increases the work of breathing which, to some degree, is minimized by both an increase in frequency of respirations and a reduction in tidal volume. In severe heart disease, usually involving elevation of both pulmonary and systemic venous pressures, hydrothorax develops, further interfering with pulmonary function and intensifying dyspnea. Less commonly, in patients with heart disease, dyspnea is due to a severely diminished cardiac output, resulting in inadequate perfusion of the respiratory muscles and hence their fatigue; dyspnea may also be associated with severe systemic and cerebral anoxia, as occurs during exertion in patients with congenital heart disease and right-to-left shunts.

Cardiac dyspnea usually begins as breathlessness on strenuous exertion and, over the course of months or years, progresses until the patient is dyspneic at rest. Occasionally, as in patients with massive acute myocardial infarction, the course may be associated with a nonproductive cough developing in the recumbent position, particularly at night.

ORTHOPNEA Orthopnea, i.e., dyspnea in the recumbent position, is characteristic of those forms of heart failure associated with elevations of pulmonary venous and capillary pressures. While orthopnea is usually a symptom of more advanced heart failure than exertional dyspnea, in patients who are physically inactive its onset may actually precede that of exertional dyspnea. Orthopnea is associated with the redistribution of blood from the lower extremities and splanchnic bed to the lungs as

the result of the alteration of gravitational forces when the recumbent position is assumed. This augmentation of intrathoracic blood volume elevates pulmonary venous and capillary pressures which increases the pulmonary closing volume and reduces the vital capacity. An additional factor associated with recumbency is the elevation of the diaphragm, which results in a lower end-expiratory lung volume. This combination of lower end-expiratory lung volume and increase in closing volume results in a significant alteration of alveolar-capillary gas exchange.

PAROXYSMAL (NOCTURNAL) DYSPNEA Also known as *cardiac asthma,* this condition is characterized by attacks of severe shortness of breath which generally occur at night and usually awaken the patient from sleep. The attack is precipitated by stimuli which aggravate the previously existing pulmonary congestion; frequently the total blood volume is augmented at night because of the reabsorption of edema from dependent portions of the body during recumbency; the redistribution of blood volume which takes place results in an increase in intrathoracic blood volume and therefore produces pulmonary congestion. A sleeping patient can tolerate relatively severe pulmonary engorgement and may awaken only when actual pulmonary edema and bronchospasm have developed, with the feeling of suffocation and with wheezing respirations.

CHEYNE-STOKES RESPIRATION See Chap. 236.

DIAGNOSIS The diagnosis of cardiac dyspnea depends on the recognition of heart disease on the basis of the history and physical examination. There may be a history of antecedent myocardial infarction, third and fourth sound gallops may be audible, and/or there may be evidence of left ventricular enlargement, jugular neck vein distention, and/or peripheral edema. Often there are radiographic signs of heart failure, with evidence of interstitial edema, pulmonary vascular redistribution, and accumulation of fluid in the septal planes and pleural cavity (Chap. 233). Cardiomegaly is often present, but the overall heart size may be normal, particularly in patients with dyspnea due to acute myocardial infarction or mitral stenosis; an enlarged left atrium is usually evident in the latter condition. The electrocardiogram (Chap. 232) is rarely specific for heart disease and cannot specifically indicate whether a patient's dyspnea is caused by heart disease; however, it is rarely normal in patients with cardiac dyspnea.

Differentiation between cardiac and pulmonary dyspnea In most patients with dyspnea there is obvious clinical evidence of disease of either heart or lungs. The dyspnea of chronic obstructive lung disease tends to develop more gradually than that of heart diseases; exceptions, of course, occur in patients with obstructive lung disease who develop an episode of infectious bronchitis, pneumonia, or pneumothorax, or an exacerbation of asthma. Like patients with cardiac dyspnea, patients with chronic obstructive lung disease may also waken at night with dyspnea, but this is usually associated with sputum production; the dyspnea is relieved after these patients rid themselves of secretions.

The difficulty in the distinction between cardiac and pulmonary dyspnea may be compounded by the coexistence of diseases involving both organ systems. Patients with a history of chronic bronchitis or asthma who develop left ventricular failure tend to develop recurrences of bronchoconstriction and wheezing in association with bouts of paroxysmal nocturnal dyspnea and pulmonary edema. This condition, i.e., cardiac asthma, usually occurs in patients with overt clinical evidence of heart disease. Acute cardiac asthma is further differentiated from acute attacks of bronchial asthma by the presence of diaphoresis, more bubbly airway sounds, and the more common occurrence of cyanosis.

It is desirable to carry out pulmonary function testing in patients in whom the etiology of dyspnea is not clear, for these tests should be helpful in determining whether dyspnea is produced by heart disease, lung disease, abnormalities of the chest wall, or anxiety. In addition to the usual means of assessing patients for heart disease (Chap. 230), the arm-to-tongue circulation time may be useful, since in patients with dyspnea on a cardiac basis it usually exceeds the upper normal limit of 16 s by 4 s or more. Careful observation during the performance of an exercise treadmill test will often help in the identification of the patient who is malingering or whose dyspnea is secondary to anxiety. Under these circumstances the patient usually complains of severe shortness of breath but appears to be breathing either effortlessly or totally irregularly.

PULMONARY EDEMA

An increase in pulmonary venous pressure, which results initially in the engorgement of the pulmonary vasculature, is common in most instances of dyspnea in association with congestive heart failure. The lungs become less compliant, the resistance of small airways increases, and there is an increase in lymphatic flow which apparently serves to maintain a constant pulmonary extravascular fluid volume. At this early stage there is usually mild tachypnea, and if arterial blood gases are measured, the arterial P_{O_2} and P_{CO_2} are both lowered with an increase in the alveolar-to-arterial oxygen difference. Tachypnea itself, which might result from stimulation of receptors in the pulmonary interstitium, apparently increases lymphatic flow by augmenting ventilatory pumping of lymphatic vessels. The changes described are seen well in advance of auscultatory findings or radiographic signs pointing to congestive heart failure. If sufficient both in magnitude and duration, the increase in intravascular pressure results in a net gain of fluid in the extravascular space despite further increases in lymphatic flow. It is at this point that symptoms worsen, tachypnea increases, gas exchange deteriorates further, and radiographic changes, such as Kerley B lines and loss of distinct vascular margins, are seen. Even at this intermediate stage, the capillary endothelial intercellular junctions have been shown to widen and allow passage of macromolecules into the interstices. Up to and including this stage, the edema is purely *interstitial*. Sufficient further elevations in intravascular pressure result in disruption of the tighter junctions between alveolar lining cells, and alveolar edema ensues with outpouring of fluid, which contains both red blood cells and macromolecules. At this point *alveolar edema* is present. Although originally considered an early and subtle radiographic sign of interstitial edema, recent evidence suggests that an antigravity redistribution of pulmonary blood flow occurs only after the onset of alveolar edema. With yet more severe disruption of the alveolar-capillary membrane, edematous fluid floods the alveoli and airways. At this point, full-blown clinical pulmonary edema with bilateral wet rales and rhonchi will occur, and the chest radiograph may show diffuse haziness of the lung fields. Typically, the patient is anxious and perspires freely, and the sputum is frothy and blood-tinged. Gas exchange is more severely compromised with worsening hypoxemia and possibly hypercapnia. Without effective treatment (Chap. 236) progressive acidemia, hypoxemia, and respiratory arrest ensue.

The earlier sequence of fluid accumulation described above follows the Starling law of capillary–interstitial fluid exchange:

$$\text{Fluid accumulation} = K[(P_c + \pi_{IF}) - (P_{IF} + \pi_{pl})] \quad Q_{lymph}$$

where K = permeability coefficient
P_c = mean intracapillary pressure
π_{IF} = oncotic pressure of interstitial fluid
P_{IF} = mean interstitial fluid pressure
π_{pl} = oncotic pressure of the plasma
Q_{lymph} = lymphatic flow

The pressures tending to move fluid out of the vessel are P_c and π_{IF}, which are normally more than offset by pressures tending to move fluid back into the vasculature, i.e., the algebraic sum of P_{IF} and π_{pl}. Implicit in the above equation is that lymphatic flow can increase in the case of imbalance of forces and result in no net accumulation of interstitial fluid. However, in later sequences, with opening of first the endothelial and then the alveolar intercellular junctions, the permeability coefficient changes strikingly. Thus, the initial process of hemodynamic pulmonary edema is one of fluid filtration and clearance. With further increasing pressures, disruption of both the structure and the function of the alveolar-capillary membrane occurs.

There are several clinical conditions which are associated with pulmonary edema based upon an imbalance of Starling forces other than through primary elevations of pulmonary capillary pressure. Although diminished plasma oncotic pressure in hypoalbuminemic states (e.g., severe liver disease, nephrotic syndrome, protein-losing enteropathy) might be expected to lead to pulmonary edema, the balance of forces normally so strongly favors resorption that even under these conditions some elevation of capillary pressure is necessary before interstitial edema develops. Increased negativity of interstitial pressure has been implicated in the genesis of unilateral pulmonary edema following rapid evacuation of a large pneumothorax. In this situation the findings are apparent only by radiography. It has been recently proposed that large negative intrapleural pressures during acute severe asthma may be associated with the development of interstitial edema. If this proposal can be supported by sufficient clinical data, then asthma would represent an additional example of edema due to increased negativity of interstitial pressure. Lymphatic blockade secondary to fibrotic and inflammatory diseases or lymphangitic carcinomatosis may lead to interstitial edema. In such instances both clinical and radiographic manifestations are dominated by the underlying disease process.

There are other conditions characterized by increases in the interstitial fluid content of the lungs which begin neither with an imbalance between intravascular and interstitial forces nor with alterations in lymphatics, but rather appear to be associated primarily with disruption of the alveolar-capillary membranes. Experimentally the prototype for such conditions is the pulmonary edema following alloxan administration. Any number of spontaneously occurring or environmental toxic insults are associated with diffuse pulmonary edema which clearly does not have a hemodynamic origin. These conditions are discussed in Chap. 271.

There are three forms of pulmonary edema which have not been clearly related to increased permeability, inadequate lymphatic flow, or an imbalance of Starling forces; hence their precise mechanism remains unexplained. *Narcotic overdose* is a well-recognized antecedent to pulmonary edema. Although illicit use of parenteral heroin has been the most frequent cause, parenteral and oral overdoses of legitimate preparations of morphine, methadone, and dextropropoxyphene have also been associated with pulmonary edema. Thus the earlier idea that injected impurities lead to the disorder is untenable. Available evidence suggests that there are alterations in the permeability of alveolar and capillary membranes rather than elevation of pulmonary capillary pressure. *Exposure to high altitude* in association with severe physical exertion is a well-recognized setting for pulmonary edema in unacclimatized, yet otherwise healthy, persons. Recent data show that acclimatized high-altitude natives also develop this syndrome upon return to high altitude after a relatively brief sojourn at low altitudes. The mechanism for high-altitude pulmonary edema remains obscure, and studies have been conflicting, some suggesting pulmonary venous constriction and others indicating pulmonary arteriolar constriction as the prime mechanisms. Neurogenic pulmonary edema has been suspected in patients with central nervous system disorders and without apparent preexisting left ventricular dysfunction. Although most experimental equivalents have implicated sympathetic nervous system activity, the mechanism whereby sympathetic efferent activity leads to pulmonary edema is a matter of speculation. It is known that a massive adrenergic discharge leads to peripheral vasoconstriction with elevation of blood pressure and shifts of blood to the central circulation. In addition, it is probable that a decrease in left ventricular compliance also occurs, and both factors serve to increase left atrial pressures sufficiently to induce pulmonary edema on a hemodynamic basis.

Treatment of pulmonary edema   See Chap. 236.

REFERENCES

CAMPBELL EJM et al: *Breathlessness.* Oxford, Blackwell, 1966
—— et al: *The Respiratory Muscles: Mechanisms and Neural Control.* Philadelphia, Saunders, 1970
FISHMAN AP, RENKIN EM (eds): *Pulmonary Edema.* Washington, DC, American Physiological Society, 1979
GOLD W: Dyspnea, in *Signs and Symptoms,* 6th ed, RS Blacklow (ed). Philadelphia, Lippincott, 1979, chap 19
MCFADDEN ER, INGRAM RH JR: Relationship between diseases of the heart and lungs, in *Heart Disease,* E Braunwald (ed). Philadelphia, Saunders, 1980, chap 53
SCOGGIN CH et al: High altitude pulmonary edema in the children and young adults of Leadville, Colorado. N Engl J Med 297:1269, 1977
STAUB NC: State of the art review: Pathogenesis of pulmonary edema. Am Rev Respir Dis 109:358, 1974
SZIDON JP et al: The alveolar-capillary membrane and pulmonary edema. N Engl J Med 286:1200, 1972

28
CYANOSIS, HYPOXIA, AND POLYCYTHEMIA

EUGENE BRAUNWALD

CYANOSIS

Cyanosis refers to a bluish color of the skin and mucous membranes resulting from an increased amount of reduced hemoglobin, or of hemoglobin derivatives, in the small blood vessels of those areas. It is usually most marked in the lips, nail beds, ears, and malar eminences. The "red cyanosis" of polycythemia vera (Chap. 320) must be distinguished from the true cyanosis discussed here. A cherry-colored flush, rather than cyanosis, is caused by carboxyhemoglobin (Chap. 224). In *argyria,* the skin is bluish because of the deposition of silver salts, and the discoloration persists despite pressure, unlike cyanotic skin which blanches. The degree of cyanosis is modified by the quality of cutaneous pigment, the color of the blood plasma, and the thickness of the skin, as well as by the state of the cutaneous capillaries. The accurate clinical detection of the presence and degree of cyanosis is difficult, as proved by oxi-

metric studies. Some observers can reliably detect central cyanosis when the arterial saturation has fallen to 85 percent; others may not detect it until the saturation has reached 75 percent.

The increase in the amount of reduced hemoglobin in the cutaneous vessels, which produces cyanosis, may be brought about either by an increase in the quantity of venous blood in the skin as the result of dilatation of the venules and venous ends of the capillaries, or by a decrease in the oxygen saturation in the capillary blood. In general, cyanosis becomes apparent when the mean capillary concentration of reduced hemoglobin exceeds 5 g per 100 ml. It is the *absolute* rather than the *relative* amount of reduced hemoglobin which is important in producing cyanosis. Thus, in a patient with severe anemia the relative amount of reduced hemoglobin in the venous blood may be very large when considered in relation to the total amount of hemoglobin. However, since the latter is markedly lowered, the absolute amount of reduced hemoglobin may still be small, and therefore patients with severe anemia and marked arterial desaturation do not display cyanosis. Conversely, the higher the total hemoglobin content, the greater the tendency toward cyanosis; thus, patients with marked polycythemia tend to be cyanotic at higher levels of arterial oxygen saturation than patients with normal hematocrit values. Likewise, local passive congestion, which causes an increase in the total amount of reduced hemoglobin in the vessels in a given area, may cause cyanosis. Cyanosis also is observed when nonfunctional hemoglobin is present in the blood; as little as 1.5 g per 100 ml methemoglobin or 0.5 g sulfhemoglobin is sufficient to produce cyanosis (Chap. 315).

True cyanosis may be subdivided into *central* and *peripheral* categories. In the *central* type, there is arterial blood unsaturation or an abnormal hemoglobin derivative, and the mucous membranes and skin are both affected. *Peripheral* cyanosis is due to a slowing of blood flow to an area and abnormally great extraction of oxygen from normally saturated arterial blood. It results from vasoconstriction and diminished peripheral blood flow, such as occurs in cold exposure, shock, congestive failure, and peripheral vascular disease. Often, in these conditions, the mucous membranes of the oral cavity or those beneath the tongue may be spared. Clinical differentiation between central and peripheral cyanosis may not always be simple, and in conditions such as cardiogenic shock with pulmonary edema there may be a mixture of both types.

DIFFERENTIAL DIAGNOSIS (See Table 28-1)   **Central cyanosis** Decreased arterial oxygen saturation results from a marked reduction in the oxygen tension in the arterial blood. This may be brought about by a decline in the tension of oxygen in the inspired air without sufficient compensatory alveolar hyperventilation to maintain alveolar oxygen tension. Cyanosis does not occur in a significant degree in an ascent to an altitude of 8000 ft but is marked in a further ascent to 16,000 ft. The reason for this becomes clear on studying the S shape of the oxygen dissociation curve (Fig. 53-4). At 8000 ft the tension of oxygen in the inspired air is about 120 mmHg, the alveolar tension is approximately 80 mmHg, and the hemoglobin is nearly completely saturated. However, at 16,000 ft the oxygen tensions in atmospheric air and alveolar air are about 85 and 50 mmHg, respectively, and the oxygen dissociation curve shows that the arterial blood is only about 75 percent saturated. This leaves 25 percent of the hemoglobin in the reduced form, an amount likely to be associated with cyanosis in the absence of anemia. Similarly, a mutant hemoglobin with a low affinity for oxygen (Hb Kansas) causes lowered arterial oxygen saturation and resultant central cyanosis (Chap. 315).

Seriously *impaired pulmonary function*, through alveolar hypoventilation or perfusion of unventilated or poorly ventilated areas of the lung, is a common cause of central cyanosis

(Chap. 255). This may occur acutely, as in extensive pneumonia or in pulmonary edema, or with chronic pulmonary diseases (e.g., emphysema). In the last situation clubbing of the fingers and polycythemia are generally present. However, in many types of chronic pulmonary disease with fibrosis and obliteration of the capillary vascular bed, cyanosis does not occur because there is relatively little perfusion of underventilated areas.

Another cause of decreased arterial oxygen saturation is shunting of systemic venous blood into the arterial circuit. Certain types of congenital heart disease are associated with cyanosis (Chap. 240). Since blood normally flows from a high-pressure to a low-pressure region, in order for a cardiac defect to result in a right-to-left shunt, it must ordinarily be combined with an obstructive lesion distal to the defect or with elevated pulmonary vascular resistance. The commonest congenital cardiac lesion associated with cyanosis is the combination of ventricular septal defect and pulmonary outflow tract obstruction (tetralogy of Fallot). The more severe the obstruction, the greater the degree of right-to-left shunting and resultant cyanosis. The mechanisms for the elevated pulmonary vascular resistance which may produce cyanosis in the presence of intra- and extracardiac communications without pulmonic stenosis are discussed elsewhere (Chap. 240). In patients with patent ductus arteriosus, pulmonary hypertension, and right-to-left shunt, differential cyanosis results; i.e., cyanosis occurs in the lower extremities but not in the upper extremities.

Pulmonary arteriovenous fistulas may be congenital or acquired, solitary or multiple, microscopic or massive. The degree of cyanosis produced by these fistulas depends upon their size and number. They occur with some frequency in hereditary hemorrhagic telangiectasia (Chap. 317). Arterial oxygen unsaturation also occurs in some patients with cirrhosis, presumably as a consequence of pulmonary arteriovenous fistulas or portal vein-pulmonary vein anastomoses.

In patients with cardiac or pulmonary right-to-left shunts, the presence and severity of cyanosis depend on the size of the shunt relative to the systemic flow as well as on the oxyhemoglobin saturation of the venous blood. In patients with central cyanosis due to arterial oxygen unsaturation, the severity of cyanosis increases with exercise. With increased extraction of oxygen from the blood by the exercising muscles, the venous blood returning to the right side of the heart is more unsaturated than at rest, and shunting of this blood or its passage through lungs incapable of normal oxygenation intensifies the cyanosis. Also, since the systemic vascular resistance normally decreases with exercise, the right-to-left shunt is augmented by

TABLE 28-1
Causes of cyanosis

I Central cyanosis
  A Decreased arterial oxygen saturation
    1 Decreased atmospheric pressure—high altitude
    2 Impaired pulmonary function
      a Alveolar hypoventilation
      b Uneven relationships between pulmonary ventilation and perfusion
      c Impaired oxygen diffusion
    3 Anatomic shunts
      a Certain types of congenital heart disease
      b Pulmonary arteriovenous fistulas
      c Multiple small intrapulmonary shunts
    4 Hemoglobin with low affinity for oxygen
  B Hemoglobin abnormalities
    1 Methemoglobinemia—hereditary, acquired
    2 Sulfhemoglobinemia—acquired
    3 Carboxyhemoglobinemia (not true cyanosis)
II Peripheral cyanosis
  A Reduced cardiac output
  B Cold exposure
  C Redistribution of blood flow from extremities
  D Arterial obstruction
  E Venous obstruction

exercise in patients with congenital heart disease and communications between the two sides of the heart. Secondary polycythemia occurs frequently in patients with arterial unsaturation and contributes to the cyanosis.

Cyanosis can be caused by small amounts of circulating methemoglobin and by even smaller amounts of sulfhemoglobin (Chap. 315). Although they are uncommon causes of cyanosis, these abnormal hemoglobin pigments should be sought by spectroscopy when cyanosis is not readily explained by malfunction of the circulatory or respiratory systems. Generally, clubbing does not occur with them. The diagnosis of methemoglobinemia can be suspected if, on mixing the patient's blood in a test tube, it remains brown.

Peripheral cyanosis Probably the most common cause of peripheral cyanosis is generalized vasoconstriction resulting from exposure to cold air or water. This is clearly a normal response to the stimulus and is transient. When cardiac output is low, as in severe congestive heart failure or shock, cutaneous vasoconstriction occurs as a compensatory mechanism, so that blood is diverted to more vital areas [central nervous system, heart (Chap. 236)], and intense cyanosis associated with cool extremities may result. Even though the arterial blood is normally saturated, the reduced volume flow through the skin and the reduced oxygen tension at the venous end of the capillary result in cyanosis.

Arterial obstruction to an extremity generally results in pallor and coldness, but there may be associated slight cyanosis. If there is venous obstruction, the extremity is usually congested and markedly cyanotic, and there is true stagnation of blood flow. Venous hypertension, which may be local (as in thrombophlebitis) or generalized (as in tricuspid valve disease or constrictive pericarditis), dilates the subpapillary venous plexuses and intensifies cyanosis.

APPROACH TO THE PATIENT WITH CYANOSIS Certain features are important in arriving at the proper cause of cyanosis:

1 The history, particularly the duration (cyanosis present since birth is usually due to congenital heart disease); possible exposure to drugs or chemicals which may produce abnormal types of hemoglobin.
2 Clinical differentiation of central as opposed to peripheral cyanosis. Objective evidence by physical or radiographic examination of disorders of the respiratory or cardiovascular systems. Massage or gentle warming of a cyanotic extremity will increase peripheral blood flow and abolish peripheral but not central cyanosis.
3 The presence or absence of clubbing of the fingers. Clubbing without cyanosis is frequent in patients with subacute bacterial endocarditis and in association with ulcerative colitis; it may occasionally occur in healthy persons, and in some instances it may be occupational, e.g., in jackhammer operators. Slight cyanosis of the lips and cheeks, without clubbing of the fingers, is common in patients with well-compensated mitral stenosis and is probably due to minimal arterial hypoxia resulting from fibrotic changes in the lungs secondary to long-standing congestion combined with reduction of cardiac output. The combination of cyanosis and clubbing is frequent in many patients with certain types of congenital cardiac disease and is seen occasionally in persons with pulmonary disease such as lung abscess or pulmonary arteriovenous shunts. On the other hand, peripheral cyanosis or acutely developing central cyanosis is not associated with clubbed fingers.

4 Determination of arterial blood oxygen tension or oxygen saturation. Spectroscopic and other examinations of the blood for abnormal types of hemoglobin.

HYPOXIA

The fundamental purpose of the cardiorespiratory system is to deliver oxygen (and substrates) to the cells and to remove carbon dioxide (and other metabolic products) from them. Proper maintenance of this function depends on intact cardiovascular and respiratory systems and a supply of inspired gas containing adequate oxygen. Changes in oxygen and in carbon dioxide tension as well as changes in the intraerythrocytic concentration of certain *organic phosphate compounds*, especially 2,3-diphosphoglyceric acid (2,3-DPG), cause shifts in the oxygen dissociation curve. These are discussed in detail in Chap. 53 and are illustrated in Fig. 53-4. When hypoxia results as a consequence of respiratory failure, arterial P_{CO_2} usually rises (Chaps. 263 and 271), and the oxygen dissociation curve tends to be displaced to the right. Under these conditions the percentage saturation of the hemoglobin in the arterial blood at a given level of alveolar oxygen tension declines. Thus arterial hypoxia and cyanosis are likely to be more marked in proportion to the degree of depression of alveolar oxygen tension when such depression results from pulmonary disease than when the depression occurs as the result of a decline in the partial pressure of oxygen in the inspired air, in which case arterial P_{CO_2} falls and the oxygen dissociation curve is displaced to the left.

DIFFERENTIAL DIAGNOSIS Anemic hypoxia Any decrease in hemoglobin concentration is attended by a corresponding decline in the oxygen-carrying power. The P_{O_2} in the arterial blood remains normal, but the absolute amount of oxygen transported per unit volume of blood is diminished. As the anemic blood passes through the capillaries, and the usual amount of oxygen is removed from it, the P_{O_2} in the venous blood declines to a greater degree than would normally be the case.

Carbon monoxide intoxication (Chap. 224) This condition is accompanied by the equivalent of anemic hypoxia in that the hemoglobin which is combined with the carbon monoxide (carboxyhemoglobin) is unavailable for oxygen transport. In addition, the presence of carboxyhemoglobin increases the affinity of normal hemoglobin for oxygen at low levels of P_{O_2} (i.e., shifts the lower portion of the dissociation curve of hemoglobin to the left), so that the oxygen can be unloaded only at lower tensions. By such formation of carboxyhemoglobin a given degree of reduction in oxygen-carrying power produces a far greater degree of tissue hypoxia than the equivalent reduction in hemoglobin due to simple anemia.

Circulatory hypoxia As in anemic hypoxia, arterial P_{O_2} is normal but venous and tissue P_{O_2} are reduced as a consequence of reduced tissue perfusion in the face of normal tissue oxygen consumption. For this reason the term *stagnant hypoxia* may be used for this condition. Generalized circulatory hypoxia occurs in heart failure, as discussed in Chap. 236.

Specific organ hypoxia Decreased circulation to a specific organ resulting in localized stagnant hypoxia may be due to organic arterial or venous obstruction or may occur as a reflex phenomenon. The latter may occur when vasoconstriction of, for instance, the limbs results from an attempt to maintain adequate perfusion to more vital organs, as in severe congestive heart failure. When organic arterial obliterative disease develops, ischemic hypoxia results, with accompanying pallor. Localized hypoxia may also result from venous obstruction which results in congestion. Edema, which increases the distance through which oxygen diffuses before it reaches the cells, can also cause localized hypoxia.

Increased oxygen requirements Even if oxygen diffusion into blood perfusing the pulmonary capillary bed is unhampered and the hemoglobin is qualitatively and quantitatively normal, the P_{O_2} in venous blood (hence, capillary and tissue P_{O_2}) may be reduced if the oxygen consumption of the tissues is elevated without a corresponding increase in volume flow per unit of time. Such a situation may be encountered in febrile states and in thyrotoxicosis. Under such conditions the circulation may be considered deficient relative to the metabolic requirements. Thus, this type of metabolic hypoxia is comparable to circulatory hypoxia, in that in both conditions the volume flow of blood is decreased relative to the needs of the tissues; the difference is that in one case the primary defect is the volume flow of blood and in the other the primary defect is an increased oxygen need by the tissues.

Ordinarily, the clinical picture of patients with hypoxia due to an elevated basal metabolic rate is quite different from that in other types of hypoxia; the skin is warm and flushed, owing to increased cutaneous blood flow which dissipates the excessive heat produced, and cyanosis is absent in these patients.

Exercise is a classic example of increased tissue oxygen requirements. The increased demands are normally met by several mechanisms: (1) increasing the cardiac output and thus oxygen delivery to the tissues; (2) preferentially directing the blood to the exercising muscles and away from resting muscles (by changing vascular resistances in various circulatory beds, in some areas by direct effects, in others reflexly); (3) increasing oxygen extraction from the delivered blood and widening the arteriovenous oxygen differences. If the capacity of these mechanisms is exceeded, then hypoxia, especially of the exercising muscles, will result.

Improper oxygen utilization The administration of cyanide (Chap. 224) and several other similarly acting poisons leads to a paradoxic state in which the tissues are unable to utilize oxygen and as a consequence the venous blood tends to have a high oxygen tension. This condition has been termed *histotoxic hypoxia*. Cyanide produces cellular hypoxia by paralyzing the electron-transfer function of cytochrome oxidase so that it cannot pass electrons to oxygen, whereas diphtheria toxin is believed to inhibit the synthesis of one of the cytochromes and thus interfere with oxygen consumption and energy production by the cells involved.

EFFECTS OF HYPOXIA When hypoxia is general, all parts of the body may suffer some impairment of function, but those parts which are most sensitive to the effects of hypoxia give rise to symptoms which dominate the clinical picture. The *changes in the central nervous system*, particularly the higher centers, are especially important. Acute hypoxia produces impaired judgment, motor incoordination, and a clinical picture closely resembling that of acute alcoholism. When hypoxia is long-standing, the symptoms consist of fatigue, drowsiness, apathy, inattentiveness, delayed reaction time, severe fatigue, and reduced work capacity. As hypoxia becomes more severe, the centers of the brainstem are affected, and death usually results from respiratory failure. With reduction of arterial oxygen tension, cerebrovascular resistance decreases and cerebral blood flow increases, which tends to minimize the cerebral hypoxia. On the other hand when the reduction of arterial P_{O_2} is accompanied by hyperventilation and diminution of P_{CO_2}, cerebrovascular resistance rises, blood flow falls, and hypoxia is enhanced. Compared with the brain, the phylogenetically older spinal cord and peripheral nerves are relatively insensitive to hypoxia. Hypoxia also causes pulmonary arterial constriction, which serves the useful function of shunting blood away from poorly ventilated areas toward better-ventilated portions of the lung. However, it has the disadvantage of causing increased pulmonary vascular resistance and an increased burden on the right ventricle.

A complex disturbance of cellular functions results from the metabolic effects of severe acute hypoxia. In liver and muscles the breakdown of the primary foodstuff, carbohydrate, normally proceeds anaerobically (i.e., without oxidation) to the stage of formation of pyruvic acid. The breakdown of pyruvate requires oxygen, and when this is deficient, increasing proportions of pyruvate are reduced to lactic acid, which cannot be further broken down (Chap. 86). Hence, there is an increase in the blood lactate, with decrease in bicarbonate and a corresponding acidosis. Under these circumstances the total energy obtained from foodstuff breakdown is greatly reduced, and the amount of energy available for continuing resynthesis of energy-rich phosphate compounds becomes inadequate. Impairment of the myriad anabolic reactions which take place in tissues follows. The deficiency of energy-rich phosphate compounds produces a complex disturbance of cellular function.

Most of the useful respiratory response to hypoxia originates in special chemosensitive cells in the carotid and aortic bodies, although the respiratory center is also stimulated directly by oxygen lack. The peripheral chemoreceptors are extremely rugged and continue to function after other tissues have been damaged by hypoxemia. The chemoreceptors are stimulated by a reduction in their oxygen supply below their needs, either by lowered arterial P_{O_2} or by lowered blood flow to them. If respiration is stimulated by hypoxia, the resulting increase in ventilation, with loss of carbon dioxide, tends to make the blood more alkaline. On the other hand, the diffusion of additional quantities of lactic acid from the tissues into the blood tends to make the blood more acid. In either case the total amount of bicarbonate, and hence the carbon dioxide–combining power, tends to be diminished. With mild hypoxia there is likely to be respiratory alkalosis; severe hypoxia is attended by metabolic acidosis.

The heart, although relatively sensitive to hypoxia as compared with most of the structures of the body, is less sensitive than the nervous system. Consequently, in the absence of severe coronary artery disease, serious manifestations arising in the nervous system dominate the picture. Diminished oxygen tension in any tissue results in local vasodilatation, and the diffuse vasodilatation which occurs in generalized hypoxia results in an elevation of total cardiac output (Fig. 53-5). In patients with preexisting heart disease, particularly coronary artery disease, the combination of hypoxia and the requirements of the peripheral tissues for an increase of cardiac output may precipitate congestive heart failure. Prolonged or severe hypoxia may also impair hepatic and renal function.

One of the important mechanisms of compensation for prolonged hypoxia is an increase in the amount of hemoglobin in the blood (Fig. 53-5). This is due not to direct stimulation of the bone marrow but to the effect of an erythropoiesis-stimulating factor (erythropoietin) which originates primarily in the kidneys. Assayable levels of erythropoietin are increased by hypoxia, and its production has been found to be regulated by the balance between tissue oxygen supply and demand.

POLYCYTHEMIA

The term *polycythemia* signifies an increase above the normal in the number of red corpuscles in the circulating blood. This increase is usually, though not always, accompanied by a corresponding increase in the quantity of hemoglobin and in the volume of packed red corpuscles. The increase may or may not be associated with an increase in the total quantity of red blood cells in the body. It is important to distinguish between *absolute* polycythemia (an increase in the total red corpuscle mass) and *relative* polycythemia, which occurs when, through loss of blood plasma, the concentration of the red corpuscles becomes greater than normal in the circulating blood. This may be the consequence of abnormally lowered fluid intake, of the loss of plasma into the interstitial fluid, and of the marked loss of body fluids, such as occurs in persistent vomiting, severe diarrhea, copious sweating, or acidosis (Chap. 85).

Because the term polycythemia is used loosely to refer to all varieties of increase in the number of red corpuscles, the terms *erythrocytosis* and *erythremia* are preferred in referring to two forms of absolute polycythemia. Erythrocytosis denotes absolute polycythemia which occurs in response to some known stimulus (secondary polycythemia); erythremia (polycythemia rubra vera) refers to the disease of unknown etiology, which is discussed elsewhere (Chap. 320). An approach to the differential diagnosis of erythrocytosis should begin with a consideration of its mechanisms (Table 28-2). Erythrocytosis develops as a consequence of a variety of factors and represents a physiologic response to conditions of hypoxia. Sojourn at high altitudes leads to defective saturation of arterial blood with oxygen and stimulates the production of more red corpuscles. The oxygen saturation, rather than oxygen tension, appears to be the more important determinant of the erythropoietic response to chronic hypoxia (Fig. 28-1). A disorder may set in insidiously after several years of continued residence at high altitudes, leading to the development of a condition known as *chronic mountain sickness* or *seroche* (Monge's disease). Prominent manifestations are a florid color which turns to cyanosis on mild exertion, mental torpor, fatigue, and headache. Those affected are usually in the fourth to sixth decades. Return to sea level promptly relieves the symptoms. *Brisket disease of cattle*, a disorder of calves grazing at high altitudes in Utah and Colorado, which is characterized by pulmonary hypertension and subsequent failure of the right side of the heart, is not a true counterpart of Monge's disease, since it is not associated

FIGURE 28-1

Relationship between mean arterial oxygen saturation (percent) and the mean hemoglobin content (grams per 100 ml) in healthy male residents at various altitudes. (From Hurtado, by permission of Annals of Internal Medicine.)

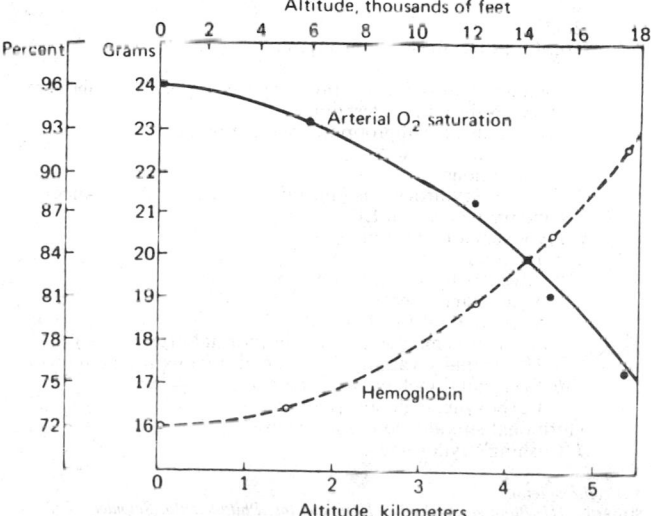

with sustained oxygen unsaturation or polycythemia. Living at high altitudes also evokes a number of compensatory reactions which act to increase oxygen delivery to the tissues. These include hyperventilation, which reduces the oxygen gradient between ambient and alveolar air, an augmentation of pulmonary capillary blood volume, a reduction of diffusing capacity, and an increase in cardiac output.

Any chronic pulmonary disease which alters ventilation-perfusion relationships or seriously impairs gas diffusion may produce chronic hypoxemia and lead to erythrocytosis. *Pulmonary arteriovenous fistulas* or *cavernous hemangioma of the lung* may lead to impaired saturation of arterial blood with oxygen, with the consequent development of erythrocytosis and of a clinical picture resembling closely that of certain types of congenital heart disease. The increased blood viscosity secondary to the polycythemia elevates pulmonary arterial pressure and, combined with the elevation of pulmonary vascular resistance resulting from hypoxia, further elevates right ventricular pressure, contributing to the development or intensification of cor pulmonale (Chap. 246).

The *abnormal ventilatory conditions* present in very obese individuals may cause alveolar hypoventilation and result in arterial unsaturation, erythrocytosis, hypercapnia, and somnolence (the Pickwickian syndrome, Chap. 270). This syndrome is observed less commonly in nonobese persons, in whom decreased sensitivity of the respiratory center to CO_2 may play a role.

The partial shunting of blood from the pulmonary circuit, such as occurs in *congenital heart disease,* causes the most striking erythrocytosis resulting from abnormalities in the heart or lungs. Erythrocyte counts as high as 13 million per mm³, which are possible only when the red corpuscles are smaller than normal, have been observed in such cases, with volumes of packed red blood cells even as high as 86 ml per 100 ml of blood. As the polycythemia develops, there is a progressive rise in blood viscosity, the sharpest increase beginning when the volume of packed red blood cells reaches 65 to 70 percent. The commonest defect producing such polycythemia is pulmonary stenosis associated with a right-to-left shunt that allows venous blood to enter the systemic arterial tree without traversing the lungs. Other conditions include transposition of the great arteries, tricuspid atresia, persistent truncus arteriosus, and other less common anomalies, discussed in Chap. 240.

Reduction in red blood cell volume (phlebotomy with reinfusion of the plasma) is sometimes performed in severely symptomatic patients with extremely high hematocrit levels, but it must be carried out slowly and with great caution. It

results in a reduction of the elevated blood viscosity which decreases the impedance to flow. When pulmonary blood flow is derived largely from the systemic circuit, as in patients with tetralogy of Fallot and severe pulmonary outflow obstruction, this maneuver reduces systemic O_2 saturation. On the other hand, if pulmonary blood flow is independent of the systemic circuit, as in D-transposition of the great arteries, an increase in pulmonary blood flow occurs.

The polycythemia of cyanotic congenital heart disease may lead to spontaneous thrombosis at any site, including the central nervous system. It may also be accompanied by a variety of blood coagulation defects, including reduced fibrinogen and prothrombin concentrations, as well as thrombocytopenia.

The excessive use of coal-tar derivatives and other forms of chronic poisoning, by producing abnormal hemoglobin pigments such as methemoglobin and sulfhemoglobin (Chap. 315), also may cause erythrocytosis. Carriers of certain abnormal hemoglobins which displace the oxygen dissociation curve to the left and interfere with oxygen unloading in the tissues stimulate the production of erythropoietin and a secondary erythrocytosis unassociated with leukocytosis or thrombocytosis (Chap. 315).

Erythrocytosis is found in *Cushing's syndrome* (Chap. 336) and can be produced by the administration of large amounts of adrenocortical steroids. Especially intriguing are the instances of polycythemia observed in association with various *tumors.* These have been chiefly of two varieties, *infratentorial* and *renal.* The tumors in the posterior fossa of the skull have usually been vascular (hemangioblastomas). The renal tumors have included hypernephroma, adenoma, and sarcoma. Other tumors that have been associated with polycythemia include uterine myoma and hepatic carcinoma. Polycythemia also has been reported in association with polycystic disease of the kidneys and hydronephrosis. However, only a small proportion (0.3 to 2.6 percent) of the various renal disorders mentioned above have been associated with polycythemia. Plasma erythropoietin levels have been found to be elevated in a number of these patients. Erythropoiesis-stimulating activity has been demonstrated in tumor extracts and in renal cyst fluid, and polycythemia has disappeared after the associated tumor was removed.

The term *stress erythrocytosis* has been applied to the polycythemia seen occasionally in very active, hard-working persons in a state of anxiety, who appear florid but who have none of the characteristic signs of erythremia—no splenomegaly or leukocytosis with immature cells in the blood. In such persons the total red blood cell mass is normal, and the plasma volume is below normal.

The differential diagnosis of polycythemia is discussed in Chap. 320. However, it should be pointed out that in secondary polycythemia with hypoxia, arterial P_{O_2} is reduced, erythropoietin levels are elevated, while levels of leukocyte alkaline phosphatase and serum vitamin B_{12} are normal. In polycythemia vera, erythropoietin levels are normal or decreased and leukocyte alkaline phosphatase and vitamin B_{12} levels are elevated.

TABLE 28-2
Differential diagnosis of erythrocytosis

I Autonomous erythroid proliferation (↓ EP*); polycythemia vera
II Secondary erythroid proliferation
   A Autonomous or inappropriate increase in EP
      1 Neoplasm
      2 Renal lesions
      3 Familial erythrocytosis (autosomal recessive inheritance)
   B Secondary increase in EP
      1 Hypoxemia (↓ arterial P_{O_2})
         a High altitude
         b Alveolar hypoventilation
         c Pulmonary disease
         d Cardiac right-to-left shunt
      2 Abnormal hemoglobin function (normal arterial P_{O_2})
         a High-affinity variants (autosomal dominant inheritance)
         b Congenital methemoglobinemia
         c Carboxyhemoglobin (smokers)
   C Hormonal stimulus to erythropoeisis
      1 Cushing's syndrome

* *Erythropoietin.*
SOURCE: *HF Bunn et al, Human Hemoglobins, Philadelphia, Saunders, 1977.*

REFERENCES

DENNIS RC et al: Improved myocardial performance following high 2,3-DPG red cell transfusions. Surgery 77:741, 1975

GOLD W: Cyanosis, in *Signs and Symptoms,* 6th ed, RS Blacklow (ed). Philadelphia, Lippincott, 1979

HARKNESS DR: The regulation of hemoglobin oxygenation, in *Advances in Internal Medicine,* GH Stollerman (ed). Chicago, Year Book, 1971, p 189

HURTADO A: Some clinical aspects of life at high altitudes. Ann Intern Med 53:247, 1960

JEPSON JH, FRANKL W: *Haematological Complications in Cardiac Practice.* Philadelphia, Saunders, 1975

ROSENTHAL A, TYLER DC: Effect of red cell volume reduction or pulmonary blood flow in polycythemia of cyanotic congenital heart disease. Am J Cardiol 33:410, 1974

SMITH JR, LANDAW SA: Smokers' polycythemia. N Engl J Med 298:6, 1978

WILLIAMS EJ (ed): Erythrocyte disorders—polycythemia, in *Hematology*, 2d ed. New York, McGraw-Hill, 1977, p 624

29
EDEMA

EUGENE BRAUNWALD

Edema is defined as an increase in the extravascular (interstitial) component of the extracellular fluid volume, which may increase by several liters before the abnormality is recognized. Therefore, a weight gain of several kilograms usually precedes overt manifestations of edema, and a similar weight loss resulting from diuresis can be induced in a slightly edematous patient before "dry weight" is achieved. *Ascites* (Chap. 40) and *hydrothorax* refer to accumulation of excess fluid in the peritoneal and pleural cavities, respectively, and are considered to be special forms of edema. *Anasarca*, or "dropsy," refers to gross, generalized edema. Depending on its etiology and mechanism, edema may be localized or have a generalized distribution; it is recognized in its generalized form by puffiness of the face, which is most readily apparent in the periorbital areas, and by the persistence of an indentation of the skin following pressure; this is known as "pitting" edema. In its more subtle form, it may be detected by the fact that the rim of the bell of the stethoscope leaves an indentation on the skin of the chest that lasts a few minutes. One of the early symptoms a patient may note is the ring on a finger fitting more snugly than in the past, or difficulty in putting on shoes, particularly in the evening.

PATHOGENESIS (A more detailed discussion of the volume and distribution of body fluids is presented in Chap. 84.) About one-third of the total body water is confined to the extracellular space. This compartment, in turn, is composed of the plasma volume and the interstitial space. Under ordinary circumstances the plasma volume represents about 25 percent of the extracellular space, and the remainder is interstitial fluid. The forces that regulate the disposition of fluid between these two components of the extracellular compartment are frequently referred to as the Starling forces (see "Pulmonary Edema" in Chap. 27). In general terms, two forces, the hydrostatic pressure within the vascular system and the colloid oncotic pressure in the interstitial fluid, tend to promote a movement of fluid from the vascular to the extravascular space. In contrast, the colloid oncotic pressure contributed by the plasma proteins, and the hydrostatic pressure within the interstitial fluid, referred to as the *tissue tension,* promote a movement of fluid into the vascular compartment. As a consequence of these forces there is a large movement of water and diffusible solutes from the vascular space at the arteriolar end of the microcirculation and back into the vascular compartment at the venous end. In addition, fluid is returned from the interstitial space into the vascular system by way of the lymphatics, and unless these channels are obstructed, lymph flow tends to increase if there is a tendency toward a net movement of fluid from the vascular compartment to the interstitium. All these forces are usually balanced so that a steady state exists in the size of the intravascular and interstitial compartments, and yet a large exchange between them is permitted. However, should any one of these factors be altered significantly, a net movement of fluid from one component of the extracellular space to the other will occur.

An increase in capillary pressure may readily result from an increase in venous pressure due to local obstruction in venous drainage, to congestive heart failure, or rarely to the simple expansion of the vascular volume by the administration of large volumes of fluid at a rate in excess of the ability of the kidneys to excrete these excesses. The colloid oncotic pressure of the plasma may be reduced, owing to any of the factors that may induce hypoalbuminemia, such as malnutrition, liver disease, and loss of protein into the urine or into the gastrointestinal tract, or to a severe catabolic state.

Edema may also result from damage to the capillary endothelium, which increases the permeability of these vessels, permitting the transfer to the interstitial compartment of a fluid containing more protein than usual. Injury to the capillary walls may be the result of chemical, bacterial, thermal, or mechanical agents. Increased capillary permeability may also be a consequence of a hypersensitivity reaction and is characteristic of immune injury. Damage to the capillary endothelium is presumably responsible for inflammatory edema, which is nonpitting, usually localized, and readily recognized by the presence of other signs of inflammation—redness, heat, and tenderness.

In an attempt to formulate a hypothesis about the pathophysiology involved in edematous states, it is important to discriminate between the *primary* events, such as venous or lymphatic obstruction, reduction of cardiac output, hypoalbuminemia, or trapping of fluid in spaces such as the peritoneal cavity, and the predictable *secondary* consequences, which include the renal retention of salt and water. There are instances in which an abnormal positive balance of salt and water may, in fact, be the primary disturbance. In these circumstances the edema is a secondary manifestation of the generalized increase in extracellular fluid volume. These special instances are usually related to conditions characterized by an acute reduction in renal function, such as acute tubular necrosis or acute glomerulonephritis (Fig. 29-1).

These circumstances aside, a hypothesis can be advanced, which, although admittedly incomplete, leads to improved understanding of the events in a variety of edematous states and enhances the perception of their pathophysiology. The basic premise is that the primary disorder concerns one or more alterations in the Starling forces so that there is a net movement of fluid from the vascular system into the interstitium or into a "third space," or from the arterial compartment of the vascular space into the chambers of the heart or into the venous circulation itself. The *effective arterial blood volume,* an as yet poorly defined parameter of the filling of the arterial tree, is reduced, and a series of physiologic responses which are designed to restore it to normal are set into motion. A key element of these responses is the retention of an increment of salt and water, and in many instances this repairs the deficit of the effective arterial blood volume; often this occurs without the development of overt edema. If, however, the retention of salt and water is insufficient to restore and maintain the effective arterial blood volume, the stimuli are not dissipated, the retention of salt and water continues, and edema develops. The sequence of events described above is operative in a variety of circumstances, including dehydration and hemorrhage. Although there is a reduction of effective arterial blood volume and activation of the entire sequence shown on the right side of Fig. 29-1, including the retention of salt and water, edema does not occur because the total extravascular fluid volume is reduced.

Certain data suggest that the increase in volume of some component(s) of the extracellular space normally promotes the secretion of a natriuretic hormone, also referred to as "third factor." The unambiguous demonstration of such a hormone, its site(s) of secretion, and its characterization is yet to be presented. The retention of sodium is accompanied by an increased reabsorption of water. This is attested to by (1) the usual failure to accumulate edema if sodium is not available in the diet, and (2) the successful use of pharmacologic agents and other measures that promote the excretion of sodium chloride in the urine. In most circumstances the mechanisms responsible for maintaining a normal effective osmolality in the body fluids continue to operate efficiently so that sodium retention promotes thirst and secretion of the antidiuretic hormone, which, in turn, lead to the ingestion and retention of approximately 1 liter of water for each 140 mmol sodium retained. Similarly, measures which promote the loss of sodium into the urine are accompanied by the net loss of an equivalent volume of water from the body.

Obstruction of venous and lymphatic drainage of a limb   In this condition the hydrostatic pressure in the capillary bed increases so that more fluid is transferred from the vascular to the interstitial space than can be reabsorbed at the venous end of the capillaries; since the alternate route (i.e., the lymphatic channels) is obstructed as well, this event must of necessity cause an increased volume of interstitial fluid in the limb, i.e.,

FIGURE 29-1
Sequence of events leading to the formation and retention of salt and water and the development of edema.

a trapping of fluid in the extremity, at the expense of the blood volume in the remainder of the body, thereby reducing effective arterial blood volume and leading to the consequences shown in Fig. 29-1.

As fluid accumulates in the interstitium of the limb, in which venous and lymphatic drainage are obstructed, tissue tension rises until it is great enough to counterbalance the primary alterations in the Starling forces, at which time no further fluid will accumulate in that limb. At this point the additional accumulation of fluid will repair the deficit in plasma volume, and the stimuli to retain more salt and water are dissipated. The net effect is an increase in the volume of interstitial fluid in a local area, and the secondary responses repair the plasma volume deficit incurred by the primary event. This same sequence may be translated to many other edematous states.

Congestive heart failure (see also Chap. 236)   In this disorder it is postulated that the defective systolic emptying of the chambers of the heart promotes an accumulation of blood in the heart and venous circulation at the expense of the arterial volume, and the aforementioned sequence of events (Fig. 29-1) is initiated. In many instances of mild heart failure a small increment of volume may be achieved, which repairs the volume deficit and establishes a new steady state because through the operation of Starling's law of the heart, up to a point an increase in the volume of blood within the chambers of the heart promotes a more forceful contraction and may thereby increase the volume ejected in systole (Fig. 235-4). However, if the cardiac disorder is more severe, retention of fluid cannot repair the deficit in effective arterial blood volume. The increment accumulates in the venous circulation, and the increase in hydrostatic pressure therein promotes the formation of ede-

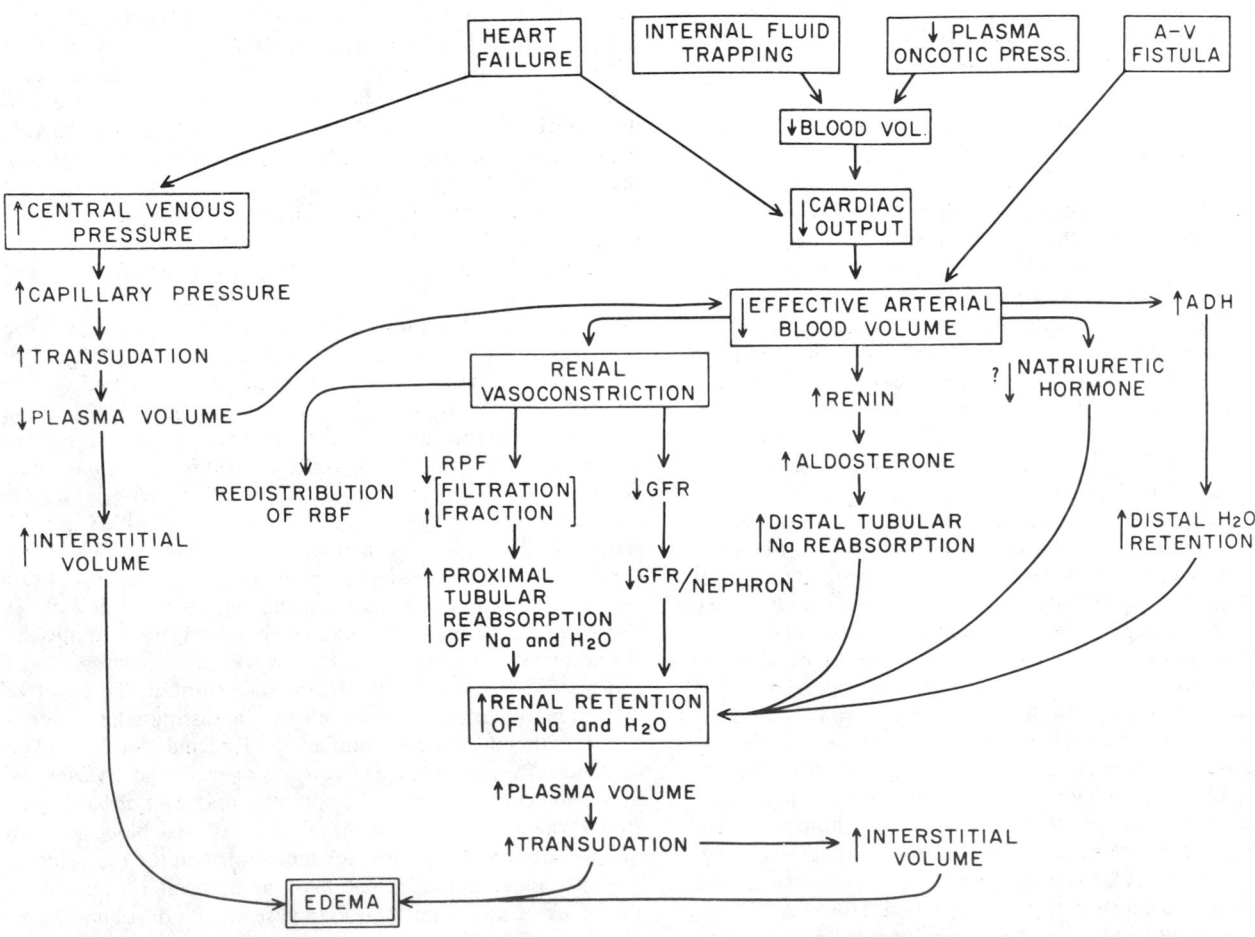

ma. The formation of edema in the lungs (Chap. 27) impairs gas exchange and may induce hypoxia, which embarrasses cardiac function still further.

In addition to the sequence shown on the right-hand side of Fig. 29-1, incomplete ventricular emptying leads to an elevation of ventricular end-diastolic pressure. If the impairment of cardiac function involves the right ventricle primarily, then incomplete ventricular emptying leads to an elevation of right ventricular end-diastolic volume and pressure; as a consequence pressures in the systemic veins and capillaries also rise, thereby augmenting transudation of fluid into the interstitial space and enhancing the likelihood of peripheral edema. If the impairment of cardiac function involves the left ventricle, then pulmonary venous and capillary pressures rise [leading in some instances to pulmonary edema (Chap. 27)], as does pulmonary artery pressure; this in turn interferes with the systolic emptying of the right ventricle, leading to an elevation of right ventricular end-diastolic and central and systemic venous pressures, enhancing the likelihood of edema formation.

A reduction of cardiac output is associated with a reduction of the effective arterial blood volume as well as of renal blood flow and an elevation of the filtration fraction, i.e., the ratio of glomerular filtration rate to renal plasma flow. In severe heart failure the blood flow to the outer renal cortex, in particular, is significantly reduced with less depression in the more central regions of the kidney, and there is a reduction in the glomerular filtration rate. This constriction of renal cortical vessels appears to play an important role in the retention of salt and water and the formation of edema in heart failure. Indirect evidence suggests that at different stages of heart failure, activation of the sympathetic nervous system and of the renin-angiotensin systems is responsible for renal vasoconstriction. Activation of the former can be counteracted by the administration of alpha-adrenergic blocking agents, a finding which indicates that the elevated renal vascular resistance in heart failure is mediated, at least in part, by sympathetic stimuli.

It is generally agreed that an increase in the tubular reabsorption of glomerular filtrate plays a principal role in the salt and water retention of heart failure. However, the precise site(s) in the system composed of the renal tubules, loops of Henle, and collective ducts which is involved is not clear, nor have the responsible mechanism(s) been identified. Alterations in intrarenal hemodynamics appear to play a significant role. Heart failure, by augmenting renal arteriolar constriction, reduces the hydrostatic pressure and raises the colloid osmotic pressure in the peritubular capillaries, thus enhancing salt and water reabsorption in the proximal tubule. The aforementioned distribution of intrarenal blood flow characteristic of heart failure may be responsible for augmentation of sodium reabsorption in the ascending limb of the loop of Henle.

In addition, the diminished renal blood flow characteristic of all states in which the effective arterial blood volume is reduced is translated by the renal juxtaglomerular cells into a signal for increased renin release (Chap. 336). The specific nature of the signal is complex. One factor involves a baroreceptor mechanism, in which reduced renal perfusion results in incomplete filling of the renal arterioles and diminished stretch of the juxtaglomerular cells, a signal that provides for the elaboration or release, or both, of renin. A second mechanism involves the macula densa; as a result of reduced glomerular filtration the sodium load reaching the distal renal tubules is reduced. This is sensed by the macula densa, which in an as yet undefined manner signals the neighboring juxtaglomerular cells to secrete renin. A third mechanism involves the sympathetic nervous system and circulating catecholamines. Activation of the beta-adrenergic receptors in the juxtaglomerular

cells stimulates them to release renin. These three mechanisms generally act in concert.

Renin, an enzyme that has a molecular weight of about 40,000, acts on its substrate, angiotensinogen, an α_2 globulin synthesized by the liver, resulting in the elaboration of angiotensin II, an octapeptide with vasoconstrictor properties. The intrarenal production of angiotensin II may also contribute to renal vasoconstriction in heart failure and to the salt and water retention in this state. Angiotensin II also passes through the circulation and stimulates the production of aldosterone by the zona glomerulosa region of the adrenal cortex. In patients with heart failure, not only is aldosterone secretion elevated, but the biologic half-life of aldosterone is prolonged, indicating a reduced catabolic rate and further increasing the plasma level of the hormone. A depression of hepatic blood flow, particularly during exercise, secondary to a reduction in cardiac output, is responsible for the reduced hepatic catabolism of aldosterone.

Although increased quantities of aldosterone have been demonstrated to be secreted during heart failure and other edematous states, augmented levels of aldosterone (or other mineralocorticoids) do not always promote the accumulation of edema, as witnessed by the lack of striking fluid retention in most instances of primary aldosteronism. Furthermore, although normal subjects will retain some salt and water under the influence of a potent mineralocorticoid, such as deoxycorticosterone acetate or 9α-fluorohydrocortisone, the accumulation appears to be self-limiting, despite continued exposure to the steroid and to salt and water. It is probable that the failure of normal subjects to accumulate large quantities of fluid is a consequence of an increase in glomerular filtration rate, other hemodynamic influences, and most importantly the increase in volume which promotes an increased excretion of salt independent of the filtered load of sodium, i.e., through the action of natriuretic substance(s). The role of aldosterone in the accumulation of fluid in edematous states may be more important because these patients are unable to repair the crucial deficit in volume.

Nephrotic syndrome and other hypoalbuminic states (see also Chap. 278) The primary alteration in this disorder is a diminished colloid oncotic pressure due to massive losses of protein into the urine. This should promote a net movement of fluid into the interstitium and hypovolemia, and initiate the sequence of events described above. As long as the hypoalbuminemia is severe, the salt and water retained cannot be restrained within the vascular compartment, and hence the stimuli to retain salt and water are not abated. A similar sequence of events occurs in other conditions which lead to severe hypoalbuminemia, including severe nutritional deficiency states, protein-losing enteropathy, congenital hypoalbuminemia, and severe, chronic liver disease.

Cirrhosis (see also Chaps. 40 and 304) The total blood volume in cirrhosis of the liver is commonly increased when the disorder is accompanied by a system of dilated venous radicles and multiple small arteriovenous fistulas. Effective systemic perfusion and the effective arterial blood volume appear to be diminished, probably as a consequence of the passage of blood through these fistulas. The enlarged abdominal venous system resulting from obstruction of the lymphatic drainage of the liver, as well as from portal vein obstruction, also promotes a deficit in the arterial component. These alterations are frequently complicated by the reduced serum albumin characteristic of cirrhosis, which tends to reduce the effective arterial blood volume even further. Initially, the excess interstitial fluid is localized preferentially behind the congested portal venous system and obstructed hepatic lymphatics, i.e., in the peritoneal cavity. In late stages of the disease, particularly when there is hypoalbuminemia, peripheral edema may also be noted.

Idiopathic cyclic edema This syndrome, which occurs predominantly in women, particularly those with psychosocial difficulties, is characterized by periodic episodes of edema, frequently accompanied by abdominal distention. Fairly large, diurnal alterations in weight occur, so that the patient may well weigh several pounds more in the evening than in the morning after having been in the upright posture most of the day. Such large diurnal weight changes suggest an increase in capillary permeability which appears to fluctuate in severity. The fact that it occurs most commonly in women and appears to have some temporal relation to the menstrual cycle suggests that there may be some hormonal influence in the permeability of the vessels which permits the loss of plasma volume into the interstitial space and the sequence of events secondary to a contraction in plasma volume.

The treatment of idiopathic cyclic edema includes a reduction in salt intake, education in the use of rest in the supine position for several hours each day, the wearing of elastic stockings which are put on before arising in the morning, and an attempt to understand the underlying emotional problems. Diuretics are initially effective but may lose their effectiveness with continuous administration; accordingly, they should be employed sparingly. It has been reported that the plasma concentration of cyclic adenosine monophosphate (AMP) is high in patients with idiopathic edema in both the recumbent and upright positions, and its renal clearance, unlike that of creatinine, is low. If a relationship between extracellular cyclic AMP and the action of hormones on beta-adrenergic receptors could be established, the favorable therapeutic effect of propranolol in cases where diuretics alone did not satisfactorily control the disease could be explained.

DIFFERENTIAL DIAGNOSIS As a rule, localized edema can be readily differentiated from generalized edema. The great majority of patients with noninflammatory generalized edema of significant degree suffer from advanced cardiac, renal, hepatic, or nutritional disorders. Consequently, the differential diagnosis of generalized edema should be directed toward implicating or excluding these several conditions.

Localized edema Edema originating from inflammation or hypersensitivity is usually readily identified. Localized edema due to venous or lymphatic obstruction may be caused by thrombophlebitis, chronic lymphangitis, resection of regional lymph nodes, filariasis, etc. Lymph edema is particularly intractable because restriction of lymphatic flow results in increased protein concentration in the interstitial fluid, a circumstance which severely impedes removal of retained fluid.

Edema of heart failure Evidence of heart disease, as manifested by cardiac enlargement and gallop rhythm together with evidence of cardiac failure, such as dyspnea, basilar rales, diminished vital capacity, prolonged circulation time, venous distention, increased venous pressure, and hepatomegaly, usually provides an indication of the pathogenesis of edema resulting from heart failure (see also Chap. 236).

Edema of the nephrotic syndrome Massive proteinuria, severe hypoproteinemia, and in some instances hypercholesterolemia are present. This syndrome may occur during the course of a variety of kidney diseases, which include glomerulonephritis,

diabetic glomerulosclerosis, and hypersensitivity reactions. A history of previous renal disease may or may not be elicited (see also Chap. 278).

Edema of acute glomerulonephritis The edema occurring during the acute phases of glomerulonephritis is characteristically associated with hematuria, proteinuria, and hypertension. Although some evidence supports the view that the fluid retention is due to increased capillary permeability, in most instances the edema in this disease results from primary retention of sodium and water by the kidneys owing to renal insufficiency. This state differs from congestive heart failure in that it is characterized by a normal or increased cardiac output, normal or diminished circulation time, a reduction in the packed cell volume, a normal arteriovenous oxygen difference, and failure to respond to a digitalis preparation. Patients commonly have evidence of pulmonary congestion on chest roentgenograms before cardiac enlargement is significant and do not develop orthopnea. If one cannot discriminate between the congested state and congestive heart failure, use of a cardiac glycoside is appropriate, but special care should be taken to avoid digitalis intoxication in a patient with impaired renal function (see also Chap. 278).

Edema of cirrhosis Ascites and evidence of hepatic disease (collateral venous channels, jaundice, and spider angiomas) characterize edema of hepatic origin. The ascites is frequently refractory to treatment because it collects as a result of a combination of obstruction of hepatic lymphatic drainage, portal hypertension and hypoalbuminemia. Edema may also occur in other parts of the body in these patients as a result of hypoalbuminemia. Furthermore, the sizable accumulation of ascitic fluid may be expected to increase intraabdominal pressure and impede venous return from the lower extremities; hence, it tends to promote accumulation of edema in this region as well (see also Chap. 304).

Edema of nutritional origin An inadequate diet over a prolonged period may produce hypoproteinemia and edema, which may be intensified by beriberi heart disease, in which multiple peripheral arteriovenous fistulas result in reduced effective systemic perfusion and effective arterial blood volume, thereby enhancing edema formation. More striking edema is commonly observed when these famished subjects are provided with an adequate diet. The mechanism responsible for this latter phenomenon is not clear, but the ingestion of more food may increase the quantity of salt ingested, which is then retained along with water. Edema of nutritional origin may be more apparent than under other circumstances, because the subcutaneous tissue is so depleted of fat that modest collections of edema may be more obvious than they would be in a well-nourished subject.

Distribution The distribution of edema is an important guide to the cause. Thus, edema of one leg or of one or both arms is usually the result of venous and/or lymphatic obstruction. Edema resulting from hypoproteinemia characteristically is generalized, but it is especially evident in the eyelids and face and tends to be most pronounced in the morning because of the recumbent posture assumed during the night. Edema associated with heart failure, on the other hand, tends to be more extensive in the legs and to be accentuated in the evening, a feature also determined largely by posture. In the rare types of cardiac disease, such as tricuspid stenosis and constrictive pericarditis, in which orthopnea may be absent and the patient actually prefers the recumbent posture, the factor of gravity may be equalized and facial edema observed. Less common causes of facial edema include trichinosis, allergic reactions, and myxedema. Unilateral edema occasionally results from lesions in the central nervous system affecting the vasomotor fibers on one side of the body; paralysis also reduces lymphatic and venous drainage on the affected side.

Additional factors in diagnosis The color, thickness, and sensitivity of the skin are significant. Local tenderness and increase in temperature suggest inflammation. Local cyanosis may signify a venous obstruction. In individuals who have had repeated episodes of prolonged edema, the skin over the involved areas may be thickened, hard, and often red.

Measurement of the venous pressure is also of great importance in evaluating edema. Elevation in an isolated part of the body usually reflects localized venous obstruction. Generalized elevation of systemic venous pressure suggests the presence of congestive heart failure, although it may be present in the congested state that accompanies acute renal insufficiency. Ordinarily, significant increase in venous pressure can be recognized by the level at which cervical veins collapse; in doubtful cases and for accurate recording, the central venous pressure should be measured. In patients with obstruction of the superior vena cava, edema is confined to the face, neck, and upper extremities, where the venous pressure is elevated compared with that in the lower extremities. Measurement of venous pressure in the upper extremities is also useful in patients with massive edema of the lower extremities and ascites; it is elevated when the edema is on a cardiac basis (e.g., constrictive pericarditis or tricuspid stenosis), but is normal when it is secondary to cirrhosis.

Determination of the concentration of serum proteins, and especially of serum albumin, clearly differentiates those patients in whom edema is due entirely or in part to diminished intravascular colloid osmotic pressure. The presence of proteinuria affords useful clues. The complete absence of protein in the urine is evidence against, but does not exclude, either cardiac or renal disease as a cause of edema. Slight to moderate proteinuria is the rule in patients with heart failure, whereas persistent massive proteinuria usually reflects the presence of the nephrotic syndrome. Valuable information can also be obtained from other features of the examination. Some of these are the presence or absence of heart disease, the character of the urinary sediment, the dietary history, and a history of alcoholism.

APPROACH TO THE PATIENT WITH EDEMA A significant question to ask is whether the edema is localized or generalized. If it is localized, those phenomena alluded to above that may be responsible should be concentrated upon. In this context, localized edema may include hydrothorax, ascites, or both, in the absence of congestive heart failure or hypoalbuminemia. Either of these collections may be a consequence of local venous or lymphatic obstruction, as in inflammatory disease or carcinoma. It is a frequent accompaniment of an inflammatory process which involves the pleura or peritoneum, and the cause of the inflammatory process may vary from bacterial invasion to infarction or underlying parenchyma to a diffuse connective tissue disease with vasculitis, etc. In instances of either hydrothorax or ascites, an examination of the characteristics of the fluid is extremely important. This should include bacterial culture, smear with stains for ordinary and less common infectious agents, determination of protein concentration, cell count, and the presence or absence of blood; the cells should be concentrated by centrifugation and preparation for histologic examination for evidences of malignancy and other characteristics.

If the edema is generalized, it should be determined, first, if there is hypoalbuminemia of significant degree, e.g., serum albumin concentration less than 2.5 g per 100 ml. If there is, a history, physical examination, and other laboratory data will help evaluate the question of cirrhosis, severe malnutrition,

protein-losing gastroenteropathy, or the nephrotic syndrome as the underlying disorder. It should then be determined if there is evidence of congestive heart failure of a severity to promote generalized edema even in the absence of hypoalbuminemia, or if there is evidence of both congestive heart failure and some degree of hypoalbuminemia. Finally, it should be ascertained whether the patient has an adequate urine output, or is there significant oliguria or even anuria? These abnormalities are discussed in Chaps. 43, 275, and 276. The major differential diagnosis in these instances is frequently the discrimination between overload with fluid and a congested state as opposed to congestive heart failure.

REFERENCES

BRAUNWALD E et al: *Mechanisms of Contraction of the Normal and Failing Heart,* 2d ed. Boston, Little, Brown, 1976

BRENNER BM, STEIN JH (eds): *Sodium and Water Homeostasis.* New York, Churchill Livingstone, 1978

COGGINS CP: Edema, in *Signs and Symptoms,* 6th ed, RS Blacklow (ed). Philadelphia, Lippincott, 1977, chap. 36

DE WARDENER HE: The control of sodium excretion, in *Handbook of Physiology,* vol 8: *Renal Physiology,* J Orloff et al (eds). Washington, The American Physiological Society, 1973, chap 21, p 677

EARLEY LE, SCHRIER RW: Intrarenal control of sodium excretion by hemodynamic and physical factors, in *Handbook of Physiology,* vol 8: *Renal Physiology,* J Orloff et al (eds). Washington, The American Physiological Society, 1973, chap 22, p 721

GUYTON AC: Edema, in *Textbook of Medical Physiology,* 5th ed. Philadelphia, Saunders, 1976, p 403

LARAGH JH, SEALEY JE: The renin-angiotensin-aldosterone hormonal system and regulation of sodium, potassium and blood pressure homeostasis, in *Handbook of Physiology,* vol 8: *Renal Physiology,* J Orloff et al (eds). Washington, The American Physiological Society, 1973, chap 26, p 831

LEVY M, SEELY J: Pathophysiology of edema formation, in *The Kidney,* 2d ed, BM Brenner, FC Rector Jr (eds). Philadelphia, Saunders, 1980, chap 15

30

HYPOTENSION AND THE SHOCK SYNDROME

KARL ENGELMAN
EUGENE BRAUNWALD

The differential diagnosis of hypotensive states and the development of a rational plan of therapy require understanding of the normal regulation of arterial pressure.

CONTROL OF ARTERIAL PRESSURE Arterial pressure must be maintained at levels sufficient to permit adequate perfusion of the extensive capillary networks in the systemic vascular bed. The level of pressure in the central arterial bed is in a large measure dependent on two factors—the volume of blood ejected by the left ventricle per unit of time, i.e., the cardiac output, and the resistance to blood flow offered by the vessels in the peripheral vascular bed. The resistance of a blood vessel, in turn, varies inversely as the fourth power of its radius, and at any given level of cardiac output arterial pressure is therefore largely dependent upon the degree of constriction of the smooth muscle in the walls of the arterioles. Though resistance to flow also varies with the viscosity of the fluid and the length of the vessels, alterations in these factors are ordinarily of only secondary importance.

Cardiac output is controlled largely by factors which regulate ventricular end-diastolic volume, the level of myocardial contractility, and heart rate (Chap. 235). The autonomic nervous system plays a major role in the maintenance of arterial pressure by its influences on the cardiac output and on the degree of constriction of the resistance (arterioles) and capacitance (venules and veins) vessels. The afferent limbs of the autonomic reflex arcs regulating arterial pressure acutely arise in stretch receptors in the carotid sinuses, the aortic arch, the chambers of the heart, and the lungs. Impulses are transmitted along afferent fibers in the glossopharyngeal and vagus nerves to extensive central autonomic connections in the medulla. Synapses connect not only the sympathetic and parasympathetic nuclei and efferent arcs, but also the cerebral cortex and hypothalamic nuclei which control hormonal secretion via the pituitary gland.

A rapid reduction of arterial pressure diminishes the stimulation of pressoreceptors, which in turn activates sympathetic outflow and inhibits parasympathetic activity. As a result, the vascular smooth muscle in arterioles and veins constricts, while heart rate and myocardial contractility are augmented. In addition, as arterial pressure falls, adrenal medullary secretion increases, along with the output of antidiuretic hormone (ADH), adrenocorticotropic hormone (ACTH), renin, and aldosterone; all these effects act to restore the arterial pressure to control levels. Opposite changes occur if arterial pressure is raised acutely. Thus, the operation of the pressoreceptor and a number of humoral systems normally serve to buffer the body from a variety of influences which would otherwise produce marked alterations in arterial pressure.

MEASUREMENT OF ARTERIAL PRESSURE Arterial pressure is determined clinically with a pneumatic cuff; ordinarily, this indirect method provides slight underestimation of the true arterial pressure. Considerable error may be introduced if proper precautions are not taken in determining blood pressure by this method. The arterial pressure may be significantly underestimated if the air in the cuff is released too rapidly, especially in the presence of bradycardia or an irregular rhythm, or if inadequate inflation of the cuff does not result in complete vascular occlusion. This indirect method is most accurate when, in normal-sized adults, cuffs 12 to 14 cm in width are employed. However, when a cuff of this size is used on children or adults with unusually thin arms, blood pressure may be seriously underestimated, or conversely, it may be overestimated when employed on an arm or thigh greater than 20 cm in girth. Marked vasoconstriction resulting in severely attenuated limb blood flow and/or marked reductions in pulse pressure may also result in serious underestimation of arterial pressure by the auscultatory method. Direct intraarterial recordings may reveal a normal or even an elevated pressure, while the absence of Korotkov sounds makes the pressure unobtainable by the indirect methods.

THE "NORMAL" BLOOD PRESSURE The "normal" blood pressure is difficult to define. Traditional statistical approaches define normality on the basis of values included within two standard deviations of the mean of pressures obtained in a large population of presumably healthy individuals. On this basis 95 percent of the population are defined as being normotensive, the remaining 5 percent evenly divided between the hypertensive and hypotensive groups. A better definition of abnormality would be based on demonstrated deleterious effects of blood pressure levels exceeding certain limits. If such criteria are used, chronic hypotension would seem to occur very rarely. However, the incidence of hypertension based on casual blood pressure levels exceeding 160/95 (widely accepted as hazardous) is estimated to be approximately 15 percent in the adult population of the United States, the incidence in the black population exceeding that in the nonblacks by 50 to 100 percent. Even these statistics may understate the prevalence of hypertension if one accepts the validity of actuarial data indicating that longevity is shortened progressively in adults whose blood pressures exceed 100/60. The hazard of hypertension and its major complication, widespread vascular disease, appears to be a function of the level of blood pressure; the hazard rises more steeply with higher levels, especially as they exceed diastolic values of 90 to 95 mmHg (Chap. 251).

ACUTE HYPOTENSION AND SHOCK

Not uncommonly, physicians are called upon to treat patients who acutely develop severe hypotension or shock. These two terms are not synonymous; although shock is usually associated with hypotension, a previously hypertensive patient may be in shock despite an arterial pressure within normal limits, and hypotension may occur in the absence of shock. Shock may be defined as a state in which there is widespread, serious reduction of tissue perfusion, which, if prolonged, leads to generalized impairment of cellular function.

CAUSES The most common clinical causes of shock are listed in Table 30-1. Since arterial pressure is dependent on

TABLE 30-1
Etiologic factors in shock

I Hypovolemia
  A External fluid losses
    1 Hemorrhage
    2 Gastrointestinal
      a Vomiting (pyloric stenosis, intestinal obstruction)
      b Diarrhea
    3 Renal
      a Diabetes mellitus
      b Diabetes insipidus
      c Excessive use of diuretics
    4 Cutaneous
      a Burns
      b Exudative lesions
      c Perspiration and insensible water loss without replacement
  B Internal sequestration
    1 Fractures
    2 Ascites (peritonitis, pancreatitis, cirrhosis)
    3 Intestinal obstruction
    4 Hemothorax
    5 Hemoperitoneum
II Cardiogenic
  A Myocardial infarction
  B Arrhythmia (paroxysmal tachycardia or fibrillation, severe bradycardia)
  C Severe congestive heart failure with low cardiac output
III Obstruction to blood flow
  A Pulmonary embolus
  B Tension pneumothorax
  C Cardiac tamponade
  D Dissecting aortic aneurysm
  E Intracardiac (ball valve thrombus, atrial myxoma)
IV Neuropathic
  A Drug induced
    1 Anesthesia
    2 Ganglion-blocking or other antihypertensive drugs
    3 "Ingestion" (barbiturates, glutethimide, phenothiazines)
  B Spinal cord injury
  C Orthostatic hypotension (primary autonomic insufficiency, peripheral neuropathies)
V Other
  A Infection
    1 Gram-negative septicemia (endotoxin)
    2 Other septicemias
  B Anaphylaxis
  C Endocrine failure (Addison's disease, myxedema)
  D Anoxia

cardiac output and peripheral vasomotor tone, marked reductions in either of these variables without a compensatory elevation of the other results in systemic hypotension. Reduction of cardiac output due to hypovolemia or acute myocardial infarction is among the most frequently encountered and easily categorized causes of shock. Failure of neurogenic mechanisms resulting in decreased vasoconstrictor impulses is another well-defined category; in many patients, particularly in the late stages of shock, multiple factors figure in the development of circulatory failure.

Hypovolemia has been studied much more extensively than any other cause of shock; the mechanism of development is usually readily evident and well understood, and therapy, i.e., restoration of blood volume, is both simple and effective if applied before irreversible tissue damage occurs. Whether the primary insult is the external loss of blood, plasma, or water and salt or the internal sequestration of these fluids in a hollow viscus or body cavity, the general effect is similar, i.e., reduced venous return and decreased cardiac output. For purposes of a general discussion of shock, hemorrhagic hypovolemia will be used as the model, but the consequences of general reduced tissue perfusion are similar in other forms of shock.

Stages of hypovolemic shock Depending upon the severity and rate of development of hypovolemia, the shock syndrome may develop abruptly or evolve gradually. If the precipitating factors progress unabated, the endogenous defense mechanisms, while initially competent to maintain adequate circulation, eventually are extended beyond their capacity for compensation. The development of the shock syndrome may be thought to evolve through several stages which merge with one another:

1 The period in which the blood volume deficit is relatively minor and in which the patient may be asymptomatic. In a previously healthy individual compensation for an acute blood loss of as much as 10 percent of the normal blood volume (as with venesection of 500 ml blood from a donor) is achieved acutely by constriction of the arteriolar bed and an augmentation of heart rate, effects mediated by reflex increases in sympathetic neural discharge of norepinephrine from sympathetic nerve endings and of both norepinephrine and epinephrine from the adrenal medulla. Other responses with more gradual effects include the increased secretion of antidiuretic hormone and the activation of the renin-angiotensin-aldosterone axis (Chap. 336). Arterial pressure is maintained and cardiac output is normal, or only slightly reduced, primarily as a consequence of selective reductions of blood flow to the skin and muscle beds.

2 With a reduction of blood volume of 15 to 25 percent, cardiac output falls markedly, and despite intense arteriolar constriction in most vascular beds, arterial pressure declines, although proportionately less than cardiac output. Generalized venoconstriction occurs, increasing the fraction of the total blood volume in the central circulation and tending to sustain venous return. Accompanying this massive reflex adrenergic discharge are tachycardia, tachypnea, intense cutaneous vasoconstriction, pallor, diaphoresis, piloerection, oliguria, apprehension, and restlessness. The latter mental signs relate to primary reduction in cerebral circulation due to decreased perfusion pressure rather than to local vasoconstriction. Angina may occur in patients who have intrinsic coronary vascular disease.

3 Once the patient has achieved this state of maximal mobilization of compensatory mechanisms, small additional losses of blood result in rapid deterioration of the circulation, with life-threatening reductions of cardiac output, blood pressure, and tissue perfusion. The duration of this shock state, the severity of tissue anoxia, and the age and underlying phys-

ical state of the patient are of primary importance in determining the ultimate outcome. If tissue perfusion is restored rapidly, recovery may be expected. However, if shock persists, the severe vasoconstriction may itself become a complicating factor, and by reducing tissue perfusion even further may initiate a vicious cycle leading to an irreversible state due to widespread cellular injury. Blood flow to the brain, heart, and kidneys is further reduced, and severe ischemia of these vital organs leads to irreversible tissue damage which may result in impaired function of the organ and, eventually, death. Impaired coronary perfusion depresses cardiac function, particularly in patients with some coronary vascular obstruction, and this may lead to further lowering of cardiac output, thus perpetuating a vicious cycle. Cardiac function is also depressed by the release of myocardial *depressant factor(s)* from other hypoperfused organs. Reduced flow to the medullary vasomotor center late in the stage of shock depresses the activity of compensatory reflexes. Anoxia, hypercapnia, and lactic acidosis result from hypoperfusion of tissues and anaerobic metabolism. These metabolic derangements ultimately result in failure of the energy-requiring active transport systems of cell membranes. The cellular high-energy phosphate reserves are depleted. The integrity of the cells is compromised, and potassium ions, intracellular lysosomal enzymes, peptides, and other vasoactive compounds are released into the circulation. The integrity of capillary membranes is disrupted, and fluid, proteins, and cellular constituents of the blood seep into the extravascular space of tissues.

In profound shock from any cause an additional important factor which may exacerbate the status of microcirculation is widespread disseminated intravascular coagulation (DIC) in the bowel, kidney, and other organs. The resultant ischemia produced in the bowel may further complicate the circulatory compensation as a result of breakdown of the mucosal barrier, leading to entry of bacteria and toxic bacterial products into the circulation. Similar changes in the capillary network of the lungs result in interstitial and alveolar edema and impaired respiratory gas transfer. Because many bacterial substances are potent vasodilators, vasoconstrictor mechanisms may be inhibited, with a further decrease in blood pressure despite intense sympathetic activity.

Just as tissue perfusion may fall to dangerous or even fatal levels because of actual fluid losses or sequestration with diminished venous return, cardiac failure or intrathoracic obstruction to blood flow may have a similar effect. Furthermore, even in the presence of a normal blood volume and cardiac function, "vasomotor collapse" due to drug-induced or neuropathic failure of sympathetic vasomotor activity can result in shock because of reduction of peripheral resistance and the pooling of blood in the venous bed.

Other forms of shock A complex form of shock may result from infection, especially gram-negative bacteremia with endotoxin release. This form of shock is associated with vascular pooling, diminished venous return, and reduced cardiac output. Sometimes there is inadequate vasoconstriction with a decline in perfusion pressures. At other stages there is intense vasoconstriction with tissue damage secondary to reduced perfusion. In anaphylactic shock, release of histamine or a histaminelike substance causes venous dilatation and an attendant increase in vascular capacity and reduction in cardiac output. Also, it results in arteriolar dilatation and a reduction of perfusion pressure, as well as increased capillary permeability with loss of intravascular volume.

TREATMENT This should be directed toward the rapid restoration of cardiac output and tissue perfusion. General supportive measures must be undertaken immediately, sometimes even before the cause of the shock state has been identified. Whether shock results from decreased cardiac output due to a primary reduction in intravascular volume or from a reduction of "effective blood volume" with pooling of blood in certain vascular beds, the most effective means of restoring adequate circulation is by the rapid infusion of volume-expanding fluids (whole blood, plasma, plasma substitutes, or isotonic electrolyte solutions). However, when shock is secondary to, or is accompanied by, cardiac failure with increased pulmonary vascular and central venous pressures, the infusion of volume-expanding fluids may result in pulmonary edema. Here attention must be directed toward restoring cardiac function with cardiotonic drugs such as digitalis glycosides and isoproterenol, and an attempt should be made to support arterial pressure at levels sufficient to maintain the coronary perfusion pressure (Chap. 245). Arrhythmias, which may also contribute to the low cardiac output, should be corrected (Chap. 237).

The appearance of the external jugular veins may be helpful in differentiating between shock with high or low central venous pressure. However, catheters inserted into the superior vena cava and, if possible, into the pulmonary artery (a Swan-Ganz balloon-tipped catheter) are the best means for continuously monitoring venous pressure and of considerable value in guiding therapy; such catheters should be inserted in patients with shock whenever possible. Serial measurements of central venous pressure, urine flow rate, heart rate, and the clinical and mental state of the patient often provide more important indexes of the efficacy of therapy than arterial pressure changes do. In patients with shock and impaired left ventricular function, e.g., cardiogenic shock due to massive acute myocardial infarction, the balloon-tipped catheter "floated" into the pulmonary artery at the bedside without the aid of fluoroscopy is essential in guiding treatment (Chap. 245).

There is considerable debate concerning the efficacy of vasoconstrictor drugs in shock. In patients with severe peripheral constriction these agents are often ineffective and may actually reduce the already lowered tissue perfusion. However, these drugs are usually helpful in patients with inadequate vasoconstrictor responses. The use of alpha-adrenergic blocking agents or massive doses of adrenal glucocorticoids in shock secondary to gram-negative septicemia with endotoxin release is also a matter of considerable controversy and cannot yet be considered a routine procedure. Following immediate attention to improvement of perfusion, attention should be directed to treating the underlying etiologic factor, such as diabetic acidosis, pneumothorax, or septicemia (Table 30-1).

CHRONIC HYPOTENSION

Although many patients have been treated for chronic "low blood pressure," most of them, with systolic pressures in the range of 90 to 110 mmHg, are normal and may actually have a greater life expectancy than those with higher pressures. Patients with true chronic hypotension may complain of lethargy, weakness, easy fatigability, and dizziness or faintness, especially if arterial pressure is lowered further when the erect position is assumed. These symptoms are presumably due to a decrease in perfusion of the brain, heart, skeletal muscle, and other organs.

Chronic hypotension occasionally results from severe reductions of the cardiac output. The major endocrine causes of chronic hypotension are associated with deficient gluco- and mineralocorticoid secretion and resultant reductions of the intravascular and interstitial fluid volume. Hypotension is usually more pronounced in patients with primary adrenocortical insufficiency than in those with hypopituitarism because secretion of the salt-retaining adrenocortical hormone, aldosterone, is partially preserved in pituitary insufficiency (Chap. 336).

Malnutrition, cachexia, chronic bed rest, and a variety of neurologic disorders may result in chronic hypotension, especially in the standing position. Interference with the neural pathways anywhere between the vasomotor center and the efferent sympathetic nerve endings on the blood vessels or heart may prevent the vasoconstriction and increase in cardiac output which occur as a normal response to a reduction in arterial pressure. Multiple sclerosis, amyotrophic lateral sclerosis, syringomyelia, syphilitic or diabetic tabes dorsalis, peripheral neuropathies, spinal cord section, diabetic neuropathy, extensive lumbodorsal sympathectomy, and the administration of drugs interfering with nerve transmission in the sympathetic nervous system are all associated with orthostatic hypotension. In addition, *idiopathic orthostatic hypotension* (primary autonomic insufficiency), a rare condition in which there is degeneration of central and/or peripheral autonomic nervous structures, may result in such severe orthostatic hypotension that syncope or seizures occur when the patient arises from recumbency. This condition is progressive and characterized by ascending anhydrosis and loss of hair, decreased basal metabolic rate (BMR), reduced norepinephrine production, deficient secretion of lacrimal and salivary glands, ileus, bladder atony, and absence of tachycardia on standing despite the marked reduction of blood pressure.

Those patients with central nervous system disease have normal resting plasma norepinephrine levels, while those with only peripheral autonomic disease have depressed levels at rest. Both groups fail to increase their circulating concentrations of the neurotransmitter during standing and exercise. Thus, it appears that patients with orthostatic hypotension and central nervous system disease have an intact peripheral sympathetic nervous system, but are unable to activate it, while those without central disease have true insufficiency of the peripheral autonomic nervous system.

Specific therapy is not available for most of the neurologic causes of orthostatic hypotension, and treatment with sympathomimetic drugs has not proved effective over prolonged periods. However, the expansion of extracellular volume, which may be achieved with a high-salt diet (10 to 20 g per day), and/or the potent synthetic salt-retaining steroid, 9α-fluorohydrocortisone (0.1 to 0.5 mg per day) may be helpful. Tight, full-length elastic supportive hose to reduce orthostatic pooling of blood in the legs may also be helpful in sustaining arterial pressure, and in the most severe cases pressurized aviator suits may be necessary to permit ambulation.

REFERENCES

ANDERSON RW: Shock and circulatory collapse, in *Gibbon's Surgery of the Chest,* 3d ed, DC Sabiston, FC Spencer (eds). Philadelphia, Saunders, 1976, chap 5, p 107

CHRISTY JH: Pathophysiology of gram-negative shock. Am Heart J 81:694, 1971

GUYTON AC: Circulatory shock and physiology of its treatment, in *Textbook of Medical Physiology,* 5th ed. Philadelphia, Saunders, 1976, chap 28, p 357

NICKERSON M: Vascular adjustments during the development of shock. Can Med Assoc J 103:853, 1971

SOBEL BE: Shock, in *Heart Disease,* E Braunwald (ed). Philadelphia, Saunders, 1980, chap 18

WEIL MH et al: Treatment of circulatory shock. JAMA 231:1280, 1975

ZIEGLER MG et al: The sympathetic nervous system defect in primary orthostatic hypotension. N Engl J Med 296:293, 1977

31
ELEVATION OF ARTERIAL PRESSURE

GORDON H. WILLIAMS
KARL ENGELMAN
EUGENE BRAUNWALD

DIAGNOSIS OF HYPERTENSION Patients with elevations of arterial pressure are usually asymptomatic, and the blood pressure abnormality often arouses attention only incidentally during military, life insurance, or other periodic physical examinations. Because hypertension results in secondary organ damage and a reduced life span, it should be evaluated fully and, when appropriate, treated.

Often, however, the first question is whether patients with a moderately elevated routine blood pressure recording are truly hypertensive. It is well established that anxiety, discomfort, physical activity, or other stress can acutely and transiently raise arterial pressure. Most persons have a higher pressure when initially examined than after several measurements made in the course of a single visit; in order to establish the diagnosis of hypertension, it is necessary to document in the course of several examinations that arterial pressure remains elevated (Chap. 251). This precaution need not be taken in patients with markedly elevated blood pressure and/or in those in whom significant target organ damage is already manifest. Patients with transient or "labile" hypertension may not require immediate treatment but should be reexamined periodically, since over the course of time they often develop sustained hypertension.

Systolic hypertension is most commonly seen in elderly patients with decreased compliance of the aortic wall and, like diastolic hypertension, is a risk factor for the development of atherosclerosis (Chap. 251). When systolic hypertension is due to an elevated stroke volume, as in patients with severe bradycardia, thyrotoxicosis, severe anemia, aortic valvular regurgitation, arteriovenous shunts or fistulae, patent ductus arteriosus, or the hyperkinetic heart syndrome, it is usually accompanied by a reduced diastolic pressure and a normal mean pressure, and under these circumstances it does not appear to be a risk factor for atherosclerosis.

Regardless of the primary cause, the hemodynamic abnormality in most patients with increased systolic, mean, and diastolic arterial pressures is increased vascular resistance, especially at the level of the smaller muscular arteries and arterioles, though a small number of patients may have an increased cardiac output, particularly in the early stages of the illness. In some patients, hypertension is associated with hypervolemia.

MECHANISM OF HYPERTENSION Arterial pressure is the product of cardiac output and peripheral resistance. Cardiac output in turn is dependent on four interrelated factors (Chap. 235): (1) myocardial contractile state (contractility, inotropic state, or the position of the heart's force-velocity curve); (2) preload—i.e., the length of cardiac muscle at the onset of contraction; (3) afterload—the tension which the muscle is called upon to develop during contraction; and (4) heart rate.

Peripheral resistance is determined by the intrinsic physical characteristics of the resistance vessels, i.e., the ratio of lumen to wall thickness, as well as the neurohumoral influences that act on vascular smooth muscle; the latter include the neurotransmitters norepinephrine, a vasoconstrictor, and in some vessels, acetylcholine, a vasodilator. Humoral and locally acting substances include angiotensin II (a vasoconstrictor) and prostaglandins and kinins (vasodilators). Hypoxia and products of metabolism, such as H^+, lactic acid, and perhaps most important, adenosine, also exert potent *local* vasodilating influences.

For arterial pressure to rise, there must be an increase either in cardiac output or peripheral resistance, or both. Theories of the pathogenesis of essential hypertension have suggested increases in either cardiac output or peripheral resistance as the initiating events.

In 1963, Borst and Borst de Geus proposed that "hypertension is part of a homeostatic reaction to deficient renal sodium output." The proposed abnormality in renal function, i.e., reduced sodium excretion at normal arterial pressure, might be secondary to (1) a primary (perhaps genetic) tubular defect, (2) mild increases in mineralocorticoid activity, (3) decreased renal kallikrein-kinin or prostaglandin activity, or (4) *local* increases in vasoconstrictor activity (angiotensin II or sympathetic nervous system), reducing renal blood flow and secondarily sodium excretion. Regardless of the mechanism of salt retention, according to this concept, blood volume rises because of the decreased sodium excretion, raising central venous pressure and preload, and thereby, cardiac output, i.e., systemic blood flow. However, tissues have the intrinsic capacity to regulate this overperfusion down to appropriate levels by increasing local vascular resistance. When resistance is increased in many vascular beds, arterial pressure rises and serves as negative feedback by increasing cardiac afterload, thereby depressing stroke volume and cardiac output (Fig. 235-6). As has been shown by Guyton, and others, the elevated arterial (renal perfusion) pressure also increases the urinary excretion of sodium, thereby serving as a source of negative feedback and reducing blood volume, central venous pressure, preload, and ultimately cardiac output. Thus, the end result of this process would be increased peripheral resistance and arterial pressure, with all other parameters, including blood volume, cardiac output, and renal sodium excretion, remaining normal. Indeed, this sequence has been documented in experimental human (desoxycorticosterone) and animal (renal artery stenosis) hypertension. However, in patients with essential hypertension, most investigations have reported only a normal cardiac output and elevated peripheral resistance, suggesting either that the studies have not been performed early enough in the course of the disease or that this theory is incorrect in that a change in peripheral resistance is actually a *primary* rather than secondary event.

Such a primary elevation in peripheral resistance can occur either because of an increase in factors tending to produce vasoconstriction, a reduction in factors producing vasodilation, or a change in the arterial smooth muscle—i.e., an increase in muscle mass or an increase in its responsiveness and/or sensitivity to vasoconstrictor stimuli. Each theory has it advocates. Thus, the hypertension associated with emotional stress, some neurologic disorders, and perhaps early essential hypertension is accompanied by increased plasma or urine levels of norepinephrine. Presumably, this reflects augmented neural releases of the vasoconstrictive adrenergic neurotransmitter which is responsible for the increased arterial pressure. Secondly, there is an increased vascular response to vasoconstrictor agents (e.g., angiotensin II, norepinephrine) in many patients with essential hypertension. Finally, since the early 1930s, hypertensive patients have been noted to exhibit a decrease in the urinary excretion of kinins, and thus it is possible that reduced vasodilator activity could also result in increased peripheral resistance and arterial pressure.

The "primary increase in peripheral resistance" hypothesis and the "deficient renal sodium output" theory are not necessarily mutually exclusive . For example, an increased retention of sodium enhances vascular reactivity, at least to angiotensin II, even in normotensive subjects. Thus, a primary defect of sodium excretion could simultaneously increase both cardiac output and peripheral resistance. It appears that all the factors mentioned above play some role in the development of essential hypertension; individual patients may differ in the relative importance of each. Thus, essential hypertension might be best regarded as a multifactorial disease related to abnormalities of the regulatory mechanisms normally concerned with the control of systemic vascular resistance, sodium excretion, blood volume, cardiac output, and ultimately arterial pressure. The specific parameter which is improperly regulated may differ from patient to patient.

ETIOLOGY OF HYPERTENSION A specific cause for the elevated arterial pressure cannot be defined for most patients with hypertension. The percentage of patients with so-called "idiopathic," essential, or primary hypertension is high, varying from 80 to 95 percent depending on both the patient population and how extensive the "routine" evaluation is.

TABLE 31-1
Classification of arterial hypertension

I Systolic hypertension with wide pulse pressure
  A Decreased compliance of aorta (arteriosclerosis)
  B Increased stroke volume
    1 Arteriovenous fistula
    2 Thyrotoxicosis
    3 Hyperkinetic heart disease
    4 Fever
    5 Psychogenic factors
    6 Aortic valvular insufficiency
    7 Patent ductus arteriosus
II Systolic and diastolic hypertension (increased peripheral vascular resistance)
  A Renal
    1 Chronic pyelonephritis
    2 Acute and chronic glomerulonephritis
    3 Polycystic renal disease
    4 Renovascular stenosis or renal infarction
    5 Most other severe renal disease (arteriolar nephrosclerosis, diabetic nephropathy, etc.)
    6 Renin-producing tumors
  B Endocrine
    1 Oral contraceptives
    2 Adrenocortical hyperfunction
      a Cushing's disease and syndrome
      b Primary hyperaldosteronism
      c Congenital or hereditary adrenogenital syndromes (17α-hydroxylase and 11β-hydroxylase defects)
    3 Pheochromocytoma
    4 Myxedema
    5 Acromegaly
  C Neurogenic
    1 Psychogenic
    2 "Diencephalic syndrome"
    3 Familial dysautonomia (Riley-Day)
    4 Poliomyelitis (bulbar)
    5 Polyneuritis (acute porphyria, lead poisoning)
    6 Increased intracranial pressure (acute)
    7 Spinal cord section
  D Miscellaneous
    1 Coarctation of aorta
    2 Increased intravascular volume (excessive transfusion)
    3 Polyarteritis nodosa
    4 Hypercalcemia
  E Unknown etiology
    1 Essential hypertension (>90% of all cases of hypertension)
    2 Toxemia of pregnancy
    3 Acute intermittent porphyria

More specific etiologic relationships have been established for a smaller group of patients with systemic hypertension (Table 31-1). Primary renal diseases associated with the development of serious hypertension (as distinguished from renal damage secondary to hypertension) have been recognized for years, although in many cases the exact mechanism of blood pressure elevation is unknown. In some instances it is due to activation of the renin-angiotensin-aldosterone axis; in others, perhaps it is related to a reduced ability to excrete sodium and the sequence already described. Hypertension may develop suddenly during the course of acute glomerulonephritis, and it is usually a prominent feature in the late stages of renal damage due to chronic glomerulonephritis or pyelonephritis. Polycystic renal disease, renal infarction, and partial occlusion of the renal artery due to congenital or acquired vascular defects are also implicated as etiologic factors, the last of these being clearly related to activation of the renin-angiotensin-aldosterone system.

The most clearly defined etiologic relationships in the development of hypertension are found among the endocrine disorders. Adrenocortical hormones have also been implicated in the hypertensive syndromes associated with tumors or hyperplasia of the anterior pituitary (Cushing's syndrome, primary hyperaldosteronism, Chap. 336), as well as with various congenital or hereditary enzyme defects (hypertensive adrenogenital syndromes). Secretion of excessive quantities of the pressor catecholamines, norepinephrine and epinephrine, associated with pheochromocytomas, i.e., chromaffin cell tumors arising from the adrenal medulla or sympathetic ganglia, is also commonly associated with hypertension (Chap. 337). Up to 50 percent of patients with acromegaly (Chap. 333) may have hypertension, but the mechanism of their blood pressure elevation is less clear. The presence of these endocrinopathies is usually readily recognizable and distinguishable from essential hypertension by their distinctive clinical and biochemical features. The clinical differences between the primary form and the various forms of secondary hypertension are detailed in Chap. 251.

EFFECTS OF HYPERTENSION For nearly 70 years it has been known that patients with hypertension die prematurely. The most common cause of death is heart disease, with strokes and renal failure also frequently occurring, particularly in those patients with significant retinopathy.

Effects on heart (see also Chap. 251) Cardiac compensation for the excessive workload imposed by increased arterial pressure is at first sustained by the development of left ventricular hypertrophy. Ultimately, the function of this chamber deteriorates; it dilates, and the symptoms and signs of heart failure appear (Chap. 236). Angina pectoris may also occur because of accelerated coronary arterial disease and/or increased myocardial oxygen requirements as a consequence of the increased myocardial mass, which exceeds the capacity of the coronary circulation. On physical examination the heart is enlarged and has a prominent left ventricular impulse. The sound of aortic closure is accentuated, and there may be a faint murmur of aortic insufficiency. Presystolic (S_3) gallop sounds appear frequently in hypertensive heart disease, and a protodiastolic (S_4, summation) gallop rhythm may be present. Electrocardiographic changes of left ventricular hypertrophy are common; evidence of ischemia or infarction may be observed late in the disease. The majority of deaths due to hypertension result from myocardial infarction or congestive heart failure.

NEUROLOGIC EFFECTS (See also Chap. 365) The neurologic effects of long-standing hypertension may be divided into retinal and central nervous system changes. Because the *retina* is the only tissue in which the arteries and arterioles can be examined directly, repeated ophthalmoscopic examination provides the opportunity to observe the progress of the vascular effects of hypertension. The Keith-Wagener-Barker classification of the retinal changes in hypertension has provided a simple and excellent means for serial evaluation of the hypertensive patient. Increasing severity of hypertension is associated with focal spasm and progressive general narrowing of the arterioles, as well as the appearance of hemorrhages, exudates, and papilledema. These retinal lesions often produce scotomata, blurred vision, and even blindness, especially in the presence of papilledema or hemorrhages of the macular area. Hypertensive lesions may develop acutely, and if therapy results in significant reduction of blood pressure, may show rapid resolution. Rarely, these lesions resolve without therapy. In contrast, retinal arteriolosclerosis results from endothelial and muscular proliferation, and it accurately reflects similar changes in other organs. Sclerotic changes do not develop as rapidly as hypertensive lesions, nor do they regress appreciably with therapy. As a consequence of increased wall thickness and rigidity, sclerotic arterioles distort and compress the veins as they cross within their common fibrous sheath, and the reflected light streak from the arterioles is changed by the increased opacity of the vessel wall.

Central nervous system dysfunction also occurs frequently in patients with hypertension. Occipital headaches, most often in the morning, are among the most prominent early symptoms of hypertension. Dizziness, lightheadedness, vertigo, tinnitus, and dimmed vision or syncope may also be observed, but the more serious manifestations are due to vascular occlusion or hemorrhage.

The pathogenesis of each of these disorders is quite different. Cerebral infarction is secondary to the increased atherosclerosis observed in hypertensive patients, while cerebral hemorrhage is the result of both the elevated arterial pressure and the development of cerebral vascular microaneurysms (Charcot-Bouchard aneurysms). Only age and increased arterial pressure are known to influence the development of the microaneurysms. Thus, it is not surprising that the correlation of arterial pressure with cerebral hemorrhage is so much better than with either cerebral or myocardial infarction. The former is two-factorial while the latter are multifactorial.

Renal effects (see also Chap. 282) Arteriolosclerotic lesions of the afferent and efferent arterioles and the glomerular capillary tufts are the most common renal vascular lesions in hypertension and result in decreased glomerular filtration rate and tubular dysfunction. Proteinuria and microscopic hematuria occur because of glomerular lesions, and approximately 10 percent of the deaths secondary to hypertension result from renal failure. Blood loss in hypertension occurs not only from renal lesions; epistaxis, hemoptysis, and metrorrhagia also occur more frequently in these patients.

APPROACH TO THE PATIENT WITH HYPERTENSION The physician's first task is to determine whether or not a patient with a given level of arterial pressure has hypertension. Then, determinations of the extent of pretreatment evaluation, whether or not to treat, how to treat, and how frequently to reevaluate are necessary. In general, it is preferable to measure arterial pressure on several occasions prior to starting therapy using a mercury sphygmomanometer with the patient seated.

Initial history, physical examination, and laboratory evaluation should be directed at (1) uncovering correctable secondary forms of hypertension (Table 31-1), (2) establishing the base-line status of the patient, and (3) assessing factors which may influence the type of therapy or which therapy may adversely modify.

An assessment of the following areas in the medical history is particularly important: family or personal history of hypertension; drugs or dietary factors which may aggravate the hypertension, e.g., high salt intake, oral contraceptives, and hormones; cardiovascular risk factors including diabetes mellitus, smoking, lipid abnormalities, or strokes; cardiac or renal disease; and symptoms suggestive of secondary forms of hypertension, e.g., muscle cramps and weakness associated with primary aldosteronism (Chap. 336) or episodic headaches, palpitations, and sweating associated with pheochromocytoma (Chap. 337).

The *physical examination* should include: a standing blood pressure, height, weight, funduscopic examination, assessment of thyroid size, bruits in neck or abdomen, peripheral pulses including determination of synchrony between upper and lower extremities, examination of the heart for size, rate, murmurs, gallops, auscultation of the lungs, examination of the abdomen for masses, and particularly kidney size, and a neurologic examination to assess the presence of deficits associated with a stroke.

The basic *laboratory evaluation* should consist of hematocrit, urinalysis, blood urea nitrogen or creatinine, serum potassium, ECG, and chest x-ray. Often blood glucose, uric acid, and cholesterol determinations and a blood count are also useful, particularly since they may be part of a battery of automated blood tests that as a group are about the same price as the individual tests listed above. Other studies to identify secondary forms of hypertension may be indicated on the basis of the initial therapy or physical examination.

If the average diastolic pressure is greater than 105 mmHg, therapy is almost always indicated. In an adult, if the diastolic pressure is less than 90 mmHg, no other therapy than a change in diet or exercise is usually needed. Individualization is necessary for patients with intermediate elevations of arterial pressures (diastolic pressure between 90 and 105 mmHg), since documentation that therapy is beneficial is lacking. Thus, ancillary factors such as age, sex, and family history need to be considered before starting therapy. In most instances, therapy is indicated in patients with pressures in this range.

Therapy should be directed at reducing the arterial pressure to or near normal levels, since studies have documented that morbidity and mortality are reduced particularly if the initial diastolic pressure is greater than 105 mmHg. In order to minimize drug side effects in achieving this goal, a "step-care approach" has been advocated. The principle involves initiating therapy with a small dose of a single drug, usually a thiazide diuretic, increasing the dose of that drug, and then adding other drugs as needed, one at a time (Chap. 251). The therapeutic regimen should be revised as dictated by the arterial pressure measured at periodic intervals. The frequency of reevaluation should be as often as weekly while blood pressure is being lowered in patients with initial diastolic pressures greater than 115, and approximately every 4 months in symptom free patients on stable treatment programs.

The specific drugs are discussed elsewhere (Chap. 251). However, it is important to emphasize here that control of arterial pressure is a lifelong endeavor the success of which is often dependent on the physician's ability to motivate the patient to adhere to the therapeutic program and to recognize the pharmacologic interactions and adverse reactions of antihypertensive agents.

REFERENCES

Borst JGG, Borst de Geus A: Hypertension explained by Starling's theory of circulatory homeostasis. Lancet 1:677, 1963

GENEST J et al: Role of the adrenal cortex and sodium in the pathogenesis of human hypertension. Can Med J 118:538, 1978

GUYTON AC: Regulation of arterial pressure, in *Textbook of Medical Physiology*, 5th ed. Philadelphia, Saunders, 1976, pp 265–294

HUNT JC: Management and treatment of essential hypertension in *Hypertension: Physiopathology and Treatment*, J Genest et al (eds). New York, McGraw-Hill, 1977, pp 1068–1085

KAPLAN NM: *Clinical Hypertension*, 2d ed. Baltimore, Williams & Wilkins, 1978

MOSER M et al: Report of the joint national committee on detection, evaluation, and treatment of high blood pressure. JAMA 237:255, 1977

PICKERING G: *Hypertension*, 2d ed. New York, Churchill Livingstone, 1974

32
SUDDEN CARDIOVASCULAR COLLAPSE AND DEATH

BURTON E. SOBEL
EUGENE BRAUNWALD

Sudden death claims more than 400,000 lives annually in the United States alone. It is a major health problem in the Western world. Despite the liberality of the definition of sudden death according to the Joint American Heart Association-International Society of Cardiology Committee (death occurring instantaneously or within an estimated 24 h of the onset of acute symptoms or signs), about half of all sudden deaths are virtually instantaneous. A brief period of time, usually only several minutes, elapses between sudden cardiovascular collapse (without effective cardiac output) and irreversible ischemic changes in the central nervous system. Prolonged survival without functional impairment may be the reward for prompt treatment of certain forms of cardiovascular collapse.

MECHANISMS Sudden cardiovascular collapse may be due to (1) dysrhythmia (Chap. 237); (*a*) most commonly, ventricular tachycardia or fibrillation, sometimes occurring following a bradyarrhythmia, or (*b*) less frequently, ventricular asystole or severe bradycardia; (2) a marked, abrupt reduction in cardiac output, such as occurs with mechanical blockade of the circulation; massive pulmonary thromboembolism (Chap. 266) and cardiac tamponade are two examples of this form; (3) sudden ventricular (pump) failure, which may occur in the presence of critical aortic stenosis (Chap. 242) or acute myocardial infarction ("nonarrhythmic cardiac death") with or without ventricular rupture (Chap. 245); (4) activation of vasodepressor reflexes, which may contribute to sudden reductions in arterial pressure and heart rate, and which are activated in diverse conditions, including primary pulmonary hypertension (Chap. 265), pulmonary thromboembolism, and the hypersensitive carotid sinus syndrome (Chap. 13).

Sudden death and coronary atherosclerosis Sudden death is primarily a complication of coronary atherosclerosis. More than two-thirds of the cases result from this disorder. In the vast majority of such patients sudden death results from precipitous ventricular fibrillation. However, evidence of coronary occlusion and, indeed, of acute myocardial infarction may not be found at autopsy; nonetheless, acute myocardial ischemia appears to be the precipitating event. Only approximately 40 percent of patients dying from coronary artery disease survive long enough to be hospitalized. The remainder (approximately

300,000 patients per year in the United States) die suddenly before they reach the hospital. In fact, in 25 percent of patients with coronary artery disease, death is the first indication of the presence of the disorder (Chap. 245). By extrapolation from experience in coronary care units, in which control of electrical activity of the heart has affected the mortality rate favorably, it would appear that the incidence of sudden death in the community might be reduced substantially by prophylactic therapy in populations at particularly high risk, if such therapy could be demonstrated to be effective, of low toxicity, and convenient to the patient. However, sudden death may be but one mode of expression of coronary artery disease, and effective prevention of sudden death will almost certainly require reduction in the incidence and severity of this disease.

Factors associated with increased risk of sudden death in nonhospitalized persons When electrocardiograms are recorded for 24 h during the course of normal activities, supraventricular premature contractions are found to occur in most American men over 50 years of age, ventricular premature contractions and complex ventricular dysrhythmias in almost two-thirds, and persistent or transient conduction defects in less than 10 percent. Supraventricular dysrhythmias do not appear to be associated with increased risk of sudden death except when they are a manifestation of ventricular dysfunction or atrial infarction accompanying extensive myocardial infarction. Conduction abnormalities and certain types of ventricular premature beats, such as those originating from the left ventricle (recognizable by their terminal anterior and rightward vectors), those occurring during the vulnerable period, and those occurring in pairs or salvos have been thought to be associated with an increased risk. However, among patients with myocardial infarction, late ventricular ectopic beats are particularly prone to be associated with complex malignant ventricular dysrhythmia.

Ventricular premature beats may precipitate ventricular fibrillation, particularly with concomitant myocardial ischemia. On the other hand, they may be manifestations of common fundamental electrophysiologic disturbances predisposing to both ventricular premature beats and ventricular fibrillation or totally independent phenomena associated with electrophysiologic mechanisms different from those responsible for fibrillation. Thus, it is not surprising that, in more than 75 percent of patients with recurrent ventricular fibrillation, after resuscitation from primary ventricular fibrillation warning ventricular dysrhythmias are absent.

In general, ventricular dysrhythmias are of greater significance and more ominous in the presence of acute ischemia than in its absence. In the asymptomatic patient, ventricular premature contractions, particularly when they are relatively frequent (more than 20 per hour), should alert the physician to look for more definitive evidence of heart disease, such as other electrocardiographic abnormalities, mitral valve prolapse, hypertension, or a history of angina.

Overt coronary artery disease, hypertension, or diabetes mellitus is present in more than 75 percent of persons dying suddenly, and perhaps more significantly, the incidence of sudden death in persons with at least one of the three abnormalities is substantially increased. Severe coronary artery disease, not necessarily accompanied by morphologic evidence of an acute event, is consistently present in victims of sudden, unexpected death. More than 75 percent of men without known prior coronary artery disease who die suddenly exhibit at least two of the following four risk factors: hypercholesterolemia, hypertension, hyperglycemia, and cigarette smoking. Obesity and electrocardiographic criteria of left ventricular hypertrophy are also associated with an increased incidence. The incidence of sudden death is higher in cigarette smokers than in nonsmokers, perhaps because of the elevation of circulating catecholamines and fatty acids and the production of increased circulating carboxyhemoglobin with consequently diminished oxygen-carrying capacity by the blood. The proclivity of cigarette smoking to cause sudden death is not cumulative and appears to be reversible when smoking is discontinued.

Ventricular premature contractions may be increased or made overt by exercise, and sudden death appears sometimes to follow unusual exertion. On the other hand, their incidence appears to be diminished in subjects engaged in regular, intermittent, strenuous physical activity in comparison with controls in the same socioeconomic group with a more sedentary existence. Cardiovascular collapse on exertion occurs only rarely in patients with ischemic heart disease undergoing exercise testing, and with appropriate personnel and facilities these episodes respond promptly to electrical defibrillation. Acute emotional stress may precipitate acute myocardial infarction and sudden death, findings which are in keeping with recent experimental observations of increased susceptibility to ventricular tachycardia and ventricular fibrillation after coronary occlusion in emotionally stressed animals or those with augmented sympathetic activity.

Two major clinical syndromes may be recognized in patients who die suddenly and unexpectedly; both are generally associated with ischemic heart disease. In the larger group, the dysrhythmia, which may be termed *primary ventricular fibrillation,* occurs totally unexpectedly and without preceding symptoms or prodromata. This form is *not* associated with acute myocardial infarction; following resuscitation, there is a propensity for early recurrence, probably reflecting the myocardial electrical instability responsible for the initial episode, and a relatively high 2-year mortality rate (approximately 50 percent). Clearly, these patients can be salvaged only by a rapidly responsive system, and pharmacologic prophylaxis is required to enhance survival. The second, smaller group consists of patients who, following resuscitation, exhibit evidence of acute myocardial infarction. These patients often exhibit prodromal symptoms—chest pain, dyspnea, and syncope—and show a much lower recurrence and 2-year mortality rate (15 percent). Survival in this subgroup is similar to that following resuscitation from ventricular fibrillation complicating acute myocardial infarction in the coronary care unit. Thus, the propensity for developing ventricular fibrillation at the time of acute infarction is of short duration, while ventricular fibrillation in the absence of acute infarction may be related to a chronic process and is likely to recur.

Other causes of sudden death   Sudden cardiovascular collapse may result from a number of disorders other than coronary atherosclerosis (Table 32-1). Severe aortic stenosis (congenital or acquired) with sudden dysrhythmias or pump failure, idiopathic hypertrophic subaortic stenosis, and myocarditis or cardiomyopathy associated with dysrhythmia may be responsible. Massive pulmonary embolism leads to circulatory collapse and death within minutes in approximately 10 percent of patients; some of the remainder succumb gradually with progressive right ventricular failure. Acute circulatory collapse may be presaged by smaller emboli occurring at variable intervals before the lethal attack. Accordingly, implementation of therapy during the premonitory sublethal phase, including anticoagulant administration, may be lifesaving (Chap. 266). Sublethal emboli are common in hospitalized patients and can be recognized in at least 40 percent of postmortem examinations when specialized pulmonary arterial injection techniques are utilized. Their clinical manifestations include unexplained or disproportionate dyspnea or tachypnea, hypoxemia, respiratory alkalosis, and hypocapnia. Sinus tachycardia is common. Atrial flutter, chaotic atrial rhythms, and multiple premature atrial beats are compatible with the diagnosis; thrombophlebi-

tis or conditions predisposing to this are also helpful, suggestive signs.

Sudden death with cardiovascular collapse is a rare but always potential complication of infective endocarditis (Chap. 243). In this condition it is usually due to relentless progression of congestive heart failure, but it may also result from ventricular fibrillation, complete atrioventricular block, rupture of a sinus of Valsalva, or a septic embolus to the cerebral or coronary vessels. Sudden, unexpected death in infants, so-called "crib death," is responsible for approximately 10,000 deaths per year in the United States. A defect in the regulation of ventilation may be responsible.

A number of less common causes of sudden death have been recognized increasingly in recent years. Primary degeneration of the atrioventricular conduction system, with or without deposition of calcium or cartilage, may lead to sudden death in the absence of severe coronary atherosclerosis. Trifascicular atrioventricular (AV) block is often seen in these conditions, which account for more than two-thirds of the cases of chronic AV block in adults (Chap. 237). Patients in whom the degree of block is unstable are particularly susceptible to more serious brady- or tachyarrhythmias. Electrocardiographic QT-interval prolongation, nerve deafness, and autosomal recessive inheritance seem to be associated with a high proportion of cases of ventricular fibrillation. The same electrocardiographic abnormality and electrophysiologic instability without nerve deafness appear to be inherited in an autosomal dominant mode. Electrocardiographic changes in these disorders may be manifest only after exercise, and so they may be more important causes of sudden death than has been generally recognized. Other conditions with QT prolongation and increased temporal dispersion of repolarization, such as hypothermia and phenothiazine, emetine, or quinidine toxicity, are rarely associated with sudden death. Sinoatrial arrest or block with depression of lower pacemakers or the sick sinus syndrome, usually accompanied by conduction system dysfunction as well, may also lead to asystole. Sudden rupture of a papillary muscle, the ventricular septum, or free wall, usually occurring within the first few days following acute myocardial infarction, occasionally causes sudden death (Chap. 245). Sudden cardiovascular collapse is also a major, and frequently the terminal,

TABLE 32-1
Conditions associated with cardiovascular collapse and sudden death in adults

Ischemic heart disease secondary to coronary atherosclerosis (including acute myocardial infarction)
Prinzmetal's variant angina; coronary artery spasm
Congenital coronary artery disease
Coronary embolism
Wolff-Parkinson-White syndrome
Hereditary QT-interval prolongation (with or without congenital deafness)
Sinoatrial node disease
Atrioventricular block (Stokes-Adams syndrome)
Secondary disease of the conduction system (e.g., amyloid, sarcoid, hemochromatosis, thrombotic thrombocytopenic purpura, myotonia dystrophica)
Drug toxicity or idiosyncrasy (e.g., digitalis, quinidine)
Valvular heart disease, especially aortic stenosis
Infective endocarditis
Myocarditis
Cardiomyopathies, particularly idiopathic hypertrophic subaortic stenosis
Pericardial tamponade
Cardiac tumor
Ruptured or dissecting aortic aneurysm
Pulmonary thromboembolism
Cerebrovascular accident, particularly hemorrhage

event in patients with major cerebrovascular accidents, sudden alterations of intracranial pressure, or lesions affecting the brainstem. It may also occur with asphyxia, and the toxicity of cardioactive drugs such as digitalis and quinidine may result in life-threatening arrhythmias, leading to sudden cardiovascular collapse and, if treatment is not immediate, to death (Chap. 238).

Electrophysiologic mechanisms underlying ventricular fibrillation Potentially lethal ventricular dysrhythmias in patients with acute myocardial infarction may result from reentry, enhanced automaticity, or both. It would appear that reentry plays a dominant role in early dysrhythmia, for example, within the first hour, and that increased automaticity is an important contributing factor later. Analysis of electrophysiologic changes after experimental coronary occlusion in dogs supports this differentiation, since slowed conduction, asynchronous depolarization, and alterations in recovery time compatible with reentry occur early in ischemic zones.

Several factors appear to set the stage for ventricular fibrillation and other rhythms dependent upon reentry early after the onset of ischemia. Local accumulation of hydrogen ions, an increased ratio of extra- to intracellular potassium, and regional adrenergic stimulation tend to shift diastolic transmembrane potentials toward zero and facilitate slow-current depolarizations. Such depolarizations, sometimes mediated by calcium currents, are characterized by a slow rate of rise of the action potential, low amplitude, diminished duration of the plateau phase of the action potential, and repetitive reponses triggered by a single depolarization. It appears likely that the prominence of depolarizations of this type within ischemic zones of myocardium, in contrast to the fast, sodium-mediated depolarizations evident under physiologic conditions, contribute to slowed conduction required for the development of reentry early after the onset of ischemia.

Another mechanism implicated in reentry early after ischemia is focal reexcitation. Anoxia results in marked abbreviation of the duration of the action potential. Accordingly, during electrical systole, cells within an ischemic zone may be repolarized before cells in adjacent nonischemic tissue. The consequent disparity between prevailing transmembrane potentials may give rise to an uneven depolarization of adjacent cells and hence contribute to dysrhythmia dependent upon reentry.

Among some patients with ischemic heart disease, concomitant pharmacologic or metabolic factors may predispose toward reentry. For example, quinidine may depress conduction velocity, thereby facilitating dysrhythmias dependent upon reentry early after the onset of ischemia.

The so-called "vulnerable period," corresponding to the ascending limb of the T wave (Chap. 239), represents that portion of the cardiac cycle when temporal dispersion of ventricular refractoriness is maximum under physiologic conditions and, accordingly, when reentrant rhythms leading to sustained, repetitive activity can be initiated most readily. In patients with severe myocardial ischemia, the vulnerable period is prolonged and the intensity of stimulus required to evoke repetitive tachycardia or ventricular fibrillation is reduced, so that a single ventricular premature contraction may initiate the rhythm. Electrical shocks of low energy or even a blow struck over the precordium ("thump version") may terminate ventricular tachycardia, presumably by interrupting a reentrant pathway. Since paroxysms of ventricular ectopic beats progressively increase asynchrony of recovery, such paroxysms frequently augur ventricular fibrillation.

Temporal dispersion of refractoriness may be increased in nonischemic tissue in the presence of a slow heart rate. Accordingly, profound bradycardia due to decreased automaticity of the sinus node or AV block may also be particularly dangerous in patients with acute myocardial infarction since it may potentiate reentry.

Malignant ventricular dysrhythmia occurring later after the onset of ischemia appears to be dependent in part on enhanced automaticity of Purkinje fibers and possibly of myocardial cells as well. Reduction of diastolic transmembrane potential in response to regional biochemical alterations induced by ischemia may contribute to the enhanced automaticity by facilitating repetitive depolarizations of Purkinje fibers triggered by a single depolarization. Since catecholamines facilitate propagation of such slow-current responses, enhanced regional adrenergic stimulation may be an important contributing factor. The apparent efficacy of beta-adrenergic blockade in suppressing some ventricular dysrhythmias and the relative inefficacy of conventional antiarrhythmic agents such as lidocaine in patients with sympathetic hyperactivity may be reflections of the importance of regional adrenergic stimulation to enhanced automaticity.

Electrophysiologic derangements tend to occur with greatest frequency early following the onset of myocardial ischemia or infarction. They may be accentuated by widely distributed ischemia, concomitant metabolic derangements, and deleterious effects of cardioactive drugs. These derangements cause the majority of instantaneous deaths, but they may also occur suddenly and unexpectedly later in the course of an otherwise uncomplicated hospitalization. Since slow-current depolarizations, mediated by calcium under some conditions, have been implicated as factors contributing to malignant ventricular dysrhythmias early after the onset of ischemia depend in part on reentry and to dysrhythmias occurring later, apparently reflecting enhanced automatcity as well, electrical stability of the ischemic heart might be enhanced by administration of antiarrhythmic agents, such as verapamil (currently under investigation in the United States), which selectively block slow-current, calcium-mediated responses.

Asystole is a less common electrophysiologic mechanism underlying sudden death due to coronary atherosclerosis. It may occur when impulse formation in the sinus node is impaired or AV block impedes transmission and subsidiary pacemakers fail to function effectively.

PREVENTION OF SUDDEN DEATH The difficulties entailed in ambulatory electrocardiographic monitoring or other procedures for mass screening to detect candidates at risk for sudden death are formidable, since the population at risk comprises more than one-third of all men 35 to 74 years of age. At greatest risk are patients who have previously experienced primary ventricular fibrillation without associated acute mycardial infarction. Also, patients with ischemic heart disease who exhibit bouts of rapid ventricular tachycardia as well as those within 6 months after recovery from acute myocardial infarction with frequent, early, and/or multifocal ventricular premature contractions at rest, during physical activity, or during psychologic stress are particularly susceptible to sudden death. Patients with prolonged QT intervals and frequent premature contractions, particularly those who present with a history of syncope, represent another vulnerable group. Although identification of patients at high risk is particularly important, selection of an effective prophylactic regimen remains difficult, and none has clearly demonstrated effectiveness in reducing the risk. For example, although procainamide is effective in suppressing ventricular dysrhythmias in patients in the coronary care unit, drug toxicity militates against its routine prolonged use in a general ambulatory population.

It is reasonable to propose a trial of prophylactic treatment, on an individual basis, for patients with known or suspected coronary artery disease with recurrent or complex dysrhythmias. Quinidine gluconate, 330 mg by mouth every 6 h, may be effective in suppressing these dysrhythmias. The dosage may be increased up to 3 g per day if found necessary, unless gastrointestinal disturbances or electrocardiographic evidence of toxicity occurs. The long-acting preparation has the obvious advantage of requiring relatively infrequent dose schedules (bid or tid). Patients who tolerate quinidine poorly may do well with procainamide, 500 mg by mouth every 4 h. Ambulatory electrocardiographic monitoring may be particularly helpful in documenting the efficacy of treatment, since the incomplete knowledge regarding the pathogenesis of sudden death makes rational prophylactic drug selection and dosage difficult and a stereotyped regimen for all patients impractical. However, since the fundamental electrophysiologic derangements underlying ventricular fibrillation and premature ventricular beats may not be the same, documented suppression of premature beats provides no real assurance of prevention of sudden death.

Decreased incidence of sudden death in a random selection of patients surviving acute myocardial infarction has been documented in prospective double-blind studies utilizing beta-adrenergic blocking agents, although the effect of treatment on dysrhythmia was not quantified and the mechanism of apparent protection has not yet been identified. Similarly, it has been suggested that sulfinpyrazone, a uricosuric agent that inhibits platelet aggregation, reduces the incidence of sudden death in patients who had experienced myocardial infarction.

Delays by the patient, physician, and transportation system and in the emergency room after the occurrence of acute myocardial infarction are significant impediments to prevention of sudden death. The median elapsed time between onset of symptoms and hospitalization averages 5 to 8 h in most areas of the United States. Denial by the patient of the seriousness of the condition and indecision by both the patient and physician contribute most to total delay.

Experience gained in Seattle, Washington, has shown that in order to deal effectively on a community-wide basis with the problem of sudden cardiovascular collapse and death, it is necessary to develop a system that provides rapid and effective response for these emergencies. Important elements of the system include a city-wide emergency call number through which the system can be activated, a well-trained group of paramedical personnel such as fire fighters to respond, a short average time of response (under 4 min), and a large number of lay people trained in techniques of resuscitation. Clearly, the success in immediate resuscitation and for long-term survival is directly related to how soon following collapse resuscitation efforts are initiated. The availability of special ambulances (mobile coronary care units) equipped and staffed to handle acute cardiac emergencies appears to reduce delay by increasing community and physician awareness of the urgency of prompt medical attention. Such a system can be effective in resuscitating more than 40 percent of patients who have undergone cardiovascular collapse, and more than 25 percent of such patients are discharged from the hospital.

Therefore, providing instructions to susceptible persons on how to seek medical care on an emergency basis upon the development of symptoms of myocardial infarction is of great importance in the prevention of sudden cardiac death. This strategy includes instructing the patient that prompt entry into an effective emergency care system is not only correct but also what the physician expects of the patient, regardless of whether symptoms suggestive of myocardial infarction occur during the day or night (Chap. 245); this concept also means instructing the patient to bypass the physician and to contact the emergency care system directly. Unsupervised physical stress, such as jogging, should be discouraged in patients with known ischemic heart disease and prohibited in those at high risk of sudden death, as defined above.

APPROACH TO THE PATIENT WITH SUDDEN CARDIOVASCULAR COLLAPSE Sudden death can often be averted even when cardiovascular collapse has occurred. In patients experiencing sudden onset of ventricular fibrillation without prior ventricular failure (primary ventricular fibrillation) while they are under observation in the operating room, the cardiac catheterization laboratory, or the coronary care unit, correction of the dysrhythmia is the rule, and the outcome is usually favorable. However, prompt application of definitive therapy for sudden cardiovascular collapse in the community entails formidable practical obstacles, as outlined above.

The development of transvenous and transthoracic cardiac pacemakers (Chap. 237) and the improvement of cardiopulmonary resuscitative maneuvers, including external cardiac massage coupled with artificial respiration, have contributed to effective therapy.

When a patient under close medical observation develops sudden collapse from a dysrhythmia, the immediate goal must be restoration of effective cardiac rhythm. Circulatory collapse must be recognized and confirmed immediately. Its cardinal features are (1) loss of consciousness, syncope, and seizures, (2) absent peripheral arterial pulses, and (3) absent heart sounds. Since external cardiac massage can provide only limited cardiac output, no more than 30 percent of the lower limit of normal, definitive restoration of effective rhythm should be the immediate goal, and in the absence of evidence to the contrary, abrupt circulatory collapse should be assumed to be due to ventricular fibrillation. If the physician sees the patient within 1 min of the collapse, time should not be wasted by attempting to achieve oxygenation. An immediate blow to the precordium ("thump version") may be attempted, since this is occasionally effective and takes only seconds. Electrical defibrillation (Chap. 239) should be attempted immediately thereafter, without necessarily even pausing first to record an electrocardiogram on separate equipment, although use of portable defibrillators capable of electrocardiographic recording directly from the defibrillating electrodes may be helpful. Maximum electrical output, usually 400 W·s, should be used. If these immediate attempts are unsuccessful, external cardiac massage and complete cardiopulmonary resuscitation should be implemented.

If collapse is due to unequivocal asystole, transthoracic or transvenous electrical pacing should be implemented immediately. Intracardiac epinephrine, 1 ml of 1:1000 solution diluted 1:10 with intracavitary blood, may facilitate the heart's response to artificial pacing or be helpful when a slow ventricular focus is present but ineffective. If these initial definitive measures fail despite adequate technical performance, prompt restitution of a favorable metabolic milieu and monitoring are necessary. This is best accomplished by these three procedures: (1) External cardiac massage. (2) Correction of acid-base balance, often requiring intravenous sodium bicarbonate administration in an initial dose of 1 mg/kg repeated once within 5 to 10 min. Administration of subsequent doses of bicarbonate should be guided by frequent determinations of arterial pH, particularly since intracellular pH may paradoxically decrease, despite a rise in extracellular pH, because permeability to carbon dioxide is so much greater than to bicarbonate. (3) Assessment and correction of electrolyte imbalance. Definitive efforts to restore an effective cardiac rhythm should be attempted again as soon as possible, certainly within minutes. When effective cardiac rhythm is restored but rapidly degenerates again into ventricular tachycardia or fibrillation, lidocaine should be administered as a bolus, 1 mg/kg intravenously, then continued by intravenous infusion at a rate up to 1 to 5 (mg/kg)/h, and countershock repeated.

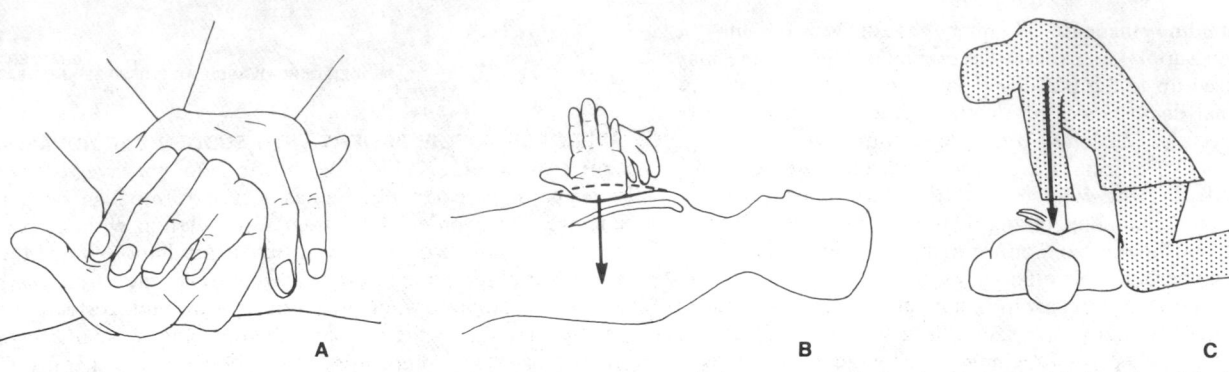

FIGURE 32-1

External cardiac massage. A. Position of hands during application of external cardiac massage. B. When pressure is applied, the lower portion *of the sternum is displaced posteriorly with the palm of the hand. C. In order to apply maximal downward pressure, the resuscitator leans forward so that both arms are at right angles to the patient's sternum.*

Cardiac massage External cardiac massage is designed to lead to the ejection of blood from the heart by manual compression of the ventricles between the sternum and the spine, and cyclic passive ventricular filling. Adherence to several aspects of technique is essential (Fig. 32-1). (1) The patient should be placed supine on a firm surface (a wooden board serves well). (2) Compression of the chest should be performed with the heel of one hand on the lower third of the sternum cephalad to the xiphoid process (to avoid lacerations of the liver) and the other hand applied on top of the first. (3) The frequency of external massage should approximate one per second to permit adequate time for ventricular filling. (4) The resuscitator's waist must be higher than the patient's chest in order to permit the resuscitator to administer the approximately 100-lb force required to depress the anterior chest wall of an adult male the necessary 5 cm per beat. (5) Depression and release of the chest wall should be smooth, with each occupying 50 percent of the cycle, since sudden compression may elicit a pressure wave palpable at the femoral or carotid artery but able to eject little blood. (6) Massage should not be interrupted, even momentarily, since cardiac output increases cumulatively during the first 8 to 10 compressions and even brief interruptions are detrimental. (7) Effective ventilation must be carried out. To accomplish this, the chin must be retracted and the neck fully extended. Mouth-to-mouth or mouth-to-nose technique must be continued throughout the resuscitative effort at a frequency of about 12 per minute and monitored by arterial blood gas analyses. If the latter are clearly abnormal, endotracheal intubation should be carried out expeditiously.

Each external cardiac compression limits venous return, and the optimal anticipated cardiac index during external massage approximates only 40 percent of the lower limit of normal, well below that seen in most patients after spontaneous ventricular contractions have returned or have been induced by ventricular pacing. Therefore, prompt restoration of effective cardiac rhythm is essential. Rarely, organized electrocardiographic activity unaccompanied by effective cardiac contraction (electromechanical dissociation) may occur and respond to intracardiac epinephrine (1 ml of 1:1000 solution diluted 1:10 with blood) or calcium gluconate (1 g). Cardiac massage should be terminated as soon as effective cardiac contractions, initiated spontaneously or by ventricular pacing, serve to produce a detectable pulse and systemic arterial blood pressure. Subsequent treatment of dysrhythmias and hypotension and adjustment of intravascular volume should be guided by the same general principles underlying their management in circulatory collapse due to cardiogenic shock (Chap. 245).

The therapeutic approach outlined above is based on several considerations: (1) irreversible brain damage often occurs after a few (approximately 4) minutes of circulatory collapse; (2) the likelihood of restoring effective cardiac rhythm and successfully resuscitating the patient diminishes rapidly with time; (3) 80 to 90 percent survival can be anticipated in patients developing primary ventricular fibrillation, as when undergoing cardiac catheterization or exercise testing, in whom definitive treatment is prompt; (4) survival rates in the general hospital setting are much lower, approximately 20 percent, depending in part on the coexisting or underlying disease process; (5) survival rates in the community approach zero, unless special emergency care systems have been perfected, probably because of unavoidable delays in initiating definitive therapy and limitations of equipment and available personnel; and (6) external cardiac massage can provide only a limited cardiac output. When ventricular fibrillation occurs, the earliest application of electrical countershock is the one most likely to succeed. Thus, when circulatory collapse is a primary event, therapy must be directed toward prompt restoration of effective cardiac rhythm.

Complications External cardiac massage is not free from significant complications, including rib fracture, hemopericardium and tamponade, hemothorax, pneumothorax, liver laceration, fat embolus, and ruptured spleen with late, occult blood loss. However, these complications can be minimized by proper technique and, if appropriately considered, can be readily recognized and often managed effectively. The decision to terminate unsuccessful cardiopulmonary resuscitation is always difficult. In general, if effective cardiac rhythm has not been restored and if the patient's pupils are fixed and dilated despite 30 min or more of cardiac massage, a successful resuscitation cannot be expected.

An important challenge to the medical system is to provide trained medical or paramedical personnel immediately for patients who develop sudden cardiovascular collapse. The development of appropriately staffed "rescue stations" in large factories, office buildings, and sports arenas is one approach that has been proposed since aggressive precoronary care can reduce the mortality rate. However, it is likely that the identification of individuals at high risk and the application of effective preventive measures to this segment of the population will be more satisfactory.

REFERENCES

THE AUTURANE REINFARCTION TRIAL RESEARCH GROUP: Sulfinpyrazone in the prevention of cardiac death after myocardial infarction. N Engl J Med 298:289, 1978

CORDAY E, DODGE HT (eds): Symposium on Identification and Management of the Candidate for Sudden Cardiac Death. Am J Cardiol 39:813, 1977

HAYNES RE et al: Repolarization abnormalities in survivors of out-of-hospital ventricular fibrillation. Circulation 57:654, 1978

KANNEL WB et al: Precursors of sudden coronary death: Factors related to the incidence of sudden death. Circulation 51:606, 1975

LOWN B: Cardiovascular collapse and sudden death, in *Heart Disease,* E Braunwald (ed). Philadelphia, Saunders, 1980, chap 22

MULTICENTRE INTERNATIONAL STUDY: Improvement in prognosis of myocardial infarction by long-term beta-adrenoreceptor blockade using practolol. Br Med J 217:35, 1975

OLDHAM HN JR: Cardiopulmonary arrest and resuscitation, in *Gibbon's Surgery of the Chest*, 3d ed, DC Sabiston, FC Spencer (eds). Philadelphia, Saunders, 1976, chap 10, pp 239-255

PANTRIDGE JF et al: *The Acute Coronary Attack*. New York, Grune & Stratton, 1975

PRINEAS RJ, BLACKBURN H (eds): Sudden coronary death outside hospital. Circulation 52(suppl 3):287, 1975

RAIZES G et al: Instantaneous nonarrhythmic cardiac death in acute myocardial infarction. Am J Cardiol 39:1, 1977

SCHULZE RA et al: Sudden death in the year following myocardial infarction. Relation to ventricular premature contractions in the late hospital phase and left ventricular ejection fraction. Am J Med 62:192, 1977

section 5 | Alterations in gastrointestinal function

33
ORAL MANIFESTATIONS OF DISEASE

PAUL GOLDHABER

DISTURBANCES OF THE TEETH AND DENTAL TISSUES

DENTAL CARIES, PULPAL AND PERIAPICAL INFECTION, AND SEQUELAE Dental caries, the principal cause of tooth loss up to the fourth decade of life, is characterized by a bacteria-induced progressive destruction of the mineral and organic components of the outer enamel and underlying dentin. Numerous long-term studies have clearly shown that the artificial fluoridation of drinking water supplies to a level of 1 part per million leads to a 50 to 75 percent reduction in the occurrence of dental caries in permanent teeth of children, presumably because of an alteration of the developing enamel crystals during tooth formation which makes them more resistant to acid dissolution.

If the carious lesion progresses unchecked, there is eventual infection of the dental pulp, giving rise to an *acute pulpitis*. During the early stages of pulpitis moderately severe pain may result from thermal changes, particularly with cold drinks. As more of the pulp becomes involved because of advanced caries, heat or reclining may stimulate the onset of even more severe and continuous pain. At this stage, damage to the pulp is irreversible, and treatment consists of either extraction or thorough removal of the remaining contents of the pulp chamber and root canals followed by sterilization and filling with an inert material (root canal therapy).

If the pulpitis is not treated, infection may spread beyond the apex of the tooth into the periodontal ligament, giving rise to pain on chewing or percussion. The most common manifestation of periapical disease is the *periapical granuloma*, a localized mass of chronic granulation tissue which slowly expands at the expense of the surrounding alveolar bone. The *chronic periapical granuloma* may present the above symptoms or may be asymptomatic. If allowed to persist untreated, the periapical granuloma may give rise to a *periapical cyst* or a *periapical abscess*—all three lesions appearing as radiolucent areas on roentgenograms. The acute periapical abscess may extend into the surrounding bone marrow, resulting in an *osteomyelitis*. More frequently, the abscess perforates the cortical plate and, following the path of least resistance, spreads through various tissue spaces, giving rise to cellulitis and bacteremia, or discharges into the oral cavity, into the maxillary sinus, or through the skin.

The symptoms produced by cellulitis depend on which tissue space is affected. For example, *Ludwig's angina* originates from an infected mandibular molar, involves the submaxillary space, and subsequently extends into the sublingual and submental spaces. Clinically, this is manifested by swelling of the floor of the mouth, elevation of the tongue, and difficulty in swallowing and breathing. With continued swelling, there may be edema of the glottis, necessitating an emergency tracheotomy. Spread of the infection to the parapharyngeal spaces may lead to cavernous sinus thrombosis.

PERIODONTAL DISEASE

After the third decade chronic destructive periodontal disease *(periodontitis)* is responsible for the loss of more teeth than dental caries. It begins as a marginal inflammation of the gingivae (gingivitis), which slowly spreads to involve the underlying alveolar bone and periodontal ligament. As the disease progresses, the alveolar bone is resorbed, resulting in loss of periodontal ligament fiber attachment from the tooth to the bone. The separation of the soft tissue from the tooth surface results in "pocket" formation, the inner aspect of which bleeds readily on probing or spontaneously during chewing. Frank pus sometimes exudes from under the gingival margin, accounting for the use of the now outmoded term "pyorrhea." With continued loss of alveolar bone the involved teeth become mobile. As the periodontal pockets deepen, the pocket orifice may become occluded, leading to the formation of a *periodontal abscess*. The prognosis for teeth with advanced bone loss, extreme mobility, and recurrent abscess formation is usually poor or hopeless, and the usual treatment is extraction.

The most important local etiologic factors associated with this disease are thought to be *poor oral hygiene*, resulting in the accumulation of grossly visible adherent masses of bacteria *(bacterial plaque)*, calculus (mineralized bacterial plaque), and food impaction. The margins of overextended fillings also play a role as local irritating factors. Occlusal trauma, particularly trauma due to grinding and clenching habits, may be involved. Therapy is aimed at elimination of these factors and the development of a local environment which can be maintained in health by good oral hygiene.

Systemic factors are thought to modify the response of the host to the local factors, but their nature is more obscure. Reduced neutrophil functions, such as chemotaxis and phagocytosis, appear to predispose to *juvenile periodontitis*, a form of periodontitis characterized by early and severe alveolar bone loss. Similar periodontal destruction is found in youngsters with the *Papillon-Lefèvre syndrome*, which includes keratotic lesions of the palms and soles. Individuals with *Down's syndrome* seem to be particularly susceptible to periodontal disease and may demonstrate advanced alveolar bone loss around the permanent mandibular incisors and maxillary first molars. Severe chronic periodontal disease may be present in uncontrolled *diabetes mellitus*. In some instances, however, there are characteristic alterations in the gingiva in response to a number of specific systemic conditions. For example, during *pregnancy* the gingiva may become edematous and friable, with a raspberry-like appearance of the interdental papillae. Occasionally, a tumorlike mass may develop in an interdental area; this usually regresses following parturition. Oral contraceptives may lead to an increase in gingival inflammation. The use of the anticonvulsant drug *phenytoin* (Dilantin) frequently results in fibrous hyperplasia of the gingiva, which may actually cover the teeth, interfere with mastication, and cause a serious aesthetic problem. A similar clinical picture, although usually more generalized and extensive, occurs in *idiopathic familial fibromatosis*. The latter condition appears to be hereditary.

A relatively common gingival disease, found predominantly in young adults, is *acute necrotizing ulcerative gingivitis* (Vincent's infection, trench mouth). This disease is characterized by tender or painful gingivae, bleeding on pressure, and the pathognomonic sign of papillary or marginal gingival necrosis and ulceration. Clinical evidence suggests that the cause of this disease has a psychosomatic component. Vincent's infection differs from *acute herpetic gingivostomatitis*, with which it is most frequently confused, in that fever or malaise rarely develops, and patients respond rapidly to penicillin or broad-spectrum antibiotics.

It should be noted that both infected periapical lesions and periodontal disease provide potential sources of infection which may spread to other sites. Transient bacteremias have been demonstrated after simple massage of inflamed gingivae or use of an oral irrigative device, as well as during tooth extraction. The frequent association of tooth extraction with the subsequent occurrence of subacute bacterial endocarditis has led to the prophylactic use of antibiotics in dental patients with a history of rheumatic fever or other evidence of valvular disease. Similar precautions should be taken with dental patients having heart valve or joint prostheses. Prophylactic extraction of healthy teeth in leukemic patients is not justified.

DISEASES OF THE ORAL MUCOSA AND TONGUE

HEMATOLOGIC DISTURBANCES Oral manifestations are common in both the acute and chronic forms of all types of leukemia, particularly *monocytic leukemia*. They consist of local gingival bleeding, enlargement, and necrosis. Petechiae and ulceration of the oral mucosa may also be evident. Extensive ulcerations of the gingivae, buccal mucosa, lips, soft palate, pharynx, and tonsils may also occur in *agranulocytosis*. In thrombocytopenic states multiple petechiae, ecchymoses, and bleeding gingivae may be observed. The mucous membranes of the oral cavity, including the papillae of the tongue, are atrophic in the *Plummer-Vinson syndrome* (see Chaps. 34 and 289). As a result, the tongue is red, smooth, and sore, and there is difficulty in swallowing. Of interest is the finding that the atrophic mucous membranes have a predisposition toward the development of oral carcinoma. The oral symptoms in *pernicious anemia* are similar (see Chap. 311). Ulceration, mucositis, xerostomia, and infection (bacterial or fungal) are relatively common oral complications among patients receiving chemotherapy and/or radiotherapy for malignancies not involving the head or neck.

VITAMIN DEFICIENCIES *The oral effects of deficiency of the B group of vitamins* involve the soft tissues primarily, giving rise to reddening and ulceration of the oral mucosa and tongue, swelling and burning of the tongue, and fissuring at the corners of the lips (*angular cheilosis*). Severe vitamin C deficiency (*scurvy*) is manifested by petechiae in the oral mucosa; swollen, ulcerated, bleeding gingivae; and loosening of teeth.

PIGMENTATIONS (See Table 33-1) The spread of irregular spots or blotches or brown pigment throughout the oral mucosa, primarily the buccal mucosa, may be the first sign of *Addison's disease*. The pigmentation associated with the *Peutz-Jeghers syndrome* is readily differentiated because of its characteristic distribution around the lips, eyes, and nostrils, as well

TABLE 33-1
Pigmented lesions of the oral mucosa

Condition	Usual location	Clinical features	Course
Black, hairy tongue	Dorsum of tongue	Elongation of filiform papillae of tongue, which take on a brown to black coloration	Long-lasting but may disappear spontaneously
Heavy metal pigmentation (bismuth, mercury, lead)	Gingival margin	Thin blue-black pigmented line along gingival margin due to prior treatment for syphilis with bismuth or mercury or from accidental absorption of lead	Long-lasting
Drug ingestion (tranquilizers, oral contraceptives, antimalarials)	Any area in mouth	Brown, black, or gray areas of pigmentation	Disappears following cessation of drug
Amalgam tattoo	Gingiva and mucobuccal fold	Small blue-black pigmented areas associated with embedded amalgam particles in soft tissues; these will show up on radiographs as radiopaque particles	Remains indefinitely
Fordyce's disease	Buccal and labial mucosa	Aggregation of numerous, small yellowish spots just beneath mucosal surface; no subjective symptoms	Remains without apparent change indefinitely
Addison's disease	Any area in mouth but mostly on buccal mucosa	Blotches or spots of bluish black to dark brown pigmentation occurring early in the disease accompanied by diffuse pigmentation of skin; other symptoms of adrenal insufficiency	Condition controlled by steroid therapy
Peutz-Jeghers syndrome	Any area in mouth	Dark brown spots on lips, buccal mucosa, and palate with characteristic distribution of pigment around lips, nose, eyes, and on hands; concomitant intestinal polyposis	Lesions remaining indefinitely
Malignant melanoma	Any area in mouth	May appear as a raised, painless, brown-black lesion or may be amelanotic; may be ulcerated and infected	Early metastasis leading to death

TABLE 33-2
Vesicular, bullous, or ulcerative lesions of the oral mucosa

Condition	Usual location	Clinical features	Course
VIRAL DISEASES			
Acute herpetic gingivostomatitis (herpes simplex, type I)	Lip and oral mucosa	Labial vesicles which rupture and crust, and intraoral vesicles which quickly ulcerate; extremely painful to pressure; acute gingivitis, fever, malaise, foul odor, and cervical lymphadenopathy; occurs primarily in infants and children	Heals spontaneously in 10–14 days unless secondarily infected
Recurrent herpes labialis	Mucocutaneous junction of lip	Eruption of groups of vesicles which may coalesce, then rupture and crust; painful to pressure or spicy foods	Lasts about 1 week, but condition may be prolonged if secondary infection occurs
Primary herpes, type II	Mouth, oral pharynx, and genitalia	Large, painful, discrete vesicles on zone of erythema; anterior cervical glands enlarged	Lasts several weeks; may recur
Herpangina (coxsackievirus A; also possibly coxsackievirus B and echovirus)	Oral mucosa, pharynx, tongue	Sudden onset of fever, sore throat, and oropharyngeal vesicles usually in children under 4 years, during summer months; diffuse pharyngeal injection and vesicles (1–2 mm), grayish white surrounded by red areola; vesicles enlarge and ulcerate	Incubation period 2–9 days; fever for 1–4 days; recovery uneventful
Hand, foot, and mouth disease (type A coxsackieviruses)	Oral mucosa, pharynx, palms, and soles	Fever, malaise, headache with oropharyngeal vesicles which become painful, shallow ulcers	Incubation period 2–18 days; lesions heal spontaneously in 2–4 weeks
Chickenpox	Gingiva and oral mucosa	Skin lesions may be accompanied by small vesicles on oral mucosa that rupture to form shallow ulcers; may coalesce to form large bullous lesions that ulcerate; mucosa may have generalized erythema	Lesions heal spontaneously within 2 weeks
Herpes zoster	Cheek, tongue, gingiva, or palate	Unilateral vesicular eruption and ulceration in linear pattern following sensory distribution of trigeminal nerve	Gradual healing without scarring
Infectious mononucleosis	Oral mucosa	Fatigue, sore throat, malaise, low-grade fever, and enlarged cervical lymph nodes; numerous small ulcers usually appear several days before lymphadenopathy; gingival bleeding and multiple petechiae at junction of hard and soft palates	Oral lesions disappear during convalescence
Warts	Any place on skin and oral mucosa, primarily lips and vestibule	Single or multiple papillary lesions, with thick, white, keratinized surfaces containing many pointed projections	Lesions grow rapidly and spread
BACTERIAL OR FUNGAL DISEASES			
Acute necrotizing ulcerative gingivitis ("trench mouth," Vincent's infection)	Gingiva	Painful, bleeding gingiva characterized by necrosis and ulceration of gingival papillae and margins plus lymphadenopathy and foul odor	Continued destruction of tissue followed by remission, but may recur
Prenatal (congenital) syphilis	Palate, jaws, tongue, and teeth	Gummatous involvement of palate, jaws, and facial bones; Hutchinson's incisors, mulberry molars, glossitis, mucous patches, and fissures of corners of mouth	Tooth deformities in permanent dentition irreversible
Primary syphilis (chancre)	Lesion appears where organism enters body; may occur on lips, tongue, or tonsillar area	Small papule developing rapidly into a large, painless ulcer with indurated border; unilateral lymphadenopathy; chancre and lymph nodes containing spirochetes; serologic tests positive by third to fourth weeks	Healing of chancre in 1–2 months, followed by secondary syphilis in 6–8 weeks
Secondary syphilis	Oral mucosa frequently involved with mucous patches, primarily on palate but also at commissures of mouth	Maculopapular lesions of oral mucosa, about 5–10 mm in diameter with central ulceration covered by grayish membrane; eruptions occurring on various mucosal surfaces and skin accompanied by fever, malaise, and sore throat	Lesions may persist from several weeks to a year
Tertiary syphilis	Palate and tongue	Gummatous infiltration of palate or tongue followed by ulceration and fibrosis; atrophy of tongue papillae may produce characteristic bald tongue and glossitis	Gumma may destroy palate, causing complete perforation
Gonorrhea	Lesions may occur in mouth at site of inoculation or secondarily by hematogenous spread from a primary focus elsewhere	Earliest symptoms are burning or itching sensation, dryness, or heat in mouth followed by acute pain on eating or speaking; tonsils and oropharynx most frequently involved; oral tissues may be diffusely inflamed or ulcerated; saliva develops increased viscosity and fetid odor; submaxillary lymphadenopathy with fever in severe cases	Lesions resolve with appropriate antibiotic therapy
Tuberculosis	Tongue, tonsillar area, soft palate	A solitary, irregular ulcer covered by a persistent exudate; ulcer has an undermined, indurated border	Lesion may persist
Cervicofacial actinomycosis	Swellings in region of face, neck, and floor of mouth	Infection may be associated with an extraction, jaw fracture, or eruption of molar tooth; in acute form resembles an acute pyogenic abscess, but contains yellow "sulfur granules" (gram-positive mycelia and their hyphae)	Acute form may last a few weeks; chronic form lasts months or years; prognosis excellent; actinomycetes respond to antibiotics (tetracyclines or penicillin) but not to antifungal drugs

TABLE 33-2 (continued)
Vesicular, bullous, or ulcerative lesions of the oral mucosa

Condition	Usual location	Clinical features	Course
BACTERIAL OR FUNGAL DISEASES (continued)			
Histoplasmosis	Any area in mouth, particularly tongue, gingiva, or palate	Numerous small nodules which may ulcerate; hoarseness and dysphagia may occur because of lesions in larynx, usually associated with fever and malaise	May be fatal
DERMATOLOGIC DISEASES			
Mucous membrane pemphigoid	Primarily mucous membranes of the oral cavity, but may also involve the eyes, urethra, vagina, and rectum	Painful, grayish white collapsed vesicles or bullae with peripheral erythematous zone; gingival lesions desquamate, leaving ulcerated area	Protracted course with remissions and exacerbations; involvement of different sites occurs slowly; corticosteroids may control severe cases
Erythema multiforme (Stevens-Johnson syndrome)	Primarily the oral mucosa and skin of hands and feet	Intraoral ruptured bullae surrounded by an inflammatory area; lips may show hemorrhagic crusts; the "iris" or "target" lesion on the skin is pathognomonic; patient may have severe signs of toxicity	Onset very rapid; condition may last 1–2 weeks; may be fatal
Pemphigus vulgaris	Oral mucosa and skin	Ruptured bullae and ulcerated oral areas; mostly in older adults	With repeated recurrence of bullae, toxicity may lead to cachexia, infection, and death within 2 years
NEOPLASTIC DISEASES			
Squamous cell carcinoma	Any area in mouth, most commonly on lower lip, tongue, and floor of mouth	Ulcer with elevated, indurated border; failure to heal, pain not prominent; lesions tend to arise in areas of leukoplakia or in smooth or atrophic tongue	Invades and destroys underlying tissues or may metastasize to regional lymph nodes
Acute leukemia	Gingiva	Gingival swelling and superficial ulcerations followed by hyperplasia of gingiva with extensive necrosis and hemorrhage; deep ulcers may occur elsewhere on the mucosa complicated by secondary infection	Fatal
Lymphosarcoma	Gingiva, palate, tongue, and tonsillar area	Elevated, ulcerated area which may proliferate rapidly, giving the appearance of a traumatic inflammatory lesion; swelling of regional lymph nodes	Fatal
OTHER CONDITIONS			
Recurrent aphthous stomatitis	Any place on oral mucosa	Single or clusters of painful ulcers with surrounding erythematous border, found anywhere on mucosa; lesions may be 1–15 mm in diameter	Lesions heal in 1–2 weeks but may recur monthly or several times a year
Behçet's syndrome	Oral mucosa, eyes, and genitalia	Multiple aphthouslike ulcers in mouth; inflammatory ocular changes and ulcerative lesions on genitalia	Ulcers may persist for several weeks and heal without scarring
Traumatic ulcers	Any place on oral mucosa; dentures frequently responsible for ulcers in vestibule	Localized, discrete ulcerated lesion with red border; produced by accidental biting of mucosa, penetration by a foreign object, or chronic irritation by a denture	Lesion usually heals in 7–10 days when irritant is removed, unless secondarily infected

TABLE 33-3
White lesions of oral mucosa

Condition	Usual location	Clinical features	Course
Pachyderma oris	Any area in mouth	Elevated white lesion due to hyperkeratosis and thickening of the oral epithelium secondary to chronic irritation	Removal of irritant leads to healing in 2–3 weeks
Leukoplakia	Any area in mouth	White patch or raised plaque with sharply defined borders; in more severe cases the lesion is indurated and rough, and may be fissured and eroded; pain not present in early lesions	Carcinoma frequently arises in the more severe type of lesion
Lichen planus	Any area in mouth but most often on buccal mucosa	Varied appearance of lesion due to arrangement of grayish white papules which coalesce to make up the pattern; a reticular network is most common; oral lesions may precede skin lesions	May disappear spontaneously
Moniliasis (thrush)	Any area in mouth	Creamy white curdlike patches which reveal a raw, bleeding surface when scraped; found in sick infants, debilitated elderly patients, or patients receiving high doses of corticosteroids or broad-spectrum antibiotics	Responds favorably to antifungal therapy after correction of predisposing causes
Chemical burns	Any area in mouth	White slough due to necrosis of epithelium and underlying connective tissue caused by contact with agents (e.g., aspirin) applied locally or the use of undiluted sodium perborate or hydrogen peroxide as a mouthwash; removal of slough leaves a raw, painful surface	Lesion heals in several weeks if not secondarily infected

as its intraoral distribution. Both *lead poisoning* and *bismuth poisoning* may be manifested by a dark line along the gingival margin, particularly in individuals who have poor oral hygiene. Bismuth poisoning may also demonstrate pigmented patches elsewhere in the oral mucosa.

INFECTIONS   See Tables 33-2 and 33-3.

DERMATOLOGIC DISEASES   See Tables 33-2 and 33-3 and Chaps. 48 to 52.

TONGUE ALTERATIONS   See Table 33-4.

MALODOROUS BREATH   A distinctly unpleasant odor of the breath (halitosis) may emanate from any patient with *infections of the upper part of the respiratory tract*, especially in bronchiectasis and lung abscess. Halitosis may occur with oral sepsis as in *stomatitis, gingivitis,* or extensive *caries.* Some persons who smoke excessively may have halitosis. Occasionally otherwise normal persons will have halitosis without obvious cause. A *fishy odor* of the breath is found in patients with hepatic failure, an *ammoniacal or urinary odor* is found in azotemia, and a *sweet, fruity odor* is typical of diabetic acidosis.

DISEASES OF THE SALIVARY GLANDS

Conditions affecting the salivary glands include mumps parotitis (Chap. 188), Mikulicz's disease, Sjögren's syndrome (Chap. 356), and sarcoidosis. Inflammation of the salivary glands (*sialadenitis*) is usually associated with the presence of a salivary stone (*sialolithiasis*) in the duct of one of the major salivary glands. The classic history of pain and swelling of the gland at mealtimes is due to the partial blockage of salivary flow by the

stone. Localization of the stone may be accomplished by palpation or by roentgenograms with or without the use of an intraductal injection of radiopaque material (*sialography*). Acute or recurrent parotitis, with or without a defined microorganism, may occur in children and is marked by sudden onset of swelling of the whole gland or side of the face, accompanied by suppuration from Stensen's duct.

Xerostomia, or dryness of the mouth, is due to salivary gland dysfunction and may be temporary or permanent. Among the factors which cause temporary dryness are emotional factors (such as fear), infection of the glands, and administration of drugs, such as atropine, antihistamines, or tricyclic antidepressants and phenothiazines. Radiation of the area may produce a more permanent xerostomia because of atrophy of the glands. A similar dryness may occur in Sjögren's syndrome. The dry mouth may give rise to rampant caries, particularly if sugar-containing candies are sucked in an attempt to stimulate salivary flow. Extensive dental caries, especially around the gum margins of the teeth, may be seen in drug addicts and alcoholics, presumably due to xerostomia and lack of oral hygiene and dental care. Xerostomia-induced caries may be prevented or arrested by the daily topical application of a 1% sodium fluoride gel.

Benign or malignant tumors may arise in the major or minor salivary glands. The benign *mixed tumor* accounts for the vast majority of all salivary gland tumors and has a relatively high recurrence rate. Malignant tumors of the parotid gland may affect the facial nerve.

ORAL CANCER

Oral cancer constitutes more than 5 percent of all human cancers. *Squamous cell carcinoma* is the most common malignant oral tumor, accounting for approximately 90 to 95 percent of all oral malignant tumors. Most of these tumors occur on the lips, primarily the lower lip, rather than intraorally. About half the intraoral tumors involve the tongue, primarily the posterior two-thirds and the lateral borders. The major etiologic factor in lip cancer appears to be exposure to intense sunlight. Predisposing factors for intraoral carcinoma include tobacco (usually in the form of cigar or pipe smoking, or snuff placed in the mucobuccal fold), excessive consumption of alcohol, syphilitic glossitis, and the atrophic mucosa of the Plummer-Vinson syndrome. Although numerous instances of carcinoma of the tongue adjacent to a sharp tooth or dental appliance have been reported, animal studies with chronic irritation per se, as well as epidemiologic studies, cast doubt on this apparent relationship. The most common *precancerous lesion* in the oral cavity is *leukoplakia,* a whitish patch on the mucosa that histologically shows hyperkeratosis, acanthosis, and dyskeratosis. Recent evidence suggests that the asymptomatic, red velvety (erythroplastic) lesion of the floor of the mouth, ventrolateral aspect of the tongue, or soft palate–anterior pillar complex is more likely to be carcinoma in situ or invasive carcinoma than is the white lesion. *All chronic ulcerative lesions which fail to heal within 1 to 2 weeks should be considered potentially malignant* and must be biopsied in order to make the definitive diagnosis. It is noteworthy that in their early stages intraoral epidermoid carcinomas are rarely painful, in contrast to similar-appearing inflammatory lesions.

The prognosis for patients with carcinoma of the lip is usually good, since these malignant tumors are noted sooner and apparently metastasize later. Patients with carcinoma of the tongue have a poorer prognosis, particularly as the tumor occurs more posteriorly on the tongue. Intraoral carcinomas may

TABLE 33-4
Alterations of the tongue

Type of change	Clinical features
SIZE OR MORPHOLOGY CHANGES	
Macroglossia	Enlarged tongue which may be part of a syndrome found in developmental conditions such as Down's syndrome; may be due to tumor (hemangioma or lymphangioma), metabolic disease (such as primary amyloidosis), or endocrine disturbance (such as acromegaly or cretinism)
Fissured ("scrotal") tongue	Dorsal surface and sides of tongue covered by painless shallow or deep fissures which may collect debris and become irritated
Median rhomboid glossitis	Congenital abnormality of tongue with ovoid, denuded area in the median posterior portion of the tongue
COLOR CHANGES	
"Geographic" tongue ("wandering rash")	Asymptomatic inflammatory condition of the tongue, with rapid loss and regrowth of filiform papillae, leading to appearance of denuded red patches "wandering" across the surface of the tongue
Hairy tongue	Elongation of filiform papillae of the medial dorsal surface area due to failure of keratin layer of the papillae to desquamate normally; brownish black coloration may be due to staining by tobacco, food, or chromogenic organisms
"Strawberry" and "raspberry" tongue	Appearance of tongue during scarlet fever due to the hypertrophy of fungiform papillae plus changes in the filiform papillae
"Bald" tongue	Complete atrophy of papillae which may occur in pernicious anemia, severe iron-deficiency anemia, pellagra, or syphilis; may be accompanied by painful, burning sensations

spread by direct invasion to the underlying bone. Depending on the site of origin of the intraoral carcinoma, metastases usually spread to the submaxillary or cervical lymph nodes. Death may result from recurrent or uncontrollable disease above the clavicles; metastatic disease beyond the neck; treatment complications; or a second primary cancer, usually in the oral cavity or the upper parts of the gastrointestinal or respiratory tract.

NEUROLOGIC DISTURBANCES

A number of neurologic disturbances have a direct effect on oral and paraoral structures. *Trigeminal neuralgia* (tic douloureux) is an example of a syndrome involving the trigeminal nerve. It is characterized by extremely severe, unilateral, lancinating pain of the face occurring spontaneously or set off by pressure on a "trigger zone" on the face (see Chap. 376). Facial palsy is a unilateral disturbance of the motor branch of the facial nerve due to either trauma, surgical sectioning, or tumor involvement. When it is of acute onset and unknown cause, possibly a localized infection in the nerve, it is called *Bell's palsy*. It may be due to cranial herpes zoster in some instances. The condition is manifested by drooping of the corner of the mouth, inability to close the eye on the same side, and difficulty in speech and eating. In mild cases the symptoms may disappear spontaneously within a month. Alteration in taste sensation in the anterior two-thirds of the tongue due to disturbance of the sensory component of the facial nerve occurs in some cases and indicates a more central location of the lesion in the nerve (see Chap. 376).

The pain associated with the *glossopharyngeal neuralgia syndrome* is similar in type and intensity to that found in trigeminal neuralgia, being set off by a trigger zone in the pharynx and affecting the posterior region of the tongue, pharynx, soft palate, and ear. Disturbance of the hypoglossal nerve leads to dysfunction of the tongue musculature and atrophy. Bilateral nerve involvement prevents protrusion of the tongue; unilateral involvement leads to deviation of the protruded tongue toward the affected side.

DISTURBANCES OF THE TEMPOROMANDIBULAR JOINT

Pain in the area of the temporomandibular joint frequently causes the patient to seek therapy. It may be due to posterior displacement of the condyle in the fossa leading to displacement of the meniscus and chronic trauma. *Dislocation of the condyle anteriorly* beyond the articular eminence due to sudden stretching or tearing of the capsular ligament may result in a locking of the mandible in an open position. In *osteoarthritis* the clinical signs and symptoms may be minimal despite extensive changes in the condyle. Temporomandibular joint involvement occurs less frequently in *rheumatoid arthritis*. When affected, the joints are swollen and painful, leading to limitation of movement, particularly on arising in the morning. In children the disease may lead to malocclusion. *Ankylosis* on the joint may occur eventually, necessitating a condylectomy (see Chap. 356).

The myofascial pain syndrome, the most common disorder of the temporomandibular joint, is characterized by facial pain and mandibular dysfunction. The pain is often localized in the ear or jaw and may extend to the neck and shoulder. The mandibular dysfunction is manifested by limitation of movement, particularly an inability to open the jaw to the fullest extent. It is thought that such patients have increased musculature tension and hyperexcitable reflexes related to emotional tension. The precipitating factor appears to be the stretching of

an abnormal focus of pain which initiates a self-sustaining pain-spasm-pain cycle. Treatment of the pain-dysfunction syndrome involves the use of drugs to relieve the pain, lessen cortical excitability, and relax the muscles. Local anesthetics are used intramuscularly in the region of the trigger zone or as superficial sprays in an attempt to break the pain-spasm-pain cycle.

REFERENCES

BHASKAR SN: *Synopsis of Oral Pathology*, 5th ed. St Louis, Mosby, 1977

CIANCIOLA LJ et al: Defective polymorphonuclear leukocyte function in a human periodontal disease. Nature 265:445, 1977

GOLDMAN HM, COHEN DW (eds): *Periodontal Therapy*, 6th ed. St Louis, Mosby, 1978

MASHBERG A: Erythroplasia: The earliest sign of asymptomatic oral cancer. J Am Dent Assoc 96:615, 1978

SHAFER WG et al: *A Textbook of Oral Pathology,* 3d ed. Philadelphia, Saunders, 1974

SHAW JH et al: *Textbook of Oral Biology.* Philadelphia, Saunders, 1978

SHKLAR G, McCARTHY PL: *The Oral Manifestations of Systemic Disease.* Woburn, Mass, Butterworths, 1976

34
DYSPHAGIA

THOMAS R. HENDRIX

Dysphagia, or difficulty in swallowing, is a most reliable symptom and indicates the presence of disease or dysfunction. Dysphagia should never be dismissed as an emotional disturbance or be confused with globus hystericus, a term used to indicate the sensation of a lump or tightness in the throat independent of swallowing.

The most characteristic manifestation of dysphagia is the sensation of food "sticking" somewhere in its passage to the stomach, usually at the level of the obstruction but sometimes referred to the suprasternal notch, even though the obstruction may be at the lower end of the esophagus. Pain may accompany dysphagia, especially if esophageal spasm is induced by the peristaltic waves attempting to force the bolus through the obstruction. If the pain is mild, it tends to be localized to the site of obstruction; if more severe, it radiates more widely, into the base of the neck, angles of the jaw, arms, epigastrium, or back. Sometimes pain, in a sense, may even cause dysphagia, as when the throat is so sore that swallowing is difficult. For further details regarding these symptoms, see Chap. 289.

Normal swallowing is a complex function dependent upon coordination of voluntary muscular structures of the oropharynx, striated muscles protecting the larynx and respiratory passages, as well as relaxation of the esophageal sphincters and the peristaltic wave itself; hence dysphagia may occur as a consequence of derangement or incoordination of any of the elements of the swallowing act as well as narrowing of the lumen by inflammatory stricture or tumor.

For clinical purposes it is useful to consider dysphagia as having either an oropharyngeal or an esophageal origin, because symptoms, etiology, and treatment are usually different for the two types.

OROPHARYNGEAL DYSPHAGIA Symptoms associated with dysphagia caused by disorders of oropharyngeal structures include aspiration with swallowing, regurgitation of fluid into the nose, pharyngeal pain with swallowing, and inability of the tongue to move the bolus into the pharynx. Dilatation and atony of piriform sinuses and pharynx and retention of contrast media in the valleculae are characteristic radiographic findings in patients with pharyngeal dysfunction. In addition, aspiration of contrast medium into the trachea or regurgitation into the nasopharynx and apparent obstruction at the upper esophageal sphincter (cricopharyngeus) may be found.

Neuromuscular disorders are the most common causes of oropharyngeal dysphagia, which, however, is usually only part of the symptom complex. Examples of these disorders are cerebrovascular accidents which cause pseudobulbar palsy (see Chap. 15) or bulbar palsy, poliomyelitis, motor system disease, diphtheritic polyneuritis, myasthenia gravis, myotonic dystrophies and restricted muscular dystrophies (oculopharyngeal and laryngoesophageal), and dermatomyositis. Ulcerative lesions such as pharyngitis, Vincent's angina, monilia stomatitis, viral infections with herpetic lesions, and retropharyngeal abscess interfere by causing pain and thereby inhibiting the initiation of deglutition. Plummer-Vinson syndrome (Paterson-Kelly syndrome, or sideropenic dysphagia) may also be listed here, since the difficulty in swallowing in this disorder resembles that due to a neuromuscular disorder, although pain may be an additional disturbing feature. Limited pathologic studies have shown both epithelial and muscle atrophy. It is clear that the dysphagia is not due to the characteristic web, or mucosal fold, of the anterior aspect of the cricopharyngeal area, because the web often persists long after the symptoms have been relieved by iron replacement.

Oropharyngeal dysphagia may be caused by narrowing of the lumen of the pharynx or upper esophagus by tumor, granulomatous disease, Zenker's diverticulum, or an enlarged thyroid.

ESOPHAGEAL DYSPHAGIA Symptoms indicating that the cause of dysphagia is to be found in the esophagus range from retrosternal fullness with swallowing to failure of the bolus to pass through the esophagus associated with pain relieved only by regurgitation of the offending bolus. Barium swallows in patients with dysphagia of esophageal origin show segmental narrowing of the esophageal lumen, failure of peristalsis, or both. Abnormalities of peristalsis may be characterized more precisely by intraluminal manometric studies.

Mechanical narrowing of the esophageal lumen is most frequently caused either by carcinoma of the squamous type, arising from the esophagus itself, or by adenocarcinoma of the cardia extending up into the esophagus. Rarely, benign tumors may reach sufficient size to cause dysphagia. Inflammatory strictures most commonly result from reflux esophagitis but are also caused by ingestion of corrosive substances, such as lye, or by trauma from foreign bodies or instrumentation. In addition, a lower esophageal ring may produce dysphagia by obstructing the esophageal lumen. Extrinsic pressure from aneurysms, vascular anomalies, mediastinal tumors, or paraesophageal diaphragmatic hernias may compress the esophageal lumen sufficiently to cause dysphagia. Finally, the motility disturbances associated with diffuse esophageal spasm, achalasia, and esophageal reflux may be the basis of dysphagia. Although esophageal peristalsis is absent in the majority of patients with scleroderma, dysphagia does not become a prominent symptom until reflux esophagitis has led to an inflammatory stricture.

DIFFERENTIAL DIAGNOSIS Determination of the basic mechanism responsible for dysphagia is usually a simple matter, but identification of the exact disorder responsible for it may be quite difficult. For example, cancer of the esophagus sometimes presents suddenly rather than gradually, and the roentgenogram may have a smooth, symmetric appearance such as is more commonly seen with benign stricture or achalasia; even esophagoscopy may be inconclusive, and biopsy

may yield deceptive results if the tissue shows only inflammatory reaction and does not include neoplastic cells. Similarly, neuromuscular disorders and disturbances of esophageal motility interfering with swallowing may be difficult to classify.

Certain symptoms associated with dysphagia, however, have diagnostic value. Hiccups, together with difficulty in swallowing, suggest a lesion at the terminal portion of the esophagus, such as carcinoma, achalasia, or hiatal hernia. Dysphagia followed, after an interval of some duration, by hoarseness usually means extension of a malignant growth beyond the walls of the esophagus and the involvement of a recurrent laryngeal nerve. When the hoarseness comes first and the dysphagia later, the primary lesion is almost always in the larynx. This combination of laryngeal and pharyngeal symptoms may also occur in polymyositis or dermatomyositis or with any disease causing bilateral involvement of vagus nerves or nuclei (poliomyelitis and polyneuritis). In motor system disease, the most common cause of a mixture of bulbar and pseudobulbar palsy, dysphagia is usually combined with dysphonia and dysarthria; the jaw jerk is hyperactive and the tongue atrophic. Dysphagia and unilateral wheezing virtually always indicate a mediastinal mass involving the esophagus and a main or large bronchus. Coughing with each swallow of food or drink means a fistulous communication between the esophagus and the trachea or a motor disorder in which the larynx is not effectively closed. Coughing occurring some time after swallowing may be due to regurgitation of food, most common in achalasia and Zenker's diverticulum.

DIAGNOSTIC PROCEDURES Examination of the mouth and pharynx should disclose those lesions which impede the transfer of food from the mouth to the esophagus, because of pain or mechanical interference. When lesions of the hypopharynx (e.g., *chronic abscess secondary to tuberculosis of the spine*) or of the larynx (e.g., *tuberculosis* or *carcinoma*) are suspected, examination with a mirror is necessary.

The most important diagnostic technique in the evaluation of dysphagia is a *barium swallow*, which makes it possible to determine whether dysphagia is caused by mechanical obstruction or by esophageal motor abnormality. Absence of esophageal peristalsis can best be demonstrated by barium swallows with the patient in Trendelenburg's position. If there is no peristalsis, barium will remain in the esophagus until the patient is tilted upright. Since the muscular action of the pharynx is so rapid, swallows must be recorded by *cineradiography*. Projection of the film at slow speed permits detection and analysis of abnormalities of pharyngeal function.

If barium swallow shows a lesion within the esophagus or a narrowing of the lumen, *esophagoscopy* is the most direct method for establishing the nature of the lesion. In addition to inspecting the lesion, one should perform biopsies and brushings of the lesion for cytologic examination to differentiate inflammatory from neoplastic lesions. A malignant stricture is not ruled out with certainty, however, if the biopsy shows only normal tissue or chronic inflammation, because tumors of the esophagus often spread beneath the mucosa and may be missed by a superficial biopsy. In such circumstances repeated biopsies or exfoliative cytologic examination is necessary. Cytologic studies by experienced personnel are very accurate in the diagnosis of esophageal cancer.

Since dysphagia usually is first experienced with solid food and only later with liquids, a normal swallow with liquid barium must not be taken as evidence that significant esophageal disease has been excluded. To simulate the situation in

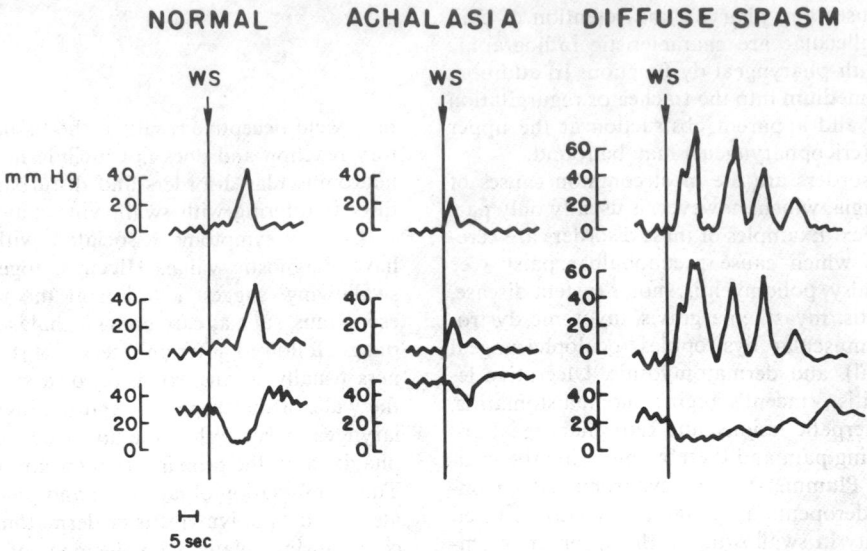

NORMAL   ACHALASIA   DIFFUSE SPASM

FIGURE 34-1

Esophageal manometric records from patients with normal esophageal function, achalasia, and diffuse esophageal spasm. Intraluminal pressure is recorded in the lower esophageal sphincter (lowest tracings) and 5 and 10 cm above the sphincter. Normally, a swallow of water (ws) is followed by relaxation of the lower esophageal sphincter, then the esophagus is cleared by a peristaltic wave proceeding abroad, and finally the sphincter closes. In achalasia, the resting pressure in the sphincter is elevated, and the sphincter does not relax completely in response to a swallow. The

simultaneous elevation of pressure in the esophagus is caused by the pharynx propelling the bolus into an esophagus that is closed because of incomplete relaxation of the sphincter. In diffuse spasm, a swallow triggers a simultaneous series of repetitive high-amplitude esophageal contractions. In this record sphincter pressure and relaxation are normal. Relaxation is prolonged in association with continuing motor activity in the body of the esophagus. Some patients with diffuse spasm have sphincter dysfunction with elevated pressure and intermittent incomplete relaxation.

which the patient experiences dysphagia, the passage of a solid bolus, such as a radiopaque marshmallow, is observed. A solid bolus swallow most often demonstrates peristaltic disorders missed by liquid swallow but occasionally provides the first indication of early cancer of the esophagus.

Motor abnormalities of the pharynx and esophagus may be suspected by viewing the movement of a swallowed radiopaque bolus by fluoroscopy, but to characterize these abnormalities definitely, the motor response of pharynx and esophagus to swallowing must be studied by recording intraluminal pressure from several points simultaneously. Records are best obtained by use of a train of water-filled, perfused catheters connected to external pressure transducers or strain gauges. Examination of manometric records of swallows will demonstrate whether the wave is normally propagated over the length of the esophagus, whether the pressure generated by the peristaltic wave is normal and sufficient to propel the bolus, and finally, whether sphincter relaxation is complete, of adequate duration, and properly coordinated with the peristaltic wave (Fig. 34-1). Combining manometric with cineradiographic techniques has added greatly to understanding pharyngoesophageal function.

REFERENCES

CASTELL DO et al: Dysphagia. Gastroenterology 76:1015, 1979

COHEN BR, WOLF BS: Cineradiographic and intraluminal pressure correlations in the pharynx and esophagus, in *Handbook of Physiology*, sec 6, vol IV, CF Code (ed). Washington, American Physiological Society, 1968, p 1841

KILMAN WJ, GOYAL RK: Disorders of pharyngeal and upper esophageal sphincter motor function. Arch Intern Med 136:592, 1976

MUKHOPADHYAY AK, GRAHAM DY: Esophageal motor dysfunction in systemic disease. Arch Intern Med 136:583, 1976

PHILLIPS MM, HENDRIX TR: Dysphagia. Postgrad Med 50:81, 1971

POPE CE: Esophageal motility—Who needs it? Gastroenterology 74:1337, 1978

35
INDIGESTION

KURT J. ISSELBACHER

Indigestion is a term frequently used by patients to describe a multitude of symptoms generally appreciated as distress associated with the intake of food. The term is thus nonspecific and may not have the same meaning for the patient and the physician. In approaching the patient with indigestion, it is important for the physician first to elicit a good description of this complaint. To some patients indigestion refers to a feeling that digestion has not proceeded naturally. They may describe a sense of abdominal fullness, pressure, or actual pain. Others may use the term to describe heartburn, belching, distention, or flatulence. These complaints are considered in this chapter. Discussed elsewhere are the closely related symptoms of dysphagia, nausea and vomiting, and anorexia (Chaps. 34 and 36).

Indigestion may occur as a result of disease of the gastrointestinal tract or in association with pathologic states in other organ systems. As a result of systematic clinical and laboratory tests, a definable pathophysiologic process often can be shown to be responsible for the symptoms in a given case of indigestion. Frequently, however, clear etiologic explanation for the patient's complaints of indigestion are not established. Such cases are often designated as "functional indigestion," with a strong implication that psychosomatic factors underlie the complaints. Although it is clear that psychic factors may lead to symptoms of indigestion, the designation of "functional indigestion" is rarely, if ever, a satisfactory explanation, serving only to rephrase the patient's description of the symptoms. A psychogenic cause should not be assumed until organic causes of indigestion have been thoroughly excluded.

After having ascertained the patient's definition of indigestion, it is also important to determine (1) the location and duration of the discomfort, (2) the temporal relation of the symptoms to the ingestion of food, and (3) the possible relation of the symptoms to the ingestion of specific types of food (e.g., fatty foods, milk, and drugs).

PAIN PATTERNS True visceral abdominal pain as seen in indigestion is mediated over visceral afferent nerves which accompany the abdominal sympathetic pathways (see Chap. 6). Visceral pain is generally described as dull and aching in nature (with a diffuse midline localization) or as fullness or pressure. The location of the discomfort corresponds generally to the segmental level of the affected organ. Abdominal visceral pain can be produced experimentally by artificially increasing pressure in a hollow viscus. Usually this pain is the result of distention or exaggerated muscular contraction of a viscus. Inflammation generally lowers the threshold to such stimuli.

The visceral pain of indigestion should be distinguished from the sharp, lateralized, and localized pain patterns seen in many acute abdominal processes involving the peritoneum. In contrast to true visceral pain, this pain is mediated over cerebrospinal afferent nerves. Again it is of a dull, aching type, whether from inflammation of the viscera or of peritoneal surfaces.

In view of the diffuse nature of true visceral abdominal pain, the main clue comes from the segmental level of the viscus; in any given segmental region there is no way of determining which of several viscera are the source of it (Table 35-1). The following rules, already given in Chap. 6, are useful: *Substernal pain* of gastrointestinal origin usually arises from disorders in the esophagus or cardia of the stomach. Because pain in this area is frequently of cardiac origin, heart disease must be considered carefully and excluded. *Epigastric pain* is generally of gastric, duodenal, biliary, or pancreatic origin. As the pathologic process in the biliary tract and pancreas becomes more intense, it tends to lateralize and localize, e.g., biliary pain to the right upper quadrant and tip of the right scapula and pancreatic pain to the epigastrium, left upper quadrant, and back. *Periumbilical pain* is generally associated with small-intestinal disease. *Pain below the umbilicus* is often of appendiceal, large-intestinal, or pelvic origin.

TEMPORAL RELATIONSHIPS OF PAIN AND INDIGESTION The unraveling of the temporal relationships of the patient's symptoms often provides the most significant diagnostic information. It is important to ascertain whether the symptoms are *constant* (continually present over extended periods of time), as may occur, for example, with an infiltrating gastric carcinoma, or *intermittent,* as in acute gastritis following an alcoholic binge or in association with the use of certain drugs. The symptoms may have a *diurnal* pattern; e.g., pain occurring *nocturnally* and with *recumbency* is seen in esophagitis and hiatus hernia. Symptoms are occasionally *seasonal;* this may occur in peptic ulcer disease, in which some patients experience more discomfort in the spring and autumn.

Another important and often diagnostic feature is the relation of pain or indigestion to ingestion of food. This relationship is especially significant or helpful if symptoms occur either during or minutes after the meal or if they occur several hours (4 or more) after eating. *Early postprandial symptoms* may reflect esophageal disease, because they may be associated with disordered swallowing function. In such instances, the distress or other symptoms of indigestion often are experienced substernally. Early postprandial complaints occur also in gastric disorders such as acute gastritis or carcinoma. *Late postprandial indigestion,* i.e., that occurring several hours after eating, may reflect failure of the stomach to empty adequately, as in pyloric stenosis or gastric atony. It may also be a symptom of duodenal ulcer, in which case it classically occurs several hours after the meal, when the ulcerated mucosa is exposed to acid secretions of the stomach unbuffered by food. Conversely,

the relief of pain following food ingestion is also seen in patients with peptic ulcer and is presumably due to the neutralization of the acid by the ingested food. Such pain also is typically alleviated quickly by oral antacids. Late postprandial indigestion also may result from impaired digestive and absorptive processes, as in pancreatic insufficiency.

FOOD INTOLERANCE In a number of situations specific foods or types of foods appear to be related to indigestion. Careful documentation of this relationship is sometimes of great help in arriving at an etiologic diagnosis.

Some foods may be poorly tolerated because of their consistency. Patients with esophageal stricture or carcinoma may tolerate liquids well, but the ingestion of solids may be associated with discomfort, especially substernal distress (see Chap. 289). Certain foods may be tolerated poorly because the intestinal tract cannot assimilate them adequately. This may occur following the ingestion of fatty foods in patients with pancreatic or biliary tract disease. Citrus fruits, with their relatively low pH, often provoke symptoms in patients with peptic ulcer disease.

Individuals may lack a specific enzyme required for assimilation of a certain nutrient. Patients may have a deficiency of the mucosal enzyme lactase, which catalyzes the hydrolysis of lactose. When lactase deficiency exists on a hereditary or acquired basis (e.g., in sprue, ulcerative colitis) (Chap. 292), the ingestion of milk (which contains lactose) results in abdominal cramps, distention, flatulence, and diarrhea.

There are a number of other conditions or disorders in which specific foods are poorly tolerated. Foods may be poorly tolerated because they initiate *allergic reactions* or exert a deleterious or *toxic effect* on the intestinal tract of susceptible persons (e.g., gluten in patients with nontropical sprue). Finally, certain substances may lead to systemic effects because of biochemical defects in the patient which render the substances particularly hazardous. An example of the latter is galactose intolerance in galactosemia (Chap. 98).

The above mechanisms do not explain the majority of clinical situations in which indigestion is associated with the eating of specific foods. For example, a history of fatty-food intolerance or an inability to eat cabbage, cucumbers, or spicy foods

TABLE 35-1
Distribution of visceral pain and examples of disorders frequently involving the specific organ

Organ	Location of referred pain	Frequent disorders
Esophagus	Substernum, epigastrium	Peptic esophagitis, hiatus hernia, stricture, carcinoma
Stomach	Epigastrium	Gastritis, peptic ulcer, carcinoma
Duodenum (first and second portions)	Epigastrium	Peptic ulcer
Duodenum (third portion, jejunum, and ileum)	Periumbilical	Regional enteritis, lymphoma, gastroenteritis (infectious), intestinal obstruction
Gallbladder	Epigastrium, right upper quadrant, right side of back	Cholelithiasis, cholecystitis
Pancreas	Epigastrium, left side of back	Pancreatitis, pancreatic carcinoma
Liver	Right upper quadrant	Passive congestion of liver, hepatitis, cirrhosis
Colon	Below umbilicus	Ulcerative colitis, carcinoma, partial obstruction

is commonly obtained from patients with indigestion. However, the mechanisms underlying the production of symptoms in these circumstances are still unclear.

ADDITIONAL SYNDROMES COMMONLY DESCRIBED AS INDIGESTION Gaseousness, flatulence, aerophagia A number of common clinical syndromes which may be described by the patient as "indigestion" appear to be related to increased quantities of gas in the intestinal tract. About 20 to 60 percent of intraluminal gas represents swallowed air. A degree of air swallowing, or *aerophagia,* occurs in normal persons, and the swallowed air can be observed at fluoroscopy. Under certain circumstances, such as chronic anxiety, poor eating habits, or actual intestinal disease itself, aerophagia may increase in magnitude and lead to symptoms in its own right.

The combination of early postprandial fullness and pressure, relieved by eructation and accompanied by a large amount of air seen in the gastric fundus on roentgenogram, is often referred to as the *magenblase* (i.e., gastric bubble) *syndrome.* Acute gastric distention by swallowed air can occasionally produce sharp pains which may mimic angina pectoris. This sequence of events may be especially perplexing in older patients with coronary artery disease, because it is well recognized that true angina pectoris may itself be precipitated by the ingestion of a large meal. Fatty meals delay gastric emptying and hence the passage of swallowed air in the intestine. This relationship may explain, in part, the prolonged sense of fullness and eructations experienced by many individuals after a fatty meal.

Swallowed air that is not eructated passes on in the intestinal tract and may either produce diffuse abdominal distention or become trapped in the splenic flexure of the colon. Distention of this segment of the colon produces a sensation of left upper quadrant fullness and pressure with radiation to the left side of the chest. This is known as the *splenic flexure syndrome.* Patients will often describe relief of pain with defecation or with the expulsion of flatus. Diagnosis may be made by demonstrating, on physical examination, a note of increased tympany in the extreme left lateral portion of the upper part of the abdomen or by the visualization of large amounts of air in the splenic flexure of the colon by radiography.

A second major source of intestinal gas is the fermentative action of bacteria on carbohydrates and proteins within the lumen. Increased amounts of intraluminal gas production due to this mechanism have been demonstrated in conditions associated with abnormal bacterial colonization of the small intestine and in patients with carbohydrate malabsorption.

Increased gas production may occur following the ingestion of certain foods (e.g., the legumes) which contain significant quantities of nonabsorbable sugars. As in the case of swallowed air, increased amounts of intraluminally produced gas can produce symptoms by causing distention, pain, increased motility (with diarrhea), or flatulence.

Heartburn Heartburn, or pyrosis, is a sensation of warmth or burning located substernally or high in the epigastrium. Experimental studies in human beings have shown that esophageal distention or increased motor activity is associated in most subjects with a feeling of fullness and burning in this area.

Heartburn may occur with organic disease of the intestinal tract and is usually associated with gastroesophageal reflux. This is frequently the case in hiatus hernia. In this setting, heartburn occurs after a large meal or with stooping or bending. Esophageal reflux of acid contents at these times leads to symptoms by either the production of abnormal motor activity or direct mucosal irritation (i.e., esophagitis). Heartburn may arise following the ingestion of certain foods or drugs (e.g.,

alcohol and aspirin). It may also be seen in the absence of a demonstrable anatomic or motor pathologic condition, in which case it is frequently accompanied by aerophagia and for lack of other explanation is often attributed to psychological factors.

INDIGESTION DUE TO DISEASE OUTSIDE THE INTESTINAL TRACT A multitude of extraintestinal disease processes may result in indigestion by mechanisms which are poorly understood. Indigestion may be the presenting complaint, for example, in congestive heart failure, uremia, pulmonary tuberculosis, and neoplastic disease. Under these circumstances the symptoms of indigestion may present with no unique features to suggest that they are in fact due to some other systemic disease process. Drugs such as aspirin, corticosteroids, indomethacin, and phenylbutazone affect gastric secretion and are ulcerogenic; thus they may lead to symptoms of indigestion.

DIAGNOSTIC APPROACH TO THE PATIENT WITH INDIGESTION Indigestion represents a challenging and difficult diagnostic problem because of the nonspecific nature of its manifestations. The evaluation of indigestion must include initially a thorough medical workup, with ultimate confirmation or exclusion of pathophysiologic derangements by the appropriate diagnostic procedures.

A careful history should include an assessment of the patient's general medical health, including the possibility of diseases in extraintestinal organ systems which may produce indigestion. Careful evaluation of psychological factors is crucial, because they often play an etiologic or contributory role in the patient's problem. Of particular importance are anxiety, depressive reactions, and hysteria (Chap. 11). Evaluation of the patient's intestinal problem must include an assessment of nutritional status, changes in weight, and appetite.

A clear and detailed description of the specific symptoms should be obtained, particularly the patient's definition of the term "indigestion." The nature of the pain, its frequency and time of occurrence, its relationship to meals, and the special circumstances which lead to its exacerbation or relief should be elicited. Associated intestinal symptoms such as nausea and vomiting, abnormal bowel habits, steatorrhea, diarrhea, and melena should also be sought. Physical examination rarely establishes the specific diagnosis, but it may be useful in detecting disease in other organ systems (e.g., congestive heart failure) which can affect intestinal physiology.

X-ray examination of the alimentary tract is crucial to the evaluation of indigestion. This may involve examination of the esophagus, stomach, small intestine, colon, and biliary tract. Esophagoscopy, gastroscopy, colonoscopy, or sigmoidoscopy also may be helpful or necessary. Stools should be examined for appearance, occult blood, fat, and muscle fibers. As stated above, careful attempts must be made to exclude nonintestinal disease, especially cardiac disease.

Unfortunately, even after completion of careful diagnostic studies, many cases of indigestion will turn out to have no clear explanation. Some of these are psychogenic and may respond to appropriate psychiatric measures. Others represent physiologic derangements which are undetectable by currently available diagnostic methods. Still others represent actual disease processes in early stages which may be diagnosable by conventional methods at a later date. The ultimate evaluation of indigestion requires, therefore, the utmost in sensitivity, diligence, and patience on the part of the examining physician.

REFERENCES

BOND JH, LEVITT MD: A rational approach to intestinal gas problems. Viewpoints Digestive Dis vol 9, no 2, 1977

COGHILL NF: Dyspepsia. Br Med J 4:97, 1967

Lasser RB et al: The role of intestinal gas in functional abdominal pain. N Engl J Med 293:524, 1975

Levitt MD: Methane production in the gut. N Engl J Med 291:528, 1974

36
ANOREXIA, NAUSEA, AND VOMITING

KURT J. ISSELBACHER

ANOREXIA Anorexia, or loss of the desire to eat, is a prominent symptom in a wide variety of intestinal and extraintestinal disorders. It must be clearly differentiated from satiety and from specific food intolerance. Anorexia occurs in many disorders and as a result *by itself is of little specific diagnostic value.* The mechanisms whereby hunger and appetite are modified in various disease states are poorly understood. Normally food intake is regulated by two hypothalamic centers—a lateral "feeding center" and a ventromedial "satiety center." The latter inhibits the feeding center following a meal leading to the sensation of satiety.

Anorexia is commonly seen in diseases of the gastrointestinal tract and liver. For example, it may precede the appearance of jaundice in hepatitis, or it may be a prominent symptom in gastric carcinoma. In the setting of intestinal disease, anorexia should be clearly differentiated from *sitophobia,* or fear of eating because of subsequent or associated discomfort. In such circumstances, appetite may persist, but the ingestion of food is curtailed nonetheless. Sitophobia may be seen, for example, in regional enteritis (especially with partial obstruction) or in patients with gastric ulcer following partial or total gastrectomy

Anorexia may also be a prominent feature of severe extraintestinal diseases. For example, anorexia may be profound in severe congestive heart failure and is often associated with cardiac glycoside intoxication. It may be a major symptom in patients with uremia, pulmonary failure, and various endocrinopathies (e.g., hyperparathyroidism, Addison's disease, and panhypopituitarism). Anorexia also often accompanies psychogenic disturbances, such as anxiety or depression. For a discussion of anorexia nervosa, see Chap. 77.

NAUSEA AND VOMITING Nausea and vomiting may occur independently of each other, but generally they are so closely allied that they may conveniently be considered together. *Nausea* denotes the feeling of the imminent desire to vomit, usually referred to the throat or epigastrium. *Vomiting* refers to the forceful oral expulsion of gastric contents; *retching* denotes the labored rhythmic respiratory activity that frequently precedes emesis. Extremely forceful *projectile vomiting* is a special form of vomiting which has significance because it connotes the presence of increased intracranial pressure.

Nausea often precedes or accompanies vomiting. It is usually associated with diminished functional activity of the stomach and alterations of the motility of the duodenum and small intestine. Accompanying severe nausea there is often evidence of altered autonomic (especially parasympathetic) activity: pallor of the skin, increased perspiration, salivation, and the occasional association of hypotension and bradycardia (vasovagal syndrome). Anorexia is also often present.

Following a period of nausea and a brief interval of retching, a sequence of involuntary visceral and somatic motor events occurs, resulting in emesis. The stomach plays a relatively passive role in the vomiting process, the major ejection force being provided by the abdominal musculature. With relaxation of the gastric fundus and gastroesophageal sphincter, a sharp increase in intraabdominal pressure is brought about by forceful contraction of the diaphragm and abdominal wall. This, together with concomitant annular contraction of the gastric pylorus, results in the expulsion of gastric contents into the esophagus. Increased intrathoracic pressure results in the further movement of esophageal contents into the mouth. Reversal of the normal direction of esophageal peristalsis may play a role in this process. Reflex elevation of the soft palate during the vomiting act prevents the entry of the material into the nasopharynx, whereas reflex closure of the glottis and inhibition of respiration help to prevent pulmonary aspiration.

Repeated emesis may have deleterious effects in a number of different ways. The process of vomiting itself may lead to traumatic rupture or tearing in the region of the cardioesophageal junction, resulting in massive hematemesis, the Mallory-Weiss syndrome. Prolonged vomiting may lead to dehydration and the loss of gastric secretions (especially hydrochloric acid), resulting in metabolic alkalosis with hypokalemia. Finally, in states of central nervous system depression (coma, etc.), gastric contents may be aspirated into the lungs, with a resulting aspiration pneumonitis.

Vomiting mechanism The act of vomiting is under the control of two functionally distinct medullary centers: the *vomiting center* and the *chemoreceptor trigger zone.* They lie close to each other near other brainstem centers regulating vasomotor and autonomic functions. The vomiting center controls and integrates the actual act of emesis. It receives afferent stimuli from the intestinal tract and other parts of the body, from higher cortical centers, especially the labyrinthine apparatus, and from the chemoreceptor trigger zone. The important efferent pathways in vomiting are the phrenic nerves (to the diaphragm), the spinal nerves (to the abdominal musculature), and visceral efferent nerves (to the stomach and esophagus).

The chemoreceptor trigger zone is also located in the medulla but by itself is incapable of mediating the act of vomiting. Activation of this zone results in efferent impulses to the medullary vomiting center, which in turn initiates the act of emesis. The chemoreceptor trigger zone can be activated by many stimuli, including drugs such as apomorphine, cardiac glycosides, and ergot alkaloids. Certain of the phenothiazine derivatives appear to antagonize the effects of the above-mentioned drugs on the chemoreceptor trigger zone.

Clinical classification Nausea and vomiting are common manifestations of organic and functional disorders. The precise mechanisms triggering vomiting in the various clinical states are poorly understood, making classification of mechanisms difficult. The categories mentioned below serve to illustrate some of the many disorders which may be accompanied by nausea and vomiting.

Many *acute abdominal emergencies* which lead to the "surgical abdomen" are associated with nausea and vomiting. Notably, vomiting may be seen with inflammation of a viscus as in acute appendicitis or acute cholecystitis, obstruction of the intestine, or acute peritonitis (see Chap. 6).

In many of the disorders involving *chronic indigestion* (see Chap. 35) nausea and vomiting may be prominent. Emesis may be either spontaneous or self-induced and may lead to relief of symptoms, as, for example, in uncomplicated peptic ulcer. Nausea and vomiting may accompany the distention and pain seen in the aerophagic syndromes. Often in patients with chronic indigestion, nausea and vomiting may be provoked by specific foods (e.g., fatty foods), for reasons that are poorly understood.

Acute systemic infections with fever, especially in young children, are frequently accompanied by vomiting and often by severe diarrhea. The mechanism whereby infections remote from the gastrointestinal tract produce these manifestations is unclear. Viral, bacterial, and parasitic infections of the intestinal tract may be associated with severe nausea and vomiting, often with diarrhea. Severe nausea and vomiting may be prominent in viral hepatitis, even before the appearance of jaundice.

Central nervous system disorders which lead to increased intracranial pressure may be accompanied by vomiting, often projectile. Brain swelling due to inflammation, anoxemia, acute hydrocephalus, neoplasms, etc., may thus be complicated by vomiting. Disorders of the labyrinthine apparatus and its central connections which underlie vertigo may be accompanied by vomiting with nausea and retching. Acute labyrinthitis and Ménière's disease are examples of such disturbances. Migraine headaches, tabetic crises, and acute meningitis are additional examples of disorders of the nervous system which may lead to vomiting. In the reactive phase of hypotension with syncope, there may also be nausea and vomiting.

Severe nausea and vomiting may be present in *acute myocardial infarction*, especially of the posterior wall of the heart. Nausea and vomiting may also be seen in *congestive heart failure*, perhaps in relation to congestion of the liver. The possibility that these symptoms may be due to drugs (e.g., opiates or digitalis) should always be borne in mind in patients with cardiac disease.

Nausea and vomiting commonly accompany several *endocrinologic disorders*, including diabetic acidosis and adrenal insufficiency, especially adrenal crises. The morning sickness of early pregnancy is another instance of nausea and vomiting possibly related to hormonal changes.

The *side effects of many drugs and chemicals* include nausea and vomiting. In some instances this is because of gastric irritation which stimulates the medullary vomiting center.

Psychogenic vomiting means vomiting which may occur as part of any emotional upset on a transitory basis or more persistently as part of a psychic disturbance. Close observation will usually disclose the condition to be one of regurgitation rather than of vomiting, and weight loss may not correspond at all to the patient's description of the frequency and severity of vomiting. As discussed in Chap. 77, anorexia nervosa is an emotional disturbance which may be associated not only with anorexia but also with vomiting. Often patients with emotional disorders and vomiting maintain a relatively normal state of nutrition because a relatively small amount of the ingested food is vomited.

Differential diagnosis Vomiting should be distinguished from *regurgitation,* which refers to the expulsion of food in the absence of nausea and without abdominal diaphragmatic muscular contraction which is part of vomiting. Regurgitation of esophageal contents may occur with esophageal stricture or diverticula. Regurgitation of gastric contents is generally seen with gastroesophageal sphincter incompetence, especially with hiatus hernia or in association with peptic ulcer, usually when pylorospasm supervenes.

The temporal relationships of vomiting to eating may be of help diagnostically. Vomiting which occurs predominantly in the morning is often seen early in pregnancy and uremia. Alcoholic gastritis is commonly accompanied by early-morning emesis, the so-called "dry heaves." Vomiting which occurs shortly after eating may suggest pylorospasm or gastritis. On the other hand, vomiting which occurs 4 to 6 h or longer after eating and involves the elimination of large quantities of undigested food

often indicates gastric retention (e.g., diabetic gastric atony or pyloric obstruction).

The character of the vomitus offers clues to the diagnosis. If the vomitus contains free hydrochloric acid, the obstruction may be due to an ulcer; absence of free hydrochloric acid is more compatible with gastric malignancy. A feculent or putrid odor reflects the results of bacterial action on the intestinal contents. Such vomiting may be seen with low-intestinal obstruction, peritonitis, or gastrocolic fistula. Bile is commonly present in gastric contents whenever vomiting is prolonged. It has no significance unless constantly present in large quantities, when it may signify an obstructive lesion below the ampulla of Vater. The presence of blood in the gastric contents usually denotes bleeding from the esophagus, stomach, or duodenum.

REFERENCES

HALL RJC: Normal and abnormal food intake. Gut 16:744, 1975

LUMSDEN K, HOLDEN SW: The act of vomiting in man. Gut 10:173, 1969

SWANSON DW et al: Persistent nausea without organic cause. Mayo Clin Proc 51:257, 1976

37
CONSTIPATION, DIARRHEA, AND DISTURBANCES OF ANORECTAL FUNCTION

STEPHEN E. GOLDFINGER

NORMAL COLONIC FUNCTION Each day one to two liters of semiliquid material composed of undigested dietary residue, intestinal secretions, and cellular debris passes across the ileocecal valve to the colon. Little of nutritional value remains following the extensive digestive processing and absorption that occurs in the small intestine. This liquid ileal effluent is converted to solid feces in the colon before it is advanced to the rectum and evacuated. To accomplish this, many important physiologic processes underly normal colonic function; among these are *absorption* of fluid and electrolytes; *peristaltic contractions* that facilitate mixing, dessication, and passage of feces to the rectum; and finally, *defecation.*

Absorption of fluid and electrolytes (see also Chap. 292) In Western societies the average daily stool weight is less than 200 g, of which 60 to 80 percent is water. Thus, the colon normally absorbs more than 90 percent of the fluid it receives, and this occurs well within its absorptive *capacity* of 6 liters water and 800 meq sodium per day. The primary absorptive sites are the ascending and transverse colon. Water absorption occurs passively, osmotically following the active transport of sodium and chloride ions. In addition, bicarbonate is secreted in exchange for chloride, and there is a small net efflux of potassium across the colonic mucosa into the lumen. The secreted bicarbonate is converted, in part, to carbon dioxide by reacting with acids produced by colonic bacteria. Analysis of fecal electrolyte concentrations in normal subjects reveals considerable variation, but average values for sodium, potassium, chloride, and bicarbonate are 32, 75, 16, and 40 meq per liter, respectively. The hyperosmolality of normal stool, which averages 375 mosmol, is largely due to osmotically active organic compounds produced by bacteria.

Factors which tend to cause diarrhea include:

1 Excessive outpouring of fluid from the small intestine into the colon. This may occur in association with viral and bacterial enteritis, various malabsorptive diseases of the small intestine, pancreatic tumors secreting gastrin or vasoactive intestinal peptide, and resection of the terminal ileum.

2 Reduced amount or deficient function of colonic mucosa (e.g., subtotal colectomy, diffuse ulcerative colitis).

3 Neural and hormonal stimuli which decrease to-and-fro peristalsis or promote massive propulsive activity (see below) and thus reduce mucosal surface contact time (e.g., exaggerated postprandial motility).

4 Impaired colonic reabsorption of water and electrolytes due to the presence of excessive bile salts and fatty acids. When ileal reabsorption of bile salts is defective (e.g., ileal resection, regional ileitis), increased amounts of dihydroxy bile salts reach the colon where they inhibit sodium absorption and promote secretion. Increased intraluminal hydroxylated fatty acids, which are present in sprue and pancreatic malabsorption, produce diarrhea by a similar effect upon mucosal cells.

5 Excessive colonic secretion distal to reabsorptive sites (e.g., villous adenoma of the rectum).

6 Increased luminal concentrations of nonabsorbed molecules exerting significant osmotic effect (e.g., magnesium-containing cathartics, lactose when individuals with lactase deficiency eat milk products).

Excessively hard stools are usually due to increased absorption of fluid as a result of prolonged contact of the luminal contents with the colonic mucosa consequent to delayed transit. In some instances ingested material such as calcium carbonate can explain "rock-like" feces.

Motility (contraction) patterns of the colon The colon and rectum are innervated by sympathetic and parasympathetic fibers, as well as by nonadrenergic, noncholinergic nerves that may release bioactive amines, peptides, or nucleotides. Impulses transmitted via these nerve fibers, local neural reflex arcs, and intrinsic contractile responses of smooth muscle all play a part in the coordination of colonic motility. Parasympathetic nerves, which stimulate peristaltic contraction, dominate the regulation of colonic motor activity; adrenergic tone inhibits cholinergic stimulation. The precise integration of all neural and nonneural mediators of colonic motility remains poorly understood.

Basal colonic motor activity consists mainly of nonpropulsive contractions of circular smooth muscle which move luminal contents back and forth across relatively short segments of bowel. Since no net aboral advance is achieved, it is presumed that the main purpose of these movements is to maximize mucosal surface contact for absorption. With increased parasympathetic tone, such as occurs postprandially, more propulsive activity occurs. This may take the form of aboral contractions across short segments of colon or involve massive peristalsis, which begins in the right or transverse colon and rapidly moves luminal contents to the sigmoid colon and rectum. Massive peristalsis may occur only several times a day. Resultant distention of the rectum initiates the defecatory urge.

Since colonic motility plays an important role in both absorption and movement of contents to the rectum, alterations of bowel tone occurring as a result of disease, stress, or various drugs tend to have an important influence on bowel movements. In view of the number of pharmacologic agents that may influence smooth muscle contractility, it is essential to take a careful drug history when evaluating patients with constipation or diarrhea of recent onset.

Defecation The defecatory reflex is initiated by acute distention of the rectum. When it is allowed to progress by supraspinal centers, sigmoidal and rectal contractions heighten the pressure within the rectum and also obliterate the rectosigmoi-

dal angle. Concomitant relaxation of the internal and external anal sphincters then permits the evacuation of feces. This can be augmented by an increase in intraabdominal pressure created by the Valsalva maneuver (i.e., voluntary closure of the glottis, diaphragmatic fixation, and abdominal-wall contraction). Conversely, defecation may be consciously prevented by the forceful contraction of the striated muscles of the pelvic diaphragm and external anal sphincter. The functional value of voluntary control of defecation requires little elaboration, but the opportunity for individuals to resist the defecatory urge, when abused, may lead to chronic rectal distention, reduced afferent signals, lax motor tone, and chronic constipation.

DIARRHEA AND CONSTIPATION The bowel habits of apparently healthy persons vary widely. For this reason, the terms *diarrhea* and *constipation* have most meaning when viewed as a change from an individual's customary pattern. Reasonably detailed information is important in evaluating either abnormality. When patients complain of diarrhea, it is important to obtain an estimate of the volume as well as frequency of fecal output and, in addition, to directly examine a stool sample for consistency, blood, oiliness, and malodor. For example, the repeated elimination of small quantities of solid material admixed with gas has a far different connotation than the same number of movements of voluminous blood-tinged feces. The term *constipation* may be used by the patient to refer to a variety of changes including reduction in frequency of defecation, a constant sensation of rectal fullness with incomplete evacuation of feces, and sometimes painful defecation due to hard stools or perianal pathology. In an assessment of complaints of diarrhea or constipation, it is important to consider the patient's emotional state since in many instances the recent onset of psychological stress is the major reason for altered bowel habits. However, it can be hazardous to assume this to be the case, even when the relationship seems convincing. For this reason, the judicious use of laboratory, proctoscopic, and radiologic procedures is recommended to make certain that organic disease will not be overlooked.

Acute diarrhea Diarrhea of abrupt onset occurring in otherwise healthy persons is most often related to an infectious process. A variety of accompanying symptoms are often observed, including fever, headache, anorexia, vomiting, malaise, and myalgia, but they cannot be used to distinguish with certainty among viral, bacterial, and protozoal causes. In most instances, identifiable pathogens are not recovered from the feces. For this reason so-called "nonspecific" diarrhea is usually considered to be of viral etiology. However, the demonstration of enterotoxins produced by strains of *Escherichia coli* and other bacteria, which are not distinguishable from "normal flora" on routine culture, suggests that this assumption may sometimes be incorrect and that these bacteria may account for a number of cases that are usually ascribed to viral infection.

Acute diarrhea presumed to be of viral etiology typically persists for a period of 1 to 3 days; death is extremely rare except in previously debilitated individuals who become severely dehydrated. Abnormal small-intestinal morphology including villous shortening, increase in the number of crypt cells, and increased cellularity of the lamina propria has been described in experimentally infected human volunteers who have also demonstrated transient malabsorption of fat and xylose. Unfortunately, immune electron microscopy, the technique frequently used for viral identification in stool, is generally not available clinically. The diagnosis of viral diarrhea is supported (but not confirmed) by the absence of polymorphonuclear leukocytes and erythrocytes in stool samples after preparation with Loeffler's methylene blue. Bacterial diarrhea may be suspected if there is a history of a similar and simultaneous illness in individuals who shared contaminated food with the patient. Diarrhea developing within 12 h of the meal is most likely due to ingestion of a preformed toxin (e.g., staphylococcal exotoxin). A lag period of up to 3 days after consumption of contaminated food can occur with salmonellosis.

The pathogenesis of bacterial diarrhea is due to two principal mechanisms, *mucosal invasion* and *enterotoxin-induced hypersecretion.* Bacterial invasion of the colonic wall leads to mucosal hyperemia, edema, leukocytic infiltration, and frank ulceration. Lower abdominal cramps and tenderness are prominent, as are tenesmus and rectal urgency. In severe cases the stool is grossly bloody. At other times, microscopic examination of the stool will reveal erythrocytes along with pus cells. In *shigellosis* diarrhea is mainly due to mucosal destruction by the invading microorganisms, but small-intestinal hypersecretion may also occur with some enterotoxin-producing strains of *Shigella.* The prototype of hypersecretory bacterial diarrhea is *cholera,* in which the organism *Vibrio cholerae* adheres to, but does not invade, the surface epithelial cells and releases an enterotoxin which stimulates massive secretion of fluid and electrolytes by the small intestine. This may be produced experimentally in animals by placing the enterotoxin, free of the organism itself, into isolated intestinal loops. Hypersecretion reaches a peak at 4 to 6 h and is mediated by the stimulation of mucosal adenylate cyclase by the toxin. It should be emphasized that in cholera, mucosal morphology is essentially normal, and intestinal absorptive capacity is preserved. This provides the basis for oral rehydration therapy with solutions containing glucose and sodium chloride, the former stimulating absorption of the latter. Because other species of bacteria, such as *E. coli, Clostridium,* and *Salmonella,* have been shown to produce enterotoxins, the finding of an exudate-free stool does not preclude bacterial infection as the cause of diarrhea.

Protozoal infections may also be responsible for acute diarrhea. *Entamoeba histolytica,* prevalent in some areas of the United States, produces an inflammatory colitis which can closely mimic idiopathic ulcerative colitis. Giardiasis is a cause of prolonged, watery diarrhea that often afflicts travelers returning from endemic areas where the water supply has been contaminated. In some patients giardiasis is associated with an underlying immunoglobulin deficiency of the IgA type. Careful examination of fresh stools by experienced technicians is required for the diagnosis of protozoal infection. Duodenal samples in the form of aspirate and biopsy touch preparations may be necessary to make the diagnosis of giardiasis.

Travelers' diarrhea may result from any one or several of the pathogens described above. However, often no known agent is identified, and the etiology is assumed to be viral or due to enterotoxin-producing coliform organisms. Not infrequently prolonged bowel irregularity will occur following the acute illness.

Ulcerative colitis and *regional enteritis* (Crohn's disease) may begin as acute diarrhea (Chaps. 293 and 294). Bloody stools and generalized abdominal cramping and tenderness are more apt to occur in the patients with ulcerative colitis; in regional enteritis, the diarrhea tends to be milder, is usually nonbloody, and is associated with right lower quadrant pain and tenderness. Diarrhea may be caused by a variety of *drugs,* including cholinergic agents, magnesium-containing antacids, antimetabolites used in cancer chemotherapy, and broad-spectrum antibiotics. Diarrhea due to *diverticulitis* is usually ac-

companied by fever, tenesmus, and rectal urgency, together with cramps and tenderness in the left lower quadrant (Chap. 294). When there is no evidence of acute inflammation, diarrhea in the presence of colonic diverticula is probably due to a spastic (irritable) colon which may set the stage for the development of diverticula. In elderly and debilitated individuals with *fecal impaction,* the presenting symptom may be the frequent expulsion of small amounts of liquid stool overflowing from colonic distention behind the impaction. Acute *psychological stress* can cause diarrhea at any age.

DIAGNOSTIC APPROACH The appropriate tempo and approach in the evaluation of acute diarrhea depend so heavily on the clinical setting in which it occurs that only very general guidelines can be offered. It is entirely reasonable to withhold studies in mild, self-limited cases such as are seen as part of an epidemic viral illness. When dealing with sporadic severe diarrhea or when a suggestive epidemiologic history is obtained, bacterial cultures and microscopic examination of the stool for parasites and inflammatory cells are appropriate. Proctoscopy is generally reserved for patients with bloody diarrhea, or those who do not show improvement within 5 days. Likewise, radiologic studies should usually be deferred until the initial course of the illness has been observed. In cases of massive fluid loss, measurement of serum electrolytes is useful to aid in determining replacement therapy.

TREATMENT General and nonspecific treatment of acute diarrhea includes rest, encouragement of fluid intake, and prescription of opiate-containing agents by mouth. Intravenous fluid and electrolyte replacement may be desirable and necessary in infants and the elderly. As a result of success achieved with cholera patients, the use of oral glucose-electrolyte solutions is being extended to the treatment of patients with acute diarrhea considered to be due to other enterotoxin-producing bacteria.

Chronic diarrhea Diarrhea persisting for weeks or months, whether constant or intermittent, may be a functional symptom or a manifestation of serious illness. For this reason, it is incumbent upon the physician to search carefully for evidence of organic disease, such as fever, weight loss, malnutrition, anemia, or an increased erythrocyte sedimentation rate. Abdominal tenderness and fever suggest the presence of inflammation. When there is involvement of the large bowel, the major diseases to be considered include ulcerative colitis, Crohn's disease of the colon, amebiasis, and diverticulitis. Crohn's disease of the small intestine may involve one or more of its segments. The ileum is most frequently affected. Other diarrheal conditions which may resemble Crohn's disease radiographically include tuberculous and fungal enteritis, lymphosarcoma, amyloidosis, and argentaffin (carcinoid) tumors of the small bowel.

Prolonged diarrhea without evidence of inflammation may reflect impairments of absorption, secretion, or digestion. Selective derangements, such as those due to *bile salt enteropathy* and *lactase deficiency,* are usually not accompanied by weight loss or malnutrition. *Mucosal disorders,* best exemplified by sprue, are frequently associated with weight loss, malodorous stools, abdominal distention, and anemia, and, when more severe, with osteomalacia, hypoprothrombinemia, avitaminotic neuropathies, and tetany. *Pancreatic insufficiency* resulting from chronic pancreatitis, carcinoma, or resection produces steatorrhea and weight loss of varying severity. A number of mechanisms may be responsible for *postgastrectomy diarrhea* (see Chap. 290). These include the dumping syndrome, postvagotomy motility derangements, inadequate stimulation of pancreatic digestive enzymes, and incomplete mixing of these enzymes with food. On rare occasions severe postgastrectomy diarrhea and malnutrition are due to the inadvertent creation by the surgeon of a gastroileostomy instead of a gastrojejunostomy. *Bacterial overgrowth* in the small intestine, as may occur with extensive diverticulosis and prolonged bowel stasis secondary to disorders of peristalsis (e.g., scleroderma, diabetic visceral neuropathy), can also lead to chronic diarrhea and weight loss. This has been attributed to bacterial deconjugation of bile salts and hydroxylation of long-chain fatty acids, to consumption of nutrients by the organisms, and to mucosal abnormalities believed to be caused by bacteria or their metabolites (see Chap. 292). At times, diarrhea may accompany stasis in the absence of bacterial overgrowth.

Endocrine disorders that may be accompanied by chronic diarrhea include thyrotoxicosis, diabetes mellitus, adrenal insufficiency, and hypoparathyroidism. The release of potent secretagogues from neoplastic tissue in the Zollinger-Ellison syndrome (gastrin), medullary carcinoma of the thyroid (calcitonin, prostaglandins), and pancreatic cholera syndrome (vasoactive intestinal peptide) makes diarrhea a prominent feature of these disorders. The passage of excessive amounts of clear liquid, at times sufficient to cause dehydration, occurs in some patients with large villous adenomas of the rectum.

Habitual *cathartic abuse* must be suspected when the cause of prolonged diarrhea remains perplexing. Even if this is denied by the patient, a stool sample should be alkalinized with sodium hydroxide; this will produce a burgundy color if phenolphthalein-containing laxatives have been surreptitiously ingested. The observation of melanosis coli by sigmoidoscopy indicates chronic usage of anthraquinone laxatives.

Constipation   Constipation is a common complaint often resulting from the inordinate expectation of "regularity" in bowel-conscious individuals. Stools are described as infrequent, incomplete, or unduly hard; unusual straining may be required to achieve defecation. A review of the patient's habits often reveals contributory and correctable causes, such as insufficient dietary roughage, lack of exercise, suppression of defecatory urges arising at inconvenient moments, inadequate allotment of time for full defecation, and prolonged travel. Appropriate adjustments of these patterns and reassurance are preferable to the prescription of laxatives and may be all that is required for improvement. When the patient also has symptoms such as fatigue, malaise, headaches, or anorexia, the possibility should be considered that such symptoms reflect an underlying depression of which constipation is but one component. Decreased colonic motility is responsible for the constipation associated with the use of parasympatholytic drugs, spinal cord injury, scleroderma, and Hirschsprung's disease.

Hemorrhoids, anal fissures, perineal abscesses, and rectal strictures often prevent easy and adequate stool evacuation. When constipation and tenesmus of recent onset are reported, the possibility of carcinoma of the rectum or descending colon must be seriously considered. In such instances sigmoidoscopic and barium enema examinations should be obtained early and are virtually obligatory if fecal blood has been observed or if occult blood is detected on any of three successive stool specimens. Stools of abnormally thin caliber occur in patients with rectal or sigmoid colon carcinoma but are even more commonly due to an irritable colon. Other mechanical causes of constipation include volvulus of the sigmoid colon, diverticulitis, intussusception, and hernias. A variety of metabolic abnormalities, such as hypothyroidism, hypercalcemia, hypokalemia, porphyria, lead poisoning, and dehydration are often associated with constipation Tremendous fecal retention and impaction may occur in certain neurologic disorders (e.g., spinal cord injury, multiple sclerosis, cerebral palsy, senility), and in these instances, when autonomous regulation of evacuation

is unachievable, vigorous and sustained enema programs are often necessary.

IRRITABLE BOWEL   The irritable bowel syndrome (also referred to as *spastic colon* and *mucous colitis*) is one of the most frequent gastrointestinal disorders (see Chap. 294). This condition is characterized by periodic or chronic symptoms of diarrhea, constipation, and abdominal pain. These symptoms are generally associated with psychologic stresses, but the anxiety produced by the bowel disturbance is sometimes regarded by the patient as the fundamental cause of the emotional upset. Stools tend to be thin, fragmented, or pelletlike, and accompanied by excessive mucus and gas. Efforts to ameliorate symptoms with mild cathartics or antispasmodic drugs may yield adverse and exaggerated responses. An increased sigmoidal motility has been demonstrated in association with the clinical pattern of pain and constipation, whereas hypomotility is characteristic of painless diarrhea. A variety of therapeutic approaches, including the avoidance of foods which tend to upset the patient, addition of bulk-forming agents, judicious use of antispasmodics and tranquilizers, and gentle psychotherapy may provide some relief. If the patient's life goals can be shifted away from the quixotic search for the perfect stool, much can be accomplished. At the same time, it must be remembered that such individuals are not exempt from developing bowel cancer, and any worrisome deviation from their general pattern of derangement must be seriously evaluated.

FLATULENCE   A significant amount of flatus is passed each day by normal persons, and the complaint of flatulence often reflects a heightened and embarrassing awareness of this natural occurrence. Many who complain of gas are, in reality, experiencing symptoms ascribable to disordered motility. Excessive passage of intestinal gas may be the result of aerophagia or the formation of increased amounts of gas by intestinal bacteria. The latter process can be associated with malabsorption syndromes or significant constipation but is more frequently a consequence of eating foods such as beans, broccoli, and cabbage which have a high content of nondigestible polysaccharides. The oligosaccharides stachyose and raffinose, isolated from beans, are particularly effective substrates for fermentation to carbon dioxide, hydrogen, and methane by colonic flora. The treatment of flatulence is generally undertaken to reduce embarrassment and consists of measures to decrease aerophagia along with avoidance of foods that cause excessive gas.

REFERENCES

DAVENPORT HW: *Physiology of the Digestive Tract*, 4th ed. Chicago, Year Book, 1977

DEBONGNIE JC, PHILLIPS SF: Capacity of the human colon to absorb fluid. Gastroenterology 74:698, 1978

DROSSMAN DA et al: The irritable bowel syndrome. Gastroenterology 73:811, 1977

GORBACH SL et al: Travellers' diarrhea and toxigenic *Escherichia coli*. N Engl J Med 292:933, 1975

LASSER RB et al: The role of intestinal gas in functional abdominal pain. N Engl J Med 293:524, 1975

PHILLIPS SF: Diarrhea: A current view of the pathophysiology. Gastroenterology 63:495, 1972

PLOTKIN GR et al: Gastroenteritis: Etiology, pathophysiology and clinical manifestations. Medicine 58:95, 1979

SCHREIBER DS et al: Recent advances in viral gastroenteritis. Gastroenterology 73:174, 1977

38

HEMATEMESIS AND MELENA

KURT J. ISSELBACHER
JOHN W. POPP, JR.

Hematemesis is defined as the vomiting of blood, and *melena* as the passage of stools rendered black and tarry by the presence of altered blood. These symptoms of gastrointestinal hemorrhage should bring the patient to medical attention and, within certain limits, suggest the anatomic site of bleeding. Exsanguinating gastrointestinal hemorrhage will rarely occur without the appearance of altered or gross blood passed by mouth or rectum. The color of vomited blood will vary depending on the concentration of hydrochloric acid in the stomach and its admixture with the blood. Thus, if vomiting occurs shortly after the onset of bleeding, the vomitus appears red; if there is a delay in vomiting, the appearance will be dark red, brown, or black. Precipitated blood clots in the vomitus will produce a characteristic "coffee grounds" appearance. Hematemesis usually indicates bleeding proximal to the ligament of Treitz, since blood entering the gastrointestinal tract below the duodenum rarely reenters the stomach.

While bleeding sufficient to produce hematemesis usually results in melena, less than half of patients with melena have hematemesis. *Melena* usually denotes bleeding from the esophagus, stomach, or duodenum, but lesions in the jejunum, ileum, and even ascending colon may cause melena provided the gastrointestinal transit time is sufficiently prolonged. Approximately 60 ml of blood is required to produce a single black stool; acute blood loss greater than this may produce melena for up to 3 days. After the stool color returns to normal, tests for occult blood may remain positive for up to a week or longer.

The black color of stools secondary to intestinal bleeding results from contact of the blood with hydrochloric acid to produce hematin. Characteristically, such stools are tarry ("sticky"). This tarry consistency is in contrast to black or dark stools occurring after the ingestion of iron, bismuth, or licorice. Similarly, red stools may result from the ingestion of beets or intravenous administration of sulfobromophthalein. Gastrointestinal bleeding, even if detected only by positive tests for occult blood, indicates potentially serious disease and must be further investigated.

Hematochezia, the passage of bright red blood per rectum, generally signifies bleeding from a source distal to the ligament of Treitz. However, since blood must remain in the gut for approximately 8 h to produce melena, rapid hemorrhage into the esophagus, stomach, or duodenum may also result in hematochezia.

The clinical manifestations of gastrointestinal bleeding depend upon the extent and rate of hemorrhage, and the presence of coincidental diseases. Blood loss of less than 500 ml is rarely associated with systemic signs; exceptions include bleeding in the elderly or in the anemic patient in whom smaller amounts of blood loss may produce hemodynamic alterations. Rapid hemorrhage of greater volume results in decreased venous return to the heart, decreased cardiac output, and increased peripheral resistance due to reflex vasoconstriction. Orthostatic hypotension greater than 10 mmHg usually indicates a 20 percent or greater reduction in blood volume. Concomitant symptoms include syncope, lightheadedness, nausea, sweating, and thirst. When blood loss approaches 40 percent of blood volume, shock frequently ensues with pronounced tachycardia and hypotension. Pallor is prominent, and the skin is cool.

It is important to recognize that the hematocrit, when determined immediately after the onset of bleeding, may not accurately reflect blood loss, since equilibration with extravascular fluid and hemodilution require several hours. Common laboratory findings include mild leukocytosis and thrombocytosis which develop within 6 h after the onset of bleeding. The blood urea nitrogen may be mildly elevated, particularly in upper gastrointestinal bleeding, due to breakdown of blood proteins to urea by intestinal bacteria as well as from a mild reduction in the glomerular filtration rate. Blood in the gut may also produce a low-grade fever.

ETIOLOGY OF UPPER GASTROINTESTINAL BLEEDING A careful history and physical examination of the oropharynx should serve to exclude swallowed blood as a source of hematemesis or melena.

The three most common causes of upper gastrointestinal hemorrhage are (1) peptic ulceration, (2) erosive gastritis, and (3) variceal bleeding. These entities account for up to 90 percent of all cases of upper gastrointestinal hemorrhage in which a definite lesion can be found.

Peptic ulcer Peptic ulcer is probably the most common cause of upper gastrointestinal bleeding; the majority of such ulcers are found in the duodenum. Approximately 20 to 30 percent of patients with documented ulcers will have significant bleeding sometime during the course of their disease. Since hemorrhage may be the initial manifestation of a peptic ulcer, this lesion should be seriously considered even when a history characteristic of ulcer disease is not obtained.

Gastritis Gastritis may be associated with recent alcohol ingestion or with the use of anti-inflammatory drugs, such as aspirin or indomethacin. Another frequent setting is the development of gastric erosions in stressful situations such as following major trauma or surgery, or in association with severe systemic disease. The occurrence of gastritis in burn victims and patients with increased intracranial pressure is also common. Since there are no characteristic physical findings, the diagnosis of gastritis must be suspected when the appropriate clinical setting is encountered. Gastroscopy is usually needed to confirm the diagnosis since radiologic examination generally lacks the sensitivity required to detect gastritis.

Variceal bleeding Variceal bleeding is characteristically abrupt and massive; chronic gastrointestinal blood loss is unusual. Bleeding from esophageal or gastric varices is usually the result of portal hypertension, secondary to hepatic cirrhosis. Although alcoholic cirrhosis is the most prevalent cause of esophageal varices in the United States, any condition producing portal hypertension, even in the absence of hepatic disease (i.e., portal vein thrombosis or idiopathic portal hypertension), may result in variceal bleeding. Further, while the presence of varices usually connotes long-standing portal hypertension, acute hepatitis or severe fatty infiltration of the liver may occasionally produce varices which disappear once the hepatic abnormality resolves. It should be emphasized that although upper gastrointestinal bleeding in a patient with cirrhosis suggests a variceal source, approximately half those patients will be bleeding from other lesions (e.g., gastritis, ulcers). Consequently, it is essential to exclude nonvariceal causes of bleeding so that the appropriate treatment can be instituted. Finally, since varices may occur at any site in the gastrointestinal tract, angiography may be required to identify hemorrhage from varices distal to the duodenum.

Other lesions With the advent of esophagogastroduodenoscopy, the Mallory-Weiss syndrome has been demonstrated with increasing frequency as a cause of acute upper gastrointestinal hemorrhage. This syndrome refers to laceration in the region of the esophagogastric junction characterized by retching or nonbloody vomiting followed by hematemesis. Less common bleeding esophageal lesions include esophagitis (with or without hiatus hernia) and carcinoma; these generally cause chronic blood loss and rarely produce massive bleeding.

Gastric carcinoma may result in chronic gastrointestinal bleeding. Lymphoma, polyps, and other tumors of the stomach and small bowel are uncommon and, consequently, are infrequent causes of hemorrhage. Leiomyoma and leiomyosarcoma are likewise rare, but they can lead to massive hemorrhage. Bleeding from duodenal and jejunal diverticula is relatively unusual. Vascular insufficiency of the mesenteric vessels, including occlusive and nonocclusive disease, may lead to bloody diarrhea.

Arteriosclerotic aortic aneurysms may rupture into the small intestine; such an event is almost always fatal. Rupture may also occur following arterial reconstructive surgery with fistula formation between synthetic graft and bowel lumen. Sudden bleeding may also occur after trauma resulting in hepatic laceration; this may result in blood loss into the bile ducts (i.e., hemobilia).

Primary blood dyscrasias, including leukemia, thrombocytopenic states, the hemophilias, and disseminated intravascular coagulation may result in significant gastrointestinal bleeding. Polycythemia vera, although associated with an increased incidence of peptic ulceration, may also result in gastrointestinal bleeding due to mesenteric or portal vein thrombosis. Periarteritis nodosa, Henoch-Schönlein purpura, and other forms of vasculitis may lead to gastrointestinal blood loss.

Mild gastrointestinal bleeding may be seen with amyloidosis, Osler-Weber-Rendu disease, pseudoxanthoma elasticum, Turner's syndrome, intestinal hemangiomas, neurofibromatosis, Kaposi's sarcoma, and Peutz-Jeghers syndrome. Uremia may produce gastrointestinal blood loss; the most common presentation is chronic, occult bleeding from diffuse involvement of the mucosa of the stomach and small bowel.

ETIOLOGY OF LOWER GASTROINTESTINAL LESIONS Anal and rectal lesions

Small amounts of bright red blood on the surface of the stool and toilet tissue are often caused by hemorrhoids; such bleeding is generally precipitated by the strained passage of a hard stool. Anal fissures and fistulas may present in a similar fashion. Proctitis is another source of rectal bleeding; it is frequently seen in young adults, especially in male homosexuals. In the latter situation, proctitis may be nonspecific or due to gonorrheal infection. Rectal trauma is a cause of hematochezia, and the placement of foreign objects in the rectal vault may precipitate perforation as well as acute rectal hemorrhage. It must be emphasized that anal pathology does not preclude other sources of blood loss, and these must be sought and excluded.

Colonic lesions

Carcinoma of the colon, as well as colonic polyps, may produce chronic blood loss. Frankly bloody diarrhea is common and may be the presenting symptom in patients with ulcerative colitis; it is less frequent in granulomatous colitis, but occult blood may be present in the stool. Bleeding may also accompany diarrhea due to infections such as shigellosis, amebiasis, and rarely, salmonellosis. In the elderly patient, ischemic colitis may be a cause of bloody diarrhea; this lesion may also be seen in the younger age group associated with the use of oral contraceptive agents. Angiodysplastic lesions, usually involving the ascending colon, can be a major source of bleeding in elderly patients, especially those with aortic stenosis; such vascular lesions can be identified by angiography or colonoscopy.

Diverticula

Colonic diverticula are most often located in the sigmoid colon; however, most episodes of diverticular bleeding originate in the ascending colon. Bleeding from colonic diverticula is one of the most common causes of massive lower gastrointestinal hemorrhage. The usual presentation of a diverticular hemorrhage is that of painless passage of a maroon-colored stool. Mild blood loss is more often associated with diverticulitis. Meckel's diverticulum, a congenital anomaly of the distal ileum, is present in about 2 percent of the population and may cause bleeding. Although only about 15 percent of these diverticula contain gastric mucosa, the lesions which cause acute bleeding contain gastric mucosa half the time. This anomaly is an important cause of acute hemorrhage in children and young adults.

APPROACH TO THE PATIENT WITH GASTROINTESTINAL BLEEDING

The approach to the bleeding patient depends upon the site, extent, and rate of bleeding. Patients with hematemesis have usually bled greater amounts (often greater than 1000 ml) than those who have melena alone (usually 500 ml or less), and mortality with the former is about twice that of the latter. When first seen, the patient may be in shock. Prior to taking a history and performing a thorough physical examination, vital signs should be noted, blood sent for typing and cross matching, and a large-bore intravenous line placed for infusion of saline or other plasma expanders. The physician initiating the evaluation of the bleeding patient must be aware that the primary consideration is the necessity of maintaining adequate intravascular volume and hemodynamic stability during the diagnostic workup.

History A history of prior ulcer disease or symptoms suggestive thereof may provide a useful clue. Similarly, recent abuse of alcohol or ingestion of anti-inflammatory drugs should make erosive gastritis more suspect. If alcohol abuse has been long-standing, esophageal varices may be a more likely source of hemorrhage. Aspirin use may also cause bleeding by aggravating a preexisting lesion (e.g., peptic ulceration). Prior history of gastrointestinal bleeding may be helpful, as may a family history of intestinal disease or hemorrhagic diathesis. Recent retching followed by hematemesis should suggest the possibility of the Mallory-Weiss syndrome. The acute onset of bloody diarrhea may indicate the presence of inflammatory bowel disease or infectious involvement of the colon. It is also important to exclude associated systemic illnesses or recent trauma, since bleeding from erosive gastritis is frequently seen under such conditions.

Physical examination Following evaluation for orthostatic changes in pulse and blood pressure and institution of volume repletion, the patient should be examined for clues to the underlying illness. A nonintestinal bleeding source should be excluded by careful examination of the nasopharynx. Dermatologic examination may disclose the characteristic telangiectasia of Osler-Weber-Rendu disease (although these will not be visible if severe anemia is present), the perioral pigmentation of Peutz-Jeghers syndrome, the dermal fibromas of neurofibromatosis, the sebaceous cysts and bony tumors of Gardner's syndrome, the palpable purpura frequently seen with vasculitis, or the diffuse pigmentation seen in hemochromatosis. Stigmata of chronic liver disease such as spider angiomata, gynecomastia, testicular atrophy, jaundice, ascites, and hepatosplenomegaly should suggest portal hypertension resulting in bleeding from esophageal or gastric varices. Significant lymph node enlargement or abdominal masses may reflect underlying intraabdominal malignancy. Careful rectal examination is important to exclude local pathology as well as to observe the color of the stool.

Laboratory studies Initial studies should include the hematocrit, hemoglobin, careful assessment of red blood cell morphologic features (hypochromic, microcytic red blood cells suggest that blood loss is chronic), white blood cell count, differential, and platelet count. Prothrombin time, partial thromboplastin time, and other coagulation studies may be in order to exclude primary or secondary clotting defects. A radiograph of the abdomen is rarely helpful in establishing a diagnosis unless a perforated viscus is suspected. Though the initial studies are valuable and essential, repeated evaluation of the laboratory data is important as one follows the clinical course of the bleeding.

Diagnostic approach The diagnostic approach to the patient with gastrointestinal hemorrhage must be individualized. The initial management of gastrointestinal bleeding may be under the direction of the internist, but it is prudent to consult a surgeon in the event that the bleeding cannot be controlled by medical means. It must be emphasized that demonstration of a lesion in a patient with gastrointestinal bleeding should also be accompanied by evidence that this lesion is the site of bleeding. In recent years the availability of experienced endoscopists as well as radiologists with facilities for selective arteriography has increased to the extent that in many medical centers it is possible to have emergency endoscopic, angiographic, and barium studies performed within hours of the patient's admission to the hospital. It is to be hoped that this "vigorous diagnostic approach" will serve to decrease the morbidity and mortality rates associated with upper gastrointestinal bleeding.

When there is a history of melena or hematemesis or the suspicion of bleeding from the upper part of the gastrointestinal tract, the patient should have a nasogastric tube passed to empty the stomach and to determine whether the bleeding is in the upper part of the gastrointestinal tract. If the initial nasogastric aspirate is clear, the tube should be left in place until bile-stained material appears, since active duodenal bleeding may occur with a clear nasogastric aspirate. The latter situation is due to failure of duodenal contents to reflux into the stomach secondary to pyloric irritability and spasm. If the aspirate is bile-stained and negative for occult blood, one can assume that active bleeding is not occurring in the gastroduodenal region, and the nasogastric tube can be removed.

If red blood or "coffee grounds" material is aspirated from the nasogastric tube, iced saline irrigation of the stomach should be initiated. Irrigation serves two purposes: it provides the clinician with an assessment of the rapidity of the bleeding, and its vasoconstricting effect often diminishes bleeding due to erosive gastritis. Subsequent diagnostic maneuvers will depend on whether bleeding continues; this can be assessed by vital signs, transfusion requirements, and the number and consistency of stools.

If the nasogastric aspirate suggests that bleeding has stopped, one may proceed with either esophagogastroduodenoscopy or upper gastrointestinal barium studies. Although *endoscopy* provides a higher diagnostic yield, it has not been proved conclusively that survival is increased by early endoscopy. *Barium examination* often identifies a potential source of hemorrhage, but there are important limitations to such x-rays. First, lesions such as erosive gastritis and Mallory-Weiss lacerations are not visualized by x-ray. Second, if the patient rebleeds following a barium exam, the retained contrast material will make endoscopy difficult and angiography impossible. Clearly the approach in this setting must be individualized. The decision to employ esophagogastroduodenoscopy or barium studies will depend on several variables, including the availability of an experienced endoscopist and the condition of the patient. The two procedures should be viewed as complementary in the diagnostic evaluation of upper gastrointestinal hemorrhage.

Persistent upper gastrointestinal hemorrhage must be viewed differently, and most clinicians would proceed immediately to esophagogastroduodenoscopy. Determination of the site and cause of bleeding is essential for appropriate therapy, particularly if varices are responsible. Such information is beneficial both to the surgeon, who may be asked to intervene, and to the angiographer, should injection of vasoconstricting agents into the artery supplying the lesion be deemed appropriate. Thus, anticipation of surgery, angiography, or the suspicion of bleeding varices are strong indications for esophagogastroduodenoscopy in the evaluation of the patient with persistent upper gastrointestinal bleeding.

In contrast, esophagogastroduodenoscopy is less vital in the evaluation of *massive* hemorrhage, since large amounts of blood obscure visualization of mucosal pathology. In such a setting, selective arteriography or surgery is more appropriate.

Should bleeding continue and gastric aspiration fail to reveal fresh blood, the site of hemorrhage may be beyond the ligament of Treitz. In this situation angiography is frequently valuable in establishing a diagnosis. Angiographic demonstration of the bleeding site requires blood loss at a rate of at least 0.5 ml/min. Clinical correlates reflecting this degree of blood loss include postural hypotension and the necessity for blood transfusion to maintain stable vital signs. Emergency angiography may localize the site of bleeding; however, the cause of the bleeding may not be determined unless varices, vascular malformations, or aneurysms are present. Therapeutic angiography is a promising approach to the control of persistent hemorrhage. Continuous intraarterial infusion of vasoconstrictor agents, such as vasopressin, is often successful in controlling hemorrhage (Fig. 38-1). Additionally, embolic material may be injected directly into the artery perfusing the bleeding site. This technique has been performed successfully with autologous clot as well as with commercially available hemostatic material such as gelatin powder (Gelfoam). At present embolization therapy is regarded as a temporizing measure for bleeding varices and peptic lesions, and eventual surgery is to be expected.

If bleeding esophageal varices are identified on upper endoscopy, peripheral infusions of vasopressin (Pitressin) may control the bleeding. The ability to respond to such therapy depends upon the general condition of the patient as assessed by certain clinical and laboratory parameters (Child's criteria). It has been shown that intraarterial vasopressin is no more effective than intravenous administration in the control of variceal bleeding. This is not the case, however, for arterial bleeding where selective angiographic catheter placement is mandatory to achieve hemostasis. Varices may also be controlled by balloon tamponade with a Sengstaken-Blakemore tube. Unlike vasopressin, this technique is generally used as a stabilizing preoperative measure which should be followed by surgical decompression of the portal system within 48 h whenever possible.

In the evaluation of *rectal* bleeding the most important procedures are the digital examination, anoscopy, and sigmoidoscopy. The last of these may identify a bleeding site or document bleeding coming from above the range of the instrument. If brisk bleeding continues, arteriography may serve to localize the bleeding site and allow local infusion of vasoconstrictor agents to control bleeding. Several investigations are currently being conducted to assess the efficacy of colonoscopy in identifying bleeding lesions proximal to the sigmoid colon. This procedure has therapeutic promise as well, since direct visualization may allow the colonoscopist to excise the bleeding lesion or cauterize it with an electrosurgical device. As with esophagogastroduodenoscopy, massive hemorrhage precludes effective use of colonoscopy, and in such instances it should not be

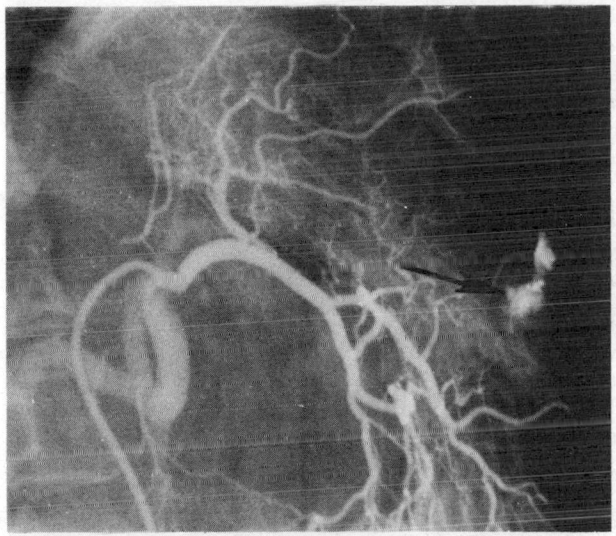

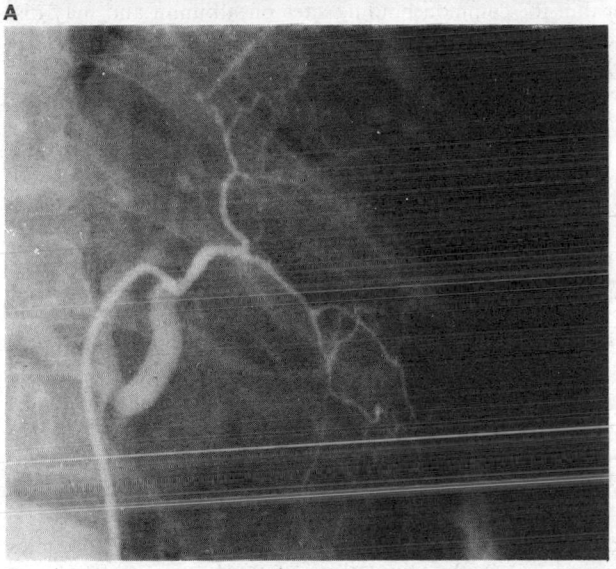

A

B

FIGURE 38-1

Angiographic findings on a patient with massive upper gastrointestinal bleeding. Angiographic studies revealed the bleeding to be secondary to hemorrhagic gastritis; it was controlled by the selective left gastric arterial infusion of vasopressin. A. Selective left gastric arteriography demonstrates massive extravasation of contrast material (arrow) from a branch of the left gastric artery. B. Selective left gastric arteriography during the infusion of 0.1 unit of vasopressin per minute demonstrates a marked decrease in the caliber of the left gastric artery and cessation of hemorrhage.

attempted. Finally, a barium enema has a limited role in the evaluation of acute rectal bleeding. A barium-filled colon may localize potential bleeding sources, but will not necessarily define the bleeding site. Furthermore, if brisk bleeding recurs, subsequent colonoscopy or angiography will be difficult to interpret due to retained contrast material. Therefore, it is advisable to withhold barium studies of both the upper and lower bowel for at least 24 h after the cessation of active bleeding.

REFERENCES

ATHANASOULIS CA: Angiography. Its contribution to the emergency management of gastrointestinal hemorrhage. Radiol Clin North Am 14:265, 1976

——: Angiodysplasia of the intestinal tract as a cause of recurrent bleeding. Prog Gastroenterol 3:857, 1977

CONN HO et al: Intraarterial vasopressin in the treatment of upper gastrointestinal hemorrhage: A prospective, controlled clinical trial. Gastroenterology 68:211, 1975

DRONFIELD MW et al: A prospective, randomised study of endoscopy and radiology in acute upper-gastrointestinal-tract bleeding. Lancet 1:1167, 1977

HASTINGS PR et al: Antacid prophylaxis of bleeding in the critically ill. N Engl J Med 298,1041, 1978

HEDBERG SE: Endoscopy in gastrointestinal bleeding. A systematic approach to diagnosis. Surg Clin North Am 54:549, 1974

TERES J et al: Upper gastrointestinal bleeding in cirrhosis: Clinical and endoscopic correlations. Gut 17:37, 1976

39
JAUNDICE AND HEPATOMEGALY

KURT J. ISSELBACHER

JAUNDICE

Jaundice, or *icterus,* refers to the yellow pigmentation of the skin or scleras by bilirubin. This in turn is a result of elevated levels of bilirubin in the bloodstream. Jaundice may be brought to clinical attention by a darkening of the urine or a yellow discoloration of the skin or sclera; the latter often is the site where clinical icterus may first be detected. Scleral pigmentation is attributed to richness of this tissue in elastin, which has a special affinity for bilirubin. Jaundice must be distinguished from other causes of yellow pigmentation such as carotenemia (see Chaps. 51, 80, and 335), which is due to carotenoid pigments in the bloodstream and is associated with a yellowish discoloration of the skin but not of the sclera. Atabrine treatment (see Chap. 200) may produce a yellow color of the skin and urine, but the scleras are usually only minimally discolored, and when pigment is present, it is seen only in the regions of the scleras exposed to light.

Normal serum bilirubin concentrations range from 0.5 to 1.0 mg per 100 ml, and normally most of this is unconjugated (see Fig. 39-1). The precise level at which jaundice becomes clinically evident varies, but usually it can be recognized when the total serum bilirubin exceeds 2 to 2.5 mg per 100 ml. Not infrequently in deep jaundice the skin may take on a greenish hue because of the conversion of bilirubin to biliverdin, an oxidation product of bilirubin. Oxidation occurs more readily with conjugated bilirubin, and hence a greenish hue is seen more frequently in conditions with pronounced conjugated hyperbilirubinemia. When bilirubin is exposed to visible light (from 430 to 470 nm) the pigment undergoes photooxidation leading to water-soluble and colorless breakdown products. Ultraviolet light can also produce isomers of bilirubin (IXα) that may not require conjugation for hepatic excretion (see below).

PRODUCTION AND METABOLISM OF BILIRUBIN Normal sources of bilirubin (Fig. 39-2) The greater part of the bilirubin is derived from the catabolism of hemoglobin present in senescent red blood cells. This normally accounts for about 80 to 85 percent of the daily bilirubin production. When a circulating red blood cell reaches the end of its normal life span of approximately 120 days, it is destroyed in the reticuloendothelial system. In the catabolism of hemoglobin, globin is first dissociated from heme, after which the heme moiety (ferroprotoporphyrin IX) is oxidatively cleaved and converted to bili-

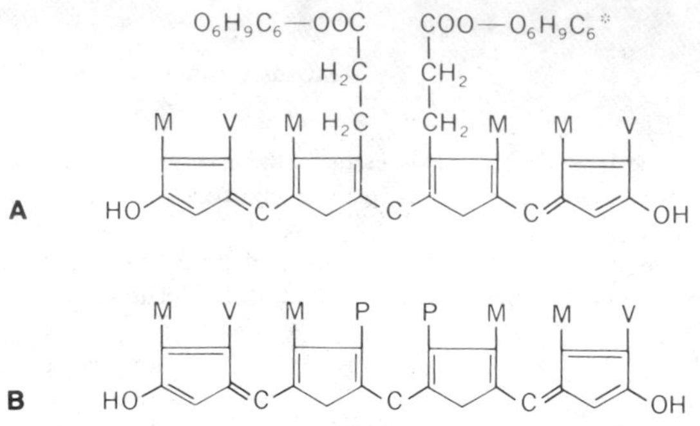

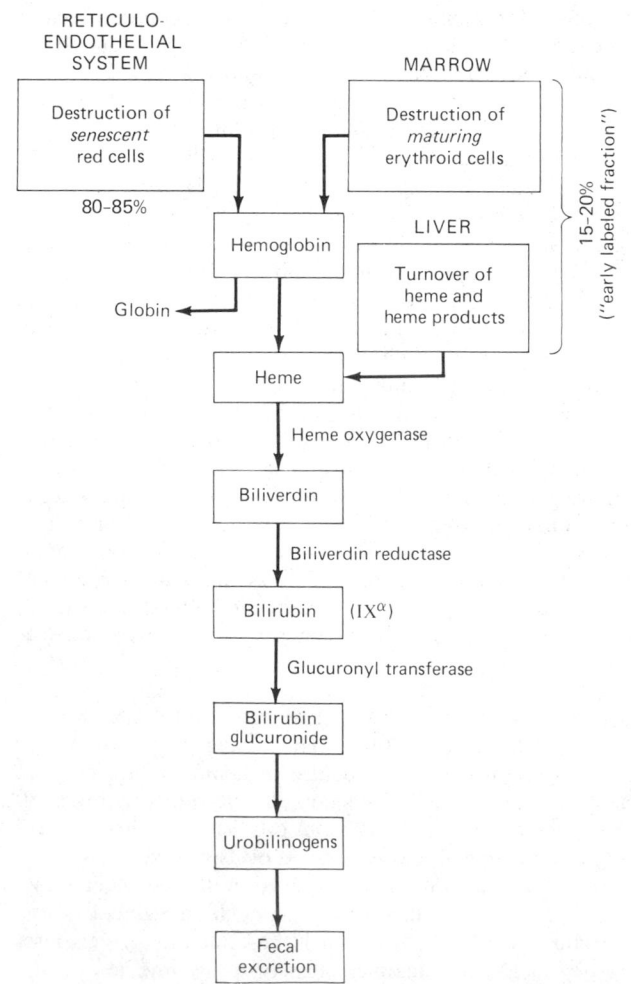

$O_6H_9C_6$—OOC   COO—$O_6H_9C_6$*

A

B

FIGURE 39-1

The chemical structures of conjugated (A) and unconjugated (B) bilirubin. Abbreviations: M = methyl, V = vinyl, P = propionic acid. The asterisk (*) refers to glucuronic acid.

verdin by a microsomal heme oxygenase. This enzyme system requires oxygen and a cofactor, reduced nicotinamide adenine dinucleotide phosphate (NADPH). Bilirubin (in the chemical form of bilirubin $IX\alpha$) is then formed from biliverdin by biliverdin reductase.

About 15 to 20 percent of the bilirubin is derived from sources other than senescent erythrocytes. One source is the *destruction of maturing erythroid cells in the bone marrow,* or so-called "ineffective erythropoiesis" (see Chap. 312). The other is *nonerythroid components,* especially in the liver, and involves

FIGURE 39-2

The sources and precursors of bilirubin and steps in its subsequent metabolism and excretion.

the turnover of heme and heme proteins (such as cytochrome, myoglobin, and heme-containing enzymes). These two sources of bilirubin are collectively referred to as the *early labeled fraction,* a term derived from experiments with labeled glycine and Δ-aminolevulinic acid (ALA). Thus when labeled glycine is administered to a normal subject, approximately 15 percent of the label appears in stool urobilinogens in the first 3 to 5 days; 85 percent of the label appears at about 120 days and reflects the bilirubin produced from the normal destruction of senescent red blood cells.

Transport of bilirubin Following liberation of bilirubin into the plasma, virtually all the pigment is tightly *bound to albumin.* The maximum binding capacity is 2 mol bilirubin per mole of albumin. Because in a normal adult this corresponds to plasma unconjugated bilirubin concentrations of 60 to 80 mg/ml, saturation of the binding capacity of the plasma almost never occurs. It is clinically relevant that certain organic anions, such as sulfonamides and salicylates, compete with bilirubin for common binding sites on albumin and may displace bilirubin from albumin, permitting it to enter tissues such as the central nervous system. Most of the evidence for albumin binding has been obtained from studies using unconjugated bilirubin. The conjugated pigment also appears to be bound primarily to albumin, although the binding to albumin is much weaker than with unconjugated bilirubin. This may account for the fact that conjugated, but not unconjugated, bilirubin may be filtered by the renal glomeruli.

Bilirubin is found in body fluids (cerebrospinal fluid, joint effusions, cysts, etc.) in proportion to the albumin content of the fluids and is absent from true secretions such as tears, saliva, and pancreatic juice. Scar tissue is rarely bilirubin-stained. The appearance of jaundice is also influenced by blood flow and edema. Paralyzed extremities and edematous areas tend to remain uncolored, and "unilateral" jaundice in patients with hemiplegia and edema may be seen if jaundice develops.

Hepatic metabolism of bilirubin (Fig. 39-3) The liver occupies a central role in the metabolism of the bile pigments. Three distinct phases are recognized: (1) *hepatic uptake,* (2) *conjugation,* and (3) *excretion* into bile. Of these three steps, excretion appears to be the rate-limiting step and the one most susceptible to impairment when the liver cell is damaged.

UPTAKE Unconjugated bilirubin bound to albumin is presented to the liver cell, and upon entry the pigment and albumin become dissociated. The uptake phase is believed to involve the binding of bilirubin to certain cytoplasmic anionic binding proteins (ligandins). Hepatic uptake appears to be reversible.

CONJUGATION Unconjugated bilirubin is water-insoluble and must be converted to a *water-soluble derivative* in order to be excreted by the liver cell into bile. This is accomplished by conjugation whereby bilirubin is predominantly converted to bilirubin glucuronide. The reaction occurs in the endoplasmic reticulum of the hepatocytes by action of bilirubin glucuronyl transferase. As shown in Fig. 39-3, this appears to be a two-step reaction, resulting first in the formation of the monoglucuronide followed by the production of the diglucuronide. It has recently been suggested that the conversion of the monoglucuronide to the diglucuronide may be mediated by a separate enzyme, a plasma membrane transesterase (or transglucuronidase), rather than glucuronyl transferase. However, other studies suggest glucuronyl transferase may also mediate the conversion of monoglucuronide to diglucuronide. Normally, bile contains 85 percent of bilirubin diconjugates and 15 percent monoconjugates. Unconjugated bilirubin usually is *not* ex-

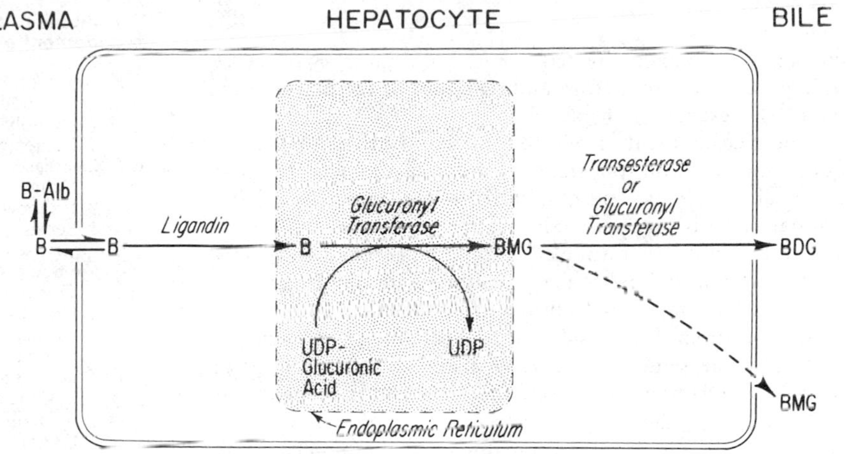

FIGURE 39-3

Scheme of bilirubin uptake, conjugation, and excretion by the liver cell. Abbreviations: B = bilirubin, BMG = bilirubin monoglucuronide, BDG = bilirubin diglucuronide, UDP = uridine diphosphate.

creted by the liver into the bile (except following photooxidation, see below). Bile also contains small amounts of bilirubin conjugated with other sugars (e.g., with xylose and aldobiuronic acid). The physiologic significance of these nonglucuronide conjugates is not known.

EXCRETION OR SECRETION INTO BILE   Normally, for bilirubin to be excreted into bile, *the pigment must be in the conjugated form.* Although the overall process is not well understood, the excretion of conjugated bilirubin into bile appears to be an energy-dependent process and the *rate-limiting* step in the hepatic metabolism of bilirubin. When this step is compromised, two consequences occur: (1) decreased excretion of bilirubin into the bile, and (2) "regurgitation," or reentry of conjugated bilirubin from the liver cells into the bloodstream.

It should be noted that bilirubin (i.e., IXα, Z isomer) is readily photooxidized to an isomer (IXα, E isomer), which does not need to be conjugated in order to be excreted by the liver cell. Hence after phototherapy unconjugated bilirubin (as the E isomer) can be excreted into bile.

Intestinal phase of bilirubin metabolism   After its appearance in the intestinal lumen, bilirubin glucuronide may be excreted in the stool or metabolized to urobilinogen and related products. Because of its polarity, *conjugated bilirubin is not reabsorbed* by the intestinal mucosa, a mechanism which may serve to rid the body of this pigment. The formation of urobilinogen from conjugated bilirubin requires the action of bacteria and occurs in the lower part of the small intestine and colon.

In contrast to conjugated bilirubin, *urobilinogen is reabsorbed* from the small intestine into the portal blood and is thus subject to enterohepatic circulation. Some urobilinogen is reexcreted by the liver into the bile; the rest is excreted in the urine in an amount usually not exceeding 4 mg daily. When the hepatic excretory mechanism is impaired (e.g., in hepatocellular disease) or the production of bilirubin is greatly increased (e.g., in hemolytic anemia), the urinary urobilinogen may increase significantly.

The normal output of fecal urobilinogen ranges from 50 to 280 mg per day. Under conditions of decreased excretion of conjugated bilirubin into the intestine (e.g., liver disease, bile duct obstruction) or suppression of intestinal flora by antibiotics, fecal output will be diminished. In hemolytic anemia, urinary and fecal urobilinogen excretion is greatly increased.

In a normal person with a blood volume of 5 liters and a hemoglobin concentration of 15 g per 100 ml, the total circulating hemoglobin is 750 g. Because approximately 0.8 percent of the red blood cells are destroyed daily, 6.3 g hemoglobin is released for catabolism. Assuming a quantitative degradation of heme to bilirubin and to urobilinogen, the expected daily output of urobilinogen would be approximately 250 mg plus

the additional 15 to 30 mg which would be derived from the other sources described above (i.e., ineffective erythropoiesis, nonhemoglobin heme precursors). Often, however, the amount excreted is considerably less, and it appears likely that there are alternative pathways for hemoglobin degradation not involving bilirubin formation.

Renal excretion of bilirubin   Normally the urine contains no bilirubin that can be detected by the methods usually employed, although traces may be detectable by sensitive spectrophotometric procedures. Unconjugated bilirubin, being tightly bound to albumin, is not filtered by the renal glomeruli, and because there is no tubular secretory process for bilirubin, *unconjugated bilirubin is not excreted in urine.* On the other hand, conjugated bilirubin is less tightly bound to albumin, and a small fraction (about 5 percent) is unbound. The unbound fraction is dialyzable and is filtered by the renal glomeruli. Thus, in contrast to the unconjugated pigment, a fraction of plasma *conjugated bilirubin appears in the urine.* Bile salts enhance the dialyzability of conjugated bilirubin, and in obstructive jaundice, the elevated level of plasma bile acids may account for an increased renal excretion of conjugated bilirubin. This may also explain why in biliary tract obstruction, serum conjugated bilirubin levels tend to plateau and not to exceed 30 to 40 mg per 100 ml, while with severe hepatocellular injury bilirubin levels higher than this may occur.

CHEMICAL TESTS FOR BILE PIGMENTS   The most widely employed chemical test for the bile pigments in serum is the van den Bergh reaction. In this reaction the bilirubin pigments are diazotized with sulfanilic acid, and the chromogenic products are measured colorimetrically. The van den Bergh reaction can be used to distinguish between unconjugated and conjugated bilirubin because of the different solubility properties of the pigments. When the reaction is carried out in an *aqueous* medium, the water-soluble conjugated bilirubin reacts to give the so-called "direct" van den Bergh reaction. When the reaction is carried out in *methanol,* both conjugated and unconjugated pigments react, giving a measure of the *total* bilirubin level. The total minus the direct-reacting bilirubin give the *indirect* value, which is a measure of the unconjugated bilirubin level.

In the direct van den Bergh reaction, the most accurate measurements are those carried out at 1 min. If the reaction is allowed to proceed longer, a small amount of the unconjugated pigment may begin to react in the aqueous medium. As a result, if the reaction is carried out at 30 min in a patient with unconjugated hyperbilirubinemia, falsely low values for the indirect-reacting bilirubin may be obtained. This serves to emphasize that the direct and indirect van den Bergh reactions represent *approximations* (not absolute measurements) of the conjugated and unconjugated pigments. A summary of the key differences in the properties and reactions of the bilirubin pigments is presented in Table 39-1.

The measurement of bilirubin in the urine may be carried out by the Harrison spot test or with Ictotest tablets. The foam test is also a simple and qualitatively valid procedure. When normal urine is vigorously shaken in a test tube, the foam is absolutely white. In a urine containing bilirubin, the foam will be yellow. This difference may be subtle and may become evident only by comparing a normal urine specimen and one containing bilirubin side by side. Urine urobilinogen may be estimated by the semiquantitative Watson-Schwartz test or the qualitative Diamond test. Fecal measurement must be quantitative to be of value.

Except for concentrated urine, the most common cause of a deep yellow-brown or dark urine is bilirubinuria. However, other mechanisms and diseases associated with a dark urine need to be considered. These include yellow urine due to drugs (e.g., sulfasalazine); red urine due to porphyria, hemoglobinuria, myoglobinuria, or drugs (e.g., pyridium); and dark brown or black urine due to homogentisic acid (in ochronosis) or melanin (with melanoma).

APPROACH TO THE PATIENT WITH JAUNDICE Once jaundice is recognized clinically or chemically, it is important to determine whether it is predominantly due to unconjugated or conjugated hyperbilirubinemia. *A simple clue in this regard is to determine whether bilirubin is present in the urine.* Its absence in the urine suggests unconjugated hyperbilirubinemia (since this pigment is not filtered by the glomerulus); its presence indicates conjugated hyperbilirubinemia. One can then proceed to the direct chemical measurement of the bilirubin pigments in the serum. In predominantly unconjugated hyperbilirubinemia, 80 to 85 percent of the total serum bilirubin is unconjugated (i.e., less than 15 to 20 percent is conjugated). The patient is considered to have predominantly conjugated hyperbilirubinemia when more than 50 percent of the serum bilirubin is of the conjugated type.

An approach to the classification of jaundice based on this important distinction is presented in Table 39-2. Derangements of bilirubin metabolism may occur through any of four mechanisms: (1) overproduction, (2) decreased hepatic uptake, (3) decreased hepatic conjugation, and (4) decreased excretion of bilirubin into bile (due to both intrahepatic and extrahepatic factors). Jaundice may also be described on the basis of the pathogenetic mechanisms or disease processes leading to increased bilirubin levels. Thus, the terms *hemolytic jaundice, hepatocellular jaundice,* and *obstructive* (or cholestatic) *jaundice* are often used.

Though these classifications and terms are helpful, in any one patient more than a single derangement or more than one "type" of jaundice may be present. For example, a patient with cirrhosis may have not only impaired liver cell function (and hence hepatocellular jaundice) but also hemolysis. Furthermore, obstructive jaundice may be due to either *mechani-*

TABLE 39-1
Comparison of the major differences between conjugated and unconjugated bilirubin

Properties and reactions	Unconjugated	Conjugated
Water solubility	0	+
Affinity for lipids	+	0
Bound to serum albumin	+ + +	+
Renal excretion	0	+
Van den Bergh reaction	Indirect (total minus direct)	Direct
Lipid membrane permeability	+	0

TABLE 39-2
Classification of jaundice based on underlying derangement of bilirubin metabolism

I Predominantly *unconjugated* hyperbilirubinemia
  A Overproduction
    1 Hemolysis (intra- and extravascular)
    2 Ineffective erythropoiesis
  B Decreased hepatic uptake
    1 Drugs (e.g., flavaspidic acid)
    2 Prolonged fasting (< 300 cal per day)
    3 Sepsis
  C Decreased bilirubin conjugation (decreased glucuronyl transferase activity)
    1 Gilbert's syndrome (*mild* decrease in transferase)
    2 Crigler-Najjar type II (*moderate* decrease in transferase)
    3 Crigler-Najjar type I (absent transferase)
    4 Neonatal jaundice
    5 Acquired transferase deficiency
      a Drug inhibition (e.g., pregnanediol, chloramphenicol)
      b Hepatocellular disease (hepatitis, cirrhosis)*
    6 Sepsis
II Predominantly *conjugated* hyperbilirubinemia
  A Impaired hepatic excretion (intrahepatic defects)
    1 Familial or hereditary disorders
      a Dubin-Johnson syndrome; Rotor syndrome
      b Recurrent (benign) intrahepatic cholestasis
      c Cholestatic jaundice of pregnancy
    2 Acquired disorders
      a Hepatocellular disease* (e.g., viral or drug-induced hepatitis)
      b Drug-induced cholestasis (e.g., oral contraceptives, methyltestosterone)
      c Sepsis
  B Extrahepatic biliary obstruction (mechanical obstruction, e.g., stones, stricture, tumor of bile duct)

* *In hepatocellular disease (hepatitis and cirrhosis) there is usually interference in the three major steps of bilirubin metabolism—uptake, conjugation, and excretion. However, excretion is the rate-limiting step and is usually impaired to the greatest extent. As a result, conjugated hyperbilirubinemia predominates.*

cal obstruction of the biliary radicles or *functional* factors causing impaired hepatic excretion of bilirubin into bile.

In the present chapter a brief description of the major types of jaundice is given. A more detailed discussion of the individual disease entities is found in Chap. 301.

Jaundice with predominantly unconjugated bilirubin in the serum OVERPRODUCTION OF BILIRUBIN When an increased amount of hemoglobin is released from red blood cells into either the bloodstream or tissues, increased bilirubin production occurs. Hyperbilirubinemia develops when the capacity of the liver to remove the pigment from the circulation is exceeded. In most cases of hemolysis, the total serum bilirubin concentration ranges from 3 to 5 mg per 100 ml. A slight increase in direct-reacting pigment may also be found, but this usually constitutes less than 15 percent of the total serum bilirubin. This finding is probably analogous to the slight elevations of direct-reacting bilirubin which occur when normal subjects are infused with unconjugated bilirubin. Both instances appear to be a reflection of the fact that the rate-limiting step in hepatic bilirubin metabolism is excretion and that when the excretory capacity of the liver is exceeded, some reentry of conjugated bilirubin into the bloodstream occurs. For a detailed description of the causes of increased bilirubin production, see Chap. 301.

IMPAIRED HEPATIC UPTAKE OF BILIRUBIN As indicated previously, the uptake of bilirubin by the liver cell involves dissociation of the pigment from albumin, and presumably binding to certain cytoplasmic proteins (i.e., ligandins). In some cases of drug-induced jaundice (e.g., due to flavaspidic acid) and possibly in some patients with Gilbert's syndrome, there may be a derangement in this phase of bilirubin metabolism (see Chap. 301).

IMPAIRED GLUCURONIDE CONJUGATION Both acquired and genetic derangements in hepatic glucuronyl transferase occur.

In the fetus and at birth, glucuronyl transferase activity is low and appears to account in part for the *neonatal jaundice* normally found between the second and the fifth days of life. *Mild* decreases in glucuronyl transferases occur in Gilbert's syndrome, *moderate* decreases are found in Crigler-Najjar syndrome type II, and the enzyme is totally absent in the rare Crigler-Najjar syndrome type I (see Chap. 301).

Acquired defects in bilirubin glucuronyl transferase activity may be produced by drugs (i.e., enzyme inhibition) or intrinsic liver disease. However, with liver cell damage, the excretory capacity of the liver is impaired to a greater extent than is the conjugating capacity. Therefore in most hepatocellular diseases, the hyperbilirubinemia is predominantly of the conjugated type (see Chap. 301).

Jaundice with predominantly conjugated bilirubin in the serum
IMPAIRED EXCRETION OF BILIRUBIN BY THE LIVER The impaired excretion of bilirubin into the biliary canaliculi, whether due to functional or mechanical factors, results in predominantly conjugated hyperbilirubinemia and bilirubinuria. The presence of *bilirubin in the urine is evidence of conjugated hyperbilirubinemia* and is a most important point in the differential diagnosis of jaundice. Such findings are identical to those occurring in complete obstruction of the bile duct, emphasizing that *jaundice due to hepatocellular disease can seldom be differentiated from that due to extrahepatic obstruction solely on the basis of changes in bile pigment metabolism.* Indeed there are often instances when the two conditions are not distinguishable by any biochemical criteria, and liver biopsy or other diagnostic procedures are needed for the definitive diagnosis.

When there is interference in the excretion of conjugated bilirubin into bile, by what mechanism does this pigment enter the systemic circulation? Several postulates have been proposed for this "reentry": (1) rupture of the bile canaliculi secondary to the necrosis of the hepatic cells that constitute their walls; (2) occlusion of the canaliculi by inspissated bile or their compression by swollen hepatic cells; (3) obstruction of the terminal intrahepatic bile ducts (cholangioles) by inflammatory cells; (4) altered hepatic cell permeability; and (5) as a result of impaired excretion, accumulation of conjugated bilirubin in the hepatocytes and secondary diffusion into the plasma. Although some of these postulates are speculative, it is likely that several of these mechanisms occur. For example, occasionally in histologic sections, escape of bile through rents in the walls of canaliculi in areas of necrosis is apparent. Also, microscopic studies of the liver of rats injected with fluorescent dyes have shown reflux of bile from canaliculi into sinusoids. However, no anatomic damage needs to be invoked, because when unconjugated bilirubin is infused into normal subjects at high rates, conjugated hyperbilirubinemia occurs; this is explained most logically by passive diffusion.

EXTRAHEPATIC BILIARY OBSTRUCTION Complete obstruction of the extrahepatic bile ducts leads to jaundice with predominantly conjugated hyperbilirubinemia, bilirubinuria, and clay-colored stools. Failure of bile to reach the intestine results in virtual disappearance of urobilinogen from the stool and urine. The concentration of bilirubin rises progressively but then usually plateaus at a level of 30 to 40 mg per 100 ml. To some extent this plateau may be explained by a balance between renal excretion and diversion of bilirubin to other metabolites. In hepatocellular jaundice, such a plateau tends not to occur, and bilirubin levels in excess of 50 mg per 100 ml may be found.

Partial obstruction of the extrahepatic bile ducts can also give rise to jaundice but only if the intrabiliary pressure is increased, because the excretion of bilirubin does not diminish until the intraductile pressure approaches the maximal secretory pressure of approximately 250 mmHg bile. Jaundice may

occur at much lower pressures if the obstruction is complicated by infection of the ducts or hepatocellular injury. Therefore, jaundice, bilirubinuria, and clay-colored stools are inconstant findings in partial biliary obstruction, and the amount of urobilinogen in urine and stool varies with the degree of occlusion.

The functional reserve of the liver is so great that *occlusion of the intrahepatic bile ducts* does not give rise to jaundice unless the drainage of bile from a large segment of the parenchyma is interrupted. Either of the two major hepatic ducts or a large number of secondary radicles may be occluded without production of jaundice. In experimental animals the ducts draining at least 75 percent of the parenchyma must be occluded before jaundice appears.

Additional points of terminology In clinical practice, a patient may be described as having *obstructive*, or *cholestatic*, jaundice. By this is meant that clinically, and especially biochemically, there is little to suggest hepatocellular damage and that the main features point to interference with, or obstruction in, the flow of bile. Typically one would expect such a patient to show (1) predominantly conjugated hyperbilirubinemia, (2) minimal biochemical changes of parenchymal liver damage, and (3) a moderate to a marked increase in the serum alkaline phosphatase level [usually three or four times normal (greater than 15 Bodansky units or greater than 250 IU per liter)]. As emphasized in Chaps. 299 and 300, an *elevated alkaline phosphatase level* in a patient with jaundice or liver disease, in the absence of other disorders such as bone disease, is most suggestive of interference with bile secretion or an infiltrative process in the liver. However, *laboratory tests alone may not permit differentiation of intrahepatic from extrahepatic cholestasis.*

Some clinicians reserve the term obstructive jaundice for those situations in which anatomic obstruction can be demonstrated and use the term cholestatic jaundice for cases of parenchymal liver disease in which the obstructive phase is on a junctional basis. Nevertheless, because these two entities frequently are indistinguishable by clinical and biochemical criteria, the terms obstructive jaundice and cholestatic jaundice are often used interchangeably.

Hepatocellular disorders in which jaundice associated with an obstructive, or cholestatic, phase occurs include (1) occasional cases of viral hepatitis, (2) drug reactions, especially those due to chlorpromazine and methyltestosterone, (3) some cases of alcoholic hepatitis or alcohol-induced fatty liver, (4) jaundice in the last trimester of pregnancy, (5) most cases of Dubin-Johnson or Rotor syndrome, (6) benign recurrent intrahepatic cholestasis, and (7) certain types of postoperative jaundice. These and other conditions are discussed in Chaps. 301 and 302.

In summary, all forms of conjugated hyperbilirubinemia have by definition an impairment in the excretion of bilirubin into bile. In most cases of parenchymal liver disease, a broad derangement is shown by the biochemical tests of liver function. However, when the major detectable alterations of liver function tests include (1) conjugated hyperbilirubinemia and (2) moderate to marked elevation of the serum alkaline phosphatase level, the terms obstructive or cholestatic jaundice may be appropriate. Additional procedures, including operation, are often needed to determine the cause of the cholestasis (see Chaps. 298 and 300).

HEPATOMEGALY

In the supine position, the major part of the liver lies beneath the right rib cage. In some normal persons the liver edge may be palpable 1 to 2 cm below the right costal margin, and a palpable liver edge by itself does not necessarily indicate hepatomegaly. In evaluating liver size by physical examination, two factors other than ability to palpate the liver edge need to be considered, namely, (1) the location of the upper border of liver dullness by percussion, and (2) the body habitus.

Normally, the upper edge of liver dullness on the right side in the midclavicular line is at the level of the fifth rib, but in asthenic habitus it may be lower. The liver edge normally descends 1 to 3 cm with deep inspiration. In hypersthenic subjects, the liver may extend over to the left side of the abdominal wall, with the lower edge high and not palpable; in hyposthenic subjects with a very acute costal angle, the liver may lie in the right half of the abdomen, the edge being palpable by as much as 6 to 8 cm below the right costal margin lateral to the right rectus abdominis muscle. Thus, palpability does not necessarily imply hepatomegaly.

In determining liver enlargement by palpation, one should be certain that the liver is being palpated rather than other right upper quadrant masses such as gallbladder, colonic neoplasm, or fecal material in the colon. Liver enlargement is often confirmed by radiologic studies, including hepatic scintiscans, celiac axis angiography, and echography.

In many cases of generalized liver enlargement, the left lobe will be felt in the epigastrium between the xiphoid and umbilicus. The liver should be carefully palpated during deep inspiration to determine whether the edge is tender, regular or irregular, firm or soft, rounded and thickened, or sharp. The edge is tender and often rounded with hepatic inflammation, as in hepatitis, or when the liver is acutely congested, as in cardiac decompensation. Pulsation of the liver may be found with tricuspid valvular incompetence. A carcinomatous liver may be rocklike in hardness; the cirrhotic liver is very firm in consistency. The largest livers are often found with carcinoma (primary or metastatic), marked fatty infiltration, congestive cardiac decompensation, Hodgkin's disease, and amyloidosis. Rapid decrease in liver size may occur with improvement of congestive failure, mobilization of fat from the liver, or massive hepatic necrosis.

TABLE 39-3
Causes of a palpable liver and hepatomegaly

I Palpable liver without hepatomegaly
  A Right diaphragm displaced downward (e.g., emphysema, asthma)
  B Subdiaphragmatic lesion (e.g., abscess)
  C Aberrant lobe of liver (Riedel's lobe)
  D Extremely thin or relaxed abdominal muscles
  E Occasionally present in normal persons
II Hepatomegaly
  A Vascular congestion (e.g., congestive heart failure, hepatic vein thrombosis)
  B Bile duct obstruction (e.g., lesion in common duct leading to hepatomegaly and subsequently biliary cirrhosis)
  C Infiltrative disorders
    1 Bone marrow and reticuloendothelial cells
      a Extramedullary hematopoiesis
      b Leukemia
      c Lymphoma
    2 Fat
      a Fatty liver (e.g., secondary to alcohol, diabetes, or toxins)
      b Gaucher's disease and some other lipidoses
    3 Glycogen (e.g., diabetes, especially after insulin excess)
    4 Amyloid
    5 Iron (hemochromatosis and hemosiderosis)
    6 Granuloma (tuberculosis, sarcoid)
  D Inflammatory disorders
    1 Hepatitis—due to drugs or infectious agents
    2 Cirrhosis—except in late stages when prolonged scarring may lead to a *small,* shrunken liver
  E Tumors—primary or metastatic
  F Cysts—polycystic disease, congenital hepatic fibrosis

In a patient with hepatomegaly, auscultation is sometimes helpful. A friction rub may be audible (and palpable) in the right upper quadrant; it is usually due to a recent biopsy, tumor, or perihepatitis. In portal hypertension a venous hum may be audible between the umbilicus and the xiphoid. An arterial murmur or bruit over the liver may indicate tumor, usually hepatoma.

Some of the causes of a palpable liver and hepatomegaly are given in Table 39-3.

REFERENCES

BERK PD et al: Inborn errors of bilirubin metabolism. Med Clin North Am 59:803, 1975

BISSELL DM: Formation and elimination of bilirubin. Gastroenterology 69:519, 1975

FEVERY J et al: Unconjugated bilirubin and an increased proportion of bilirubin monoconjugates in the bile of patients with Gilbert's syndrome and Crigler-Najjar disease. J Clin Invest 60:970, 1977

GORESKY CA, FISHER MM: *Jaundice.* New York, Plenum, 1975

SCHMID R: Bilirubin metabolism: State of the art. Gastroenterology 74:1307, 1978

SCHMID R, McDONAGH AF: Hyperbilirubinemia, in *The Metabolic Basis of Inherited Disease,* 4th ed, JB Stanbury et al (eds). New York, McGraw-Hill, 1978

40
ABDOMINAL SWELLING AND ASCITES

ROBERT M. GLICKMAN
KURT J. ISSELBACHER

ABDOMINAL SWELLING Abdominal swelling or distention is a common problem in clinical medicine and may be the initial manifestation of a systemic disease or of otherwise unsuspected abdominal disease. *Subjective* abdominal enlargement, often described as a sensation of fullness or bloating, is usually transient and is often related to a functional gastrointestinal disorder when it is not accompanied by objective physical findings of increased abdominal girth or local swelling. *Obesity* and lumbar lordosis, which may be associated with prominence of the abdomen, may usually be distinguished from true increases in the volume of the peritoneal cavity by history and careful physical examination.

Clinical history Abdominal swelling may first be noticed by the patient because of a progressive increase in belt or clothing size, the appearance of abdominal or inguinal hernias, or the development of a localized swelling. Often, considerable abdominal enlargement has gone unnoticed for weeks or months, either because of coexistent obesity or because the ascites formation has been insidious, without pain or localizing symptoms. Progressive abdominal distention may be associated with a sensation of "pulling" or "stretching" of the flanks or groins and vague low back pain. Localized *pain* usually results from involvement of an abdominal organ (e.g., a passively congested liver, large spleen, or colonic tumor). Pain is uncommon in cirrhosis with ascites and when it is present pancreatitis, hepatoma, or peritonitis should be considered. Tense ascites or abdominal tumors may produce increased intraabdominal pressure, resulting in *indigestion* and *heartburn* due to gastroesophageal reflux or *dyspnea, orthopnea,* and *tachypnea* from elevation of the diaphragm. A coexistent pleural effusion, more commonly on the right, presumably due to leakage of ascitic fluid through lymphatic channels in the diaphragm, may also contribute to respiratory embarrassment. The patient with diffuse abdominal swelling should be questioned about increased alcoholic intake, a prior episode of jaundice or hematuria, a change in bowel habits, or a past history of rheumatic heart disease. Such historic information may provide the clues that will lead one to suspect an occult cirrhosis, a colonic tumor with peritoneal seeding, congestive heart failure, or nephrosis.

Physical examination A carefully executed *general physical examination* can yield valuable clues concerning the etiology of abdominal swelling. Thus palmar erythema and spider angiomas suggest an underlying cirrhosis, while supraclavicular adenopathy (Virchow's node) should raise the question of an underlying gastrointestinal malignancy. *Inspection* of the abdomen is an important but often cursorily performed aspect of the abdominal examination. By noting the abdominal contour, one may be able to distinguish localized from generalized swelling. The tensely distended abdomen with tightly stretched skin, bulging flanks, and everted umbilicus is characteristic of ascites. A prominent abdominal venous pattern with the direction of flow away from the umbilicus often is a reflection of portal hypertension; venous collaterals with flow from the lower part of the abdomen toward the umbilicus suggests obstruction of the inferior vena cava; flow downward toward the umbilicus suggests superior vena cava obstruction. "Doming" of the abdomen with visible ridges from underlying intestinal loops is usually due to intestinal obstruction or distention. An epigastric mass, with evident peristalsis proceeding from left to right, usually indicates underlying pyloric obstruction. A liver with metastatic deposits may be visible as a nodular right upper quadrant mass moving with respiration.

Auscultation may reveal the high-pitched, rushing sounds of early intestinal obstruction or a succussion sound due to increased fluid and gas in a dilated hollow viscus. Careful auscultation over an enlarged liver occasionally reveals the harsh bruit of a vascular tumor, especially a hepatoma, or the leathery friction rub of a surface nodule. A venous hum at the umbilicus may signify portal hypertension and an increased collateral blood flow around the liver. A fluid wave and flank dullness which shifts with change in position of the patient are important signs that indicate the presence of peritoneal fluid. In obese patients, small amounts of fluid may be difficult to demonstrate; on occasion the fluid may be detected by abdominal percussion with patients on their hands and knees. Doubt about the presence of peritoneal fluid may be resolved by careful paracentesis with a small-gauge (No. 19 or 20) needle. Careful percussion should serve to distinguish generalized abdominal enlargement from localized swelling due to an enlarged uterus, ovarian cyst, or distended bladder. Percussion can also outline an abnormally small or large liver. Loss of normal liver dullness may result from massive hepatic necrosis; it may also be a clue to free gas in the peritoneal cavity, as from perforation of a hollow viscus.

Palpation is often difficult with massive ascites, and ballottement of overlying fluid may be the only method of palpating the liver or spleen. A slightly enlarged spleen in association with ascites may be the only evidence of an occult cirrhosis. When there is evidence of portal hypertension, a soft liver suggests that obstruction to portal flow is extrahepatic; a firm liver suggests cirrhosis as the likely cause of the portal hypertension. A very hard or nodular liver is a clue that the liver is infiltrated with tumor, and when accompanied by ascites, it suggests that the latter is due to peritoneal seeding. A pulsatile liver and ascites may be found in tricuspid insufficiency.

An attempt should be made to determine whether a mass is solid or cystic, smooth or irregular, and whether it moves with respiration. The liver, spleen, and gallbladder should descend with respiration unless they are fixed by adhesions or extension of tumor beyond the organ. A fixed mass not descending with respiration may indicate that it is retroperitoneal. Tenderness, especially if localized, may indicate an inflammatory process

such as an abscess; it may also be due to stretching of the visceral peritoneum or tumor necrosis. Rectal and pelvic examinations are mandatory; they may reveal otherwise undetected masses due to tumor or infection.

Radiographic and laboratory examinations are essential for confirming or extending the impressions gained on physical examination. Upright and recumbent films of the abdomen may demonstrate the dilated loops of intestine with fluid levels characteristic of intestinal obstruction or the diffuse abdominal haziness and loss of psoas margins suggestive of ascites. A plain film of the abdomen may reveal the distended colon of otherwise unsuspected ulcerative colitis and give valuable information as to the size of the liver and spleen. An irregular and elevated right side of the diaphragm may be a clue to a liver abscess or hepatoma. Studies of the gastrointestinal tract with barium or other contrast media are usually necessary in the search for a primary tumor.

ASCITES In most cases the clinical and laboratory evaluation of the patient with ascites is sufficient to reveal the cause of the fluid accumulation. Often the ascites is a component or complication of cirrhosis, congestive heart failure, nephrosis, or disseminated carcinomatosis. However, even when the cause of ascites seems obvious, it is often important to determine whether another separate or related disease process has supervened. For example, when the patient with compensated cirrhosis and minimal ascites develops progressive ascites that is increasingly difficult to control with sodium restriction or diuretics, the obvious temptation is to attribute the worsening of the clinical picture to progressive liver disease. However, an occult hepatoma, portal vein thrombosis, spontaneous bacterial peritonitis, or even tuberculosis may be responsible for the decompensation. The disappointingly low success of diagnosing tuberculous peritonitis or hepatoma in the patient with cirrhosis and ascites reflects the too-low index of suspicion for the development of such superimposed conditions. Similarly, the patient with congestive heart failure may develop ascites from a disseminated carcinoma with peritoneal seeding. The thorough evaluation of each patient with ascites, even in the presence of an "obvious" cause, will help avoid these errors.

Diagnostic paracentesis (50 to 100 ml) should be part of the routine evaluation of the patient with ascites. The fluid should be examined for its gross appearance, protein content, cell count, and differential cell count, as well as Gram's and acid-fast stains and culture. Cytologic and cell-block examination may disclose an otherwise unsuspected carcinoma. Table 40-1 presents some of the features of ascitic fluid typically found in various disease states. In some disorders, such as cirrhosis, the fluid has the characteristics of a transudate (less than 2.5 g protein per 100 ml and a specific gravity less than 1.016); in others, such as peritonitis, the features are those of an exudate. Although there is variability of the ascitic fluid in any given disease state, some features are sufficiently characteristic to suggest certain diagnostic possibilities. For example, blood-stained fluid with more than 2.5 g protein per 100 ml is unusual in uncomplicated cirrhosis but is consistent with tuberculous peritonitis or neoplasm. Cloudy fluid with a predominance of polymorphonuclear cells and a positive Gram stain are characteristic of bacterial peritonitis; if most cells are lymphocytes, tuberculosis should be suspected. The complete examination of each fluid is most important, for occasionally only *one* finding may be abnormal. For example, if the fluid is a typical transudate but contains more than 250 white blood cells per cubic millimeter, the finding should be recognized as

TABLE 40-1
Ascitic fluid characteristics in various disease states

| Condition | Gross appearance | Specific gravity | Protein, g/100 ml | Cell count | | Other tests |
				Red blood cells, >10,000/mm³	White blood cells, per mm³	
Cirrhosis	Straw-colored or bile-stained	<1.016 (95%)*	<2.5 (95%)	1%	<250 (90%);* predominantly endothelial	
Neoplasm	Straw-colored, hemorrhagic, mucinous, or chylous	Variable, >1.016 (45%)	>2.5 (75%)	20%	>1000 (50%); variable cell types	Cytology, cell block, peritoneal biopsy
Tuberculous peritonitis	Clear, turbid, hemorrhagic, chylous	Variable, >1.016 (50%)	>2.5 (50%)	7%	>1000 (70%); usually >70% lymphocytes	Peritoneal biopsy, stain and culture for acid-fast bacilli
Pyogenic peritonitis	Turbid or purulent	If purulent, >1.016	If purulent, >2.5	Unusual	Predominantly polymorphonuclear leukocytes	+Gram's stain, culture
Congestive heart failure	Straw-colored	Variable, <1.016 (60%)	Variable, 1.5–5.3	10%	<1000 (90%); usually mesothelial, mononuclear	
Nephrosis	Straw-colored or chylous	<1.016	<2.5 (100%)	Unusual	<250; mesothelial, mononuclear	If chylous, ether extraction, Sudan staining
Pancreatic ascites (pancreatitis, pseudocyst)	Turbid, hemorrhagic, or chylous	Variable, often >1.016	Variable, often >2.5	Variable, may be blood-stained	Variable	Increased amylase in ascitic fluid and serum

* Since the conditions of examining fluid and selecting patients were not identical in each series, the percentage figures (in the parentheses) should be taken as an indication of the order of magnitude rather than as the precise incidence of any abnormal finding.
SOURCES: *Berner et al; Borhanmanesh et al; Coder and Olander; Malagelada et al.*

atypical for cirrhosis, nephrosis, or congestive heart failure and should warrant a search for tumor or infection. This is especially true in the evaluation of cirrhotic ascites where occult peritoneal infection may be present with only minor elevations in the white blood cell count of the peritoneal fluid (300 to 500 cells per cubic millimeter). Since Gram's stain of the fluid may be negative in a high proportion of such cases, careful culture of the peritoneal fluid is mandatory.

Chylous ascites refers to a turbid, milky, or creamy peritoneal fluid due to the presence of thoracic or intestinal lymph. Such a fluid shows Sudan-staining fat globules microscopically and an increased triglyceride content by chemical examination. A turbid fluid due to leukocytes or tumor cells may be confused with chylous fluid, and it is often helpful to carry out alkalinization and ether extraction of the specimen. Alkali will tend to dissolve cellular proteins and thereby reduce turbidity;

FIGURE 40-1
Starch peritonitis. Examination of ascitic fluid under polarized light reveals doubly refractile starch granules.

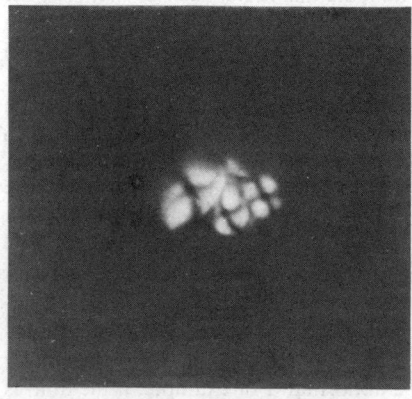

ether extraction will lead to clearing if the turbidity of the fluid is due to lipid. Chylous ascites is most often the result of lymphatic obstruction from trauma, tumor, tuberculosis, filariasis (see Chap. 209), or congenital abnormalities. It may also be seen in the nephrotic syndrome.

Rarely, ascitic fluid may be *mucinous* in character, suggesting either pseudomyxoma peritonei (Chap. 297) or rarely a colloid carcinoma of the stomach or colon with peritoneal implants.

On rare occasions a syndrome may be seen of fever and ascites, without infection, occurring several weeks after abdominal surgery. This seems to result from starch (from surgical gloves) introduced into the peritoneum at the time of surgery, with a subsequent foreign-body reaction and ascites formation. Given the proper index of suspicion, diagnosis can be made by paracentesis and finding double refractile particles (i.e., starch) when polarized light is used (Fig. 40-1).

The etiology of ascites may remain uncertain even after the all these conditions pronounced weight loss, wasting, anorexia, and fever may be found, and hepatomegaly, splenomegaly, and deranged liver function tests may be present. Procedures such as peritoneal biopsy, peritoneoscopy, liver biopsy, splenoportography, or laparotomy may be necessary to provide the diagnosis. Other less common causes of ascites include constrictive pericarditis, hepatic vein obstruction, myxedema and benign tumors of the ovary, particularly fibroma (Meigs's syndrome, with ascites and hydrothorax). The physiologic and metabolic factors involved in the production of ascites are described in Chap. 304.

REFERENCES

BAR-MEIR S: Analysis of ascitic fluid in cirrhosis. Dig Dis Sc 24:136, 1979
BERNER C et al: Diagnostic probabilities in patients with conspicuous ascites. Arch Intern Med 113:687, 1964

BORHANMANESH F et al: Tuberculous peritonitis: Prospective study of 32 cases in Iran. Ann Intern Med 76:567, 1972

CODER DM, OLANDER GA: Granulomatous peritonitis caused by starch glove powder. Arch Surg 105:83, 1972

CONN HO: Spontaneous bacterial peritonitis: Multiple revisitations. Gastroenterology 70:455, 1976

————, FESSEL JH: Spontaneous bacterial peritonitis in cirrhosis: Variations on a theme. Medicine 50:161, 1971

MALAGELADA JR et al: Origin of fat in chylous ascites of patients with liver cirrhosis. Gastroenterology 67:878, 1974

WARSHAW AL: Diagnosis of starch peritonitis by paracentesis. Lancet 2:1054, 1972

section 6 | Alterations in body weight

41
GAIN AND LOSS IN WEIGHT

DANIEL W. FOSTER

GENERAL PRINCIPLES

In normal persons weight is maintained stable because caloric intake is matched to caloric expenditure by the coordinated activities of the feeding and satiety centers located in the brainstem. Energy costs fall into three categories: (1) calories needed for maintenance of basal metabolism, (2) calories necessary for food absorption (specific dynamic action), and (3) calories required for physical activity. *Basal metabolism* is defined as the total caloric requirement when the body is in the supine position, motionless except for quiet respiration. It can be translated as the energy required to maintain structural and functional integrity of the organism in the absence of physical activity. Under normal circumstances about half the total daily caloric intake is consumed by basal processes. In nonobese, nonsedentary subjects another 10 percent of the total intake is used for food absorption. The remainder is spent in physical activity. In active persons this represents about 40 percent of daily intake, though athletes may use greater than 50 percent of calories for physical activity.

Gain or loss in tissue mass is determined by the net balance between caloric intake and caloric expenditure. Change in body weight as a consequence of voluntary alteration in diet or exercise is never worrisome; change in weight that is not deliberately sought, on the other hand, is a frequent reason for consultation with the physician and often indicates the presence of disease. It is important to recognize that changes in weight may reflect alteration in either tissue mass or body fluid content. Rapid swings almost always indicate the latter. Even when tissue mass is changing, fluid loss or gain plays a major role in the measured change in weight, particularly over the short run. This point is well illustrated by the data of Table 41-1 where the composition of weight loss was estimated during a 24-day period of semistarvation in 13 normal soldiers (daily intake 1010 cal). During the first 3 days 70 percent of the weight loss was due to water, while in subsequent stages protein and fat accounted for essentially all the decreased mass. This varying contribution of fluid accounts for the fact that one cannot use a fixed formula for predicting weight loss or gain. It is frequently stated that a net change of 7700 cal will be accompanied by a 1-kg change in body mass (3500 cal/lb). While this figure is reasonable as an estimate for long-term

changes in caloric intake, obviously the apparent caloric cost per kilogram of weight lost or gained will vary with the accompanying fluid shifts. In the experiment summarized in Table 41-1, for example, a negative balance of only 2596 cal resulted in the loss of a kilogram of weight between days 1 and 3, while between days 22 and 24, loss of a kilogram required a deficit of 8700 cal. In general if weight loss or gain has occurred over a period of weeks or months, it is safe to assume that change in tissue mass has occurred; weight loss or gain limited to a several-day period may be due to fluid shifts alone. Occasionally true loss of tissue mass is obscured by fluid retention as in the case of the cirrhotic patient who develops ascites or the patient with anorexia nervosa and edema.

WEIGHT GAIN

While obesity is a major public health concern (see Chap. 76), its diagnosis is usually uncomplicated. Obese subjects often deny overeating, but the true situation can usually be assessed either by tabulating actual food intake and determining its caloric content from standard tables or by interviewing the patient's family and friends. Regardless of history, excess caloric intake is the cause of obesity in the overwhelming majority of cases. Pathological causes of obesity are rare. In the adult, Cushing's syndrome can result in acquired obesity in a previously nonobese patient, but usually the diagnosis suggests itself by the pattern of fat distribution and the clinical picture. Other endocrine diseases such as hypothyroidism, hypogonadism, and insulin-secreting tumors are frequently listed in the differential diagnosis of acquired obesity but in fact do not represent significant diagnostic problems. Congenital diseases such as the Prader-Willi and Laurence-Moon-Biedl syndromes are usually readily recognizable and appear early in life. Rarely neoplastic disease involving the hypothalamus, particularly

TABLE 41-1
Percentage composition of mean daily weight loss in 13 young men during caloric restriction for 24 days

Days	Mean weight loss, kg/day	Water, %	Fat, %	Protein, %	Calorie equivalents of weight loss, cal/kg
1–3	0.80	70	25	5	2596
11–13	0.23	19	69	12	7043
22–24	0.17	0	85	15	8700

SOURCE: *After Brožek et al.*

craniopharyngioma, may be a cause of acquired obesity. Extensive workup of the central nervous system in obesity is not indicated, however, in the absence of suspicious symptoms (headache, visual difficulties, vomiting, or endocrine changes).

WEIGHT LOSS

Weight loss in the absence of deliberate dieting is a more serious problem than weight gain simply because there is a high chance that organic disease is present. Mechanisms include decreased appetite, accelerated tissue metabolism, and loss of calories in urine or stool, acting singly or in combination. No attempt will be made to list all the diseases capable of causing weight loss. The majority of cases will fall into one of the seven following categories.

DIABETES MELLITUS Initial weight loss with the onset of diabetes is largely fluid and is due to the osmotic diuresis induced by hyperglycemia. Subsequently loss of tissue mass occurs in the insulin-dependent form of the disease due to both caloric wastage (the consequence of glycosuria) and the hormonal abnormalities that characterize the illness. Insulin deficiency and glucagon excess result in impaired synthesis of protein and fat and simultaneously cause accelerated proteolysis and lipolysis such that the net energy state is catabolic. Weight loss in diabetes is frequently associated with increased food intake.

ENDOCRINE DISEASE The most important endocrine disease causing weight loss is thyrotoxicosis. While weight loss is not inevitable (indeed, thyrotoxicosis may rarely be found in a patient who has gained weight), it is extremely common. Increased appetite and food intake are the rule, and patients often spontaneously choose a very high carbohydrate diet. Caloric expenditure is enormous, primarily because of an increased metabolic rate, but increased motor activity also plays a role. The molecular mechanism whereby thyrotoxicosis causes weight loss is not settled, but thyroid hormone is thought to increase sodium-potassium adenosine triphosphatase (ATPase) activity in many tissues, suggesting that the diminished efficiency of ingested calories is due to a futile cycle of adenosine triphosphate (ATP) synthesis and breakdown with energy lost as heat. Panhypopituitarism and adrenal insufficiency may also be associated with weight loss, probably primarily as a consequence of diminished appetite secondary to cortisol deficiency.

GASTROINTESTINAL DISEASE A variety of gastrointestinal diseases may cause weight loss. Overt or occult steatorrhea due to sprue, chronic pancreatitis, or cystic fibrosis may produce wasting despite major increases in food intake. Chronic diarrhea due to inflammatory bowel disease (with or without fistulas) or parasites, esophageal disease with reflux or vomiting, even ordinary peptic ulcer have to be considered in the differential diagnosis. The mechanism of weight loss in alimentary tract disease is generally either decreased food intake or malabsorption, though inflammation per se probably plays a major role in ulcerative colitis and regional enteritis.

INFECTION Hidden infection must always be sought in patients with unexplained weight loss. Tuberculosis, fungal diseases, amebic abscess, and subacute bacterial endocarditis should be high on the list of suspects. The mechanism probably involves both anorexia and inflammation-induced acceleration of cellular metabolic demands. It has been suggested that glucagon plays a major role in the induction of negative nitrogen balance and tissue wastage in inflammation, but it is likely that the catabolic state also requires changes in a number of other hormones.

MALIGNANCY Occult malignancy is probably the number one cause of weight loss occurring in the absence of major signs and symptoms. In the search for malignancy particular emphasis must be placed on the gastrointestinal tract, pancreas, and liver. Lymphoma and leukemia should also be considered. While silent (except for weight loss) malignancy can occur in any organ, statistically the gastrointestinal tract is the most common site.

PSYCHIATRIC DISEASE The classic psychiatric illness associated with profound weight loss is anorexia nervosa (Chap. 77). However, anorexia may also occur in depressive states and schizophrenia. The presence of anorexia is usually clear from the history. While organic disease causing both anorexia and depression has to be ruled out, ordinarily the psychiatric nature of the problem will be clear.

RENAL DISEASE One of the earliest manifestations of uremia is anorexia. As a consequence all patients with unexplained weight loss should be given screening renal function tests.

SUMMARY

Weight loss is more often a diagnostic problem than weight gain and much more often a sign of serious organic illness. If the weight loss is associated with increased food intake, the diagnosis will likely be diabetes, thyrotoxicosis, or a malabsorption syndrome. If food intake is normal or decreased, malignancy, infection, renal disease, psychiatric syndromes, or endocrine deficiency will more commonly be found.

REFERENCES

BROŽEK J et al: Changes in body weight and body dimensions in men performing work on a low calorie carbohydrate diet. J Appl Physiol 10:412, 1957

KONISHI F: Food energy equivalents of various activities. J Am Diet Assoc 46:186, 1965

RUNCIE J, HILDITCH TE: Energy provision, tissue utilization and weight loss in prolonged starvation. Br Med J 2:352, 1974

YANG M-U, VAN ITALLIE TB: Composition of weight loss during short-term weight reduction. Metabolic responses of obese subjects to starvation and low calorie ketogenic and non-ketogenic diets. J Clin Invest 58:722, 1976

42

PROTEINURIA, HEMATURIA, AZOTEMIA, AND OLIGURIA

FREDRIC L. COE

PROTEINURIA

Normal adults may excrete up to 150 mg protein daily. Of this, only 10 to 15 mg is albumin; the rest is composed of over 30 different plasma proteins and of glycoproteins that derive from the renal cells. Tamm-Horsfall mucoprotein, the most prevalent of the urine proteins that do not arise from plasma, is produced by the cells of the ascending limb of the loop of Henle and is excreted at the rate of 25 mg per day. Daily excretion of more than 150 mg protein is properly termed *pathological proteinuria*, but in common usage the word *proteinuria* suffices. Protein excretion above 3.5 g per 24 h is termed *massive* proteinuria and usually occurs when glomeruli have been damaged enough to allow plasma proteins, especially albumin, to enter the urine. Urinary albumin loss lowers serum albumin concentration, and the consequent fall in intracapillary oncotic pressure fosters the accumulation of tissue edema (Chap. 29); serum lipids rise. The combination of *massive proteinuria, hypoalbuminemia, edema,* and *hyperlipidemia* is often called the *nephrotic syndrome,* but this term is becoming synonymous with massive urinary protein loss alone. Hypoalbuminemia, elevated blood lipids, and edema are pathophysiologic consequences of massive proteinuria and occur only when hepatic albumin synthesis, though normal or even increased, fails to compensate for urine albumin losses; they are not a direct result of renal disease.

DETECTION OF PROTEINURIA Detection of proteinuria is usually by urine "dipsticks" that register a trace result in response to as little as 50 mg protein per liter, and a distinct color change of the 1+ level at about 300 mg per liter. Since proteinuria can be missed if the urine is very dilute, fasting morning samples that tend to be concentrated are usually studied. Dipsticks respond best to albumin, so that a negative result can occur when large amounts of other protein, or protein fragments such as light chains, are being excreted. Dipstick proteinuria requires additional evaluation by the measurement of 24-h excretion rate. If total protein excretion is abnormal, it is helpful to characterize the proportions of albumin and globulins in the urine by cellulose acetate electrophoresis or other methods. Immunoelectrophoresis is required to identify immunoglobulin fragments, kappa or lambda light chains, when their presence is suggested by a monoclonal peak on routine urine electrophoresis.

MECHANISMS OF PROTEINURIA Tubular proteinuria Normal low-molecular-weight serum proteins below 40,000 daltons, such as β_2 microglobulin (11,600 mol wt), lysozyme (14,000 mol wt), or light chains (22,000 mol wt) are readily filtered by the glomeruli but are normally present in urine in only trace amounts because tubular reabsorption of them is very efficient. Diseases that selectively damage the tubules more than glomeruli (Chap. 281) cause excessive excretion of these small proteins with little or no increase in albumin excretion. The resulting proteinuria is usually between 1 and 3 g per 24 h, and edema and lipid disorders do not occur because albumin losses are small. Bence-Jones protein, which is probably a dimer of two light chains, light chains themselves, and myoglobin are examples of proteins whose plasma concentrations may increase as a consequence of disease. If their filtered load rises enough to exceed tubular reabsorptive capacity, "overflow" proteinuria may occur.

Glomerular proteinuria When glomerular damage is present, albumin and even larger globulin molecules may be filtered excessively because normal selective filtration is lost. The glomerular capillary endothelial cells form a barrier penetrated by pores of about 1000 Å diameter that holds back cells and other particles but offers no impediment to most proteins. The glomerular basement membrane traps molecules above 50 Å in effective radius. These usually have a molecular weight above 100,000 daltons. The *foot processes (podocytes)* of the visceral epithelial cells (Fig. 42–1) cover the urinary aspect of the glomerular basement membrane and produce a series of narrow channels through which molecules that traverse the basement membrane must pass. Anionic molecules, like albumin, are filtered less freely than are neutral or positively charged molecules of the same size, so little albumin enters the filtrate. This charge selectivity appears to be due to anionic glycoproteins that cover the surfaces of the foot processes and contribute to the matrix structure of the basement membrane (Chap. 274). The glycoproteins are anionic because they contain the dicarboxylic amino acids, glutamic and aspartic acid, and sialic acid. At the pH of blood (7.4) or urine (4.5 to 7.5) carboxylic and sialic acid residues are dissociated and, therefore, have a negative charge. Albumin also carries an overall negative charge. The negatively charged portions of the glycoproteins repel those of albumin and retard filtration.

Glomerular disease can disrupt any of these filtration barriers. Injury limited to the polyanion glycoproteins would tend to produce selective losses of anionic proteins, such as albumin, that would be filtered more completely by the normal glomerulus but for their charge. Extensive injury that involves the entire basement membrane, not only its polyanion components, may increase losses of very large proteins, as well as albumin.

The selectivity of proteinuria varies with the extent of glomerular injury. However, the clinical value of measuring selectivity has not been fully defined. The basis of such measurements is to express the excretion rate of a protein as a fraction of its theoretical maximum filtered load, which is the product of its serum concentration and the glomerular filtration rate (GFR). This fraction must reflect the relative filtration efficiency of the protein to that of a completely filtered GFR marker, usually inulin or creatinine, provided that tubular reabsorption and renal production or catabolism are negligible. The slope of a plot of such a clearance ratio against molecular weight for a variety of serum proteins is one index of filtration selectivity. A more practical version of this test is based upon the ratio of the clearance fractions of two proteins of different molecular weight. For example, the IgG transferrin clearance fraction ratio is below 0.1 in most children with lipoid nephrosis, a proteinuric disorder in which fusion of foot processes is the only detectable glomerular abnormality (Chap. 278). In chronic membranous glomerulopathy (Chap. 278) the basement membrane is filled with immune complex deposits, and progressive renal failure occurs. Here, the clearance ratio usually is between 0.1 and 0.2. The ratio usually is above 0.2 in membranoproliferative glomerulonephritis, a severe renal disease that can progress rapidly to renal failure and in which glomerular architecture is severely disturbed (Chap. 278). These and other aspects of the relationship between glomerular pathology and proteinuria are considered in greater detail in Chaps. 277 to 279.

APPROACH TO THE PATIENT WITH PROTEINURIA Given dipstick proteinuria of the 1+ level or more, 24-h urine protein excretion must be measured. If it is above 150 mg, electrophoresis should be carried out to determine the proportions of albumin and other proteins. Excretion mainly of albumin signifies a glomerular lesion. When the total daily protein excretion exceeds 3.5 g, by definition the nephrotic syndrome is considered to be present; milder albuminuria is called an *asymptomatic urinary abnormality*. Tubular proteinuria usually reflects a hereditary or acquired tubular disorder or tubulointerstitial nephropathy (Chap. 281). The presence of large amounts of Bence-Jones protein suggests that multiple myeloma may be present (Chap. 63).

ISOLATED HEMATURIA Urinary tract bleeding from the urethra to the renal pelvis produces isolated hematuria, without significant proteinuria, cells, or urinary casts. Total hematuria, which occurs evenly throughout voiding, means that blood has had the opportunity to mix fully with the bladder urine. When bleeding occurs mainly at the beginning or end of micturition, a prostatic or urethral origin is more likely.

Common causes of *isolated* hematuria are urinary tract stones, benign and malignant neoplasms of the urinary tract, tuberculosis, trauma, and prostatitis; few primary renal diseases cause it. As discussed in Chaps. 273 and 278, *focal glomerulitis,* in the syndrome of benign recurrent hematuria or in Berger's disease, i.e., IgA nephropathy, is usually associated with red blood cell casts. Analgesic nephropathy and sickling states cause isolated hematuria, but modest proteinuria, papillary necrosis, or azotemia often is present and suggests a renal origin. Hemoglobin electrophoresis is appropriate whenever a sickling disorder is suspected.

Prostatic and external urethral examination is the basic first step in the evaluation of isolated hematuria. Intravenous pyelography is the next. If no lesion is found, cystoscopy and retrograde pyelography may become necessary. At cystoscopy, blood may be found to issue from only one ureter, a helpful clue which indicates a localized lesion rather than a primary renal disease. Disorders of coagulation, and thrombocytopenia, as well as urinary infection, must be excluded. Because

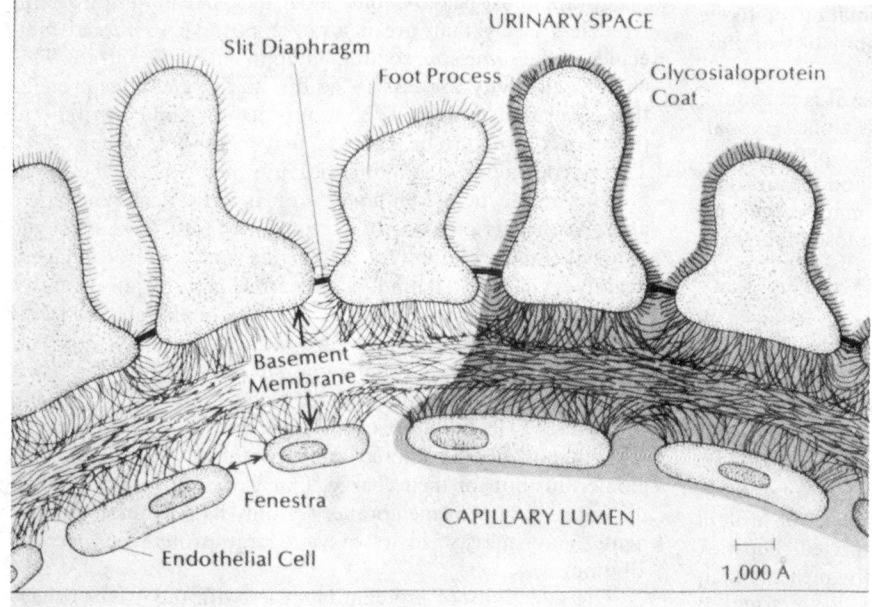

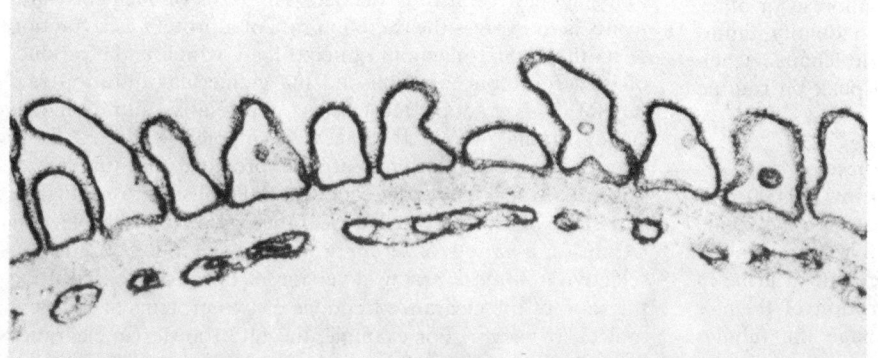

FIGURE 42-1

Top. Diagram showing normal structures separating the capillary lumen and urinary space in the glomerulus. In the process of glomerular filtration, an ultrafiltrate of plasma traverses the glomerular capillary wall through endothelial fenestrae, basement membrane, and slit diaphragms. Macromolecules in the plasma are believed to be restricted from entry into glomerular urine by each of these wall structures. In addition, circulating polyanions (e.g., albumin) are thought to be retarded by negatively charged glycosialoproteins, which, as shown by the shaded area in the upper panel, are distributed throughout the glomerular wall. Bottom. A corresponding electron micrograph of the same structures. (Drawing by NL Gahan from BM Brenner, R Beeuwkes, Hosp Prac, vol 13, no 7, 1978. Reproduced with permission.)

infection with tuberculosis and fungi may be difficult to detect, multiple urine samples must be cultured and examined by microscopy.) Renal arteriography may be needed to disclose anatomic lesions such as cysts or tumors.

HEMATURIA ASSOCIATED WITH URINARY TRACT INFECTION

Bacterial infection of the lower urinary tract or of the kidneys occasionally causes hematuria. The presence of associated pyuria suggests the diagnosis of infection and the demonstration of pathogenic bacteria in concentrations above 10^5 colonies per milliliter of urine establishes it. Acute cystitis or urethritis in women is an especially common cause of gross hematuria. Urinary tuberculosis can produce isolated hematuria, but pyuria often is present as well.

HEMATURIA WITH EVIDENCE OF RENAL DISEASE   Nephronal

hematuria Blood may enter the tubular fluid anywhere along the nephron, from the glomerulus to the end of the collecting duct. Tamm-Horsfall protein tends to gel when concentrated at a low pH, as occurs during dehydration, or when exposed to myoglobin, hemoglobin, albumin, Bence-Jones protein, and pyelographic contrast media. Red blood cells in the tubule lumens can be trapped in a cylindrical mold of the gelled protein to produce red blood cell casts, which provide conclusive evidence of bleeding into the nephron. Degenerated red blood cells and clumps of hemoglobin can produce deeply pigmented casts that have the same significance as red blood cell casts.

Bleeding from the nephron itself, like glomerular proteinuria, always connotes significant renal disease such as glomerulonephritis, tubulointerstitial injury, or a vasculitis that has damaged the circulation of the nephron. Glomerular or tubular proteinuria often accompanies renal bleeding, as a consequence of nephron injury. (As a rule, renal bleeding or proteinuria alone arises from diseases that have a better prognosis than those in which proteinuria and hematuria occur in combination.)

Hematuria with proteinuria or casts Frequently, hematuria is accompanied by proteinuria, but red blood cell and deeply pigmented granular casts are absent. The presumption then is that bleeding is of nephronal origin, but a coincident independent lesion of the urinary tract must always be considered, because common renal diseases, such as diabetic glomerulosclerosis and arteriolar nephrosclerosis associated with hypertension, produce mainly proteinuria.

Heavy albuminuria or dehydration can cause showers of transparent, refractile "hyaline" casts. During heavy proteinuria tubule cells fill with cholesterol-rich lipid droplets that display a Maltese-cross appearance in polarized light. Casts that incorporate these cells are called *fatty casts* because the lipid droplets are prominent. The same lipid-rich cells free in urine are called *oval fat bodies.*

White blood cell and *epithelial cell casts* can occur in any inflammatory state that involves the nephrons. White blood cell casts are particularly common in pyelonephritis, nephritis associated with systemic lupus erythematosus, and during transplant rejection. When white blood or epithelial cells degenerate, they form granular nonpigmented casts that contain cellular debris and aggregated proteins. So-called *waxy* casts, with few granules and very distinct margins, arise when cell debris has broken down to a fine dispersion so that granules are no longer visible.

Broad casts, of unusual width, are thought to arise in the dilated tubules of enlarged nephrons that have undergone compensatory hypertrophy in response to a reduction of functioning renal mass. A urine sample that contains a combination of broad and waxy casts as well as cellular or granular casts or red blood cells indicates a chronic smouldering process and has been termed a *telescoped* urine. This abnormality, first

described in polyarteritis nodosa and systemic lupus erythematosus, can also be found in many chronic forms of glomerulonephritis with active glomerulitis.

APPROACH TO THE PATIENT WITH HEMATURIA The most important step is to determine whether the hematuria is isolated or associated with other features of primary renal disease, i.e., cells, casts, or proteinuria. Many urinalyses may be needed to define the casts, cells, and proteins which accompany the hematuria, and the magnitude and type of associated proteinuria should be determined. As a general rule intravenous pyelography should be performed, if it can be done safely, even when the hematuria is of definite nephronal origin. Not only lesions of the urinary tract, but renal tumors or cysts, discrete areas of papillary necrosis, or signs of renal venous obstruction may be present. The source of isolated hematuria must always be ascertained, and this means a progressively detailed examination of the urinary tract by cystoscopy, retrograde pyelography, and arteriography to disclose tumor, stone, cysts, or other cause. If all the studies disclose normal structures, a nephronal origin of hematuria is likely even if no red blood cell casts are present. Hematuria with infection or overt renal disease usually requires no steps beyond intravenous pyelography.

AZOTEMIA, OLIGURIA, AND ANURIA

AZOTEMIA Measurements of urea and creatinine concentrations in serum are often obtained to assess the GFR. Both substances are produced at a reasonably constant rate, by the liver and muscles, respectively. As discussed in Chap. 274, they undergo complete glomerular filtration and are not reabsorbed extensively by the renal tubules; hence their clearances tend to reflect the GFR. An increase in their serum concentrations, termed *azotemia* (*azo,* "containing nitrogen"), occurs as the GFR falls. Renal failure is reflected by a high blood nitrogen level. Of the two substances, creatinine is a more reliable index of GFR because of its lower back diffusion from tubule lumen to peritubular blood. Although azotemia is a laboratory finding, rather than a symptom, it is an almost universal clue to the presence of abnormal renal function and often of renal disease, now that multiple-test biochemical screening of blood has become a common practice.

Glomerular filtration rate may be reduced by a fall in the filtration rates of individual functioning nephrons, or by a reduction in the total number of functioning nephrons. (See Table 42-1.)

Reduced single-nephron glomerular filtration rate TUBULAR FUNCTION NORMAL The physiological response of the normal kidney to a sodium-conserving stimulus is reduction of the single-nephron glomerular filtration rate (SNGFR) and subsequent reabsorption of an increased fraction of the reduced amounts of NaCl and water that enter the tubules. Depletion of extracellular fluid volume is a most instructive example of such a stimulus. Azotemia occurs and urine Na concentration falls below 20 (often below 1 meq per liter). Secretion of vasopressin is stimulated by depletion of extracellular fluid volume, and as a consequence, the distal tubules and collecting ducts become fully permeable to water. The concentrating mechanisms in the inner medulla (Chap. 274) are very efficient when flow rates through the loops of Henle and the collecting ducts are low. As a result, the filtrate that escapes reabsorption in the proximal tubule undergoes maximal osmotic concentration, the urine volume becomes small, and it has a high osmolality, above 500 mosmol per kilogram of water. Most of the filtered creatinine escapes tubular reabsorption, and so the ratio of the urine-to-plasma (U/P) creatinine concentrations is very high, 40 or more. Because urea can back-diffuse more completely than creatinine, the urea U/P ratio is less elevated, above 8, and the blood urea nitrogen (BUN) level rises more than the serum creatinine concentration. Normally, the ratio of BUN to serum creatinine concentration is 10:1; with depletion of the extracellular fluid volume the ratio rises.

The pattern of renal response to extracellular fluid volume depletion appears in any edema-forming condition during the phase of NaCl and water accumulation. Typical examples include the nephrotic syndrome and hepatic cirrhosis with ascites (Chaps. 29 and 278). When a diuretic is being administered to inhibit the tubular reabsorption of NaCl, urine volume and sodium concentration may be normal or elevated, even though SNGFR falls in response to the combination of the underlying edema-forming stimulus and further extracellular fluid volume depletion from the drug. Severe oliguria may appear upon withdrawal of the drug as the renal tubules resume intense reabsorption of NaCl and water. The pattern of low SNGFR with well-preserved tubule function may also be seen when renal blood flow is reduced, by systemic hypotension, incomplete renal arterial or venous occlusion, or other cause (Chap. 282). Acute incomplete obstruction of the ureter and acute glomerular injury may also reduce SNGFR and leave tubule function relatively intact, but whenever chronic obstruction or glomerulonephritis damages nephrons extensively, the high urinary osmolality, U/P ratios for creatinine or urea, and low urinary sodium concentrations disappear.

TUBULAR FUNCTION IMPAIRED   Certain acute renal diseases which produce azotemia lower SNGFR and at the same time damage the tubules sufficiently to reduce or even abolish their reabsorptive functions. Acute tubular necrosis, exposure to nephrotoxic agents, and all forms of acute tubulointerstitial disease are excellent examples. Azotemia and oliguria appear, but the urine sodium concentration is above 20 meq per liter and usually above 40 meq per liter, the U/P ratios for urea and creatinine are below 2 and 20, respectively, and urine osmolality is below 350 mosmol per kilogram of water. The ratio of BUN to serum creatinine is not elevated.

Reduced nephron number   INCREASED SNGFR   If one kidney is removed, the other grows larger, its nephrons enlarge, and the SNGFR increases until the total GFR becomes nearly normal for two kidneys. The tubules are overperfused with filtrate, but they appear to cope well with their increased reabsorptive burdens, perhaps in part because they are longer and wider and possess more cells. If more kidney tissue is removed, the remnant nephrons enlarge further, and their SNGFR rises. Extreme overperfusion of the tubules interferes with sodium conservation. At the same time, total GFR comes to depend more and more upon expansion of the extracellular fluid volume largely because the increase in SNGFR is due not only to anatomic growth of the glomeruli but also to a relatively high rate of blood flow per glomerulus.

Azotemia occurs because the total GFR, the product of the elevated SNGFR and the markedly reduced nephron number, is low. The ratio of BUN to serum creatinine concentration is approximately 10. Urine-to-plasma ratios for creatinine and urea are usually between 3 and 10, urine sodium concentration is above 40 meq per liter, and urine osmolality approaches that of plasma. Tubule conservation of filtered water and sodium conservation are poor, so fluid and salt intake must be liberal. Clinical states that produce this picture include surgical loss of renal substance because of trauma, neoplasm, stone, and destruction of kidneys by bacterial infection or tuberculosis, polycystic and medullary cystic renal diseases, and all the

TABLE 42-1
Pathophysiologic mechanisms of azotemia

Mechanism of reduced GFR	Clinical examples	Laboratory findings					
		Oliguria	Urine osm, mosmol/kg	Urine [Na$^+$], meq/L	$\left(\dfrac{U}{P}\right)_{creat}$	$\left(\dfrac{U}{P}\right)_{urea}$	$\dfrac{BUN}{Serum\ creat}$
REDUCED SNGFR							
Tubules normal	Severe dehydration, edema-forming states, diuretic agents, systemic hypotension, acute glomerular disease, acute urinary obstruction, incomplete renal vascular obstruction	Often present	>500	<20	>40	>8	>10
Tubules damaged	Acute tubular necrosis, nephrotoxic agents, glomerulonephritis with tubule injury	Usually present	<350	>40	<20	<2	10
REDUCED NEPHRON NUMBER							
Elevated SNGFR	Chronic tubulointerstitial/renal disease Surgical loss of renal tissue	Rare*	290	>40	3–10	3–10	10
Normal SNGFR	Diffuse chronic glomerulonephritis Diabetic nephropathy	Rare†	100–350‡	10–100‡	>3	>20	>10
Reduced SNGFR	Any of the factors that can reduce SNGFR (listed above) may lower SNGFR in a patient who has a reduced number of functioning nephrons	Usually present	290	>20	<10	<3	>20

* Occurs only when total GFR is below 5% normal.
† Rare as long as GFR is above 5% normal.
‡ Varies with diet and with the level of GFR. When GFR is below 20% normal, osmotic concentration of the urine is usually impossible.
NOTE: osm = osmolality; creat = creatinine concentration; U = urine; P = plasma.

chronic tubulointerstitial nephropathies (Chaps. 281 and 283). In each of these disorders, the nephrons that remain viable are either fully intact or behave as though the SNGFR is better preserved than tubule function.

SNGFR NORMAL The SNGFR does not appear to increase despite a reduction of nephron number in diseases such as glomerulonephritis and diabetic glomerulosclerosis, where the glomerulus is the primary site of damage. In these diseases total GFR falls directly with nephron number and is not supported by elevated SNGFR. Since the tubules are not confronted with an excessive reabsorptive burden, sodium conservation is adequate. In these disorders, superimposed conditions that lower SNGFR, such as depletion of extracellular fluid volume, can cause oliguria with low urine sodium concentration and U/P ratios for creatinine and urea above 3 and 20, respectively. The serum urea to creatinine ratio will rise distinctly.

SNGFR REDUCED In patients with chronic renal disease in whom total GFR has been sufficient to support life only because of a very high SNGFR, inadvertent dehydration or any other factor that lowers the SNGFR can provoke oliguria and severe azotemia. Under these circumstances, urine sodium concentration will fall, but not below 20 meq per liter, as in the normal person, because SNGFR, though reduced, may still be above normal. The U/P ratios for creatinine and urea will be low, usually below 3 and 10, respectively, despite oliguria, and urine osmolality will not rise above the plasma level. The serum urea to creatinine ratio may rise, but not above 20. In less extreme situations, reduction of SNGFR will worsen azotemia and alter urine chemistry in the same directions but to a lesser extent.

OLIGURIA In this condition urine volume is insufficient to sustain life in a steady state; it is usually less than 400 ml per 24 h (16.6 ml/h) in an adult of average size. Daily urine volume is difficult to measure when flow rate is low, because small absolute errors of volume measurement, in the range of 50 to 100 ml of urine each day, or of timing of collection, may represent large percentage errors.

APPROACH TO THE PATIENT WITH AZOTEMIA OR OLIGURIA Clinical history, physical examination, and urinalysis often disclose an obvious reason for azotemia or oliguria. The most discriminating additional measurements include serum urea and creatinine concentrations, and the sodium, urea, and creatinine concentrations and osmolality of a concurrent urine sample. Reduction of SNGFR with well-preserved tubular function is usually present when urine osmolality exceeds 500 mosmol per kilogram of water, sodium is below 20 meq per liter, the U/P ratios for urea and creatinine exceed 8 and 40, respectively, and the BUN is more than 10 times the serum creatinine concentration. The prognosis for recovery of adequate GFR is good, if the cause of reduced SNGFR can be reversed. When urine osmolality is below 350 mosmol per kilogram of water, sodium is above 40 meq, the U/P values for urea and creatinine are below 2 and 20, respectively, and the BUN exceeds the serum creatinine by only tenfold, tubule function has been lost, and some form of acute or chronic renal failure usually is present.

ANURIA This extreme condition is uncommon. Urinary obstruction is the main cause and must be excluded as a first step (Chap. 285). Complete renal arterial and venous occlusion are other important causes. Few severe renal diseases produce anuria in the adult, and anuria should never be ascribed to a primary renal disease until patency of the urinary tract and major renal blood vessels has been established.

REFERENCES

BRENNER BM et al: Molecular basis of proteinuria of glomerular origin. N Eng J Med 298:826, 1978

DE WARDENER HE: Tests of glomerular functional integrity, in *The Kidney*, IIE de Wardener (ed). London, Churchill Livingstone, 1973

GLASSOCK RJ, BENNETT CM: The glomerulopathies, in *The Kidney*, BM Brenner, FC Rector Jr (eds). Philadelphia, Saunders, 1980

MORRISON RBI: Urinalysis and assessment of renal function, in *Renal Disease*, D Black (ed). Oxford, Blackwell, 1972

POLLAK VE, PESCE AJ: Proteinuria: A review of glomerular permeability in the normal and in various disease states, in *Seminars in Nephrology*, E Becker (ed). New York, Wiley, 1977

43
POLYURIA AND NOCTURIA

FREDRIC L. COE

Though considered together in this chapter because they are superficially similar, polyuria and nocturia have little in common pathophysiologically. True polyuria that is not due to a deliberate, habitual high fluid intake always points to an important defect of renal water handling or of the secretion of vasopressin. Nocturia is less specific. It can arise from defective renal water conservation, excretion of an abnormal fraction of the daily salt load at night, low bladder capacity, irritable bladder, or partial bladder obstruction.

Patients cannot always distinguish urinary frequency from polyuria. Voiding of small volumes is typical of frequency, whereas large volumes characterize the polyuric states. Since voiding volumes may not be clear from the history, polyuria must be substantiated by 24-h urine collection before beginning an investigation of causes. The presence of nocturia is best established by the history alone.

POLYURIA

PHYSIOLOGY OF URINE FORMATION Adaptation to life on dry land requires efficient renal water conservation, and even though modern life no longer requires it, the normal person enjoys the convenience of a modest urine volume. When an individual is in water balance, urine volume is the difference between water intake and insensible water losses. Polyuria implies the production of more urine than normal; if it is chronic, there is also high water intake. A reasonable definition of polyuria is a urine volume above 3 liters per day, but should be qualified to exclude normal individuals who desire a large fluid intake and therefore form large volumes of urine.

NORMAL RENAL WATER CONSERVATION (See also Chap. 274) Between 20 and 30 percent of NaCl and water filtered at the glomerulus reach the thick ascending limb of Henle's loop in the outer medulla where NaCl is reabsorbed but most of the water and urea are not. As a result of this process, the outer medullary interstitial fluid becomes hypertonic to plasma, about 400 mosmol/kg compared with 290 mosmol/kg, as NaCl is transported from the tubular lumen of the thick ascending limb of Henle's loop without a corresponding transport of water. Therefore, the fluid that leaves the thick ascending limb of Henle's loop to enter the distal convoluted tubule is hypotonic to plasma.

The dilute tubular fluid equilibrates to isotonicity with plasma by losing water into the cortical interstitium as it traverses the terminal portion of the distal convoluted tubule and cortical collecting tubule, provided that vasopressin is present. Without vasopressin the water permeability of the entire distal convoluted tubule is low. Though it becomes isotonic to plasma, late distal convoluted tubule fluid has a composition different from that in the thick ascending limb of Henle's loop. Much of its osmolality is due to urea, not to NaCl, because urea is lost from the fluid to only a small extent whereas NaCl is reabsorbed in the thick ascending limb of Henle's loop and beginning of the distal convoluted tubule. By the time it reaches the end of the distal convoluted tubule the fluid is appreciably reduced in volume. Like the end of the distal convoluted tubule, the cortical collecting tubule in the presence of vasopressin is permeable to water but not to urea (Fig. 274-2).

The urea-rich fluid then enters the inner medulla in the papillary portion of the collecting duct. The inner medullary interstitium is very hypertonic to plasma because of high urea and NaCl concentrations. Water is extracted from the papillary collecting duct segments to create the final urine. Unlike the thick ascending limb of Henle's loop, distal convoluted tubule, and cortical collecting tubules, the permeability to urea of the papillary portion of the collecting duct epithelium is high, but urea losses from the tubule are low because of a high prevailing interstitial urea concentration.

How the inner medulla comes to have an interstitium so hypertonic is still a matter of controversy, but a *passive counterflow model* seems reasonable and is widely accepted as a working hypothesis at present. If the medullary interstitium were empty, without an accumulation of surplus urea or NaCl urea would diffuse out of the papillary collecting duct and enter the interstitium, because the luminal fluid has been rendered hypertonic in the outer medulla. The urea would be removed by the ascending vasa recta, but counterflow exchange between ascending and descending vasa recta lowers the efficiency of solute removal and allows a high interstitial urea concentration to develop. The urea concentration will be distributed as a gradient, with a peak level at the papillary tips. This is true because the trapping efficiency of the counterflowing vasa recta loop increases with its length. In other words, the concentration of solute in vasa recta can exceed that in the blood that enters the vasa recta more and more as the solute approaches the tip of the loop.

Given a urea gradient, NaCl accumulation could be passive. The descending limb of the loop of Henle appears very permeable to water, less so to urea, and even less to NaCl. Water can leave the descending limb because of the urea gradient in the medullary interstitium, so that intratubular NaCl concentration rises progressively down to the bend of the loop. The thin ascending limb appears to very permeable to NaCl, less so to urea, and least to water, so that in the presence of a favorable electrochemical gradient, the accumulated NaCl can diffuse into the interstitium until its interstitial concentration rises to the equilibrium dictated by its entry and washout rates. In other words, transport of NaCl in the thick ascending limb of Henle's loop can lead to urea and NaCl accumulation in the inner medulla.

When the process is fully established, the inner medulla is in a complex steady state. Urea and NaCl deliveries from papillary collecting ducts and descending limbs balance total washout in the thin ascending limb of Henle's loop and the vasa recta. Water that is lost from papillary collecting ducts in the process of creating an osmotically concentrated urine must be carried away in the ascending vasa recta, so that total flow in the ascending vasa recta must exceed that in the descending vasa recta. The process can be disrupted by changes in tubular or vascular flow rates, or by structural abnormalities that prevent normal equilibration between capillary loops, tubules, and interstitium. In particular, increased rates of blood flow diminish the efficiency of solute trapping by the vasa recta and promote medullary washout. Excessive delivery of water into the papillary collecting ducts or into the descending limb of Henle's loop has the same effect.

CAUSES Polyuria can arise from inadequate secretion of vasopressin, failure of the renal tubules to respond to vasopressin, solute diuresis, or natriuresis (Table 43-1). It may also occur as a physiological adaptation to deliberate excessive water drinking.

Diabetes insipidus (see also Chap. 334) The term *diabetes insipidus* is applied to situations in which renal water conservation is so inadequate that polyuria occurs. Either vasopressin insufficiency (central diabetes insipidus) or renal unresponsiveness to vasopressin (nephrogenic diabetes insipidus) produces severe polyuria and secondary thirst. In both, water reabsorption is reduced all along the distal nephron, because passive water movement from tubules into the hypertonic outer and inner medullary interstitium is slow. But even though the rate of water movement out of the collecting ducts is low for a given osmotic difference between the tubule lumen and interstitial fluid, the fluid that enters the collecting ducts is so abnormally dilute and copious in volume that more water enters the inner medulla than under normal circumstances and medullary solutes are washed out into the vasa recta. Washout is incomplete and vasopressin administration can lead to formation of an osmotically concentrated urine, but the maximum urine osmality that can be attained is below normal.

Vasopressin-sensitive (central) diabetes insipidus may be idiopathic or secondary to hypophysectomy or trauma or to neoplastic, inflammatory, vascular, or infectious causes (Table 43-1). Idiopathic diabetes insipidus can be familial, and then it is usually inherited as an autosomal dominant trait; but more commonly it is sporadic and appears in childhood. In both forms there is selective destruction of the neurons that produce vasopressin in the supraoptic nucleus.

Failure of the kidney to respond to vasopressin, i.e., nephrogenic diabetes insipidus, may be acquired or congenital. Nephrogenic diabetes insipidus acquired from renal disease (Table 43-1) probably is the most common form; the familial form is rare. Hypercalcemia and hypokalemic nephropathy are important reversible causes of nephrogenic diabetes insipidus.

TABLE 43-1
Causes of polyuria

I Inadequate renal water conservation
  A Diabetes insipidus
    1 Vasopressin-sensitive (posthypophysectomy; posttrauma; postpituitary ablation; idiopathic, supra- or intrasellar tumors or cysts; histiocystosis or granuloma; encroachment by aneurysm; Sheehan's syndrome, meningoencephalitis; Guillain-Barré's syndrome; fat embolus; empty sella)
    2 Nephrogenic
      a Acquired tubulointerstitial renal disease (pyelonephritis, analgesic nephropathy, multiple myeloma, amyloidosis, obstructive uropathy, sarcoidosis, hypercalcemic or hypokalemic nephropathy, Sjögren's syndrome, sickle cell anemia, renal transplantation)
      b Drugs or toxins (lithium, demeclocycline, methyoxyflurane, ethanol, diphenylhydantoin, propoxyphene, amphotericin)
      c Congenital (hereditary nephrogenic diabetes insipidus, polycystic or medullary cystic disease)
  B Solute diuresis (glucosuria, high-protein tube feedings, urea or mannitol infusion, radiographic contrast media, chronic renal failure)
  C Natriuretic syndromes (salt-losing nephritis, diuretic phase of acute tubular necrosis, diuretic agents)
II Primary polydipsia

Lithium carbonate, methoxyflurane (1,1-difluoro-2,2-dichlor-ethyl methyl ether) anesthetic, and demeclocycline, a tetracycline derivative, can also produce nephrogenic diabetes insipidus.

Solute diuresis Excessive filtration of a poorly resorbed solute such as glucose, mannitol, or urea can depress reabsorption of NaCl and water in the proximal tubule and cause their loss in the urine, producing polyuria. Urine sodium concentration is below that of blood, so that more water than salt is lost from the body and serum hypertonicity can be produced. Glucosuria in diabetes mellitus is a common cause of solute diuresis. Iatrogenic solute diuresis may arise from mannitol infusion, angiographic contrast media, and high-protein gavage feedings, which produce excessive excretion of urea.

Natriuretic syndromes Excessive chronic sodium loss may occur during the course of tubulointerstitial or cystic renal diseases. Polyuria and polydipsia are accompanied by an unusually large daily sodium requirement. Examples of this phenomenon include medullary cystic disease, Bartter's syndrome, and the diuretic phase of acute tubular necrosis, in which sodium and water losses are very large.

Primary polydipsia Whether because of habit, predilection, psychiatric disorder, or a specific lesion in the brain, some people drink enough water every day to produce polyuria. The body and the kidneys rarely if ever are injured by chronic polydipsia, but the condition can be confused with diabetes insipidus, which it resembles closely. During deliberate polydipsia, extracellular fluid volume is normal or high, and vasopressin secretion is reduced to a basal level because serum osmolality tends to be near the lower limits of normal. Reabsorption of water from the end distal convoluted tubule and collecting ducts is reduced so that all the surplus water can be excreted into the urine. The inner medulla loses its urea and NaCl gradients because of washout, as in diabetes insipidus. Washout may be more severe than in diabetes insipidus because primary polydipsia tends to cause expansion of the extracellular fluid volume, whereas primary renal water loss does the opposite. Volume expansion raises total delivery of NaCl and water to the thick ascending limb of Henle's loop and therefore to the inner medulla, all things being equal. It also raises renal blood flow, and increased flow through the vasa rectae reduces their ability to trap solutes in the medulla.

APPROACH TO THE PATIENT Solute diuresis and natriuretic syndromes usually are apparent from the history, physical examination, urinalysis, clinical setting, blood count, and serum creatinine or the BUN. Diagnostic problems occur mainly when stable, chronic polyuria and polydipsia of uncertain origin are present. Here, one must try to distinguish between vasopressin-sensitive diabetes insipidus, nephrogenic diabetes insipidus, and primary polydipsia; and the best way to do this is by measuring the response of urine osmolality to water deprivation and the administration of vasopressin.

The patient should have free access to water and receive a normal diet that provides approximately 100 mmol NaCl per day for 3 days; then a total fast is instituted. During the fast, pulse and blood pressure should be measured every 30 min and body weight every hour, using an accurate balance. When 3 percent of the initial body weight has been lost or 14 h has elapsed, urine and serum osmolality are measured. A normal subject will lower urine volume below 0.5 ml/min and raise urine osmolality to above 700 mosmol per kilogram of water. In complete diabetes insipidus, nephrogenic or vasopressin-sensitive, the urine osmolality will remain below 200 mosmol/kg and urine flow will remain above 0.5 ml/min, but some rise in osmolality and fall in flow will occur given incomplete dia-

betes insipidus. If urine osmolality is below 700 mosmol/kg, by the end of the fasting period, 5 milliunits per minute of aqueous vasopressin is administered by intravenous drip. Patients with complete or partial vasopressin-sensitive diabetes insipidus will raise their urine osmolality above the level achieved by fasting alone. No increase will occur given complete nephrogenic diabetes insipidus, although incomplete forms of nephrogenic diabetes insipidus will permit some response to vasopressin.

The response of patients with primary polydipsia is quite different. During fluid restriction the secretion of vasopressin increases, and at the completion of the test the flow rate and osmolality of the urine will reflect a physiological level of vasopressin acting upon normal tubules that traverse a medullary interstitium whose urea and NaCl concentrations have been reduced by chronic washout. In other words, the washout will set the upper limit on urine osmolality, and patients with primary polydipsia thus demonstrate a submaximal concentrating ability in spite of intact vasopressin secretion. Exogenous vasopressin can increase urine osmolality very little, if at all, because medullary washout, not vasopressin insensitivity, is the main limiting factor. Usually the urine osmolality will be above 400 mosmol/kg by the end of the fluid deprivation test, in contrast to the lower values of approximately 200 mosmol/kg encountered in patients with nephrogenic diabetes insipidus; but it may be impossible to distinguish incomplete nephrogenic diabetes insipidus from primary polydipsia, in some cases, by using the fluid deprivation test alone.

NOCTURIA

Whether an individual sleeps through the night without urinating depends upon a diurnal rhythm in which the volume of urine formed during sleep does not exceed bladder capacity. Nocturia results when nocturnal urine volume exceeds bladder capacity, or it results from reduced renal osmotic concentration, high sodium excretion, solute diuresis, or low bladder capacity.

All the polyuric states may cause nocturia. Urinary concentrating ability falls in most renal diseases (Chap. 274), often at an early stage. Even though overt polyuria may be absent, overnight urine volume frequently exceeds bladder capacity. Nocturia also occurs in edema-forming states. In congestive heart failure, nephrotic syndrome, and hepatic cirrhosis with ascites, fluid accumulates preferentially in dependent portions of the body during the day. At night, with recumbency, tissue capillary forces change and some edema fluid is mobilized, producing the effect of an intravenous saline infusion. Venous insufficiency may produce dependent edema of the legs that is often also mobilized at night, causing nocturia.

Reduced bladder capacity is present when infection, tumor, or stone, causes inflammation or increased irritability. Chronic partial bladder-outflow obstruction, from prostatic hypertrophy, urethral stricture, or benign or malignant neoplasm or stone, causes a frequent stimulus to void and also a thickening of the muscular wall that reduces its compliance. Frequent small voidings may be a clue to this lower urinary tract cause of nocturia, but in its earlier phases chronic obstruction may lead to only one nocturnal voiding of reasonable volume.

REFERENCES

ANDREOLI TE et al (eds): *Disturbances in Body Fluid Osmolality.* Baltimore, Williams & Wilkins, 1977

KLEEMAN CR: Water metabolism, in *Clinical Disorders of Fluid and Electrolyte Metabolism*, MH Maxwell, CR Kleeman (eds). New York, McGraw-Hill, 1972

HAYS RM, LEVINE SD: Pathophysiology of water metabolism, in *The Kidney*, 2d ed, BM Brenner, FC Rector Jr (eds). Philadelphia, Saunders, 1980

BERL T et al: Clinical disorders of water metabolism. Kidney Int 10:117, 1976

44
DYSURIA, INCONTINENCE, AND ENURESIS

WILLIAM GILL
FREDRIC L. COE

NORMAL BLADDER FUNCTION

The detrusor muscle, which provides the propulsive force for emptying the bladder, consists of interlacing fibers of smooth muscle that are under parasympathetic autonomic control through the pelvic nerves from sacral spinal cord segments S2, S3, and S4. The smooth muscle of the trigonal portion of the bladder, between the ureteral orifices and the posterior area of the bladder outlet, is innervated by motor fibers from thoracolumbar segments (T11 to L2) of the sympathetic nervous system, in which alpha receptor sites predominate. This layer of muscle extends into the posterior urethra and acts as an involuntary internal sphincter that helps maintain urinary continence even in the absence of voluntary control. The external urethral sphincter and perineal muscles are under voluntary control via the pudendal nerves.

Sensory tracts for pain, temperature, and distention pass from the bladder via the pelvic nerves to sacral spinal levels S2, S3, and S4, creating a simple spinal voiding reflex between the bladder and the sacral spinal cord. The sensory tracts from the bladder further ascend through sacrobulbar pathways to the medulla of the brain and ultimately to cortical centers (superomedial portion of the frontal lobes), from which impulses arise, pass back down the lateral and ventral reticulospinal tracts, and normally suppress the sacral spinal reflex arc controlling bladder emptying.

The normal adult bladder can accommodate as much as approximately 400 ml fluid without a significant increase in intravesical pressure (< 20 cmH$_2$O). Above this point, sensations of fullness are transmitted to the sacral cord. If not suppressed by cortical control, the sacral cord reflexly discharges motor impulses that cause powerful sustained detrusor contraction. Urination can be prevented by cortical suppression of the reflex arc or by voluntary contraction of the external sphincter and perineal muscles. Infants, and adults with spinal cord damage above S2, urinate spontaneously when the bladder fills sufficiently.

Normal micturition is initiated by voluntary suppression of cortical inhibition of the reflex arc and by relaxation of the muscles of the pelvic floor and the external sphincter. The base of the bladder falls; then the trigone contracts, an action that occludes the ureters as they pass through the bladder wall and helps to prevent vesicoureteral reflux of urine during voiding. Finally, the detrusor contracts and voiding occurs.

DYSURIA

Dysuria refers to anything abnormal having to do with urination, such as urinary frequency, nocturia, hesitancy in starting urination, straining to urinate, burning upon urination, urgency, decreased size of urinary stream, dribbling at the end of urination, and combinations of these symptoms. Some clinicians restrict the use of the term dysuria to burning or pain upon urination, but the broader definition is preferable.

MECHANISMS OF DYSURIA Reduced bladder compliance When the bladder has a decreased ability to expand, frequency, nocturia, and urgency usually result. When decreased expansion is due to inflammation of the mucosa (cystitis) from infection, radiation, chemicals, or foreign bodies (catheters, stones), burning usually is more prominent than when it is due to infiltration of the muscle by tumors of the bladder or from adjacent organs (prostate, rectum, uterus). Any upper motor neuron lesion that interferes with cortical inhibition of the voiding reflex produces a spastic hypertonic bladder, and incontinence is then a frequent manifestation.

Impaired bladder emptying Increased outflow resistance because of obstruction of the bladder neck or urethra causes hesitancy, reduced caliber of the stream, and dribbling. Damage to the sacral nerves involved in vesical emptying can produce a completely autonomous bladder, or a sensory paralytic or motor paralytic neurogenic bladder. Thus, the individual whose bladder has lost all sensory and motor innervation must rely for emptying upon distention of the organ leading to muscle stretching and automatic contraction, because the sacral voiding reflex is absent. Hesitancy, incomplete emptying, and even gross retention of urine can result. Symptoms of bladder fullness will depend upon whether the sensory tracts are intact. Since the bladder cannot empty itself properly in the worst cases of deficient innervation, gross overflow incontinence occurs.

CAUSES OF DYSURIA Infection *Acute bacterial cystitis*, which occurs more frequently in women, usually causes great frequency day and night, burning on urination, and, not infrequently, gross hematuria. *Prostatitis* or *prostatocystitis* in men can cause a picture similar to acute cystitis in women. When only the prostate is involved, milder symptoms such as vague pain or discomfort in the lower abdomen, groin, perineum, rectum, testes, or penis occur. The symptoms may be associated with urination, but more frequently are noticed at times other than during micturition or ejaculation.

Benign prostatic hypertrophy This condition afflicts upwards of 75 percent of older men. It is manifested by nocturia, reduced size and force of the urinary stream, straining to urinate, and terminal dribbling, all due to outflow obstruction.

Psychosomatic cystitis The functional bladder syndrome and chronic glandular urethrotrigonitis are synonyms for a very common but poorly understood affliction of middle-aged and older women, in which pain is usually vague, aching in nature, and in the lower abdomen or vagina. There is daytime frequency without nocturia; pyuria is absent. A complete urological evaluation usually becomes necessary because symptoms are chronic and hard to eradicate. The functional bladder syndrome must be distinguished from the effects of a cystocele, which can be repaired surgically. (See also Chap. 280.)

APPROACH TO THE PATIENT The medical history should focus on past as well as present urinary problems. A pelvic examination in women and prostatic examination in men are necessary components of the physical examination. Microscopic examination of a two-glass urinary sediment in all patients and of the prostatic fluid in men is also necessary. The first 20 ml of a voiding, if collected separately, may contain a higher concentration of leukocytes and bacteria than the remainder of the voided urine, when the urethra is the principal site of inflammation or infection. Normal prostatic fluid, not subjected to centrifugation, contains less than 10 leukocytes per high-power field; excessive leukocytes in the prostatic fluid are an important clue to prostatitis and may, when prostatitis is chonic, be the only detectable abnormality. Further diagnostic studies will depend upon such positive findings as a history of chronic or recurrent episodes or associated fever, which are rare in lower urinary tract infections except in acute prostatitis, or an abnormality on physical examination such as a pelvic or rectal mass or tenderness, hematuria or pyuria, or excessive leukocytes and macrophages in the prostatic fluid. Serum acid phosphatase may be elevated when carcinoma of the prostate has extended beyond the boundary of the prostatic capsule.

Additional evaluation of dysuria, when the cause is not evident from clinical examination, may include cultures of urine and prostatic fluid for aerobic and anerobic bacteria, tubercle bacilli, and mycoplasma, excretory urography and voiding cystourethrography. If these examinations do not reveal the diagnosis, but the symptoms are sufficiently troublesome, urologic consultation should be sought. The urologist may carry out cystoscopy and urethroscopy with endoscopic biopsies where abnormalities are found. Functional urodynamic studies, gas cystometry, sphincter electromyography, urethral pressure profile, uroflometry, and urine spectrometry may be needed in special cases.

INCONTINENCE

Incontinence refers to the inability to retain urine in the bladder. The diagnostic approach to the evaluation of the patient should be the same as that used for dysuria.

Stress incontinence is common in postmenopausal parous women. The structures of the female urethra atrophy when deprived of estrogen and many become unable to resist the passage of urine under the stress of increased intraabdominal pressure during coughing, sneezing, climbing stairs, and other physical activity. Parturition may damage the pelvic support of the bladder so that the bladder and urethra can slip downward from their normal position above the pelvic diaphragm. As they do, the urethra shortens, and the normal urethrovesical angle, important in closing the urethral sphincter, is lost. In men, stress incontinence usually is secondary to prostatic surgery for benign prostatic hypertrophy or prostatic carcinoma. If the external sphincter has also been damaged during operation, total, complete incontinence may result.

Inflammatory lesions of the bladder mucosa, especially in the trigone area, can cause uncontrollable detrusor contractions and unwanted passage of urine, often called *urgency incontinence*. Common inflammatory lesions include infection, stones in the intravesical ureter, bladder tumors, and catheters in the bladder. Upper motor neuron lesions of the spinal cord or brain may produce a hypertonic, spastic, neurogenic bladder with frequent, uncontrollable, urgency incontinence.

Overflow or paradoxical incontinence arises from large residual volumes of urine secondary to obstruction at the bladder neck or along the urethra (urethral stricture) or from neurological damage. Hypotonic neurogenic bladders may occur in diseases which produce autonomic peripheral neuropathy, such as diabetes mellitus, uremia, hypothyroidism, chronic alcoholism, Guillain-Barré syndrome, collagen vascular diseases, and toxic neuropathies associated with some carcinomas (espe-

cially lung and kidney). It may also occur because of prolonged overdistention of the bladder. Hydronephrosis and impaired renal function can occur in patients with chronic overflow incontinence.

Some congenital anomalies, extrophy of the bladder, patent urachus, and ectopic ureteral openings distal to the vesical neck cause *mechanical incontinence*. Acquired mechanical incontinence can follow transurethral resection of the prostate in which damage has occurred to both the internal and external sphincter mechanisms. Pelvic surgery or irradiation of the uterus or rectum may cause incontinence because of vesicovaginal, ureterovaginal, vesicoperineal, or ureteroperineal fistulae.

Children, and even some young adults, draw attention to themselves by feigning incontinence and thereby derive some secondary emotional satisfaction. A complete diagnostic evaluation usually is necessary to rule out organic disease even when *psychogenic incontinence* is strongly suspected.

ENURESIS

Enuresis refers to the involuntary passage of urine at night or during sleep—hence, the synonym *bed-wetting*. Some clinicians reserve the term enuresis for those bed-wetters who have no gross urological abnormalities, but it should be used for bed-wetting in general.

The sacral spinal reflex arc alone controls urination in the infant; therefore, enuretic incontinence is normal under the age of 2 years. As the nervous system matures, cortical control over the spinal reflex arc results in the voluntary control over urination and defecation by the age of 2½ years. Even so, enuresis beyond the age of 3 years occurs to some degree in approximately 10 percent of all otherwise normal children and probably is due to a delay in maturation of bladder control, which may be familial.

Although the majority of bed-wetters will be dry by the age of puberty, organic diseases, especially infections of the urinary tract, obstructive lesions with overflow incontinence, neurovesical dysfunction, and polyuric conditions that overload the bladder must be suspected in any child who is enuretic beyond the age of 3 years. Patients with organic disease usually, but not always, are incontinent during the day as well as at night. The approach to the patient with enuresis is the same as that used for dysuria or incontinence.

REFERENCES

BRADLEY WE: Autonomic neuropathy and the genitourinary system. J Urol 119:299, 1978

——, SCOTT FB: Physiology of the urinary bladder, in *Urology*, 4th ed, JH Harrison et al (eds). Philadelphia, Saunders, 1978, vol 1, chap 4, p 87

HARRISON JH et al (eds): Infections and inflammations of the genitourinary tract, in *Urology*, 4th ed. Philadelphia, Saunders, 1978, vol 1, sec IV, p 451

LAPIDES J (ed): *Symposium on Neurogenic Bladder: The Urologic Clinics of North America*. Philadelphia, Saunders, 1974

WHITESIDE CG, ARNOLD EP: Persistent primary enuresis: A urodynamic assessment. Br Med J 1:364, 1975

45
DISTURBANCES IN MENSTRUATION, SEXUAL FUNCTION, AND REPRODUCTION IN WOMEN

JAMES D. MADDEN
JEAN D. WILSON

Since normal reproductive physiology depends upon the integrated action of the central nervous system, the endocrine glands, and the reproductive organs, it is to be expected that abnormalities in the menstrual cycle, sexual function, and reproductive capacity occur in association with a variety of systemic and psychological disorders as well as with primary disease in the endocrine system and reproductive organs.

MENSTRUATION

MENARCHE During the prepubertal years, the anterior pituitary can respond to hypothalamic luteinizing hormone-releasing hormone (LHRH) by secreting gonadotropins [follicle-stimulating hormone (FSH), luteotropic hormone (LH)]. The prepubertal ovaries are capable of responding to exogenous gonadotropin stimulation as evidenced by maturation of follicles and production of estrogen. Puberty in the female probably commences as a result of increased synthesis and release of LHRH and the subsequent increase in the secretion of ovarian hormones. Sexual maturation occurs as an orderly sequence beginning with breast development, early growth of genital and axillary hair, and increase in the rate of growth. There is ordinarily a 2-year interval between the commencement of sexual maturation and menarche.

During early puberty gonadotropins are released principally during sleep (see Chap. 342). There appears to be a relationship between the onset of the pubertal process and a "critical body weight." For American girls of European ancestry, the average weight at which menarche occurs is 48 kg. However, weight increase alone is not sufficient, and a critical combination of weight and percent body fat is required. In some unknown manner the amount of body fat determines the minimum weight for height necessary for the onset and maintenance of menstrual cycles. Earlier acquisition of the critical body composition, the result of improved nutrition, is believed to have led to earlier sexual maturation in recent generations. In the United States menarche now occurs on the average approximately two years earlier than at the beginning of this century. It is uncertain whether the critical changes in body composition are the cause or only a correlate of the neuroendocrine events initiating puberty.

THE NORMAL CYCLE At the time of menarche, the increase in gonadotropin release is no longer limited to the time of sleep. FSH and LH are secreted episodically by the anterior pituitary throughout the day. A young woman enters reproductive life with approximately 300,000 follicles in the ovaries. The normal menstrual cycle is discussed in Chap. 342. In brief, owing to the precise biochemical messages conveyed to the gonad by FSH and LH, a cohort of follicles within one ovary begins to mature in each cycle. It is uncertain what determines which follicles will mature, nor is it known why a single member of the cohort gains ascendancy (becoming the "dominant follicle") while the remainder of the follicles in the cohort undergo atresia. A burst of estradiol secreted from the mature "dominant follicle" operating through a positive feedback mechanism causes a surge in the secretion of LH from the anterior pituitary. The latter begins approximately 24 h prior to ovulation and is responsible for the release of the ovum and its surrounding cumulus mass from the ovary. LH also causes luteinization of the ovarian granulosa and theca cells remaining behind in the follicle after ovulation. This collection of luteinized cells, known as the *corpus luteum,* secretes progesterone at an increasing rate for approximately one week. Progesterone, in addition to causing qualitative changes in the endometrium favorable for implantation of a fertilized ovum, causes elevation of basal body temperature and an increase in breast volume. The life span of the corpus luteum appears to be fixed (14 ± 3 days) unless it is "rescued" by the luteotropin human chorionic gonadotropin (HCG) arising from the implanting trophoblast. Thus, pregnancy is the only normal cause of a persistent corpus luteum. The corpus luteum continues to produce progesterone for the first 8 weeks of pregnancy and thus maintains a secretory endometrium as well as ensures myometrial quiescence. The placenta then takes over the task of progesterone production and retains this function for the remainder of the pregnancy.

Corpus luteum death and progesterone/estrogen withdrawal lead to spasm of the spiral arterioles of the endometrium. It is likely that prostaglandins and related metabolites formed in the endometrium cause myometrial contractions during menstruation. Such contractions cause discomfort but are likely useful in expelling the menstrual content. Menstrual blood does not normally clot, and the amount of blood lost per spontaneous cycle varies from 10 to 80 ml in normal women. The duration of menses varies from 2 to 8 days.

As judged by relative infertility and the relative infrequency of biphasic basal body temperature patterns in early postmenarchal girls, many of the cycles in early reproductive life are anovulatory. A similar pattern is characteristic of the perimenopausal woman.

DISORDERS OF MENSTRUATION **Primary amenorrhea** The average age of menarche in the United States is 12½ years with a range of 9 to 16 years. Constitutional delay of menarche often correlates with delay in acquisition of critical body composition. The age at which the diagnosis of primary amenorrhea should be made is arbitrary. Evaluation should be performed by age 14 when primary amenorrhea is associated with a failure of breast development or at any age when the lack of menstruation becomes of concern to a patient or her parents, recognizing that many such patients will prove to have only a delayed onset of puberty. The two most common causes of true primary amenorrhea at age 18 (gonadal dysgenesis and congenital absence of the uterus and vagina) can both be diagnosed by physical examination and laboratory tests several years before that age. Other causes of primary amenorrhea in declining order of frequency are polycystic ovarian disease, CNS disorders that interfere with gonadotropin secretion (such as craniopharyngioma or pituitary tumor), male or female pseudohermaphroditism, and pregnancy.

Secondary amenorrhea Cessation of menses in a woman who has previously experienced spontaneous vaginal bleeding is termed *secondary amenorrhea*. Any disruption in the hypothalamic-pituitary-ovarian-uterine interrelationships described above may lead to secondary amenorrhea, but the disorder must be considered to be due to pregnancy until proved otherwise. In the past it was common to attempt to induce withdrawal bleeding with progestational agents to rule out pregnancy. This procedure is to be discouraged because of the increase in congenital malformations (limb reduction defects, congenital heart disease, hypospadias, and neural tube defects) that appear to be associated with the use of progestational agents during pregnancy.

The common causes of secondary amenorrhea are conveniently categorized as chronic acyclic endogenous estrogen production and a profound deficiency of estrogen production. In the former category are patients with partial (often temporary) disruption in the hormonal relationships between the brain and ovary leading to ovarian estrogen production but not ovulation. Also in this category are patients with the rare granulosa–theca cell tumors of the ovary which secrete estradiol. The remaining patients in this category are victims of excessive extraglandular estrogen production and include those with polycystic ovarian disease (Stein-Leventhal syndrome), liver disease, and obesity (see dysfunctional uterine bleeding below).

Those patients with absence of estrogen production have either primary or secondary ovarian failure. The former situation is termed *premature menopause* and is diagnosed by detecting castrate levels of FSH and LH in serum. The cause of primary ovarian failure is seldom apparent, and there is little hope for fertility in these patients. Secondary ovarian failure is the result of decreased gonadotropin production and is caused by psychogenic (stress) and organic/endocrinologic disorders influencing hypothalamic pituitary function (craniopharyngioma, prolactin-secreting pituitary microadenoma, severe systemic illness, malnutrition, "post-pill oversuppression").

Rarely secondary amenorrhea may be the consequence of loss of functioning endometrium, due to endometrial tuberculosis or endometrial scarring following pregnancy-related uterine curettage (Asherman's syndrome). Occasional cases of secondary amenorrhea are accompanied by acquired virilization, and the cause of ovarian or adrenal androgen excess must be sought (Chap. 46).

Abnormal uterine bleeding Any woman in the reproductive age group with abnormal uterine bleeding has a pregnancy-associated disorder (abortion, ectopic pregnancy) until proved otherwise. Continuing improvements in the specificity and sensitivity of pregnancy tests make it easier for the clinician to exclude complications of pregnancy as a cause of abnormal bleeding. The second major cause is iatrogenic due to exogenous hormone administration.

Organic lesions of the uterus (submucous leiomyoma, adenomyosis, endometritis, endometrial polyp) usually produce menorrhagia (heavier bleeding than usual at the expected time of menses). Carcinoma of the endometrium is primarily a disease of postmenopausal women but should also be considered in cases of abnormal bleeding during the "perimenopause" or in individuals with predisposing conditions such as morbid obesity, liver disease, chronic oligoanovulation from the time of puberty, or a strong family history of cancer. In the woman who has never had a previous episode of abnormal menstruation, the possibility of a bleeding diathesis (e.g., idiopathic thrombocytopenic purpura, acute leukemia) must be considered.

The term *dysfunctional uterine bleeding* is intended to describe bleeding from an endometrium which has not progressed through full maturation under the influence of a dominant ovarian follicle that passes through full follicular and luteal phases. This is "anovulatory bleeding" and is seen in two broad classes of patients: (1) Individuals who usually ovulate but who have suffered a transient disruption in the synchronous hypothalamic-pituitary-ovarian relationships that are necessary for monthly ovulation; this occurs most commonly at the extremes of reproductive life but may occur at any time. (2) Patients with *chronic estrus*. The most common entity in this group is patients with polycystic ovarian disease (Stein-Leventhal syndrome). Characteristically, these patients give a history of relative infertility and oligoanovulation dating from puberty and often exhibit cutaneous manifestations of androgen excess (hirsutism, acne). A predominant feature of the pathophysiology of this disorder is increased ovarian production of androstenedione which is converted to estrone in extragonadal sites, resulting in chronic excess endogenous estrogen production. Since androstenedione is also a precursor of testosterone, overproduction of androstenedione is also ultimately responsible for the androgenic manifestations. Two other causes of a chronic estrous state due to excessive estrogen (estrone) production at extragonadal sites are liver disease and obesity. In these two disorders the production of androstenedione is normal, but the extent of conversion to estrone is increased. It should be noted that certain previously designated "nonendocrine" epithelial, germ cell, or metastatic ovarian neoplasms (e.g., mucinous cystadenoma, mature teratoma, or Krukenberg tumor) can also secrete excessive androstenedione which may lead to overproduction of testosterone. Infrequently (since it is an uncommon tumor, occurring most often in postmenopausal women), unilateral granulosa–theca cell tumors of the ovary secrete estradiol and cause premenopausal women to present with chronic estrus and abnormal bleeding. These tumors are usually sizable and, therefore, palpable on bimanual examination.

Ordinarily a careful history and physical examination will disclose the likely etiology of the anovulatory bleeding. Endometrial biopsy is not part of the standard management of patients with dysfunctional uterine bleeding. The only exceptions are individuals who are at high risk for endometrial carcinoma.

PAIN   Mittelschmerz The term applied to ovulatory pain is *mittelschmerz*. This is typically a dull aching pain at midcycle in one lower quadrant lasting from a few minutes to 8 h. The etiology of the pain is unknown but may be inflammation of the ovulation site itself or peritoneal irritation from follicular fluid released at ovulation. The principal clinical importance of mittelschmerz is that it must be distinguished from more serious organic diseases such as appendicitis, pelvic inflammatory disease, and ectopic pregnancy.

Premenstrual syndrome The premenstrual syndrome consists of a variety of somatic symptoms occurring in the postovulatory phase of the cycle and ordinarily terminating with the onset of menses. These symptoms include edema, breast engorgement, abdominal bloating, headache, and exacerbation of acne. There is, in addition, a psychological component known colloquially as "premenstrual tension" consisting of cyclic irritability, depression, and lethargy. The severity varies. The biochemical events responsible for the somatic symptoms and for the psychological component are not known.

Painful menstruation Virtually all menses subsequent to ovulation are associated with some pelvic discomfort if only for the first few hours of bleeding. This is so because myometrial contraction is an essential part of the process. *Dysmenorrhea* refers to excessive and incapacitating pain at the time of menstruation. In patients with such complaint, careful search for congenital uterovaginal malformation, pelvic infection, tumor, endometriosis, or other pelvic nongenital pathology should be made. The majority of cases of dysmenorrhea are deemed "primary" in that no discernible organic cause for the pain can be discovered. It is likely that primary dysmenorrhea is caused by an exaggeration of the biochemical events leading to the synthesis of prostaglandin and related uterotonic metabolites and their action on the myometrium or by an alteration in the individual's response to the genuine discomfort of myometrial contraction—or a combination of the two. Careful inquiry will often disclose precipitating or aggravating psychological factors.

Explanation of the physiology of primary dysmenorrhea, reassurance, and general measures such as rest and local heat will suffice in many instances. More potent analgesics and sedatives are sometimes required. Prostaglandin inhibitors such as aspirin may be useful if begun during the week prior to menses. In cases where the episodes are recurrent and the degree of incapacitation is significant, low-dose, combination oral contraceptive therapy (estrogen plus progestin) is ordinarily effective. Such therapy probably reduces the amount of prostaglandin precursors present in the endometrium at the end of the cycle and decreases the volume of blood lost during menses with the consequence that myometrial contractions are reduced.

MENOPAUSE Cessation of menstruation is a significant event in the life of most women. The loss of this physiologic function is a dramatic reminder that aging is relentless, and the psychological impact is maximal in a culture that prizes youth. The term *climacteric* refers to the time of life during which menopause occurs. Many other significant events relating to a woman's career or her role as spouse and parent may occur during the climacteric.

The average age of menopause is 47 years. The postmenopausal ovary is on an average two-fifths of its previous weight, is virtually devoid of follicles, and no longer secretes estrogen. An auxiliary mechanism of estrogen production becomes manifest during the postmenopausal years. Androgens of adrenal origin are converted in peripheral tissues to estrone. While estrone is a less potent estrogen than estradiol, it is nonetheless biologically active. Thus, the postmenopausal woman is only *relatively* deficient in estrogen. The efficiency of this mechanism of estrogen production increases with aging and with excess weight. Estrogen therapy is indicated only in the postmenopausal woman with complaints of vasomotor instability or urogenital atrophy. The role of estrogens in the prevention of osteoporosis in postmenopausal women remains controversial. Ordinarily estrogens should be given orally and in the smallest effective dose for the shortest possible time. Personality change, easy fatigability, insomnia, and depression are symptoms more likely related to events in the climacteric other than ovarian failure.

SEXUAL FUNCTION

Patients consult physicians more and more frequently because of disturbances in sexual function. In general, women request help more frequently than men, and they usually complain of lack of arousal during intercourse or failure to achieve orgasm. (See also Chap. 345, "Sexual Counseling.") The term *frigidity* has been used for centuries in connection with female sexual problems. Recent classifications of female sexual problems have moved away from the term because of its imprecision.

LIBIDO Libido or sexuality is not governed exclusively by sex hormones. While the normal action of certain hormones appears to be important for human libido, cultural, emotional, and other influences on behavior affect sexuality to variable degrees. A reduction in libido is rarely caused solely by ovarian or adrenal insufficiency. Augmented or diminished libido is most often the consequence of psychological events rather than an endocrinopathy.

SEXUAL RESPONSE The female sexual response consists of two distinct components: (1) a local genital vasocongestive response analogous to erection in the male and (2) orgasm. Vasocongestion of the vagina, under autonomic nervous control, leads to vaginal lubrication in preparation for intromission. The lubrication is due principally to a transudate from the glandless vaginal mucosa. There is also a general increase in pelvic and vulvar vascularity. Healthy vaginal tissue is a prerequisite to normal lubrication, but the neurogenic reflex leading to genital congestion and vaginal lubrication is initiated by psychic sexual stimuli. Fatigue, interpersonal conflicts between the couple, depression, anxiety, or stress may lead to failure of the vasocongestive response.

Orgasm is a cortical sensory phenomenon in which involuntary rhythmic contractions of skeletal muscles and engorged tissues surrounding the vaginal outlet as well as some deeper pelvic muscles are perceived as pleasurable. Direct or indirect stimulation of the clitoris is as critical in producing female orgasm as stimulation of the penis for male orgasm. The female can physically participate in sexual intercourse without experiencing either component of sexual response and may enjoy nonorgasmic sexual encounters particularly with a loving partner, presumably because of the pleasure derived from physical closeness in a cherished relationship. Exploitation of a woman's capacity to participate in sexual intercourse without sexual response can, however, be destructive to a couple's general relationship and may be a source of frustration manifested on occasion by psychosomatic complaints. Failure of orgasm in spite of normal vaginal lubrication is most often the consequence of insufficient clitoral stimulation. Organic diseases that preclude normal vascularity and sensation in the genitalia may also cause failure of sexual response. (See Chap. 345.)

DYSPAREUNIA Painful intercourse is termed *dyspareunia;* it can ordinarily be localized by the patient to the vagina or deeper within the pelvis. Dyspareunia is most commonly due to the failure of vaginal lubrication but may be due to organic pathology of the vagina or pelvis. Failure of the appearance of the vaginal transudate may be the result of estrogen deficiency or failure of the autonomic nervous mechanisms which lead to vasocongestion. The latter is analogous to male impotence and like impotence most often indicates a psychological conflict. Pelvic dyspareunia may be due to pathology such as infection, endometriosis, or tumor. In instances where relief cannot be anticipated as a result of restoration of more normal pelvic anatomy, changes in coital technique which limit the extent of vaginal penetration may prevent the discomfort.

VAGINISMUS Vaginismus is the painful, involuntary contraction of the musculature surrounding the entrance to the vagina. This rare but disabling disorder prohibits intromission and usually is a conditioned response related to some previous real or imagined adverse sexual experience. Treatment consists of eliminating the conditioned response by progressive dilation of the vaginal entrance by the patient. In only the most recalcitrant cases is it profitable to subject a patient to psychotherapy in search of the etiologic sexual conflict.

REPRODUCTION

The scarcity of infants for adoption has aggravated the plight of couples in whom the reproductive process has failed. While not an illness, infertility can be devastating in that it is the unexpected denial of the personal and often powerful drive to reproduce. A systematic approach to the problem in an atmosphere of empathy and honesty will be most rewarding to infertile couples.

Infertility is always a problem involving two people. The physician's initial encounter with an infertile couple should be used to gather historical data relative to the reproductive process. Frequency of intercourse, relationship of time of intercourse to time of ovulation, use of potentially spermicidal lubricants, general health of the individuals, and use of medications that might be detrimental to the reproductive process should be reviewed.

Because it is the simplest, safest, and least expensive part of an infertility evaluation, a semen analysis is the first laboratory test performed (see Chap. 341). Unfortunately, there is no opportunity to scrutinize directly the female germ cells.

The preovulatory postcoital test is a second useful procedure for the evaluation of infertility; during the immediate preovulatory time of the cycle an aspirate of cervical mucus is taken within 2 h after intercourse. A normal test should disclose several motile spermatozoa per high-power microscopic field and implies successful male erection, intromission, and ejaculation, as well as presumably normal cervical function. Infections or alterations in cervical mucus production subsequent to surgery or cryotherapy of the cervix are the most common causes of abnormal postcoital tests when the male is normal.

Basal body temperature graphs, endometrial biopsy, and plasma progesterone 1 week prior to expected menses are indirect methods useful for determining ovulation and the adequacy of corpus luteum function. An occasional short luteal phase is likely a normal event in many women; it remains conjectural whether repeated corpus luteum insufficiency can be responsible for infertility or repeated spontaneous abortion. The list of therapeutic alternatives useful in inducing ovulation in some ovulatory disorders is slowly expanding and includes clomiphene citrate, human menopausal gonadotropins, bromocriptine mesylate, and wedge resection of the ovary.

Hysterosalpingography is the accepted method of determining tubal patency. The oviduct plays several roles in the reproductive process including pickup of the ovum from the site of ovulation, spermatozoan and ovum transport to the site of fertilization in the ampullary portion of the oviduct, and nourishment and transportation of the early zygote. A radiographic study showing patency of the oviduct does not assess these aforementioned aspects of tubal function. Infection, endometriosis, and adhesions due to previous pelvic surgery are the most frequent causes of distortions of tubal anatomy and function. Though recent advances in microsurgical techniques have improved the likelihood of reversing surgical sterilization, surgical restoration of normal tubal function in the aforementioned disorders is less than satisfactory. Pharmacological superovulation of a female who had no oviducts, harvesting of the ovum through laparoscopy, in vitro fertilization, and transfer of the embryo to the mother's uterus resulted in the delivery of an apparently normal infant in England in 1978. It remains to be seen whether this technique in the coming decade will continue to be a medical curiosity or will have widespread application in the management of the infertile couple.

We understand only a small part of the story of reproduction, and our diagnostic tests are inadequate to perceive many impediments to conception (for example, to assess tubal function). These limitations likely account for the fact that at least 10 percent of barren couples have no discernible cause for infertility. In some of these the impediment is relative, for after a variable and sometimes lengthy period of time, conception may occur.

REFERENCES

AIMAN J et al: The origin of androgen and estrogen in a virilized postmenopausal woman with bilateral benign cystic teratomas. Obstet Gynecol 49:695, 1977

FORDNEY DS: Dyspareunia and vaginismus. Clin Obstet Gynecol 21:205, 1978

FRISCH RF, MCARTHUR JW: Menstrual cycles: Fatness as a determinant of minimum weight for height necessary for their maintenance or onset. Science 185:949, 1974

KAPLAN HS: *The New Sex Therapy: Active Treatment of Sexual Dysfunctions.* New York, Brunner/Mazel, 1974

LEVINE SB, ROSENTHAL M: Marital sexual dysfunction: Female dysfunctions. Ann Intern Med 86:588, 1977

SHOEMAKER E et al: Estrogen treatment of postmenopausal women, benefits and risks. JAMA 238:1524, 1977

SIITERI PK, MACDONALD PC: Role of extraglandular estrogen in human endocrinology, in *Handbook of Physiology: Endocrinology II,* part I, RO Greep, EB Astwood (eds). Washington, DC, The American Physiological Society, 1973, chap 28, p 615

46
HIRSUTISM AND VIRILIZATION

JEAN D. WILSON

Hirsutism in women, the growth of hair in a pattern characteristic of men, is a common and perplexing problem in medicine. Numerous factors—genetic, endocrine, and undefined—influence the growth and distribution of hair so that there is considerable overlap between normal men and women. As a consequence abnormal hair growth is difficult to define; an unbearable burden to one woman may be an unnoticed amount of hair in another. However, if the patient thinks that hair growth is excessive, no amount of reassurance, persuasion, or argument will convince her otherwise. The central issue in dealing with such patients is the separation of those infrequent instances in which hirsutism is one manifestation of an underlying virilizing or defeminizing syndrome from the vast majority of individuals in which it is fundamentally a cosmetic problem.

CONTROL OF NORMAL HAIR GROWTH AND DISTRIBUTION
Endocrinology There are three principal circulating androgens in women—dehydroepiandrosterone derived from the adrenal, androstenedione derived equally from adrenal and ovary, and testosterone which is both secreted from the ovary and formed by peripheral conversion from circulating dehydroepiandrosterone and androstenedione. The production of adrenal androgen is regulated primarily by adrenocorticotropic hormone (ACTH), while ovarian androgen secretion is regulated by the gonadotropins. Dehydroepiandrosterone and androstenedione are weak androgens, but they can be converted into physiologically potent hormones in nonendocrine (peripheral) tissues; by this process dehydroepiandrosterone is converted to androstenediol, and androstenedione is transformed into testosterone and dihydrotestosterone. Androgens are the major determinants of hair distribution in both sexes.

In simple terms four types of androgen response can be defined:

1 No androgen dependence: lanugo, eyebrows, eyelashes
2 Dependence upon adrenal androgen and hence equal growth in men and women: axillary and lower pubic hair
3 Dependence upon testicular androgen: upper pubic, facial, ear, extremity, and truncal hair
4 Inhibition by testicular androgen: scalp hair

Why different body regions respond differently to the same or similar androgen is uncertain. Theoretically, the metabolism of androgens might differ in the various sites, or hormone receptors might vary. Evidence against the former possibility comes from studies of patients with single gene mutations influencing androgen action (Chap. 344). The hair follicle, like other androgen-responsive cells, requires conversion of testosterone to dihydrotestosterone for expression of testicular androgen action, and hair follicles from all regions of the body perform this conversion equally well. Moreover, the same cytoplasmic receptor that is essential for androgen action in other cells (Chap. 341) is necessary for the action of adrenal and testicular androgens in the hair follicle. Genetic disorders with normal testosterone production but absent receptor have deficient or absent axillary, pubic, facial, truncal, and limb hair. Regional differences in androgen responsiveness of hair are probably the consequence of regional differences in the level of androgen receptor in hair follicles.

Genetic factors Despite similar hormone levels, there is considerable diversity in the distribution of hair among individuals and among racial groups in regard to facial, truncal, and pubic hair. It is generally agreed that dark-haired, darkly pigmented whites of either sex tend to be more hirsute than blonde or fair-skinned persons. Orientals, American Indians, and blacks are less hirsute than whites. Orientals rarely have facial or body hair except in the pubic and axillary regions, and American Indians, in addition, rarely develop baldness in either sex. There is also considerable heterogeneity of hair patterns within family groups. The inheritance of hair patterns is obviously complex and is probably polygenic in nature.

Other factors Aging is a prerequisite for the expression of some types of hair development, whether mediated by androgens or otherwise. For example, in men hair on the trunk and extremities frequently increases for several years after maximal levels of plasma androgens have been reached. Conversely, loss of androgens rarely results in diminution of normal hair or reverses hirsutism. The appearance of pubic hair is frequently the heralding event of puberty in females. Women in the first trimester of pregnancy commonly observe increased hairiness of the face, extremities, and breasts. Menopause is often associated with the loss of hair in the pubic area, axillae, and extremities, whereas growth of hair on the face increases in postmenopausal women. The physiological basis for these changes is unclear and cannot be explained entirely by changes in androgen levels.

PATHOLOGICAL HAIR GROWTH OR DISTRIBUTION Drugs Drug-induced hirsutism is a frequent complication of modern therapy. It may be an isolated symptom or part of a virilizing syndrome. If the onset is subtle, it may go unrecognized by the physician. Drugs that produce hirsutism without actual virilization include phenytoin, Minoxidil, diazoxide, hexachlorobenzene, and ACTH. Steroidal drugs that are capable of inducing virilization as well as hirsutism include progestins (which may also cause virilization of infants born to mothers given them) and androgens.

Virilizing syndromes In an evaluation of patients for hirsutism, the most important feature is whether virilization or defeminization is also present (Table 46-1). In patients with androgen overproduction defeminizing signs are more consistent than are the signs of virilization, although the latter, if present, are valuable, since they indicate either ovarian or adrenal pathology. Two reservations should be kept in mind in interpreting the presence or absence of virilization. First, virilization is indicative of androgen excess at some time in the patient's life but does not mean that active disease is present at the time of evaluation. This can be ascertained by measurement of plasma androgen levels and/or production rates. Second, severe over-androgenization may exist in the absence of a true virilization syndrome; i.e., at the same level of androgen production clitoromegaly may be present in one patient and not another.

Two types of virilizing syndromes can occur—ovarian and adrenal—but it should be emphasized that these disorders account for only a small fraction of patients who complain of hirsutism.

OVARIAN ANDROGENIZATION Polycystic ovary disease is the commonest cause of ovarian hyperandrogenism (see Chap. 342). The disorder has a wide clinical spectrum that varies from apparently normal menses and mild hirsutism to complete amenorrhea and virilization; hyperthecosis of the ovary characterized by the presence of luteinized theca-like cells in the ovarian stroma is a varient of the disorder. Luteinizing hormone (LH) is almost invariably elevated, and there is considerable overproduction of androgens by the ovary. Other causes of ovarian virilization include stromal hyperplasia, luteomas, hilar-cell hyperplasia, and a variety of androgen-secreting tumors including arrhenoblastoma and Krukenberg tumor; in these disorders plasma testosterone levels are elevated, frequently to the male range; the tumors may be so small as to be undetectable by pelvic examination or laparoscopy.

ADRENAL ANDROGENIZATION Adrenal androgen-secreting tumors (adenoma or carcinoma) are generally accompanied by elevated urinary 17-ketosteroid excretion. Plasma testosterone levels may be elevated but not as high as in ovarian disease. Hirsutism can also be a manifestation of congenital adrenal hyperplasia and Cushing's disease.

Idiopathic or simple hirsutism This term applies to those hirsute women in whom a specific etiologic diagnosis cannot be made. The diagnosis should be restricted to patients in whom the urinary 17-ketosteroid level is not elevated, the ovaries are not enlarged, adrenal function is normal, there is no evidence of an adrenal or ovarian tumor, and menstruation is normal. Slight elevations of plasma androstenedione and/or testosterone are usual, and testosterone secretion rates may be increased above the mean; whether these abnormalities represent the extreme end of a normal continuum or a distinct pathological group is unclear. However, substantial evidence indicates that in the majority of such women the increased plasma androgens are derived from the ovaries. In some the underlying diagnosis may be mild or early polycystic ovarian

TABLE 46-1
Clinical signs of defeminization and virilization

Signs of defeminization	Signs of virilization
Amenorrhea	Frontal balding
Decrease in breast size	Increase in size of shoulder
Loss of female body contours	girdle muscles
	Clitoromegaly
	Coarsening of the voice
	Acne

SOURCE: *After Karp and Herrmann.*

disease, but in most the hormone abnormalities are not accompanied or followed by signs of ovarian dysfunction. Thus, it is possible that these patients are variants of normal. Since androgens are a major determinant of hair distribution and growth, it is to be expected that within the normal range higher androgen levels would be associated on average with greater androgen-mediated hair growth. Therefore, the belief of many endocrinologists that the majority of hirsute women have no associated endocrinopathy may still be valid.

TREATMENT In the case of drugs and tumors of the ovaries or adrenal glands, treatment is straightforward—stop the drugs or remove the tumors. In polycystic ovarian disease and idiopathic hirsutism, effective therapy is ovarian suppression using a combination-type oral contraceptive; improvement in hirsutism can frequently be documented in 6 months to a year. Whether the risks of contraceptive therapy are justified in simple hirsutism is an individual judgment. If fertility is desired, other forms of therapy are indicated (Chap. 342). Since coarsened hairs usually do not return completely to normal, local therapy for hirsutism including depilatory agents, shaving, tweezing, and electrolysis is often required. Other evidences of virilization such as balding, clitoromegaly, and coarsening of the voice rarely improve following cure of the overandrogenization.

REFERENCES

GIVENS JR: Hirsutism and hyperandrogenism. Adv Intern Med 21:221, 1976

KARP L, HERRMANN WL: Diagnosis and treatment of hirsutism in women. Obstet Gynecol 41:283, 1973

KIRSCHNER MA, BARDIN CW: Androgen production and metabolism in normal and virilized women. Metabolism 21:667, 1972

MULLER SA: Hirsutism. Am J Med 46:803, 1969

ROSENFIELD RL: Relationship of androgens to female hirsutism and infertility. J Reprod Med 11:87, 1973

47
DISTURBANCES OF SEXUAL FUNCTION AND REPRODUCTION IN MEN

PATRICK C. WALSH
JEAN D. WILSON

A coordinated sequence of physiological events (psychic, endocrine, vascular, and neurological) controls normal sexual and reproductive function in men. In this chapter, the discussion is focused on the clinical presentation of sexual disorders in men. (Also see Chaps. 341, "Diseases of the Testis," and 345, "Sexual Counseling.")

SEXUAL FUNCTION

NORMAL SEXUAL FUNCTION Simply stated, normal male sexual function can be divided into five phases, each of which is under diverse regulation: libido, erection, ejaculation, orgasm, and detumescence.

The first, sexual desire or libido, is regulated by poorly understood psychic factors and by testicular androgens. Castration produces a decline in libido that can be restored by treatment with testosterone.

The second phase, erection, is primarily a neurological event that results in modification of the vascular supply to the penis, causing it to become engorged with blood. The neurological aspect of erection is controlled by both reflex and psy-

chic stimuli. The sensory portion begins with fibers that originate in pacinian corpuscles of the penis and pass via the pudendal nerve to the S_2 to S_4 dorsal root ganglia. The efferent limb begins with parasympathetic preganglionic fibers from the S_2 to S_4 dorsal root ganglia, which synapse in the perivesicular, prostatic, and cavernous plexuses. From there, postganglionic fibers pass to blood vessels of the corpora cavernosa. Efferent fibers from S_3 and S_4 ganglia also travel in the pudendal nerve to the ischiocavernosus and bulbocavernosus muscles. There is also sympathetic innervation of the male genitalia. These fibers originate from the lateral columns of the spinal cord at the levels of T_{12} and L_1, the so-called "thoracolumbar erection center," and synapse in the pelvic and perivesicular plexuses. Postganglionic fibers innervate the smooth muscle of the vas deferens, seminal vesicle, and internal sphincter of the bladder. Sympathetic innervation can act synergistically with the sacral parasympathetics to mediate erection initiated by psychic stimuli. For example, some patients with sacral cord transection who cannot have erection with tactile "reflex" stimulation can become erect in response to psychic stimuli. On the other hand, sympathetic innervation is not mandatory for erection. This is demonstrated by continued potency in most patients after bilateral complete sympathectomy. The central nervous system modulates erectile response via pathways thought to descend in the lateral columns of the spinal cord. The effect of the central nervous system on erection can be either stimulatory or inhibitory; thus the importance of psychic stimulation for erection.

While erection is primarily controlled by the parasympathetic system, the transformation of the penis from a flaccid to an erect state is a vascular phenomenon. Blood reaches the penis via terminal branches of the right and left internal pudendal arteries. The erectile tissue of the penis consists of two corpora cavernosa lying side by side on the dorsal aspect of the penis and the corpus spongiosum that surrounds the urethra. This tissue consists of an irregular sponge-like system of valvular spaces interspersed between arteries and veins. These valve-like structures (called *polsters*) are located in the arterioles, and in the flaccid state are constricted, causing blood to be shunted away from the corpora directly into the veins. Under the influence of the autonomic erection centers, the polsters relax and allow blood to fill the vascular spaces of the corpora and expand the penis to the erect state. It is not clear whether venous valves impede flow and thus further promote erection. Passive venous obstruction undoubtedly occurs.

The third phase, ejaculation, is under control of the sympathetic nervous system and consists of two processes, seminal emission and true ejaculation. Emission results from the contraction of the vas deferens, prostate, and seminal vesicles which causes seminal fluid to enter the urethra. True ejaculation results from contraction of the muscles of the pelvic floor including the bulbocavernosus and ischiocavernosus muscles. Retrograde ejaculation is prevented by partial bladder neck closure mediated by the sympathetic nerves.

The fourth phase, orgasm, is a cortical sensory phenomenon in which the rhythmic contraction of the bulbocavernosus and ischiocavernosus muscles is perceived as pleasurable. It is purely psychic. The fact that orgasm can occur without either ejaculation or bladder neck closure explains why some drugs that prevent ejaculation do not interfere with erection or orgasm.

The mechanism for detumescence after orgasm and ejaculation is poorly understood but may be related to vasoconstriction of the arterioles supplying blood to the erectile tissue, thus allowing venous drainage to empty the sinuses and the penis to become flaccid. Following orgasm, there is a refractory period that varies with age, physical condition, and psychic factors during which erection and ejaculation are inhibited.

IMPOTENCE Male sexual dysfunction, often termed *impotence*, may be manifested in various ways: loss of desire, inability to obtain or maintain an erection, premature ejaculation, absence of emission, inability to achieve orgasm. Many subjects complain of more than one abnormality simultaneously. These complaints can be secondary to other chronic or debilitating diseases, the consequence of specific disorders of the urogenital or endocrine systems, or the result of psychiatric disturbance. It is mandatory in all instances to exclude organic (and in some instances potentially correctable or treatable) causes.

Loss of desire Because androgens have a major influence on sexual desire in men, a decrease in libido may indicate androgen deficiency arising from either pituitary or testicular disease. This possibility can be tested by the measurement of plasma testosterone and gonadotropins. However, since the testosterone required to maintain libido is usually less than the amount necessary for full stimulation of the prostate and seminal vesicles, the patient should also complain of absence of emission when the loss of libido is on an endocrine basis. Conversely, if patients have normal semen volume, it is unlikely that endocrine factors are responsible for their sexual dysfunction.

Loss of erection Some of the organic causes of erectile impotence are listed in Table 47-1. Several types of neurological disorders can cause impotence including lesions in the anterior temporal lobe, spinal cord disorders, insufficiency of sensory input as can occur in diabetic neuropathy and tabes dorsalis, or damage to parasympathetic nerves, for example following surgical procedures such as total prostatectomy. Transurethral prostatectomy, in contrast, probably does not cause organic impotence. If spinal cord injury is above the thoracolumbar region, reflex erections may occur. Injury at the level of the

TABLE 47-1
Some organic causes of erectile impotence in men

I Neurological diseases
  A Anterior temporal lobe lesions
  B Diseases of the spinal cord
  C Loss of sensory input
    1 Diabetes mellitus and various polyneuropathies
    2 Tabes dorsalis
    3 Disease of dorsal root ganglia
  D Disease of nervi erigentes
    1 Complete prostatectomy
    2 Rectosigmoid operations
    3 Aortic bypass surgery
II Endocrine causes
  A Testicular failure (primary or secondary)
  B Hyperprolactinemia
III Drugs
  A Phenothiazines
  B Thioridazine
  C Imipramine
  D α-Methyldopa
  E Guanethidine
  F Reserpine
  G Spironolactone
  H Alcohol
  I Heroin, methadone
  J Estrogen
IV Vascular diseases: Leriche syndrome
V Failure of detumescence, priapism
VI Penile diseases
  A Previous priapism
  B Penile trauma
  C Peyronie's disease

sacral cord or cauda equina does not interfere with psychogenic erections but prevents reflex or tactile erections. Diffuse injury of the spinal cord results in total impotence. Diabetes mellitus deserves special comment. As many as half of diabetic men develop impotence within 6 years of the onset of diabetes, and impotence may be the first clinical manifestation of diabetic neuropathy. However, when careful neurological examination is performed including the cystometrogram, other evidences of neurological disturbance are usually uncovered. Many of the other polyneuropathies described in Chap. 377, and the paralytic states of the autonomic nervous system described in Chap. 13, have similar effects.

Endocrine causes of testicular failure that result in impotence usually bring about such profound changes that the disorders are not difficult to recognize (Chap. 341). Recent studies suggest that hyperprolactinemia may be a cause for impotence in some patients with pituitary tumors (see Chap. 333). As many as 90 percent of men with increased prolactin levels are impotent; gonadotropins and testosterone values are in the low normal range, and there is a normal pituitary response to luteinizing hormone–releasing hormone (LHRH). Bromocriptine mesylate, a dopamine agonist, lowers prolactin levels and reverses impotence in most such patients.

Drugs are a common cause of impotence. The usual explanation is neurological blockade, and this may well be the case for those drugs with peripheral parasympatholytic actions such as the tricyclic antidepressants. Others may act by enhancing prolactin secretion. In addition, the drugs of addiction such as alcohol, methadone, and heroin frequently lead to impotence. Whether the impotence in the latter instances is caused by reduced testosterone levels or the general condition of the patient is unclear.

One can readily understand vascular causes of impotence since continued high flow into the vascular network of the penis is necessary to maintain the erect state. The prototype of impaired penile blood supply is the Leriche syndrome. Here impedance to the blood flow into the penis occurs as the result of obstruction of the distal aorta at the bifurcation of the common iliacs. This usually presents as claudication and impotence; either can occur separately. Likewise, occlusion in smaller vessels supplying the penis can also lead to impotence. Recently several noninvasive methods have been devised to detect decreased blood flow to the penis using the Doppler technique. Differences between brachial pressure and systolic pressure in the penis should not be greater than 30 to 40 mmHg. There is a good correlation between vascular obstruction as the cause for impotence and failure to meet these criteria.

Premature ejaculation This disorder seldom has an organic cause. It is usually related to anxiety in the sexual situation, unreasonable expectations about performance, or an emotional disorder. A variety of successful therapeutic modalities have been described by Levine.

Absence of emission Three disorders may produce this symptom: (1) retrograde ejaculation, (2) sympathetic denervation, or (3) androgen deficiency. Retrograde ejaculation may occur following surgery on the bladder neck or may develop spontaneously in diabetic men. Examination of a postcoital urine specimen will establish the diagnosis. Following sympathectomy or occasionally after extensive retroperitoneal surgery, the autonomic innervation of the prostate and seminal vesicles is lost, resulting in absence of smooth-muscle contraction at the time of ejaculation. Finally, androgen deficiency may lead to absence of secretions from the prostate and seminal vesicles.

Absence of orgasm If libido and erectile function are normal, the absence of orgasm is almost always due to a psychiatric disorder.

Failure of detumescence *Priapism* is a persistent painful erection, often totally unrelated to sexual activity. The etiology of priapism is usually idiopathic, but the disorder can be associated with sickle-cell anemia, chronic granulocytic leukemia, or spinal cord injury. The disorder is thought to be secondary to clotting within the penile vascular network. The persistent erection disrupts this network and can lead to fibrosis and subsequent erectile impotence.

Penile diseases Finally, in addition to priapism, penile trauma and Peyronie's disease of the penis can also cause impotence (Table 47-1).

Evaluation of impotence Although the failure of erectile function is frequently the result of psychological disturbances, every effort must be made to exclude a remedial, organic cause (Table 47-1). Usually, the history is informative. Normally, from early childhood through the eighth decade, erections occur during sleep. This phenomenon, termed *nocturnal penile tumescence* (NPT), occurs during rapid eye movement sleep, and the total time of NPT usually averages 100 min per night. Consequently, if the patient gives a history of turgid erections under any circumstances (often when awakening in the early morning), the psychic, efferent neurological, and circulatory systems that mediate erection are intact, and dysfunction is probably due to a psychiatric disorder. In these patients the physical and laboratory examinations should be limited. (Occasional patients with sensory neuropathy may have nocturnal erections.) If the history of nocturnal erections is questionable, measurements of NPT can be made with the use of a strain gauge attached to a recorder.

Factors in favor of organic impotence include a similar degree of erectile dysfunction under all circumstances, onset not associated with any particular psychiatric symptomatology, a previous uninterrupted period of normal erectile function, and persistent sexual desire. Questions should be directed toward specific etiologies. These should include symptoms of diabetes, symptoms of peripheral neuropathy or bladder dysfunction, and symptoms referable to the vascular system such as intermittent claudication or history of priapism. A thorough drug history should be obtained, and inquiry concerning past operations that may have produced neurological damage should be made.

Physical examination should include a thorough genital examination to rule out any abnormalities of the penis itself. The testes should be palpated for size or abnormal masses; if the length is less than 4 cm, hypogonadism should be considered. Evidence of feminization should be looked for such as gynecomastia and abnormal body hair distribution. All pulses should be palpated, including the penile pulse, which can be felt by pressing both corpora between the thumb and forefinger and palpating to either side of the midline. If possible, penile blood pressure should be measured. If there is an indication from either history or physical examination of a vascular etiology, an aortogram may be indicated.

A neurological examination to evaluate the erectile reflex is advisable including anal sphincter tone, perineal sensation, and the bulbocavernosus reflex. This reflex is obtained by squeezing the glans penis and noting the degree of anal sphincter constriction. An examination for peripheral neuropathy, including distal muscle weakness, loss of tendon reflexes in the legs, and tests for impairment of vibratory, position, tactile, and pain sensation, should also be performed (see Chap. 377).

A frequent cause of prolonged impotence is an anxiety or depression state. These closely related conditions can be diagnosed by the criteria enumerated in Chaps. 11 and 25. Other psychological factors such as disinterest in the sexual partner, fear of sexual incompetence, marital discord, deviant sexual

attitudes, worry, fatigue, and ill health often operate in various combinations to reduce sexual impulse.

Laboratory evaluation is probably of minimal value. Measurement of serum testosterone in the absence of evidence of feminization or hypogonadism is seldom helpful.

Treatment of impotence Medical therapy with androgens offers little more than placebo benefit except in hypogonadal men. If a pituitary tumor producing high prolactin levels is present, however, either surgical removal or treatment with bromocriptine mesylate will usually result in return of potency. Surgical therapy may be useful in the treatment of decreased potency related to aortic obstruction; however, potency can be lost rather than improved after aortic operation if the autonomic nerve supply to the penis is damaged. This complication is minimized if an endarterectomy is done or, if a graft is required, the reconstruction of the distal end is performed above the origin of the external iliac arteries. Early surgical relief of priapism by shunting procedures, such as corpora spongiosum shunting, might prevent subsequent impotence.

A useful surgical technique for improvement of potency in refractory patients such as individuals with diabetic neuropathy is the implantation of a penile prosthesis, that is, the insertion within the corpora of a small, blunt silastic rod. The patient must be made aware that full erection is not produced and that the device only prevents buckling during intercourse. More recently, an inflatable prosthetic device has been devised for implantation on either side of the corpora. A connecting reservoir of material is placed in the perivesicular space, and pumps are located in the scrotum. By means of these pumps the penis can be made to become nearly fully erect at the appropriate time and then be made to relax after intercourse.

In the larger group of anxiety states and depressive illnesses measures directed at their alleviation will usually restore sexual potency, and sexual counseling, education, and psychotherapy are beneficial in alleviating psychogenic factors.

REPRODUCTION

Approximately a tenth of marriages in the United States are barren, and another tenth result in fewer children than desired. The husband is the cause of the infertility in about a third of these marriages.

Infertility in the male can be due to disorders of the hypothalamic-pituitary system, disorders of the testes, or abnormalities of the ejaculatory system (Table 341-1). When a history is obtained, information should be sought about the duration of infertility, fertility in other marriages of either the husband or wife, acquired or congenital disease that may lead to infertility, technique and frequency of intercourse, and family history of infertility. To exclude the presence of gross abnormalities of the endocrine system, the physical examination should evaluate the distribution of body hair, the presence of gynecomastia, the development of the scrotum and penis, the location of the urethral meatus, and the presence of normal vasa deferentia and epididymides. The size of each testis should be estimated with care. Because the seminiferous tubules account for more than 75 percent of the testicular mass, a reduction in testicular size (less than 4 cm in length) indicates a severe deficiency in the spermatogenic function of the testis. Finally, with the patient standing in the upright position, the Valsalva maneuver should be utilized to test for the presence of a varicocele.

The next step in the evaluation of the male partner is the semen analysis. This provides a semiquantitative estimation of the severity of the dysfunction. The findings are usually considered normal if: the semen coagulates and then liquefies, the volume is 2 to 5 ml, the spermatozoa count is greater than 20 million per milliliter, more than 60 percent of the spermatozoa are actively motile, and more than 60 percent have normal morphology. If no spermatozoa are present, the term *azoospermia* is used; if spermatozoa are present but the count is less than 20 million per milliliter, the patient is considered to have oligospermia. In the azoospermic male with normal-sized testes, the differential diagnosis includes hyalinization of the seminiferous tubules, Sertoli cell–only syndrome, gonadotropin deficiency, ductal obstruction, or maturation arrest. Plasma testosterone and serum LH and follicle-stimulating hormone (FSH) measurements are helpful in distinguishing among these conditions. In patients with hyalinization of the seminiferous tubules LH and FSH are elevated, and plasma testosterone is low or borderline normal. Patients with Sertoli cell–only syndrome usually have normal LH and testosterone levels, but FSH levels are characteristically elevated. In gonadotropin deficiency LH, FSH, and testosterone are low, and in ductal obstruction or maturation arrest all studies are normal. To differentiate between the last two disorders, a testicular biopsy is necessary. In oligospermic patients, if the history

and physical examination are normal, it is unlikely that any further laboratory investigation will be useful in defining the etiology. These patients are usually classified in the large group having *idiopathic oligospermia.*

REFERENCES

AMELAR RD et al: *Male Infertility.* Philadelphia, Saunders, 1977, p 153

FITZPATRICK T: A cavernosogram study on the valvular competence of the deep human dorsal vein. J Urol 113:497, 1975

FURLOW WL: Surgical management of impotence using the inflatable penile prosthesis: Experience with 103 patients. Br J Urol 50:114, 1977

KARACAN I et al: Sleep-related penile tumescence as a function of age. Am J Psychiatry 132:9, 1975

KOLODNY RC et al: Sexual dysfunction in diabetic men. Diabetes 23:306, 1974

LAROCQUE M et al: Priapism: A review of 46 cases. J Urol 112:770, 1974

LEVINE SB: Marital sexual dysfunction: Ejaculation disturbances. Ann Intern Med 84:575, 1976

WEISS H: The physiology of human penile erection. Ann Intern Med 76:793, 1972

section 9 | Alterations in the skin

48
INTERPRETATION OF ALTERATIONS IN THE SKIN

THOMAS B. FITZPATRICK
HARLEY A. HAYNES

CLINICAL EXAMINATION OF THE SKIN

The identification of skin lesions, or alterations, is a problem similar to the recognition of cells in a blood smear: the minute details are of the greatest importance. The individual type of skin lesion (e.g., papule, nodule) can be considered as a letter in the alphabet, forming the basic element for the identification of the pathologic change and often leading to the clinical diagnosis. Lesions may be the presenting complaint of the patient or may be incidental findings during the routine physical examination; or they may be incidental to some major presenting complaint such as fever, cough, arthralgia, and the like. The recognition of the important and nonimportant skin lesions commonly encountered during the routine physical examination of the skin is a requisite part of the physician's task (Plates 1 to 6).

Inasmuch as the identification of skin lesions is the *sine qua non* of dermatologic diagnosis, the examiner's eye is undoubtedly the most valuable instrument at his or her disposal. Adequate illumination, preferably with natural light, is necessary. The observation of the skin should begin with an overall, "low-power" general assessment of the completely disrobed patient. The systematic approach to the examination of skin should be as follows: first the fingernails and then the anterior and posterior aspects of the arm; then, in sequence, the scalp, the face, the trunk, the lower extremities and the skin between the toes;

and then the mucous membranes, including the mouth and anogenital areas. The examiner of dermatologic lesions should consider: (1) the specific *type* of lesion, (2) the *configuration,* or *shape* of the lesion, and (3) the *arrangement* of the groups of lesions, such as linear, arciform, annular, polycyclic, herpetiform, zosteriform, and serpiginous.

Types of skin lesions can be classified by determining the topographic level of the lesions in relation to the normal skin (Table 48-1). For example, it is possible to distinguish lesions that are in or that protrude or are superimposed above or below the level of the normal skin. The lesions that are encom-

TABLE 48-1
Types of skin lesion

Flat lesions (in plane of skin)	Elevated lesions (above plane of skin)	Depressed lesions (below plane of skin)
Macule	Vesicle and bulla	Atrophy§
Infarct*	Pustule	Sclerosis§†
Sclerosis*†	Abscess‡	Erosion
Telangiectasia†	Cyst†	Excoriation
	Papule	Scar†
	Wheal	Ulcer
	Plaque	Sinus‡
	Nodule‡	Gangrene§
	Vegetation	
	Keratosis	
	Desquamation (scales)	
	Exudate* (crusts)	
	Lichenification	

* *May also be below the plane of the skin.*
† *May also be above the plane of the skin.*
‡ *May also be in or below the plane of the skin.*
§ *May also be in the plane of the skin.*
SOURCE: *TB Fitzpatrick, in Dermatology in General Medicine, 2d ed, TB Fitzpatrick et al (eds), New York, McGraw-Hill, 1979.*

passed within the scope of dermatology are listed in Fig. 48-1 and Table 48-1, and the histologic aspects are illustrated in Figs. 48-2 through 48-13.

The *shape* of the individual lesion and the *arrangement* of two or more lesions in relation to each other sometimes constitute important diagnostic clues. A linear arrangement of lesions often is indicative of an exogenous cause; also, linear lesions may occur because the pathologic process involves a vein, a lymphatic component, or an arteriole. Linearity can often be seen in various types of cutaneous hamartoma involving epidermal cells or melanocytes or even dermal connective tissue. In contrast, annular and arciform lesions and annular and arciform arrangements are relatively common and therefore only rarely lead to a specific diagnosis. The *iris* lesion, however, a special and important type of annular lesion, is an erythematous annular macule or papule with either a purplish papule or vesicle in the center. Iris lesions are characteristic of the erythema-multiforme syndrome. Annular macules may be observed in drug eruptions, secondary syphilis, and lupus erythematosus. Annular lesions with scale often suggest dermatophytosis or pityriasis rosea or psoriasis. The wheals that occur in creeping eruptions as well as the nodules in the late syphilis are arranged in a *serpiginous* (snake-like) pattern.

Lesions that are contiguous are described as *grouped,* and are of relatively little diagnostic value except in the special pattern, *herpetiform,* which is pathognomonic for herpes simplex or herpes zoster. Similarly, the special arrangement, *zosteriform,* follows a dermatome in a bandlike pattern and is characteristically seen in herpes zoster; a zosteriform arrangement of skin nodules is occasionally seen in metastatic carcinoma of the breast. A *reticular* arrangement often results from vascular dilatation and is observed in cutis marmorata and livedo reticularis.

The *distribution* of sites of localization of skin eruptions has been greatly overemphasized in dermatologic diagnosis; of far more importance are the type, shape, and arrangement of the lesions. The distribution of eruptions can be classified as *isolated, regional,* or *generalized;* the term *total* (universal) denotes an involvement of all the skin, including the hair and the nails.

When the eruption occurs in a bilateral and symmetric distribution, the pathologic stimulus is usually endogenous or is hematogenously disseminated. Bilateral symmetry is characteristic of hypersensitivity and is a common response to a drug. In photosensitivity eruptions, lesions are localized to the parts of the body that are exposed to sunlight. The exposed areas of the face that are usually spared include the fold of skin in the upper eyelids, the skin of the hair-covered scalp, and the region below the chin.

LABORATORY AND OTHER AIDS IN EXAMINATION OF THE SKIN

There are certain technical, clinical, and laboratory aids and procedures that are indispensable in the clinical examination and interpretation of skin conditions.

VISUAL AIDS Magnification Certain diagnostic signs can be revealed only by magnification of the skin lesions, e.g., the follicular plugging indicative of lupus erythematosus, the fine telangiectasia and raised border indicative of basal cell carcinoma, and, if present, the bluish color indicative of early primary malignant melanoma. A pocket magnifier (2 to 7×) is necessary for proper identification.

Transillumination Transillumination, or sidelighting, of skin lesions, which is done in a darkened room, is often required to detect slight degrees of elevation or depression, and is also sometimes useful in estimating the extent of the eruption.

Diascopy Diascopy is an essential technique for the examination of skin because it permits the differentiation of purpura from erythematous macules. Diascopy consists of firmly press-

FIGURE 48-1

Common lesions, shown on anterior and posterior views of the patient, encountered during the physical examination of the skin. See also Plates 1 to 6. [From TB Fitzpatrick, DP Johnson, in Dermatology in General Medicine, TB Fitzpatrick et al (eds), New York, McGraw-Hill, 1971.]

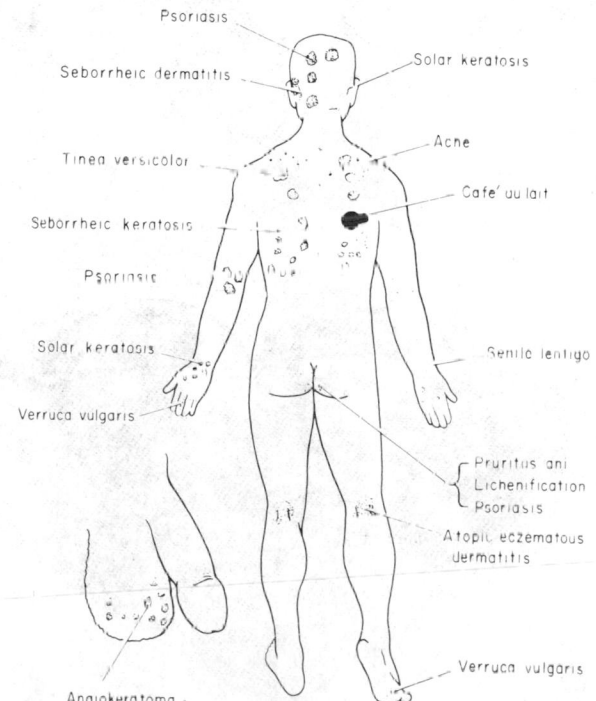

Verruca vulgaris
Xanthelasma
Melasma
Solar keratosis (in exposed areas)
Spider angioma
Rosacea, Acne
Seborrheic dermatitis
Solar keratosis
Perlèche
Senile angioma (blue)
Acrochordon (skin tags)
Senile angioma
Atopic eczematous dermatitis
Fungal infection
Dermatofibroma
Racial pigmentation
Tobacco reactive hyperkeratosis
Leukoplakia
Fungal infection
Eczematous dermatitis
Psoriasis
Geographic tongue
Fungal infection (between toes)
Scrotal tongue

Psoriasis
Seborrheic dermatitis
Solar keratosis
Tinea versicolor
Acne
Cafe' au lait
Seborrheic keratosis
Psoriasis
Solar keratosis
Senile lentigo
Verruca vulgaris
Pruritus ani
Lichenification
Psoriasis
Atopic eczematous dermatitis
Verruca vulgaris
Angiokeratoma

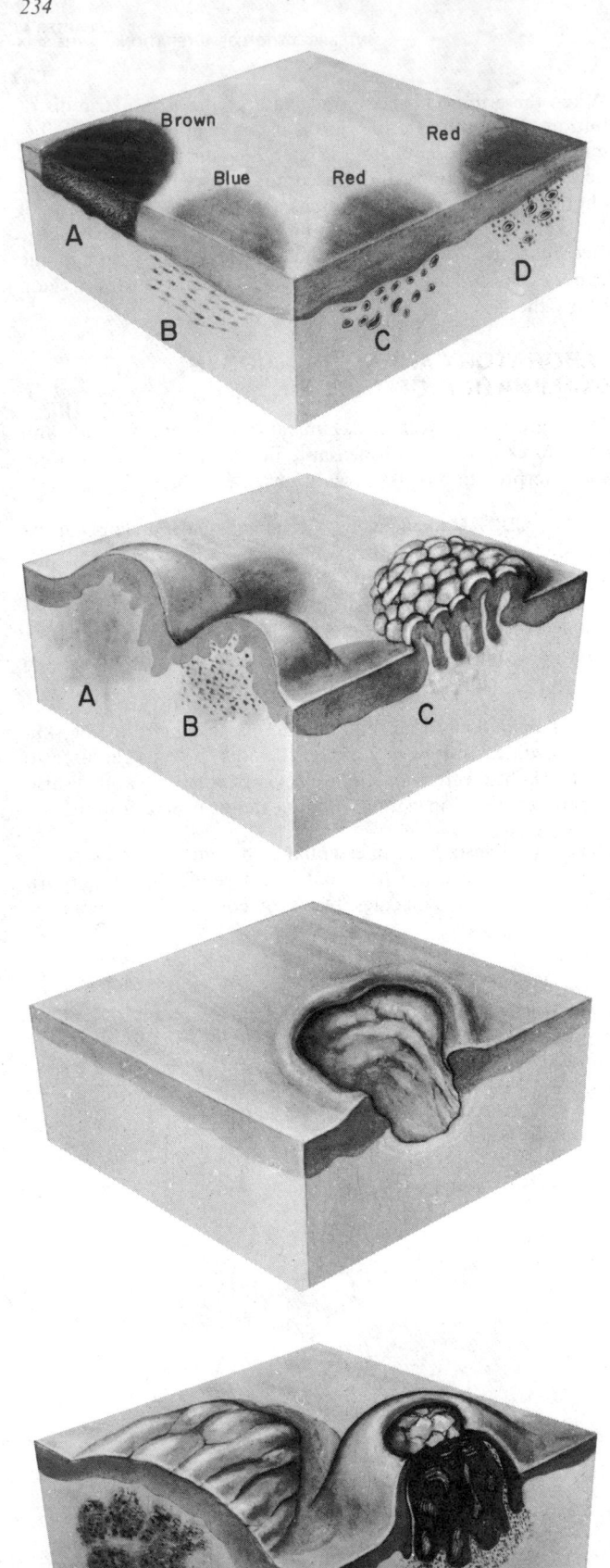

MACULE

FIGURE 48-2

A macule is a circumscribed area of change in normal skin color without elevation or depression of the surface relative to the surrounding skin. The macules may be of any size and are the result of hypopigmentation (e.g., vitiligo) or hyperpigmentation—melanin (A) or hemosiderin (D)—such as café au lait spots and Mongolian spots (B), or permanent vascular abnormalities of the skin, as in a capillary hemangioma or transient capillary dilation (erythema) (C). Pressure of a glass slide (diascopy) on the border of a red lesion is a simple and reliable method for detecting the extravasation of red blood cells. If the redness remains under the pressure of the slide, the lesion may be purpuric (D); if the redness disappears, the lesion is erythematous and is due to vascular dilation (C).

PAPULE

FIGURE 48-3

A papule is a solid lesion, generally considered as less than 1 cm in diameter. Most of it is elevated above, rather than deep within, the plane of the surrounding skin. The elevation is caused by metabolic deposits (A) in the dermis or by localized infiltrates (B) in the dermis or by localized hyperplasia of cellular elements (C) in the dermis or epidermis. Superficial papules with distinct borders are seen when the lesion is the result of an increase in the number of epidermal cells (C) or melanocytes. Deeper dermal papules resulting from cellular infiltrates have indistinct borders. The topography of a papule or plaque may consist of multiple, small, closely packed, projected elevations that are known as a vegetation (C).

ULCERS

FIGURE 48-4

An ulcer is a lesion in which there has been destruction of the epidermis and the upper papillary layer of the dermis. Certain features that are helpful in determining the cause of ulcers include location, borders, base, discharge, and any associated topographic features of the lesions, such as nodules, excoriations, varicosities, hair distribution, presence or absence of sweating, and adjacent pulses.

NODULE

FIGURE 48-5

A nodule is a palpable solid, round, or ellipsoidal lesion deeper than a papule and is in the dermis or subcutaneous tissue (A) or in the epidermis (B). The depth of involvement rather than the diameter primarily differentiates a nodule from a papule. Nodules result from infiltrates (A), neoplasms (B), or metabolic deposits in the dermis or subcutaneous tissue and often indicate systemic disease. Late syphilis, tuberculosis, the deep mycoses, lymphoma, and metastatic neoplasms, e.g., can present as cutaneous nodules. Therefore, biopsy should be performed on unidentified persistent nodules, and a portion of excised tissue should be ground in a sterile mortar and cultured for fungi. Nodules can develop as a result of a benign or malignant proliferation of keratinocytes, as in keratoacanthoma (B), verruca vulgaris, and squamous-cell and basal-cell carcinoma.

Types of skin lesion (continued)

WHEAL

FIGURE 48-6

A wheal is a rounded or flat-topped, pale-red elevation in the skin that is characteristically evanescent, disappearing within hours. Observation of the borders of wheals that have been traced with a skin-marking pencil reveals that the wheals shift relatively rapidly from the involved to the uninvolved adjacent areas. Wheals are the result of edema in the upper layer of the dermis.

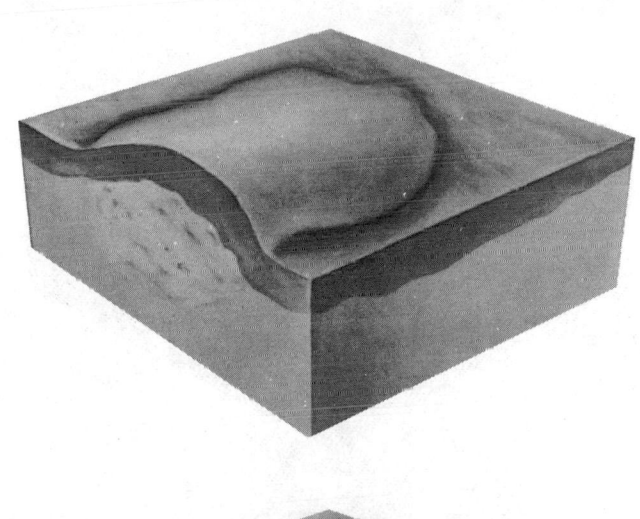

VESICLE

FIGURE 48-7

A vesicle (less than 0.5 cm) or a bulla (more than 0.5 cm) is a circumscribed elevated lesion containing fluid. Often the walls are so thin that they are translucent, and the serum, lymph fluid, blood, or extracellular fluid can be seen. Vesicles and bullae arise from a cleavage at various levels of the skin; the cleavage may be within the epidermis (i.e., intraepidermal vesication), or at the epidermal-dermal interface (i.e., subepidermal).

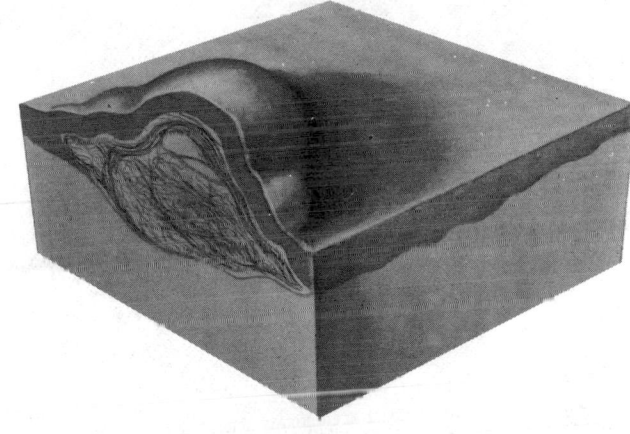

BULLA (A, subcorneal; B. spongiotic)

FIGURE 48-8

When the cleavage is just beneath the stratum corneum, a subcorneal vesicle or bulla results (A), as seen in impetigo and subcorneal pustular dermatosis. Intraepidermal vesication may result from intercellular edema, or spongiosis (B), as characteristically seen in delayed hypersensitivity reactions of the epidermis (e.g., in contact eczematous dermatitis), and in dyshidrotic eczema (B). Spongiotic vesicles may or may not be seen clinically as vesicles.

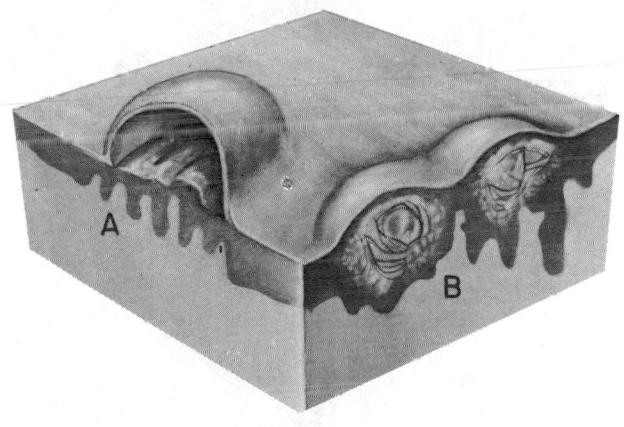

VESICLE (A, acantholytic; B, viral)

FIGURE 48-9

Loss of intercellular bridges, or desmosomes, is known as acantholysis (A), and this type of intraepidermal vesication is seen in the vesicles or bullae of pemphigus vulgaris; the cleavage is usually just above the basal layer, as in pemphigus vulgaris, but may occur just below the subcorneal layer, as in pemphigus foliaceus. Viruses cause a curious "ballooning degeneration" of epidermal cells (B), as in herpes zoster, herpes simplex, variola, and varicella. Vital bullae often have a depressed ("umbilicated") center.

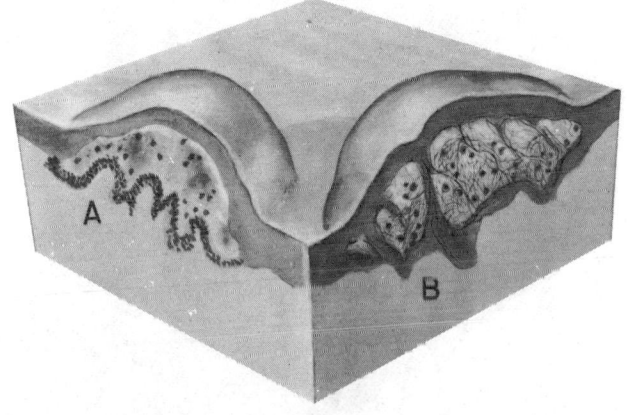

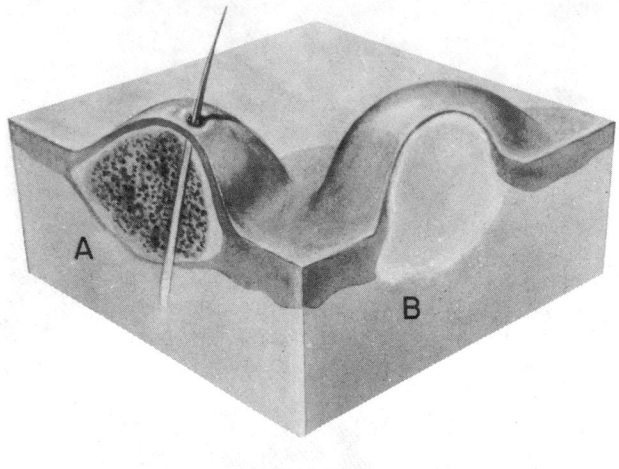

PUSTULE

FIGURE 48-10

A pustule is a circumscribed elevation of the skin that contains a purulent exudate that may be white, yellow, or greenish yellow. This process may arise in a hair follicle (A) or independently (B). Pustules may vary in size and shape; follicular pustules, however, are always conical and usually contain a hair in the center. The vesicular lesions of the viral diseases (varicella, variola, vaccinia, herpes simplex, and herpes zoster) may secondarily become pustular. A Gram's stain and culture should be done on all pustules.

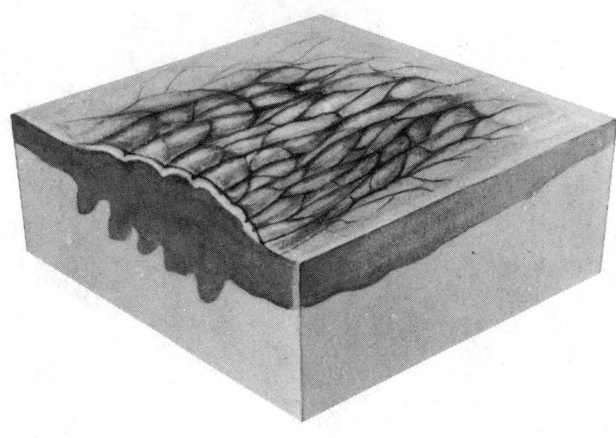

PLAQUE

FIGURE 48-11

A plaque is an elevation above the skin surface that occupies a relatively large suface area in comparison with its height above the skin. Frequently, it is formed by a confluence of papules, as in psoriasis and mycosis fungoides. Lichenification is a proliferation of keratinocytes and stratum corneum forming a plaquelike structure. The skin appears thickened, and the skin markings are accentuated. The process results from repeated rubbing, and frequently develops in persons with atopy. Lichenification occurs in eczematous dermatitis.

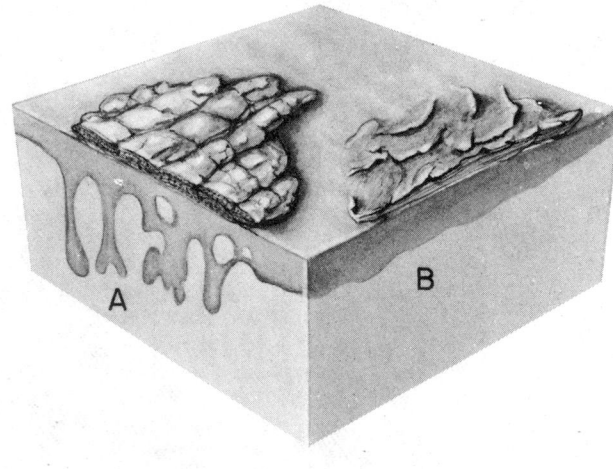

SCALES

FIGURE 48-12

Epidermal cells are completely replaced every 27 days. The end product of this holocrine process is the stratum corneum. This outermost layer of skin, the stratum corneum, normally does not contain nuclei and is imperceptibly lost. With an increased rate of proliferation of epidermal cells, as in psoriasis, the stratum corneum is not formed normally, and the outermost layers of the skin retain the nuclei. These desquamating layers of skin are seen clinically as scales. *Densely adherent scales that have a gritty feel (like sandpaper) result from a localized increase in the stratum corneum and are typically seen in solar keratosis (B).*

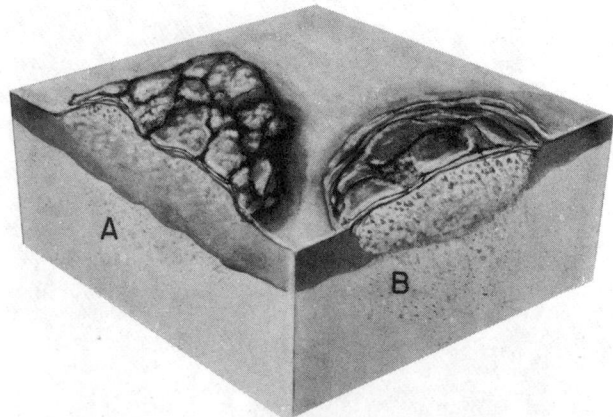

CRUSTS

FIGURE 48-13

Crusts, *resulting when serum, blood, or purulent exudate dries on the skin surface, are the hallmark of pyogenic infection. Crusts may be thin, delicate, and friable (A) or thick and adherent (B). Crusts are yellow when formed from dried serum, green or yellow-green when formed from purulent exudate, or brown or dark red when formed from blood. Superficial crusts occur as honey-colored, delicate, glistening particulates on the surface (A) and are typically seen in impetigo. When the exudate involves the entire epidermis, the crusts may be thick and adherent, and this condition is known as ecthyma (B).*

ing a microscope slide or a piece of clear plastic over the skin lesion; if the lesion is erythematous, the pressure will reveal capillary dilatation rather than an extravasation of blood. Sarcoidosis, lymphoma, and tuberculosis of the skin are suggested if diascopy of the nodules shows either a characteristic hyaline, yellowish brown, or an "apple-jelly" appearance.

Long-wave ultraviolet light, or Wood's lamp Long-wave ultraviolet light (360 nm), or Wood's lamp, is a necessary source of illumination for examination of the skin. Wood's lamp consists of a high-pressure mercury arc lamp with a specially compounded glass filter made of nickel oxide and silica (Wood's filter). This filter permits the passage of a band of radiation of 360 nm, which will reveal fluorescence when light passed through the filter impinges upon certain structures.

Wood's lamp is important for the detection of the pinkish red fluorescence of the urine of patients with porphyria cutanea tarda; the addition of 5% hydrochloric acid greatly intensifies the fluorescence, owing to the oxidation of porphyrin precursors to porphyrins.

Wood's lamp is also a great help in estimating variation in the pigmentation of the skin; it reveals both increased and decreased pigmentation. Inasmuch as melanin is a universal absorber of ultraviolet light, areas of increased melanin will show an increased intensity under Wood's lamp; conversely, areas of decreased melanin will show a decrease in intensity (or an increased reflection) because the ultraviolet light is not absorbed. In this respect, Wood's lamp may be the only means of recognizing the sometimes indistinguishable hypomelanotic macules in tuberous sclerosis, a dominantly inherited trait associated with mental retardation and seizures. The white spots are present at birth and remain throughout life, and therefore represent important markers of this serious genetic disorder. The Wood's lamp can be used in mass screening for detection of the fluorescence of dermatophytosis *in the hair shaft* in ringworm of the scalp.

CLINICAL TESTS **Patch testing** Patch testing is primarily used by dermatologists to detect contact sensitivity. The contactants are listed in Fisher's 1973 monograph on the subject.

Darier's sign One very useful clinical response of the skin, Darier's sign, is used as a test for urticaria pigmentosa, and is evoked by the vigorous rubbing of a pigmented macule with the blunt end of a pen. In urticaria pigmentosa (mastocytosis), a palpable red wheal occurs within a few minutes after the physical trauma, owing to the release of histamine by the mast cells in the skin.

LABORATORY PROCEDURES **Examination for bacteria in crusts and biopsy specimens** Gram's stains and bacterial cultures of exudates should be performed on all lesions consisting of crusts and purulent exudates. Ulcers and nodules should be biopsied by removal of a wedge of tissue that extends from the surface down to the subcutaneous fat. The biopsy specimen should be minced in a sterile mortar and cultured for bacteria (including typical and atypical mycobacteria) and fungi.

Examination for mycelia The presence of mycelia may be ascertained by the application of 10% potassium hydroxide to a single tiny portion of scale, which is then gently heated. For fungi and yeasts, scales and hair should be cultured on Sabouraud's medium.

Tzanck test The Tzanck test, or the microscopic examination of cells from the base of vesicles, determines the presence of giant epithelial cells and multinucleated giant cells that occur in herpes simplex, herpes zoster, and varicella. Material taken from the base of a vesicle by gentle curettage with a scalpel is

spread gently on a glass slide and prepared with Giemsa's or Wright's stain for the examination.

Dark-field examination of serum for *Treponema pallidum* Dark field examination of serum from ulcers and erosions on the male and female genitalia is essential for the detection of *Treponema pallidum*. Dark-field examination of material obtained from the oral cavity is not diagnostic because of the presence of nonpathogenic treponemas that are indistinguishable from *T. pallidum*.

BIOPSY Microscopic examination of tissue is particularly applicable in dermatology because biopsies of the lesions can be easily obtained. Although the classic method is an elliptical incision followed by suturing, a satisfactory method for diagnostic purposes is "punch" biopsy. Biopsy of the skin enables correlation of gross and microscopic pathology. For punch biopsy, a small, 3.0- to 4.0-nm, disposable tubular blade is rotated between the thumb and index finger to cut through the entire thickness of the abnormal skin; the resulting cylinder of

TABLE 48-2
Approach to dermatologic diagnosis

I Initial clinical impression.
II Physical examination.
  A Detailed examination of skin, hair, nails, and mucous membranes, including transillumination and disascopy.

> Seven cardinal signs:
> *1* *Type of lesion:* macule, papule, nodule, vesicle, etc.?
> *2* *Color:*
>   *a* *If diffuse:* red, brown, gray-blue, white, purple, orange-yellow?
>   *b* *If circumscribed:* red, orange, yellow, brown, blue or white? (Use Wood's lamp.)
>   *c* Does color blanch with diascopy?
> *3* *Palpation of lesion:* soft, doughy, firm, hard, "infiltrated," dry, moist, change in temperature?
> *4* *Shape of individual lesion:* round, oval, ash-leaf, annular, iris, arciform, linear, umbilicated?
> *5* *Arrangement of multiple lesions:* isolated, grouped, herpetiform, zosteriform, annular, arciform, linear, reticular?
> *6* *Distribution* (examine scalp and mouth):
>   *a* *Extent of involvement:* circumscribed, regional, generalized, universal?
>   *b* *Pattern and location:* symmetry, exposed areas, sites of pressure, intertriginous areas?
>   *c* *Characteristic patterns:* scabies, secondary syphilis, erythema multiforme, psoriasis, seborrheic dermatitis, atopic dermatitis, lichen planus, pityriasis rosea, dermatitis herpetiformis?
> *7* *Morphologic component of skin primarily affected* (see Table 48-3).

  B Does the patient appear ill?
  C Examination for lymphadenopathy and hepatosplenomegaly.
III History of skin lesions and system review as indicated by differential diagnosis. Two key questions:
  A How long?
  B Does it itch?
IV Laboratory procedures.
  A Special.
    1 Material (crusts, scales, or exudate) for Gram's stain for bacteria and KOH preparation for yeast or fungi.
    2 If vesicle, direct smear of base for giant cells (herpes simplex or varicella zoster).
    3 Biopsy: for an inflammatory nodule, obtain tissue for mycologic and bacterial culture.
    4 Wood's lamp examination of urine for porphyrins, and of hair for fluorescence.
    5 Hematologic, chemical, urine, serologic, and roentgenologic studies.
    6 Reexamination over *time* and a biopsy of the skin may be required for definitive diagnosis.
  B General.
V Final diagnosis.

SOURCE: *TB Fitzpatrick, in Dermatology in General Medicine, 2d ed, TB Fitzpatrick et al (eds), New York, McGraw-Hill, 1979.*

TABLE 48-3

Clinical classification of skin lesions and syndromes according to the component of the skin primarily involved

  I Epidermis (keratinocytes and melanocytes)
  A Keratinocytes
    1 Scaling macules, papules, or plaques
    2 Vesicles and bullae
    3 Pustules
    4 Exudative (impetiginized) lesions
    5 Eczematous dermatitis
    6 Erythroderma syndrome (exfoliative dermatitis)*
    7 Atrophy, diffuse* or circumscribed
  B Melanocytes
    1 Hypomelanotic macules
    2 Diffuse hypomelanosis*
    3 Hypermelanotic (brown) macules
    4 Diffuse brown hypermelanosis*
 II Dermis (connective tissue and blood vessels)
  A Connective tissue component
    1 Papules and nodules (with and without inflammation)
    2 Ulcers
    3 Sclerosis, diffuse* or circumscribed
    4 Edema*
    5 Atrophy, diffuse* or circumscribed
  B Blood vessels
    1 Morbilliform and scarlatiniform eruptions
    2 Urticarial syndromes
    3 Erythema multiforme syndrome
    4 Purpura (with and without inflammation)
    5 Infarcts
    6 Telangiectasia
III Panniculus adiposus (connective tissue and blood vessels)
  A Connective tissue component
    1 Nodules, noninflammatory, usually nontender
    2 Atrophy
  B Blood vessels
    1 Nodules, inflammatory, usually tender and red
      a Erythema nodosum syndrome

* *Pathologic changes affect large areas of skin, and there are no discrete, circumscribed lesions.*
SOURCE: *TB Fitzpatrick, in Dermatology in General Medicine, 2d ed, TB Fitzpatrick et al (eds), New York, McGraw-Hill, 1979.*

---

skin is then lifted out with forceps, and the skin is cut off at its base with a pointed scissors. This simple operation is done under local anesthesia, and the bleeding can be stopped by the use of pressure or absorbable foam; suturing is not usually necessary. This technique is as harmless and simple as a venipuncture, and supplies enough tissue to permit a definitive histologic diagnosis in most cases.

APPROACH TO DIAGNOSIS In Tables 48-2 and 48-3 an orderly sequence is suggested as a method of establishing a diagnosis in a patient presenting with skin lesions.

REFERENCES

FISHER AA: *Contact Dermatitis.* Philadelphia, Lea & Febiger, 1973
FITZPATRICK TB et al (eds): *Dermatology in General Medicine,* 2d ed. New York, McGraw-Hill, 1979
ROOK A, WILKINSON DS: The principles of diagnosis, in *Textbook of Dermatology,* A Rook et al (eds). Oxford, Blackwell Scientific Publications, 1972, p 37

49
SKIN LESIONS OF GENERAL MEDICAL SIGNIFICANCE

THOMAS B. FITZPATRICK
HARLEY A. HAYNES

The skin is one of the best indicators of serious disease; even an untrained eye can recognize the ashen pallor of shock, or cyanosis, or jaundice. The competent physician must be able to detect the subtle skin signs of life-threatening diseases and the skin clues to diseases in other organs. Skin lesions are frequently critical in the final resolution of puzzling diagnostic medical problems.

The skin (Fig. 49-1) is composed of three layers: (1) the *epidermis,* the outermost part, which consists of two main cell types, keratinocytes and melanocytes; (2) the *dermis,* upon which the epidermis rests, which is composed of a mélange of connective tissue elements, nerves, blood and lymph vessels, glands, appendages, and a few cells (mast cells, histiocytes); and (3) the *panniculus adiposus* (subcutaneous tissue), which acts as a cushion between the epidermis and dermis and the underlying bone. The specialized cells of the epidermis, the keratinocytes, produce and retain in their cytoplasm the scleroprotein keratin. They are constantly turning over, about 27 days being required to complete differentiation and maturation. Maturation of keratinocytes consists of loss of the nucleus, leaving only the cytoplasm. The latter is made up of a highly ordered, two-phase system of keratin filaments embedded in an amorphous matrix, much like the cellulose-lignin system of wood fiber, which is known to be well adapted to withstand shearing and compression forces. The anucleate outermost portion of the epidermis is the *stratum corneum,* which acts as a tough, keratinous membrane. The stratum corneum functions structurally as a "waterproof" wall between the internal fluid milieu and the environment, and is the major barrier of the skin, protecting the body against loss of fluids and entrance of toxic agents. It also serves as a passive membrane—substances move across the skin by passive diffusion in the direction of the concentration gradient.

The skin has a relatively limited number of pathologic responses. If the letters of the alphabet are taken to represent individual skin lesions (see Table 48-1), then words or phrases can be said to represent groups of lesions. The lesions in the majority of patients seen by the general physician can be classified in one of the groups of clinical reactions (see Table 48-3) or types of skin lesions listed in Table 48-1. These skin lesions

FIGURE 49-1

Anatomy of the skin. (Copyright 1967 CIBA Pharmaceutical Company, division of CIBA-Geigy Corporation. Reproduced, with permission from the Clinical Symposia, illustrated by Frank H. Netter, M.D. All rights reserved.)

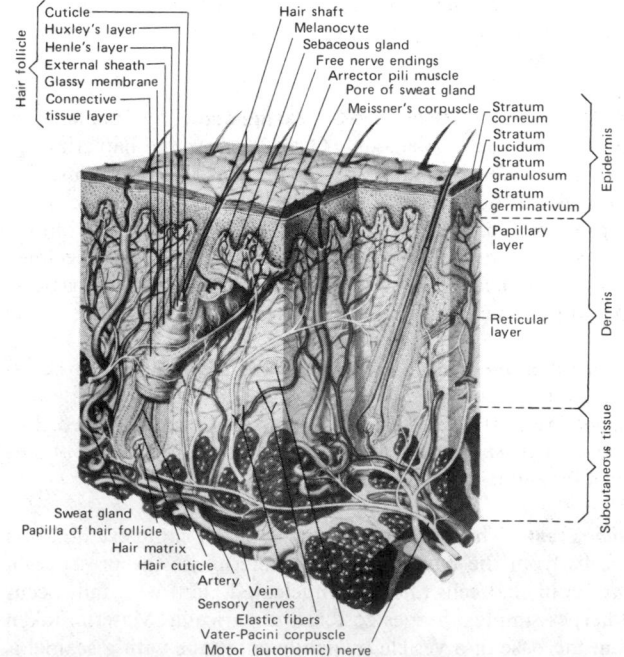

or clinical reactions may consist of one type of lesion, such as a vesicle or a nodule, or aggregates of various types of lesions, such as papules or vesicles, as in erythema multiforme. Just one lesion or several solitary lesions or one or more groups of lesions may be distributed any place on the body. A pathologic process may involve the skin in the form of isolated lesions, as just mentioned, or the pathologic process may involve all the skin so that the borders of the lesions may not be defined; this latter type of diffuse involvement occurs in systemic sclerosis and in pigmentation disorders.

In the physician's attempts to identify the specific types of lesions, it is therefore essential to try to estimate the component of the skin that is *primarily* affected, as the epidermis, the dermis, the blood vessels, or the panniculus adiposus. Inasmuch as there are a finite number of disorders that produce pathologic changes in the various individual components, this method of approach will improve the physician's diagnostic acumen. For example, even though erythema multiforme involves the dermis and the epidermis, the *primary component* affected is the blood vessel, and it is this involvement that explains the erythematous macules; the inflammatory process leads subsequently to the development of the cellular infiltrates seen clinically as papules and to destruction of the basement membrane and the development of bullae.

CLASSIFICATION OF LESIONS ACCORDING TO THE COMPONENT OF THE SKIN PRIMARILY AFFECTED

EPIDERMIS Scaling macules, papules, or plaques Generalized scaling macules, papules, or plaques are frequent and important diagnostic problems and are usually a presenting complaint of the patient (see Figs. 48-2, 48-3, and 48-11).

Sudden onset of symmetrical, scaling, erythematous macules or papules should suggest that drugs are the etiologic agents. Scaling erythematous papules on the scalp and extensor aspects of the arms and legs are suggestive of *psoriasis;* psoriatic lesions often are accentuated on the sites of repeated trauma, such as the elbows and knees. The papules or plaques of psoriasis often contain a silvery white micaceous scale that is relatively easily removed in layers (see Plate 2-6). In psoriasis, there is a severalfold increase in the normal number of the basal cells of the epidermis. This increase in the basal cell population reduces the turnover time of the epidermis from the normal 27 days to 3 to 4 days. With this shortened interval of epidermal cell migration from the basal layer to the skin surface, the normal events of cell maturation and keratinization do not occur (see A in Fig. 48-12); this failure of maturation is reflected by an array of abnormal morphologic and biochemical changes. In association with the basal cell hyperplasia, there is enhanced metabolism and accelerated synthesis and degradation of nucleoproteins, resulting in an elevated urinary excretion of nucleic acid metabolites such as uric acid. In addition, there is a proliferation of the subepidermal vasculature that is necessary to support the increased rate of cell division. These numerous cytologic, histologic, histochemical, and biochemical alterations are now known to be the result, rather than the cause, of the disease process. The only main fact known at this time about the fundamental cause of psoriasis is that the predisposition to its development is genetically transmitted. An erosive joint disease, *psoriatic arthritis,* is discussed in Chap. 358.

The treatment of psoriasis still remains the province of the dermatologist. The most effective treatment in the control of localized psoriasis, for most patients, is the use of topical corticosteroids with plastic wrap, topical coal-tar preparations, and ultraviolet light or sunlight exposures. Corticosteroids can also be injected directly into small, resistant plaques. Systemic corticosteroids not only are ineffective in psoriasis but may cause generalization of the process and are absolutely contraindicated. With certain patients who are resistant to topical therapy, it has been necessary to use a variety of systemic chemotherapeutic agents, especially methotrexate; the latter has the capacity to inhibit cell replication without a proportionate inhibition of cell function, i.e., keratinization. In 1974, a new form of photochemotherapy was introduced which uses oral methoxsalen and a high-intensity, long-wave ultraviolet light source. This approach may replace many of the other forms of therapy.

In this so-called "PUVA" treatment, psoralen (P) is administered by mouth 2 h before total-body irradiation with a special light system that emits predominantly long-wave (320- to 400-nm) ultraviolet light (UV-A). The light alone is ineffective in producing erythema or remission of psoriatic lesions; however, in the presence of one of the psoralens (methoxsalen) the UV-A becomes a potent photoactive agent and produces an erythematous response and a remission of psoriatic lesions after several exposures. The mechanism of action is probably related in part to the binding of psoralen to DNA by the action of UV-A. Large, multicenter, clinical trials involving over 3000 patients have shown that oral methoxsalen photochemotherapy is highly effective in the control of severe psoriasis; in over 80 percent of such patients the psoriasis completely cleared in 3 to 4 weeks of treatment using two or three exposures per week. After clearing, the patients were given maintenance exposures once per week or less frequently. While methoxsalen photochemotherapy is effective, it requires specialized knowledge and lighting systems, delivering precise measured amounts of UV-A. Therefore, the treatment is available at present in only a few hundred centers in the United States and Europe, and PUVA treatment is recommended only for patients with disabling psoriasis because long-term sequelae will not be known for a decade; such adverse effects could include skin cancers, skin aging, and cataracts.

The general physician does not always appreciate the impact of psoriasis as a major cause of disability and of disfigurement. Psoriasis affects between 4 and 8 million persons in the United States.

Psoriasiform lesions occurring on the face, lower abdomen, buttocks, groin, perineum, and legs occur in *glucagonoma syndrome.* The lesions may be almost indistinguishable from subacute psoriasis, but often they have necrosis in the center of the plaques; also stomatitis, anemia, and marked weight loss are present. Hyperglycemia may or may not be present. The eruption disappears rapidly on removal of the glucagon-secreting tumor of the pancreas.

Symmetrical scaling macules or papules localized on the palms and soles often are presenting signs of *secondary syphilis;* very frequently there is generalized lymphadenopathy and there may be mouth lesions occurring as erosions.

A relatively common and often baffling generalized scaling eruption is seen in *pityriasis rosea.* In this condition, the scale at the periphery of the lesion is very thin and forms a collarette; the center of the lesion may or may not be scaly. Pityriasis rosea typically has a "fir-tree" type of distribution, especially evident on the back. Very often, but not always, a preceding, single, isolated scaling lesion is present for several days before generalization of the lesions.

Scaling macules and papules are seen in *dermatophytosis* (Plate 2-1) and *candidiasis,* and it is therefore necessary that some of the scales be examined for the presence of mycelia (see "Laboratory Procedures" in Chap. 48).

From the clinician's point of view, *mycotic infections of the skin* may be separated into two major categories, each of which has a different etiology, associated systemic disease, and response to treatment, with only one category responding to the oral antifungal, griseofulvin.

The various types of *dermatophytosis* (so-called "ringworm" infections) constitute one category, and all (except tinea versicolor) respond to oral griseofulvin and are confined to the epidermis, hair, toenails, and fingernails. Dermatophytosis is due to three types of fungus: *Microsporum, Epidermophyton,* and *Trichophyton. Microsporum audouini,* a parasite of humans, is the principal pathogen causing epidemic urban fungous infection of the scalp. *Microsporum canis,* which affects the scalp and also the face, where it causes boggy nodules, is a parasite of animals and originates largely from young (usually) farm animals and pets (kittens, puppies, and calves). *Trichophyton rubrum, T. mentagrophytes,* and *E. floccosum,* which also are parasites of humans, are the agents usually causing dermatophytosis of the feet, the most common site of mycotic infection. The type of fungus infecting upper extremities, face, and trunk can be *Trichophyton* or *Microsporum* or *Epidermophyton.*

Inasmuch as *Trichophyton, Microsporum,* and *Epidermophyton* are parasites in humans, factors other than mere contact might be implicated. Variation in the host response, for instance, based on hereditary factors and mediated, possibly, through increased susceptibility or related to immune factors, has yet to be clearly defined.

The response of these three types of fungus to oral griseofulvin varies. Griseofulvin is effective, even in short courses, in fungous infection of the scalp, trunk, and groin, but even prolonged therapy rarely controls infection of the hands, fingernails, or toenails. Topical treatment with any of the antifungals is quite effective in infection of the feet, trunk, and groin, but is ineffective for infections of the fingernails or toenails.

The other major category of mycotic infections is represented by candidiasis (monilial infections). These infections do not respond at all to oral griseofulvin and are caused chiefly by *Candida albicans,* although occasionally by *C. tropicalis, C. krusei,* and *C. stellatoidea. C. albicans* can exist as a harmless saprophyte in the gastrointestinal tract and in the vagina. It is more common in females, and is most often present in those who are pregnant or who are taking oral contraceptives or broad-spectrum antibiotics. The association with diabetes mellitus, however, is so common that all patients (regardless of sex) with candidiasis should be screened for this disease.

Despite the fact that *C. albicans* is a normal saprophytic fungus in the vagina and gastrointestinal tract, it is rarely isolated from the exposed surface of the normal skin. *C. albicans* can invade the epidermis when the skin is exposed to high humidity and when the skin becomes macerated; therefore, candidiasis commonly occurs in the intertriginous areas (under the breasts and in the umbilicus, groin, and axillae) and in the oral, as well as the vaginal, mucous membranes. Chronic paronychia is usually caused by *C. albicans.* Candidiasis also may involve the lungs, urinary tract, and heart (see Chap. 158).

The treatment of candidiasis of the skin and mucous membranes depends on the site of the infection and the type of lesion. Maceration of the skin should be treated by air-drying of the area. Lotions and dusting powders containing nystatin are also very useful for intertriginous areas. Oral administration of nystatin is not of value in cutaneous moniliasis. Unless the sexual partner is treated when candidiasis is present, there will be constant retransfer of the infection. For monilial paronychia, 2% alcohol solutions of gentian violet are still the best treatment.

Differentiation between dermatophytosis caused by any of the three types of fungus already mentioned and candidiasis may be difficult, if not impossible, without cultures of the fungus. Direct examination of the scales from a scaling eruption in the intertriginous area is not diagnostic because it may reveal mycelia in both dermatophytosis and candidiasis; spores, however, are seen only in candidiasis. Too often, the general physician starts treatment with topical antifungal agents or with griseofulvin without establishing whether the eruption is a type of dermatophytosis or candidiasis. Inasmuch as candidiasis does not respond to systemic griseofulvin or to most of the topical antifungal agents, prescribing these agents for an eruption that is actually candidiasis results in prolonged disability for the patient. Newer agents such as haloprogin and miconazole are effective against both dermatophytosis and candidiasis.

In the past few years, fungous diseases have assumed a new significance in medicine because of the increased number of patients under treatment with chemotherapeutic agents for leukemia and other neoplasms. Almost all of the saprophytic fungi are now known to invade the tissues of patients who are being treated with chemotherapeutic agents or who have had kidney transplants.

Vesicles and bullae Some diseases may occasionally be associated with vesicles or bullae, such as erythema multiforme or porphyria cutanea tarda, but blisters (vesicles and bullae) are the major feature of a number of disorders: certain bacterial and viral infections; allergic contact dermatitis (such as poison ivy); trauma from mechanical, thermal, or chemical agents; and most important, the bullous diseases of unknown cause (such as pemphigus and pemphigoid).

Grouped vesicles occur in herpes zoster and herpes simplex, whereas scattered, discrete vesicles occur in varicella. A helpful sign in determining the nautre of the vesicles is the Tzanck test (see "Laboratory Procedures" in Chap. 48). In herpes simplex, herpes zoster, and varicella, there will be clusters of epithelial giant cells, which are absent in vaccinia and variola. Skin biopsy will also establish the nature of the vesicle or bulla; that is, whether it is an intraepidermal (as seen in virus infections and pemphigus) or a subepidermal bulla (as seen in bullous pemphigoid) (see Figs. 48-7 to 48-9).

Vesicles arranged in linear streaks are characteristic of poison ivy dermatitis. The most reliable clue to the diagnosis of both allergic and primary-irritant contact dermatitis is the localization of vesicles to the skin areas likely to have been exposed to the agent in question. Isolated vesicles and bullae on the pressure areas of the dorsa of the hands and the face may be the only sign of porphyria cutanea tarda; the diagnosis is immediately confirmed by examination of the urine, using the Wood's lamp. These patients do not present with photosensitivity.

Scattered, isolated bullae in adults represent a special and serious problem in diagnosis and treatment. *Bullous pemphigoid* and *pemphigus* are chronic and occur primarily in adults; one of them, pemphigus, has serious consequences for the patient. These two disorders need to be distinguished by biopsy of the skin and by the newly available immunofluorescence techniques. It is impossible on the basis of clinical diagnosis alone to distinguish between bullous pemphigoid, which is a chronic and relatively benign disorder and often of limited duration, and *pemphigus vulgaris,* which is a serious disease leading in a relentless course to death, unless treatment with immunosuppressive agents or steroids is instituted. Pemphigus has been divided into four separate entities, but pemphigus vulgaris is the most important for the general physician to recognize. Pemphigus vulgaris may begin in the nasal or oral mucous membrane, and the patient may consult the dentist or otolaryngologist first for persistent erosions of the larynx (hoarseness), the mouth, or a bloody nasal discharge. The lesions tend to involve in an unpredictable fashion other parts of the body, but localize chiefly on the umbilicus, scalp, and trunk, although there is no specific distribution pattern. Pemphigus vulgaris affects primarily the middle-aged, particularly between the ages of 40 and 60. It rarely occurs before the age of 17 or after the age of 75. The clinical lesions appear as flaccid bullae from the beginning; they break easily and rarely become very large. The denuded areas that form at the site of the ruptured bullae increase in size as the epidermis detaches itself. Occasionally, almost the entire surface may be involved by large, denuded areas; this involvement represents a serious problem in the management of secondary infection and in maintenance of fluid balance—more or less the same problems that occur in a severely burned patient. Oral or nasal mucosal lesions occur in nearly all the patients, and more than half have lesions in the mucous membrane of the mouth as the first manifestation of the disease. The disease often starts with only a few lesions in the mouth and may remain limited in extent for several weeks; it then gradually spreads to other parts of the body.

The diagnosis of pemphigus is made on the basis of the light-microscopic examination of the biopsy of an early vesicle. The earliest change in pemphigus vulgaris consists of intercellular edema followed by disappearance of intercellular bridges in the lower epidermis (see A in Fig. 48-9). This results in loss of cohesion between the epidermal cells (acantholysis) and leads to the formation of clefts and then bullae that are predominantly in the suprabasal locations; in other words, the basal cells, although separated from one another, remain attached to the dermis much like a "row of tombstones."

Immunofluorescence allows detection of IgG antibodies specific for an intercellular substance of the skin and mucosa in the serum of patients with pemphigus, and makes possible a differentiation of pemphigus and pemphigoid by the localization of the antibody. The antibodies, which are in the IgG fraction of serum, react with a specific intercellular antigen. The fluorescence is localized precisely to the site of acantholysis in pemphigus; IgG is confined to the glycocalyx of epidermal cells. In bullous pemphigoid, however, the antibodies react with the basement membrane, and the fluorescence is localized there.

Treatment of pemphigus with systemic corticosteroids, sometimes in combination with azathioprine, is quite successful. Azathioprine alone can control the disease in some patients.

Pustules This skin reaction (see Fig. 48-10) may result from infections or from sterile inflammation. Pustules may arise from preexisting vesicles of any etiology. Infection by pyogenic bacteria, especially staphylococci, as well as by certain fungi and mycobacteria, can produce pustules without a preceding vesicular stage. Noninfectious causes of pustules include acne, pustular psoriasis, and hypersensitivity to drugs, particularly sulfonamides, iodides, or bromides.

Exudative (impetiginized) lesions Acute infection with gram-positive cocci can occur as a primary process or may be superimposed on eczematous dermatitis or occasionally on any of the vesicular bullous diseases, and is characterized by the presence of crusts (see Fig. 48-13). Such infection on the skin has the same implications as a streptococcal pharyngitis, inasmuch as acute glomerular nephritis develops in a significant percentage of patients with impetiginized dermatitis. Patients with impetiginized dermatitis must be treated with full courses of systemic antibiotics.

Eczematous dermatitis Eczematous dermatitis (Plates 2-2 and 5-6) is not a specific disease entity but a characteristic inflammatory response of the skin due to both endogenous and exogenous agents that cause a delayed hypersensitivity reaction. Eczematous dermatitis therefore requires a qualifying etiologic term, e.g., atopic eczematous dermatitis. Eczematous dermatitis is sufficiently serious to account for the highest incidence of

skin disease, being responsible for incalculable losses of time and productivity in industry; approximately one-third of all patients in the United States seen by dermatologists have eczema. In Tables 49-1 and 49-2 some of the types of eczematous dermatitis are summarized (see also B in Fig. 48-8 and Fig. 48-11). For the general physician, atopic eczematous dermatitis is the most important disease of this group of disorders. Over 30 percent of patients develop respiratory allergic manifestations. Furthermore, the disease may persist for 15 to 20 years. Cataracts develop in 15 percent of young patients. Finally, patients with atopic eczematous dermatitis are susceptible to infections with herpes simplex and vaccinia. The majority of patients with severe atopic eczematous dermatitis have elevated serum levels of IgE. The control of the intractable pruritus in this disease is difficult, and best results are obtained by judicious use of topical corticosteroids, tar gels, oil baths, lubrication with emollients, and limitation of emotional stress.

Erythroderma syndrome (exfoliative dermatitis) The erythroderma syndrome is an important dermatologic complication that may occur as the result of an extension of a drug reaction, as a generalized spreading of a preexisting dermatitis, such as psoriasis or atopic dermatitis, or in association with lymphoma and leukemia. This syndrome consists of a generalized, erythematous, scaling eruption involving all of the skin surface, and has important implications in general medicine because of the systemic effects occasioned by the massive and continuous exfoliation of the skin. The severity of the metabolic response to exfoliation depends on the duration and severity of the process itself. Patients with extensive exfoliative dermatitis may have negative nitrogen balance, edema, hypoalbuminemia, and loss of muscle mass. Another salient feature in these patients is the large extrarenal water loss, due to the defective cutaneous barrier that leads to markedly increased transepidermal water loss. Serious metabolic effects of chronic exfoliative dermatitis occur when the rate of scaling reaches 17 g/m^2 per 24 h. The etiology of exfoliative dermatitis determines its course: the disease eventually clears in patients with psoriasis or atopic dermatitis, whereas the prognosis is relatively poor in patients with lymphoma and leukemia. Approximately 60 percent of patients with exfoliative dermatitis recover within 8 to 10 months, 30 percent die, and 10 percent have a persistent problem unresponsive to therapy.

Atrophy, diffuse or circumscribed Epidermal atrophy is manifested by an almost transparent epidermis and is associated with a decrease in the number of epidermal cells. An atrophic epidermis may or may not retain the normal skin markings. Circumscribed epidermal atrophy occurs in discoid lupus erythematosus, in necrobiosis lipoidica diabeticorum, and in striae cutis distensae; diffuse epidermal atrophy occurs with aging and in scleroderma.

The most important atrophic-type disorder is *necrobiosis lipoidica diabeticorum* (NLD) (Plate 5-1). These lesions, which are usually asymptomatic, occur more frequently in women and *on the areas subject to trauma* such as the anterior and lateral surfaces of the lower legs. Lesions may also occur on the arms and even on the face. The lesion begins as a small, reddish, elevated nodule with a sharply circumscribed border, gradually enlarges, and becomes flattened and depressed as the skin becomes atrophic. The brownish yellow color is prominent, and blood vessels are readily seen because of the atrophic epidermis that is smooth and loses its skin markings entirely. The lesions of NLD are extremely indolent, and shallow ulcerations that are very slow to heal may develop. NLD may apparently occur when diabetes mellitus cannot be detected, but in these patients full tests of glucose tolerance, such as the cortisone-glucose tolerance test, have not been done. It is characterized by focal changes in the dermis that present as acellular and intense eosinophilic areas of necrosis bordered by inflammation. The inflammatory cells are granulomatous and include epithelioid cells, histiocytes, and multinucleated giant cells. The blood vessels are always involved, with endothelial proliferation and sometimes even occlusion of the arterioles and arteries deep within the dermis; the capillary walls are thickened with focal deposits of PAS-positive material. NLD can be controlled with intralesional injections of suspensions of triamcinolone acetonide in some patients.

Hypomelanotic macules See Chap. 51.

Diffuse hypomelanosis See Chap. 51.

Hypermelanotic macules See Chap. 51.

Diffuse brown hypermelanosis syndrome See Chap. 51.

DERMIS Papules and nodules (with and without inflammation)
Papules and nodules without epidermal change (i.e., scaling) may be either skin color, erythematous, or even slightly pigmented (yellow or brown). Dermal papules and all nodules require a biopsy for definitive diagnosis because they often represent either processes that have general medical significance, such as sarcoidosis or histiocytosis X, or tuberculosis or lymphoma. Inasmuch as dermal nodules may be present in deep mycotic infections such as coccidioidomycosis, it is necessary to obtain a biopsy, not only to rule out malignancy but to culture a portion of the excised tissue for fungi. Cultures of nodules must be made from minced tissue. The histologic specimen should be carefully studied for the presence of acid-fast bacilli, since nodules are the presenting feature of leprosy

or tuberculosis; nodules removed from the common areas of localization for leishmaniasis (face and arms) should be carefully examined for the presence of parasites.

Papules and nodules with and without inflammation can occur in disorders of the sebaceous glands. Sebaceous glands are distributed largely on the face and scalp, although they can also occur in the labia minora and on the scrotal skin, trunk, nipples, and eyelids. The sebaceous gland is a holocrine gland in which the entire cell is cast off into the excretory stream. Sebum is a complex lipid mixture of squalene (a major product of the steroid pathway), triglycerides, and wax ester. Sebaceous glands are controlled by direct hormonal stimulation with androgens, derived largely from the gonads in both sexes; in the female, but not in the male, adrenal androgens may be important factors in maintaining sebum production. The major disease of the sebaceous gland in humans is *acne vulgaris* (Plate 1-5), which occurs predominantly on the face and, to a lesser degree, on the back, chest, and shoulders. It is characterized by a variety of clinical lesions. These lesions may be either noninflammatory or inflammatory papules and nodules. The noninflammatory papules are called comedones, and these may be either open (blackheads) or closed (whiteheads). The closed comedones are the precursors of large inflammatory nodules and of papules and pustules. In addition, cysts and scars of various sizes may occur, the typical acne scar being a sharply punched-out pit. In the pustular and cystic lesions, despite a large amount of purulent exudate that may be recovered following incision, the lesions are usually sterile but may contain *Propionibacterium acnes*. It is believed that acne develops as a result of a primary inflammation in the follicle wall, and that the follicle partly ruptures, leading to a spilling out of its components and the development of a perifollicular inflammatory process. The inflammatory infiltrate is lymphocytic, but later, as a result of the presence of keratinous material, gram-positive diphtheroids, and sebum, the infiltrate consists essentially of a foreign-body giant-cell reaction.

The initial stimulus to the formation of comedones (both

TABLE 49-1
Various types of eczematous dermatitis* of uncertain etiology

Clinical type	Suspected pathogenesis	Diagnostic considerations
Atopic eczematous dermatitis	Hereditary predisposition plus precipitating factors	Eczematous dermatitis, especially localized to the antecubital and popliteal fossae and to the face
Lichen simplex chronicus	Hereditary predisposition plus repeated local trauma	One or more lichenified plaques (see Fig. 48-11), especially on neck
Prurigo nodularis	Repeated local trauma	One or more nodules, especially on extremities
"Neurodermatitis"	Hereditary predisposition plus repeated scratching	Generalized or localized eczematous eruption at sites of repeated trauma
Stasis dermatitis	Chronic venous insufficiency	Signs of venous insufficiency
Nummular eczematous dermatitis	Various precipitating factors (contact irritants, xerosis, emotional stress, etc.)	Discrete coin-shaped patches, usually on extremities and trunk
"Dyshidrotic" eczematous dermatitis	Emotional stress plus other factors‡	Vesicles and bullae on palms and soles
Seborrheic dermatitis	Constitutional diathesis	Greasy scaling patches on scalp, eyebrows, and nasolabial area
Various patterns of eczematous dermatitis	Association with gastrointestinal malabsorption	Eczematous eruption in patient with steatorrhea and abnormal biopsy specimens of the jejunal mucosa
"Eczematous-like eruptions"† with systemic disease: Wiskott-Aldrich syndrome X-linked agammaglobulinemia Phenylketonuria Ahistidinemia Hurler's syndrome Hartnup disease Acrodermatitis enteropathica	Metabolic and immunologic disorders	Related features of clinical syndrome plus immunologic deficiency or biochemical abnormality

* *This term is used by many clinicians for at least four types of eczematous dermatitis that may be exclusively localized to the hands (atopic eczematous dermatitis, allergic contact eczematous dermatitis, nummular eczematous dermatitis, and "dyshidrotic" eczematous dermatitis). Possibly, contact irritants to which the hands are frequently exposed may precipitate or aggravate one of the above-mentioned basic types of eczematous dermatitis.*
† *These eruptions are reported in the literature as eczematous dermatitis, but clear, careful clinical descriptions with cutaneous biopsy specimens are frequently lacking.*
‡ *Such as constitutional diathesis and contact dermatitis.*

the closed and open types) is not precisely known at this time, but the initial histologic event in comedone formation is excessive keratinization within the follicular canal. It is currently believed that *Propionibacterium acnes* is responsible for lipolysis with a release of fatty acids; it is thought that these fatty acids are capable of producing an inflammatory process in the follicle wall. Acne vulgaris is a serious problem, especially common during adolescence, and its therapy is complex and prolonged. Moderate to severe acne vulgaris is best treated by a dermatologist who has a number of modalities: topical agents, incision and drainage of the cystic lesions, ultraviolet light therapy, and judicious use of systemic antibiotics; x-ray therapy has no place in the treatment of acne vulgaris.

The mechanism of action of antibiotics such as tetracycline is not completely understood, but these drugs are known to suppress the number of propionibacteria and to cause a reduction of free fatty acids recoverable from the skin. Because the organisms have been shown to have lipolytic activity in vitro, it is presumed that the antibiotic causes this reduction of free fatty acids. Benzoyl peroxide lotions and gels probably act as antibacterial agents and decrease the bacterial population; these agents are very effective and are widely used by dermatologists.

Estrogens combined with progestins (oral contraceptives) were initially considered to be effective in controlling acne; however, they have been of only limited value in the treatment of acne in females and cannot be given to males. There is no evidence suggesting that diet has any effect on the course or severity of acne vulgaris. Acne vulgaris may begin as early as the eighth year or may not appear until the twentieth. It lasts for several years and then subsides spontaneously, usually when the patients are in their early twenties. In some patients, however, acne vulgaris may continue into the third and fourth decades. Topical antibiotic solutions such as clindamycin or erythromycin are effective new agents for treatment of acne vulgaris.

Pretibial myxedema (PM) also may cause nodules on the legs and dorsa of the feet (Plate 5-2). The lesions are usually bilateral and consist of elevated, firm, dermal nodules and plaques that are not easily movable. They may be skin color, pink, or, rarely, brown, and, when diascoped, appear yellow and waxy. The epidermis over the nodules may appear normal or may have a marked verrucous (warty) surface. The pathogenesis of pretibial myxedema is not clear. Pretibial myxedema may occur with or without hyperthyroidism (Graves' disease) or before or after treatment of hyperthyroidism, and its development does not parallel the ocular changes (if present). The nodules in pretibial myxedema are accumulations of mucopolysaccharides, which can be demonstrated by special staining of the histopathologic material. LATS (long-acting thyroid stimulator), which is associated in the plasma with immu-

noglobulin G (7S gamma globulin), has been implicated in the pathogenesis of pretibial myxedema, exophthalmos, and acropachy; the role of LATS in the pathogenesis of pretibial myxedema has not been established.

Ulcers Ulcers occur as a result of destruction of the epidermis and, at least, the papillary layer of the dermis (see Fig. 48-4). All ulcers of the skin that do not heal within a period of a month must be assumed to be carcinoma until proved otherwise, and it is essential that a biopsy be obtained to rule out malignancy. Ulcers can be divided into two categories: lesions that occur on the legs and feet, and lesions that occur elsewhere on the body. Ulcers not occurring on the legs are rather rare except in primary cancer of the skin or in malignant metastases to the skin. Ulcers arising in nodules with inflammation should be approached in the manner suggested previously for nodules—that is, a biopsy should be obtained, and the tissue examined for bacterial, mycotic, and parasitic diseases. Chancre-like ulcerations and noduloulcerative lesions with regional lymphadenopathy may occur in primary syphilis and primary tuberculosis and in tularemia, anthrax, glanders, and bubonic plague. Isolated noduloulcerative lesions may be seen in sporotrichosis, coccidioidomycosis, leishmaniasis, cryptococcosis, and tertiary syphilis. Serologic studies are necessary in the diagnosis of syphilis.

The most prominent etiologic factors in ulceration on the legs and feet are disturbances of circulation. Chronic venous insufficiency leads to ulceration, especially on the medial aspect of the ankle or lower leg, and the ulcers develop in areas of skin with brownish hemosiderin pigmentation and occasionally where there is edema or sclerosis of the area. Hypertensive or ischemic ulcerations tend to start on the lateral aspect of the ankle. Ulceration can also occur as a result of tissue infarction in areas supplied by either large or small blood vessels (arteries, arterioles); this infarction may occur as the result of occlusion or constriction due to a variety of etiologic factors, in addition to those already mentioned; emboli, thrombosis, cryoagglutinins, macroglobulinemia, cryoglobulinemia, thrombotic thrombocytopenic purpura, polycythemia, systemic lupus erythematosus, Raynaud's phenomenon, arteriosclerosis obliterans, and thromboangiitis obliterans. Ulceration of the lower extremities also occurs in hemolytic anemia, including sickle-cell anemia, thalassemia, and hereditary spherocytosis.

Some ulcers show extensive necrosis of the edges, such as those in *pyoderma gangrenosum* (Plate 5-3), an indolent ulcer usually on the lower extremities and often associated with ulcerative colitis or regional ileitis. The ulcers in pyoderma gan-

TABLE 49-2
Various types of eczematous dermatitis* of known etiology

Clinical type	Pathogenesis	Diagnostic considerations
Allergic contact eczematous dermatitis	Chemical allergens (plants, medicaments, cosmetics, metals, fabrics, etc.)	Site and configuration are clues to causal agent; patch tests may confirm diagnosis; avoidance of cause cures eruption
Photoallergic contact eczematous dermatitis	Ultraviolet radiation plus topical chemicals (in soaps, perfumes, citrus fruits, etc.), which then become allergens	Occurs on exposed skin; photopatch tests confirm diagnosis
Polymorphous light-induced eruption—eczematous type	Ultraviolet radiation; sometimes visible light	Occurs on exposed skin; diagnosis implies that all known causes of light-induced eruptions have been eliminated
"Infectious eczematoid dermatitis"	Bacterial products from draining focus (e.g., ear infection)	Occurs near site of infection; responds to treatment of primary infection
Eczematous dermatophytosis	Fungus	Fungi demonstrated in scales or exudate

* *This term is used by many clinicians for at least four types of eczematous dermatitis that may be exclusively localized to the hands (atopic eczematous dermatitis, allergic contact eczematous dermatitis, nummular eczematous dermatitis, and "dyshidrotic" eczematous dermatitis). Possibly, contact irritants to which the hands are frequently exposed may precipitate or aggravate one of the above-mentioned basic types of eczematous dermatitis.*

grenosum have ragged bluish red overhanging edges and a necrotic base. These lesions often start as pustules or tender red nodules at the site of trauma, and then gradually increase in size until liquefaction necrosis occurs and an irregular ulcer develops. The ulcers are often multiple and may cover large areas of the leg. The histopathologic findings are not specific. The healing of the ulcers usually parallels the activity of the ulcerative colitis, and, inasmuch as the ulceration extends into and involves the reticular layer of the dermis and the subcutis, scarring occurs.

The term *"tropical" ulcer,* in addition to cutaneous leishmaniasis, now also includes ulceration due to cutaneous diphtheria, treponemal disorders (syphilis, yaws, and bejel), and phagedenic ulcer, a chronic ulcer of the feet and legs caused by mixed bacteria that occurs in persons suffering from starvation and neglect.

Ulcers can be associated with peripheral neuropathy ("neuropathic" ulcer, or malum perforans) seen in diabetes mellitus, tabes dorsalis, polyneuritis, leprosy, congenital anesthesia, or hereditary sensory radicular neuropathy.

Anal and perianal ulcers are seen in histiocytosis X and in amebiasis. A hanging-drop preparation is necessary to detect *Entamoeba histolytica.*

Ulcers with artificial and bizarre shapes must be suspected of being self-induced by means of destructive agents such as acid and lighted cigarettes. Factitial ulcers are overstudied and, unfortunately, underdiagnosed by most physicians.

Stony-hard, noduloulcerative lesions, particularly around joints (elbows, knees, and fingers) are suggestive of calcinosis cutis or gout; roentgenographic examination enables the detection of calcinosis cutis but shows no opaque bodies in gout.

Sclerosis, diffuse or circumscribed Diffuse sclerosis of the skin is most often seen on the upper extremities, chest, and face in systemic scleroderma (sometimes called progressive systemic sclerosis). Initially, the skin appears yellowish and shows slight nonpitting edema; later, however, it becomes indurated, bound down, and may be markedly hyperpigmented. Calcinosis cutis and Raynaud's phenomenon commonly occur.

Circumscribed sclerosis occurs in *morphea,* which consists of one or more round or oval, firm, reddish plaques up to several centimeters in diameter that become white or yellow centrally, often with a lilac-colored, telangiectatic border. This disorder is not associated with any other organ involvement and is a localized cutaneous form of scleroderma. Another type of localized scleroderma is *linear scleroderma,* in which the morphologic change is the same as that seen in morphea except that the process occurs in bands extending parallel to the long axis of the extremity or along the paramedian line of the forehead and scalp. This form of scleroderma has no relationship to progressive systemic sclerosis.

Edema In addition to the various causes of localized edema and generalized edema, there is a type of edema of the lower extremities that is not often recognized by the physician. This is a bilateral pedal edema which is common in patients with subacute or chronic dermatitis of the lower extremities. This type of edema is most often seen with chronic eczematous dermatitis but is unrelated to cardiac failure or lymphatic obstruction. It is most probably due to an increased permeability as a result of local capillary damage, which is part of the inflammatory process in the skin. The increased capillary permeability leads to an increased transfer of fluid from the intravascular to the extravascular component of the extracellular fluid space. This type of pitting edema disappears completely when the dermatitis has resolved.

Atrophy, diffuse or circumscribed Dermal atrophy results from a decrease of the papillary or reticular connective tissue and is manifested in the skin as a depression. Circumscribed dermal atrophy may follow trauma, or may occur in association with epidermal atrophy, as in the striae of pregnancy or in Cushing's disease.

PANNICULUS ADIPOSUS (SUBCUTIS) Nodules (inflammatory, usually tender, red) Nodules in the subcutis may be recognized by the fact that the skin is usually movable over the nodule; occasionally, however, in inflammatory processes, the nodule may involve both the dermis and panniculus adiposus, and the skin will then not be movable over the nodule. Acute, tender, red nodules on the leg are characteristically found in two disorders: *erythema nodosum syndrome* and *nodular subcutaneous fat necrosis* associated with pancreatitis.

The erythema nodosum syndrome refers to the occurrence of multiple bilateral tender nodules appearing principally on the anterior aspect of the lower extremities and occasionally on the upper extremities and face. The erythema nodosum syndrome is associated with a number of disorders that are unrelated to each other.

The nodules in erythema nodosum are only slightly elevated, edematous, and sometimes exquisitely tender. Bruising is a characteristic feature of the disease and is due to hemorrhage, leading to the formation of contusions. The lesions never ulcerate or become indurated and very seldom leave any scarring or atrophy. Erythema nodosum is associated with primary tuberculosis and primary coccidioidomycosis, histoplasmosis, *Yersinia* infection, beta-hemolytic streptococcal infections, lymphogranuloma venereum, leprosy, sarcoidosis, ulcerative colitis, Crohn's disease, regional enteritis, drugs (penicillin, sulfonamides, bromides, iodides), and oral contraceptives containing ethynylestradiol and norethynodrel.

Tender, red subcutaneous nodules may also appear on the legs in association with acute pancreatitis and with pancreatic neoplasms and are often erroneously called erythema nodosum. This disorder has been termed *nodular liquefying panniculitis* (NLP). These lesions are distinctive. Their morphologic features are different from those of classic erythema nodosum. The lesions in NLP vary in size from a few millimeters to several centimeters, and, in contrast to the lesions of erythema nodosum, are movable. The lesions of NLP involute in 2 to 3 weeks and may leave a hyperpigmented scar that is slightly depressed. The nodules are often associated with abdominal pain and may also be accompanied by fever and arthralgia. Rarely, lesions may be present on other parts of the body besides the legs. Some of the larger nodules may undergo an abscess-like change, becoming fluctuant, and may rupture, exuding a whitish, creamy, or oily viscous material; abscess formation with drainage rarely, if ever, occurs in erythema nodosum. The most common pancreatic neoplasm associated with NLP is an acinous adenocarcinoma of the pancreas. In *Weber-Christian panniculitis,* the subcutaneous nodules, which at first are slightly mobile, become adherent to the overlying skin; then, as the edema subsides in the area of induration, a central depression occurs.

In addition to the above-mentioned entities, various types of vasculitis may also produce tender subcutaneous nodules. Therefore, diagnosis of these lesions often requires an excisional or incisional biopsy.

Nodules (noninflammatory, usually nontender, nonerythematous) Movable, painless, noninflammatory-appearing nodules occur around joints in rheumatic fever, rheumatoid arthritis, and in certain metabolic diseases such as xanthoma, gout, and calcinosis. Metastatic carcinoma or metastatic malignant melanoma may appear as movable, nontender subcutaneous nodules. Sarcoidosis may be manifested in the skin solely as subcutaneous nodules on the lower extremities. Subcutaneous nodules also occur in onchocerciasis and loiasis. *Lipomas*, relatively common causes of subcutaneous nodules, are benign tumors composed of adipose tissue and may be single or multiple and are frequently lobulated; they are often rubbery or compressible and occur most often on the trunk and back of the neck and forearms. Occasionally, subcutaneous lipoma may be painful and associated with marked obesity; this condition, known as *Dercum's disease*, is most common in middle-aged females.

Atrophy, diffuse or circumscribed Atrophy of the panniculus adiposus produces depressions in the skin; these depressions are seen in progressive lipodystrophy, in liquefying panniculitis, and in the localized fat atrophy that occurs at the site of injections of insulin. About 25 percent of diabetics who receive insulin (most often females under the age of 20) have this type of atrophy. The depressed areas of localized fat atrophy show a complete absence of the panniculus, and there is no inflammation. In lipodystrophy, diffuse atrophy of the skin may involve large portions of the body.

BLOOD VESSELS Morbilliform and scarlatiniform eruptions Morbilliform (measlelike) and scarlatiniform eruptions are macular and papular exanthems and can be due to drug hypersensitivities, measles, German measles, erythema infectiosum, viral exanthems, rickettsial diseases including endemic murine typhus and Rocky Mountain spotted fever, scarlet fever, and secondary syphilis. Many of the diseases manifested by macules or papules and occurring in acutely ill patients with a fever are listed in Table 49-3.

TABLE 49-3
Rash and fever in the acutely ill patient: Diagnosis according to type of lesion

DISEASES MANIFESTED BY MACULES OR PAPULES

Drug hypersensitivities	Rocky Mountain spotted fever (early lesions)*
Scarlet fever	
Erythema infectiosum (fifth disease)	Pityriasis rosea
Measles (rubeola)	Erythema multiforme
German measles (rubella)*	Erythema marginatum
Enterovirus (echo- and coxsackievirus) infections	Systemic lupus erythematosus*
	Dermatomyositis
Adenovirus infections	"Serum sickness" (manifested only as wheals)
Typhoid fever	
Secondary syphilis	Urticaria, acute (viral hepatitis)
Typhus, murine (endemic)	

DISEASES MANIFESTED BY VESICLES, BULLAE, OR PUSTULES

Drug hypersensitivities	Eczema vaccinatum†
Dermatitis from plants	Variola†
Rickettsialpox	Enterovirus (echo- and coxsackievirus) infections, including hand-foot-mouth disease
Varicella (chickenpox)†	
Generalized herpes zoster†	
Disseminated herpes simplex†	Toxic epidermal necrolysis
Eczema herpeticum†	Staphylococcal scaled-skin syndrome
Disseminated vaccinia†	Erythema multiforme bullosum

DISEASES MANIFESTED BY PURPURIC MACULES, PURPURIC PAPULES, OR PURPURIC VESICLES

Drug hypersensitivities	Enterovirus (echo- and coxsackievirus) infections
Bacteremia:‡	
Meningococcemia (acute or chronic)*	Rickettsial diseases:
Gonococcemia*	Rocky Mountain spotted fever*
Staphylococcemia	Typhus, louse-borne (epidemic)
Pseudomonas bacteremia	
Subacute bacterial endocarditis	"Allergic" vasculitis*,‡
	Purpura fulminans‡

* May have arthralgia or musculoskeletal pain.
† One characteristic lesion of these exanthems is an umbilicated papule or vesicle.
‡ Often present as infarcts.
SOURCE: TB Fitzpatrick, RA Johnson, in *Dermatology in General Medicine*, 2d ed, TB Fitzpatrick et al (eds), New York, McGraw-Hill, 1979.

Urticaria Urticaria is characterized by wheals, of which the outstanding feature is their persistence for only a few hours (see Fig. 48-6). This short duration differentiates urticarial wheals from the otherwise almost identical papules of erythema multiforme, which persist for more than 1 or 2 days rather than for a few hours. An acute onset of urticaria is usually related to ingestion of drugs or certain types of foods (shellfish, fresh berries).

Chronic recurrent urticaria is a special problem, and its causes are not easily established. Most patients with this disorder require a careful examination for cryptic diseases such as lymphoma, systemic lupus erythematosus, primary or metastatic carcinoma, intestinal parasites, acute hepatitis, systemic vasculitis, or dermatomyositis. It is especially important, even in chronic urticarias, to carry out a painstaking interrogation of the patient in search of a history of drugs. Aspirin is one of the most common causes of chronic urticaria and can often be missed even in a careful drug history because many patients do not consider aspirin a drug. It is probably true that some patients with chronic urticaria can relate their problem to emotional stress, but this should be considered only after excluding all possible organic causes.

Erythema multiforme syndrome Erythema multiforme syndrome is a characteristic response of the skin and mucous membranes that is related to a number of possible etiologies, including infectious agents (herpesvirus hominis, *Mycoplasma pneumoniae*) and drugs (especially penicillin, antipyretics, barbiturates, hydantoins, and sulfonamides). In 50 percent of patients no etiology is ascertained. The major pathologic change is an acute lymphohistiocytic inflammatory infiltrate around blood vessels and may include degenerative changes in the endothelial cells of the capillaries and marked papillary dermal edema. There is some evidence for an immune-complex etiology with hypocomplementemic vasculitis.

The lesions occur in a characteristic symmetrical distribution and favor the extensor areas of the distal parts of the limbs, the backs of the hands, and the dorsa of the feet; the palms and soles are often involved, even to the exclusion of the dorsal surfaces. Oral lesions, first as blisters and then erosions, occur on the buccal mucous membrane, gums, and tongue, and there is often swelling and crusting of the lips. The syndrome may also include severe toxemia and prostration, high fever, cough, and "patchy" inflammation of the lungs. The skin lesions are often characterized by a vivid redness that gradually becomes duller, and they become more indurated, with the development of centers that are pale or may have bullae; these "target" or "iris" lesions, which are characteristic of erythema multiforme but do not invariably occur, are identified by the clear red area at the periphery that surrounds a pale pink zone and a central livid area, which may contain a bulla. The efficacy of systemic corticosteroids has not been proved, but this therapy is commonly used.

Purpura (with and without inflammation) A purpuric eruption demands immediate exploration for its etiology. Purpura arises in the skin of the vascularized dermis and is almost always confined to the dermis. The purpuric macules gradually disappear after days or weeks, depending on their size. Punctate or tiny purpuric spots are termed *petchiae*, larger (>2.0 cm) macules are spoken of as *suggillations*, and extensive purpuric macules are called *ecchymoses* (see D in Fig. 48-2).

Purpura with inflammation is usually "palpable," i.e., papular, and is seen in systemic vasculitis and in bacteremias such as staphylococcemia, gonococcemia (Plate 5-4), and meningococcemia. In these bacteremias and in vasculitis, the examination of biopsied skin may establish a diagnosis within 8 h (the time required for processing the tissue). Gentle scraping of the purpuric lesions will produce enough material for a Gram's stain; intracellular gram-negative diplococci are occasionally found in the lesions in acute, but not in chronic, meningococcemia, and are rarely found in acute gonococcemia. The differential diagnosis of papable purpuric lesions and infarcts occurring in *systemic vasculitis* (necrotizing vasculitis) as compared with those in chronic meningococcemia is not easy. The skin lesions in systemic vasculitis are usually bilateral, and almost symmetrical, in their distribution. They tend to be concentrated on the lower extremities, especially on the lower portion and around the ankles and the dorsa of the feet. The lesions in chronic meningococcemia are more randomly distributed, with occurrence on the trunk, lower and upper extremities, and face. Nevertheless, in meningococcemia, lesions can occur in a bilateral distribution, which makes the distinction between chronic meningococcemia and systemic vasculitis difficult, if not impossible, at times. The individual lesions in both chronic meningococcemia and systemic vasculitis may be identical, consisting of a mixture of palpable purpura and urticarial-type papules without purpura. Unfortunately, the histologic findings in biopsy specimens of the lesions in both diseases do not permit a distinction. Therefore, a patient with bilaterally distributed palpable purpuric lesions and fever is best treated with antibiotics before the results of blood cultures are available.

Purpura without inflammation is completely macular, and examination of a blood smear can quickly establish the presence of platelets; if platelets are seen in the smear, thrombocytopenic purpura can be safely ruled out as a possibility.

On the lower legs of older people, a great variety of inflammatory skin diseases, including various types of contact dermatitis, may be associated with purpura; under these circumstances, the purpura does not have the same importance as it does when present on the trunk or upper extremities. Perifollicular purpura, however, on the lower extremities (usually accompanied by a follicular hyperkeratosis) is almost pathognomonic of scurvy.

Purpura frequently develops in amyloidosis when the lesions (waxy macules and papules) are pinched. This "pinch" purpura, however, may also occur in the normal skin of patients with thrombocytopenic purpura or in the skin of apparently normal elderly persons. (For a full discussion of the classification and differential diagnosis of purpura, see Chaps. 54 and 316.)

Infarcts Infarcts in the skin are usually not pale like those that occur in the kidney but have a variegated dusky red, grayish hue. They are irregularly shaped macules, sometimes slightly depressed below the plane of the skin, and often surrounded by a pink zone of hyperemia. Infarcts are usually slightly tender.

Cutaneous infarctions are important and often diagnostic signs of serious multisystem disease, including both acute and chronic meningococcemia, streptococcal and staphylococcal septicemia, gonococcemia, pseudomonas septicemia, systemic vasculitis, purpura fulminans, systemic lupus erythematosus, and, rarely, dermatomyositis.

Telangiectasia Redness of the skin is most frequently caused by transient dilatation of blood vessels (erythema). In contrast to the color produced by fixed blood pigments, as in purpura, the erythema will disappear under the pressure of a glass or plastic slide (see "Diascopy" in Chap. 48). Telangiectasia is the condition in which the redness of the skin is the result of a permanent enlargement in the caliber of the blood vessels (which will be revealed by examination with a hand lens) and an increase in the number of the vessels. Telangiectasia may be composed of fine linear branches of blood vessels appearing distinctly red (i.e., not blue), which are often seen on the nose and face, or of confluent macular areas that appear as a permanent erythema. Telangiectasia is the cause of the erythema in discoid and systemic lupus erythematosus, dermatomyositis, and psoriasis.

Telangiectasia may also occur in a scattered, discrete fashion on the upper trunk or on the extremities and is seen characteristically in progressive systemic sclerosis (systemic scleroderma). Telangiectasia occurring around the nail beds, i.e., periungual telangiectasia, is an important diagnostic sign in lupus erythematosus (both discoid and systemic) and in dermatomyositis; these lesions are seen rarely, if at all, in systemic scleroderma or rheumatoid arthritis.

Sharply outlined, red macules or papules 1 to 2 mm in diameter, with an area of radiating telangiectasia, are seen in *hereditary hemorrhagic telangiectasia* (Chap. 318). These occur on the lips, tongue, nasal mucosa, face, and hands.

Generalized telangiectasia occurring in the form of red macules over most of the body surface may be the presenting sign of mastocytosis or urticaria pigmentosa.

Telangiectasia is a prominent and diagnostic feature of *ataxia telangiectasia,* or Louis-Bar syndrome. Telangiectasia may be present as early as the second year of life but usually develops by the fifth year; it appears first on the bulbar conjunctiva and subsequently involves the ears, the eyelids, the butterfly area of the face, the upper aspect of the chest, and the extremities.

Telangiectasia may occur in a characteristic form known as the *arterial spider,* or spider nevus, spider angioma, or naevus araneus. The main vessel of the spider is an arteriole, and it is usually faintly pulsating, which will show under the diascope. A less common skin lesion usually found with vascular spiders in liver disorders is the telangiectatic *mat* or net, a small red patch composed of intermeshed fine vessels that blanch on pressure. Spider angiomas, usually three or fewer, occur not infrequently in normal children and adults. Numerous spider angiomas often develop during pregnancy or after the ingestion of progestational agents or in rheumatoid arthritis or thyrotoxicosis. Most patients with numerous and prominent vascular spiders, however, have some form of underlying diffuse liver disease, e.g., alcoholic cirrhosis. The progression of subacute hepatitis is often paralleled by the appearance of crops of spiders, and in alcoholic and postnecrotic cirrhosis, almost half the patients have multiple vascular spiders. The mechanism responsible for the development of spider angiomas in liver disease is not known, nor has it been firmly established that the lesions result from disordered metabolism of estrogens by the liver.

REFERENCES

FARBER EM, COX AJ (eds): *Psoriasis: Proceedings of the Second International Symposium.* New York, Yorke Medical Books, 1977

FITZPATRICK TB: Fundamentals of dematologic diagnosis, in *Dermatology in General Medicine,* 2d ed, TB Fitzpatrick et al (eds). New York, McGraw-Hill, 1979

———, JOHNSON RA: Atlas of differential diagnosis of rashes in the acutely ill febrile patient and in life-threatening diseases, in *Dermatology in General Medicine,* 2d ed, TB Fitzpatrick et al (eds). New York, McGraw-Hill, 1979

PARRISH JA et al: Photochemotherapy of psoriasis with oral methoxsalen and longwave ultraviolet light. N Engl J Med 291:1207, 1974

WOLFF K et al: Photochemotherapy for psoriasis with orally administered methoxsalen. Arch Dermatol 67:669, 1976

THOMAS B. FITZPATRICK
HARLEY A. HAYNES

Generalized pruritus is a frequent and important problem in differential diagnosis for the general physician. In many patients, intense generalized pruritus is the only symptom. Unfortunately, there are no good studies that have described in detail the special qualities of pruritus that permit a specific diagnosis; in other words, it is not really known what type of pruritus is seen, for example, in obstructive biliary disease as opposed to lymphoma. In the absence of these data, the clinician must rely on the history, physical examination, and laboratory studies to establish the nature of the pruritus.

An important cause of pruritus is psychogenic, that is, a reaction to stress and strain. This type of pruritus often affects the skin of the scalp, and may be associated with other sensory complaints such as a bitter taste in the mouth or burning of the tongue. Some patients with psychogenic pruritus are convinced that the itching is caused by some sort of parasite in their skin that cannot be seen by themselves or the physician. Such patients may scratch their skin until the lesions become excoriated, and then assert that the itching has disappeared, owing, they believe, to removal of the parasite or "germ" by the appearance of bleeding.

Older persons in whom dry skin is a common occurrence may have generalized pruritus unrelated to multisystem disease. Some other older persons, however, usually more than 60 years of age, who do not have obvious dry skin may also have generalized ("senile") pruritus that is intense and does not seem to be caused by emotional stress. This pruritus is usually most severe when the patients disrobe to go to bed, and usually begins in one area, particularly the back, and spreads to involve the entire body. Neither psychogenic nor senile pruritus leads to a loss of sleep.

A subtle and important cause of pruritus without a visible rash may be a reaction to drugs, such as aspirin and, especially, opiates and their derivatives, and quinidine.

The itching that is associated with pediculosis corporis may be so intense that it will interfere with the patient's sleep. This type of eruption is usually relatively easy to diagnose by the linear excoriations that occur along the back and often the insect can be found in the clothing, particularly along the seams.

For a list of conditions in which generalized pruritus occurs without any evidence of primary skin disease, see Table 50-1.

The pruritus in hepatic disease has no special qualities. Generalized pruritus may frequently be the first sign of biliary cirrhosis and may occur many months before the onset of jaundice. It may be the first sign also of lymphoma, and, rarely, of carcinoma. The pruritus may be of sudden onset and may be very severe from the beginning.

Patients with pruritus associated with obvious skin lesions, such as vesicles and papules, should be referred to a dermatologist. Some of the dermatologic disorders in which pruritus is a common symptom include scabies, dermatitis herpetiformis, lichen planus, urticaria, mycosis fungoides, insect bites, psoriasis, and eczematous dermatitis including atopic dermatitis. Many of these disorders require specialized dermatologic approaches, particularly biopsy of the skin, in order to establish the diagnosis.

The itching patient without an apparent skin eruption, with or without the sequelae of chronic scratching (linear excoriations) and rubbing (lichenification, polished nails), poses a diagnostic challenge. Initially, a search should be undertaken for subtle evidence of a cutaneous disorder.

Thorough evaluation of the patient with generalized pruritus in an attempt to discover an underlying systemic disease should include, in addition to history and physical examination, the following basic laboratory screening tests: complete blood count; sedimentation rate; urinalysis; blood glucose; liver, thyroid, and renal function tests; chest x-ray; Papanicolaou smear; and stool test for ova, parasites, and occult blood. Additional tests such as serum protein electrophoresis, serum calcium, and radiologic surveys should be performed when indicated. A psychological assessment is helpful. Attributing generalized pruritus of uncertain etiology to a psychological disturbance is hazardous.

The treatment of generalized pruritus is unsatisfactory. Not one of the systemic medications has been shown to be effective in generalized pruritus. A topical preparation containing 0.5% menthol and 1% phenol in Nivea oil is somewhat helpful in relieving pruritus temporarily. The topical anesthetics containing benzocaine should be avoided because of the high risk of allergic sensitization. When the patient with pruritus also has insomnia, a hypnotic or a sedative should be prescribed. Antihistamines are of little value except in pruritus due to urticaria. It is a general clinical impression that aspirin is helpful in pruritus of any origin, but this has not been proved. The development of drugs that control pruritus remains one of the great challenges of medical research, and it is paradoxical that, at this juncture, severe pain can be immediately controlled with a variety of agents but there is not one single agent that is so effective for generalized pruritus. The receptors for the itch stimuli reside in the papillary layer of the dermis, but there are

TABLE 50-1

Conditions with generalized pruritus without diagnostic skin lesions

Psychogenic states:
    Transitory: periods of emotional stress
    Persistent: delusions of parasitosis
Metabolic and endocrine conditions:
    Hyperthyroidism
    Diabetes mellitus*
    Carcinoid syndrome
Malignant neoplasms:
    Lymphoma and leukemia
    Abdominal cancer*
    CNS tumors*
    Multiple myeloma*
Drug ingestion:
    Opium derivatives
    Subclinical drug sensitivities
Infestations:
    Pediculosis corporis
    Scabies†
    Hookworm (ancylostomiasis)
    Onchocerciasis
Renal disease:
    Chronic renal failure
Hematologic disease:
    Polycythemia vera‡
Hepatic disease:
    Obstructive biliary disease
    Pregnancy (intrahepatic cholestasis)
Miscellaneous conditions:
    Dry skin§
    "Senile" pruritus§

* *Not definitely proved.*
† *Diagnostic lesions may be present.*
‡ *Especially after a bath.*
§ *Unexplained intense pruritus in patients over 65 years old without obvious "dry skin" and with no apparent emotional stress.*
SOURCE *TB Fitzpatrick, in Dermatology in General Medicine, 2d ed, TB Fitzpatrick et al (eds), New York, McGraw-Hill, 1979.*

no specific end organs for itching. Itching is a sensation carried principally by unmyelinated slowly conducting fibers of the C group to central neuronal pools in the spinal cord. The stimuli are then carried by the posterior roots of the spinal nerves, and, from the anterolateral spinothalamic tracts, enter the thalamus and then proceed to the sensory area of the gyrus postcentralis of the cortex.

REFERENCE

CAIRNS RJ: The skin and the nervous system, in *Textbook of Dermatology*, A Rook et al (eds). Oxford, Blackwell Scientific Publications, 1972, p 1791

51
PIGMENTATION OF THE SKIN AND DISORDERS OF MELANIN METABOLISM

THOMAS B. FITZPATRICK
DAVID B. MOSHER

THE MELANOCYTE SYSTEM

DEFINITION OF MELANIN The presence of melanin, oxyhemoglobin, reduced hemoglobin, and carotene accounts for the kaleidoscope of normal human skin colors, but melanin is the principal pigment responsible for the color of human skin, hair, and eyes. Melanin is also a filter that decreases the harmful effects of ultraviolet light on the dermis and thereby provides protection against acute sunburn reaction and chronic actinic damage, including skin cancer.

Derived from the Greek word *melas,* "black," melanin is a protein-bound polymer formed by the oxidation of tyrosine by tyrosinase to dihydroxyphenylalanine (dopa) within melanocytes, which are specialized epidermal dendritic cells of neural crest origin. The precise chemical nature of melanin is unknown because it is so insoluble that all attempts to degrade it into identifiable fragments have failed. However, all animal melanins are known to contain indoles and are composed basically of indole 5,6-quinone units, in contrast to plant melanins which contain catechols. Radioactive dopa studies have shown that melanin is a copolymer of dopa quinone, indole 5,6-quinone, and indole 5,6-quinone 2-carboxylic acid in a ratio of 3:2:1.

Skin color is derived from the presence of melanin within the keratinocytes, which are receptor cells for melanocyte-formed melanin-containing organelles called *melanosomes.* Normal skin color is "constitutive"—that of habitually unexposed skin, as the buttocks—and "facultative"—that resulting from the sun-induced tanning reaction or from increased pigmentation by pituitary melanocyte-stimulating hormones (MSH).

BIOSYNTHESIS OF MELANIN The melanocyte system is composed of melanocytes found at the dermoepidermal interface, in the hair bulb, uveal tract, retinal pigment epithelium, inner ear, and leptomeninges (Fig. 51-1). The melanocyte system is analogous to, but not known to be related to, the chromaffin system, the cells of which are also derived from the neural crest and which possess biochemical mechanisms for the hydroxylation of tyrosine to dopa. However, in the latter system the enzyme is not tyrosinase but tyrosine hydroxylase, and dopa is converted to adrenochrome and not to tyrosine melanin.

The melanocytes present in the epidermis at the dermoepidermal interface are dendritic cells that are functionally linked to a number of keratinocytes; they constitute the epidermal melanin unit (Fig. 51-2). This functional unit permits organized transfer of specialized tyrosinase-containing organelles, or melanosomes, to associated keratinocytes. Melanosomes are spherical vesicles which are thought to arise in the area of the endoplasmic reticulum and Golgi apparatus; they are formed as unmelanized spherical structures that darken and become more dense and oval in shape with increasing melanization.

Tyrosinase is one of a large group of copper-containing aerobic oxidases that catalyze the oxidation of both monohydroxy and *o*-dihydroxy phenols to orthoquinones. In humans and other mammals, this oxidase catalyzes the hydroxylation of the melanin precursor, tyrosine, to dopa and dopa quinone (Fig. 51-3). Tyrosinase is required only for the first step in the biosynthesis of tyrosine melanin, i.e., the orthohydroxylation of tyrosine. It is noteworthy that zinc ions catalyze the conversion of dopachrome to 5,6-dihydroxyindole and that melanosomes have been shown to contain high concentrations of zinc.

BIOLOGY OF MELANIN PIGMENTATION Melanin pigmentation (Fig. 51-4), from the clinical point of view, results from the melanin present in the keratinocytes and also in the melanocytes. Inasmuch as the ratio of keratinocytes to melanocytes in the epidermis is 36:1, it is apparent that the amount of melanin present in the keratinocytes must be the predominant factor in the determination of skin color. The relationship of skin color

FIGURE 51-1

Diagram showing the embryonic origin, dispersal, and developmental fate of melanocytes in humans. (By permission from JB Stanbury et al (eds), The Metabolic Basis of Inherited Disease, 2d ed, New York, McGraw-Hill, 1966.)

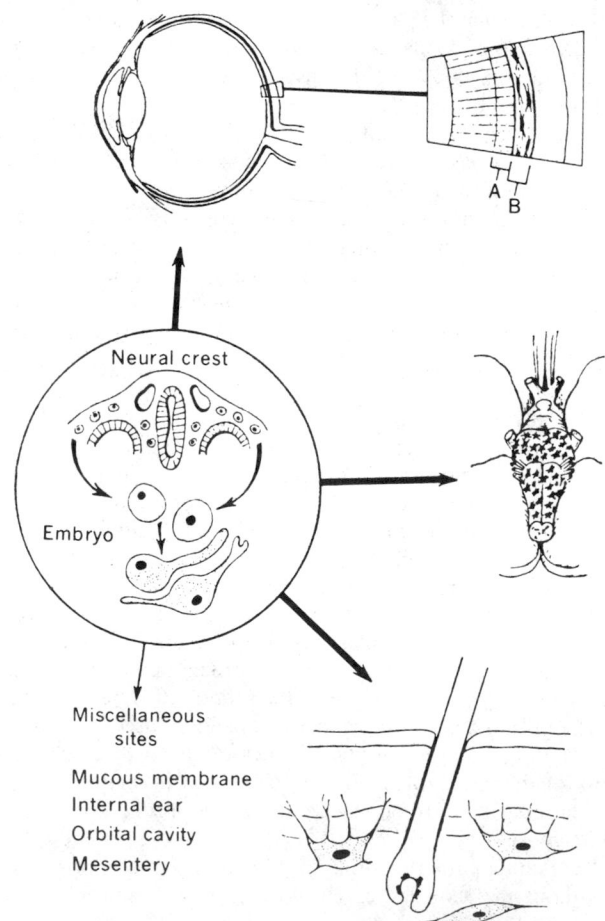

Neural crest

Embryo

Miscellaneous sites

Mucous membrane
Internal ear
Orbital cavity
Mesentery

to the location of melanin in the epidermis was studied with the light microscope in Negro Americans of various hues of brown coloration. In lightly pigmented skin, there was a great variation in both the number and location of melanin particles within the epidermis; only scanty melanin deposits were in the malpighian layer, and no deposits were in the stratum corneum. In fact, in the most lightly pigmented skin, the only melanin particles were in the keratinocytes of the basal layer.

FIGURE 51-2

Epidermal melanin unit. Four biologic processes in melanin pigmentation underscore the differences in melanosome formation and packaging between Negroes and Caucasians: (1) Formation of melanosomes in melanocytes; (2) melanization of melanosomes in melanocytes; (3) secretion of melanocytes by keratinocytes; and (4) transport of melanocytes by keratinocytes, either with degradation of melanosomes within lysosome-like organelles (in Caucasoids) or without apparent degradation of melanosomes (in Negroids). Note the difference in size between the melanosomes in the Negroid and Caucasoid epidermal keratinocytes. In the Negroid keratinocytes, the melanosomes are nonaggregated. In the Caucasoid keratinocytes, groups of several melanosomes are aggregated within membrane-limited lysosome-like organelles, and the melanosomes often appear fragmented (G, Golgi apparatus; N, nucleus; I to IV, the four stages in the development of the melanosome). The epidermal melanin unit is shown at the top. The melanocyte supplies melanosomes to a group of keratinocytes.

In the most heavily pigmented skin, there were melanin particles in the keratinocytes of the basal layer, throughout the malpighian cells, and in the stratum corneum.

It is apparent, therefore, from studies of normal skin and of pigmentary disorders, that the intensity of pigmentation, as viewed clinically, depends not only on the rate of melanosome production but also on the number of melanosomes that are transferred to the keratinocytes (Fig. 51-2). Another factor that determines normal and abnormal melanin pigmentation is the degree of melanization of the individual melanosomes. Until recently, three factors—melanosome formation, melanosome melanization, and melanosome secretion—were considered to be the major variables in normal and abnormal melanin pigmentation. In the past few years, however, a fourth variable has been implicated in melanin pigmentation, i.e., the phenomenon of aggregation and degradation of melanosomes that occurs during their transport in the keratinocytes.

Melanosomes are present in melanocytes mainly as nonaggregated (single), membrane-delimited, discrete organelles. In keratinocytes, however, melanosomes occur either as single, or nonaggregated, particles or as aggregates of three or more within a membrane-delimited organelle. These melanosome-containing organelles resemble the melanosome-containing organelles within macrophages that have been identified as lysosomes. In the epidermal keratinocyte, melanosomes appear to undergo a gradual degradation. In heavily pigmented skin, however, intact melanosomes remain in the stratum corneum, indicating that some melanosomes are apparently not degraded with the lysosomes in the epidermis. Numerous studies in recent years have shown that there appears to be a considerable variation in the arrangement of melanosomes in the

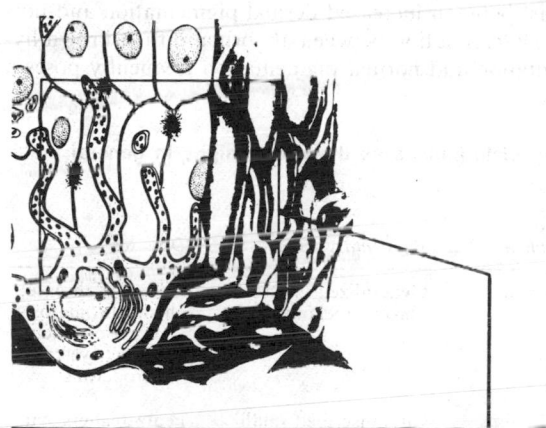

FIGURE 51-3

Biosynthesis of tyrosine melanin.

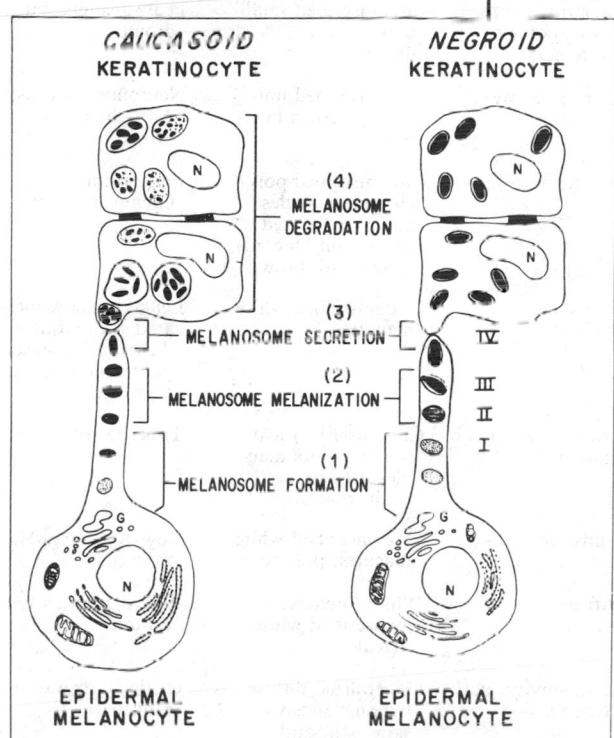

Tyrosine

↓(O)

Dopa

Tyrosinase

↓(O)

Melanin

5,6,-Dihydroxyindole

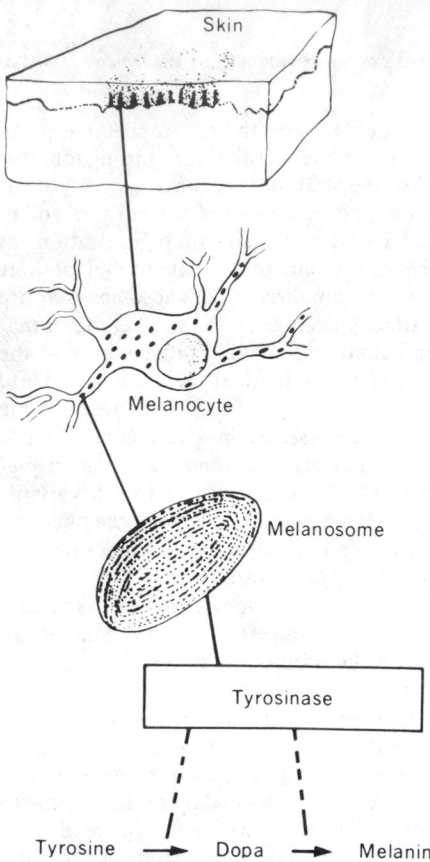

FIGURE 51-4

Melanogenesis in human skin, as seen in the light and the electron microscopes and at the molecular level.

nonfollicular keratinocytes in different racial groups. In the keratinocytes of the hair follicle in all racial groups, there are, in the growing phase of the hair growth cycle, single, or nonaggregated, melanosomes. In Negroids and Australian aborigines, however, melanosomes are found, in the epidermal keratinocytes, to be nonaggregated (single), whereas in Caucasoids, Mongoloids, and American Indians, melanosomes are found, in the keratinocytes, to be mostly aggregated, and there is often a suggestion of fragmentation of the melanosomes within these lysosome-like organelles. Some recent observations have shown that the size of the melanosome determines whether a melanosome becomes aggregated in the keratinocytes. Melanosomes that are smaller than 1 μm can aggregate in the form of a phagosome and undergo degradation—a process that could gradually decrease the intensity of the coloration.

Melanin pigmentation of the skin is related to 11 biologic processes as shown in Fig. 51-5. Aggregation[1] and dispersion of melanosomes probably play little part in the pigmentary anomalies of humans. Such movement has thus far been observed only in specialized effector cells, *melanophores*, present only in vertebrates below mammals in the phylogenic scale; this movement of melanosomes is under neural and hormonal control in these animals.

DISORDERS OF THE MELANOCYTE SYSTEM; HYPOMELANOSES AND HYPERMELANOSES

Disorders of melanin pigmentation have been increasingly found to be markers for diseases of other organ systems (Table

[1] *Aggregation in this sense refers to the clustering of melanosomes around the nucleus of the melanocyte, e.g., the phenomenon that occurs when a frog is placed on a white background; when the frog is placed on a dark background, however, there is movement, or dispersion, of the melanosomes into the dendrites.*

51-1). Such disorders (Table 51-2) may be classified as hypomelanoses (decreased or absent epidermal melanin) or hypermelanoses (increased epidermal or dermal melanin). Hypomelanoses, in general, result from the absence of melanocytes, failure of formation of normal melanosomes, or failure of transfer of melanosomes to keratinocytes. The hypermelanoses are further classified as epidermal disorders which present as brown, or as dermal disorders which are blue, blue-gray, or gray. Brown hypermelanoses arise from increased melanin in the epidermis, resulting from increased melanocyte activity, increased numbers of secretory melanocytes, increased numbers of melanosomes, or increased size of melanosomes. The blue-gray hypermelanoses represent a virtual "melanin tattoo"—the presence of melanin in the dermis in ectopic dermal melanocytes or in dermal macrophages which, because of the Tyndall effect, imparts a characteristic slate, blue, or gray color to the skin. Blue or slate-gray coloration of the skin may also arise from nonmelanin sources—ochronosis, tattoos, and deposition of other foreign materials in the dermis.

Clinical recognition of hypomelanosis and of gray or slate or blue hypermelanosis is usually not difficult. When the degree of hypomelanosis is very slight, when the patient's normal skin color is very light, or when the patient's skin is untanned, the lesions may be inapparent, and the diagnosis may be facilitated by the use of black light (Wood's lamp; see Chap. 48). This maneuver will heighten the contrast between abnormal epidermal pigmentation and normal skin but will not increase the contrast between increased dermal pigmentation and normal skin. Differentiation between abnormal diffuse brown hyperpigmentation and normal pigmentation frequently poses a

TABLE 51-1

Pigmentary disturbances as diagnostic signs in general medicine

Complaint or presenting problem	Pigmentary change	Diseases
Darkening skin	Generalized diffuse brown melanosis	Addison's disease; hemochromatosis; ACTH-producing tumors; systemic scleroderma
Abdominal pain; brown spots on lips, fingers	Circumscribed small dark brown macules	Peutz-Jeghers syndrome
Brown spots; hypertension	Circumscribed uniformly brown macules	Neurofibromatosis; Albright's syndrome
Mole	Circumscribed polychromic macules and papules (red, white, and blue admixed with brown)	Early primary malignant melanoma
White spots	Circumscribed white macules	Leukoderma associated with vitiligo, Addison's disease, pernicious anemia, thyrotoxicosis
Seizures; mental retardation	Circumscribed leaf-shaped white macules present at birth; poliosis	Tuberous sclerosis
Uveitis; deafness	Circumscribed white macules; poliosis	Vogt-Koyanagi-Harada disease
Deafness	White forelock; circumscribed white macules	Waardenburg's syndrome
Sun sensitivity; decreased vision	Generalized diffuse hypomelanosis of skin, hair, and uveal tract	Oculocutaneous albinism

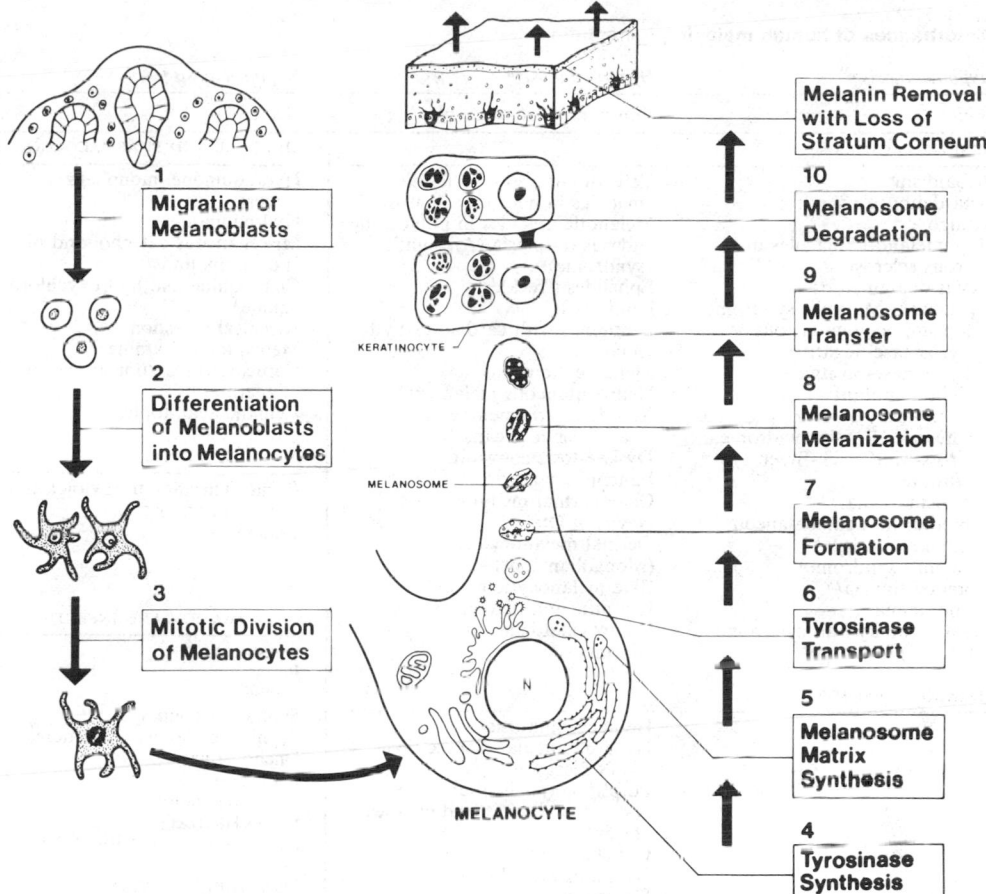

FIGURE 51-5
Morphological and metabolic pathway of epidermal melanin pigmentation.

Labels in figure:
1. Migration of Melanoblasts
2. Differentiation of Melanoblasts into Melanocytes
3. Mitotic Division of Melanocytes
4. Tyrosinase Synthesis
5. Melanosome Matrix Synthesis
6. Tyrosinase Transport
7. Melanosome Formation
8. Melanosome Melanization
9. Melanosome Transfer
10. Melanosome Degradation
Melanin Removal with Loss of Stratum Corneum

KERATINOCYTE
MELANOSOME
MELANOCYTE

problem because there is such a wide range of skin coloration in normal individuals. Diffuse color changes may be insidious; often patients themselves have been unaware of an unusual or unexplained progressive or gradual deepening of their skin color, such as a summer tan which is fading. The degree of hypermelanosis that develops pathologically appears to be related to the basic skin color of the patient involved. With the onset of primary Addison's disease, a patient of Mediterranean extraction (such as Italian, French, or Spanish) may become intensely pigmented, whereas a light-skinned individual may have only a minimal degree of hypermelanosis that may or may not be apparent. Localized pigmentation that develops in mucous membranes and in specific areas, such as axillae and palmar creases, is usually easier to identify as an abnormality than is generalized brown hyperpigmentation.

GENETIC FACTORS *Oculocutaneous albinism* is an autosomal recessive trait characterized by congenital, decreased, uniform hypomelanosis of skin and hair; albinism involving the skin alone has not been reported, but ocular albinism with minimal or no cutaneous involvement has been observed. The classic constellation of findings in oculocutaneous albinism includes marked hypomelanosis or amelanosis of skin, white or faintly blondish hair, photophobia, nystagmus, hypopigmented fundus oculi, and translucent irides. Oculocutaneous albinism may be classified according to the presence or absence of tyrosinase in plucked hair follicles of the scalp (the hair bulb incubation test). In normal individuals hair bulbs darken when incubated with tyrosine; in some persons with oculocutaneous albinism the hair follicles darken when incubated in tyrosine, i.e., *tyrosinase-positive*, while in others no such darkening occurs, i.e., *tyrosinase-negative*. These two types of albinism are known to have separate gene loci. In oculocutaneous albinism melanocytes are present, but formation of melanosomes is interrupted in the early stages so that few mature melanosomes

are present in albino skin or hair. Whatever tyrosinase is present must be functionally defective and unable to convert enzymatically tyrosine to dopa. Other variants of oculocutaneous albinism include yellow mutant, Cross-McKusick-Breen syndrome (oculocerebral-hypopigmentation syndrome), Hermansky-Pudlak syndrome (hemorrhagic diathesis secondary to storage pool platelet defect), and Chédiak-Higashi syndrome (recurrent infections, hematologic and neurologic abnormalities, and early death from lymphoma). The deficiency of melanin in oculocutaneous albinism has two disturbing consequences for humans: decreased visual acuity and an abnormal degree of intolerance to sunlight. The sensitivity of human albinos to ultraviolet light often leads to the development of carcinoma in exposed areas of the skin. Nearly all albinos in the tropics are said to have actinic keratoses or skin cancers by the third decade. Daily use of effective topical sunscreens and avoidance of unnecessary sun exposure are indicated for all albinos.

Phenylketonuria is an autosomal recessive disorder of phenylalanine metabolism in which there is a single metabolic block in the conversion of phenylalanine to tyrosine. There is pigmentary dilution of the skin, hair, and irides. The lightening of hair, which is characteristically light blond to dark brown, may be appraised only by comparison with uninvolved siblings. The melanocytes are normal but lack a full complement of melanosomes. Decreased melanin formation results from the fact that excess phenylalanine and its metabolites, present in serum and extracellular fluid, act as competitive inhibitors of tyrosinase and block melanin synthesis. Institution of universal screening programs of neonates has resulted in early detection of cases of phenylketonuria. Early treatment with a low phenylalanine diet prevents development of mental retardation which, once established, is not reversible.

Vitiligo is an idiopathic, acquired, circumscribed hypomelanosis which is familial in about 30 percent of cases and is

TABLE 51-2
Disturbances of human melanin pigmentation

Hypomelanosis[a] White	Hypermelanosis[a] Brown, gray, slate, or blue[b]
GENETIC FACTORS	

Piebaldism[c]
Waardenburg's syndrome[c]
Vitiligo[c,d]
Hypomelanotic macules in tuberous sclerosis[c,e]
Nevus depigmentosus[c,e]
Ziprkowski-Margolis syndrome[c]
Albinism, oculocutaneous:[f,g]
  Tyrosinase-negative
  Tyrosinase-positive
  Yellow mutant
  Hermansky-Pudlak syndrome
  Chédiak-Higashi syndrome
  Cross-McKusick-Breen syndrome
Albinism, ocular[c,g,h]
Albinoidism, oculocutaneous[f,g,h]
Phenylketonuria[f,g,h]
Fanconi's syndrome[h]
Homocystinuria[f,h]
Histidinemia[f]
Menkes' kinky hair syndrome[h]
Canities, premature[h]
	Café au lait and freckle-like macules in neurofibromatosis[c]
	Melanotic macules in polyostotic fibrous dysplasia (Albright's syndrome)[c]
	Ephelides (freckles)[c]
	Lentigines[c]
	Lentigines with cardiac arrhythmias[c]
	Melanocytic nevus[c]
	Neurocutaneous melanosis[c]
	Xeroderma pigmentosum[c]
	Acanthosis nigricans[c]
	Dyskeratosis congenita[c]
	Fanconi's syndrome[c]
	Oculodermal melanocytosis
	Nevus of Ota[b,c]
	Dermal melanocytosis (Mongolian spot)[b,c]
	Blue melanocytic nevus[b,c]
	Incontinentia pigmenti[b,c]
	Franceschetti-Jadassohn syndrome[b,c]

METABOLIC FACTORS	
	Hemochromatosis[f] Hepatolenticular disease (Wilson's disease)[f] Porphyria (congenital erythropoietic, variegata and cutanea tarda)[f] Gaucher's disease[i] Niemann-Pick disease[i] Hemochromatosis[f] Amyloidosis, cutaneous macular[b,c]
ENDOCRINE FACTORS	
Hypopituitarism[f] Addison's disease[c] Hyperthyroidism[c]	ACTH-producing and MSH-producing pituitary and other tumors[f] ACTH therapy[f] Pregnancy[i] Addison's disease[f] Estrogen therapy[j] Melasma[c,k]
NUTRITIONAL FACTORS	

Chronic protein deficiency or loss:[h,l]
  Kwashiorkor
  Nephrosis
  Ulcerative colitis
  Malabsorption
Vitamin B$_{12}$ deficiency[h]
	Kwashiorkor[c]
	Pellagra[i]
	Sprue[i]
	Vitamin B$_{12}$ deficiency[i]
	Chronic nutritional insufficiency[c]

CHEMICAL AND PHARMACOLOGIC AGENTS	
Hydroquinone, monobenzyl-ether[c] Hydroquinone[c,e] Miscellaneous catechol and phenol compounds[c] Chloroquine and hydroxychloroquine[h] Arsenical ingestion[c] Mercaptoethyl amines[c] Corticosteroids, topical and intradermal[c,e] Retinoic acid, topical[c,e]	Arsenical intoxication[f] Busulfan administration[f] Photochemical agents (topical or systemic drugs)[c] 5-Fluorouracil, systemic[f] Cyclophosphamide[f] Nitrogen mustard, topical[c] Bleomycin[c] Fixed (drug) eruption[b,c]
PHYSICAL AGENTS	
Burns: Thermal, ultraviolet, ionizing radiation[c,m] Trauma[c,m]	Ultraviolet light (suntanning)[c] Thermal radiation[c] Alpha, beta, and gamma ionizing radiation[c] Trauma (e.g., chronic pruritus)[c]
INFLAMMATION AND INFECTION	
Sarcoidosis[c,e] Pinta[c] Yaws[c] Syphilis, secondary[c] Syphilis, endemic, nonvenereal[c] Onchocerciasis[c] Leprosy[c,e] Tinea versicolor[c,e] Post-kala azar[c] Eczematous dermatitis[c,e] Psoriasis[c] Discoid lupus erythematosus[c] Vagabond's leukoderma[c] Miscellaneous postinflammatory hypomelanoses[c,e]	Postinflammation melanoses (exanthems, drug eruptions)[c] Lichen planus[c] Lupus erythematosus, discoid[c] Lichen simplex chronicus[c] Atopic dermatitis[i] Psoriasis[c] Tinea versicolor[c] Pinta in exposed areas[b,c] Erythema dyschromicum perstans[c,n]
NEOPLASMS	
Leukoderma acquisitum centrifugum (including halo nevus)[c] Malignant melanoma Around primary neoplasms[c] Vitiligo-like hypomelanosis[c,e] Around nevi and metastatic melanoma[c]	Malignant melanoma[c,h] Mastocytosis (urticaria pigmentosa)[c] Acanthosis nigricans, with adenocarcinoma and lymphoma[c] Slate-gray dermal pigmentation with metastatic melanoma and melanogenuria[f]
MISCELLANEOUS FACTORS	
Vogt-Koyanagi-Harada syndrome[c] Scleroderma, circumscribed or systemic[c] Canities[h] Alopecia areata[o] Horner's syndrome, congenital and acquired[g] Idiopathic, guttate hypomelanosis[c]	Scleroderma, systemic[f] Chronic hepatic insufficiency[f] Whipple's syndrome[f] Encephalitis, chronic[c] Lentigo, senile ("liver spots")[c] Cronkhite-Canada syndrome[c] Catatonic schizophrenia[c]

[a] Listing includes the pigmentation disorder itself or the condition with which it is associated.
[b] Gray, slate, or blue color results from the presence of dermal melanocytes or phagocytized melanin in the dermis.
[c] Pigment change is circumscribed.
[d] Total loss of pigment in the skin and hair may occur.
[e] Loss of pigmentation is usually partial (hypomelanosis); viewed with Wood's lamp, the lesions are not completely devoid of pigment (amelanosis), as in vitiligo.
[f] Pigment change is diffuse, not circumscribed, and there are no identifiable borders.
[g] Pigment is decreased in the iris.
[h] Pigment is decreased in the hair.
[i] Pigment change may be diffuse or circumscribed.
[j] Nipples are affected.
[k] Idiopathic or due to progestational agents.
[l] Hair is gray or reddish.
[m] There is a loss of melanocytes.
[n] Areas of brown may be admixed with the slate-gray and blue discoloration.
[o] Regrown hair is white.

SOURCE: DB Mosher et al, in Dermatology in General Medicine, 2d ed, TB Fitzpatrick et al (eds), New York, McGraw-Hill, 1979.

characterized by progressively enlarging amelanotic macules (Table 51-3). Vitiligo may be localized, segmental (one or more dermatomes), or generalized. On occasion, vitiligo may become so extensive that all or nearly all the skin becomes white. Characteristic distribution patterns of vitiligo involve extensor surfaces and bony prominences (elbows, knees), the small joints in the hands, and the area around the eyes and mouth. The low back, axillae, and flexor wrists may also be involved. Genitalia, palms and soles, and mucous membranes are often affected. Typically, the vitiligo macules gradually enlarge centrifugally, and new macules appear. In up to 30 percent of cases some minimal spontaneous repigmentation occurs, particularly in sun-exposed areas of skin. White hairs are common in macules of vitiligo, but may also be seen on normally pigmented skin and scalp. Most vitiligo patients are generally healthy, although thyroid disease, diabetes mellitus, Addison's disease, and pernicious anemia occur with increased frequency. Thyroid disease—hyperthyroidism, thyroiditis, hypothyroidism, and nontoxic goiter—may, in fact, be a common coexisting disorder with vitiligo in patients over the age of fifty. Syndromes with multiple endocrinopathies and with hyperthyroidism, hypoparathyroidism, Addison's disease, chronic mucocutaneous candidiasis, and alopecia areata have been described. Circulating complement-binding antimelanocyte antibodies have been found in two such patients.

Electron microscope studies show a total absence of melanocytes in the white vitiligo macules and decreased numbers of melanocytes in trichrome areas (macules or margins of vitiligo patches in which a color intermediate between the normal skin color and the vitiligo white is present).

In over half the patients treated with psoralens and ultraviolet A [UV-A (sunlight or an artificial UV-A light system; see Chap. 52)] significant repigmentation occurs, particularly on the face and neck, and usually on the trunk, upper arms, and legs. Up to 200 or more treatments may be required, however. In some older patients with extensive areas of depigmentation, irreversible depigmention with topical monobenzylether of hydroquinone cream is a more practical and feasible approach. These persons look essentially normal but need to use sun-protective lotions.

Piebaldism is a congenital, autosomal dominant, stable, circumscribed hypomelanosis which resembles vitiligo except that it has a characteristic distribution pattern different from vitiligo and does not usually progress or resolve over time. The hypomelanosis in piebaldism occurs in circumscribed areas on the extremities and anterior surface of the thorax. A white forelock is typical. The eyes are normal, and the patients are otherwise healthy.

Waardenburg's syndrome, an autosomal dominant trait, has a characteristic appearance similar to that of piebaldism, but also present are congenital deafness, wide-spaced inner canthi, heterochromia irides, and hypertelorism. Electron microscope studies of the white macules in piebaldism and in Waardenburg's syndrome show an absence of identifiable melanocytes.

Tuberous sclerosis is an autosomal dominant disease which manifests itself by the presence of congenital, circumscribed, white macules in up to 98 percent of cases, and classically by the development by the fourth year of seizures, mental retardation, and adenoma sebaceum. The white macules are characteristically on the trunk or buttocks, hypomelanotic, number from 3 to 100, and of typical shape—oval, lance-ovate, or polygonal, like a "thumbprint." The most characteristic, though not the most frequent, is the lance-ovate or American mountain "ash-leaf" macule, which is usually less than 3 cm in its longest dimension and off-white, not pure white, in color. The macules are usually oriented transversely on the trunk and axially on the extremities. The size and color of these lesions do not change over time. The presence of three or more circumscribed macules in a patient is strongly suggestive of tuberous sclerosis. Examination with Wood's lamp is often necessary to visualize the lesions. Histologically, these macules contain melanocytes which have decreased numbers of small melanosomes. All persons with unexplained seizures or mental retardation should be screened with a Wood's lamp examination for the presence of white spots to exclude tuberous sclerosis. In addition, examination of parents and siblings is necessary for genetic counseling.

Neurofibromatosis (von Recklinghausen's disease) is an autosomal dominant trait characterized by the appearance, usually by the age of three and primarily on the trunk and the extremities, of numerous pale yellow-brown macules (Plate 1-4), or café au lait spots, that vary in diameter from less than 1 cm to more than 15 cm. Spotty generalized pigmentation and axillary freckling may also be present. Often, a few or many soft, rounded, cone-shaped, or pendulous cutaneous tumors covered by normal skin appear by the second or third decade.

The presence of six or more café au lait spots—which are uniformly hypermelanotic, circumscribed, oval macules with a diameter greater than 1.5 cm—is characteristic of neurofibromatosis even in the absence of a positive family history. In *Albright's disease* (polyostotic fibrous dysplasia), however, there are rarely more than three or four such macules, which are usually unilaterally distributed on the buttocks or cervical areas. A single, large, isolated café au lait spot of neurofibromatosis resembles the macule of Albright's disease. It is possible, however, using light microscopy, to detect large pigmented globules in whole amounts of epidermis prepared from café au lait macules of neurofibromatosis; these pigmented globules, or macromelanosomes, are usually not found in the macular pigmented areas present in Albright's disease or in the café au lait macules observed in 10 percent of the normal population. Café au lait spots have also been associated with pulmonic stenosis (Watson's syndrome).

Generalized *lentigines* may be a feature of Moynahan's syndrome, or the "leopard" syndrome, which is an autosomal dominant trait in which the diffuse presence of multiple, small, circumscribed hypermelanotic macules has been associated with ECG abnormalities and, in its fully expressed form, with other findings (lentigines, ECG abnormalities, ocular hypertel-

TABLE 51-3
Circumscribed vitiligo-type hypomelanosis of skin

Presentation	Delayed onset
ASSOCIATED WITH GENETIC DISORDERS	
Piebaldism	Vitiligo
Waardenburg's syndrome	
Nevus depigmentosus	
Tuberous sclerosis	
Neurofibromatosis	
Ataxia telangiectasia	
ASSOCIATED WITH CHEMICALS (OCCUPATIONAL OR THERAPEUTIC)	
Phenolic germicides (O-Syl, Phebocide, etc.)	
Hydroquinone	
Hydroquinone, monobenzylether of	
Hydroquinone, monomethylether of	
ASSOCIATED WITH METABOLIC OR ENDOCRINE DISORDERS	
Addison's disease	
Hyperthyroidism	
Pernicious anemia	
Hypoparathyroidism-Addison's disease-candidiasis syndrome	
ASSOCIATED WITH NEOPLASMS	
Malignant melanoma (in sites of regression)	
Melanocytic nevi (halo nevi)	
ASSOCIATED WITH INFECTIONS	
Leprosy	
Pinta	
Tinea versicolor	
ASSOCIATED WITH IDIOPATHIC CONDITIONS	
Vogt-Koyanagi-Harada syndrome	
Postinflammation: atopic dermatitis, pityriasis alba, psoriasis	
Sarcoidosis	

orism, *p*ulmonary stenosis, *a*bnormal genitalia, *re*tardation of growth, and *deaf*ness).

Peutz-Jeghers syndrome is an autosomal dominant disorder in which hyperpigmented, brown to blue macules on the lips and buccal mucosa are associated with similar cutaneous lesions and gastrointestinal polyps. The cutaneous macules may fade by adulthood. Chronic gastrointestinal blood loss may occur.

METABOLIC FACTORS Generalized brown hypermelanosis of the skin is a characteristic manifestation of hemochromatosis and of porphyria cutanea tarda. The hyperpigmentation observed in hemochromatosis may be grayish brown or brown and indistinguishable from that of Addison's disease. The diagnosis of hemochromatosis may be established from a skin biopsy which shows hemosiderin deposition in the sweat glands of the skin. Porphyria cutanea tarda may be diagnosed by the clinical presence of vesicles, bullae, atrophic macules, sclerodermoid changes, and milia on the skin of the dorsal hands and face, and in the laboratory by red fluorescence of acidified urine, or the presence of increased urinary uroporphyrins (uroporphyrin to coproporphyrin ratio usually is greater than 3:1). Similar changes may be seen in patients with variegate porphyria which has a distinctive porphyrin profile including a urinary uroporphyrin to coproporphyrin ratio around 1:1.

NUTRITIONAL FACTORS In chronic nutritional deficiency, in general, splotches of dirty-brown hyperpigmentation appear, especially on the trunk. In selective deficiencies, such as protein deficiency in kwashiorkor, or when there is protein loss as in chronic nephrosis, ulcerative colitis, and malabsorption syndrome, there is sometimes dilution of hair color so that the hair becomes a reddish brown and eventually gray. In other selective deficiencies, such as sprue, there may be a brown hypermelanosis over any area of the body. In pellagra, however, the abnormality is limited to areas of skin exposed to light or to irritation. In vitamin B_{12} deficiency, there is premature graying of hair and a hypermelanosis most apparent overlying the small joints of the hands.

ENDOCRINE FACTORS Diffuse brown hypermelanosis is a striking feature of primary adrenocortical insufficiency (Addison's disease). There is a marked accentuation of pigmentation over certain areas, namely, the pressure points (vertebrae, knuckles, elbows, and knees), and in body folds, palmar creases, and gingival mucous membrane. An identifiable type of diffuse hyperpigmentation has also been reported to follow adrenalectomy in patients with Cushing's disease. In these patients, there usually are signs and symptoms of pituitary tumors; all tumors recorded have been chromophobe adenomas. A third example of the Addisonian type of melanosis has also been observed in patients with pancreatic and lung tumors. The generalized brown hypermelanosis found in all these conditions results from overproduction of melanocyte-stimulating hormone (MSH) and adrenocorticotropic hormone (ACTH), which share common amino acid sequences. It appears that an excess of α-MSH plays a dominant role in the abnormal pigmentation that occurs in Addison's disease. Both MSH and ACTH are increased in adrenal insufficiency as a result of decreased output of cortisol by the adrenals. Hypermelanosis of the Addisonian type can be produced in adrenalectomized human subjects by the administration of large amounts of homogeneous ACTH and α-MSH.

Melasma, or the "mask of pregnancy," is found in pregnant women, women on oral contraceptives, and in some otherwise normal women and men. This is a circumscribed hypermelanosis, usually of the forehead, cheeks, upper lip, and chin, probably secondary to progestational effects. MSH levels are normal in these patients. Melasma-like hyperpigmentation has also been observed in patients taking phenytoin or mesantoin.

CHEMICAL FACTORS Use of various chemicals, particularly phenol derivatives and sulfhydryl compounds, may cause depigmentation. Topical use of hydroquinone induces a temporary lightening which may be useful in some patients with melasma; monobenzylether of hydroquinone, however, causes a permanent vitiligo-like leukoderma, even remote from the site of application, and is used only to depigment completely the normal skin in patients with extensive vitiligo. Addisonian-like hypermelanosis of the skin follows busulfan therapy, and hypermelanosis may also be seen after use of cyclophosphamide and nitrogen mustard. Inorganic trivalent arsenicals may also produce generalized Addisonian-like hypermelanosis as well as scattered macular hypomelanosis and punctate keratosis of the palms and soles.

PHYSICAL FACTORS Mechanical trauma, as well as burns caused by heat, ultraviolet light, or alpha, beta, and gamma radiation, can lead to hypomelanosis or hypermelanosis. The effects of these physical agents on pigmentation are determined by the intensity and duration of exposure and are limited to the site of injury. Hypomelanosis results from destruction of melanocytes.

INFLAMMATORY AND INFECTIOUS FACTORS Many epidermal proliferative processes resolve and leave aberrations of pigmentation at the sites of involvement; both postinflammatory hypermelanosis (blue-gray, brown, or both) and hypomelanosis may occur following resolution of eczema, psoriasis, lichen planus, drug reactions, pemphigus, viral exanthems, etc. Usually these hypermelanoses disappear spontaneously within several months. White halos surrounding psoriatic plaques (Wornoff rings) are a result of abnormal prostaglandin synthesis and are not an abnormality of melanin biology.

Tinea versicolor, a hypomelanotic, not amelanotic, scaling, circumscribed eruption of the upper anterior and posterior chest in young people, results from the presence in the skin of *Pityrosporum orbiculare* which contains an enzyme that forms azelaic acid, a tyrosinase inhibitor, and results in decreased melanin pigmentation. Repigmentation with sun exposure follows appropriate topical therapy.

Tuberculoid and lepromatous leprosy have hypomelanotic macules that are anesthetic. The color, unlike vitiligo, is not pure white, rather, off-white, and the margins of these macules are characteristically indiscrete.

NEOPLASTIC FACTORS Disorders of melanin pigmentation are uncommon features of neoplasms. Hypomelanosis has been found around benign nevi (halo nevi) in healthy patients but may also be found in or around malignant melanoma, primaries, or metastases; vitiligo-like hypomelanotic macules remote from the melanoma may also occur. A Vogt-Koyanagi-Harada syndrome has been reported following bacillus Calmette-Guérin (BCG) therapy of melanoma. During terminal stages of malignant melanoma, striking development of blue hypermelanosis may be observed, associated with large amounts of a conjugated derivative of 5,6-dihydroxyindole excreted in the urine (melanogenuria). This intermediate in the metabolic pathway from tyrosine to melanin can be oxidized to melanin in the absence of tyrosinase; therefore, melanin can be synthesized at almost any site in which oxidation can take place. Consequently, diffuse black pigmentation may develop

Atlas of common lesions encountered during the physical examination of the skin

The skin and mucous membrane may frequently contain a variety of lesions that are rarely a major complaint (see Fig. 48-1). They are, therefore, incidental findings in the general physical examination. The recognition of "bumps and blemishes" is a necessary first step for physicians inasmuch as they will be required to distinguish the trivial from the serious and important skin changes. For example, such a serious lesion as a malignant melanoma may be incidentally discovered during a routine physical examination (see Plates 6-1 to 6-4 and the discussion in Chap. 330).

The common disorders of the skin that every physician should be able to recognize are presented in this series of color photographs (Plates 1 to 4).

1-1 **Dermatofibroma** is especially common in middle life and in women. The lesions, when pigmented, are occasionally confused with malignant melanoma. They appear as isolated, slightly elevated, hard, button-like nodules *(A)*. In fair-skinned persons, the lesions are not usually skin color, but are pink or dark red, yellowish brown, or gray-black. They are usually less than 1 cm in diameter. A diagnostic sign is that a dermatofibroma dimples or becomes depressed *(B)* when it is laterally compressed; melanocytic nevus and melanoma, however, with which dermatofibroma may be easily confused, become elevated with lateral compression.

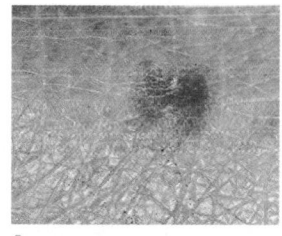 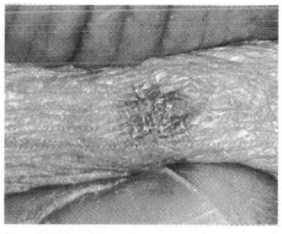

A   **B**

1-2 **Acrochordon** (skin tag) is very common after middle life and appears on the neck, especially in women, in the axillae, and on the upper part of the trunk. The lesions are small (1 to 5 mm), soft, pedunculated papules, usually of normal skin color.

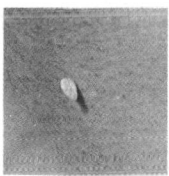 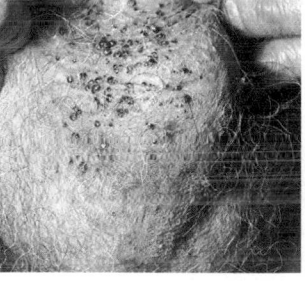

1-3 **Angiokeratomas** are bizarre vascular dilatations that occur under the tongue and on the scrotum and consist of myriads of 2- to 3-mm purplish red papules. They are of no known significance. When they occur on the trunk and extremities, a biopsy is indicated to rule out glycolipid lipidosis or Fabry's disease.

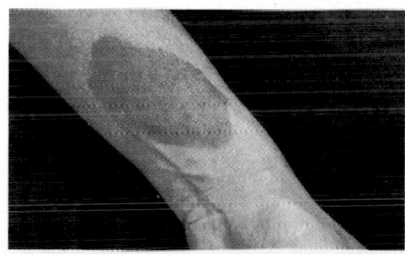

1-4 **Café au lait macules** are found in about 10 percent of the normal population and, in fair-skinned persons, are light yellowish brown macules, which may also be markers of neurofibromatosis and polyostotic fibrous dysplasia (Albright's syndrome). The presence of six or more café au lait macules with a diameter of 1.5 cm or greater is diagnostic of neurofibromatosis.

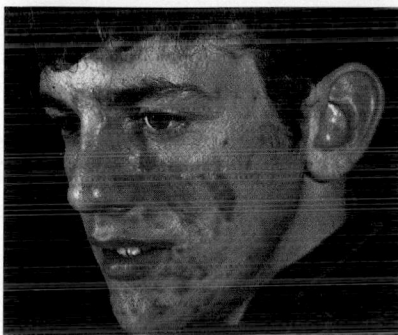

1-5 **Acne** is a condition in which the most characteristic lesion is the comedo, or "blackhead," that later becomes a conical erythematous papule or pustule. A third type of lesion is the "blind boil," which is a dermal cyst without an orifice. This lesion is often associated with atrophic or hypertrophic scarring. Cystic acne may appear with only a very few comedones; also, comedo-like acne may occur with few cysts or erythematous papules.

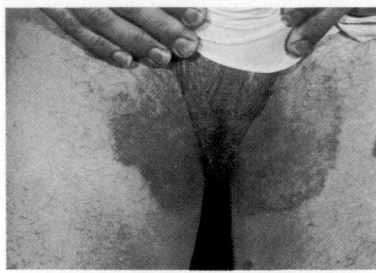

2-1 **Dermatophytosis** is identified by the striking polycyclic, annular shape of the scaling, especially on the feet and hands, where there is often a scalloped pattern. A positive diagnosis of dermatophytosis is quickly established by direct examination of scales from the advancing border; the mycelia are revealed when the scales are immersed in 10% potassium hydroxide or Swartz stain.

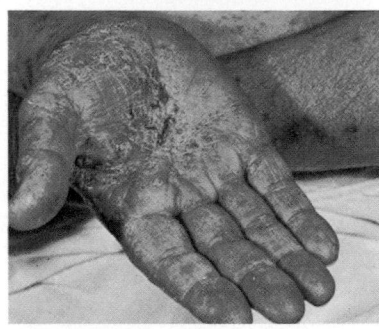

2-2 **Eczematous dermatitis** is a very common cutaneous reaction that is localized to the hands of housewives, to the legs in patients with chronic venous insufficiency, and behind the ears in patients with seborrheic dermatitis. In subacute eczematous dermatitis, there are mild erythema, dry scales, and often small red papules, many of which are excoriated. In chronic eczematous dermatitis, lichenification is the most prominent feature.

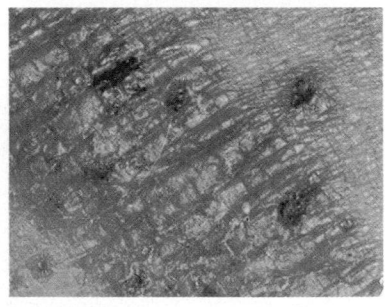

2-3 **Localized lichenification** results from repeated rubbing of the skin and consists of isolated, circumscribed plaques. These single lesions vary in size from 2 to 10 cm and occur most often on the extensor aspect of the forearm and in the scrotal, nuchal, inguinal, and anogenital areas. The perianal and vulvar areas may become diffusely lichenified. Lichenification is thought to be more frequent in persons with an atopic background.

2-4 **Melasma (chloasma)** is the so-called "mask" of pregnancy, but it also occurs in men and in women taking progestational agents. The pigmentation is uniform and is limited to the exposed areas of the face. There is no scaling or epidermal change. In fair-skinned persons, the pigment may be any shade from light tan to a very dark brown. It is most often seen on the cheeks and upper lip, as here, and on the forehead.

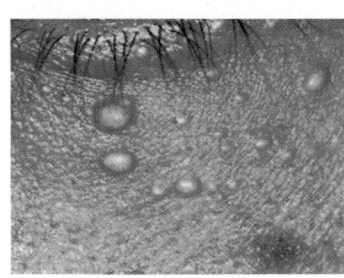

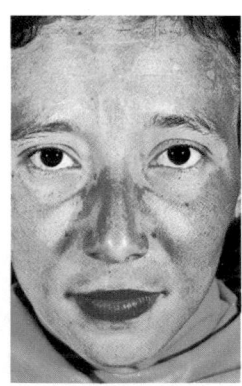

2-5 **Milia** are a collection of lesions, occurring most commonly on the face, and consist of tiny (1 to 2 mm), white, hard, rounded, superficial papules. There is no orifice, and the keratinous contents are easily expressed by lateral compression after the making of a tiny incision in the dome of the lesion.

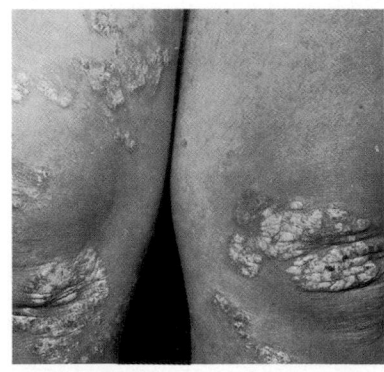

2-6 **Psoriasis,** affecting more than 2 percent of the population, consists of isolated scaling papules or plaques and is quite commonly observed in the routine physical examination. The lesions occur most frequently on the scalp, elbows, and knees. The color and type of scales are the identifying features of the lesions. The scales are either dense and lamellated with peripherally detached edges or loose and branny. The plaques are pink to deep red, and the borders are distinct.

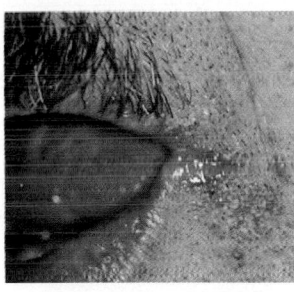

3-1 **Perlèche** consists of painful small fissures at the angles of the mouth, often covered with yellow crusts. Perlèche most often occurs with poorly fitting dentures and in moniliasis and secondary syphilis.

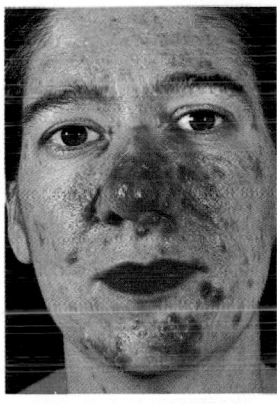

3-2 **Rosacea,** usually limited to the face, consists of tiny, erythematous papules and pustules 1 to 5 mm in size. The pustules, often tiny and sometimes hardly visible, sit on the dome of the papules. The diffuse redness of the face is due to vasodilatation, as well as to myriad telangiectases. In men, rhinophyma, a disfiguring enlargement of the nose, may occur.

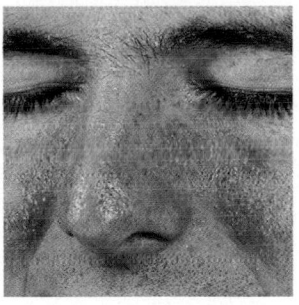

3-3 **Seborrheic dermatitis,** a common disorder found in all age groups, occurs most frequently on the scalp, eyebrows, and nasolabial folds and behind the ears. Scaling is the prominent feature and is loose and branny; it may be yellow and oily or dry and white. The lesion may become exudative and crusted or eczematous.

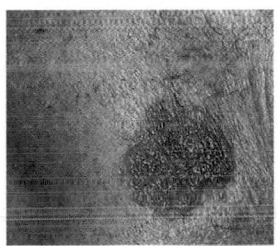

3-4 **Seborrheic keratosis** appears in middle life and may occur on exposed or unexposed areas but is especially common on the trunk. The lesions are irregularly round or oval flat-topped papules or plaques that seem "stuck" on the skin. The margins are distinct, and the surface is often warty or consists of multiple tiny projections (vegetation). In fair-skinned persons, the lesions are light brown at first but, enlarging, become more heavily pigmented and may be confused with malignant melanoma.

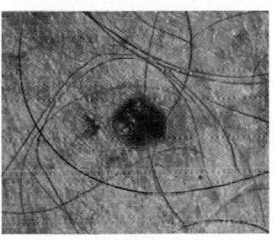

3-5 **Senile angioma ("cherry red spot")** appears in the third decade. On the lip, the lesion is usually singular and consists of a bluish red round nodule. On the trunk, the lesions are small (2 to 3 mm), bright red, globular papules.

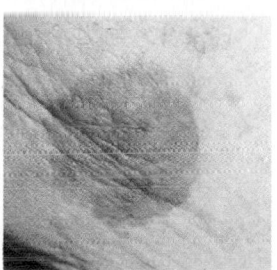

3-6 **Senile lentigo** occurs as a single macule or as a group of isolated, sharply circumscribed macules on the exposed areas, especially on the dorsal surfaces of the hands and arms and on the forehead and cheeks. The macules are usually light yellowish brown, but may be dark brown; the color is somewhat variegated, rather than uniform as it is in a café au lait macule. Rarely, dark brown *papules* develop in these lesions, and then the condition is called *lentigo maligna,* which may slowly develop, over a period of years, into a melanoma *(lentigo maligna melanoma).*

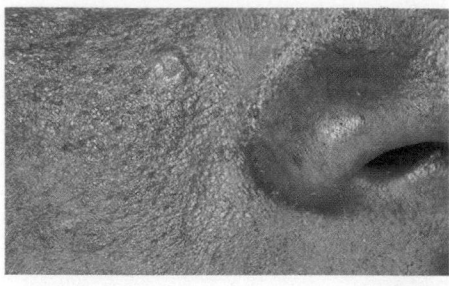

4-1 **Senile sebaceous adenoma** occurs on the face in patients over 40 and is often diagnosed as basal-cell carcinoma. The lesions are soft, small, flat-topped papules, varying in size from 1 to 8 mm, and are characterized by a minute central depression from which sebaceous material can be exuded by lateral compression.

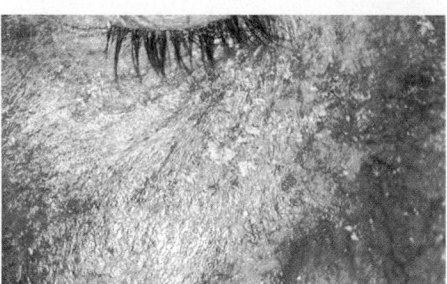

4-2 **Solar keratosis** (1) occurs usually in persons with light skin prone to sunburn or with darker skin after chronic excessive exposure; (2) is strictly limited to exposed skin, especially on the face and dorsal surfaces of the hands; (3) is more easily felt than seen (gritty and sandpaperish); (4) in fair-skinned persons, consists of skin-colored or light brown macules or slightly raised papules with superficial adherent scales not easily removed; and (5) is associated with marked wrinkling, telangiectasia, and often diffuse, tiny, pale yellow papules indicating solar degeneration of connective tissue ("turkey skin").

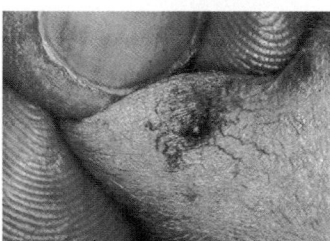

4-3 **Spider nevus** consists of a central, punctate, bright red macule or papule (the body) from which fine red lines radiate like spider legs. There is often a red flare between the radiating vessels. On diascopy, the central body pulsates.

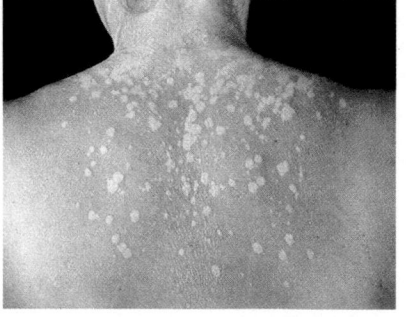

4-4 **Tinea versicolor** is a relatively common disorder occurring primarily on the trunk and appearing in two forms: as scattered, 3- to 5-mm, very slightly scaling brown macules or as whitish macules that may be confused with vitiligo. The fungal spores and hyphae can be easily demonstrated on direct examination of the scales using Swartz stain.

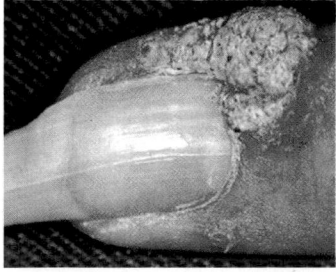

4-5 **Verruca vulgaris** may occur at any age, but it is most common in children. The lesions, which vary in size from 0.5 to 2.0 cm, are round or oval, firm, skin-colored papules with multiple tiny keratotic, rounded or filiform projections covering the surface (vegetation). They occur most frequently on the hands and soles.

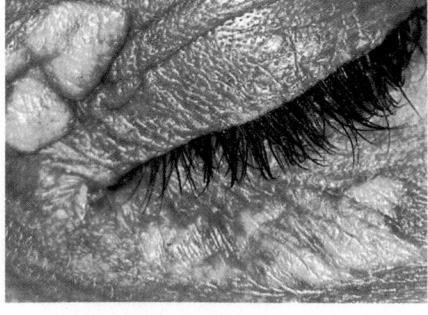

4-6 **Xanthelasma** consists of one or more bright yellow, sharply marginated plaques with no epidermal change, usually occurring on the eyelids, All patients with xanthelasma should be investigated for evidence of plasma lipid abnormalities.

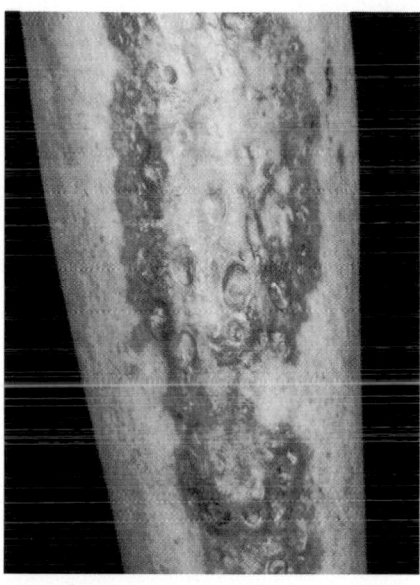

5-1 **Necrobiosis lipoidica diabeticorum** Note the vivid colors (brown and yellow) and fine, arborizing blood vessels traversing the atrophic skin.

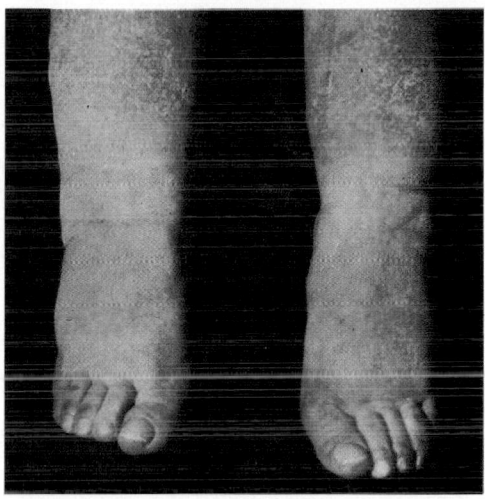

5-2 **Pretibial myxedema.**

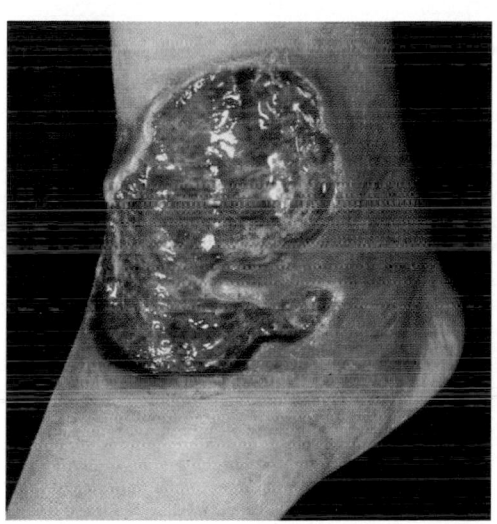

5-3 **Pyoderma gangrenosum** in a patient with ulcerative colitis.

5-4 **"Palpable" purpura with inflammation occurring in gonococcemia.** An identical lesion may be seen in meningococcemia, staphylococcemia, and systemic vasculitis.

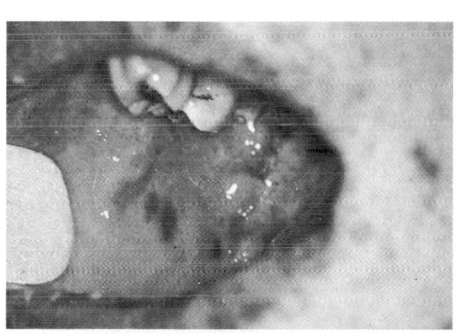

A   **B**

5-5 **Peutz-Jeghers syndrome.** *A*. Macules on the buccal mucosae that are blue or blue-black and are pathogonomonic. *B*. Punctate dark brown macules that typically occur on the lips, around the mouth, and on the fingers. The pigmented macules may disappear on the lips but not on the buccal mucosa.

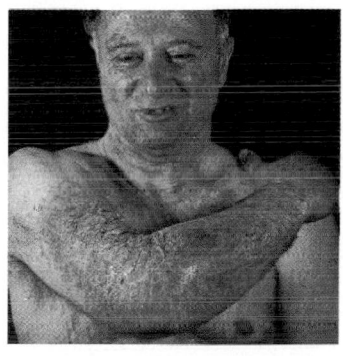

5-6 **Contact eczematous dermatitis.** The diagnosis is made by detailed history in the manner of a detective and also by the periodicity of the attacks. The artificial configuration (sharp borders, etc.) indicates an "outside job."

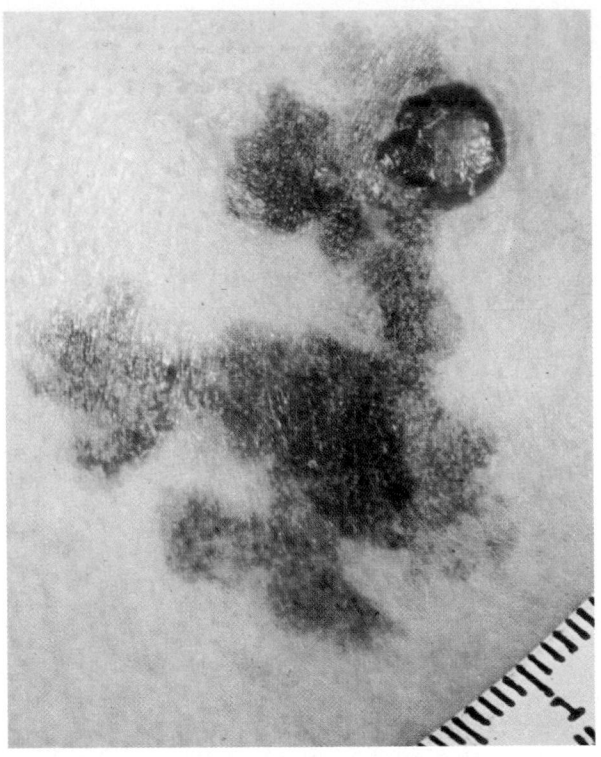

6-1 In **lentigo maligna melanoma,** the lesion is predominantly flat, but there may be a few nodules or papules. The color consists mainly of shades of brown and black, admixed with whitish gray and, occasionally, with reddish brown, bluish gray, and bluish black.

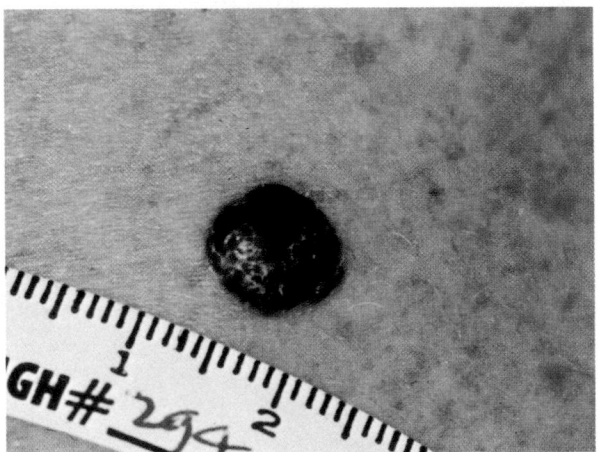

6-3 In **nodular melanoma,** the lesion is always raised and may be dome-shaped or polypoid. The color is usually uniform bluish black, but there may rarely be shades of reddish blue (purple) or an admixture of bluish black with brown or black.

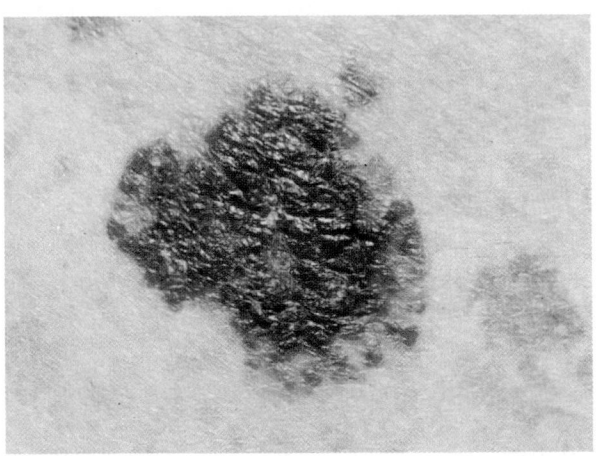

6-2 In **superficial spreading melanoma,** the lesion is usually slightly raised in its entirety and is punctuated with papules and, sometimes, nodules. The color consists mainly of brown and black, admixed with bluish red (violaceous), bluish gray, bluish black, reddish brown, and often whitish pink. The presence of a notched border is distinctive.

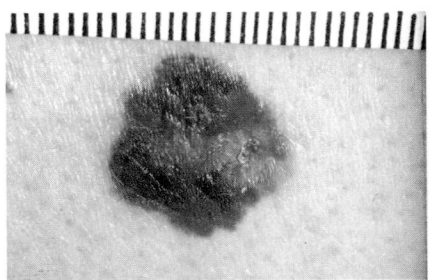

6-4 **Superficial spreading melanoma, superficially invasive.** At this very early stage in the evolution of this tumor, the variegation of color is the clue to the diagnosis.

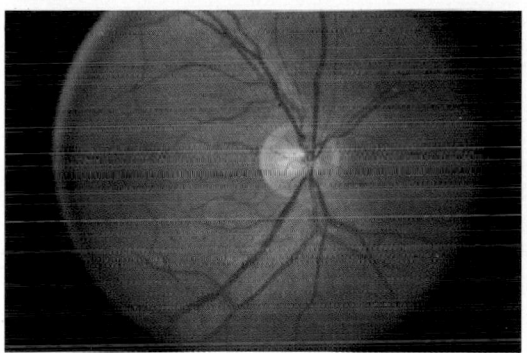

7-1 **Normal optic nerve and retina.**

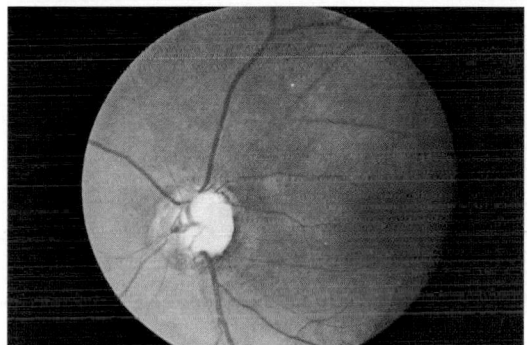

7-2 **Glaucomatous optic disk with secondary atrophy.**

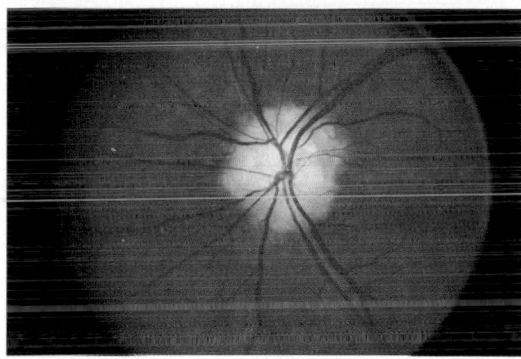

7-3 **Drusen of the optic nerve head.**

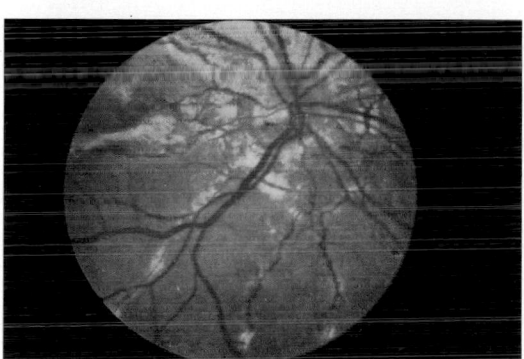

7-4 **Angioid streaks.**

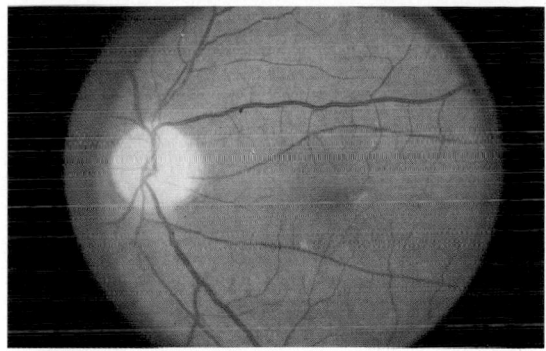

7-5 **Primary optic atrophy.**

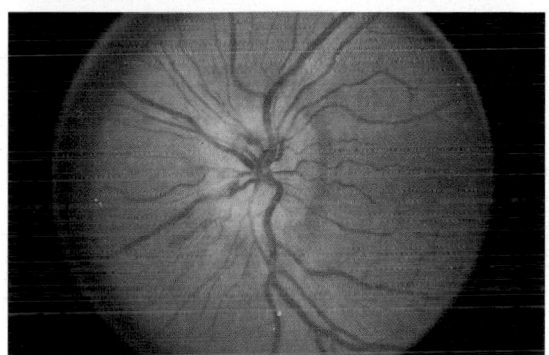

7-6 **Early papilledema.**

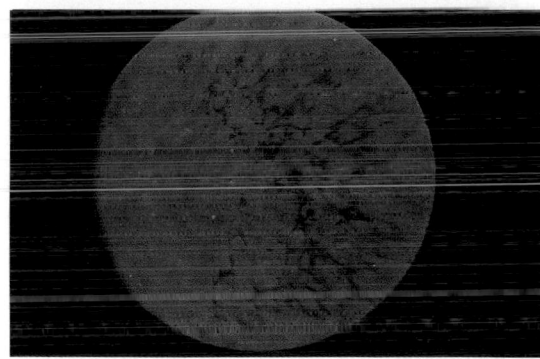

7-7 **Retentive pigmentosa.**

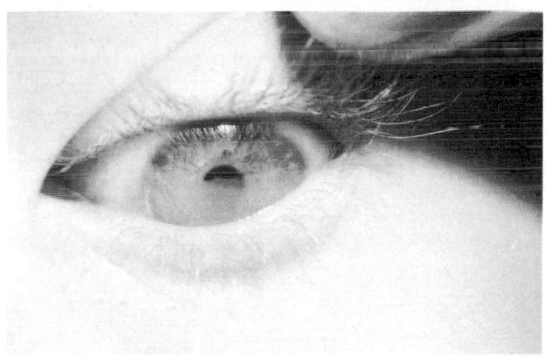

7-8 **Band keratopathy.**

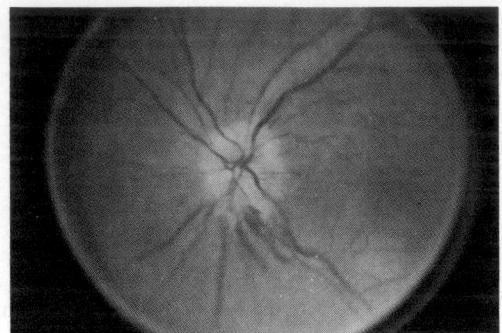

8-1 **Schemic optic neuritis with temporal arteritis.**

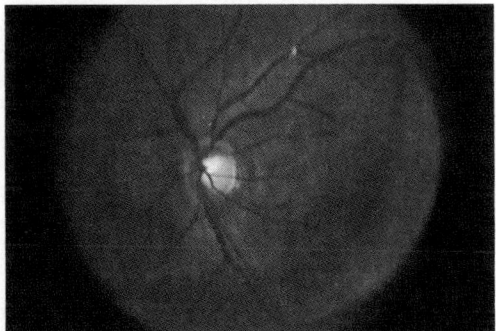

8-2 **Cholesterol embolus in retinal arteriole.**

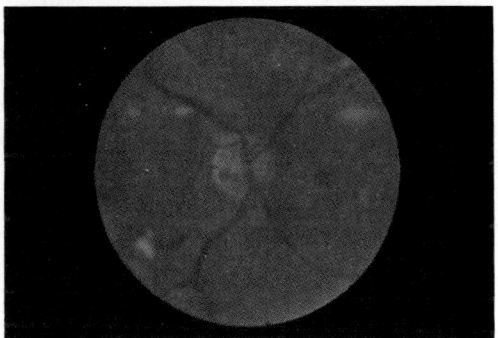

8-3 **Diabetic retinopathy microaneurysm.**

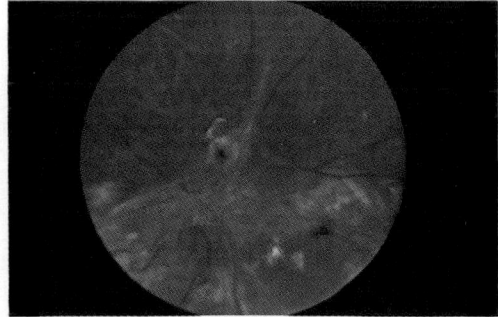

8-4 **Retinitis proliferans in diabetes mellitus.**

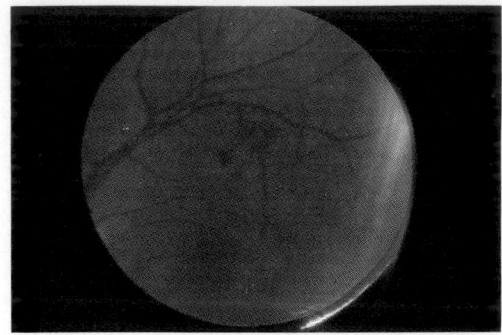

8-5 **Roth spot with subacute bacterial endocarditis.**

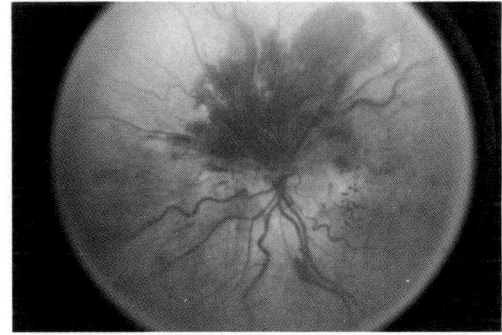

8-6 **Central retinal vein thrombosis.**

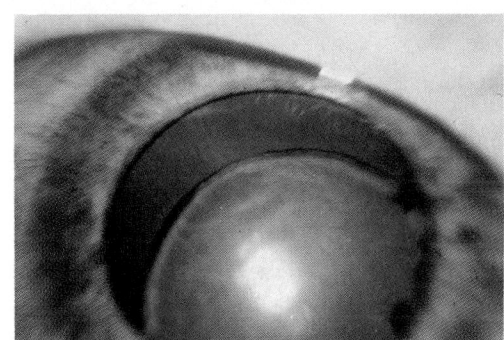

8-7 **Dislocated lens in Marfan's disease.**

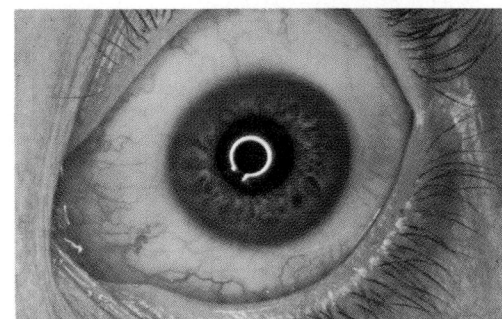

8-8 **Kayser-Fleischer ring in Wilson's disease.**
(*Note:* The ring is the golden brown pigment at the periphery of the cornea and is characteristically broader superiorly and inferiorly than it is medially and laterally.)

in peritoneum, liver, heart, muscle, and dermis of patients during the late stages of malignant melanoma. The brown melanin in the dermal phagocytes appears clinically as blue in the skin because of the Tyndall light-scattering phenomenon. Velvety textured hypermelanotic (brown) macules, representing acanthosis nigricans, may be found in the axillae and other areas in patients with various carcinomas, particularly adenocarcinomas of the gastrointestinal tract. Acanthosis nigricans may also be congenital or benign and associated with diabetes mellitus, Cushing's disease, Addison's disease, pituitary adenoma, and other disorders.

The multiple, irregular, round or oval, yellowish brown to reddish brown macules and papules characteristic of urticaria pigmentosa are related to the presence of melanin in the epidermis overlying clusters of mast cells. Vigorous stroking of such lesions results in the development of urticarial wheals. Systemic mastocytosis, in which mast cells infiltrate diffusely into the liver, spleen, gastrointestinal system, and bones, is a rare condition. Mast-cell leukemia occasionally develops. In children, the skin lesions usually appear in infancy and often spontaneously disappear in several years. The usual course is quite benign, but symptoms of flushing, itching, and urticaria occur in about 30 percent of patients; less than 15 percent experience vomiting, syncope, or shock. The symptoms are presumed to be due to histamine release from mast cells and often coincide with increased urinary excretion of free histamines and metabolites. Urinary levels of 5-hydroxyindoleacetic acid are normal. Antihistamines are of little value.

UNKNOWN CAUSES Generalized brown hypermelanosis of the type seen in Addison's disease may be associated with systemic scleroderma, even early in the course of the disorder. Generalized hyperpigmentation occasionally develops in patients with chronic hepatic insufficiency, especially that due to portal cirrhosis. The pathogenesis of the pigmentation in both conditions is unknown; MSH levels are not elevated. Hypomelanotic macules may also be found in a small percentage of patients with sarcoidosis. These macules are characteristically not pure white and are circumscribed with indiscrete margins. They may overlie dermal nodules, particularly on the extremities but also at times on the trunk.

REFERENCES

Demis DJ: Mast cell disease (urticaria pigmentosa), in *Clinical Dermatology*, DJ Demis et al (eds). New York, Harper & Row, 1974, vol 1, units 4–11, p 1

Fitzpatrick TB et al: Biology of the melanin pigmentary system, in *Dermatology in General Medicine*, 2d ed, TB Fitzpatrick et al (eds). New York, McGraw-Hill, 1979

Jimbow K et al: Congenital circumscribed hypomelanosis: A characterization based on electron microscopic study of tuberous sclerosis, nevus depigmentosis, and piebaldism. J Invest Dermatol 64:50, 1975

Mosher DB et al: Abnormalities of pigmentation, in *Dermatology in General Medicine*, 2d ed, TB Fitzpatrick et al (eds). New York, McGraw-Hill, 1979

Toda K et al: Alteration of racial differences in melanosome distribution in human epidermis after exposure to ultraviolet light. Nature [New Biol] 236:143, 1972

Witkop CV et al: Albinism, in *The Metabolic Basis of Inherited Diseases*, 4th ed, JB Stanbury et al (eds). New York, McGraw-Hill, 1978, p 283

52

PHOTOSENSITIVITY AND OTHER REACTIONS TO LIGHT

MADHUKAR A. PATHAK
THOMAS B. FITZPATRICK
JOHN A. PARRISH

Humans have evolved in sunlight and depend upon it for much more than an indirect source of food and maintenance of the earth's temperature. The natural light has always been recognized for, and endowed with, health-giving powers. Our skin, eyes, blood vessels, and certain endocrine gland functions respond to radiation from the electromagnetic spectrum of the sun. The formation of vitamin D from sterol precursors in the skin by solar ultraviolet (UV) exposure has long been recognized in the management of rickets. Certain of our daily biorhythms are dependent upon the cycles of sunlight. Yet, sunlight can be harmful and damage or kill living cells. Sunlight causes sunburn, damage to deoxyribonucleic acid (DNA), skin cancer, wrinkling and aging of the skin, eye inflammation, and possibly cataracts. During the last decade, interest in the reaction of human skin to light has been renewed as a result of (1) the public's obsession with sunbathing, resulting in premature "aging" of the skin (solar elastosis); (2) demographic data indicating that exposure to sunlight is an important cause of basal-cell and squamous-cell carcinoma and even melanoma of the sun-exposed parts of the body; (3) the widespread use of certain drugs such as phenothiazines, thiazides and related sulfonamide diuretics, and antibiotics (demethylchlortetracycline), which alter the cutaneous responses to sunlight and cause undesirable photosensitivity reactions; (4) the increased recognition of, and better diagnostic and therapeutic approaches to, various skin eruptions (papules, plaques, and eczematous and urticarial reactions) of unknown cause and differing morphologic features (i.e., polymorphic photodermatitis) that follow exposure to UV and visible light; and (5) increased awareness that sunlight is a major cause of discomfort and photosensitivity reactions in patients with certain types of porphyria, especially for those with erythropoietic protoporphyria.

In spite of these negative factors, UV radiation and visible light can be advantageously used in phototherapy and control of certain skin diseases and to prevent brain damage (kernicterus) due to neonatal hyperbilirubinemia. Considerable interest has been generated in recent years in a new type of treatment called *photochemotherapy;* this involves the oral or systemic administration of a drug (methoxsalen) and subsequent exposure of skin to UV radiation (320 to 400 nm). This regimen has been found to be highly effective in clearing psoriasis in over 90 percent of persons treated.

There are more than 25 human disorders that are either caused by or aggravated by exposure of the skin to sunlight. These range from degenerative and neoplastic changes to disability and discomfort associated with chemically induced photosensitivity reactions. These abnormal reactions to light in humans are briefly presented in Table 52-1.

This chapter will be concerned with (1) common conditions such as sunburn, the degenerative and neoplastic conditions associated with solar radiation [basal-cell carcinoma, squamous-cell carcinoma, malignant melanoma, solar keratoses (Plate 4-2)] and chronic sun-induced degeneration; (2) photosensitivity related to drugs and to increased blood or plasma levels of photosensitizing porphyrins in patients with all types of porphyria (except acute intermittent porphyria); (3) photochemotherapy; and (4) photoprotection.

The unit of wavelength most commonly used to measure

and express nonionizing UV radiation or visible light is the nanometer (1 nm = 10^{-9} m = 10 Å). Electromagnetic emanations from the sun comprise a wide range of radiation and include electric waves, radio waves, infrared rays, visible light, UV radiation, roentgen rays (x-rays), gamma rays, and cosmic rays. The shortest wavelengths that reach the surface of the earth through the atmosphere are about 286 to 290 nm. Wavelengths shorter than 286 nm are principally absorbed by ozone in the stratosphere. The solar radiation that reaches the earth's surface ranges from around 286 nm in the UV region, through the visible (400 to 760 nm) and infrared region and well beyond to include electric and radio waves. The solar spectrum that can affect human skin includes wavelengths of 290 to 720 nm; however, infrared radiation (1.5 to 1000 μm) can produce thermal effects (including burn) and potentiate the photochemical and biologic reactions initiated by UV or visible radiation.

For practical reasons, UV radiation is often arbitrarily subdivided into three bands designated as (1) UV-A (320 to 400 nm or long-wave ultraviolet), (2) UV-B (290 to 320 nm or sunburn spectrum), and (3) UV-C (below 290 nm or germicidal radiation).

The amount and type of solar radiation that may reach a given part of the earth at any given time are determined by a great variety of factors, including latitude, time of day, season, altitude, local atmospheric conditions (smog, cloudiness, haze, smoke, dust, fog, humidity, aerosol particles), variations in the thickness of the ozone layer, and height of the sun above the horizon.

Approximately 50 percent of the sun's radiant energy is in the visible portion of the spectrum (400 to 760 nm), about 40 percent in the infrared region, and about 10 percent in the UV region. The damage to skin (sunburn, skin cancer) is evoked by 3 percent of the ultraviolet radiation wavelengths, namely, from 290 to 320 nm.

The transmission of radiant energy varies with wavelength and different areas of the human skin; it may range from 0 to 70 percent. Shorter wavelengths (< 285 nm) are mostly absorbed by the dead-cell layer of the stratum corneum; wavelengths that produce sunburn (290 to 315 nm) are also mostly absorbed in the epidermis. Longer wavelengths (320 to 760 nm) penetrate more deeply into the dermis. Transmission of different wavelengths depends upon (1) the regional thickness of the epidermis, (2) the degree of hydration, (3) the concentration of UV and visible light-absorbing components such as melanin, proteins (keratin, elastin, collagen), nucleic acid, urocanic acid, carotenoids, and hemoglobin, and (4) the number and spatial arrangement of melanosomes and of blood vessels. In fair-skinned individuals, about 85 to 90 percent of 290- to 315-nm radiation is absorbed by the epidermis and only about 10 to 15 percent can penetrate through the epidermis to reach the dermis. In dark-skinned individuals, nearly 90 to 95 percent of 290- to 315-nm radiation is absorbed by the epidermis. The transmission through the epidermis of long-wave UV radiation (320 to 400 nm) and visible radiation (400 to 760 nm) may range from 20 to 70 percent.

The most detrimental effect of UV radiation is cell death. Other effects include mutagenesis, carcinogenesis, interference or inhibition in the synthesis of DNA, ribonucleic acid (RNA), and protein. The mutagenic and carcinogenic effects appear to be mediated largely though the action of UV-B radiation on DNA. The most common reactions, such as sunburn, tanning or melanin pigmentation, keratosis, and skin aging are also caused by UV-B radiation. Although the longer wavelengths (UV-A or 320 to 400 nm and visible or 400 to 760 nm) penetrate more deeply into the skin, they are much less effective at causing these types of photobiologic phenomena. However, in the presence of certain chemical agents (e.g., drugs that are given orally or endogenous porphyrins in certain porphyrias), these wavelengths become highly damaging and cause severe skin photosensitization reactions.

Protection against this damage to the "normal" skin has been the subject of much investigation, and many commercially available sunscreens can be recommended in the prevention of sunburn, skin cancer, aging of skin, and in various types of photosensitivity disorders.

SUNBURN AND TANNING

CLINICAL CHANGES **Erythema, or sunburn reaction** Erythema is caused principally by 290- to 320-nm radiation, maximum solar effectiveness being from 300 to 307 nm. Ultraviolet radiation, emitted by artificial light sources, produces erythema maximally at 297 and 254 nm. Light of wavelengths greater than 320 nm (320 to 760 nm) is generally considered to be nonerythemogenic, although prolonged exposure to radiation of 320 to 400 nm (2 h of midday summer sun in northern latitudes) can produce mild sunburn in normal subjects. Wavelenths of 290 to 320 nm are thought to accelerate aging (wrinkling) of the skin and to lead to the development of solar keratoses, carcinoma, and, possibly, some types of malignant melanoma.

The sunburn reaction is a complex inflammatory process. The observed histologic changes include the appearance of dyskeratotic cells (containing pyknotic nuclei), spongiosis, vacuolation of keratinocytes, and edema. The dermal changes include an inflammatory infiltrate (mostly neutrophils), endothelial swelling, and capillary leakage manifested by extravasation of red blood cells. The severity of these changes and the rate at which they evolve depend on the exposure dose, the incident wavelength, and the type of skin. Hypopigmented, fair-skinned individuals (e.g., red-haired, freckled individuals such as the Irish or Scottish) are more susceptible than pigmented individuals who tan well. The nature of the chromophore that absorbs the light energy which initiates the primary photochemical responses is not well established, although the bulk of evidence suggests that nucleic acids (DNA) are primary targets for the absorption of the 290- to 320-nm radiation. Vasodilatation which accompanies the sunburn reaction

TABLE 52-1
Diseases induced or exacerbated by light

I By light alone
  A Genetic: ephelides (freckles)
  B Idiopathic
    1 Acute solar skin damage (sunburn)
    2 Connective tissue degeneration (wrinkling)
    3 Telangiectasia
    4 Solar keratoses and solar lentigo
    5 Basal-cell carcinoma
    6 Squamous-cell carcinoma
    7 Malignant melanoma
    8 Polymorphous photodermatosis
    9 Solar urticaria
II By light plus exogenous agents
  A Chemical or drug
    1 Phototoxic reactions
    2 Phytophotodermatitis
    3 Lupus erythematosus (with hydralazine, procainamide)
  B Chemical and immunologic: photoallergic reactions
III By light plus metabolite(s)
  A Porphyrias
  B Porphyria cutanea tarda associated with hexachlorobenzene, estrogens, alcohol
IV By light plus preexisting disease
  A Genetic
    1 Xeroderma pigmentosum
    2 Oculocutaneous albinism
    3 Vitiligo
    4 Hartnup syndrome
  B Nutritional or metabolic
    1 Pellagra
    2 Malignant carcinoid
  C Viral: herpes simplex
  D Unknown: lupus erythematosus (cutaneous, systemic)

appears to result from the activation and release of one or more chemical mediators (e.g., kinins, serotonin, histamine).

There has been considerable focus on the role of prostaglandins and related derivatives of arachidonic acid. These are low-molecular-weight, oxygenated, fatty acid structures synthesized by microsomal enzymes present in all mammalian cells, including epidermal cells. Increased levels of prostaglandins (PGE series) have been observed in widely different types of inflammation, including the UV-induced sunburn reaction. Indomethacin, a nonsteroidal anti-inflammatory agent, when applied topically or given intradermally, can decrease a delayed sunburn response of human skin produced by UV-B radiation. Since indomethacin is known to inhibit prostaglandin synthesis, these findings support the possible role of prostaglandins as mediators of the delayed erythemal response to UV-B radiation. Ultraviolet radiation may also have a direct effect on the blood vessels of the upper layer of the dermis (capillaries, venules, and arterioles). The formation of peroxides or free radicals may play an important role in the damage to lysosomal membranes associated with lipid peroxidation. In fair skin 290- to 320-nm spectrum is known to produce damaging free radicals (molecules with unpaired electrons).

Melanin pigmentation, or tanning Tanning (increase in melanin pigment) that follows exposure of the skin to solar radiation involves two distinct photobiologic processes. The first, *immediate pigment darkening* (IPD), or darkening of preformed pigment in the epidermis, is elicited by wavelengths of 320 to 720 nm. The second, *melanogenesis*, is an intricate process that consists of the *erythema response (sunburn)* followed usually in 3 to 4 days by formation of new pigment. Immediate pigment darkening results from oxidation of melanin through the production of semiquinone-like free radicals in the melanin polymer; transfer of melanosomes from melanocytes and redistribution of already existing melanosomes within the keratinocytes also may occur.

Melanogenesis involves (1) an increase in the number of functional melanocytes, resulting from increased proliferation of melanocytes, and activation of dormant melanocytes; (2) increased arborization of melanocytic dendrites; (3) an increase in the number of melanosomes in proliferating melanocytes; (4) an increase in tyrosinase activity; and (5) an increase in the transfer of melanosomes from melanocytes to keratinocytes. The degree of melanin pigmentation, however, that can be achieved in an individual by exposure to solar radiation is genetically predetermined. People with fair skin who burn easily but do not tan or tan poorly (skin types I and II) cannot with repeated sun exposures achieve that degree of tanning which can be easily achieved by someone genetically able to tan profusely with minimal exposure.

CELLULAR AND MOLECULAR CHANGES Hyperplasia Within 72 h after exposure, there is an increase in the number of epidermal cells with a high rate of mitotic activity. The rate of cell proliferation decreases after 7 to 10 days, and the thickness of the epidermis gradually returns to normal within the next 30 to 60 days.

DNA and RNA changes Damage to DNA by sunburn-producing UV light (290 to 320 nm) may result in cell death. The principal epidermal DNA photoproducts are pyrimidine dimers (e.g., thymine dimers); these are of the cyclobutane type and are formed between adjacent pyrimidine bases. DNA and RNA synthesis in the epidermis is inhibited within 1 h after irradiation. New synthesis is evident by 24 h and is maximal by 60 to 70 h.

Mitosis Inhibition of epidermal mitosis and retardation of basal-cell turnover occur within 1 h after irradiation. The epidermal cell cycle is interrupted at the S phase of DNA synthesis. Inhibition of mitosis can persist for 7 to 24 h; it is followed by an acceleration of mitotic rate and basal-cell turnover that reaches a peak by 48 to 72 h and is associated with epidermal hyperplasia. The mitotic cycle appears to be interrupted in the G_2 stage, in the prophase stage, or in both. The increased mitotic activity and the associated hyperplasia may last for 30 to 60 days. This hyperplasia appears to be due to a combination of the removal of the epidermal mitotic inhibitors (chalones) and stimulation of growth by the action of cyclic adenosine monophosphate (AMP) and guanosine 5'-monophosphate (GMP).

SUN-INDUCED CARCINOMA

Epidemiologic evidence clearly implicates solar radiation as a factor in the induction of human skin cancer. Some studies have established that carcinoma of the skin occurs more frequently on the parts of the body habitually exposed to sunlight; thus, the lesions of the head and hands are concentrated on the nose, central portions of the cheeks, eyelids, and dorsum of the hands. In fair-skinned Caucasoids who sunburn easily, these cancers are limited almost exclusively to the exposed portions of the face, head, neck, arms, and hands. Negroid skin, on the other hand, is remarkably resistant to the development of skin cancer on the exposed surfaces, and a similar resistance is seen among the pigmented Caucasoids (e.g., East Indians), American Indians, and Asiatics.

Carcinoma of the exposed skin is more prevalent among persons who are outdoors a great deal and is the common cause of cancer in Caucasoids in Australia, South Africa, and the southern parts of the United States. The action spectrum for photocarcinogenesis is similar to that of sunburn reaction.

Several studies based on the distribution of local populations in the United States, Australia, and Ireland have emphasized that skin cancer develops earlier and more frequently in people who have light skin and freckles, who burn easily and do not tan on exposure to the sun, and who are of mostly Celtic ancestry (people with skin types I and II). *Australia, with the highest reported incidence of skin cancer* in the world, has a population largely descended from British stock, with about 25 percent claiming Celtic (i.e., Irish, Scottish, and Welsh) extraction. In all three countries surveyed, persons of Celtic ancestry were found to have a disproportionately high incidence of skin cancer. Dark-pigmented races and people who tan well (skin types IV to VI) are least susceptible to skin cancer.

All varieties of skin cancer develop in patients with *xeroderma pigmentosum*, an autosomal recessive disorder. This rare defect represents, in the extreme, the basic problem of solar radiation and skin cancer. Patients with this disease have a greatly increased susceptibility to malignant tumors of the skin in the light-exposed areas. The characteristic skin manifestations are atrophy, telangiectasia, hyperpigmented macules, keratoses, and ulcerations, all occurring in sun-exposed areas. Within the first few years of life, basal-cell or squamous-cell carcinomas or sarcomas or malignant melanomas develop. An inherited enzyme defect may be responsible, at least in part, for the cancer-forming potential in patients with xeroderma pigmentosum. Cultured fibroblasts from patients with xeroderma pigmentosum are incapable of releasing thymine dimers from DNA and, in consequence, are deficient in their ability to repair their UV-damaged DNA. Xeroderma pigmentosum is the most notable human disease in which there is a defect in the excision repair process involving the removal of UV-induced dimers followed by the synthesis and re-forming of new segments of DNA. This enzymatic deficiency may result in a high somatic mutation rate of skin cells after sun exposure and, eventually, in cancer formation.

DEGENERATIVE CHANGES OF THE SKIN

Degenerative skin changes (wrinkling, telangiectasia, keratoses) are more frequent in white-skinned people living in areas where the intensity of UV radiation is great (e.g., southwestern United States, Australia, South Africa). The term *solar degeneration* implies a group of changes in the exposed areas of the skin, including wrinkling, atrophy, hypermelanotic and hypomelanotic macules, telangiectasia, yellow papules and plaques, and keratoses. The furrowed and leathery condition of the skin is seen particularly in persons who have fair skin and poor tanning ability and are constantly exposed to the sun. The most conspicuous and characteristic change may result from biochemical and structural alterations of connective tissue (elastin as well as collagen). The generative changes are caused by sunburn-producing (290 to 320 nm) and UV-A (320 to 400 nm) radiation that can penetrate deeply into the dermis.

Chronically light-damaged human epidermis shows shortening or flattening of the rete ridges, thinning of the epidermis (decrease in malpighian cells), and many abnormal cells in disorderly arrangement. There is a progressive degeneration in the papillary and subpapillary zones of the dermis. Other changes include (1) the development of vascular ectasia, (2) accumulation of acid mucopolysaccharides, (3) appearance of abnormal fibrocytes, (4) loss of collagen, (5) degeneration of elastic tissue ("actinic elastosis") and disorganization of the connective tissue into amorphous masses. These changes are irreversible and can be minimized by daily topical application of effective sunscreens.

PHOTOTOXICITY AND PHOTOALLERGY

Sensitivity to sunlight is a common clinical problem. Continuous daily exposure to sun alone may be the major factor responsible for irreversible skin changes (e.g., freckles, telangiectasia, wrinkling, keratoses, atrophy, hypermelanotic and hypomelanotic macules, and carcinomas in the sun-exposed regions). Apart from these chronic changes, human skin can also become hypersensitive to UV and visible light. The interface between humans and their environment is the skin, and the physical (light) and chemical agents acting directly on it are important etiologic or precipitating factors in photosensitivity disorders.

EFFECT OF DRUGS AND OTHER CHEMICALS IN ASSOCIATION WITH LIGHT EXPOSURE Some chemicals and drugs by themselves may not act as contact irritants and are generally innocuous to skin in the absence of light exposure. However, when the skin is challenged with proper concentrations of the agent and the appropriate light wavelengths, these agents can induce undesirable skin reactions.

Cutaneous photosensitivity is a general term used to refer to the abnormal reaction of the human skin to the stimulus of light. Drug photosensitivity reactions may be defined clinically as adverse skin responses resulting from the combination of exposure to certain therapeutic or chemical agents and UV radiation of 320 to 400 nm. Adverse cutaneous reactions can occur in some individuals who either have ingested certain drugs or have been in contact with certain chemicals (Tables 52-2 and 52-3). These reactions may include an acute, abnormal sunburn response, namely, edema, papules, macules, vesicles, bullae, or acute eczematous or urticarial reactions. There may be desquamation and hyperpigmentation or hypopigmentation. These adverse photosensitivity reactions are classified into two broad categories: (1) phototoxic reactions and (2) photoallergic reactions.

TABLE 52-2
Contact photosensitizers: Chemicals that induce photosensitivity reactions in humans

Name	Use	Reported clinical observations
Halogenated salicylanilides; 3,3',4',5-tetrachlorosalicylanilide; 3,4',5- and 3,3',5-trichlorosalicylanilide; 3,4',5- and 3,3',5-tribromosalicylanilide; 3,5- and 4,5'-dibromosalicylanilide	Deodorant, bacteriostatic agents in soaps	Phototoxic and eczematous photoallergic reactions, burning, itching, cross-photosensitivity reactions
Hexachlorophene	Antimicrobial, antiseptic	Phototoxic reactions
Bithionol or bis(2-hydroxy-3,5-dichlorophenyl) sulfide	Antimicrobial, antiseptic	Photoallergic reactions
Fentichlor (2,2'-dihydroxy-5,5'-dichlorodiphenyl sulfide); multifungin (bromochlorosalicylanilide); Jadit (4-chloro-2-hydroxybenzoic acid *N-n*-butylamide)	Antifungal	Phototoxic and photoallergic reactions
5-Flurouracil	Antineoplastic	Acceleration of inflammatory process
p-Aminobenzoic acid (PABA) and esters of PABA	Sunscreen	Photoallergic reactions
4,4'-Bis(3-phenylureido)-2,2'-stilbenedisulfonic acid or blankophor	Fluorescent brightening agent for cellulose, nylon, or wool fibers	Phototoxic and photoallergic reactions
Cadmium sulfide	In tattoos	Erythema
Furocoumarins: psoralen, 8-methoxypsoralen, 5-methoxypsoralen, 4,5',8-trimethylpsoralen	In vitiligo for increased pigment formation and sun tolerance	Marked erythema, vesicles, bullae, hyperpigmentation
Essential oils: oil of bergamot, oil of lime, oil of cedar, oil of lavender, oil of citron, oil of sandalwood	Cosmetics and beauty aids	Phototoxic reactions and postinflammatory hyperpigmentation
Plants: Umbelliferae, Rutaceae	Used in perfumes or flavorings or as spices	Phytophotodermatitis, hyperpigmentation, vesicles, bullae
Dyes: fluorescein, rose bengal, eosin, erythrocine, trypaflavin, orange red, paraphenylenediamine, methylene blue, toluidine blue, trypan blue	Cosmetics and dye industry	Erythema, edema, vesicles, pigmentation, phototoxic reaction
Coal tar and coal tar derivatives containing anthracene, phenanthrene, naphthalene, thiophene, and many phenolic agents; pitch	In therapy for psoriasis and chronic eczema; in hair shampoos	Smarting, exaggerated sunburn, urticarial wheals, tar melanosis

SOURCE: *TB Fitzpatrick et al, in Sunlight and Man: Normal and Abnormal Photobiologic Responses, MA Pathak et al (eds), Tokyo, University of Tokyo Press, 1974.*

Phototoxic reactions are those that can be elicited in almost everyone with enough light energy of the appropriate wavelengths and when appropriate concentrations of the agent are either applied topically or given orally. Light plus the offending agent leads to an exaggerated sunburn reaction, with or without painful edema. The reaction can occur within 5 to 18 h after exposure to the sun and is usually maximum at 36 to 72 h. Hyperpigmentation and desquamation can also occur. The reaction is usually confined to the site of exposure. If the applied concentration of the implicated agent is high, bullae or small vesicles may develop.

Certain *phototoxic reactions* require the presence of molecular oxygen (e.g., hematoporphyrin, several dyes). The oxygen-dependent reactions are referred to as *photodynamic reactions*. On the other hand, many phototoxic reactions can occur in the absence of oxygen (e.g., psoralen photosensitization). Most reactions have been reported to require UV-A (320 to 400 nm) radiation; however, certain phototoxic reactions can be initiated by the UV-B (290 to 320 nm) as well as by the visible (400 to 700 nm) spectra. The phototoxic reactions in general should be regarded as the undesirable sequelae of augmentation of the primary photochemical reactions that underlie the inflammatory response of skin evoked by UV radiation. It is believed that a deleterious amount of radiant energy is absorbed by the skin and the photosensitizing agents. This absorbed energy can directly cause cell damage by creating a covalent linking of the sensitizing molecule to the pyrimidines (e.g., thymine) in the cellular DNA. This linkage (the formation of cyclobutane photoadducts of the sensitizer and the pyrimidines) can be lethal to the cell. Photosensitizers like the psoralens selectively intercalate between two base pairs and produce interstrand cross-links with epidermal DNA. In addition, the photosensitizing molecule can transfer the absorbed energy and promote formation of free radicals (molecules with unpaired electrons that are highly reactive) and cause damage to the cell membranes and lysosomes. In the presence of certain porphyrins (e.g., hematoporphyrin, protoporphyrin), a reactive singlet form of oxygen can be generated by these photosensitizing molecules. Drug-induced phototoxic reactions may thus involve damage to the DNA, RNA, lysosomes, cell membranes, and other organelles.

Photoallergy to drugs is an acquired and altered capacity of the skin to respond to light in the presence of a photosensitizer, and involves the immune system. The absorbed light energy seems to promote a photochemical reaction between the drug and the skin proteins. The drug acts to form a haptenic group and either combines directly with the protein to form a photoantigen or is altered by the absorbed energy; this altered haptenic group then reacts with the proteins to form an antigen.

The clinical manifestations in drug-induced photoallergic reactions may range from acute urticarial lesions, developing

TABLE 52-3
Systemic photosensitizers: Chemicals that induce photosensitivity reactions in humans

Name	*Uses*	*Clinical observations*	*Action spectrum, nm*
SULFONAMIDES			
Sulfanilamide, sulfathiazole, sulfapyridine, sulfamethazine, sulfaguanidine, sulfisoxazole, monochlorphenamide	Chemotherapy, antibacterial agents	Phototoxic and photoallergic reactions	290–320
SULFONYLUREA			
Carbutamide, tolbutamide (Orinase), chlorpropamide (Diabinese)	Hypoglycemic or antidiabetic drugs	Phototoxic reactions	290–360
CHLORTHIAZIDES			
6-Chloro-7-sulfamyl-3,4-dihydro-1,2,4-thiodiazine 1,1-dioxide (HydroDiuril)	Diuretics, antihypertensive	Papular and edematous eruption, plaques	290–320
Quinethazone (Diuril)	Antihypertensive	Phototoxic and photoallergic reactions	320–400
PHENOTHIAZINES			
Chlorpromazine (Thorazine), promethazine (Phenergan), mepazine, Stelazine, trimeprazine, Compazine, promazine (Sparine)	Tranquilizer, nematode infestation agent, urinary antiseptic, antihistamine	Exaggerated sunburn, maculopapular and urticarial eruptions, gray-blue hyperpigmentation	290–400
ANTIBIOTICS			
Demethylchlortetracycline (Declomycin), chlortetracycline, oxytetracycline, doxycycline	Broad-spectrum antibiotic	Exaggerated sunburn, phototoxic reaction	320–400
Griseofulvin	Antimycotic	Exaggerated sunburn, phototoxic and photoallergic reactions	320–400
Nalidixic acid (NegGram)	Antibacterial	Erythema, bullae	320–400
FUROCOUMARINS			
4,5′,8-Trimethylpsoralen (trioxsalen), 8-methoxypsoralen (methoxsalen), psoralen	In photochemotherapy of psoriasis and vitiligo; for sun tolerance and increased pigment formation	Erythema, bullae, hyperpigmentation	320–400
ESTROGENS AND PROGESTERONES			
Mestranol and norethynodrel, diethylstilbesterol	Oral contraceptives	Melasma, phototoxic reactions	?290–320
Chlordiazepoxide (Librium)	Tranquilizer, psychotropic	Eczematous eruption	290–360
Triacetyldiphenolisatin	Laxative	Eczematous photoallergic reaction	290–320
Cyclamates, calcium cyclamate, sodium cyclohexylsulfamate	Artificial sweeteners	Phototoxic and photoallergic reactions	?290–360

SOURCE: *TB Fitzpatrick et al, Sunlight and Man: Normal and Abnormal Photobiologic Responses, MA Pathak et al (eds), Tokyo, University of Tokyo Press, 1974.*

within a few minutes after exposure, to eczematous or papular lesions appearing within 24 h or later. The eruption may extend beyond the exposed areas. In recurrent cases, flare-ups of distant, previously uninvolved sites may also occur. Some edema and vasodilatation are common in most of these eruptions. The action spectrum is generally in the long-wave range (320 to 400 nm), and less energy is required than is necessary for the production of phototoxic reactions.

The various systemic therapeutic agents and their effects on the skin in the presence of light (whether phototoxic or photoallergic reactions) are listed in Table 52-3. The biologic action spectra that induce either the phototoxic or photoallergic reactions are also given.

EFFECT OF PLANTS PLUS LIGHT *Phytophotodermatitis* (phototoxic reactions) can develop as the result of contact with many plants (belonging principally to the families Rutaceae and Umbelliferae, e.g., certain limes, parsley, celery, bishop's weed, figs) and subsequent exposure of the skin to sunlight. The photodermatitis involves a mild-to-severe erythematous reaction with or without vesicles or bullae. Dense postinflammatory hyperpigmentation is visible within 3 to 5 days. Perfumes and colognes containing oil of bergamot are also known to induce hyperpigmentation with or without erythema. The pigmentation in berloque dermatitis occurs in configurations that seem bizarre but actually represent the areas to which the scent was applied; sometimes the hyperpigmentation may be droplike or pendant-like, and has therefore been named accordingly (*berloque* or *berlock,* meaning trinket or pendant). This phytophotodermatitis, as well as that which follows contact with various other plants, is thought to be caused by furocoumarins (e.g., 5-methoxypsoralen, 8-methoxypsoralen, and other psoralens) characteristically present in these plants. The combination of exposure to long-wave UV radiation (320 to 400 nm) and furocoumarins greatly enhances the erythema and the pigmentation response.

Treatment Therapy of acute phototoxic reactions induced by topical or systemic agents is best achieved by removal of the offending agent and avoidance of exposure to the sun, or both. If necessary, the usual dermatologic procedures for minimizing the discomforts of the inflammatory response should be undertaken. However, in instances in which continued systemic use of the drug is vital, cutaneous photoreactions can be prevented by instructing the patient to remain indoors or by avoiding exposure to sunlight between 10 A.M. and 4 P.M. Generally the problem subsides within a week after discontinuation of the stress (sun and the drug). Sunscreens listed in Table 52-4 also should be prescribed.

EFFECT OF LIGHT PLUS ENDOGENOUS PHOTOSENSITIZERS This category includes several photosensitivity reactions in patients with various types of porphyria (see Chap. 96). The photosensitivity reactions are related to the overproduction in vivo of either photo-, uro-, or coproporphyrins and their precursors.

TABLE 52-4
Topical sunscreens

Formulation ingredient	Concentration	Commercial name	PF*	Recommended for skin type nos.
PABA SUNSCREENS				
Aminobenzoic acid in 50–70% ethyl alcohol	5%, clear lotion	PreSun	>10–15	I and II
		Pabanol	>10–15	I and II
		Coppertone SuperShade	6	III and IV
ESTERS AND DERIVATIVES OF PABA				
Isoamyl-*p*-*N*,*N*-dimethyl aminobenzoate (Escalol 506, Padimate A)	2.5% or 3.3%, clear lotion	Block Out	6	III and IV
		PABA Film	6	III and IV
		Spectraban	6	III and IV
Glyceryl PABA + octyldimethyl PABA or 2-ethyl-hexyl ester of dimethylaminobenzoate (Escalol 507)	2.5% + 2.5%, milky lotion	Eclipse	>8–10	I and II
Escalol 507 + dioxybenzone	2.5% + 3%, clear lotion	Sungard	6	III and IV
Escalol 507 (octyldimethyl PABA) in ammonium acrylate–acrylate polymer	3.3%, milky lotion	Sundown	4–5	IV
Homomenthyl salicylate + *p*-dimethylaminobenzoate	5%, clear lotion	Aztec	6	III and IV
NON-PABA CHEMICAL SUNSCREENS				
2-Hydroxy-4-methoxybenzophenone 5-sulfonic acid	10%, milky lotion	UVAL	7	III and IV
Ethylhexyl-*p*-methoxycinnamate + 2-hydroxy-4-methoxybenzophenone + 2-phenylbenzamidazole sulfonic acid (G6)	5% + 3% + 4%, cream	Piz Buin Exclusiv Piz Buin Extrem Cream	11	I and II
Ethylhexyl-*p*-methoxycinnamate	4%–4.5% cream or lotion	Piz Buin	>6	I and II
Ethylhexyl-*p*-methoxycinnamate + 2-hydroxy-4-methoxybenzophenone	5% + 3% milky lotion	Piz Buin	>8	I and II
PHYSICAL SUNSCREENS				
Titanium dioxide, zinc oxide, kaolin, talc, iron oxide, etc.	Heavy cream or paste	A-fil RVPaque Shadow Reflecta Covermark	>4–8	All skin types—protection against UV-A, UV-B, and visible light.

* PF = Protection factor established under field conditions with natural sunlight.
NOTE: Eyes should be always protected with ultraviolet-opaque goggles or sunglasses while sunbathing or skiing.

In the prophyrias, endogenously synthesized porphyrin molecules, when exposed to light, cause burning, itching, urticaria, edema, crusting and scarring, vesiculation, atrophy, and many other disabling cutaneous changes. The light-absorbing molecules involved in evoking the cutaneous reactions are the irreversibly oxidized porphyrins present in abnormal amounts in red blood cells, plasma, skin, liver, stool, and urine. The photodermatitis is produced by a narrow band of light in the region of 400 to 410 nm, which corresponds to one of the absorption peaks of porphyrins. Patients, however, are sensitive to wavelengths from 380 to 600 nm. The most disabling type of photosensitivity reactions are encountered in erythropoietic (congenital) porphyria and in erythropoietic protoporphyria (Chap. 96). Symptoms and signs of sensitivity to sunlight occur in early childhood.

The adverse cutaneous responses to sunlight in patients with erythropoietic protoporphyria (EPP) have been found to be ameliorated by oral ingestion of β-carotene (Chap. 96). Patients who take β-carotene are able to withstand prolonged exposures to sunlight and experience relief from their usual photosensitivity reactions. A recommended treatment is the daily oral ingestion of β-carotene (Solatene) sufficient to maintain blood levels of 600 to 800 μg per 100 ml (usually adults receive a dose of 120 to 180 mg per day; children under 12 years receive 30 to 90 mg per day). Photoprotective effect of β-carotene is observed after 4 to 6 weeks, and the therapy is generally continued throughout the year. In vitro, β-carotene has been found to be an effective quencher for the "singlet" oxygen generated in certain photosensitivity reactions. During porphyrin-mediated photosensitivity reactions, peroxides are generated which damage the lipid membranes. It is presumed that β-carotene is preferentially oxidized and that by quenching the "singlet" oxygen, it inhibits lipid peroxide formation.

POLYMORPHOUS LIGHT ERUPTIONS

Polymorphous light eruption (PMLE) is an idiopathic, acquired syndrome characterized by a delayed abnormal response to light and varied morphology. The clinical patterns are pleomorphic or polymorphic in nature. The most common pattern consists of multiple small papules, or papules and vesicles that may become confluent and present at times an eczematous clinical picture. Lichenification due to scratching of the pruritic lesions commonly supervenes. Less frequently, the primary lesion is a large papule that may present an erythema multiforme-like pattern or become confluent to form plaques. This variety is usually, but not exclusively, confined to the face and neck. The only consistent histologic feature in all cases is a dense perivascular infiltrate in the upper and middle dermis. Typically the lesions appear in early spring and after each exposure. The latent period between exposure and the appearance of rash may range from a few hours to 2 days, with the most common interval being 24 to 36 h. Itching is frequent and may occur during sun exposure and even preceding the eruption.

The sunburn-producing spectrum (UV-B, or 290 to 320 nm) is the most effective waveband for eliciting abnormal PMLE responses. However, in many instances, the action spectrum may extend into the UV-A (320 to 400 nm) region; in some instances it may extend into the visible region. Even alpha particles, x-rays, and germicidal radiation (290 nm) may produce PMLE. Although the mechanisms underlying these reactions are not known, the evidence suggests a delayed hypersensitivity reaction to an antigen induced by radiation.

TREATMENT Photoprotection, either through avoidance or with the use of highly effective sunscreens (Table 52-4), may be adequate to control symptoms and appearance of new lesions. The synthetic antimalarials are effective in PMLE, but they must be used with great caution to prevent retinopathy and optic nerve atrophy. The lesions of PMLE are often responsive to topical corticosteroids; systemic steroids are rarely indicated. Desensitization by repeated graduated exposure to sunlight or to artificial radiation (UV-A) in combination with psoralens (methoxsalen) has been successful in a limited number of cases. Oral administration of β-carotene (Solatene) has been found to be of limited value.

PHOTOTHERAPY AND PHOTOCHEMOTHERAPY

Phototherapy refers to the therapeutic effectiveness of UV (usually 290 to 320 nm) or visible radiation without the systemic use of a drug. Photochemotherapy, on the other hand, involves the combination of nonionizing electromagnetic radiation and a systemically administered, photochemically reactive agent. Generally in the doses used, neither the drug alone nor the radiation alone has any therapeutic response; only the combination of the photoactive drug and the radiation, administered at the appropriate time, is therapeutic. Indications for phototherapy include various dermatoses, uremic pruritus, and neonatal hyperbilirubinemia. Phototherapy with blue visible light (430 to 500 nm) enhances the photodegradation and excretion of bilirubin in neonatal jaundice. Psoriasis, eczema, and pityriasis rosea may improve with controlled sun exposures. UV-B radiation (290 to 320 nm) is, therefore, a part of the therapeutic regimen for these dermatoses.

The treatment of psoriasis and other proliferative diseases of the skin has involved attempts to inhibit cellular proliferation and DNA synthesis.

The topical application of crude coal tar products followed by subsequent UV exposure has been a standard treatment for severe generalized psoriasis. Although tar-induced phototoxicity affecting DNA synthesis is believed to be responsible for therapeutic effects, it is not yet clear whether the beneficial effects are due to the chemical ingredients of tar alone or the photosensitizing action of UV-A (320 to 400 nm) or UV-B.

ORAL PSORALEN PHOTOCHEMOTHERAPY Psoralens are naturally occurring furocoumarins that are tricyclic compounds, many of which are photochemically reactive [e.g., 8-methoxypsoralen (methoxsalen) and 4,5',8-trimethylpsoralen (trioxsalen)]. It has been shown that in the presence of psoralen irradiation with UV-A (320 to 400 nm) can result in covalent binding of psoralens to pyrimidine bases in DNA. This photoconjugation may lead to interstrand cross-linking of psoralen between base paired strands of DNA, inhibition of DNA synthesis, and cell death. Methoxsalen is now widely used in treating psoriasis, vitiligo, eczema, and mycosis fungoides. Two hours after ingestion of methoxsalen (0.6 to 0.9 mg/kg), patients are exposed to a measured dose of UV-A radiation. The initial dose depends on the patient's skin reactivity to ultraviolet radiation (sunburn history) and degree of melanin pigmentation of skin. Repeated psoralen plus UV-A treatments cause disappearance of psoriatic lesions; a total of 10 to 20 treatments given two or three times weekly will usually result in clearance of psoriasis. Maintenance treatments are recommended, and it appears that gradually tapering the frequency of treatments is most effective. The scalp and areas to which UV-A does not penetrate do not respond to therapy.

In vitiligo, a disease characterized by amelanotic macules of varying sizes and absence of melanocytes, methoxsalen plus UV-A treatment can be used in restoring the normal skin color to pigmentless areas of vitiligo macules. Over 100 to 200 treatments are needed, and this long duration of treatment can often be frustrating, especially when the pigment response is slow, unpredictable, and subject to the presence of functional melanocytes.

The long-term concerns of photochemotherapy include premature aging (irreversible changes in connective tissue, blood vessels, and keratinocytes), cataract, and skin cancer. Oral methoxsalen photochemotherapy using long-wave UV radiation sources is a new approach. Although over 2000 patients with psoriasis and thousands of patients with vitiligo have been treated, well-documented examples of actinic keratoses or early squamous-cell carcinoma have been observed. However, there is no evidence of cataractogenesis in humans treated with psoralens and sunlight or high-intensity ultraviolet radiation over the past 25 years. Photochemotherapy is an effective treatment which, when compared with other available treatments for generalized psoriasis or vitiligo, appears to have the most acceptable risk/benefit ratio.

TOPICAL SUNSCREENS IN HEALTH AND DISEASES

Sunscreens protect viable cells of the skin by absorbing and reflecting the radiation impinging on the skin. The majority of sunscreens are designed to protect the user against UV-B (290 to 320 nm). In counseling people in the prevention of sunburn, skin cancer, aging of the skin, actinic elastosis, and various forms of sun sensitivity, the choice and recommendations of sunscreen depend upon several factors. The most important consideration should be the individual's reactivity to sunlight. People with fair skin, blue eyes, with or without freckles, who burn easily and tan poorly (skin types I and II) should be given those sunscreens that have a high protection index (Table 52-4) i.e., a protection factor of 6 or more. Individuals with skin types III and IV, who burn moderately or minimally but tan well, may be recommended sunscreens with a protection factor of 4.

For the greatest protection patients should apply 5.0 percent p-aminobenzoic acid (PABA) lotions in 50 to 70 percent ethyl alcohol 1 h before exposure. PABA esters in 2.5 percent concentration in ethanol are less effective than PABA. Most sunscreens should be reapplied after swimming or during prolonged sunbathing. In many instances patients may be exquisitely sensitive, irrespective of skin type, and they may require combination therapy with two or more sunscreens (preferably an opaque sunscreen). The drug-induced photosensitization reactions can be minimized or prevented by prescribing topical sunscreens containing benzophenones (Table 52-4). Sunscreens containing PABA or its derivatives should *not* be prescribed for individuals who are photosensitive to certain drugs and manifest phototoxic or cell-mediated delayed hypersensitivity reactions. In patients receiving antihypertensive thiazide diuretics or sulfonamides there may be a cross-reaction with PABA leading to eczematous dermatitis. These patients should be prescribed sunscreens containing benzophenones or opaque sunscreens containing zinc oxide, titanium oxide, and other light-scattering agents such as kaolin.

Individuals with acute sunburn reaction manifesting severe erythema, edema, and painful blistering reaction may be treated with systemic corticosteroids. Oral prednisone, beginning with 40 to 60 mg and tapering over 4 to 8 days, will help to control the severe sunburn reaction.

REFERENCES

MAGNUS IA: *Dermatological Photobiology.* Oxford, Blackwell, 1976

PARRISH JA et al: Photomedicine, in *Dermatology in General Medicine,* 2d ed, TB Fitzpatrick et al (eds). New York, McGraw-Hill, 1979

PATHAK MA et al (eds): *Sunlight and Man: Normal and Abnormal Photobiologic Responses.* Tokyo, University of Tokyo Press, 1974

——, EPSTEIN JH: Normal and abnormal reactions of man to light, in *Dermatology in General Medicine,* TB Fitzpatrick et al (eds). New York, McGraw-Hill, 1971

—— et al: Evaluation of topical agents that prevent sunburn. N Engl J Med 280:1459, 1969

section 10 | Hematologic alterations

53
PALLOR AND ANEMIA

H. FRANKLIN BUNN

PALLOR

Pallor is the physical finding most commonly associated with anemia. However, the usefulness of this sign is limited by other factors that affect the color of the skin. The thickness and texture of the skin vary widely among individuals. Furthermore, the blood flow to the skin can undergo wide fluctuations. Normal individuals will appear sallow when blood is shunted away from the skin, whereas anemic patients may appear flushed when overheated or during periods of excitement. The concentration of melanin in the epidermis is another important

determinant of skin color. Individuals with a fair complexion may look pale even though they are not anemic. Conversely, pallor is difficult to detect in deeply pigmented individuals. Furthermore, acquired disorders of melanin pigmentation (e.g., Addison's disease, hemochromatosis) or jaundice may interfere with detection of pallor. Nevertheless, even in blacks, the presence of anemia may be suspected by the color of the palms or of noncutaneous tissues such as oral mucous membranes, nail beds, and palpebral conjunctivas. The color of the creases of the palm is a useful sign. When they are as pale as the surrounding skin, the patient usually has a hemoglobin of less than 7 g per 100 ml.

Two factors contribute to the development of pallor in patients with anemia. There is, of course, a decrease in the hemoglobin concentration of blood perfusing the skin and mucous membranes. Also, blood is shunted away from the skin and other peripheral tissues, permitting enhanced blood flow to vital organs. Redistribution of blood flow is an important mode of compensation in anemia (see Fig. 53-5).

ANEMIA

By definition patients with anemia have a significant reduction in red cell mass and a corresponding decrease in the oxygen-carrying capacity of the blood. Normally, blood volume is maintained at a nearly constant level. Therefore, anemia entails a decrease in the concentration of red cells or hemoglobin in peripheral blood. Measuring the packed cell volume (PCV) or hematocrit is the simplest and one of the most precise ways to ascertain the concentration of red cells in the blood; the result is termed the *hematocrit*. Generally, a small sample of anticoagulated blood is drawn into a capillary tube which is sealed at one end and centrifuged. The PCV is the ratio of the volume of packed red cells to the total volume. Alternatively, the concentration of hemoglobin can be determined spectrophotometrically from the absorbance of the cyanmethemoglobin form at a specific wavelength. With the advent of automated red blood cell counting technology, very precise measurements became readily available in nearly all hospitals and well-equipped clinical laboratories. The electronic counter makes a direct measurement of the red cell count (RBC/µl) and the mean red cell volume (MCV):

$$MCV \text{ (fl)} = \frac{PCV \text{ (liters/liters)}}{(RBC/\mu l) \times 10^{-9}}$$

This instrument calculates the PCV from the direct measurement of MCV and RBC/µl. In addition, hemoglobin concentration is measured directly on a separate channel. The mean corpuscular hemoglobin concentration (MCHC) is then computed as follows:

$$MCHC \text{ (g per 100 ml)} = \frac{Hb \text{ (g per 100 ml)}}{PCV \text{ (liters/liters)}}$$

A third red blood cell index, the mean corpuscular hemoglobin (MCH), is determined as follows:

$$MCH \text{ (pg)} = \frac{Hb \text{ (g per 100 ml)}}{(RBC/\mu l) \times 10^{-7}}$$

Generally, an automated system provides a printout which includes hemoglobin concentration, red cell count, packed cell volume, and the three red cell indexes (MCV, MCHC, and MCH). Normal values for individuals of various ages are shown in the Appendix. In women in the childbearing age group the normal blood values are 10 percent lower than in men. At high altitudes, higher values are found, roughly in proportion to the elevation above sea level. Anemia may be defined as a reduction of more than 10 percent below the mean values for the sex. However, since the variations in normal hemoglobin values approach this limit, the documentation of mild anemia may be uncertain.

RED BLOOD CELL PRODUCTION   Red cells are derived from an undifferentiated progenitor cell in the bone marrow called the *pluripotent stem cell* (Fig. 53-1). A stem cell is one which is capable of both self-renewal and differentiation. *Pluripotent* implies that granulocytes, monocytes, and platelets also evolve from this ancestor cell. The pluripotent stem cell probably has the morphological characteristics of a mature lymphocyte. The control of proliferation into differentiated cell lines is poorly understood. Experiments have been hampered by difficulty in isolating early red cell precursors from the bone marrow. However, in the past 5 years, considerable advances have been made in culturing erythroid progenitor cells in vitro. As Fig. 53-1 shows, the most primitive erythroid progenitor which has been cultured from both bone marrow and peripheral blood is called the *erythroid burst-forming unit* (BFU$_e$). After 10 to 15 days in tissue culture it produces a large colony of recognizable red cell precursors. The BFU$_e$ is responsive only to high doses of the erythroid-promoting hormone, erythropoietin. A more developed cell, the *erythroid colony-forming unit* (CFU$_e$), develops a smaller clone of erythroid cells after 4 to 7 days in culture and is very sensitive to erythropoietin. A number of other factors have been proposed to influence erythroid cell differentiation including catecholamines, steroids, thyroid hormone, growth hormone, and cyclic nucleotides. In addition, helper T lymphocytes may also play a role. Well-designed experiments involving erythroid cells in culture should provide considerably more information about the mechanism underlying the differentiation and maturation of erythroid cells, as well as insights into certain disorders involving erythroid precursor cells.

Erythropoietin, a glycoprotein having a molecular weight of about 32,000 has been purified nearly to homogeneity. Original experiments indicated that this hormone is produced primarily by the kidneys. Alternatively, the kidneys may produce a substance, renal erythropoietic factor, which converts a biologically inactive plasma protein into erythropoietin, analogous to the formation of angiotensin. Erythropoietin production is stimulated by hypoxia. Currently, erythropoietin is

FIGURE 53-1
Differentiation and morphological maturation of erythroid cells. Erythroid cells are derived from pluripotent stem cells shown on left. Under the influence of erythropoietin, erythroid stem cells (BFU$_e$ → CFU$_e$) differentiate into proerythroblasts, the earliest recognizable red blood cell precursor in the bone marrow. During further maturation, globin mRNA accumulates, directing the cell to synthesize hemoglobin. (After Nienhuis and Benz.)

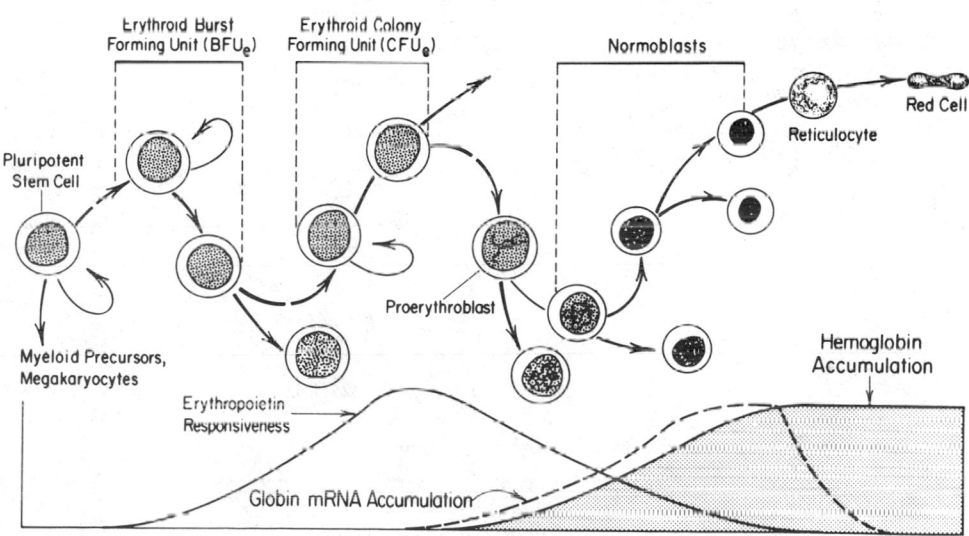

measured by rather crude bioassays. Its recent purification should permit the development of a more accurate and sensitive radioimmune assay. Reliable measurements of erythropoietin would have a number of diagnostic applications and also provide new information about the pathogenesis of several types of anemias.

Erythropoietin probably interacts with specific receptors on the surfaces of committed erythroid stem cells, inducing them to differentiate into pronormoblasts, the earliest red cell precursor that can be recognized on examination of the bone marrow. In addition, erythropoietin acts on later red cell precursors, stimulating cell division as well as hemoglobin synthesis. Normally the transition from the proerythroblast to the most mature normoblast involves three or four cell divisions over a 4-day period (Fig. 53-1). During this time, the nucleus becomes smaller, and an increasing amount of hemoglobin is produced in the cytoplasm. Following the last division, the pyknotic nucleus is removed from the normoblast, forming the reticulocyte which stays in the bone marrow for about two days. The reticulocyte is then released into the general circulation, where it remains for another 24 h before it loses its mitochondria and ribosomes and assumes the morphologic appearance of a mature red cell.

Erythroid precursor cells ranging from the pronormoblast to the reticulocyte possess a specific surface receptor for the iron-transferrin complex, enabling them to incorporate sufficient iron for hemoglobin production (Fig. 53-2). Normally, about 80 percent of circulating iron bound to plasma transferrin goes to erythroid cells in the marrow. After 4 to 6 days the iron reappears in circulating erythrocytes. The use of a radioactive iron label such as ^{59}Fe permits a quantitative assessment of erythropoiesis. From the rate at which injected ^{59}Fe-labeled transferrin disappears from the plasma, plasma iron turnover can be calculated. This parameter is generally proportional to the total developing erythroid cell mass. The extent to which circulating red cells acquire the label provides an index of the efficiency or effectiveness of erythropoiesis.

Under maximal stimulation, the normal marrow is capable of increasing its red cell production about six- to eightfold. As the erythroid marrow expands, fat is replaced by erythroid cells, and formerly inactive or "yellow" marrow becomes active or "red."

HEMOGLOBIN BIOSYNTHESIS Erythroid cell development is directed toward the production of hemoglobin-containing cells. About 98 percent of the protein in the cytoplasm of circulating red cells is hemoglobin. This protein is a tetramer composed of two pairs of polypeptide chains designated α, β, γ, and δ, each of which is covalently linked to a heme group. The synthesis of a particular globin subunit is directed by a corresponding gene inherited from each parent. As shown in Fig. 53-1, there is a marked amplification in the transcription of globin chain mRNA during the development of proerythroblasts.

In the red cells of normal adults, hemoglobin A ($\alpha_2\beta_2$) composes about 97 percent of the total hemoglobin. The remaining 3 percent is primarily hemoglobin A$_2$ ($\alpha_2\delta_2$). As discussed in Chap. 315, this minor component is increased in patients with β thalassemia. Hemoglobin F or fetal hemoglobin ($\alpha_2\gamma_2$) is found in trace amounts in adult red cells localized to about 1 to 7 percent of red cells. It is the main hemoglobin component of fetal red cells. During the last 3 months of gestation, γ-chain synthesis switches to β-chain synthesis. However, in certain types of congenital hemolytic anemias such as the β thalassemias and sickle-cell anemia, the production of γ chains (and therefore of hemoglobin F) persists. In addition, increased levels of hemoglobin F may also be encountered in certain acquired anemias in which there is disordered red cell proliferation.

Normally α- and β-chain synthesis in erythroid precursors is evenly balanced. The thalassemias (Chap. 315) are characterized by imbalance in globin chain synthesis.

The synthesis of *heme* in red cell precursors is closely matched to globin chain production. As shown in Fig. 53-3 the initial and rate-limiting step is the condensation of succinyl CoA and glycine to form δ-aminolevulinic acid. This reaction which takes place in mitochondria requires that glycine be activated by pyridoxal phosphate. Accordingly, patients with sideroblastic anemia in whom heme synthesis is usually defective may sometimes respond to pyridoxine therapy (Chap. 310). The next steps of heme synthesis take place in the cytosol. Two molecules of δ-aminolevulinic acid condense to form a ring structure, porphobilinogen. The concentration of this colorless pyrrole is elevated in acute intermittent porphyria and can be detected in urine by the Watson-Schwartz test. The subsequent steps in porphyrin synthesis are also shown in Fig. 53-3. The

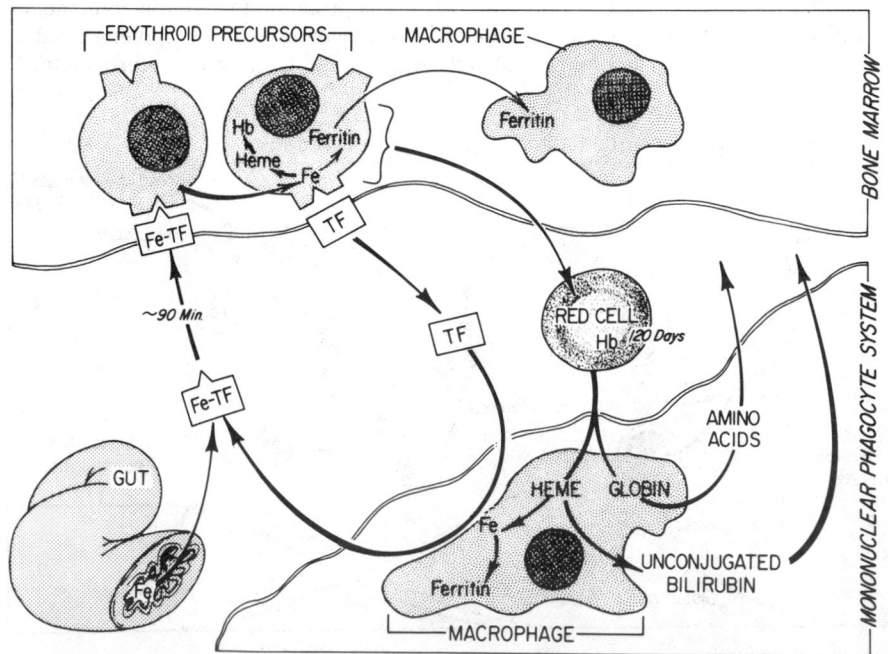

FIGURE 53-2

Erythrocyte production, circulation, and destruction. Circulating iron-bound transferrin (TF) is bound to specific receptors on the surface of red blood cell precursors in the marrow. Most of this iron is incorporated into hemoglobin; the remainder is stored as ferritin. Following maturation of the erythroid precursor, the nucleus is shed and the red blood cell emerges from the marrow into the plasma where it circulates for approximately 120 days. The senescent red blood cell is taken up by the mononuclear-macrophage system and is destroyed. The heme-iron is initially incorporated into ferritin. This storage iron is available for transport to the marrow via transferrin.

last three reactions take place in mitochondria. Iron is inserted into protoporphyrin IX to form heme. In iron deficiency, as well as in lead poisoning, increased levels of protoporphyrin can be detected in red cells. Disorders of porphyrin synthesis and metabolism are discussed in Chap. 96.

HEMOGLOBIN STRUCTURE AND FUNCTION The primary role of red cells is to transport oxygen from lungs to tissues and to transport carbon dioxide in the reverse direction. Both of these functions are assumed by hemoglobin. The three-dimensional structure of human hemoglobin has been determined from x-ray crystallographic analysis. The important functional properties of hemoglobin such as heme-heme interaction, the pH dependency of oxygen affinity (the Bohr effect), and the interaction with 2,3-diphosphoglycerate can now be understood on a stereochemical basis. This structural information has also been useful in explaining the abnormal functional properties of a number of human hemoglobin variants which are associated with clinical and hematologic manifestations (see Chap. 315).

During the circulation through the lungs, hemoglobin becomes almost fully saturated with oxygen (1.34 ml O_2 per gram of hemoglobin). As red cells perfuse the capillary beds, oxygen is extracted. Efficient unloading of oxygen at relatively high oxygen tensions is possible because of the sigmoid shape of the oxygen dissociation curve (heme-heme interaction) (see Fig. 53-4). The affinity of hemoglobin for oxygen is modified by three intracellular cofactors: hydrogen ion, carbon dioxide, and 2,3-diphosphoglycerate (2,3-DPG). Increasing concentrations of each of these three effectors results in a "shift to the right" in the oxygen dissociation curve. In human red cells, 2,3-DPG appears to be an important regulator of hemoglobin

function. One molecule of 2,3-DPG binds to the β chains of deoxyhemoglobin, thereby decreasing oxygen affinity. Elevated levels of 2,3-DPG have been noted in various states of hypoxia. The resulting decrease in oxygen affinity permits enhanced oxygen release. The oxygenation of a particular organ or tissue depends on three main factors (depicted in Fig. 53-5): blood flow, oxygen-carrying capacity of the blood (hemoglobin concentration), and the difference between arterial and venous oxygen saturation. The last factor is dependent on the shape and position of the oxygen dissociation curve. Patients with a primary abnormality of one of these three factors depend on adjustments in one or both of the other two in order to maintain optimal tissue oxygenation. For example, patients with anemia have two available modes of compensation: enhanced blood flow and decreased oxygen affinity, mediated by increased levels of 2,3-DPG. Conversely, individuals with a hemoglobin variant having increased oxygen affinity have a primary defect in oxygen unloading. As discussed in Chap. 315, such patients compensate by developing secondary erythrocytosis.

RED BLOOD CELL METABOLISM As the red cell emerges from the bone marrow, it loses its nucleus, ribosomes, and mitochondria and therefore all capability for cell division, protein synthesis, and oxidative phosphorylation. Compared with other cells, the erythrocyte has a rather simple scheme of intermediary metabolism. Glucose is virtually the only fuel utilized

FIGURE 53-3

The biosynthesis of heme. The following abbreviations are used: CoA, coenzyme A; GTP, guanosine triphosphate; GDP, guanosine diphosphate; Pi, inorganic phosphorus; GSH, glutathione; Δ-ALA-DH, Δ-aminolevulinate dehydrase; UIS, uroporphyrinogen I synthetase; UIII CoS, uroporphyrinogen III cosynthetase; UD, uroporphyrinogen decarboxylase; CO, coproporphyrinogen oxidase; HS, heme synthetase. Enzymatic steps that occur in mitochondria are shown.

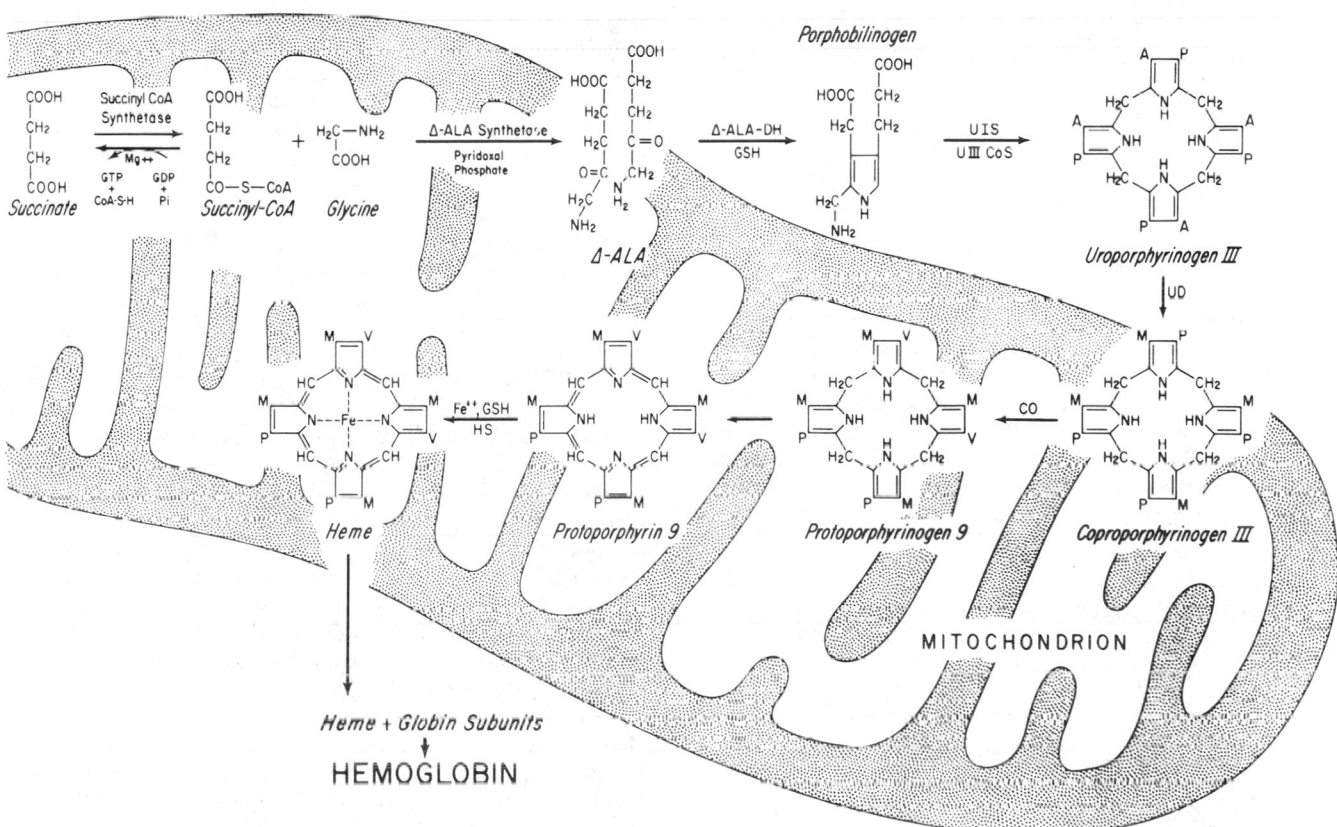

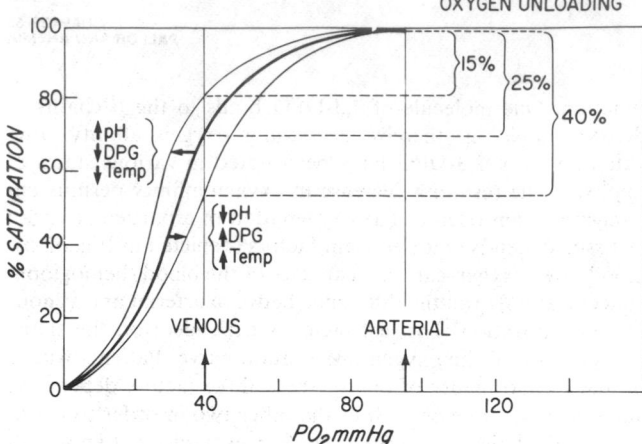

OXYGEN UNLOADING

FIGURE 53-4

The oxyhemoglobin dissociation curve of normal blood. The major factors influencing the position of the curve are pH, temperature, and the intracellular concentration of 2,3-DPG. An increase in plasma pH or a decrease in temperature and 2,3-DPG causes an increase in oxygen affinity (shift to the left) and a relative decrease in oxygen unloading when going from an arterial P_{O_2} of 95 mmHg to a venous P_{O_2} of 40 mmHg. Conversely, a decrease in pH or an increase in temperature and 2,3-DPG causes a decrease in oxygen affinity (shift to the right) and a relative increase in oxygen unloading.

by the red cell. It readily enters the red cell by facilitated diffusion and is then phosphorylated to glucose 6-phosphate. There are two major pathways available for glucose 6-phosphate (Fig. 314-2). About 80 to 90 percent of this intermediate is converted to lactate by means of the glycolytic (or Embden-Meyerhof) pathway. Two moles of adenosine triphosphate (ATP) are generated for every mole of glucose that is metabolized. The intracellular mediator of hemoglobin function, 2,3-diphosphoglycerate, is synthesized in a side reaction shown in Fig. 314-2. About 10 percent of intracellular glucose 6-phosphate may undergo oxidation by means of the hexose-monophosphate shunt. This pathway maintains glutathione in the reduced form, thereby protecting sulfhydryl groups in hemoglobin and the red cell membrane from oxidation by peroxides and superoxide as well as by certain drugs and toxins. Such oxidant stress can compromise red cell function and viability in patients with a deficiency in glucose 6-phosphate dehydro-

FIGURE 53-5

Oxygen delivered to an organ or tissue is directly proportional to (1) blood flow, (2) hemoglobin concentration, and (3) the difference in oxygen saturation of the arterial and venous blood. Patients with various types of hypoxia may compensate in the following ways: (1) The distribution of blood flow is altered to maintain oxygenation of vital organs; total cardiac output increases when hypoxia is severe. (2) Increased erythropoietin production stimulates erythropoiesis. (3) Oxygen unloading is enhanced by a shift to the right in the oxygen dissociation curve, mediated by red blood cell pH and 2,3-DPG.

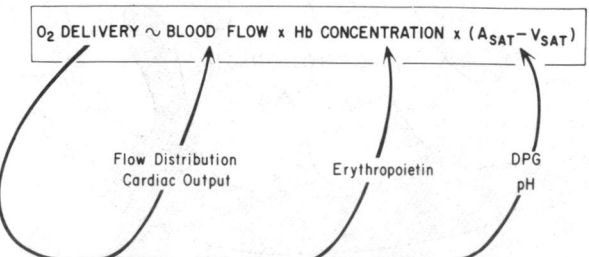

genase, the first enzymatic step in the hexose monophosphate shunt (see Chap. 314). Less commonly, individuals may have a deficiency in one of the enzymes of the glycolytic pathway or in one of the other enzymes of the hexose monophosphate shunt.

The red cell has rather modest metabolic obligations in keeping with its simplified structure. A significant portion of the ATP generated by glycolysis is spent in operating the sodium-potassium pump, necessary to preserve the ionic milieu in the cytoplasm and prevent colloid osmotic lysis. In addition, some metabolic energy is expended on maintenance and repair of the red cell membrane. Certain proteins in the membrane become phosphorylated by means of ATP and protein kinases, but the physiologic significance of this process is not yet understood. Finally, a small amount of metabolic currency is spent on maintaining hemoglobin iron atoms in the reduced form (Fe^{2+}).

The 120-day survival of the circulating red cell is dependent on preservation of the pliability of its membrane. The red cell membrane is composed of 50 percent protein, 40 percent lipid, and 10 percent carbohydrate. According to the most widely accepted model, it is a bilayer consisting of molecules of phospholipid and cholesterol in a 1.2:1 molar ratio oriented in a stacked array so that the hydrophobic portions of the molecules are oriented toward the interior while the polar side groups are either on the external surface of the cell (the plasma membrane) or on the inner cytoplasmic surface (see Fig. 53-6). The distribution of phospholipids differs significantly in the two portions of the bilayer. The outer surface is relatively rich in lecithin and sphingomyelin while the inner surface has relatively more phosphatidyl serine and phosphatidyl ethanolamine. The lipids on the outer surface exchange freely with plasma lipids.

The red cell membrane contains about eight major proteins (depicted in Fig. 53-6) and a large number of minor components. These proteins can be divided into two groups. A few span the lipid bilayer so that one end of the polypeptide is on the external cell surface and the other is on the inner surface. Examples include glycophorin which contains a number of polysaccharide blood group antigens and band 3, which serves as a channel for the passage of anions in and out of the red cell. Other proteins bind only to the inner surface of the red cell membrane. These include several enzymes as well as two structural proteins, spectrin and actin, which interact to form a meshwork that laminates the cytoplasmic surface of the membrane.

It is likely that the physiologic demise of 120-day-old red cells is due to a loss of membrane flexibility preventing them from negotiating the narrow-bore channels of the microcirculation including the sinusoids of the spleen. The factors responsible for red cell senescence are poorly understood. Experimental evidence indicates that deterioration of the red cell's metabolic machinery, sufficient to deplete it of ATP, can cause the cell to become spiculated (ecchinocytic) and lose its normal pliability. Depletion of ATP disrupts the spectrin and actin meshwork lining the inner membrane surface, resulting in aggregation of these proteins. Other factors such as enhanced rigidity due to accumulation of calcium and, perhaps, alterations in charge on the external surface of the membrane may also contribute to the recognition of the senescent red cell by the mononuclear-phagocyte system. In contrast to normal red cells, there is a large and well-documented body of information on the mechanisms responsible for red cell destruction in various hemolytic anemias. These will be discussed in Chap. 314.

Once the senescent red cell is sequestered (Fig. 53-2), hemoglobin is readily catabolized. Amino acids are released by proteolytic digestion and subsequently neutralized or metabolized. The heme group is catabolized by a microsomal oxidizing system. The porphyrin ring is converted to bile pigments which are excreted almost quantitatively by the liver. One mole of carbon monoxide is formed per mole of heme that is broken down. Measurement of endogenous carbon monoxide production is a rather precise indication of erythroid cell destruction. As Fig. 53-2 shows, the iron that is released during heme catabolism may be initially incorporated into the storage protein, ferritin, but it is eventually transported to marrow erythroid precursors by transferrin, the plasma-iron-binding protein.

If red cell production is disordered, there may be significant destruction of erythroid cells within the bone marrow. A number of anemias are characterized by *ineffective erythropoiesis*, particularly those in which erythroid maturation is morphologically abnormal and the circulating red cells are abnormal in size. Examples discussed in detail elsewhere include megaloblastic anemias, sideroblastic anemias, and β-thalassemia major. Such disorders are characterized by erythroid hyperplasia in the bone marrow and rapid uptake of labeled iron into the marrow but a low recovery of the labeled iron in circulating red cells. Endogenous carbon monoxide production and plasma levels of unconjugated bilirubin are generally elevated in ineffective erythropoiesis.

SIGNS AND SYMPTOMS OF ANEMIA The clinical presentation of the anemic patient depends on the underlying disease as well as on the severity and chronicity of the anemia. The manifestations of anemia per se can be explained by the pathophysiologic principles outlined in this chapter. Most of these signs and symptoms represent cardiovascular and ventilatory adjustments which compensate for the decrease in red cell mass.

The degree to which symptoms occur in an anemic patient depends on several contributing factors. If the anemia has developed rapidly, there may not be adequate time for compensatory adjustments to take place, and the patient may have more marked symptoms than if an anemia of equivalent severity had developed insidiously. Furthermore, the patient's complaints may depend on the presence of local vascular disease. For example, angina pectoris, intermittent claudication, or transient cerebral ischemia may be unmasked by the development of anemia.

Individuals with mild anemia are often asymptomatic.

They may complain of fatigue as well as dyspnea and palpitation, particularly following exercise. Severely anemic patients will often be symptomatic at rest and unable to tolerate significant exertion. When the hemoglobin concentration falls below 7.5 g per 100 ml, resting cardiac output rises significantly with an increase in both heart rate and stroke volume. The patient may be aware of this hyperdynamic state and complain of palpitation or a pounding pulse. Symptoms of cardiac failure may develop if the patient's myocardial reserve is reduced.

The clinical manifestations of severe anemia extend to other organ systems. Patients often complain of dizziness and headache and may experience syncope, tinnitus, or vertigo. Many patients are irritable and have difficulty sleeping or concentrating. Because of decreased blood flow to the skin, patients may become hypersensitive to cold. Gastrointestinal symptoms such as anorexia, indigestion, and even nausea or bowel irregularity are attributable to shunting of blood away from the splanchnic bed. Females commonly develop abnormal menstruation, both amenorrhea and increased bleeding. Males may complain of impotence or loss of libido.

The *physical findings* associated with anemia include pallor, discussed at the beginning of the chapter, tachycardia, wide pulse pressure, and a hyperdynamic precordium. A systolic ejection murmur is often heard over the precordium, particularly at the pulmonic area. In addition, a venous hum may be detected over the neck vessels. These cardiac findings disappear when the anemia is corrected. Patients with hemolytic anemia often have icterus and splenomegaly and occasionally develop superficial skin ulceration over the ankle bones.

APPROACH TO THE PATIENT WITH ANEMIA

In evaluating the anemic patient, the physician should proceed in an orderly fashion so that the correct diagnosis can be established with a minimum of laboratory tests and procedures. As in other clinical disciplines, a comprehensive history and meticulous physical examination are of paramount importance in

FIGURE 53-6
Diagram of a cross section of the red blood cell membrane. Spectrin and actin form a meshwork which laminates the inner surface of the membrane. Several other proteins of varying sizes including the enzyme glyceraldehyde 3-phosphate dehydrogenase (G3PD) also bind to the inner surface. In contrast, other proteins such as the glycophorins A and B (GP–A and GP–B) and the anion transport protein traverse the lipid bilayer.

Long polysaccharide chains are covalently attached to these proteins on the outer surface of the cell and also to glycolipid. Phospholipids include phosphatidyl choline (PC) and sphingomyelin (SM), which are located primarily on the outer surface of the membrane, and phosphatidyl serine (PS) and phosphatidyl ethanolamine (PE), which are located primarily on the inner surface of the membrane. (This figure was prepared by Dr. Samuel Lux IV.)

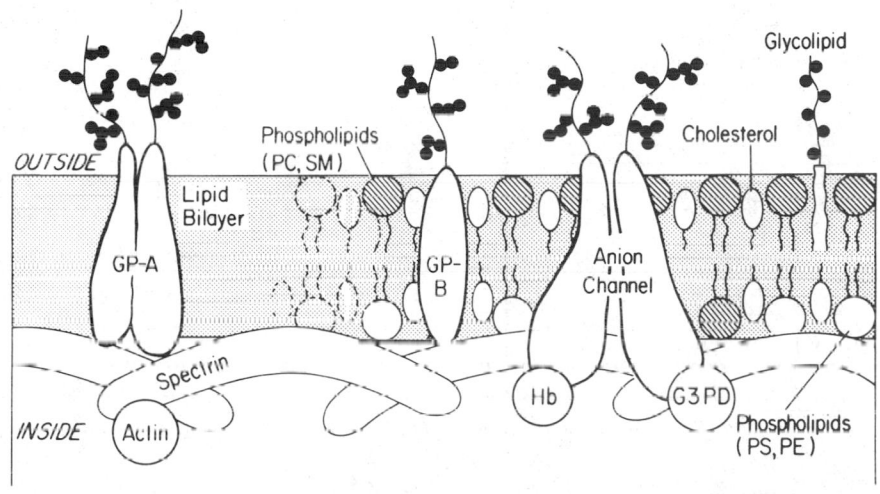

the initial work-up of the anemic patient. For example, a family history which reveals a dominant inheritance pattern provides strong support for the diagnosis of hereditary spherocytosis. The discovery of a heart murmur and splenomegaly raises the possibility that the anemic patient may have subacute bacterial endocarditis.

The work-up of the anemic patient should be based on a firm understanding of the pathophysiologic principles outlined earlier in this chapter. Table 53-1 shows an overview of the laboratory tests that are useful in the diagnosis of anemias. The clinician must first ask whether the anemia is due to a decreased production of red cells or enhanced destruction. In addition, the possibility of blood loss either as the sole etiology or as a contributing factor must always be considered. At this crossroad, laboratory information can be gathered which will establish whether the patient is failing to produce an adequate number of red cells or is undergoing accelerated cell breakdown.

The *reticulocyte count* is the most useful laboratory test in answering this question. When an appropriate supravital stain is applied to a sample of peripheral blood, the 1- to 2-day-old red cells exhibit a network of purple strands, which are aggregates of ribosomes. On a routinely prepared peripheral smear, these young red cells appear larger than average and have a purplish hue, so-called polychromatophilia. Reticulocytosis is a reflection of the release of an increased number of young cells from the bone marrow. The degree of increased erythropoiesis can be assessed more quantitatively by determining the

reticulocyte index, which uses the hematocrit or PCV and is calculated as follows:

$$\text{Reticulocyte index} = \text{reticulocyte \%} \times \frac{\text{patient's PCV}}{\text{normal PCV}}$$

This measure fails to consider the distribution of reticulocytes between the bone marrow and the peripheral blood. When the marrow is greatly stimulated, marrow reticulocytes enter the circulation prematurely. Since the circulation of these "shift reticulocytes" in the peripheral blood is prolonged, the reticulocyte index should be divided by 2. This correction should always be made if normoblasts are encountered in the peripheral blood since this finding indicates the premature release of red cell precursors into the circulation.

A failure to produce red cells is reflected in an inappropriately low reticulocyte count. In contrast, a significant elevation of reticulocytes is suggestive of hemolysis. Exceptions include (1) the brisk reticulocyte response that is seen in a patient with hemorrhage, (2) reticulocytosis encountered in patients recovering from a suppression of erythropoiesis (e.g., an individual with pernicious anemia who received an injection of vitamin B_{12} 1 week earlier), and (3) mild to moderate elevations in reticulocytes (3 to 7 percent) encountered in myelophthisic anemia in which cells may be prematurely released because of irritative foci within the bone marrow such as tumor or granulomata. These exceptions are often readily appreciated in the initial evaluation of the patient. Furthermore, a number of ancillary laboratory tests described below are useful in determining to what extent hemolysis is occurring. The measurement of unconjugated bilirubin in the serum is a particularly

TABLE 53-1
Laboratory evaluation of anemias

	Reticulocytes	Peripheral smear	Marrow	Additional lab tests	Diagnosis
↓ Hematocrit	Normal, decreased	Hypochromic: Microcytic	0 Iron	↓ Fe, ↑ TIBC	Iron deficiency
			+ Iron	↑ Hb A₂, ↑ Hb F	β thalassemia
			Ring sideroblasts	↓ Hb A₂	Sideroblastic anemia
		Macrocytic	Megaloblastic	↓ Serum B₁₂ achlorhydria	Vitamin B₁₂ deficiency, pernicious anemia
				↓ Serum folate	Folic acid deficiency
		Normochromic: Normocytic	Normal	↓ Fe, ↓ TIBC	Anemia of chronic inflammation
				↑ Creatinine	Anemia of uremia
				Abnormal LFT	Anemia of liver disease
				↓ T₄	Anemia of myxedema
			Aplastic		Aplastic anemia
		Normoblasts, teardrops	Infiltrated: Tumor, lymphoma, etc.		Myelophthisic
			Fibrosis	↑ LAP	Myeloid metaplasia
	Increased	Polychromatophilia +	Erythroid hyperplasia	+ Sucrose lysis	Paroxysmal nocturnal hemoglobinuria
		Schistocytes, helmet cells			Traumatic hemolytic anemia
		Spherocytes		+ Coombs' test	Immunohemolytic anemia
				↑ Osmotic fragility	Hereditary spherocytosis
		Spur cells		Abnormal LFT	Spur-cell anemia
		Sickle cells		Positive sickle prep	Sickle-cell syndromes
		Target cells		Abnormal Hb electrophoresis	Hb C, D, etc.
		Heinz bodies		Abnormal Hb electrophoresis	Congenital Heinz body hemolytic anemia
				↓ G6PD	G6PD deficiency
				Blood in stomach, stool	Blood loss anemia

NOTE: *Fe, iron; TIBC, total iron-binding capacity; Hb, hemoglobin; LAP, leukocyte alkaline phosphatase; G6PD, glucose 6-phosphate dehydrogenase, LFT, liver function tests.*

useful guide to the presence of accelerated red blood cell breakdown. Once this information is obtained, the work-up can be directed toward the establishment of a specific etiology.

Four additional base-line studies are of critical importance in the initial work-up of the patient with anemia: *measurement of red cell indexes, examination of the peripheral blood smear, testing the stool for occult blood,* and, in many patients, *bone marrow examination.*

RED CELL INDEXES   As Table 53-2 shows, two indexes, the MCV and MCHC, are particularly useful in classifying the anemias due to decreased red cell production. Microcytic, hypochromic anemias have low values for MCV. On microscopic examination, the red cells appear small and pale. In contrast, in the macrocytic anemias the MCV is elevated and large oval cells (macroovalocytes) are seen on microscopic examination. Unlike the anemias of underproduction, nearly all the hemolytic anemias are normochromic and normocytic. Exceptions include the severe forms of thalassemias in which hypochromic microcytic red cells are accompanied by brisk hemolysis. In addition, hereditary spherocytosis is the one commonly encountered hemolytic anemia in which red cells are hyperchromic with a significantly increased MCHC.

EXAMINATION OF THE BLOOD SMEAR   In the evaluation of patients with anemia, the physician should take the time to examine a well-stained peripheral blood film. Plate 9 shows examples of abnormalities in red cell morphology encountered in various types of anemia. Many subtleties escape the attention of the technologist whose primary purpose in examining the slide is to obtain a white cell differential count. Furthermore, the clinician can approach the specimen with a prepared mind and can scrutinize it for specific abnormalities. As suggested above, the examination can confirm the size and color of red cells as estimated by RBC indexes. Furthermore, while these indexes provide mean statistical values, the microscopic examination can reveal variation in red cell size (anisocytosis) or shape (poikilocytosis), changes which are helpful in the diagnosis of specific anemias. Examination of the blood smear is particularly important in evaluating a patient with hemolysis. Most hemolytic anemias have characteristic morphologic abnormalities. Finally, this practice may yield unexpected dividends. The finding of rouleaux may indicate the presence of dysproteinemia as occurs in multiple myeloma. The examination may provide the initial clue that the patient has significant thrombocytopenia.

TABLE 53-2
Anemias due to decreased red cell production

   I Microcytic-hypochromic anemias
     A Iron deficiency (Chap. 310)
     B Sideroblastic anemias (Chap. 310)
     C Thalassemias (Chap. 314)
  II Macrocytic (megaloblastic) anemias (Chap. 311)
     A Vitamin B_{12} deficiency, including pernicious anemia
     B Folic acid deficiency
     C Others: Drug-induced, orotic aciduria, some refractory anemias, erythroleukemia
 III Normocytic-normochromic anemias
     A Primary bone marrow failure (Chap. 312)
       1 Aplastic anemia
         (rare: pure red cell anemia)
       2 Myelophthisic anemias: leukemia and lymphoma, other neoplasms, myelofibrosis, granulomas
     B Secondary anemias (Chap. 313)
       1 Anemias of chronic inflammation
         (infections, connective tissue disorders, etc.)
       2 Anemia of uremia
       3 Anemias associated with endocrinopathies
       4 Anemia of chronic liver disease

BONE MARROW EXAMINATION   A microscopic examination of the bone marrow is generally indicated in the work-up of any *unexplained* anemia. The more severe the anemia, the more likely that the procedure will be informative. An assessment of the quantity and quality of red cell precursors may determine whether there is a primary defect in cell production. A marrow biopsy is particularly useful in estimating overall cellularity. The normal differential of nucleated cells in the marrow is shown in the Appendix. The ratio of myeloid (M) to erythroid (E) precursors is normally 3:1. The ratio is increased in patients with infection, a leukemoid reaction, or neoplastic proliferation of myeloid cells. Rarely, a high M:E ratio is due to selective aplasia of the red cell precursors. A decreased M:E ratio indicates erythroid hyperplasia (seen in hemolysis or hemorrhage) or ineffective erythropoiesis (megaloblastic and sideroblastic anemias). The morphology of the precursors may reveal a maturation deficit such as megaloblastic anemia. The bone marrow examination is also important in demonstrating the presence of cellular infiltrates such as those found in leukemia, lymphoma, or multiple myeloma. The demonstration of tumor, fibrosis, or granulomata usually requires a biopsy. A portion of the marrow specimen should routinely be stained with Prussian blue. In addition to providing an assessment of iron stores, the iron stain is required for the identification of sideroblasts.

ANEMIA DUE TO BLOOD LOSS   This form of anemia varies considerably in its clinical presentation depending upon the site, severity, and rapidity of the hemorrhage. At opposite extremes are acute fulminant bleeding producing hypovolemic shock and chronic occult blood loss leading to iron-deficiency anemia.

Patients who have sustained an acute hemorrhage generally present with signs and symptoms secondary to hypoxia and hypovolemia. Depending on the severity of the process, the patient will have weakness, fatigue, light-headedness, stupor, or coma. He will often appear pale, diaphoretic, and irritable. Vital signs are a reflection of cardiovascular compensation to the acute blood loss. The patient will have hypotension and tachycardia in proportion to the degree of hemorrhage. Elicitation of postural signs is useful in the initial evaluation of patients with acute blood loss. If the pulse rises 25 percent or more, or the systolic blood pressure falls 20 torr or more upon going from a supine to sitting position, the patient is likely to have significant hypovolemia (blood loss > 1000 ml) and requires prompt replacement. Acute blood loss in excess of 1500 ml usually leads to cardiovascular collapse.

If the blood loss has been acute and recent, the peripheral blood may not reveal a significant decrease in packed cell volume or hemoglobin, since the red cell mass and plasma volume are contracted in parallel. There often is a moderate leukocytosis and a "shift to the left" in the white cell differential count. Thrombocytosis may be encountered in both acute and chronic blood loss. During the first few days following an acute hemorrhage there is usually an increase in reticulocytes. Occasionally nucleated red cells may appear in the peripheral blood. Since young red cells are larger than old ones, the patient may develop slightly macrocytic red cell indexes (MCV = 100 to 105 fl). As mentioned above, sustained reticulocytosis will be seen if significant blood loss continues, until iron stores have been exhausted. Internal bleeding may be accompanied by an increase in unconjugated bilirubin and even in methemalbumin (see below). These abnormalities are a reflection of an increase in catabolism of heme from extravasated red cells.

Patients with large amounts of blood in the gut will often have an elevation of blood urea nitrogen.

It is of critical importance to assess these patients promptly and institute treatment without delay. A large-bore intravenous line should be placed. While blood is being typed and cross matched, saline, Ringer's lactate, or, preferably, a colloid such as 5% albumin should be infused to correct hypovolemia. Whole blood is then administered as soon as it is available. Monitoring of vital signs and central venous pressure is useful in determining the appropriate amount of volume replacement. During and following these emergency measures, diagnostic studies may reveal the site or sites of bleeding. If there appears to be generalized hemorrhage from skin, mucous membranes, urine, etc., an emergency coagulation profile should be obtained. Demonstration of bleeding from the gastrointestinal tract may require the insertion of a nasogastric tube. Appropriate radiologic studies may be indicated to determine sites of internal bleeding such as retroperitoneal hemorrhage.

Chronic blood loss is usually due to lesions in the gastrointestinal tract or the uterus. The testing of stool specimens for occult blood is an essential, though frequently overlooked, part of the evaluation of anemia. It may be necessary to examine serial specimens over a prolonged period of time since gastrointestinal bleeding is often intermittent. The hematologic manifestations of chronic blood loss are those of iron-deficiency anemia, discussed in detail in Chap. 310.

ANEMIAS DUE TO DECREASED RBC PRODUCTION As shown in Table 53-2, red cell indexes are useful in classifying the anemias due to underproduction of red cells. They can be conveniently grouped into three major categories: microcytic-hypochromic, macrocytic (normochromic), and normocytic-normochromic.

The *microcytic-hypochromic* anemias include iron-deficiency anemia (Chap. 310), some sideroblastic anemias (Chap. 310), and the thalassemias (Chap. 314). Collectively, they represent a decrease in the availability or synthesis of one of the three major constituents of the hemoglobin molecule: iron, porphyrin, and globin. Since hemoglobin composes over 90 percent of the protein within the erythrocyte, it is not surprising that these defects in hemoglobin synthesis result in the formation of small, pale red cells. As mentioned above, these disorders involve a variable degree of ineffective erythropoiesis. In addition, the anemias of chronic inflammation and malignancy may be slightly microcytic and hypochromic (Chap. 313). This phenomenon may be due to a poorly understood defect in the availability of iron. However, these disorders are more often normocytic-normochromic and have been so classified in Table 53-2. As shown in Table 53-1, measurement of serum iron and iron-binding capacity and evaluation of marrow iron stores are particularly useful in distinguishing between these anemias.

The *macrocytic* anemias generally are associated with megaloblastic morphology in the bone marrow. In most cases, a deficiency of either vitamin B_{12} or folic acid results in an impairment of the replication of DNA, particularly in cells having a high turnover rate. Because nuclear maturation lags behind cytoplasmic development, large red cells tend to be produced in the bone marrow. Megaloblastic anemias are discussed in detail in Chap. 311. Like the microcytic-hypochromic anemias, these disorders are maturation defects associated with ineffective erythropoiesis. Macrocytosis, generally of a lesser degree, may also be encountered in patients with liver disease and hypothyroidism. However, in these two conditions, the red cell precursors in the bone marrow do not appear megaloblastic. The macrocytes in liver disease and hypothy-

roidism may be related to an increased deposition of lipid in the red cell membrane.

The *normocytic-normochromic* anemias of underproduction[1] comprise a diverse group of disorders. As shown in Table 53-2, this group can be conveniently subdivided into two categories: those due to intrinsic pathology within the bone marrow and those secondary to some other underlying disease.

The primary disorders of the bone marrow are best approached by microscopic examination of a marrow aspirate. In addition, biopsy of the bone marrow is particularly useful in the evaluation of these patients. For example, a biopsy may reveal the presence of fibrosis, granulomata, or tumor deposits which may not be detected in a marrow aspirate. This group of anemias is often accompanied by leukopenia and thrombocytopenia. Pancytopenia, usually to a lesser degree, can also be seen in hypersplenism and in the megaloblastic anemias. Aplastic anemia and the myelophthisic anemias are discussed in Chap. 312.

The diagnosis of anemia secondary to some underlying disease is usually quite straightforward. Conversely, the presence of an unexplained normocytic-normochromic anemia should prompt the search for an underlying disorder such as chronic renal failure, infection, or myxedema. If the presence of such an illness is established, the physician is obliged to investigate whether other factors such as blood loss or a nutritional deficiency contribute to the patient's anemia. Generally, the anemias due to liver disease, chronic inflammation, or an endocrinopathy are of only moderate severity. Unlike the other "secondary" anemias, that due to chronic renal failure can be severe. All these anemias are discussed in more detail in Chap. 313.

HEMOLYTIC ANEMIAS Hemolytic anemias are encountered much less frequently than the anemias due to decreased red cell production. Although they are a diverse group, the hemolytic anemias have a number of clinical features in common. Signs and symptoms of patients with hemolysis are discussed above.

A number of laboratory tests are available to establish the presence of accelerated breakdown of red cells. This group of tests, shown in Table 53-3, is useful in determining the extent of hemolysis but provides no information on specific etiology.

[1] *As mentioned above, the hemolytic anemias are also normocytic-normochromic.*

TABLE 53-3
Laboratory evaluation of hemolysis

	Moderate hemolysis (RBC life span 20–60 days)	Severe hemolysis (RBC life span 5–20 days)
HEMATOLOGIC		
Routine blood film	Polychromato-philia	Polychromato-philia
Reticulocyte index	↑	↑↑
Bone marrow examination	Erythroid hyperplasia	Erythroid hyperplasia
PLASMA OR SERUM		
Bilirubin	↑ Unconjugated	↑ Unconjugated
Haptoglobin	↓, absent	Absent
Hemopexin	Normal, ↓	↓, absent
Plasma hemoglobin	↑	↑↑
Lactate dehydrogenase	↑ (variable)	↑↑ (variable)
Methemalbumin	0	+ (intravascular)
URINE		
Bilirubin	0	0
Urobilinogen	Variable	Variable
Hemosiderin	0	+
Hemoglobin	0	+ (intravascular)

As mentioned previously, the reticulocyte count is the single most useful test in the initial work-up. Patients with hemolytic anemia generally have a brisk reticulocytosis. The bone marrow predictably reveals erythroid hyperplasia. Since it seldom provides useful additional information, a bone marrow examination is generally not indicated in the evaluation of a patient with hemolytic anemia, unless an associated disorder such as lymphoma is suspected.

A variety of serum tests are useful in establishing the presence of hemolysis (see Table 53-3), among them the test for bilirubin, a tetrapyrrole formed from the oxidative catabolism of heme. *Unconjugated* or *"indirect" bilirubin* circulates in the plasma in transit from the mononuclear-phagocyte system to the liver where it is conjugated. When measured accurately, unconjugated bilirubin is a very reliable guide to the presence of increased heme catabolism and is predictably elevated in patients with hemolysis. The serum level of conjugated or "direct" bilirubin is normal unless the patient has associated hepatic or biliary dysfunction. Unconjugated bilirubin is also increased in patients with ineffective erythropoiesis where there is enhanced destruction of red cell precursors within the bone marrow. Since circulating unconjugated bilirubin is tightly bound to albumin, it does not pass through renal glomeruli. Thus, patients with hemolytic anemia have acholuric jaundice, whereas the hyperbilirubinemia of liver disease is associated with bilirubin in the urine.

Other serum tests are also useful in the assessment of hemolysis. *Haptoglobin* is an α globulin which is present in high concentration (~100 mg per 100 ml) in the plasma (and serum). It binds specifically and tightly to the protein (globin) in hemoglobin. The hemoglobin-haptoglobin complex is cleared within minutes by the mononuclear-phagocyte system, while free haptoglobin has a prolonged circulation time ($T_{1/2}$ = 4 days). Thus, patients with significant hemolysis, either intravascular or extravascular, have low or absent levels of serum haptoglobin. Haptoglobin synthesis is decreased in patients with hepatocellular disease. Conversely, synthesis is enhanced in inflammatory states. Haptoglobin, like $α_1$-antitrypsin, orosomucoid, and the third component of complement are acute phase reactants. These facts must be considered in the interpretation of serum haptoglobin. *Hemopexin* is a plasma β globulin which binds specifically to heme. It becomes depleted in patients with moderate and severe hemolysis. The usefulness of the test is limited by the fact that in vitro hemolysis during the collection of the specimen will give a falsely elevated result. In addition to that bound by hemopexin, some of the heme from circulating free hemoglobin is transferred to albumin, resulting in the formation of *methemalbumin*. This complex is encountered only in severe intravascular hemolysis.

The urine should be tested in patients suspected of having intravascular hemolysis. Once the haptoglobin binding capacity of the plasma is exceeded, free hemoglobin will permeate renal glomeruli, primarily as αβ dimers with a molecular weight of 32,000. This filtered hemoglobin is reabsorbed by the proximal tubule. The molecule is catabolized in situ, and the heme iron is incorporated into storage proteins, ferritin and hemosiderin. The presence of hemosiderin in the urine, detected by staining the sediment with Prussian blue, indicates that a significant amount of circulating free hemoglobin has been filtered by the kidneys. When the absorptive capacity of the tubular cells is exceeded, hemoglobinuria will ensue. The presence of hemoglobinuria indicates severe intravascular hemolysis. Sometimes the clinician is faced with the dilemma of whether benzidine-positive heme pigment in the urine is hemoglobin or myoglobin. The easiest way to distinguish between these alternatives is to examine an anticoagulated blood specimen after centrifugation. Patients with myoglobinuria have normal-appearing plasma. Conversely, the plasma of patients with hemoglobinuria always has a reddish brown color. Be-

cause of its higher molecular weight, hemoglobin has a lower glomerular permeability than myoglobin and is less rapidly cleared by the kidneys.

Tagging red cells with an appropriate isotopic label provides the most direct and precise measure of cell survival. The most commonly used labels are sodium [^{51}Cr]chromate and diisopropylfluoro[^{32}P]phosphate. Such studies are not necessary or indicated in the diagnostic work up of the majority of patients with hemolytic anemia. However, scanning with a collumnated detector can be employed to monitor the sequestration of ^{51}Cr-tagged red cells in the liver and spleen. This approach has proved useful in evaluating patients for possible splenectomy.

Classification of hemolytic anemias A large battery of laboratory tests is available for establishing the specific diagnosis in a patient with hemolytic anemia. No other area of internal medicine is better suited to detailed and fruitful diagnostic probing. In the interest of time and money, the clinician should use the available tests in an orderly fashion. This complex group of disorders is easier to approach diagnostically if a concise and workable classification is used. The hemolytic anemias can be grouped in several ways: congenital versus acquired, intracorpuscular versus extracorpuscular, or by anatomic site of the erythrocyte defect. In Table 53-4, all three ways of classifying these anemias are shown. As stressed earlier in this chapter, the laboratory work-up should begin with careful scrutiny of a well-stained peripheral blood smear. All the hemolytic anemias are normocytic-normochromic except for the thalassemias. However, many of the hemolytic anemias have characteristic red cell morphology. Often the information gleaned from a careful history and physical examination coupled with an inspection of the blood film is sufficient to suggest a working diagnosis which can then be confirmed by appropriate laboratory tests. In this way, a large number of unnecessary diagnostic studies can be circumvented. The various kinds of hemolytic anemia are discussed in Chap. 314.

THERAPEUTIC CONSIDERATIONS The effective treatment of anemia, like other disorders, is predicated upon a thorough diagnostic evaluation. There is no reason to administer hematinics such as iron, vitamin B_{12}, or folic acid unless a specific deficiency of these substances has been demonstrated or is anticipated. Although the indiscriminate administration of vitamin B_{12} is not deleterious per se, it lulls both the patient and the physician into false security. In contrast, the inappropriate use of iron preparations over a prolonged period of time can be

TABLE 53-4
Hemolytic anemias

Extracorpuscular	*I* Environmental factors
	  A Antibody: Immunohemolytic anemias
	  B Mechanical trauma: Microangiopathic hemolytic anemia
	  C Direct toxic effect: Malaria, clostridial infection, etc.
	II Membrane abnormalities
	  A Spur-cell anemia
		Acquired

Intracorpuscular	*B* Paroxysmal nocturnal hemoglobinuria
	  C Hereditary spherocytosis (rare: elliptocytosis, stomatocytosis)
	III Abnormalities of red blood cell interior
	  A Enzyme defects
	  B Hemoglobinopathies
		Hereditary

directly harmful, leading to a state of iron overload. Pyridoxine is indicated only in the treatment of sideroblastic anemias.

Many kinds of anemias can be corrected if a precipitating cause can be uncovered and reversed. If a drug or toxin can be incriminated, its withdrawal may allow full recovery. The outcome of the "secondary" anemias is dependent on whether the underlying condition can be corrected. Anemias due to an endocrinopathy or infection should respond favorably to appropriate treatment. Occasionally, the anemia of malignancy is corrected by the removal of the primary tumor. One of the most dramatic sequelae of a successful renal transplant is the prompt correction of the "anemia of uremia." In chronic disorders such as hepatic cirrhosis or rheumatoid arthritis, the anemia is likely to persist, along with the underlying disease.

Primary disorders of the bone marrow such as aplastic anemia or myelophthisic anemia are often irreversible and are treated with supportive measures. *Androgens* are sometimes employed in this group of anemias, but their efficacy is marginal. Many of these patients require transfusions of red cells and platelets. Because prognosis is so bleak in these disorders, a radical approach to treatment seems justified. As described in Chap. 312, bone marrow transplantation is now a reasonable therapeutic alternative in selected cases of severe aplastic anemia and possibly in refractory leukemia.

Several factors should be weighed in determining whether an anemic patient should be transfused. The risks and complications of the administration of blood products are discussed in Chap. 319. Patients with chronic or long-standing anemias are able to compensate in several ways, discussed earlier in this chapter. A considerable reduction in red cell mass can be surprisingly well tolerated, especially if the patient is young or sedentary. Transfusion is seldom indicated in a patient with a chronic anemia whose hemoglobin is 9 g per 100 ml or greater. Those who are expected to respond to the administration of a specific agent such as iron, folic acid, or vitamin B_{12} can usually be spared transfusions. If the anemia has precipitated an episode of congestive heart failure or myocardial ischemia, prompt but cautious administration of packed red cells is indicated. In general, whole blood should be given only if the patient is hypovolemic.

Corticosteroids have only a limited role in the treatment of anemia. These agents are not effective in stimulating erythropoiesis. High doses of a glucocorticoid are indicated in the treatment of immunohemolytic anemia, thrombotic thrombocytopenic purpura, and pure red cell anemia. Otherwise, steroids should be prescribed sparingly unless some coexisting condition dictates their use.

Splenectomy is indicated in the treatment of certain hemolytic anemias. The efficacy of splenectomy correlates with the degree to which the abnormal or defective red cells are sequestered. Splenectomy is virtually curative in hereditary spherocytosis. The operation may be beneficial in selected patients with immunohemolytic anemia, congestive splenomegaly, spur-cell anemia, and certain hemoglobinopathies and enzymopathies. Splenectomy has also been recommended early in the treatment of thrombotic thrombocytopenic purpura. The operative morbidity and mortality from elective splenectomy is very low. Occasional patients develop a left subphrenic abscess. Following splenectomy, young children are at risk of developing overwhelming septicemia. This complication is much rarer in adults. Thrombocytosis generally develops promptly following splenectomy. However, in most cases, it is transient. In patients with continued hemolysis, the thrombocytosis usually persists and may occasionally be associated with thromboembolic phenomena.

REFERENCES

BUNN HF et al: *Human Hemoglobins*. Philadelphia, Saunders, 1977

ERSLEV AJ, GABUZDA TG: *Pathophysiology of Blood*. Philadelphia, Saunders, 1975

HARRIS JW, KELLERMEYER RW: *The Red Cell*. Cambridge, Harvard University Press, 1970

HILLMAN RS, FINCH CA: *Red Cell Manual*. Philadelphia, Davis, 1974

NIENHUIS AW, BENZ EJ: Regulation of hemoglobin synthesis during the development of the red cell. N Engl J Med 297:1318, 1371, 1430, 1977

RAPAPORT SI: *Introduction to Hematology*. New York, Harper & Row, 1971

SCHMID R (ed): Physiology and disorders of hemoglobin degradation. Semin Hematol 9:1, 1972

WEED RI: *Hematology for Internists*. Boston, Little, Brown, 1971

WINTROBE MM: *Clinical Hematology,* 7th ed. Philadelphia, Lea & Febiger, 1974

54
BLEEDING

HYMIE L. NOSSEL

Bleeding is one of the most serious and significant of the cardinal manifestations of disease. It may occur from a local site or may be generalized. Bleeding associated with a local lesion may be superimposed on either a normal or a defective hemostatic mechanism; in contrast, general bleeding is usually associated with a hemorrhagic diathesis. Spontaneous bleeding also suggests defective hemostasis.

LOCAL BLEEDING

In the evaluation of local bleeding, the site, appearance of the blood, signs of blood loss, and evidence for disordered hemostasis should be considered. The sites and common causes of bleeding are listed in Table 54-1. The appearance of the blood may provide a clue as to the cause of the bleeding. Bleeding from the lungs and bronchi is influenced by the degree of aeration and the presence of mucus and pus. In pneumococcal pneumonia the sputum is characteristically rusty. In tuberculosis it is usually bright red. Pus is usually mixed with the blood when infection is present. Massive hemorrhage occasionally occurs in mitral stenosis when a bronchial varicosity ruptures or in tuberculosis when a vessel is eroded. In pulmonary infarction the blood is usually dark red. Blood derived from the gastrointestinal tract may be darkened because of conversion of hemoglobin to brown hematin by gastric acid. Blood vomited from the stomach may be dark ("coffee ground") or bright red if the vomiting is sufficiently rapid. When it appears in the stool, it may be pitch black (melena). Blood derived from the colon is red or brown, and, if inflammation is the cause, mucus or pus is mixed with it (see Chap. 38). If bleeding from the urinary tract is profuse, clots or bright blood may be present in the urine. Small amounts of blood impart a smoky appearance to urine, whereas lesser degrees of hematuria may be detected only by microscopy.

The signs and symptoms of blood loss depend on the amount and rate of bleeding. If very acute, syncope occurs rapidly; with a slower rate of loss, signs and symptoms of peripheral circulatory collapse occur. Shock may occur without external blood loss if a large amount of blood is lost into a serous cavity. Slow and prolonged blood loss will gradually result in symptoms of iron-deficiency anemia.

TABLE 54-1
Causes of localized bleeding

Locations	Commonest causes
Skin (petechiae, purpura, ec-chymoses)	Thrombocytopenia
Limbs:	
Joints	Hemophilia
Intramuscular and subcutane-ous hematomas	Hemophilia
Central nervous system	Trauma, hypertension, congen-ital vascular malformations
Head and neck:	
Nose and sinuses	Trauma, inflammation, hyper-tension, polyps and tumors, hereditary telangiectasia
Ears	Trauma
Optic fundi	Hypertension, nephritis, diabe-tes, thrombocytopenia, trauma
Chest:	
Respiratory tract	Tumors, infections, bronchiec-tasis, pulmonary embolism, mitral stenosis
Serous cavity	Tumors, tuberculosis, pulmo-nary infarction
Nipples	Fissure, tumor
Gastrointestinal tract	Esophageal varices, hiatal her-nia, peptic ulcer, gastritis, tu-mors, colitis, hemorrhoids, hereditary telangiectasia
Abdominal cavity	Trauma, splenic rupture, ec-topic gestation
Urinary tract	Calculi, infections, glomerulo-nephritis, tumors, cystitis, prostatic hypertrophy
Vagina	Obstetric and endocrine disor-ders, tumors

Local bleeding which is out of proportion to the injury sug-gests a hemostatic defect. For example, when a patient suffers bleeding following dental extraction sufficient to require blood transfusion, a defect of the coagulation or platelet systems can almost always be defined.

HEMOSTASIS AND ITS DISORDERS

The successful management of patients with a disorder of the hemostatic mechanism depends on accurate diagnosis. Correct diagnosis and rational therapy depend on an understanding of the normal mechanisms for preserving hemostasis.

Normal hemostasis comprises mechanisms operative imme-diately following an injury and those acting over a longer pe-riod to maintain hemostasis. The immediate mechanism con-sists principally of two components: *vasoconstriction* due to active contraction of the smooth muscle of the vessel wall, and *plug formation* by masses of aggregated platelets. The mainte-nance mechanism consists of the *fibrin* (and fibrin clot) pro-duced by the coagulation system.

Platelet plug formation is especially important in capillary hemostasis, while vasoconstriction and fibrin formation seem to be more important in larger vessel hemostasis. These several mechanisms involved in achieving normal hemostasis are in-terconnected at several points, but for the sake of clarity they will be described as separate entities.

PLATELETS The normal platelet count is 150,000 to 400,000 per cubic millimeter. The most accurate method of counting platelets is by electronic particle counting or by phase-contrast microscopy. An estimate of platelet number may be made by examination of the stained peripheral blood smear. With a normal platelet count, several (3 to 10) platelets (individually or in small clumps) should be visible in each oil-immersion field.

Structure Normal platelets are anucleate bodies 2 to 3 μm in diameter which appear light blue and contain small purple-red granules when stained with Giemsa's solution. With the elec-tron microscope, three distinct structural zones may be identi-fied in the platelet, each related to specific platelet functions. The unique quality of the platelet is its ability to adhere to foreign surfaces and form aggregates in response to a variety of stimuli including thrombin, adenosine diphosphate (ADP), and catecholamines. The *peripheral* zone is involved in adhe-sion, the *cytoplasm* (sol-gel zone) in contraction, and the *organ-elle* zone in secretion.

The peripheral zone comprises a surface coat of acid muco-polysaccharides (the glycocalyx) and glycoproteins, the tri-laminar plasma unit membrane, and a submembranous area. The surface coat is involved in adhesion, and the membrane provides a trigger mechanism whereby stimuli are transmitted from the exterior into the interior. Specific binding sites for thrombin and ADP are present.

The submembranous area and cytoplasmic zone contain the contractile protein *actomyosin* (also termed *thrombosthenin*) in the form of a number of fibrous elements. In the submem-branous area, bundles of microtubules encircle the platelet forming a cytoskeleton that stabilizes the cell, permitting it to circulate as a flattened disk. The microtubules are composed of subfilaments which are indistinguishable from microfilaments present in the cytoplasm. The microfilaments are responsible for the centripetal movement and coalescence of granules oc-curring during platelet aggregation, the contraction of pseudo-pods, and clot retraction.

Distinct components in the organelle zone include granules, mitochondria, glycogen-containing particles, and, in an occa-sional platelet, stacks of flattened saccules resembling a Golgi apparatus. Three types of membrane-enclosed granules can be distinguished: (1) alpha granules which contain a number of proteins including platelet factor 4 which has heparin-neutral-izing activity, beta thromboglobulin, fibrinogen, and a factor(s) which stimulates the mitosis of smooth muscle cells and fibro-blasts; (2) dense granules in which calcium, ADP, serotonin, and catecholamines are localized; and (3) lysosomal granules with enzymes such as phosphatase, β glucuronidase, and ca-thepsin. The three granule populations constitute the secretory organelles of the platelet and release their contents in response to stimuli such as thrombin, collagen, ADP, and epinephrine. The threshold for release for each type of granule is different; the sequence in order of increasing threshold is alpha granules, dense granules, and lysosomal granules. Active intermediary metabolism occurs in the mitochondria. ATP is generated from both glycolysis and the tricarboxylic acid cycle. Glycogen and lipid are also synthesized.

Distribution and fate Platelets are formed in the marrow and released into the circulation. At any moment, about 80 percent of the platelets are in the circulation and 20 percent are in the spleen; free movement occurs between these two pools. If the spleen enlarges markedly, the distribution shifts and up to 80 percent of the platelets may be pooled in the spleen. Survival curves of ^{51}Cr-labeled platelets are linear and suggest that most platelets become senescent and die after a life span of about 10 days.

Some platelets appear to be consumed in repairing the mi-nor vascular injuries of daily life. There is evidence that youn-ger platelets are physiologically more active and have higher enzyme concentrations than old platelets. This distinction is most apparent when thrombopoiesis is accelerated in response to increased platelet destruction. Senescent platelets are probably removed by the reticuloendothelial system. In thrombocytopenia due to increased platelet destruction, the destruction is random. Damaged platelets may be removed primarily in the spleen or in both the spleen and the liver. The bone marrow does not contain a reserve of platelets, and if circulating platelets are rapidly destroyed or lost, thrombocytopenia persists for several days until enough new platelets are formed. Governing normal platelet production are one or more humoral factors that appear to regulate platelet production.

Function in hemostasis   The platelet contributes to hemostasis by forming platelet plugs and by promoting thrombin production. Platelet plug formation may be divided into a number of stages (Fig. 54-1).

ADHESION   Platelets adhere to subendothelial structures exposed by trauma. Such structures include collagen fibers and basement membranes. Regularly spaced free amino groups on the collagen molecule are required for platelet adhesion. In addition, a number of plasma proteins, including fibrinogen and von Willebrand factor, are required for normal platelet adherence.

RELEASE REACTION   Following adherence to collagen, platelets extrude the contents of their granules—a process termed the *release reaction*. This reaction is also induced by thrombin, and in physiologic hemostasis very likely both collagen and throm-

bin initiate release. Epinephrine and ADP also promote platelet aggregation and release.

Detailed understanding of the mechanism of release is incomplete, but certain facts are clear. The reaction has an absolute requirement for energy derived from glycolysis and the Krebs cycle. A major control mechanism for both aggregation and release is the platelet concentration of cyclic adenosine 3′, 5′-monophosphate (AMP) which is produced from ATP by adenylate cyclase and degraded by phosphodiesterase. Release is inhibited by substances which increase the platelet concentration of cyclic AMP. These agents include prostacyclin (PGI_2, a potent prostaglandin produced only in endothelial cells and not in platelets), which stimulates adenylate cyclase, and theophylline, which inhibits phosphodiesterase. Epinephrine, on the other hand, lowers platelet cyclic AMP levels and promotes release.

It has been shown that an intermediate of platelet prostaglandin synthesis plays a major role in mediating the release reaction (Fig. 54-2). When platelets are stimulated by a release-inducer, such as thrombin or ADP, phospholipase A_2 cleaves free arachidonic acid from platelet phospholipids. Arachidonic acid, under the influence of a cyclooxygenase, is sequentially converted to the cyclic endoperoxides PGG_2 and PGH_2, the latter of which is transformed to thromboxane A_2 by thromboxane synthetase. Thromboxane A_2 directly induces the release reaction but is unstable and is rapidly transformed to thromboxane B_2, which is inactive. Aspirin leads to acetylation of cyclooxygenase, rendering it inactive; thus aspirin inhibits formation of endoperoxide and thromboxane A_2. Inhibition of cyclooxygenase prevents platelet release resulting from

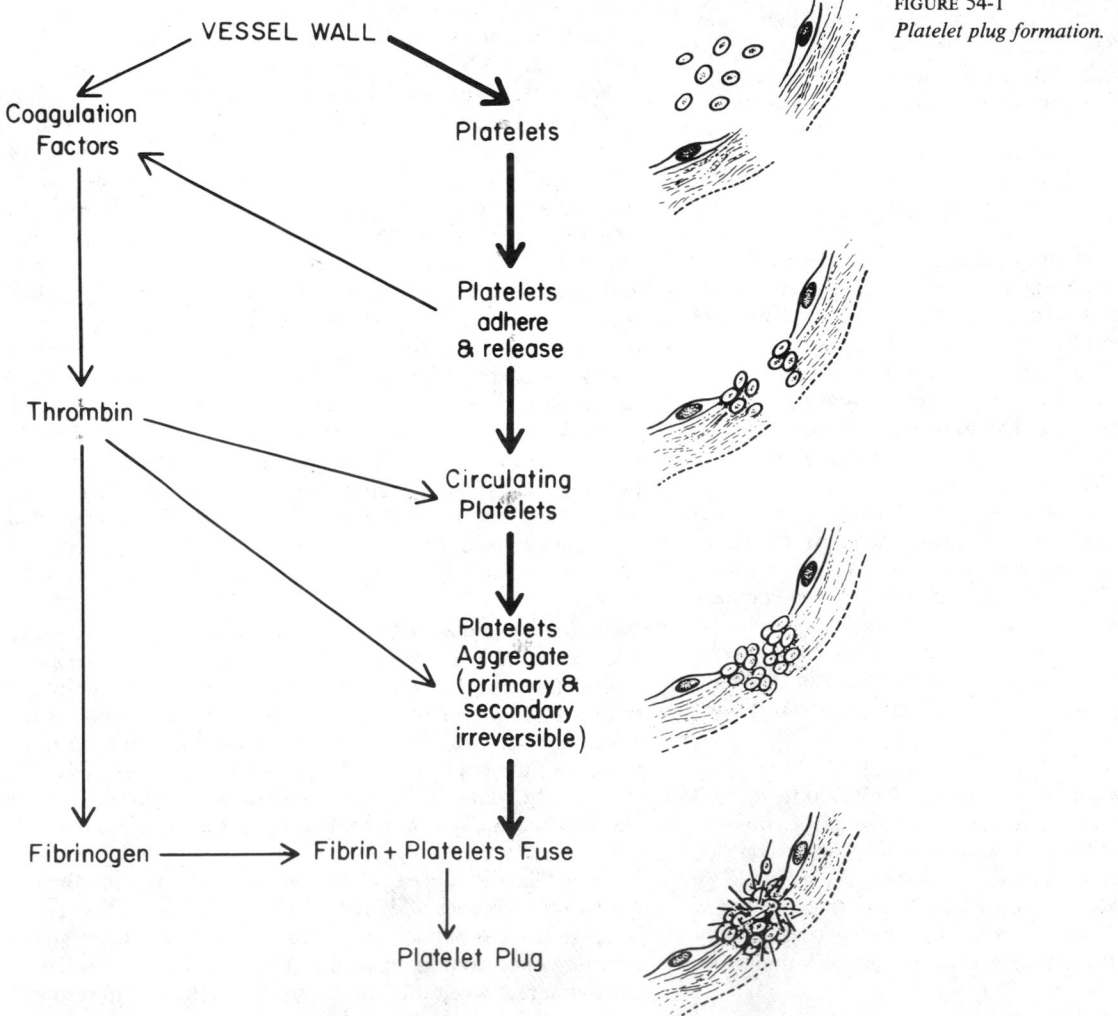

FIGURE 54-1
Platelet plug formation.

weak or moderate stimulation. High concentrations of collagen or thrombin will overcome the inhibitory effect of aspirin and produce full release, indicating the presence of an alternative release mechanism. Calcium ionophores, which allow movements of calcium ions between subcellular compartments, may induce release by still another mechanism.

AGGREGATION The released ADP causes additional platelets to aggregate and is thus a key component for amplifying the extent of platelet aggregation. How ADP produces aggregation is as yet unclear. Low concentrations of ADP ($\sim 10^{-6}$ M) cause only primary platelet aggregation, which is reversible, whereas two- to threefold higher concentrations of ADP produce irreversible aggregation. Low concentrations of thrombin or collagen, in addition to causing primary aggregation, stimulate the release of ADP, which promotes secondary irreversible aggregation.

Platelets participate in coagulation factor reactions leading to thrombin formation by providing a lipoprotein surface (so-called "platelet factor 3") on which coagulation enzymes and substrates interact. Factor X_a is bound via factor V to the platelet lipoprotein membrane and there activates prothrombin. "Activation" of the platelet is necessary for factor X_a binding and consequent promotion of coagulation (Fig. 54-5). Hence, a defect in platelet activation will be detected as a defect in the activity of platelet factor III coagulant activity.

FUSION The action of thrombin produced by the coagulation mechanism leads to coalescence. Fibrin (also a product of thrombin action) and fused platelets form a stable hemostatic plug.

CLOT RETRACTION Following in vitro coagulation of blood or platelet-rich plasma, platelets retract the fibrin threads of the clot into a contracted volume and express the fluid trapped in the clot. It is uncertain to what extent clot retraction is a necessary component of hemostasis, but the test is simple to do and provides useful information. Clot retraction is readily tested in whole blood or by adding thrombin to platelet-rich plasma and noting the extent of clot retraction 1 h later. Clot retraction is defective in a severe congenital defect of platelet function termed *thrombasthenia,* or when either the platelet count or the fibrinogen concentration is very low.

Tests of platelet function Platelet plugs rapidly stop bleeding from ruptured capillaries and small vessels. The integrity of the platelet plug-forming mechanism is tested by measuring the *bleeding time.* This is most commonly determined by the Ivy bleeding time technique, in which the time is measured for bleeding to cease from three incisions 1 cm long and 1 mm deep in an avascular area of the forearm. Venous return is obstructed by a blood pressure cuff set at 40 mmHg pressure over the upper forearm. The bleeding time is normal in disorders of the coagulation system but is abnormal in the presence of severe thrombocytopenia, defects of platelet function, deficiency of the von Willebrand plasma protein, or total absence of blood fibrinogen. Generally, clinically significant defects in platelet function are found only if the bleeding time is prolonged. Platelet aggregation, a measure of platelet function, may be studied by recording the increase in light transmitted through a cuvette containing continuously stirred platelet-rich plasma when aggregating agents are added to the plasma. The aggregating agents usually tested are collagen, epinephrine, adenosine diphosphate, thrombin, and ristocetin.

FIGURE 54-2

Generation of thromboxane A_2 in platelets and prostacyclin PGI_2 in endothelial cells and effects on platelet activation and release.

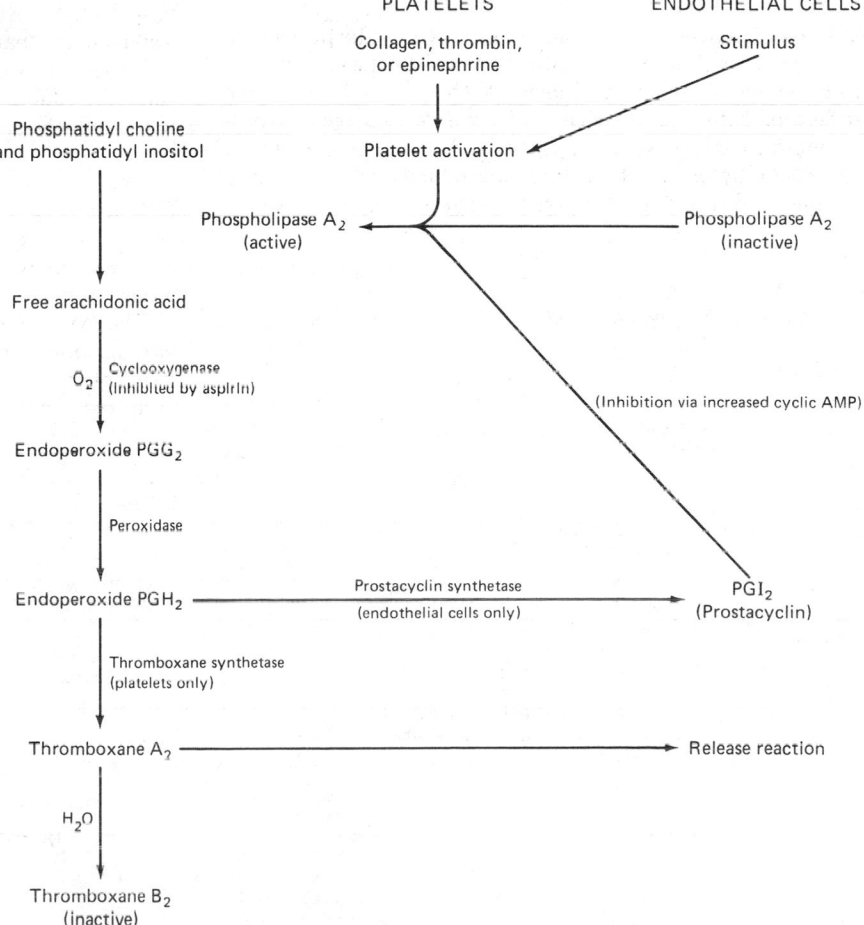

BLOOD COAGULATION: MECHANISM AND FUNCTION The two main functions of the blood coagulation mechanism are as follows:

1 Production of thrombin which stabilizes the platelet plug
2 Formation of fibrin which, by rendering the platelet plug permanent, mechanically blocks the flow of blood through ruptured vessels

A number of discrete proenzymes and proteins (termed *coagulation factors*), platelets, and calcium participate in the coagulation process. The process consists of several stages and ends with fibrin formation.

Fibrin formation Fibrinogen is a 340,000-dalton dimeric protein, each half of which contains three polypeptide chains termed Aα, Bβ, and γ. The first step in fibrin formation is cleavage by thrombin of fibrinopeptides A and B from the fibrinogen molecule to produce fibrin monomer (Fig. 54-3). Fibrinopeptide A is cleaved first, and following its release, the fibrin molecules polymerize to form visible coagulum. When the concentration of fibrin relative to fibrinogen is low, the fibrin forms a complex with fibrinogen and remains in solution. When the ratio of fibrin to fibrinogen molecules becomes greater, the fibrin precipitates to form the clot. The approximate ratio above which clot formation occurs is one fibrin molecule per five fibrinogen molecules.

Polymerized fibrin is soluble in acid and concentrated urea solutions and is hemostatically ineffective. Fibrin polymer is cross-linked by the action of activated factor XIII, which, in the presence of calcium, forms covalent peptide bonds between glutamyl and lysyl amino acid residues of adjacent molecules. The resulting product is highly insoluble and is hemostatically very effective.

Prothrombin activation Thrombin is formed by the proteolytic cleavage of a proenzyme, prothrombin. The process results from the action of activated factor X (X_a) which binds to the surface of activated platelets via factor V and cleaves prothrombin in the presence of calcium. Activation of factor X may occur by either of two separate pathways, the extrinsic and the intrinsic. Clinical experience suggests that effective he-

FIGURE 54-3
Steps in cross-linked fibrin formation.

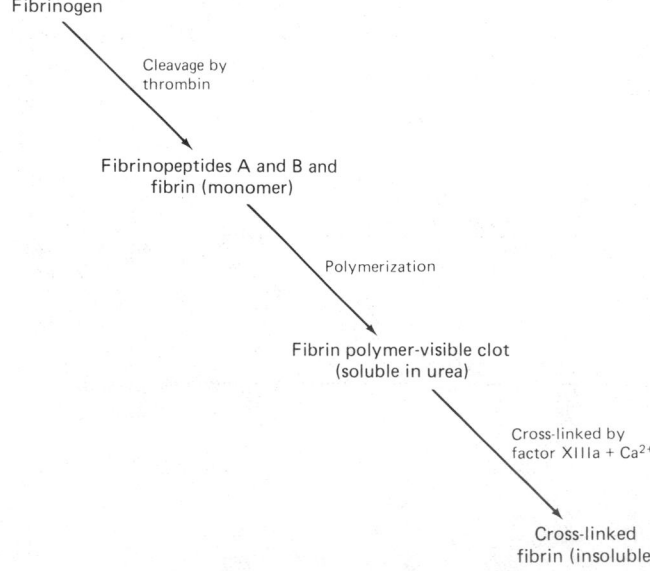

Fibrinogen

Cleavage by thrombin

Fibrinopeptides A and B and fibrin (monomer)

Polymerization

Fibrin polymer-visible clot (soluble in urea)

Cross-linked by factor XIIIa + Ca²⁺

Cross-linked fibrin (insoluble)

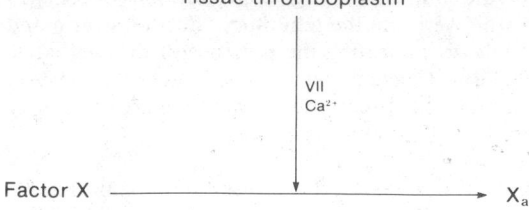

Tissue thromboplastin

VII
Ca²⁺

Factor X ————————————————→ X$_a$

FIGURE 54-4
Activation of factor X by steps in the extrinsic coagulation pathway.

mostasis requires the participation of both. In the *extrinsic pathway,* a tissue factor (tissue thromboplastin), released from damaged cells, activates factor X in the presence of factor VII and calcium (Fig. 54-4). In the *intrinsic* or *cascade pathway* (Fig. 54-5), the contact of blood with a "foreign" surface, such as collagen or skin, activates factor XII. Activated factor XII, in the presence of prekallikrein and high-molecular-weight kininogen, activates factor XI which, in the presence of calcium, cleaves a peptide from factor IX producing activated factor IX. Activated factor IX proteolytically converts factor X into the activated form (X_a) in the presence of platelet membrane lipoprotein, factor VIII, and calcium.

Tests of the coagulation mechanism The intrinsic pathway of blood coagulation including fibrin polymerization is tested by measuring the *whole-blood clotting time* and *partial thromboplastin time* (Fig. 54-6). The whole-blood clotting time is the time taken for 1 ml of whole blood to clot at 37°C with controlled temperature and exposure of the blood to the glass surface of the test tube. The test is influenced by gross defects in the intrinsic clotting system. The partial thromboplastin time (celite or kaolin cephalin time) is the time required for recalcified citrated plasma to clot. A standardized platelet substitute (cephalin or "partial thromboplastin") and standard surface activation (provided by celite or kaolin) are used to eliminate variability due to the platelet count and surface factors. The test is influenced by moderate defects in the intrinsic clotting system.

The activity of any of the coagulation factors involved in the intrinsic pathway (i.e., factors XII, XI, IX, and VIII) may be measured by comparing the ability of control and test plasma samples to shorten the partial thromboplastin time of a plasma sample known to be deficient in the specific factor.

The extrinsic clotting system is tested by the *one-stage prothrombin time*. In this test, the time taken for recalcified citrated plasma to clot in the presence of tissue thromboplastin is measured. The test is sensitive to defects in the extrinsic clot-

FIGURE 54-5
Activation of factor X by the steps in the extrinsic coagulation pathway.

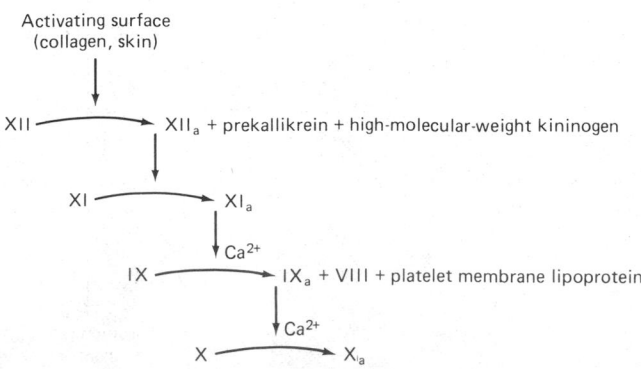

Activating surface (collagen, skin)

XII ——→ XII$_a$ + prekallikrein + high-molecular-weight kininogen

XI ——→ XI$_a$

Ca²⁺

IX ——→ IX$_a$ + VIII + platelet membrane lipoprotein

Ca²⁺

X ——→ X$_a$

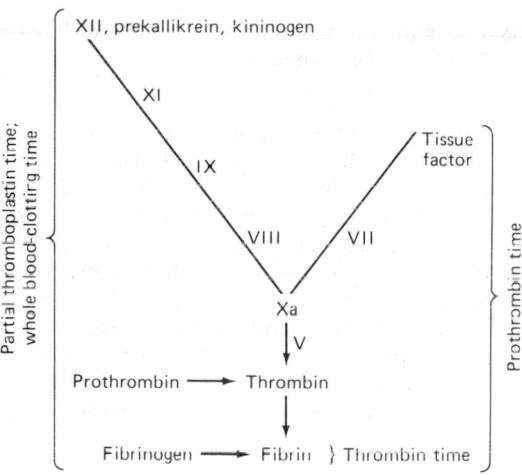

FIGURE 54-6
Coagulation tests.

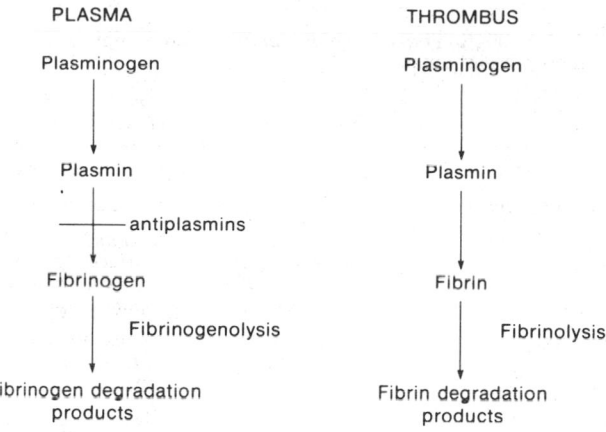

FIGURE 54-7
Plasminogen activation in plasma and in a thrombus and digestion of fibrinogen and fibrin.

ting system (Figs. 54-4 and 54-6). The activity of factor VII and the common pathway coagulation factors (factors II, V, and X) may be measured by comparing the ability of control and test plasma samples to shorten the prothrombin time of plasma deficient in the specific factor.

The polymerization of fibrinogen is tested by measuring the *thrombin clotting time.* This test measures the time for citrated plasma to clot in the presence of added thrombin. The test is abnormal in the presence of heparin or of congenital or acquired abnormalities of the fibrinogen molecule such as disseminated intravascular coagulation.

Blood fluidity system (regulator mechanisms) In addition to the coagulation factors, several mechanisms exist in the circulation for maintaining the blood in a fluid state. In the absence of this system, sufficient thrombin would be generated by the clotting of only 1 ml blood to coagulate all the fibrinogen in 3 liters blood. The fluidity-maintaining system consists of both cellular and humoral components.

The cellular component comprises the reticuloendothelial system and the liver, both of which specifically remove activated clotting factors and fibrin without affecting precursor (unactivated) coagulation factors. The humoral component consists of several proteins which specifically inactivate the activated coagulation factors. These proteins include antithrombin III and α_2 macroglobulin. Antithrombin inactivates thrombin and each of the activated intermediates of the clotting mechanism.

The humoral system also includes the fibrinolytic mechanism for dissolving fibrin. Fibrinolysis is produced by the action of an enzyme, plasmin, which is formed from a precursor, plasminogen. Plasminogen is proteolytically converted to plasmin by an extrinsic system in which the activator is supplied by damaged cells present in the blood vessel wall or by an intrinsic system in which the components are all present in the blood. The intrinsic plasmin system is initiated by the contact of factor XII with a foreign surface; by way of a number of intermediates, including prekallikrein and high-molecular-weight kininogen, an activator is formed which converts plasminogen to plasmin (Fig. 54-7).

Initially polypeptides from the C-terminal part of the Aα chain and from the N-terminal part of the Bβ chain are cleaved. The remaining part of the molecule is often termed *fragment X* and is still clottable by thrombin. Subsequent stages of digestion are not clottable. An intermediate stage is often termed *fragment Y,* and final stages are termed *D* and *E.* These products of plasmin digestion are termed *fibrinogen fi*

brin degradation products. The degradation products have significant physiologic effects. They inhibit the clotting of normal blood by acting as anticoagulants. They delay the polymerization of fibrin and thus prolong the thrombin clotting time. The fibrinogen-fibrin degradation products may also interpose between fibrin polymers as they are forming. This results in a weak, disordered fibrin clot. Platelet aggregation by ADP is also inhibited. Plasmin also digests factors V and VIII. A number of powerful inhibitors are present in normal blood, and these control plasmin action and prevent proteolysis of fibrinogen. The most important of these inhibitors is a 63,000-dalton α_2 globulin which rapidly and irreversibly inactivates plasmin.

As fibrin is deposited, plasminogen becomes incorporated in the growing thrombus, and is thereby separated from the circulating inhibitors of plasminogen activation so that the plasmin formed is localized at the site of fibrin formation. Thus freed from the inhibitors, it is able to digest fibrin. In this way, discrete local lysis of fibrin can occur without proteolysis of circulating fibrinogen. Clot lysis following fibrin deposition results in release of *fibrin degradation products* into the blood. In those pathologic conditions with extensive intravascular clotting, fibrin degradation products may accumulate in the blood without detectable plasmin levels in the blood sampled from a distant site such as an arm vein.

Production, distribution, and life span of coagulation factors Because the concentrations of all plasma clotting factors, except factor VIII, are depressed in patients with massive liver necrosis, it is thought that hepatic parenchymal cells synthesize all factors except factor VIII. There is evidence that von Willebrand protein, which is closely related to factor VIII, is synthe-

TABLE 54-2
Properties of coagulation factors

Factor	Plasma concentration, µg/ml	Hemostatic level, % of normal	In vivo recovery, % of infused material	$T_{1/2}$, h
Fibrinogen	3000	100 mg per 100 ml	50	100
Prothrombin	150	?40	50	72
V	10	25	?50–100	16
VII	0.5	10	?100	6
VIII (antihemophilic)	?	30	80	12
IX	3	25	50	24
X	15	20	50 100	48
XI	6	?25	100	60
XII	29	—	—	60
XIII	20	3	50 100	120

TABLE 54-3
Clinical distinction between blood coagulation defects and capillary and platelet defects

	Coagulation defects	Capillary and platelet defects
Family history	Usually positive	Usually negative
Sex predominance	Males	Females
Type of bleeding	Visceral and intramuscular deep hematomas; usually after trauma	Skin and mucosal surfaces; petechiae and ecchymoses; spontaneous
Duration	Delayed after trauma and persistent	Immediate after trauma; short-lived
Local pressure	Not effective	May stop bleeding

sized by endothelial cells. It is not known where factor VIII coagulant activity is synthesized. It does not appear to be made in endothelial cells. Levels of factor VIII rise sharply after a burst of muscular exercise or an infusion of epinephrine. The rise apparently reflects the release of stores of factor VIII into the circulation. Stress, fever, and infection elevate fibrinogen and factor VIII levels by an unknown mechanism. Gram-negative bacterial endotoxin also stimulates fibrinogen production. Levels of factors VII, VIII, and X and fibrinogen are elevated in pregnancy and in patients using oral contraceptives.

The plasma clotting factors have short intravascular half-lives compared with other plasma proteins. These can be grouped (in order of decreasing intravascular half-life) as follows (see also Table 54-2):

1 Fibrinogen, factor XIII: 4 to 5 days
2 Prothrombin, factors V, IX, X, XI, and XII: 1 to 3 days
3 Factor VIII: 12 h
4 Factor VII: 5 h

Because of these relatively short half-lives, postoperative prophylaxis or control of bleeding following trauma in a patient with a severe clotting-factor deficiency usually requires repeated replacement therapy during the period of healing.

DIAGNOSTIC APPROACH TO DISORDERS OF HEMOSTASIS

The diagnosis of coagulation disorders is based on both clinical and laboratory evidence. A careful and knowledgeably col-

lected history is essential if the results obtained from laboratory studies are to be properly interpreted.

CLINICAL HISTORY (Table 54-3) A history taken to evaluate hemostasis should answer these questions: (1) Has *abnormal bleeding* or *bruising* occurred either spontaneously or after injury, dental extraction, or surgery? Was there *delayed* or *prolonged* bleeding, suggesting a coagulation disorder, or immediate and transient bleeding, suggesting a platelet disorder? (2) Was there bleeding from the umbilical stump or after circumcision? (3) Is there a history of *prolonged nose bleeds?* Brief epistaxis, stopping within minutes, even if frequent, is usually associated with normal tests of hemostasis.

One should try to determine the degree and frequency of the following:

1 Bruising. Spontaneous bruises larger than the palm of the hand are generally significant; a history of hematomas and bruises at the sites of injections or immunizations may likewise be suggestive of a hemostatic disorder.
2 Excessive bleeding from small cuts. Specific details as to the size of laceration and duration of bleeding should be elicited.

One should question the patient for (1) evidence of an underlying *systemic disorder* that may be accompanied by defective hemostasis, such as liver disease, systemic lupus erythematosus, uremia, or a hematologic malignancy; (2) a *family history* of bleeding and, if present, the hereditary pattern of transmission; and (3) *drug ingestion.* Drugs that interfere with hemostasis fall into two categories: (1) drugs that impair formation of the hemostatic plug by inhibiting platelet function or causing thrombocytopenia and (2) drugs that interfere with blood coagulation.

Drugs that impair plug formation include aspirin in ordinary doses, but such prolongation in bleeding time usually remains within the normal range unless platelet function is already abnormal; aspirin should be discontinued several days before surgery. Other drugs which interfere with platelet function are dipyridamole, clofibrate, phenylbutazone, antihistamines, and tranquilizers. The clinical significance of these drugs with respect to hemostasis has yet to be clearly documented.

Drugs that interfere with blood coagulation include heparin and the oral coumarin drugs. Although preoperative patients are rarely receiving parenteral heparin, patients on long-term oral anticoagulant therapy are frequently encountered.

TABLE 54-4
Diagnosis of bleeding disorders involving coagulation

Disorders	Tests					
	Prothrombin time	Partial thromboplastin time	Thrombin time	Fibrinogen concentration	Fibrinogen proteolysis	Factor assays
Congenital deficiency of factor VII	Abnormal	Normal	Normal	Normal	Normal	Specific factor abnormal
Congenital deficiency of factors VIII, IX, XI, XII, high-molecular-weight kininogen or prekallikrein	Normal	Abnormal	Normal	Normal	Normal	Specific factors abnormal
Deficiency of prothrombin, factor V, factor X, or vitamin K; or coumarin or warfarin effect	Abnormal	Abnormal	Normal	Normal	Normal	Specific factor abnormal
Dysfibrinogenemia, heparin effect	Abnormal	Abnormal	Abnormal	Normal	Normal	Normal
Disseminated intravascular coagulation, liver failure, congenital hypofibrinogenemia	Abnormal	Abnormal	Abnormal	Decreased	Abnormal	Abnormal

TABLE 54-5
Diagnosis of bleeding disorders involving platelets

	Tests				
			Platelet function		
Disorders	Bleeding time	Platelet count	Clot retraction	PF III*	Platelet aggregation
Thrombocytopenia	Prolonged	Decreased	Abnormal		
Thromboasthenia	Prolonged	Normal	Abnormal	Abnormal	Abnormal with ADP and other aggregating agents
Release defects	Prolonged	Normal	Normal	Abnormal	Primary normal, secondary abnormal
von Willebrand's disease (also has low factor VIII coagulant activity and antigenic activity)	Prolonged	Normal	Normal	Normal	Abnormal only with ristocetin, normal with ADP, epinephrine, thrombin, collagen

* *Activity of platelet factor III.*

PHYSICAL FINDINGS   The patient should be examined for the following.

1 *Abnormal bleeding in the skin.* Ecchymoses suggest abnormal bleeding from relatively large vessels due to a defect in blood clotting. Petechiae, which may be small, require a careful search, particularly around the ankles. Petechiae suggest increased vascular fragility secondary to thrombocytopenia.
2 *Mucosal bleeding.* Look for purpura of the buccal mucosa and the conjunctival surfaces of the eyelids. Hemorrhagic bullae in the mouth are found only in the presence of thrombocytopenia. Hemorrhages in the optic fundi, however, may reflect local eye disease, hypertension, diabetes, severe anemia, or thrombocytopenia. The presence of telangiectasia on or under the tongue should be noted.
3 *Hemarthrosis and ankylosis.* These suggest a deficiency of factor VIII or IX.
4 *Hereditary connective tissue disorder.* Abnormal elasticity of the skin and hyperextensibility of the joints (Ehlers-Danlos syndrome) may be associated with vascular bleeding.
5 *Chronic liver disease,* including spider angiomas, palmar erythema, dilated abdominal veins, hepatomegaly, or splenomegaly.

LABORATORY STUDIES   Screening tests   A careful history is the best screening test. Nevertheless, laboratory tests for the integrity of the coagulation and platelet components of the hemostatic mechanism are indicated under a number of circumstances, including (1) historical or physical evidence of abnormal hemostasis; (2) family history of abnormal hemostasis; (3) presence of a disorder which may be associated with abnormal hemostasis, e.g., liver disease, systemic lupus erythematosus; and (4) prior surgical procedures known to be associated with a high incidence of hemorrhage.

Coagulation system tests   (Table 54-4) A commonly used set of screening tests for coagulation defects include (1) *prothrombin time,* (2) *partial thromboplastin time,* (3) *thrombin clotting time,* and (4) *fibrinogen concentration* (most tests of fibrinogen depend on measuring the concentration of thrombin-clottable protein in the plasma). If one or more of these tests are abnormal, an assessment is made, based on the history as well as the test results, as to the most likely defect. The factor(s) most likely to be abnormal should be specifically assayed, including factor XIII. If all the coagulation system screening tests are normal, no further tests are necessary unless the history strongly suggests abnormal hemostasis.

Platelet system tests   (Table 54-5) Basic screening tests include (1) the *bleeding time* and (2) the *platelet count.*
Tests which screen for defects of platelet function include (1) clot retraction; (2) activity of platelet factor III; and (3) platelet aggregation.
If the bleeding time is prolonged and thrombocytopenia is detected, the etiology of the thrombocytopenia should be pursued by a careful history of drug or toxin exposure, physical examination for splenomegaly and systemic disease, a complete blood count, examination of the bone marrow, and tests for systemic lupus erythematosus and platelet antibodies. If the bleeding time is prolonged and the platelet count is normal, tests for von Willebrand's disease and for platelet function should be undertaken (see Chaps. 316 and 318).

REFERENCES

BIGGS R (ed): *Human Blood Coagulation, Haemostasis and Thrombosis,* 2d ed. Oxford, Blackwell, 1976
Haemostasis. Br Med Bull, vol 33, no 3, 1977
MONCADA S, VANE JR: Arachidonic acid metabolites and the interactions between platelets and blood vessel walls. N Engl J Med 300:1142, 1979
WILLIAMS WJ et al (eds): *Hematology,* 2d ed. New York, McGraw-Hill, 1977, chaps 128–162

55

ENLARGEMENT OF LYMPH NODES AND SPLEEN

ALEXANDER FEFER

LYMPH NODES

STRUCTURE AND FUNCTION   The principal cells in lymph nodes are the lymphocytes in the lymphoid follicles and the reticuloendothelial cells which line nodal sinuses. Each follicle, located in the cortex of the node, has a germinal center which contains rapidly dividing large lymphocytes (B cells) and macrophages. Surrounding the germinal center is a cuff of densely packed small lymphocytes (T cells) which proliferate at a slower rate and which ultimately leave the node. The chief function of lymphocytes is to respond to antigens presented to the node from the structures being drained. The cells either differentiate into plasma cells and produce antibody (B cells) or enlarge, proliferate, and generate a T-cell-mediated response. The reticuloendothelial cells (histiocytes or macrophages), which can also proliferate, participate in immunity but function chiefly in the phagocytosis of cellular debris and foreign material such as microorganisms which may have gained access to the node from the area being drained by it.

MECHANISMS OF LYMPH NODE ENLARGEMENT Lymphadenopathy may be due to an increase in the number and size of lymphoid follicles with proliferation of lymphocytes or reticuloendothelial cells or to infiltration of the node by cells normally not present in it. Nodal cells proliferate in response to antigens, to other stimuli which evoke greater phagocytic activity, and to unknown stimuli which cause nodal cells to become transformed to lymphoma cells and to proliferate autonomously. Nodes can be infiltrated by leukemia or metastatic carcinoma cells, by polymorphonuclear cells in lymphadenitis, or by metabolite-laden macrophages in the lipid storage diseases.

SIGNIFICANCE OF LYMPHADENOPATHY In normal persons nodes are not palpable or barely palpable. Whether a palpable node is clinically significant depends partly on its location and on the age and occupation of the patient. The number and size of nodes are greater at puberty. Children are far more likely than adults to respond with lymphoid hyperplasia and generalized adenopathy even to relatively minor stimuli, such as mild infections of the upper respiratory tract or skin, and develop appendicitis, mesenteric adenitis, and tonsillitis far more often than do adults.

Lymphadenopathy reflects significant disease more often in adults than in children. However, palpable nodes do not always connote serious disease. They may reflect merely minor trauma to and infections of the structures being drained, such as the hands of a manual laborer (epitrochlear nodes), the upper extremities (axillary), upper respiratory tract and teeth (cervical), and, most frequently, the lower extremities (inguinal). Although usually benign, enlargement of the inguinal nodes may at times reflect significant disease, and enlarged posterior auricular, supraclavicular, epitrochlear (not in a manual laborer), popliteal, mediastinal, and abdominal nodes must always be considered pathological.

DISEASES ASSOCIATED WITH LYMPHADENOPATHY Enlarged nodes may reflect no significant disease, a self-limited benign disease, or a severe or even fatal one. Table 55-1 presents a partial list of the conditions associated with enlarged nodes. The likelihood of each diagnosis varies with age, sex,

TABLE 55-1
Conditions associated with lymph node enlargement

I Neoplastic
  A Hematologic: Lymphomas, acute leukemia, chronic lymphocytic leukemia, myeloproliferative syndromes, histiocytoses
  B Nonhematologic: Carcinomas of head and neck, lung, breast, kidney
II Immunologic or inflammatory
  A Infections: Pyogenic streptococcal, staphylococcal, and salmonella infections, brucellosis, tuberculosis, syphilis, infectious mononucleosis, cytomegalovirus, infectious hepatitis, rubella, lymphogranuloma venereum, toxoplasmosis, histoplasmosis, coccidioidomycosis, malaria
  B Connective tissue diseases: Rheumatoid arthritis, systemic lupus erythematosus, dermatomyositis
  C Serum sickness
  D Reaction to hydantoins
  E Sarcoidosis
  F Miscellaneous: Giant (angiofollicular) lymph node hyperplasia, sinus histiocytosis, dermatopathic lymphadenitis, immunoblastic lymphadenopathy
III Endocrine: Hyperthyroidism, Addison's disease
IV Lipid storage diseases: Gaucher's and Niemann-Pick's diseases

and geography. Although most patients with significant adenopathy will have either a malignancy, an infection, or a connective tissue disease, the likelihood of each of those conditions is greatest, respectively, in the old, the young, and the female.

PHYSICAL CHARACTERISTICS OF ENLARGED NODES Some nodal characteristics provide clues to the diagnosis. Nodes involved by lymphomas or by chronic lymphatic leukemia tend to be large, symmetric, rubbery, firm, movable, discrete, and nontender, whereas nodes in acute leukemia are often tender because of rapid enlargement and concurrent infection. Nodes containing metastatic carcinoma are stony-hard, nontender, well-localized, and bound to surrounding tissues and, therefore, nonmovable. In acute infections, nodes are firm, tender, asymmetric and matted, and the overlying skin may be red and edematous, whereas in chronic infections the nodes are nontender and there is no edema. However, these nodal characteristics are only modestly helpful clues, not pathognomonic signs.

LOCATION OF ENLARGED NODES The extent and location of enlarged nodes also provide diagnostic clues. Generalized adenopathy, i.e., involving more than two separate node groups, is common in non-Hodgkin's lymphomas, chronic lymphocytic leukemia, the histiocytoses, and immunoblastic lymphadenopathy but not with nonhematologic malignancies. Generalized adenopathy is uncommon in adults with infections except in infectious mononucleosis, brucellosis, cytomegalovirus, tuberculosis, infectious hepatitis, secondary syphilis, toxoplasmosis, and histoplasmosis.

In the absence of generalized adenopathy, enlargement of specific lymph node groups can be helpful diagnostically. Posterior auricular adenopathy suggests rubella. Unilateral anterior auricular adenopathy is associated with lesions of the conjunctiva and eyelids with a resultant oculoglandular syndrome as is seen with trachoma, tularemia, cat-scratch fever, tuberculosis, syphilis, epidemic keratoconjunctivitis, and swimming pool outbreaks of adenovirus type III pharyngoconjunctival fever. Oropharyngeal or dental infections can occasionally cause cervical adenopathy. Bilateral cervical adenopathy is prominent in tuberculosis, coccidioidomycosis, infectious mononucleosis, toxoplasmosis, sarcoid, lymphomas, and leukemias. However, a unilateral cervical mass often represents a metastasis from an undetected asymptomatic nasopharyngeal tumor. In one study of 1600 patients admitted to surgery with a nonthyroid neck mass, 88 percent of the patients had a malignancy, most often a metastatic tumor or a lymphoma. Therefore, a nonthyroid neck mass in adults, but not children, should be considered neoplastic until proved otherwise and is a strong indication for examination of the mouth, pharynx, nasopharynx, and larynx in search of a malignancy.

Palpable supraclavicular nodes are always abnormal and, in the absence of generalized adenopathy, reflect neoplastic disease in the abdomen or chest. The right node drains parts of the lungs and mediastinum and is involved by intrathoracic lesions especially of the lung and esophagus, whereas the left (Virchow's) node is close to the thoracic duct and is involved by intraabdominal tumor, especially from the stomach, ovary, testis, and kidney. Axillary nodes drain part of the breast and are favorite sites for metastatic breast carcinoma. Epitrochlear nodes often are chronically enlarged bilaterally in secondary lues. Inguinal adenopathy is especially common in lymphogranuloma venereum, chancroid, and syphilis.

Enlarged nodes in certain areas cannot be palpated but are suspected in the presence of characteristic clinical problems. For example, enlarged mediastinal or hilar nodes detectable on routine chest x-ray may be asymptomatic or may cause tracheobronchial compression with cough and wheezing, recurrent laryngeal nerve compression with hoarseness and stridor, paralysis of the left leaf of the diaphragm, esophageal compression with dysphagia, superior vena caval compression with swelling of the neck and face, and subclavian vein compression with swelling of the arm. Hilar nodes are often asymmetrically involved by metastatic carcinoma from the lungs and, rarely, from the testis and kidney. Bilateral asymmetric mediastinal adenopathy is common with non-Hodgkin's lymphomas and is characteristic of nodular sclerosing Hodgkin's lymphoma. Hilar adenopathy is rarely associated with bacterial or viral pneumonias. It is seen, however, in tuberculosis (usually unilateral) and in coccidioidomycosis (usually bilateral). Bilateral hilar adenopathy is characteristic of sarcoidosis, although tuberculous involvement must be excluded. One study of 100 patients with bilateral hilar adenopathy documented its very frequent association with sarcoidosis and revealed that such adenopathy in patients without symptoms or only with erythema nodosum or uveitis was nearly diagnostic for sarcoidosis. Unlike lymphomatous nodes, hilar nodes in sarcoidosis, coccidioidomycosis, and tuberculosis often show roentgenographically detectable calcification.

Abdominal nodes can enlarge in any disorder which causes generalized adenopathy. However, the cause of intraabdominal or retroperitoneal adenopathy in adults is most often neoplastic, especially lymphomatous. The nodes may cause abdominal pain, nausea, constipation, intestinal obstruction, urinary complaints, backache, fever, ascites, or peripheral edema. If sufficiently large, they can be detected by abdominal, pelvic, or rectal examination, but they are most often detected only by lymphangiography; ultrasonography and, more particularly, computerized tomography (CT) scan are often helpful in detecting abdominal and retroperitoneal lymph nodes.

APPROACH TO THE PATIENT WITH ENLARGED LYMPH NODES
In most patients, a diagnosis can be made by a careful history and physical examination, hematologic and other laboratory tests, skin tests, and routine x-rays. The association of some diagnoses with age and sex is helpful, e.g., systemic lupus erythematosus in the young female, breast carcinoma in the older female, infectious mononucleosis in the young adult, and chronic lymphocytic leukemia in the old. A history of exposure to potential sources of infection, and of constitutional complaints such as fever, malaise, fatigue, and weight loss, which accompany hematologic malignancies and systemic infections, is important. The duration of symptoms and signs is suggestive. Patients whose nodes are neoplastic tend to present with a longer history—often months—of adenopathy, whereas patients with painful infectious or inflammatory adenopathy often present within days after the nodes appear.

Physical examination should include a search for associated findings of special significance, e.g., splenomegaly for its myriad implications (see below), hepatomegaly for hepatitis and malignancies, skin rashes for viral infections, heart murmurs as in subacute bacterial endocarditis, and evidence of local infection such as chancre. An oral and nasopharyngeal examination for tumor is essential in any patient with a neck mass.

Routine hematologic studies may be diagnostic. The immature cells of leukemia or the atypical lymphocytes of infectious mononucleosis and other viral infections may be detected. A chest x-ray might reveal mediastinal nodes with or without pulmonary nodules or infiltrates. A liver and spleen scan using radioactive material might reveal increased size and defects associated with neoplasia. Cultures of blood, throat, sputum, urine, bone marrow, and other possible infectious sites should be obtained when appropriate, as should special serologic tests such as a test for syphilis, antibody titers for toxoplasmosis and cytomegalovirus, and a heterophil test for infectious mononucleosis. A marrow aspiration is indicated for anemia, thrombocytopenia, or leukopenia and may reveal leukemia or metastatic carcinoma or, when cultured, tuberculosis or other

infections. A marrow biopsy is more likely than an aspirate to reveal a lymphoma.

If the above work up is not diagnostic and a neoplasm or infection for which treatment should not be delayed is suspected, then a lymph node should be biopsied, examined, and cultured. It is best to biopsy cervical or supraclavicular nodes and to avoid axillary or inguinal nodes which are subject to local trauma and infections. Excision biopsy of an entire node provides a look at the nodal architecture. A node biopsy can be diagnostic in lymphoma, carcinoma, immunoblastic lymphadenopathy, infections such as tuberculosis or histoplasmosis, or a granuloma without caseation suggestive of sarcoidosis.

However, in 40 to 60 percent of patients the node biopsy will reveal only reactive hyperplasia and will not yield a specific diagnosis. This failure has been attributed to inability to differentiate histologically conditions such as hydantoin-induced hyperplasia from a true lymphoma, to noninvolvement of the node obtained, or to distortion of the involved node by other processes. If another node is palpable or detectable on chest x-ray, an open biopsy or biopsy via mediastinoscopy should be obtained. If no nodes are evident and lung carcinoma, sarcoidosis, or tuberculosis is considered likely, a biopsy of the scalene node and fat pad in the supraclavicular area should be obtained. However, if despite a nondiagnostic biopsy lymphoma remains a strong possibility, no other nodes are accessible, and progressive disease is apparent, a lymphangiogram is indicated. If abnormal abdominal or retroperitoneal nodes are detected, abdominal laparotomy may be necessary for diagnostic biopsies. However, if the patient with the nondiagnostic biopsy is otherwise well or improving and has no other accessible nodes, watchful waiting is acceptable. Adenopathy secondary to infections will almost always regress within 2 to 3 weeks. However, in several long-term follow-up studies, 25 to 60 percent of patients with nondiagnostic lymph node biopsies were found within a very few months to have lymphomas or carcinomas and, less often, connective tissue disease or infection. The need for careful and frequent follow-up evaluations of such patients and for a node biopsy as nodes become available is obvious.

Lymph node syndromes In addition to the diagnostic entities cited, several new diseases of lymph nodes, with or without involvement of other organs, have been discovered. These include the combination of fever, rash, and lymphadenopathy, also termed the *mucocutaneous lymph node syndrome* (*Kawasaki's disease*), in children (Chap. 180) and a lymphoproliferative and granulomatous disease involving predominantly the lungs called *lymphomatoid granulomatosis*. This process usually spares the lymph nodes, spleen, and bone marrow, although sometimes generalized atypical lymphoid hyperplasia may antedate for pulmonary lesions.

IMMUNOBLASTIC LYMPHADENOPATHY   This is a disease characterized by the morphological triad of (1) predominant infiltration of immunoblasts, (2) proliferation of arborizing small blood vessels, and (3) deposition of acidophilic material in the lymph nodes, liver, spleen, and other organs. Clinically, the disease is characterized by weakness, fever, sweats, weight loss, generalized lymphadenopathy, and often hepatosplenomegaly. Rashes, which vary from maculopapular to urticarial, are common. An autoimmune hemolytic anemia is a commonly associated finding as is polyclonal hypergammaglobulinemia, involving at one time or another gamma-G, gamma-M, and gamma-A immunoglobulins. One report describes a subset of these patients who also have interstitial pulmonary infiltrates, vasculitis, and hypocomplementemia. Most of these patients are elderly; the majority have had progressive disease and have died within 18 months but, in a few, the course has been much more benign, and they have done well with modest doses of steroids. According to some authors, aggressive chemotherapy is contraindicated in these patients.

The pathophysiology of this process remains a matter of speculation. Because many cases have followed in the wake of drug ingestion, it has been suggested that this disease is a hyperimmune response of the B-cell system, which escapes from T-cell suppressor control resulting in an exaggerated transformation to immunoblasts and plasma cells. This hypothesis remains to be confirmed.

ENLARGEMENT OF THE SPLEEN

STRUCTURE OF THE SPLEEN Splenic function reflects the specialized cells and unique circulation of this organ. The spleen has a capsule and trabeculae which enclose the white and red pulp. The white pulp consists of periarterial sheaths of lymphocytes with follicles containing germinal centers in which there are plasma cells and macrophages. The red pulp consists of cords of reticulum containing phagocytic macrophages separated from sinuses by a basement membrane. The narrow, tortuous splenic circulation sequesters blood within the pulp and exposes the traversing blood cells to phagocytic cells and to metabolic and immunologic hazards, as well as to barriers which make it necessary for the cells to change their size and shape in order to squeeze through the cords and sinuses and return into the circulation.

FUNCTION OF THE SPLEEN The spleen functions as the largest lymph node. It responds to antigens with proliferation of T lymphocytes in the lymphatic sheath and of the antibody-forming B cells in the germinal centers, as well as with proliferation of phagocytic cells. The phagocytic function of the spleen includes "culling" and "pitting" which occur mostly in the tortuous red pulp. Culling refers to phagocytosis of abnormal whole red blood cells which have been damaged physically or immunologically and of cells containing nuclei or Howell-Jolly bodies, reticulocytes, siderocytes, target cells, and spherocytes. Pitting refers to the removal of inclusions, e.g., red blood cell nuclei, Heinz bodies, and malarial parasites from red blood cells without destroying the cells. The spleen serves as a reservoir of platelets but not of red blood cells or leukocytes. It normally sequesters 30 to 40 percent of the blood platelets. The spleen is normally the site of blood formation through the fifth fetal month, but not after birth—except in some abnormal conditions.

MECHANISMS OF SPLENIC ENLARGEMENT Like other lymph nodes, the spleen enlarges with reactive hyperplasia in infection and inflammation and with proliferation of lymphoma cells or with infiltration by other neoplastic cells, mostly in chronic leukemias, or by lipid-laden macrophages. The spleen also enlarges with extramedullary hemopoiesis, with proliferation of phagocytic cells in response to increased destruction of blood cells, and, uniquely, by vascular congestion in the presence of portal hypertension.

DISEASES ASSOCIATED WITH SPLENOMEGALY Table 55-2 lists the principal conditions associated with splenomegaly, some of which require a brief comment. Any condition which causes generalized lymphadenopathy can cause splenomegaly.

TABLE 55-2
Conditions associated with splenomegaly

I Immunologic-inflammatory *[→ ROCKY MOUNTAIN SPOTTED FEVER]*
  A Infections: Subacute bacterial endocarditis, brucellosis, tuberculosis, infectious mononucleosis, cytomegalovirus, syphilis, histoplasmosis, malaria, kala azar, schistosomiasis
  B Connective tissue diseases: Rheumatoid arthritis, Felty's syndrome, systemic lupus erythematosus
  C Sarcoidosis
II Hematologic disorders
  A Neoplastic: Lymphomas, histiocytoses, myeloproliferative syndromes (chronic myelocytic leukemia, polycythemia vera, myelofibrosis, and myeloid metaplasia), chronic lymphocytic leukemia, acute leukemia
  B Nonneoplastic: Hemolytic anemias, e.g., hereditary spherocytosis, autoimmune hemolytic anemia, hemoglobinopathies, immunoblastic lymphadenopathy
III Congestive splenomegaly due to portal hypertension: Hepatic cirrhosis, portal or splenic vein thrombosis or stenosis, myeloid metaplasia, vinyl chloride
IV Metabolic-infiltrative: Gaucher's and Niemann-Pick's disease, amyloidosis
V Miscellaneous: Cyst, splenic abscess, aneurysm of splenic artery, cavernous hemangioma

Splenomegaly is frequent in infectious mononucleosis, subacute bacterial endocarditis, brucellosis, histoplasmosis, malaria, kala azar, and other parasitic infections. It occurs in 10 to 20 percent of patients with systemic lupus erythematosus and in rheumatoid arthritis which, when associated with splenomegaly and anemia, thrombocytopenia, or, most often, leukopenia, is designated *Felty's syndrome*. The cytopenia often responds to splenectomy. Splenomegaly also occurs in most patients with immunoblastic lymphadenopathy.

Lymphomas often involve the spleen even when it is not palpable, and laparotomy to determine the extent of a lymphoma—especially in Hodgkin's disease—always includes splenectomy. The spleen is massively enlarged in myeloproliferative syndromes, especially chronic myelogenous leukemia and myelofibrosis. Splenomegaly may also be prominent in chronic lymphocytic leukemia and may be associated with autoimmune hemolytic anemia. Splenomegaly associated with increased destruction of red blood cells occurs with many hemolytic anemias some of which like hereditary spherocytosis and, sometimes, autoimmune hemolytic anemia, respond dramatically to splenectomy.

Chronic congestive splenomegaly due to portal hypertension (Banti's syndrome; see Chap. 322) is associated with gastrointestinal bleeding and pancytopenia. It is usually secondary to cirrhosis of the liver or, less commonly, to portal vein thrombosis. Splenomegaly is often accompanied by the syndrome of hypersplenism (Chap. 322), consisting of a large spleen, anemia, leukopenia or thrombocytopenia, and hyperactivity of the bone marrow. It is often reversed by splenectomy. Hypersplenism may occur in most splenomegalic states (Table 55-2). Its severity does not correlate with the degree of splenic enlargement. However, splenomegaly does not always cause hypersplenism.

APPROACH TO THE PATIENT WITH AN ENLARGED SPLEEN
Splenomegaly is common, yet a palpable spleen in an adult is almost always clinically significant. In one study, the spleen was palpable in only 3 percent of students entering an American college and persisted in only a third of them. The spleen is even less likely to be palpable in normal persons beyond college age. Therefore, patients with a palpable spleen but without other signs or symptoms should have at least a spleen scan and complete blood count. Colloid tagged with technetium 99 injected intravenously is taken up by reticuloendothelial cells and visualizes splenic size, shape, and defects suggestive of tumor or abscess. The scan is the best method for detecting an

enlarged spleen and for ruling out a nonsplenic mass, e.g., cyst or metastatic tumor, which might cause splenic displacement rather than enlargement. A complete blood count and smear are often helpful or even diagnostic in asymptomatic splenomegalic patients with chronic myelogenous or lymphocytic leukemia.

Since most conditions which cause splenomegaly also cause lymphadenopathy, the approach to diagnosis is that presented in the section on adenopathy (above). The cause of splenomegaly should be determined not by tests on the spleen itself but by tests—possibly including a lymph node biopsy—for diseases known to cause splenomegaly and lymphadenopathy. Splenomegaly in acute leukemia is usually a minor clinical feature—the diagnosis is made by blood count and marrow examinations. Splenomegaly in lymphomas is almost always associated with adenopathy, and the diagnosis made by node biopsy or at laparotomy.

Most conditions which cause splenomegaly without adenopathy can also be suspected and diagnosed by history and physical and laboratory examination. For example, a hemolytic anemia is detectable by routine laboratory tests for anemia and for hemolysis, including reticulocyte counts and serum bilirubin. Specific causes for hemolysis can then be determined by other procedures such as Coombs' test, osmotic fragility, and hemoglobin electrophoresis. Similarly, splenomegaly and hypersplenism secondary to portal hypertension caused by cirrhosis of the liver are readily diagnosed by a history of alcoholism or previous liver disease, physical signs of liver dysfunction and portal hypertension, laboratory abnormalities consistent with liver dysfunction and hypersplenism, and radiological evidence of esophageal varices. The diagnosis of the rare vascular causes of portal hypertension requires angiography.

Some patients with splenomegaly may have systemic symptoms but no nodes available for biopsy. If an underlying lymphoma or serious infection is considered likely but is not detected by the usual examinations, including lymphangiograms,

a laparotomy with biopsy of the liver and abdominal nodes, and splenectomy, may be necessary. Appropriate cultures and pathological examinations are essential. Such laparotomies on patients with splenomegaly of unknown cause have revealed lymphoma in one-third, congestive splenomegaly in one-fourth, and inflammatory disease in one-fifth of patients.

REFERENCES

CHRISTENSEN BE: Pathophysiology of "hypersplenism syndrome." Scand J Haematol 11:5, 1973

FRIZZERA G et al: Angio-immunoblastic lymphadenopathy. Am J Med 59:803, 1975

LIEBOW AA et al: Lymphomatoid granulomatosis. Hum Pathol 3:457, 1972

LUKES RJ, TINDLE BH: Immunoblastic lymphadenopathy. N Engl J Med 292:1, 1975

MCINTYRE OR, EBAUGH FG JR: Palpable spleens in college freshmen. Ann Intern Med 66:310, 1967

SINCLAIR S et al: Biopsy of enlarged, superficial lymph nodes. JAMA 228:602, 1974

SKANDALAKIS JE et al: Tumors of the neck. Surgery 48:375, 1960

WEINSTEIN IM: Lymph node enlargement and splenomegaly, in *Hematology*, WJ Williams et al (eds). New York, McGraw-Hill, 1977, chap 106, p 950

WEISENBURGER D et al: Immunoblastic lymphadenopathy with pulmonary infiltrates, hypocomplementemia and vasculitis. Am J Med 63:849, 1977

WINTERBAUER RH et al: A clinical interpretation of bilateral hilar adenopathy. Ann Intern Med 78:65, 1973

WINTROBE MM et al: *Clinical Hematology*, 7th ed. Philadelphia, Lea & Febiger, 1974

ZUELZER WW, KAPLAN J: The child with lymphadenopathy. Semin Hematol 12:323, 1975

---

section 11 | Alterations in laboratory findings

56
ABNORMALITIES OF LEUKOCYTES

DAVID C. DALE

Alterations of leukocyte counts and functions occur in a wide variety of hematologic, infectious, inflammatory, metabolic, and neoplastic diseases. Because leukocytes are affected by so many diseases, the routine laboratory evaluation of many patients begins with determination of the leukocyte count and the examination of a stained blood smear. From the clinical examination and these blood studies, certain diagnoses can be made or strongly suspected, e.g., leukemia, agranulocytosis, infectious mononucleosis, systemic mastocytosis, and the Chédiak-Higashi syndrome. In patients with infectious and inflam-

matory diseases, the leukocyte count usually serves as a useful guide to the severity of the disease process. The leukocyte count and blood smear examination plus special studies of leukocyte function also will identify certain patients with heightened susceptibility to infections.

Five types of circulating leukocytes can be identified by their morphology on blood smears: neutrophils, lymphocytes, monocytes, eosinophils, and basophils. It is generally accepted that all these leukocyte types, along with erythrocytes and platelets, derive from a common pluripotent stem cell. However, beyond this common origin, independent regulatory mechanisms govern the production, distribution, and function of each type of leukocyte. For simplicity, inferences are often made about the presence or severity of illness from the total leukocyte count and the differential leukocyte count expressed as a percentage. It is more precise to express the counts of each type of leukocyte in terms of the concentration or absolute count per cubic millimeter of blood. This is usually determined simply by multiplying the total leukocyte count by the percent value. Normal values for blood leukocyte counts are shown in Table 56-1.

NEUTROPHILS

NORMAL PHYSIOLOGY The primary function of neutrophils is phagocytosis, killing, and digestion of microorganisms. The cells develop the capacity to perform these special functions in the bone marrow. Early neutrophil precursors, myeloblasts and promyelocytes, differentiate from hematopoietic stem cells by developing an active Golgi apparatus and endoplasmic reticulum and beginning the formation of cytoplasmic granules. The initial or *primary granules* stain reddish-purple with azure dyes; hence they are also called *azurophilic granules*. They contain myeloperoxidase, acid hydrolases, lysozyme, and cationic antibacterial proteins. With further development the cells become myelocytes. At this stage the cytoplasm becomes packed with characteristic secondary or *specific granules* which stain faintly pink with the usual blood stains. These granules contain alkaline phosphatase, collagenase, lactoferrin, lysozyme, and aminopeptidase. Beyond the myelocyte stage, neutrophilic cells do not divide; instead their nuclear chromatin becomes condensed, the cell diminishes modestly in size, and cytoplasmic glycogen accumulates. Normally neutrophils are not released to the blood until the nucleus is segmented, that is, the cells have matured beyond the metamyelocyte and "band" stages.

Approximately 8 to 14 days are required for a cell to move through the sequence of four to six cell divisions and complete maturation, that is, from the myeloblast stage to a mature blood neutrophil. Measurement of the time required for the early developmental stages is difficult, but it is clear that there are normally 3 to 4 days of neutrophil maturation after cell division is finished. During this time the maturing cells can be released from the bone marrow to the blood under sufficient stress, and therefore they are described as being in the marrow neutrophil reserves. Morphologic and radioisotopic studies on bone marrow indicate that there are normally about 10 times as many nearly mature neutrophils in the marrow as in the blood. The size of the marrow neutrophil reserves can be estimated by administration of endotoxin, etiocholanolone, or glucocorticosteroids and measuring the increase in the neutrophil counts. In normal individuals, these agents roughly double the count or increase blood neutrophils by a minimum of 2000 cells per cubic millimeter.

The regulation of neutrophil production and release remains poorly understood. Normal individuals maintain their own characteristic neutrophil count, but this is subject to substantial day-to-day variation and is greatly affected by activity and many other factors. A humoral substance has been identi-

fied which will stimulate neutrophil release from the bone marrow (neutrophilia-inducing factor). Colony-stimulating factor, a substance present in serum and urine which will stimulate neutrophilic bone marrow cells to grow in tissue culture systems, is another possible neutrophil regulator. The precise physiologic role of these substances is not clear.

The blood serves to transport neutrophils to areas of acute inflammation as well as to the mucosal surfaces of the body where these cells serve to maintain the normal defensive barrier to microbial invasion. Normally only about half of the neutrophils in the vascular system are circulating freely and are described as being in the circulating neutrophil pool. Only these cells are counted in routine blood samples. The other half of the blood neutrophils are loosely adherent to the walls of blood vessels throughout the body in the marginal neutrophil pool. In response to inflammation, neutrophils are shifted to the marginal pool. Certain drugs, i.e., epinephrine, glucocorticosteroids, and other anti-inflammatory agents, may reduce margination.

The neutrophil blood half-disappearance time (blood half-life) is only about 6 to 7 h. Neutrophils leave the vascular compartment by passing between endothelial cells presumably because they are attracted to sites of inflammation by chemotactic factors. Bacteria can release low molecular weight chemotactic substances. A well-characterized chemotactic factor, C5a, is generated from the complement system when plasma reacts with endotoxin, antigen-antibody complexes, and other foreign substances. Kallikrein, plasminogen activator, transfer factor, and other substances will also attract neutrophils.

At the inflammatory site, phagocytosis is facilitated by humoral substances, opsonins, which have coated the surface of the foreign material to be ingested. Immunoglobulins (IgG) and complement (C3) are the best-characterized opsonins. Phagocytosis stimulates numerous intracellular events including increased oxygen consumption, glycogenolysis, glucose oxidation via the hexosemonophosphate shunt, and hydrogen peroxide production. Within the cell, the phagocytized particle is held in a vacuole, and the contents of the secondary and then the primary granules are sequentially emptied into this vacuole. The vacuolar pH is dramatically lowered, and the granule enzymes are activated. The neutrophil possesses a variety of bactericidal mechanisms giving it an "overkill" capacity. The best characterized bactericidal mechanism involves myeloperoxidase, hydrogen peroxide, and a halide such as iodide or chloride. The highly reactive oxygen derivatives, superoxide (O_2^-), singlet oxygen ($^1O_2$), and hydroxyl radical (OH·) may also participate in the microbicidal system of the cell. An interesting result of the cell's respiratory burst and the generation of these oxygen derivatives is the emission of light, or chemiluminescence. The neutrophil usually degenerates after it digests the phagocytized material. Neutrophils, cellular debris, and digested foreign matter become the pus which characterizes acute inflammation, and to which the residual myeloperoxidase imparts the slightly greenish color.

NEUTROPHIL DISORDERS

A branching diagram for evaluating patients with neutrophil disorders is shown in Fig. 56-1. Neutrophil abnormalities are readily separated into those in which the number or morphology of the cells is abnormal and those in which the cell number and morphology are usually normal. The data base for evaluating disorders of neutrophils includes a complete history, with particular emphasis on drug usage and the frequency and severity of infections, and physical examination, especially noting the presence or absence of lymphadenopathy, splenomegaly, bone tenderness, and signs of inflammation. Basic laboratory data should include complete blood counts with

TABLE 56-1
Normal values for concentration of blood leukocytes*

Cell type	Mean, cells/mm³	95% confidence limits, cells/mm³
Neutrophil	3650	1830–7250
Lymphocyte	2500	1500–4000
Monocyte	430	200–950
Eosinophil	150	0–700
Basophil	30	0–150

* *Total leukocyte counts from venous blood samples were done in a Coulter counter, and 200 leukocytes were differentiated on Wright-stained blood smears made on cover glass.*

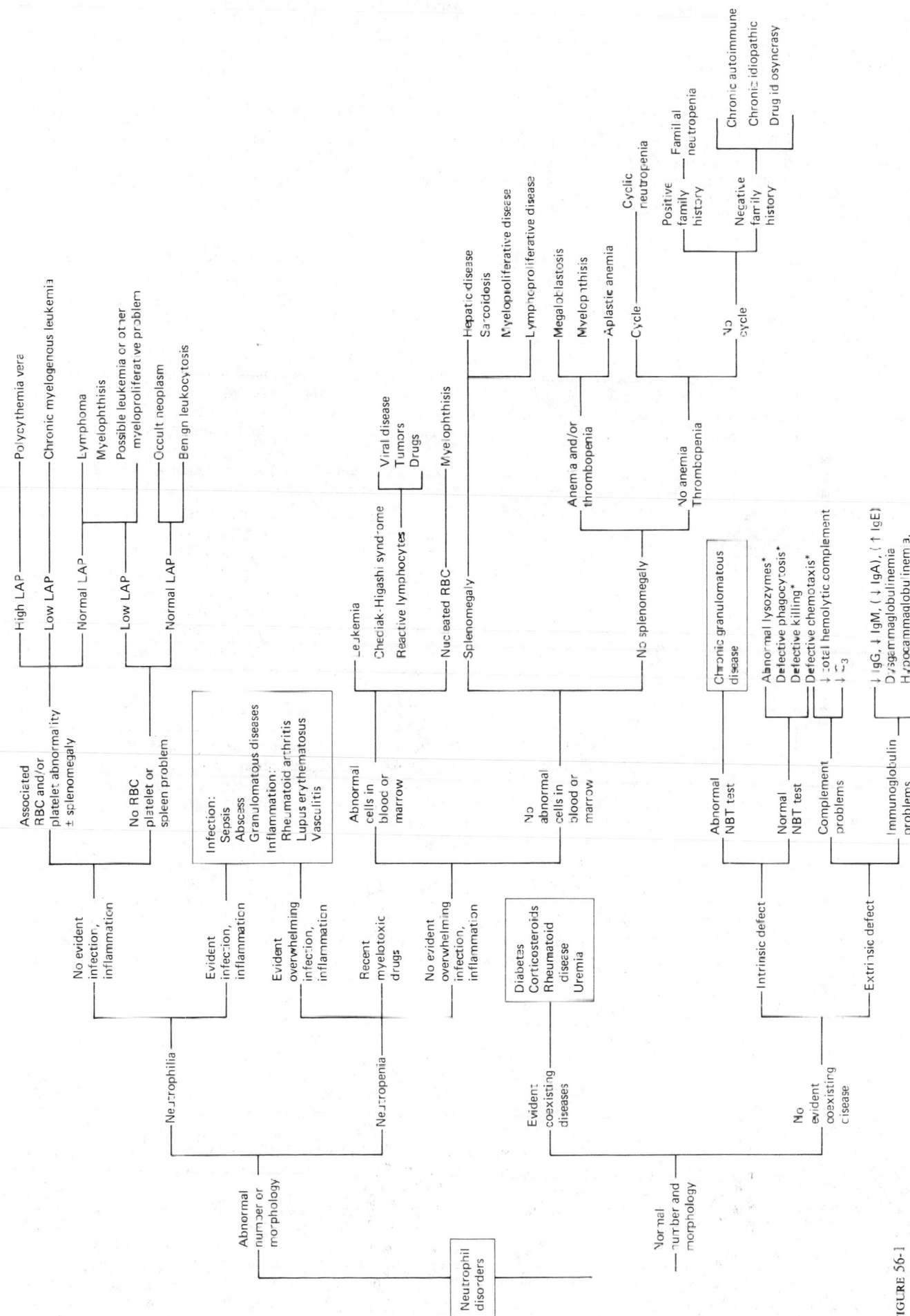

FIGURE 56-1

Diagnostic evaluation of neutrophil disorders.

*Special research techniques required

careful observation of leukocyte morphology and bone marrow aspirate and biopsy. In patients with neutrophilia, measurement of the leukocyte (neutrophil) alkaline phosphatase activity is very helpful for distinguishing between leukemoid reactions, chronic myelogenous leukemia, and other myeloproliferative states. In patients with frequent infections, immunoglobulins and complement are measured and nitroblue tetrazolium reduction (NBT) tests are done as base-line investigations before other studies of neutrophil function are made.

NEUTROPHILIA An absolute neutrophil count of greater than 10,000 per cubic millimeter should be regarded as elevated in most patients, although for a few individuals neutrophil counts of 10,000 to 15,000 per cubic millimeter are normal. The causes of neutrophilia are listed in Table 56-2. Exercise, excitement, epinephrine administration, or stress of any sort will increase the count up to twice the resting level within a few minutes. The duration of this neutrophilia is brief. It is largely due to a shift of cells from the marginal to circulating pool and is not accompanied by an increase in the number of nonsegmented blood neutrophils. Most acute bacterial infections are associated with neutrophilia, especially those that are accompanied by bacteremia, involve substantial amounts of tissue, and are localized in a closed space. This neutrophilia initially occurs because of accelerated release of cells from the bone marrow reserves and is often accompanied by an increase in the number of nonsegmented neutrophils in the blood, i.e., a "shift to the left." With prolonged inflammation from any cause, neutrophil production is stimulated and the bone marrow shows granulocytic hyperplasia. Toxic granulation, due to increased staining of the primary granules, and cytoplasmic vacuolization also occur under these circumstances. In all the usual conditions causing neutrophilia, the counts are generally between 10,000 and 25,000 per cubic millimeter. Persisting neutrophilia with counts greater than 30,000 to 50,000 per cubic millimeter is called a *leukemoid reaction*. This term is sometimes used to describe any persisting high leukocyte count because this degree of leukocytosis suggests leukemia. Characteristically in a leukemoid reaction the raised count is due predominantly to an increase in mature neutrophils with some increase of band neutrophils and metamyelocytes. Blood myelocytes are rare. The leukocyte alkaline phosphatase is generally high, and the cells do not contain Auer rods. The erythrocyte and platelet counts also are usually not strikingly abnormal. The differentiation between leukemoid reactions, leukemia, and myeloproliferative diseases is discussed further in Chaps. 321 and 326.

NEUTROPENIA Neutrophil counts of less than 2000 per cubic millimeter are relatively uncommon in normal individuals although some healthy resting adults, particularly black persons and Yemenite Jews, may have counts as low as 1000 per cubic

TABLE 56-2
Causes of neutrophilia

Physiologic: Exercise, excitement, stress, epinephrine
Infections: Chiefly bacterial, also fungal, parasitic, and some viral diseases
Inflammation: Burns, tissue necrosis as in myocardial and pulmonary infarction, collagen vascular diseases, hypersensitivity states, other inflammatory diseases
Metabolic disorders: Ketoacidosis, acute renal failure, eclampsia, acute poisoning
Myeloproliferative diseases: Myelocytic leukemia, myeloid metaplasia, polycythemia vera
Other: Metastatic carcinoma, acute hemorrhage or hemolysis, glucocorticosteroids, lithium therapy, idiopathic

TABLE 56-3
Clinical conditions characterized by neutropenia

Hematologic diseases: Chronic idiopathic neutropenias; cyclic neutropenia, lazy-leukocyte syndrome; Chédiak-Higashi syndrome; leukemia; aplastic anemia
Drug-induced conditions: Agranulocytosis; myelotoxic drugs
Nutritional deficiencies: Vitamin B_{12}; folate, especially in alcoholics; copper
Secondary to other diseases: Infections including typhoid, infectious mononucleosis, malaria, overwhelming sepsis; diseases with splenomegaly, Felty's syndrome, congestive splenomegaly, Gaucher's disease, sarcoidosis; malignancies with marrow infiltration

millimeter with no apparent disease. Neutropenia occurs in a wide variety of clinical circumstances (Table 56-3). In general, as the count declines below about 1000 per cubic millimeter, the risk of infection increases. However, the risk of infection is related to both the nature of the primary disease process and the cell count. For instance, many patients with chronic idiopathic neutropenia have counts of less than 500 per cubic millimeter for years without infections, whereas few patients with leukemia or aplastic anemia will survive for even a few weeks at these levels without developing an infection.

It is not possible to describe the neutropenias on the basis of kinetic mechanisms analogous to the mechanisms of anemia and thrombocytopenia. Most patients encountered will fit into the following general clinical categories.

Chronic neutropenia without splenomegaly (Chronic idiopathic neutropenia or granulocytopenia, familial benign neutropenia, chronic hypoplastic neutropenia, and chronic benign neutropenia of childhood) Isolated individuals and families are occasionally observed with neutropenia as their sole hematologic abnormality. Characteristically, the spleen is not enlarged. Onset may occur at any age; frequently, the syndrome is recognized on an incidental blood count. In adults, there is a striking female predominance, whereas in children both males and females are affected. Neutrophil counts may be as low as 50 to 200 per cubic millimeter with only infrequent infections, usually involving the upper respiratory tract. Bacteremia is rare. The blood usually contains normal-appearing mature neutrophils in reduced numbers; blood monocytes are often increased, and hypergammaglobulinemia may be present. The marrow is normocellular and shows few or no mature neutrophils. In a few cases, not readily distinguished from the rest of these patients on clinical grounds, leukoagglutinating antibodies to normal neutrophils have been detected and may be of etiologic significance (chronic idiopathic immunoneutropenia). The disease mechanisms otherwise remain largely unknown. In periods of observation up to 25 years, evolution to leukemia has been reported only extremely rarely. A few children with this disorder have had spontaneous remissions. In a few patients with frequent infections and extremely low counts, alternate-day glucocorticosteroids have elevated the neutrophil counts and reduced infections.

Several other groups of patients with chronic neutropenia without splenomegaly can be recognized which have distinctly different clinical characteristics. *Infantile genetic agranulocytosis* is usually a rapidly fatal disorder associated with anemia and atypical, vacuolated marrow precursor cells. *Neutropenia associated with hypogammaglobulinemia* leads to fatal infections at an early age. In *cyclic neutropenia, lazy-leukocyte syndrome,* and *Chédiak-Higashi syndrome,* chronic neutropenia is present but additional neutrophil abnormalities have been observed. Other patients are occasionally encountered with episodic severe neutropenia associated with febrile illnesses. Many other unusual neutropenic disorders have been observed; undoubtedly these neutropenias will be categorized further as their etiologies are better understood.

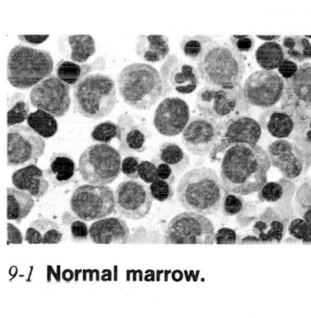

9-1 **Normal marrow.**

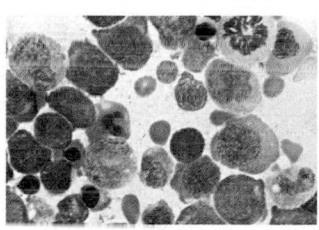

9-2 **Megaloblastic marrow.**

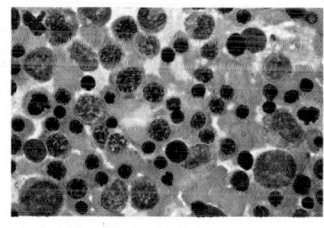

9-3 **Erythroid hyperplasia.**

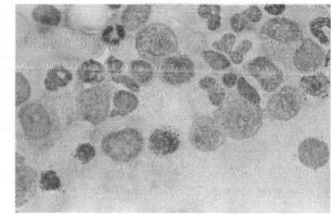

9-4 **Sideroblastic anemia.**

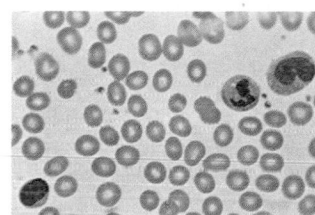

9-5 **Normal blood smear.**

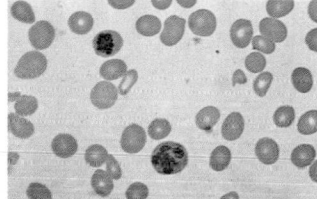

9-6 **Megalobastic anemia.**

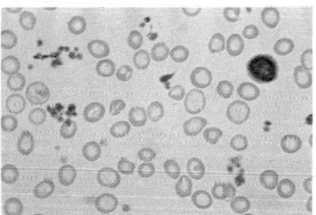

9-7 **Iron-deficiency anemia.**

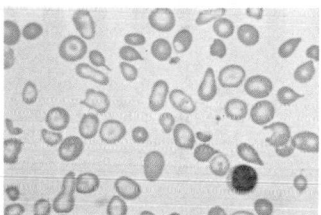

9-8 **β thallasemia intermedia.**

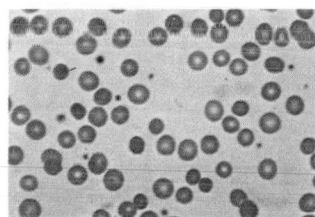

9-9 **Myeloid metaplasia.**
HEREDITARY SPHEROCYTOSIS

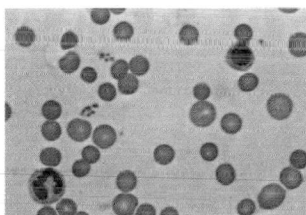

9-10 **Uremia.**
IMMUNOHEMOLYTIC ANEMIA

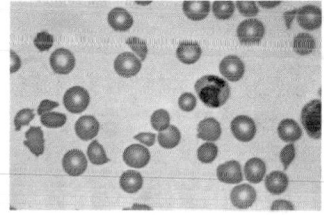

9-11 **Liver disease.**
TRAUMATIC HEMOLYSIS

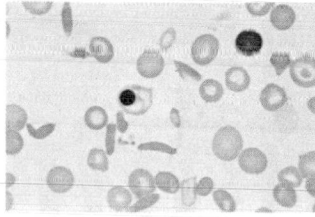

9-12 **Spur-cell anemia.**
SICKLE-CELL ANEMIA

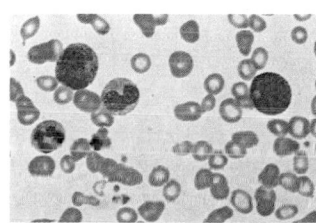

9-13 **Hereditary spherocytosis.**
MYELOID METAPLASIA

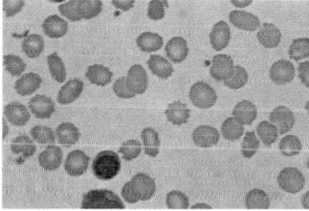

9-14 **Immunohemolytic anemia.**
UREMIA

9-15 **Traumatic hemolysis.**
LIVER DISEASE

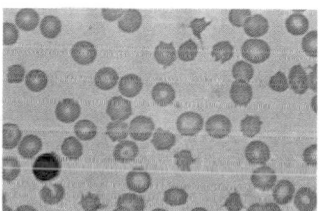

9-16 **Sickle-cell anemia.**
SPUR-CELL ANEMIA

PLATE 9

Normal and abnormal bone marrow smears (top row) and peripheral blood smears (bottom three rows). The size of normal red blood cells is about the same as that of the nucleus of a mature lymphocyte. Cell specimens were prepared with Wright's stain except the sideroblastic anemia marrow (9-4) which was stained with Prussian blue. 760×. (Courtesy of C von Kapff.)

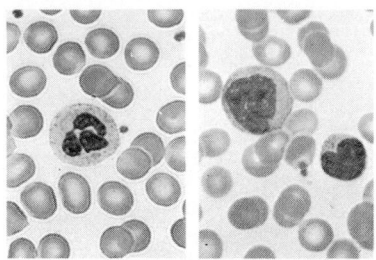

10-1 A. **Normal granulocyte.** B. **Normal monocyte and lymphocyte.**

10-2 A. **Normal eosinophil.** B. **Normal basophil.**

10-3 **Normal granulocyte precursors in marrow.**

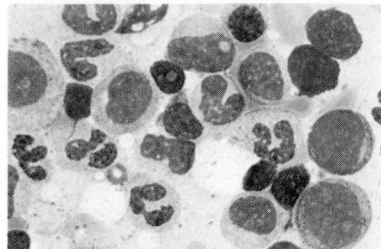

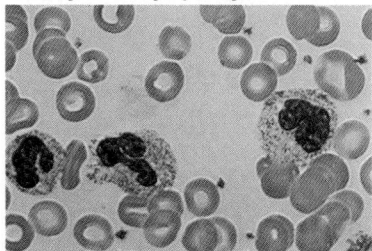

10-4 **Neutrophils with toxic granulation.**

10-5 **Band with Döhle body** (center).

10-6 **Hypersegmentation.**

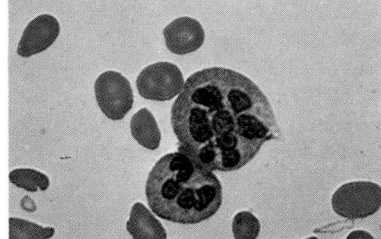

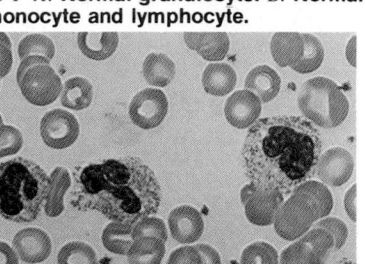

10-7 A. **Chédiak-Higashi anomaly.** B. **Pelger-Hüet anomaly.**

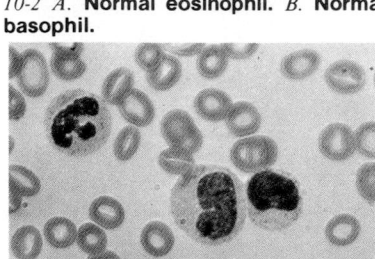

10-8 **Reactive lymphocytes** (infectious mononucleosis).

10-9 **Chronic granulocytic leukemia.**

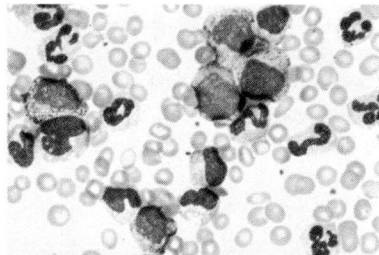

10-10 **Acute myelogenous leukemia:** myeloblast with Auer rod (center).

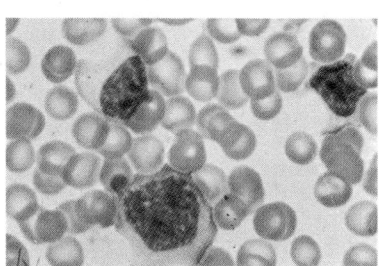

10-11 **Chronic lymphocytic leukemia.**

10-12 **Acute lymphoblastic leukemia** (marrow).

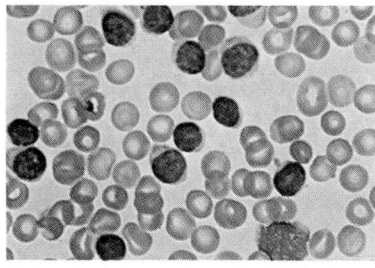

10-13 **Hodgkin's disease:** Reed-Sternberg cell in marrow (center).

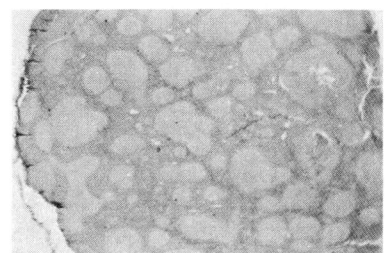

10-14 **Non-Hodgkin's nodular lymphoma** (lymph node).

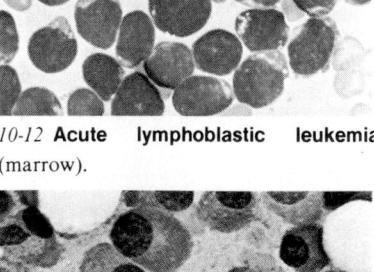

10-15 **Multiple myeloma** (marrow).

PLATE 10

Normal and abnormal leukocytes. (From American Society of Hematology Slide Bank, 2d ed, 1977. Used with permission.)

Cyclic neutropenia This disorder is characterized by the periodic absence of neutrophils from the blood and bone marrow associated with fever, malaise, mouth ulcers, and cervical adenopathy. These findings recur regularly at approximately 21-day intervals. Between episodes the patients are usually well. Symptoms characteristically begin in early childhood, although adult onset has been described. Cyclic fluctuations of other blood leukocytes, platelets, and reticulocytes occur, and bone marrow investigations indicate that the disease is due to a defect in the regulation of hematopoietic cell proliferation. Treatment with glucocorticosteroids, androgens, or splenectomy is not of predictable benefit, although cases improving with each of these treatments have been reported. Early recognition and prompt treatment of infectious complications are very important.

Neutropenia in the leukemias and aplastic anemia In leukemia, particularly the acute leukemias, neutropenia is frequently present at the time the disease is recognized. The predisposition to infection is severe, in part because the neutrophils which are present may not be functionally normal. The number of neutrophils and other host defenses are further suppressed by chemotherapy. When the neutrophil count is less than 500 per cubic millimeter, especially in patients in relapse, fever and infection should be expected (Chap. 107).

In aplastic anemia, the infection risk is probably roughly proportional to the neutrophil count with the chance of a severe and possibly fatal infection being substantially increased with neutrophil counts below 500 per cubic millimeter. The monocytopenia observed in these patients coupled with their neutropenia contributes substantially to the predisposition to infection.

Agranulocytosis (Schultz syndrome) Severe neutropenia occurs as an occasional or rare reaction to a great variety of drugs (Table 56-4). In most instances the patient is seen by the physician several weeks or months after beginning the offending agent and presents acutely ill with fever, sore throat, and oral or perianal ulceration. The total leukocyte count is often 1000 to 2000 per cubic millimeter, and neutrophils are absent from the blood and bone marrow. Marrow examination generally will exclude leukemia as the cause. Marrow recovery is the rule if the patient can be sustained long enough after the drug is discontinued. The pathophysiologic mechanisms for these reactions remain poorly understood. Both toxic effects of drugs on neutrophil formation and immunologic mechanisms causing accelerated cell destruction have been proposed and demonstrated in a few instances.

With some drugs, e.g., chloramphenicol, phenothiazines, carbamazepine (Tegretol), and propylthiouracil, patients may have a gradually declining neutrophil count, probably due to suppressed neutrophil production. It is not absolutely certain

TABLE 56-4
Drugs producing neutropenia

INFREQUENTLY CAUSE NEUTROPENIA

Analgesics: Aminopyrine, dipyrone, salicylates
Anticonvulsants: Dilantin, carbamazepine
Anti-inflammatory drugs: Phenylbutazone
Antimicrobial agents: Chloramphenicol, penicillins, sulfonamides, organic arsenicals
Antithyroid agents: Propylthiouracil, methimazole
Phenothiazine: Chlorpromazine, promazine
Tranquilizers: Meprobamate

REGULARLY CAUSE NEUTROPENIA

Alkylating agents: Nitrogen mustard, busulfan, chlorambucil, cyclophosphamide
Antibiotics: Daunomycin
Antimetabolites: Methotrexate, 6-mercaptopurine, 5-fluorocytosine

that these patients will develop agranulocytosis if the drug is not discontinued. However, as a rule, the presumed offending agent should be discontinued if the neutrophil count falls below 3000 per cubic millimeter.

Neutropenia and hematotoxic drugs In sufficient doses, a great number of therapeutic agents predictably cause leukopenia and neutropenia. This is particularly true for the agents used in cancer chemotherapy and for immunosuppressive therapy of nonmalignant, inflammatory diseases (Chap. 324). These drugs reduce neutrophil production. If the neutrophil count is not allowed to drop below 1000 to 2000 cells per cubic millimeter or if the period of neutropenia is brief, infectious complications are infrequent.

Neutropenia and nutritional deficiencies Vitamin B_{12} and folic acid deficiencies are sometimes accompanied by neutropenia as well as neutrophil hypersegmentation, particularly when folate deficiency is coupled with alcoholism. Copper deficiency, which may occur with chronic hyperalimentation, also reduces blood neutrophils.

Neutropenia with infections Certain infections may be accompanied by neutropenia. These include typhoid and paratyphoid fevers (Chap. 123), brucellosis (Chap. 127), tularemia (Chap. 128), infectious mononucleosis (Chap. 195), infectious hepatitis (Chap. 302), yellow fever (Chap. 190), measles (Chap. 181) and many other viral infections, malaria (Chap. 200), kala azar (Chap. 201), and rickettsial diseases (Chaps. 163 to 171). For the most part, these neutropenias are mild and their precise mechanisms are not known. It is postulated that they are largely due to redistribution of cells out of the circulating pool into an enlarged marginal pool. In certain overwhelming infections, for example, gram-negative bacteremia, pneumococcal pneumonia, and miliary tuberculosis, the occurrence of neutropenia portends a poor prognosis. This is particularly true in alcoholics, malnourished individuals, and patients with preexisting hematopoietic diseases.

Neutropenia with splenomegaly Neutropenia occurs in Felty's syndrome (Chap. 55), congestive splenomegaly (Chap. 55), Banti's syndrome (Chap. 55), Gaucher's disease (Chap. 102), and sarcoidosis (Chap. 216) as well as in infectious diseases with splenomegaly. There are often an associated mild thrombocytopenia and anemia. Splenic sequestration, as well as increased peripheral utilization, are proposed mechanisms. The predisposition to infection with these disorders is quite variable. Splenectomy to attempt to alter the neutropenia should be reserved for patients with repeated severe infections.

NEUTROPHIL DYSFUNCTION The normal functions of mature neutrophils are chemotaxis, phagocytosis, microbicidal action, and digestion of foreign material. There are a few specific diseases and syndromes in which these functions are abnormal. More commonly, defects in neutrophil function are observed which are secondary to other diseases such as alcoholism, diabetes mellitus, uremia, rheumatoid arthritis, and lupus erythematosus. Other defects occur secondary to abnormalities of complement and immunoglobulin metabolism.

Chemotaxis Accumulation of neutrophils in response to inflammation is most often deficient because of neutropenia. The tissue neutrophil response is also reduced by drugs, such as alcohol and glucocorticosteroids, which impair neutrophil adherence to the vascular endothelium. Chemotactic defects due to complement abnormalities have been observed chiefly in patients with either C3 or C5 deficiency. In general, defects permitting complement activation and C3 generation by the alternate complement pathway, for example, C1r, C2, and C4 deficiency, are associated with only a temporary delay in generation of chemotactic factor, and these patients have comparatively few infections. Defects in chemotaxis also may occur because of complement depletion in essential C3 hypercatabolism and possibly in acute glomerulonephritis and systemic lupus erythematosus. Chemotactic factor inactivators and inhibitors have been described in Hodgkin's disease, cirrhosis, uremia, and a few other circumstances. In patients with these complement-related disorders, the cells are usually normal when tested with normal serum. Cellular defects in chemotaxis have been described in the Chédiak-Higashi syndrome, lazy-leukocyte syndrome, newborn infants, and some patients with congenital ichthyosis, diabetes mellitus, rheumatoid arthritis, burns, hypogammaglobulinemia, and acute infections. In the *lazy-leukocyte syndrome,* the patients have gingivitis, stomatitis, and otitis with relatively few severe infections. They also have severe neutropenia, but the bone marrow shows ample mature neutrophils. The marrow neutrophils are not mobilized with endotoxin administration, and the cells show defective chemotaxis and random migration in vitro. In *Job's syndrome,* characterized by recurrent staphylococcal abscesses, eczema, and high IgE levels, a cellular defect in chemotaxis is also observed. Abnormal chemotaxis and defective phagocytosis have been recognized with hypophosphatemia and consequently diminished intracellular ATP. A specific chemotactic defect has been described resulting from the lack of the normal cellular contractile proteins necessary for cell movement.

Phagocytosis Reduced serum opsonic activity is the best-known cause for abnormal phagocytosis. This occurs in hypo- and agammaglobulinemia and certain complement disorders, including most of those with reduced chemotaxis, especially if activated C3 is not generated normally. Defective opsonic activity has been documented in premature infants, sickle-cell anemia, lupus erythematosus, and cirrhosis.

Microbicidal defects A few patients have reduced killing mechanisms because of isolated lysozomal enzyme deficiencies. In hereditary and acquired myeloperoxidase deficiency the leukocytes are morphologically normal except that specific staining shows decreased or absent myeloperoxidase. Eosinophil peroxidase is normal. The bactericidal and fungicidal defect is not as severe as in chronic granulomatous disease, and severe infections have been infrequent. Neutrophil lysozyme deficiency and total absence of secondary granules have been described with accompanying subnormal bactericidal activity.

CHRONIC GRANULOMATOUS DISEASE (CGD) This inherited disorder is characterized by severe recurrent infections of the skin, lymph nodes, lungs, liver, and bones. The infections are caused chiefly by staphylococci and certain gram-negative bacteria (particularly *Escherichia coli, Serratia marcescens,* and *Salmonella*). Histologically the tissues usually show a granulomatous reaction, lipid-filled macrophages, and multiple small abscesses. The neutrophils are morphologically normal. Neutrophil production, blood counts, and chemotaxis are also normal. Other measures of host defenses, including delayed hypersensitivity and lymphocyte functions, are normal, but immunoglobulins may be increased. The neutrophils, as well as the monocytes, have a greatly impaired ability to kill the types of microorganisms with which these patients usually become infected. Phagocytosis of bacteria is normal, but the metabolic burst which follows ingestion is markedly blunted. Superoxide

and H_2O_2 are not generated normally, and chemiluminescence is not observed. When CGD neutrophils phagocytize streptococci or pneumococci, these bacteria are killed normally because the bacteria contribute reactive oxygen derivatives from their own metabolism to the intracellular environment. This observation emphasizes the key role of oxygen and its derivatives in the intracellular bactericidal mechanism. Chronic granulomatous disease is most easily diagnosed by determining the amount of nitroblue tetrazolium (NBT) reduction which occurs when the patient's cells are incubated with this dye. Normally NBT is reduced intracellularly to a blue-black substance, blue formazan, which precipitates in the cell and can be seen as black intracellular particles. In CGD cells this reaction does not occur. The diagnosis is confirmed by observing that postphagocytic O_2 consumption, glucose C-1 oxidation, or the iodination reaction is reduced.

NADPH oxidase is probably the critically deficient enzyme in CGD. However, deficiencies of NADH oxidase and glutathione peroxidase, have been described in patients having typical CGD. The genetic heterogeneity indicated by family studies and the variable clinical presentations of CGD suggest that several different molecular lesions may result in this clinical picture. In *familial lipochrome histiocytosis* the neutrophils have a similar defect, but this disorder is described only in women, has a late onset, and presents very striking lipid-laden histiocytes in many tissues. Severe *deficiency of leukocyte glucose 6-phosphate dehydrogenase* with G6PD levels less than 5 percent of normal is also accompanied by neutrophil dysfunction similar to CGD. The management of CGD and its variants depends upon careful observation and detection of infections as early as possible. Cultures of affected tissues are critical for the correct diagnosis and selection of the appropriate antibiotic. Prophylactic antibiotics have probably been useful for some cases but may be accompanied by the usual problems of superinfections and emergence of resistant organisms (Chap. 114).

CHÉDIAK-HIGASHI SYNDROME This rare autosomal recessive disease is characterized by partial albinism, giant lysosomal granules in most granule-containing cells (neutrophils, monocytes, hepatocytes, renal tubular cells), and increased susceptibility to infections. The abnormal blood cells are readily seen on routine blood smears. The disease is usually recognized in children. There are several neutrophil abnormalities including moderately severe neutropenia, reduced marrow neutrophil reserves, and reduced neutrophil chemotaxis. In addition, in microbicidal studies, the giant primary granules are observed to degranulate slowly and thereby delay the killing of phagocytized bacteria. The disease is also accompanied by an accelerated phase with lymphohistiocytic infiltration in the liver, spleen, nerves, and other tissues with accompanying dysfunctions. Treatment is limited to prompt antimicrobial therapy of infections which usually resolve slowly. In the accelerated phase, vincristine and prednisone have been used to retard organ infiltration.

Other neutrophil abnormalities Unusual morphologic abnormalities of neutrophils include hereditary hyposegmentation (Pelger-Huet anomaly); hereditary hypersegmentation; retained remnants of endoplasmic reticulum, chiefly composed of RNA (May-Hegglin anomaly and Doehle bodies); and abnormally large azurophilic granules (Alder-Reilly anomaly). These abnormalities apparently do not interfere with neutrophil function.

OTHER LEUKOCYTIC CELLS

LYMPHOCYTES The chief functions of lymphocytes are production of immunoglobulins and expression of cellular immunity. Immunoglobulins react directly with foreign substances,

TABLE 56-5
Characteristics of T and B cells

	T cells	B cells
Origin	Bone marrow (with thymic influence)	Bone marrow
Life span	Long (months to years)	Short (probably days to weeks)
Circulating pattern	Chiefly recirculating	Chiefly nonrecirculating
Major location		
Lymph nodes	Deep cortical Perifollicular	Germinal centers Subcapsular
Spleen	Periarteriolar	Red pulp
Receptors	Sheep erythrocyte (rosettes) Mitogens (phytohemagglutinin)	Immunoglobulin (Fc) Complement (C3)
Functions		
Cellular immunity	4+	±
Antibody synthesis	0	4+

hastening their removal from the body by many mechanisms (Chap. 61). Cellular immunity is involved in delayed hypersensitivity and homograft rejection. Lymphocytes also can directly damage some foreign cells (cellular cytotoxicity).

On the blood smear, lymphocytes are a reasonably homogeneous collection of mononuclear cells with a small amount of blue cytoplasm containing a few granules. Through the analysis of surface receptors and responses to antigenic and mitogenic stimuli, it has been learned that there are two main types of lymphocytes, T and B cells, with strikingly different biological properties (Table 56-5). Approximately 80 percent of blood lymphocytes are T cells and 12 to 15 percent are B cells in normal individuals; these percentages are altered in many disease states. Different proportions of T and B cells are found also in the various lymphoid organs, i.e., lymph nodes, spleen, and bone marrow. Human lymphocytes are formed chiefly in the bone marrow. Normal T cells develop only in the presence of a normally functioning thymus (Chap. 62). Labeling studies indicate that there is a huge overproduction or ineffective production of lymphocytes by the lymphoid organs but that a substantial portion of the cells which reach the blood may live for years. These long-lived cells are principally T cells. They recirculate through the spleen and lymph nodes, thoracic duct, and bone marrow, leaving and reentering the circulation repeatedly. There are subpopulations of T cells which serve to enhance (helper T) or reduce (suppressor T) B-cell responses. It is not yet known precisely how the various surface receptors on T and B cells influence cell function, but they are probably involved in antigen recognition and cell-to-cell interactions with macrophages and other lymphocytes.

Lymphocytosis An increase in the absolute lymphocyte count occurs in certain infections: infectious mononucleosis, infectious hepatitis, infectious lymphocytosis, pertussis, tuberculosis, brucellosis, syphilis, thyrotoxicosis, and adrenal insufficiency. A lymphocyte count of greater than 10,000 per cubic millimeter usually indicates chronic lymphocytic leukemia especially in older patients (Chap. 326). The term "relative lymphocytosis" is sometimes used to describe situations where neutrophils are decreased with an increase in the percentage, but not absolute number, of lymphocytes. This term is misleading and should not be used.

Lymphocytopenia An absolute lymphocyte count of less than 1000 per cubic millimeter is observed in less than 5 percent of normal individuals but commonly occurs with acute, stressful illnesses such as myocardial infarction, pneumonia, or sepsis.

A transient lymphocytopenia regularly occurs even with very small doses of glucocorticosteroids. Chronic lymphocytopenia occurs in a variety of malignancies, uremia, congestive heart failure, lymphomas (especially Hodgkin's disease), aplastic anemia, lupus erythematosus, intestinal lymphangiectasia, and other immunologic deficiency syndromes (Wiskott-Aldrich syndrome, ataxia telangiectasia, Di George's syndrome, Swiss-type agammaglobulinemia, and thymic alymphoplasia) (Chap. 62). It also occurs following treatment with antilymphocyte globulin and certain chemotherapeutic agents.

MONOCYTES Monocytes are phagocytic cells with bactericidal capacities similar to neutrophils but with distinctive physiologic characteristics. They form in the bone marrow from promonocytes and have lysosomal granules containing myeloperoxidase, lysozyme, and acid phosphatases. They spend less time in the marrow than neutrophils and enter the blood with mitochondria and protein synthetic capacity intact, able to complete their differentiation as the circumstances demand. Monocytes leave the blood more slowly than neutrophils with a half-disappearance time estimated to be 12 to 24 h. They accumulate after neutrophils in acute inflammations in response to monocyte chemotactic factors.

In response to pinocytosis of serum proteins or ingestion of foreign material, monocytes enlarge and synthesize increased amounts of lysosomal enzymes and thereby are transformed to more active phagocytes called *macrophages*. Blood monocytes are the precursors of the pulmonary alveolar macrophages, spleen macrophages, and fixed macrophages of the monocyte-macrophage system (sometimes less precisely called the *reticuloendothelial system*). This system serves chiefly to remove foreign matter from the blood, e.g., bacteria, fungi, injected colloidal substances, and damaged or effete blood cells. During differentiation in each tissue site, monocytes acquire unique characteristics for that particular site. For instance, alveolar macrophages utilize chiefly oxidative phosphorylation to meet energy requirements, whereas peritoneal macrophages may chiefly utilize glycolysis. Generally, in all tissue sites these cells maintain the capacity to divide.

Monocytes have surface receptors for IgG, IgM, and complement, form rosettes with antibody-coated (IgG) erythrocytes, and are capable of synthesizing components of the complement system, transferrin, interferon, endogenous pyrogen, and colony-stimulating factor. In chronic inflammation they are probably responsible for the high serum and urine lysozyme concentrations. Monocytes serve a critical role in processing of antigen essential for both cellular and humoral immunity. They respond to lymphocyte-derived chemotactic and immobilizing factors (migration inhibitory factor, MIF). The incompletely catabolized endogenous materials generated in Gaucher's, Niemann-Pick's, and Fabry's diseases also accumulate in monocytes.

Monocytosis Increases in blood monocytes are observed in certain infections: tuberculosis, subacute bacterial endocarditis, brucellosis, Rocky Mountain spotted fever, malaria, and kala azar; in granulomatous diseases: sarcoidosis, regional enteritis; in some collagen vascular diseases; and in malignancies. Monocytosis may occur in leukemia and preleukemia, lymphomas, myeloproliferative syndromes, hemolytic anemias, and chronic idiopathic neutropenia.

Monocytopenia Reduced blood monocyte counts are seen acutely with stress and following glucocorticosteroid administration. Monocytopenia is observed in many acute infections, with aplastic anemia and acute leukemia, and as a direct effect of myelotoxic and immunosuppressive drugs.

EOSINOPHILS Many diseases are encountered where blood or tissue eosinophils are increased (Table 56-6). Eosinophils develop in the bone marrow similar to neutrophils. Their characteristic red-staining granules contain a unique peroxidase. Eosinophils have microbicidal capacities, and although these cells are chiefly involved in allergic and immune responses, their precise function in these responses is not known. Eosinophils are selectively attracted by an eosinophilic chemotactic factor elaborated by lymphocytes in response to certain stimuli. Eosinophils also accumulate in the skin in response to the topical application of allergens in allergic individuals. Animal studies indicate that the blood pool of eosinophils is relatively small compared with the number of these cells in various tissues. Significant tissue eosinophilia may occur in many inflammatory states, not necessarily accompanied by marked blood eosinophilia.

Eosinophilia More than 500 eosinophils per cubic millimeter of blood is infrequent in normal individuals. The most common cause for mild eosinophilia in hospitalized patients is probably some form of drug allergy. Parasitic infections, principally helminthic infections, cause eosinophilia, especially during the invasive phase. Some parasites may be difficult to recognize, e.g., strongyloides (Chap. 207), trichinella (Chap. 208), toxocara (Chap. 207), and filariae (Chap. 209). In these diseases the eosinophil count is rarely greater than 25,000 per cubic millimeter with the highest counts probably occurring in trichinosis. Protozoan infections generally do not cause eosinophilia. Eosinophilia is usually mild and irregularly present in allergic and collagen vascular diseases and malignancies and is not necessarily a clear guide to disease activity. The hypereosinophilic syndromes cause the highest eosinophil counts, occasionally in the 50,000 to 100,000 per cubic millimeter range or higher. Many tissues become infiltrated by eosinophils, a condition leading to organ dysfunction, particularly congestive heart failure.

Eosinopenia A reduction in eosinophils occurs with any stress or following corticosteroid administration. No known adverse effects result.

BASOPHILS These are the least common blood leukocytes; usually none are seen in the routine examination of a blood smear. The distinctive deep-blue granules, characteristically obscuring the cell nucleus, are rich in histamine. These cells are thought to be involved in certain acute allergic responses. Basophils are increased in chronic myelogenous leukemia, myelofibrosis, and polycythemia vera. This finding helps to distinguish these diseases from leukemoid reactions. Basophilia

may also be observed occasionally in some chronic inflammatory conditions.

REFERENCES

BABIOR BM: Oxygen dependent microbial killing by phagocytes. N Engl J Med 298:659, 721, 1978

CHUSID MJ et al: The hypereosinophilic syndrome. Medicine 54:1, 1975

CRADDOCK CG et al: Lymphocytes and the immune response. N Engl J Med 285:324, 1971

DALE DC et al: Chronic neutropenia. Medicine 58:128, 1979

GOLDE DW, CLINE MJ: Regulation of granulopoiesis, N Engl J Med 291:1388, 1974

KLEBANOFF SJ: Antimicrobial mechanisms in neutrophilic polymorphonuclear leukocytes. Semin Hematol 12:117, 1975

MORETTA L et al: Functional analysis of two human T cell subpopulations: Help and suppression of B-cell responses by T cells bearing receptors for IgM or IgG. J Exp Med 146:184, 1977

PRICE TP, DALE DC: The selective neutropenias. Clin Hematol 7:501, 1978

QUIE PG: Pathology of bactericidal power of neutrophils. Semin Hematol 12:143, 1975

ROWLANDS DT, DANIELE RP: Surface receptors in the immune response. N Engl J Med 293:26, 1975

STOSSEL TP: Phagocytosis. N Engl J Med 290:717, 774, 833, 1974

VAN FURTH R (ed): *Mononuclear Phagocytes in Immunity, Infection and Pathology.* Oxford, Blackwell, 1975

WILLIAMS WJ et al: *Hematology.* New York, McGraw-Hill, 1977

WINTROBE MM et al: *Clinical Hematology,* 7th ed. Philadelphia, Lea & Febiger, 1974

57
BIOCHEMICAL ABNORMALITIES AS A PRESENTING COMPLAINT

JEAN D. WILSON

INTRODUCTION Until a few years ago the majority of laboratory tests were performed at the discretion of clinicians. In the recent past the use of routine laboratory screening procedures has become more widespread, and the measurement of a biochemical profile, which includes some assays made formerly on a discretionary basis, is now a standard part of the clinical evaluation of patients.

Problems inherent in the interpretation of such screening tests constitute only a magnification of issues inherent in the understanding of all laboratory tests. Indeed, the unsuspected, unexplained abnormal laboratory result is a common, recurring problem in practice. It is also true that performing tests for which there is no obvious clinical indication is not solely a concern of laboratory medicine; the routine taking of blood pressure, examination of the heart, and roentgenography of the chest also fall into the category of screening procedures. However, the implications of admission biochemical profiles for the identification of asymptomatic disease constitute a particular challenge. [The problems inherent in population screening and of screening groups at high risk for certain diseases are beyond the scope of this discussion (see Chaps. 87 to 90).]

The vast majority of unanticipated abnormal results in medicine can be explained as due to laboratory error, a lack of recognition of the so-called "normal" range of values, or the presence (or presumed presence) of previously unrecognized disease.

LABORATORY ERROR One reason for unexpected, unexplained abnormal results is laboratory error, either random or

TABLE 56-6
Causes of blood eosinophilia

Drug reactions: Iodides, aspirin, sulfonamides, nitrofurantoin (see Chap. 71)
Parasitic infections: Hookworm disease, strongyloidiasis, toxocariasis, trichuriasis, trichinosis, filariasis, schistosomiasis, echinococcosis, cysticercosis
Allergic diseases: Hay fever, asthma, angioedema, serum sickness, allergic vasculitis, eczema, pemphigus
Collagen vascular diseases: Rheumatoid arthritis, dermatomyositis, periarteritis nodosa
Malignancy: Hodgkin's disease, carcinomatosis, mycosis fungoides, chronic myelogenous leukemia
Hypereosinophilic syndromes: Loeffler's syndrome, Loeffler's endocarditis, eosinophilic leukemia

systematic. The random error may be caused by incorrect labeling, switching of specimens, or error at any stage in the process of reception, analysis, or reporting; the frequency of random error is difficult to assess, but it may occur in 1 percent or more of analyses. Systematic error is more common; it may represent a generalized decrease in or general lack of precision within the laboratory. Lack of precision may be due to poorly trained personnel, but even in well run laboratories systematic errors occur from time to time and may carry whole groups of measurements from the normal to the abnormal range. Constant vigilance is required to detect the appearance of such errors.

LACK OF UNDERSTANDING OF NORMAL VALUES   There is no absolute method for defining either normal values or normal ranges for laboratory tests. For example, if a normal population is surveyed for 16 independent factors, each of which is normally distributed (gaussian), and if the limit of normal is accepted as ±2 standard deviations (SD) of the mean, then 40 percent of the population will have at least one abnormally high result. In practice many factors are not normally distributed, and a range of normal greater than ±2 SD is used. Furthermore, so-called "normal" values are usually not corrected for age or sex (glucose, albumin, uric acid, calcium, creatinine, alkaline phosphatase, bilirubin, cholesterol, potassium). Changes with age are a particular problem, since mean values may either increase (glucose, alkaline phosphatase) or decrease (calcium) in the elderly. If the whole distribution of values shifts to a different mean with age while the standard deviation remains unchanged, it can be assumed that the increase in the number of elevated or lowered values is due to a physiological change rather than to more frequent disease in the older population. Abnormal results due to failure to correct for age and sex usually fall just outside the normal range.

Another factor that influences interpretation of normal values is lack of appreciation of the magnitude of variation with time in the same individual. These variations are often due to the operation of a series of biological rhythms that influence the levels of plasma constituents, particularly hormones. Such rhythms operate over a period of minutes (plasma luteinizing hormone, testosterone), as diurnal or sleep-related variations during a 24-h cycle (cortisol, growth hormone, luteinizing hormone), or as monthly cycles (estradiol, progesterone, gonadotropins in women). Furthermore, biological rhythms may be more significant at certain times of life (secretion of growth hormone and luteinizing hormone at night in adolescents and preadolescents).

Other plasma constituents are subject to major day-to-day variations of unknown cause and without evident rhythmicity (urea, uric acid, phosphate, bilirubin, creatine kinase, and calcium). Although the magnitude of such changes is usually less than differences between individuals, in specific instances it may be the source of confusion. The degree of intraindividual variation in disease can be either less than normal (serum cortisol in Cushing's disease) or greater than normal (serum calcium in hyperparathyroidism).

DETECTION OF DISEASE   In instances in which an unanticipated laboratory result is truly abnormal, such a finding may have any of several diagnostic implications.

Expansion of understanding in a recognized disease   Analyses of biochemical profiles have provided insights into certain diseases that are not afforded by discretionary measurements. For example, in the past, serum uric acid was measured only in those patients with suspected gout, whereas determination of uric acid in all patients entering the hospital has led to elucidation of the pathophysiology of uric acid changes in many disorders other than gout (see Chap. 92). Likewise, as the result of

routine measurements, it is now clear that serum alkaline phosphatase is frequently elevated in hyperthyroidism.

Suspected but undocumented disease   Abnormal tests may be found in patients who have no evidence of disease; this may pose little problem. In one 5-year follow-up of 241 patients with asymptomatic monoclonal elevations of serum globulins, development of associated disease was documented in only 18 percent. The presence of such an abnormality in the asymptomatic individual requires long-term follow-up, but no therapeutic intervention is indicated when disease is suspected but not proved.

Presymptomatic disease or disease with early manifestations
In some patients biochemical abnormalities are initially unaccompanied by symptoms or signs but later prove to be early evidence of a specific disease. Examples include high serum transaminase in patients with unsuspected hepatitis, elevated blood urea in patients with unrecognized renal failure, and elevated serum alkaline phosphatase values in patients who have unsuspected liver or bone disease. Diagnosis by serendipity has always been a part of medicine.

The therapeutic implications of such a diagnosis depend on the disease in question, the extent of the manifestations, and the treatment modalities available. For example, in a 4-year follow-up of 20 patients with elevated serum alkaline phosphatase values who proved to have asymptomatic biliary cirrhosis, only half developed symptoms of the disease. Thus, in this case long-term follow-up is warranted, but since no effective treatment is available, the recognition of asymptomatic disease is probably of no benefit to the patient.

In other instances the issues are more complicated, as is perhaps best illustrated by the problem of hyperparathyroidism (see Chap. 350). Whereas previously only about 1 percent of cases were considered to be asymptomatic, with the widespread use of the biochemical profile large numbers of patients with unanticipated, persistent hypercalcemia are now being detected. In one large series only about 15 percent of such hypercalcemic patients developed symptomatic hyperparathyroidism over a 3-year period, and consequently many patients with hypercalcemia must be classified as having suspected but undocumented hyperparathyroidism.

Nevertheless, the fortuitous finding of hypercalcemia is so common that the 15 percent who do have hyperparathyroidism now constitute a significant fraction of patients in whom the diagnosis is made. Some of these patients are clinically asymptomatic but have biochemical or roentgenographic evidence of the disease (change in bone density or hypercalciuria) on careful examination. When a potentially serious disorder such as hyperparathyroidism is metabolically manifest—even mildly—it is generally assumed that surgical intervention is indicated. Such patients with purely laboratory manifestations now account for one-fifth or more of patients coming to surgery in many hospitals. Whether routine intervention in such cases is appropriate will not be clear until more is known about the natural history of the process.

In *summary,* the finding of unanticipated abnormal laboratory results is increasingly common because of the availability of routine laboratory screening procedures. In some instances, the presence of disease is established after a complete evaluation, and therapeutic intervention is warranted; in other cases, patients have either suspected disease or asymptomatic disease and should simply be followed closely long term. In still other instances, particularly in that group of borderline patients who are clinically asymptomatic but have some laboratory or metabolic evidence of disease, therapy is commonly undertaken. Whether this is actually justified is unknown.

REFERENCES

BARZEL US: The changing face of hyperparathyroidism. Hosp Prac 12:89, November 1977

KYLE RA: Monoclonal gammopathy of undetermined significance. Natural history in 241 cases. Am J Med 64:814, 1978

LONG RG et al: Presentation and course of asymptomatic primary biliary cirrhosis. Gastroenterology 72:1204, 1977

MARTIN HF et al: *Normal Values in Clinical Chemistry*. New York, Marcel Dekker, 1975

MURPHY EA, ABBEY H: The normal range—a common misuse. J Chron Dis 20:79, 1967

SUNDERMAN FW JR: Current concepts of "normal values," "reference values," and "discrimination values" in clinical chemistry. Clin Chem 21:1873, 1975

WHITEHEAD TP: Multiple analyses and their use in the investigation of patients. *Advan Clin Chem* 14:389, 1971

WILSON JMG: Current trends and problems in health screening. J Clin Pathol 26:555, 1973

WINKEL P, STATLAND BE: Using the subject as his own referrent in assessing day-to-day changes of laboratory test results, in *Contemporary Topics in Analytical and Chemical Chemistry*, DM Hercules et al (eds). New York, Plenum, 1977, p 287

PART THREE | BIOLOGICAL CONSIDERATIONS IN THE APPROACH TO CLINICAL MEDICINE

section 1 | Genetics and human disease

58
GENETIC ASPECTS OF HUMAN DISEASE

JOSEPH L. GOLDSTEIN
MICHAEL S. BROWN

GENETIC PRINCIPLES

More than one-fifth of the proteins (and hence genes) in each human being exist in a form that differs from the one present in the majority of the population. This remarkable degree of genetic variability, or polymorphism, among "normal" people accounts for much of the naturally occurring variation in body traits such as height, intelligence, and blood pressure. Moreover, these genetic differences produce marked variations in the ability of individuals to handle every environmental challenge, including those that produce disease. Thus, every human disease can be considered to occur as a result of an interaction between a given individual's genetic makeup and the environment. In certain diseases, however, the genetic component is so overwhelming that it expresses itself in a predictable manner without a requirement for extraordinary environmental challenges. Such diseases are termed *genetic disorders*.

MOLECULAR BASIS OF GENE EXPRESSION All hereditary information is transmitted from parent to offspring through the inheritance of specific molecules of deoxyribonucleic acid (DNA). DNA is a linear polymer composed of purine and pyrimidine bases whose sequence ultimately determines the sequence of amino acids in every protein molecule made by the body. The four types of bases in DNA are arranged in groups of three, each group forming a code word, or codon, that signifies a particular amino acid. A *gene* represents the total sequence of bases in DNA that specifies the amino acid sequence of a single polypeptide chain of a protein molecule.

In order to be translated into a polypeptide, each DNA region corresponding to a gene must first be transcribed within the cell nucleus into a molecule called *messenger ribonucleic acid* (mRNA). The mRNA represents a sequence of purine and pyrimidine bases that is "complementary" to that of the DNA. Hence, each adenine of DNA becomes a uridine of RNA, each cytosine of DNA becomes a guanine of RNA, each thymine of DNA becomes an adenine of RNA, and each guanine of DNA becomes a cytosine of RNA. Figure 58-1 shows the DNA and mRNA code words for each of the 20 amino acids that are utilized to form proteins.

The mRNA leaves the cell nucleus and enters the cytoplasm where it becomes associated with *ribosomes* and thereby serves as a template for the ribosomal synthesis of proteins. Each of the 20 precursor amino acids for protein synthesis is attached in the cell cytoplasm to specific molecules called *transfer RNA* (tRNA). Each tRNA contains a sequence of purine and pyrimidine bases that is "complementary" to a specific codon in the mRNA. These tRNA molecules with their attached amino acids line up along the mRNA molecule in the precise order dictated by the mRNA code. Under the action of a variety of cytoplasmic enzymes (initiation factors, elongation factors, and termination factors), peptide bonds are formed between the various amino acids, and the completed protein is released from the ribosome. A schematic diagram of the genetic control of protein synthesis is shown in Fig. 58-2.

MAINTENANCE OF GENETIC DIVERSITY THROUGH TRANSMISSION AND SEGREGATION OF GENES It is estimated that the amount of DNA in the nucleus of each human cell is sufficient to code for more than 100,000 genes and hence to specify more than 100,000 polypeptide chains. The genes are arranged in a linear sequence of DNA that together with certain histone proteins form rod-shaped bodies called *chromosomes*. Each somatic cell contains 46 chromosomes, arranged in 23 pairs, one of each pair derived from each of the individual's parents. Thus, each individual inherits two copies of each chromosome and hence two copies of each gene. The chromosomal location of the two copies of each gene is termed the *genetic locus*. When a gene occupying a genetic locus exists in two or more different forms, these alternate forms of the gene are referred to as *alleles*.

In humans, a given gene resides at a specified genetic locus on one particular chromosome. For example, the genetic locus for the Rh blood group is on chromosome 1; at this chromosomal site there are two Rh genes, one on chromosome 1 derived from the mother and the other on chromosome 1 derived from the father. When two genes at the same genetic locus are identical, the individual is a *homozygote*. When the two genes differ (i.e., two alleles are present at the locus), the individual is a *heterozygote*. Each normal human is heterozygous at approximately 20 percent of genetic loci and homozygous at 80 percent. Figure 58-3 shows a map of human chromosome 1, illus-

Second nucleotide

First nucleotide	A or U		G or C		T or A		C or G		Third nucleotide
A or **U**	**AAA** *UUU*	} Phe	**AGA** *UCU*		**ATA** *UAU*	} Tyr	**ACA** *UGU*	} Cys	**A** or **U**
	AAG *UUC*		**AGG** *UCC*	} Ser	**ATG** *UAC*		**ACG** *UGC*		**G** or **C**
	AAT *UUA*	} Leu	**AGT** *UCA*		**ATT** *UAA*	} Stop	**ACT** *UGA*	Stop	**T** or *A*
	AAC *UUG*		**AGC** *UCG*		**ATC** *UAG*		**ACC** *UGG*	Trp	**C** or **G**
G or **C**	**GAA** *CUU*		**GGA** *CCU*		**GTA** *CAU*	} His	**GCA** *CGU*		**A** or **U**
	GAG *CUC*	} Leu	**GGG** *CCC*	} Pro	**GTG** *CAC*		**GCG** *CGC*	} Arg	**G** or **C**
	GAT *CUA*		**GGT** *CCA*		**GTT** *CAA*	} Gln	**GCT** *CGA*		**T** or *A*
	GAC *CUG*		**GGC** *CCG*		**GTC** *CAG*		**GCC** *CGG*		**C** or **G**
T or *A*	**TAA** *AUU*		**TGA** *ACU*		**TTA** *AAU*	} Asn	**TCA** *AGU*	} Ser	**A** or **U**
	TAG *AUC*	} Ile	**TGG** *ACC*	} Thr	**TTG** *AAC*		**TCG** *AGC*		**G** or **C**
	TAT *AUA*		**TGT** *ACA*		**TTT** *AAA*	} Lys	**TCT** *AGA*	} Arg	**T** or *A*
	TAC *AUG*	Met	**TGC** *ACG*		**TTC** *AAG*		**TCC** *AGG*		**C** or **G**
C or **G**	**CAA** *GUU*		**CGA** *GCU*		**CTA** *GUA*	} Asp	**CCA** *GGU*		**A** or **U**
	CAG *GUC*	} Val	**CGG** *GCC*	} Ala	**CTG** *GAC*		**CCG** *GGC*	} Gly	**G** or **C**
	CAT *GUA*		**CGT** *GCA*		**CTT** *GAA*	} Glu	**CCT** *GGA*		**T** or *A*
	CAC *GUG*		**CGC** *GCG*		**CTC** *GAG*		**CCC** *GGG*		**C** or **G**

Note: The DNA codons appear in boldface type; the complementary RNA codons are in italics. A = adenine, C = cytosine, G = guanine, T = thymine, U = uridine (replaces thymine in RNA). In RNA, adenine is complementary to thymine of DNA; uridine is complementary to adenine of DNA; cytosine is complementary to guanine, and vice versa. "Stop" = termination. The amino acids are abbreviated as follows:

Ala = alanine	*Cys = cysteine*	*His = histidine*	*Met = methionine*	*Thr = threonine*
Arg = arginine	*Gln = glutamine*	*Ile = isoleucine*	*Phe = phenylalanine*	*Trp = tryptophan*
Asn = asparagine	*Glu = glutamic acid*	*Leu = leucine*	*Pro = proline*	*Tyr = tyrosine*
Asp = aspartic acid	*Gly = glycine*	*Lys = lysine*	*Ser = serine*	*Val = valine*

FIGURE 58-1

The genetic code.

trating the location of those genes that have been assigned loci on this chromosome.

The genetic information carried on chromosomes is transmitted to daughter cells under two different sets of circumstances. One of these occurs whenever a somatic cell (i.e., a nongerm cell) divides. This process, called *mitosis,* functions to transmit identical copies of each gene to each daughter cell, thus maintaining a uniform genetic makeup in all cells of a single organism. The other set of circumstances prevails when genetic information is to be transmitted from one individual to an offspring. This process, called *meiosis,* functions to produce germ cells (i.e., ova or spermatozoa) that possess only one copy of each parental chromosome, thus allowing for new combinations of chromosomes to occur when ovum and sperm cell fuse during fertilization.

During the process of meiosis, the 46 chromosomes of an immature germ cell arrange themselves in 23 pairs at the center of the nucleus, each pair being composed of one chromosome derived from the mother and its homologous chromosome derived from the father. At a specified point in the meiotic process, the two partner chromosomes separate, only one of each pair going into each daughter cell, or gamete. Thus, meiosis produces gametes with a reduction in the number of chromosomes from 46 to 23, each gamete having received one chromosome from each of the 23 pairs. The assortment of the chromosomes within each pair is random so that each germ cell receives a different combination of maternal and paternal chromosomes. During the process of fertilization,

FIGURE 58-3

Gene map of human chromosome 1. The black bands represent those genetic regions of the chromosome that stain brightly by a fluorescent dye such as quinacrine; the white bands are the negatively staining regions; the hatched area is a variable region that stains differently (i.e., either brightly or negatively) in the chromosomes of different individuals. Each gene that has been localized to this chromosome is listed opposite its genetic locus on the right. (Data provided by FH Ruddle and VA McKusick.)

FIGURE 58-2

A schematic diagram of the genetic control of protein synthesis, illustrating the flow of genetic information from DNA to messenger RNA (mRNA) to the polypeptide chain of a protein molecule. Although DNA exists in a double-stranded form, only one of the two strands is used as a template for transcribing mRNA.

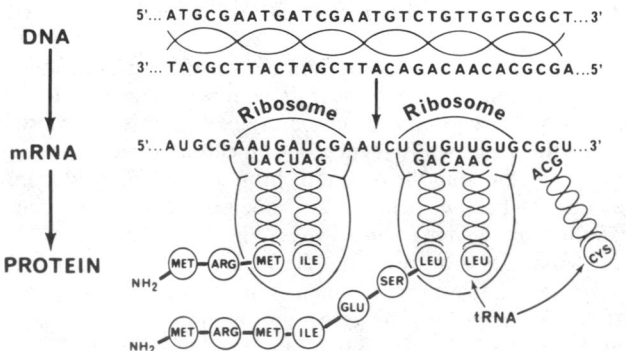

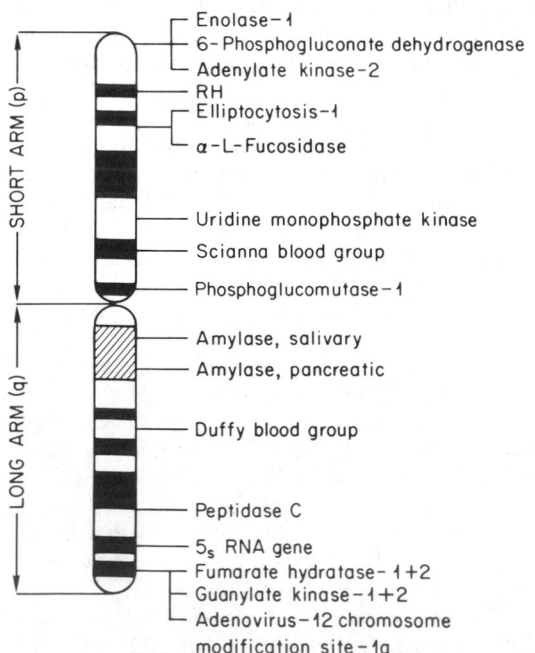

the fusion of ovum and sperm cell, each of which has 23 chromosomes, results ultimately in an individual with 46 chromosomes.

The independent assortment of chromosomes into gametes during meiosis produces an enormous diversity among the possible genotypes of the progeny. For each 23 pairs of chromosomes, there are 2^{23} different combinations of chromosomes that could occur in a gamete, and the likelihood that one set of parents will produce two offspring with the identical complement of chromosomes is one in 2^{23} or one in 8.4 million (assuming no monozygotic or identical twins).

RECOMBINATION Adding even further to the enormous genetic diversity in humans is the phenomenon of *genetic recombination*. During meiosis, when homologous chromosomes are paired, bridges frequently form between corresponding regions of the chromosome pair. These bridges, or *chiasmata*, are regions in which the two chromosomes break at identical points along their length and subsequently rejoin, the distal segments having been switched from one homologous chromosome to another. This process is designated *crossing over*. Although no net change in the amount of genetic material occurs during crossing over, a recombination of genes does occur. For example, consider a chromosome with two loci, A and B, located at opposite ends of the same chromosome. On this particular chromosome, the A locus has a rare allele *x* and the B locus also has a rare allele *y*. Without the phenomenon of recombination every offspring that inherited the *x* allele at the A locus would also inherit the *y* allele at the B locus. However, if recombination occurs, the A locus with the *x* allele would then be on the opposite chromosome from the B locus with the *y* allele. In this case any offspring that inherited the *x* allele at the A locus could not inherit the *y* allele at the B locus.

Crossing over in humans occurs with great frequency in every meiosis, and the resultant recombination of genes may occur at any point on a chromosome. The farther apart two genes are on the same chromosome, the greater is the likelihood that a crossing over will occur in the space between them. When two genes are on the opposite ends of a long chromosome, the probability of recombination is so great that their respective alleles are transmitted to offspring almost independently of one another, just as if the two gene loci were on different chromosomes. On the other hand, gene loci that are close together on the same chromosome are said to be *linked* so that there is a great likelihood that offspring will inherit the same combination of alleles that are present on the parental chromosome.

Several examples of *gene linkage* can be seen from the map of human chromosome 1 (Fig. 58-3). For example, the locus for the gene specifying the Rh blood group factor and the locus for the gene producing one form of the dominant trait, hereditary elliptocytosis, occur in close proximity on this chromosome. Thus, if a subject with hereditary elliptocytosis transmits the disease to an offspring, the offspring will usually inherit the allele that is present at the Rh locus on this chromosome. If the Rh allele happens to be a rare one in the population (such as *r'*), one can assume that whichever offspring inherits the *r'* allele at the Rh locus will also inherit the abnormal allele at the elliptocytosis locus. On the other hand, if an offspring does not exhibit the *r'* allele, he or she will not usually have elliptocytosis. The concept of linkage does not imply an association between any particular set of Rh alleles and the disease state elliptocytosis, rather between the two genetic loci. Thus, in different families the abnormal elliptocytosis allele may be linked to the R^1, R^0, r_2, or any other allele at the Rh locus, depending on the allele that happened to be at that locus when the elliptocytosis mutation occurred. Stated another way, the elliptocytosis locus is linked to the Rh locus in every family,

but the particular Rh allele with which it is associated will differ from family to family.

MUTATION Broadly defined, a *mutation* is a stable, heritable alteration in DNA. Although the causes of mutation in humans are largely unknown, a variety of environmental agents, such as radiation, viruses, and chemicals, are among the factors that are implicated.

Mutations can involve a visible alteration in the structure of a chromosome, such as a deletion or translocation of a portion of a chromosome, or they can involve a minute change in one of the purine or pyrimidine bases of a single gene. Most commonly, such "point" mutations consist of the substitution of one base for another, changing the meaning of the codon containing that base, hence their designation as *missense mutations*. For example, in the gene coding for the β chain of hemoglobin, the sixth position normally contains either the nucleotide triplet CTT or CTC, both of which code for the amino acid glutamic acid (Fig. 58-1). The mutation that gives rise to hemoglobin C produces a change of the first base of this triplet from cytosine to thymine, changing the triplet to TTT or TTC, either of which codes for lysine. On the other hand, the mutation that gives rise to hemoglobin S produces a change in the second base of the same triplet (from thymine to adenine), producing either CAT or CAC, which codes for valine. Thus, in the sixth position of the β chain of hemoglobin, the normally occurring glutamic acid may be replaced with either lysine (producing hemoglobin C) or valine (producing hemoglobin S). More than 84 such single-base mutations in the hemoglobin β chain have been identified in different population groups, and many of these mutations produce distinct clinical syndromes. Of all the mutations so far elucidated in humans, the vast majority involve such single-base changes.

Besides producing an amino acid substitution, a single-base substitution can also cause another abnormality in protein synthesis—premature chain termination. Three mRNA code words (UAA, UAG, and UGA) normally do not specify an amino acid but constitute the signal that the message has ended and that the protein chain should be released from the ribosome (Fig. 58-1). If a change occurs in DNA that produces one of these mRNA code words [for example, a switch in an mRNA triplet from UAU (tyrosine) to UAA (termination)], the polypeptide chain would be terminated prematurely when translation had reached that point. Such mutations, called *nonsense mutations*, produce short fragments of proteins that have reduced function.

CELLULAR MECHANISM BY WHICH MUTANT GENES PRODUCE DISEASES Critical to the modern understanding of heredity is the concept that the only information transmitted from generation to generation is the sequence of bases in DNA and that these sequences in turn specify only the primary structure of RNA and protein molecules. All other chemical reactions within a cell—such as the synthesis of complex lipids and carbohydrates, the formation of membranes and other cellular organelles, and the accumulation and partitioning of inorganic ions—occur as a secondary consequence of the action of specific proteins. Many of these proteins are enzymes that catalyze the biochemical conversion of one molecule into another. Others are structural proteins such as collagen and elastin, and still others are regulatory proteins that dictate how much of each enzyme and each structural protein is to be made.

Since proteins are the cellular molecules whose structures are encoded by genes, mutations in genes exert their deleterious effects by altering the structure of enzymes, structural proteins, or regulatory proteins. For example, in a disease such as glycogen storage disease, type I (von Gierke's disease), massive accumulation of glycogen in the liver is due not to a primary structural abnormality in the polysaccharide glycogen but to a structural abnormality in a protein, glucose 6-phosphatase, an enzyme that is required to liberate glucose from glycogen. Other examples of the biochemical mechanisms by which mutant genes alter cellular metabolism are discussed below in "Simply Inherited Disorders."

GENETIC HETEROGENEITY When two or more mutations can produce a similar clinical syndrome, genetic heterogeneity is said to exist. Hemophilia is one example of such a genetically heterogeneous syndrome. A clinically similar bleeding disorder can be caused by mutations at either of two different loci on the X chromosome, one leading to a deficiency of factor VIII (classic hemophilia) and the other causing a deficiency of factor IX (Christmas disease). It is now generally believed that most, if not all, hereditary diseases, when carefully analyzed, will be shown to be genetically heterogeneous.

Genetic heterogeneity may result from the existence of a series of different mutations at a single genetic locus (allelic mutations) or from mutations at different genetic loci (nonallelic mutations). For example, drug-induced hemolysis of red blood cells can occur in patients with several different types of allelic mutations at the glucose 6-phosphate dehydrogenase locus. On the other hand, hemophilia is an example of a syndrome in which nonallelic mutations can produce a similar clinical picture (see above).

In some cases of heterogeneity, both the genetic locus and the mode of inheritance will differ, depending on the mutation. Diseases such as spastic paraplegia, Charcot-Marie-Tooth peroneal muscular atrophy, and retinitis pigmentosa are inherited as autosomal dominant traits in some families, as autosomal recessives in others, and as X-linked recessives in still others. The identification of such genetic heterogeneity in these disorders is of obvious importance for correct genetic counseling.

TAKING THE FAMILY HISTORY

The investigation of a patient with a possible genetic disorder begins with the *family history*. The first step in obtaining an accurate family history involves obtaining certain information on the *proband* or *index case* (i.e., the clinically affected person who has brought the family to attention) and on each of the *first-degree relatives* (i.e., the parents, siblings, and offspring of the proband). This information includes the given name, surname, maiden name, birth date or current age, age at death, cause of death, and name or description of any disease or defect.

The second step includes asking six questions designed to survey the family for the presence of disease or defect. (1) Has any relative an identical or similar trait? (2) Has any relative a trait that is absent in the proband but is known to occur in some patients with the same disease? This question requires that the physician have some knowledge about the manifestations of the disease in question. For example, when obtaining the family history from a proband with dissecting aneurysm caused possibly by Marfan's syndrome, one should ask about the occurrence of eye abnormalities, cardiac abnormalities, and skeletal abnormalities in the proband's relatives. (3) Has any relative a trait that is recognized to be genetically determined? The purpose of this question is to ascertain the occurrence of hereditary disease in the family even though the particular patient may not be involved. (4) Has any relative an

unusual disease, or has any relative died of a rare condition? The purpose of this question is to identify a condition that might be genetically determined though not recognized as such by the informant. In addition, this question may help to identify conditions in relatives that might be etiologically related to the patient's problem. For example, a patient with pheochromocytoma should be suspected of having von Recklinghausen's disease who has a brother with scoliosis and mental retardation, both of which can be manifestations of the neurofibromatosis (von Recklinghausen's) gene. (5) Is there any consanguinity in the family? This inquiry should be made directly, but in addition one should ask whether common last names appear in the families of husband-wife pairs. Consanguineous marriage may be the source of a rare autosomal recessive syndrome, and sometimes its presence in the family may not be known by the proband. (6) What is the ethnic origin of the family? Persons of various ethnic origins, such as blacks, Jews, and Greeks, have increased chance of specific genetic diseases. Table 58-1 lists examples of simply inherited disorders that are found with increased frequency in various ethnic groups.

CATEGORIES OF GENETIC DISORDERS

Genetic diseases generally fall into one of three categories: (1) *Chromosomal disorders* involve the lack, excess, or abnormal

TABLE 58-1
Examples of simply inherited disorders that occur with increased frequency in specific ethnic groups

Ethnic group	Simply inherited disorder
African blacks	Hemoglobinopathies, especially Hb S, Hb C, persistent Hb F, α and β thalassemias Glucose 6-phosphate dehydrogenase deficiency
Armenians	Familial Mediterranean fever
Ashkenazi Jews	Abetalipoproteinemia Bloom's syndrome Dystonia musculorum deformans (recessive form) Factor XI (PTA) deficiency Familial dysautonomia (Riley-Day syndrome) Gaucher's disease (adult form) Neimann-Pick disease Pentosuria Tay-Sachs disease
Chinese	α thalassemia Glucose 6-phosphate dehydrogenase deficiency Adult lactase deficiency
Eskimos	Pseudocholinesterase deficiency Adrenogenital syndrome
Finns	Congenital nephrosis Mulibrey nanism
French Canadians	Tyrosinemia
Japanese	Acatalasemia
Lebanese	Homozygous familial hypercholesterolemia
Mediterranean peoples (Italians, Greeks, Sephardic Jews)	β thalassemia Glucose 6-phosphate dehydrogenase deficiency Familial Mediterranean fever Glycogen storage disease, type III
Northern Europeans	Cystic fibrosis
Scandinavians	α_1-Antitrypsin deficiency LCAT (lecithin: cholesterol acyltransferase) deficiency
South African whites	Porphyria variegata

SOURCE: *After McKusick.*

arrangement of one or more chromosomes, producing excessive or deficient genetic material. (2) *Mendelian or simply inherited disorders* are determined primarily by a single mutant gene. This is indicated by the fact that these disorders display simple (mendelian) inheritance patterns which can be classified into autosomal dominant, autosomal recessive, or X-linked types. (3) *Multifactorial disorders* are caused by an interaction of multiple genes and multiple exogenous or environmental factors. Although many of these multifactorial disorders, such as essential hypertension and cleft lip and palate, are said to run in families, the inheritance pattern is complex and the risk to relatives is much less than that seen in the single-gene (mendelian) disorders. Each of these three categories of genetic disease presents different problems with respect to causation, prevention, diagnosis, genetic counseling, and treatment.

CHROMOSOMAL DISORDERS The karyotype of an individual (i.e., the number and structure of the chromosomes) can be ascertained from readily accessible body tissues, such as peripheral blood lymphocytes or skin, by growing them in tissue culture until active cell proliferation occurs and then preparing single cells for examination of chromosomes by microscopy. Recent developments have made it possible to identify accurately each individual chromosome by special staining of DNA sequences, by the affinity of fluorescent dyes (such as quinacrine hydrochloride) for certain chromosomal segments that can be visualized by fluorescence microscopy, and by treatment with special dyes (Giemsa) and proteolytic enzymes (trypsin). These techniques produce characteristic *banding patterns* for each chromosome (Fig. 58-4).

The number of chromosomes in normal individuals is 46, of which 44 are the 22 pairs of *autosomes* and the other two are the *sex chromosomes*. Females have two X chromosomes (XX), and males have one X chromosome and one Y chromosome (XY). Each of the 22 pairs of autosomes and the two sex chromosomes can be distinguished on the basis of size, location of the centromere (which divides the chromosome into arms of equal or unequal length), and the unique banding pattern (Fig. 58-4). The relative length of the arms and the position of the centromere are used as further criteria to divide the human

FIGURE 58-4

The karyotype of a normal male showing the chromosomes of a single somatic cell in the metaphase stage of cell division. The photographic images of the chromosomes have been cut out and arranged according to descending length and varying arm ratio. The chromosomes have been stained by the Giemsa technique, which allows each chromosome pair to be identified by its unique banding pattern. Chromosomes 1 to 22 are the autosomes. The sex chromosomes in this normal male are an X and a Y. The normal female has an identical karyotype except for the absence of the Y chromosome and the presence instead of a second X chromosome. (Courtesy of K Hirschhorn.)

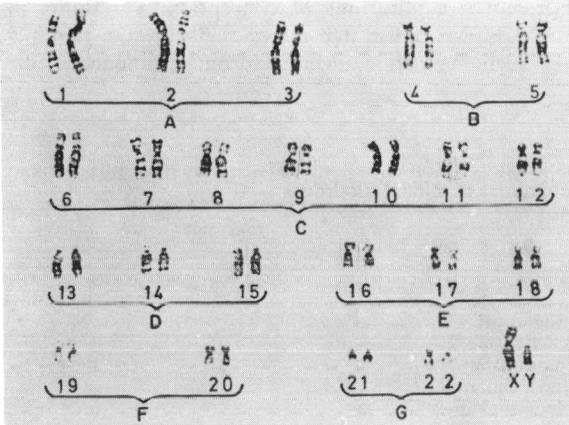

chromosomes into seven groups (designated A to G) (Fig. 58-4).

For a complete discussion of the etiology and clinical features of chromosomal abnormalities affecting humans, the reader is referred to Chap. 60.

SIMPLY INHERITED DISORDERS Disorders caused by the transmission of a single mutant gene show one of three simple (or mendelian) patterns of inheritance: (1) autosomal dominant, (2) autosomal recessive, or (3) X-linked. The distinction between "dominant" and "recessive" is one of convenience in pedigree analysis and does not imply a fundamental difference in genetic mechanism. The term *dominant* implies that a mutation will be clinically manifest when an individual has a single dose of this mutation (or is *heterozygous* for it), while *recessive* implies that a double dose (or *homozygosity*) is required for clinical detection. Genes are never dominant or recessive; their effects, however, produce clinical patterns that are classified as dominant or recessive. Despite their overall clinical "normality," individuals who are heterozygous for "recessive" genes often have biochemical abnormalities that are demonstrable in the laboratory; on the other hand, those who are homozygous for "dominant" genes are usually more severely affected than are the heterozygotes.

With few exceptions, each of the approximately 1200 or so mendelian diseases is rare. However, as a group these disorders constitute an important cause of morbidity and death, accounting directly for more than 5 percent of all hospital admissions.

The demonstration that a particular disease or syndrome shows one of the three mendelian patterns of inheritance implies that its pathogenesis, no matter how complex, is due to an abnormality in a single protein molecule. For example, in sickle-cell anemia, the entire clinical syndrome, including such seemingly unrelated disturbances as anemia, pain crises, nephropathy, and predisposition to pneumococcal infections, are all the physiologic consequences of having thymine instead of adenine at a specific site in the gene that codes for the β chain of hemoglobin, producing a substitution of a valine for a glutamic acid in the sixth amino acid position in the protein sequence.

In many mendelian disorders, especially in those with dominant inheritance, it is not possible to demonstrate directly the protein that is primarily altered by the mutation. In such cases (e.g., adult polycystic kidney disease and tuberous sclerosis) only the distal physiologic effects of the mutation are recognizable. Nevertheless, it is safe to assume that a single primary defect exists whenever a disease is transmitted by a single gene mechanism and that the various manifestations of the disease all can be related to the mutational event by a more or less complicated "pedigree of causes." Table 58-2 lists the most commonly encountered mendelian disorders affecting adults.

Autosomal dominant disorders Dominant diseases are those manifest in the heterozygous state, that is, when only one abnormal gene (*mutant allele*) is present and the corresponding partner allele on the homologous chromosome is normal. The gene responsible for an autosomal dominant disorder is located on one of the 22 autosomes, and both males and females can be affected. Since alleles segregate independently at meiosis, there is a 1 in 2 chance that the offspring of an affected heterozygote will inherit the mutant allele and, similarly, a 1 in 2 chance of the offspring inheriting the normal allele.

Figure 58-5 shows a typical pedigree involving an autosomal dominant trait. The following features are characteristic:

TABLE 58-2
Some relatively frequent mendelian disorders affecting adults

AUTOSOMAL DOMINANT DISORDERS

Familial hypercholesterolemia
Hereditary hemorrhagic telangiectasia
Marfan's syndrome
Hereditary spherocytosis
Adult polycystic kidney disease
Huntington's chorea
Acute intermittent porphyria
Osteogenesis imperfecta tarda
von Willebrand's disease
Myotonic dystrophy
Hemochromatosis
Idiopathic hypertrophic subaortic stenosis (IHSS)
Noonan's syndrome
Neurofibromatosis
Tuberous sclerosis

AUTOSOMAL RECESSIVE DISORDERS

Deafness
Albinism
Wilson's disease
Sickle-cell anemia
β thalassemia
Cystic fibrosis
Hereditary emphysema (α_1-antitrypsin deficiency)
Homocystinuria
Familial Mediterranean fever
Friedreich's ataxia
Phenylketonuria

X-LINKED DISORDERS

Hemophilia A
Glucose 6-phosphate dehydrogenase deficiency
Fabry's disease
Ocular albinism
Testicular feminization
Chronic granulomatous disease
Hypophosphatemic rickets
Color blindness

(1) Each affected individual has an affected parent (unless the condition arose by a new mutation in the given individual or is mildly expressed in the affected parent); (2) an affected individual will bear, on the average, both normal and affected offspring in equal proportions; (3) normal children of an affected individual will have only normal offspring; (4) males and females are affected in equal proportions; (5) each sex is equally likely to transmit the condition to male and female offspring, with male-to-male transmission occurring; and (6) vertical transmission of the condition through successive generations occurs, especially when the trait does not impair reproductive capacity.

While half of the offspring of an individual with an autosomal dominant condition will inherit the disease, it is not necessarily true that each affected person must have an affected

FIGURE 58-5

Pedigree pattern of an autosomal dominant trait. Note the vertical *pattern of inheritance.*

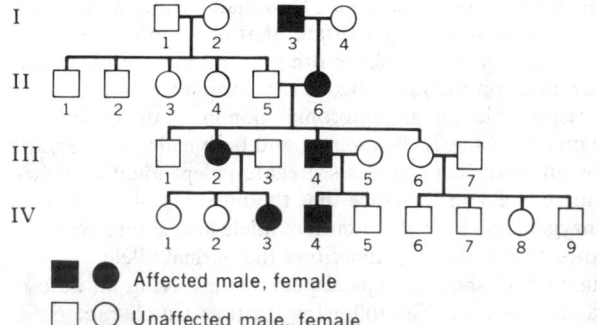

parent. In every autosomal dominant disease a certain proportion of affected persons owe their disorder to a new mutation rather than to an inherited mutation. Since the estimated frequency of mutation is 5×10^{-6} mutations per gene per generation and since a dominant trait, by definition, requires a mutation in only one of a pair of alleles, one would expect that about 1 in 100,000 newborn persons would possess a new mutation at any given genetic locus. Many of these mutations either will not impair the function of the gene product or will involve a recessive function so that the mutation will be clinically silent. Others, however, will cause a defective gene product that gives rise to a dominant trait. The parent in whose germ cells the mutation arose will be clinically normal. Likewise, the siblings of the affected individual will be normal since the mutation will affect only a single germ cell. However, the affected individual will be able to transmit the disease, and half of his or her children will be affected.

The proportion of patients with dominant disorders who represent new mutations is inversely proportional to the effect of the disease in question on biologic fitness. The term *biologic fitness* refers to the ability of an affected individual to produce children who survive to adult life and reproduce. In the extreme case, if a dominant mutation produced absolute infertility, then all observed cases would of necessity represent new mutations, and it would be impossible to prove the genetic transmission of the trait. In less severe disorders, as in tuberous sclerosis, the severe mental retardation reduces biologic fitness to about 20 percent of normal, and the proportion of cases due to new mutations is about 80 percent. Other examples of the relation between biologic fitness and the proportion of new mutations in dominant disorders are shown in Table 58-3.

Many new mutations appear to occur in the germ cells of fathers who are of relatively advanced age. Such a "paternal age effect" is seen, for example, in Marfan's syndrome in which the average age of fathers of sporadic or "new mutation" cases (37 years) is in excess of the mean age of fathers generally (30 years) and also in excess of the age of fathers who transmit Marfan's disease due to an inherited mutation (30 years).

Before one concludes that a dominant disorder in a given patient with unaffected parents is the result of a new mutation, it is important to consider two other possibilities: (1) that the gene may be carried by one parent in whom the disease is of low expressivity (discussed below), and (2) that extramarital paternity may have occurred, since such is found in about 3 to 5 percent of randomly studied children in the United States.

Most autosomal dominant disorders show two characteristic features that are not usually seen in recessive syndromes: (1) *delayed age of onset* and (2) *variability in clinical expression.* Delayed age of onset is seen in disorders such as Huntington's chorea and adult polycystic kidney disease. These disorders do not manifest clinically until adult life, even though the mutant gene is present from the time of conception. Variability in clinical expression is illustrated dramatically by the multiple endocrine adenoma–peptic ulcer syndrome. Patients in the

TABLE 58-3
Approximate proportion of patients affected by new mutations in some autosomal dominant disorders

Disorder	Percentage
Achondroplasia	80
Tuberous sclerosis	80
Neurofibromatosis	40
Marfan's syndrome	30
Myotonic dystrophy	25
Huntington's chorea	4
Adult polycystic kidney disease	1
Familial hypercholesterolemia	Very low

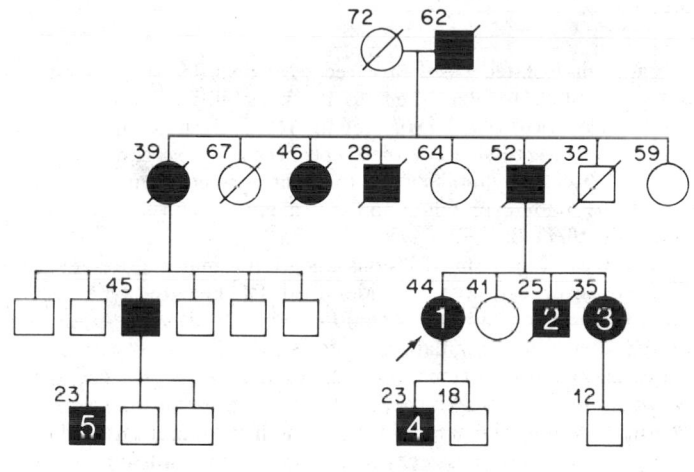

FIGURE 58-6

Pedigree of a family affected with the multiple endocrine adenoma–peptic ulcer syndrome, a disorder inherited as an autosomal dominant trait. Circles denote females; squares, males. Open circles and squares denote unaffected relatives; closed circles and squares denote affected relatives. Deceased relatives are indicated by the oblique line. The age of each relative is indicated above his or her symbol. Note the marked variation in clinical expression among living affected heterozygotes.

1 Islet cell adenomas
   Parathyroid adenomas
   Lipomas

2 Lipomas, kidney stones

3 Islet cell adenomas
   Parathyroid adenomas
   Pituitary adenoma
   Lipomas

4 Peptic ulcer
   disease

5 Pituitary
   adenoma

same family inheriting the same abnormal gene may have hyperplasia or neoplasia of one or all of a wide variety of endocrine tissues such as the pancreas, parathyroid glands, pituitary gland, or adipose tissue. The resulting clinical manifestations are extremely diverse; different members of the same family may develop peptic ulcers, hypoglycemia, kidney stones, multiple lipomas of the skin, or bitemporal hemianopsia. The recognition that each family member suffers from the same genetic abnormality can be very difficult, as illustrated by the family pedigree in Fig. 58-6.

Since dominant mutations involve a type of gene product that in a 50 percent deficiency is capable of producing clinical symptoms in heterozygotes, the responsible mutations are likely to involve abnormalities in two classes of proteins: (1) those that regulate complex metabolic pathways, such as membrane receptors and rate-limiting enzymes in pathways under feedback control, and (2) key structural proteins, such as hemoglobin or collagen.

The basic biochemical defects have been identified in only a handful of the approximately 600 autosomal dominant disorders. These include familial hypercholesterolemia (abnormal cell surface receptor that binds plasma low-density lipoprotein and thereby regulates cholesterol metabolism); hereditary methemoglobinemia and several hemolytic anemias due to unstable forms of hemoglobin (abnormal hemoglobin molecule); hereditary angioneurotic edema (abnormal protein inhibitor of an enzyme involved in the serum complement system); and acute intermittent porphyria (abnormal enzyme that catalyzes a rate-limiting step in the heme biosynthetic pathway).

Autosomal recessive disorders Autosomal recessive conditions are those that are clinically apparent only in the homozygous state, that is, when both alleles at a particular genetic locus are mutant alleles. By definition, the gene responsible for an autosomal recessive disorder must be located on one of the 22 autosomes; thus, both males and females can be affected.

Figure 58-7 shows a pedigree in which an autosomal recessive trait is present in the family. The following features are characteristic: (1) the parents are clinically normal; (2) only siblings are affected, and vertical transmission does not occur; and (3) males and females are affected in equal proportions.

The relative infrequency of recessive genes in the population and the requirement for two abnormal genes for clinical expression combine to create special conditions for autosomal recessive inheritance: (1) the more infrequent the mutant gene in the population, the stronger the likelihood that affected individuals are the product of consanguineous matings (see below); (2) if a husband and a wife are both carriers for the same autosomal recessive gene, 25 percent of the children will be normal, 50 percent will be heterozygous carriers, and 25 percent will be homozygous and affected with the disease; (3) if an affected individual marries a heterozygote (as may occur with consanguineous marriage), half the children will be affected, and a pedigree simulating dominant inheritance will result; and (4) if two individuals with the same recessive disease marry, all their children will be affected.

The clinical picture in autosomal recessive disorders tends to be more uniform than that of dominant diseases, and the age of onset is often early in life. As a general rule, recessive disorders are more commonly diagnosed in children, while dominant diseases are more frequently encountered in adults.

Since with recessive inheritance only one of four children in a sibship is expected to be affected, multiple cases in a family may not occur. This is especially true in a society in which small families are common. Consider, for example, 16 families in which both parents are heterozygous for the same recessive disorder. If each family has two children, 9 of the families will have no affected children, 6 will have one affected and one normal child, and only 1 of the 16 families will have two affected children. In the United States physicians usually see

FIGURE 58-7

Pedigree pattern of an autosomal recessive trait. Note the horizontal pattern of inheritance.

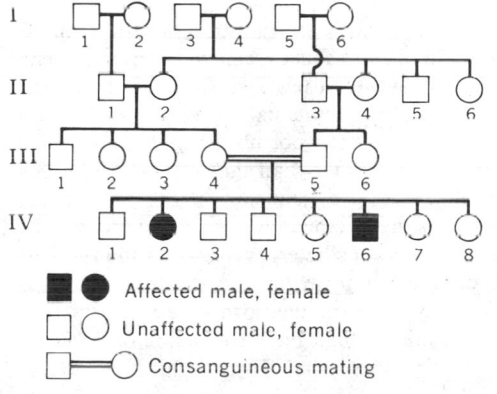

sporadic or isolated cases of a recessive disorder without an affected sibling to alert them to the possibility of a genetic disorder. Fortunately, because of the relatively uniform clinical picture of recessive disorders and because most can be diagnosed directly by biochemical tests, the correct diagnosis can usually be made even when no other members of a family are clinically affected.

The basic biochemical lesions underlying many autosomal recessive disorders have been identified. Of the three types of proteins in which mutations could occur (i.e., enzymes, structural proteins, and regulatory proteins), the one most easy to study has been the enzymes. A mutation that destroys the catalytic activity of an enzyme generally does not impair the health of a heterozygote (i.e., an individual who has one mutant allele specifying a functionless enzyme and one normal allele on the partner chromosome specifying a normal enzyme). In this situation each cell in the body usually produces about 50 percent of the normal number of active enzyme molecules. However, normal regulatory mechanisms function to avert any clinical consequences of this 50 percent deficiency, and so heterozygotes usually are clinically normal. On the other hand, when an individual inherits functionless alleles at both loci specifying an enzyme, the reduction in enzyme activity is too great for a compensatory mechanism to overcome the deficiency, and a disease results. For example, heterozygotes for phenylketonuria who have half the normal activity of phenylalanine hydroxylase are clinically asymptomatic because the body compensates for the half-normal level of the enzyme by raising the substrate concentration approximately twofold. Under these conditions a normal amount of phenylalanine can be metabolized with no symptoms. On the other hand, the homozygote for phenylketonuria has such a severe reduction in phenylalanine hydroxylase activity that enormous levels of phenylalanine and its derivatives accumulate, causing detrimental brain development. As in the case of phenylketonuria, the majority of enzyme deficiency states produce *simultaneously* both a simple accumulation of one or more metabolites preceding the enzymatic block and a deficient production of other metabolites distal to the block in the metabolic pathway.

Most of the genetic enzyme deficiencies that have been elucidated are not only inherited as recessive traits, but also tend to involve enzymes that participate in catabolic pathways. Frequently these enzymes degrade organic molecules that are ingested in the diet, such as galactose (galactosemia), phenylalanine (phenylketonuria), and phytanic acid (Refsum's syndrome). A special class of such catabolic diseases is that in which the deficiency affects an acid hydrolase that occurs within lysosomes. In these *lysosomal storage disorders* the substrate, usually a complex lipid or polysaccharide, accumulates within swollen lysosomes in specific organs, giving the cells a foamy appearance. Examples of such lysosomal diseases include the mucopolysaccharidoses such as Hurler's syndrome (α-iduronidase deficiency) and the lipid storage diseases such as Gaucher's disease (glucocerebrosidase deficiency).

In general, recessive diseases are rare because the reduced biologic fitness of homozygotes acts to remove the mutant gene from the population. However, a few recessive disorders, such as cystic fibrosis and sickle-cell anemia, are very common. To explain this paradox, it has been postulated that the biologic fitness of heterozygotes is greater than that of noncarriers for these genes. In such a case the frequency of the gene in the population depends on the balance between the increased fitness of the relatively numerous heterozygotes and the reduced fitness of the less common homozygotes. A small selective advantage of the heterozygote over the normal results in a high gene frequency and hence a high birth frequency of homozygotes even when the disease is lethal. Thus, about 1 in 22 Caucasians is a heterozygous carrier for the genetically lethal disease cystic fibrosis, and the disease occurs in about 1 in 2000 Caucasian births. In order to maintain such a high gene frequency, heterozygotes for cystic fibrosis must have a definite reproductive advantage over noncarriers, but the nature of this advantage is unknown. However, in sickle-cell anemia, another recessive disorder with high frequency among certain populations, heterozygotes appear to have increased resistance to malaria.

Inasmuch as recessive diseases require the inheritance of a mutation at the same genetic locus from each parent, when the genes are rare, the likelihood of any two parents being carriers for the same defect becomes very small. However, if the parents have a common ancestor and if that ancestor was a carrier for the same recessive gene, then the likelihood that two of the descendants would each have inherited the gene becomes relatively great. The rarer the recessive gene, the stronger becomes the likelihood that an affected individual will have resulted from such a consanguineous mating. On the other hand, certain recessive genes are so common in the population that the likelihood of two random parents being carriers is great enough to eliminate the need for consanguinity. For common traits such as sickle-cell anemia, phenylketonuria, cystic fibrosis, and Tay-Sachs disease, all of which have a high carrier frequency in certain populations, consanguinity is usually not present in the parents.

In general, consanguinity is an infrequent finding clinically in families with recessive diseases in the United States. This is because the background rate of consanguinity in the general population is very low. In most of the United States (as opposed to areas with relative geographic isolation such as northern Norway and Switzerland), a disorder must indeed be rare before it is associated with an important frequency of consanguinity. For example, consanguinity is expected in a large proportion of families having children with very rare disorders such as the Laurence-Moon-Biedl syndrome and abetalipoproteinemia.

Genetic compounds represent a special type of recessively inherited disorder in which the affected individual's two mutant genes, although derived from the same genetic locus, are not identical. The mutations in the paternal and maternal alleles presumably involve different alterations in the DNA of the same gene. Sickle-cell-C hemoglobinopathy is an example of such a *heteroallelic* compound state in which individuals have a gene for sickle-cell hemoglobin on one chromosome and a gene for hemoglobin C on the homologous chromosome.

X-linked disorders The genes responsible for X-linked disorders are located on the X chromosome; therefore, the clinical risk and severity of the disease are different for the two sexes. Since a female has two X chromosomes, she may be either heterozygous or homozygous for a mutant gene, and the trait may therefore demonstrate either recessive or dominant expression. Males, on the other hand, have only one X chromosome, so they can be expected to display the full syndrome whenever they inherit the gene regardless of whether the gene behaves as a recessive or as a dominant trait in the female. Thus, the terms *X-linked dominant* or *X-linked recessive* refer only to the expression of the gene in women.

An important feature of all X-linked inheritance is the absence of male-to-male (i.e., father-to-son) transmission of the trait. This follows because a male must always contribute his Y chromosome to his sons; hence, he can never contribute his X chromosome. On the other hand, a male contributes his one X chromosome to all his daughters.

The pedigree in Fig. 58-8 illustrates the characteristic features of X-linked recessive inheritance. (1) In contrast to the vertical transmission in dominant traits (parents and children affected) and the horizontal transmission in autosomal reces-

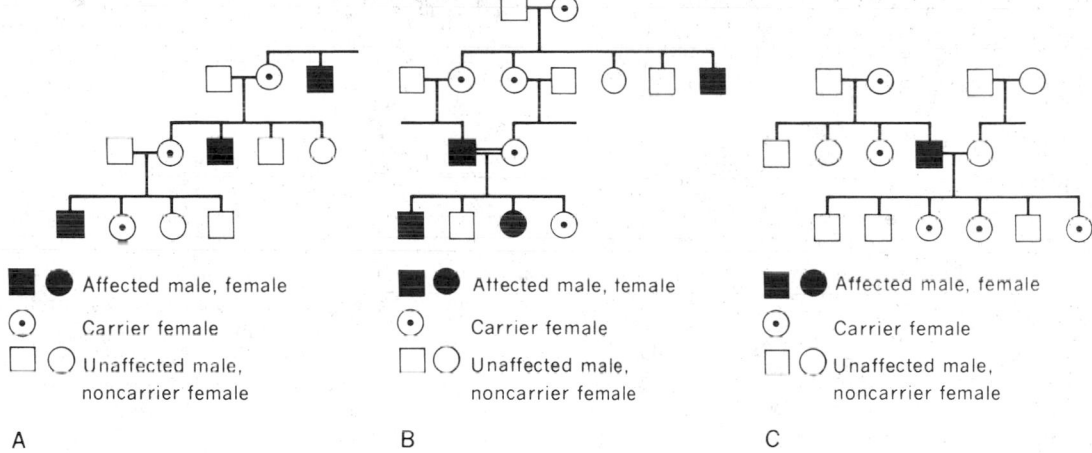

■ ● Affected male, female	■ ● Affected male, female	■ ● Affected male, female
⊙ Carrier female	⊙ Carrier female	⊙ Carrier female
□ ○ Unaffected male, noncarrier female	□ ○ Unaffected male, noncarrier female	□ ○ Unaffected male, noncarrier female
A	B	C

FIGURE 58-8

Pedigree patterns of an X-linked recessive trait. A. Note the oblique pattern of inheritance. B. An affected female can result from the mating of an affected male and a carrier female, as in the consanguineous marriage shown here. C. An affected male mating with a normal noncarrier female has all normal sons and all carrier daughters. (Courtesy of VA McKusick.)

sive traits (siblings affected), the pedigree pattern in X-linked recessive traits tends to be oblique because of the occurrence of the trait in the sons of normal carrier sisters of affected males (uncles and nephews affected) (Fig. 58-8A); (2) male offspring of carrier women have a 50 percent chance of being affected; (3) all female offspring of affected males are carriers, and affected males do not transmit the disease to their sons (Fig. 58-8C); (4) unaffected males do not transmit the trait to any offspring; and (5) affected homozygous females occur only when an affected male fathers the child of a carrier female (Fig. 58-8B).

Examples of X-linked recessive disorders in humans include hemophilia A, nephrogenic diabetes insipidus, the Lesch-Nyhan syndrome, Duchenne form of muscular dystrophy, glucose 6-phosphate dehydrogenase deficiency, testicular feminization, and Fabry's disease. Color blindness is also inherited as an X-linked recessive trait, but it is sufficiently frequent (occurring in about 8 percent of Caucasian males) that the occurrence of homozygous color-blind females is no rarity.

X-linked dominant inheritance is illustrated by the pedigree in Fig. 58-9. Its characteristic features are as follows: (1) Females are affected about twice as often as males; (2) an affected female transmits the disorder to half of her sons and half of her daughters; (3) an affected male transmits the disorder to all his daughters and to none of his sons; and (4) the syndrome

is more variable and less severe in heterozygous affected females than in hemizygous affected males. One common trait, the Xg(a+) blood group, is inherited as an X-linked dominant trait, as are diseases such as vitamin D-resistant rickets (hypophosphatemic rickets) and pseudohypoparathyroidism.

Some rare conditions may be inherited as X-linked dominant traits in which there is lethality in the hemizygous male. The characteristics of this form of inheritance are illustrated by the pedigree in Fig. 58-10: (1) The disorder occurs only in females who are heterozygous for the mutant gene; (2) an affected mother transmits the trait to half of her daughters; (3) an increased frequency of abortions occurs in affected women, the abortions representing affected male fetuses. Conditions that appear to be transmitted by this mode of inheritance include incontinentia pigmenti, focal dermal hypoplasia, orofaciodigital syndrome, and hyperammonemia due to ornithine transcarbamylase deficiency.

Understanding of the mechanisms of gene expression of X-linked traits in females has been greatly advanced by the so-called "Lyon hypothesis" or "X-inactivation hypothesis." (The term *hypothesis* is used for historical reasons only; Lyon's hypothesis can now be regarded as proved fact.) This hypothesis states that early in embryonic development one of the two X chromosomes in each somatic cell of a female is inactivated. The inactivation process is random, so that for each cell there

FIGURE 58-9

Pedigree pattern of an X-linked dominant trait.

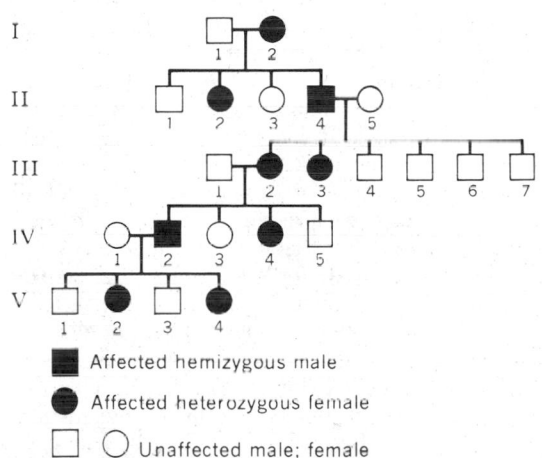

■	Affected hemizygous male
●	Affected heterozygous female
□ ○	Unaffected male; female

FIGURE 58-10

Pedigree pattern of an X-linked dominant trait lethal in the hemizygous male.

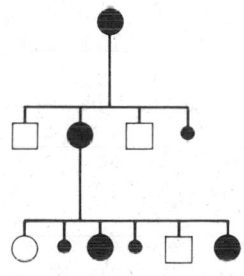

● ◌	Affected and unaffected female
□	Unaffected male
●	Abortion

is an equal probability that the paternally or maternally derived X chromosome will be inactivated. The inactivated X chromosome is rendered permanently nonfunctional, so that all progeny of the initial cell inherit the same active and inactive X chromosomes. Thus, each female is a mosaic; on the average, half of her cells express the X chromosome of the father, and half express the X chromosome of the mother. If a mutation in a gene is carried on one of her X chromosomes, about one-half of the cells in each tissue will be normal and the other half will manifest the mutant phenotype. However, chance or selection of one or the other set of clones of cells may disturb these proportions in any given individual. Depending on the proportions of mutant and normal X chromosomes in each tissue, a genetically heterozygous female may either be clinically normal or have mild or severe manifestations of the disease. To illustrate, mothers of boys with the X-linked recessive Duchenne form of muscular dystrophy may occasionally show mild manifestations of the disease, such as limb girdle weakness or hypertrophied calves.

In each female cell the nonfunctional X chromosome can be visualized by several techniques. By ordinary staining, the inactivated X chromosome in metaphase appears heteropyknotic (very condensed in appearance), and it replicates late in the mitotic cycle ("late-labeling" with tritiated thymidine). In nondividing cells the inactivated X chromosome can be observed as a clump of chromatin at the periphery of the nucleus—the so-called "X chromatin" or "Barr body." In abnormal states with more than two X chromosomes such as 47 XXX, all but one of the X chromosomes are inactivated, so female cells may have multiple X chromatin bodies (see Chap. 60).

Since a single mutant allele is sufficient for the expression of X-linked recessive disorders, consanguinity does not increase the likelihood of expression in males, unlike the case in the rare autosomal recessive disorders. On the other hand, just as in the dominantly inherited disorders, new mutations can be a factor. In general, if an X-linked recessive condition reduces biologic fitness to zero, one-third of affected males will be born as a result of new mutations and an additional one-third will be born to mothers who themselves are carriers as a result of a new mutation. Thus, only one-third will come from a classic pedigree manifesting oblique transmission. An example of such a disease is the Duchenne form of muscular dystrophy in which affected hemizygous males are so severely disabled that they never reproduce. In hemophilia A, in which the biologic fitness is greater than zero, about 20 percent of affected males represent new mutations.

In families in which only one male is affected with an X-linked recessive disease and there is no other family history of the trait, it is essential for proper genetic counseling that the mother undergo biochemical tests or other relevant studies to determine whether she is a carrier. If she is a carrier, half of her daughters will be carriers and half of her sons will be affected. On the other hand, if her affected son represents a new mutation, only his daughters will inherit the gene. At present, biochemical tests can identify female carriers for several X-linked diseases including the Lesch-Nyhan syndrome, Fabry's disease, Hunter's syndrome, hemophilia, and the Duchenne form of muscular dystrophy.

The distinction between X-linked inheritance and *sex-influenced autosomal dominant inheritance* is important. Both baldness and hemochromatosis are probably inherited as autosomal dominant traits, yet both disorders occur mainly in men and rarely in women. Heterozygous females rarely manifest the hemochromatosis gene because of menstruation and pregnancy, which mitigate against the overaccumulation of iron, and they express the baldness gene only when a source of testosterone becomes available as occurs with a masculinizing tumor of the ovary.

MULTIFACTORIAL GENETIC DISEASES The common chronic diseases of adults (such as essential hypertension, coronary heart disease, diabetes mellitus, peptic ulcer disease, and schizophrenia) as well as the common birth defects (such as cleft lip and palate, spina bifida, and congenital heart disease) have been long known to "run in families." They fit best into the category of *multifactorial genetic diseases*. The genetic element in these disorders rarely manifests itself in an all-or-none fashion as it does in the simply inherited (mendelian) disorders and in chromosomal aberrations. Instead, it is the interaction of multiple genes with multiple environmental factors that produces the familial aggregation.

In the multifactorial genetic diseases, there is a *polygenic component* consisting of a series of genes that interact in a cumulative fashion. An individual who inherits just the right combination of these genes passes beyond a "threshold of risk," at which point an *environmental component* determines whether and to what extent that person is clinically affected. In order for another individual in the same family to express the same syndrome, the same or a very similar combination of genes must be inherited. Since the first-degree relatives of an affected individual (i.e., parents, siblings, and offspring) each share half of that person's genes, they are all at increased risk of exhibiting the same polygenic syndrome. Second-degree relatives (uncles, aunts, and grandparents) share on the average one-fourth of an individual's genes $(\frac{1}{2})^2$, and third-degree relatives (cousins) share one-eighth $(\frac{1}{2})^3$. Thus, as the degree of relation becomes more distant, the likelihood of a relative inheriting the same combination of genes becomes less. Moreover, the chances of any relative inheriting the right combination of risk genes decrease as the number of genes required for the expression of a given trait increases.

Since the precise number of genes responsible for polygenic traits is unknown, the risk of inheritance for a relative of an affected individual is difficult to calculate, and the standard is based on empiric risk figures (i.e., a direct tally of the proportion of affected relatives in previously reported families). In contrast to the simply inherited disorders in which 25 or 50 percent of the first-degree relatives of an affected proband are at genetic risk, multifactorial genetic disorders are generally observed empirically to affect no more than 5 to 10 percent of first-degree relatives. Moreover, in contrast to mendelian traits, the recurrence risk of multifactorial conditions varies from family to family, and its estimation is significantly influenced by two factors: (1) the number of affected persons already present in the family, and (2) the severity of the disorder in the index case. The greater the number of affected relatives and the more severe their disease, the higher the risk to other relatives. For example, the risk of cleft lip in the siblings of a child with unilateral cleft lip is about 2.5 percent, but if the lesion in the index case is bilateral, the risk in the siblings rises to 6 percent. Table 58-4 lists the empirical risk figures for the familial recurrence of a number of multifactorial genetic diseases.

The hypothesis of a polygenic component in the inheritance of multifactorial diseases has been given a sound basis in recent years by the demonstration that at least one-third of all gene loci harbor polymorphic alleles that vary among individuals. Such a large degree of variation in normal genes undoubtedly provides the substrate for variations in genetic predisposition with which environmental factors can interact. So far, the genetic loci most strikingly associated with predisposition to specific diseases are those that constitute the HLA system. The HLA gene complex is located on the short arm of chromosome 6. It consists of four closely linked but distinct

TABLE 58-4
Empiric risks for some common multifactorial genetic diseases affecting adults

Disorder in index case	Estimated absolute risk for first-degree relatives, %
Cleft lip and/or palate	3
Congenital heart disease	4
Coronary heart disease	8 for male relatives 3 for female relatives
Diabetes mellitus	5–10
Epilepsy	5–10
Hypertension	10
Manic-depressive psychosis	10–15
Psoriasis	10–15
Schizophrenia	15
Thyroid disease (autoimmune disorders including hyperthyroidism, thyroiditis, primary myxedema, simple goiter)	10

TABLE 58-5
Alleles at the HLA loci associated with multifactorial genetic diseases

Disease	HLA locus	Specific allele	Relative risk*
Ankylosing spondylitis	B	B27	121
Reiter's syndrome	B	B27	40
Psoriasis with arthritis	B	B27	5
Celiac disease	B	B8	10
Chronic active hepatitis	B	B8	4
Myasthenia gravis	B	B8	4
Diabetes mellitus (insulin-dependent)	B	B8, B15	3
	D	D3	3
Hyperthyroidism	D	D3	4
Addison's disease	B	B8	7
	D	D4	10
Multiple sclerosis	D	D2	7

* Relative risk *is the probability of the disease developing in an individual with the specific allele, divided by the probability of its development in an individual who does not possess this specific allele.*

loci (A, B, C, and D). The products of these genes are proteins that are found on the surface of body cells and that enable an individual's immune system to distinguish its own cells from those of someone else. Each HLA locus in the population consists of multiple alleles, each of which produces an immunologically distinct protein. For example, an individual may inherit any 2 of 20 alleles at the HLA-B locus.

An important observation of recent years has been the finding that certain alleles at the HLA loci predispose individuals to certain specific diseases. For example, if the B27 allele at the HLA-B locus is inherited by an individual, that person has a

121-fold greater chance of developing ankylosing spondylitis than an individual who lacks this allele (Table 58-5). Ankylosing spondylitis remains a multifactorial disease, however, because its development clearly requires one or more other factors in addition to the B27 allele. Thus, less than 15 percent of people who inherit this allele develop this disease. Table 58-5 lists some of the diseases associated with alleles at the HLA loci. Several of them in the past have been suspected to be of viral etiology, suggesting that the HLA loci may dictate the mode of expression of certain viral diseases.

Multifactorial disorders are heterogeneous in the sense that

TABLE 58-6
Examples of inherited disorders involving an abnormal response to drugs

Disorder	Molecular abnormality	Mode of inheritance	Frequency	Clinical effect	Drugs producing abnormal response
Slow inactivation of isoniazid	Isoniazid acetylase in liver	Autosomal recessive	~50% of U.S. population	Polyneuritis	Isoniazid, sulfamethazine, sulfamaprine, phenelzine, dapsone, hydralazine
Suxamethonium sensitivity	Pseudocholinesterase in plasma	Autosomal recessive	Several mutant alleles; most common affects 1 in 2500	Apnea	Suxamethonium, succinylcholine
Coumadin	? Altered receptor or enzyme in liver with increased affinity for vitamin K	Autosomal dominant	Rare	Inability to achieve anticoagulation with usual doses of drug	Coumadin
Glaucoma	Unknown	? Autosomal dominant	Common	Increased intra-ocular pressure	Corticosteroids
Malignant hyperthermia	Unknown	Autosomal dominant	~1 in 20,000 anesthesized patients	Severe hyperpyrexia, muscle rigidity, death	Such anesthetics as halothane, succinylcholine, methoxyfluorane, ether, cyclopropane
Unstable hemoglobins: Hemoglobin Zurich	Arginine substitution for histidine at sixty-third position of β chain of hemoglobin	Autosomal dominant	Rare	Hemolysis	Sulfonamides
Hemoglobin H	Hemoglobin composed of four β chains	Autosomal dominant	Rare	Hemolysis	Sulfisoxazole
Glucose 6-phosphate dehydrogenase deficiency	Glucose 6-phosphate dehydrogenase in erythrocytes	X-linked recessive	~ 1×10^8 affected persons in world; common in persons of African, Mediterranean, Asiatic origin; multiple mutant alleles	Hemolysis	Analgesics, sulfonamides, antimalarials, nitrofurantoin, other drugs

SOURCE: *ES Vesell, N Engl J Med 287:904, 1972.*

the relative contribution of the polygenic factors ("risk genes") and environmental factors to the etiology will vary greatly from patient to patient. However, it is important to remember that among common phenotypes which are largely multifactorial, often a small proportion will be created by major mutant genes. For example, although coronary heart disease is usually of multifactorial etiology, about 5 percent of subjects with premature myocardial infarctions are heterozygotes for familial hypercholesterolemia, a single-gene disorder that produces atherosclerosis in the absence of any other predisposing factor. Similarly, in a small proportion of patients with other common diseases such as peptic ulcer disease or "essential" hypertension, the condition is not multifactorial but determined by a single gene, as in the multiple endocrine adenoma–peptic ulcer syndrome or the medullary thyroid carcinoma–pheochromocytoma syndrome, respectively.

INTERACTION BETWEEN SINGLE GENETIC AND ENVIRONMENTAL FACTORS

Many diseases are now recognized to result from an interaction between a specific genotype and a specific environmental factor. In particular, inherited single-gene mutations have been shown to produce clinically significant and often life-threatening idiosyncratic responses to certain drugs.

Table 58-6 lists the most important of these *pharmacogenetic disorders,* which encompass all the mendelian modes of inheritance. Perhaps the most common is glucose 6-phosphate dehydrogenase deficiency, an X-linked recessive trait in which a variety of drugs may precipitate a hemolytic anemia. Plasma pseudocholinesterase deficiency and hepatic transacetylase deficiency are examples of autosomal recessive traits which alter drug catabolism so that when the muscle relaxant suxamethonium or the antituberculous drug isoniazid is administered, apnea or peripheral neuropathy, respectively, may ensue. Malignant hyperthermia is an autosomal dominant trait in which acute hyperpyrexia, muscle rigidity, and hyperkalemic cardiac arrest may be induced by administration of any one of several anesthetic agents. Acute intermittent porphyria is another example of a genetic disorder that is exacerbated by drugs, such as barbiturates.

Misinterpretation of adverse drug reactions may result in serious harm to patients. In general, all unusual idiosyncratic reactions should be considered to be genetically determined until proved otherwise. Fortunately, the pharmacogenetic disorders are a group of diseases for which therapy is straightforward: avoidance of the noxious drug by patient and relatives.

In addition to drugs, other factors in the environment may aggravate specific genetic traits. Cigarette smoke may have deleterious effects on persons homozygous and possibly heterozygous for α_1-antitrypsin deficiency, who are predisposed to the development of emphysema. Patients with xeroderma pigmentosa and anhydrotic ectodermal dysplasia are unusually sensitive to sunlight and high temperatures, respectively. Avoidance of milk at an early age prevents many of the complications ordinarily seen in persons with galactosemia.

Genetic-environmental interactions are particularly important in pregnancy. Women who are affected with phenylketonuria may develop high plasma phenylalanine levels during pregnancy, and thus their offspring may suffer from a variety of phenylalanine-induced birth defects even though the offspring may not themselves have phenylketonuria. Other examples of diseases resulting from an adverse genetic relation between the mother and fetus include erythroblastosis caused by Rh incompatibility and diabetic embryopathy, a term that re-

fers to a series of major birth defects occurring in about 5 percent of the offspring of women who are clinically diabetic during pregnancy.

REFERENCES

BROWN MS, GOLDSTEIN JL: New directions in human biochemical genetics: Understanding the manifestations of receptor deficiency disorders. Prog Med Genet 1:103, 1976

CARTER CO: Genetics of common disorders. Br Med Bull 25:52, 1972

CAVALLI-SFORZA LL, BODMER WF: *The Genetics of Human Populations.* San Francisco, Freeman, 1971

CHILDS B, DER KALOUSTIAN VM: Genetic heterogeneity. N Engl J Med 279:1205, 1267, 1968

HARRIS H: *The Principles of Human Biochemical Genetics,* 2d ed. New York, American Elsevier, 1975

MCKUSICK VA: *Mendelian Inheritance in Man: Catalogs of Autosomal Dominant, Autosomal Recessive and X-linked Phenotypes,* 5th ed. Baltimore, Johns Hopkins, 1978

———, CLAIBORNE R: *Medical Genetics.* New York, HP Publishing, 1973

NORA JJ, FRASER FC: *Medical Genetics: Principles and Practice.* Philadelphia, Lea & Febiger, 1974

SCHALLER JG, OMENN GS: The histocompatibility system and human disease. J Pediat 88:913, 1976

STANBURY JB et al: *The Metabolic Basis of Inherited Disease,* 4th ed. New York, McGraw-Hill, 1978

WATSON JD: *Molecular Biology of the Gene,* 3d ed. New York, Benjamin, 1976

59

PREVENTION AND TREATMENT OF GENETIC DISORDERS

JOSEPH L. GOLDSTEIN
MICHAEL S. BROWN

APPROACHES TO PREVENTION

In view of the present trend for couples to have smaller families, there is increasing concern that children should be healthy and free of genetic diseases, and primary-care physicians are called upon to play a more active role in the prevention and treatment of hereditary diseases. In most clinical situations, genetic advice can be given by the primary physician once the relatively simple principles of medical genetics (Chap. 58) and genetic counseling (discussed below) have been mastered.

RETROSPECTIVE GENETIC COUNSELING The prevention of genetic diseases requires the identification of matings that are capable of producing defective genotypes. These may involve matings in which one of the two individuals is carrying a dominant or X-linked gene mutation or a balanced translocation, or matings in which both individuals are carriers of a deleterious recessive gene. Such individuals are usually identified through an affected child or near relative, in which case retrospective genetic counseling can be provided.

When advising family members about the risk of transmitting a disorder that has already affected someone in the family, the counselor's first step is to be certain of the *correct diagnosis*—in particular, to make certain that the problem in question is really of genetic origin. This is especially important in disorders that may have either a genetic or a nongenetic etiology, such as deafness or mental retardation. Second, if the disease has a hereditary element, the possibility of *genetic heterogeneity,* i.e., a situation in which clinically similar genetic disorders show varying patterns of inheritance, must be considered. For example, there are two types of hereditary methemoglobinemia that resemble each other quite closely, but one shows autosomal recessive and the other autosomal dominant inheritance.

To estimate the *recurrence risk,* one must initially determine what is known of the genetic mechanisms controlling the relevant disorder. When more than one genetic mechanism exists, or when environmental factors can cause clinically indistinguishable traits, the *relative probabilities* of the different mechanisms operating in the particular family are computed. For conditions determined by simple mendelian inheritance, there is no difficulty in predicting the probability of an offspring being affected, provided that the genotypes of the parents can be recognized. Identification of the parental genotype is easiest for autosomal recessive and X-linked disorders since the basic lesions in these two forms of mendelian inheritance usually

involve simple enzyme deficiencies for which biochemical tests are now available.

For autosomal dominant disorders, identification of the parental genotype is considerably more difficult since the basic defect is known for only a few of these disorders, and the diagnosis of the heterozygote for a dominant disorder depends almost exclusively on the clinical evaluation and a careful pedigree analysis. In counseling a family in which one relative is affected with a dominant disorder, it is important that appropriate clinical examination of all first-degree relatives and appropriately selected distant relatives be carried out. If relatives appear unaffected, there is the possibility that the clinical symptoms may be masked by *delayed age of onset* and *variability in expression.* When no relatives are affected, the possibility of a new dominant mutation must be entertained. Table 59-1

TABLE 59-1
Methods for detection of asymptomatic heterozygotes in frequently encountered dominantly inherited disorders

Disorder	*Method of heterozygote detection*		*Therapeutic advantage of early diagnosis*
	Physical findings	*Laboratory tests*	
GASTROINTESTINAL, LIVER, AND PANCREAS			
Hemochromatosis		Serum iron	Prevent cirrhosis, heart failure, and diabetes
Gilbert's disease		Serum bilirubin	Avoid confusion with more serious forms of liver disease
Peutz-Jeghers syndrome	Melanin spots on lips, buccal mucosa, and digits	X-ray of small intestine	Clarify cause of gastrointestinal bleeding
Familial polyposis		X-ray of colon; colonoscopy	Prevent colon carcinoma
Gardner's syndrome	Multiple sebaceous cysts; lipomas; fibromas; osteomas; dental abnormalities; desmoid tumors	X-ray of colon and small intestine; colonoscopy	Prevent colon carcinoma
METABOLIC AND ENDOCRINE			
Medullary thyroid carcinoma-pheochromocytoma syndrome		Serum calcitonin; measurement of blood pressure	Prevent thyroid carcinoma and complications of hypertension
Multiple endocrine adenomatosis	Multiple lipomas	Serum calcium, gastrin, blood sugar; x-rays of sella turcica, stomach, and small intestine	Prevent complication of hyperparathyroidism, hypoglycemia, peptic ulcer, metastatic cancer
Familial hyperparathyroidism		Serum calcium, parathyroid hormone	Prevent renal damage and other complications of hypercalcemia
Familial hypercholesterolemia	Tendon xanthomas, xanthelasma, arcus corneae	Serum cholesterol; low-density lipoprotein receptor activity of cultured fibroblasts	Prevent premature coronary heart disease
HEART AND VASCULAR			
Holt-Oram syndrome	Abnormality of thumb and carpals; murmur of atrial septal defect	X-ray of hands; cardiac evaluation	Prevent complications of atrial septal defect
Noonan's syndrome	Hypertelorism; small chin; low-set ears; ptosis; pectus deformity; cryptorchidism; murmur of pulmonic stenosis	Cardiac evaluation; x-ray of skeleton; intravenous pyelogram (renal anomalies)	Prevent heart failure
Idiopathic hypertropic subaortic stenosis (asymmetric septal hypertrophy)	Presystolic gallop; characteristic carotid arterial pulse	ECG; echocardiogram	Prevent sudden death, syncope, angina, heart failure
Dominantly inherited form of atrial septal defect	Heart murmur	ECG showing first degree heart block, right bundle branch block, right axis deviation	Prevent complications of atrial septal defect
HEMATOLOGIC			
Hereditary spherocytosis	Splenomegaly; jaundice	Blood smear; reticulocyte count; hemoglobin; osmotic fragility test	Prevent anemia, cholethiasis
Hereditary hemorrhagic telangiectasia	Telangiectasia of tongue, lips, conjunctiva, ears, fingers; pulmonary AV fistula	X-ray of lungs	Clarify cause of nosebleeds and gastrointestinal bleeding

TABLE 59-1 *(continued)*
Methods for detection of asymptomatic heterozygotes in frequently encountered dominantly inherited disorders

Disorder	Physical findings	Laboratory tests	Therapeutic advantage of early diagnosis
Method of heterozygote detection			
HEMATOLOGIC *(continued)*			
Von Willebrand's disease		Immunologic and functional assays of plasma antihemophilic globulin levels; bleeding time	Prevent gastrointestinal and urinary bleeding
CONNECTIVE TISSUE AND BONE			
Ehler-Danlos syndromes (types I, II, III)	Loose-jointedness; fragile, stretchable, bruisable skin; subcutaneous calcified spherules		
Marfan's syndrome	Ectopic lens; mitral and aortic murmurs; excessive length of extremities	Slit-lamp examination; metacarpal index by x-ray	Reduce risk of aortic dissection; prevent blindness
Osteogenesis imperfecta	Multiple fractures; loose-jointedness; blue scleras; deafness; aortic regurgitation	X-ray of bones	
RENAL			
Alport's syndrome	Nerve deafness; cataracts, lenticonus, spherophakia	Urinalysis, slit-lamp examination	Prevent uremia
Nail-patella syndrome	Dysplastic nails; absent patellas	X-ray of pelvis (iliac horns); urinalysis	Clarify cause of hematuria and azotemia
Polycystic kidney disease		Urinalysis; intravenous pyelogram; renal arteriogram; measurement of blood pressure	Prevent uremia and complications of hypertension
Renal tubular acidosis		X-ray of kidneys (nephrocalcinosis); urine pH, calcium; serum electrolytes, calcium	Prevent acidosis, osteoporosis, kidney stones
RESPIRATORY			
Hereditary angioneurotic edema		Serum level of Cl esterase inhibitor of complement	Reduce risk of sudden death caused by laryngeal edema and clarify cause of acute abdominal pain
DERMATOLOGIC			
Neurofibromatosis	Café au lait spots; neurofibromas; scoliosis		Prevent malignant degeneration of neurofibromas
Waardenburg syndrome	Wide bridge of nose; frontal white blaze of hair; heterochromia iridis; white eyelashes; deafness		Clarify cause of deafness
Basal-cell nevus syndrome	Multiple basal-cell carcinomas; jaw cysts; pits on palms and soles; skeletal defects (ribs, spina bifida, scoliosis)	X-rays of skull (calcification of falx cerebri) and skeleton	Removal of cutaneous cancers; provide cosmetic surgery
NEUROLOGIC			
Charcot-Marie-Tooth disease	Pes cavus; atrophy of anterior tibial and calf muscles ("stork legs"); absence of deep tendon reflexes	Biopsy of muscle and of sural cutaneous nerve	Improve walking by corrective shoes and orthopedic measures
Myotonic dystrophy	Myotonia; muscle wasting of temporal and sternocleidomastoid muscles; cataracts; frontal baldness; signs of hypogonadism	Slit-lamp examination; electromyography; measurement of serum immunoglobulins; electrocardiogram	Anticipate complete heart block
Acute intermittent porphyria		Measurement of uroporphyrinogen synthetase activity in red blood cells	Reduce risk of neuropathic attacks by avoidance of aggravating drugs such as barbiturates
Tuberous sclerosis	Adenoma sebaceium; cutaneous white macules; shagreen patch; periungual fibromas		Prevent seizures
Huntington's chorea	Paranoia, other personality changes; choreic movements; dementia		
Periodic paralysis syndromes (hypo-, hyper-, and normokalemic types)	Cold-induced myotonia	Electromyogram; serum potassium	Reduce frequency of attacks by avoidance of aggravating agents such as high-carbohydrate diet and exposure to cold
PHARMACOGENETIC			
Malignant hyperthermia		Serum creatine phosphokinase	Prevent fatal episode of hyperthermia induced by general anesthesia

lists the most commonly encountered dominant disorders affecting adults and the best clinical methods currently available for detection of the heterozygote.

When advising families about multifactorial genetic diseases, such as diabetes mellitus, in which the inheritance pattern is not clear-cut, the physician must resort to empiric risk estimates that have been derived from retrospectively assembled data (Table 58-4).

Once the parental genotypes are determined, the genetic prognosis is usually presented in terms of probability that a given couple will produce an affected offspring. The physician providing genetic counseling must make certain that the couple understands not only the meaning of such absolute risk figures, but also the severity of the disease and the variability in clinical expression. In other words, in dealing with a disorder such as neurofibromatosis, it is important for the parents to realize not only that they have a 50 percent risk of producing a child with this disorder but also that a certain proportion of patients with the disorder have severe disease, a certain proportion have mild disease, etc. They should also have an understanding of the potential impact of the disease on their family; a disease that is lethal at birth might be classified by some as more "severe" than one that is lethal at age 16, but the latter is likely to have a much more profound impact on the family.

Although different families initially react in different ways to the same risk, most couples who seek genetic advice can be expected to take a responsible course of action that is based on the information quoted. Generally, the physician should avoid giving direct advice to the couple as to whether they "should" or "should not" have children. For serious genetic disease, with a recurrence risk equal to or greater than 1 in 10, most parents are usually deterred from planning further children. When the risk is less than 1 in 10, most parents usually continue with additional pregnancies.

PROSPECTIVE GENETIC COUNSELING In contrast to retrospective genetic counseling in which advice is given after the birth of at least one affected family member, in prospective genetic counseling advice is provided to possible carriers of recessive genes before an affected individual is born. As a first step, this requires the identification of heterozygous individuals by a population-screening procedure. Second, unmarried heterozygotes are instructed about the risk of their having affected children if they marry another heterozygote for the same gene. Finally, if two heterozygotes are already married, there is the possibility of interrupting the birth of affected infants if the disease can be diagnosed in utero by amniocentesis.

Population screening for heterozygote detection is possible for several autosomal recessive disorders (such as sickle-cell anemia, thalassemia major, and Tay-Sachs disease) that occur in certain populations with high frequency. For example, 8 percent of the American black population are carriers of the sickling gene, and 4 percent of the American Jewish population of Eastern and Central European extraction are carriers of the Tay-Sachs gene.

Screening programs raise many ethical and social problems. Informing a healthy person that he or she is carrying a specific mutant gene that may cause disease in the children if a certain type of mate is chosen differs from counseling parents who have already had an affected child. Very little is known about the social and psychologic effects as well as occupational discrimination that may result from discovering that a person carries a "bad" gene.

PRENATAL DIAGNOSIS The use of transabdominal amniocentesis permits diagnosis of certain genetic diseases at a stage early enough to terminate a pregnancy and to prevent the birth of a defective child. This procedure gives high-risk couples the opportunity to have unaffected children provided they are willing for the pregnancy to be terminated in the event that an abnormal fetus is detected. Amniocentesis consists of the transabdominal aspiration of amniotic fluid from the uterus. The procedure is preferably performed between the fourteenth and sixteenth weeks of pregnancy. When performed by a trained gynecologist, the technique is relatively safe for both mother and fetus.

Direct examination of the amniotic fluid itself may be diagnostic. For example, an elevated level of α-fetoprotein is a relatively good indicator of the presence of spina bifida or some other related neural tube abnormality. More frequently, prenatal diagnosis requires culture of the fetal cells in vitro, a process which usually takes 3 weeks. By this means the karyotype of the fetus can be determined, to ascertain fetal sex and to detect various chromosomal aberrations. Moreover, many inborn errors of metabolism can be detected by suitable assays of specific enzyme activities in the cultured fetal cells. Table 59-2 lists those enzyme deficiency states for which prenatal diagnosis is currently feasible. More disorders are constantly being added to this list.

TABLE 59-2
Inborn errors of metabolism for which prenatal diagnosis is feasible

LIPIDOSES

Cholesteryl ester storage disease
Fabry's disease
Gaucher's disease
Krabbe's disease (globoid cell leukodystrophy)
Metachromatic leukodystrophy
Neimann-Pick disease
Refsum's syndrome
Tay-Sachs disease and other gangliosidoses
Wolman's syndrome

MUCOPOLYSACCHARIDOSES

β-Glucuronidase deficiency
Hunter's syndrome
Hurler's syndrome
Sanfilippo's syndrome
Scheie's syndrome

AMINO ACID AND RELATED DISORDERS

Argininosuccinicaciduria
Citrullinemia
Cystathionine synthetase deficiency (homocystinuria)
Cystinosis
Histidinemia
Maple syrup urine disease
Methylmalonic aciduria

DISORDERS OF CARBOHYDRATE METABOLISM

Fucosidosis
Galactosemia
Glucose 6-phosphate dehydrogenase deficiency
Glycogen storage diseases, types II, III, and IV
Mannosidosis

MISCELLANEOUS DISORDERS

Adenosine deaminase deficiency
Familial hypercholesterolemia, homozygous form
Hypophosphatasia
I-cell disease
Lesch-Nyhan syndrome
Lysosomal acid phosphatase deficiency
Orotic aciduria
Sickle-cell anemia
Testicular feminization
Thalassemia
Xeroderma pigmentosa

SOURCE: *Milunsky.*

TABLE 59-3
Major indications for prenatal diagnosis

Clinical situation	Estimated risk to fetus, %	Method of detection of abnormal fetus
Couples having a previous child with spina bifida or anencephaly	5	Measurement of α-fetoprotein in amniotic fluid
Couples having a previous child with a chromosomal disorder such as the trisomy 21 form of Down's syndrome	2	Chromosomal analysis of cultured amniotic fluid cells
Couples in whom either the husband or wife carries a balanced translocation for Down's syndrome	5-20	Chromosomal analysis of cultured amniotic cells
Pregnant women 38 years of age and older whose risk of having a child with Down's syndrome is increased	1-2	Chromosomal analysis of cultured amniotic fluid cells
Couples at risk for having a child with a detectable inborn error of metabolism (see Table 59-2)	25 or 50	Biochemical analysis of cultured amniotic fluid cells

Prenatal diagnosis by amniocentesis is currently indicated in the following high-risk situations: (1) couples having a previous child with spina bifida or anencephaly, (2) couples having a previous child with a chromosomal aberration such as the trisomy 21 form of Down's syndrome, (3) couples in whom either the husband or wife carries a balanced translocation

TABLE 59-4
Some treatable hereditary disorders affecting adults

Method of treatment	Disorder
REDUCTION OF TOXIC FOOD	
Lactose	Lactase deficiency
Galactose	Galactosemia
Fructose	Fructose intolerance
Neutral fats	Familial lipoprotein lipase deficiency
Cholesterol and saturated fats	Familial hypercholesterolemia
Phytanic acid	Refsum's syndrome
Phenylalanine	Phenylketonuria
METABOLIC SUPPLEMENTATION	
Vitamin D and phosphate	Hypophosphatemic rickets
Gamma globulin	Agammaglobulinemia
Factor VIII (AHG)	Hemophilia
Cortisol	Adrenogenital syndromes
Thyroxine	Familial goiters
Growth hormone	Pituitary dwarfism
REMOVAL OF TOXIC PRODUCT	
Cystine removal by D-penicillamine	Cystinuria
Copper removal by D-penicillamine	Wilson's disease
Iron removal by phlebotomy	Hemochromatosis
SURGERY	
Splenectomy	Hereditary spherocytosis
Portacaval shunt	Glycogen storage disease, type I
Colectomy	Familial polyposis of the colon
Thyroidectomy	Medullary thyroid carcinoma syndrome
ORGAN TRANSPLANTATION	
Kidney	Fabry's disease
Kidney	Adult polycystic kidney disease

chromosome for Down's syndrome, (4) couples at high risk for having a child with a detectable inborn error of metabolism, and (5) pregnant women 38 years of age and older. Table 59-3 lists the major indications for prenatal diagnosis, the risks involved, and methods by which the abnormal fetus can be detected.

APPROACHES TO TREATMENT

The goal of treatment for genetic diseases is to modify the natural history of the genetic trait so that an affected person may live a comfortable and healthy life despite a mutant genotype. Such treatment can be achieved for a number of inherited diseases using a variety of approaches, including (1) the exclusion or restriction of toxic foods, (2) metabolic supplementation, (3) removal of toxic products, (4) surgery, and (5) organ transplantation. Table 59-4 lists examples of hereditary diseases affecting adults that can be successfully treated at the present time.

REFERENCES

EPSTEIN CJ: Prenatal diagnosis of genetic disorders. Adv Intern Med 20:325, 1975

MILUNSKY A: *The Prevention of Genetic Disease and Mental Retardation.* Philadelphia, Saunders, 1975

STANBURY JB et al: *The Metabolic Basis of Inherited Disease,* 4th ed. New York, McGraw-Hill, 1978

WORLD HEALTH ORGANIZATION: *Genetic Disorders: Prevention, Treatment, and Rehabilitation.* WHO Tech Rep 497, 1972

60
CYTOGENETIC ASPECTS OF HUMAN DISEASE

JAMES GERMAN

The chromosome complement of humans, like that of other species, is guarded carefully against change; most chromosome mutations, either structural or numerical, are deleterious. Only rarely is a balanced structural rearrangement (one that results in neither deficiency nor duplication of significant chromosome segments) introduced into the population and transmitted from generation to generation. (Figure 60-1 shows the normal human chromosome complement. In the legend of the figure several terms used in human cytogenetics are defined.) As a rule an abnormal number of autosomes results in early death, except for trisomy of the shortest chromosome. In contrast, an abnormal number of sex chromosomes is often tolerated reasonably well, although infertility or subfertility usually is present. Nevertheless, among human embryos abnormalities in chromosome structure and number are common and are, in fact, the major known cause of embryonic and early fetal wastage. However, not every fetus with an abnormal chromosome complement is aborted, and those that survive constitute the material of medical cytogenetics.

Clinical disorders resulting from chromosome imbalance present varying features including abnormal anatomic development, mental retardation, behavioral disorders, and disturbances in growth and sexual development. Sometimes infertility, repeated abortion, or the birth of malformed children is the presenting complaint of persons with abnormal chromosome complements whose own general development is normal.

The disorders just referred to are due to chromosome imbalance that affects tissues throughout the body. In addition, change can occur in the chromosome complement in a single cell of some somatic tissue. Such a mutant cell may have a proliferative advantage over normal cells, in which case a clone bearing the abnormal chromosome complement can develop amid otherwise normal cells. Although such mutant clones are in many cases clinically insignificant, much evidence suggests that they are also important in the etiology of cancer.

This chapter is addressed to those aspects of normal chromosome structure and function that constitute the basis for an understanding of the chromosome alterations in human disease. In addition, the classes of alterations important in adult medicine and their consequences are summarized.

CHROMOSOME STRUCTURE AND FUNCTION The human autosomes are numbered 1 through 22, and the sex chromosomes are denoted X and Y (Fig. 60-1). Each is recognizable microscopically by morphological features such as relative length and position of the centromere and by staining characteristics (banding pattern). Each mammalian chromosome is believed to be composed of one double-stranded chain of deoxyribonucleic acid (DNA) that extends from one end through the centromere to the other end.

FIGURE 60-1

Normal human lymphocyte chromosomes arrested in metaphase and stained for G bands (G standing for Giemsa). The inset shows the arrangement of chromosomes in an intact cell, and the remainder of the figure shows their ordered arrangement into a karyotype. By the time mitosis begins, each chromosome consists of two identical parts called sister chromatids and is identified by the relative length, the location of the centromere, and a distinctive sequence of bands of varying lengths and depth of staining. Normally, the G-band patterns of the two chromosomes of a pair are alike, with the exception of certain polymorphic regions, examples of which are shown in Fig. 60-3.

The centromere of a chromosome divides it into a short arm (p) and a long arm (q). Numbers 13 to 15, 21, 22, and Y are called acrocentric because of the nearly terminal positions of their centromeres; the minute p of each acrocentric autosome bears a nucleolus-organizing region which

often causes a secondary constriction in the metaphase chromosome (the constriction at the centromere is the primary constriction). Telomeres are the nonvisible, somewhat theoretical, "structures" at the ends of each chromosome.

By standard nomenclature, this karyotype is described as 46,XY, indicating that its chromosome number is 46, its sex chromosomes are an X and a Y, and the autosomes (those besides the X and Y) number 44. The following examples show the general use of this nomenclature: A normal female karyotype is described as 46,XX. A female cell with an extra chromosome 18 (trisomic for 18) would be described as 47,XX,+18. A cell with only one sex chromosome, an X, and with deletion in the short arm of chromosome 5 would be described as 45,X,5p−. A male cell with a translocation between the long arm of chromosome 2 and the short arm of chromosome 3 would be described as 46,XY,t(2q;3p); exact breakpoints could be indicated by additional characters and symbols.

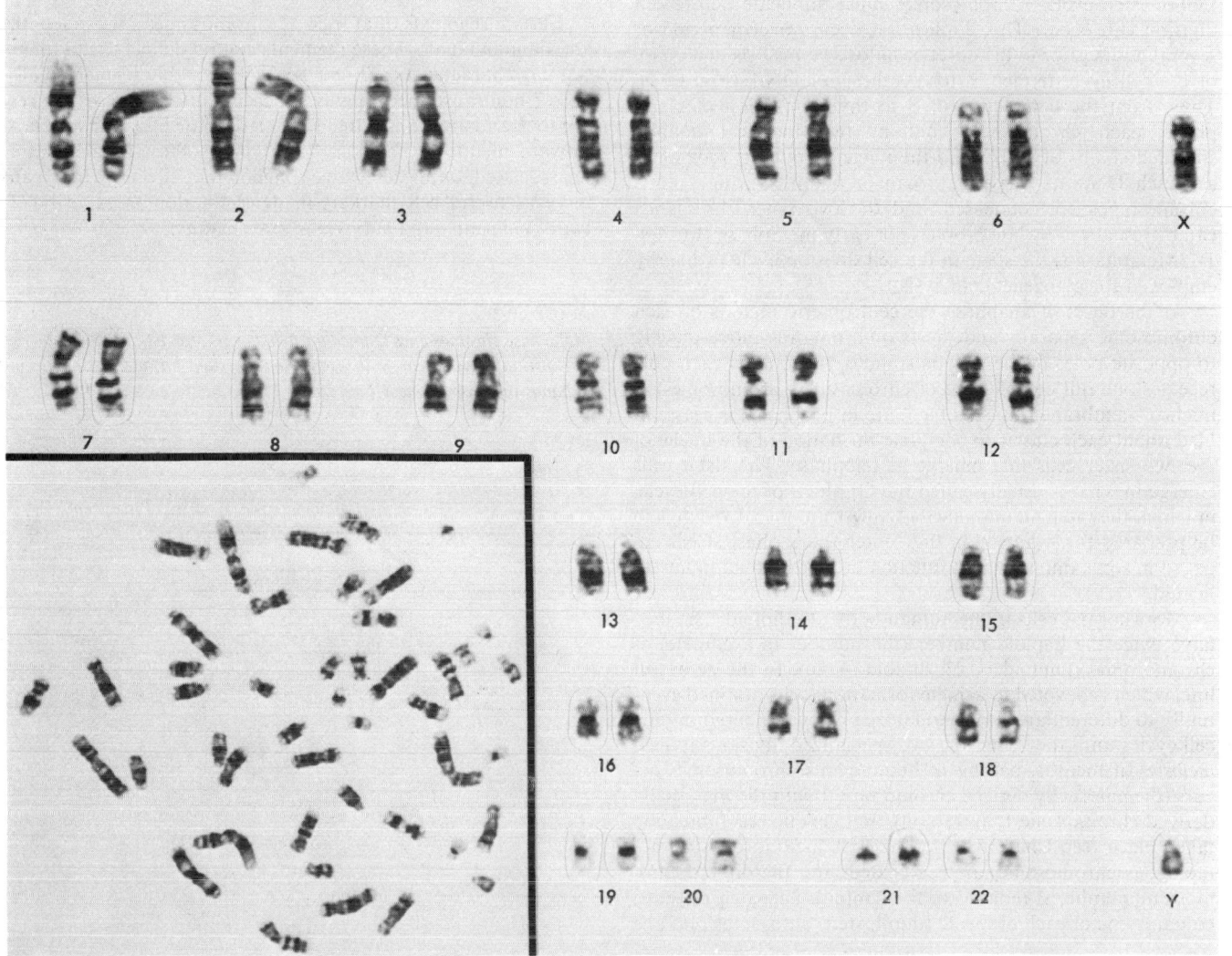

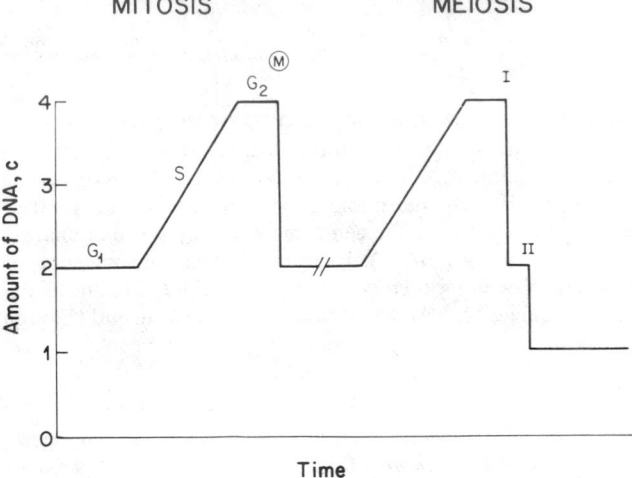

FIGURE 60-2

Schematic representation of the mitotic and meiotic cell division cycles, as described in the text. G_1 and G_2 = time gaps before and after S, the period in which DNA replicates. Each of these intervals is several hours in duration; together they constitute interphase. M = mitosis; I and II = the two divisions of meiosis. The DNA content of the cycling cells is indicated on the vertical axis: $1c$ = the content in a gamete; $2c$ = that in either an egg immediately postfertilization or a somatic cell emerging from mitosis; $4c$ = the amount in a cell which has completed chromosome duplication and is ready to enter mitosis or meiosis.

Cell division cycle Chromosomes must duplicate before cell division can occur. This duplication occurs over a period of several hours prior to the onset of mitosis or meiosis in a phase of the cell cycle termed S, for synthesis of DNA (Fig. 60-2). Thus, from the completion of S to the completion of metaphase, each chromosome contains two identical double-stranded chains of DNA, and the nucleus contains four times as much DNA as a spermatozoan or ovum. During mitosis chromosomes are condensed, and the two sister chromatids can be visualized by late prophase or early metaphase (Fig. 60-1). (Metaphase is the stage in the cell division cycle ordinarily employed for cytogenetic analysis.)

At the onset of anaphase the centromeric regions of each chromosome separate, and the two chromatids move quickly to opposite poles of the mitotic spindle. As soon as each pole receives one full complement of chromatids (chromosomes), a nuclear membrane (disassembled late in prophase) is reassembled about each cluster to complete formation of the nuclei of the two sister cells that emerge at telophase. The sister cells emerge in what is usually called the G_1 phase of the cell cycle, in which they remain unreplicated unless another division is to be prepared for, whereupon they enter the S phase. Cells engaged in some differentiated function ordinarily remain unreplicated.

Most normal cells in the human body are diploid; i.e., they have twice the haploid number (the number in a gamete) of chromosomes (haploid = 23, diploid = 46). In the germ cell line, which is devoted to gamete formation, cells destined eventually to differentiate into spermatozoa or ova undergo mitotic cell cycles until they enter the two specialized divisions termed *meiosis*. In meiosis, pairing of homologous chromosomes occurs (the paternally derived chromosome 1 with the maternally derived chromosome 1, and so on), and genetic recombination takes place (see Chap. 58). At the first meiotic division homologous chromosomes are segregated, and the diploid chromosome number is reduced to the haploid; i.e., each cell then contains one of each of the 22 (duplicated) autosomes plus one

(duplicated) sex chromosome. No S phase takes place between the first and second meiotic divisions (depicted in Fig. 60-2, right) so that at the second division, in which sister chromatids separate, emerging cells maintain the haploid number of chromosomes but are reduced in their content of DNA to half the amount of diploid G_1 cells of somatic tissues. With fertilization of an ovum by a spermatozoan, both the chromosome constitution and the DNA content of the zygote are restored to that of a G_1 somatic cell. An S period in the zygote then permits reinstitution of regular cell-division cycles characteristic of the somatic cells.

Chromosome differentiation A chromosome is differentiated along its length, and some aspects of this differentiation are resolvable in the light microscope. The DNA is complexed with a number of proteins in a highly specific way. The DNA-protein complex together with some associated ribonucleic acid (RNA) is referred to as *chromatin*. The fine structure and the manner in which the DNA is compacted and interacted with proteins are thought to pertain to the control of RNA production and DNA replication, perhaps to cellular differentiation itself.

The sequences of nucleotide bases in DNA that constitute the genes and that can be transcribed into messenger RNA are distributed throughout the length of the various chromosomes. (These sequences are too short to be resolved microscopically.) Over a hundred genes have been mapped to specific chromosomes, in many cases to specific regions of a chromosome; for example, the Rh blood group locus is on the short arm of chromosome 1, and the ABO blood group locus has been assigned to a band near the end of the long arm of chromosome 9.

Certain segments of at least 12 chromosomes vary in length among individuals. These segments can be delineated by their staining characteristics (Fig. 60-3). The variable segments consist of nontranscribed, highly repetitive nucleotide sequences of DNA and are transmitted from parent to child in a straightforward mendelian fashion. Variations in these segments are unassociated with detectable phenotypic effect. (They can serve as useful cell markers in determination of zygosity of twins, paternity, and survival of transplants.)

FIGURE 60-3

Metaphase chromosomes stained for C bands (C standing for centromeric or constitutive heterochromatin), showing inherited variation in lengths of C bands in chromosome 1 (arrows).

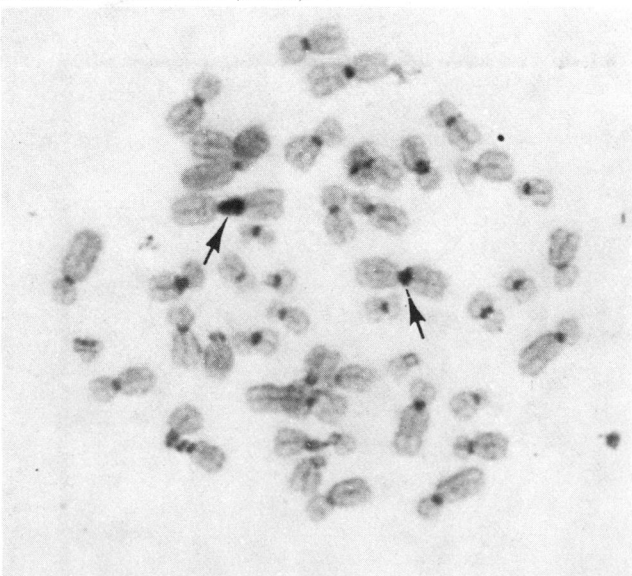

Other microscopically recognizable segments in the short arms of the acrocentric autosomes are devoted to the production of ribosomal RNA and nucleoli. As mitosis progresses, these nucleolus-organizer regions tend to remain relatively uncondensed later than other regions. Consequently, at metaphase they appear understained and thereby demarcate condensed segments of chromatin distal to them on the chromosome arms—*satellites*. (Satellites are examples of the polymorphic segments just mentioned.) Other examples of segmental specialization along the chromosome include regions known as *telomeres* and *centromeres*. Telomeres, the distal termini of each arm, have some relationship to the nuclear membrane and probably are important in the maintenance of the order of the interphase nucleus; centromeric regions are sites of microtubule attachment at metaphase.

A further example of chromosome differentiation is the established sequence by which various segments replicate during S; certain segments replicate early, others late. In general, late replication of a chromosome segment correlates with genetic inertness. This correlation is exemplified by one of the two X chromosomes in female cells; the chromosome inactivated by the Lyon effect is almost entirely late-replicating (see Chap. 58 for an explanation of the Lyon hypothesis).

A little-understood type of chromatin is that which has long been referred to as *heterochromatin*. It is tightly condensed, not just at metaphase but throughout interphase. Such condensation of chromatin correlates positively with genetic inactivity and also with late replication. Some regions are condensed and inactive in all cells (constitutive heterochromatin), while others, for example, the X chromosome, may be either condensed and inactive or unwound and active (facultative heterochromatin). Many chromosome imbalances that permit viability beyond intrauterine life involve chromosome segments that are rich in this apparently inactive, or inactivatable, type of chromatin, e.g., chromosomes that can be trisomic in live-born individuals or, in the case of X, monosomic. The activity of genes can sometimes be affected, even inactivated, if they are positioned near regions of heterochromatin.

Therefore, in chromosomal imbalance both the specific genetic loci and the particular types of chromatin deleted or duplicated are important. Also, the significance of a structural rearrangement probably depends on the new and abnormal positioning of structural and regulatory genes in relation to each other and to heterochromatin.

Fortunately for the cytologist, several differentiated features of the chromosome correlate with cytological artifacts that can be produced and visualized in the laboratory. A number of techniques are now in use to display a pattern of bands of various lengths and staining characteristics (Figs. 60-1 and 60-3). These patterns are identical in each chromosome 1, each chromosome 2, etc., varying only in the inert polymorphic regions mentioned above, so that they can be used in clinical cytogenetics to identify chromosomes and to detect and define structural rearrangements.

Sources of error   Every aspect of the cell division cycle is complicated. Doubtless a large number of genetic loci must be active to produce the numerous enzymes and structural proteins required to initiate and complete a cycle. Remarkable precision and accuracy are demanded over and over in matters such as the passage of a cell from G_1 into S, orderly progression of replication, assembly of the mitotic spindle, and spindle function in segregating chromatids during mitosis. An additional battery of loci is activated to permit a cell of the germ line to pass successfully through the complicated stages of meiotic prophase, including pairing of homologous chromosomes, genetic recombination, and then disjoining of chromosomes. Probably all these mechanisms and processes are subject to

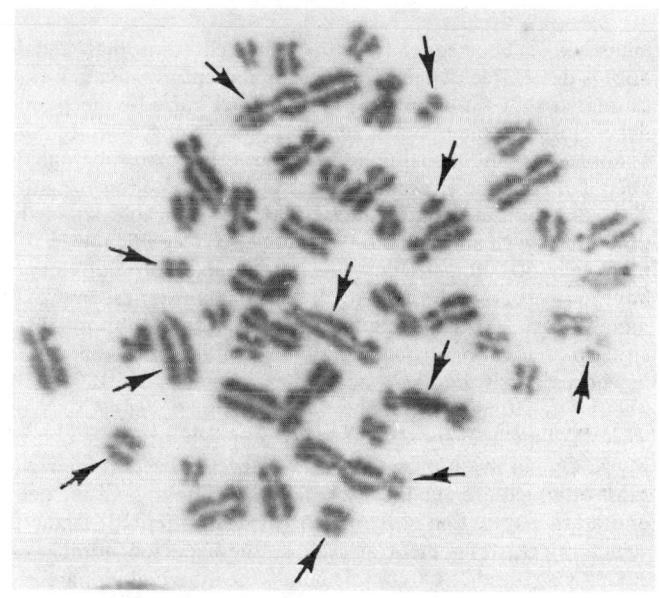

FIGURE 60-4

Breaks and rearrangements (arrows) in metaphase chromosomes of a blood lymphocyte that received γ-ray irradiation before being stimulated by phytohemagglutinin to enter S and divide.

errors, some spontaneous, others promoted by some unfavorable environmental influence (Fig. 60-4) or by the presence of deleterious mutations involving one of the many steps just mentioned. Furthermore, the genetic material itself is subject to damage, and an unrepaired or erroneously repaired lesion in DNA theoretically may predispose to chromosome rearrangement. Errors at many of these steps lie behind chromosome imbalance. Errors that occur in germ cells, during fertilization, and in early postfertilization divisions are important in relation to embryonic maldevelopment and infertility; errors in somatic cells may be important in relation to neoplasia.

CHROMOSOME ABNORMALITIES   Mutations of a single base in a gene and small chromosome deletions and duplications are not visible to the cytogeneticist. In fact, for the normal chromosome banding pattern to be detectably disturbed, a lengthy segment of DNA must be deleted, duplicated, or transposed. This means that a microscopically detectable chromosome mutation must involve relatively huge amounts of DNA. It is noteworthy, however, that the same environmental agents known to produce point mutations (mutagens in the usual sense) are in general also chromosome breaking agents and vice versa. Thus, it seems safe to assume the existence of a spectrum extending from mutations visible to the cytogeneticist to those that must be defined by nucleotide sequencing. Mutations visible to the cytogeneticist ordinarily exert a more widespread effect on development than do point mutations; ordinary genes—often many of them—as well as other specialized types of chromatin, whose function is unknown, are involved in cytologically visible mutations.

If an entire chromosome is affected in an imbalance, the genome is said to be either trisomic or monosomic for the chromosome (thus, trisomy 13, monosomy X). Genes and chromatin carried on the affected chromosome then are present in triple or single dose, respectively, rather than the normal double dose. Abnormal dosage affecting less than an entire chromosome, the result of chromosome breakage and rearrangement, is often termed *partial trisomy* or *partial monosomy*, to indicate that segments rather than entire chromosomes are involved (thus, partial trisomy 13q, partial monosomy 4p).

Incidence The frequency with which chromosomal imbalance is detectable depends on the population investigated. It is estimated that a minimum of 1 in 10 recognized conceptions has a chromosome abnormality. In human embryos and fetuses aborted spontaneously, the incidence of chromosome imbalance is higher the earlier in pregnancy the sampling is made. The contribution of imbalance to late abortion and stillbirth, though not well studied yet, probably also is significant. In the more than 50,000 consecutive or random live-born babies that have now been examined in different laboratories, approximately 1 in 200 has a significant chromosome abnormality, either numerical or structural. In such studies, at least 1 in 700 newborns is trisomic for one of the autosomes 21, 18, or 13; about 1 in 350 newborn males has the complement 47,XXY or 47,XYY. One in every several thousand newborns has monosomy X. One in five hundred has some structural rearrangement, most of which are genetically balanced. Samplings of the general adult population reveal an occasional inherited balanced structural rearrangement as well as the expected number of XXY, XYY, and XXX complements; the inherited, apparently innocuous segmental polymorphisms (e.g., Fig. 60-3) and minor structural rearrangements demonstrable by banding techniques are found in abundance.

In populations of individuals with mental retardation, 10 to 15 percent have a chromosome abnormality, the proportion being greater if there also are anatomic malformations. In some groups of male criminals and in all infertile men, an increased incidence of individuals with an extra sex chromosome, an X or a Y, is found. Infertile women also include many individuals with extra or missing sex chromosomes and an appreciable number with structural chromosome rearrangement; approximately one-fourth of women with primary amenorrhea have some abnormality of the X chromosome. Among infertile men and women, individuals with genes that interfere with meiosis, so-called "meiotic mutants," are also found occasionally.

Numerical abnormalities Trisomy (47 chromosomes) is the most common chromosome imbalance in early spontaneous abortuses, followed by monosomy (45 chromosomes) and triploidy (69 chromosomes). The extra or missing chromosomes can be either paternal or maternal in origin, and the error in segregation of chromosomes can occur in the germ line, fertilized egg (zygote), or early embryo. Trisomy of every chromosome has been observed in spontaneous abortions, trisomy 16 most frequently.

Sex chromosomal trisomy (XXY, XYY, and XXX) is compatible with intrauterine survival; in contrast, autosomal trisomy rarely permits survival to term. However, a small proportion of autosomal trisomics is live-born. For practical purposes these are only trisomy 21, 18, and 13, in decreasing frequency. Trisomies 18 and 13 cause death during infancy. Trisomies of significance in adults are trisomy 21, XXY, XXX, and XYY. A few other autosomal trisomies, such as trisomy 8, have occasionally been reported, usually in mosaicism with a normal cellular component. (Mosaicism is the coexistence of multiple, genetically different populations of cells, derived originally from a single zygote.)

Autosomal monosomy is rare even among abortion material. In contrast, monosomy X (45,X) occurs in approximately 1.5 percent of recognized conceptions. It is common (approximately 10 percent) among spontaneously aborted human embryos and is present in one in every several thousand live-born babies. The reason for the death of 45,X embryos and fetuses is unknown, although developmental abnormalities doubtless contribute to it; cardiovascular and renal anomalies are common in the few that survive. In monosomy X, the missing sex chromosome can be either a Y or an X and is either paternal or maternal in origin. Often the second sex chromosome is not completely absent but is replaced by a structurally rearranged Y or X. Mosaicism is common in live-borns with monosomy X; here, tissues are populated not only by cells with a 45,X complement but by other cells, perhaps with a normal complement, either 46,XY or 46,XX, or with a complement in which the second sex chromosome is rearranged in some way.

Triploidy is rare in live-born babies and usually leads to early death, even when in a mosaicism with normal cells: 46,XY/69,XXY. The phenotypic effects of the autosomal trisomies, of 47,XXY, and of monosomy X (45,X) are characteristic and well defined so that their diagnosis usually is not difficult. The effects of the 47,XYY and 47,XXX constitutions are less striking, and therefore these complements are underdiagnosed. Mosaicism with coexistence of abnormal and normal populations of cells can cause an abnormal phenotype to approach the normal.

The mechanisms responsible for the numerical abnormalities are undefined and may be multiple. A striking but unexplained maternal age effect exists in trisomies 21, 18, 13, XXY, and XXX. Over one-third of babies with trisomy 21 are born to women over 35, whereas only one-tenth of all births occur in this group. The frequency of trisomy 21 rises from 0.5 to 0.7 per 1000 live births between ages 21 and 23 to 3.1 per 1000 at age 35, 10.5 per 1000 at age 40, and 33.6 per 1000 at age 45. (A paternal age effect may also exist in trisomy 21.) Maternal x-ray irradiation in low dosage is also associated with an increased incidence of trisomy 21. After a child with trisomy 21 is born, the risk to the parents of recurrence in future pregnancies is increased to approximately 1 percent. As to the etiology of monosomy X, the frequent association of the 45,X complement in mosaicism with normal complements and with structural rearrangements of the X and Y suggests that the zygote or early embryo may often be the target of a chromosome-breaking event.

Structural abnormalities Some structural chromosome rearrangements are inherited, and others represent new mutations. The etiology of the new rearrangements is unknown, although they are assumed to be partly spontaneous and partly the effect of environmental agents such as mutagenic chemicals or ionizing radiation acting on the germ line, zygote, or early embryo (Fig. 60-4).

Many of the known chromosome rearrangements have been detected only once or a few times. Others are detected repeatedly, the same one occurring in unrelated individuals and families. For example, the commonest translocation, one that can occur either as a result of de novo mutation or by inheritance, affects one chromosome 13 and one 14 at or near their centromeres. In this translocation, only inert chromatin is lost from the tiny short arms. A similar translocation affecting chromosomes 14 and 21 is also common.

Chromosome complements bearing rearrangements can be genetically balanced or effectively so, thus imparting no unfavorable phenotypic effect to their bearers; about two-thirds of rearrangements detected during surveys of consecutive live-born babies are balanced. Or the complement can be unbalanced and affect development unfavorably, the usual case when rearrangements are detected during surveys of spontaneous abortuses or of individuals with multiple anomalies and mental retardation.

Some balanced rearrangements are transmitted from generation to generation without producing clinical effects. In other cases, however, they are profoundly important to members of the kindred transmitting them, by being responsible for the conception of embryos with unbalanced genomes. For example, bearers of some 13;14 translocations are at risk of having children with the trisomy 13 syndrome, and inherited translocations involving chromosome 21 predispose to the trisomy 21 syndrome. Approximately 5 percent of live-borns with the trisomy 21 syndrome have a translocation, and in about a fifth of those it is detectable in one of the parents. Because most babies with the trisomy 21 syndrome due to translocation are born to women under 30, a search for a translocation is important when a child with this clinical syndrome is born to young parents.

Different translocations bestow on their carriers different risks of having offspring with unbalanced rearrangements. These risks cannot be predicted on the theoretical basis of the way the translocation might be expected to behave during meiosis. Useful empiric risk figures have been accumulated for common translocations; e.g., the 14;21 translocation bestows a 2 percent risk on a balanced male carrier and more than a 10 percent risk on a female carrier of having a child with the trisomy 21 syndrome. In contrast, the balanced carrier of a 21;21 translocation can expect only unbalanced offspring. Information of this type is indispensable to those undertaking genetic counseling in relation to chromosome disorders.

Although the phenotypic effects of many of the different segmental chromosome imbalances which can occur are varied and nonspecific, the resulting anomalies sometimes compose a recognizable clinical syndrome. Two examples are the following: (1) If a rearrangement causes partial trisomy of the distal band of the long arm of 21, the clinical features composing the full syndrome associated with an extra chromosome 21 develop. (A triple dose of other segments of the long arm of chromosome 21 also produces adverse effects but not the trisomy 21 syndrome.) (2) Partial monosomy of a short segment within the short arm of chromosome 5 causes mental retardation, a characteristic facies, and a characteristic cry during infancy. This group of signs is known as the *5p−* or *cri-du-chat syndrome.*

Because of the large number of karyotype-phenotype correlations made in recent years, additional specific syndromes produced by imbalance of many different segments now are known, e.g., the 4p−, 9p partial trisomy, 13q−, and 18q− syndromes, to name a few. Rearrangements not previously described and their corresponding clinical syndromes are still being recognized. Any of these syndromes may appear as result either of de novo chromosome rearrangement or through formation of a genetically unbalanced gamete in a person carrying in balanced state a rearrangement affecting the segment involved. Families transmitting an unusual rearrangement in balanced form are said, because of the recurrence of individuals with the same specific imbalance, to have *private syndromes.*

In most individuals with chromosome imbalance, regardless of which segments are affected, a degree of phenotypic similarity is present. These recurring and nonspecific features include mental retardation, growth retardation, dysmorphic ears, nose, and mouth, cardiac malformations of standard types, abnormalities of dermal ridges and creases, and dysmorphic digits. (As a rule, autosomal imbalance need not be considered in the etiology of anatomic defects unaccompanied by mental retardation.) Why similar abnormalities occur with so many different segmental imbalances is unknown, but when several such features are observed in a single individual, they can be a valuable clinical indication for cytogenetic analysis. Imbalance affecting certain segments also causes specific phenotypic changes; an example is the anomalous cry in the 5p− syndrome mentioned above. Another example of specificity is retinoblastoma, which may develop when one particular band of chromosome 13 is present in single dose. Whereas the nonspecific changes serve to call the clinician's attention to the possibility of some chromosome imbalance, the specific features can suggest the exact segment of the genome affected.

DISEASE ASSOCIATIONS Various combinations of abnormalities in malformed and defective individuals have been correlated with variations in the chromosome complement. In this way, clinical syndromes due to specific chromosome imbalances have been defined. (Many of the pediatric conditions are of little significance in adult medicine because of their lethality in infancy or early childhood.)

Autosome imbalance Of the three autosomal trisomies found in live-born babies, only trisomy 21 is compatible with survival past infancy. The phenotype produced by the presence of an extra chromosome 21, formerly known as *mongolism* but now termed the *Down syndrome* or *trisomy 21 syndrome,* is characteristic and easily diagnosed from birth: mental retardation, short stature, muscular hypotonia, brachycephaly, short neck, typical facies (oblique orbital fissures, flat nasal bridge, small simple or folded ears, nystagmus, mouth hanging open), narrow palate, short broad hands with incurving fifth fingers, gaps between the first and second toes, and characteristic dermatoglyphics. Additional findings may include congenital heart disease, blepharitis and conjunctivitis, Brushfield's spots of the iris, straight pubic hair, abnormal teeth, protruding furrowed tongue, high-arched palate, loose skin of the neck, transverse palmar creases, and hyperflexibility of the joints. Cardiac malformations lead to death in infancy in a third of individuals with trisomy 21, and other malformations and infections may also cause early death. However, subjects who survive infancy often reach adulthood, and some even old age. The proneness to develop leukemia in affected infants is not maintained in later life. Females occasionally become pregnant and, as expected, approximately half their children have trisomy 21.

Mosaicism of trisomy 21 with normal cells (46/47,+21) may occur in individuals with modified features of the trisomy 21 syndrome, and it is probable that many individuals with this mosaicism go unrecognized. The risk of such persons having trisomic children is increased, but unfortunately their mosaicism is usually detected only after they have had an affected child. Partial trisomy, partial monosomy, or a combination of the two explains many of the instances in both children and adults of multiple developmental defects combined with mental retardation. Sometimes a balanced autosomal translocation is detected in normally developed adults who have repeated spontaneous abortion or subnormal fertility, with or without abnormal live-born children.

Sex chromosome imbalance (see also Chap. 344) In contrast to autosome imbalance, sex chromosome imbalance has relatively mild phenotypic effects. This is because X chromosomes beyond one in the complement of somatic cells are usually inactivated and because the Y chromosome bears few if any genes other than the testis determinants. X-linked loci (in contrast to autosomal loci) function normally in single dose: the male is hemizygous for X-linked genes, having only one X chromosome (with the possible exception of a few loci on the Y that may be homologous to a segment on the X); the female is functionally hemizygous through the Lyon effect. The addition of an extra sex chromosome to the normal male or female complement has a phenotypic effect but insufficient to interfere with intrauterine survival. Since major anatomic defects are usually absent, individuals with the complements 47,XXY and 47,XYY, both of whom are males, and 47,XXX, who are females, ordinarily go unrecognized till adolescence or later, often never to be diagnosed at all.

The *Klinefelter syndrome* (Chap. 344), which in classic form consists of small testes, infertility, gynecomastia, and variable degrees of underandrogenization, sometimes with mild mental retardation, antisocial behavior, or both, is the consequence of the addition of an extra X to the male complement: 47,XXY. The extra X interferes in some way with the survival of germ cells, and atrophy of the spermatogenic tubules and azoospermia are the consequence. Sometimes the phenotypic effects are surprisingly mild, the testicular atrophy being the only noteworthy feature in otherwise healthy and socially well-adjusted men. The mosaicism 46,XY/47,XXY sometimes occurs and may ameliorate the phenotypic effect of the extra X. More extreme phenotypic effects and mental retardation result when more than one extra sex chromosome is added to the normal male complement: 48,XXXY or 49,XXXXY.

The phenotypic effect of 47,XYY is less well defined; although increased height, behavioral difficulties, and infertility are common, the extra Y is sometimes found in otherwise normal men. The rare complement 48,XXYY results in infertility, probably because of the extra X, as in the 47,XXY Klinefelter's syndrome. The phenotype associated with 47,XXX is also poorly defined, but women with mild mental retardation, psychosis, and menstrual abnormalities are increased in frequency; this complement is sometimes detected in normal, healthy women. Further clarification is needed concerning the effects on personality and behavior of all three complements: 47,XXY, 47,XYY, and 47,XXX.

Loss of the Y or of the second X has drastic effects on development. If it does not cause abortion, it may or may not be recognizable at birth. Loose nuchal folds and edema of the hands and feet in a newborn girl, with or without renal or cardiovascular anomalies, may point to the diagnosis of the 45,X complement. The *Turner syndrome* is the manifestation in subsequent life (Chap. 344): short stature resistant to all treatment, infantilism of otherwise normal female external and internal genitalia, germ-cell-free gonads referred to as *gonadal streaks,* and variable renal, cardiovascular, skeletal, and ectodermal anomalies. Without estrogen administration breast development remains infantile, and menstruation does not occur. Although mental retardation is not a feature, a poorly defined emotional immaturity and difficulty with spatial perception are common.

The Turner syndrome may be the developmental consequence of several chromosome constitutions besides 45,X. Mosaicism as well as structural abnormalities of a second sex chromosome, either a Y or an X, cause a spectrum of disorders at both the clinical and cytogenetic levels. A normal male or normal female cellular component may be present along with the 45,X cellular component, or one component may bear a structurally abnormal chromosome. Common abnormalities of the Y and X are isochromosome formation (one arm deleted and the other duplicated) or deletion of part of or all one arm. In some affected individuals, all cells have 46 chromosomes, with one normal X plus an abnormal Y or X, for example, 46,XXp− deletion from the short arm of one of the X chromosomes. In others, a second or third cellular component may be present as well, for example, 45,X/46,XX/46,XXp−. Clinically pure Turner syndrome may be found in association with various combinations of these karyotypes if one of them is either monosomic or partially monosomic for X. However, when Y-bearing cells coexist with the 45,X cells, for example, 45,X/46,XY, genital ambiguity often develops, and gonads may vary from streaks to functional testes (the syndrome of *mixed gonadal dysgenesis*); here the risk of malignant gonadal tumors is significant. When 46,XX cells coexist with 45,X, varying degrees of ovarian function may be maintained, including ovulation. Although the phenotype may approach a normal male or female pattern when normal and abnormal

cells coexist, the effects of mosaicism are unpredictable. Thus, the clinical syndrome associated with monosomy X and structurally abnormal Ys or Xs ranges from a predominantly male phenotype through Turner syndrome to an almost normal female phenotype.

Two other rare conditions deserve mention—*true hermaphroditism* and the *46,XX male* (see also Chap. 344). *True hermaphroditism* is present when both testicular and ova- and follicle-containing ovarian tissue exist in the same individual. In most cases, 46,XX is the chromosome complement, and it appears normal by banding; here the most plausible explanation is that an occult translocation of the testis-determining segment of the Y to an X or autosome has occurred. Sometimes true hermaphrodites have the complement 46,XY; rarely the chimerism 46,XY/46,XX is found, the two cellular components having been derived from two zygotes.

Males occasionally have the complement 46,XX. As in 47,XXY men, the second X interferes with meiosis, and azoospermia results. In both the 46,XX true hermaphrodite and the *46,XX male* the rule that a Y is required for testicular differentiation appears to break down. However, the two conditions may have the same etiologic basis, undetected translocation of Y material onto another chromosome.

Chromosome change in cancer The theory that an alteration in the chromosomal complement may be the cause of cancer was advanced almost seven decades ago, but the matter is still unsettled. Chromosome changes are plentiful in cancer, but this very fact—too many changes—has been a major reason many have rejected them as of etiologic significance. However, support for the idea that chromosome alteration is significant in the etiology of human cancer has come from two observations: (1) the known environmental "causes" of human cancer (carcinogenic chemicals and ionizing radiation) are also chromosome-breaking agents (Fig. 60-4); and (2) three recessively inherited disorders result in increased chromosome breakage and rearrangement in cells in culture, and in each the risk of cancer is increased—Bloom's syndrome, Fanconi's anemia, and ataxia-telangiectasia (the Louis-Bar syndrome). Thus, the known environmental and the known genetic causes of increased chromosome mutation all predispose to cancer.

Many human cancers have altered chromosome complements. In the leukemias, lymphomas, and certain myeloproliferative disorders, the alterations are less extensive than in solid tumors and, therefore, easier to define. In certain lymphomas, chromosome 14 is often found to have undergone structural rearrangement. In over 80 percent of chronic granulocytic leukemias, a translocation affecting chromosome 22 (usually chromosome 9 is the other chromosome affected) is detected, the so-called "Ph¹ chromosome"; if the disease progresses into a "blastic" phase, the karyotype often evolves, certain additional chromosome changes being added stepwise in a nonrandom sequence. In this leukemia and in a few others, the various chromosome changes appear to have some value in prognosis and choice of therapy. In most other leukemias, detectable karyotypic specificity is less impressive so far.

Solid tumors, which generally are studied later in their course than conditions affecting the bone marrow, show extensive karyotypic changes, both structural and numerical. Different cells from a single tumor have similar numerical changes and structural rearrangements, but in the same type tumor from another person the changes are usually different. This apparent lack of specificity is partly due to the complexity of the changes, however, and a few examples of chromosome alterations specific for a solid tumor are known; for example, meningiomas are associated with a deletion of chromosome 22 in almost every case. The findings in both solid tumors and leukemias demonstrate the clonal nature of human cancer.

Human metaphase chromosomes can be examined in any tissue in which sufficient cells are cycling. Preparations can therefore be made directly from almost any embryonic tissue and from adult bone marrow, lymphoid tissue, and malignant tissues. In searches for mosaicism, the study of multiple tissues is often required. Some tissues unlikely to yield cells in metaphase can be placed in culture, and chromosome preparations can be made after many cells have been brought into mitosis. Blood lymphocytes stimulated to enter cell division cycles by phytohemagglutinin are the standard material for diagnosing constitutional chromosome imbalance. In some myeloproliferative disorders and leukemias, unstimulated circulating blood cells divide spontaneously after a few hours in culture. Long-term cultures of fibroblasts can be derived from minute skin biopsies or from most any tissue, although more elaborate laboratory facilities and a longer period of time are required before cytogenetic preparations can be made. Amniotic fluid is among the sources of cells suitable for culture, and these embryonic cells are widely used in the diagnosis of fetal chromosome imbalance.

Nucleated cells in interphase can be used for the study of sex chromatin. Cells from buccal mucosa and hair follicles are perhaps the most readily obtained, but surgical and autopsy specimens or cells in culture are at times useful also. X chromatin (formerly called the Barr body), a condensed body of chromatin characteristically apposed to the nuclear membrane, is present in normal female cells. The X responsible for X chromatin in any particular cell is the one genetically inactivated and late-replicating. The number of X-chromatin masses is an indication of the number of X chromosomes in excess of 1. Y chromatin, a condensed segment of the Y demonstrated by quinacrine staining and fluorescence microscopy, is present in interphase nuclei of Y-bearing cells (for example, 48,XXYY cells contain one X-chromatin plus two Y-chromatin masses).

Meiotic chromosome preparations from testicular biopsies are sometimes useful in obscure cases of infertility. Here translocations and genetically determined disturbances in meiotic pairing may be identified.

section 2 | Clinical immunology

61

INTRODUCTION TO CLINICAL IMMUNOLOGY

BRUCE C. GILLILAND

Clinical immunology is a rapidly expanding field with increasing practical application to medicine. The scope of immunology covers defense against infections, prevention of diseases by immunization, organ transplantation, blood banking, deficiencies of the immune system, and a variety of disorders that are mediated by immunologic mechanisms. Besides the clinical relevance of immunology, immunologic techniques are frequently used in the clinical laboratory, as in the measurement of hormones and drugs.

The intent of this chapter is to provide the reader with a review of the essential fundamentals of immunology. The cellular components of the immune system, lymphocytes, plasma cells, and macrophages, along with their role in antibody-mediated or humoral immunity and in cell-mediated or cellular immunity, will be discussed first. This will be followed by a review of the immunoglobulins, cellular immunity, the interrelationship of the B and T lymphocytes and macrophages in the immune response, tolerance, and autoimmunity. The last sections cover the complement system and types of immunologically mediated inflammation and tissue damage.

CELLS OF THE IMMUNE SYSTEM

The principal cells of the immune system are lymphocytes, plasma cells, and macrophages which are collectively organized into lymphoid tissue. The thymus, lymph nodes, and spleen are examples of highly developed lymphoid tissues. Other lymphoid tissue is found along the gastrointestinal tract (tonsils, Peyer's patches, appendix) and also may accumulate at sites of inflammation.

The large body of experimental evidence has affirmed the existence of two populations of lymphocytes. These two populations were first demonstrated in chickens by removal of the thymus or by removal of the bursa of Fabricius (a lymphoid organ near the cloaca) during the neonatal period. Excision of the bursa resulted in low immunoglobulin levels and impaired antibody synthesis. Lymphoid nodules did not develop in lymph nodes and spleen, and only a few plasma cells were present. Cell-mediated immunity, however, remained intact as demonstrated by delayed hypersensitivity and allograft rejection. Evidence for two populations of immunocompetent cells in humans has largely come from study of congenital and acquired defects of immunity (Chap. 62) and from development of techniques for identification of populations of lymphocytes. These observations clearly indicate the existence of two separate systems for the differentiation of lymphoid cells involved in humoral and cellular immunity (Fig. 61-1). The two populations of immunocompetent lymphocytes are referred to as B cells and T cells (Table 61-1). The designation *B cell* was used originally because these cells depend for their development on the presence of the bursa in birds or its equivalent in humans. The equivalent of the bursa in humans remains unknown but might be the fetal liver, spleen, or bone marrow. The designation *T cell* connotes the role of the thymus in the development of these cells.

B CELLS B cells represent approximately 15 to 20 percent of the normal peripheral blood lymphocytes, 50 percent of the splenic lymphocytes, and 75 percent of the lymphocytes in the bone marrow. They are the principal cells in the cortical germinal centers and medullary cords of lymph nodes. Their chief role is the production of antibodies.

The B cells carry membrane-bound immunoglobulins as demonstrated by immunofluorescence staining with anti-immunoglobulin antiserum. The main immunoglobulin classes on

TABLE 61-1
Characteristics of T and B lymphocytes

	T cells	B cells
Function	Delayed hypersensitivity	Humoral immunity
Product	Lymphokines	Immunoglobulins
Identification	Sheep RBC rosettes	Surface Ig Fc and activated complement receptors
Assessment	Proliferative response to PHA, Con A Delayed skin test	Immunoglobulin levels Antibody response to immunization Blastogenic response to PWM

NOTE: *Ig, immunoglobulin; PHA, phytohemagglutinin; Con A, concanavalin A; PWM, pokeweed mitogen.*

the surface of peripheral blood B cells are IgM, present in the low-molecular-weight (7S subunit) monomeric form, and IgD. Approximately three-quarters of the peripheral blood B cells carry these two immunoglobulins; the remaining cells stain mostly for IgG, while about 1 percent stain for IgA. The membrane-bound immunoglobulin molecule is attached by its crystallizable fragment (Fc) portion to the plasma membrane, leaving the antigen-binding sites freely available. Upon contact with specific antigen and with modulatory signals from other cells, B cells bearing the complementary antigen binding site will evolve through a series of events leading to clonal expansion and differentiation into antibody-synthesizing plasma cells.

The most widely accepted theory of antibody formation is clonal selection, which suggests that there are large numbers of precommitted lymphocytes, each with its specific membrane receptor capable of reacting with specific immunogen. The selective binding of immunogens is followed by clonal expansion and antibody production.

Most of the B cells have a membrane receptor for the Fc portion of IgG in the form of either antigen-antibody complexes or aggregated IgG. Approximately one-half of the B cells also carry membrane receptors for the activated third component of complement (C3b). Receptors for other complement components (C3d, C4, and Clq) have also been identified on B cells. These various membrane receptors and membrane-bound immunoglobulins have membrane mobility and can undergo redistribution and capping. For example, when membrane-bound immunoglobulin binds with specific antigen, the immunoglobulin molecules reorganize into patches on the membrane and then these molecules localize at one pole of the

cell (capping). The polar cap of molecules is interiorized by endocytosis. As this process is occurring, the B cell is synthesizing new immunoglobulins for insertion into its membrane. These events may be important in the initiation of cell proliferation and antibody production. It has also been suggested that the capping process may serve only to remove excess antigen from the cell surface.

T CELLS   Approximately 70 to 80 percent of normal peripheral blood lymphocytes and 90 percent of lymphocytes in thoracic duct fluid are T cells. They circulate primarily as long-lived small lymphocytes. These cells are the principal lymphocytes in the deep cortical areas of lymph nodes and in the periarteriolar areas of the splenic white pulp. The T cells are the main effectors of cell-mediated immunity and also are involved as helper or suppressor cells in modulating the immune response.

The T cells possess antigens that are identified with specific anti-T-cell antiserum by use of immunofluorescence or cytotoxic assays. The similarity of a T-cell antigen to the theta antigen identified on the lymphocyte in the thymus of mice has led to the following concept of T-cell differentiation in humans. Stem cells proliferate in the bone marrow and migrate to the thymus, where, under the influence of the epithelial cells of thymus, they acquire the characteristics of T cells, including the theta antigen or its equivalent in humans. Once the T cell has left the thymus, this gland may continue to exert an effect on T cells by secretion of thymic hormones.

The T cells in humans are usually identified by the presence of membrane receptors for sheep red blood cells which form rosettes around T cells when they are incubated together. Several subpopulations of T cells are recognized on the basis of differences in function, surface antigens, and membrane receptors for immunoglobulins. The various subsets of T cells function as helper cells, suppressor cells, or cytotoxic effector cells (see "Immune Response" below). The nature of the antigen-binding receptor on T cells is uncertain. One candidate for antigen receptor is a monomeric IgM-like molecule which has been identified on the T-cell membrane by some investigators. Other candidates include the cell membrane product of histocompatibility genes and the membrane product of immune response genes (Ir genes).

A small number of lymphocytes in blood (2 to 10 percent) do not have the usual surface membrane markers for B or T cells and are referred to as *null cells*. Some of these cells may represent incompletely differentiated B or T cells. Others have an Fc receptor for IgG and are referred to as *K* or *killer cells*,

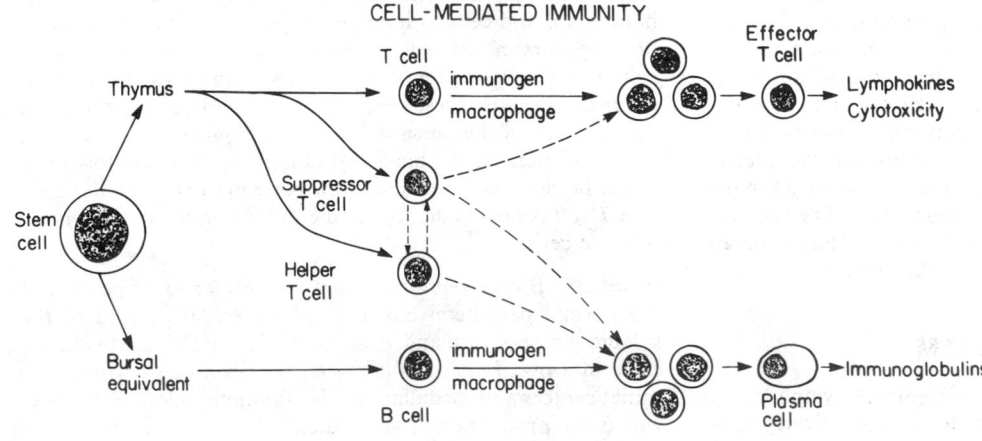

CELL-MEDIATED IMMUNITY

HUMORAL IMMUNITY

FIGURE 61-1

Schematic representation of the development of the immune system and the immune response. Upon exposure to immunogen, T cells proliferate and become sensitized lymphocytes that form the basis of cell-mediated immunity. The B cells proliferate and evolve to antibody-synthesizing plasma cells that constitute the basis of humoral immunity. Macrophages process and present immunogen to T and B cells. Subsets of T cells function as helper T cells which stimulate B-cell activity, or as suppressor T cells which suppress humoral and cell-mediated immune responses.

since they are the effector cell in antibody-dependent cell-mediated cytotoxicity (see "Immune Mechanisms of Tissue Injury" below).

MACROPHAGES Macrophages originate from promonocytes in the bone marrow and are released into the circulation as monocytes. Monocytes comprise 3 to 8 percent of the circulating leukocyte population. An even greater number of monocytes, estimated to be approximately three times the circulating population, exists in a marginal pool consisting of monocytes adhering to endothelial surfaces. Upon entering tissue, monocytes develop into macrophages. Tissue sites where macrophages are commonly found include the liver (where they are called *Kupffer cells*), peritoneum, lung, spleen, and lymph nodes. Macrophages have surface receptors for IgG1 and IgG3, and also a receptor for C3b. Through these receptors, macrophages can effectively bind and interiorize antigen-antibody complexes consisting of IgG antibodies or immune complexes which contain activated C3. Macrophages kill bacteria, fungi, and tumor cells. They also function in the induction of the immune response by processing and presenting immunogenic material to lymphocytes (see "Immune Response" below).

IMMUNOGLOBULINS

Immunoglobulins are synthesized by the B-cell series and have common structural features and structural units. Immunoglobulin molecules are composed of two kinds of polypeptide chains (Fig. 61-2); each molecule consists of larger identical polypeptide chains referred to as *heavy chains* (H chains) and two identical smaller ones referred to as *light chains* (L chains). These polypeptide chains are held together by disulfide bonds and by noncovalent bonds, which are primarily hydrophobic. The heavy and light polypeptide chains are synthesized on separate ribosomes, assembled in the cell, and secreted as an intact molecule. A slight to moderate excess of light chains is synthesized and secreted as free light chains.

The understanding of the structure and function of immunoglobulins was facilitated by studies of fragments produced by enzymatic cleavage of the antibody molecule (Fig. 61-3). For example, treatment of antibody molecules with papain results in two Fab fragments, which are the antigen binding fragments of the molecule, and one Fc fragment, which is responsible for the biologic activities discussed below. The amino-terminal half of the light chains and the amino-terminal quarter of the heavy chains of the immunoglobulin molecules vary in their amino acid sequence and are termed the *variable region* (V region) of the polypeptide chains. Portions of the V region of one heavy and one light polypeptide chain contribute the site for antigen binding. Considerable variation of the amino acid sequence must exist in this portion of the immunoglobulin molecule in order to explain the estimated 1 million antibody specificities. The constant region of H chains allows their differentiation into a class or subclass and confers to the immunoglobulins certain biological properties such as the ability to activate complement, to cross the placenta, and to bind to polymorphonuclear leukocytes or macrophages.

Five immunoglobulin classes (IgG, IgA, IgM, IgD, and IgE) are recognized on the basis of structural differences of their heavy chains including the amino acid sequence and length of the polypeptide chain. The antigenic determinants on the heavy chains also permit the identification and quantitation of the immunoglobulin classes by immunochemical techniques. On protein electrophoresis at a pH of 8.6, the immunoglobulins migrate mainly in the gamma region. Significant amounts of immunoglobulins also may be found in the beta region. The bulk of the gamma globulin consists of IgG immunoglobulin. The wide range in which immunoglobulins can migrate on protein electrophoresis is due to amino acid differences in the variable region of the molecules. A narrow band of protein staining in the gamma to beta region usually indicates the presence of a monoclonal population of immunoglobulins, the product of a single clone of cells as in multiple myeloma or macroglobulinemia (Chap. 63). Antibodies to a given antigen may be detected in all or several classes of immunoglobulins or may be restricted to a single class or subclass of immunoglobulin. Autoantibodies likewise may belong to one or several classes of immunoglobulins. For example, rheumatoid factors (antibodies to IgG) are most often recognized as an IgM immunoglobulin, but can also consist of IgG or

FIGURE 61-2

Schematic model of the variable and constant regions of an antibody molecule. The blackened areas represent the variable regions in the amino terminal half of each L chain and the amino terminal quarter of each H chain. The remainder of the molecules constitutes the constant regions. Amino acid sequences in the variable regions provide the basis for antibody specificity.

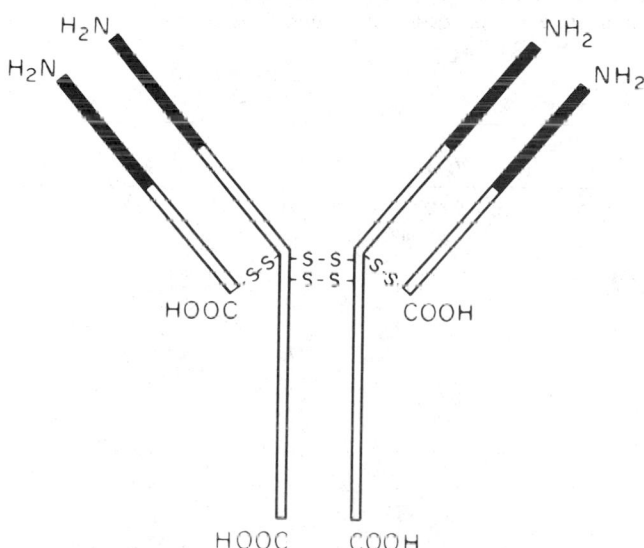

FIGURE 61-3

Schematic representation of enzyme cleavage of immunoglobulin molecules. Papain cleaves the molecule into three parts, two Fab fragments with antigen-binding sites and one Fc fragment. Pepsin produces a bivalent F(ab')₂ fragment, and the Fc portion is cleaved into small peptides.

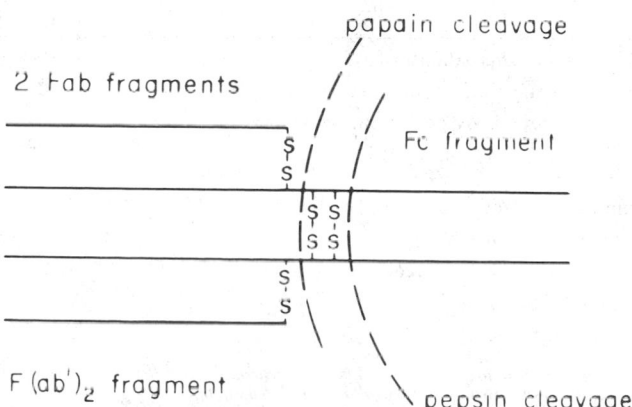

IgA. The physical and biologic properties of immunoglobulins are listed in Table 61-2.

IgG The most abundant immunoglobulin is IgG; approximately 50 percent of its distribution is in the intravascular compartment. It has a molecular weight of 150,000 daltons. IgG is the only immunoglobulin that crosses the placenta and thereby provides maternal antibodies to the neonate. The structural features that mediate the transport across the placenta reside in the Fc fragment of IgG molecules. Four subclasses of IgG have been defined. While each has a common antigenic determinant for IgG, some differences in their amino acid sequences provide antigens that permit separation into subclasses. IgG1 and IgG3 are able to activate the complement system upon formation of immune complexes and to react with IgG receptors on monocytes and polymorphonuclear leukocytes. Both of these properties of IgG reside in the Fc portion of the molecule. Approximately 70 percent of the total IgG is IgG1, 18 percent is IgG2, 8 percent is IgG3, and 4 percent is IgG4.

IgA The predominant immunoglobulin in external secretions of the respiratory tree, gastrointestinal tract, and genitourinary system, and in tears, saliva, and colostrum is IgA. The IgA-producing plasma cells are the predominant plasma cells in the submucosa. For example, in the lamina propria of the intestine, approximately 20 IgA-producing plasma cells exist for each IgG-producing cell, compared with a 1:3 ratio in the peripheral lymph nodes and spleen. Secretory IgA is composed of two IgA molecules bound to a secretory piece by disulfide bonds. The secretory piece is a polypeptide chain with a molecular weight of 70,000 daltons that is synthesized by epithelial cells. The dimeric IgA is held together by a single J chain which is also synthesized by submucosal plasma cells and has a molecular weight of 15,000 daltons. Once the dimeric IgA leaves the plasma cell, it enters the epithelial cell and becomes covalently bound to a secretory piece. It is then secreted into the lumen. Secretory IgA has a molecular weight of approximately 400,000 daltons. Low concentrations of secretory IgA sometimes are found in the normal serum. Secretory IgA is more resistant to digestion by most proteolytic enzymes than monomeric IgA. An IgA protease that specifically cleaves human IgA in secretions has been discovered. This protease occurs in certain microorganisms such as *Neisseria gonorrhoeae* and *Streptococcus sanguis,* both of which are known to invade mucosal membranes in spite of prior immunity. Secretory IgA

can have antibody activity to bacterial and viral antigens, toxins, and dietary macromolecules. Secretory antibodies bind microorganisms and prevent their attachment to epithelial cells, and administration of antigens by either the gastrointestinal or respiratory route results in enhanced production of secretory IgA in these organ systems.

In the serum, IgA exists as a monomer with a molecular weight of 160,000 daltons, and to a lesser extent in polymeric forms. Two subclasses of IgA have been identified; approximately 75 percent of the total IgA is IgA1, and 25 percent IgA2. No biological differences are known to exist between IgA1 and IgA2 except that IgA2 appears to be resistant to cleavage by the specific IgA proteases.

IgM Approximately 10 percent of the serum immunoglobulins are IgM, which is a pentamer of the usual four polypeptide chain structure of immunoglobulins, having a molecular weight of 900,000 daltons. The five IgM subunits are linked by disulfide bonds in association with a single J chain to constitute the IgM molecule. While the J chain apparently assists in the polymerization of IgM, polymers form in the absence of the J chain. Even though the pentameric IgM has 10 antigen binding sites, these antibodies have a functional valence of 5 with large antigenic molecules. The distribution of IgM is predominantly intravascular. Activation of the complement system requires only one molecule of IgM antibody to react with antigen. IgM antibody is prominent in the early immune response and is the major class of antibodies to blood group substances A and B. Autoantibodies, such as rheumatoid factor (anti-IgG) and cold agglutinins, are also predominantly IgM immunoglobulins. A natural subunit of IgM is called *low-molecular-weight IgM* and has a molecular weight of 180,000 daltons. It is found on the surface of B cells, in fetal blood, and in certain diseases such as rheumatoid vasculitis, systemic lupus erythematosus, ataxia telangiectasia, progressive muscular atrophy and idiopathic chronic neuropathy, Waldenström's macroglobulinemia, and lymphoma. The biological significance of this molecule in the circulation is not known.

IgD IgD has a molecular weight of 180,000 daltons and is found mainly in the intravascular space and on resting B cells as a cell surface immunoglobulin. IgD is easily degraded by proteolytic enzymes and by heat. The function of free IgD in blood is not known, but the IgD on B cells may, in association with monomeric IgM, play an important role in the binding of antigen to B cells.

IgE The distinctive biological feature of IgE is its role in the immediate allergic or hypersensitivity reaction (reagenic prop-

TABLE 61-2
Properties of immunoglobulins

	IgG	*IgA*	*IgM*	*IgD*	*IgE*
Molecular weight, daltons	150,000	160,000	900,000	180,000	190,000
Average serum concentration, mg per 100 ml	1200	280	100	3	0.025*
Percent of total body pool in intravascular compartment	50	40	75	75	
Half-life days	23	5.5	5.1	2.8	2.3
Complement fixation by classic pathway	Yes†	No‡	Yes	No	No
Reagenic properties	No	No	No	No	Yes
Selective secretion by mucous membranes	No	Yes	No	No	No
Placental transfer	Yes	No	No	No	No
Macrophage binding	Yes¶	No	No	No	No

* *Serum concentration in normal nonatopic individuals is less than 0.025 mg per 100 ml.*
† *IgG4 does not activate complement and IgG2 only weakly.*
‡ *IgA activates complement system only by the alternative pathway.*
¶ *Only IgG1 and IgG3.*

erty) (Chap. 65). IgE has a molecular weight of 190,000 daltons and binds to basophils and mast cells through its Fc region. When a specific antigen combines with the antigen-binding sites on IgE, histamine and serotonin are released from these cells. The allergen must bind to two or more adjacent molecules of IgE to evoke the release of histamine. These pharmacological mediators lead to the characteristic wheal and flare reaction in the skin. In the lung, the same sequence of events leads to the release of slow reactive substance of anaphylaxis. The bulk of the body's pool of IgE is bound to basophils and mast cells, and the serum concentration of this immunoglobulin is extremely low, in the order of 0.1 to 0.2 $\mu g/ml$.

CELL-MEDIATED IMMUNITY (DELAYED TYPE OF HYPERSENSITIVITY)

The principal effectors of cell-mediated immunity are T cells that have become sensitized to foreign substances. These specifically sensitized T cells, along with macrophages, play a very important role in the defense of the host against a variety of infectious microorganisms including *Mycobacterium tuberculosis*, fungi, viruses, and protozoa. Cell-mediated immunity is most prominent in infections due to intracellular organisms. The killing of tumor cells and rejection of allografts such as kidney transplants are also expressions of cell-mediated immunity (Chap. 69).

Cell-mediated immunity is exemplified by the delayed type of hypersensitivity reaction in skin. The intradermal or subcutaneous injection of antigen into an individual previously sensitized to that antigen results in a reaction that consists of erythema followed by induration and reaches a peak in approximately 2 days. Lymphocytes and macrophages are the predominant cells in the lesion. If the inflammation is intense, necrosis of the skin may occur. Cell-mediated immunity can be transferred to a previously unimmunized individual with T cells but not with serum. In addition, cell-mediated immunity can also be transferred to a normal recipient with *transfer factor*, a low-molecular-weight material derived from disrupted sensitized lymphocytes or from the supernatant of a stimulated lymphocyte culture.

The events of cell-mediated immunity are initiated as the result of interaction of antigen with a few specifically sensitized T cells. The sensitized T cells, activated by antigen, elaborate soluble products referred to as *lymphokines*, which have several biological activities. Lymphokines mediate and amplify cell-mediated immune reactions by affecting the activities of macrophages, polymorphonuclear leukocytes, B cells, and other T cells. Several of the products of activated lymphocytes are listed in Table 61-3. While the T cell is considered the principal cell in cell-mediated immunity, the concept of cell-mediated immunity has taken on a broader connotation with the observation that B cells also release lymphokines, including macrophage chemotactic factor, macrophage activating factor, and macrophage inhibitory factor.

The development of the cell-mediated immune reaction in vivo may occur as follows: Antigen activates specifically sensitized T cells resulting in the elaboration of lymphokines. One of these factors, macrophage chemotactic factor, attracts macrophages to the site of immunologically induced inflammation where they are activated by macrophage-activating factor which is either identical or similar to macrophage migration inhibitory factor (MIF). Properties of the activated macrophages include an increase in their size and number of lysosomes, greater phagocytic ability, and enhanced killing of bacteria or tumor cells. The biological property of MIF is most likely to reduce the random migration of macrophages, thereby keeping them at the site of inflammation. Mitogenic factors amplify the response by increasing the number of acti-

vated lymphocytes. The sensitized T cells kill antigen-specific target cells, such as tumor cells, either by direct cell-to-cell contact or by the elaboration of lymphotoxin. Bacteria or tumor cells are also killed by macrophages, and polymorphonuclear leukocytes are then attracted to the site of inflammation.

For the clinical assessment of cell-mediated immunity, skin tests continue to be useful. The diagnosis of several infectious diseases is aided by the finding of a positive skin test which indicates prior exposure and T-cell sensitization to the particular organisms but not necessarily active disease. Since at least 80 percent of the population have been sensitized to *Candida*, *Trichophyton*, or streptokinase-streptodornase, these antigens are suitable for determining the general status of cell-mediated immunity. The absence of a response to a battery of antigens that previously elicited a cell-mediated immune response is termed *anergy* and may signify an underlying disorder such as lymphoma or sarcoidosis. Several drugs, diseases, and other conditions may suppress skin tests of the delayed type. These include glucocorticosteroids, malignant diseases such as Hodgkin's disease or lymphoma, sarcoidosis, infections (measles, infectious mononucleosis, miliary tuberculosis), old age, malnutrition, acquired and congenital immunodeficiency disorders, and, in some instances, fever.

The ability of an individual to develop cell-mediated immunity de novo can be determined by applying directly to the skin a chemical such as dinitrochlorobenzene (DNCB) to which the individual has not been previously exposed. The chemical combines with skin proteins to form an immunogenic substance that stimulates the sensitization of T cells to DNCB. Ten to fourteen days following this initial exposure to DNCB, the reapplication of DNCB on the skin will result in a positive skin test if cell-mediated immunity is intact. In suspected anergic patients, a negative test with DNCB confirms a cutaneous anergic state.

Cell-mediated immunity can be assessed in vitro by stimulating lymphocytes with specific antigens, unrelated lymphocytes, or nonspecific substances such as the plant lectins, phytohemagglutinin or concanavalin A. The functional capacity of T cells is determined by culturing lymphocytes with phytohemagglutinin or concanavalin A. These lectins bind to the carbohydrate moieties of cell membrane receptors and stimulate transformation or blastogenesis of lymphocytes which is measured by the incorporation of radioactive precursors (tritiated thymidine) into DNA. These two lectins are primarily T-cell mitogens; however, they stimulate different subsets of T cells.

T cells previously sensitized to an antigen will also undergo blastogenesis when cultured with the specific antigen. The blastogenic response of T cells on exposure to antigen in vitro

TABLE 61-3
Products of activated lymphocytes

I Affecting macrophages
  A Migration inhibitory factor (MIF)
  B Macrophage-activating factor (identical to MIF?)
  C Chemotactic factor for macrophages
II Affecting lymphocytes
  A Mitogenic factor
  B Transfer factor
III Affecting polymorphonuclear leukocytes
  A Chemotactic factors for neutrophils, eosinophils, and basophils
  B Migration-inhibiting factor
IV Affecting other cell types
  A Cytotoxic factors (lymphotoxin)
  B Interferon
  C Growth inhibitory factors (inhibits proliferation of target cells)
  D Osteoclast activation factor

corresponds fairly well with the in vivo skin tests of delayed hypersensitivity. The response of T cells to specific antigens can also be determined by measuring the biologic activity of the various soluble mediators or lymphokines released from the activated T cells (e.g., quantitating the amount of inhibition of macrophage migration resulting from the release of MIF). The release of soluble mediators from T cells may occur without the cells undergoing blastogenesis.

The mixed lymphocyte culture (MLC) is an assay widely used in the field of transplantation for the typing of histocompatibility antigens (Chap. 69). The test is usually performed in unidirectional method by treating the stimulating lymphocyte population with either radiation or mitomycin C which prevents these cells from responding without affecting their stimulatory properties. When the lymphocytes from a normal individual are cultured with these treated lymphocytes, the individual's T cells will undergo blastic transformation if the antigens on the stimulatory cells are sufficiently different. The cell antigens recognized in the MLC reaction are the products of genes at the HLA-D locus. The absence of a response indicates the presence of identical antigens in the two cell populations. The MLC reaction can also be used to assess the functional capacity of T cells.

IMMUNE RESPONSE

Upon exposure to a foreign substance, an individual can respond by producing specific antibodies, by developing cell-mediated immunity (delayed hypersensitivity), or by becoming immunologically unresponsive. The substances that elicit an immune response are termed *immunogens,* and their ability to evoke this response is called *immunogenicity.* Antigens are substances that will react specifically with available antibodies or sensitized lymphocytes. Certain small molecules with molecular weights of less than 1000 daltons usually are not capable of inducing an immune response but can interact as antigens with available antibodies and are called *haptens.* However, an immune response can be elicited with haptens if they are coupled to a larger carrier molecule which is immunogenic in the host.

The route of administration, the dose of the immunogen, and the response of the host are all factors determining the immune response. For example, the oral administration of poliomyelitis virus leads to effective immunization by stimulating the production of IgA antibodies in the gastrointestinal tract. Skin contact with chemicals (e.g., resins of poison ivy) evokes primarily a cell-mediated or delayed hypersensitivity reaction involving the skin. The dose of immunogen also affects the immune response. Both very high doses and low doses of immunogen may produce tolerance. The failure to detect an immune response, therefore, is not conclusive, since a substance may be immunogenic at a different dose or by a different route of administration.

One of the most exciting areas in immunology is the role of genetic factors in the immune response. Evidence for a genetic influence on the immune response to a given immunogen is based on studies in inbred strains of mice and other laboratory animals. Genetic differences within a species are associated with an immune response to a given immunogen in one strain and with no response in another. These differences may also lead to a high level of antibody production in one strain and to low levels in another strain. In several species including humans, the ability of an individual to respond to a specific immunogen is under the control of immune response genes that are located in the chromosomal region referred to as *major histocompatibility gene complex.* Genes within this region code for molecules that are involved in the initiation, stimulation, and suppression of the immune response.

CELL COOPERATION Many immunogens require an interaction of B and T cells to generate a humoral immune response. These immunogens are referred to as being *thymus dependent.* Examples of some thymus-dependent antigens are glycoproteins, natural proteins, heterologous serum proteins, and erythrocytes. The interaction of T cells with B cells is termed *cooperation,* and the T cells that function in this context are called *helper T cells.* Other immunogens, referred to as being *thymus independent,* are able to initiate B-cell proliferation and antibody production without the help of T cells. The biochemical characteristics that differentiate thymus-independent from thymus-dependent immunogens have not been fully identified, but some differentiating features are the repeating linear polymeric structure of the thymus-independent immunogens and the slow degradation of these molecules in the host. Examples of thymus-independent immunogens include pneumococcal polysaccharides, polymerized *Salmonella* flagellin, dextran, and lipopolysaccharides.

T cells play a central role in the induction and regulation of the immune response. Various subsets of T cells function as helper cells, suppressor cells, or cytotoxic cells. In mice, these functions of T cells have been shown to be genetically programmed. The subsets of T cells are identified by surface antigens belonging to the Ly system of T-cell alloantigens. T cells expressing the surface phenotype Ly1$^+$ are helper cells and cooperate with B cells to induce antibody production. They also stimulate proliferation of T cells expressing the surface phenotype Ly2, 3$^+$ which function as cytotoxic effector cells in cell-mediated immunity. Other Ly2, 3$^+$ cells have suppressor activity. The third subset of T cells, Ly1, 2, 3$^+$, represents resting cells that have receptors for antigen but are not yet committed to either helper or suppressor activity. A set of these resting Ly1, 2, 3$^+$ cells can be activated by antigen-stimulated Ly1$^+$ helper cells to produce suppressor activity. These observations suggest that Ly1$^+$ helper cells, when activated by specific antigen, induce B cells to produce antibody and also stimulate Ly1, 2, 3$^+$ to exert suppression of helper T cell activity. The suppression of helper T cell activity, in turn, would lead to a reduction in antibody formation as well as suppressor cell activity. The interaction of these subsets of T cell provides a mechanism for self-regulation and homeostasis of the immune response. Similar systems of immunoregulation are undoubtedly present in humans. In them, a subpopulation of T cells that carry receptors for the Fc portion of IgM and that may represent helper T cells has been recognized. Another group has membrane receptors for the Fc portion of IgG and may represent suppressor T cells. The distinguishing features of helper and suppressor T cells are being investigated intensively, and the field is very much in flux. In a clinical context, hyperactivity of the suppressor T-cell system in patients with common variable hypogammaglobulinemia may induce low levels of immunoglobulins by suppressing B-cell proliferation and antibody production (Chap. 62). Hypergammaglobulinemia, on the other hand, may represent too much helper T cell activity owing to loss of suppressor T cell function.

Macrophages are also critical cells in the immune response and especially involve thymus-dependent antigens. An important function of the macrophage is the presentation of immunogenic material to B and T cells. In this setting, immunogens may interact directly with the surface of macrophages. Macromolecules or particulate substances, however, require digestion by macrophages to become immunogenic. A few immunogenic molecules of the digested material are retained on the surface of the macrophages. Macrophages also elaborate soluble biologic substances that stimulate both T and B cells.

MODELS OF ANTIBODY PRODUCTION Several models of antibody production involving T and B cell cooperation have emerged from studies in animals. In one such model, immunogenic material may be initially processed by macrophages or may directly bind with a specific antigen receptor on T cells. As mentioned above, the nature of the antigen receptor on T cells may be an IgM-like molecule. This T cell antigen receptor and the antigen dissociate as a complex from the T cell and bind to the macrophage, perhaps through the Fc receptor on the macrophage. As a result of this binding, the necessary density and frequency of antigenic determinants are created for the interaction with antigen receptors on B cells and subsequent stimulation of antibody production. The antigen-activated T cells may also elaborate nonspecific factors that stimulate antibody production.

Other models for antibody production take into greater consideration the genetic control of the immune response. The antigen receptor on T cells in one such model is referred to as the *T-cell recognition factor* and is coded for by an immune response gene. The T cell, through its recognition factor, can directly bind immunogen or can interact with immunogen presented on the surface of a macrophage. The recognition factor is associated with an interaction factor which is coded for by an I-region gene. I-region genes are located within the major histocompatibility complex and control immune responsiveness. The complex of antigen, recognition factor, and interaction factor dissociates from the T cell and binds to B cells carrying the specific immunoglobulin receptor for antigen and the complementary receptor site for interaction factor. The receptor site for interaction factor on these B cells is also coded for by the same I-region gene. Antigen-stimulated T cells may also react directly with the B cells carrying the complementary antigen receptor and site for interaction factor. The interactions between T cells, B cells, and macrophages may depend on the sharing of common histocompatibility antigens.

PRIMARY AND SECONDARY IMMUNE RESPONSES   On a first exposure to a new immunogen, several days are required before humoral and cell-mediated immunity are detected. This initial response to a new immunogen is termed the *primary* immune response. When the immunogen is thymus dependent, IgM and IgG classes of antibody are initially secreted by the B cells, and IgM appears first. As the titer of IgG rises during the second week following immunogenic stimulation, the IgM titer falls. The antibody titer reaches a peak in approximately two weeks and then falls gradually. However, low levels of antibody can be demonstrated for months and even years. The switch from IgM synthesis to predominantly IgG synthesis in B cells requires T-cell cooperation. The synthesis of IgA and IgE also is dependent on T-cell cooperation. In the absence of T-cell cooperation, the B cells stimulated by thymus-dependent antigens produce low levels of antibody belonging to the IgM classes. The thymus-independent immunogens such as pneumococcal polysaccharides and *Salmonella* O stimulate the production of antibodies belonging to the IgM class even after repeated injections.

Following a second exposure to the same immunogen, heightened cell-mediated or humoral responses are observed. This is termed a *secondary* or *anamnestic* response. These responses occur sooner than the primary response, usually in 4 to 5 days in humans, and depend on a marked proliferation of antibody-producing cells or effector T cells of cell-mediated immunity. The antibody produced is of the IgG class and has a greater affinity for antigen than the antibody synthesized initially during the primary immune response. The secondary response depends on immunologic memory that must be demonstrated by both T and B cells.

TOLERANCE   A state of specific immunologic unresponsiveness to substances that would normally evoke an immune response is termed *tolerance*. It is an active physiologic process and not merely the lack of an immune response. Humoral immunity, cell-mediated immunity, or both may be suppressed. Tolerance provides the essential mechanism for the prevention of immunologically induced self-injury. The impairment of self-tolerance is presently considered the basic pathogenic mechanism in autoimmune diseases.

Tolerance can be induced in several ways. The physical form and dose of an antigen are important factors determining whether tolerance or an immune response develops. In experimental models, the administration of soluble antigen in monomeric form produces tolerance, while the same antigen in aggregated or polymeric form leads to an immune response. High doses of antigen lead to tolerance of both B and T cells. In comparison with B cells, tolerance in T cells is induced with lower doses of antigen and persists longer. Tolerance is more readily achieved in the neonate than in the adult. The maintenance of tolerance requires repeated or chronic exposure to the tolerogenic antigen. Tolerance may also be induced and maintained by the stimulation of suppressor T-cell activity which can suppress both humoral and cell-mediated immunity.

Immunologic unresponsiveness also can be caused by antibody. Antibody binding to antigen may produce conformational changes in the antigen, preventing its interaction with lymphocytes. Antibody in the form of an immune complex can also suppress the immune response by interacting with suppressor T cells enhancing suppressor activity.

AUTOIMMUNITY   The development of immunologic responsiveness to self is called *autoimmunity* and reflects the impairment of self-tolerance. Immunologic, environmental, and genetic factors are closely interrelated in the pathogenesis of autoimmunity. Clinical disorders in which autoimmune responses play a role in the pathogenesis of the illness are referred to as *autoimmune diseases*. Autoantibodies, however, are found in some normal persons without evidence of autoimmune disease. The frequency of autoantibodies in the general population increases with age, suggesting a breakdown of self-tolerance with aging. Autoantibodies also may develop as an aftermath of tissue damage. The spectrum of autoimmune disorders ranges from thyroiditis, which is organ specific, to systemic lupus erythematosus, which is characterized by an array of autoantibodies to cell and tissue antigens.

The development of autoimmunity usually involves the breakdown or circumvention of self-tolerance. The potential for the development of autoantibodies probably exists in most individuals. For example, normal human B cells are capable of reacting with several self-antigens (e.g., thyroglobulin) but are suppressed from producing autoantibodies by one or more mechanisms of tolerance. Precommitted B cells in tolerant individuals can be stimulated in several ways. Tolerance involving only T cells, induced by persistent low levels of circulating self-antigens, may be circumvented by substances such as endotoxin. Such substances would stimulate the B cells directly to produce autoantibodies, thus obviating the need for helper T cells. A decrease in suppressor T cell activity could also lead to production of autoantibodies (see below).

Autoimmunity may develop to antigens that were sequestered or anatomically separated from the immune system during embryonic development. For example, in the absence of low levels of circulating antigen, both B and T cells are immunocompetent. In later life, exposure to such antigens through trauma or infection results in autoimmune responses (e.g., release of myelin in experimental allergic encephalomyelitis).

Viruses also play an important role in the pathogenesis of autoimmunity. Several animal models of autoimmunity such as F_1 hybrids of the New Zealand black (NZB) and white (NZW) mice have persistent viral infections from birth (Chap. 68). It is difficult to determine whether the viral infection interferes with the immune system or if preexisting abnormal immunity permits chronic viral infection. In any event, these animals develop circulating immune complexes, composed of antibodies to nuclear antigens and to viral antigens, which deposit in the glomerular basement membrane and other tissue sites, leading to the manifestations of immune complex disease. The expression of viral antigens on the surfaces of the host's cells may elicit autoantibodies to cell membrane antigens. Furthermore, autoantibodies may develop from exposure to exogenous viral antigens that cross-react with autoantigens. Bacteria or other foreign substances may also act as cross-reacting antigens.

It has been proposed that autoimmunity is a disorder of abnormal immunologic regulation resulting in excessive B-cell activity and diminished T-cell activity. A decrease in suppressor T-cell activity or an increase in helper T-cell activity would result in uncontrolled excessive production of autoantibodies. The strongest support for this concept of autoimmunity comes from studies in animal models and human autoimmune disorders in which the loss of suppressor T-cell function and excessive B-cell antibody production can be demonstrated.

A role for genetic factors in the pathogenesis of autoimmunity has been clearly demonstrated in animal models and clinical autoimmune disorders. New Zealand black mice manifest autoimmune hemolytic anemia, whereas the NZB/NZW F_1 hybrids develop a disease analogous to systemic lupus erythematosus (SLE). The relatives of patients with SLE may have clinical and serologic abnormalities of SLE: a high concordance of SLE is also found in monozygotic twins. Associations with histocompatibility antigens are noted in several clinical autoimmune disorders. Chronic active hepatitis, Graves' disease, and Addison's disease occur more often in individuals who are HLA-B8 positive. An association with genes located at the HLA-D locus has been noted in adult rheumatoid arthritis, Sjögren's syndrome, and multiple sclerosis. These associations may be significant because of the close relationship between genes determining histocompatibility antigens and genes controlling the type and magnitude of the immune response.

COMPLEMENT SYSTEM The complement system consists of a group of at least 15 plasma proteins which interact sequentially, producing substances that mediate several functions of inflammation (see Table 61-4). The activated complement components and the enzymatically cleaved fragments of components exert many of their biologic activities by interaction with cell membranes. The actions of complement system include cell lysis, release of histamine from mast cells and platelets, vascular permeability, contraction of smooth muscle, chemotaxis of leukocytes, and neutralization of certain viruses. The complement system also is interrelated with the coagulation, fibrinolytic, and kinin systems. Complement is involved in the pathogenesis of tissue injury observed in many immuno-

logically mediated diseases which include SLE, rheumatoid arthritis, glomerulonephritis, and immunohemolytic anemia.

The activation of complement is initiated either by the classic pathway or by the alternative (properdin) pathway (Fig. 61-4). Both pathways lead to activation of a common terminal sequence of complement components. The complement components of the classic pathway are C1, C4, and C2. C1 is composed of three subunits, C1q, C1r, and C1s, which are held together by calcium. The classic pathway is activated by immune complexes containing IgG or IgM, and by aggregates of IgG (IgG1, IgG3, and IgG2), which bind to C1q by their Fc fragments. The binding of C1q activates C1r, which in turn activates C1s, resulting in formation of an esterase. The esterase cleaves C4 into a small fragment, C4a, and a large fragment, C4b, which binds to the immune complex or cell membrane. Activated C1s and C4b act together to split C2 into a small fragment, C2a, which has kinin-like properties and a larger fragment. The larger fragment of C2 combines with C4b to form C3 convertase, a magnesium-dependent enzyme that acts on C3.

The alternative (properdin) complement pathway produces activation of C3 by a series of reactions that bypass C1, C4, and C2. The components of the alternative complement system include factor D, which is an esterase similar to C1s, factor B, properdin, and C3. This pathway is activated by endotoxin, other polysaccharides, aggregated IgA, immune complexes, or nephritic factors. The latter are most likely IgG immunoglobulins which function by binding to the alternative pathway C3 convertase and may be autoantibodies to this enzyme complex. Nephritic factors are present in the serum of some patients with membranoproliferative glomerulonephritis or with partial lipodystrophy. The C3 convertase of the alternative pathway is formed by the interaction of factor D or nephritic factors, factor B and C3, and requires divalent Mg^{2+} ions. The C3 convertase is stabilized by properdin. Cleavage of C3 by either pathway results in a small peptide, C3a, and a large molecule, C3b. The latter interacts with components of the alternative complement pathway, resulting in C3 activation with formation of C3b which leads to more activation of C3, and amplification of complement activity. Regulators of this pathway are C3b inactivator and its cofactor, $\beta 1H$.

The two complement pathways converge at C3. Activation of the terminal complement components (C5 to C9) is initiated by C5 convertase, which consists of C3b in association with C3 convertase from either pathway. The C5 convertase cleaves a small fragment C5a from C5, and the remaining larger fragment C5b along with C6 to C9 self-assemble on the cell membrane. The insertion of these components into the membrane results in hydrophobic characteristics and reorientation of the lipid bilayer leading to membrane injury and disruption of the cell.

The regulation of the complement system is through the rapid decay of C2 to C5 once they have been activated. There is also decay of C3 convertase of both the classic and alternative pathways. C1 inhibitor (C1 INH) inhibits activated C1r and C1s by combining with these enzymes. The inactivation of C3b by C3b inactivator and its cofactor $\beta 1H$ is important in preventing the continued formation of C3b which interacts with components of the alternative pathway to produce a functional C3 convertase and thus more cleavage of C3 to C3b.

The peptides C3a and C5a are referred to as *anaphylatoxins*. C5a and the trimolecular complex of C5 to C7 are chemotactic for neutrophils, eosinophils, and monocytes. The presence of C3b on the cell membranes enhances phagocytosis by interaction with phagocytic cells possessing receptors for C3b. The interaction of C5b with neutrophils causes these cells to become adherent and to release lysosomal enzymes. Neutralization of certain viruses, such as herpes simplex, occurs by coating the virus with C1, C4, and C2. A peptide generated from

TABLE 61-4
Biological functions of complement

Biological function	Complement components
Chemotaxis	C3a, C5a, $\overline{C5}$, $\overline{C6}$, $\overline{C7}$
Histamine release (anaphylatoxin)	C3a, C5a
Opsonization	C3b
Cytolytic	C5 to C9
Kinin-like activity	C2 fragment
Viral neutralization	C1, C4

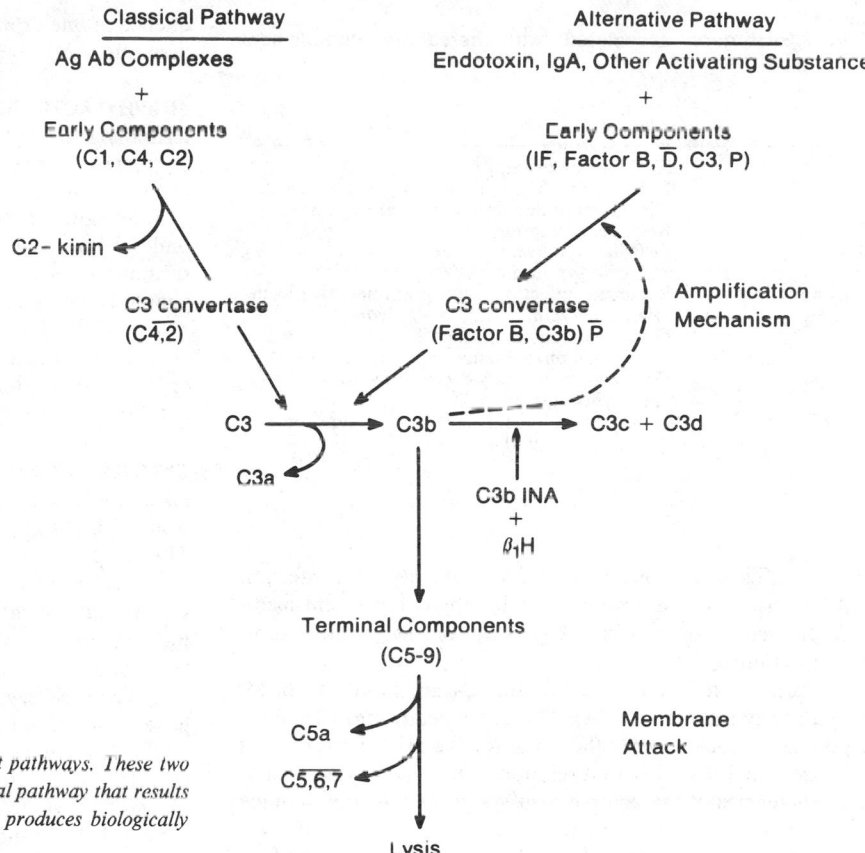

Classical Pathway

Ag Ab Complexes
+
Early Components
(C1, C4, C2)

Alternative Pathway

Endotoxin, IgA, Other Activating Substances
+
Early Components
(IF, Factor B, $\overline{D}$, C3, P)

C2– kinin

C3 convertase
($C\overline{4,2}$)

C3 convertase
(Factor $\overline{B}$, C3b) $\overline{P}$

Amplification
Mechanism

C3 ⟶ C3b ⟶ C3c + C3d

C3a

C3b INA
+
β_1H

Terminal Components
(C5-9)

C5a

Membrane
Attack

C5,6,7

Lysis

FIGURE 61-4

Diagram of the classic and alternative complement pathways. These two pathways converge at C3 to form a common terminal pathway that results in cell lysis. Cleavage of complement components produces biologically active fragments. (See text for details.)

activated C2 has been shown to have kinin-like properties and is probably responsible for the swelling observed in hereditary angioedema.

The complement system interacts with the coagulation, fibrinolytic, and kinin-generating systems. The activation of Hageman factor (factor XII) not only leads to clotting but also to the formation of plasmin, a fibrinolysin. Plasmin also activates C1 and cleaves C3 to produce C3a (anaphylatoxin). Plasmin also cleaves Hageman factor to produce Hageman factor fragments which convert prekallikrein to kallikrein. Kallikrein cleaves kininogen to bradykinin. Lysosomal enzymes can activate C1 and cleave C5 to form C5a.

Measurement of complement may be useful in diagnosis, assessment of disease activity, and evaluation of treatment. The serum level of complement depends on the balance of synthesis, catabolism, and consumption of the various complement components. Evidence for complement activation may be reflected in a low hemolytic complement level, decreased levels of individual components, or the finding of cleavage fragments of complement components. Low complement levels, however, may be the result of decreased synthesis or an inherited deficiency of a complement component. Normal or elevated complement levels do not exclude the participation of complement since synthesis of complement may equal or exceed consumption. Serum complement levels do not necessarily reflect intense local consumption of complement as might occur in synovial and pleural fluid. Further evidence of complement activation in disease can be adduced by the demonstration of complement components in lesions by immunofluorescence microscopy.

Complement is measured by its hemolytic activity expressed in CH_{50} units. Normal hemolytic activity depends on optimum concentrations of all the major components, C1 through C9. If any one component is markedly reduced or absent, little or no hemolytic activity is measured. The C3 and C4 components are readily measured immunochemically. In most instances, the measurements of C3 and C4 and hemolytic complement activity provide sufficient clinical information. Measurements of C1q and factor B may also be useful. For example, low levels of C1q, C4, C3, and CH_{50} indicate activation of complement primarily through the classic pathway. Immune complex disease such as systemic lupus erythematosus may show this complement profile. Reduced C3, CH_{50}, and factor B with a normal C4 reflect activation of complement by the alternative complement pathway, and may be seen in patients with membranoproliferative glomerulonephritis and in patients with bacterial endotoxin shock. The absence of CH_{50} may signify a hereditary deficiency of a complement component.

HEREDITARY DEFICIENCIES OF COMPLEMENT The most common hereditary deficiency of complement is C2 deficiency which is inherited as an autosomal recessive trait (Table 61-5). Homozygous C2 deficiency has been recognized in normal individuals and in patients with SLE and other syndromes with a comparable clinical picture. Heterozygous C2 deficiency may also be associated with rheumatic disorders. Inherited as well as acquired deficiencies of the early components (C1, C4, C2) appear to be more common in diseases resembling SLE. Lupus-like illness has also been noted in persons with hereditary angioedema who lack C1 inhibitor. Serum levels of C4 and C2 are often low in these individuals. Systemic lupus erythematosus has been observed in patients with the homozygous deficiency of C5 or C8. Severe recurrent bacterial infections occur in patients with homozygous C3 deficiency and in those patients with low levels of C3 secondary to the absence of C3b inactivator. In addition, acquired or hereditary deficiencies of early complement components may predispose individuals to infection because of inefficient activation of C3. The homozygous deficiency of a terminal complement component (C5 to C8) has been noted in patients with disseminated *Neisseria*

TABLE 61-5
Clinical disorders associated with hereditary complement deficiencies

Complement component	Clinical disorders
Clr, Cls	SLE-like syndrome
C2	SLE-like syndrome, dermatomyositis, vasculitis, glomerulonephritis, normal persons
C3	Recurrent infections
C4	SLE-like syndrome
C5	SLE-like syndrome
C5 dysfunction	Recurrent infections with gram-negative bacteria and eczema (Leiner's syndrome)
C6	Gonococcal, meningococcal infections
C7	Raynaud's phenomenon, normal persons
C8	Gonococcal, meningococcal infections, SLE-like syndrome
C1 inhibitor	Hereditary angioedema, SLE-like syndrome
C3b inactivator	Recurrent infections

NOTE: *SLE, systemic lupus erythematosus.*

infections. These persons may be more susceptible to infection with bacteria which are normally killed by complement-mediated cell lysis, a function which depends on the terminal complement components.

Hereditary deficiencies of C2 and C4 are linked to histocompatibility antigens (HLA). The genes determining immune responses are located near the genes for the HLA system. This has raised the possibility that relationships exist between inherited deficiencies of the complement system, HLA, the immune response, and the development of SLE or lupus-like illnesses. In view of the current hypothesis of a viral etiology for SLE, it has been suggested that the inherited deficiencies of early complement components predispose these individuals to viral infections. The development of lupus-related illnesses in patients with acquired deficiencies of early complement components also supports this notion and makes the possibility less likely that a direct causative relationship exists between HLA and SLE. Another explanation is that inherited deficiency of C2 or C4 is more closely associated with a particular type of immune response that predisposes these individuals to autoimmune disease. Further work is needed to elucidate the meaning of the associations between complement synthesis and SLE or lupus-like illnesses.

Hereditary angioedema is characterized by acute episodes of circumscribed edema involving skin, gastrointestinal tract, and upper respiratory tract and an imminent danger of life-threatening laryngeal edema. The basic abnormality is the absence of C1 inhibitor. The disorder has an autosomal dominant pattern of inheritance, and the affected heterozygote has low levels of C1 inhibitor. In approximately 10 to 15 percent of these individuals, normal amounts of C1 inhibitor can be measured immunochemically, but the protein does not possess C1 inhibitor activity (Chap. 65).

IMMUNE MECHANISMS OF TISSUE INJURY

The immune system protects the individual from the attacks of microorganisms by preventing their entry or facilitating their removal. The same immunologic mechanisms that protect the individual, however, may cause damage to normal tissue, especially if the immune response is excessive or prolonged. Moreover, damage to normal cells and tissue occurs in autoimmune disorders because immune responses are directed against autoantigens. The mechanisms of immune injury have been divided into four types: anaphylactic (type I), cytotoxic (type II), immune-complex-mediated (type III), and cell-mediated reactions (type IV). An additional mechanism interferes with the function of biologically active substances and is referred to as type V. Clinical manifestations of disease may be the conse-

quence of one or any combination of these five mechanisms of tissue injury.

ANAPHYLACTIC REACTION (TYPE I) This reaction is characterized by the release of pharmacologically active substances from mast cells or basophils as a result of the binding of antigen to IgE antibody attached to the surface of these cells. Histamine, slow-reacting substances of anaphylaxis, and eosinophil chemotactic factor of anaphylaxis are the major substances released from the mast cells in this reaction. The anaphylactic reaction is also referred to as *immediate hypersensitivity*. Clinical features of the anaphylactic reaction include generalized anaphylaxis, urticaria, angioedema, and atopic disorders (allergic rhinitis or hay fever, bronchial asthma, atopic dermatitis) (Chap. 65).

CYTOTOXIC REACTIONS (TYPE II) In the cytotoxic mechanism of injury, antibodies belonging to either IgG or IgM class react with antigenic determinants on cell membranes or tissue. The antigens may be intrinsic or result from the firm binding of free antigens to cell membranes or tissues. The ensuing tissue damage from antigen-antibody reactions occurs through the activation of the complement system when the antibody belongs to the IgM class. Receptors for IgM are not present on phagocytic cells, and complement activation is necessary for generation of inflammation. Antigen-antibody reactions involving IgG antibodies, however, can lead to tissue damage with or without the activation of complement. Since macrophages and neutrophils have receptors for IgG, these phagocytic cells will bind to the IgG antibodies that are attached to cell membranes or tissue. Examples of type II reactions include immune hemolytic anemia, transfusion reactions, erythroblastosis fetalis, immune thrombocytopenia, and Goodpasture's syndrome. In immune hemolytic anemia of the warm antibody type, IgG antibody coated red blood cells become bound to macrophages mainly in the spleen and in other reticuloendothelial tissues. A portion of the red blood cell membrane is removed by the macrophage. The red blood cell with its decreased membrane returns to the circulation as a spherocyte which has both increased mechanical and osmotic fragility. Penicillin-induced hemolytic anemia is an example of a cytotoxic reaction in which free antigen (penicillin) becomes firmly bound to the red blood cell membrane. If patients on high doses of penicillin form anti-penicillin antibodies of the IgG class, these antibodies will react with the penicillin antigens bound to the red blood cell membrane and lead to increased red blood cell destruction by the process of erythrophagocytosis. In Goodpasture's syndrome, antibodies develop that are specific for antigens intrinsic to the glomerular basement membrane and for antigens in the walls of pulmonary blood vessels. The inflammation generated by these antigen-antibody reactions leads to glomerulonephritis and pulmonary vasculitis, and these patients often present with hemoptysis as their initial complaint.

ANTIGEN-ANTIBODY COMPLEX-MEDIATED REACTIONS (TYPE III) The deposition of circulating antigen-antibody complexes in tissue leads to inflammation (Chap. 66). An understanding of immune complex disease has come largely from studies of experimental serum sickness. Many human diseases in which immune complexes play a pathogenetic role are now recognized. Circulating immune complexes have been identified in SLE, subacute bacterial endocarditis, and malignancies, to name only a few. Immune complex disease may develop locally at a tissue site such as in the rheumatoid joint or in the lung in patients with hypersensitivity pneumonitis. The systemic form of immune complex disorders such as SLE is characterized by deposition of circulating immune complexes in various sites such as the glomerular basement membrane, pleura, pericardium, synovium, and in cutaneous blood vessels. The process by which immune complexes generate inflammation involves the following steps: (1) antigen-antibody complexes deposit at tissue sites, (2) complement activation provides chemotactic factors and vasoactive peptides which dilate blood vessels and attract neutrophils, and (3) interaction of phagocytic cells with immune complexes leads to release of lysosomal enzymes which damage surrounding tissue.

CELL-MEDIATED REACTIONS (TYPE IV) This form of immune injury, also referred to as *delayed type of hypersensitivity,* centers on the role of the cytotoxic effector T cell (see "Cell-mediated Immunity" above). Sensitized T cells activated by antigen become cytotoxic cells capable of killing bacteria, tumor cells, or other target cells. They also release lymphokines, which stimulate macrophages, neutrophils, and other lymphocytes. The T cell is also capable of inducing cytotoxicity. Macrophages attracted to the site of immunologically mediated inflammation by T cells also cause tissue damage. Cell-mediated reactions play a significant role in the development of immunity and/or formation of lesions in tuberculosis, mycotic infections, and certain viral infections such as mumps, hepatitis, vaccinia, and herpes. Cell-mediated reactions are also involved in the pathogenesis of rheumatoid synovitis, Hashimoto's thyroiditis, and contact dermatitis resulting from exposure to oily resins of plants (e.g., poison oak) or to a variety of simple chemicals in the home or work environment. Renal allograft rejection and the graft versus host reaction observed in bone marrow transplantation are also in part a consequence of cell-mediated reactions (Chap. 69).

Another form of cell-mediated tissue injury is antibody-dependent cell-mediated cytotoxicity (ADCC). First, antibodies of the IgG class react with antigens on target cells such as tumor cells. Effector lymphocytes or macrophages through their receptors for the Fc portion of IgG then bind to IgG antibodies on the target cells without involving immunologic specificity. This interaction of lymphocytes or macrophages with target cells results in the killing of target cells. Only small amounts of antibody are required to initiate this form of immune injury. The type of lymphocyte participating in ADCC is not clear. While these cells have receptors for the Fc fragment of IgG, other markers that would distinguish them as B or T cells are absent. As noted in the description of T cells (above), these lymphocytes are referred to as *K* or *killer cells* and may be the same as the null cell which lacks T- and B-cell markers.

INTERFERENCE WITH FUNCTION OF BIOLOGICALLY ACTIVE SUBSTANCES (TYPE V) The interaction of antibodies with biologically active substances can interfere with their function. Antibodies to clotting factors, in particular factor VIII, may lead to serious bleeding abnormalities. Antibodies to intrinsic factors in patients with pernicious anemia may interfere with the absorption of vitamin B_{12}. In patients with myasthenia gravis, antibodies to acetylcholine neural receptors may be responsible for the block of neural transmission. In most diabetic patients receiving foreign insulin, antibodies to insulin develop. Anti-insulin antibodies are responsible for the insulin resistance observed in some patients. In other patients, antibodies to cell membrane receptors for insulin produce severe insulin resistance. These examples illustrate the potential clinical importance of recognizing this form of immune reaction.

REFERENCES

BELLANTI JA (ed): *Immunology II.* Philadelphia, Saunders, 1978

FUDENBERG HH et al (eds): *Basic & Clinical Immunology.* Los Altos, Lange, 1978

ROITT IM: *Essential Immunology.* Philadelphia, Lippincott, 1977

SAMTER M (ed): *Immunological Diseases.* Boston, Little, Brown, 1979

TALAL N (ed): *Autoimmunity. Genetic, Immunologic, Virologic and Clinical Aspects.* New York, Academic, 1977

Diseases of under- and overproduction of immune globulins

62
IMMUNE DEFICIENCY DISEASES

ALEXANDER R. LAWTON III
MAX D. COOPER

INTRODUCTION Immunologic functions are mediated by two developmentally divergent, but functionally interacting, families of lymphocytes. The activities of B and T lymphocytes, and their products, in host defense are closely integrated with the functions of other cells of the reticuloendothelial system. Fixed and wandering macrophages play an important role in the trapping and processing of antigens and become effector cells, especially when activated by products of T lymphocytes. The scavenger activity of polymorphonuclear leukocytes is directed and made specific by antibodies in concert with products of the complement system (Chap. 61). The interaction of basophils and tissue mast cells with IgE antibodies in causation of immediate hypersensitivity is discussed in Chap. 65. Consideration of these interrelationships is an important part of the analysis of patients with suspected immune deficiency.

CLINICAL DISEASE FEATURES COMMON TO IMMUNE DEFICIENCY Immunodeficiency syndromes, whether congenital, spontaneously acquired, or iatrogenic, are characterized by unusual susceptibility to infection and, sometimes, to autoimmune disease and lymphoreticular malignancies. The types of infection often provide the first clue to the nature of the immunologic defect.

Patients with defects in humoral immunity have recurrent or chronic sinopulmonary infection, meningitis, and bacteremia, most commonly caused by pyogenic bacteria such as *He-*

mophilus influenzae, Streptococcus pneumoniae, and staphylococci. This spectrum of infections is similar to that occurring in patients with normal immune responses, but with either neutropenia or a deficiency of the pivotal third component of complement (C3), suggesting that a tripartite collaboration involving antibody, complement, and phagocytes exists as the chief mechanism of host defense against pyogenic organisms. Binding of antibody to the bacterial surface causes activation of the complement system. One cleavage product of activated C3 serves as a chemotactic factor for polymorphonuclear leukocytes. Activated C3b fixed to bacterial surfaces facilitates phagocytosis by interaction with C3b receptors on neutrophils.

Agammaglobulinemic patients in whom cell-mediated immunity is intact have an interesting response to viral infections. The clinical course of primary infection with viruses such as varicella zoster or rubeola, unless complicated by bacterial infection, does not differ significantly from that of the normal host. However, long-lasting immunity may not develop, and as a result multiple bouts of chickenpox and measles may occur. Such observations suggest that intact T cells may be sufficient for control of established viral infections, while antibodies are primarily important in limiting the initial dissemination of virus. Exceptions to this generalization are becoming more widely recognized. Agammaglobulinemic patients fail to clear hepatitis B virus from their circulation and have a progressive, and often fatal, course. Chronic encephalitis, which may progress over a period of months to years, is being observed with apparently increasing frequency. Echoviruses and adenoviruses have been isolated from brain biopsies or spinal fluid from some patients; in others no agent has been detected. Immunologic injury resulting from a partial and ineffective immune response may contribute as much to the pathogenesis of these diseases as the direct effects of the viruses.

The occurrence of unusual serious infection, for example, *H. influenzae* meningitis in an older child or adult, warrants consideration of humoral immune deficiency. Bacterial infections in certain sites may also suggest this possibility. Chronic otitis media occurs frequently in patients with hypogammaglobulinemia, and is significant because of its relative rarity in normal adults. Pansinusitis, although almost invariably present in immunoglobulin deficiency, is a less helpful finding because it is not rare in apparently normal people. Bacterial infections of the skin or urinary tract are less frequent problems in hypogammaglobulinemic patients.

Abnormalities of cell-mediated immunity predispose to *disseminated virus infections,* particularly with latent viruses such as herpes simplex (Chap. 193), varicella zoster (Chap. 185), and cytomegalovirus (Chap. 195). Patients so affected also almost invariably develop mucocutaneous candidiasis and frequently acquire widely disseminated fungal infections.

Pneumonia caused by the protozoan *Pneumocystis carinii* is also common (Chap. 204).

Infestation with the intestinal parasite *Giardia lamblia* is a frequent enough cause of diarrhea in antibody-deficient patients to warrant diagnostic duodenal aspiration and intestinal biopsy when the organism cannot be demonstrated in the stool.

T-cell deficiency is probably always accompanied by some abnormality of antibody responses, although this may not be reflected by hypogammaglobulinemia. This may explain in part why patients with primary T-cell defects are also subject to overwhelming bacterial infection.

The most severe form of immune deficiency occurs in individuals, usually infants, who lack both cell-mediated and humoral immune functions. They are susceptible to the whole range of infectious agents including organisms not ordinarily considered pathogenic. Multiple infections with viruses, bacteria, and fungi occur, often simultaneously. Because donor lymphocytes cannot be rejected by the recipients, blood transfusions can produce fatal graft-versus-host disease.

DIFFERENTIATION OF T AND B CELLS The functional deficits which occur in both congenital and acquired immunodeficiencies are most usefully viewed as defects at various points along the differentiation pathways of immunocompetent cells. For this reason certain features of the development and differentiation of T and B cells that are especially relevant to the analysis of immunodeficiency are briefly presented here; Chap. 61 provides a general account of their roles in cellular and humoral immunity.

A subpopulation of hematopoietic stem cells may become restricted to lymphoid differentiation prior to migration to the thymus, where T cells are generated, or to the fetal liver and adult bone marrow, where B-cell development occurs (Fig. 62-1). A major function of central lymphoid tissues is to generate the clonal diversity characteristic of the immune system. Each T or B lymphocyte is induced to express surface receptor molecules of a unique specificity for antigen. The receptors of B lymphocytes are immunoglobulins. The nature of T-cell receptors is not yet precisely defined, but they may be similar or identical to the variable regions of immunoglobulins. Generation of clonal diversity depends upon cellular proliferation, such that each of the different receptor specificities encoded in the genome comes to be expressed in individual cells. Thus a clone contains all cells that express the identical antigen-binding receptors. Estimates for the total number of B-cell clones usually vary between 1 and 100 million. This process of clonal development is independent of antigen and reflects a genetically programmed sequence of differentiation analogous to that of primary erythropoiesis or myelopoiesis. This phase, termed *primary differentiation,* begins early in human fetal development but probably continues into adult life.

The first recognizable step in development of B cells is the emergence of lymphoid cells which contain small amounts of intracytoplasmic IgM but lack the surface immunoglobulin receptors characteristic of mature B lymphocytes. These pre-B cells are found almost exclusively in the bone marrow of adults but are first generated in fetal liver. Pre-B cells proliferate rapidly and spawn immature B lymphocytes which express surface IgM receptors and divide rarely. Young B lymphocytes differ from their more mature counterparts in an important physiologic characteristic; they are highly susceptible to inactivation when their receptors bind antigen. This phenomenon almost certainly is an important mechanism in the development of tolerance to self-antigens.

The developmental sequence for expression of diverse immunoglobulin classes by human B lymphocytes begins with expression of IgM. The expression of IgD on IgM-bearing cells occurs later. Lymphocytes committed to synthesis of IgG, IgA, and IgE are all derived from IgM-bearing precursors through a genetic switch mechanism.

There is increasing evidence suggesting that the diversity of T-lymphocyte function is associated with developmentally divergent subpopulations of T cells. T lymphocytes which, as helpers or suppressors, regulate B-lymphocyte differentiation are distinguishable by the presence of cell surface receptors which bind IgM or IgG antibodies, respectively, and also on the basis of histochemical markers and fine-structural features. Membrane antigenic differences, recognized by antiserums prepared in animals or by antibodies occurring in certain autoimmune states, are also being used to identify subpopulations of T cells having different functions. This developmental heterogeneity may explain some immunodeficiencies in which T-cell functions are impaired selectively.

In addition to generating T cells, the thymus apparently secretes hormonal products which regulate cellular maturation

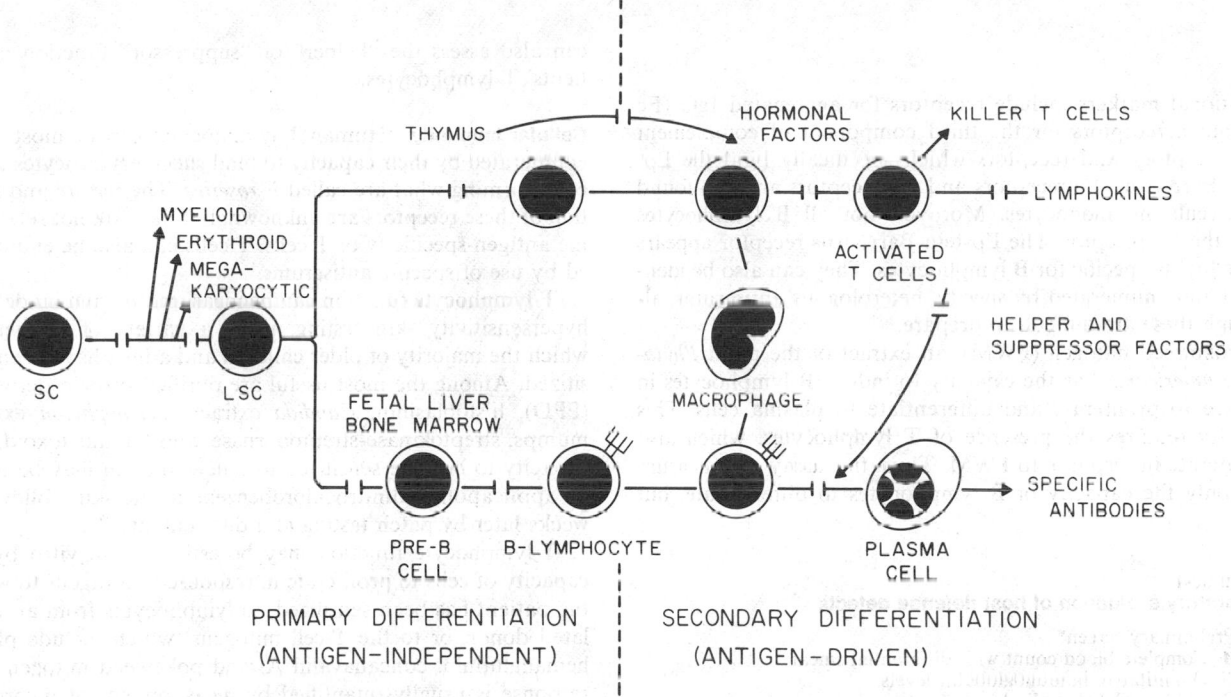

PRIMARY DIFFERENTIATION
(ANTIGEN-INDEPENDENT)

SECONDARY DIFFERENTIATION
(ANTIGEN-DRIVEN)

FIGURE 62-1

Failure to develop T and B cells may result from defective stem cells or from inborn metabolic errors affecting both cell types. Rarely, other hematopoietic cell lines are also absent. Absence of either T or B cells suggests malfunction of central lymphoid tissues, including the thymus and the fetal liver–bone marrow complex. B-cell deficiency may result from failure to generate pre-B cells from their stem-cell precursors or from failure of pre-B cells to give rise to their B-lymphocyte progeny. Agammaglobulinemia and deficiencies of some T-cell functions may occur despite the presence of normal numbers of B or T cells in the circulation. Failure of B lymphocytes to differentiate to plasma cells can be due to intrinsic cellular abnormalities or to faulty T-cell regulation.

in peripheral lymphoid tissues. These hormones have been called *thymosin* or *thymopoietin*, deficiencies of these factors have been implicated in some immunodeficiencies.

The events designated *secondary differentiation* (Fig. 62-1) follow stimulation of specific clones of lymphocytes by antigen. These processes are synonymous with the immune response (Chap. 61). Particularly important in consideration of immunodeficiencies are the collaborative interactions among macrophages, T cells, and B cells. B lymphocytes can proliferate in response to thymus-dependent antigens without the help of T cells, and may differentiate to IgM-secreting plasma cells when stimulated by thymus-independent antigens such as polysaccharides. However, production of normal quantities of antibodies, particularly those of the IgA and IgG classes, requires the collaboration of T cells.

Differentiation of T or B cells may be arrested at either the primary or secondary stage (Fig. 62-1). Reflecting the complex cellular interactions involved in immune responses and the pivotal role played by T lymphocytes, immune deficiencies primarily involving T cells are usually also associated with abnormal B-cell function. Conversely, immunodeficiencies manifested primarily by inability to produce antibodies may be caused by T-cell defects not associated with abnormal cell-mediated immunity.

EVALUATION OF IMMUNODEFICIENT PATIENTS Many of the laboratory assays used for precise evaluation of immunologic functions in humans are available only in specialized centers; nevertheless, most immunodeficiencies may be diagnosed by thoughtful use of tests available in most clinical laboratories. Table 62-1 presents a résumé of laboratory investigations roughly in order of increasing complexity.

A careful history will usually indicate whether the major problem involves the antibody-complement-phagocyte system or cell-mediated immunity. A history of a normal response to smallpox vaccination or of contact dermatitis due to poison ivy suggests intact cellular immunity. Lymphopenia and the absence of palpable lymph nodes may be important findings. However, patients with profound immunodeficiency may have diffuse lymphoid hyperplasia.

Humoral immunity With rare exceptions, deficiency of humoral immunity is accompanied by diminished serum concentration of one or more classes of immunoglobulin. Normal values vary with age, and adult concentrations of IgM (100 mg per 100 ml) are reached at about 1 year, of IgG (1000 mg per 100 ml) at 5 to 6 years, and of IgA (200 mg per 100 ml) at puberty (Chap. 61). Also, the wide range of values among normal adults creates difficulty in defining the lower limits of normal. Reasonable estimates for low normal values are 40 mg per 100 ml for IgM, 500 mg per 100 ml for IgG, and 50 mg per 100 ml for IgA. In the presence of borderline hypogammaglobulinemia, assessing the patient's capacity to produce specific antibodies becomes particularly important. Most hospital laboratories can measure isohemagglutinins, antistreptolysin O, and "febrile agglutinins." Typhoid H and O agglutinins can be measured before and after immunization with standard typhoid vaccine. Many state public health laboratories can perform titrations for antibodies to common viral agents.

Since antibody deficiency may be mimicked clinically by deficiency of complement components, measurement of total hemolytic complement (CH_{50}) should be a part of the evaluation of host defense. Measurement of C3 ($\beta 1C$) alone is inadequate for screening, since deficiencies of both early and late complement components may predispose to bacterial infection (Chap. 61). Estimation of numbers of circulating B lymphocytes has been of great value in determining the pathogenesis of certain types of immune deficiency. B lymphocytes are identified by the presence of membrane-bound immunoglobulins;

additional markers include receptors for aggregated IgG (Fc receptor), receptors for the third component of complement (C3 receptor), and receptors which specifically bind the Epstein-Barr virus. Fc receptors and C3 receptors are also found on circulating monocytes. Morover, not all B lymphocytes bear the C3 receptor. The Epstein-Barr virus receptor appears to be highly specific for B lymphocytes. They can also be identified and enumerated by specific heterologous antiserums, although these are difficult to prepare.

Pokeweed mitogen (PWM), an extract of the plant *Phytolacca americana,* has the capacity to induce B lymphocytes in culture to proliferate and differentiate to plasma cells. This activity requires the presence of T lymphocytes, which also proliferate in response to PWM. Thus, this assay can measure not only the capacity of B lymphocytes to differentiate, but

TABLE 62-1
Laboratory evaluation of host defense defects

I Preliminary screen*
  A Complete blood count with differential smear
  B Quantitative immunoglobulin levels
II Readily available studies†
  A B-cell function
    1 Natural or commonly acquired antibodies: isohemagglutinins, "febrile" agglutinins, antibodies to common viruses (rubella, rubeola, influenza), and toxins (diphtheria, tetanus)
    2 Response to immunization (typhoid, polio, diphtheria-tetanus vaccines)
  B T-cell function
    1 Skin tests (PPD, mumps, *Candida, Trichophyton,* histoplasmin), streptokinase-streptodornase (Varidase, 1:200), tetanus toxoid
    2 Contact sensitization with dinitrochlorobenzene
    3 Chest x-ray (thymus shadow in infants, thymoma in adults)
  C Complement
    1 C3 (β1C globulin)
    2 CH_{50} (total hemolytic complement)
  D Phagocyte function
    1 Reduction of nitroblue tetrazolium
    2 Inflammatory skin window (Rebuck)
III In-depth investigation
  A B cell
    1 Pre-B cell examination in bone marrow samples
    2 B-lymphocyte membrane markers: IgM, IgD, IgG, IgA; receptors for aggregated IgG (Fc receptor), C3, Epstein-Barr virus; antigens detected by anti-B antiserum
    3 Induction of B-lymphocyte differentiation in vitro stimulated by pokeweed mitogen
    4 Kinetics and immunoglobulin class of antibody produced in response to specific primary and secondary immunization
    5 Measurement of IgG subclasses and κ/λ ratio
    6 Histologic and immunofluorescent examination of biopsy specimens (intestinal mucosa, lymph node, bone marrow)
  B T cell
    1 Surface markers: binding of sheep erythrocytes (E rosettes), anti-T antiserum, T cells bearing receptors for IgM (T_M) and IgG (T_G)
    2 In vitro correlates of delayed hypersensitivity
      a Proliferative response to mitogens: phytohemagglutinin, concanavalin A specific antigens (PPD, *Candida*); allogeneic cells (one-way mixed lymphocyte response)
      b Quantification of lymphokines (migration inhibitory factor, etc.)
      c Induction of killer cells by stimulation with allogeneic lymphocytes
    3 Measurement of thymus hormones
    4 Assays for T-cell "helper" function using supernatants of antigen-activated T cells or T cells plus PWM or antigens to trigger B-lymphocyte differentiation
    5 Skin graft rejection
  C Phagocytes and complement
    1 Chemotactic response in vitro
    2 Bactericidal function
    3 Classic and alternative complement components
  D Miscellaneous: lymphocytotoxic antibodies to T or B cells

* *Together with a history and physical examination, these tests will identify more than 95 percent of patients with primary immunodeficiencies.*
† *These assays are generally available in either hospitals or state public health laboratories. With rare exceptions, information gained from tests in categories I and II is sufficient to diagnose and treat those immunodeficiencies amenable to conventional treatment with gamma globulin or plasma.*

can also assess the "helper" or "suppressor" function of patients' T lymphocytes.

Cellular immunity Human T lymphocytes can be most easily enumerated by their capacity to bind sheep erythrocytes in the cold, forming what are called *E rosettes.* The nature and function of these receptors are unknown, but they are not related to the antigen-specificity of T cells. T cells can also be enumerated by use of specific antiserums.

T-lymphocyte function can be measured in vivo by delayed hypersensitivity skin testing, using a variety of antigens to which the majority of older children and adults have been sensitized. Among the most useful are purified protein derivative (PPD), histoplasmin, *Candida* extract, *Trichophyton* extract, mumps, streptokinase-streptodornase, and tetanus toxoid. The capacity to become sensitized to a new antigen may be tested by application of dinitrochlorobenzene to the skin, followed 2 weeks later by patch testing at a different site.

T-lymphocyte function may be estimated in vitro by the capacity of cells to proliferate in response to antigens to which the patient has been sensitized, to lymphocytes from an unrelated donor, or to the T-cell mitogens, which include phytohemagglutinin, concanavalin A, and pokeweed mitogen. The response is usually quantified by measurement of incorporation of radioactive thymidine into newly synthesized DNA. It is also possible to measure the production of lymphokines, particularly migration inhibition factor, by activated T cells. Finally, the ability of T cells activated in mixed lymphocyte culture to lyse target cells sensitized by phytohemagglutinin can be measured.

The capacity of T lymphocytes from immunologically normal persons to be activated in vitro with antigens or mitogens may be abolished or markedly diminished by acute febrile illness, treatment with corticosteroids, or stress. Except for these situations, there are relatively few instances in which normal numbers of T lymphocytes, as measured by the E rosette test, are not associated with relatively normal function in the aforementioned in vitro assays.

CLASSIFICATION Primary immunodeficiencies may be either congenital or acquired, and are currently classified according to mode of inheritance and whether the defect involves T cells, B cells, or both. Unfortunately, the best current classification, established by an expert committee of the World Health Organization, still places the majority of immunodeficiency diseases in an undefined category called *common variable immunodeficiency.* In general, this classification will be followed in the following discussion, which emphasizes three related concepts; first, that immunodeficiencies are most logically viewed as defects of cellular differentiation; second, that these defects may involve either primary development of T or B cells or the antigen-dependent phase of their differentiation; and third, that defects of secondary B-cell differentiation may in some instances reflect T-cell abnormalities resulting from faulty T-B collaboration.

Secondary immunodeficiencies are those not caused by intrinsic abnormalities in development or function of T and B cells. Examples are immune deficiency associated with malnutrition, protein-losing enteropathy, and intestinal lymphangiectasia. Also considered secondary are immunodeficiencies resulting from hypercatabolic states such as occur in myotonic dystrophy, immunodeficiency associated with lymphoreticular malignancy, and immunodeficiency resulting from treatment with x-rays, antilymphocyte serum, or cytotoxic drugs.

Incidence As a group, the immunodeficiency syndromes discussed in this chapter are relatively common. Isolated IgA deficiency occurs in approximately 1 in 600 individuals; no other specific category approaches this frequency, but the cumulative total is not insignificant. The incidence of diagnosed immunodeficiency diseases is clearly a function of the awareness of physicians in a community. An epidemic of immunodeficiency diseases commonly follows the addition of a clinical immunologist to a medical center staff.

The more severe forms of primary immunodeficiency have their onset early in life and all too frequently result in death during childhood. Immunodeficiencies may be acquired at any age, however, and a substantial number of patients with congenital hypogammaglobulinemia survive to middle age or beyond. In a referral center for patients with immunodeficiency diseases, approximately two-thirds of the immunodeficient patients under care are adults. Improved methods of diagnosis and treatment can be expected to increase this ratio in the future.

Severe combined immunodeficiency (SCID) This syndrome is characterized by gross functional impairment of both humoral and cell-mediated immunity. It is usually congenital, may be inherited either as an X-linked or autosomal recessive defect, or may occur sporadically. Affected infants rarely survive beyond one year. This syndrome has been associated with a diversity of defects in development of immunocompetent cells, some of which may be related to specific enzymatic abnormalities.

The classic example of SCID, *Swiss-type agammaglobulinemia*, is characterized by severe lymphopenia involving both T and B cells, and is inherited with an autosomal recessive pattern. Rarely, other hematopoietic cell lines fail to develop. The cellular defect in these forms of SCID logically rests with the precursor common to both T and B cells. The immunologic defects in a few of these patients have been repaired following transplantation of fetal liver as a source of stem cells, confirming the hypothesis that they have a thymus and bursa equivalent capable of supporting differentiation of normal stem cells. About half of patients with autosomal recessive SCID are deficient in an enzyme involved in purine metabolism, adenosine deaminase (ADA). These patients have varying degrees of lymphopenia, T cells usually being more deficient than B cells. The pathophysiologic relationship of ADA deficiency to lymphoid differentiation is slowly being unraveled. The best current evidence suggests that intracellular accumulation of deoxy-ATP, by inhibiting ribonucleotide reductase enzymes, interferes with synthesis of DNA precursors, particularly deoxycytidine. Improvement of both clinical status and immunologic function has occurred in some but not all patients treated with a source of exogenous ADA; therapy with deoxynucleosides is currently being investigated.

SCID may also occur with an X-linked inheritance pattern. Affected boys may not have severe lymphopenia; some have had normal numbers of B lymphocytes with few or no circulating T lymphocytes. This developmental pattern (which may also occur with autosomal recessive inheritance) suggests the possibility of a faulty thymus epithelium. Mononuclear cells from such patients have been induced to express T-cell characteristics by coculture on normal thymus epithelium or by treatment with thymus hormones.

A number of individuals with SCID have been successfully treated by transplantation of histocompatible bone marrow from sibling donors. The same treatment has been used in children and adults with leukemia or aplastic anemia (Chaps. 69 and 312) following purposeful destruction of the immune system by irradiation and cytotoxic drugs. Other modes of treatment, including fetal liver and thymus transplants, have been successful in restoring immunocompetence, but as yet there are only short-term survivors. Treatment of these patients should probably be attempted only in centers with a strong research interest in this problem. It is crucial that these patients be recognized early and not be given blood transfusions which may cause fatal graft-versus-host disease.

T-cell immunodeficiency Primary T-cell defects are extremely difficult to define. Reflecting the diversity of T-cell functions, abnormalities of T-cell development may be responsible for a wide spectrum of immune deficiencies including severe combined immunodeficiency, apparently isolated defects in cell-mediated immunity, and syndromes presenting as antibody deficiency with apparently normal cell-mediated immunity. These defects may be acquired as well as congenital. Until very recently, laboratory assays of T-lymphocyte function were limited to correlates of cell-mediated immunity; no means were available for studying T-cell regulation of B-cell differentiation. With the development of appropriate methodology it will undoubtedly be found that clinically significant abnormalities of T cells are much more common and heterogeneous than is now appreciated.

DI GEORGE SYNDROME This is the classic example of isolated T-cell deficiency and results from maldevelopment of organs derived embryologically from the third and fourth pharyngeal pouches. Affected infants usually present with congenital cardiac defects, particularly those involving the great vessels, hypocalcemic tetany due to failure of parathyroid development, and absence of the thymus. Other associated abnormalities may include abnormal ears, shortened philtrum, and hypertelorism. Serum immunoglobulin concentrations are usually normal. Lymphocyte counts may be normal, but virtually all the lymphocytes are B cells. Carefully performed autopsies have often revealed a tiny, histologically normal thymus, usually in an ectopic location. With time, a few patients developed functional T cells. Patients with Di George's syndrome have had transplants of fetal thymus and subsequently have developed normal cell-mediated immunity, associated with T cells of host origin.

Children lacking the congenital anomalies associated with Di George's syndrome may present with severe impairment of cell-mediated immunity. Some have normal or even increased immunoglobulin levels, while others have selective deficiencies of one or more immunoglobulin classes. Specific antibody responses are usually impaired even in patients with normal concentrations of immunoglobulins. This ill-defined entity has been called the *Nezelof syndrome*.

Inherited deficiency of the enzyme purine nucleoside phosphorylase (PNP) is associated with an often severe and selective deficiency of T-lymphocyte function. This enzyme functions in the same purine salvage pathway as ADA; toxic effects of its deficiency are attributed to reduction in synthesis of deoxycytidine by mechanisms similar to those involved in ADA deficiency.

A few patients with isolated T-cell deficiency have been treated with fetal thymus grafts. Some have shown improvement in numbers of circulating T cells, in vitro reactivity to mitogens, and clinical condition, while others have had no change in status. A patient treated with thymosin developed increased numbers of circulating T cells and delayed hypersensitivity skin reactions associated with clinical improvement. Transfer factor has been reported to benefit a few patients.

ATAXIA-TELANGIECTASIA This is an autosomal recessive genetic disorder characterized by cerebellar ataxia, oculocutaneous telangiectasia, and immunodeficiency. Onset of truncal ataxia usually occurs in infancy and is progressive. Immunodeficiency is clinically manifest by recurrent and chronic sinopulmonary infection leading to bronchiectasis. The two most frequent causes of death are chronic pulmonary disease and malignancy. Lymphomas are most common, although carcinomas have also occurred.

The immunologic abnormalities seem to be related to maldevelopment of the thymus. If found at all, the thymus in autopsied patients has been markedly hypoplastic and similar in appearance to an embryonic thymus. Patients' lymphocytes frequently respond poorly to T-cell mitogens in vitro. Cutaneous anergy and delayed rejection of skin grafts are common. Although the number and class distribution of B lymphocytes are usually normal, most patients are deficient in serum IgE and IgA, and a smaller number have reduced serum levels of IgG. IgM and IgD are usually normal. This suggests a maturational arrest of B lymphocytes secondary to T-cell dysfunction. Indeed, in one IgA-deficient patient, peripheral lymphocytes were triggered by pokeweed mitogen to develop into IgA-synthesizing plasma cells.

There is circumstantial evidence that ataxia-telangiectasia may involve a generalized defect in cellular differentiation. Ovarian agenesis occurs frequently. Persistence of very high levels of oncofetal proteins, including α-fetoprotein and carcinoembryonic antigen, has been found in patients' serum. At the other end of the age spectrum are signs of progeria, including premature graying and early development of senile keratoses and vitiligo. These patients may have a defect in DNA repair mechanisms. Such a defect might underly their unusual susceptibility to irradiation injury, a high frequency of chromosomal breaks in some patients, and the increased incidence of malignancy.

Only symptomatic treatment is available. Unless severe deficiency of IgG is present, therapy with gamma globulin is not indicated. Transplantation with histocompatible bone marrow was followed in one patient by increased synthesis of IgA and transient improvement of cellular immune responsiveness, but chimerism could not be demonstrated. Unusual sensitivity to x-irradiation should be kept in mind in planning therapy for patients who develop cancer.

Immunoglobulin deficiency syndromes X-LINKED AGAMMA-GLOBULINEMIA This syndrome was long thought to represent a central failure of development of all elements of the B-cell lineage. Recent evidence has modified this concept. Affected males have very few immunoglobulin-bearing B lymphocytes in their circulation and lack primary and secondary lymphoid follicles. However, pre-B cells are found in normal frequency in their bone marrow. This developmental block contrasts with earlier and later arrests in B-cell differentiation characterizing other immunodeficiencies (see below and Fig. 62-1). Patients usually have a substantial number of small mononuclear cells bearing receptors for aggregated immunoglobulin and C'3. Although resembling B lymphocytes, these cells have been shown to have markers characteristic of the monocyte line and to lack the B-lymphocyte specific surface antigen(s) and receptors for Epstein-Barr virus. A few patients with well-documented X-linked agammaglobulinemia have had a normal number of B lymphocytes, suggesting that there may be two distinct forms of this disease.

Agammaglobulinemia is a misnomer, as most patients with this and other forms of severe panhypogammaglobulinemia synthesize some immunoglobulins, primarily of the IgG class. Within the same family some affected males have had substantial levels of IgM, IgG, and IgA, while others have been nearly agammaglobulinemic. All these patients were markedly deficient in circulating B lymphocytes. This observation suggests that the few B lymphocytes which are generated are fully capable of differentiating to plasma cells and secreting immunoglobulins. A form of arthritis with some of the features of rheumatoid disease occurs in some of these patients and may remit following treatment with gamma globulin.

TRANSIENT HYPOGAMMAGLOBULINEMIA OF INFANCY This is a reversible syndrome in which normal physiologic hypogammaglobulinemia of infancy is unusually prolonged and severe. IgG levels of normal-term infants commonly drop to levels of 300 to 400 mg per 100 ml between 3 and 6 months of age as maternally derived IgG is catabolized; levels subsequently rise reflecting the infants' increased synthetic capacity. In transient hypogammaglobulinemia, the rate of synthesis of IgM, IgG, and IgA remains low for long periods. Some of these infants have a reduced number of B lymphocytes while others have a normal number.

ISOLATED DEFICIENCY OF IgA This is by far the most commonly encountered immunodeficiency, occurring with a frequency of approximately 1 in 600 individuals. With rare exceptions, both serum and secretory IgA are involved. Many adults with isolated IgA deficiency do not seem to have unusual problems with infection. Nevertheless, this condition is not benign. A substantial proportion of IgA-deficient individuals develop precipitating antibodies to IgA. These patients may have severe anaphylactic reactions when transfused with normal blood from a blood bank.

As a group, individuals with IgA deficiency have an increased number of respiratory infections of varying severity, and a few have had severe pulmonary disease such as bronchiectasis. Chronic diarrheal disease also occurs. The incidence of asthma and other atopic diseases among IgA-deficient patients is high, and, conversely, the incidence of IgA deficiency among atopic children has been found to be twenty to forty times that in the normal population. In one study it was found that combined deficiency of IgE and IgA (or IgE deficiency alone) did not predispose to recurrent respiratory infections, while IgA-deficient patients with normal or elevated IgE had recurrent sinopulmonary disease. IgA deficiency is also significantly associated with autoimmune diseases such as rheumatoid arthritis and systemic lupus erythematosus.

IgA deficiency may be familial, but no single pattern of inheritance has been encountered consistently. It has occurred in association with congenital intrauterine infections, such as toxoplasmosis, rubella, and cytomegalovirus infection. Several patients with abnormalities of chromosome 18 have had isolated IgA deficiency. Most commonly, the syndrome appears as a sporadic defect. It may be transient or acquired late in life.

The pathogenesis of IgA deficiency, whether genetic or caused by environmental insult, apparently involves a block in terminal differentiation of B lymphocytes. The great majority of patients studied have had normal numbers of circulating B lymphocytes bearing surface IgA determinants. In vitro stimulation with pokeweed mitogen cells from some patients has resulted in differentiation of IgA-secreting plasma cells, while in others selective T-cell suppression of IgA plasma cell differentiation may exist. Although peripheral lymphocytes from IgA-deficient patients generally respond normally to T-cell mitogens, diminished numbers of circulating T cells as detected by the E rosette test and abnormal production of lymphokines by stimulated T cells have been described. Thus, it seems likely that the failure of IgA-bearing B lymphocytes to mature to secretory plasma cells in many patients may reflect abnormalities in T-cell function, the nature of which could reflect either deficiencies in helper T cells or excessive activity of suppressor T cells. A primary T-cell defect, rather than IgA deficiency per se, may help to explain the striking association of IgA deficiency with other immunologically related diseases.

Treatment of IgA deficiency is symptomatic. IgA cannot be effectively replaced by exogenous gamma globulin or plasma, and use of either would greatly increase the risk of development of antibodies to IgA. IgA-deficient patients in need of transfusion should be screened for the presence of antibodies to IgA, and ideally should be given blood only from IgA-deficient donors. All patients known to be IgA-deficient should be warned of the risk of severe transfusion reactions which may occur following infusion of only a few milliliters of blood.

X-LINKED IMMUNODEFICIENCY WITH INCREASED LEVELS OF IgM This is a specific syndrome only because of its inheritance pattern. IgG levels are usually very low, and IgA low or undetectable, while IgD levels may be high. The clinical patterns of infection are similar to those occurring with other hypogammaglobulinemic states. The number and distribution of B lymphocytes bearing IgM, IgG, and IgA have been normal, suggesting that this type of immunodeficiency may also involve a block in terminal differentiation of B lymphocytes. Neutropenia often occurs in affected males and can increase their vulnerability to infections.

ISOLATED DEFICIENCY OF IgM This syndrome has been reported rarely in this country but was detected frequently in a British population. Approximately 20 percent of these patients were asymptomatic while 60 percent had severe recurrent infections, often with bacteremia. Pneumococcal pneumonia and meningitis have often been noted in IgM-deficient patients. Other associated conditions included gastrointestinal disease, atopy, splenomegaly, and development of malignancy. The condition was frequently familial, and was four times more common in males than females. The number of circulating B lymphocytes has varied from very low to normal.

Common variable immunodeficiency This represents a heterogeneous group of syndromes which may be congenital or acquired, sporadic or familial, and which occur in both males and females. These patients have in common the clinical manifestations of antibody deficiency associated with panhypogammaglobulinemia, with deficiency of IgG and IgA, or rarely, with selective IgG deficiency.

Approximately one-third of these patients have few or no circulating B lymphocytes, suggesting a central failure of development of this cell line. The remainder have B lymphocytes, and more than half have a normal number and class distribution. In the few patients studied, B lymphocytes capable of binding specific antigens were present and increased in frequency following immunization. Consistent with the evidence that B lymphocytes in these patients are able to recognize antigens and proliferate, but fail to differentiate to plasma cells, is the fairly common finding of lymphoid hyperplasia, including splenomegaly and nodular lymphoid hyperplasia of the gut.

In agammaglobulinemic patients having B lymphocytes, the pathogenesis of immune deficiency must involve the failure of these cells to differentiate to plasma cells. By use of assays capable of measuring B-lymphocyte differentiation to plasma cells in vitro, three major types of defect have been tentatively identified. First, and most common, is an intrinsic abnormality of B lymphocytes. B lymphocytes from these patients cannot differentiate into immunoglobulin-secreting plasma cells even when provided with help from normal T cells. In other instances, plasma cells containing intracytoplasmic immunoglobulin develop but fail to secrete this product. Second, there is evidence that in some patients the T cells, or their products, may actively suppress terminal differentiation of autologous or normal B lymphocytes. The increase in suppressor activity could be either a primary or secondary abnormality; the latter could explain the increase in T-cell suppressor activity in patients with abnormal B lymphocytes and others in whom B lymphocytes are congenitally absent. Third, quantitative deficiency of helper T-cell function has been observed in some

patients, usually also in association with defective B-cell function.

Cells from some agammaglobulinemic patients having normal B-lymphocyte numbers respond normally to pokeweed mitogen in vitro. Studies of their separated T and B lymphocytes have shown no distinctive abnormalities of the types described above.

Patients with common variable immunodeficiency may present with signs and symptoms highly suggestive of lymphoid malignancy, including fever, weight loss, splenomegaly, generalized lymphadenopathy, and lymphocytosis. Routine histologic examination of lymphoid tissues usually reveals germinal center hyperplasia which may be extremely difficult to distinguish from nodular lymphoma (Chapter 327). Demonstration of a normal distribution of immunoglobulin isotypes and light chain classes on circulating and tissue B lymphocytes can serve to distinguish these patients from those having a monoclonal B-cell malignancy with secondary hypogammaglobulinemia. Treatment of several patients with gamma globulin has resulted in relief of symptoms and reversal of lymphoid hyperplasia.

IMMUNODEFICIENCY WITH THYMOMA Recognition of this condition provided one of the early clues as to the role of the thymus in immunobiology. Although T-cell numbers and cell-mediated immunity are frequently intact, several T-cell abnormalities have been identified. Patients' T cells suppress differentiation of normal B lymphocytes in the pokeweed mitogen assay and may also suppress development of erythroid precursors. Suppressor T-cell activity is mediated by the subset of T cells bearing receptors for IgG, which are found in increased numbers. These patients are very deficient in circulating B lymphocytes, frequently have eosinopenia, and may develop erythroid aplasia. Failure to produce B lymphocytes has been traced to the stem-cell level, since pre-B cells could not be found in their bone marrow. The relationship between the thymoma, T-cell dysfunction, and apparent abnormalities of hematopoietic stem cells remains conjectural.

WISKOTT-ALDRICH SYNDROME This is an X-linked genetic disease characterized by eczema, thrombocytopenia, and repeated infections. Affected boys often present with bleeding in infancy. Most do not survive childhood, dying of complications of bleeding, infection, or lymphoreticular malignancy. The immunologic defects in this disease are well characterized but poorly understood. Serum concentrations of IgM are usually decreased, while IgA and IgG are normal. However, synthetic rates for all three classes may be elevated, indicating a significant element of hypercatabolism. The number and class distribution of B lymphocytes usually have been normal. Some patients acquire a diminished number of T cells as evaluated by the E rosette test and appraisal of lymph node biopsies. Functionally, these boys are unable to make antibodies to polysaccharide antigens normally; responses to protein antigens are often not impaired. They are frequently anergic, and their T cells do not respond normally to challenge with ubiquitous antigens. However, responses to T-cell mitogens, such as phytohemagglutinin, are generally normal. Serial appraisal of affected males suggests that the defects in T-cell function are secondary. It is possible that the Wiskott-Aldrich syndrome reflects a primary defect in the B lymphocyte.

A number of patients with this syndrome have been treated with transfer factor obtained from leukocytes of normal donors. About half appear clinically improved, as judged by a decreased number of infections, clearing of eczema, and, in a few, increased platelet counts. Clinical improvement has been correlated with transfer of delayed hypersensitivity skin reactions to antigens to which the donor was sensitive. It has been difficult to assess the value of transfer factor in the treatment of patients with this syndrome because controlled studies are only now being done. However, fatal infections, severe eczema, hemolytic anemia, nephrotic syndrome, and development of lymphoreticular malignancy have all occurred in patients with and without transfer factor treatment. Greater success has been obtained with transplantation of histocompatible sibling bone marrow in a few patients. The first, treated nearly 10 years ago, has sustained marked improvement in immunologic function but remains thrombocytopenic. Two other boys have apparently had both hematologic and immunologic abnormalities corrected by elimination of their own lymphopoietic system before matched marrow transplantation.

Miscellaneous immunodeficiency syndromes Infection with *Candida albicans* is the almost universal accompaniment of severe deficiencies in cell-mediated immunity. The syndrome of *chronic mucocutaneous candidiasis* is different because superficial candidiasis is usually the only major manifestation of immunodeficiency. These patients rarely develop systemic infection with *Candida* or other fungal agents and are not unusually susceptible to virus or bacterial disease. The syndrome is often congenital and may be associated with single or multiple endocrinopathies as well as iron deficiency. Treatment of associated conditions may lead to improvement or even cure of *Candida* infection.

No uniformity of immunologic defects has been identified in these patients, although defects of antibody formation have been detected occasionally. Humoral immunity, including ability to make specific anti-*Candida* antibodies, is usually normal. Many patients are anergic, some to a variety of antigens and some only to *Candida;* anergy in some patients has been related to inability of their lymphocytes to produce migration inhibition factor.

Results of treatment with antifungal agents, such as amphotericin B, have been variable but generally not encouraging. In some patients, clearing of the *Candida* lesions by treatment with antifungal agents has been maintained sometimes with surgical removal of affected nails and sometimes without periodic administration of transfer factor.

IMMUNODEFICIENCY ASSOCIATED WITH SERUM LYMPHOCYTO-TOXINS This syndrome has been reported in a few patients with recurrent bacterial and fungal infections. Most have had fluctuating lymphopenia. Both cellular immunity and specific antibody responses were impaired, although immunoglobulin levels were usually normal. Antibodies specific for B-cell antigens have also been reported as a cause of selective elimination of B cells and resultant hypogammaglobulinemia.

IMBALANCES OF IgG SUBCLASSES Some patients with repeated infections and only moderately decreased serum IgG levels may have an imbalance of IgG subclasses. A few such patients appeared to benefit from administration of gamma globulin. *Kappa light-chain deficiency* has also been reported in association with recurrent infections, and doubtless many more subtle gaps in antibody diversity, which may be clinically significant, will be elucidated.

Metabolic abnormalities associated with immunodeficiency The relation of deficiencies of the purine salvage enzymes, adenosine deaminase and purine nucleoside phosphorylase, to immunodeficiency was discussed earlier. Other inherited metabolic defects should be briefly mentioned because of their po-

tential importance in understanding the molecular basis of immunologic function. Inherited *deficiency of transcobalamin II,* the serum carrier molecule responsible for transport of vitamin B_{12} to tissues, was associated with failure of immunoglobulin production as well as megaloblastic anemia, leukopenia, thrombocytopenia, and severe malabsorption. All abnormalities were reversed by administration of pharmacologic doses of vitamin B_{12}. The syndrome of *acrodermatitis enteropathica* includes severe desquamating skin lesions, intractable diarrhea, bizarre neurologic symptoms, variable combined immunodeficiency, and an often fatal outcome. This disease is apparently caused by an inborn error of metabolism resulting in malabsorption of dietary zinc, and can be effectively treated by parenteral or large oral doses of zinc. Similar disease manifestations have occurred in mice and cattle with different inherited defects leading to zinc malabsorption. Zinc deficiency might in part account for the immunodeficiency which accompanies severe malnutrition.

TREATMENT OF IMMUNODEFICIENCIES Treatment of immunodeficiency diseases involving severe abnormalities of T-cell function, with or without hypogammaglobulinemia, is currently limited in effectiveness and extremely complicated. Experimental approaches, including transplantation of bone marrow, fetal liver, and thymus, were mentioned in preceding sections. Also under investigation is the use of thymic hormones and of pharmacologic agents which may correct defects in lymphoid function caused by inherited metabolic disorders.

Replacement therapy with human gamma globulin should be used in patients who have recurrent bacterial infections and are deficient in IgG. Maintenance of serum IgG levels between 100 and 300 mg per 100 ml is sufficient to prevent most overwhelming infections, although chronic sinusitis, otitis media, and bronchitis often persist. These serum levels usually can be achieved by intramuscular injection of IgG, 100 mg/kg, at monthly intervals, following a loading dose of twice this amount given over a period of several days. Forty milliliters of 16% gamma globulin, given in two or more sites at one time, is about the maximum tolerable in adults. If more is needed, it is preferable to increase the frequency of injections. Many hypogammaglobulinemic patients and their physicians normally prefer division of the monthly doses into bimonthly injections. In patients with mild to moderate IgG deficiency (300 to 400 mg per 100 ml), the decision to treat must be based on clinical symptoms and on failure to respond to antigenic challenge, because injection of gamma globulin at the recommended doses will not significantly elevate serum IgG levels. Gamma globulin treatment is of no value in patients with deficiencies of immunoglobulins other than IgG. This form of treatment is not benign. Many patients become intolerant, having symptoms of diaphoresis, tachycardia, and hypotension immediately following injections. This reaction is thought to be mediated by aggregates of IgG in the gamma globulin preparation, but why it develops after years of treatment in some patients, and never in others has not been adequately explained. Most patients intolerant of gamma globulin injections can be treated successfully with plasma.

Infusion of fresh plasma, 10 to 20 ml/kg at intervals of 3 to 4 weeks, has the advantages of being less painful and of replacing IgM and IgA as well as IgG; however, both IgM and IgA have a half-life of only a few days. The major disadvantage of plasma is the risk of transmitting hepatitis, which is particularly devastating in immunodeficient patients. This risk can be minimized by use of selected donors, usually family members, carefully screened for the absence of Australia antigen or antibody.

Therapy with exogenous IgG usually does not prevent chronic sinopulmonary infection and its all too frequent progression to pulmonary fibrosis and bronchiectasis. Therefore, maintenance of good pulmonary toilet with regular postural drainage is an especially important part of patient management. The principles of antibiotic therapy are not different in these than other patients, except that the index of suspicion of bacterial infection should remain very high.

REFERENCES

AIUTI F et al: Identification, enumeration, and isolation of B and T lymphocytes from human peripheral blood. Scand J Immunol 3:521, 1974

BERGSMA D et al (eds): *Immunodeficiency in Man and Animals, Birth Defects,* Original Article Series, vol XI, no 1. The National Foundation–March of Dimes, Sunderland, Mass, Sinauer Associates, 1975

COOPER MD et al: Meeting Report 2nd International Workshop on Primary Immunodeficiency Diseases in Man. Clin Immunol Immunopathol 2:416, 1974

JAPAN MEDICAL RESEARCH FOUNDATION (eds): *Immunodeficiency: Its Nature and Etiological Significance in Human Disease.* Tokyo, University of Tokyo Press, 1978

MEISCHER PA, MÜLLER-EBERHARD HJ (eds): *Seminars in Immunopathology,* vol 1: *Immunodeficiency Diseases.* Berlin, Springer-Verlag, 1978

STIEHM ER, FULGINITI VA (eds): *Immunologic Disorders in Infants and Children,* 2d ed. Philadelphia, Saunders, 1979

63
PLASMA CELL NEOPLASMS AND RELATED DISORDERS

RAYMOND ALEXANIAN

Plasma cell diseases constitute a group of related disorders in which a single clone of cells produces large quantities of an immunoglobulin molecule that is usually recognized as a peak on serum or urine electrophoresis. The most important entity is multiple myeloma; other related conditions include Waldenström's macroglobulinemia, idiopathic monoclonal gammopathy, primary amyloidosis, and the heavy-chain diseases. A combination of clinical and electrophoretic studies is necessary to distinguish these entities, to stage the extent of disease, and to evaluate change in tumor mass with or without therapy.

The distinction between these disorders requires an understanding of normal and abnormal immunoglobulin synthesis. Normal immunoglobulins are produced by differentiated plasma cells and consist of two heavy chains linked to two light chains by disulfide bonds. In normal humans, a very large number of different plasma cells produce a wide range of different immunoglobulins that have been grouped into five major classes depending on their heavy chain type: IgG, IgA, IgM, IgD, and IgE. Light chains are of either kappa or lambda type; because of a slightly excessive rate of light chain synthesis, normal humans excrete in urine up to 10 mg per day of a mixture of kappa and lambda light chains. Fig. 63-1 depicts the electrophoretic pattern of normal serum and urine.

Among the different plasma cell disorders, the frequency of a specific abnormality in a globulin is proportional to the number of cells producing that particular type of protein and is reflected by the concentration of the different immunoglobulins in serum. Monoclonal gammopathies of IgG type are more common than those of IgA or IgM classes. A monoclonal gammopathy is usually recognized on electrophoresis when about 10^{11} cells of a single clone are present, as in idiopathic gammopathy or primary amyloidosis. Tumor growth usually occurs when about 10^{12} malignant cells are produced, as in multiple myeloma, macroglobulinemia, or the heavy chain

diseases. In addition to the markedly increased production of a monoclonal protein, the quality of immunoglobulin synthesis may also be defective. For example, there may be a markedly excessive rate of monoclonal light chain production, and some patients excrete up to 40 g protein (Bence-Jones protein) a day in the urine. In fact, about 20 percent of the patients with multiple myeloma show only light chain production, although immunofluorescent studies of the involved cells indicate that a low level of heavy chain synthesis also may occur. Some patients produce only the Fc fragments of heavy chains, and have heavy chain disease. Others with myeloma or macroglobulinemia have smaller deletions of segments of their heavy or light chains. The autonomously proliferating cells in these malignant disorders are capable of producing immunoglobulins that are structurally normal in some patients, and a few even demonstrate immunological reactivity. In contrast, still other patients produce a distorted proportion of heavy and light chains, or an excessive quantity of defective globulins.

MULTIPLE MYELOMA Multiple myeloma is a disseminated malignancy of plasma cells that may be associated with bone destruction, bone marrow failure, hypercalcemia, renal failure, and recurrent infections. The disease is most common in the middle-aged and elderly; the median age of occurrence is 60 years. Males are affected slightly more frequently than females. The annual incidence of the disease is about 3 per 100,000 population.

Clinical and laboratory findings The clinical manifestations of multiple myeloma result primarily from the damage produced by plasma cell tumors in the bone marrow and from the effects of abnormal proteins. There is a wide spectrum of pathologic features, and the complications of the disease as well as the modes of therapy required vary markedly among patients.

FIGURE 63-1

Electrophoretic patterns of normal serum and urine. Normal humans produce a mixture of gamma globulins with different heavy and light chain types. In hypergammaglobulinemia, an increased number of plasma cells produce larger quantities of different globulins so that a broad elevation is apparent.

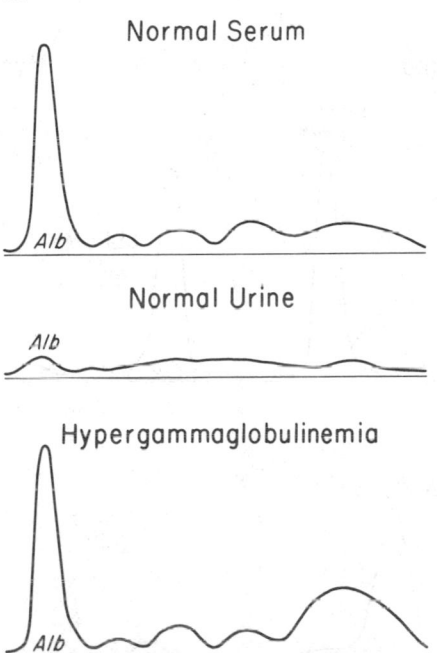

Normal Serum

Alb

Normal Urine

Alb

Hypergammaglobulinemia

Alb

Bone pain from pathologic fractures constitutes the most common symptom and usually is due to compression fractures of the thoracic or lumbar spine. Typically, the pain is well localized, sometimes radicular, and is usually aggravated by movement, as on arising. In about 5 percent of patients, extradural plasmacytomas arising from a vertebra may produce spinal cord compression, paraplegia, and bladder dysfunction. Pathologic fractures of the ribs and proximal bones of the extremities are common. In about two-thirds of the patients, skeletal radiographs demonstrate punched-out lesions that are best seen on lateral skull films, but demineralization without focal destruction or even a normal skeletal structure may be present. Isotopic bone scans are sometimes useful when radiographic bone surveys fail to demonstrate bony lesions and vice versa. Osteolysis appears to result from the increased production by the malignant plasma cells of a factor that stimulates osteoclast proliferation. Rarely, a diffuse osteoblastic bone reaction may occur. In about 15 percent of patients, firm plasmacytomas grow from areas of underlying bone destruction; these lesions usually develop over the skull, sternum, and clavicles where the skin is contiguous to the involved bones. Multiple vertebral compression fractures frequently result in a painless kyphosis of the dorsal spine and a diminution in height of as much as 6 in.

In about 90 percent of patients, the bone marrow infiltration by plasma cells produces a normochromic, normocytic anemia at the time of diagnosis, and the anemia becomes more severe as the number of malignant cells increases. Other factors that contribute to anemia include the hypoferremia of chronic disease, renal failure, chemotherapy, and radiotherapy. The globulins of myeloma may coat the red blood cells, causing rouleaux formation, a markedly increased erythrocyte sedimentation rate, and increased hemolysis. When there is marked hyperglobulinemia the plasma volume may be increased to an extent to reduce the hematocrit by as much as 6 volume percent lower than the value expected for the red blood cell volume. Occasionally, plasma cells may be present in the peripheral blood, but plasma cell leukemia with more than 1000 cells per cubic millimeter is unusual. Granulocytopenia or thrombocytopenia occurs in less than 10 percent of untreated patients. Some myeloma globulins may produce an increased bleeding tendency by interfering with platelet function or by interactions with specific coagulation factors. When

present in high concentrations, IgG or IgA myeloma globulins may result in a symptomatic hyperviscosity syndrome or in cold hypersensitivity from cryoglobulinemia.

Bone marrow aspirates usually contain prominent focal collections of immature plasma cells. The cells are usually large, ovoid, and basophilic, and contain an eccentric nucleus with finely clumped chromatin. Multinucleated cells, prominent nucleoli, and intracytoplasmic deposits of protein may be present. Electron microscopy always reveals a highly developed endoplasmic reticulum characteristic of cells elaborating extracellular protein, even in those few patients without apparent evidence of a monoclonal globulin on electrophoretic studies. Yet, there are no pathognomonic cytologic features that will always distinguish malignant from normal plasma cells.

A variety of chemical abnormalities may result from bone or kidney damage. Hypercalcemia with levels in excess of 11.5 mg per 100 ml is found in about one-fourth of the patients at the time of diagnosis and is due to increased bone resorption. Symptoms due to hypercalcemia, such as nausea, mental confusion, and constipation, may constitute the patient's major complaint. Mild or severe renal failure with elevations of blood urea nitrogen to more than 40 mg per 100 ml is a serious complication that occurs in about 20 percent of the patients. Although tubular damage from large quantities of filtered light chains is considered the major factor, other important causes include hypercalcemia, uric acid nephropathy, and amyloidosis. Renal failure may be precipitated by dehydration, as is induced by some radiographic procedures. In rare patients, an adult Fanconi syndrome may result from derangement of specific tubular functions. An elevated serum uric acid level may occur as a consequence of an increased plasma cell turnover, increased cell destruction from chemotherapy, and/or decreased uric acid clearance from renal impairment. A symmetrical peripheral neuropathy that most frequently involves the lower extremities has been described in some patients. An increased susceptibility to bacterial infection results primarily because the levels of normal immunoglobulins are decreased in about 85 percent of the patients. Cell-mediated immunity is also impaired. Pneumonia, urinary tract infection, and bacteremia may develop, particularly when the myeloma has not been controlled by chemotherapy. Herpes zoster occurs in about 10 percent of the patients.

One of the major features of the disease that is seen in about 98 percent of patients is a homogeneous globulin peak on electrophoresis of the serum, urine, or both (Fig. 63-2). This

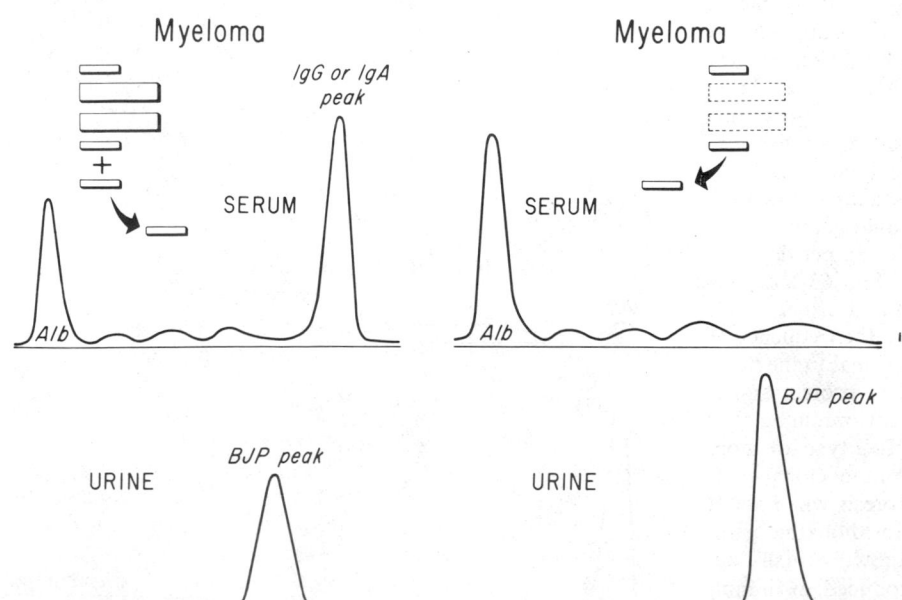

FIGURE 63-2
Serum and urine electrophoresis in upper and lower panels from two patients with multiple myeloma. On the left, increased production of a complete monoclonal globulin is reflected in a serum peak; excessive light chains are excreted and produce a urine peak of different mobility. A second patient on the right has a normal serum electrophoresis with evidence only of light chain excretion in the urine.

is present in the serum of about 80 percent of patients and is usually a complete gamma globulin, with immunoelectrophoresis usually revealing monoclonal IgG or IgA heavy chains combined with either kappa or lambda light chains (for example, IgGK, IgAL). Abnormal globulins of IgG type are about three times more frequent than those of IgA type. Monoclonal globulins of IgD or IgE heavy chain type are rare, and Bence-Jones proteinemia has been detected primarily when renal failure inhibits the normal catabolism and excretion of monoclonal light chains. In about 20 percent of patients, only the light chain portion of a gamma-globulin molecule is evident —Bence-Jones protein. Because of its lower molecular weight of about 20,000, light chains of either kappa or lambda type are excreted in the urine and detected as a monoclonal peak on urine electrophoresis (Fig. 63-2). All patients suspected of having multiple myeloma or one of its variants should have electrophoretic studies of both serum and urine. In about 2 percent of patients, a monoclonal globulin cannot be detected in either serum or urine, but immunofluorescent studies almost always confirm the production of a monoclonal globulin by plasma cells.

Diagnosis The diagnosis should be suspected when one or more of the following abnormalities is present: bone pain from pathologic fractures of the spine or ribs, anemia, proteinuria, azotemia, hypercalcemia, recurrent infection, or spinal cord compression. In patients with severe bone pain and anemia who demonstrate bone marrow plasmacytosis, the presence of lytic bone lesions and a peak on serum or urine electrophoresis is diagnostic. Both serum and urine electrophoresis must be evaluated in patients suspected of having myeloma, and electrophoresis of concentrated urine may be necessary for the detection of small amounts of light chains. Examination of the marrow alone may not distinguish the plasma cell infiltration of multiple myeloma from the reactive plasmacytosis found in chronic infection, chronic liver disease, or collagen diseases. In these disorders, the generalized plasma cell reaction will usually produce a diffuse hypergammaglobulinemia on electrophoresis (Fig. 63-1). The occurrence of hypercalcemia or azotemia is also not specific, but the finding of markedly depressed normal immunoglobulins may help to distinguish myeloma from other nonmalignant plasma cell dyscrasias. In patients with equivocal findings, the presence of large IgG or IgA peaks in the serum (>3.0 g per 100 ml), depressed values of normal serum immunoglobulins, or a detectable quantity of Bence-Jones protein in the urine supports the diagnosis of myeloma. The excretion of monoclonal light chains of either kappa or lambda type usually signifies myeloma, macroglobulinemia, or primary amyloidosis, but the patient may not be clinically symptomatic for a prolonged period when this is the only abnormality. Diseases that must be distinguished from myeloma include idiopathic monoclonal gammopathy, primary amyloidosis, Waldenström's macroglobulinemia, the heavy chain diseases, and metastatic bone tumors. In addition, patients with localized plasmacytoma or indolent multiple myeloma need to be identified because in them chemotherapy is not indicated.

Treatment and prognosis The best treatment for multiple myeloma requires the prevention and control of the complications of this disease, as well as simultaneous efforts to reduce the number of malignant plasma cells. In disabled patients, increased physical activity should be encouraged by the rational use of analgesics, corsets, and walkers. Radiation therapy is useful for disabling bone pain from pathologic fractures, particularly when there is little improvement after the first course of chemotherapy. Immediate radiotherapy to areas of spinal cord compression may prevent the need for decompressive laminectomy after tumor masses are identified by prompt my-

elography. Adequate hydration is essential in order to prevent and control renal complications from the precipitation of Bence-Jones protein in the renal tubules; dehydration must be avoided in preparing patients for radiologic procedures. For patients with severe renal failure, hemodialysis may maintain life for the period required to reduce Bence-Jones protein production with chemotherapy. Hypercalcemia in previously untreated patients is almost always reversible with fluids, increased activity, and chemotherapy with drug combinations that include prednisone. If a bacterial infection develops, prompt and rational use of antibiotics is essential. Prophylactic gamma globulin has no value, and vaccinations with live organisms must be avoided in these immunosuppressed patients.

For symptomatic patients with multiple myeloma and asymptomatic patients with rising myeloma proteins or progressive lytic bone lesions, chemotherapy is required in order to reduce the number of plasma cells. Serial assessments of myeloma protein levels in serum and/or urine are essential for evaluating changes in tumor mass. Before each course of drug therapy, blood counts must be monitored to ensure adequate recovery of granulocytes to a level of 2000 per cubic millimeter and platelets to a level of 100,000 per cubic millimeter. Intermittent courses of an alkylating agent–corticosteroid combination, repeated at 4- to 6-week intervals, will produce tumor reductions of greater than 75 percent in about one-half of previously untreated patients. Melphalan (8 mg/m^2 per day for 4 days) and prednisone (60 mg/m^2 per day for 4 days) are the drugs most commonly used for patients with multiple myeloma. The addition of intravenous vincristine (1.0 mg) with a 3-week treatment interval may produce a 15 percent higher response rate and a median survival time about 5 months longer than previously achieved. Recalcification of lytic bone lesions and an elevation of low immunoglobulin levels occur in 15 percent of patients who respond. Intermittent treatment should be continued for at least 18 months because many patients respond slowly. After 18 months, patients who have responded and whose abnormal globulins have disappeared from the serum can be followed without chemotherapy. Serial electrophoretic measurements must continue to be made because tumor recurrence, recognized by the reappearance of myeloma proteins, can usually be controlled with chemotherapy. When relapses fail to respond despite continued treatment with alkylating agents and steroids, repeated courses of doxorubicin (Adriamycin) combinations can produce significant tumor reductions in about 25 percent of patients resistant to alkylating agents. A representative program consists of intravenous vincristine (1.0 mg) and intravenous doxorubicin (25 mg/m^2 on day 1) combined with cyclophosphamide (100 mg/m^2 per day) and prednisone (60 mg/m^2 per day for 4 days). Patients who have not responded previously to an alkylating agent–corticosteroid combination rarely respond to doxorubicin.

The median survival time for patients who receive combinations of alkylating agents, corticosteroids, and vincristine is about 30 months. But there is a wide variation in prognosis that depends on the extent of tumor mass at the time of diagnosis and the maximum degree of tumor reduction with chemotherapy. The pretreatment tumor mass can be estimated from such laboratory data as the degree of anemia, hypercalcemia, and bone lesions; the degree of tumor mass reduction can be assessed by the rate of reduction in myeloma proteins. The median survival is less than 1 year for patients with a high cell mass and no response, about 4 years for those with a low tumor mass and a marked response, and various intermediate responses depending on the number of plasma cells. When severe irreversible renal failure is present, the median survival is short regardless of the tumor mass and the degree of remission. About 2 percent of all patients and about 6 percent of responding patients who live longer than 2 years will develop acute myelogenous and monocytic leukemia; the long-term treatment with alkylating agents is probably the major cause.

INDOLENT MYELOMA An increasing number of asymptomatic patients with multiple myeloma in an indolent phase have been recognized. In many patients, the diagnosis was first suspected after routine biochemical studies revealed an elevated total protein level which on serum electrophoresis is found to be due to a monoclonal gammopathy. Further studies usually confirm bone marrow plasmacytosis and depressed normal immunoglobulins; mild anemia and lytic bone lesions may also be present. Chemotherapy should be withheld in patients unlikely to experience major morbidity, but changes in the level of myeloma protein, hemoglobin, and bone lesions must be monitored to detect tumor mass progression. Patients with Bence-Jones proteinuria, compression fractures of the vertebrae, recurrent infection, or rising myeloma proteins should receive chemotherapy without delay.

LOCALIZED MYELOMA In occasional patients considered to have a localized plasmacytoma, only one or two plasma cell tumors can be identified without other areas of bone destruction or bone marrow plasmacytosis. All the major disease complications usually associated with myeloma, such as severe anemia and hypercalcemia, are absent. About one-half of the patients do not show a monoclonal globulin peak in the serum or urine; even when present, the level is always low. Normal serum immunoglobulins are usually not depressed. Local radiotherapy in a dose of about 4000 rads is recommended for treatment, but prophylactic chemotherapy is not indicated. Periodic evaluation of serum and urine globulins and of skeletal radiographs in those without abnormal globulins is necessary to detect the presence of multiple myeloma.

WALDENSTRÖM'S MACROGLOBULINEMIA Waldenström's macroglobulinemia is a chronic lymphoproliferative disorder with a wide range of manifestations. This disease affects the middle-aged and elderly and has a slightly higher frequency in men than women. The presence of a monoclonal peak on electrophoresis which is found to be of IgM type by immunoelectrophoresis is a prerequisite for the diagnosis (Fig. 63-3). Aside from uncommon patients with idiopathic IgM peaks, most patients have evidence of an underlying lymphoma which is characterized by bone marrow infiltration, enlargement of lymph nodes and/or spleen, chronic lymphocytic leukemia, or a combination of these features. Conversely, in about 80 percent of patients with chronic lymphocytic leukemia or lymphocytic lymphoma, the affected cells show evidence of monoclonal IgM production by immunofluorescent studies; about 5 percent of patients with these diseases also have an IgM peak on serum electrophoresis.

Clinical and laboratory features The most common clinical presentations include anemia, lymphadenopathy, chronic lymphocytic leukemia, and the hyperviscosity syndrome. The anemia usually results from a marked bone marrow infiltration by lymphocytes, plasma cells, and lymphocytes that resemble plasma cells. Histologically, the nodes are infiltrated diffusely in a pattern that resembles a lymphocytic lymphoma, although the picture may be closer to that of a histiocytic lymphoma. Because of the large molecular weight of the pentametric IgM molecule (Fig. 63-3), increased serum concentrations of mono-

clonal IgM may produce marked hyperviscosity of the blood. The symptoms of the hyperviscosity syndrome are most commonly lassitude and confusion, segmental dilatation of retinal veins with retinal hemorrhages, and an increased bleeding tendency due to an interaction of the monoclonal IgM with coagulation factors and interference with platelet function. Sometimes the macroglobulin may show the characteristics of a cold agglutinin and produce a chronic hemolytic anemia. Renal failure is rare in macroglobulinemia, probably because Bence-Jones proteinuria is absent or the protein is excreted at low levels. About 2 percent of patients show lytic bone destruction, as seen in myeloma. Normal IgG and IgA are usually not reduced to the degree found in multiple myeloma. Cryoglobulins have been described in patients who have both macroglobulinemia and multiple myeloma. These consist of monoclonal globulins that precipitate at temperatures below 37°C (98.6°F). Raynaud's phenomenon, ulcers of the fingers and toes, and other manifestations of cold sensitivity may develop. In the work-up of patients with cryoglobulinemia, serum should be collected and separated at warm temperatures before precipitation is studied in the cold.

Treatment For most patients, the best management includes the reduction of the tumor mass with chemotherapy and the simultaneous control of complications. Red blood cell transfusions should be given only after considering that a markedly increased plasma volume due to the IgM globulin may produce severe hemodilution and reduce the hematocrit up to 6 volume percent and that raising the hematocrit with transfusions may increase blood viscosity to symptomatic levels. For patients with symptoms due to cryoglobulinemia, protection of the extremities from the cold is necessary. When fatigue or neurologic changes occur, and serum viscosity measurements

FIGURE 63-3

In macroglobulinemia, the excessive production of a single pentameric globulin is demonstrated as a peak and requires immunoelectrophoretic studies for identification. With heavy chain disease, IgG heavy chains are present in serum and urine without monoclonal kappa or lambda light chains.

Macroglobulinemia

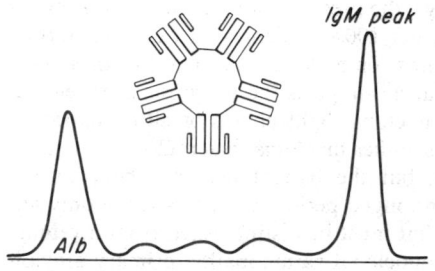

Heavy Chain Disease

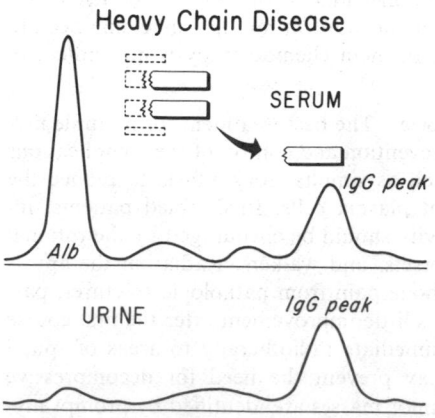

that exceed five times normal are present, plasmapheresis is indicated. This procedure is carried out most expeditiously with an automatic blood cell separator. Because about 80 percent of the macroglobulin is located within the circulation, efficient removal of IgM molecules is possible.

Intermittent courses of a chlorambucil (8 mg/m² per day for 10 days) and prednisone (30 mg/m² per day for 10 days) combination, repeated at 6-week intervals, are effective in reducing the tumor mass by at least 50 percent in approximately three-fourths of the patients. As in myeloma, periodic monitoring by serum electrophoresis is necessary because changes in the monoclonal IgM concentration are helpful in assessing the change in tumor mass. Irradiation may be necessary for aggregates of large lymph nodes. After 18 months, chemotherapy can be withheld from selected patients who achieve a marked reduction in tumor and can be resumed should relapse occur. When there is progressive tumor growth despite repeated courses of alkylating agents and prednisone or when the histologic features of a histiocytic lymphoma are present, other drug combinations that include doxorubicin (Adriamycin) and bleomycin may be helpful. The prognosis is considered slightly better than for multiple myeloma; the median survival is about 3 years.

IDIOPATHIC MONOCLONAL GAMMOPATHY About 0.5 percent of normal individuals over the age of 40 years show a small monoclonal peak on serum electrophoresis. The incidence increases with advancing age so that about 3 percent of individuals over the age of 70 show this abnormality. Usually, monoclonal gammopathy is not suspected when the electrophoresis is ordered, and none of the laboratory or radiographic abnormalities associated with myeloma are present. The concentration of the monoclonal protein is almost always less than 3.0 g per 100 ml, and Bence-Jones proteinuria is rarely present. The protein consists of IgG in about 85 percent of patients, and IgA and IgM globulins account for the remainder. In contrast to myeloma, immunoglobulin levels are usually normal.

When a peak is detected, appropriate studies should rule out the presence of myeloma, macroglobulinemia, or amyloidosis. Most authorities agree that any relationship between monoclonal peaks and other specific underlying diseases, such as an occult solid tumor, is probably coincidental. Periodic long-term follow-up usually shows no changes in the level of the abnormal globulin for the remainder of the patient's life. Less than 20 percent of these individuals have developed multiple myeloma, lymphoma, or amyloidosis after many years of evaluation. Prophylactic chemotherapy, as is used in myeloma, is unjustified. Some benign peaks are transient, particularly those associated with acute hepatitis and other viral infections.

PRIMARY AMYLOIDOSIS (Chap. 64) Amyloidosis is a disease in which major organs become damaged by a homogeneous material that probably results from the interaction of light-chain fragments with tissue polysaccharides. The organs most commonly affected are the kidneys (nephrotic syndrome), heart (congestive failure), joints (carpal tunnel syndrome), tongue (macroglossia), nerves (peripheral neuropathy), and gastrointestinal tract (malabsorption syndrome). "Secondary" amyloidosis occurs in association with prolonged chronic infection or inflammation, such as familial Mediterranean fever or rheumatoid arthritis. "Primary" amyloidosis with the organ involvement described above has no apparent inflammatory basis and occurs in about 15 percent of patients with overt myeloma or macroglobulinemia; usually it is recognized in these patients only on postmortem examination. In addition, about 90 percent of patients with primary amyloidosis and without evidence of myeloma have a small monoclonal peak on serum or urine electrophoresis. Fragments of light chains are present in amyloid fibrils both in myeloma-associated and

in primary amyloidosis without myeloma. Therefore, primary amyloidosis must be considered a monoclonal gammopathy. The disease apparently results from a single clone of plasma cells that has expanded to a stable size of about 10¹¹ cells, as in idiopathic monoclonal gammopathy, but with an excess secretion of free light chains that produces tissue damage in the form of amyloidosis. Biopsies of skin lesions, gums, and rectum provide the best histologic evidence for the disease. All histologic material should be stained with Congo red, and the presence of green birefringence should be sought by polarized microscopy. Because of the risks of hemorrhage, liver and renal biopsies should be employed only when biopsies of other sites are negative. In patients with a monoclonal gammopathy, the excretion of more than 1.0 g albumin in the urine should suggest the diagnosis of amyloidosis. Chemotherapy with melphalan and prednisone is ineffective in resolving amyloid infiltration but may slow the rate of amyloid production by reducing the size of the plasma cell clone.

HEAVY CHAIN DISEASES These rare malignant disorders are characterized by an excessive production of heavy chain fragment, related mainly to the Fc portion of the gamma-globulin molecule. Each of the three described types (gamma, alpha, and mu) have different clinical features and requires immunoelectrophoretic and other special studies for diagnosis.

Patients with *gamma heavy chain disease* are elderly and have easy fatigability, recurrent infections, lymphadenopathy, and splenomegaly. The clinical picture resembles a diffuse lymphoma. Palatal edema may be present because the nodes of Waldeyer's ring are frequently enlarged. Anemia, thrombocytopenia, and eosinophilia are often present, and the bone marrow and lymph nodes are replaced by plasma cells or lymphocytes that resemble plasma cells. The diagnosis requires the demonstration of a monoclonal globulin in both serum and urine of identical electrophoretic mobility and a positive immunoelectrophoretic reaction to IgG antibody (Fig. 63-3). An IgG globulin is present simultaneously in both serum and urine because the Fc fragment of the heavy chain molecule has a molecular weight of about 60,000. No light chains are present. In the presence of a monoclonal peak in serum the diagnosis should be considered when a monoclonal urine globulin does not react with antibody to kappa or lambda light chains. Chemotherapy has usually been ineffective and the prognosis is poor; most patients die of infection within a year of the diagnosis.

Alpha chain disease is the most common of the heavy chain diseases, and afflicted patients have an extensive plasmacytic infiltrate throughout the small intestinal mucosa. The result is a severe malabsorption syndrome with all its attendant complications. Chronic diarrhea, abdominal pain, nausea, and weight loss are common. Young adults between 20 and 30 years of age who live in the Mediterranean region are affected most commonly. There is no sexual preponderance. The diagnosis requires the demonstration of a monoclonal gammopathy in serum or urine that consists only of alpha heavy chains and that is devoid of light chains. Because serum electrophoresis may appear normal, sensitive immunoelectrophoretic procedures and other special studies are often necessary to establish the diagnosis. The disease is progressive in most patients, although spontaneous remissions in some patients have suggested that the disease may represent an unusual reaction to infection.

Very few patients with *mu chain disease* have been described. Most have had a chronic lymphocytic leukemia with a small monoclonal component that is usually difficult to detect on serum electrophoresis. The diagnosis requires the demonstration by serum immunoelectrophoresis of an IgM monoclonal globulin that is devoid of light chains, although free light chains may be present in the urine. Insufficient data are available to determine whether the natural history of this disease differs from that of chronic lymphocytic leukemia.

REFERENCES

ALEXANIAN R et al: Prognostic factors in multiple myeloma. Cancer 36:1192, 1975

————: Combination therapy for multiple myeloma. Cancer 40:2765, 1977

AXELSSON U et al: Frequency of pathologic proteins (M-components) in 6995 sera from an adult population. Acta Med Scan 179:235, 1966

FRANGIONE B, FRANKLIN EC: Heavy chain diseases: Clinical features and molecular significance of the disordered immunoglobulin structure. Semin Hematol 10:53, 1973

ISOBE T, OSSERMAN EF: Patterns of amyloidosis and their associations with plasma cell dyscrasia, monoclonal immunoglobulins and Bence-Jones proteins. N Engl J Med 290:473, 1974

KYLE RA, BAYRD ED: Amyloidosis: Review of 236 cases. Medicine 54:271, 1975

————, ————: The Monoclonal Gammopathies. Springfield, Ill, Charles C Thomas, 1977

MacKENZIE MR, FUDENBERG HH: Macroglobulinemia: An analysis of 40 patients. Blood 39:874, 1972

64
AMYLOIDOSIS

ALAN S. COHEN

DEFINITION AND CLASSIFICATION   Amyloidosis may be defined as the extracellular deposition of the fibrous protein amyloid in one or more sites of the body. This protein has unique ultrastructural, x-ray diffraction, and biochemical characteristics. It can be deposited locally where it has no clinical consequences or may involve virtually any organ system of the body leading to severe pathophysiologic changes, or the disease may fall between these two extremes. The natural history of amyloidosis is poorly understood, and the clinical diagnosis is often not made until the disease is far advanced. The following classification is clinically the most useful: (1) primary amyloidosis (no evidence for preexisting or coexisting disease); (2) amyloid associated with multiple myeloma; (3) secondary amyloidosis associated with chronic infectious diseases (e.g., osteomyelitis, tuberculosis, leprosy) or chronic inflammatory diseases (e.g., rheumatoid arthritis and ankylosing spondylitis); (4) heredofamilial amyloidosis, the amyloidosis associated with familial Mediterranean fever and a variety of neuropathic, renal, cardiovascular, and other syndromes; (5) local amyloidosis (local, often tumor-like, deposits occur in isolated organs without evidence of systemic involvement); and (6) amyloidosis associated with aging.

PATHOLOGY AND STRUCTURE   Amyloid is amorphous, eosinophilic, hyalin, extracellular, and ubiquitous in distribution. The involved organs may have a rubbery firm consistency and a waxy, pink or grey appearance. Organ enlargement, especially of the liver, kidney, spleen, and heart, may be prominent.

Microscopically, amyloid stains pink with the hematoxylin-eosin stain and shows metachromasia with crystal violet or methyl violet. The Congo red stain imparts a unique green birefringence when sections are viewed in the polarizing microscope. This is the single most useful procedure for establishing the presence of amyloid. Amyloid deposits may be focal in almost any area of the body but are most often perivascular.

The heart may show focal or diffuse interstitial deposits in the myocardium, endocardium, or pericardium.

In the kidney, the glomerulus is primarily affected although interstitial, peritubular, and vascular amyloid occur. In early lesions, small nodular or diffuse deposits appear near the basement membrane and, as the disease progresses, the glomerulus may be massively laden with amyloid, and its capillary bed will be occluded.

In the gastrointestinal tract, there may be perivascular deposits only, or irregular or diffuse deposits may be found in the submucosa, in the muscularis mucosa, or subserosa. The amyloid may appear at any level or portion of the gastrointestinal tract including the gallbladder and pancreas.

In the nervous system, amyloid has been described along peripheral nerves, in autonomic ganglia, and in senile plaques as well as blood vessels of the central nervous system. It may be found in any portion of the orbit including the vitreous humor and cornea.

In summary, there is virtually no area of the body that is spared. This ubiquitous distribution elicits a wide variety of clinical symptoms and signs.

All types of human amyloid consist of fine, nonbranching rigid fibrils that in tissue sections measure approximately 100 Å in diameter. The amyloid fibrils are usually seen earliest in the mesangial cell in the kidney and Kupffer cell in the liver. Isolated amyloid fibrils have a delicate, thin, nonbranching fibrous character. The individual fibril (or filament) has a diameter of about 70 Å and tends to aggregate laterally. Each fibril (filament) has subunit protofibrils of 30 to 35 Å diameter.

A second component, the plasma component or pentagonal unit (P component) with a different ultrastructure, x-ray diffraction pattern, and chemical characteristics, has also been isolated from amyloid and is identical with a circulating α globulin present in very minute amounts. It is not responsible for the characteristic tinctorial properties or ultrastructure of amyloid.

BIOCHEMISTRY OF AMYLOID FIBRILS   The bulk of amyloid deposits consists of fibrils. The homology of the fibril of primary and myeloma amyloid to the N-terminal region of the variable fragment of an immunoglobulin light chain and subsequently, in a limited number of cases, to a homogeneous light polypeptide chain, has been demonstrated. These light chain–related proteins range in size from about 5000 to 25,000 daltons and are now termed amyloid light chain (AL) or A_κ or A_λ (Table 64-1). Amino acid sequence analysis indicates that most primary amyloid proteins contain the N-terminal amino acid residue identical to the variable regions of the light chain (Asp-Ile-Gln-Ser-Pro-Ser-Ser-Leu- . . .).

Another protein that is unrelated to any known immunoglobulin has been described in the secondary amyloid deposits. This protein, amyloid A (AA) protein, can be isolated from the amyloid of patients with secondary amyloidosis and from that associated with familial Mediterranean fever. It is a unique protein with a molecular weight of about 8500 daltons made up of 76 amino acid residues arranged in a single chain, and an amino acid sequence beginning with Arg-Ser-Phe . . . .

Antiserums to alkali-degraded amyloid fibrils of the AA protein have detected an antigenically related serum component, SAA. Amino acid analysis, peptide maps, and sequence studies suggest that AA protein is an amino terminal fragment of SAA and is derived from it by proteolysis. SAA appears to behave as an acute phase reactant and is elevated in infection, inflammation, and with aging. In addition, SAA is elevated in amyloid-resistant animals suggesting that the appearance of

TABLE 64-1
Helsinki nomenclature of amyloid

Current usage	New nomenclature
TISSUE ISOLATES	
Amyloid fibril protein related to immunoglobulin light chains	AL (or A_κ or A_λ) subtype when known, for example, A_{KI}
Amyloid of unknown origin, nonimmunoglobulin amyloid, amyloid A, A protein	AA
Pentagonal unit of amyloid, plasma component of amyloid, P component	AP
SERUM ISOLATES	

To designate the serum-related component, simply add S as a prefix; i.e., the serum-related AA would now be SAA (instead of amyloid serum component, ASC, etc.). It is recognized that the serum-related component of AL may simply be designated as kappa or lambda light chains or Bence-Jones proteins.

SOURCE: *Cohen AS, Rheumatology-Immunology: The Scientific Basis of Clinical Medicine, New York, Grune & Stratton, 1979, with permission.*

amyloid is not solely determined by the level of SAA. SAA appears to suppress antibody response, suggesting that it might act as an immune regulator.

P component of amyloid In addition to the characteristic fibrils described above, a minor second component, the P component, has been noted in most amyloid deposits. P component (AP) has been recognized by electron microscopy as a pentagonal-shaped structured unit having an outside diameter of about 90 Å and an inside diameter of about 40 Å. On immunoelectrophoresis it migrates as an alpha globulin, and it possesses antigenic identity with a constituent of normal human plasma. The amino acid sequence is distinct from that of the amyloid fibrils. Its pentagonal ultrastructure is similar to C-reactive protein (CRP), but the latter is one-half the molecular weight of AP and has other well-defined differences despite a similar amino acid sequence.

IMMUNOBIOLOGY OF AMYLOID The etiology and pathogenesis of amyloidosis are unknown. Electron microscopic autoradiographic studies have revealed high concentrations of fibrils adjacent to reticuloendothelial cells, suggesting that these cells may synthesize as well as degrade the fibrils.

An excess antigenic stimulus has been shown to induce amyloid in animals. However, the basic conditions for the experimental induction of amyloidosis have not been clearly defined. Marked depression of T cells with maintenance of normal or hyperactive B-cell function has been described. These findings suggest that disturbances in immunoregulatory mechanisms may be an important step in the pathogenesis of amyloid disease.

CLINICAL MANIFESTATIONS The clinical manifestations of amyloidosis are varied and depend entirely on the area of the body which is involved.

Kidney Renal involvement may consist of mild proteinuria or frank nephrosis. In some cases, the urinary sediment may show only a few red blood cells. The renal lesion is usually not reversible and in time leads to progressive azotemia and death. The prognosis does not appear to be related to the degree of the proteinuria; when azotemia finally develops, the prognosis is grave. In one series the mean survival of patients with renal amyloid from the time of biopsy was 29 months, but in a few cases there was presumptive evidence of regression of the renal amyloid. Hypertension is rare except in long-standing amyloi-

dosis. Renal tubular acidosis or renal vein thrombosis may occur. Localized accumulation of amyloid may be noted in the ureter, bladder, or other parts of the genitourinary tract.

Liver While hepatic involvement is common, liver function abnormalities are minimal and occur late in the disease. The two tests most useful in indicating hepatic amyloid are the Bromsulphalein (BSP) extraction and serum alkaline phosphatase activity. Liver scans produce variable and nonspecific results. Portal hypertension occurs but is uncommon. In a series of 54 patients in which liver tissue was available for examination, all 54 had some amyloid present either in the parenchyma or blood vessels, irrespective of the type of amyloidosis (primary or secondary). Amyloidosis of the spleen characteristically is not associated with leukopenia and anemia.

Heart Cardiac manifestations consist primarily of congestive failure and cardiomegaly (with or without murmurs) and a variety of arrhythmias. Although the cardiac manifestations reflect predominantly diffuse myocardial amyloid, the endocardium, the valves, and the pericardium may be involved as well. Pericarditis with effusion is very rare, although the differential diagnosis of constrictive pericarditis versus restrictive cardiomyopathy frequently arises. Echocardiography has demonstrated symmetrical thickening of left ventricular wall, hypokinesia and decreased systolic thickening of the interventricular septum and left ventricular posterior wall, and left ventricular cavities of small to normal size. Hearts which are heavily infiltrated with amyloid may or may not show an enlarged silhouette. Fluoroscopy usually shows decreased mobility of the ventricular wall; angiographic studies usually demonstrate thickened ventricular wall, decreased ventricular mobility, and absence of rapid ventricular filling in early diastole. Cardiac amyloidosis can present as intractable heart failure. Electrocardiographic abnormalities include a low-voltage QRS complex and abnormalities in atrioventricular and intraventricular conduction, often resulting in varying degrees of heart block. Owing to their propensity to develop conduction defects and arrhythmias, patients with cardiac amyloidosis appear to be especially sensitive to digitalis, and this drug should be used with caution.

Skin Involvement of the skin is one of the most characteristic manifestations of so-called "primary" amyloidosis. The lesions may consist of slightly raised, waxy papules or plaques which usually are clustered in the folds of the axillae, anal, or inguinal regions, the face and neck, or mucosal areas such as ear or tongue. The lesions are seldom pruritic. Involvement of the skin or mucosa may not be apparent clinically but may be disclosed by biopsy. Gentle rubbing of the skin may induce bleeding into the skin, leading to purpura. Cutaneous involvement also can occur in secondary amyloidosis; in one series it was found in 42 percent of such patients, in 55 percent of a group of patients with primary disease, and in all eight patients with hereditary amyloid neuropathy.

Gastrointestinal tract Gastrointestinal symptoms are common in amyloidosis. They may result from direct involvement of the gastrointestinal tract at any level or from infiltration of the autonomic nervous system with amyloid. The symptoms include those of obstruction, ulceration, malabsorption, hemorrhage, protein loss, and diarrhea. Infiltration of the tongue occasionally leads to macroglossia. When not enlarged, the tongue may become stiffened and firm to palpation. While infiltration of the tongue is characteristic of primary amyloidosis or amyloidosis accompanying multiple myeloma, it is occasionally seen in the secondary form of the disease.

Gastrointestinal bleeding may occur from any of a number of sites, notably the esophagus, stomach, or large intestine, and may be severe. Amyloid infiltration of the esophagus may lead to abnormal motility patterns. Small-bowel lesions may lead to clinical and x-ray changes of obstruction. A malabsorption syndrome is seen at times. Amyloidosis may develop in association with other entities involving the gastrointestinal tract, especially tuberculosis, granulomatous enteritis, lymphoma, and Whipple's disease; differentiation of these conditions, which give rise to secondary amyloidosis, from diffuse primary amyloidosis of the small bowel may be difficult. Similarly, amyloidosis of the stomach may closely mimic gastric carcinoma, with obstruction, achlorhydria, and the radiologic appearance of tumor masses.

Nervous system Neurologic manifestations may include peripheral neuropathy, postural hypotension, inability to sweat, Adie pupil, hoarseness, and sphincter incompetence. These manifestations are especially prominent in the heredofamilial amyloidoses. The cranial nerves are generally spared except for those involving the pupillary reflexes. The protein concentration in the cerebral spinal fluid may be increased. Infiltrates of the cornea or vitreous body may be present in hereditary amyloid syndromes. Certain of these syndromes are characterized by a bilateral scalloping appearance of the pupil. Amyloid may infiltrate the thyroid or other endocrine glands but rarely causes endocrine dysfunction. Local amyloid deposits almost invariably accompany medullary carcinoma of the thyroid. Amyloid infiltration of muscle may lead to a pseudomyopathy.

Joints Amyloid can directly involve articular structures by its presence in the synovial membrane and synovial fluid or in the articular cartilage. Amyloid arthritis can mimic a number of rheumatic diseases because it can present as a symmetrical arthritis of small joints, including nodules, morning stiffness, and fatigue. Most patients with amyloid arthropathy eventually are found to have multiple myeloma. The synovial fluid usually has a low white blood cell count, a good to fair mucin clot, a predominance of mononuclear cells, and no crystals.

Respiratory system The nasal sinuses, larynx, and trachea may be involved by accumulations of amyloid which block the ducts, in the case of the sinuses, or the air passages. Amyloidosis of the lung involves the bronchi and alveolar septa diffusely. The lower respiratory tract is affected most frequently in primary amyloidosis and in the disease associated with dysproteinemia. Pulmonary symptoms attributable to amyloid are present in about 30 percent of these patients and in some are the most serious manifestations of the disease. In secondary amyloidosis, pulmonary disease is a frequent histopathologic accompaniment but seldom gives rise to clinically significant symptoms. Amyloid may also be localized in the bronchi or pulmonary parenchyma and may resemble a neoplasm. In these cases, local excision should be attempted and, when successful, may be followed by prolonged remissions.

Hematopoietic system Hematologic changes may include fibrinogenopenia, increased fibrinolysis, and selective deficiency of clotting factors.

HEREDOFAMILIAL AMYLOIDOSIS There is no generally accepted nosology for the heredofamilial amyloid syndromes. Some reports emphasize the site of predominant organ involvement as neuropathic, nephropathic, or cardiopathic amyloidosis, while others stress the genetic aspects. To date, virtually all analyses of pedigrees have shown that, with one major exception, the mode of inheritance is autosomal dominant. The exception is amyloidosis of familial Mediterranean fever which is inherited as an autosomal recessive disorder (Chap. 217). Since there are no specific biochemical, hematologic, or immunologic tests that enable the differentiation of one type of amyloid from another, the specific and recognizable clinical patterns form the basis for classification. Table 64-2 proposes a tentative classification and is based largely on the major site of organ involvement, in addition to genetic data and ethnic background.

The heredofamilial amyloidoses include a group primarily involving the nervous system. Among these are lower limb neuropathy, first described in Portugal, which has a poor prognosis and is characterized by progressively severe neuropathy including marked autonomic nervous system involvement. This variety also has been described in Japan and in a family of Greek origin in the United States and probably exists in several other kinships. In some of these individuals, bilateral "scalloped" pupils are pathognomonic of the disease. The second type of neuropathy has been found in families of Swiss origin in Indiana and of German origin in Maryland. It is a milder disease and is often associated with a carpal tunnel syndrome and vitreous opacities. A more severe variety of generalized neuropathy associated with renal amyloidosis has been described in Iowa in a family of English-Irish-Scottish ancestry.

Several types of severe familial renal disease in association with amyloid have been described. Possibly the most remarkable is familial Mediterranean fever (FMF), a disorder subdivided into phenotype I, with irregularly occurring fever and abdominal, chest, or joint pain, preceding or accompanying renal amyloid, and phenotype II, in which amyloidosis is the first or only manifestation of the disease (Chap. 217). Sporadically, other hereditary forms of renal amyloidosis have been described, including the curious association of urticaria, deafness, and renal amyloid.

Severe familial amyloid heart disease has been described in a Danish family, and familial persistent atrial standstill with amyloid in a family of Mexican-American origin. Miscellaneous hereditary amyloid syndromes include hereditary multiple endocrine neoplasms type II (including medullary carcinoma of the thyroid with amyloid) as well as others listed in Table 64-2.

DIAGNOSIS The specific diagnosis of amyloidosis depends upon obtaining a tissue specimen by biopsy and the demonstration of amyloid with appropriate stains. First, of course, the disease must be suspected. When a patient with a chronic disorder predisposing to amyloid such as rheumatoid arthritis,

TABLE 64-2
Heredofamilial amyloidoses

I Neuropathy
   A Lower limb (Portuguese, Japanese, Swedish, other)
   B Upper limb (Swiss-Indiana, German-Maryland)
II Nephropathy
   A Familial Mediterranean fever
   B Fever and abdominal pain (Swedish, Sicilian)
   C Urticaria, deafness, and renal disease
   D Renal disease and hypertension
III Cardiopathy
   A Progressive heart failure (Danish)
   B Persistent atrial standstill (Mexican-American)
IV Miscellaneous
   A Medullary carcinoma of the thyroid
   B Lattice corneal dystrophy and cranial neuropathy (Finland)
   C Cerebral hemorrhage (Iceland)

SOURCE: *Cohen AS, Rheumatology-Immunology: The Scientific Basis of Clinical Medicine, New York, Grune & Stratton, 1979, with permission.*

tuberculosis, paraplegia, multiple myeloma, bronchiectasis, or leprosy develops hepatomegaly, splenomegaly, malabsorption, cardiac disease, or, most importantly, proteinuria, amyloid should come to mind. In addition, in any heredofamilial syndromes, especially those which have a dominant autosomal mode of inheritance and are characterized by peripheral neuropathy, nephropathy, or cardiopathy, the diagnosis of amyloid should be considered. Finally, primary systemic amyloid should be considered in any individual with a diffuse noninflammatory infiltrative disease involving either mesenchymal tissues—blood vessels, heart, gastrointestinal tract—or parenchymal tissues—kidney, liver, spleen, adrenal.

When the diagnosis is suspected, it is good practice to perform a rectal biopsy. If there is a specific reason for not carrying out this procedure, other sites including skin, gums, or the suspected organ—kidney, liver—may be biopsied. All tissues obtained must be stained with Congo red and examined in the polarizing microscope for green birefringence.

In order to establish the relationship of immunoglobulin-related amyloid to multiple myeloma, electrophoretic and immunoelectrophoretic studies on serum or urine should be performed, when the biopsy reveals amyloid deposition. Most of these patients will have only relatively small paraprotein components and only a few will have frank multiple myeloma. The therapeutic implications of these findings are discussed in greater detail in Chap. 63.

PROGNOSIS AND TREATMENT The course of amyloidosis is difficult to document since dating the time of origin of the disease is rarely possible. When amyloidosis develops in patients with rheumatoid arthritis, it seldom becomes evident when the arthritis is less than 2 years in duration. The mean duration of arthritis before amyloidosis was detected was 16 years in one series. When amyloidosis develops in patients with multiple myeloma, manifestations leading to initial hospitalization are more apt to be related to amyloid disease than to myeloma. In these cases prognosis is very poor, and life expectancy is usually less than 6 months.

Instances have been reported of amyloidosis accompanying treatable infections, such as osteomyelitis, in which at least partial remission has occurred following treatment of the primary disease. There have been similar experiences following successful treatment of tuberculosis or drainage of chronic empyema. However, many such reports are not substantiated by biopsy proof of resorption.

Generalized amyloidosis is usually a slowly progressive disease and leads to death in several years, but it may have a better prognosis than was suspected in the past. The average survival in most large series is 1 to 4 years, but a number of individuals with amyloid have been followed 5 to 10 years and longer.

The major cause of death is renal failure. Sudden death, presumably due to arrhythmias, is also quite common. Occasionally, gastrointestinal hemorrhage, respiratory failure, intractable heart failure, and superimposed infections are the terminal events.

There is no specific therapy for any variety of amyloidosis. Rational therapy should be directed at (1) decreasing chronic antigenic stimuli that produce amyloid, (2) inhibition of the synthesis and extracellular deposition of amyloid fibrils, and (3) promoting lysis or mobilization of existing amyloid deposits.

A variety of agents have been used to treat amyloidosis. Proof of their efficacy is not available. The finding that a portion of the immunoglobulin light chain is incorporated in the amyloid of patients with primary amyloidosis and its presumed synthesis by plasma cells has led to the use of alkylating agents. However, these agents cause bone marrow depression, and there are reports of acute leukemia developing in patients receiving melphalan. Moreover, there is experimental evidence that immunosuppressive agents may enhance the deposition of preexisting amyloid. Hence, conservative and supportive measures provide the mainstay of management. It is important to provide these patients with a more optimistic outlook.

Two patients with severe renal amyloidosis and azotemia were subjected to bilateral nephrectomy and renal transplantation followed by immune therapy. One patient died of infection 5 months after surgery. The donor kidney showed no evidence of amyloidosis. The second patient is in clinical remission 7 years after receiving a transplanted kidney. Notwithstanding the hazards of operating upon patients with systemic amyloidosis who may have cardiac involvement, carefully selected azotemic patients could benefit from transplantation.

Colchicine has been shown to be effective in preventing acute attacks in patients with familial Mediterranean fever, and two groups of investigators independently have reported the inhibition of amyloid deposition in the mouse model by colchicine. It is conceivable, therefore, that colchicine is effective in blocking amyloid deposition. However, the exact mechanism of its action is unknown, and no controlled human clinical study has been reported.

REFERENCES

COHEN AS: Amyloidosis. N Engl J Med 277:522, 1967

———: Diagnosis of amyloidosis, in *Laboratory Diagnostic Procedures in the Rheumatic Diseases*, 2d ed, AS Cohen (ed). Boston, Little, Brown, 1975, p 395

——— et al: Amyloidosis: Current trends in its investigation. Arthritis Rheum 21:153, 1978

FRANKLIN EC, ZUCKER-FRANKLIN D: Current concepts of amyloid. Adv Immunol 15:249, 1972

GLENNER GG et al: Amyloid fibril proteins: Proof of homology with immunoglobulin light chains. Science 172:1150, 1971

Diseases of immune-mediated injury

65
DISEASES OF IMMEDIATE TYPE HYPERSENSITIVITY

K. FRANK AUSTEN

INTRODUCTION The capacity of a toxic substance, when injected repeatedly, to elicit an adverse reaction rather than a protected state was recognized and designated *anaphylaxis* by Portier and Richet in 1902. Von Pirquet, perceiving that immunity and hypersensitivity were intimately linked, coined the term *allergy* in 1906 to imply a state of changed reactivity. The inadvertent passive transfer of the capacity to develop an acute allergic response to horses by blood transfusion from an allergic to a nonallergic subject was recognized in 1919 by Ramirez. Passive transfer of serum from a patient allergic to fish to the skin of a normal recipient followed by the antigen-induced appearance of wheal and flare at that site was accomplished by Prausnitz and Küstner in 1921, and this technique became the reference for defining a specific allergy. The association of allergic rhinitis and asthma in the same patient, often with a familial background, and the presence in serum of passive transfer activity to the clinical allergen led Coca and Cooke in 1923 to introduce the concept of *atopy* to imply a propensity to develop the altered state without an unusual exposure to the relevant allergens. As presently used, the term *atopic allergy* implies a familial tendency to manifest alone or in combination such conditions as asthma, rhinitis, urticaria, and eczematous dermatitis (atopic dermatitis). However, individuals with an atopic background may also develop hypersensitivity reactions, particularly urticaria and anaphylaxis, associated with the same class of antibody found in atopic individuals. Thus, the designation *diseases of immediate type hypersensitivity* presents a more suitable framework than the broad term *allergy* or the restrictive definition of atopy.

The passively transferred activity in human serum belongs to a unique immunoglobulin class, IgE; a myeloma protein with skin-fixing capacity was independently recognized and shown to be of the same class. The fixation of IgE to human basophils has been demonstrated by radioautography and electron microscopy and to intraepithelial and perivenular mast cells in tonsils, adenoids, and nasal polyps of humans by immunofluorescence. The biochemical characteristics of mast-cell activation, mediator generation, and secretion of both preformed and newly derived mediators are considered elsewhere (Chap. 61) utilizing information gained from studies with human lung slices or peripheral blood leukocytes rich in basophils. IgE-dependent mediator generation and release also occur in the mast cells of human nasal polyps or skin and thus have been observed in those tissues most involved in diseases of immediate type hypersensitivity.

The physicochemically and functionally diverse mast-cell–derived mediators, presented in Chap. 257 include: histamine, which increases venular permeability and elicits both direct and reflex alterations in pulmonary mechanics; eosinophil chemotactic factor of anaphylaxis (ECF-A) which contains acidic tetrapeptides with preferential chemotactic activity for eosinophils; slow-reacting substance of anaphylaxis (SRS-A) with permeability-enhancing and smooth-muscle–contracting activity; platelet activating factors (PAFs), lipids capable of initiating platelet secretion and aggregation; a heparin proteoglycan; and diverse enzymes with degradative capacity, including a chymotrypsin-like protease termed chymase. Thus the mast cell, bearing a specific recognition unit in the form of IgE, and positioned in tissues, has the capacity to respond to a foreign substance by eliciting a local increase in venular permeability and by initiating the influx of certain cell types from the marginated cell pool; this response allows plasma proteins such as antibody and complement and various phagocytic cells to be recruited to the reaction site without the necessity for extensive local tissue injury. On the other hand, an uncontrolled response could proceed from a physiologic local reaction to a self-perpetuating inflammatory state.

Consideration of the mechanism of immediate type hypersensitivity diseases in the human has focused largely on the IgE-dependent recognition of otherwise nontoxic substances. Support for this thesis has come from the finding that clinical atopic allergy is associated with elevated total levels of IgE and in some instances with a specific immune response that is linked to the histocompatibility locus. Populations of allergic Caucasians have a significantly higher total serum level of IgE than nonallergic individuals, and highly atopic persons with asthma have significantly higher serum levels of IgE than those with fewer allergic manifestations. Further, IgE distribution in families is consistent with the dominant inheritance of the low IgE phenotype. Thus, as a result of the action of a single IgE regulator gene the majority of family members would have elevated IgE levels as a possible basis for their atopic state. The association between HLA histocompatibility type and the immediate hypersensitivity response has been noted in persons of the low IgE phenotype who were studied with highly purified allergens, generally of small size. Such presumptive evidence of immune response (Ir) genes by linkage disequilibrium, that is, the association of the hypersensitivity response with a particular histocompatibility haplotype, represents an additional element in the polygenic atopic allergic state. Nonetheless, all the studies taken together, both of families and of populations, seem to indicate that the genetically determined elevated IgE levels found in about three-fourths of atopic allergic subjects exert the predominant influence on most specific IgE responses. It is also likely that diseases of immediate type hypersensitivity may occur because of deficient intracellular controls of mediator generation or release, or both, or that the extracellular controls directed against mediator inactivation may be impaired.

ANAPHYLAXIS **Definition** The life-threatening anaphylactic response of a sensitized human appears within minutes after administration of specific antigen and is manifested by respiratory distress often followed by vascular collapse, or shock without antecedent respiratory difficulty. Cutaneous manifestations exemplified by pruritus and urticaria with or without angioedema are characteristic of such systemic anaphylactic reactions.

Predisposing factors and etiology   There is no convincing evidence that age, sex, race, occupation, or geographic location predisposes a human being to anaphylaxis except through exposure to some immunogen. According to some studies, but not others, atopy predisposes individuals to penicillin anaphylaxis.

The materials capable of eliciting the systemic anaphylactic reaction in the human include the following: heterologous proteins in the form of antiserum, hormones, enzymes, *Hymenoptera* venom, pollen extracts, and foods; polysaccharides such as iron dextran; and most commonly diagnostic agents and drugs such as antibiotics and even vitamins. The diagnostic and therapeutic agents are generally of low molecular weight and are considered to function as haptens which form immunogenic conjugates with host proteins. The conjugating hapten may be the parent compound, a nonenzymatically derived storage product, or a metabolite formed in the host.

Pathophysiology and manifestations   Individuals differ in the time of appearance of perception of symptoms and signs, but the hallmark of the anaphylactic reaction is the onset of some manifestation within seconds to minutes after introduction of the antigen, generally by injection or less commonly by ingestion. There may be upper or lower airway obstruction or both. Laryngeal edema may be experienced as a "lump" in the throat, hoarseness, or stridor, while bronchial obstruction is associated with a feeling of tightness in the chest or audible wheezing. A particularly characteristic feature is the eruption of well-circumscribed, discrete cutaneous wheals with erythematous, raised, serpiginous borders and blanched centers. These urticarial eruptions are intensely pruritic and may be localized or distributed. They may coalesce to form giant hives, and seldom persist beyond 48 h. A localized, nonpitting, deeper edematous cutaneous process, angioedema, may also be present. It may be asymptomatic or cause a burning or stinging sensation.

In fatal cases with clinical bronchial obstruction, the lungs show marked hyperinflation on gross and microscopic examination. The microscopic findings in the bronchi, however, are limited to luminal secretions, peribronchial congestion, submucosal edema, and eosinophilic infiltration, and the acute emphysema is attributed to intractable bronchospasm which subsides with death. The angioedema resulting in death by mechanical obstruction occurs in the epiglottis and larynx, but the process is also evident in the hypopharynx and to some extent the trachea; on microscopic examination there is wide separation of the collagen fibers and the glandular elements; vascular congestion and eosinophilic infiltration are also present. Patients dying of vascular collapse without antecedent hypoxia from respiratory insufficiency have visceral congestion but no major shift in the distribution of blood volume. Whether the associated electrocardiographic abnormalities, with or without infarction, noted in such patients reflect a primary cardiac event or are secondary to a critical reduction in plasma volume has not been established.

The manifestations of the anaphylactic syndrome have been attributed to release of endogenous histamine. The role of SRS-A in altering pulmonary mechanics by causing marked bronchiolar constriction awaits further definition. Vascular collapse without respiratory distress in response to experimental challenge with the sting of a hymenopteran was associated not only with marked and prolonged elevations in blood histamine but also with evidence of intravascular coagulation.

Diagnosis   The diagnosis of an anaphylactic reaction depends largely upon an accurate history revealing the onset of the appropriate symptoms and signs within minutes after the responsible material is encountered. When only a portion of the full syndrome is present, such as isolated urticaria, sudden bronchospasm in an asthmatic patient, or vascular collapse after intravenous administration of an agent it is difficult to exclude a nonimmunologic, toxicologic, or idiosyncratic response. For example, intravenous administration of a chemical mast-cell degranulating agent elicits generalized urticaria, angioedema, and a sensation of retrosternal oppression without clinically detectable bronchoconstriction or hypotension. Furthermore, nonsteroidal anti-inflammatory agents such as indomethacin, aminopyrine, mefenamic acid, and acetylsalicylic acid may precipitate a life-threatening episode of obstruction of upper or lower airways in asthmatic subjects which is clinically reminiscent of anaphylaxis but is not associated with a detectable IgE response.

The presence of a labile reagin (IgE) in the heart blood of a patient dying of systemic anaphylaxis has been demonstrated at postmortem by passive transfer of the serum intradermally into a normal recipient, followed in 24 h by antigen challenge into the same site, with subsequent development of a wheal and flare, the Prausnitz-Küstner reaction. Indeed, such a reagin can be transiently identified in the serum of most patients who develop systemic anaphylaxis to a variety of different agents. In order to avoid the hazards of transferring hepatitis to the recipient in the Prausnitz-Küstner reaction, it is preferable to employ the less sensitive monkey recipient or a human leukocyte suspension enriched with basophils for subsequent antigen challenge. It is presumed that the activity responsible for most cases of systemic anaphylaxis resides with the IgE class, since the Prausnitz-Küstner activity in the serums of patients with systemic reactions to Hymenoptera venom or human seminal plasma protein can be removed by IgE immunosorbent columns. Furthermore, radioimmunoassays have demonstrated specific IgE antibodies in patients with anaphylactic reactions to insulin and to parathromone, but such approaches require purified antigens. In the transfusion anaphylactic reaction which occurs in patients with IgA deficiency, the responsible specificity resides in IgG anti-IgA rather than in IgE; the mechanism of the reaction is presumed to be complement activation with secondary mast cell participation.

Treatment and prevention   Early recognition of an anaphylactic reaction is mandatory, since death occurs within minutes to hours after the first symptoms. Mild symptoms such as pruritus and urticaria can be controlled by administration of 0.2 to 0.5 ml of 1:1000 epinephrine subcutaneously, with repeated doses as required at 3-min intervals for a severe reaction. If the antigenic material was injected into an extremity, the rate of absorption may be reduced by prompt application of a tourniquet proximal to the reaction site, administration of 0.2 ml of 1:1000 epinephrine into the site, and removal without compression of an insect stinger, if present. An intravenous infusion should be initiated to provide a route for administration of epinephrine, diluted 1:50,000, volume expanders, and vasopressive agents if intractable hypotension occurs. Whether epinephrine acts to prevent mediator release, to reverse the action of mediators on target tissues, or both is not established; but its early administration appears critical. When epinephrine fails to control the situation, hypoxia due to airway obstruction or related to a cardiac arrhythmia, or both must be considered. Oxygen via a nasal catheter or intermittent positive pressure breathing of oxygen with 0.5 ml isoproterenol diluted 1:200 in saline may be helpful, but either endotracheal intubation or a tracheostomy is mandatory if progressive hypoxia exists. Ancillary agents such as the antihistamine diphenhydramine, 50 to 80 mg intramuscularly or intravenously, and aminophylline, 0.25 to 0.5 g intravenously, are appropriate for urticaria-angioedema and bronchospasm, respectively. Intravenous corticosteroids are not effective for the acute event but may be considered for persistent bronchospasm and hypotension.

Prevention of anaphylaxis must take into account the sensitivity of the recipient, the dose and character of the diagnostic or therapeutic agent, and the effect of the route of administration on the rate of absorption. If there is a definite history of a past anaphylactic reaction, even though mild, it is advisable to select another agent or procedure. A skin test should be performed before the administration of certain materials producing a high incidence of anaphylactic reactions, such as horse serum or allergenic extracts, or when the nature of the past adverse reaction is unknown. Since even a skin or conjunctival test can produce a serious reaction, a scratch test should precede these tests in a high-risk situation. With regard to penicillin, two-thirds of patients with a positive reaction history and positive intradermal skin tests to benzylpenicilloyl-polylysine (BPL) and/or the minor determinant mixture (MDM) of benzylpenicillin products experience allergic reactions with treatment, and these are almost uniformly of the anaphylactic type in those patients with minor determinant reactivity. Even patients without a history of previous clinical reactions have a 6 percent incidence of positive skin tests to the two test materials, and about 3 per 1000 with a negative history experience anaphylaxis with therapy with a mortality of about 1 per 100,000. The value of skin testing is both to permit therapy with the agent in question when the risk does not exist and to emphasize the hazards where the sensitivity is confirmed. In the event that an agent must be used despite a positive history, a positive skin test, or both, the following precautionary measures should be taken. An intravenous infusion should be started, with intubation equipment and a tracheostomy set at hand; the material should be given intradermally, then subcutaneously, and then intramuscularly in increasing doses at 20- to 30-min intervals so that the initial dose by the next route does not exceed the final dose by the previous route. It is difficult to be certain that the mediator-containing cells have been exhausted, and therapeutic use of the agent may be accompanied by untoward consequences. It may be critical to give the therapeutic agent at regular intervals to prevent the reestablishment of a sensitized cell pool of large size. A different form of protection involves the development of blocking antibody of the IgG class which is protective against Hymenoptera venom–induced anaphylaxis by interacting with antigen so that less reaches the sensitized tissue mast cells; to be effective this immunotherapy requires the use of specific or cross reacting Hymenoptera venom rather than whole insect body extracts.

URICARIA AND ANGIOEDEMA **Definition** Urticaria and angioedema may appear separately or together as cutaneous manifestations of localized nonpitting edema; a similar process may occur at mucosal surfaces of the upper respiratory or gastrointestinal tract. *Urticaria* involves only the superficial portion of the dermis presenting as well-circumscribed wheals with erythematous raised serpiginous borders with blanched centers which may coalesce to become giant wheals. *Angioedema* is a well-demarcated localized edema involving the deeper layers of the skin including the subcutaneous tissue. Recurrent episodes of urticaria and/or angioedema of less than 6 weeks duration are considered acute, while attacks persisting beyond this period are designated chronic.

Predisposing factors and etiology The occurrence of urticaria and angioedema is probably more frequent than usually described because of the evanescent, self-limited nature of such eruptions, which seldom require medical attention when limited to the skin. Although persons in any age group may expe-

rience acute or chronic urticaria and/or angioedema, these lesions increase in frequency after adolescence, with the highest incidence occurring in persons in the third decade of life; indeed, one survey of college students indicated that some 15 to 20 percent had experienced a pruritic wheal reaction.

The classification of urticaria/angioedema presented in Table 65-1 focuses on the different mechanisms for eliciting clinical disease. Only the IgE-dependent and the IgG-mediated reactions in IgA-deficient persons should be considered immediate hypersensitivity. However, the other mechanisms are important for differential diagnosis, and most cases of chronic urticaria are idiopathic. The appearance of urticaria and angioedema in atopic persons in the absence of a specific exposure is attributed to the atopic diathesis and implies an IgE mechanism. Urticaria and/or angioedema occurring during the appropriate season in patients with seasonal respiratory allergy or as a result of exposure to animals or molds is attributed to inhalation of pollens, animal dander, and mold spores, respectively. However, urticaria and angioedema secondary to inhalation are relatively uncommon compared with ingestion of fresh fruits, shellfish, chocolate, nuts, tomatoes, and various drugs, including penicillin-contaminated milk products, which may elicit not only the anaphylactic syndrome with prominent gastrointestinal complaints but also chronic urticaria. Additional etiologies include physical stimuli such as cold, solar rays, exercise, and mechanical irritation (dermographism). Angioedema without urticaria occurs with C1 inhibitor (C1 INH) deficiency that can be inborn as an autosomal dominant characteristic or can be acquired in association with lymphoproliferative disorders. The urticaria and angioedema associated with classical serum sickness or with idiopathic cutaneous necrotizing angiitis is believed to be an immune complex disease when hypocomplementemia is a concomitant. The idiosyncratic drug reactions to mast cell granule-releasing agents and to nonsteroidal anti-inflammatory drugs can be systemic, resembling anaphylaxis, or limited to cutaneous sites.

Pathophysiology and manifestations Urticarial eruptions are distinctly pruritic, involve any area of the body from the scalp to the soles of the feet, and appear in crops of 24- to 72-h duration with old lesions fading as new ones appear. The most common sites are the extremities, external genitalia, and face, particularly the region of the eyes and lips. Although self-limited in duration, angioedema of the upper respiratory tract may be life-threatening due to laryngeal obstruction, while gastrointestinal involvement may present with abdominal colic, with or without nausea and vomiting, and may precipitate unnecessary surgical intervention. No residual discoloration occurs with either urticaria or angioedema unless there is an underlying process leading to superimposed extravasation of erythrocytes.

TABLE 65-1
Classification of urticaria with angioedema

I IgE-dependent
  A Atopic diathesis
  B Specific antigen sensitivity (pollens, foods, drugs, therapeutic agents, Hymenoptera venom, helminths)
  C Physical: dermographism; cold; light; cholinergic; vibratory
II Complement-mediated urticaria
  A Hereditary angioedema
  B Acquired angioedema with lymphoproliferative disorders
  C Necrotizing vasculitis
  D Serum sickness
  E Reactions to blood products
III Nonimmunologic urticaria
  A Direct mast cell–releasing agents: opiates; antibiotics; curare, D-tubocurarine; radiocontrast media
  B Agents which presumably alter arachidonic acid metabolism: aspirin and nonsteroidal anti-inflammatory agents; azo dyes and benzoates
IV Idiopathic urticaria

The pathology of urticaria and angioedema is usually characterized by massive edema of the dermis in urticaria, and the subcutaneous tissue as well as dermis in angioedema. Collagen bundles in affected areas are widely separated, and the venules are sometimes dilated. The perivenular infiltrate may consist of lymphocytes, eosinophils, and neutrophils that are present in varying combination and number throughout the dermis. Allergen-induced wheal and flare reactions are characterized by mast-cell degranulation and an accumulation of eosinophils over hours to days. The elicitation of a wheal and flare response upon injection of the relevant allergen into a patient with urticaria and/or angioedema, or into a site in a normal recipient prepared with serum from the patient, the Prausnitz-Küstner reaction, indicates an IgE-dependent, mast-cell–mediated reaction.

Perhaps the best-studied example of mast-cell–mediated urticaria and angioedema is *cold urticaria*. Acquired cold urticaria is a disorder in which patients exposed to cold experience an urticarial eruption that may evolve into angioedema and be associated with syncope. Cryoglobulins, cryofibrinogens, cold agglutinins, or hemolysins may be recognized, but not in the majority of patients. The finding in a number of patients of a serum factor, characterized as being of the IgE class, that is capable of transferring the cold urticaria reaction to a skin site of a normal recipient has focused attention upon the mast cell in this condition. Immersion of an extremity in an ice bath precipitates angioedema of the distal portion with urticaria at the air interface within minutes of the challenge. Histologic studies reveal marked mast cell degranulation with associated edema of the dermis and subcutaneous tissues. The venous effluent of the cold-challenged and angioedematous extremity reveals a marked rise in plasma content of histamine, low-molecular-weight eosinophilotactic activity, and high-molecular-weight neutrophil chemotactic activity which are presumably of mast cell origin, whereas the venous effluent of the contralateral normal extremity contains none of these mediators.

Diagnosis The rapid onset and self-limited nature of urticarial and angioedematous eruptions are distinguishing features. Additional characteristics are the occurrence of the urticarial crops in various stages of evolution and the asymmetric distribution of the angioedema. Urticarial and/or angioedema involving IgE-dependent mechanisms are often appreciated by historical considerations implicating specific allergens, by seasonal incidence, by exposure to certain environments, or by physical stimuli such as cold, exercise, sunlight (solar urticaria), or trauma (dermographism). Direct reproduction of the lesion with physical stimuli is particularly valuable because it so often establishes the cause of the lesion. The diagnosis can be confirmed by careful testing with the putative foreign substance to determine if a local wheal and flare results, and by passive transfer of such a reaction with serum of the patient to a skin site in a normal recipient, the Prausnitz-Küstner phenomenon. Passive transfer to the skin of a nonhuman primate or in vitro to human basophils may also be attempted. IgE-mediated urticaria and/or angioedema may or may not be associated with an elevation of total IgE or with peripheral eosinophilia. Fever, leukocytosis, or an elevated sedimentation rate are characteristically absent.

The classification of urticarial and angioedematous states noted in Table 65-1 in terms of possible mechanisms necessarily includes some differential diagnostic points. Hypocomplementemia is not observed in IgE-mediated mast cell disease and can reflect either an acquired abnormality generally attributed to the formation of immune complexes or a genetic deficiency of C1 INH. Chronic recurrent urticaria and angioedema, generally in females, associated with arthralgias, an elevated sedimentation rate, and hypocomplementemia suggest an underlying cutaneous necrotizing angiitis. Confirmation depends upon a biopsy which reveals cellular infiltration, nuclear debris, and fibrinoid necrosis of the venules.

Hereditary angioedema is an autosomal dominant state associated with the absence of functional C1 INH. The diagnosis is suggested not only by family history but also by the lack of urticarial lesions, the prominence of recurrent gastrointestinal attacks of colic, and episodes of laryngeal edema. Laboratory diagnosis depends upon demonstrating the antigenic lack of C1 INH in most kindreds, but some kindreds have an antigenically intact nonfunctional protein and require a functional assay to establish the diagnosis. The natural substrates of uninhibited C1̄, C4, and C2 are chronically depleted but fall further during attacks due to the activation of additional C1 to C1̄. The pathogenetic peptide is cleaved from the C2 substrate and then fully activated by the additional proteolysis of plasmin. An acquired form of C1 INH deficiency, associated with lymphoproliferative disorders, has the same clinical manifestations and differs only in the lack of a familial element and in the reduction of C1̄/C1̄ as well as C1 INH, C4, and C2.

Urticaria and angioedema must be differentiated from contact sensitivity, an acute vesicular eruption that progresses to chronic thickening of the skin with continued allergenic exposure. They must also be differentiated from atopic dermatitis, a condition that may present as erythema, edema, papules, vesiculation, and oozing proceeding to a subacute and chronic stage in which vesiculation is less marked or absent, and in which scaling, fissuring, and lichenification predominate in a distribution that characteristically involves the flexor surfaces.

Prevention and treatment Identification of the etiologic factor(s) and their elimination provide the most satisfactory therapeutic program; this approach is feasible to varying degrees with IgE-mediated allergens or physical stimuli. Topically applied steroids are of no benefit in the management of urticaria and/or angioedema, and while systemic steroids have no proved value, they are helpful in an occasional patient with necrotizing cutaneous angiitis or even ordinary urticaria and angioedema. Antihistamines and sympathomimetic agents often provide symptomatic relief; cyproheptadine, hydroxyzine, and similar drugs are held to be even more beneficial. The therapy of C1 INH deficiency has been simplified by the finding that attenuated androgens correct the biochemical defect and afford prophylactic protection. Since the use of such agents for children and pregnant women is not yet accepted, the antifibrinolytic agent ε-aminocaproic acid may be used to control spontaneous attacks or for preoperative prophylaxis in some patients.

ALLERGIC RHINITIS Definition Allergic rhinitis is characterized by sneezing, rhinorrhea, obstruction of the nasal passages, conjunctival and pharyngeal itching, and lacrimation. Although commonly seasonal owing to its relation to airborne pollens, other patterns and etiologies occur. The use of the term "hay fever" to describe seasonal allergic rhinitis is a common convention but is literally inappropriate because the symptom complex is neither produced by hay nor associated with fever.

Predisposing factors and etiology Allergic rhinitis generally presents in atopic individuals, that is, in persons with a family history of a similar or related symptom complex and a personal history of collateral allergy expressed as eczematous dermatitis, urticaria, and/or asthma (Chap. 257). Symptoms generally appear before the fourth decade of life and tend to diminish gradually with aging, although complete spontaneous remissions are uncommon. A relatively small number of weeds which depend upon wind rather than insects for cross-pollination, as well as certain grasses and trees, produce sufficient quantities of pollen suitable for wide distribution by air currents to elicit seasonal allergic rhinitis. The dates of pollination of these species generally vary little from year to year in a particular locale but may be quite different in another climate. Molds, which are widespread in nature because they occur in soil or decaying organic matter, may propagate spores in a pattern dependent upon climatic conditions. Perennial allergic rhinitis occurs in response to allergens that are present throughout the year such as in desquamating epithelium in animal dander, the plant materials processed or chemicals utilized in an industrial setting, or the dust accumulating at work or at home. Dust has a diverse content including mites, and many patients with allergic rhinitis are sensitive only to house dust. Moreover, in many patients with this disease, no clear-cut allergen can be demonstrated. When present, the ability of allergens to cause rhinitis rather than lower respiratory symptoms may be attributed to their size, 10 to 100 μm. When inhaled, they are retained within the nose without progressing to the lower respiratory tract.

Pathophysiology and manifestations Episodic rhinorrhea, sneezing, and obstruction of the nasal passages with lacrimation and pruritus of the conjunctiva, nasal mucosa, and oropharynx are the hallmarks of allergic rhinitis. The nasal mucosa is pale and boggy, but the nares are not reddened or excoriated. The conjunctiva may be congested and edematous; the pharynx is generally unremarkable but may appear injected. Swelling of the turbinates and mucous membranes with obstruction of the sinus ostia and eustachian tubes precipitates secondary infections of the sinuses and middle ear, respectively, commonly in perennial but rarely in seasonal disease. Nasal polyps often arise concurrently with edema and/or infection within the sinuses and increase obstructive symptoms.

The nose presents a large mucosal surface area through the folds of the turbinates and thus serves to adjust the temperature and moisture content of inhaled air and to filter out particulate materials. The convoluted nasal passages readily filter out particles above 10 μm in size by impingement in a mucous blanket at bends in their course; ciliary action then moves the entrapped particles toward the pharynx. Entrapment of pollen and digestion of the outer coat by mucosal enzymes such as lysozymes release protein allergens generally of 10,000 to 40,000 molecular weight. Although the initial interaction occurs between the allergen and intraepithelial mast cells sensitized with specific IgE, the bulk of the mast cells are located beneath the mucosal surface and are recruited secondarily. During the symptomatic season when the mucosa are already swollen and hyperemic, there is enhanced adverse reactivity to the seasonal pollen as well as to antigenically unrelated pollens for which there is underlying hypersensitivity. This priming effect is attributed to improved penetration of the allergens to the deeper perivenular mast cells. Biopsy specimens of nasal mucosa during an episodic allergic reaction show profound submucosal edema with infiltration predominantly by eosinophils, although some neutrophil polymorphonuclear leukocytes are present. Polyps, a feature in perennial rhinitis, are mucosal protrusions containing chiefly edema fluid with variable degrees of eosinophilic infiltration.

The muccosal surface fluid contains not only IgA that is present preferentially because of its secretory piece, but also IgE, which apparently arrives by diffusion from plasma cells distributed in proximity to mucosal surfaces. IgE fixes to mucosal and submucosal mast cells, and the intensity of the clinical response to inhaled allergens is quantitatively related to the naturally occurring or experimentally defined pollen dose. Specific IgE is distributed not only to tissue mast cells but also to circulating basophilic leukocytes; patients with more severe clinical disease have basophils which release histamine in response to lesser concentrations of allergen in vitro than do cells from patients with milder disease. Human nasal polyps from ragweed-sensitive patients release histamine, ECF-A, and SRS-A upon challenge with ragweed allergen in vitro. Polyps from nonallergic patients with cystic fibrosis or chronic sinusitis, passively sensitized by interaction with serum of a ragweed-sensitive patient, release the same mediators upon challenge with the allergen. Thus, the mast cells of nasal polyp tissue, and presumably of the nasal mucosa and submucosa, generate and release mediators through IgE-dependent reactions which are capable of producing tissue edema and eosinophilic infiltration.

Diagnosis The diagnosis of seasonal allergic rhinitis depends largely upon an accurate history of occurrence coincident with the pollination of the offending weeds, grasses, or trees. The continuous character of perennial allergic rhinitis due to contamination of the home or place of work makes historical analysis difficult, but there may be a variability in symptoms that can be related to animal exposure or work habits. Patients with perennial rhinitis commonly develop the problem in adult life, are more often women than men, and manifest nasal polyps and thickening of the sinus membranes by x-ray. The term *vasomotor rhinitis* designates a symptom complex resembling perennial allergic rhinitis without an established allergic basis. Other entities to be excluded are exposure to irritants, upper respiratory infection, pregnancy with prominent nasal mucosal edema, prolonged topical use of alpha-adrenergic agents in the form of nose drops, and the use of certain therapeutic agents such as rauwolfia. Nasal polyps are a characteristic of perennial allergic rhinitis and are often associated with sinus infection.

The nasal secretions of allergic patients are rich in eosinophils, and peripheral eosinophilia with elevations in relation to clinical exacerbations is a common feature. Local or systemic neutrophilia implies infection. Total serum IgE is frequently elevated, but the demonstration of immunologic specificity for IgE is critical to an etiologic diagnosis. Some normal individuals will exhibit a wheal and flare skin response to intracutaneous inoculation of high concentrations of common airborne allergens. The diagnosis rests not only on the skin test alone, but also on the correlation of the clinical history with skin reactivity to concentrations of allergen selected by controlled testing. This provides the best balance of selectivity with specificity. Scratch tests with food allergens are unreliable but are not dangerous, while intracutaneous testing may be, and elimination diets are the best approach to the diagnosis. Regardless of method of testing, food allergy is uncommon as a significant cause of allergic rhinitis.

Although standard radioimmunodiffusion techniques can be used to screen for patients with markedly elevated levels of IgE, their sensitivity of less than 1000 ng/ml is insufficient to detect the elevations in most atopic allergic patients. A commonly employed technique, sensitive to about 50 ng/ml, is known as the competitive radioimmunosorbent test (RIST). In this procedure, the IgE of the serum competes with radiolabeled IgE for solid-phase-bound anti-IgE; the displacement of radiolabeled IgE is compared to a standard curve to yield the IgE concentration of the serum. Other assays, such as the noncompetitive RIST and double antibody radioimmunoprecipitin test (RIP), have greater sensitivity and reproducibility, respectively, and, like the competitive RIST, establish a normal geometric mean serum IgE for nonallergic Caucasians of less than 120 ng/ml. Even more useful is the measurement of specific anti-IgE in serum by its binding to a solid-phase allergen and quantitation by the subsequent uptake of radiolabeled anti-IgE. This radioallergosorbent technique (RAST) correlates satisfactorily with the bioassay of specific IgE by skin test or histamine release from peripheral blood leukocytes and is convenient for the patients; however, it requires defined allergens and full standardization.

Prevention and treatment Avoidance of exposure to the offending allergen is the most effective means of controlling allergic diseases; removal of pets from the home to avoid animal danders, utilization of air filtration devices to minimize the concentrations of airborne pollens, travel to nonpollinating areas during the critical periods, and even a change of domicile to eliminate a mold spore problem may be necessary. *Immunotherapy*, often termed *hyposensitization* consists of repeated subcutaneous injections of gradually increasing concentrations of the allergen(s) considered to be specifically responsible for the symptom complex. Controlled studies in ragweed and grass allergic rhinitis have established that patients are partially relieved of their symptoms by such treatments applied over a period of years. Improvement appears to be dose-related, and the end point is based either on severe adverse local or systemic reactions to the allergen injection or on satisfactory relief of symptoms. The immunologic characteristics of a response include a rise in antibodies of the IgG class, a small increase in specific IgE early in the treatment course followed by a plateau or decline, and a decline in the percentage of histamine released from peripheral blood basophilic leukocytes challenged with a fixed concentration of the allergen. The antibodies of the IgG class might well reduce or neutralize the quantity of allergen available for interaction with the tissue mast cells but, more importantly, could modify the seasonal booster response in specific IgE synthesis. None of the individual parameters of the response to immunotherapy correlates well with the assessments of clinical efficacy, suggesting that benefit is derived from a complex of effects. Immunotherapy should be reserved for clearly documented seasonal diseases that cannot be managed with drugs because of their side effects.

Management with pharmacologic agents offers a diverse approach. Antihistamines are the only specific end-organ antagonists available for control of a mast-cell–derived reaction and are limited to competition with but one mediator. Nonetheless, antihistamines are very effective for some patients, and the side effects such as drowsiness and gastrointestinal distress, which limit the dosage of a particular preparation, can sometimes be circumvented by use of an agent of different structure. An orally active agent with alpha-adrenergic activity is often employed for its decongestant effects and to partially counteract the drowsiness produced by antihistamines. Topical administration of alpha-adrenergic agents may be helpful but has the immediate disadvantage of rebound vasodilatation and prolonged usage may produce a chronic rhinitis. The topically active steroids of the beclamethasone class ameliorate symptoms of both seasonal and perennial rhinitis without detectable adrenal suppression and may represent a major advance in therapy in view of the earlier favorable results with certain other steroids which were more readily absorbed. Cromolyn sodium inhaled nasally has also given encouraging prophylactic results and is of particular merit because it acts to prevent mast-cell activation.

REFERENCES

AUSTEN KF: Systemic anaphylaxis in the human being. N Engl J Med 291:277, 1973

BIAS WB, MARSH DG: The genetic basis of asthma: current studies of the genetics of the IgE-mediated immune response in man, in *Asthma: Physiology, Immunopharmacology and Treatment. Second*

International Symposium, LM Lichtenstein, KF Austen (eds). New York, Academic, 1977, p 21

GREEN GR et al: Evaluation of penicillin hypersensitivity: value of clinical history and skin testing with penicilloyl-polylysine and penicillin G. J Allerg Clin Immunol 60:339, 1977

KALINER M et al: Immunologic release of chemical mediators from human nasal polyps. N Engl J Med 289:277, 1973

KAPLAN AP et al: In vivo studies of mediator release in cold urticaria and cholinergic urticaria. J Allergy Clin Immunol 55:394, 1975

LICHTENSTEIN LM, NORMAN PS: Pathogenesis of allergic rhinitis, in *Immunological Diseases*, 2d ed, M Samter (ed). Boston, Little, Brown, 1971, p 825

NORMAN PS, LICHTENSTEIN LM: Allergic rhinitis: Clinical course and treatment, in *Immunological Diseases*, 2d ed, M Samter (ed). Boston, Little, Brown, 1971, p 840

SOTER NA et al: Urticaria and arthralgias as manifestations of necrotizing angiitis (vasculitis). J Invest Dermatol 63:485, 1974

66
IMMUNE-COMPLEX DISEASES

BRUCE C. GILLILAND
MART MANNIK

DEFINITION Immune-complex diseases are characterized by the deposition of antigen-antibody complexes in vascular and glomerular basement membranes and by the presence of these complexes in the circulation and in other body fluid compartments. The localization of immune complexes in tissues initiates immunologically mediated inflammation with resultant tissue damage. Immune-complex diseases have a common pathogenic mechanism, but the etiology is variable since the sources of antigens differ from disease to disease. The immune-complex diseases constitute a clinical syndrome which includes glomerulonephritis, arthritis, skin eruptions, pericarditis, pleuritis, and vasculitis at diverse sites.

PATHOGENESIS Upon the first exposure to a foreign substance, the host develops an antibody response after a week or 10 days. The synthesized antibodies result in formation of antigen-antibody complexes, which facilitate removal of the antigen. Normally, the majority of immune complexes are removed by cells in the reticuloendothelial system (also called the mononuclear phagocyte system). However, when complexes are deposited at other sites, such as along vascular and glomerular basement membranes, inflammation may develop at these sites, leading to the signs and symptoms of immune-complex disease.

The concepts of immune-complex disease in humans have evolved largely through study of animal models, including both spontaneous and experimentally induced disease. Acute serum sickness can be induced in experimental animals by injection of a foreign protein such as bovine serum albumin. Antigen disappears from the circulation in three phases: the first represents equilibration of the antigen between the intra- and extravascular compartments; the second is produced by catabolism of the antigen; the third involves the immune clearance of the antigen due to newly made specific antibodies. During the initial part of the immune-clearance phase, small circulating immune complexes are formed. As more antibody is synthesized, the lattice structure of the immune complexes increases until the complexes reach a critical lattice structure. Then the complexes are rapidly removed from the circulation by the reticuloendothelial system in the liver and elsewhere. Once the circulating immune complexes reach a critical size, the complement system is activated. This is manifested by a decrease in total hemolytic complement or individual complement components. This event does not ensue if the complexes are formed by antibodies incapable of complement activation. The overwhelming bulk of the antigen in the form of immune complexes is removed from the circulation by the reticuloendothelial system. For example, in experimental animals less than 1 percent of the circulating immune complexes becomes entrapped in the kidneys as determined in chronic serum sickness models or by intravenous injection of preformed immune complexes. Yet these small quantities of immune complexes suffice to cause glomerulonephritis. In human diseases no data are available on the total burden of circulating immune complexes or on the amount deposited in kidneys. The exact nature of the complexes that become deposited in the vascular or glomerular basement membranes is not certain, but persistence of complexes in the circulation is a requirement for development of renal disease. In rabbits, the release of vasoactive amines facilitates the deposition of immune complexes in the glomeruli, but in humans this mechanism has not been demonstrated. Coincident with circulating immune complexes and complement utilization, clinical abnormalities develop in experimental animals (Fig. 66-1). These abnormalities include glomerulonephritis, vasculitis, arthritis, skin eruptions, pleuritis, and pericarditis. Once the antigen is completely cleared, the complement levels return to normal, and gradually the lesions in target organs subside. Thus, acute serum sickness is a limited disease and progresses only as long as antigen persists in the recipient.

In experimental animals the acute serum sickness model can be converted to a chronic serum sickness or immune-complex disease model by repeated administration of antigen. The development of clinical abnormalities in such models can be achieved by frequent (daily or several times a week) administration of an appropriate dose of antigen. For development of maximal lesions the total dose of antigen should result in slight antigen excess in relation to the specific antibody pool. In such a model, renal failure due to chronic proliferative glomerulonephritis can be achieved. These animals also develop vasculitis in other locations, and extensive antigen, antibody, and C3 deposits are identifiable.

A chronic immune-complex disease can develop spontaneously in animals with viral or other microbial infection that provides a continued source of antigen for immune-complex formation. Glomerulonephritis develops in mice with persistent lymphocytic choriomeningitis virus, Maloney sarcoma virus, or lactic dehydrogenase virus infection and in Aleutian disease of mink. Immune complexes consisting of antivirus antibody, virus antigen, and complement components (mainly C3) can be identified in the kidney and serum of these animals. Immune-complex nephritis resembling closely that of systemic lupus erythematosus occurs in the F_1 hybrid of New Zealand black and New Zealand white mice. Deoxyribonucleic acid (DNA), antibodies to DNA, and C3 deposits are found in the glomerular basement membrane. The role of viruses in the etiology and pathogenesis of this disease model remain under investigation.

A localized experimental immune-complex disease can be generated by repeated injection of a foreign substance into the same location of an immunized animal. For example, rabbits immunized with a foreign protein, such as bovine serum albumin, develop arthritis when the same protein is injected into the joint cavity. Intense inflammation can be induced in a similar manner in the pericardial and pleural cavities. Again, the local immunologically induced inflammation progresses as long as antigen is present. The synovitis of rheumatoid arthritis appears to be a local immune-complex disease of joints.

Immune complexes activate complement components, leading to formation of vasoactive peptides and chemotactic factors. Neutrophils accumulate in the involved area and phagocytize the immune complexes, resulting in release of lysosomal enzymes and subsequent damage to structural components of tissue. Later in the course of the lesions monocytes, T cells, and B cells accumulate because of specific chemotactic factors. Newly arrived B cells evolve to plasma cells that synthesize antibodies to the antigen present at the site. For example, if bovine serum albumin is used to induce arthritis in the rabbit, the bulk of plasma cells in the synovium of this animal will synthesize antibodies to bovine serum albumin.

PATHOLOGY Light microscopy of the renal lesion of acute serum sickness or immune-complex disease reveals swelling of endothelial cells and the presence of a few leukocytes. In the chronic form, thickening of the basement membrane is accompanied by accumulation of neutrophils and proliferation and swelling of endothelial cells. Epithelial cells proliferate to form crescents with eventual obliteration of Bowman's space. The renal lesions may be classified as showing mesangioproliferative, focal proliferative, diffuse proliferative, or membranous glomerular involvement, depending on the extent of the disease and the characteristics of the inflammatory response. Immunofluorescent studies of the kidney in both the acute and chronic forms of disease reveal granular deposits of immunoglobulin and complement (C3) in the mesangial matrix or along the glomerular basement membrane. Transmission electron microscopy shows electron-dense deposits in the mesangial matrix, the subendothelial space, the subepithelial space, and the glomerular basement membrane.

This history of the vascular lesion initially shows accumulation of neutrophils and proliferation of endothelial cells. This is followed by disruption of the internal elastic lamina and fibrinoid necrosis of the vessel wall. Mononuclear cells appear later. The vasculitis may vary from an intense inflammatory lesion consisting mainly of polymorphonuclear cells to one in which only perivascular cuffing with mononuclear cells is seen at the time of biopsy. If the examination is made early in the

FIGURE 66-1

Schematic presentation of events in experimental acute serum sickness. In this experimental animal, antibody production began on the eighth day with the appearance of circulating immune complexes and subsequent decrease in serum complement (C). Vasculitis, glomerulonephritis, and arthritis develop after deposition of immune complexes. With the clearance of immune complexes by the reticuloendothelial system, the pathogenic process ceases, free antibody can be detected, and the inflammatory events run their course and gradually abate.

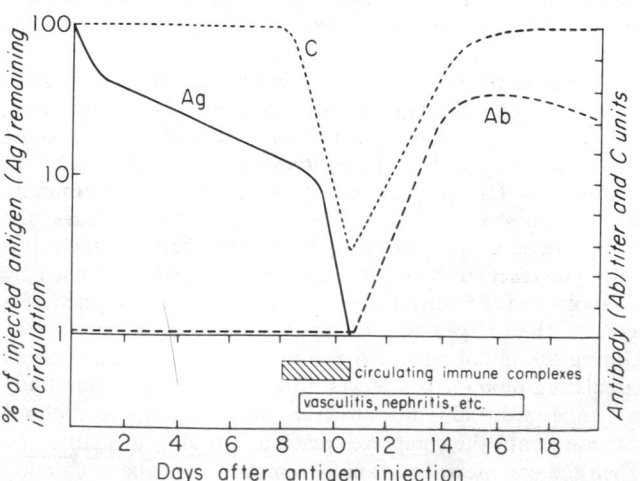

course, granular deposits of immunoglobulin and complement may be identified by immunofluorescence. However, within hours, these immune deposits are removed by the inflammatory response.

ETIOLOGY For any given immune-complex disease the etiology depends on the nature and source of the antigens that form immune complexes as well as the immunogens that incite the immune response. In most immune-complex diseases the antigen and immunogen are the same substance, but in certain autoimmune diseases they may differ. Thus, in immune complex diseases the etiologic factors may be drugs, microorganisms, tumors, or the host's own tissues. If strict criteria are employed, the etiology of an immune-complex disease is defined when the specific antigens and antibodies causing the tissue inflammation are identified. This has been achieved largely by elution of antigens and antibodies from the target tissues or by immunofluorescent microscopy using specific antigens and antibodies. The list of established immune-complex diseases has grown steadily (Table 66-1). A number of diseases, particularly glomerulonephritis and vasculitis, have all the hallmarks of immune-complex diseases in terms of the clinical pattern of the disorder and the deposition of immunoglobulins at sites of inflammation, but the involved antigens are not defined—therefore, these disorders are often listed as "probable" immune-complex diseases.

Drugs produce immune complex disease either by acting as immunogens or by inducing synthesis of autoantibodies by an unknown mechanism. Numerous drugs and foreign proteins (e.g., penicillins, sulfonamides, horse antitoxin to tetanus, and horse antihuman lymphocyte serum) are potentially immunogenic and cause immune-complex disease. Binding of a drug or its metabolite to a serum protein may be necessary for its immunogenicity.

A form of immune-complex disease restricted to the destruction of platelets or red blood cells is occasionally observed after administration of stibophen, phenacetin, quinine, or quinidine. Antibodies made in response to one of these drugs combine with the drug to form immune complexes. These complexes are absorbed to the blood cell surface and activate complement, leading to either hemolytic anemia or thrombocytopenia. Some drug-induced neutropenias may also develop by this mechanism.

Other drugs do not act as immunogens but instead stimulate the synthesis of autoantibodies, especially those with specificity to nuclear antigens. Patients receiving drugs such as procainamide, hydralazine, or hydantoins may form antibodies to nuclear antigens and manifest features of systemic lupus erythematosus. Several months of drug administration may be required before the onset of symptoms. The autoantibodies persist for months after administration of the drug has been discontinued.

Several types of infections are accompanied by immune-complex disease, and many have glomerulonephritis as a common feature. Antigens derived from the responsible microorganisms are presumed to be released at the site of bacterial growth and then are deposited as immune complexes in glomeruli. Examples include poststreptococcal glomerulonephritis, the glomerulonephritis of bacterial endocarditis, infected ventriculoatrial shunt, osteomyelitis, quartan malaria, and hepatitis B infection.

Manifestations of immune-complex disease may accompany viral infections. For example, the preicteric phase of hepatitis B infection can be recognized by the appearance of fever, arthritis, and skin eruptions along with low serum complement and circulating hepatitis-associated antigen. As the arthritis and rash subside and complement levels return to normal, the hepatitis-associated antigen disappears from the circulation, and antibodies to the antigen can then be demonstrated

with the onset of clinical manifestations of hepatitis. In this disorder the immune complexes consist of viral surface antigens (HBsAg) and the specific antibody.

Fungal diseases such as coccidioidomycosis may be accompanied by erythema nodosum and arthritis, most likely due to immune complex deposition.

Patients with malignancies may develop arthritis, arthralgia, and skin eruptions. Renal biopsies in some patients with nephrotic syndrome associated with adenocarcinoma of the colon have shown IgG, complement components, and carcinoembryonic antigen in the glomerular basement membrane. As methods are developed for identifying other tumor antigens, examples of immune complex disease will increase.

The autoimmune group of disorders is characterized by immune complexes composed of autologous antigens and their specific antibodies. The prototype of this group is systemic lupus erythematosus characterized by formation of antibodies to nuclear antigens (Chap. 68). In particular, deposition of immune complexes consisting of native DNA, and antibodies to native DNA, in the glomerular basement membrane and other tissue leads to inflammation at these sites. Another example is mixed cryoglobulinemia in which immune complexes composed of IgG anti-IgG can be identified in the cryoprecipitate. The antibody in these immune complexes consists of IgG, IgA, or IgM, and the antibody specificity is directed to IgG. These complexes are soluble at body temperatures and show progressive insolubility as the temperature is lowered. Upon deposition, they produce glomerulonephritis, arthritis, and vasculitis. Cutaneous lesions may also develop owing to precipitation of complexes at reduced temperatures in the extremities. Immune complexes of IgG-anti-IgG are also found in rheumatoid arthritis and in hypergammaglobulinemic purpura of Waldenström, in which joint inflammation, pleuritis, pericarditis, and vasculitis are not uncommon.

Autologous antigens may be released by prior tissue damage to serve first as immunogens and later as antigens in the generation of immune-complex disease. For example, in sickle-cell disease, renal tubular cell antigens are released from damaged tubular cells, antibodies to these antigens are synthesized, and the resultant immune complexes are deposited in the glomerular basement membrane.

Many forms of vasculitis, especially small-vessel vasculitis, are caused by deposition of immune complexes (Chap. 67). Biopsy of an involved site may reveal immunoglobulins along

TABLE 66-1
Immune-complex diseases in humans

I Administered (exogenous) antigens
  A Serum sickness (animal antitoxins, antiserums, hormones, drugs)
  B Drug-induced hemolytic anemia and thrombocytopenia (stibophen, quinine, quinidine, phenacetin)
  C Hypersensitivity pneumonitis (e.g., farmer's lung)
II Microbial antigens
  A Poststreptococcal glomerulonephritis
  B Glomerulonephritis of bacterial endocarditis, infected ventriculoatrial shunts, syphilis, typhoid fever, toxoplasmosis, quartan malaria, schistosomiasis, infectious mononucleosis
  C Arthritis, polyarteritis, glomerulonephritis of hepatitis B infection
III Autologous antigens
  A Systemic lupus erythematosus
  B Rheumatoid arthritis
  C Mixed cryoglobulinemia
  D Thyroiditis
  E Glomerulonephritis due to renal tubular antigen
IV Tumor antigens
  A Glomerulonephritis with colonic carcinoma, bronchogenic carcinoma, clear-cell renal carcinoma

with complement components. The absence of these substances, however, does not exclude an immune-complex pathogenesis because immune complexes may be destroyed by the inflammatory process within hours of their deposition. The nature and source of antigens that lead to immune-complex–induced vasculitis are largely unknown. In some patients with periarteritis nodosa, hepatitis-associated antigen is found in the serum. Furthermore, the antigen, antibodies, and complement components are present in the involved vessel wall, suggesting a pathogenic role for these specific immune complexes.

A localized form of immune-complex disease occurs when antibodies come in contact with their antigens at or near the site where antigen is being released or where it is being absorbed. The gingivitis of periodontal disease is thought to be generated by complexes composed of bacterial antigens from the plaque and the specific antibodies. Studies of experimental thyroiditis indicate that antibodies specific to thyroglobulin react with this antigen as it is released from the follicular cells. Immune complexes are formed between the follicular basement membrane and the follicular cells, leading to interstitial inflammation. Thyroiditis in humans may be produced by a similar mechanism. The synovitis of rheumatoid arthritis also represents a localized immune-complex disease, in part attributed to antibodies to IgG (rheumatoid factors) that are produced in the synovium. Hypersensitivity pneumonitis, such as pigeon breeder's lung and farmer's lung, results from antibodies uniting with the respective inhaled antigen in the alveolar wall (Chap. 258).

CLINICAL MANIFESTATIONS Since immune-complex diseases have a common pathogenic mechanism, many of the clinical manifestations are similar even though the responsible antigens may be quite different. Glomerulonephritis, arthritis, and skin lesions are frequently observed, either individually or in various combinations. The characteristics of skin lesions can be indicative of the size of involved blood vessels. The involvement of small vessels causes palpable purpura, urticaria, morbilliform eruptions, and maculopapular eruptions. The inflammation of arterioles and small arteries leads to small infarcts, ulcerations, and bullous lesions. The involvement of even larger vessels leads to digital gangrene. Renal involvement may not be apparent clinically or by urinalysis; however, biopsy may show immune deposits in the mesangium or in the glomerular capillary loop. Pleuritis, pericarditis, and small-vessel vasculitis also occur. The number and severity of clinical manifestations vary among patients, even when the disorder is produced by a single etiologic agent. The reasons for this variability are not apparent.

The clinical manifestations and course of the acute, self-limited form of immune-complex disease are best exemplified by serum sickness following injection of a foreign protein such as horse antitoxin to diphtheria or tetanus. In the person who has not been previously exposed to the antitoxin, the first manifestation is reddening and swelling at the site of injection, occurring 1 to 2 weeks after antitoxin administration. This is followed within a few days by fever, myalgia, skin lesions, arthralgias or arthritis, gastrointestinal symptoms, and lymphadenopathy including nausea, vomiting, and abdominal pain. The skin lesions are most commonly urticarial; but petechial, erythematous, macular, or morbilliform lesions may be seen. Arthritis usually begins in one or two joints and rapidly progresses to include many joints. The wrists, ankles, knees, and small joints of the hand are most commonly involved. Acute glomerulonephritis with red blood cell casts, proteinuria, and decreasing renal function may develop. Vasculitis of the vasa nervorum produces peripheral neuropathy. Rarely meningoencephalitis may develop. In a person with previous exposure to

the antitoxin, the above manifestations may appear 3 to 4 days following exposure. The same syndrome may occur after administration of a drug or in association with infection.

An anaphylactoid reaction may follow administration of a drug or foreign protein in a previously immunized patient who has preformed circulating antibodies to the specific antigen (Chap. 65). This reaction begins minutes after exposure and is characterized by urticaria, bronchospasm, dyspnea, diarrhea, hypotension, and shock. This reaction may be fatal. It is caused by the release of large amounts of vasoactive peptides.

Chronic forms of immune-complex disease occur in patients who have prolonged or repeated availability of the antigen. Such conditions are seen when the antigen is released from a persistent microorganism or a persistent tumor, or when the antigen is a normal constituent of the host. Examples include bacterial endocarditis, adenocarcinoma of the colon, and systemic lupus erythematosus.

DIAGNOSIS Immune-complex disease should be suspected in a patient presenting with arthritis, skin eruptions, and glomerulonephritis. It should also be considered in patients with pericarditis, pleuritis, vasculitis, and/or neuropathy. When the presence of an immune-complex disease is suspected, the offending antigen must be identified by historical or laboratory inquiry. A detailed history of drug exposure is extremely important. The presence of chronic bacterial or viral infections must be sought by history and by physical and laboratory examinations.

Several diseases with diffuse vascular involvement in many organ systems may mimic immune-complex disease. Patients with a left atrial myxoma may have showers of skin lesions due to small emboli of myxomatous tissue. Similarly, patients with nonbacterial thrombotic endocarditis have peripheral embolization to small blood vessels. These patients may also have arthralgias. Patients with thrombotic thrombocytopenic purpura develop skin lesions, arthralgias, or arthritis, central nervous system abnormalities, and renal failure. The severity of the thrombocytopenia and absence of an inflammatory component in the purpuric skin lesions help to distinguish this entity from immune-complex disease.

LABORATORY FINDINGS The laboratory abnormalities in patients with immune-complex disease include an elevated erythrocyte sedimentation rate, anemia, mild leukocytosis, and occasionally eosinophilia. The cerebrospinal fluid often shows pleocytosis. The urine may contain protein, red blood cells, and red blood cell casts. Serum complement may be low. Conduction abnormalities may be present on the electrocardiogram.

In the patient suspected of having immune-complex disease, the search for antigen should include blood cultures for detection of bacteria that may release the antigens and serologic tests for viral antigens, such as the hepatitis B antigen. Serologic tests for detection of antibody to microbial antigens may be useful in detecting the underlying etiology. These include heterophil, antistreptolysin O, and fluorescent treponemal antibody absorption tests, to mention just some. Tumor antigens, such as the carcinoembryonic antigen, should be sought. In the autoimmune diseases, antibodies to nuclear antigens and antibodies to IgG (rheumatoid factors) point to the underlying disorder. Tests for cryoglobulins should be performed; if they are found, specific antigens and antibodies can be characterized. Measurements of serum complement can be helpful in supporting the diagnosis initially and in following the course of immune-complex diseases. Since immune complexes primarily activate the classic complement pathway, both the early and late components of complement will be consumed. A normal complement level does not exclude the presence of immune-complex disease because the rate of synthesis may compensate for the degree of complement consumption.

The biopsy and routine histological examination of suspected vasculitic skin lesions is relatively innocuous and useful in the diagnosis of immune-complex diseases with vasculitis (Chap. 67). Examination of tissue by immunofluorescence or by electron microscopy may be helpful in establishing the diagnosis of immune-complex disease. Demonstration of IgG and complement components in the glomerular basement membrane by immunofluorescence indicates deposition of immune complexes. They stain in a granular or "lumpy" pattern. In contrast, a linear pattern of staining is seen when antibody is directed to antigens of the glomerular basement membrane (e.g., in Goodpasture's syndrome). Also, the detection of immunoglobulin and complement in the wall of involved blood vessels suggests an immune-complex etiology. Phagocytosis of these deposited complexes results in the finding of immunoglobulins and complement in the phagolysosomes of neutrophils and macrophages.

The finding of decreased total hemolytic complement, decreased complement components, immunoglobulin and complement tissue deposits, or elevated titers of specific antibodies provides only inferential evidence for the presence of circulating immune complexes.

The detection and quantification of circulating immune complexes is possible with specialized techniques. Immune complexes can be identified by analytical ultracentrifugation, but this technique is insensitive. Certain monoclonal rheumatoid factors (anti-IgG antibodies) are effective in combining and precipitating with immune complexes containing IgG. Also, the first component of complement (Clq) can be used to detect complexes containing IgG since this molecule combines firmly with IgG in large-latticed immune complexes. It is also possible to detect circulating immune complexes by the use of a human lymphoblastoid cell line (called the Raji cell line). Complement-fixing immune complexes bind to these cells through complement (C3b, C3d, and Clq) receptors. These techniques are limited by the requirement to form an immune complex lattice of a critical size, in order to facilitate binding of complement or interaction with cell receptors, and by the subclass of antibody. The presence of antibodies to lymphocytes may cause false-positive tests for immune complexes in the Raji cell assay. The presence of circulating DNA or endotoxin may cause false-positive tests for immune complexes in the assay with Clq.

TREATMENT The principles of therapy for immune-complex diseases are to remove the offending antigen and to reduce the inflammation when it threatens to compromise organ function. When a drug is suspected of causing immune-complex disease, its administration should be stopped immediately. In patients with immune-complex disease associated with an infection, such as bacterial endocarditis, adequate doses of the appropriate antibiotic should be given.

The treatment of anaphylactic reactions is considered in Chap. 65.

In acute or subacute immune-complex disease, anti-inflammatory drugs such as salicylates will usually reduce joint pain. Antihistamines or small doses of epinephrine will relieve urticaria. In some patients the severity of disease warrants the use of corticosteroids which help to minimize clinical manifestations. Prednisone, 40 mg per day, can be given over a 2-week period with gradual tapering. Tissue damage may be slowed in chronic immune-complex disease by the use of corticosteroids alone or in combination with immunosuppressive drugs. Treatment of the chronic forms of immune-complex disease is discussed in detail in the chapters dealing with the specific disorders.

REFERENCES

BEAUFILS M et al: Glomerulonephritis in severe bacterial infections with and without endocarditis. Adv Nephrol 7:217, 1978

COCHRANE CB, KOFFLER D: Immune complex disease in experimental animals and man. Adv Immunol 16:185, 1963

HAAKENSTAD AO, MANNIK M: The biology of immune complexes, in *Autoimmunity*, N Talal (ed). New York, Academic, 1977

KENNETH SR et al: Application of the solid phase Clq and Raji cell radioimmune assay for the detection of circulating immune complexes in glomerulonephritis. J Clin Invest 62:61, 1978

LAMBERT PH et al: A WHO collaborative study for the evaluation of eighteen methods for detecting immune complexes in serum. J Clin Lab Immunol 1:1, 1978

ROY LP et al: Etiologic agents of immune deposit disease, in *Progress in Clinical Immunology*, RS Schwartz (ed). New York, Grune & Stratton, 1972

THEOFILOPOULOS AN et al: The Raji cell radioimmune assay for detecting immune complexes in human sera. J Clin Invest 57:169, 1976

ZUBLER RH, LAMBERT PH: Detection of immune complexes in human diseases. Prog Allergy 24:1, 1978

67
VASCULITIS

MART MANNIK
BRUCE C. GILLILAND

Many clinical syndromes of necrotizing inflammation of blood vessels exist. In most of these conditions the etiology is not known, but several descriptive classifications have been offered, depending on the size of the involved blood vessels, the anatomic sites, the stage of the inflammation, and the histologic characteristics of the lesions. In these conditions cellular infiltration, necrosis, and fibrinoid deposits are present in the walls of blood vessels and perivascular areas. The cellular infiltrates are composed of polymorphonuclear leukocytes in acute stages; with progression of the lesion, monocytes, lymphocytes, and plasma cells appear. Giant cells are encountered in some types of vasculitis. Endothelial edema and proliferation, together with hemorrhage, contribute to diminution or occlusion of the vascular lumen and subsequent ischemic symptoms and signs.

Most forms of vasculitis are thought to be caused by immunologic phenomena. Multiple reasons exist for this belief. Necrotizing inflammation of blood vessels is a common finding in experimentally induced immune-complex diseases (Chap. 66). Vasculitis is a known manifestation of human serum sickness and occurs frequently in several known immune-complex diseases. For example, in systemic lupus erythematosus DNA, antibodies to DNA and complement components have been identified in vascular lesions. In mixed cryoglobulinemia IgG, antibodies to IgG and complement components have been seen in involved vessels. Furthermore, in some patients with polyarteritis the hepatitis-associated antigen has been implicated as the causative agent with the finding of antigen, immunoglobulins, and complement in the lesions. In other types of necrotizing inflammation, immunoglobulins and complement components have been visualized with immunofluorescence microscopy, but antigens have not been identified. Future work should identify the etiologic factors in many forms of vasculitis. Until then, however, the histologic and clinical features of the vasculitides serve to classify them.

Periarteritis nodosa was delineated by Kussmaul and Maier in the last century. In the early 1950s Zeek's careful descriptive work laid the foundation for most of the classifications of vasculitides. The descriptive classifications of vasculitides have been helpful in predicting the prognosis and response to therapy of individual patients. Upon careful microscopic examination of the lesions, the vasculitides can usually be placed in one of the five categories indicated in Table 67-1. However, at times the clinical problem defies categorization, and even within each of these categories variability from patient to patient is common. The nature of the antigen, the type of antibodies produced, the size of immune complexes formed, and cellular immunity are factors that may play a role in the pleomorphism of the clinical picture in the various vasculitides.

PERIARTERITIS NODOSA **Pathology** In periarteritis nodosa (polyarteritis nodosa) the necrotizing inflammation involves medium and small arteries, adjacent veins, occasionally arterioles and venules, but not capillaries. The lesions involve segments of vessels, at times affecting only part of the circumference, and there is a predilection for the bifurcation of arteries. These areas may form small aneurysms, which may rupture. During the active disease each patient has acute lesions that show predominantly polymorphonuclear leukocytic infiltration of the vessel walls and perivascular areas, as well as chronic lesions with mononuclear cell infiltration and partial healing. These observations suggest that the disease process is continuous, with repeated insults, and if it is caused by immune mechanisms, there must be repeated or continuous availability of antigen(s).

The lesions of periarteritis nodosa are widespread throughout the body; they are commonly found in such places as the coronary arteries, mesenteric arteries, kidneys, muscles, and vasa nervorum. The extent and location of lesions dictate the severity of clinical symptoms. Central nervous system involvement is unusual. The lungs are usually not involved, but this question has caused controversy and confusion among those contributing to literature in the field. Necrotizing inflammation and granuloma formation in blood vessels accompanied by lung involvement and eosinophilia should be classified as allergic granulomatosis.

Clinical manifestations Periarteritis nodosa is usually a disease of adulthood, but it occurs in childhood and senescence.

It affects two to three men for every woman. The onset of the disease is extremely variable. Often an antecedent history of upper respiratory tract infection or reaction to drugs is recorded.

The early complaints of patients with polyarteritis nodosa include fever, weakness, anorexia, weight loss, myalgias, and arthralgias. With the progression of the disease several organs may show involvement. Small, 5- to 10-mm nodules occur along the course of the arteries as a result of aneurysm formation. Involvement of vessel walls leads to occlusion, ecchymoses, ulceration (often secondarily infected), and gangrene of fingers or toes. Muscle weakness may evolve. Arthralgias are common, but severe and persistent arthritis is uncommon. Mononeuritis multiplex develops because of involvement of the vasa nervorum. Asymmetric and multiple nerve trunks may be involved. Retinal exudates and hemorrhages may occur.

Pericarditis and pleuritis, with or without effusions, are common. Involvement of coronary arteries may lead to myocardial ischemia or infarction, but electrocardiographic abnormalities may be recorded in the absence of symptoms.

Abdominal complaints are frequent (in 60 to 70 percent of patients) and include abdominal pain, nausea, vomiting, diarrhea, and bleeding. All these symptoms are related to the involvement of the mesenteric arteries. The mesenteric vasculitis may lead to mucosal ulceration, with hemorrhage, perforation, and infarction. The acute abdominal symptoms early in the disease lead to erroneous diagnoses of intraabdominal catastrophies of other causes, often resulting in unavoidable but unnecessary laparotomy. The liver may be involved, and massive hepatic infarction has been reported. Periarteritis of the gallbladder may cause cholecystitis and perforation.

Renal involvement occurs in over half the patients, and affects predominantly arteries and arterioles. Glomerulosclerosis occurs with severe involvement. Hypertension may evolve along with renal failure. However, hypertension may occur early in the disease when renal function is normal. Rupture of intrarenal aneurysms may cause renal infarcts or perinephric hematomas.

The causes of death in polyarteritis nodosa include renal failure, myocardial infarction, infections, congestive heart failure, and gastrointestinal bleeding.

Laboratory findings and diagnosis No specific chemical or serologic tests exist for periarteritis nodosa. The leukocyte count is elevated in about 80 percent of patients, principally because

TABLE 67-1
Classification of vasculitis

Periarteritis nodosa	Allergic granulomatosis	Wegener's granulomatosis	Hypersensitivity vasculitis	Giant-cell arteritis
SIZE OF INVOLVED BLOOD VESSELS				
Medium and small arteries, adjacent veins	Small arteries, adjacent veins, occasional arterioles	Small arteries, arterioles, venules, some capillaries	Arterioles, venules, capillaries	Large and medium arteries
HISTOLOGY AND STAGE OF LESIONS				
Necrotizing inflammation, coexistence of acute and healing lesions, no giant cells	Necrotizing inflammation with extravascular granulomas, coexistence of acute and healing lesions, giant cells in granulomas, abundant eosinophils	Necrotizing inflammation with granulomas, coexistence of acute and healing lesions, giant cells in granulomas	Necrotizing inflammation, all lesions in same stage, no giant cells	Inflammation without necrosis, no neutrophils, giant cells present
ANATOMIC PREDILECTIONS				
Widespread, common to branching points of arteries; lungs rarely involved	Widespread, but lungs frequently involved	Upper and lower respiratory tract involved; necrotizing glomerulitis	Widespread but common to skin, serosal surfaces, glomeruli	All large arteries, including aorta, coronary, vertebral, carotid, temporal, mesenteric

of neutrophilia. Anemia may be present because of blood loss and the inflammatory process. The erythrocyte sedimentation rate is often elevated. Other abnormalities depend on the organ involvement, e.g., hematuria, proteinuria, and decreased renal function due to kidney involvement or abnormal electrocardiogram (ECG) due to coronary artery vasculitis.

Angiography has become useful in documenting the diagnosis of periarteritis nodosa. The characteristic aneurysms at branching points of arteries occur in the kidneys, mesentery, liver, pancreas, and elsewhere during the acute phase of the disease. In late stages of the disease narrowing and thrombosis of arteries predominate in the same areas. In a number of reports the finding of arterial aneurysms on angiography has been employed to support the diagnosis of periarteritis nodosa. A large-scale study of the prevalence of these aneurysms during the course of the disease has not been reported.

The diagnosis of periarteritis nodosa often causes difficulties. This disease should be suspected in patients with involvement in several of the systems mentioned above, particularly in adult males. Infections, systemic lupus erythematosus, trichinosis, heart failure, Hodgkin's disease, and most other syndromes can be ruled out. Histologic examination of tissue is essential for proper diagnosis and for distinction from other vasculitides. Clinically involved tissue is best for histologic examinations, and tender subcutaneous nodules, tender muscles, and skin infarcts are suitable. Each tissue should be examined thoroughly because of the segmental nature of the lesions. Blind muscle biopsy has yielded positive information only in one-third of patients shown to have periarteritis later. Since vasculitis may involve the testes, testicular biopsy may be of diagnostic value.

Hepatitis-associated antigen has been found in the circulatory systems of 30 to 40 percent of patients with periarteritis nodosa. The same substance has been identified in vascular lesions along with immunoglobulins and complement, suggesting that in these patients the vasculitis is caused by immune complexes containing the hepatitis antigen. The liver involvement in these patients may be mild and overlooked unless liver function studies are performed. Some patients with this form of vasculitis have chronic liver disease, which may progress to hepatic failure. The evaluation of a patient with polyarteritis should include a search for the hepatitis B antigen.

In some patients the necrotizing vasculitis appears to follow a bout of serous otitis media. The basis of this association has not been established.

Treatment The prognosis of periarteritis nodosa with involvement of many organ systems is grim. Hypertension and renal involvement are thought to predict rapid progression of the disease. In untreated patients one-half to two-thirds have died within a year, but these statistics are heavily biased by postmortem studies and selective inclusion of severely ill patients. Treatment with corticosteroids frequently leads to rapid symptomatic improvement (initial dose 40 to 60 mg prednisone or prednisolone per day, tapered subsequently). In one study 5-year survival in untreated patients was estimated at 13 percent. Controlled studies on the use of cytotoxic (immunosuppressive) drugs have not been recorded, but some experiences suggest that these agents may help when other drugs have failed.

ALLERGIC GRANULOMATOSIS Allergic granulomatosis is separated from periarteritis nodosa because of prominent eosinophilia in the lesions, the presence of perivascular granulomas, and the clinical association with bronchial asthma.

Pathology In allergic granulomatosis small arteries and veins are most commonly involved in segmental fashion. Prominent eosinophilia is seen, epithelioid cells are numerous, giant cells

are present, and a marked accumulation of inflammatory cells occurs, thus leading to the granulomatous appearance. At times extravascular granulomas are present. The organ involvement is comparable to that of periarteritis nodosa, except that pulmonary involvement is seen with granuloma formation in the vessel walls and perivascular areas.

Manifestations Patients with allergic granulomatosis frequently give a history of an antecedent respiratory infection. Many have asthma that precedes evidence of vasculitis. In contrast to polyarteritis nodosa, fever is common. Fifty-four percent of these patients have peripheral eosinophilia, with eosinophils in excess of 1500 per cubic millimeter. The radiologic examination is not diagnostic, but parenchymal lung lesions include consolidation in small and large areas. Pleural effusions are not common.

The clinical findings due to involvement of other organs is quite similar to that in periarteritis nodosa, and includes the heart, kidneys, intestine, and peripheral nerves.

Treatment This has not been evaluated systematically. Sporadic reports and analogy to other forms of necrotizing vasculitis indicate that corticosteroids, in the same doses used for periarteritis, are the drugs of choice. Cytotoxic (immunosuppressive) drugs might be tried in patients unresponsive to corticosteroids.

WEGENER'S GRANULOMATOSIS See Chap. 218.

HYPERSENSITIVITY VASCULITIS (SMALL-VESSEL VASCULITIS) Hypersensitivity vasculitis has been given many names because of its varied clinical picture. The role of immunity in its pathogenesis is inferred by similarity to experimental models, and in some patients with this disorder the involvement of antigen-antibody complexes is documented. Basically, the arterioles, venules, and capillaries of many organs are involved by necrotizing inflammation. All lesions tend to be of the same age. The clinical picture depends on the extent of the disease and on the primary target organ. Systemic lupus erythematosus, rheumatoid arthritis, and mixed cryoglobulinemia are excellent examples of this type of vasculitis in which immune mechanisms have been implicated in the pathogenesis of the blood vessel inflammation. The finding that the cryoprecipitates from many patients with mixed cryoglobulinemia contain the hepatitis B surface antigen or its antibody suggests that this syndrome may be related to hepatitis B virus. Drugs and microbial infections have also been implicated as the causative agents. Small-vessel vasculitis is also seen in some patients with hyperglobulinemic purpura of Waldenström. These patients have characteristic purpura of the lower extremities, marked elevation of gamma globulin on serum protein electrophoresis, and intermediate complexes on ultracentrifugation of serum.

Pathology Hypersensitivity vasculitis (small-vessel vasculitis) is the most frequently encountered vasculitis. The inflammation and necrosis involve arterioles and capillaries, and not medium and large arteries. In some studies the lesions have been confined to venules. As a result, the clinical symptoms do not evolve from large vessel ischemia and infarction but result from hemorrhagic and exudative lesions and microinfarcts. Many organs may be involved, including skin, mucous membranes, brain, lungs, heart, gastrointestinal tract, kidneys, and muscle. Neutrophils have accumulated in small-vessel walls and in perivascular areas. Necrosis, edema, and extravasation of blood are present. Many neutrophils are fragmented; hence some prefer to call this form of vasculitis "leukocytoclastic angiitis." These patients may have detectable hypocomplementemia. In contrast, when the inflammatory lesions consist entirely of lymphocytes during the active phase of the disease, the serum complement levels are normal. Healing and hyalinization occur late. Focal or diffuse glomerulonephritis occurs in some patients. Characteristically all vascular lesions are in the same stage of evolution, in contrast to what occurs in periarteritis nodosa. This observation suggests episodic, rather than continuous, exposure to immune complexes, if indeed this is the mechanism of injury. Immunopathologic studies have shown deposits of immunoglobulins and complement components in active vasculitic skin lesions, if examined within 24 h of their development.

Clinical manifestations The clinical manifestations and onset of hypersensitivity vasculitis are variable, and the reasons for this variability are not known. In some patients the skin manifestations are extensive; systemic manifestations and involvement of other organs predominate throughout the course of the illness in others. In some the disease follows a quick course that leads to death, but most patients survive for years and may recover without recurrences.

In youngsters and in some adults hypersensitivity vasculitis may present as the Henoch-Schönlein syndrome, with prodromal headache, anorexia, fever, abdominal pain and bleeding, arthralgias, purpuric eruptions, and evidence of renal involvement. In adults the criteria for the Henoch-Schönlein syndrome are not usually fulfilled; however, in a group of adults with refractory urticaria and arthralgias, small-vessel vasculitis was present in the skin lesions.

The history of an antecedent respiratory infection may be obtained; drugs may have been ingested. (The list is long and includes penicillin, sulfonamides, other antibiotics, salicylates, phenylbutazone, phenacetin, propylthiouracil, busulfan, iodides, vaccines, and phenothiazines.) Fever is a common systemic symptom. The skin lesions include urticaria, purpura, ecchymoses, papules, nodules, vesicles, and necrotic ulcerations. Lesions may occur anywhere, but they tend to have some symmetry, and the lesions predominate in lower extremities—the legs, ankles, and feet. Patients frequently complain of itching, burning, stinging, and pain in the skin lesions. They may have myalgia, arthralgia, and arthritis. The joints may be warm, red, and painful with acute effusions. However, synovitis of long duration with synovial hypertrophy is unusual, and bony erosions do not develop, unless rheumatoid arthritis is present. Pulmonary infiltrates and pleural effusions may be found on chest roentgenograms. Pericarditis and myocarditis may develop, accompanied by electrocardiographic abnormalities. These patients may have peripheral neuropathy and encephalopathy, manifested by confusion, delirium, and coma. Diffuse electroencephalographic abnormalities may be present. Renal involvement becomes apparent, with microscopic hematuria, proteinuria, and decreasing renal function. Abdominal and gastrointestinal bleeding pain occur.

Similar clinical manifestations accompany the vasculitis associated with systemic lupus erythematosus, rheumatoid arthritis, and mixed cryoglobulinemias. Patients with subacute bacterial endocarditis may have small-vessel vasculitis, as manifested by the Osler's nodes, Roth's spots, arthralgias, and glomerulonephritis, although some of these lesions may be embolic in origin.

Laboratory findings Elevation of the erythrocyte sedimentation rate is the most common abnormality. Mild anemia and moderate leukocytosis occur. Complement levels may be reduced, particularly when neutrophilic infiltrates predominate

in the lesions. The finding of a positive test for antibodies to nuclear antigens suggests that the vasculitis is a feature of systemic lupus erythematosus. Similarly, the finding of a positive test for rheumatoid factor might indicate underlying rheumatoid arthritis, mixed cryoglobulinemia, or subacute bacterial endocarditis with vasculitis. Examination of the urinary sediment and evaluation of proteinuria and renal function are indicated for initial evaluation and follow-up of these patients. Biopsy of lesions is important.

Treatment The mortality figures for this disorder are variable because many series are based on autopsy findings. Spontaneous improvement occurs in some patients; in others the disease lingers. If drugs, toxins, or other environmental factors are suspected, all these exposures should be eliminated. If this disorder is immunologically mediated, then removal of the antigen would be the best treatment. Uncontrolled observations suggest that corticosteroids favorably influence the course of this disorder. The optimal dosages have not been determined; 40 to 60 mg prednisone or prednisolone seems reasonable at the onset, but the dose should be reduced when symptoms, signs, and laboratory tests show improvement. The dose should be increased when flare-ups occur. By analogy to systemic lupus erythematosus and Wegener's granulomatosis, cytostatic (immunosuppressive) drugs might be used in desperate situations. However, the results of controlled clinical trials with this therapy are not yet available.

GIANT-CELL ARTERITIS Giant-cell arteritis (also called *temporal or cranial arteritis*) is an inflammation of arteries in elderly persons. The cause of the disorder is unknown, and the pathogenesis of arterial inflammation has not been elucidated. However, some evidence for both humoral and cellular immunity to elastic arterial tissue has been presented. Any large or medium-sized artery may be involved, including the superficial temporal artery. Giant-cell arteritis responds dramatically to treatment with corticosteroids.

Pathology The inflammatory changes of giant-cell arteritis affect the large and medium-sized arteries without involving the arterioles and capillaries. Histiocytes, epithelioid cells, multinucleated giant cells, lymphocytes, and plasma cells accumulate in the intima and media adjacent to the internal elastic lamina of medium-sized arteries. The elastic lamina is highly fragmented and absent in some areas. In large arteries and the aorta, the media tends to be prominently involved with inflammation and fragmentation of the elastic fibers. The intima is thickened more than expected from age alone. The lesions are spotty and do not involve long stretches of the arteries. Thrombosis may occur at sites of inflammation.

The segmental lesions of giant-cell arteritis may involve any arteries, including the superficial temporal artery. The aorta is frequently involved, and aneurysms and dissection have been recorded. The external and internal carotid arteries and the vertebral artery systems are involved. Inflammation and occlusion of the ophthalmic or central retinal artery lead to blindness. Involvement of iliac, femoral, mesenteric, and coronary arteries may cause ischemia and infarction in the respective sites. The distribution and histopathology of the lesions in giant-cell arteritis resemble the pathology of pulseless disease or Takayasu's syndrome (see Chap. 252), but in the latter the lesions tend to be confined to the aorta and the disease starts in early life, particularly in women during the second and third decade.

Clinical manifestations Giant-cell arteritis is a disease of the elderly that affects both sexes nearly equally. This illness has rarely been diagnosed before the age of 50 or 60, and it is rare among blacks. The symptomatic involvement of arteries is frequently preceded by systemic symptoms, including fever, sweats, malaise, fatigue, anorexia, and weight loss. The fever tends to be low grade but may be striking. A fever of unknown origin in an elderly person, accompanied by a very high erythrocyte sedimentation rate, should always raise the diagnostic possibility of giant-cell arteritis.

Patients with giant-cell arteritis often have the *polymyalgia rheumatica* syndrome. This is characterized by an aching pain and stiffness in the neck and shoulders, which may extend to the upper arms and less frequently to the forearms. The hips and thighs may be similarly involved. Aching is increased with motion. Marked morning stiffness may be present. The muscles may be tender, and disuse atrophy may ensue. Joint pain in the shoulders, hips, and, less commonly, peripheral joints is reported, but objectively the joints are usually not inflamed and do not show synovial hypertrophy, even though small effusions may be present. Biopsy of asymptomatic temporal arteries will establish a histologic diagnosis of giant-cell arteritis in some patients with polymyalgia rheumatica. The segmental occurrence of the lesions must be considered in interpreting the results of the biopsies. The frequency of positive temporal artery biopsies varies from series to series, but the true prevalence of giant-cell arteritis in polymyalgia rheumatica remains unknown.

Headache is a frequent symptom, particularly in patients who have clinical temporal arteritis, with tender and thickened temporal arteries. The headache has no typical pattern, but marked scalp tenderness is often prominent. Furthermore, these patients may complain of intermittent claudication of the jaws and tongue upon mastication or talking.

Loss of vision is a serious complication of giant-cell arteritis. Blindness usually develops suddenly without significant warning, but mild visual disturbances may herald total visual loss. Usually for months or weeks these patients will have had other complaints suggestive of giant-cell arteritis or polymyalgia rheumatica. Aortic aneurysms, aortic dissection, mesenteric arteritis, myocardial ischemia, and infarction and claudication of the lower extremities have been attributed to giant-cell arteritis.

Laboratory findings The significant abnormalities in laboratory tests include a very high erythrocyte sedimentation rate (ESR), mild to moderate hypoproliferative anemia, and elevation of the α globulins and fibrinogen. The ESR exceeds 50 mm/h (by Westergren's method) and often reaches values above 100 mm/h. Important negative findings include normal serum levels of muscle enzymes and normal electromyograms, even in the presence of severe polymyalgia. Muscle biopsies disclose no characteristic changes.

In the absence of specific diagnostic tests, the diagnosis of giant-cell arteritis or polymyalgia rheumatica has to rest on clinical findings and a positive biopsy. Any one of the symptoms discussed above, in the presence of a high ESR in an elderly person, should raise the question of giant-cell arteritis or polymyalgia rheumatica. A temporal artery biopsy should be considered early in the evaluation of such patients. Other causes of high ESR must, of course, be considered, including occult neoplasms and chronic infections.

Treatment Though patients with the polymyalgia rheumatica syndrome and giant-cell arteritis may obtain some relief from their symptoms with salicylates, indomethacin, or phenylbutazone, the basic process of arteritis does not seem to improve. Patients with this disorder, however, have a remarkable response to corticosteroid treatment. The clinical symptoms abate in a few days, the ESR and the hypoproliferative anemia return toward normal within 2 weeks, and the reversal of arterial lesions has been documented by arteriography. Several dosage schedules have been recommended. For patients with proved giant-cell arteritis a daily starting dose of 60 mg prednisone is recommended. A dramatic improvement in symptoms can be expected in a few days. The dose should be reduced gradually when symptoms have abated and the ESR has decreased. The maintenance dose is usually 10 mg prednisone per day or less. In patients with polymyalgia rheumatica a starting dose of prednisone from 10 to 20 mg per day can give striking relief of symptoms. Higher doses can be considered if fever, anemia, or profound symptoms are debilitating to the patient. Alternate-day corticosteroids are not useful for patients with these disorders. Ultimately, corticosteroids can be discontinued in the majority of patients. The hazards of corticosteroids should be considered, and the prolonged use of high doses of corticosteroids should be discouraged.

REFERENCES

CHUMBLEY LC et al: Allergic granulomatosis and angiitis (Churg-Strauss syndrome): Report and analysis of 30 cases. Mayo Clin Proc 52:477, 1977

CHURG J, STRAUSS L: Allergic granulomatosis, allergic angiitis and periarteritis nodosa. Am J Pathol 27:277, 1951

FISHER RG et al: Polyarteritis nodosa and hepatitis-B surface antigen: Role of angiography in diagnosis. Am J Roentgenol 129:77, 1977

HAMILTON CR JR et al: Giant cell arteritis: Including temporal arteritis and polymyalgia rheumatica. Medicine 50:1, 1971

HAMRIN B: Polymyalgia arteritica. Acta Med Scand (suppl): 533, 1973

KLEIN RG et al: Large artery involvement in giant cell (temporal) arteritis. Ann Intern Med 83:806, 1975

LEVO Y et al: Association between hepatitis B virus and essential mixed cryoglobulinemia. N Engl J Med 296:1501, 1977

MICHALAK T: Immune complexes of hepatitis B surface antigens in the pathogenesis of periarteritis nodosa. Am J Pathol 90:619, 1978

PARK JR, HAZLEMAN BL: Immunological and histological study of temporal arteries. Ann Rheum Dis 37:238, 1978

SERGENT JS, CHRISTIAN CL: Necrotizing vasculitis after acute serous otitis media. Ann Intern Med 81:195, 1974

SOTER NA et al: Two distinct cellular patterns in cutaneous necrotizing angiitis. J Invest Dermatol 66:344, 1976

ZEEK PM: Periarteritis nodosa and other forms of necrotizing angiitis. N Engl J Med 148:764, 1953

68
SYSTEMIC LUPUS ERYTHEMATOSUS

MART MANNIK
BRUCE C. GILLILAND

INTRODUCTION Systemic lupus erythematosus (SLE) is a disease of unknown cause. However, abundant evidence shows that immunologic mechanisms of tissue injury are important in its pathogenesis. The clinical presentation and the course of SLE are variable. A hallmark of this disease is the presence of a number of antibodies to nuclear components, but other immunologic abnormalities exist as well. Some patients with SLE have spontaneous remissions, others respond favorably to treatment with corticosteroids, and in some patients the course is unresponsive to available medications. On the basis of detailed studies of animal models that resemble SLE, viral infections and genetic predisposition appear etiologically important.

PATHOGENESIS The serum of patients with SLE contains many antibodies; among them are the antibodies to deoxyribonucleic acid (DNA), nucleoprotein, histones, nuclear ribonucleoprotein, and other nuclear constituents. These antibodies are collectively termed antibodies to nuclear antigens (ANA). The antibodies to nuclear antigens alone are harmless; their presence in vivo or in tissue cultures does not harm living cells, since antibodies do not penetrate the membrane of living cells. However, the ANA participate in the pathogenesis of SLE by forming antigen-antibody complexes with their specific antigens. DNA and antibodies to DNA, nucleoprotein and antibodies to nucleoprotein, as well as complement components, have been demonstrated in the renal glomerular basement membrane and in the vascular basement membrane of patients with SLE. These observations resemble the findings in experimental serum sickness (Chap. 66). During the active phase of SLE, serum complement is decreased and circulating immune complexes can be detected with sensitive techniques. For these reasons SLE has been classified as an immune-complex disease. Even though DNA and nucleoprotein have been identified in tissue lesions, the source of these antigens has not been clarified. Other antigen-antibody systems may also be involved.

In experimental immune-complex diseases of animals and in human serum sickness, inflammation of joints, pleura, and pericardium occurs because of the presence of antigen and subsequent immune-complex formation. Similar mechanisms may well explain the multitude of clinical manifestations in patients with SLE.

ETIOLOGY The reasons for development of the antinuclear and other antibodies in SLE are not clear. Furthermore, the origin of the antigens in tissue lesions has not been elucidated—they may be autologous nuclear components, or they may originate from invading microorganisms. The hypothesis that SLE results from a viral infection in genetically predisposed persons is supported by several observations. The strongest support for this hypothesis comes from studies on the F_1 hybrids of New Zealand black (NZB) and white (NZW) mice that develop a syndrome analogous to SLE. These mice develop among other manifestations renal lesions, antinuclear antibodies, antibodies to DNA, and decreased serum complement. DNA and antibodies to DNA exist in the renal deposits of immune complexes. Furthermore, in certain colonies of dogs SLE-like disease can be transmitted with cell-free extracts, and C-type viruses have been identified in these animals in association with the disease. In a very high percentage of patients with SLE, cytoplasmic virus-like tubuloreticular structures are found by electron microscopy in endothelial cells of glomerular and other capillaries. These structures initially were thought to represent viruses, but now are thought to represent an unidentified response to cell injury. Similar inclusions are seen in other disorders, but with lesser frequency.

In humans and mice with SLE, abnormalities exist in the regulatory mechanisms of the immune response. A suppression of cell-mediated immunity is apparent with an enhanced activity of humoral immunity. These observations suggest a diminution of the T-cell suppressor mechanism on B-cell functions. These abnormalities may account for the multitude of antibodies to intracellular components as mentioned above, but the reasons for the existence of these abnormalities remain obscure.

A genetic predisposition for SLE has been suggested by the subclinical abnormalities in relatives of patients with SLE and by the high concordance of clinical SLE in monozygotic twins. On the other hand, the finding of a high prevalence of lymphocytotoxic antibodies among household contacts, including but not limited to blood relatives, raises the possibility of nongenetic transmission of SLE. The occurrence of SLE and lupus-like syndromes in patients with several inborn errors of complement (predominantly deficiencies of C1, C4, and C2) has been noted but not explained.

PATHOLOGY The pathologic changes in SLE are variable and depend on the stage of the disease. Fibrinoid deposits are commonly seen in blood vessels, among collagen fibers, and on serosal surfaces. Hematoxylin bodies are specific for SLE and are defined as hematoxylin-stained round or oblong masses in areas of inflammation. Hematoxylin bodies are thought to represent degenerated nuclei that have interacted with antibodies to nuclear antigens.

The renal lesions in patients with SLE have been classified into *focal glomerulonephritis, diffuse glomerulonephritis,* and *membranous lupus nephritis.* In focal glomerulonephritis some glomeruli show focal hypercellularity, accumulation of inflammatory cells, and thickening of the basement membrane. Immunofluorescence microscopy shows the presence of immunoglobulins and the third component of complement (C3) in involved areas as well as in the mesangium of uninvolved areas. In diffuse glomerulonephritis the same changes are present in all glomeruli, but frequently in an uneven manner. The basement membrane may be considerably thickened. On immunofluorescence microscopy, extensive "lumpy-bumpy" deposits of immunoglobulin and C3 are seen along the basement membrane. On electron microscopy, the electron-dense deposits are found on the endothelial side of the basement membrane and in the mesangium.

In membranous lupus nephritis hypercellularity is not present, but the basement membrane is diffusely thickened. Immunofluorescence microscopy discloses granular deposits of immunoglobulins and C3. By electron microscopy these deposits are localized on the epithelial side of the basement membrane and within the basement membrane. The mechanisms for these differences in renal involvement have not been elucidated.

Over the years a number of lupus patients with normal renal function and normal urine have had renal biopsies. Histologically these specimens may be normal, show increased mesangial cellularity, or have minimal glomerulonephritis. On immunofluorescence microscopy mesangial deposits of immunoglobulins and complement components are commonly seen. By electron-microscopic examination, electron-dense deposits are in the mesangial matrix and to a small extent in the subendothelial area of the glomerular basement membrane. These observations indicate that glomerular abnormalities are ubiquitous in patients with SLE, even when renal function and urine sediment are entirely normal by the usual clinical criteria. With follow-up only some of these patients progress to overt renal involvement and renal failure.

In addition to glomerular damage, immune complexes also lead to interstitial nephritis in SLE. Over half of biopsied patients show focal or diffuse interstitial cellular infiltrates, tubular damage, or interstitial fibrosis. The finding of immunoglobulins, complement components, and electron-dense deposits along the tubular basement membrane and in the interstitium indicate that immune complexes initiate these lesions. The immune-complex interstitial nephritis is most common in patients with diffuse proliferative glomerulonephritis and less frequent in the other glomerulonephritides associated with SLE.

The pathological findings in skin lesions vary according to the clinical stage of the lesions. The histology of the erythematous, maculopapular eruptions, as seen in the butterfly distribution on the face, are not diagnostic. Edema, extravasation of red cells, and some perivascular inflammation are early alterations. More chronic lesions show hyperkeratosis, epidermal atrophy, and small vessel inflammation in the dermis. The lesions in discoid lupus erythematosus will show atrophy, epidermal hyperkeratosis, and keratotic plugging. The dermis is edematous and infiltrated variably with lymphocytes, plasma cells, and histiocytes. On immunofluorescent staining, the epidermal-dermal junction of patients with SLE has IgG and C3 deposits. Similar changes are frequently present in clinically uninvolved skin. The mechanism for development of these deposits has not been clarified, but antibodies to nuclear antigens, including antibodies to DNA, have been identified in these deposits.

Widespread small-vessel vasculitis may be present in many organs. Such lesions exist in the synovium and show both mononuclear and polymorphonuclear infiltration. Autopsy studies on SLE patients with central nervous system abnormalities may show necrotizing vasculitis of arterioles and capillaries in many parts of the brain. Microinfarcts of brain tissues may be apparent. In some patients abundant deposits of immunoglobulins and complement components occur at the basement membrane of vessels in the choroid plexus analogous to glomerular deposits of immune complexes. The spleen shows marked intimal proliferation of penicillar and central arteries, which gives an "onion skin" appearance to these vessels. The heart valves and chordae tendineae have at times nonbacterial verrucous vegetations (Libman-Sacks endocarditis).

CLINICAL MANIFESTATIONS SLE is predominantly a disease of women (9 women to 1 man) in the second to fifth decades of life, but it spares neither children nor persons of advanced age. The prevalence of SLE is 2 to 3 per 100,000. Most recent estimates indicate that 77 percent of patients with SLE survive 5 years. The presence of renal disease and central nervous system involvement decrease survival. The most frequent causes of death are uremia, heart failure, hemorrhage, central nervous system disease, and intercurrent bacterial infections. Patients with SLE may present with a variety of abnormalities, including arthritis and arthralgias, cutaneous manifestations, nephritis, fever, central nervous system manifestations, Raynaud's phenomenon, pleurisy, pericarditis, hemolytic anemia, leukopenia, or thrombocytopenia (Table 68-1).

The course of SLE is highly variable from patient to patient. The observations on outcome and prognosis are largely based on patient populations studied at medical centers and therefore would exclude patients with mild and uncomplicated disease. SLE is not always a fatal disease as was thought years ago.

Arthritis and *arthralgias* are the most frequent presenting as well as the most common complaints during the course of the illness. The arthralgias are fleeting; they involve the hands or feet and also large joints. Redness, warmth, tenderness, and synovial effusions are frequently present. However, deformities are rare, and the erosions so characteristic of rheumatoid arthritis are unusual. The synovial fluid white blood cell counts are relatively low (less than 3000 per mm³), and mononuclear cells predominate. Aseptic necrosis may occur, in part because of therapy with corticosteroids. Profound muscle weakness and tenderness reflect myositis in some patients.

Fever is frequent during the course of SLE. Fatigue, malaise, anorexia, and weight loss also occur. However, systemic complaints may be totally absent in some patients.

Cutaneous manifestations of SLE include a variety of lesions. A facial eruption, with butterfly distribution over the malar areas and bridge of the nose, consists of erythema and edema during the acute phase; atrophy and telangiectasia appear in chronic lesions. This characteristic rash occurs in about 40 percent of patients. Similar eruptions may occur in other parts of the body, particularly in the exposed areas. At times skin eruptions are precipitated or worsened by exposure to ultraviolet rays. Patchy alopecia occurs with similar frequency and is found only if sought under coiffures or wigs. Patients with SLE may have short broken hairs above the forehead, the

so-called "lupus hairs." Dermal vasculitis can be found in about 20 percent of patients, usually as small infarcts of the digital skin. In some patients only erythema due to excessively large or numerous capillaries around the digits and fingernails is seen. Ulcers may be encountered on nasal or oral mucous membranes. Other cutaneous manifestations include purpura, bullae, hives, and angioneurotic edema. Raynaud's phenomenon is seen in about one-fifth of patients with SLE.

Discoid lupus is a chronic skin ailment with lesions usually confined to face, neck, arms, and scalp. Scaling is prominent, with atrophy, telangiectasia, and keratotic plugging. Deep scars remain when the lesions subside. Only a few of these patients go on to develop systemic lupus erythematosus. On the other hand, some patients with SLE also have discoid lesions.

Renal involvement is one of the most serious manifestations in SLE. Clinically detectable evidence of renal involvement is seen in about one-half of all patients with SLE. These abnormalities extend from minimal proteinuria and few red blood cell casts to massive hematuria, proteinuria, and frank nephrotic syndrome. In some patients renal involvement goes on to total renal failure; in others there is a course of exacerbations and remissions, with eventual renal failure. Some patients respond well to treatment or improve spontaneously, but minimal proteinuria and decreased creatinine clearance may persist as evidence of irreversible damage.

The development of superimposed urinary tract infection should always be kept in mind, since these patients seem liable to such infections.

Cardiopulmonary abnormalities are moderately frequent in patients with SLE. Symptoms and signs of pericarditis or other cardiac abnormalities are encountered in almost 50 percent of them. Pericarditis may be the presenting complaint, with the usual physical and electrocardiographic findings. Tamponade due to SLE pericarditis is unusual. Myocarditis may occur. The nonbacterial verrucous endocarditis is rarely diagnosed clinically but should be suspected when new murmurs develop in the absence of bacterial endocarditis. Symptomatic or asymptomatic pleural involvement occurs in nearly half the patients. Patchy and transient parenchymal infiltrates have been noted, and occasionally severe lupus pneumonitis may occur. The cause of these abnormalities is not known, and they are difficult to distinguish from infiltrates caused by infections.

Neurologic manifestations represent another serious aspect of SLE. A variety of central nervous system manifestations has been noted in 20 to 50 percent of patients. Among these are convulsive disorders, followed in frequency by abnormalities in mental functions and cranial nerves and by transverse myelitis. Peripheral neuropathies are infrequent. Occasionally pa-

TABLE 68-1
Clinical manifestations during the course of systemic lupus erythematosus

Manifestation	Cumulative percentage of patients
Arthritis and arthralgias	92
Fever	84
Skin eruptions	72
Lymphadenopathy	59
Renal involvement	53
Anorexia, nausea, vomiting	53
Myalgia	48
Pleuritis	45
Central nervous system abnormalities	26

SOURCE: *After Dubois.*

tients present with primarily mental dysfunction, e.g., emotional lability, psychosis, or organic brain syndrome, without other significant symptoms. Cerebrospinal fluid of patients with central nervous system involvement may show slight to moderate increase in protein concentration and mild increase in lymphocytes; usually these occur late in the disease. The electroencephalogram is abnormal, with diffuse nonspecific changes. The brain scan may show focal increased uptake of isotope during active central nervous system involvement. Computerized tomography may reveal infarcts due to cerebral vasculitis.

Lymph node enlargement occurs in many patients with SLE. Such abnormalities may be diffuse or local. Characteristically the nodes are not tender. The enlargement of nodes is thought to occur because of increased activity of the immune system. Splenomegaly occurs in about 10 percent of patients and may be associated with hemolytic anemia. *Hepatomegaly* is found in about 25 percent of patients. Lupoid hepatitis is a syndrome of chronic active hepatitis associated with positive tests for LE cells or antibodies to nuclear antigens (Chap. 303).

LABORATORY FINDINGS A variety of abnormalities in *hematologic* and *immunologic* tests may be encountered in SLE (Table 68-2).

A mild, normochromic, normocytic *anemia* is seen frequently. Most likely this is the hypoproliferative anemia that accompanies many inflammatory processes. Less frequently patients have severe immune-hemolytic anemia that requires steroid therapy or splenectomy. *Leukopenia* is seen in over half the patients. The mechanisms for leukopenia and thrombocytopenia are not fully delineated, but intravascular immune complexes as well as antibodies directed to leukocytes and platelets may contribute to these abnormalities. A potentially serious but infrequent problem is the occurrence of *clotting defects* due to antibodies to factors VII, IX, or X or to the presence of an inhibitor to prothrombin activation. Prior to a renal biopsy, the integrity of the clotting mechanism must be evaluated.

Urinalysis and renal function studies indicate that over half the patients with SLE have mild to severe damage to the kidneys. With early or focal glomerulonephritis the creatinine clearance may be normal, and only mild proteinuria and microscopic hematuria may exist. With more extensive renal involvement proteinuria may become significant (>0.5 per day), and the urine sediment may contain abundant red and white blood cells and red blood cell casts as indicators of glomerular damage.

The serum albumin/globulin ratio becomes reversed because of an increase in immunoglobulins, particularly IgG. Serum electrophoresis reveals that the major elevation is in globulin. Small amounts of cryoglobulins, composed of immunoglobulins and complement components, may be present. The erythrocyte sedimentation rate (ESR) tends to be high in patients with active disease.

The most characteristic laboratory abnormalities in SLE are the autoantibodies. The presence of antibodies to nuclear antigens (ANA) in a patient with active SLE is almost a sine qua non for the diagnosis. These tests are now widely available as a diagnostic aid. The ANA are usually detected by rat or mouse liver sections (other tissues with nucleated cells may also be used); the test serum is applied to the tissue section, antibodies to nuclear antigens interact with the nuclei, other proteins are washed away, and the ANA are detected with an antiserum to human immunoglobulins (these antibodies are coupled with fluorescein isothiocyanate that permits their detection with appropriate microscopy). The patterns of nuclear staining were attributed to the presence of specific antibodies to certain nuclear antigens. These interpretations, however, were fraught with difficulties and tests are now available for specific antibodies. The ANA include antibodies to single-stranded DNA, double-stranded (native) DNA, deoxyribonucleoprotein, histones, nuclear ribonucleoprotein (abbreviated RNP), and an acidic nuclear protein (also called the Sm antigen). Patients with SLE also have antibodies to RNA, ribosomes, lysosomes, and other cytoplasmic constituents. The reasons for such a large number of antibodies are not clear. Many of these antibodies persist even when the disease is quiescent, except that the titers of antibodies to native DNA tend to be higher during exacerbations of the disease. Antibodies to native DNA in high titers are most specific for SLE with a low prevalence in other disorders. The lupus erythematosus cell test (LE cell test) is positive less frequently than the test for ANA because more antibodies are required for positivity. The listed antibodies to nuclear antigens are not specific for SLE, but when three or more of these antibodies are present, the likelihood of SLE in a given patient is very high. In end-stage renal disease due to SLE, the tests for ANA may become negative.

During flare-ups of SLE the total serum hemolytic complement (expressed in 50 percent hemolytic units—CH_{50}) or individual components of complement are decreased owing to activation by immune complexes. The most frequently used measurements of complement components are the immunochemically determined C3 and C4 levels. These measurements are useful in following the response to therapy or for detecting exacerbations. Occasionally the complement levels remain low in spite of apparent full clinical remission; the reasons for this are not known. In addition, during clinically active disease, circulating immune complexes can be detected.

About 20 percent of patients with SLE develop positive tests for rheumatoid factors, but the titers tend to be lower than in rheumatoid arthritis. False positive tests for syphilis are encountered, at times prior to clinical onset of SLE. Antibodies to nuclear antigens occur in many other diseases (rheumatoid arthritis, 20 percent; Sjögren's syndrome, 60 percent; scleroderma, 40 percent) and are induced by several drugs (see below).

DIAGNOSIS The possibility of SLE should be considered in any young or middle-aged female in the presence of three or four of the symptoms or signs listed in Table 68-1 or in the presence of glomerulonephritis, hemolytic anemia, leukopenia, or thrombocytopenia. A positive test for ANA is essential for diagnosis. Other diseases that cause positive tests for ANA must be considered, and they must often be excluded on the basis of clinical observations alone. Major consideration must be given to rheumatoid arthritis, scleroderma, Sjögren's syndrome, and the history of ingestion of drugs that might have

TABLE 68-2
Laboratory abnormalities in systemic lupus erythematosus

Abnormality	Percent of patients
HEMATOLOGIC	
Anemia (Hb $<$ 11 g/100 ml)	72
Leukopenia (WBC $<$ 4500/mm³)	61
Thrombocytopenia (platelets $<$ 100,000/mm³)	15
Positive direct Coombs test	14
Circulating anticoagulants	Rare
IMMUNOLOGIC	
Positive tests for ANA	99
Positive LE cell tests	60–80
Hypocomplementemia	75
Increased γ globulin ($>$ 1.5 g/100 ml)	60–77
Positive tests for rheumatoid factors	20
Biologic false positive tests for syphilis	15

induced a positive test for ANA. The mixed connective tissue disease (Chap. 362) is distinguished from SLE by sclerodermatous skin changes, active myositis, lack of significant glomerulonephritis, and cerebritis. The finding of very high titers of antibodies to nuclear ribonucleoprotein is the most helpful distinguishing characteristic.

Drug-Induced SLE Hydralazine and procainamide clearly induce a syndrome similar to SLE in some patients. This syndrome includes arthralgias, arthritis, myalgias, pleurisy, pericarditis, fever, skin eruptions, lymphadenopathy, and positive tests for ANA. Renal disease and central nervous system involvement are very unusual in drug-induced SLE. Prospective studies have shown that about 70 percent of patients receiving procainamide develop positive tests for ANA within weeks or months. A much smaller proportion become symptomatic. Once the drug is discontinued, the symptoms abate in a few weeks but occasionally may smolder on for months; recovery may be hastened by treatment with corticosteroids. The ANA tests revert to negative in a few months. Isoniazid alone or with p-aminosalicylic acid (PAS), several anticonvulsants (Dilantin, Mesantoin), phenothiazine derivatives, γ-methyldopa, and levodopa have also been associated with positive tests for ANA. In some patients the administration of sulfonamides, penicillin, and oral contraceptives has been associated with exacerbations of SLE.

TREATMENT A cure for SLE is not available. However, abundant experience indicates that appropriate therapy may suppress flare-ups and prolong life. The optimal treatment programs for various manifestations of SLE have not been defined. Adequately designed studies have been difficult to perform because of the variability in the manifestations and course of the disease and the lack of adequate prognostic parameters. Corticosteroids remain the cornerstone of therapy, even though the "immunosuppressive" drugs seem to be helpful in some patients.

Arthralgias, arthritis, myalgias, and fever may respond adequately to rest and salicylates. Antimalarials have been used successfully for the same symptoms, as well as for control of skin eruptions. Chloroquine was used widely in mild SLE, but potential retinal toxicity has decreased its usage. Hydroxychloroquine in small dosages (200 mg per day) seems safe, but the patient should be cautioned about potential toxicity, and careful examination by the ophthalmologist should be conducted at least twice a year. Exposure to ultraviolet light should be avoided, particularly with active and recurrent skin lesions. If skin involvement becomes debilitating and does not respond to conservative therapy, corticosteroids in small to moderate dosages should provide relief.

Central nervous system involvement, pericarditis, myocarditis, pleurisy, severe myositis, severe hemolytic anemia, clotting problems, significant leukopenia, and thrombocytopenia are indications for use of corticosteroids. In desperate situations, particularly in central nervous system involvement with seizures or psychosis, relatively high doses should be used (even up to 2 mg prednisone or prednisolone per kg body weight). With central nervous system involvement a high (60 mg or more per day) dose of prednisone should be used up to about 2 weeks. Once improvement has occurred, the dose should be tapered and adjusted to maintain control of symptoms. Many of the above manifestations can be controlled with 10 mg prednisone or less per day as a maintenance dose. If a flare-up occurs and is recognized by the patient and the physician, only a moderate (5 to 10 mg) increase of the prednisone dose may provide control of symptoms. Careful follow-up of patients, with judicious use of laboratory tests, is essential in treatment of the above manifestations of SLE. Psychosis or other mental disturbances may be difficult to evaluate in a

patient who is receiving steroids for SLE, since such symptoms may be caused by the steroids or by the SLE. No single laboratory test, including cerebrospinal fluid complement levels, can distinguish between these two possibilities. With further increase of the steroid dosage the symptoms should decrease if they are due to central nervous system involvement by SLE. In the use of corticosteroids the side effects, such as increased risk of infections and osteopenia, must always be considered in relation to the anticipated benefits.

Several approaches to the treatment of SLE nephritis have been advocated, but no currently available program is useful in all patients. Renal biopsy is recommended for establishing the nature of glomerular lesions, since those with focal lupus glomerulonephritis respond to treatment well or improve spontaneously. Perhaps the most useful program is to start with 40 to 60 mg prednisone or prednisolone per day until all clinical symptoms have abated. This may take a few weeks; the urinary sediment should improve, and complement should return toward normal. Thereafter the steroid dose should be reduced gradually to the minimal dose to keep the patient free of symptoms. With severe focal involvement and with diffuse lupus glomerulonephritis or membranous glomerulonephritis, higher doses (up to 150 to 200 mg prednisone or prednisolone) have been tried and found helpful for some patients, with subsequent improvement of renal function. However, the diffuse and membranous lesions do not respond well. For these reasons azathioprine (1 to 2 mg per kilogram of body weight) or cyclophosphamide (100 to 150 mg per day) has been added to prednisone. Cyclophosphamide and prednisone appear to be the most effective combination, but many serious side effects are encountered, including marrow toxicity, hemorrhage cystitis, alopecia, and sterility; their long-term risks are not fully known. The search for better combinations of drugs and new medications for treatment of severe SLE continues.

Plasmapheresis has been suggested as an adjunct to treatment with corticosteroids. The rationale for plasmapheresis is to remove sufficient immune complexes from the circulation to allow endogenous clearance mechanisms to cope with the load of immune complexes until other forms of therapy control the disease manifestations.

Any intercurrent infections must be recognized and treated with appropriate therapy. Patients with SLE, either because of their disease or as a consequence of treatment, are liable to bacterial infections, which are a leading cause of death among them.

Exacerbations of SLE tend to occur during the third trimester of pregnancy or in the immediate postpartum period. Nevertheless, many patients with SLE can be carried to term and successful delivery with appropriate therapy. Therefore, SLE is not an absolute indication for therapeutic abortion, but the procedure is recommended during life-threatening active disease.

REFERENCES

BRENTJENS JR et al: Interstitial immune complex nephritis in patients with systemic lupus erythematosus. Kidney Int 7:342, 1975

CAVALLO T et al: Immunopathology of early and clinically silent lupus nephropathy. Am J Pathol 87:1, 1977

DECKER JL et al: Cyclophosphamide or azathioprine in lupus glomerulonephritis. A controlled trial: Results at 28 months. Ann Intern Med 83:606, 1975

DUBOIS EL (ed): Lupus Erythematosus, 2d ed. Los Angeles, University of Southern California Press, 1974

FRIES JF, HOLMAN HR: Systemic Lupus Erythematosus: A Clinical

Analysis, vol 6: *Major Problems in Internal Medicine,* LH Smith (ed). Philadelphia, Saunders, 1975

GRIGOR R et al: Systemic lupus erythematosus: A prospective analysis. Ann Rheum Dis 37:121, 1978

NOTMAN DD et al: Profiles of antinuclear antibodies in systemic rheumatic diseases. Ann Intern Med 83:464, 1975

PHILLIPS PE: The virus hypothesis in systemic lupus erythematosus. Ann Intern Med 83:709, 1975

POLLACK VE et al: The clinical course of lupus nephritis: Relationship to the renal histological findings, in *Perspectives in Nephrology and Hypertension,* P Kincaid-Smith et al (eds). New York, Wiley, 1973, vol 1, p 1167

STEINMAN CR et al: Binding of synthetic double-stranded DNA by serum from patients with systemic lupus erythematosus: Correlation with renal histology. Am J Med 62:319, 1977

VERRIER-JONES J et al: Plasmapheresis in the management of acute systemic lupus erythematosus? Lancet 1:709, 1976

69
HISTOCOMPATIBILITY AND TRANSPLANTATION

CHARLES B. CARPENTER
JOHN P. MERRILL

INTRODUCTION Transplantation of the human kidney is now a justified procedure for the treatment of advanced chronic renal failure. Tens of thousands of such procedures have been performed, and occur at the rate of 50 or more per year in some medical centers. The results with properly matched familial donors are superior to those obtained with organs from cadaveric donors, with 75 to 80 percent compared to 45 to 50 percent graft survival rates at 1 year, respectively. Grafts functioning at 1 year are rejected at a much slower rate over the subsequent years, although occasionally a graft may suffer an acute irreversible rejection episode after many months of good function. The most striking improvement in clinical renal transplant results in recent years is in patient morbidity and mortality, the latter declining to less than 5 percent in a number of units. These findings represent an increasing tendency on the part of transplant teams to decrease immunosuppressive therapy so that in the case of severe rejection the kidney rather than the patient may be lost. The figures for graft survival, however, show no improvement since 1970, suggesting that methods of immunosuppressive therapy which have been uniformly utilized from 1970 to the present time remain inadequate. There are increasing numbers of second and even third transplants being performed, and the overall results are comparable to those with first transplants; in other words, rejection of a graft does not necessarily prejudice the results of another transplant attempt. Human liver, pancreas, bone marrow, heart, and endocrine glands have been transplanted, but with less success. The results of cardiac transplantation in one of the largest and best-studied series in the United States show a better than 50 percent 1-year survival.

IMMUNOLOGIC CONSIDERATIONS Necessary to the understanding of transplantation immunity are the following terms: *autograft*—the transplantation of tissue from one part of an individual to another part of the same individual; *isograft*—the transplantation of tissues between two individuals of the same inbred strain. Because in these cases the antigens of the donor and recipient are identical, no histocompatibility difference exists and no immune response to the graft occurs. A case in

point in humans is transplantation between identical twins. In an *allograft,* i.e., a graft of tissues between two individuals of the same species, histocompatibility differences may be strong or weak, depending on the individual and the species. A *xenograft* is a graft between individuals of two different species. The term "heterograft" is still used synonymously with xenograft.

NATURE AND ROLE OF THE MAJOR HISTOCOMPATIBILITY GENE COMPLEX (HLA) The fate of transplanted tissues and organs depends upon a number of factors, but the recipient's immune response to graft antigens is the central event. Definition of antigenic systems which serve as strong barriers to transplantation has therefore become a major investigative interest, having both practical application in clinical transplantation and theoretical value in understanding the natural role of the histocompatibility antigens in immunobiology.

A single chromosomal gene complex codes for the major histocompatibility antigens in all vertebrate species investigated so far. The mouse is the most completely studied species because of the availability of numbers of inbred and recombinant strains which can be employed in studies to determine the precise role of each of the gene products of the histocompatibility (H-2) chromosomal segment. Except for some details of the ordering of the genes on the chromosomal segment, the human HLA system is thus far quite analogous to the H-2. In a general sense, incompatibility for major locus antigens constitutes a strong barrier to transplantation of tissues and organs, and in clinical experience matching for major locus antigens affords excellent transplantation results, since the minor mismatches are easily suppressed by immunosuppressive drug therapy. The HLA gene complex is a portion of the short arm of the C6 human chromosome and consists of several series of paired alleles which are inherited from generation to generation in a dominant fashion, segregating randomly from other important antigens such as the ABH red blood cell type groups.

Antigens of the HLA system CLASS I The development of antileukocyte antibodies after multiple blood transfusions and as a result of pregnancy was first recognized as involving a series of antigens distinct from red cell blood group antigens. HLA antigens are defined serologically by serums from human sources, principally multiparous females, and are present in varying densities in most body tissues, including B cells, T cells (see "Immunology of Rejection," below), and platelets but not in mature red blood cells. The number of serologically defined specificities is very large, and the HLA system is at present the most polymorphic genetic system known in humans. There are known to be three clearly defined loci within the HLA complex for class I serologically defined (SD), HLA antigens. Each class I antigen consists of an 11,600-dalton β_2 microglobulin subunit and a 44,000-dalton heavy chain which carries the antigenic specificity (Fig. 69-1). The A and B loci were recognized as such in 1970, and the C locus shortly thereafter. There are over 50 clearly defined A and B specificities, while over five C-locus specificities are known. Antigens of the major complex are all prefixed by HLA, but this may be omitted when the context is clear. Antigens tentatively accepted as a result of World Health Organization workshops have a w after the locus designation. The HLA antigens of African, Asian, and Oceanic peoples are not as well defined at present, although they include some of the antigens commonly found in Caucasians. The distribution of HLA antigens is distinctive for certain racial groups and can serve as anthropologic markers in the study of migration patterns.

Since chromosomes are paired, each individual has six serologically defined HLA-A, HLA-B, and HLA-C antigens, three from each parent. Each of these chromosomal sets is termed a

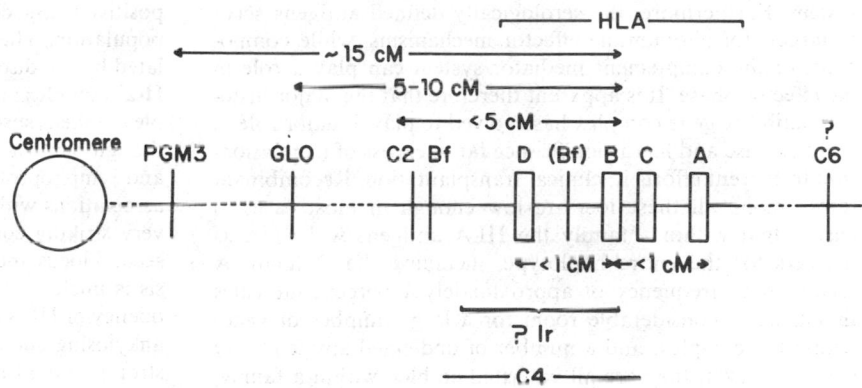

FIGURE 69-1
Short arm of the human sixth chromosome. The HLA region contains genes for three class I loci (A, B, C) and the D locus region defined by the mixed lymphocyte reaction (MLR). Class II serologically defined antigens on B lymphocytes and monocytes exist which are D-related (DR). Some of the enzyme and complement polymorphisms are also shown. C2 and C4 deficiency and allotypic variants of C2 and Bf are HLA-linked. C6 linkage is suggested by some data, but not established. (cM = centimorgan map unit.) (From CB Carpenter, in Kidney International, New York, Springer-Verlag, 1978.)

haplotype, and by simple mendelian inheritance 25 percent of siblings will have identical haplotypes, 50 percent will share a haplotype, and the remaining 25 percent will be completely incompatible (Fig. 69-2). Evidence that this gene complex plays the major role in the transplantation response comes from the fact that haplotype-matched sibling donor-recipient combinations show excellent results in kidney transplantation, in the vicinity of 85 to 90 percent long-term survival.

CLASS II   Linked to the serologically defined antigens, but distinct from them, is another locus which determines the in vitro proliferative response of lymphocytes to mismatched haplotypes. Because haplotype-matched identical siblings have negative mixed lymphocyte culture responses, it was initially assumed that the antigens were responsible for the proliferative response of lymphocytes mixed in tissue culture. However, a number of recombinants in families have shown clearly that a distinct locus, called D, exists for the mixed lymphocyte response (MLR), and is responsible for a vigorous mixed lymphocyte culture (MLC) proliferative response, even in the presence of HLA-A, HLA-B, and HLA-C antigen identity (Fig. 69-2). The recombinant rate in human families is around 1

FIGURE 69-2
Inheritance of HLA haplotypes. Each chromosomal segment of linked genes is termed a haplotype, and each individual inherits one haplotype from each parent. The A, B, C, and D antigens of haplotypes a and b are shown for this hypothetical individual in chromosomal order on the diagram, and also below as they would be written in text. If individual ab were to marry cd, their offspring would be of four types only, as far as HLA is concerned. Occasionally (dotted cross) recombination occurs in the germ line (meiosis) of a parent, resulting in an altered haplotype. The frequency of recombinant children is a measure of the map distance (1 percent recombination frequency = 1 cM; see Fig. 69-1). (From CB Carpenter, in Kidney International, New York, Springer-Verlag, 1978.)

HLA REGION, CHROMOSOME 6

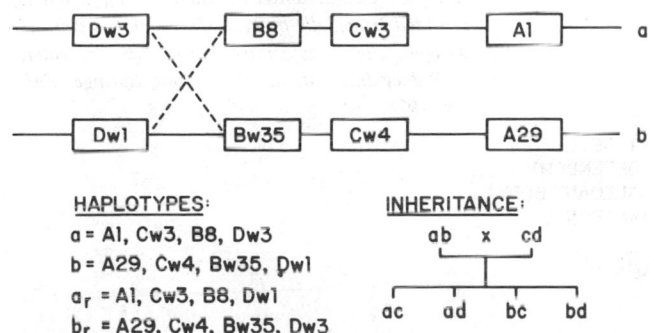

HAPLOTYPES:
a = A1, Cw3, B8, Dw3
b = A29, Cw4, Bw35, Dw1
a_r = A1, Cw3, B8, Dw1
b_r = A29, Cw4, Bw35, Dw3

INHERITANCE:
ab   x   cd

ac   ad   bc   bd

percent between B and D loci, and it is also approximately 1 percent between the A and B loci. HLA-D antigens are defined by reference stimulating lymphocytes which are homozygous for HLA-D, and inactivated by x-irradiation or mitomycin C to make the reaction unidirectional. Although D-locus antigens, sometimes called MLF-S (stimulating), are not as yet clearly identifiable by serotyping techniques, serologically defined specificities closely related to the D locus have been defined. They have the special property of not being expressed on platelets or T lymphocytes. These specificities are termed class II, having two glycoprotein chains of 29,000 and 34,000 daltons, and lacking β_2 microglobulin. They are termed HLA-DR (D-related), and are markers for closely linked D-locus determinants and putative immune response (Ir) genes. The precise relationship between HLA-D and class II serologically defined antigens (HLA-DR) has yet to be established. They could be part of the same molecule, or the products of closely linked genes. In addition, preliminary evidence exists for class II antigens unrelated to HLA-D type; hence, a complex series of loci encompassing the HLA-D region may be ultimately discerned. Two additional methods are under investigation for defining histocompatibility antigens. In the primed lymphocyte test (PLT), responder cells which have completed a proliferative response in MLC are restimulated with the same or different stimulating cells. The secondary response of primed lymphocytes is rapid (24 to 36 h, instead of 5 to 6 days), and the specificity of restimulation is a test for antigenic similarity between priming and restimulating cells. Data thus far indicate that PLT antigens are more closely related to class II HLA-DR than to HLA-D. In the cell-mediated lympholysis (CML) test the specificity of killer T cells, which arise as a result of proliferation in MLC, is determined upon target cells from donors other than those providing the MLC-stimulating cells. Antigen systems defined by this method show a close, but imperfect, correlation with class I antigens. Since killer T cells may play a crucial role in some types of allograft rejection, the definition of CML antigens may prove to be of some practical importance in clinical transplantation (Fig. 69-3).

Other sixth chromosome genes   There are at least two additional major classes of genes within the HLA region; one is for complement, with structural genes for C2 and C4 and factor B (GBG), and the other involves immune responsiveness to ragweed antigen and possibly to measles virus and *Mycobacterium leprae*. The latter findings are of enormous importance in relation to the analogy to mouse H-2 systems where the MLR region is closely linked to a number of genes responsible for certain immune responses (Ir region). There are, therefore, a number of genes in this complex which are related to the immune response, ranging from the immunogenicity of certain antigens to the proliferative response (MLR) of the immune system. Furthermore, the serologically defined antigens serve as targets for alloimmune effector mechanisms, while components of the complement mediator system can play a role in the effector phase. It is apparent therefore that the major histocompatibility gene complex has evolved to play a major role in body defense and has a significance far in excess of its relationship to current efforts in clinical transplantation. Recombinant rates among all these loci are low enough in most cases to ensure that within a family the HLA antigens will serve as markers for the entire haplotype, including the D locus. A recombinant frequency of approximately 1 percent indicates that there is considerable room for a large number of genes within the complex, and a number of undefined antigens may exist. However, they are all inherited en bloc within a family, and HLA serotyping is therefore a valuable system for marking family haplotypes. In the outbred human population, however, HLA antigens are much less likely to predict compatibility for other genes in the complex.

Disease associations If the major histocompatibility complex serves a critical natural biological function, what might that be? Hypotheses have been put forth relating to immune surveillance against neoplastic cells which develop in the course of an individual's lifetime. It is apparent also that the system could play an important role in pregnancy because of the histoincompatibility that always exists between the mother and the fetus. Work in inbred mouse models indicates the importance of some of the gene products of this locus during the phase of antigen recognition of cell-to-cell cooperation in initiation of an immune response. It is possible also that the high degree of polymorphism present ensures the survival of the species in relation to the large numbers of microbiological agents present in the environment. Self-tolerance which happens to cross react with microbiological agents would produce a high degree of susceptibility, resulting in lethal infection, whereas the high degree of polymorphism present in the HLA system provides assurance that segments of the population will recognize the offending agent as foreign and initiate the appropriate response. All these hypotheses relate to the survival value of the system under selective evolutionary pressures, and there is some evidence for each of them.

The most striking circumstantial evidence of the role of the major histocompatibility complex in human immunobiology comes from the finding that a number of disease processes are positively associated with certain HLA antigens within the population. The search for such associations has been stimulated by the discovery of immune response genes linked to the H-2 complex in the mouse, and also by the H-2 complex-linked susceptibility to murine oncogenic viruses. Although surveys of human malignancies, including leukemias and lymphoproliferative disorders, have not shown consistent associations with serologically defined HLA phenotypes, some very striking correlations exist between HLA antigens of the second locus and a number of diseases in which the pathogenesis is unclear (Table 69-1). Most striking is the increased frequency of HLA-B27 in certain rheumatic diseases, particularly ankylosing spondylitis, a condition already known to have a strong familial tendency. B27 is present in about 7 percent of the Caucasian population, while it appears in 87 percent of 286 patients combined from five studies. Expressed as a relative risk, the antigen B27 confers a susceptibility to the development of ankylosing spondylitis which is 127 times that in the general population. Similarly, Reiter's syndrome and reactive arthritis to at least three bacterial infections (yersinia, salmonella, and gonococcus) show a high degree of association with B27. Furthermore, acute anterior uveitis has a similar high association with the same antigen. Since it is well known that significant overlap exists among these three conditions (spondylitis, Reiter's syndrome, and uveitis), it seems likely that B27 is a marker for a clustering of connective tissue responses to a number of infectious agents, or unknown environmental factors. It was suggested initially that juvenile rheumatoid arthritis (JRA) might also show a similar B27 association, but this is due in part to inclusion of coexistent spondylitis in these studies. Nevertheless, true JRA does show some B27 association. The increased incidence of B27 in cases of psoriatic arthritis is also highly significant and contrasts with the increased incidence of HLA-B13 and HLA-Bw17 in psoriasis per se. Patients with degenerative arthritis or gout show no alteration in antigen frequencies. Rheumatoid arthritis patients show an association with Dw4.

Gluten-sensitive enteropathy (celiac disease, nontropical sprue) in both children and adults shows a clear-cut association with HLA-B8. The actual percentage of such patients having this antigen ranges from 66 to 88 percent in five studies in which B8 was present in 16 to 29 percent of controls. The same antigen is also present in increased frequency in patients

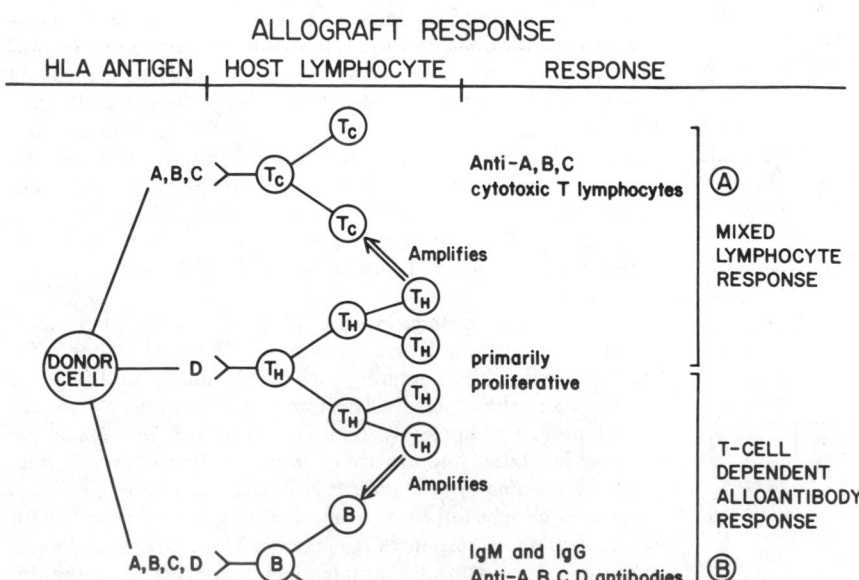

ALLOGRAFT RESPONSE

FIGURE 69-3
Schema of the relative roles of HLA-A, HLA-B, HLA-C, and HLA-D antigens in initiation of the alloimmune response and in the development of effector cells and antibodies. Two main classes of T lymphocytes recognize antigens: T_c, the precursors to the cytotoxic "killer" cells, and T_H, the helper cells for amplification of the cytotoxic response. T_H also provide help to B lymphocytes for production of a fully mature IgG response. Note that T_c generally recognize class I antigens, while the T_H signal is provided principally by HLA-D, which has class II antigens closely associated. (From CB Carpenter, in Kidney International, New York, Springer-Verlag, 1978.)

TABLE 69-1

363

CHAPTER 69
HISTOCOMPATIBILITY AND TRANSPLANTATION

Associations between HLA antigens and disease

Disease	Antigen	Relative risk*
RHEUMATIC		
Ankylosing spondylitis	B27	127
Reiter's syndrome	B27	71
Acute anterior uveitis	B27	31
Psoriatic arthritis	B27	4.7
Reactive arthritis (yersinia, salmonella, gonococcus)	B27	150 (estimated)
Rheumatoid arthritis	Dw4	6.1
	DRw4	6.0
GASTROINTESTINAL		
Gluten-sensitive enteropathy	B8	9.5
Chronic active hepatitis	B8	3.6
Hemachromatosis	A3	8.2
	B14	26.7
	A3, B14	90
SKIN		
Dermatitis herpetiformis	B8	4.3
Psoriasis vulgaris	B13, Bw17	4.3
Pemphigus	A10	3.1
ENDOCRINE		
Juvenile diabetes mellitus	B8	3.3
	Bw15	3.0
	Dw3	4.5
	Dw4	3.7
	DRw3	2.8
	DRw4	5.3
Graves's disease	B8	3.6
Addison's disease	B8	6.4
	Dw3	10.5
NEUROLOGIC		
Myasthenia gravis	B8	4.4
Multiple sclerosis	Dw2	5.0
	DRw2	3.9

* $\text{Relative risk} = \dfrac{(\%\text{ antigen-positive patients}) \ (\%\text{ antigen-negative controls})}{(\%\text{ antigen-negative patients}) \ (\%\text{ antigen-positive controls})}$

with chronic active hepatitis or dermatitis herpetiformis. Pemphigus is a disease in which a first-series antigen, HLA-A10, has shown an increased incidence.

Three endocrinopathies have been under intensive investigation following initial reports of increases in HLA-B8 frequency. Juvenile (insulin-dependent) diabetes mellitus has also shown an HLA-Bw15 association. With techniques for typing of D-locus antigens by performance of mixed lymphocyte cultures with homozygous stimulating cells and by serologic DR typing, a greater degree of association with the HLA-Dw3, DRw3, Dw4, and DRw4 has been reported. These antigens are often linked to HLA-B8 and HLA-Bw15, respectively, but these results would indicate that the loci related to juvenile diabetes are closer to the D locus than to B. Similar results have been obtained with Addison's disease. MLR typing has revealed an association with HLA-Dw2 and multiple sclerosis, while the frequently linked HLA-B7 antigen is less frequently associated.

Hence, disease associations with the HLA complex describe a spectrum, ranging from an extremely high degree of correlation with a serologically defined B locus HLA antigen, through diseases in which both B- and D-locus markers correlate, to a disease in which only the D-locus determinant is disease-associated. It is clear that definition of this spectrum is still in its early stages. It is likely that the development of more precise typing systems for identification of products of genes of the "left" of the B locus series, encompassing the D and related regions, may mark susceptibility in a number of diseases, such as leukemia, lymphoma, other malignancies and lupus erythematosus, in which HLA typing has been inconclusive.

LINKAGE DISEQUILIBRIUM Before reviewing the possible mechanisms of HLA gene complex influences in disease susceptibility, it is necessary to point to the most salient feature of the population genetics of HLA antigens, namely, the presence of linkage disequilibria among certain antigens of the A and B, B and C, and B and D loci. A linkage disequilibrium means that antigens of closely linked loci appear together more frequently than predicted by random association. The classic example is the linkage disequilibrium present between the A-locus antigen, HLA-A1, and B-locus antigen, HLA-B8, in Caucasian populations of Western Europe and America. One expects the coincidence of A1 and B8 to be the product of their individual gene frequencies, or 0.17 times 0.11 equals approximately 0.02. The observed frequency of A1 and B8 in Caucasians is 0.06, three times that expected, and an increase of 0.04 The latter value is termed Δ (delta), and is a measure of the disequilibrium. Other A and B locus haplotype disequilibria have been recognized, and include (A3, B7), (A2, B12), (A29, B12), and (A11, Bw35). Furthermore, some D-locus determinants are now known to be in linkage disequilibrium with second-series antigens (for example, Dw3 and B8), and C-locus antigens often have a Δ with B-locus antigens. Just as the serologically defined HLA antigens can serve as markers for the genes of an entire haplotype within a family, they may also serve as markers within a whole population for specific genes, but only where a linkage disequilibrium exists.

The development of linkage disequilibria is a matter of some importance because such gene associations may have some bearing on their function. For example, it has been proposed that selective pressures during the course of evolution have been the major factor in the survival of certain gene combinations in a haplotype. Such a theory would suggest, for example, that A1 and B8, along with certain D-locus and other determinants, conferred a selective advantage in the face of epidemics such as the plague or smallpox. It would go on to conclude that the descendants of the survivors now display susceptibility to certain diseases because of their unique gene complex which happens to confer an abnormal response to nonlethal environmental agents. The major difficulty with this hypothesis is the assumption that selection would have to work on several genes simultaneously in order to account for the observed deltas; however, the need for complex interactions among the products of the several loci of the major histocompatibility complex is only beginning to be appreciated, and it is possible that selection could force multiple linkage disequilibria.

On the other hand, one does not require the selection hypothesis to establish deltas in a population. With fusion of a population lacking certain antigens with one having a high frequency of antigens in equilibrium, a Δ can develop within a very small number of generations. For example, the increasing Δ value for A1, B8, found as one samples populations from East to West, from India to Western Europe, can be explained on the basis of migration and fusion. In smaller groups, consanguinity, a founder effect, and gene drift may account for disequilibria. Finally, certain linkage disequilibria could occur as a result of a nonrandomness in crossing over during gametic meiosis, because of chromosomal segments which are either more or less likely to break. In any event, the facts strongly suggest that a large number of nonrandom associations exist throughout the HLA gene complex, and the reasons for their existence, when they are better understood, may relate closely to the mechanism underlying certain disease susceptibilities.

MECHANISMS There are three main hypotheses regarding the mechanisms by which histocompatibility complex genes influence disease susceptibility. The first is termed *molecular mimicry* and would propose that immunochemical similarities between HLA glycoproteins and microbiologic agents result in an impaired immune response because of cross-reacting tolerance of self-antigens. In order to be consistent with the observed facts of the dominance of disease susceptibility in the heterozygous state (e.g., ankylosing spondylitis occurs with B27 on one haplotype only), such a hypothesis would lead to the conclusion that the diseases in question are the result of chronic infection with a depressed immune response. However, there are no clearly demonstrated HLA and microbial cross-reactions. Most telling with regard to B27 and ankylosing spondylitis is the finding that B27 usually associates with this disease only when it is on a haplotype with the first series antigens, A2 or A9, providing evidence that B27 per se is most likely a marker for a linkage disequilibrium with other HLA region genes.

The second hypothesis suggests that HLA antigens may serve as *receptors for specific viruses,* resulting in an increased susceptibility to infection. This hypothesis has problems similar to the first, and direct attempts to show predilections for cell invasion by a variety of known viruses and cells of various HLA types have been unrewarding to date.

The third hypothesis, one which is gaining increased acceptance, is that important *immune response (Ir) genes* are present in the HLA gene complex, and that HLA antigens are markers for genes in linkage disequilibrium with them. The degree of association would then depend upon the distance between the marker and disease genes on the chromosome, and the degree to which crossing over between them may be restricted. An example is the finding that dermal responsiveness to ragweed antigen segregates with HLA haplotypes in atopic families, although the HLA antigens themselves may not be the same. A suggestive association with a D-locus gene and ragweed antigen E reactivity now exists, indicating that the gene(s) for a heightened immediate hypersensitivity response is placed far enough into the putative Ir region so that B-locus series HLA antigens are not good markers. When one considers the association of HLA-B8 and HLA-Dw3 markers with so many diseases (juvenile diabetes, Addison's disease, Graves' disease, gluten sensitivity, myasthenia gravis), it is tempting to conclude that a control mechanism for immune responsiveness, particularly with regard to autoimmunity, is involved. Since the etiologic agent is known in one of these diseases (gluten), and suspected in another (viral infection in juvenile diabetes mellitus), carefully designed studies should provide evidence regarding immune responsiveness to the agent versus an exaggerated secondary response to damaged tissue antigens. The distinction between association and linkage of a disease to HLA needs emphasis. The population studies summarized in Table 69-1 show associations to varying degrees, but linkage is not proved until family studies show segregation of the disease with HLA haplotypes. There is increasing evidence that at least some forms of juvenile-onset diabetes mellitus are not only linked to HLA, but that a recessive mode of inheritance may be involved, since there is a preponderance of HLA haplotype identical siblings among diabetic children, indicating that an HLA-linked gene(s) is required from both parents. A similar situation exists with idiopathic hemochromatosis and also 21-hydroxylase deficiency (Chap. 336 and Table 69-1) in which a preponderance of HLA identity among affected siblings also exists. The latter diseases illustrate the fact that an HLA-linked gene need not be an antigen of the HLA system itself, nor even related to any currently understood parameter of the immune response. The numbers of genes involved and the variety of ways in which the final patterns of various diseases present may well be highly variable. Nevertheless, the way is now open to a better understanding of the genetic control of immune responsiveness in disease states.

Tissue typing for transplantation Study of the HLA gene complex has, at present, limited direct clinical application, but its relationship to transplantation efforts is central. Siblings matched for the major antigens are easily treated with conventional drug therapy, and renal transplant results are in the range of 85 to 90 percent long-term success. A small number of A- and B-locus identical, but D-locus incompatible, transplants have been performed, and although not statistically significant, the majority of these have been rejected. The general experience in bone marrow transplantation also emphasizes the importance of matching for the D-locus region even when, due to recombination, the serologically defined A- and B-locus antigens are mismatched. Since the degree of linkage disequilibrium between HLA serologically defined antigens and other genes, including the D locus, is variable, and in many cases absent, matching of HLA-A and -B antigens for cadaveric renal transplantation is poorly predictive of graft success. Some series in Europe have provided evidence for improved survival with increasing numbers of A- and B-locus antigen matches, but these results have not been completely confirmed in North America, possibly because the greater degree of racial inhomogeneity in the New World reduces the amount of linkage disequilibrium between A, B, D, and other loci of the major histocompatibility gene complex. In contrast, some evidence exists for the importance of D-locus matching as assessed by retrospective results in MLC responses between cadaver and recipient lymphocytes. Since the MLC takes 5 to 7 days for the development of measurable degrees of proliferation ([³H]thymidine incorporation), more rapid means (<24 h) of typing for these antigens are needed. Typing for DR antigens allows for rapid assessment of the D region and may prove to be useful in cadaveric organ matching.

HLA serologically defined A- and B-locus differences are clearly of major importance once an alloimmune response has been initiated, as these determinants are the major, though not the sole, targets for both humoral and cellular effector mechanisms. Forty to fifty percent of patients exposed to blood products while on chronic hemodialysis develop complement-dependent cytotoxic antibodies to allogenic lymphocytes. The "high responder" sensitized patients may make a selective response against certain HLA antigens, or may develop such a polyspecific response that they react with 90 to 100 percent of a randomly selected population. Transplants are not performed when the specific cross matches of recipient serums with donor lymphocytes are positive, because of a very high likelihood of an immediate "hyperacute" rejection. Furthermore, sensitized patients receiving cadaveric renal grafts may have a high failure rate, even though the specific donor cross match is negative, indicating either a lack of sensitivity in the test or the absence of the relevant antibodies at that particular time. Evidence for the latter comes from the reported improvement in kidney survival rates when additional serums, obtained at monthly intervals while on dialysis, are used at the time of cross match, or if analyses of anti-HLA specificities in the serums are made. Either way, mismatches can be avoided by assessment of past, as well as present, reactivities. In other words, a profile of the patient's immunologic memory is developed in order to avoid anamnestic responses. Further improvement in practical matching techniques, employing more sensitive cross matches and techniques for assessment of direct and antibody-dependent, cell-mediated cytotoxicity may offer further refinement in solving this major problem in cadaveric renal transplantation. Avoidance of sensitization would appear to offer a logical approach; however, a number of female patients have been sensitized by prior pregnancies, and occasionally the development of such cytotoxins is not explained by either pregnancy or blood transfusion. More important is the absence of data to confirm the notion that patients who never receive blood will have improved graft results; in fact, several studies show an increased failure rate in nontransfused patients. Taken together, these results suggest that genetic control of the alloimmune response also exists in humans, although no correlation can be made with HLA phenotypes. Prior exposure to alloantigens provides a definition of who is a "low responder" and who is a "high responder," and in the latter case it is now possible to avoid, in many instances, the specific mismatches to which a response has already been made, selecting a "new" incompatibility which, as a primary response, is more amenable to conventional drug therapy. The clinical significance of preexisting antidonor B-cell antibodies, generally though not exclusively anti-DR, is unclear. Several units report no deleterious effect when this cross-match barrier is crossed, while others find that true anti-DR responses may be harmful, although other specificities are not. The latter antibodies are usually reactive only in the cold (4 to 20°C), are of the IgM class, and frequently behave as autoantibodies.

Although minor transplantation antigen incompatibilities may on occasion be of importance in renal transplantation, the only other major antigenic system of proved importance is the ABH red blood cell system, a genetic system which segregates randomly from HLA. For example, HLA identical siblings can be mismatched for ABH. The rules of blood transfusion apply with regard to group O being a universal donor and group AB being a universal recipient. The clinical importance of non-HLA, non-ABH systems in bone marrow transplantation is greater than with organ grafts because of the graft-versus-host reactivity which commonly occurs in HLA-matched marrow recipients, and, in fact, has become the major limiting factor in clinical marrow grafting.

Another important application of HLA typing is in matching for platelet transfusions in individuals sensitized by prior blood component exposure. Platelets express most of the HLA serologic specificities (A and B loci), but not the D- and DR-locus antigens. Matching donor and recipient lymphocyte HLA-A and -B loci is of proved value in improving survival of transfused platelets in sensitized recipients.

IMMUNOLOGY OF REJECTION Knowledge of the immunology of tissue transplantation stems largely from animal experimentation. However, enough evidence has accumulated in humans, particularly in kidney transplantation, to indicate that the evidence is similar though not identical for the different species. The following observations describe reasonably accurately the events that transpire during the rejection of most human tissue transplants. Spleen and bone marrow grafts differ because in these instance cells capable of reacting against the recipient (graft-versus-host reaction) are transplanted.

From data derived both from animal and human experience, it appears that the rejection of transplanted tissue results from the antigenic stimulus of a two-component lymphoid system (Fig. 69-4). The lymphocytes involved are the offspring of marrow-derived stem cells. As these stem cells mature under the direct or humoral influence of (1) the thymus or (2) a human equivalent to the cells of the avian bursa, they develop antigen receptors so that they can respond in a cooperative manner to make an immune response when stimulated by antigen. The mature lymphocytes comprising the two distinct populations are for convenience abbreviated as (1) thymus-dependent (T) and (2) bone marrow (bursa)-dependent (B). Cooperative interaction between T and B cells, through the mediation of a factor furnished by the T cells after antigenic stimulation, is necessary for initiation of the immune response.

This cell interaction may take place upon the dendrites of tissue macrophages. In the case of the renal allograft, donor antigen may stimulate either T or B cells by way of antigen liberated from the kidney and reaching the lymphocytes by the bloodstream or lymphatics; or by contact between the recipient's lymphocytes and donor antigen as the former circulate through the kidney.

Some T cells are long-lived, circulating in the peripheral blood but "homing" in on lymphoid organs. They are responsible for cell-mediated immunity (CMI) such as graft rejection, delayed hypersensitivity (tuberculin skin test), the immune response to intracellular organisms, and possible "surveillance" which protects against growth of spontaneously occurring neoplasia. B cells are shortlived, noncirculating cells, largely responsible for the production of immune globulins, often referred to as "circulating antibody" or "humoral antibody" (Fig. 69-3). Both cell types are involved in immunity to transplants. A third effector system, involving the cooperative effort of graft-specific IgG antibodies and a nonimmune non-T cell, tentatively called a K cell, is now recognized. These effector cells are distinct from the specifically sensitized "killer" T cells. K cells interact with the Fc portion of the target-cell-bound IgG to mediate antibody-dependent cell-mediated cytotoxicity. Both lymphocytes and monocyte subpopulations may have K-cell activity. Even the polymorphonuclear leukocyte can damage IgG-coated target cells. Allografts to recipients previously unexposed to donor antigen are rejected as a "first-set" graft, largely through the T-cell system. Recipients who have previously been immunized to donor allografts by exposure to donor antigens by blood transfusions or by a previous transplant, or who have been the recipients of xenografts, have circulating preformed humoral antibody, and such grafts undergo "humoral rejection" in which the B-cell mechanism predominates. Because unrelated individuals may share one or more specific HLA determinants, a recipient may become immunized to the tissues of a donor by previous exposure to transfused white blood cells or platelets from another individual whose tissues contain the same antigens as the allograft donor. Once a kidney has been in place for several days in a previously unsensitized recipient, humoral immunity may become superimposed upon the cellular rejection; therefore, both types of immune processes may mediate the rejection of an allograft, with one or the other predominating; furthermore, the K-cell mechanism provides a potential link between humoral and cell-mediated immunity.

The rejection of an allograft by an individual who has not previously been exposed to donor antigens occurs first by way of the CMI pathways in which the sensitized T lymphocytes predominate. In the case of the kidney, the sensitized lymphocyte first combines with an antigen on vascular endothelium. Very early in the rejection process cells can be seen in contact with the small venules. The precise mechanism of the damage induced by the sensitized "killer" T lymphocytes awaits elucidation, but immunoglobulins and complement are not required. Rather, a cyclic nucleotide (cAMP and cGMP)-dependent process which follows direct cell-to-cell contact has been implicated. Similarly, the interaction of sensitized lymphocytes and antigens at the graft site is likely to release migration inhibitory factor (MIF) which may account for the accumulation of mononuclear (histiocytic) cells at the graft site. Some of these cells migrate through the vessel wall and are seen as perivascular accumulations. Intravascular accumulations result in slowing of flow, stasis, and graft ischemia. B lymphocytes, specifically sensitized, or K cells nonspecifically recruited by the prior formation of immune complexes of antibody and histocompatibility antigens, may also appear in the graft along the endothelial lining of vessels. Recovery of infiltrating cells from rejecting organs for study has shown that B cells, T cells, K cells, and monocytes may all be present. Of importance is the fact that donor-specific "killer" cells have been recovered from both animals and human allografts. When significant amounts of circulating antibodies, principally IgG and IgM, appear, the complement sequence is initiated. If intense, such activation may release significant amounts of polymorphonuclear (PMN) chemotactic factors, and PMNs are attracted to the graft, where the release of lysosomal enzymes from the leukocytes may result in damage to the vascular wall. In addition, the deposition of platelets is facilitated, with the release of vasoactive kinins and the deposition of fibrinogen and fibrin. This sequence of events is corroborated by histologic observations of rejection demonstrating interstitial infiltration of cells and damage to vascular endothelium with the deposition of fibrin, complement, and immune globulins. It can be shown also that the earliest evidence of renal allograft rejection is redistribution of blood flow from the cortex to the corticomedullary area, reflecting the primary role of the influence of vascular damage in the rejection process.

When a kidney is transplanted into a heterologous species or an individual previously sensitized to donor antigen, it is immediately perfused by "preformed" humoral antibody directed specifically against graft antigen. Again, the sequence of events which takes place reflects primarily the vascular site of injury. In such an instance little cellular infiltrate may be seen, but destruction to the vessel wall is violent and immediate, occurring in a matter of minutes in some instances. Platelet thrombi, the deposition of fibrin, and necrosis of vascular endothelium are prominent, and flow through the graft may cease within minutes or hours. Presumably, the same humoral mechanisms discussed above participate, but the sequence of events is accelerated; thus, the term "hyperacute rejection" has been applied.

The failure of transplanted kidneys after 2 or even 3 years of adequate function is due to a form of "chronic rejection." In such kidneys the development of nephrosclerosis, with proliferation of the vascular intima of renal vessels, and intimal fibrosis with marked decrease in the lumen of the vessels take place (Fig. 69-5). The result is renal ischemia, hypertension, widespread tubular atrophy, interstitial fibrosis, and glomerular atrophy with eventual renal failure. Occasionally, lobular or proliferative glomerulonephritis may be the initiating factor and may progress to renal failure. Most long-term vascular lesions and glomerular lesions are probably the result of subclinical episodes of rejection with damage to capillary and vascular epithelium and resultant healing fibrosis and sclerosis.

Finally, there is evidence that humoral antibody, in all probability some fraction of IgG, may actually play a role in promoting the *survival* of the allograft. This enhancing anti-

FIGURE 69-4

Overall scheme of the development of effector mechanisms in graft rejection. Bone marrow stem cells differentiate under the influence of the thymus gland into mature thymus-derived (T) lymphocytes, or under the influence of an equivalent to the avian bursa of Fabricius into mature bone-marrow-derived (B) lymphocytes. Exposure to antigen (Δ) results in an interaction between T cells and B cells, and often involves macrophages. The sensitized B cells, after mitoses, develop into immunoglobulin-secreting cells (e.g., plasma cells), illustrated here by IgG and IgM. Such immunoglobulins may form immune complexes with antigen in the circulation which activate the complement sequence, or they may react directly with antigens on the blood vessel surface. Elaboration of secondary mediators, including the products of complement activation, results in vascular damage as illustrated. Sensitized T lymphocytes are the primary effector cells in cell-mediated immunity (CMI) and may react directly with antigens in the graft to exert a cytotoxic effect. In addition, T cells release factors, such as macrophage migration inhibition factor (MIF) which may accelerate the rate of mononuclear cell infiltration. It has also been shown that unsensitized non-T cells (K cells) can be activated to exert cytotoxic effects by the fixation of IgG to target cells, followed by interaction of the IgG (Fc portion) with a receptor on the K cell. Nonimmune B cells may have K-cell activity, but since other mononuclear cells can react with IgG on target cells, the K cell is shown as having a separate lineage. Finally, platelet aggregation and thrombosis can occur following the endothelial damage induced by any of these mechanisms.

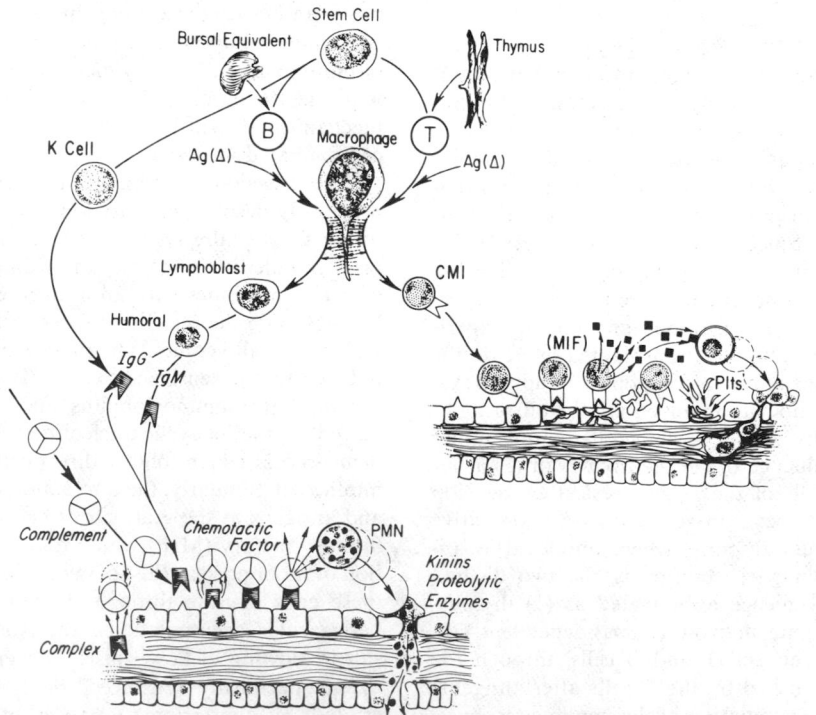

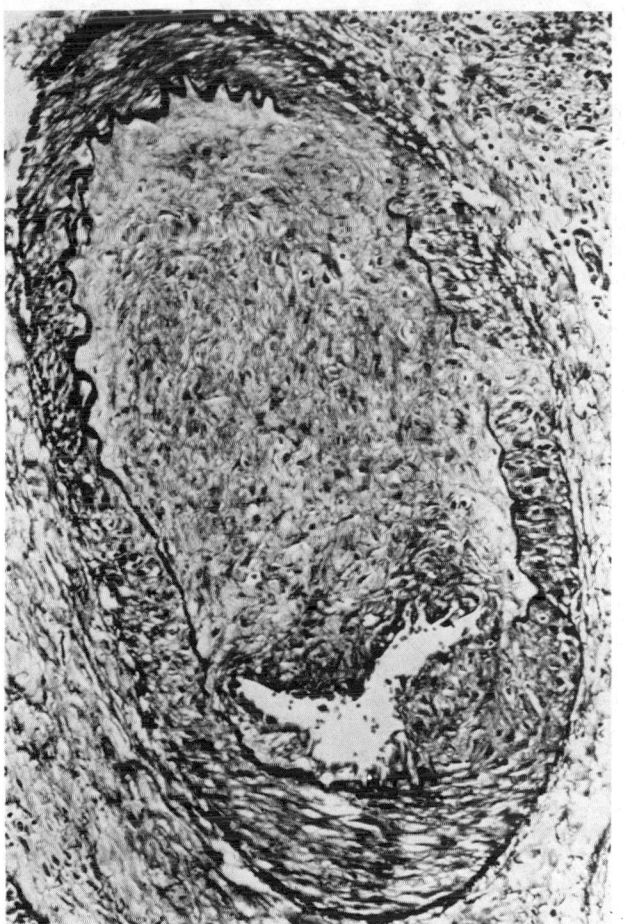

FIGURE 69-5

Biopsy of the renal cadaveric allograft illustrating obliterative endarteritis. Loss of the media is associated with intimal thickening. The elastic tissue shows dissolution of the elastica. The evidence for arteritis with subsequent thrombosis is typically the gaps in the elastica and media. The intimal thickening probably represents organization of a thrombus formed in response to the arteritis. [From GJ Dammin, JP Merrill, in Structural Basis for Renal Disease, EL Becker (ed), New York, Hoeber-Harper, 1968.]

body may block the action of cytotoxic "killer" lymphocytes, thus preventing the disastrous effects of the immune onslaught against the graft or may alter the presentation of antigen to responding B and T cells (Fig. 69-3).

IMMUNOSUPPRESSIVE TREATMENT When histocompatibility differences exist between donor and recipient, it is necessary to modify or suppress the immune response in order to enable the recipient to accept a graft. Immunosuppressive therapy in general suppresses all immune responses, including those to bacteria, fungi, and even malignant tumors. Agents used in humans to suppress the immune response are the following:

Drugs *Azathioprine (Imuran)*, an analogue of 6-mercaptopurine, is the keystone to immunosuppressive therapy in humans. This agent can inhibit synthesis of deoxyribonucleic acid (DNA), ribonucleic acid (RNA), or both. Because cell division and proliferation result as part of the immune response to antigenic stimulation, suppression may be mediated by the inhibition of mitosis of immunologically competent lymphoid cells interfering with synthesis of DNA. Alternatively, inhibition may be brought about by blocking the synthesis of ribonucleic acid (possibly messenger RNA), which is thought to play an

immunologic role in the processing of antigens prior to lymphocyte stimulation. Therapy with azathioprine is generally instituted 2 to 5 days prior to transplantation in the recipient of a living donor kidney and on the day of transplantation in the case of a cadaver donor kidney recipient. The drug is continued at levels of 2 to 3 mg/kg per day, as long as the allograft functions. Because the drug is rapidly metabolized by the liver, its dose need not be varied directly in relation to renal function, even though renal failure results in retention of the metabolites of azathioprine. Some patients are unusually sensitive to this drug, particularly when renal function is compromised, and reduction in dosage is required because of leukopenia and occasionally thrombocytopenia. Excessive amounts of azathioprine may also cause jaundice, anemia, and alopecia.

The *corticosteroids*, usually in the form of prednisone, are important adjuncts to immunosuppressive therapy. Of all the agents employed, prednisone has effects that are easiest to assess, and in large doses it is unquestionably the most effective agent for the reversal of rejection. In general, 150 to 200 mg prednisone is given immediately prior to or at the time of transplantation, and the dosage is reduced to maintenance levels over a period of 2 weeks. The well-known side effects of the corticosteroids, particularly impairment of wound healing and predisposition to infection, make it desirable to taper the dose as rapidly as possible in the immediate postoperative period. Customarily methylprednisolone, 1 to 2 g, intravenously, is administered immediately upon diagnosis of beginning rejection. When the drug is effective, the results are usually apparent within 48 to 96 h, and the dose may be subsequently tapered over a 5-day period and oral prednisone resumed. Such "pulse" doses are less effective in the slow rejection process which may not become apparent until 2 to 3 years after transplantation. Although most patients whose renal function is stable after 6 months or a year do not require large doses of prednisone, maintenance doses of 20 mg per day are the rule. Many patients tolerate an alternate-day course of steroids better without an increased risk of rejection.

When jaundice or nephritis appears in patients maintained on azathioprine, *cyclophosphamide* may be substituted. It appears to be as effective in the maintenance of renal allografts as Imuran and somewhat more effective in hepatic allografts. Leukopenia, alopecia, cystitis, ovarian fibrosis, and aspermia may result if the dosage is not carefully regulated. In one series of cadaver allografts the prospective donor was treated with massive doses of cyclophosphamide and methylprednisolone in an attempt to decrease the antigenicity of the graft by eliminating "passenger leukocytes." The preliminary results of this technique are encouraging.

Antilymphocyte globulin (ALG) When serums from animals made immune to host lymphocytes are injected into the recipient, a marked suppression of cellular immunity to the tissue graft results. The action upon CMI is considerably more effective than upon humoral immunity. A globulin fraction of the serum is the agent generally employed. For use in humans, peripheral human lymphocytes, thymocytes, lymphocytes from cadaver spleens, or those harvested from thoracic duct fistulas have been utilized. More recently, cultured human lymphoblasts, which can be produced in large quantities, offer the advantage of availability. These cells are injected into horses, rabbits, or goats to produce antilymphocyte serum, from which the globulin fraction is then separated. The globulin is injected intramuscularly, or preferably intravenously, 5 days to 1 week prior to transplantation and continued for 2 to 3 weeks thereafter. Although ALG, or ATG (antithymocyte globulin) is unquestionably effective in prolonging grafts in experimental animals, its efficacy in the transplantation of human tissue is somewhat less clear, even though an effective preparation of ALG may result in the disappearance of a previously positive delayed type of skin reaction. ALG should be used with caution in human beings; it cannot now be considered part of routine immunosuppressive therapy. Further exploration of this preparation, particularly employing larger doses, may result in the development of an effective agent which can be used with relatively little hazard of serum sickness or nephrotoxic nephritis.

Other techniques Of the alternate techniques of immunosuppression, thymectomy and splenectomy have not favorably influenced the course of human kidney transplants. Local irradiation to the transplanted kidney in two or three doses of 350 rads each has also been utilized. This technique may result in fewer early rejection episodes in cadaveric transplants than in nonirradiated controls.

COMPLICATIONS OF RENAL TRANSPLANTATION The complications of human renal transplantation often result from the use of *immunosuppressive therapy*. Wound infection with gram-negative organisms is common, as is breakdown of wounds, particularly the ureteral anastomosis. Pulmonary infections with a variety of unusual organisms, including *Candida* (Chap. 158), *Aspergillus* (Chap. 159), *Nocardia* (Chap. 152), *Pneumocystis* (Chap. 204), and cytomegalovirus (Chap. 194) also occur. Their relationship to a general defect in immunologic integrity is clear. The complications of *corticosteroid* therapy are well known and include gastrointestinal bleeding, hemorrhagic pancreatitis, impairment of wound-healing, osteoporosis, diabetes, and cataract formation. Leukopenia, anemia, and jaundice may occur as a result of azathioprine administration.

Even identical twins who do not require immunosuppressive therapy develop complications. In 18 sets of identical twins whose original disease was glomerulonephritis, 11 developed a similar histologic lesion in the transplanted kidney. The glomerular lesion is not, however, limited to the isograft, nor is it necessarily a question of "catching" the disease in the transplant because of continuing antiglomerular activity. A number of patients with true allografts treated with immunosuppressive therapy have developed typical glomerular lesions over a period of years. One patient who received a successful allograft from his mother developed a classic nephrotic syndrome with glomerulonephritis 2½ years after transplantation. Because the reason for transplantation initially was the accidental removal of a single normal ectopic kidney, the development of glomerulonephritis in the transplant cannot be attributed to "continuing activity."

Glomerular lesions occur in some 10 to 15 percent of allografts. In many of these the lesions so resemble those of the patient's own original disease that they must be considered recurrences of the original disease. The recurrence of the nephrotic syndrome with "nil disease" in transplanted kidneys whose recipient's original nil disease has progressed to renal failure with focal sclerosis, the recurrence in renal allografts of the classic lesions of IgA nephropathy, and those of membranoproliferative glomerulonephritis with electron-dense deposit disease are classic examples. In the last of these, the incidence of recurrence has been reported as high as 30 to 40 percent. In many instances, however, the recurrence of the original renal lesions may represent no threat to the patient's immediate prognosis, and an established diagnosis of glomerulonephritis is rarely taken as a contraindication to transplantation. Finally, in at least one case, glomerulonephritis has developed apparently de novo in a patient who has survived 5 years with a normally functioning allograft.

Sensitization of the human recipient to the antigens of the renal allograft may occur because of exposure to these antigens via blood transfusions or pregnancy. When the cytotoxic antibodies are directed against the antigens of the donor, rapid rejection of the graft occurs, and even when the cytotoxic antibodies in the recipient's serum are not specific for those of the donor, the prognosis for graft survival is poorer than in unsensitized individuals. This is discussed elsewhere in this chapter.

The incidence of *tumors* arising in patients on immunosuppressive therapy in one well-studied group was 5.6 percent, or approximately 100 times greater than that observed in the general population in the same age range. These figures correspond with those in the world experience in well over 27,000 cases. The most common lesions were cancer of the skin and lips and carcinoma in situ of the cervix. These lesions were easily treated. There was a high incidence of lymphomas, particularly reticulum cell sarcoma of the nervous system. The prognosis was poor when these lesions occurred. Two possibilities are suggested for the high incidence of cancer in transplant recipients: (1) immunosuppressive therapy impairs the "immunologic surveillance" of the lymphoreticular system, in consequence of which potentially malignant cellular mutations are not detected and destroyed; (2) immunosuppressed individuals frequently harbor viruses, some of which may be oncogenic. The chronic immunostimulation produced by the resident allograft may be more important than the drug-induced immunosuppression, particularly since such stimulation may activate some viruses.

Tumor cells have been transplanted inadvertently with kidneys taken from cadaver donors and occasionally from living donors. The immunosuppressive therapy which allows the kidney to be tolerated in the recipients also apparently permits survival and propagation of the malignant tumor. In two instances cessation of immunosuppressive therapy resulted in rejection of both the graft and the tumor with its metastases.

Urinary fistula requiring nephrostomy may be the result of rejection of the ureter, disruption of the ureteral blood supply, infection, or a combination of all three. Wound infection and failure of the wound to heal are not uncommon, particularly when the higher doses of steroids are required.

Hypercalcemia may develop within days or weeks after transplantation and persist for as long as 7 years. In many instances this appears to be due to markedly enlarged parathyroid glands which have developed during the uremic phase and do not spontaneously regress with the resumption of normal renal function. In other instances no elevation of blood levels of parathyroid hormone can be found. Although several instances of renal and vascular calcification have been reported, renal function in general does not appear to suffer. However, when bone disease occurs or persists in the presence of hyperparathyroidism, subtotal parathyroidectomy is indicated. Glucocorticoid administration may contribute to the hypercalcemia.

Aseptic necrosis of the head of the femur has been reported in 10 to 20 percent of the posttransplant patients. This complication is probably due to preexisting uremic bone disease or hyperparathyroidism, plus the large doses of corticosteroid. With improved management of calcium and phosphorus metabolism during periods of dialysis, however, the incidence of aseptic necrosis following transplantation has fallen dramatically.

There has been considerable improvement in patient morbidity and mortality rates during the mid-1970s, attributable to more judicious use of immunosuppressive agents and antibiotics. It is customary now to use steroid pulses only twice, or rarely three times, and to allow the patient to return to dialysis. Although graft survival is not improved by this protocol, it has not worsened, while patient mortality has dropped from around 20 percent to less than 5 percent per year, a rate which is comparable to that for hemodialysis. Urinary fistulae are also much less common, partly because aberrant polar arteries which nourish the renal pelvis and upper ureter are no longer ligated, but are anastomosed by microsurgical techniques. Concomitant with improved mortality, the incidence of bacterial infection has declined to less than 15 percent, and units which formerly had major problems with fungal and viral diseases now must deal with these in only a small minority of transplant recipients.

The incidence of death from *myocardial infarction* and *cerebrovascular accidents* is considerably higher in transplant recipients than in the population at large. The contributing factors are preexisting hypertension, vascular disease, and hypertriglyceridemia, which occurs in uremic patients and persists in the posttransplant period. There is possibly a contribution by hypercalcemia. *Gastrointestinal hemorrhage* is also a complication.

SELECTION OF RECIPIENTS FOR KIDNEY TRANSPLANTATION
Table 69-2 lists practical considerations in the selection of a recipient for a human renal allograft. Such a procedure should be undertaken only when conservative treatment has failed, when there are no reversible elements in the patient's renal failure, and when the patient is too sick to be maintained comfortably with the usual methods of treatment. However, the considerable success with kidneys transplanted from blood relatives, reports of success with second or third kidney transplants, and the ability to maintain patients who have had transplant failures on hemodialysis justify consideration of kidney transplantation before the patient is critically ill and possibly even before it is obvious that hemodialysis is the only other course. Transplantation should not be utilized in an attempt to salvage patients from failure to thrive on dialysis. On the other hand, when no well-matched related donor is available, the patient and physician should carefully consider the relative risks against those of continued dialysis. Approximately 10 percent of dialysis patients receiving cadaver transplants cannot be successfully returned to dialysis if the graft fails. The attrition rate in most well-run dialysis programs is about 4 to 7 percent per year. Each case, of course, must be individualized before the statistics have pertinence. The recipient should be free of life-threatening extrarenal complications such as cancer, severe coronary artery disease, and cerebrovascular disease. Provided that diffuse vascular involvement is not present, diabetes itself is not a contraindication. Although age may be a limiting factor, the "physiologic" age rather than the chronologic age contraindicates transplantation. A cadaver transplant into an 82-year-old patient is on record, and adult renal allografts have been transplanted into recipients as young as 3. Although abnormalities of the bladder and urethra present additional hazards, successful renal allografts have been placed in individuals with these abnormalities by prior construction of an artificial bladder (i.e., ileal conduit) into which the donor ureter is placed. The demonstration of "preformed antibodies" in the potential recipient prior to transplantation is a contraindication when in the standard lymphocytotoxicity test these antibodies react specifically to donor cells.

DONOR SELECTION Donor sources are cadavers or volunteer blood-related living donors. Living volunteer donors should be found completely normal on physical examination and should be of the same major ABO blood group, because there is good evidence that crossing major blood group barriers prejudices survival of the allograft. It is, however, possible to transplant a kidney of a type O donor into an A or B recipient. Selective renal arteriography should be performed on volunteer donors to rule out the presence of multiple or abnormal renal arteries, because the surgical procedure is inordinately difficult and the ischemic time of the normal kidney prohibitively long when vascular abnormalities exist. Cadaver donors should be free of malignant neoplastic disease because of possible transmission of cancer to the recipient.

Although tissue typing for A- and B-locus HLA antigens is of limited value for cadaver donors, direct cross matching for the presence of preformed antibodies against specific donor tissue is mandatory. The chances of finding a perfect A- and B-locus 4-antigen match between unrelated donor and recipient are calculated to be between 1 in 300 and 1 in 1000, varying with the incidence of HLA antigens in the population. If, in addition, antigens of the D locus are found to be of practical importance, matching will require a large recipient pool, maintained on hemodialysis. A coordinated regional or national system of computerized information sharing and logistical support for the transportation of cadaver kidneys to the suitable recipient is under development. It is now possible to remove cadaver kidneys and to maintain them up to 48 h on cold pulsatile perfusion or simple flushing and cooling. This should permit adequate time for various typing, cross matching, transportation, and selection problems to be solved.

CLINICAL COURSE AND MANAGEMENT OF THE RECIPIENT
Bilateral nephrectomy at some point prior to transplantation is performed for specific cause but not as a routine. Hypertension which is difficult to control or infection involving the end-stage kidneys are the two most common indications. Nephrectomized patients maintain a much lower hematocrit level, but this is no longer considered a disadvantage per se, because blood transfusions are not to be avoided in preparation for transplantation. When comparing the overall results with nephrectomized vs. nonnephrectomized recipients, no significant difference has emerged, except for the fact that nontransfused recipients of cadaveric grafts are more likely to reject their grafts. It should be ascertained also that the recipient has a normally functioning bladder and lower outflow tract.

Adequate hemodialysis should be performed within 48 h prior to surgery, and care should be taken that the serum potassium level is not markedly elevated so that intraoperative cardiac arrhythmias can be averted. In patients who have been presensitized to donor tissue, hyperacute rejection may take place on the operating table. Within minutes the kidney will become swollen, tense, and a mottled purple in color, and blood flow may cease soon thereafter. Thrombotic obliterative lesions may be seen by frozen section, and if they are extensive the kidney should be removed. Postoperatively the diuresis that occurs must be carefully monitored; in many instances it

TABLE 69-2
Contraindications to human kidney transplantation

I Absolute contraindications:
 A Reversible renal involvement
 B Ability of conservative measures to maintain useful life
 C Major extrarenal complications (cerebrovascular or coronary disease; neoplasia)
 D Active infection
 E Active glomerulonephritis
 F Previous sensitization to donor tissue
II Relative contraindications (see text):
 A Age
 B Presence of vesical or urethral abnormalities
 C Iliofemoral occlusive disease
 D Diabetes mellitus
 E Inactive lupus erythematosus
 F Psychiatric problems

may be massive, reflecting the inability of ischemic tubules to regulate sodium and water excretion. Massive potassium losses may occur and occasionally result in cardiac arrhythmias. The chronically uremic patient undoubtedly has some excess of extracellular fluid, and some degree of negative balance should be accomplished provided circulatory hemodynamics remain stable.

Although immunosuppressive regimens vary, a typical program would be the following:

Azathioprine in a dose of 4 mg/kg is given for 2 days preoperatively to recipients of a living donor transplant; on the day of operation it is administered by the intravenous route, and it is continued for about 1 week, depending upon renal function. It is then reduced to 3 mg/kg, and the maintenance dose is 1½ mg/kg by mouth. In recipients of kidneys from living donors the equivalent of 300 to 500 mg cortisone is given on the day of operation; this dose is maintained for 2 days and is decreased gradually to a maintenance dose of 50 to 100 mg cortisone, usually administered as the prednisone equivalent. For rejection episodes, 1 to 2 g soluble corticosteroid in the form of methylprednisolone is administered intravenously daily for a 3-day period. This is decreased to 800, 600, and 400 mg over the next 10-day period while oral prednisone dosage is maintained at 25 to 50 mg.

The rejection episode Early diagnosis of rejection is imperative, because prompt institution of vigorous therapy may reverse renal function and prevent irreversible damage due to fibrosis. Clinical evidence of rejection is characterized by fever, swelling, and tenderness over the allograft, and by significant reduction in urine volume. In patients whose renal function is good initially, oliguria may be accompanied by decreased urinary sodium concentration and increased osmolarity. These changes may not be present in the more chronic stages of rejection or when renal function is impaired at the onset of rejection. A transplanted cadaver kidney frequently undergoes a period of anuria which may last as long as 3 weeks without prejudicing the eventual function of the graft. In this instance, the reversible lesion is presumably due to ischemia, and the diagnosis of rejection becomes more difficult. Renal arteriography and radioactive Hippuran renograms may be useful in ascertaining changes in the renal vasculature and in renal blood flow, even in the absence of urinary flow. Diagnostic ultrasound has become the procedure of choice to rule out urinary obstruction or to confirm the presence of perirenal collections of urine, blood, or lymph. When renal function has been good initially, a rise in the serum creatinine level and a decrease in the creatinine clearance may herald the onset of rejection. The serum creatinine or its clearance is more reliable than the blood urea nitrogen because fever and the administration of prednisone may influence the concentration of blood urea nitrogen without necessarily reflecting a decrease in urea clearance. Increase in the 24-h excretion of urinary lysozyme has been helpful. Increase in proteinuria may reflect rejection, but when it occurs later in the course of the postoperative period, predominant glomerular disease may be present. Hypertension is also a concomitant of rejection. When hypertension responds to prednisone, it is likely that rejection has been responsible for the elevation of blood pressure, because other forms of hypertension usually do not improve with corticosteroid therapy. A number of tests have been posed for the diagnosis of rejection which depend upon the measurements of variation in expressions of cellular or humoral immunity; persistent antidonor antibody activity, as detected by complement-dependent cytotoxicity or by antibody-dependent cell-mediated cytotoxicity (K cells), often correlates with irreversible rejection with vasculitis in the graft. Appearance of circu-

lating cytotoxic T cells ("killer" cells) is more likely to relate to a cell-mediated rejection process. Other tests, such as the measurement of lysozyme excretion and that of fibrin-split products reflect nonspecific renal damage, although the latter test may have somewhat more pertinence to the rejection mechanism.

Modification of the usual clinical manifestations of infection by immunosuppressive therapy is a major problem in the posttransplant period. The signs and symptoms of infection may be masked and distorted, and fever without obvious cause is common. Only after days or weeks will it become apparent that it has a viral or fungal origin. The importance of blood cultures in such patients cannot be overemphasized, because systemic infection without obvious external foci is frequent. Particularly important are rapidly occurring pulmonary lesions, which may result in death within 5 days of onset. When these become apparent, immunosuppressive agents should be discontinued except for maintenance doses of prednisone. In the case of *Pneumocystis carinii*, trimethoprim-sulfa or pentamidine is the treatment of choice; amphotericin B has been used effectively in systemic fungal infections. Involvement of the oropharynx with *Candida* may be treated with local nystatin. Small doses (a total of 300 mg) of amphotericin given over a period of 2 weeks may be effective in refractory oral candidiasis. The treatment of jaundice in transplant patients should include cessation of azathioprine therapy. It is surprising that total cessation of azathioprine therapy often does not result in rejection of a graft. In some instances of jaundice, cyclophosphamide may be substituted for azathioprine. Antiplatelet agents and anticoagulants, although effective in theory, have not been strikingly successful in the prevention of the chronic vascular lesion.

The condition of patients who have been discharged from the hospital should be closely observed in a specialized outpatient clinic whose physicians are familiar with the problems and complications of the posttransplant patient. When, in spite of repeated efforts to reverse the rejection, renal function progressively fails, the philosophy should be to save the patient, not the graft. Excessive immunosuppressive therapy may lead to fatal infection or bleeding. A biopsy of the graft may establish the irreversibility of the lesion. When such irreversibility is established, the graft should be removed and the patient started again on hemodialysis. Infection and hemorrhage at the operative sites days and even months following removal of the graft occasionally occur and must be carefully watched. Psychological complications following transplantation are common. Depression and anxiety may reflect both the difficult, stressful postoperative course and the anxiety and uncertainty of the physician.

In spite of the potential teratogenic effects of immunosuppressive agents, both women and men have become parents after transplantation. The incidence of congenital abnormalities in the offspring is not unusual. The major problems with pregnancy are related to the concomitant development of rejection activity in the graft causing uremia and hypertension. In one series of over 400 pregnancies in transplant recipients 25 percent required therapeutic abortion. Although one-half of the live births had no complications, the others were either premature or underweight, and there was an increased incidence of the respiratory distress syndrome. There is an impression that pregnancy may provoke rejection activity in some previously stable patients, a point of interest because the fetus itself is an allograft. Although obstruction of the transplant ureter by extrinsic compression is a potential problem, its actual incidence is rare; furthermore, urinary infections do not seem to be more frequent in pregnant transplant recipients.

It is evident that immunosuppressive therapy as currently used in renal transplantation is inadequate. What is badly needed is a solution to the problem of producing specific immunologic unresponsiveness to the antigens of the donor without affecting the recipient's immune potential for infective agents. Such techniques have been successfully developed for the experimental animal, and their safe application to humans is eagerly awaited.

TRANSPLANTATION OF OTHER TISSUES Organs other than the kidney which have a potential for clinical transplantation are the liver and heart. Two possible indications for *liver transplantation* are chronic hepatic failure and malignancy which is localized to the liver. Two techniques for liver transplantation have been utilized in humans: (1) *orthotopic*—the recipient's own liver is removed and the transplant is substituted for it in the anatomic positon; (2) *auxiliary*—the recipient's liver is left in place and the allograft is placed in the right paravertebral gutter. The donor's vena cava then is interposed in the recipient terminal inferior vena cava, and the hepatic artery is anastomosed to the right common iliac artery. Finally, the end of the allograft portal vein is anastomosed to the recipient's superior mesenteric vein.

Immunosuppressive regimens are similar to those in kidney transplantation. There is some suggestion that the use of antilymphocyte globulin is more effective in liver allografting. Obviously, the donor source must be a cadaver. Complications of liver transplantation have been strikingly different from those encountered with renal allografts. In many instances an initial hemorrhagic diathesis with fibrinolysis occurs. This is followed by a phase of hypercoagulability in the successfully transplanted recipient, which in one instance resulted in fatal pulmonary emboli. Infections also seem to present a greater problem than with renal allografts. These complications are not insurmountable, however, and there are now a number of liver-transplant recipients who have survived for 2 years or more. Although at this time liver transplantation is not as clinically feasible a procedure as kidney grafting, in a few centers with expertise and experience in this technique liver transplants continue to be performed. It is hoped with steady improvement in the results.

Transplantation of the heart has been accomplished successfully in humans in a number of instances. Current results suggest that it is comparable to transplantation of the cadaver kidney and that results probably will improve. Indications for cardiac transplantation are myocardial insufficiency, usually due to severe coronary artery disease and myocardial fibrosis, and failure to respond to the most rigorous medical measures. The donor must be a cadaver and is usually an individual whose death has resulted from trauma or suicide. The question of the ethics and morals raised by the removal of a heart capable of sustaining life in another individual has been discussed by many medical and lay authors. It seems eminently reasonable that if "death" of the brain has occurred, as evidenced by lack of electrical activity in the electroencephalogram over a period of 24 to 36 h, dilated pupils, failure of spontaneous respiration, and lack of peripheral reflexes, the ability to maintain respiration or cardiac output by artificial methods is academic. Nevertheless, the decision as to when to discontinue these efforts should be made independently by the physician caring for the prospective donor in consultation with one or two colleagues. The question whether the heart is to be used for transplantation should not affect this decision. Once the decision has been made, the donor can be maintained until the recipient is prepared for operation. Recently a human "auxiliary heart" has been transplanted with initial success. The anastomosis of the donor heart to that of the recipient is made in such a way that the normal left ventricle of the donor assists the failing left ventricle of the recipient while the hypertrophied right ventricle of the recipient is allowed to continue to function in the pulmonary circuit, thus eliminating the sudden load imposed upon the normal right ventricle by the preexist-

ing pulmonary hypertension. At present, cardiac transplantation is and should be done only in specialized centers with highly skilled and experienced teams. Its future as an important therapeutic procedure is still unclear.

Human *spleen* and *pancreas* have been transplanted with limited success. If it could be shown that normal spleen can produce a useful amount of antihemophilic globulin (AHG), transplantation of that organ to some patients with hemophilia would provide a distinct advantage over standard substitution therapy. Transplantation of lymphoid tissue (including spleen) for total agammaglobulinemia has resulted in temporary improvement, but eventually the transplanted lymphoid tissue rejects the host (graft-versus-host reaction). Temporary success in transplanting pancreas in diabetics also has been reported, but substitution therapy seems more feasible.

Various other *endocrines*, including parathyroid, adrenal, and thyroid, have all been transplanted with only temporary success. A large percentage of *corneal grafts* survive as allografts in humans primarily because the cornea is not vascularized and excludes immunologically competent cells. Grafts of bone and blood vessels do not survive as living allografts but act as a "scaffolding" over which host tissue may grow.

Transplantation of allogenic bone marrow in humans (Chap. 312) is of particular interest to patients with leukemia and aplastic anemia and has resulted in a number of attempts to modify these diseases by this means. Similarly, the reconstitution of the defect in congenital or acquired agammaglobulinemia or alymphocytosis has been attempted by grafting into such recipients cells competent to produce cell-mediated immunity or humoral immunity. When the recipient and donor are identical twins, no immunosuppressive therapy is necessary, and 50 percent of the recipients transplanted have done well. Aplastic anemia has also been treated by marrow-grafting between siblings who are 4-antigen HLA matches and MLC-negative. In this case the recipient is prepared with cyclophosphamide and total body irradiation, while methotrexate is given after grafting. Some 50 percent of these patients have also done well. In the treatment of acute leukemia the object is to destroy as many of the malignant cells as possible; therefore, 1000 rads total body irradiation plus cyclophosphamide is given, and, in one protocol, in order to enhance the immune reaction of donor cells against malignant antigens, the recipient is immunized by radiation-killed malignant cells. In the instances where this was accomplished between identical twins, 10 remissions longer than 3 months and 1 greater than 49 months have occurred. The recipients of matched allogenic marrow, similarly prepared, have done increasingly well, and the probability of being in remission at 2 years is about 30 percent. Immune-competent donor cells reacting against the antigens of the host result in a "graft-versus-host reaction" in some 70 percent of the cases. This may be acute or indolent and is characterized by involvement of the skin, liver, and gastrointestinal tract. Infection, similar to that seen in kidney transplant recipients, is common. Methotrexate, cyclophosphamide, and antithymocyte globulin have been used in the treatment of this syndrome with some success. A striking and unexpected phenomenon has been malignant transformation of donor cells in two instances.

Transplantation of a normal allogenic liver to repair the metabolic defect in Wilson's disease has been reported in two instances with some preliminary success, and the transplantation of the kidney not as a functioning excretory organ but as a source of the congenitally absent enzyme has been attempted in Fabry's disease and oxalosis. The long-term results are disappointing.

ORGAN PRESERVATION If it were possible to remove cadaver organs and to store them for a period of weeks or longer under conditions permitting their successful replantation, one of the difficult problems in organ procurement would be solved. Bone marrow is the only organ that can be stored easily for prolonged periods.

XENOGRAFTS Kidneys, lungs, and hearts have been transplanted to human beings from various primates, including chimpanzees and baboons. Although one chimpanzee kidney graft functioned well for more than 7 months, clinical efforts in this area have been abandoned.

REFERENCES

CARPENTER CB (ed): *Clinical Histocompatibility Testing,* vol 2. New York. Grune & Stratton, 1978
——— et al: The role of antibodies in the rejection and enhancement of organ allografts. Adv Immunol 22:1, 1976

DEGOS L, DAUSSET J: Human migrations and linkage disequilibrium of HLA system. Immunogenetics 3:195, 1974
GALE RP, OPELZ G (eds): *Immunobiology of Bone Marrow Transplantation.* New York, Grune & Stratton, 1978
GOTTLIEB MN et al: Bone disease following renal transplantation, in *Calcium and Bone Metabolism in Renal Disease,* DS David (ed). New York, Wiley, 1977, p 279
JERSILD C et al: The HLA system and inherited deficiencies of the complement system. Transplant Rev 32:43, 1976
MERRILL JP: Dialysis versus transplantation in the treatment of end-stage renal disease. Annu Rev Med 29:343, 1978
STRAFFON RA (ed): Renal transplantation. Urol Clin North Am 3:3, 1976
SVEJGAARD A et al: HLA and disease associations—a survey. Transplant Rev 22:3, 1978
TERASAKI PI et al: Summary of kidney transplant data, 1977—factors affecting graft outcome. Transplant Proc 10:417, 1978
——— et al: Microdroplet testing for HLA-A, B, C and D antigens. Am J Clin Pathol 69:103, 1978
VAN ROOD JJ et al: B-cell antibodies, Ia-like determinants in man. Transplant Rev 30:122, 1976

section 3 | Clinical pharmacology

70
PRINCIPLES OF DRUG THERAPY

JOHN A. OATES
GRANT R. WILKINSON

QUANTITATIVE DETERMINANTS OF DRUG ACTION

Safe and effective therapy with drugs requires their delivery to target tissues in concentrations within the narrow range that yields efficacy without toxicity. Optimal precision in achieving concentrations of drug within this therapeutic "window" can be achieved with regimens that are based on the kinetics of the drug's availability to target sites. This chapter deals with the principles of drug elimination and distribution that form the basis for loading and maintenance regimens for the average patient and considers instances in which elimination of the drug is impaired (e.g., renal failure). The kinetic basis for optimal utilization of plasma level data is also discussed.

PLASMA LEVELS AFTER A SINGLE DOSE The levels of lidocaine (Chap. 238) in plasma following intravenous administration decline in two phases as illustrated in Fig. 70-1; such a biphasic decline is typical for many drugs. Immediately following rapid injection, all the drug is in the plasma compartment, and the high initial plasma level reflects its confinement to this small volume. Subsequently, the drug is rapidly distributed from plasma into the extravascular compartment, and the period of time during which this is occurring is referred to as the *distribution phase.* For lidocaine this distribution phase is virtually complete within 30 min; then there is a slower rate of fall, referred to as the *equilibrium phase* or the *elimination phase.* During this latter phase, the drug levels in plasma and those in the tissues of the body are in pseudoequilibrium.

Distribution phase Pharmacological events during the distribution phase depend on whether the level of drug at the receptor site closely reflects that in the plasma. If this is the case, the pharmacological effects, whether favorable or adverse, may be inordinately great during this period. For example, following a small bolus dose (25 mg) of lidocaine, antiarrhythmic effects may be evident during the early distribution phase but disappear as levels rapidly fall below those that are minimally effective and even before equilibrium between plasma and tissue is reached. Thus, larger single doses or multiple small doses must be administered in order to achieve an effect that is sustained into the equilibrium phase. The toxicity of high levels of some drugs during the distribution phase precludes administration of a single intravenous loading dose that will achieve therapeutic levels during the equilibrium phase. For example, the administration of a loading dose of the anticonvulsant, phenytoin (diphenylhydantoin) as a single intravenous bolus can cause cardiovascular collapse due to the high levels during the distribution phase. For this reason, if a loading dose of phenytoin is administered intravenously, it must be given in fractions (10 to 15 percent of the total loading amount) at intervals sufficient to permit substantial distribution of the prior dose before the next is given. For similar reasons, the loading dose of many potent drugs that rapidly equilibrate with their receptors is divided into fractional doses for intravenous administration.

After an oral dose that delivers an equivalent amount of drug into the systemic circulation, plasma levels during the distribution phase do not rise nearly as steeply as they do after an intravenous bolus dose. Because the drug is not absorbed instantly after oral administration, it is delivered into the systemic circulation more slowly, and much of the drug is already distributed by the time absorption is complete. Thus, procainamide, which is almost totally absorbed after oral administration, can be given as a single 750-mg loading dose with little risk of hypotension; in contrast, loading of the drug by the

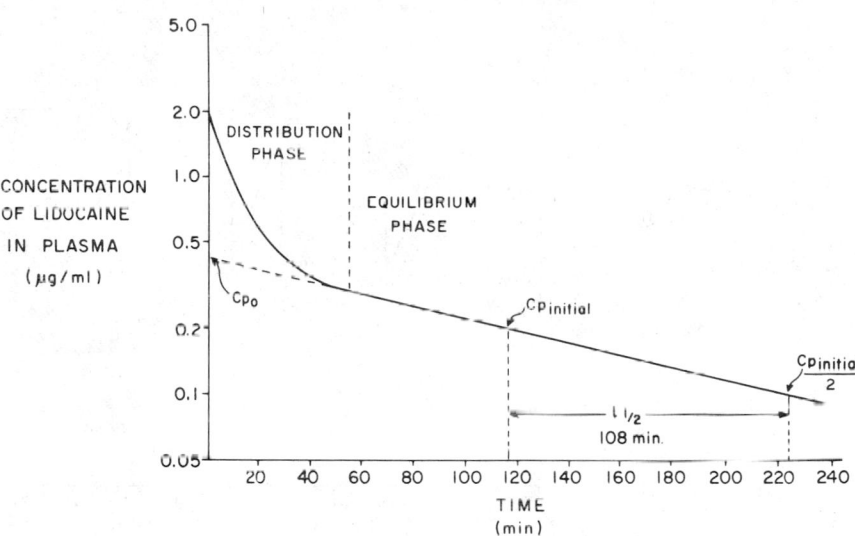

FIGURE 70-1

Concentrations of lidocaine in plasma following the administration of 50 mg intravenously. The half-life of 108 min is computed as the time required for levels to fall from any given value during the equilibrium phase ($C_{P_{initial}}$) to one-half that level. C_{P_0} is the hypothetical concentration of lidocaine in plasma at time zero if equilibrium had been achieved instantly.

intravenous route is more safely accomplished by giving the loading dose in fractions of about 100 mg at 5-min intervals in order to avoid the hypotension that would ensue during the distribution phase in some patients if the entire loading dose were given as a single bolus.

In contrast, other drugs are distributed to their sites of action only slowly during the distribution phase. For example, levels of digoxin at the receptor site (and its pharmacological effect) do not reflect plasma levels during the distribution phase (Chap. 238). Digoxin is transported (or bound) to its cardiac receptors more slowly by a process that proceeds throughout distribution. Thus, plasma levels during a distribution phase of several hours are falling while levels at the site of action and pharmacological effect are increasing. Only at the end of the distribution phase when the drug has reached equilibrium with the receptor does the concentration of digoxin in plasma reflect pharmacological effect. For this reason, there should be a 6- to 8-h wait after the distribution phase before samples for plasma levels of digoxin that are to be used as a guide to therapy are obtained.

Equilibrium phase After distribution has proceeded to the point where the concentration of drug in plasma is in equilibrium with that in the tissues outside the vascular compartment, the levels in plasma and tissues fall in parallel as the drug is eliminated from the body. Thus, the equilibrium phase is sometimes also referred to as the *elimination phase.*

Most drugs are eliminated as a first-order process. During the equilibrium phase, a characteristic of the first-order process is that the time required for the level of drug in plasma to fall to one-half the original value (the half-life) will be the same regardless of which point on the plasma level curve is chosen as a starting point for the measurement. Another characteristic of the first order process is that a plot of the concentrations in plasma versus time during the equilibrium phase is linear on a semilogarithmic graph. From such a plot (Fig. 70-1) it can be seen that the half-life of lidocaine is 108 min.

One can readily calculate what amount of the administered dose remains in the body at any multiple of the half-life interval following administration:

Number of half-lives	Amount of dose remaining in the body, %
1	50
2	25
3	12.5
4	6.25
5	3.13

In theory, the elimination process never reaches comple-

tion. From a clinical standpoint, however, elimination can be considered as being essentially complete when it has reached 90 percent. Therefore, for practical purposes, *a first-order elimination process can be said to reach completion after 3 to 4 half-lives.*

DRUG ACCUMULATION—LOADING AND MAINTENANCE DOSES With repeated administration of a drug, the amount in the body will accumulate if the elimination of the first dose is incomplete when the second dose is given, and both the amount of drug in the body and its pharmacological effect will increase with continuing administration until they reach a plateau. The accumulation of digoxin administered in repeated maintenance doses (without a loading dose) is illustrated in Fig. 70-2. As digoxin's half-life is about 1.6 days in a patient with normal renal function, 65 percent of digoxin remains in the body at the end of 1 day. Thus, the second dose will raise the amount of digoxin in the body (and average plasma level) to 165 percent of that following the first dose. Each subsequent dose will result in greater amounts in the body until a plateau is attained. At the plateau, or *steady state,* drug intake per unit of time is the same as the rate of drug elimination. For *all* drugs with first-order kinetics, the time required to accumulate to steady-state levels can be predicted from the half-life because accumulation also is a first-order process with a half-life identical to that for elimination. Hence, accumulation will reach 90 percent of steady-state levels at the end of 3 to 4 half-lives. For digoxin, with a half-life of 1.6 days (with normal renal function), accumulation thus will be practically complete in 5 days (Chap. 238). Continuing infusion of the drug at a constant rate also will result in progressive accumulation to a steady state over a time course predictable from the elimination curve for that drug (Fig. 70-3).

When the time required to reach steady-state levels is longer than one wishes to wait, plasma levels may be achieved more rapidly by the administration of a *loading dose.* Loading entails the administration of an amount that will bring the concentration in plasma (at equilibrium) to the level present during steady state. This may be accomplished by the administration of the loading amount as a single dose, or in the case of drugs with low therapeutic indexes (the therapeutic index is the ratio of the toxic dose to the therapeutic dose) the loading amount is given in a series of fractions of the total loading amount. As the accumulation of procainamide to 90 percent of steady state by infusion would require approximately 10 h (3.3 × the half-life of 3 h), a loading regimen is almost always desirable. The load required to suppress an arrhythmia, how-

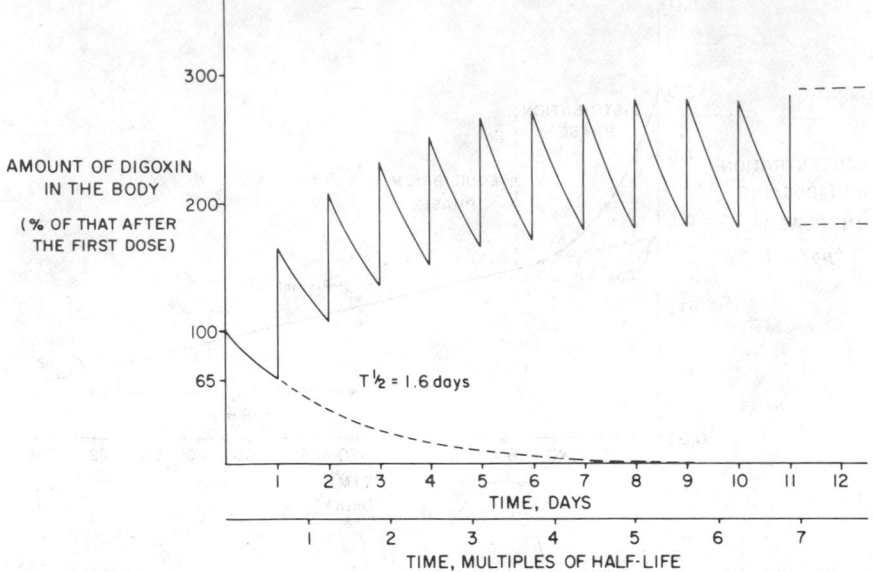

FIGURE 70-2
The time course of digoxin accumulation when a single daily maintenance dose is given without a loading dose. Note that accumulation is more than 90 percent complete by the end of 4 half-lives.

ever, varies among individuals from 300 to 1000 mg, and rapid intravenous administration of the *average loading dose* would cause hypotension during the high plasma levels in the distribution phase in some patients. Therefore, the intravenous loading dose of procainamide is given in fractions (e.g., 100 mg every 5 min) until the arrhythmia is controlled or adverse effects such as hypotension signal that no further drug should be given. Dividing the loading dose into fractions is appropriate for most drugs that, like procainamide, have a low therapeutic index. This permits better individualization of the loading amount and avoids needless adverse effects that might occur during the distribution phase of a single large dose.

The size of loading dose required to achieve the plasma levels present at steady state can be determined from the fraction of drug eliminated during the dosage interval and the maintenance dose (in the case of intermittent drug administration). For example, if the fraction of digoxin eliminated daily is 35 percent and the planned maintenance dose is to be 0.25 mg daily, then the loading dose to achieve steady-state levels should be 100/35 times the maintenance dose, or approximately 0.75 mg. Thus,

$$\frac{\text{Loading}}{\text{dose}} = \frac{100}{\%\text{ of drug eliminated per dosage interval}} \times \text{maintenance dose}$$

The fraction of drug eliminated during any dosage interval can be determined from a semilogarithmic graph, in which the total body dose at time zero is set at 100 percent and the fraction remaining at the end of 1 half-life is 50 percent.[1] Conversely, if the loading dose is known, the maintenance dose can be similarly calculated.

Regardless of the size of the loading dose, *after maintenance*

FIGURE 70-3
The time course of plasma levels of a drug following a single intravenous dose (——) compared with those during a constant intravenous infusion (----). This relationship applies to all drugs that rapidly achieve equilibrium between plasma and tissues.

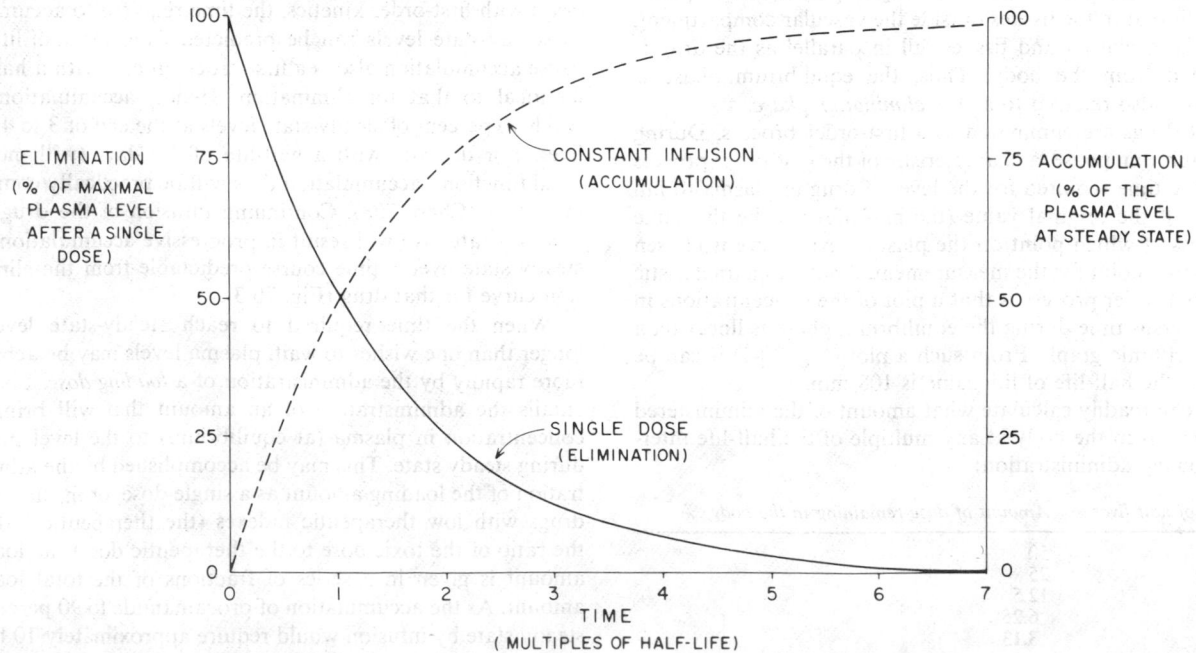

therapy has been given for 3 to 4 half-lives, the amount of drug in the body is determined only by the maintenance dose. The independence of the plasma levels at steady state from the load is illustrated in Fig. 70-3, which indicates that the elimination of any drug given at time 0 (elimination curve) would be practically complete after 3 to 4 half-lives.

DETERMINANTS OF PLASMA LEVELS DURING THE EQUILIBRIUM PHASE An important determinant of the level of drug in plasma during the equilibrium phase after a single dose is the extent to which the drug has distributed outside the plasma compartment. For example, if the distribution of a 3-mg dose of a large macromolecule is confined to a plasma volume of 3 liters, then the concentration in plasma will be 1 mg per liter. However, if a different drug is distributed so that 90 percent of it leaves the plasma compartment, then only 0.3 mg will remain in the 3-liter plasma volume, and the concentration in plasma will be only 0.1 mg per liter. The extent of extravascular distribution at equilibrium can be expressed by the term *apparent volume of distribution*, or V_d. More precisely, V_d expresses the constant relationship between the amount of drug in the body and the plasma concentration at equilibrium:

$$V_d = \frac{\text{amount of drug in body}}{\text{plasma concentration}}$$

The amount of drug in the body is expressed as mass (e.g., milligrams), and the plasma concentration is expressed as mass per volume (e.g., milligrams per liter). Thus V_d is a hypothetical volume into which a quantity of drug would distribute if its concentration in the entire volume were the same as that in plasma. Although it does not represent a real volume, it is an important quantity because it determines the fraction of total drug which is in the plasma and therefore the fraction available to the organs of elimination. An approximation of V_d in the equilibrium phase can be obtained by estimating the concentration of drug in plasma at time zero (C_{p0}) by a back-extrapolation of the equilibrium phase plot to zero time as illustrated in Fig. 70-1. Then, after intravenous administration when the amount in the body at time zero is the dose, we have

$$V_d = \frac{\text{dose}}{C_{p0}}$$

For the administration of the large macromolecule mentioned above, the measured C_{p0} of 1 mg per liter after a 3-mg dose indicates a V_d that is a real volume, the plasma volume. This example is the exception, however, for the V_d of most drugs does not relate to any real volume; many drugs are so extensively taken up by cells that cellular levels greatly exceed those in plasma water. For such drugs, the hypothetical V_d will be large, even greater than the volume of body water. For example, Fig. 70-1 indicates that the C_{p0} obtained by extrapolation following 50 mg lidocaine is 0.42 mg per liter, yielding a V_d by the above equation of 119 liters.

As elimination is carried out largely by individual organs such as the kidney and liver, it is useful to consider the elimination of drugs by these organs according to the *clearance*

concept. For example, in the kidney, regardless of the extent to which removal of drug is determined by filtration, secretion, or reabsorption, the net result is that drug removal results in a reduction of the concentration of drug in plasma as it passes through the organ. The extent to which the concentration is reduced is expressed as the *extraction ratio*, or E.

$$E = \frac{C_a - C_v}{C_a}$$

where C_a = arterial plasma concentration
C_v = venous plasma concentration

If the extraction is complete, $E = 1$. If the total plasma flow to the kidneys is Q (ml/min), the total volume of plasma from which drug is completely removed in a unit time (clearance) is determined as

$$Cl_{renal} = QE$$

If the extraction ratio of penicillin is 0.5 and renal plasma flow is 680 ml/min, then penicillin's renal clearance will be 340 ml/min. If the extraction ratio of a compound is high, as is the case for renal extraction of *p*-aminohippuric acid (PAH) or hepatic extraction of propranolol, then clearance becomes primarily a function of organ blood flow.[2]

Clearance from the total body (Cl) is the sum of clearance from all organs of elimination and is the best measure of the efficiency of the elimination processes. If a drug is removed by both renal excretion and hepatic metabolism, then

$$Cl = Cl_{renal} + Cl_{hepatic}$$

Thus, if penicillin is eliminated by both renal clearance (340 ml/min) and hepatic clearance (36 ml/min) in a normal individual, total clearance will be 376 ml/min. If renal clearance is reduced to half, total clearance = 170 + 36 = 206 ml/min. In anuria, total clearance will equal hepatic clearance.

Only the drug in the vascular compartment can be cleared during each passage through an organ. To ascertain the effect of a given plasma clearance by one or more organs on the rate of removal of drug from the body, the clearance must be related to the volume of "plasma equivalents" to be cleared, that is, the volume of distribution. If the volume of distribution is 10,000 ml and clearance is 1000 ml/min, then one-tenth of the drug in the body is eliminated per minute. This fraction, Cl/V_d, is known as a *fractional elimination constant* and is designated as k:

$$k = \frac{Cl}{V_d}$$

If the fraction k is multiplied by the total amount of drug in the body, the actual rate of elimination at any given time can be determined:

$$\text{Rate of elimination} = k \times \text{amount in body} = Cl\,C_p$$

This is the general equation for all first-order processes and expresses the fact that rate is proportional to the declining quantity in a first-order process.

---

[1] *Alternatively, the fraction of drug lost from the body during a dosage interval can be determined nongraphically from this equation*

$$\text{Fraction of drug lost from body} = 1 - e^{-kT}$$

Values for e^{-kT} can be obtained from a table of natural exponential functions or by a calculator, where k ($= 0.693/T_{1/2}$) is the fractional elimination constant (described in the next section) and T is the time interval after drug administration.

[2] *When drug is present in the formed elements of blood, then calculation of extraction and clearance from blood is more physiologically meaningful than from the plasma.*

As half-life is a temporal expression of the exponential first-order process, half-life ($T_{\frac{1}{2}}$) can be related to k as follows:

$$T_{\frac{1}{2}} = \frac{0.693}{k}$$

Because $\quad k = \dfrac{\text{Cl}}{V_d}$

then $\quad T_{\frac{1}{2}} = \dfrac{0.693 V_d}{\text{Cl}}$

As will be seen in the following discussion on drug dosage in renal failure, the linear relationship of k to creatinine clearance makes k a more useful parameter upon which to base calculations of the changes in drug elimination that occur with a known reduction in creatinine clearance in renal insufficiency. Half-life is not linearly related to clearance.

The important relationship

$$T_{\frac{1}{2}} = 0.693 V_d / \text{Cl}$$

expresses clearly that half-life is determined by both clearance and volume of distribution. Thus, for example, half-life is shortened when phenobarbital induces the enzymes responsible for hepatic clearance of a drug, and half-life is lengthened when a drug's renal clearance is attenuated in renal failure. Also, the half-life of some drugs is shortened when their volume of distribution is reduced. If, as in the case of cardiac failure, the volume of distribution is reduced at the same time that clearance is reduced, there may be little change in drug half-life to reflect the impaired clearance, but plasma levels will be increased. In treating patients after an overdose, expectations of how hemodialysis will affect the drug's elimination are dependent on its volume of distribution. When the volume of distribution is very large, as is the case with tricyclic antidepressants (V_d of nortriptyline equals more than 2000 liters), the removal of drug, even with a high-clearance dialyzer, will proceed slowly.

The extent to which a drug is bound to plasma protein also determines the fraction of drug extracted by the organ(s) of elimination. Altered binding will change the extraction ratio significantly, however, only when elimination is limited to the free drug in plasma. The extent to which binding influences elimination depends on the relative affinity of the plasma binding versus the affinity of the drug for the extraction process. The high affinity of the renal tubular anion transport system for many drugs will lead to extraction of both bound and free drug, and the efficient process by which the liver removes propranolol will result in extraction of most of this highly bound drug from blood.

STEADY STATE With a constant infusion of drug, the infusion rate equals elimination rate at steady state. Therefore,

$$\begin{array}{ccc} \text{Infusion rate} & = & C_p & \times & \text{Cl} \\ \text{(amt/unit time)} & & \text{(amt/vol)} & & \text{(vol/unit time)} \end{array}$$

when the units for amount, volume, and time are consistent.

Thus, if clearance (Cl) is known, the infusion rate required to achieve a given plasma level can be calculated. An approach to estimating the clearance of a number of drugs is discussed below in the section on renal disease.

When the dose is given intermittently instead of by infusion, the above relationship between plasma concentration and the dose administered at each dosage interval can be expressed as

$$\text{Dose} = C_{p\text{av}} \times \text{Cl} \times \text{dosage interval}$$

The average plasma concentration ($C_{p\text{av}}$) implies that, as seen in Fig. 70-2, levels can be considerably higher and lower than the average during the dosage interval.

When a drug is given orally and is not completely absorbed, the calculated dose must be corrected by the fraction (F) of drug that reaches the systemic circulation following oral administration:

$$\frac{\text{Oral}}{\text{dose}} = \frac{C_{p\text{av}} \times \text{Cl} \times \text{dosage interval}}{F}$$

DRUG ELIMINATION THAT IS NOT FIRST ORDER The elimination of some important drugs such as phenytoin and salicylate does not follow first-order kinetics when amounts of drug in the body are in the therapeutic range. For these drugs, the clearance is not a constant value but changes as levels in the body fall during elimination or after changes in dose. This pattern of elimination is said to be *dose-dependent*. Accordingly, the time for the concentration to fall to one-half becomes less as plasma levels fall; this halving-time is not truly a half-life, however, because the term *half-life* applies to first-order kinetics and is a constant. The elimination of phenytoin is dose-dependent, and when very high levels are present (in the toxic range), the halving time may be longer than 72 h, whereas after the concentration in plasma has declined to lower levels, the clearance increases and the concentration in plasma will halve in 20 to 30 h.

When drug is eliminated by first-order kinetics, the plasma level at steady state is directly related to the amount of the maintenance dose, and a doubling of the dose should lead to doubling of the steady-state plasma level. However, for phenytoin and other drugs with dose-dependent kinetics, increases in the dose may be accompanied by disproportionately large increases in plasma level. Thus, if the daily dose of phenytoin is increased from 300 to 400 mg, plasma levels rise by considerably more than 33 percent. Unfortunately, the extent of increase is not predictable because of the wide interpatient variability in the extent to which clearance deviates from first order. Salicylates are eliminated by dose-dependent kinetics at high plasma levels, and in children particular caution must be taken with the administration of high doses. Ethanol metabolism also is dose-dependent, with obvious implications. The mechanisms involved in dose-dependent kinetics may include the saturation of the rate-limiting step in metabolism or a feedback inhibition of the rate-limiting enzyme by a product of the reaction.

INDIVIDUALIZATION OF DRUG THERAPY

Recognition of factors modifying drug action is essential for therapy that provides optimal benefit with minimal risk to each individual patient. Certain disease states can modify the delivery of a drug to its site of action.

RENAL DISEASE Where urinary excretion is an important route of elimination, renal failure results in decreased drug clearance and therefore slower removal of the drug from the body, so that administration according to the usual dosage regimen leads to greater accumulation and an increased likelihood of toxicity. A reasonable therapeutic goal in such cases is to modify the dosage schedule so that the average drug concentration in the plasma of the patient with renal insufficiency is the same, and steady state is reached after a similar time interval, as in the patient with normal renal function.

One approach to dosage alteration in renal insufficiency is to calculate the *fraction of the normal dose* that is to be given at the usual dosage interval. This fraction can be determined from data on either drug clearance (Cl) or the fractional rate

TABLE 70-1
Clearance of drugs

Drug	Renal clearance,* ml/min	Nonrenal clearance, ml/min
Ampicillin†	340	12
Carbenicillin	68	10
Digoxin†	110	36
Gentamicin	78	3
Kanamycin	60	0
Penicillin G‡	340	36

* The "normal" renal clearances are those associated with a clearance of creatinine of 100 ml/min.
† The fraction of digoxin absorbed after an oral dose (F) is approximately 0.6 and F for ampicillin is 0.5.
‡ One microgram of penicillin G = 1.6 units.

constant (k), based on the fact that both renal clearance and renal k are directly proportional to creatinine clearance (Cl_{cr}). Thus, the dose in renal insufficiency ($dose_{ri}$) is

$$Dose_{ri} = dose \times \frac{Cl_{ri}}{Cl}$$

where ri = renal insufficiency
Cl = clearance from the whole body with normal renal function
Cl_{ri} = clearance from the whole body with renal insufficiency
Dose = maintenance dose with normal renal function ($Cl_{cr} \approx 100$ ml/min)

The normal clearance and that in renal impairment can be obtained by employing the data in Table 70-1 in the following equations:

$$Cl = Cl_{renal} + Cl_{nonrenal}$$

$$Cl_{ri} = Cl_{renal} \times \frac{measured\ Cl_{cr}}{100\ ml/min} + Cl_{nonrenal}$$

As the Cl_{renal} values in Table 70-1 are those found with

FIGURE 70-4

Nomogram for estimation of the dose fraction (k_{ri}/k) in patients with renal insufficiency. The application of the nomogram is described in the text.

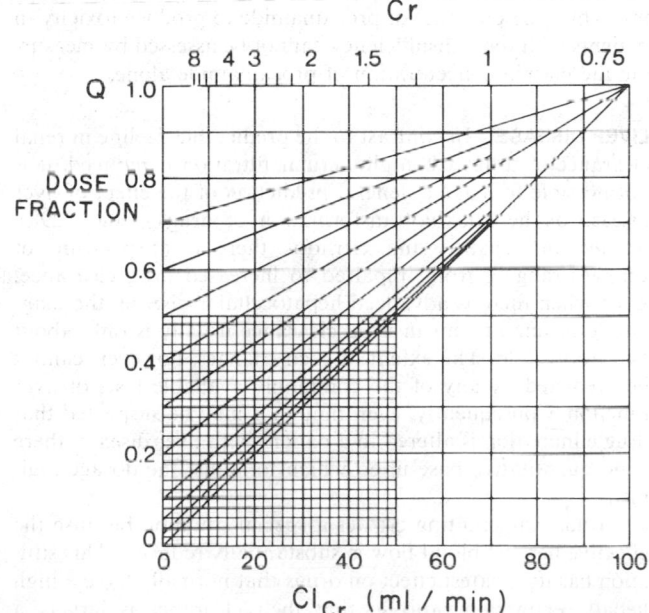

TABLE 70-2
Estimated fraction of usual dose of drug required for a patient with a creatinine clearance of zero (dose fraction₀) and average overall fractional elimination rate constant for a patient with normal renal function (k)

Drug	Dose fraction₀	k, per hour
ANTIBIOTICS		
Amikacin	0.01	0.4
Amoxicillin	0.15	0.7
Ampicillin	0.1	0.6
Carbenicillin	0.1	0.6
Cephalexin	0.04	0.7
Cephaloridine	0.08	0.4
Cephalothin	0.02	1.4
Cephazolin	0.06	0.35
Chloramphenicol	0.8	0.3
Clindamycin	0.8	0.2
Cloxacillin	0.25	1.2
Colistimethate	0.3	0.2
Dicloxacillin	0.5	1.2
Doxycycline	0.8	0.03
Erythromycin	0.7	0.5
Gentamicin	0.02	0.3
Isoniazid:		
Fast inactivators	0.8	0.5
Slow inactivators	0.5	0.25
Kanamycin	0.03	0.35
Lincomycin	0.4	0.15
Methicillin	0.12	1.4
Minocycline	0.9	0.06
Nafcillin	0.4	1.2
Oxacillin	0.25	1.4
Oxytetracycline	0.2	0.08
Penicillin G	0.1	1.4
Polymyxin B	0.12	0.15
Rifampin	1.0	0.25
Streptomycin	0.04	0.25
Sulfadiazine	0.45	0.7
Sulfamethoxazole	0.85	0.07
Tetracycline	0.12	0.08
Tobramycin	0.02	0.35
Tricarcillin	0.1	0.6
Trimethoprim	0.45	0.06
Vancomycin	0.03	0.12
MISCELLANEOUS DRUGS		
Chlorpropamide	0.4	0.02
Lidocaine	0.9	0.4
Sulfinpyrazone	0.55	0.3

Drug	Dose fraction₀	k, per day
CARDIAC GLYCOSIDES		
Digitoxin	0.7	0.1
Digoxin	0.3	0.45

Cl_{cr} = 100 ml/min, then the renal clearance of drug in renal insufficiency is obtained by multiplying Cl_{renal} by the ratio of measured Cl_{cr} (in milliliters per minute) to 100 ml/min.

For gentamicin, with a normal Cl_{renal} of 78 ml/min and $Cl_{nonrenal}$ of 3 ml/min, Cl = 81 ml/min. Therefore, with a Cl_{cr} of 12 ml/min, Cl_{ri} = 78 × (12/100) + 3 = 12.4 ml/min. If the dose of gentamicin for a given infection should be 1.5 mg/kg per 8 h in the presence of normal renal function, then

$$Dose_{ri} = \frac{1.5\ mg/kg}{8\ h} \times \frac{12.4\ ml/min}{81\ ml/min} = \frac{0.23\ mg/kg}{8\ h}$$

In the patient with renal insufficiency, this computation will yield an average plasma level during a dosage interval that is the same as the average plasma level during the dosage interval with normal renal function; the fluctuations between peaks and troughs, however, will be less pronounced.

All calculation of dosage is most accurately based on the clearance of a drug, because this is a direct measure of the efficiency of drug removal. However, clearance data are not available for some drugs, in which case [if it is assumed that renal disease does not affect the distribution of the drug (V_d)], the dosage fraction can be approximated from the ratio of the fractional rate constant for elimination from the total body in renal failure (k_{ri}) to that with normal renal function (k). The approach is the same as that employed with clearance data:

$$\text{Dose}_{ri} = \text{dose} \times \frac{k_{ri}}{k}$$

As the ratio k_{ri}/k is the fraction of the usual dose employed in a given degree of renal insufficiency, it is termed the *dose fraction* and may be readily estimated from the information in Table 70-2 and the nomogram (Fig. 70-4). Table 70-2 gives the fraction of the usual dose of a drug required at a creatinine clearance of zero (dose fraction$_0$). The nomogram presents the dose fraction as a linear function of creatinine clearance.

To calculate the dose fraction$_{ri}$, the dose fraction$_0$ is obtained from Table 70-2, plotted on the left ordinate of the nomogram, and connected by a straight line to the upper right hand corner of the nomogram. This line describes the dose fraction over a range of creatinine clearances from 0 to 100 ml/min. The point of intersection between the patient's measured creatinine clearance (on the lower abscissa) with this dose fraction line is a coordinate with the dose fraction (on the left ordinate) corresponding with that particular creatinine clearance. For example, if a patient with a creatinine clearance of 20 ml/min requires penicillin G for an infection that would be treated with 10 million units daily in patients with normal renal function, then an appropriate dose would be 2.8 million units daily. This estimated dose is obtained by plotting the dose fraction$_0$ for penicillin G (0.1) on the left-hand ordinate and connecting it to the top right-hand corner of the nomogram (Fig. 70-4). On this dose fraction line for penicillin G, the coordinate for a creatinine clearance of 20 ml/min corresponds on the left ordinate with a dose fraction of 0.28. Hence, the dose is 0.28 × 10 million units daily.

In some instances it may be desirable to calculate a dose that will yield a certain plasma level at steady state. This approach is most appropriate for constant intravenous infusions where 100 percent of the dose is delivered to the systemic circulation. When clearance of a drug in a patient with renal insufficiency is calculated as above, then

$$\begin{array}{ccc} \text{Dose}_{ri} & = & \text{Cl}_{ri} & \times & C_p \\ \text{(amt/unit time)} & & \text{(vol/unit time)} & & \text{(amt/vol)} \end{array}$$

where the time, amount, and volume terms are uniform.

If a plasma concentration of carbenicillin of 100 μg/ml is the therapeutic objective in a patient with a creatinine clearance of 25 ml/min, the infusion rate is calculated as follows. Carbenicillin clearance is

$$\text{Cl}_{ri} = 68 \times \frac{25}{100} + 10 = 27 \text{ ml/min}$$

Therefore, carbenicillin should be infused at a rate of 2700 μg/min.

Should the method of calculating dose based on the desired plasma level be applied to intermittent-dose therapy, particular attention should be given to the fact that the calculation is based on an *average* plasma level and that peak plasma levels will obviously be higher. In addition, if a drug is given orally and is not completely absorbed, the computed dose must be divided by the fraction of drug which reaches the systemic circulation following oral administration (F) (see "Steady State" above).

In all the above calculations, it is assumed that the nonrenal clearance and nonrenal k are constant in renal failure. In fact, when cardiac failure accompanies renal failure, metabolic clearance for many drugs is reduced. Accordingly, when a drug with a narrow therapeutic index, such as digoxin, is used in cardiac failure, an appropriate precaution would be to reduce the value for nonrenal clearance (or k) to about one-half.

In addition to adjusting the maintenance dose in patients with renal failure, consideration must also be given to the necessity of a loading dose. Since this dose is designed to bring the plasma concentration, or more particularly the amount of drug in the body, rapidly to the level that is reached at steady state, there is no need to modify the usual loading dose, if one is normally used. For many drugs, however, their elimination is sufficiently rapid that the time required to reach steady state is not clinically significant and no loading dose is usually used. On the other hand, in renal failure where the half-life may be significantly prolonged, this accumulation period may become unacceptably long. In such a case, for a drug given intermittently, a loading dose may be calculated as described in "Drug Accumulation" above. For an infusion, the loading dose may be approximated (when all units are consistent)

$$\text{Loading dose}_{ri} = \frac{\text{infusion rate}_{ri}}{k_{ri}}$$

Because of the considerable individual differences in volumes of distribution and rates of metabolism, the above calculations of drug dose for patients in renal failure must be viewed as valuable approximations which prevent the use of doses that are grossly excessive or inadequate for most patients. However, *maintenance dosages are most accurate when plasma level data are employed as a feedback to enable adjustment of the dose where necessary*.

Active or toxic metabolites of drugs also may accumulate in renal failure. Meperidine, for example, is cleared largely by metabolism, and its concentration in plasma is little altered by renal insufficiency. However, the plasma concentration of one of its metabolites, normeperidine, is substantially increased when its renal elimination is impaired. As normeperidine has more convulsant activity than meperidine, its accumulation in patients with renal failure probably accounts for the signs of central nervous system excitation such as irritability, twitching, and seizures that result from the administration of multiple doses of meperidine to patients in renal insufficiency.

The metabolite of procainamide, *N*-acetylprocainamide, has cardiac effects that are similar to those of the parent drug. As *N*-acetylprocainamide is eliminated almost entirely by the kidney, its concentration in plasma is increased by renal failure. Thus, the potential of procainamide to produce toxicity in patients with renal insufficiency cannot be assessed by measuring the plasma concentration of procainamide alone.

LIVER DISEASE In contrast to the predictable decline in renal clearance of drugs when glomerular filtration is reduced, it is not possible to make a general prediction of the effect of liver disease on hepatic biotransformation of drugs (Chap. 298). Rather, in hepatitis and cirrhosis there is a spectrum of changes ranging from impaired to increased drug clearance. Even when there is advanced hepatocellular disease, the magnitude of impairment in drug clearance usually is only about two- to fivefold. The extent of such changes, however, cannot be predicted by any of the commonly available tests of liver function. Consequently, even though it may be suspected that drug elimination is altered in a patient with liver disease, there is no quantitative base upon which to adjust the dosage regimen.

Portacaval shunting creates a special situation because the effective hepatic blood flow is substantially reduced. This situation has its greatest effect on drugs that normally have a high hepatic extraction ratio so that their clearance is largely a function of blood flow; thus the clearance of such drugs (e.g., propranolol and lidocaine) will be remarkably reduced by portacaval shunting. In addition, the fraction of an administered oral dose reaching the systemic circulation will be significantly increased, because drug that is shunted around the liver during the absorption process will escape the efficient first-pass metabolism by this organ.

CIRCULATORY INSUFFICIENCY—CARDIAC FAILURE AND SHOCK Under conditions leading to decreased tissue perfusion, redistribution of the cardiac output occurs to preserve blood flow to the heart and brain at the expense of other tissues (Chap. 30). As a result, the drug is distributed into a smaller volume of distribution, higher drug concentrations are present in the plasma, and the vital organs are exposed to these higher concentrations. If either the brain or heart is sensitive to the pharmacological effect of the drug, an alteration in response will occur.

Furthermore, the decreased perfusion of the kidney and liver may impair drug clearance by these organs either directly or indirectly. Thus, in severe congestive heart failure, in hemorrhagic shock, and particularly in cardiogenic shock, the response to the usual dose of the drug may be excessive, and dosage modification may be necessary. For example, the clearance of lidocaine is reduced by about 50 percent in cardiac failure, and consequently therapeutic plasma levels are achieved at infusion rates of only about half of those usually required. In cardiac failure there also is a significant reduction in lidocaine's volume of distribution which results in the requirement of a smaller loading dose. Similar situations are thought to exist for procainamide, theophylline, and possibly quinidine. Unfortunately, predictors of these types of pharmacokinetic alterations are unavailable. Therefore, loading doses should be conservative, and continued therapy should be monitored closely, following clinical indicators of toxicity and plasma levels.

DISEASE-INDUCED CHANGES IN PLASMA BINDING Many drugs circulate in the plasma partly bound to the plasma proteins and other constituents. Since only the unbound or free drug can distribute to the site of pharmacological action, the therapeutic response should be related to the free rather than the total circulating plasma drug concentration. In most cases the degree of binding is fairly constant across the therapeutic concentration range so that significant error is not caused by individualizing therapy on the basis of measuring levels of total drug in plasma. However, several clinical states such as hypoalbuminemia, liver disease, and renal disease can decrease the extent of drug binding so that at any total plasma level there is a greater concentration of free drug and a risk of increased response and toxicity. The drugs for which such changes are important are those which are normally highly bound in the plasma ($>$ 90 percent) because a small alteration in the extent of binding produces a large relative increase in the fraction of drug in the unbound form.

The binding of phenytoin is altered in patients with chronic renal failure by several mechanisms; the percentage of unbound drug increases about fourfold from a normal of approximately 7 percent to as high as 25 to 30 percent. Similar, but less pronounced, changes are also seen in patients with viral hepatitis, jaundice, and the nephrotic syndrome, and with other drugs such as diazoxide, digitoxin, clofibrate, and certain sulfonamides.

The pharmacokinetic consequences of these binding changes, particularly with respect to total drug levels, depend on whether the clearance and distribution are dependent on the unbound or total drug. For many drugs, including those cited above, elimination and distribution are largely restricted to the free fraction, and therefore a decrease in binding leads to an increase in the clearance and distribution of the total drug. The relative magnitudes of these changes are such that the net effect is to shorten the half-life. For example, in uremia the half-life of phenytoin may be as low as 6 to 8 h compared with a normal value of about 20 to 30 h. However, the clearance of *free* drug is unaffected, and the average steady-state plasma concentration of unbound drug is unaltered. Accordingly, the appropriate modification of the dosage regimen in clinical conditions with reduced drug binding is simply to administer the usual daily dose of the drug, but in divided doses at more frequent intervals. Individualization of therapy can then be based on either the clinical response or the plasma concentration of unbound drug. It is critical that the patient not be titrated into the usual therapeutic range for concentration of *total* drug in plasma since this will inevitably lead to supraeffective response and toxicity.

INTERACTIONS BETWEEN DRUGS

The effect of some drugs can be altered markedly by the administration of other agents. Such interactions can sabotage therapeutic intent by producing excessive drug action (with adverse effects) or decreasing the action of a drug, rendering it ineffective. Drug interactions must be considered in the differential diagnosis of unexpected responses to drugs, taking into account that ambulatory patients often come to the physician with a legacy of drugs acquired during their previous medical experiences. A meticulous drug history will minimize the unknown elements in the patient's therapeutic milieu; it should include examination of the patient's medications and calls to the pharmacist to identify prescriptions, if necessary.

There are two principal types of interactions between drugs. *Pharmacokinetic interactions* result from alteration in the delivery of drugs to their sites of action. *Pharmacodynamic interactions* are those in which the responsiveness of the target organ or system has been modified by other agents.

An index of the drug interactions discussed in this chapter is provided in Table 70-3. Included are a selected group of interactions which have verified significance in patients and a few which are of such potential danger to the patient that cognizance should be taken of experimental data or case reports suggesting their likely occurrence.

I PHARMACOKINETIC INTERACTIONS CAUSING DIMINISHED DRUG DELIVERY

A Impaired gastrointestinal absorption Aluminum ions, present in antacids, form insoluble chelates with the tetracyclines, thereby preventing absorption of these drugs. Ferrous ions similarly block tetracycline absorption. Cholestyramine, an ionic exchange resin, binds thyroxine, triiodothyronine, and the cardiac glycosides with sufficiently high affinity to impair their absorption from the gastrointestinal tract. This resin probably also interferes with the absorption of other drugs, and it is safest not to give it within 2 h of their administration. Oral administration of *p*-aminosalicylate interferes with the absorption of rifampin by a mechanism not yet determined.

All the above instances of impaired absorption result in a reduction in the total amount of drug absorption, with reduced area under the plasma level curve and reduced peak plasma levels, as well as lower steady-state concentrations of the drug involved.

B Induction of hepatic drug-metabolizing enzymes When the elimination of the drug proceeds largely via biotransformation, an increase in the rate at which it is metabolized reduces its availability to sites of action. The biotransformation of most drugs occurs largely in the liver, because of its mass, high blood flow, and concentration of enzymes that metabolize drugs. The initial step in metabolism of many drugs is executed by the mixed-function oxidase enzymes located in the hepatic endoplasmic reticulum. These enzyme systems containing cytochrome P_{450} oxidize the molecule by a variety of reactions including aromatic hydroxylations, N-demethylations, O-demethylations, and sulfoxidations. The products of these reactions are usually more polar (and more readily excreted by the kidney).

The number of mixed-function oxidase enzyme units in the liver can be increased by treatment with enzyme inducers, of which phenobarbital is the prototype. Almost all the barbiturates in clinical use increase the mixed-function oxidase enzymes. Induction with phenobarbital can occur with doses of as little as 60 mg daily. Mixed-function oxidases are also induced by glutethimide, phenytoin, and rifampin, and by occupational exposure to chlorinated insecticides such as DDT, as well as by alcohol.

The actions of a number of drugs are inhibited by treatment with inducing agents. Phenobarbital and other inducers lower plasma levels of warfarin, bishydroxycoumarin, digitoxin, quinidine, dexamethasone, and metyrapone. These interactions all

TABLE 70-3
Drug interaction index

Drug	Section of chapter describing interaction
Acetohexamide	IIB
Allopurinol	IIA
p-Aminosalicylate	IA
Amphetamine	IC, III
Antidepressants, tricyclic (desipramine, nortriptyline, imipramine, doxepin, protriptyline, amitriptyline)	IC
Aspirin	IIB, III
Azathioprine	IIA
Barbiturates (class)	IB
Bethanidine	IC
Bishydroxycoumarin	IB, IIA, IIB
Chloral hydrate	IIC
Chloramphenicol	IIA, III
Chlorpromazine	IC
Cholestyramine	IA
Clofibrate	IIA
Clonidine	IC
Cyclophosphamide	IIA
Dexamethasone	IB
Digitoxin	IB
Diphenylhydantoin (see phenytoin below)	
Disulfiram	IIA
Ephedrine	IC, III
Ethanol	IIA
Furazolidone	III
Guanethidine	IC
Isoniazid	IIA
6-Mercaptopurine	IIA
Methotrexate	IIB
Metyrapone	IB
Monoamine oxidase inhibitors	III
Pargyline	III
Phenobarbital	IB
Phenylbutazone	IIA, IIB
Phenylpropanolamine	III
Phenytoin (diphenylhydantoin)	IB, IIA
Potassium	III
Quinidine	IB
Rifampin	IA, IB
Spironolactone	III
Tetracycline	IA, III
Tolbutamide	IIA
Triamterene	III
Warfarin	IB, IIA, IIC, III

have obvious clinical significance. With the coumarin anticoagulants, the major risk occurs when an appropriate level of anticoagulation is achieved while the coumarin drug is coadministered with an inducing agent. When the inducer is discontinued, e.g., following discharge from the hospital, plasma levels of the coumarin anticoagulant will rise as the induction effect wears off, leading to excessive anticoagulation. Barbiturates have been shown to lower the plasma levels of phenytoin in some patients, but the clinical effect of reduced phenytoin levels is probably counter-balanced by the anticonvulsant effects of phenobarbital.

There is considerable variation among individuals in the extent to which drug metabolism can be induced. In some patients phenobarbital leads to marked acceleration in the rate of drug metabolism, whereas little induction is seen in others. This variability in the extent of induction of mixed-function oxidases is largely genetically determined.

In addition to inducing the mixed-function oxidase enzymes, phenobarbital has a number of other effects on hepatic function. It increases liver blood flow, bile flow, and the hepatocellular transport of organic anions. The conjugation of drugs and bilirubin is also enhanced by inducing agents.

C Inhibition of cellular uptake or binding   The guanidinium antihypertensives, guanethidine and bethanidine, are transported to their site of action in adrenergic neurons by an energy-requiring membrane transport system for biogenic monoamines. Although the physiological function of the transport system is re-uptake of the adrenergic neurotransmitter, it also transports a variety of ring-substituted bases, including guanethidine and bethanidine, into the adrenergic neuron against a concentration gradient. Inhibitors of norepinephrine uptake will prevent the uptake of the guanidinium antihypertensives into adrenergic neurons and will thereby block their pharmacological effects. The tricyclic antidepressants are potent inhibitors of norepinephrine uptake. Consequently, concomitant administration of clinical doses of tricyclic antidepressants including desipramine, protriptyline, nortriptyline, and amitriptyline will almost totally abolish the antihypertensive effects of guanethidine and bethanidine. Although they are less potent inhibitors of norepinephrine uptake, doxepin and chlorpromazine, when given in doses of greater than 100 mg daily, produce dose-related antagonism of the action of the guanidinium antihypertensives. In patients with severe hypertension, the loss of control of blood pressure resulting from these drug interactions can lead to serious clinical complications such as stroke and malignant hypertension.

Amphetamine also antagonizes the antihypertensive effect of guanethidine by displacing it from its site of action within the adrenergic neuron (Chap. 251). Ephedrine, a component of many drug combinations used in asthma, also antagonizes the effect of guanethidine, probably by both inhibition of uptake and displacement from the neuron.

The antihypertensive effect of clonidine in humans is partially antagonized by the tricyclic antidepressants. Clonidine lowers arterial pressure by reducing sympathetic outflow from the blood-pressure-regulating centers in the hindbrain (Chap. 251). This central hypotensive action is antagonized by the tricyclic antidepressants.

II PHARMACOKINETIC INTERACTIONS CAUSING INCREASED DRUG DELIVERY

A Inhibition of drug metabolism   If the active form of a drug is cleared largely by biotransformation, inhibition of its metabolism will lead to a prolonged half-life and to accumulation of the drug during maintenance therapy. Excessive accumulation due to inhibited metabolism leads to significant adverse effects in the case of several drugs.

The metabolism of phenytoin is inhibited by a number of drugs. Clofibrate, phenylbutazone, chloramphenicol, disulfiram, bishydroxycoumarin, and isoniazid can raise the steady-state plasma levels of phenytoin by more than two-fold. In the case of isoniazid, the extent of inhibition of phenytoin metabolism is a function of the genetically determined rate of isoniazid acetylation; substantial inhibition of phenytoin metabolism and resultant clinical toxicity are seen only in those individuals who are slow acetylators. Inhibited metabolism may lead to abrupt development of symptoms such as somnolence, mental confusion, and disturbance of gait in patients who have not changed their phenytoin dosage.

Impaired metabolism of tolbutamide with severe hypoglycemia has resulted from coadministration of clofibrate, phenylbutazone, chloramphenicol, and bishydroxycoumarin. Excessive anticoagulation by warfarin may result from inhibition of its metabolism by disulfiram or phenylbutazone, or by concurrent and copious ingestion of ethanol. Warfarin is administered as a racemic mixture, and its $S(-)$ isomer has five times the anticoagulant potency of the $R(+)$ isomer. Phenylbutazone selectively inhibits the metabolism of the $S(-)$ isomer, and only when this isomer is examined specifically can the substantial reduction in its metabolism produced by phenylbutazone be unmasked.

Azathioprine is readily converted in the body to an active metabolite, 6-mercaptopurine, which in turn is inactivated in part by xanthine oxidase which sequentially oxidizes it to 6-thiouric acid. When allopurinol, a potent inhibitor of xanthine oxidase, is administered concurrently with standard doses of azathioprine or 6-mercaptopurine, life-threatening toxicity (bone marrow suppression) can result. Therefore, it has been recommended that the doses of azathioprine and 6-mercaptopurine be reduced to one-third or one-fourth the usual amounts when allopurinol is given at the same time. These are rough approximations of the dose modifications, and the quantitative aspects of this interaction have not been determined.

B Inhibition of renal secretion A number of drugs are secreted by the renal tubular transport systems for organic ions. Inhibition of this tubular transport system can cause excessive accumulation of a drug when this is the major pathway of its elimination. Several drugs, including phenylbutazone, probenecid, salicylates, and bishydroxycoumarin, will competitively inhibit this transport system. Patients receiving the oral antidiabetic acetohexamide have developed profound hypoglycemia when phenylbutazone was added to their drug regimen. This exaggerated hypoglycemia resulted from the inhibition by phenylbutazone of the tubular secretion of hydroxyacetohexamide, an active metabolite which is responsible for most of the hypoglycemic effect that ensues from acetohexamide administration. Renal tubular secretion contributes substantially to the elimination of penicillin, which can be inhibited by probenecid.

C Inhibition of plasma protein binding When the binding of a drug to plasma protein is reduced by another agent, more unbound drug will be made available to receptor sites for any given level of total drug. Reduction in the binding of a drug does not have significance in vivo unless the drug is very highly bound (more than 90 percent) and the volume of distribution is small. A drug may alter the binding of another by competitive displacement or by an interaction with protein (usually albumin) to decrease binding affinity. Reduction in the extent of binding also will make more drug available to the organs of clearance, and if the drug normally has a low extraction ratio because binding sequesters the drug in plasma, then reduction of binding will increase its clearance. As a result, following a binding displacement interaction, total and free-drug levels at steady state will fall until free-drug concentration returns to the previous levels; at steady state, the average unbound warfarin levels should be independent of the degree of binding. Therefore, in most instances, any enhancement of the pharmacological effect will be transient.

Although reduction of the binding of many drugs by others has been demonstrated in vitro, the only instance where clinical significance has clearly been linked to reduced binding is the potentiation of the anticoagulant effect of warfarin by chloral hydrate in high dosage. Chloral hydrate is converted in the body to trichloroacetic acid, which displaces warfarin from albumin-binding sites. As a result there is a transient increase in the anticoagulant effect of warfarin, persisting for only a few days until the concentration of free warfarin returns to previous levels.

III PHARMACODYNAMIC AND OTHER INTERACTIONS BETWEEN DRUGS Therapeutically useful interactions in which the combined effect of two drugs is greater than that of either drug alone are numerous. These favorable drug combinations are covered extensively in specific therapeutic sections in this text, and the following is directed toward those pharmacodynamic interactions that create unwanted effects. Two drugs may act on separate components of a common process and yield effects greater than either drug alone. For example, small doses of aspirin (less than 1 g daily) will not alter the prothrombin time appreciably in patients who are stabilized on warfarin therapy. However, the addition of aspirin to patients therapeutically anticoagulated with warfarin increases the risk of bleeding because aspirin inhibits platelet aggregation. Thus the combination of impaired functions of both the platelets and the fluid-phase clotting system increases the potential for hemorrhagic complications in patients receiving warfarin therapy.

The administration of supplemental potassium leads to more frequent and more severe hyperkalemia when potassium elimination is reduced by concurrent treatment with spironolactone or triamterene.

Occasionally, the addition of bacteriostatic antibiotics such as the tetracyclines and chloramphenicol to bactericidal agents (e.g., penicillin) may impair the cure of infections. In vitro, the combination of bacteriostatic and bactericidal agents yields a combined effect resembling that of the bacteriostatic agent alone. This may have clinical significance in meningitis, and, on the basis of studies in experimental animals, it is suggested that when bactericidal drugs need to be used, the administration of the static drug be delayed 1 h after initiating the bactericidal agent.

VARIABLE ACTIONS OF DRUGS CAUSED BY GENETIC DIFFERENCES IN THEIR METABOLISM

ACETYLATION Isoniazid, hydralazine, procainamide, and a number of other drugs are metabolized by acetylation of a hydrazino or amino group. This reaction is catalyzed by N-acetyl transferase, a nonmicrosomal (soluble) enzyme in the liver that transfers an acetyl group from acetyl coenzyme A to the drug. Individuals differ markedly in the rate at which drugs are acetylated, and there is a bimodal distribution of the population into "rapid acetylators" and "slow acetylators." The rate of acetylation is under genetic control; rapid acetylation is an autosomal dominant trait.

The toxic, sometimes fatal, hepatitis that occurs in about 1 percent of patients on isoniazid occurs predominantly in rapid acetylators. The greater hepatotoxicity in rapid acetylators appears to result from the synthesis of more acetylisoniazid which is further metabolized to acetylhydrazine, a potent hepatotoxin. Acetylhydrazine exerts its toxic effect through an active metabolite that binds covalently to macromolecules in the hepatic cells that produce it. Conversely, the lupus erythematosus-like syndrome produced by hydralazine (Chap. 251) occurs only in individuals who are slow acetylators.

Because these important toxic drug effects are largely predictable from the acetylation phenotype, it may in certain instances be of value to determine the rate of acetylation in patients who are to receive isoniazid, or those who would benefit from doses of hydralazine above the 200 mg per day dose that can be safely employed in the population at large. Acetylation phenotype can be determined by measuring the ratio of acetylated to nonacetylated dapsone or sulfamethazine in plasma or urine following administration of a test dose of these acetylation substrates. The ratio of monoacetyldapsone to dapsone in plasma at 6 h after dapsone administration is less than 0.35 for slow acetylators and greater than 0.35 for rapid acetylators. At 6 h following the administration of sulfamethazine, less than 25 percent of the drug in the plasma is in the acetylated form in slow acetylators (rapid acetylators, more than 25 percent); in the urine collected in the 5- to 6-h interval after administration, less than 70 percent of the drug is in the acetylated form in slow acetylators (rapid acetylators, more than 70 percent).

METABOLISM BY MIXED-FUNCTION OXIDASES In healthy individuals taking no other medications, the major determinant of the rate of metabolism of drugs by the hepatic mixed-function oxidases is genetic. In contrast to the bimodal distribution of individuals with respect to acetylation rates, there is a unimodal distribution for most drugs metabolized by enzymes of the hepatic endoplasmic reticulum, indicating control by multiple genes. The genetically controlled variation in hepatic clearance is marked for some of these drugs. Steady-state plasma levels of nortriptyline, propranolol, and chlorpromazine vary by more than tenfold among individuals. This has obvious consequences in attempting to predict effect from a given dose in those individuals who differ markedly from the average.

CONCENTRATION OF DRUGS IN PLASMA AS A GUIDE TO THERAPY

Optimal individualization of therapy is assisted by measuring the concentration of certain drugs in plasma. Genetic variation in elimination rates, interactions with other drugs, disease-induced alterations in elimination and distribution, and other factors combine to yield a wide range of plasma levels in patients given the same dose. Furthermore, the problem of noncompliance with prescribed regimens during continuing therapy is an endemic and elusive cause of therapeutic failure. There are clinical indicators that assist the titration of some drugs into the desired range, and no chemical determination is a substitute for careful observations of the patient's response to treatment. However, the therapeutic and adverse effects are not precisely quantifiable for all drugs, and in complex clinical situations estimates of the action of a drug may be misleading. For example, previously existing neurological disease may obscure the neurological consequences of intoxication with phenytoin. Because clearance, half-life, accumulation, and steady-state plasma levels are difficult to predict, the measurement of plasma levels is often useful as a guide to the optimal dose. This is particularly so when there is a narrow range between the plasma levels yielding therapeutic and adverse effects. The concept of the average dose will not benefit the patient whose levels are inadequate for therapeutic effect or in the toxic range. Adjustment of dosage based on creatinine clearance in

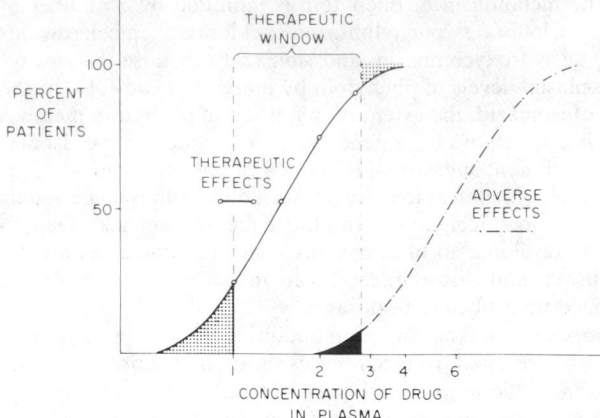

FIGURE 70-5

The cumulative percentage of patients responding to increasing levels of drug in plasma with both therapeutic and adverse effects. The therapeutic "window" defines the range of concentrations of drug that will achieve therapeutic effects in most patients with adverse effects in only a small percentage.

renal insufficiency will minimize gross over- and undertreatment, but still it is a calculation based on an average and will not yield ideal treatment for all patients.

Data on concentrations of drugs in plasma are utilized most effectively in the framework of the known kinetics of the drug, including consideration of whether the levels are likely to reflect the steady state, whether they represent the equilibrium phase (cf., the distribution phase discussed above), and the extent to which disease-induced changes in the drug binding can influence the concentration of total (bound plus unbound) drug. In addition, the variability among individual responses to given plasma levels must be recognized. This is illustrated by a hypothetical population dose-response curve (Fig. 70-5) and its relationship to the therapeutic range or therapeutic "window" of desired plasma levels. The defined therapeutic window should include the levels at which the majority of patients will achieve the intended pharmacological effect. However, there are a few people who are quite sensitive to the therapeutic effects of most drugs, responding to lower levels, whereas others are sufficiently refractory as to require levels that impose an increased likelihood of adverse effects as a potential price for therapeutic benefit. For example, a few pa-

TABLE 70-4
Concentrations of drugs in plasma: relation to efficacy and adverse effects

Drug	Efficacy*	Adverse effects†
Carbenicillin	100 µg/ml‡	300 µg/ml
Digitoxin	12 ng/ml	25–30 ng/ml
Digoxin	0.8 ng/ml	2.0 ng/ml
Gentamicin	4 µg/ml§	12 µg/ml
Lithium	0.5 meq/liter	1.3 meq/liter
Penicillin G	1–25 µg/ml¶	
Phenytoin (diphenylhydantoin)	10 µg/ml	20 µg/ml
Procainamide	4 µg/ml	8 µg/ml
Quinidine	3 µg/ml	7 µg/ml
Theophylline	8 µg/ml	20 µg/ml

* The therapeutic effect is infrequent or slight at levels below these.

† The frequency of adverse effects increases sharply when these levels are exceeded.

‡ Minimal inhibitory concentration (MIC) for most strains of Pseudomonas aeruginosa. MIC for other, more sensitive, organisms is less.

§ Dependent on the MIC. Higher levels (up to 8 µg/ml) may be desired when host defenses are impaired.

¶ There is a wide range of MIC of penicillin for various organisms, and the MIC of all those for which penicillin is used is < 20. "Massive" penicillin therapy with 20 million units daily achieves levels of 20 to 25 µg/ml in patients with clearance of creatinine of 100 ml/min.

tients with strong seizure foci will require plasma levels of phenytoin exceeding 20 μg/ml in order to control their seizure disorders. Increments in dosage to achieve this effect may be appropriate. However, with an elevation in dose that yields levels at which adverse effects become more frequent, one must exercise heightened sensitivity for subtle changes in higher integrative function. In addition, because phenytoin has dose-dependent kinetics, it is essential to monitor carefully the possibly large variations of plasma levels that can accompany small increases in the dosage as levels exceed 20 μg/ml.

As also illustrated in Fig. 70-5, some patients may be prone to adverse effects at levels which are well tolerated by most of the population, and therefore elevation of levels to those achieving a high probability of therapeutic effect may bring on unwanted actions in the exceptional patient.

Table 70-4 presents for a number of drugs the concentrations in plasma that are associated with probable adverse and therapeutic effects in most patients. Its use within the guidelines discussed should permit more effective and safer therapy for those patients who are not "average."

REFERENCES

DETTLI L: Elimination kinetics and dosage adjustment of drugs in patients with kidney disease. Prog Pharmacol, vol 1, no 4, 1977

SHAND DG et al: Pharmacokinetic drug interactions, in *Handbook of Experimental Pharmacology*, vol 28: *Concepts in Biochemical Pharmacology*, JR Gillette, JR Mitchell (eds). New York, Springer-Verlag, 1975, p 272

SHEINER LB, TOZER TN: Clinical pharmacokinetics: The use of plasma concentrations of drugs, in *Clinical Pharmacology: Basic Principles in Therapeutics*, 2d ed. New York, Macmillan, 1978, p 71

WILKINSON GR, SHAND DG: A physiological approach to hepatic drug clearance. Clin Pharmacol Ther 18:377, 1975

71
ADVERSE REACTIONS TO DRUGS

ALASTAIR J. J. WOOD
JOHN A. OATES

The beneficial effects of drugs are coupled with the inescapable risk that they may also cause untoward effects. The morbidity and mortality that result from these untoward effects often present diagnostic problems, for these drugs can involve every organ and system of the body.

Major advances in the investigation, development, and regulation of drugs ensure in most instances their uniformity, claims of effectiveness, and relative safety, as well as identify their recognized hazards. However, the extremely large number and variety of drugs and drug products available over the counter (OTC) or by prescription from a physician make it impossible for patient or physician to obtain or retain the knowledge necessary to use all these drugs well. It is understandable, therefore, that many OTC drugs are used unwisely by the public and that restricted drugs may be prescribed incorrectly by physicians.

Most physicians use no more than 50 drug products in their practice, gaining familiarity with their effectiveness and safety. Most patients probably use only a limited number of OTC drugs. Nevertheless, many patients receive care and drug prescriptions from more than one physician, and surveys have shown that in any 30-day period patients may consume more than three different OTC drug products containing nine or more different chemical agents.

Twenty-five to fifty percent of patients may make errors in self-administration of prescribed medicines, and this can be responsible for adverse drug effects. Elderly patients are most likely to commit such errors. One-third or more of patients also may not take their prescribed medications. It also seems likely that many patients commit similar errors in taking OTC drugs by not reading or following the directions for use of the medicines provided on the containers. Physicians must recognize that providing directions with prescriptions does not always guarantee their patients' compliance.

Every drug can produce untoward consequences, even when used according to standard or recommended methods of administration. When used incorrectly, the drug's effectiveness may be reduced, or adverse reactions can be expected to occur more frequently. The administration of several drugs during the same period of time also may result in adverse interactions between drugs (see Chap. 70).

In the hospital all the drugs a patient is given should be under the control of a physician, and patient compliance is, in general, ensured. Errors may occur nevertheless, in that the wrong drug or dose may be given, or the drug may be given to the wrong patient, although systems improving drug distribution and administration in hospitals have reduced this problem. On the other hand, there are no means for controlling how ambulatory patients take prescription or OTC drugs.

EPIDEMIOLOGY Epidemiologic studies of adverse drug reactions have been helpful in evaluating the magnitude of the overall problem, in calculating the rate of reactions to individual drugs, and in characterizing some of the determinants of adverse drug effects.

Patients receive on the average 10 different drugs while hospitalized. The sicker the patient, the more drugs are given, and as expected, there is a corresponding increase in the likelihood of adverse drug reactions. When fewer than six different drugs are given to hospitalized patients, the probability of an adverse reaction is about 5 percent, but if more than 15 drugs are given, the probability is over 40 percent. Retrospective analysis of ambulatory patients has revealed a history of some adverse drug effects in 20 percent of them.

Thus, the magnitude of the problem posed by drug-induced disease has become exceedingly large. Two to five percent of patients are admitted to the medical and pediatric services of general hospitals because of illnesses attributed to drugs. Five to thirty percent of patients experience adverse reactions to drugs during hospitalization. The case/fatality ratio from drug-induced disease in hospitalized patients varies from 2 to 12 percent. An unknown proportion of fetal or neonatal abnormalities may be due to medicines taken by the mother during pregnancy or parturition. An undetermined number of illnesses caused by drugs are responsible for visits of patients to physicians' offices.

Epidemiologic studies revealing the rates of adverse drug reactions are limited by the availability of suitable controls. Hence, both major and minor manifestations of presumed drug-induced illness are difficult to establish. Gastrointestinal signs and symptoms, particularly vomiting and diarrhea, account for approximately one-third; neurologic manifestations account for about one-fifth; cardiovascular, metabolic, and cutaneous manifestations each account for about one-tenth; and hematologic and other manifestations each account for about one-twentieth of adverse drug reactions. Women experience twice as many gastrointestinal manifestations of adverse drug effects as do men.

A small group of widely used drugs account for a disproportionate number of reactions. A number of studies have shown that aspirin, digoxin, anticoagulants, diuretics, antimicrobials, steroids, and hypoglycemic agents account for as many as 90 percent of all reactions.

ETIOLOGY Most adverse reactions to drugs may be classified into two groups. The most frequent are those that result from the exaggerated but predicted pharmacologic action of the drug. Other adverse reactions ensue from toxic effects on cells that result from mechanisms unrelated to the intended pharmacologic actions. These therefore are often unpredictable, are frequently severe, and result from a number of recognized as well as undiscovered mechanisms. Some of the mechanisms of extrapharmacologic toxicity include direct cytotoxicity, the initiation of abnormal immune responses, and the perturbation of metabolic processes in individuals rendered susceptible by genetic enzymatic defects.

EXAGGERATION OF THE INTENDED PHARMACOLOGIC EFFECT By prior consideration of the known factors that modify drug action, these adverse reactions often are preventable.

Abnormally high drug concentration at the receptor site (site of action) due to the pharmacokinetic variability discussed in Chap. 70 is the usual cause. For example, reduction in the volume of distribution, in the rate of metabolism, or in the rate of excretion all will result in higher than expected concentration of the drug at the receptor site with consequent increase in pharmacologic effect.

Alteration in the dose-response curve due to increased receptor sensitivity will result in an increase in drug effect at the same concentration. An example of this is seen in the excessive response to the anticoagulant warfarin at normal and lower than normal blood levels in the elderly.

The shape of the dose-response curve itself also determines the likelihood of the development of adverse drug reactions. These drugs with a steep dose-response curve are more likely to be associated with dose-related toxicity because of the small increase in dose required to produce a large change in pharmacologic effect. An increase in the dose of drugs which exhibit nonlinear kinetics, such as phenytoin (see previous chapter) may produce a proportionately greater increase in the blood level, resulting in toxicity.

Concomitant drug therapy may affect the pharmacokinetics or pharmacodynamics of other drugs. Pharmacokinetics may be affected by alterations in bioavailability, protein binding, or the rate of metabolism or excretion. Pharmacodynamics may be altered by competition for receptor sites, by prevention of the drug's reaching its site of action, or by antagonism or enhancement of the drug's pharmacological effect. These subjects are discussed in detail in the previous chapter.

TOXICITY UNRELATED TO A DRUG'S PRIMARY PHARMACOLOGIC ACTIVITY **Cytotoxic reactions** Our understanding of these so-called "idiosyncratic" reactions has greatly improved recently as it has become clear that many of these reactions are due to irreversible binding of drug or metabolites to tissue macromolecules by shared electron (covalent) bonds. Some chemical carcinogens such as the alkylating agents combine directly with DNA. However, it is more commonly only after metabolic activation to chemically reactive metabolites that covalent binding occurs. This metabolic activation usually occurs in the microsomal mixed-function oxidase system, the hepatic enzyme system which is responsible for the metabolism of many drugs (Chap. 70). During the course of drug metabolism by these pathways, reactive metabolites of some drugs may be produced which covalently bind to tissue macromolecules, causing tissue damage. Because of the highly reactive nature of these metabolites covalent binding often occurs close to the site of production, such as the liver, but the mixed-function oxidase system is found in other tissues as well.

An example of this type of adverse drug reaction is the hepatotoxicity associated with isoniazid, which is metabolized principally by acetylation (Fig. 71-1) to acetylisoniazid, which is then hydrolyzed to acetylhydralazine. The further metabolism of acetylhydralazine by the mixed-function oxidase system liberates reactive metabolites which covalently bind to liver macromolecules, causing hepatic necrosis. The rate of acetylation shows a bimodal distribution, the population dividing into slow and fast acetylators. Fast acetylators predominate in Orientals, who have been shown to be particularly susceptible to isoniazid hepatoxicity. The administration of drugs known to increase the activity of the mixed-function oxidase system, such as phenobarbital or rifampin, together with isoniazid, is associated with the production of increased amounts of reactive metabolites, increased covalent binding, and hepatic damage.

The liver necrosis produced by overdosage of acetominophen is caused by the covalent binding of reactive electrophilic metabolites to liver macromolecules. Normally these reactive metabolites are detoxified by combining with hepatic glutathione. When glutathione becomes exhausted, the metabolites bind instead to liver macromolecules with resultant hepatocyte damage. The hepatic necrosis produced by the ingestion of large quantities of acetaminophen can be prevented, or at least attenuated, by the administration of substances such as cysteamine, which bind the electrophilic metabolites and prevent them from reacting with hepatic proteins with resultant hepatic necrosis. The risks of hepatic necrosis are increased in patients also receiving drugs such as phenobarbital which increase the rate of drug metabolism and rate of production of toxic metabolites.

It is likely, though as yet unproved, that other "idiosyncratic" reactions are caused by the covalent binding of reactive metabolites to tissue macromolecules, with either direct cytotoxicity or via the initiation of an immunologic response.

FIGURE 71-1

Biotransformation of isoniazid to a hepatotoxic metabolite.

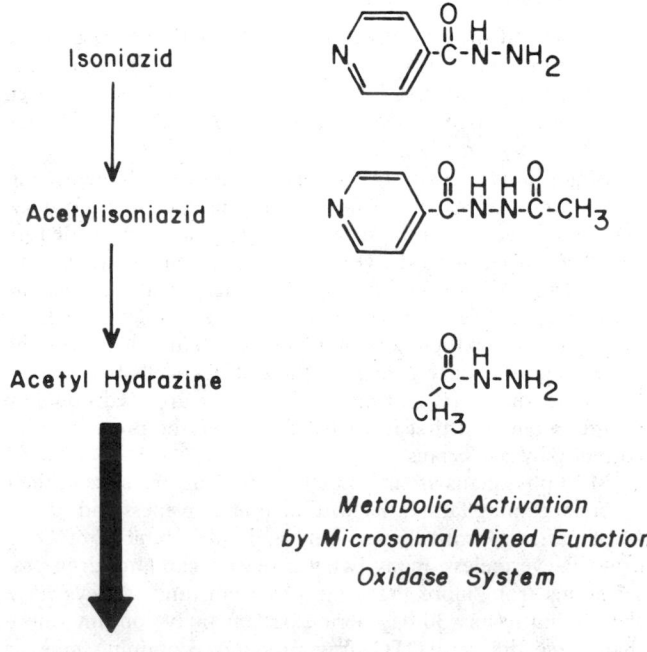

Immunologic mechanisms Most pharmacologic agents are poor immunogens since they consist of small molecules with molecular weights less than 2000. Stimulation of antibody synthesis or sensitization of lymphocytes by a drug or one of its metabolites usually requires in vivo activation and covalent linkage to protein, carbohydrate, or nucleic acid.

Drug stimulation of antibody production may mediate tissue injury by one of several mechanisms. The antibody may attack the drug affixed to a cell by covalent linkage and thereby destroy the cell, as occurs in penicillin-induced hemolytic anemia. Complexes of antibody-drug-antigen may be passively adsorbed by a bystander cell which is destroyed by activation of complement; this occurs in Sedormid-induced thrombocytopenia. Drugs or their reactive metabolites may alter host tissue, rendering it antigenic, and stimulate autoantibodies; for example, hydralazine and procainamide can chemically alter nuclear material, stimulate formation of antinuclear antibodies, and occasionally cause lupus erythematosus. Autoantibodies may be stimulated by drugs which neither interact with the host antigen nor have any chemical similarity to the host tissue; for example, alpha methyldopa frequently stimulates formation of antibodies to host erythrocytes, yet the drug does not itself attach to the erythrocyte nor share any chemical similarities with the antigenic determinants on the erythrocyte.

Serum sickness (Chap. 65) results from deposition of circulating drug-antibody complexes on endothelial surfaces. Complement activation occurs, chemotactic factors are generated locally, and an inflammatory response appears at the site of complex entrapment. Arthralgias, lymphadenopathy, glomerulonephritis, or cerebritis may result. Penicillin is the most common cause of serum sickness today. Many drugs, particularly the antimicrobial agents, induce production of IgE, which affixes to mast cell membranes. Contact with a drug antigen initiates a series of biochemical events within the mast cell and results in the release of mediators which may produce urticaria, wheezing, rhinorrhea, and occasionally hypotension characteristic of anaphylaxis.

Drugs may also excite cell-mediated immune responses. Topically administered substances may interact with sulfhydryl or amino groups in the skin and react with sensitized lymphocytes to produce the rash characteristic of contact dermatitis. Other types of rashes may also appear from the interaction of serum factors, drugs, and sensitized lymphocytes. The role of drug-activated lymphocytes in the immune mechanisms governing destruction of visceral tissue is unknown.

Toxicity associated with genetically determined enzymatic defects In the porphyrias, any drugs that accelerate the activity of enzymes proximal to the deficient enzyme in the biosynthetic pathway of porphyrins can increase the quantity of porphyrin precursors that accumulate proximal to the deficient enzyme (Chap. 96). These drugs are listed in Table 71-1.

Patients with a deficiency of glucose 6-phosphate dehydrogenase (G6PD) will develop hemolytic anemia on primaquine and a number of other drugs (Table 71-1) which do not cause hemolysis in patients who have adequate quantities of this enzyme (Chap. 314).

Diagnosis The manifestations of drug-induced diseases frequently resemble those associated with other diseases, and may be produced by different and dissimilar drugs. Recognition of the role of a drug or drugs responsible for illness is dependent upon appreciation of the possible implication of adverse reactions to drugs in any disease, identification of a temporal relationship between drug administration and development of illness, and familiarity with the manifestations most often caused by particular drugs. Although specific reactions have been described as resulting from the use of particular drugs, there is always a "first," and any drug should be suspected of causing an adverse effect if the clinical setting is appropriate.

Illness related to a drug's pharmacologic action may be more easily recognized than illness attributable to immunologic or other mechanisms. For example, side effects such as cardiac arrhythmias in patients receiving digitalis, hypoglycemia in patients given insulin, and bleeding in patients receiving anticoagulants are more easily related to the prescribed drug than are symptoms like fever or rash, which may be caused by many drugs or by other factors.

Once an adverse reaction is suspected, discontinuance of the suspected drug followed by disappearance of the reaction is presumptive evidence of a drug-induced illness. Reappearance of the reaction upon cautious readministration of the drug may provide confirmatory evidence of the relationship if such confirmation adds useful information to the future management of the patient without entailing undue risk. With concentration-dependent adverse reactions, lowering the dosage may also be followed by disappearance of the reaction, and increasing the dose may cause it to reappear. When the reaction is thought to be allergic, however, readministration of the drug may be hazardous, since anaphylactic shock may develop. Readministration is unwise under these conditions unless alternate drugs are not available and treatment is mandatory.

If the patient is receiving many different drugs when an adverse reaction is suspected, the drugs most likely to be incriminated can usually be identified. All drugs may be discontinued at once, or if this is not practical, then drugs should be discontinued one at a time, starting with the drug under greatest suspicion, and the patient observed for signs of improvement. It must be remembered that the time taken for the disappearance of a concentration-dependent adverse effect will depend on the time taken for the concentration to fall below the range associated with the adverse effect, and this in turn will depend on the initial blood level and on the rate of elimination or metabolism of the drug. Adverse effects of drugs such as phenobarbital which have long half-lives will take a considerable time to disappear.

To assist in the identification of adverse reactions, a table of the drugs recognized as producing a number of reactions appears in this chapter (Table 71-1). This table is not intended to be exhaustive but rather includes well-documented reactions and some less well-documented reactions whose effects are sufficiently devastating as to require their consideration. It should be used to suggest the likely causative drug, but the absence of a drug from the table should not be interpreted to mean that it is not responsible for the reaction.

Serum antibody has been demonstrated in some persons with drug allergy involving cellular blood elements, as in agranulocytosis, hemolytic anemia, and thrombocytopenia. In other types of drug allergy, precipitation, hemoagglutination, or complement-fixation tests with drugs or drug degradation products have only rarely been clearly related to adverse reactions. Skin tests with the drug or its degradation products are often of little value in identifying the allergic individual. These poor results testify to the inadequacy of present methods of testing and are not an argument against an immunologic basis for allergic drug reactions.

Eliciting a drug history from patients is important for diagnosis. Attention must be directed to nonprescription, or OTC, as well as to prescription drugs. Each type can be responsible for adverse drug effects, and frequently adverse interactions occur between drugs purchased by patients over the counter and those prescribed by physicians. In addition, it is common for patients to be cared for by several physicians; and duplicative, additive, counteractive, or synergistic drugs may therefore

TABLE 71-1
Clinical manifestations of adverse reactions to drugs

I Multisystem
  A Fever
    1 Penicillins
    2 Novobiocin
    3 p-Aminosalicylic acid
    4 Amphotericin B
    5 Antihistamines
    6 Cephalosporins
    7 Barbiturates
    8 Phenytoin
    9 Quinidine
    10 Sulfonamides
    11 Iodides
    12 Thiouracil
    13 Phenolphthalein
    14 Methyldopa
    15 Procainamide
  B Drug-induced lupus erythematosus
    1 Hydralazine
    2 Procainamide
    3 Isoniazid
  C Serum sickness
    1 Aspirin
    2 Penicillins
    3 Streptomycin
    4 Sulfonamides
    5 Propylthiouracil
  D Anaphylaxis
    1 Bromsulphothalein
    2 Penicillins
    3 Cephalosporins
    4 Streptomycin
    5 Dextran
    6 Iron Dextran
    7 Procaine
    8 Insulin
    9 Demeclocycline
    10 Iodinated drugs or contrast media
    11 Lidocaine
II Endocrine
  A Disorders of thyroid function tests
    1 Oral contraceptives
    2 Bromsulphalein
    3 Phenindione
    4 Iodides
    5 Tolbutamide
    6 Chlorpropamide
    7 Lithium
    8 Acetazolamide
    9 Gold salts
    10 Dimercaprol
    11 Clofibrate
    12 Phenothiazines (long term)
    13 Phenylbutazone
    14 Sulfonamides
    15 Phenytoin
  B Addisonian-like syndrome
    1 Busulfan
  C Gynecomastia
    1 Estrogens
    2 Testosterone
    3 Spironolactone
    4 Digitalis
    5 Reserpine
    6 Methyldopa
    7 Isoniazid
    8 Ethionamide
    9 Griseofulvin
  D Galactorrhea (may also cause amenorrhea)
    1 Methyldopa
    2 Phenothiazines
    3 Reserpine
    4 Tricyclic antidepressants
    5 Dexamphetamine
  E Sexual dysfunction
    1 Impaired ejaculation
      a Guanethidine
      b Debrisoquin
      c Bethanidine
      d Thioridazine
    2 Decreased libido and impotence
      a Oral contraceptives
      b Sedatives
      c Major tranquilizers
      d Lithium
      e Methyldopa
      f Clonidine
III Metabolic
  A Hyponatremia
    1 Dilutional
      a Vincristine
      b Cyclophosphamide
      c Chlorpropamide
      d Diuretics
    2 Salt wasting
      a Diuretics
      b Corticosteroid (withdrawal)
      c Enemas
      d Mannitol
  B Hyperkalemia
    1 Spironolactone
    2 Triamterene
    3 Amiloride
    4 Cytotoxics
    5 Corticosteroid (withdrawal)
    6 Succinylcholine
    7 Digitalis overdose
    8 Potassium salts of drugs
    9 Potassium preparations including salt substitute
    10 Lithium
  C Hypokalemia
    1 Diuretics
    2 Laxative abuse
    3 Corticosteroids
    4 Amphotericin B
    5 Alkali-induced alkalosis
    6 Insulin
    7 Osmotic diuretics
    8 Carbenoxolone
    9 Gentamicin
    10 Degraded tetracycline
    11 Vitamin B_{12}
  D Metabolic acidosis
    1 Paraldehyde (degraded)
    2 Phenformin
    3 Acetazolamide
    4 Spironolactone
    5 Salicylates
  E Hypercalcemia
    1 Antacids with absorbable alkali
    2 Vitamin D
    3 Thiazides
  F Hyperuricemia
    1 Thiazides
    2 Chlorthalidone
    3 Ethacrynic acid
    4 Furosemide
    5 Aspirin
    6 Cytotoxics
    7 Hyperalimentation
    8 Fructose (IV)
  G Hyperglycemia
    1 Corticosteroids
    2 Oral contraceptives
    3 Chlorthalidone
    4 Ethacrynic acid
    5 Thiazides
    6 Furosemide
    7 Diazoxide
    8 Growth hormone
  H Porphyria exacerbation
    1 Barbiturates
    2 Chlordiazepoxide
    3 Meprobamate
    4 Sulfonamides
    5 Estrogens
    6 Oral contraceptives
    7 Chlorpropamide
    8 Phenytoin
    9 Glutethimide
    10 Griseofulvin
    11 Rifampin
  I Hyperbilirubinemia
    1 Rifampin
    2 Novobiocin
IV Dermatologic
  A Exfoliative dermatitis
    1 Penicillins
    2 Sulfonamides
    3 Barbiturates
    4 Phenytoin
    5 Phenylbutazone
    6 Gold salts
    7 Quinidine
  B Toxic epidermal necrolysis (bullous)
    1 Barbiturates
    2 Phenylbutazone
    3 Phenytoin
    4 Sulfonamides
    5 Phenolphthalein
    6 Penicillins
    7 Allopurinol
    8 Iodides
    9 Bromides
    10 Nalidixic acid
  C Erythema multiforme or Steven-Johnson syndrome
    1 Sulfonamides
    2 Barbiturates
    3 Phenylbutazone
    4 Chlorpropamide
    5 Thiazides
    6 Sulfones
    7 Phenytoin
    8 Ethosuximide
    9 Salicylates
    10 Tetracyclines
    11 Codeine
    12 Penicillins
  D Erythema nodosum
    1 Penicillins
    2 Sulfonamides
    3 Oral contraceptives
  E Fixed drug eruptions
    1 Phenolphthalein
    2 Barbiturates
    3 Sulfonamides
    4 Salicylates
    5 Phenylbutazone
    6 Quinine
  F Photodermatitis
    1 Tetracyclines, particularly demeclocycline
    2 Griseofulvin
    3 Sulfonamides
    4 Sulfonylureas
    5 Thiazides
    6 Furosemide
    7 Phenothiazines
    8 Nalidixic acid
    9 Oral contraceptives
    10 Chlordiazepoxide
  G Urticaria
    1 Aspirin
    2 Penicillins
    3 Sulfonamides
    4 Barbiturates
  H Nonspecific rashes
    1 Ampicillin
    2 Barbiturates
    3 Allopurinol
    4 Phenytoin
    5 Methyldopa
  I Pigment changes (hyperpigmentation)
    1 ACTH
    2 Busulfan
    3 Phenothiazines
    4 Hypervitaminosis A
    5 Oral contraceptives
    6 Gold salts
    7 Chloroquine and other antimalarials
    8 Cyclophosphamide
    9 Bleomycin
  J Alopecia
    1 Cytotoxics
    2 Ethionamide
    3 Heparin
    4 Oral contraceptives (withdrawal)
  K Purpura (see also thrombocytopenia)
    1 Corticosteroids
    2 Aspirin
  L Lichenoid eruptions
    1 Chlorpropamide
    2 Gold salts
    3 Antimalarials
    4 PAS

TABLE 71-1 *(continued)*
Clinical manifestations of adverse reactions to drugs

5 Methyldopa
6 Phenothiazines
M Eczema (contact dermatitis)
  1 Topical antimicrobials
  2 Topical local anesthetics
  3 Topical antihistamines
  4 Cream and lotion preservatives
  5 Lanolin
N Acne
  1 Anabolic and androgenic steroids
  2 Corticosteroids
  3 Bromides
  4 Iodides
  5 Oral contraceptives
  6 Isoniazid
  7 Troxidone
V Hematologic
 A Pancytopenia (aplastic anemia)
  1 Chloramphenicol
  2 Phenytoin
  3 Mephenytoin
  4 Trimethadione
  5 Phenylbutazone
  6 Oxyphenbutazone
  7 Gold salts
  8 Mepacrine
  9 Quinacrine
  10 Potassium perchlorate
  11 Cytotoxics
 B Agranulocytosis (see also pancytopenia)
  1 Chloramphenicol
  2 Sulphonamides
  3 Phenylbutazone
  4 Oxyphenbutazone
  5 Gold salts
  6 Indomethacin
  7 Propylthiouracil
  8 Methimazole
  9 Carbimazole
  10 Phenothiazines
  11 Cytotoxics
  12 Tolbutamide
  13 Cotrimoxazole
  14 Tricyclic antidepressants
 C Thrombocytopenia (see also pancytopenia)
  1 Quinidine
  2 Quinine
  3 Furosemide
  4 Chlorthalidone
  5 Thiazides
  6 Gold salts
  7 Cotrimoxazole
  8 Aspirin
  9 Indomethacin
  10 Phenylbutazone
  11 Oxyphenbutazone
  12 Chlorpropamide
  13 Acetazolamine
  14 Phenytoin and other hydantoins
  15 Methyldopa
  16 Carbamazepine
  17 Digitoxin
  18 Novobiocin
 D Megaloblastic anemia
  1 Folate antagonists
  2 Cotrimoxazole
  3 Phenytoin
  4 Primidone
  5 Phenobarbital
  6 Triamterene
  7 Trimethoprim
  8 Oral contraceptives
 E Hemolytic anemia
  1 Methyldopa
  2 Levodopa
  3 Mefenamic acid
  4 Melphalan
  5 Isoniazid
  6 Rifampin
  7 Sulfonamides
  8 Penicillins
  9 Cephalosporins
  10 Insulin
  11 Quinidine
  12 Chlorpromazine
  13 Phenacetin

14 p-Aminosalicylic acid
15 Dapsone
F Hemolytic anemia (in G6PD deficiency)
  1 Antimalarials, e.g., primaquine
  2 Chloramphenicol
  3 Dapsone
  4 Nalidixic acid
  5 Nitrofurantoin
  6 Sulfonamides
  7 Aspirin
  8 Phenacetin
  9 p-Aminosalicylic acid
  10 Quinidine
  11 Vitamin C
  12 Vitamin K
  13 Cotrimoxazole
  14 Probenecid
  15 Procainamide
G Lymphadenopathy
  1 Phenytoin
  2 Primidone
H Leukocytosis
  1 Lithium
  2 Corticosteroids
I Eosinophilia
  1 Erythromycin estolate
  2 Sulfonamides
  3 Chlorpropamide
  4 p-Aminosalicylic acid
  5 Imipramine
  6 Nitrofurantoin
  7 Procarbazine
  8 Methotrexate
VI Cardiovascular
 A Exacerbation of angina
  1 Vasopressin
  2 Oxytocin
  3 Ergotamine
  4 Methysergide
  5 Propranolol withdrawal
  6 Excessive thyroxin
  7 Alpha blockers
  8 Hydralazine
 B Cardiomyopathy
  1 Emetine
  2 Sympathomimetics
  3 Phenothiazines
  4 Lithium
  5 Sulfonamides
  6 Daunorubicin
  7 Adriamycin
 C Pericarditis
  1 Procainamide
  2 Hydralazine
  3 Methysergide
  4 Emetine
 D Fluid retention or congestive heart failure
  1 Estrogens
  2 Steroids
  3 Carbenoxolone
  4 Phenylbutazone
  5 Indomethacin
  6 Propranolol
  7 Mannitol
  8 Diazoxide
 E Arrhythmias
  1 Sympathomimetics
  2 Thyroid hormone
  3 Digitalis
  4 Quinidine
  5 Procainamide
  6 Verapamil
  7 Atropine
  8 Propranolol
  9 Guanethidine
  10 Emetine
  11 Propellants in aerosols
  12 Tricyclic antidepressants
  13 Phenothiazines, particularly thioridazine
  14 Lithium
  15 Anticholinesterases
  16 Papaverine
  17 Daunomycin
  18 Adriamycin
  19 Lincomycin (intravenous)

F Hypotension (see also arrythmias)
  1 Nitroglycerin
  2 Phenothiazines
  3 Morphine
  4 Diuretics
  5 Citrated blood
  6 Levodopa
G Hypertension
  1 Oral contraceptives
  2 Sympathomimetics
  3 Clonidine withdrawal
  4 Monoamine oxidase inhibitors with sympathomimetics
  5 Tricyclic antidepressants with sympathomimetics
  6 Corticosteroids
  7 ACTH
  8 Phenylbutazone
II Thromboembolism
  1 Oral contraceptives
VII Respiratory
 A Nasal congestion
  1 Reserpine
  2 Guanethidine
  3 Isoproterenol
  4 Oral contraceptives
  5 Decongestant abuse
 B Respiratory depression
  1 Aminoglycosides
  2 Polymixins
  3 Trimethaphan
  4 Opiates
  5 Sedatives
  6 Hypnotics
 C Airway obstruction (bronchospasm, asthma; see also anaphylaxis)
  1 Beta blockers
  2 Nonsteroidal anti-inflammatory drugs, e.g., aspirin, indomethacin
  3 Cholinergic drugs
  4 Tartrazine (drugs with yellow dye)
  5 Penicillins
  6 Cephalosporins
  7 Streptomycin
  8 Pentazocine
 D Pulmonary infiltrates
  1 Nitrofurantoin
  2 Methysergide
  3 Chlorambucil
  4 Procarbazine
  5 Busulfan
  6 Melphalan
  7 Cyclophosphamide
  8 Azothioprine
  9 Bleomycin
  10 Methotrexate
  11 Sulfonamides
 E Pulmonary edema
  1 Heroin
  2 Methadone
  3 Hydrochlorthiazide
  4 Propoxyphene
  5 Contrast media
VIII Gastrointestinal
 A Dental discoloration
  1 Tetracycline
 B Gingival hyperplasia
  1 Phenytoin
 C Oral ulceration
  1 Aspirin
  2 Isoproterenol (sublingual)
  3 Cytotoxics
  4 Pancreatin
  5 Gentian violet
 D Taste disturbances
  1 Penicillamine
  2 Biguanides
  3 Griseofulvin
  4 Metronidazole
  5 Lithium
  6 Rifampin
 E Dry mouth
  1 Anticholinergics
  2 Levodopa
  3 Tricyclic antidepressants
  4 Clonidine
  5 Methyldopa

TABLE 71-1 *(continued)*
Clinical manifestations of adverse reactions to drugs

F Swelling of salivary gland
  1 Phenylbutazone
  2 Guanethidine
  3 Bethanidine
  4 Bretylium
  5 Clonidine
  6 Iodides
G Peptic ulceration or hemorrhage
  1 Aspirin
  2 Phenylbutazone
  3 Indomethacin
  4 Ethacrynic acid
  5 Reserpine (large doses)
H Intestinal ulceration
  1 Enteric-coated potassium chloride
I Nausea or vomiting
  1 Digitalis
  2 Opiates
  3 Estrogens
  4 Levodopa
  5 Potassium chloride
  6 Ferrous sulfate
  7 Aminophylline
  8 Tetracyclines
J Diarrhea or colitis
  1 Lincomycin
  2 Clindamycin
  3 Broad-spectrum antibiotics
  4 Magnesium in antacids
  5 Guanethidine
  6 Debrisoquin
  7 Methyldopa
  8 Reserpine
  9 Digitalis
  10 Colchicine
  11 Purgatives
  12 Lactose excipients
K Constipation or ileus
  1 Ganglionic blockers
  2 Tricyclic antidepressants
  3 Phenothiazines
  4 Opiates
  5 Aluminum hydroxide
  6 Calcium carbonate
  7 Barium sulfate
  8 Ion exchange resins
  9 Ferrous sulfate
L Malabsorption
  1 Broad-spectrum antibiotics
  2 Neomycin
  3 Cholestyramine
  4 Colchicine
  5 *p*-Aminosalicylic acid
  6 Biguanides
  7 Phenytoin
  8 Primidone
  9 Phenobarbital
  10 Cytotoxics
M Pancreatitis
  1 Corticosteroids
  2 Thiazides
  3 Azathioprine
  4 Oral contraceptives
  5 Sulfonamides
  6 Opiates
  7 Furosemide
  8 Ethacrynic acid
N Diffuse hepatocellular damage
  1 Halothane
  2 Methoxyflurane
  3 Methyldopa
  4 Isoniazid
  5 Rifampin
  6 Aminosalicylic acid
  7 Ethionamide
  8 Phenytoin and other hydantoins
  9 Acetaminophen (paracetamol)
  10 Salicylates
  11 Allopurinol
  12 Sulfonamides
  13 Tetracyclines
  14 Erythromycin estolate
  15 Propylthiouracil
  16 Methimazole
  17 Oxyphenisatin
  18 Methotrexate
  19 Pyridium

  20 Propoxyphene
  21 Monoamine oxidase inhibitors
O Cholestatic jaundice
  1 Phenothiazines
  2 Androgens
  3 Anabolic steroids
  4 Oral contraceptives
  5 Erythromycin estolate
  6 Chlorpropamide
  7 Gold salts
  8 Methimazole
  9 Acetohexamide
IX Urinary tract
A Nephrotic syndrome
  1 Penicillamine
  2 Gold salts
  3 Phenindione
  4 Probenecid
B Tubular necrosis
  1 Amphotericin B
  2 Aminoglycosides
  3 Polymixins
  4 Cephaloridine
  5 Tetracyclines
  6 Colistin
  7 Sulfonamides
  8 Radioiodinated contrast medium
  9 Methoxyflurane
C Interstitial nephritis
  1 Penicillins, particularly methicillin
  2 Sulfonamides
  3 Phenindione
  4 Furosemide
  5 Thiazides
D Nephropathies due to analgesics (e.g., phenacetin)
E Concentrating defect with polyuria (or nephrogenic diabetes insipidus)
  1 Vitamin D
  2 Lithium
  3 Demeclocycline
  4 Methoxyflurane
F Renal tubular acidosis
  1 Degraded tetracycline
  2 Amphotericin B
  3 Acetazolamide
G Calculi
  1 Acetazolamide
  2 Vitamin D
H Obstructive uropathy
  1 Intrarenal: cytotoxics
  2 Extrarenal: methysergide
I Hemorrhagic cystitis
  1 Cyclophosphamide
J Bladder dysfunction
  1 Anticholinergics
  2 Monoamine oxidase inhibitors
  3 Tricyclic antidepressants
  4 Disopyramide
X Genital (see also endocrine)
A Vaginal carcinoma
  1 Diethylstilbestrol (administered to mother)
B Impairment of spermatogenesis or oogenesis
  1 Cytotoxics
XI Neurologic
A Peripheral neuropathy
  1 Isoniazid
  2 Hydralazine
  3 Nitrofurantoin
  4 Vincristine
  5 Mustine
  6 Streptomycin
  7 Polymixin, colistan
  8 Clioquinol
  9 Phenelzine
  10 Tricyclic antidepressants
  11 Chloramphenicol
  12 Procarbazine
  13 Ethambutol
  14 Ethionamide
  15 Glutethimide
  16 Demeclocycline
  17 Nalidixic acid
  18 Tolbutamide
  19 Chlorpropamide

  20 Methysergide
  21 Phenytoin
B Exacerbation of myasthenia
  1 Aminoglycosides
  2 Polymixins
C Extrapyramidal effects
  1 Butyrophenones, e.g., haloperidol
  2 Phenothiazines
  3 Tricyclic antidepressants
  4 Methyldopa
  5 Levodopa
  6 Reserpine
  7 Metoclopramide
D Seizures
  1 Amphetamines
  2 Analeptics
  3 Phenothiazines
  4 Isoniazid
  5 Lidocaine
  6 Theophylline
  7 Penicillins
  8 Nalidixic acid
  9 Physostigmine
  10 Tricyclic antidepressants
  11 Vincristine
  12 Lithium
E Stroke
  1 Oral contraceptives
F Pseudotumor cerebri (or intracranial hypertension)
  1 Corticosteroids
  2 Oral contraceptives
  3 Tetracyclines
  4 Hypervitaminosis A
G Headache
  1 Hydralazine
  2 Bromides
  3 Glyceryl trinitrate
  4 Ergotamine (withdrawal)
  5 Indomethacin
XII Ocular
A Corneal opacities
  1 Vitamin D
  2 Mepacrine
  3 Chloroquine
  4 Indomethacin
B Corneal edema
  1 Oral contraceptives
C Cataracts
  1 Phenothiazines
  2 Corticosteroids
  3 Busulfan
  4 Chlorambucil
D Glaucoma
  1 Mydriatics
  2 Sympathomimetics
E Retinopathy
  1 Chloroquine
  2 Phenothiazines
F Optic neuritis
  1 Clioquinol
  2 Chloramphenicol
  3 Streptomycin
  4 Isoniazid
  5 Ethambutol
  6 Quinine
  7 Phenothiazines
  8 Penicillamine
  9 PAS
  10 Phenylbutazone
G Alteration in color vision
  1 Troxidone
  2 Sulfonamides
  3 Streptomycin
  4 Methaqualone
  5 Barbiturates
  6 Digitalis
  7 Thiazides
XIII Ear
A Vestibular disorders
  1 Aminoglycosides
  2 Quinine
  3 Mustine
B Deafness
  1 Aminoglycosides
  2 Ethacrynic acid
  3 Furosemide

4 Quinine
5 Bleomycin
6 Chloroquine
7 Mustine
8 Aspirin
9 Nortriptyline
XIV Musculoskeletal
  A Myopathy or myalgia
    1 Corticosteroids
    2 Chloroquine
    3 Clofibrate
    4 Oral contraceptives
    5 Amphotericin B
    6 Carbenoxolone
  B Bone disorders
    1 Osteoporosis
      a Corticosteroids
      b Heparin
    2 Osteomalacia
      a Anticonvulsants
      b Glutethemide
      c Aluminum hydroxide
XV Psychiatric disorders
  A Schizophrenic-like or paranoid reactions
    1 Amphetamines
    2 Lysergic acid

    3 Levodopa
    4 Tricyclic antidepressants
    5 Monoamine oxidase inhibitors
    6 Bromides
    7 Corticosteroids
  B Depression
    1 Centrally acting antihypertensives (reserpine, methyldopa, clonidine)
    2 Propranolol
    3 Corticosteroids
    4 Amphetamine withdrawal
    5 Levodopa
  C Hypomania, mania or excited reactions
    1 Levodopa
    2 Sympathomimetics
    3 Corticosteroids
    4 MAO inhibitors
    5 Tricyclic antidepressants
  D Hallucinatory states
    1 Amantadine
    2 Narcotics
    3 Pentazocine
    4 Propranolol
    5 Levodopa
    6 Tricyclic antidepressants

    7 Meperidine
  E Delirious or confusional states
    1 Digitalis
    2 Anticholinergics
    3 Bromides
    4 Sedatives and hypnotics
    5 Phenothiazines
    6 Antidepressants
    7 Corticosteroids
    8 Isoniazid
    9 Levodopa
    10 Amantadine
    11 Penicillins
    12 Aminophylline
    13 Methyldopa
  F Sleep disturbances
    1 Anorexiants
    2 Levodopa
    3 Monoamine oxidase inhibitors
    4 Sympathomimetics
  G Drowsiness
    1 Anxiolytic drugs
    2 Major tranquilizers
    3 Tricyclic antidepressants
    4 Antihistamines
    5 Methyldopa
    6 Clonidine
    7 Reserpine

be taken if the physicians are not aware of the patients' drug histories. Every physician should determine what drugs a patient has been taking, at least during the preceding 30 days, before prescribing any medications. A history of previous adverse drug effects in patients is common. Since these patients have a predisposition to other drug-induced illnesses, familiarity with such a history should dictate added caution in prescribing drugs.

Patients with biochemical abnormalities such as erythrocyte G6PD deficiency can be identified; patients with the defect are usually blacks or of Mediterranean extraction. Drug-induced hemolytic crisis can be avoided by testing for the enzyme defect before administering these drugs. Similarly, persons with an abnormal serum pseudocholinesterase may have abnormally prolonged apnea when given succinylcholine.

General comments No drug is completely without side effects, and it is important to remember that a side effect in one patient may be the desired pharmacologic effect in another. Recent improvements in drug regulation allow physicians to prescribe drugs with considerable confidence in their purity, bioavailability, and effectiveness. However, while regulatory bodies try to ensure that drugs with serious toxic potential are not marketed, they have to constantly weigh the potential toxicity against the possible benefits. Thus toxicity which would be acceptable for an effective antineoplastic agent would not be permitted in, for example, an oral contraceptive. In addition, because of the necessarily small number of patients treated in premarketing studies, rare adverse reactions cannot be identified, so that the first responsibility for identifying and reporting these effects must rest with the practicing clinician through the use of the various national adverse reaction reporting systems, such as those operated by the Food and Drug Administration in the United States and the Committee on Safety of Medicines in Great Britain. The publication of a newly recognized adverse reaction can in a short time stimulate a very large number of similar such reports which previously had gone unrecognized.

The prevention of adverse drug reactions must first involve a high index of suspicion that the development of a new symptom or sign may be drug-related. Reduction of the dose or discontinuation of the suspected agent will usually clarify the position in concentration-dependent toxic reactions. Physi-

cians should be familiar with the common adverse effects of the drugs they use, and if they are in doubt, should consult the literature.

REFERENCES

Cluff LE et al: *Clinical Problems with Drugs*. Philadelphia, Saunders, 1975

————, Johnson JE: Drug fever. Prog Allergy 8:149, 1964

Davies DM: *Textbook of Adverse Drug Reactions*. New York, Oxford University Press, 1977

Dowling HF: *Medicines for Man*. New York, Knopf, 1970

Gardner P, Cluff LE: The epidemiology of adverse drug reactions: A review and perspective. Johns Hopkins Med J 126:77, 1970

Hurwitz N: Predisposing factors in adverse reactions to drugs. Br Med J 1:536, 1969

Mitchell JR et al: Toxic drug reactions, in *Handbook of Experimental Pharmacology*, vol 28, no 3: *Concepts in Biochemical Pharmacology*, JR Gillette, JR Mitchell (eds). New York, Springer Verlag, 1975

72

CLINICAL PHARMACOLOGY OF THE AUTONOMIC NERVOUS SYSTEM

DAVID G. SHAND
JOHN A. OATES

FUNCTION OF THE AUTONOMIC NERVOUS SYSTEM

The autonomic nervous system comprises a series of reflex arcs which control or modulate involuntary functions, such as blood pressure, heart rate, glandular secretions, the release of renin, intestinal motility, and bladder function. The efferent nerves comprise two systems, the sympathetic and parasympathetic, that receive impulses arising in the central nervous system. Both systems form synapses at autonomic ganglia in the periphery before innervating their target tissues. The preganglionic fibers of both parasympathetic and sympathetic systems which arise in the central nervous system stimulate the ganglionic cells by releasing acetylcholine (ACh); that is, they are cholinergic. The sympathetic ganglia form a chain along the spinal column extending from the cervical to the lumbar regions. The postganglionic sympathetic fibers are adrenergic and mediate their effects by releasing norepinephrine. While most sympathetic responses are adrenergic, two exceptions exist in that the nerves stimulating the sweat glands and those causing vasodilation in skeletal muscle are both cholinergic. The final component of the sympathetic nervous system is the adrenal medulla which is derived from the same embryonic tissue as autonomic ganglia (the neural crest) and releases epinephrine into the general circulation following stimulation. This, together with the neural links in the sympathetic chain, accounts for the generalized nature of some responses to sympathetic activation. In contrast, the parasympathetic ganglia usually are situated near or in the organs they innervate, so that responses tend to be more discrete, subserving local functions, for example, in the pupil and urinary bladder. Parasympathetic postganglionic fibers are cholinergic.

The brain regulates the degree of sympathetic and parasympathetic traffic by integrating a number of input signals including those from the baroreceptors, from the perception of pain and emotional stress, and from mental and physical effort. Although a rather generalized response of the sympathetic nervous system may occur with severe stress, more often the brain controls specific autonomic functions discretely, for example, the parasympathetic control of pupillary constriction or the sympathetic reflex that evokes sexual ejaculation.

The brain plays a key role in the control of arterial pressure by regulating cardiac output, renin release, and sympathetically mediated vasoconstriction. The sympathetic impulses that lead to vasoconstriction arise from the vasomotor center in the medulla, which is the major site for integrating the excitatory and inhibitory inputs that determine the final level of traffic in peripheral sympathetic neurons. The vasomotor center is under constant stimulation by fibers arising from higher centers of the brain including the hypothalamus. This tonic level of *excitatory* impulses is heightened by wakefulness, pain, mental and muscular effort, or emotional stress. Angiotensin II also elicits stimulation of the vasomotor center by its action on neurons arising from areas in the vicinity of the third ventricle. A major *inhibitory* regulator of sympathetic activity is the baroreceptor system. With a rise in arterial pressure and accompanying stretch of the baroreceptors in the carotid sinus and aortic arch, the afferent baroreceptor fibers fire more rapidly. These baroreceptor impulses travel to the medulla where the afferent fibers form synapses with interneurons that inhibit sympathetic outflow from the vasomotor center. The synapse of these afferent baroreceptor fibers with inhibitory neurons takes place in the nucleus tractus solitarius, an area of the medulla which is a major source of the inhibitory impulses that regulate vasoconstrictor sympathetic outflow. Afferent impulses from the baroreceptors to the nucleus tractus solitarius also result in inhibition of sympathetic output to the heart and to an increase in cardiac vagal tone. Any rise in arterial pressure, therefore, results in stimulation of the nucleus tractus solitarius, which in turn inhibits the resting level of sympathetic output to resistance vessels and to the heart. In addition to the afferents from the baroreceptors, the nucleus tractus solitarius also receives fibers from other neurons, many of which are adrenergic in type. Like the baroreceptors, these adrenergic fibers also stimulate the interneurons that *inhibit* sympathetic outflow. The neurotransmitter from these neurons, either norepinephrine or epinephrine, acts through an alpha receptor to elicit inhibition of the vasomotor center. Thus, stimulation of this alpha receptor in the nucleus tractus solitarius lowers blood pressure, quite in contrast to the pressor effect of stimulating alpha receptors on arterial smooth muscle.

THE ADRENERGIC NEURON

The normal transmitter, norepinephrine, is synthesized from tyrosine by a series of steps (Fig. 72-1). The first, hydroxylation to form dihydroxyphenylalanine (dopa), is catalyzed by tyrosine hydroxylase and is rate-limiting. Dopa is then decarboxylated by aromatic L-amino acid decarboxylase to form dopamine which is taken up into the specialized neurosecretory vesicles and hydroxylated to form norepinephrine. Following stimulation, the secretory vesicles discharge their soluble contents, including norepinephrine and dopamine β-hydroxylase. The exact mechanism of this excitation-secretion coupling is unclear but involves Ca^{2+}. The nerve terminals have receptors modulating transmitter release, with stimulation of alpha receptors (alpha$_2$) decreasing and stimulation of beta receptors increasing transmitter release. It has also been postulated that prostaglandins exert a negative feedback inhibition of adrenergic transmission.

The effects of norepinephrine are terminated by three mechanisms. The first and most important involves re-uptake

FIGURE 72-1

Synthesis, storage, secretion, and disposition of the adrenergic neurotransmitter, norepinephrine (NE). A varicosity of the adrenergic neuron is depicted diagrammatically. The terminal segments of peripheral adrenergic neurons have multiple varicosities along their course which are in juxtaposition with effector sites within target organs. Tyrosine is transported into the adrenergic neuron to provide substrate for the synthesis of NE. The rate-limiting enzyme is tyrosine hydroxylase, and the final enzyme, dopamine β-oxidase, is located within the neurosecretory vesicles.

1 *Depolarization of the neuron leads to release of NE by a calcium-dependent process of "excitation-secretion coupling" in which the neurosecretory vesicle fuses with the neuronal membrane and by exocytosis discharges its soluble contents that include NE and dopamine β-oxidase.*

2 *Much of the NE released into the synaptic cleft between the neuron and effector cell is removed from this area by a specialized membrane transport system known as the NE pump, which transports NE back into the neuron against a concentration gradient. This transport system is relatively unspecific and is responsible for the uptake of a number of ring-substituted amines such as tyramine, ephedrine, and guanethidine. It is competitively inhibited by the tricyclic antidepressants.*

3 *The major pathway for intraneuronal bioinactivation of NE (and dopamine) is via monoamine oxidase (MAO).*

4 *Extraneuronally, a major pathway of NE metabolism is via catechol-o-methyl transferase (COMT) to which NE is exposed at some effector cells and in remote organs such as the liver.*

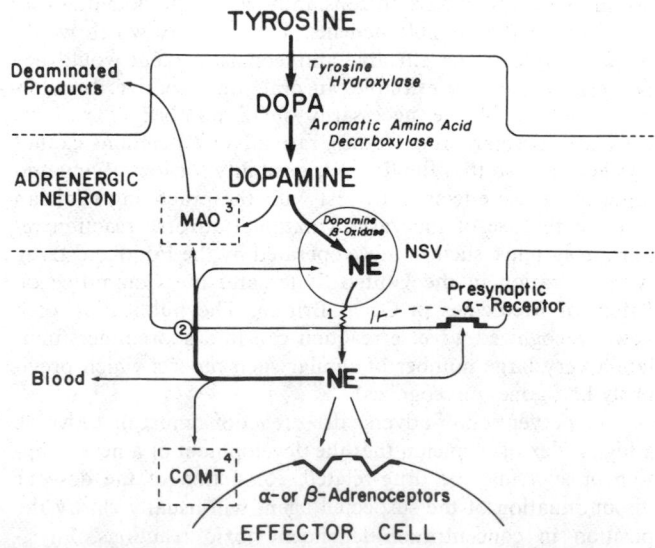

into the adrenergic neuron by means of an energy-dependent norepinephrine pump. Once inside the neuron, much of the transmitter is again taken up into the neurosecretory granules and is reused. Norepinephrine which escapes into the circulation is metabolized by catechol-*o*-methyl transferase (COMT) to normetanephrine, some of which is converted to vanillylmandelic acid (VMA) via the action of monoamine oxidase (MAO) and aldehyde dehydrogenase (Fig. 72-2). Finally, some norepinephrine is converted intraneuronally to 3,4-dihydroxymandelic acid and then to VMA by COMT. In the adrenal medulla, norepinephrine is metabolized to epinephrine; adrenal cells do not have a re-uptake system for epinephrine which, after release, is metabolized similarly by MAO and COMT to form VMA and metanephrine. Measurement of the urinary catecholamines and their metabolites forms the basis for detecting enhanced catecholamine production in patients with pheochromocytoma (Chap. 337).

EFFECTS OF DRUGS Many drugs are available which affect the synthesis, release, metabolism, and re-uptake of norepinephrine. Inhibition of tyrosine hydroxylase by α-methyl-*p*-tyrosine can profoundly depress catecholamine synthesis, a property that may be useful in patients with pheochromocytoma. Competitive inhibitors of aromatic L-amino acid decarboxylase have little effect on the endogenous synthesis of norepinephrine because this enzymatic step is not rate-limiting, and almost complete inhibition of the enzyme would be required to block norepinephrine synthesis. One decarboxylase inhibitor, carbidopa, has been used clinically to prevent the breakdown of L-dopa by peripheral tissues and thereby to reduce the dosage of the latter required in the treatment of parkinsonism. As carbidopa does not gain access to the brain, it does not prevent the beneficial central effects of L-dopa in parkinsonism.

Release of the adrenergic neurotransmitter from peripheral adrenergic neurons is blocked by *guanethidine* and *bethanidine* (Chap. 251). These adrenergic neuron blockers act in part by replacing norepinephrine in the neurosecretory vesicles. Blockade of the peripheral adrenergic neuron produces a reduction in blood pressure that is much greater in the standing position and also may be associated with exercise-induced hypotension.

FIGURE 72-2
The metabolism of norepinephrine.

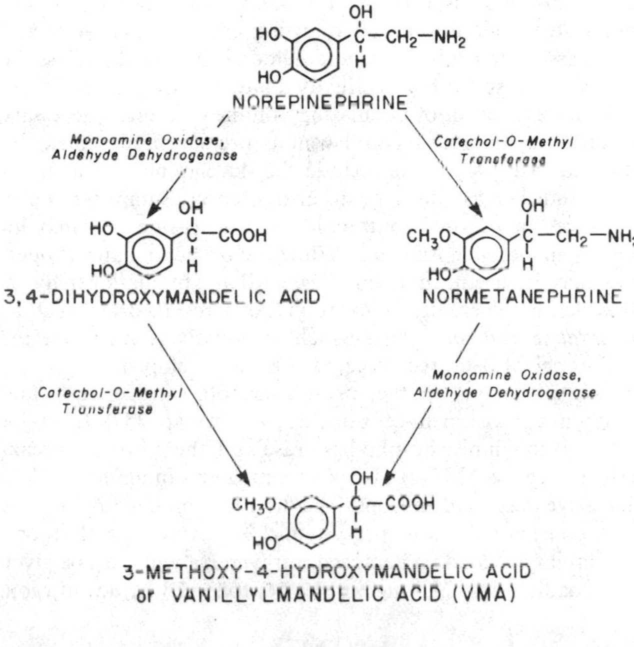

NOREPINEPHRINE

Monoamine Oxidase, Aldehyde Dehydrogenase

Catechol-O-Methyl Transferase

3,4-DIHYDROXYMANDELIC ACID

NORMETANEPHRINE

Catechol-O-Methyl Transferase

Monoamine Oxidase, Aldehyde Dehydrogenase

3-METHOXY-4-HYDROXYMANDELIC ACID
or VANILLYLMANDELIC ACID (VMA)

These highly polar drugs do not enter the central nervous system to any appreciable degree, and their use is generally devoid of side effects attributable to the central nervous system.

A state of pseudotolerance to guanethidine may develop as a result of fluid retention, and the drug is most effective when given with a diuretic together with restriction of dietary sodium. The drug has a long persistence within the adrenergic neuron and accordingly has a long half-life (about 5 days). Thus, guanethidine may be given only once daily in doses ranging upward from 10 mg. Guanethidine's action is selectively targeted to the peripheral adrenergic neuron because it is transported into the adrenergic neuron against a concentration gradient by the relatively nonspecific norepinephrine pump. The dependence of the pharmacological effects of guanethidine upon its concentration within the adrenergic neuron by the norepinephrine pump has two important clinical consequences: (1) Virtually all the actions of the drug in the body are targeted to the peripheral adrenergic neuron; thus, most of the side effects of guanethidine, including failure of ejaculation, result from the blockade of peripheral adrenergic neurons, and the drug is devoid of any toxic effects exclusive of this action. (2) Drugs that competitively inhibit the norepinephrine pump such as the tricyclic antidepressants, ephedrine, and the phenothiazines will compete with guanethidine's uptake and, therefore, counteract its antihypertensive action.

Reserpine is another antihypertensive which blocks adrenergic transmission, in this case by preventing norepinephrine incorporation into the neurosecretory vesicles. A similar effect in the central nervous system probably accounts for its most serious side effect, that of producing psychic depression. This effect is insidious in onset and is dose-dependent, so that only relatively mild degrees of hypertension can be treated with less than the greatest recommended dose (0.5 mg daily).

Inhibitors of MAO, such as *pargyline,* are occasionally used as antihypertensive agents chiefly in patients who also have psychic depression. As a result of MAO inhibition several amines as well as norepinephrine accumulate. One of these, octopamine, accumulates in and is released from the granules. As it has only 1 percent of the potency of norepinephrine, it serves as an inactive false transmitter. In addition to the accumulation of this false neurotransmitter in peripheral adrenergic neurons, actions of the MAO inhibitors in the central nervous system also may contribute to the inhibition of sympathetic reflexes.

ADRENERGIC RECEPTORS

The peripheral effects of the sympathetic nervous system are diverse. The integrated cardiovascular response of arteriolar constriction, tachycardia, enhanced cardiac contractility, and renin release maintains or raises arterial pressure. Metabolic functions including lipolysis, glycogenolysis, and release of antidiuretic hormone are stimulated by the sympathetic nervous system, as is mydriasis, ejaculation, and bronchodilatation. The sympathetic nervous system also participates in the regulation of body temperature and salivary secretion.

The peripheral effects mediated by catecholamine release have been classified as alpha or beta (Table 72-1). An important effect of norepinephrine is to cause vasoconstriction, an action on postsynaptic alpha receptors on vascular smooth muscle. Following the release of norepinephrine from the adrenergic neuron, it acts not only on postsynaptic alpha receptors, but also on receptors located on the neuron terminal itself. These presynaptic alpha receptors act to reduce the release of neurotransmitter. Thus, presynaptic alpha receptors

TABLE 72-1
Effects of peripheral postsynaptic adrenergic receptors

Alpha receptor	Beta$_1$ receptor	Beta$_2$ receptor
Vasoconstriction	Cardioacceleration	Vasodilatation
Pupil dilatation	Positive inotropy	Bronchial relaxation
Relaxation of gut		Uterine relaxation

serve as feedback inhibitors of the release of norepinephrine from the neuron terminal. Because of the differing potency of agonists and antagonists for these alpha receptors, it has been suggested that the postsynaptic receptor on vascular smooth muscle be designated an alpha$_1$ receptor and that the presynaptic receptor on the neuron terminal be designated an alpha$_2$ receptor.

Beta adrenoceptors are also divided into two types: beta$_1$ (mediating increased heart rate and contractility and probably renin release) and beta$_2$ (mediating relaxation of bronchial, uterine, and vascular smooth muscle). The metabolic responses to catecholamines, including hyperglycemia, are not well categorized according to receptor type. It is generally felt that stimulation of the beta receptor activates adenylate cyclase with a subsequent increase in intracellular concentrations of cyclic adenosine monophosphate (AMP). Cyclic AMP is thought to mediate the cellular response by activating protein kinases which phosphorylate intracellular proteins that control the cellular response. The enzyme phosphodiesterase catalyzes the breakdown of cyclic AMP to 5'-AMP.

The effect of norepinephrine and other beta-adrenergic agonists on cardiac rate is mediated by an increased rate of diastolic depolarization in the sinoatrial node as well as in other pacemaker cells, including those in the His-Purkinje system which pace the heart during atrioventricular block.

There is some evidence that both alpha and beta receptors can be regulated at the membrane level. For example, exposure to a stimulant such as isoproterenol may decrease the number of receptors (down regulation) by a process not involving protein synthesis. Conversely, reduced transmitter release or exposure to antagonists may increase receptor number. The relationship between these findings and denervation supersensitivity or withdrawal rebound phenomena is unclear.

SYMPATHOMIMETIC AGENTS

In addition to the catecholamines many drugs are available which mimic the effects of the sympathetic nervous system and act either directly to stimulate adrenergic receptors or indirectly by releasing stored norepinephrine. The directly acting drugs vary with respect to the preponderance of alpha or beta actions. *Phenylephrine* and *methoxamine* are almost pure alpha stimulators, and their major action is to produce arteriolar vasoconstriction. They may be used in the unusual hypotensive state (as occurs during spinal anesthesia) when increasing peripheral resistance without cardiac stimulation is required. These agents used alone are generally not considered beneficial in situations when depressed cardiac contractility contributes to hypotension, for example, in shock due to myocardial infarction. Alpha agonists also may be employed in the treatment of paroxysmal atrial tachycardia (see "Parasympathetic Regulation of Normal and Abnormal Cardiac Rhythm" below). Sympathomimetic vasoconstrictors are frequently employed as local nasal decongestants.

Norepinephrine, being the natural transmitter for sympathetic neurons, has both alpha and beta properties. When given systemically, the alpha vasoconstrictor effect seems to predominate, and the elevation in blood pressure causes reflex bradycardia. Stroke volume is increased and cardiac output is unchanged. Coronary blood flow is generally increased, but

flow to kidney, brain, gut, and skeletal muscle falls as a result of vasoconstriction. Prolonged infusions can lead to hypovolemia and tachyphylaxis which, together with the tendency to produce oliguria, require close attention to fluid balance, especially during weaning from the drug when the dose may have to be tapered and volume expanded to prevent hypotension. When extravasation from an intravenous infusion occurs, tissue necrosis and sloughing may occur. Infiltration with an alpha-blocking drug (see below) may counteract the vasoconstriction and prevent tissue necrosis. *Epinephrine* also has combined alpha and beta actions, but its beta effects are more striking than those of norepinephrine, especially in low doses. Vasoconstriction is produced in the skin and kidneys, while skeletal muscle vessels dilate and tachycardia is usual. Epinephrine may be injected directly into the cardiac ventricles during the treatment of cardiac arrest. It is also given subcutaneously to reverse anaphylaxis, urticaria, and angioneurotic edema, probably by increasing cyclic AMP levels in mast cells, thus inhibiting the release of allergic mediators. *Dopamine* is the third naturally occurring catecholamine which is thought to subserve a transmitter function in the CNS. Although it has not been established as a transmitter in the periphery, it produces some of its effects by stimulating what appear to be specific dopamine receptors, in addition to having both alpha and beta effects. Its effects are dose-dependent. At low doses [1 to 5 (μg/kg)/min, administered intravenously], it dilates mesenteric and renal vessels, producing increased renal blood flow and sodium excretion by its action on dopamine receptors. At intermediate doses [5 to 10 (μg/kg)/min)] beta stimulation increases cardiac output with relatively little tachycardia. Finally at higher doses alpha stimulation occurs, leading to obvious vasoconstriction which can compromise the circulation of the limbs and reverse renal vasodilation and naturesis. The combination of cardiac stimulation and renal vasodilation makes dopamine particularly useful in the treatment of a variety of hypotensive states and in the treatment of congestive heart failure.

Isoproterenol is a synthetic compound with pure beta-agonist activity causing a reduction in peripheral vascular resistance with an increase in heart rate and contractility and, thus, an increase in cardiac output. Isoproterenol is indicated in the treatment of a number of arrhythmias characterized by reduced automaticity and conductivity. It may be administered as a continuous intravenous infusion (1 to 6 μg/min) or sublingually (10 to 20 mg every 2 to 4 h) in patients with sinus arrest, sinoatrial block, sinus bradycardia, various forms of atrioventricular conduction defects, and Stokes-Adams attacks (Chap. 237). This amine is also useful in a variety of low cardiac output states, including those following cardiac operations and those associated with septic and hemorrhagic shock, unless the peripheral vascular bed is already dilated; during isoproterenol infusion expansion of circulating volume it is often necessary in order to maintain central venous pressure and ventricular preload. Adverse effects include the development of arrhythmias and increase in myocardial oxygen consumption due to enhanced myocardial contractility and heart rate; this may intensify myocardial ischemia. While the bronchodilator properties may be useful in asthmatics, cardiac stimulation may be troublesome even after inhalation. As a result, drugs such as *terbutaline* and *salbutamol* which are relatively more specific for bronchial beta$_2$ receptors have been developed.

Theophylline is another drug used both intravenously and orally in the treatment of bronchospasm (Chap. 257). Its major action is to inhibit phosphodiesterase and, therefore, the breakdown of cyclic AMP. It also causes cardiac stimulation and, in excessive doses, convulsions. The drug is eliminated by hepatic metabolism with little presystemic extraction, so that oral availability is good. When used intravenously, it may be given as a loading dose (5.6 mg/kg slowly) followed by an infusion.

In young adults an average rate of infusion of 0.7 to 0.9 (mg/kg)/h usually gives levels in the therapeutic range of 8 to 20 μg/ml. The infusion rate should be reduced to 70 percent of this rate in neonates and the elderly, and reduced to an even greater extent in patients with cardiac failure or liver disease. Somewhat higher doses may be needed in young children and in patients exposed to enzyme-inducing agents, including cigarettes. Because of considerable variation among individuals in the clearance of theophylline, the concentration of drug in plasma should be measured when infusions extend for more than 12 h, recognizing that a concentration obtained after 12 to 18 h of infusion may not reflect the steady-state concentration, but may provide a warning of excessive accumulation.

Certain sympathomimetic drugs act indirectly by releasing norepinephrine from storage sites as well as having some direct actions. Examples include *metaraminol* and *mephentermine*. Because they eventually cause depletion of the active chemical, norepinephrine, their prolonged use is not recommended and may explain in part the difficulties of weaning patients from these drugs. *Tyramine* acts only indirectly.

SYMPATHOLYTIC AGENTS

ALPHA-ADRENOCEPTOR BLOCKING DRUGS The use of the alpha blockers phentolamine and phenoxybenzamine is largely confined to the diagnosis and treatment of pheochromocytoma (Chap. 337), though phentolamine also has been used to reduce afterload, i.e., the impedance to left ventricular emptying in the treatment of heart failure (Chap. 236). Phentolamine has a relatively rapid onset and evanescent action, and has been used as a test for pheochromocytoma in which hypertension is caused by catecholamine excess. Chronic treatment with alpha blockers is used to control hypertension prior to the operative treatment of pheochromocytoma or in the rare patient with metastatic pheochromocytomas.

Whereas phentolamine and phenoxybenzamine block both pre- and post synaptic alpha receptors, prazosin blocks primarily the postsynaptic (alpha$_1$) receptors on arteriolar and venous smooth muscle. Thus, the feedback inhibition of neurotransmitter release at the presynaptic (alpha$_2$) receptor is less impaired. This may account for the lesser degree of cardiac sympathetic stimulation evoked by prazosin. By reducing both arteriolar and venous tone, prazosin lowers both the venous return and filling of the heart, i.e., the preload, as well as the impedance to left ventricular emptying, i.e., the afterload (Chap. 235) in patients who receive it for the treatment of cardiac failure or hypertension (Chap. 251).

BETA-ADRENOCEPTOR BLOCKING DRUGS The beta-blocking drugs have enjoyed widespread use in the treatment of hypertension, angina pectoris, and certain arrhythmias. Blockade is of the competitive type and antagonizes the effects of catecholamines and sympathetic-nerve stimulation on heart rate, cardiac output, and contractility. Therefore, it tends to reduce resting heart rate and cardiac index in normal subjects, but impairment of cardiac performance is even more pronounced during muscular exercise because of the blockade of the augmented sympathetic activity which occurs during exercise.

Propranolol, the initial beta-adrenoceptor blocker to be widely used clinically, is the prototype for this class. Subsequently, many other beta-adrenoceptor antagonists have been introduced. A number of differences between these beta blockers have been demonstrated, including relative selectivity for the beta$_1$ receptors, the presence or absence of a "membrane-stabilizing" effect, partial beta-agonist activity, and penetration of the blood-brain barrier. The difference which clearly has been shown to have clinical significance is that the relatively selective beta$_1$ antagonists produce less bronchospasm in asthmatic patients at the lower end of the effective dose range, even though higher doses will block bronchial beta receptors as well. Beta agonists such as isoproterenol or salbutamol can more readily surmount the blockade of bronchial beta$_2$ receptors during treatment with the relatively selective beta$_1$ antagonists. Metoprolol, atenolol, tolamolol, and acebutolol are relatively selective beta$_1$ blockers, whereas propranolol, timolol, oxprenolol, alprenolol, sotalol, and pindolol produce essentially equivalent blockade of beta$_1$ and beta$_2$ adrenoceptors. As the brain is the target for some of the adverse effects of the beta-receptor antagonists, the lack of distribution of atenolol into the central nervous system may also be of clinical significance.

In patients with impaired myocardial function and cardiac failure, there is a compensatory reflex sympathetic stimulation of myocardial contractility (Chap. 236). In some patients with severe underlying myocardial dysfunction or excessive volume or pressure overloads, the contribution of the beta-adrenergic system to maintaining cardiac performance is critical, and beta blockade may cause serious deterioration of cardiac output and even profound hypotension. The *intravenous* administration of beta blockers is particularly dangerous in patients with compromised cardiac function. On the other hand, if the major cause of the patient's cardiac failure can be corrected, as is usually the case in hypertension, the use of beta blockers may be considered. Where there is any doubt regarding the underlying myocardial function, beta-blocking drugs should be initiated with small, orally administered doses and under careful observation, as any major problem with reduced cardiac output will be evident immediately upon absorption of the first dose.

Indications Beta-adrenoceptor antagonists, alone or in combination with nitroglycerin or long-acting nitrates, are often effective in patients with angina pectoris in whom nitrates alone have failed to provide relief (Chap. 244). Propranolol with isosorbide dinitrate is one such combination which is felt to be effective. The beneficial effects of beta blockers in angina pectoris probably are achieved by preventing the increased myocardial oxygen requirements induced by sympathetic nervous discharge during physical activity, cold, or emotion. The reduced demand for oxygen allows more prolonged exercise before pain occurs.

A second major use of beta-blocking drugs is the treatment of cardiac arrhythmias, particularly in the abolition and prevention of paroxysmal supraventricular and ventricular tachycardias. They are also useful in reducing excessive ventricular rate in patients with atrial fibrillation (Chap. 237). Their beneficial effects result from prolongation of the refractory period of the atrioventricular junction by blocking adrenergic influences on this system, and this effect of propranolol is additive to that of digitalis. Beta blockade is also efficacious in sinus tachycardia and in the ventricular arrhythmias in pheochromocytoma (Chap. 337). In patients with pheochromocytoma it is important that alpha blockade be present before propranolol administration, otherwise blocking the beta vasodilation due to epinephrine may lead to unopposed alpha vasoconstriction by the catecholamines and subsequent paradoxical hypertension. The mechanism in ventricular arrhythmias is not clearly defined, but in low doses, beta blockade is probably responsible. In some patients who require higher plasma levels, electrophysiologic effects independent of beta blockade may contribute.

Propranolol has been shown to be effective in relieving

many of the symptoms of idiopathic hypertrophic subaortic stenosis (Chap. 247). Its effects are related to a depression of myocardial contractility leading to lessening of the severity of outflow obstruction.

Finally beta blockers are useful in the treatment of hypertension, their particular advantage being to lower pressure equally well in both supine and upright positions (Chap. 251). Their mechanism of action is poorly understood, but several effects may be involved including a reduction in cardiac output and inhibition of renin release leading to a fall in the vasoconstrictor hormone, angiotensin II. The drugs appear particularly useful in young patients with high cardiac output and labile or early hypertension. High-renin essential hypertensives respond well to low doses, while low-renin patients appear to need larger doses (up to 960 mg daily) when propranolol is used as the sole drug. In clinical practice, however, such large doses are seldom required as propranolol in doses up to 240 or 320 mg daily is very effective in combination with diuretics or diuretics plus a vasodilator (Chap. 251).

Pharmacokinetics Propranolol is very efficiently cleared by the liver, so that after intravenous administration its elimination depends on liver blood flow. During chronic oral therapy hepatic extraction is somewhat less, but remains relatively high (65 percent or so), and the half-life is from 3 to 6 h. Hepatic extraction is reduced in patients with liver disease. Much larger doses are required after oral than intravenous administration, because, despite complete alimentary absorption, the drug is extracted presystemically by the liver (Chap. 70). There is considerable variation in clinical response because of differing plasma levels (up to tenfold) due to genetic variation in hepatic extraction as well as the effects of other drugs, age, and smoking habits. Variable plasma binding and the generation of active metabolites may also contribute to the differences in response. All these factors necessitate an exploration of the dose-response curve in clinical practice beginning with 40 to 80 mg daily. Although the half-life is relatively short, propranolol can be given as infrequently as twice daily in the treatment of hypertension, provided the same total daily dose is administered. Metoprolol also is eliminated primarily by hepatic metabolism, having a high degree of presystemic elimination after oral administration and variable concentration in plasma. The half-life is 3 to 4 h.

Adverse effects These occur infrequently (2 to 5 percent) and in addition to precipitation of heart failure (see above) include bizarre vivid dreams, weakness, lethargy, easy fatigability, and occasional exacerbation of psychic depression. Clinically important hypoglycemia may occur in insulin-dependent diabetics in whom the sympathetic defense of hypoglycemia has been blunted and the early warning sign of palpitation is obscured. Beta blockers are specifically contraindicated in patients with impaired cardiac impulse generation or conduction. In patients with second- or third-degree atrioventricular block, they may produce serious bradycardia or even asystole, and in the presence of slowed impulse generation within or conduction from the sinoatrial node (the "sick-sinus syndrome") removal of the influence of norepinephrine can lead to sinoatrial arrest or severe bradycardia. Nonselective beta-blocking drugs are contraindicated in patients with asthma or bronchial constriction, where relatively selective $beta_1$ antagonists are preferred, though these drugs may cause some bronchospasm. Since these drugs are competitive antagonists, their effects can be counteracted by increasing sympathetic activity with isoproterenol, employing larger than usual doses to overcome the competitive beta blockade.

Another adverse reaction is the withdrawal syndrome in which severe angina, arrhythmias, and infarction may occur in patients with angina within 1 to 2 weeks of suddenly stopping the administration of propranolol. This is more common outside the hospital in patients who have gained maximum benefits. Treatment is by bed rest and reinstitution of the drug. If the discontinuation of propranolol in such patients is required, it should be tapered over 1 to 2 weeks.

REDUCTION OF ARTERIAL PRESSURE BY DRUGS ACTING ON THE CENTRAL NERVOUS SYSTEM Two antihypertensives, *methyldopa* and *clonidine*, exert their effect on the central nervous system (Chap. 251). Methyldopa itself has no direct effect on blood pressure regulation. However, it readily crosses the blood-brain barrier and enters adrenergic neurons. Intraneuronally, methyldopa is decarboxylated to form methyldopamine, which in turn is converted by dopamine β-oxidase to α-methylnorepinephrine. α-Methylnorepinephrine, like norepinephrine itself, is stored in the neurosecretory vesicles in adrenergic neurons, and when the nerve is stimulated, this metabolite of methyldopa is released in place of the normal transmitter. In the nucleus tractus solitarius, α-methylnorepinephrine acts as a potent transmitter, stimulating the alpha receptors that evoke an inhibitory effect on sympathetic outflow. Studies with inhibitors suggest that these receptors most closely resemble alpha$_2$ receptors. Because the drug must be metabolized and transported into the granules, it takes some 4 to 6 h to have a maximal effect. Doses of the order of 500 to 2000 mg daily may be required, and a continuing control of blood pressure may be achieved by administration as infrequently as twice daily. Methyldopa does produce some orthostatic hypotension, but this is less marked than with the adrenergic neuron blockers. During treatment renal blood flow is better preserved with this than other antihypertensives. Side effects referable to the central nervous system, including drowsiness, fatigue, impotency, and depression, are usual only with larger doses and are less severe than with reserpine. The most serious toxicities are drug fever and hepatotoxicity which may on rare occasions progress to necrosis. Although 25 percent of patients receiving more than 1 g daily for greater than 6 months will develop a reversible positive direct Coombs' test, fewer than 1 percent will develop frank hemolysis. Although its potential for toxicity requires vigilance, methyldopa is a useful agent.

Clonidine acts to stimulate central alpha receptors directly, and its spectrum of activity is very similar to methyldopa, including a modest orthostatic component and preservation of renal blood flow. Common side effects include sedation, dry mouth, and impotence. The most serious adverse effect is rebound hypertension on cessation of therapy occurring 8 to 36 h later. Characteristic anxiety, headache, sweating, tachycardia, and nausea occur which mimic the sympathetic overactivity seen with pheochromocytoma. Treatment is with alpha blockade.

PARASYMPATHETIC NERVOUS SYSTEM

Drugs that act directly on the efferent limb of the parasympathetic nervous system generally have the disadvantage of acting on the diverse organs which this system innervates. Acetylcholine released from parasympathetic nerves acts on receptors that slow sinoatrial rate and atrioventricular conduction, stimulate salivary, bronchial, and gastric secretion, contract the iris and the ciliary muscle, stimulate bronchial smooth muscle contraction and intestinal motility, sustain penile erection, and promote sweating with attendant heat loss. Thus, atropine, which blocks the action of acetylcholine on parasympathetic receptors (muscarinic receptors), impairs all the above functions to varying degrees, accounting for the side effects that result from its administration.

Acetylcholine also is the neuromuscular transmitter for skeletal muscle as well as the transmitter for preganglionic autonomic neurons, acting on the nicotinic type of receptors in these locations. Thus, the therapeutic use of acetylcholine esterase inhibitors (neostigmine, pyridostigmine) to enhance neuromuscular transmission in myasthenia gravis carries with it attendant side effects on the muscarinic or parasympathetic receptors (Chap. 381). These adverse effects such as gastrointestinal cramping and bronchoconstriction can be attenuated by a careful titration of atropine or other muscarinic receptor blockers. Tolerance is developed to the muscarinic side effects so that parasympathetic receptor blockers may usually be progressively withdrawn.

In contrast to the rather general enhancement of parasympathetic activity achieved with acetylcholine esterase inhibitors, some direct muscarinic-cholinergic agonists possess a relative degree of selectivity within the parasympathetic nervous system. Thus, *bethanechol* in the usually employed doses of 5 mg subcutaneously or 10 mg orally has a relative selectivity for muscarinic receptors in the bladder and the gastrointestinal tract, providing the basis for its use in selective disorders of bladder and gastrointestinal dysfunction.

PARASYMPATHETIC REGULATION OF NORMAL AND ABNORMAL CARDIAC RHYTHM Release of acetylcholine from vagal parasympathetic fibers slows the heart rate by reducing the rate of diastolic depolarization in sinoatrial pacemaker cells, an effect which counters the action of norepinephrine on sinoatrial rate. Similarly, acetylocholine prolongs atrioventricular conduction and the atrioventricular functional refractory period in opposition to the effects of norepinephrine.

Parasympathetic impulses are delivered to the heart via the vagus nerve which arises in the nucleus of the vagus in the medulla. Here, the baroreceptor reflex regulates vagal impulses to the heart in a reciprocal direction from the sympathetic outflow. The afferent baroreceptor fibers entering the nucleus tractus solitarius synapse with interneurons that *stimulate* the vagal nucleus with a resultant increase in efferent vagal traffic and cardiac slowing.

Activation of parasympathetic stimulation of the heart by the baroreceptor reflex can be employed in the treatment of some patients with paroxysmal atrial tachycardia (Chap. 237). There is evidence that a large subset of patients with atrial tachycardia has a sustained reentry pathway that involves vagal-sensitive fibers in the atrioventricular node. In such patients, reversion of the arrhythmia may be accomplished by stimulating the afferent limb of the baroreceptor reflex to evoke parasympathetic stimulation of the heart and reciprocal sympathetic withdrawal with resultant reversion of the arrhythmia. This sometimes may be achieved by a brief Valsalva maneuver or by unilateral massage of the carotid sinus area (only in young patients). If these simple measures are ineffective, elevation of arterial pressure by intravenous administration of alpha-adrenergic agents can be employed to produce a more predictable parasympathetic stimulation of the heart. For example, methoxamine may be given slowly intravenously in doses from 2 to 10 mg with the objective of cautiously elevating systolic pressure by 20 to 40 mmHg. Such maneuvers to evoke an increase in vagal tone by baroreceptor stimulation should be reserved for patients whose left ventricular function is judged adequate to sustain the increased afterload. Cholinergic slowing of conduction in the reentrant pathways associated with paroxysmal atrial tachycardia also can be achieved by blocking the metabolism of acetylcholine released from the vagal parasympathetics. The acetylcholine esterase inhibitor most suited for this purpose is *edrophonium* which has a very brief duration of action. A total of 10 mg edrophonium is given intravenously; an initial test dose of 1 mg may be followed in 2 min by the remaining 9 mg.

Parasympathetic receptor blockers are used to counteract severe bradycardias and atrioventricular block. *Methylscopolamine* appears to have advantages over atropine for this purpose as it does not cause bradycardia at low doses (as has been reported after small intravenous doses of atropine), and it does not cause effects related to blockade of central muscarinic receptors (e.g., delirium). *Methylscopolamine bromide* may be titrated giving 0.75 μg/kg intravenously as the initial dose and repeating 0.75 or 1 μg/kg every 5 min until it is effective or to a total dose of 6 μg/kg.

GANGLION BLOCKING DRUGS

Drugs which block transmission through autonomic ganglia produce the predicted effects of both sympathetic and parasympathetic blockade. The principal drug of this class currently used in therapy is *trimethaphan* which, in addition to lowering blood pressure, also diminishes myocardial contractility and consequently reduces the rate of rise of the arterial pulse, properties that are useful in the medical treatment of aortic dissection (Chap. 252). Side effects include paralytic ileus and urinary retention. High infusion rates (more than 5 mg/min) should be avoided, because such large doses may lead to respiratory depression. Tachyphylaxis may occur if large volumes of fluid are infused concomitantly.

ASSESSMENT OF SYMPATHETIC FUNCTION IN HUMANS

The pathogenesis of sympathetic insufficiency is varied (see Chap. 30). Impairment of the sympathetic nervous system may be suspected on the basis of a substantial drop in blood pressure after 2 to 5 min of standing. Patients with a marked deficiency in blood volume also have orthostatic hypotension, but usually will have a compensatory rise in the heart rate on standing. However, as the heart rate also increases following the withdrawal of parasympathetic stimulation, some disturbances of sympathetic reflex function may be accompanied by a modest increase in cardiac rate upon standing.

The diagnosis of impaired sympathetic function may be approached with some precision, allowing an assessment not only of the intactness of baroreceptor reflex function, but also of whether the lesion resides in the peripheral adrenergic neuron or in the central nervous system. Intactness of baroreceptor reflexes may be assessed by measuring both target organ response and neurotransmitter release. The vasoconstrictor response to hypotension may be assessed by the Valsalva maneuver, in which transient hypotension is produced by increased intrathoracic pressure which diminishes filling of the right side of the heart. In the supine position, the patient exhales into a manometer, maintaining a forced expiratory pressure of 40 mmHg for 10 s. The hypotension developing at the end of the maneuver normally generates a pronounced sympathetic discharge that causes a rebound pressor overshoot in which the diastolic pressure (measured via arterial needle) rises to levels higher than in the pretest period after the hypotensive stimulus is removed. The diastolic pressor overshoot should be proportional to the reduction in pulse pressure at the end of the maneuver, and its attenuation reflects an impaired sympathetic reflex arc. As a result of the pressor overshoot, a vagally mediated reflex bradycardia also occurs normally.

Interruption of the baroreceptor reflex either at the peripheral adrenergic neuron or within the central nervous system also impairs the release of neurotransmitter and is reflected by failure of the concentration of norepinephrine in plasma to rise appropriately with upright posture or exercise. When the deficit is located in the peripheral adrenergic neuron, there also is a reduced level of circulating norepinephrine in the supine position. When the baroreceptor reflex is interrupted by processes that damage the peripheral adrenergic neuron, indirectly acting sympathomimetic amines such as tyramine are ineffective pressor agents, because they act by releasing neuronal norepinephrine. Tyramine will evoke a pressor response when the only abnormality in the sympathetic reflex arc is located proximally to the peripheral adrenergic neuron in the central nervous system as is the case in the Shy-Drager syndrome, or within the afferent limb of the baroreceptor reflex.

The afferent limb of the baroreceptor reflex may be bypassed in assessing the efferent system by employing other stimuli to pressure elevation, as in the cold pressor test. When one hand is immersed in ice-cold water for 1 min, there normally is an increase in blood pressure which averages 16/12 mmHg. An abnormal Valsalva maneuver in the presence of normal cold pressor response suggests an abnormality in the afferent limb of the baroreceptor reflex. The integrity of the efferent pathway also can be tested by measuring the pressor and cardioaccelerator effects of mental arithmetic which does not require either baroreceptor or pain afferents.

REFERENCES

GOLDBERG LI: Dopamine—clinical uses of an endogenous catecholamine. N Engl J Med 291:707, 1974

GROSS, F (ed): *Antihypertensive Agents*. Berlin, Springer-Verlag, 1977

SHAND DG: Propranolol. N Engl J Med 299:280, 1975

TARAZI RC: Sympathomimetic agents in the treatment of shock. Ann Intern Med 81:364, 1974

section 4 | Nutritional disorders

73
NUTRITIONAL REQUIREMENTS

DANIEL RUDMAN

ESSENTIAL AND NONESSENTIAL NUTRIENTS AND THEIR THRESHOLDS (REQUIREMENTS, ALLOWANCES, AND TOLERANCES)

Over the past few decades diverse factors, including increased personal income, expanded public assistance programs, and vitamin and mineral enrichment of food, have reduced the prevalence of the classic nutritional deficiency diseases in the United States. Nevertheless, malnutrition, both overt and subclinical, remains a major problem, especially among the poor, the elderly, alcoholics, the chronically ill, and hospital populations. All too often the patient's nutritional status is ignored during the initial clinical evaluation, and complete nutritional needs are not met during hospitalization. To approach nutritional care rationally, the physician must assess the preexisting nutritional status, calculate the needs for maintenance and repletion, and understand how diseases influence these needs.

The body contains many thousands of species of organic molecules but requires for health the intake of only 21 organic compounds in addition to a source of calories: eight essential amino acids, one fatty acid, eleven vitamins, and water. The vast majority of organic molecules in food, although metabolized or assimilated by the body, are "nonessential" in the sense that their deletion from the diet does not cause illness. The simplicity of the *nutritional requirements* of the healthy subject, compared with the complexity of his *chemical composition,* is the result of the remarkable capacity for endogenous biosynthesis.

Of the limited number of *inorganic* compounds in food, the majority of their constituent elements, that is, 15, are believed to be nutritionally essential: calcium, phosphorus, iodine, iron, magnesium, zinc, copper, potassium, sodium, chloride, cobalt, chromium, manganese, molybdenum, and selenium.

The *minimal daily requirement* of an essential nutrient is the smallest quantity that maintains normal mass, chemical composition, morphology, and physiological functions of the various tissues and organs of the body and prevents any clinical or biochemical sign of the corresponding deficiency state. In children, an additional criterion is a normal rate of growth. Tables 73-1 to 73-3 list the minimal requirements of the 36 essential nutrients (21 organic, 15 inorganic) needed by adults, and Table 73-4 describes the main features of the illness which ensues when each essential nutrient is deficient. In children, two additional amino acids, arginine and histidine, are required. "Macro-" and "micronutrients" are defined on the basis of a daily requirement greater or less than 100 mg, respectively.

Minimal daily requirements are determined as follows:

1 In healthy adults the minimal daily requirement of protein (or its constituent amino acids) and macrominerals can be assessed by the elemental balance technique. Daily balance of each element equals intake minus output (urinary plus fecal). The requirement of each amino acid or macromineral is the smallest intake that maintains zero balance for nitrogen or for the mineral under study. Negative balance of any essential element, if it persists long enough, leads to illness and death.

2 In the infant or growing child the requirement of calories and essential nutrients is the smallest amount of each that maintains an optimal rate of growth while all others are fed in adequate amounts.

3 For micronutrients the requirement is the smallest daily intake that prevents eventual appearance of the nutrient-specific deficiency state.

The *recommended daily allowances* (RDA) of each nutrient range from 1.5 to 10 times the minimal daily requirements. Because the requirements vary among individuals due to numerous genetic and environmental circumstances, the minimal daily requirement may provide a *suboptimal* amount of a nutrient for a substantial minority of the healthy population. Accordingly, RDAs provide a margin of safety sufficient to meet

TABLE 73-1
Adult minimal daily requirements* for "reference man"† and "reference woman"‡

Nutrient	Requirements
Water	1–5 liters
Energy	2000–2700 kcal
Protein	28–33 g
Linoleic acid	3 g
Retinol equivalents	390
Vitamin D	Sunlight
Vitamin E activity	3–6 IU
Ascorbic acid	10 mg
Folacin§	50 µg
Niacin¶	9–12 mg
Riboflavin	1–1.4 mg
Thiamine	0.7–0.9 mg
Vitamin B$_6$	0.6–1.3 mg
Vitamin B$_{12}$	1 µg
Pantothenic acid	5 mg
Calcium	200–400 mg
Phosphorus	400 mg
Iodine	58–70 µg
Iron	6.5–9 mg
Magnesium	200 mg
Zinc	8–10 mg
Copper	2 mg
Potassium	2500 mg
Sodium	400 mg
Chloride	500 mg
Cobalt	0–1 µg
Chromium	200–290 µg
Manganese	2.5–2.7 mg
Molybdenum	45–500 µg
Selenium	0.1 µg

* *No minimum presently recognized for cholesterol, biotin, vitamin K, choline, cadmium, fluoride, nickel, tin, vanadium, silicon, and boron.*
† *"Reference man": 35 years old, 70 kg in weight, 172 cm tall, moderately active, temperate climate.*
‡ *"Reference woman": 35 years old, 58 kg in weight, 162 cm tall, moderatively active, temperate climate.*
§ *The folacin allowance refers to dietary sources as determined by* Lactobacillus casei *assay. Pure forms of folacin may be effective in doses one-fourth of the requirement listed here.*
¶ *One milligram of niacin may be derived from every 60 mg dietary tryptophan.*
SOURCE: *RS Goodhart, E Shils, Modern Nutrition in Health and Disease, 5th ed, Philadelphia, Lea & Febiger, 1973.*

the needs of virtually the entire healthy population (Table 73-2).

Another nutritional threshold is the maximal daily tolerance of a nutrient. Just as intake of any essential nutrient *below* a specific level causes disease, likewise intake *above* a certain level for many nutrients (either essential or nonessential) disturbs body structure or function (Table 73-5). A physiologic diet provides intakes of each nutrient between the two thresholds of minimal requirement and maximal tolerance. The recognition that tolerance for a nutrient can be exceeded is particularly important during parenteral nutrition, when the gastrointestinal mechanisms (emesis, incomplete absorption, diarrhea) that ordinarily protect the patient at least partially from the ill effects of excessive nutrient intake are bypassed. Unfortunately, although requirements and allowances have been established for each of the 31 essential nutrients, the maximal tolerance for most nutrients is uncertain.

FACTORS ALTERING NUTRITIONAL THRESHOLDS

Both the minimal requirement and maximal tolerance of each essential nutrient are influenced by a host of factors: rate of growth, age, exercise, pregnancy and lactation, chemical composition of the diet, diseases, drugs. In addition, the route, rate, and timing of alimentation influence requirements and tolerances. As the "distance" between requirement and tolerance narrows, nutritional management of the patient becomes more

difficult (e.g., protein intake of a cachectic, encephalopathic, cirrhotic patient).

PHYSIOLOGICAL FACTORS Growth, exercise, pregnancy, and lactation (Table 73-2) increase the daily requirements per kilogram of body weight for calories and most essential nutrients. Caloric requirement declines with age.

COMPOSITION OF THE DIET Given diets with identical contents of nitrogen, digestible carbohydrates, fat, vitamins, and minerals, the metabolic availability of the nutrients may vary widely. Thus all proteins are not equally effective in meeting the daily requirement because of differences in digestibility or in content of essential amino acids. Gastrointestinal absorption of some minerals is influenced by the presence in the diet of other reactive components; the utilization of vitamins may be influenced by level of intake of organic macronutrients. Examples are given in Table 73-6.

ROUTE, RATE, AND TIMING (See Chap. 78) The requirements and allowances listed in Tables 73-1 to 3 apply to *enteral* nutrition. For some nutrients, different values will be required for *parenteral* nutrition. Net gastrointestinal absorption of ingested amino acids, carbohydrates, fats, sodium, chloride, and potassium normally is greater than 90 percent (Table 73-7), and these nutrients from this point of view have the same RDAs for the intravenous as for the enteral route. For the remaining essential minerals, however, net absorption is only 50 percent or less (Table 73-7); consequently the intravenous requirement is only a fraction of the oral one. It is also likely that the requirements of amino acids are not identical by enteral and parenteral routes. After ingestion and absorption into the portal venous system, a portion of the absorbed amino acids is catabolized during the "first pass" through the liver, where many of the enzymes of amino acid degradation are located. Intravenously infused amino acids, in contrast, can bypass these catabolic pathways and directly perfuse sites of protein synthesis in muscle and other extrahepatic tissues.

Timing can be important. For example, all essential amino acids must be supplied simultaneously to support protein synthesis. If even one of the essential amino acids is administered at a different time than the other essential and nonessential acids, assimilation of all into protein is curtailed. Similarly, when amino acids, glucose, lipids, and minerals are infused at separate times during the day or week, as often happens in parenteral feeding, assimilation may be impaired. Thus omission of phosphorus or potassium from central hyperalimentation solutions impairs retention of the nitrogen furnished by the same fluid. For these reasons the requirements of several essential nutrients by the *parenteral route* remain uncertain even though parenteral nutrition is a major component of clinical therapeutics.

DISEASE Nutritional requirements and tolerances may be altered by disease through at least seven mechanisms (see also Table 73-8):

1 Increased utilization of nutrients. Fever, infection, and trauma increase resting metabolic rate and, as a consequence, daily caloric requirement. Folate is utilized more rapidly in patients with hemolysis and increased cell turnover (hemolytic anemia, psoriasis, cancer). Many nutritional

TABLE 73-2
Recommended daily dietary allowances[a]

Age, years	Weight, kg	Height, cm	Energy, kcal	Protein, g	Fat-soluble vitamins		Vitamin D, IU	Vitamin E activity,[c] IU
					Vitamin A activity			
					RE[b]	IU		
INFANTS								
0.0–05	6	60	kg × 117	kg × 2.2	420	1400	400	4
0.5–1.0	9	71	kg × 108	kg × 2.0	400	2000	400	5
CHILDREN								
1–3	13	86	1300	23	400	2000	400	7
4–6	20	110	1800	30	500	2500	400	9
7–10	30	135	2400	36	700	3300	400	10
MALES								
11–14	44	158	2800	44	1000	5000	400	12
15–18	61	172	3000	54	1000	5000	400	15
19–22	67	172	3000	54	1000	5000	400	15
23–50	70	172	2700	56	1000	5000		15
51+	70	172	2400	56	1000	5000		15
FEMALES								
11–14	44	155	2400	44	800	4000	400	12
15–18	54	162	2100	48	800	4000	400	12
19–22	58	162	2100	46	800	4000	400	12
23–50	58	162	2000	46	800	4000		12
51+	58	162	1800	46	800	4000		12
PREGNANCY								
			+300	+30	1000	5000	400	15
LACTATION								
			+500	+20	1200	6000	400	15

[a] The allowances are intended to provide for individual variations among most normal persons as they live in the United States under usual environmental stresses. Diets should be based on a variety of common foods in order to provide other nutrients for which human requirements have been less well-defined. Adult RDA for water, 1 ml/cal; for linoleic acid, 1 to 2 percent of total caloric intake.

[b] Retinol equivalents (RE): Assumed to be all as retinol in milk during the first 6 months of life. All subsequent intakes are assumed to be half as retinol and half as β-carotene when calculated from international units. As retinol equivalents, three-fourths are as retinol and one-fourth as β-carotene.

[c] Total vitamin E activity, estimated to be 80 percent as α-tocopherol and 20 percent as other tocopherols.

requirements are greater during repletion from cachexia than during maintenance of normal nutriture. In this respect, the repletion process in adults resembles growth in children.

2 *Malabsorption.* For each nutrient absorbed less efficiently than normal in malabsorption states, the daily requirement is increased correspondingly.

3 *Impaired ability to activate a nutrient.* The requirement for vitamin D is increased by renal disease which impairs hydroxylation of the vitamin; requirements for folate, thiamine, and pyridoxine in cirrhotics may be greater than normal because of impaired hepatic capacity to transform these vitamins into their active forms.

4 *Abnormally large losses of nutrients.* Impaired conservation of sodium, phosphorus, or amino acids because of renal disease, burns, blood loss, nasogastric suction, diarrhea, or hemodialysis leads to loss of nutrients. One criterion of normal nutriture for nitrogen and minerals in the adult is zero elemental balance, i.e., enteral or parenteral intake equal to urinary plus fecal output. If output of nitrogen or mineral is increased by abnormal renal or extrarenal loss, then intake must be correspondingly higher to maintain zero balance.

5 *Impaired catabolic or excretory pathways.* Metabolic defects can reduce both requirement and tolerance, because the rate

of degradation or excretion of a nutrient is slowed. In children with phenylketonuria or maple syrup urine disease, the requirements for phenylalanine or branched-chain amino acids, respectively, are less than in normals. Patients with uremia have a reduced dietary requirement for nonessential amino acids.

6 *Hyperabsorption.* Increased absorption can result in a decrease in both requirement and tolerance. Examples are calcium in hyperabsorptive hypercalciuria, iron in hemochromatosis, and copper in Wilson's disease.

7 *Drugs.* Pharmacological agents can alter nutritional requirements by causing malabsorption or renal loss of a nutrient, by preventing its metabolic utilization, or by accelerating its degradation (Table 73-9).

INDIVIDUAL ESSENTIAL NUTRIENTS

WATER A reasonable allowance is 1 ml/cal for adults and 150 ml/kg for infants. The minimal daily requirement, considerably less than the customary allowance, depends on the preformed and potential solutes ingested (largely protein, sodium, chloride, and potassium), the concentrating ability of the kidney, and extrarenal losses. Normally 50 to 100 ml per day is excreted in the feces, 400 to 600 ml is lost by exhalation and

Water-soluble vitamins							Minerals[f]					
Ascorbic Acid, mg	Folacin,[d] µg	Niacin,[e] mg	Riboflavin, mg	Thiamine, mg	Vitamin B_6, mg	Vitamin B_{12}, µg	Calcium, mg	Phosphorus, mg	Iodine, µg	Iron, mg	Magnesium, mg	Zinc, mg
35	50	5	0.4	0.3	0.3	0.3	360	240	35	10	60	3
35	50	8	0.6	0.5	0.4	0.3	540	400	45	15	70	5
40	100	9	0.8	0.7	0.6	1.0	800	800	60	15	150	10
40	200	12	1.1	0.9	0.9	1.5	800	800	80	10	200	10
40	300	16	1.2	1.2	1.2	2.0	800	800	110	10	250	10
45	400	18	1.5	1.4	1.6	3.0	1200	1200	130	18	350	15
45	400	20	1.8	1.5	2.0	3.0	1200	1200	150	18	400	15
45	400	20	1.8	1.5	2.0	3.0	800	800	140	10	350	15
45	400	18	1.6	1.4	2.0	3.0	800	800	130	10	350	15
45	400	16	1.5	1.2	2.0	3.0	800	800	110	10	350	15
45	400	16	1.3	1.2	1.6	3.0	1200	1200	115	10	350	15
45	400	14	1.4	1.1	2.0	3.0	1200	1200	115	18	300	15
45	400	14	1.4	1.1	2.0	3.0	800	800	100	18	300	15
45	400	13	1.2	1.0	2.0	3.0	800	800	100	18	300	15
45	400	12	1.1	1.0	2.0	3.0	800	800	80	18	300	15
60	800	+ 2	+0.3	+0.3	2.5	4.0	1200	1200	125	10	300	20
80	800	+ 4	+0.5	+0.3	2.5	4.0	1200	1200	250	18+[g]	450	25

[d] The folacin allowances refer to dietary sources as determined by Lactobacillus casei assay. Pure forms of folacin may be effective in doses less than one-fourth of the recommended dietary allowance.

[e] Although allowances are expressed as niacin, it is recognized that on the average 1 mg niacin is derived from each 60 mg dietary tryptophan.

[f] Reasonable guides for intake of the other essential minerals, expressed as milligrams per day, are: potassium, 2500; chloride, 2000; sodium, 2500; copper, 2.

[g] This increased requirement cannot be met by ordinary diets; therefore, the use of supplemental iron is recommended.

SOURCE: Food and Nutrition Board.

evaporation (insensible loss), and the remainder is excreted in the urine. Water intake must equal these losses for the subject to maintain water balance and avoid under- or overhydration.

Maximal tolerance normally is more than 5 liters daily because of the kidney's large capacity for free water clearance. Water requirement and tolerance are increased by factors that cause increased losses in urine, feces, or sweat. The obligatory urinary loss is proportional to the excretion of solutes (largely urea, Na^+, K^+, and Cl^-) and the kidney's concentrating capacity; it is increased in proportion to intake of protein, Na^+, K^+, and Cl^-. Water requirements are increased by deficiency of antidiuretic hormone and decreased when the hormone is secreted inappropriately. Fecal loss of water may increase to over 5 liters per day in severe diarrhea. Nasogastric suction, ileostomy, gastrointestinal fistulas, and burns similarly increase daily water requirements. Water loss is excessive during fever, heavy exercise, or exposure to high environmental temperature. Each degree Celsius of fever causes an obligatory loss of about 200 ml water per day.

CALORIES To maintain stable weight, caloric intake must equal caloric output. The output can be divided into *basal* and *activity* components. Basal metabolic rate (BMR) is usually measured in the fasting, resting subject immediately after awaking. Standard values are given in Table 73-10; values during sleep are about 10 percent less. After each meal, metabolic rate increases up to 30 percent; during each day, this "specific dynamic action" amounts to about 6 percent of the basal caloric expenditure. BMR declines with age by about 3 to 10 percent per decade. It is rarely measured except for experimental purposes.

Activity increases caloric demands. Mild, moderate, or severe exercise raises caloric expenditure by roughly 30, 50, or 100 (or more) percent, respectively. Caloric expenditures in specific types of activity are described in Chap. 76.

TABLE 73-3
Minimal daily requirements for young adult male subjects of the essential amino acids

Amino acid	Requirement, mg
L-Threonine	500
L-Valine	800
L-Methionine	1100
L-Isoleucine	700
L-Leucine	1100
L-Phenylalanine	1100
L-Lysine	800
L-Tryptophan	250

TABLE 73-4
Syndromes of undernutrition

Nutrient	Signs and symptoms of deficiency	Laboratory tests
Water	Thirst, poor tissue turgor, dry mucous membranes, vascular collapse, altered mental status	Serum electrolytes ↑, serum osmolarity ↑, total body water ↓
Calories (energy)	Weakness and physical inactivity, loss of subcutaneous fat, muscle wasting, bradycardia	Weight loss, TSF ↓, MAMC ↓, creatinine/ht ↓, BMR ↓
Protein	Psychomotor change, dyspigmented, sparse, and easily plucked hair, "flaky-paint" dermatitis, edema, muscle wasting, hepatomegaly	MAMC ↓, serum albumin and transferrin ↓, anemia, creatinine/ht ↓, serum nonessential/essential amino acids ↑, urine urea/creatinine ↓
Linoleic acid	Xerosis	Serum ratio of triene to tetraene fatty acids ↑
Sodium	Muscle weakness and cramps, confusion, apathy, anorexia, hypotension, oliguria	Serum Na^+ ↓, BUN/creatinine ↑
Chloride	Muscle cramps, apathy, anorexia	Serum Cl^- ↓
Potassium	Lassitude, polyuria, ileus, muscular weakness	Serum and urine K^+ ↓, body ^{40}K ↓, abnormal ECG
Calcium	Stunted growth, rickets, osteomalacia, convulsions	Osteopenia by x-ray, serum Ca^+ ↓
Phosphorus	Weakness, osteomalacia	Osteopenia by x-ray, serum P ↓
Magnesium	Growth failure, behavioral disturbances, weakness, tremor, tetany, seizures, cardiac arrhythmias	Serum, urine, and RBC Mg ↓
Iron	Pallor, weakness, reduced resistance to infection, angular stomatitis, atrophic lingual papillae, koilonychia	Plasma and marrow iron ↓, microcytic hypochromic anemia
Fluorine	Higher frequency of tooth decay	
Zinc	Growth restriction, hypogonadism, delayed puberty, slow wound healing, hypogeusia	Plasma, hair, and 24-h urine zinc ↓
Copper	Pallor	Hypochromic microcytic anemia, osteopenia, plasma and urine copper ↓
Iodine	Goiter, symptoms of hypothyroidism	TSH ↑, T_4 and T_3 ↓, 24-h urine iodine ↓, RAI uptake ↑
Thiamine (vitamin B_1)	Beriberi, muscle tenderness and weakness, hyporeflexia, hypesthesia, tachycardia, cardiomegaly, congestive heart failure	Erythrocyte thiamine pyrophosphate and transketolase activity ↓ and in vitro effect thereon of thiamine pyrophosphate ↑; urinary thiamine ↓, blood pyruvate, α-ketoglutarate levels ↑
Riboflavin (vitamin B_2)	Angular stomatitis (or angular scars), cheilosis, magenta tongue, atrophic lingual papillae, corneal vascularization, angular blepharitis, dyssebacia, scrotal (vulvar) dermatosis	EGR activity ↓ and in vitro effect on EGR activity of flavin adenine dinucleotide ↑
Niacin (vitamin B_3)	Pellagra, scarlet and raw tongue, atrophic lingual papillae, tongue fissuring, mental disorders, pellagrous dermatosis, diarrhea	Urinary N^1-methylnicotinamide ↓
Pyridoxine (vitamin B_6)	Nasolabial seborrhea, glossitis, kidney stones, peripheral neuropathy, muscular twitching, convulsions, microcytic anemia	EGOT activity ↓ and in vitro effect of pyridoxal phosphate on EGOT activity ↑; tryptophan load test ↓ (urinary excretion of xanthurenic and quinolinic acids); urinary vitamin B_6 excretion ↓
Pantothenic acid	Fatigue, sleep disturbances, impaired coordination, nausea	
Folic acid	Pallor, glossitis, stomatitis, diarrhea, anemia	Erythrocyte and serum folate concentration ↓; urine forminiglutamic acid excretion ↑ after histidine load; macrocytic anemia, polymorphonuclear leukocytes hypersegmented, megaloblastic bone marrow
Vitamin B_{12}	Pallor, mild icterus, anorexia, diarrhea, paresthesia, ataxia, optic neuritis, mental changes	Serum vitamin B_{12} ↓; peripheral blood and bone marrow morphology
Biotin	Fatigue, depression, nausea, dermatitis, muscular pains	
Vitamin C	Scurvy, petechiae, ecchymoses, perifollicular hemorrhage, spongy and bleeding gums (if not edentulous)	Ascorbic acid concentration in plasma, platelets, whole blood, and white blood cells ↓; urinary ascorbic acid ↓
Vitamin A	Xerosis of eye and skin, xerophthalmia, Bitot's spot, follicular hyperkeratosis	Plasma vitamin A ↓ Dark adaptation time ↑
Vitamin D	Rickets and growth failure in children, osteomalacia in adults	Serum alkaline phosphatase concentration ↑; plasma 25-hydroxycholecalciferol ↓; serum Ca and P ↓
Vitamin E	Anemia	
Vitamin K	Bleeding diathesis	Prothrombin time ↑

NOTE: *BMR = basal metabolism rate; BUN = blood-urea nitrogen; creatinine/ht = 24-h urine creatinine/height ratio; ECG = electrocardiogram; EGOT = erythrocyte glutamic-oxaloacetic transaminase; EGR = erythrocyte glutathione reductase; MAMC = midarm muscle circumference; RAI = radioactive iodine; RBC = red blood cell; T_3 = triiodothyronine; T_4 = thyroxine; TSF = triceps skin fold; TSH = thyroid-stimulating hormone.*

TABLE 73-5
Syndromes which can result from excessive intake or absorption of nutrients by oral route, or excessive infusion by parenteral route

Nutrient	Manifestation of overnutrition
Water	Edema, headache, nausea, hypertension
Calories	Obesity
Protein	Exacerbation of inborn errors in amino acid catabolism or "nitrogen accumulation diseases"; hepatic encephalopathy
Calcium	Hypercalcemia, mental and renal dysfunction
Potassium	Muscular weakness, arrhythmia, death
Sodium chloride	Hypertension, edema, heart failure
Magnesium	Diarrhea
Iron	Siderosis, hemochromatosis
Fluorine	Mottling of teeth, increased bone density, neurological disturbances
Zinc	Fever, nausea, vomiting, diarrhea
Copper	Wilson's disease
Manganese	Generalized disease of nervous system
Iodine	Depression of thyroid activity, goiter, occasional hyperthyroidism
Ascorbic acid (vitamin C)	Hyperoxaluria, destruction of vitamin B_{12}
Retinol (vitamin A)	Headache, vomiting, peeling of skin, anorexia, swelling of long bones, cirrhosis
Phylloquinone (vitamin K)	At high doses may cause jaundice
Vitamin D	Hypercalcemia, nephrolithiasis, impaired renal function

The daily energy requirement equals the sum of expenditures incurred by basal metabolism, specific dynamic action, and physical activity. The requirement can be estimated by assessing basal caloric expenditure per day from the subject's surface area (Table 73-10), using ideal body weight in this calculation. Subtract 10 percent from basal during the sleeping hours. Add 6 percent to the 24-h basal estimate to cover the specific dynamic action of meals. From an activity-calorie chart, such as is given in Chap. 76, calculate the caloric expenditure of the subject's physical activities during a typical day. The daily caloric output can be estimated as the sum of basal requirements (minus correction for sleep) plus specific dynamic action plus caloric requirement for physical activity. Since on average 93 percent of caloric intake is utilized and 7 percent is

TABLE 73-6
Some essential nutrients for which the daily dietary requirement is influenced by other dietary components

Nutrient	Influence by other dietary component
Calcium, magnesium, iron	Absorption decreased by phytates
Calcium	Urinary excretion increased by high protein intake
Essential amino acids	Utilization curtailed if any essential amino acid is deficient
Nonheme iron	Absorption improved by vitamin C or meat
Folic acid	Protected from destruction during cooking by ascorbic acid
Vitamin B_6	Requirement increased by protein
Vitamin E	Requirement proportional to intake of essential fatty acids
Thiamine	Requirement proportional to calories
Protein	Requirement inversely related to calories when the latter are deficient
Niacin	Requirement inversely related to tryptophan intake
Phenylalanine	Requirement inversely related to tyrosine intake
Methionine	Requirement inversely related to cystine intake
Valine, leucine, isoleucine	Requirement of each is increased by excess of the other branched chain amino acid(s)

TABLE 73-7
Net absorption of nutrients by normal adults

Element	Percent	Element	Percent
Protein	>90	Cu	~30
Carbohydrate	>90	Co	20–95
Fat	>95	Mn	<5
Na	>95	Se	40–70
K	80–90	F	80–90
Cl	>95	Cr	1–3
Ca	5–40	Mo	40–50
Mg	25–50	Zn	33
P	50–60	I	>90
Fe	5–15		
Cu	~30		

lost in feces and urine, the estimated caloric requirement for zero balance equals 107 percent of the calculated output.

In actual practice, a simpler formula can be used. Twenty-two calories per kilogram of ideal body weight are allowed for basal metabolism. For sedentary, moderate, or heavy activity, add 30, 50, or 100 percent, respectively. Weight is monitored weekly, and if weight increases or decreases, calories are adjusted accordingly.

Caloric expenditure is increased by fever (about 13 percent over basal per degree Celsius), burns (10 to 100 percent), trauma (40 to 100 percent), and hyperthyroidism (10 to 100 percent). Hypometabolism, whether of thyroidal or other cause, lowers the energy expenditure and, therefore, the energy requirement.

Patients with severe malabsorption may absorb as little as 25 percent of their ingested calories (fat, carbohydrate, protein) compared with the normal value of over 95 percent. In these patients, oral caloric requirement is higher than normal and may prove impossible to achieve if diarrhea is aggravated by increased nutrient intake. In such patients only parenteral nutrition can prevent progressive starvation.

PROTEIN Dietary protein provides the body a mixture of amino acids for endogenous protein synthesis and is also a metabolic fuel for energy (see Chap. 85). Healthy adults require eight essential amino acids in amounts varying from 250 to 1100 mg per day. About 30 g of nonessential amino acids is

TABLE 73-8
Diseases which alter nutrient requirements by the oral route

Nutrient	Increases dietary requirement	Reduces dietary requirement
Calories	Fever, hyperthyroidism, trauma, malabsorption	Coma, hypothyroidism
Protein	Fever, hyperthyroidism, trauma, azotorrhea	Nitrogen accumulation diseases, inborn errors of urea synthesis
Phenylalanine		Phenylketonuria
Branched-chain amino acids		Maple syrup urine diseases
Linoleic acid and fat-soluble vitamins	Malabsorption syndromes	
Calcium	Malabsorption syndromes	Hyperabsorptive hypercalciuria
Magnesium	Malabsorption syndromes	
Iron	Malabsorption syndromes	Hemochromatosis
Copper		Wilson's disease
Phosphorus	Malabsorption syndromes	Renal insufficiency
Folic acid	Increased cell turnover	
Carnitine*	Advanced cirrhosis	

* No requirement normally.

TABLE 73-9
Drugs capable of causing undernutrition

Drug	Nutrient	Mechanism
Diuretics	Water, Na, Cl, Ca, Mg, K	↑ renal excretion
Neomycin	Protein, Ca, Mg, linoleic acid	Malabsorption
Colchicine, cholestyramine	Fat-soluble vitamins, Fe, vitamin B_{12}	Malabsorption
Aluminum hydroxide, calcium carbonate (antacids), calomel (laxative)	P	Decreased intestinal absorption
Anticonvulsants (phenobarbital, phenytoin primidone, glutethimide, diphosphonates)	Vitamin D, Ca, folic acid	Altered metabolism
Alcohol	Folic acid, Mg, protein, thiamine	Malabsorption, anorexia, magnesuria
Chelating agents (D-penicillamine, EDTA)	Zn, Cu, Fe, Ca, Mg	↑ renal excretion
Isoniazid	Pyridoxine	Hydrazide formation
Potassium chloride	Vitamin B_{12}	Malabsorption
Mineral oil	Fat-soluble vitamins	Malabsorption

TABLE 73-11
Biologic value of food proteins*

Protein source	Biologic value
Milk	93
Egg	93
Beef	76
Peanut meal	74
Corn	72
Potato	69
Oat	65
Rice	65
Corn	50
Soy flour	41
Wheat gluten	40

* As determined from nitrogen balance studies conducted in the rat, generally at a dietary protein concentration of 5 percent. Tests in the rat at other concentrations, or in other species, give generally similar but not identical biologic values.

also required for protein synthesis. The requirement and allowance of dietary protein depend on the biologic value of the proteins ingested. *Biologic value* is defined as the proportion of absorbed protein retained by the body under standard test conditions. It is primarily dependent on the content of essential amino acids. Nearly optimal ratios of the eight essential and twelve nonessential amino acids are present in egg and milk proteins, which consequently have the highest biologic values for the diet, viz., 90 to 95 (Table 73-11). The biologic value of proteins in the world's major food products follows the general order: animal products > cereals (rice, wheat, corn) > legumes > roots. The adult RDA for protein given in Table 73-2, about 50 g per day, assumes a biologic value of about 80, a characteristic value when animal products are the major protein source. The lower the biologic value, the higher the daily protein requirement.

Plant proteins have low biologic value because one or more essential amino acids are deficient. Thus for corn (maize), lysine, threonine, and tryptophan are limiting; for soy beans and green peas, methionine; for rice, lysine and threonine; for wheat, lysine. Therefore, mixtures of two "complementary" vegetable proteins deficient in different essential amino acids have a higher biologic value than either protein separately.

While the usual reason for low biologic value of a particular protein or mixture of proteins is limiting content of one or

TABLE 73-10
Basal caloric requirements of normal subjects

Age, years	Males, $(cal/m^2)/h$	Females, $(cal/m^2)/h$
14–16	46.0	43.0
16–18	43.0	40.0
18–20	41.0	38.0
20–30	39.5	37.0
30–40	39.5	36.5
40–50	38.5	36.0
50–60	37.5	35.0
60–70	36.5	34.0
70–80	35.5	33.0

SOURCE: *EF DuBois, Basal Metabolism in Health and Disease, 3d ed, Philadelphia, Lea & Febiger, 1936, p 151.*

more essential amino acids, excess of an amino acid can also impair the value. For example, excessive intake of leucine increases the requirement for isoleucine; this type of influence is termed *amino acid imbalance* and is an important consideration in planning the composition of mixtures of synthetic amino acids for parenteral or enteral feeding. In addition, certain amino acids may be "spared" by chemically related amino acids. For example, tyrosine and cystine are in part converted to phenylalanine and methionine, respectively, and therefore spare the latter substances.

The daily requirement of a protein, or its constituent amino acids, is also influenced by caloric intake; the values for protein requirement and allowance given in Tables 72-1 to 72-3 assume adequate caloric intake. When the caloric requirement is met by nonprotein calories, a substantial portion of ingested amino acids is utilized for protein synthesis. If calories are deficient, amino acids are diverted from protein synthesis into pathways of oxidative metabolism and gluconeogenesis. Under these circumstances, the daily protein requirement is inversely proportional to the caloric intake. Thus, caloric undernutrition makes a person more vulnerable to protein starvation, an interaction which accounts for the high prevalence of the combined deficiency state *protein-energy undernutrition* (see Chap. 75).

The daily protein requirement per unit body weight is increased by growth, pregnancy, lactation, repletion after cachexia, fever, infection, trauma, and malabsorption.

To understand how the "nitrogen accumulation diseases," hepatic and renal insufficiency, alter the requirements and tolerances of dietary protein, consider the scheme of amino acid metabolism shown in Fig. 73-1. The daily adult requirement of about 50 g protein serves to maintain reaction 2, that is, protein synthesis, at a rate equal to protein breakdown (reaction 3). Tolerance for protein is greater than 250 g per day because of the high capacity of the degradative pathway (reactions 4, 6, 7, and 9). Note that 20 to 40 percent of urea formed in the liver is hydrolyzed by microbes within the colon and recycles at least once as ammonia (reaction 8). When step 10 is blocked (uremia), the requirement for nonessential nitrogen is reduced. Urea, instead of being excreted, recycles as ammonia and remains available for synthesis of nonessential amino acids; the carbon skeletons of these acids are readily produced by the intermediary metabolism of glucose. This pathway for endogenous synthesis of nonessential amino acids is the basis for the Giovanetti diet in uremia. If the uremic patient is fed the carbon skeletons (α-keto derivatives) of the *essential* amino acids, the requirement of the latter nutrients (except for threonine and lysine) is also reduced because of the reversibility of transamination, i.e., reaction 5 in Fig. 73-1. Similar considerations apply in advanced cirrhosis and in hereditary disorders of urea synthesis.

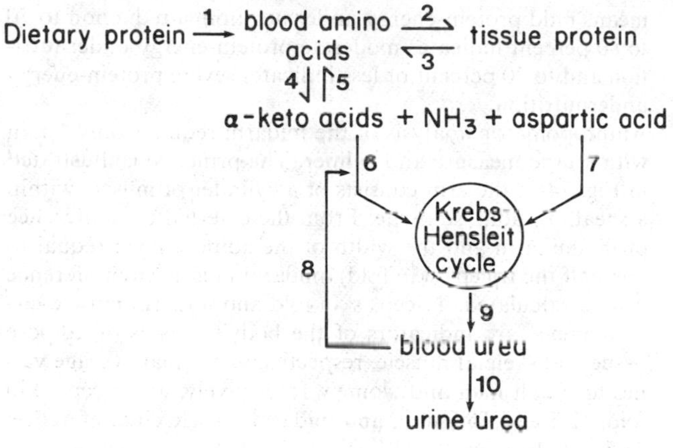

Dietary protein →(1) blood amino acids →(2)/(3) tissue protein

(4)↓↑(5)

α-keto acids + NH$_3$ + aspartic acid

(6) (7)

Krebs Hensleit cycle

(8)

(9)↓

blood urea

(10)↓

urine urea

FIGURE 73-1
Overview of amino acid metabolism.

Not only is the daily requirement for protein in some uremics and cirrhotics lower than normal, but the maximal tolerance is curtailed as well. As little as 20 g protein a day can precipitate or aggravate symptoms of hepatocerebral disease in the susceptible hepatic patient. Intakes of protein customary for healthy subjects in the United States (80 to 100 g per day) can also intensify the uremic syndrome.

FAT While the average adult in the United States eats 70 to 120 g fat per day, the only actual requirement is for about 3 g linoleic acid per day. Within the range 3 to 120 g fat, it is unclear what intake to recommend, except as dictated by body weight considerations. Palatability requires a minimum of 40 g. In patients predisposed to hyperlipoproteinemia by heredity or obesity, the distribution of calories between fat and carbohydrates influences the severity of the lipemia.

MINERALS AND VITAMINS The daily requirements/allowances and the influence of physiological and pathological circumstances on these thresholds are listed in Tables 73-1, 73-2, 73-6, and 73-8. The deficiency syndromes corresponding to each nutrient are listed in Table 73-4, and some clinical effects of exceeding the daily tolerance are given in Table 73-5 (see also Chaps. 79 to 82).

REFERENCES

FOOD AND NUTRITION BOARD: *Recommended Dietary Allowances.* Washington, DC, National Academy of Sciences, 1974

HERBERT V: The five possible causes of all nutrient deficiency: Illustrated by deficiencies of vitamin B$_{12}$ and folic acid. Am J Clin Nutr 26:77, 1973

ROE D: Drug-induced nutritional deficiencies. Westport, Conn, Avi Publishing Company, 1976

SCRIMSHAW NW, YOUNG UR: The requirements of human nutrition. Sci Am 235:50, September 1976

SHILS E: Nutrition and neoplasia, in *Modern Nutrition in Health and Disease,* 5th ed, RS Goodhart, ME Shils (eds). Philadelphia, Lea & Febiger, 1973, pp 981-996

74
ASSESSMENT OF NUTRITIONAL STATUS

DANIEL RUDMAN

Undernutrition is a common contribution to morbidity and mortality in most hospitals. As a peculiar discrepancy, however, undernutrition rarely appears on charts in the list of diagnoses or in the progress notes. Consequently, quantitative tests of nutritional status are rare in the initial clinical workup, and the progress of the nutritional state is not monitored regularly during the course of illness. As a result, undernutrition tends to be recognized late, when it is severe and difficult to treat. This chapter defines feasible methods for identifying and quantifying the deficiency syndromes, for investigating their cause, and for monitoring their course.

MASS AND COMPOSITION OF THE BODY COMPARTMENTS
Consideration must first be given to the normal mass and chemical composition of the major body compartments, since these compartmental properties are altered by nutritional deficiencies in characteristic ways. The body can be viewed as consisting of four compartments: extracellular fluid, protoplasm (intracellular compartment), bone, and adipose tissue. The first three make up the *lean body mass*.

The mass and elemental composition of the body compartments of a healthy "reference man," 70 kg in weight, 172 cm tall, 35 years old, are shown in Table 74-1. Typical masses of extracellular fluid, protoplasm, bone, and adipose tissue are 17, 35, 5, and 13 kg, respectively. Chloride is localized almost exclusively in the extracellular fluid, where its average concentration is 96 meq per liter; nitrogen and potassium are largely located in protoplasm, with normal concentrations of 27 and 150 meq per kilogram of wet weight, respectively; calcium is found primarily in bone, where its concentration averages 260 g per kilogram of wet weight. The adipose tissue contains insignificant levels of these elements.

DIRECT AND INDIRECT METHODS FOR MEASURING MASS OF BODY COMPARTMENTS If one assumes that the concentrations of chloride, nitrogen, potassium, phosphorus, and calcium remain normal in extracellular fluid, protoplasm, and bone during a period of observation involving expansion or contraction of these compartments, and if one knows the balance (i.e., intake and output) of each element (termed Δ nitrogen, Δ phosphorus, etc.) during this period, then from the equations in Table 74-2 one can calculate the change (Δ) in the mass of each of these three compartments during the period under consideration. The change in adipose mass can then be estimated as

Δ body weight − (Δ protoplasm
+ Δ extracellular fluid + Δ bone)

TABLE 74-1
Approximate mass and major elemental composition of body compartments in a 70-kg healthy "reference man"

	Protoplasm	Extracellular fluid	Bone	Adipose tissue
Mass	35 kg	17 kg	5 kg	13 kg
Body weight	50%	24%	7%	19%
Elemental composition, per kg wet wt	27 g N 97 mmol P 150 meq K	140 meq Na 96 meq Cl	260 g Ca 115 g P	

TABLE 74-2
Reifenstein equations for determining change in mass of body compartments

Δ Protoplasm (g) $= 27 \times \Delta$ N (g)

Δ ECF* (g) $= 9.6 \times \Delta$ Cl (meq)

Δ Bone (g) $= 0.1 \times \Delta$ Ca (meq)

Δ Adipose tissue (g) $= \Delta$ BW† (g) $-$ [Δ protoplasm (g)
$\qquad\qquad\qquad\qquad\qquad\qquad\qquad$ $+ \Delta$ ECF (g) $+ \Delta$ bone (g)]

* *Extracellular fluid.*
† *Body weight.*

The equation is based on the fact that each kilogram of extracellular fluid, protoplasm, or bone gained or lost by the body contains a characteristic amount of chloride, nitrogen, or calcium, respectively.

Metabolic balance techniques of this type provide estimates of the change in mass of each compartment during the period of observation but provide no information about the absolute mass of the compartment at the beginning and end. Several methods capable of such absolute measurements are available: whole-body counting of potassium (total body protoplasm); measurement of extracellular fluid by isotope dilution; measurement of total body water by isotope dilution; calculation of intracellular water (closely related to protoplasmic mass) as total body water minus extracellular water; measurement of adipose mass by determining whole-body density. These various methods are largely restricted to research units. Fortunately, several indirect methods for estimating the mass of body compartments are available to the clinician:

1 In the nonedematous patient, body weight as percent of ideal is a useful indicator of adipose tissue plus lean body mass. Reduction of the ratio, body weight/ideal body weight, to 80 percent in nonedematous patients usually means mild protein-energy undernutrition, a reduction to 70 to 80 percent indicates moderate protein-energy undernutrition and to 70 percent or less indicates severe protein-energy undernutrition.

2 Anthropometric analysis of the midarm requires only 1 min with a tape measure and caliper. The principle is illustrated in Fig. 74-1; the arm consists of a cylinder of muscle within a sheath of adipose tissue. From the external circumference of the midarm and the width of the adipose layer (equal to one-half the triceps skin fold), midarm muscle circumference can be calculated. Triceps skin fold and midarm muscle circumference are indicators of the body's masses of adipose tissue and skeletal muscle, respectively. Normal average values for adult men and women, respectively, are triceps skin fold, 12.5 and 16.5 mm, and midarm muscle circumference, 25.3 and 23.2 cm.

3 The ratio of 24-h creatinine excretion (in grams) to height (in centimeters), is a more accurate measure of muscle mass. Urine creatinine is related to lean body mass by the equation

Lean body mass (kg) $= 21.0 + 21.5 \times$ (g creatinine/24 h)

The creatinine/height ratio is the best clinical laboratory test for protein starvation. In normal men and women, the ratio averages 10.5 and 5.8 mg/cm, respectively. In men, ratios in the ranges 8.4 to 9.5, 7.4 to 8.4, and less than 7.4 mg/cm signify mild, moderate, and severe degrees of protein starvation, respectively.

4 Sagittal or horizontal radiograms of an extremity also provide quantitative information about the mass of representative skeletal muscles but are more expensive.

FIGURE 74-1

Anthropometric measurement of muscle and adipose compartments of the mid-upper arm. Midarm circumference is measured with a tape measure and triceps skin fold with a caliper. (After Butterworth and Blackburn.)

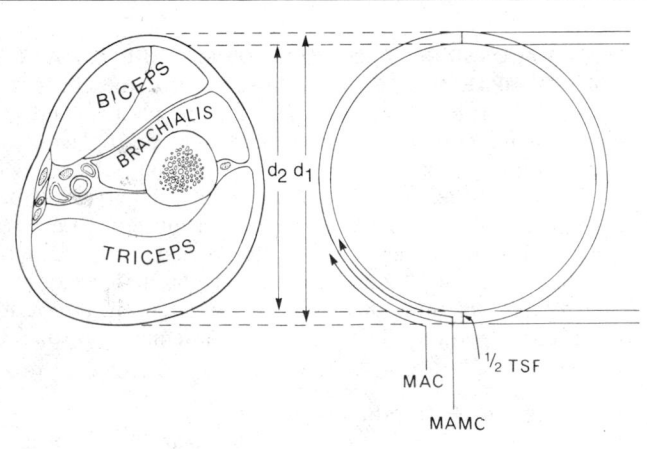

Calculation of mid upper arm muscle circumference

C_1 = mid upper arm circumference in centimeters

S = triceps skinfold in centimeters

d_1 = arm diameter

d_2 = muscle diameter

Skinfold (S) = 2 $\times$ subcutaneous fat

$\qquad$ = $d_1 - d_2$

Circumference (C_1) = πd_1

Muscle circumference (C_2) = πd_2

$\qquad\qquad$ = $\pi [d_1 - (d_1 - d_2)]$

$\qquad\qquad$ = $\pi d_1 - \pi (d_1 - d_2)$

$\qquad\qquad$ = $C_1 - \pi S$

Midarm circumference (adults), cm

Sex	Normal	>90% normal	90-60% normal	<60% normal
Male	29.3	>26.3	26.3-17.6	<17.6
Female	28.5	>25.7	25.7-17.1	<17.1

Midarm muscle circumference (adults), cm

Sex	Normal	>90% normal	90-60% normal	<60% normal
Male	25.3	>22.8	22.8-15.2	<15.2
Female	23.2	>20.9	20.9-13.9	<13.9

Triceps skinfold (adults), mm

Sex	Normal	>90% normal	90-60% normal	<60% normal
Male	12.5	>11.3	11.3-7.5	<7.5
Female	16.5	>14.9	14.9-9.9	<9.9

Skeletal muscle makes up about 30 percent of the lean body mass. This organ atrophies progressively in protein-energy starvation, the most common deficiency state in American hospitals (see Chap. 75). By monitoring the creatinine/height ratio and midarm muscle circumference, the clinician can identify protein-energy starvation easily and inexpensively and monitor its course.

SYNDROMES OF UNDERNUTRITION When any of the 36 essential nutrient requirements (Chap. 73) are not met, undernutrition syndromes result. Undernutrition of such macronutrients as nitrogen, sodium, chloride, potassium, calcium, and phosphorus reduces the mass of one or more body compartments, often with associated abnormalities in compartmental chemistry, structure, and function. For example, deficiencies of nitrogen (protein), sodium, and calcium erode protoplasm, extracellular fluid, and bone, respectively. Undernutrition of a micronutrient tends to cause a specific morphological or functional abnormality in certain tissues without alteration in compartmental mass or elemental composition. While in theory there are 36 different types of human malnutrition, undernutrition syndromes usually occur in groups rather than in "pure" form.

Deficiency of each essential nutrient can be characterized in terms of symptoms, signs, and chemical and radiographic abnormalities, but deficiency syndromes have several principles in common:

1 Undernutrition can be either primary or secondary in origin. The primary form is due to inadequate supply of food containing the essential nutrients. In secondary undernutrition adequate diet is available but, because of illness or medical treatment, nutrients cannot be ingested, absorbed, or metabolized adequately, or the rate of utilization or external losses is excessive. Primary and secondary mechanisms frequently reinforce each other; for example, the hypermetabolism and anorexia of infection precipitate nutritional deficiencies more rapidly in patients who previously subsisted on marginal diets than in well-nourished individuals. To determine whether undernutrition in a particular patient is primary or secondary, the physician must obtain a dietary history, assess personal income and living conditions, and examine the patient for organic disease.
2 Nutritional deficiency syndromes tend to evolve through three stages. Many essential nutrients are stored in the tissues of the well-nourished subject: for example, iron, folate, thiamine, pyridoxine, and vitamins B_{12}, A, and D in liver; essential fatty acids in adipose tissue; nitrogen in a labile reserve in muscle and liver. When intake falls below the daily requirement, these reserves temporarily forestall deficiency manifestations and maintain normal blood levels (stage 1). In stage 2, blood levels of the nutrient or nutrient-dependent metabolic products decline, but the patient continues to be asymptomatic. In stage 3, clinical signs and symptoms develop. Methods for assessing the nutritional status should ideally be capable of detecting all three stages of each deficiency syndrome. Available techniques, however, usually reveal only stages 2 and 3.
3 Because anorexia is a major mechanism in the current endemic of protein-energy undernutrition in hospitals in the United States, the intake of nutrients must be measured in one of three ways: by recall, by diary (outpatient), or by observation (inpatient).
4 Change in weight is ambiguous. In the absence of edema various proportions of weight loss are adipose tissue and lean body mass. In the presence of edema body weight changes are even more difficult to interpret. Gain in weight

can reflect accumulation of edema, masking erosion of protoplasm; loss of weight can reflect diuresis with simultaneous expansion of the protoplasmic compartment. An initially obese patient can lose 30 lb because of chronic wasting illness and present for the first medical examination with a normal body weight, the still substantial adipose organ masking a shrinkage in the lean body mass. For these reasons, direct or indirect estimation of the size of the protoplasmic compartment is essential as described above.
5 The undernourished patient is usually deficient in several nutrients. Common patterns are deficiency of both protein and energy, deficiency of two or more water-soluble vitamins (usually including folate, vitamin C, and/or thiamine), and deficiency of both Ca^{2+} and Mg^{2+} in patients with malabsorption.

The various physical, chemical, and radiographic characteristics of each type of undernutrition are summarized in Table 73-4. The most commonly used chemical indexes of nutrient deficiency are listed in Table 74-3, which gives three average concentration ranges for each test: normal, subnormal without clinical manifestations, and subnormal with clinical signs or symptoms of deficiency. Although these tests are of value in population surveys and in following the response of patients to therapy, the variation is such that they have limited diagnostic value (Chaps. 79 to 82).

The clinician must select a reasonable number of historical, physical, and laboratory items to use as a "nutritional data base" to screen patients for undernutrition. Table 74-4 presents a selection of historical and physical items that would reveal most deficiency states in hospital patients.

INVESTIGATING THE CAUSE OF MALNUTRITION The first issue is to distinguish between primary and secondary malnutrition. Socioeconomically determined primary malnutrition is the major variety worldwide. With improving socioeconomic conditions, primary malnutrition sufficient to cause symptoms is now uncommon in the United States. Subclinical deficiencies of protein, iron, folate, and ascorbate are still detectable in up to 40 percent of the population in some regions (see Chap. 75).

The prevalence of primary malnutrition is closely related to the nutrient density of the population's diet. A child or adult generally cannot ingest more than about 3000 g (or ml) of food, or 3500 cal, per day. To forestall a deficiency syndrome, recommended daily allowance (RDA) quantities of the 36 essential nutrients must be available in the food ingested. Foods meeting this requirement are said to have satisfactory nutrient density. The alarming prevalence of protein starvation (kwashiorkor) in certain African nations has been attributed to the critically low protein "density" in the bulky, root-based diet which is often available in large quantity but which can be consumed up to a limit of only about 3000 g per day. The quantity and quality of protein in this volume of root-based food are insufficient to prevent negative nitrogen balance and eventual protein starvation. Similarly, the substantial prevalence of subclinical primary nutritional deficiency in the United States may be related to the growing consumption of "snack foods" with low nutrient density ("empty calories"). Alcohol represents another type of "low nutrient density" food. For these reasons, evaluation of the undernourished patient's habitual dietary intake at home is of central importance

TABLE 74-3
Interpretation of laboratory tests for the evaluation of nutritional status (adults)

Test	Deficient (often with clinical manifestations)	Low (usually without clinical manifestations)	Acceptable	Nutrient evaluation
Serum iron, μg per 100 ml	<30	30–60	>60	Iron
Serum albumin, g per 100 ml	<3.0	3.0–3.5	>3.5	Protein
Plasma retinol, μg per 100 ml	<10	10–20	>20	Vitamin A
Serum folate, ng/ml	<3	3.0–6.0	>6.0	Folate
Erythrocyte folate, ng/ml	<140	140–160	>160	Folate
Serum vitamin B_{12}, pg/ml	<150	150–200	>200	Vitamin B_{12}
Serum ascorbic acid, mg per 100 ml	<0.20	0.20–0.30	>0.30	Vitamin C
Erythrocyte transketolase (% thiamine diphosphate stimulation)	>20	15–20	<15	Thiamine
Erythrocyte glutathione reductase activity coefficient	>1.40	1.20–1.40	<1.20	Riboflavin
Erythrocyte aminotransferase activity coefficients:				
EGPT	>1.25		<1.25	Vitamin B_6
EGOT	>2.0		<2.0	Vitamin B_6
Tryptophan load test (xanthurenic acid), mg per day	>50	25–50	<25	Vitamin B_6
N^1-Methylnicotinamide excretion, mg/g creatinine	<0.5	0.5–1.59	>1.6	Niacin
Serum Ca $\times$ P product, mg per 100 ml	<40		>40	Vitamin D
Alkaline phosphatase, King-Armstrong units per 100 ml	>40	15–40	8–14	Vitamin D
Hemoglobin, g per 100 ml	<12	12–14	>14	Protein, Fe, folate, vitamin B_{12}, pyridoxine, Cu
24-h urine K$^+$, meq	<20	20–40	>40	K
24-h urine Mg^{2+}, meq	<4	4–8	>8	Mg
24-h urine Ca^{2+}, mg	<50	50–100	>100	Ca
24-h urine Na$^+$, meq	<20	20–40	>40	Na
24-h urine P, mg	<100	100–300	>300	P
24-h urine urea N, g	<6	6–10	>10	Protein
Creatinine/height ratio	<90% of standard	90–95%	>95%	Protein

in searching for a possible primary etiology of the deficiency state.

In secondary undernutrition, a diet furnishing all the RDAs is available, but the patient becomes undernourished because of one or more problems: (1) inadequate intake (anorexia, dysphagia, coma, intestinal obstruction); (2) malabsorption; (3) inadequate utilization of nutrients (e.g., failure to activate vitamin D in renal or hepatic disease); (4) increased requirement (e.g., increased requirement for calories in fever or for folate in psoriasis or hemolytic anemia); (5) increased loss (iron in bleeding, electrolytes and calories in diarrhea); or (6) drug-nutrient interactions (see Chap. 73).

MONITORING THE COURSE OF MALNUTRITION Besides defining the type, severity, and mechanism for the development of undernutrition, it is important to ascertain its rate of pro-

FIGURE 74-2

Monitoring the course of a patient with protein-calorie depletion during repletion by nasogastric hyperalimentation.

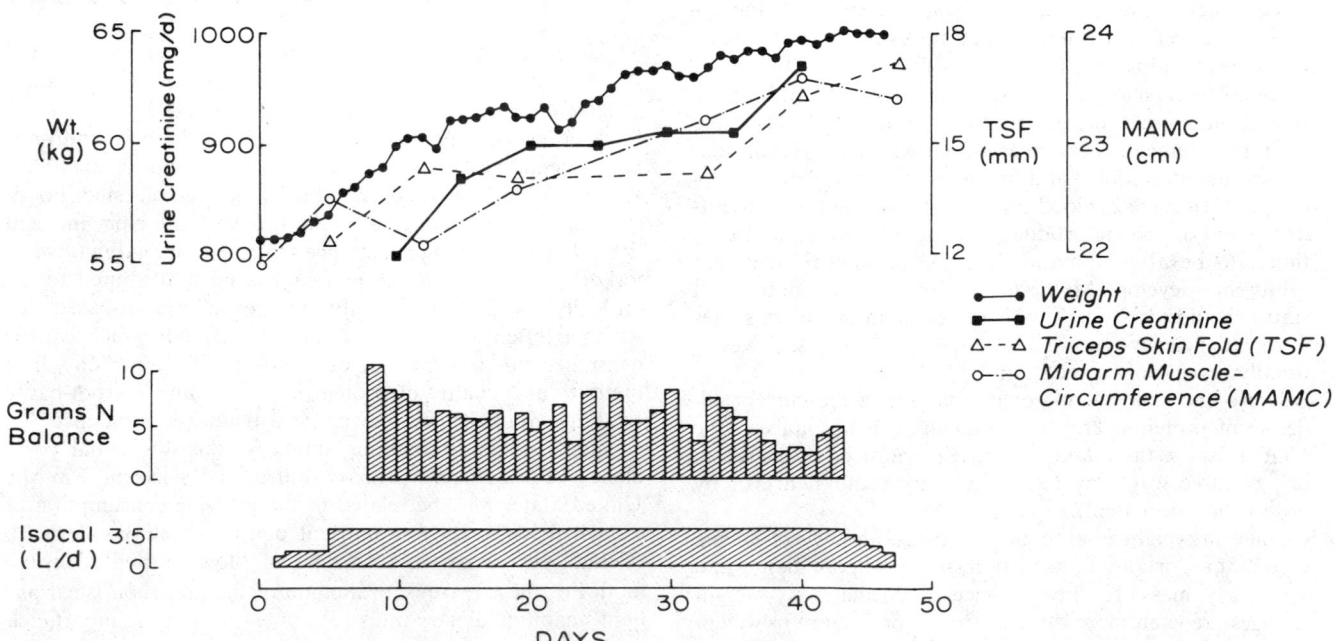

TABLE 74-4
Nutritional data base

HISTORY

Previous weight curve
Dietary intake by retrospective recall and prospective diary
Alcohol
Socioeconomic and family status, including income
Anorexia, vomiting, diarrhea
Blood loss
Pregnancy, lactation, menses
Vitamin and mineral supplements
Use of drugs which might affect nutrition

PHYSICAL EXAMINATION

General: Weight as percent of ideal body weight; triceps skin fold; midarm muscle circumference
Skin: Xerosis, follicular hyperkeratosis, pellagrous dermatitis, petechiae, ecchymoses, perifollicular hemorrhages, flaky paint dermatitis, pallor
Hair: Dyspigmentation, easy pluckability, thinning, straightening
Head: Temporal wasting, parotid enlargement
Eyes: Bitot's spots, conjunctival and scleral xerosis, keratomalacia, corneal vascularization, angular palpebritis
Mouth: Cheilosis, angular stomatitis, magenta tongue, atrophic lingual papillae, tongue fissuring, glossitis, spongy gums
Heart: Cardiomegaly, findings of congestive heart failure
Abdomen: Hepatomegaly
Extremities: Edema, koilonychia
Neurological: Irritability, weakness, calf tenderness, loss of deep tendon reflexes

gression. This is accomplished by periodic monitoring of body weight, albumin, hematocrit, creatinine excretion, midarm muscle circumference, triceps skin fold, and appropriate blood or urine concentrations of nutrition-dependent variables. An example of monitoring the course of progressive protein-energy malnutrition is shown in Fig. 74-2. A bedside estimate of daily nitrogen balance in grams can be made as follows:

$$\tfrac{1}{6} [\text{Daily protein intake in grams (estimated by hospital dietician)}] - (\text{24-h urine urea nitrogen in grams}) + 4 \text{ g}^1$$

The more negative the nitrogen balance, the more rapidly protein depletion progresses.

REFERENCES

ARROYAVE G et al: Assessment of protein nutritional status. Am J Clin Nutr 23:807, 1970

BUTTERWORTH CE, BLACKBURN GL: Hospital malnutrition and how to assess the nutritional status of a patient. Nutr Today 10:8, March/April 1974

JELLIFFE DB: *The Assessment of the Nutritional Status of the Community.* Geneva, World Health Organization, 1966

REIFENSTEIN EC JR et al: The accumulation, interpretation and presentation of data pertaining to metabolic balances, notably those of calcium, phosphorus and nitrogen. J Clin Endocrinol Metab 5:367, 1945

SAUBERLICH HE et al: *Laboratory Tests for the Assessment of Nutritional Status: Critical Reviews in Clinical Laboratory Sciences*, JW King, R Faulkner (eds). Cleveland, CRC Press, 1973, vol 4, no 3, pp 215–340

VITERI FE, ALVARADO J: The creatinine height index: Its use in the estimation of the degree of protein depletion and repletion in protein caloric malnourished children. Pediatrics 46:696, 1970

---

¹ *Four grams is the approximate sum of urinary nonurea nitrogen plus fecal and integumentary losses of nitrogen.*

75

PROTEIN-ENERGY UNDERNUTRITION

DANIEL RUDMAN

RELEVANCE TO CONTEMPORARY MEDICINE

Attention was focused on this deficiency state in the 1930s by physicians in developing nations. The syndrome affects structure and function of every organ in the body. The causes, manifestations, and treatment have been intensively studied in African and Asian children, in whom the prevalence of the primary form of the disease averages 25 percent. It is recognized that the secondary varieties of protein-energy deficiency are common within hospital populations in developed nations. Subacutely or chronically ill patients living longer under the protection of modern therapeutics but handicapped by anorexia, hypermetabolism, or malabsorption may rapidly develop protein-calorie deficiency.

DEFINITION AND ETIOLOGY

The syndrome consists of progressive loss of both lean body mass and adipose tissue. It results from insufficient consumption of protein and calories, although one or the other may play the dominant role in a given individual. The inadequate intake may be primary or secondary, as discussed in Chap. 74. Synergism between the two mechanisms is common. Patients with scanty reserves of protein and energy develop clinical protein-energy starvation more rapidly than well-nourished subjects when challenged by the hypermetabolism, catabolism, and anorexia of infection or other illnesses.

On a global basis, the primary mechanism predominates. Socioeconomic factors that limit the quantity and quality of the diet are paramount. Particularly important is the poor biologic value of many vegetable proteins. The problem is accentuated if calories are deficient, because a large proportion of the dietary amino acids must then be oxidized as fuel instead of used to synthesize tissue and plasma protein. In developed countries poverty is the most important cause of the syndrome, but the low nutrient densities of alcohol and snack foods play an important role in subclinical protein deficiency regardless of economic status.

EPIDEMIOLOGY

The prevalence of protein-energy undernutrition can be assessed by measuring percent reduction from normal in triceps skin fold, midarm muscle circumference, 24-h urinary creatinine/height ratio, and serum albumin (see Chap. 74).

Estimates of prevalence of protein-energy depletion in various population groups are given in Table 75-1. It is much more prevalent in Africa than in the United States. In the United States, subclinical protein deficiency is more common in the South than in the North and in blacks and Latin Americans than in whites. In contrast to developing nations, protein-energy depletion in the general population of the United States tends to be mild and subclinical. In hospitals, on the other hand, severe as well as mild deficiencies are frequently encountered. Protein-energy starvation is frequently associated with other types of malnutrition.

PATHOPHYSIOLOGY

Calorie and protein undernutrition have been studied most extensively in children of developing nations in whom inadequate or marginal diets, the augmented nutritional require-

TABLE 75-1
Prevalence of protein-energy malnutrition in selected groups

Group	Criterion of deficiency	Prevalence of deficiency, %
Pregnant or lactating women, United States*	<3.5 g albumin per 100 ml serum	50
Children <5 years, 28 developing countries†	Body weight <80% (kwashiorkor) or <60% of standard (marasmus)	25
General surgical patients 1 week post-operative, Leeds, England‡	Midarm muscle circumference, triceps skin fold, serum albumin more than two standard deviations below normal mean	50
Heart valve recipients, postoperative, London§	Total body ⁴⁰K less than 87% of standard	40
General surgical patients, Boston City Hospital¶	Midarm muscle circumference, triceps skin fold, serum albumin more than two standard deviations below normal mean	48

* J Carter, US Department of Health, Education, and Welfare Publication no (HSM) 72-8132, 1971.
† JM Bengou, J Trop Pediatr 13:169, 1967.
‡ GL Hill et al, Lancet 1:689, 1977.
§ RK Walesby, Lancet 1:76, 1978.
¶ BR Bistrain et al, JAMA 230:858, 1974.

ments of infancy, and frequent episodes of infectious disease combine to cause florid deficiency manifestations. Two syndromes have been distinguished: (1) *marasmus,* caused primarily by deficiency of calories and manifested by stunted growth, loss of adipose tissue, and generalized wasting of lean body mass without edema; and (2) *kwashiorkor,* in which calories are adequate but protein is deficient. This syndrome is manifested by growth failure (in children), hypoalbuminemia, edema, fatty liver, and preservation of adipose tissue. Mixed forms (kwashiorkor-marasmus) are common. It is likely that similar principles apply to protein-energy malnutrition in adults.

METABOLIC AND ENDOCRINE ASPECTS   Calorie deficiency When the intake of calories falls below the daily requirement, the body responds with an orderly physiologic adaptation (see Chap. 86), engineered in large part by a reduced secretion of insulin, augmented plasma levels of glucagon and cortisol, and curtailed hepatic production of triiodothyronine (T_3) from thyroxine (T_4). The fall in plasma insulin permits free fatty acids and amino acids to be mobilized from adipose tissue and muscle to provide carbon for the continuing oxidative metabolism of the body. When energy balance is negative, oxidative metabolism claims first priority in the utilization of dietary protein. During starvation, the carbon chains of amino acids also provide substrate for gluconeogenesis, since a continuing supply of glucose is required by the central nervous system. As amino acids are diverted from protein synthesis into oxidative metabolism and gluconeogenesis, protein synthesis in the body is curtailed, particularly in muscle. The metabolic rate gradually declines, because of diminished extrathyroidal conversion of T_4 to T_3, decreased synthesis of the T_3 receptor, curtailed production and turnover of catecholamines, and loss of the specific dynamic action of the dietary components. During partial or total deprivation of calories, both lean body mass and adipose tissue contract, but the latter does so more rap-

idly. The progress of the consumption of adipose tissue and muscle can be followed at the bedside by such clinical indicators as measurement of the triceps skin fold, midarm muscle circumference, and creatinine/height ratio.

During the first week of total starvation, the average patient loses 4 to 5 kg of body weight which consists of about 25 percent adipose tissue, 35 percent extracellular fluid, and 40 percent protoplasm. Losses of nitrogen, potassium, sodium, and chloride represent 3 to 8 percent of the body content of each element. Negative balances of magnesium, phosphorus, and calcium are also considerable. During ensuing weeks, as further adaptive endocrine and enzymatic adjustments occur, losses of nitrogen and other elements continue but at a slower rate. The intracellular compartment does not contract at the same rate in all tissues. The central nervous system does not lose weight. Skeletal muscle atrophies more rapidly than cardiac muscle, while gastrointestinal tract and liver lose mass more rapidly than kidneys. Mobilization of amino acids from muscle to liver permits the latter organ to continue to synthesize some albumin and lipoproteins; as a consequence hypoalbuminemia and fatty liver are not conspicuous.

Protein deficiency   Frequently the intake of protein is more limited than that of calories. This occurs because dietary protein is more expensive than carbohydrate or fat; because protein of high biologic value (chiefly animal) is more expensive than protein of low biologic value (chiefly vegetable); because high-calorie, low-protein foods (many snack foods, ethanol, starchy root-based vegetables) are in frequent use in the United States and abroad; and because physicians often use glucose as the sole organic nutrient in the intravenous feeding of the patient who cannot eat. The deficiency state under these conditions is analogous to kwashiorkor in children. The reduction of insulin secretion, which is a central mechanism in the adaptation to energy starvation, is circumvented. Insulin secreted in response to the dietary or intravenous carbohydrate promotes lipogenesis and retards lipolysis; adipose tissue is well-preserved, and free fatty acids are not available for oxidation in place of amino acids. The high-plasma insulin also impairs mobilization and redistribution of muscle amino acids from skeletal muscle to liver. Plasma amino acids fall, and the total body rate of protein synthesis declines. Fatty infiltration of the liver is common. Two biochemical mechanisms are probably involved: (1) lack of methionine limits phospholipid synthesis, secondarily impairing lipoprotein formation, and (2) hepatic synthesis of triglycerides from glucose continues. In the blood decreased concentrations of albumin, transferrin, and hemoglobin reflect severe protein starvation. Edema is characteristic of this stage.

Variable degrees of calorie and protein starvation occur together.

Mineral metabolism   Protein-energy undernutrition is generally associated with depletion of body minerals. In part this reflects the contraction of protoplasmic and extracellular fluid compartments with their constituent elements (nitrogen, phosphorus, potassium, and magnesium within cells; sodium and chloride in extracellular fluid) being excreted into the urine in the same proportions as in the lean body mass. However, mineral losses are often out of proportion to the contraction of lean body mass. One reason is a shift of potassium and magnesium from muscle to plasma in exchange for sodium. In addition, potassium, magnesium, phosphorus, and calcium intakes may be even less adequate than those of protein and calories (e.g., during prolonged intravenous nutrition with magnesium- or phosphorus-free solutions). Finally, renal and extrarenal losses of these elements may be significant (diuresis, diarrhea, fistulas, etc.).

CARDIOVASCULAR-RESPIRATORY AND RENAL RESPONSES

The heart and kidneys lose mass progressively during the course of protein-energy starvation. These losses are generally proportional to the erosion of lean body mass, so that ratios of heart mass/lean body mass and kidney mass/lean body mass remain normal. Consequently functional insufficiency of these two shrunken organs is not a usual feature of protein-energy depletion. Cardiac output declines in parallel with the falling metabolic rate. Blood pressure is reduced by the fall in cardiac output. The ventilatory response to hypoxia is blunted. Glomerular filtration rate and renal blood flow are lowered. The ability of the kidney to excrete an acid load or to respond to antidiuretic hormone may be impaired. Although these changes in cardiac and renal structure and function are appropriate to the reduced lean body mass and hypometabolic state, they may become important handicaps during vigorous nutritional repletion, acute infection, or other circumstances that require rapid increases in cardiac output, metabolic rate, and urinary excretion of solutes.

BLOOD

Reduced blood volume, hematocrit, albumin, and transferrin are characteristic in the wasted patient. The anemia of "pure" protein-energy depletion is normocytic and normochromic and usually results from decreased production of red blood cells, perhaps reflecting the protein requirement for globin synthesis. Frequently deficiencies of iron, folate, or pyridoxine contribute to the anemia.

STRUCTURE AND FUNCTION OF GASTROINTESTINAL TRACT AND PANCREAS

The gastrointestinal tract and pancreas atrophy. In the small intestine, villous height, mitotic index, and content of disaccharidases and dipeptidases all decline. Exocrine elements of the pancreas atrophy as well, and the production of digestive enzymes is reduced. Bacterial overgrowth may occur in the small intestine. These factors combine to produce malabsorption and lactose intolerance. The structural and functional regression of the small intestine results, at least in part, from decreased oral feeding rather than systemic malnutrition, since patients fully nourished by the parenteral route exhibit the same lesion.

IMMUNE SYSTEM

Lymphatic tissues atrophy. Impaired cell-mediated immunity is evident by all standard tests (blastogenic response of lymphocytes to mitogens, total lymphocyte count, and skin testing with recall antigens). Bactericidal activity of polymorphonuclear leukocytes is decreased. Plasma immunoglobulin concentrations and humoral responses to antigens are preserved. Protein-energy starved patients experience increased morbidity and mortality during common infections compared with well-nourished groups and are subject to infection by opportunistic organisms (gram-negative bacteria, *Candida*, herpes simplex). Cachectic patients do not manifest the usual reactions to infection; hypothermia, delayed healing of wounds, paucity of polymorphonuclear cells, and increased degree of tissue necrosis at sites of infection are all characteristic.

WOUND HEALING

The fibroblastic response to surgical wounds is impaired by protein-energy depletion. Consequently, incisions and enteric anastomoses heal more slowly in undernourished patients; wound dehiscence is common.

TEMPERATURE REGULATION

In severe protein-energy starvation in the absence of fever, basal metabolic rate is reduced. Hypothermia is frequent. The underlying mechanisms are reduced heat production due to exhaustion of carbohydrate and fat reserves, low plasma T_3, possible decreased adrenergic function, and loss of thermal insulation when subcutaneous adipose tissue is gone. Hypoglycemia is occasionally seen (see Chap. 340).

REPRODUCTION

Nearly every phase of the reproductive process is impaired by protein deficiency in the mother's diet. Fertility is reduced. If implantation occurs, there is a high risk of early fetal resorption. If gestation is completed, the progeny are substandard in weight and length. Lactation is impaired by protein starvation, so that undernutrition is common postnatally. Even if postnatal nutrition is adequate, stunted growth in the infant is in part irreversible, and life-long impairment in learning capacity may result.

PATHOLOGICAL CHANGES

In the child growth is stunted, weight more than height. At all ages the body is wasted and may be edematous. Ascites is common. Subcutaneous fat may be totally absent (advanced calorie depletion) or variably preserved (protein starvation). Involution is most pronounced in adipose tissue, thymolymphatic system, spleen, exocrine glands, skeletal muscle, gastrointestinal tract, and pancreas. The gastrointestinal tract is thin and distended; rectal prolapse is common. The size and fat content of the liver are variable. Heart and kidney size are decreased in proportion to the loss of nonedematous body weight. Pituitary, thyroid, and adrenal glands are atrophic. Muscle atrophy is invariable. Terminal infection is common, often with opportunistic organisms; there is less inflammatory reaction and more tissue necrosis, including gangrenous ulcers, than in well-nourished cadavers bearing evidence of terminal infection.

Skin is atrophic, dyspigmented, scaly, and frequently ulcerated. The cornea is dry, atrophic, and often ulcerated.

No microscopic lesions are specific in protein-energy starvation. Adipose tissue is atrophic. Mitotic figures in proliferating tissues are decreased compared with those of patients who die with normal nutriture. Enzyme granules and ribosomes are less prominent in exocrine glands. The liver is often fatty. Muscle and kidney show nonspecific hyalinization and cloudy swelling. Germinal centers are absent in lymph nodes. Columnar epithelium tends to become cuboidal, villi are flat, and the brush border atrophies in many cells.

CLINICAL MANIFESTATIONS

HISTORY

A primary component in the etiology can be uncovered only by reviewing the intakes of protein and calories and the biological quality of the dietary protein during the months before the clinical examination. Suggestive of a primary component are poverty, alcoholism, habitual consumption of "low nutrient density" foods, solitary life-style, and old age. Suggestive of a secondary etiology are the presence of a known chronic medical problem, anorexia or other gastrointestinal symptoms (including lack of teeth), or prolonged fever.

In children, failure to gain height and weight is an early sign. In adults, weight loss usually occurs. However, in the adult a body weight equal to or greater than ideal does not rule out the presence of deficiency of calories, protein, or both. Thus progressive loss of protoplasm and adipose tissue may be masked by accumulating edema; or the patient may have been previously obese, and a substantial loss of lean body mass during the current illness may be masked by a residue of obesity. Listlessness, easy fatigability, sensation of coldness, swollen ankles, and dry, cracked skin are frequent symptoms in patients eating insufficient protein or calories.

PHYSICAL SIGNS

The facies is drawn, temporal regions are concave and fleshless, intercostal spaces are excavated, and the skin hangs in folds on the wasted extremities. "Flaky paint" dermatitis and dyspigmentation of skin and hair are common. The patient is pale and may be edematous. Signs of deficiency of water-soluble or fat-soluble vitamins may be present. Decubiti and skin ulcers are typical in advanced stages.

VITAL SIGNS Blood pressure is decreased. Pulse is slow, and extremities are cool; central temperature may be decreased.

ANTHROPOMETRICS Triceps skin fold and midarm muscle circumference are reduced in varying ratios dependent on preillness nutritional state and relative severity of the energy and protein deficiencies.

LABORATORY AND X-RAY FINDINGS Twenty-four-hour urinary creatinine/height ratio is decreased. This is the most sensitive and practical clinical indicator of protein starvation and should be monitored at weekly intervals in the chronically ill hospital patient. The excretion of 3-methylhistidine has similar significance but is more difficult to measure. These analyses should be done only in afebrile patients, since urinary excretion of both creatinine and 3-methylhistidine is increased by fever. Other signs include decrease in serum albumin, serum transferrin, and hematocrit, but these changes are less specific. Nevertheless, protein depletion may be the most common cause of hypoalbuminemia in hospitalized patients, even in patients with hepatic disease. Serum essential and nonessential amino acid concentration and urine urea and creatinine levels are reduced. T-lymphocyte cell function is decreased, as revealed by cutaneous anergy and peripheral lymphopenia (absolute lymphocyte count < 1200 cells per cubic millimeter). Glucose tolerance is impaired. Plasma cortisol is often increased (in part because of retarded metabolic clearance). T_3 is decreased, reverse T_3 may be increased, and basal metabolic rate is low. Heart size is small on chest film. Echocardiography shows a small heart with decreased cardiac output. Sagittal or cross-sectional x-rays of arm show diminished muscle mass.

COURSE A typical case is illustrated in Fig. 75-1. In children, an early manifestation is slowing of growth. As the protein-energy depletion becomes more severe, pallor, fatigue, and

FIGURE 75-1
Course of a typical case of progressive protein-energy starvation.

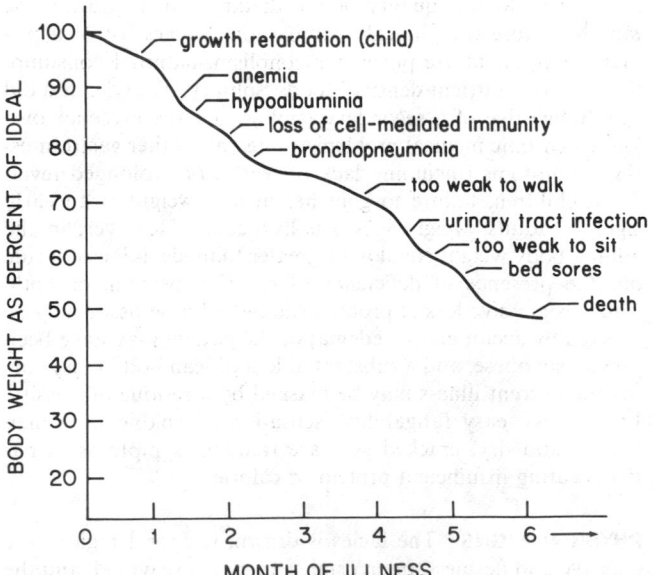

TABLE 75-2
Undesirable practices affecting the nutritional health of hospital patients

1 Failure to record height and weight on admission.
2 Lack of a weight curve in the hospital chart.
3 Prolonged use of glucose and saline intravenous feedings.
4 Failure to measure patient's food intake.
5 Withholding meals because of diagnostic tests.
6 Use of tube feedings of inadequate amount and uncertain composition.
7 Ignorance of the composition of nutritional products.
8 Failure to recognize increased nutritional needs due to injury or illness.
9 Delay of nutrition support until the patient is in an advanced state of depletion.
10 Limited availability of laboratory tests to assess nutritional status; failure to use those that are available.
11 Failure to correct inadequate dentition or the edentulous state.

SOURCE: *After Butterworth.*

amenorrhea appear. Loss of cell-mediated immunity predisposes to infections. The hypermetabolism and anorexia of intercurrent infection accelerate the progress of the cachexia. In advanced undernutrition (triceps skin fold < 3 mm, creatinine/height ratio < 60 percent of standard), decubiti, hypothermia, and terminal infection are the rule.

RELATION TO OTHER DEFICIENCY STATES Usually other nutrients are also depleted. Folic acid, thiamine, riboflavin, nicotinic acid, pyridoxine, ascorbic acid and vitamin A deficiencies are relatively common in hospital populations in the United States (see Table 75-2). Body content of most minerals is also reduced, but a distinction must be made between absolute and relative decreases. As protoplasmic protein is consumed to supply metabolic fuel and substrate for gluconeogenesis in the underfed patient, the intracellular minerals potassium, phosphorus, magnesium and perhaps some of the microminerals are excreted in parallel with the nitrogen. Such loss is absolute but not relative, since the intracellular and extracellular concentrations of potassium, phosphorus, and magnesium usually remain normal. If the diet is specifically deficient in potassium, phosphorus, or magnesium, a further relative deficiency occurs, with the intracellular and perhaps the extracellular and urinary concentrations becoming subnormal. Similar considerations apply to the body content of essential fatty acids. Whether the depletion of potassium, phosphorus, magnesium, or essential fatty acids is absolute or relative, repletion with a feeding solution that contains little or none of that nutrient may lead to chemical and clinical manifestations of the corresponding deficiency state within a few days. Life-threatening hypokalemia, hypophosphatemia, or hypomagnesemia can occur. By similar mechanisms, plasma levels of trace minerals regularly decline during hyperalimentation if adequate rations of these nutrients are not provided.

REFERENCES

ALLEYNE GAO et al: *Protein-Energy Malnutrition.* London, Butler & Tanner, 1977
BISTRIAN BR et al: Protein status of general surgical patients. JAMA 230:858, 1974
——— et al: Prevalence of malnutrition in general medical patients. JAMA 235:1567, 1976
BOLLET AJ, OWENS S: Evaluation of nutritional status of selected hospitalized patients. Am J Clin Nutr 26:931, 1973
BUTTERWORTH CE: The skeleton in the hospital closet. Nutr Today 9:4, March/April 1974
———, BLACKBURN GL: Hospital malnutrition and how to assess the nutritional status of a patient. Nutr Today 10:8, March/April 1975

CAHILL GF: Starvation in man. N Engl J Med 282:668, 1970

GEEFHUYSEN J et al: Impaired cellular immunity in kwashiorkor with improvement after therapy. Br Med J 27:527, 1971

HANSEN RG: An index of food quality. Nutr Rev 31:1, 1973

LAW DK et al: Immunocompetence of patients with protein-calorie malnutrition. Ann Intern Med 79:545, 1973

LEEVY CM et al: Incidence and significance of hypovitaminemia in a randomly selected municipal hospital population. Am J Clin Nutr 17:259, 1965

NICOL BM: Protein and calorie concentration. Nutr Rev 29:83, 1971

Ten-State Nutrition Survey, 1968-1970, US Department of Health, Education, and Welfare Publication no (HSM) 72-8131, 1972

WHITEHEAD RG ALLEYNE GAO: Pathophysiological factors of importance in protein-calorie malnutrition. Br Med J 28:72, 1972

76
OBESITY

JERROLD M. OLEFSKY

The ability to store food energy as fat has provided significant survival value to organisms living in environments in which food supply is scarce or sporadic. Unlike glycogen or protein, triglyceride does not require water or electrolytes for storage purposes and can be retained essentially as pure fat; 1 g adipose tissue yields close to the full theoretical equivalent of 9 kcal. Because of the efficient storage of energy in adipose tissue, an individual of normal weight can survive up to 2 months of total starvation. However, Western society is generally not characterized by periodic or insufficient food supply but rather by constant and abundant food. As a consequence, the ability to store fat all too frequently becomes of negative survival value because of overconsumption and the resulting obesity.

DEFINITION AND INCIDENCE Obesity can most easily be assessed using a subject's height and weight. One way to do this is to relate the patient's weight to an average range for his height and age. This measure of relative weight leads to an underestimation of the problem, however, since in the United States the "average" individual is somewhat obese. Tables of ideal or desirable weight provide more meaningful information and are based on actuarial estimates of what is consistent with normal life expectancy. Such tables are more useful if adjusted for differences in body build. Although relative weight correlates fairly well with the degree of adiposity, excess poundage can be either lean or fat tissue. Obviously, with this measurement, heavily muscled individuals would be considered obese. More precise measurements of obesity are based on body density or isotopic dilution methods, but these are too complicated for routine clinical use. Anthropometry is a simpler but accurate method for measuring the degree of adiposity. Skin fold thickness can be measured over various areas of the body and along with height, weight, and age can be used to assess the degree of adiposity. Triceps and subscapular skin folds are most commonly employed (see Chap. 74).

Obesity is often defined as an excess of adipose tissue, but the meaning of *excess* is hard to define. Aesthetic considerations aside, the clinical diagnosis of obesity can best be viewed as the degree of excess adiposity that imparts a health risk. This cutoff can only be approximated. The Framingham study demonstrated that a 20 percent excess over ideal weight imparted a health risk; by use of that criterion 20 to 30 percent of men and 30 to 40 percent of women are obese.

ETIOLOGY When caloric intake exceeds expenditure, the excess calories are stored as fat tissue; the net balance between these two variables regulates the amount of adipose tissue in the body. Many obese patients firmly believe they suffer from a "metabolic problem," but this is rarely the case. Abnormal eating behavior is the essential cause of the problem.

The regulation of eating behavior is incompletely understood. To some extent, appetite is controlled by discrete areas in the hypothalamus. A feeding center is located in the ventrolateral nucleus of the hypothalamus (VLH), and a satiety center is present in the ventromedial hypothalamus (VMH). The cerebral cortex receives positive signals from the feeding center that stimulate eating (Fig. 76-1), and the satiety center modulates this process by sending inhibitory impulses to the feeding center. Destruction of the feeding center in animals results in decreased food intake, while destruction of the satiety center leads to overeating and gross obesity. Several regulatory processes have been proposed as modulators of these hypothalamic centers. The satiety center may be activated by the surges in plasma glucose and/or insulin that follow a meal. It is of interest that the VMH contains insulin receptors and is insulin-sensitive. Meal-induced gastric distention is another possible inhibitory factor. The total adipose tissue mass may also influence the activity of the hypothalamic centers; i.e., there is a relatively fixed "set point" for the body's degree of adiposity. An elevated set point may account for the frequent recidivism in obese patients who have lost weight. How the "set point" is established and the mechanism by which the hypothalamus senses total fat stores are unknown. Glycerol release from fat cells and ascending neural impulses have been

FIGURE 76-1

The regulation of eating. The ventromedial satiety center is considered to be inhibitory, and the ventrolateral feeding center stimulatory. See text for discussion.

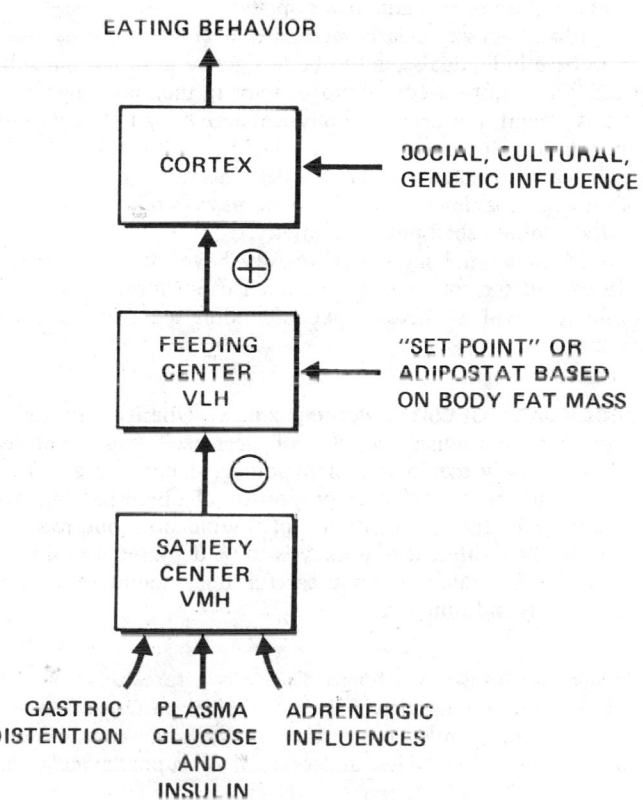

suggested as signals of adipose tissue size. Additionally, the hypothalamic centers are sensitive to catecholamines, and beta-adrenergic stimulation inhibits eating behavior. This provides at least one rationale for the anorexant effects of amphetamines.

Ultimately, the cerebral cortex controls eating behavior, and impulses from the feeding center to the cerebral cortex are only one input. Psychological, social, and genetic factors also influence food intake. In many obese subjects these influences are overriding; indeed, obese patients usually respond to external signals such as time of day, social setting, and smell or taste of food to a greater extent than do normal persons.

Although overeating is the cause of obesity in the majority of patients, other factors may participate—at least in certain individuals. Daily caloric needs range between 31 and 35 kcal per kilogram of body weight; this figure is somewhat higher in active and somewhat lower in sedentary individuals. With rare exceptions overly efficient utilization of food energy or decreased metabolic rate have not been documented in obesity. However, a distinction must be made between *static obesity* and the actual *process of gaining weight*. When normal subjects consume hypercaloric diets, less weight is gained than would be predicted on the basis of the excess calories ingested. This effect is most marked when carbohydrate is consumed and disappears when the excess calories consist of fat. Thus, humans can apparently adapt to chronic excessive carbohydrate and protein intake, and this protective effect attenuates the weight gain. Part of this adaptive response is related to an increase in thermogenesis. The mechanism of the increase in thermogenesis is unknown, but overeating of carbohydrate or mixed nutrients leads to increased plasma levels of triiodothyronine (T_3) and decreased levels of reverse T_3 (rT_3). A converse effect is seen in starvation with decreased T_3 and increased rT_3 levels. The conversion of thyroxine to T_3 occurs largely in the liver; excess food may induce adaptive thermogenesis by increasing the concentration of T_3 relative to that of T_4 and rT_3. An interesting postulate is that in certain individuals obesity results from a failure of this adaptive response.

Physical activity clearly modulates overall caloric balance, and obese individuals tend to be less active than normal subjects. This can be a contributory factor in the maintenance of excess weight, but decreased physical activity is unlikely to be important as a *cause* of major weight gain. Rather, obesity itself leads to inactivity. The modest increase in weight that often accompanies the middle years may be related more directly to diminished physical activity.

Certain animal models of obesity have clear-cut genetic causes, but the role of genetic influences in human obesity is difficult to evaluate because of confounding social and cultural factors.

SECONDARY OBESITY Hypothyroidism

Obesity can result from hypothyroidism because of decreased caloric needs. However, only a minority of hypothyroid patients are truly obese, and an even smaller proportion of obese patients are hypothyroid. Indiscriminate use of thyroid hormone replacement in the treatment of obesity is to be deplored and should never be instituted without careful documentation of decreased thyroid function.

Cushing's disease Cushing's disease is a rare cause of obesity. Hyperadrenocorticism elicits a typical pattern of obesity with predominantly centripetal fat stores, characteristic rounded or moon facies, and cervical or supraclavicular fat deposits.

Insulinoma Hyperinsulinemia, secondary to an insulinoma, can occasionally cause obesity, presumably because of increased caloric intake secondary to recurrent hypoglycemia. Most patients with islet-cell tumors and hypoglycemia are not obese.

Hypothalamic disorders Froehlich's syndrome is characterized by obesity and hypogonadotrophic hypogonadism in boys with other variable features such as diabetes insipidus, visual impairment, and mental retardation. The anterior pituitary is usually normal, and the syndrome is thought to be the result of hypothalamic dysfunction. Occasionally pituitary tumors are present (as in Froehlich's original case) which may physically impair the hypothalamus. Most likely this syndrome includes a number of overlapping disorders having in common a hypothalamic lesion that leads to overeating and to hypogonadotrophism.

Other rare diseases include the Laurence-Moon-Biedl syndrome characterized by retinitis pigmentosa, mental retardation, skull deformities, polydactyly and syndactyly, and the Prader-Willi syndrome which is associated with hypotonia, mental retardation, and a predilection for diabetes mellitus. Both of these disorders also feature obesity and hypogonadism that are thought to be hypothalamic in origin.

PATHOLOGICAL SEQUELAE

Increased adipose tissue stores are deposited subcutaneously around all internal organs, throughout the omentum, and in the intramuscular spaces. Obese individuals also have an expansion of lean body mass as evidenced by increased size of the kidneys, heart, liver, and skeletal muscle mass. Fatty livers are common in extreme obesity.

Adipocyte size and number Obese individuals can be classified on the basis of the relative degree of *adipocyte hypertrophy* versus *hyperplasia*. In several rodent species and in humans the capacity to increase adipocyte number exists for only a limited period in early life. Sometime prior to reaching adulthood the organism's ability to increase the number of adipocytes ceases, and after this time expansion of adipose tissue mass is accomplished solely by an increase in fat-cell size. Thus, overnutrition during the time of preadipocyte proliferation leads to a permanent change in cell number and an increase in cell size; later nutritional alterations influence only cell size. Cross-sectional studies in humans have demonstrated that *individuals with severe obesity have both increased adipocyte size and number* with a tendency toward onset of obesity early in life. Patients having mild to moderate obesity show *only fat-cell hypertrophy,* and the onset of obesity is during adult life. Impressive supporting evidence for this formulation has been provided by studies showing that when adult men are made experimentally obese by purposeful overfeeding, fat-cell size, but not number, increases. Weight reduction is accompanied only by a decrease in adipocyte size. It is possible that preadipocyte proliferation from adipoblasts, usually a phenomenon of early life, can also occur at additional critical points such as puberty and early adolescence.

METABOLIC SEQUELAE

Obesity has a profound impact on diabetes mellitus and various hyperlipoproteinemias primarily through its influences on insulin secretion and insulin sensitivity (see Chaps. 100 and 338).

Hyperinsulinemia: insulin resistance Increased insulin secretion is a well-characterized feature of obesity. It occurs in the basal state and in response to a wide variety of insulinogenic agents. A correlation exists between the degree of obesity and the magnitude of the hyperinsulinemia—particularly the basal insulin levels. Some obese patients exhibit hyperglycemia or frank diabetes in the face of hyperinsulinemia. The combination of hyper- or euglycemia and hyperinsulinemia indicates an insulin-resistant state, and decreased hypoglycemic responses to insulin are common in obese humans and animals. Insulin resistance could be due to an abnormal beta-cell product, circulating insulin antagonists, or tissue insulin insensitivity. Since abnormal islet secretory products or circulating antagonists have not been identified, it is thought that the insulin resistance of obesity is primarily due to tissue insensitivity. The initial step in the cellular action of insulin involves binding to specific cell surface receptors located in target tissues. After the formation of the plasma membrane–insulin receptor complex, insulin's biological effects are initiated. Cells from obese animals and humans contain decreased numbers of insulin receptors, and this decrease in insulin receptors doubtless plays an important role in the insulin resistance of obesity. However, other factors may participate. The enlarged adipocytes of obese rats have a decrease in insulin receptors but an even greater defect in the capacity to metabolize glucose, suggesting a major biochemical abnormality distal to the receptor mechanism. Since adipose tissue accounts for only a small ($<$ 5 percent) portion of total body glucose metabolism, a similar intracellular defect presumably exists in other major insulin target tissues such as muscle and liver. Both decreased insulin receptors and intracellular defects in glucose metabolism probably contribute to the overall tissue insulin resistance in obesity.

Diabetes mellitus Although only a minority of obese patients are diabetic, the converse is not the case. Nonketotic, insulin-independent patients compose about 90 percent of the diabetic population in the United States, and 80 to 90 percent of nonketotic diabetics are obese. Obesity is an important contributory factor in these patients, predominantly through its influences on insulin sensitivity. Obesity exacerbates the diabetic state, and in many cases diabetes can be ameliorated by weight reduction.

Hyperlipoproteinemia (see also Chap. 100) Most plasma cholesterol circulates in the low-density lipoprotein (LDL) fraction, and, in the fasting state, very low density lipoproteins (VLDL) contain most of the circulating triglyceride. The association between obesity and elevated LDL levels is modest at best, and this is especially true when the relationship is corrected for other factors such as age. Total body cholesterol is increased in obesity, but this is mainly accounted for by adipose tissue cholesterol stores. Cholesterol turnover may be increased in obesity, leading to increased biliary excretion of cholesterol. This may contribute to the increased incidence of gallstone formation in obese individuals. Obesity has a more clear-cut and pronounced effect on VLDL metabolism. Hypertriglyceridemia is frequent, and the degree of obesity correlates with the level of hypertriglyceridemia. The increased triglyceride levels are due to increased hepatic VLDL production with no defect in the removal of VLDL from plasma. As discussed above, plasma insulin levels are greatly elevated in obesity, particularly in the portal blood. Hyperinsulinemia can promote increased hepatic VLDL synthesis and secretion. In addition, increased plasma free fatty acid (FFA) turnover exists in obesity, and FFA extracted by the liver provides an important precursor for hepatic triglyceride synthesis. Thus, the hypertriglyceridemia in obesity may be secondary to increased hepatic VLDL secretion due to hyperinsulinemia and augmented FFA availability.

MANIFESTATIONS AND COMPLICATIONS Gross obesity produces mechanical and physical stresses that aggravate or directly cause a number of disorders including osteoarthritis (es-

pecially the hips) and sciatica. Additionally, varicose veins, thromboembolism, ventral and hiatal hernias, and cholelithiasis are more common than in individuals of normal weight.

Hypertension In significantly obese persons, use of the standard size blood pressure cuff leads to readings which are erroneously high; an oversize cuff should always be used. A strong association between hypertension and obesity is observed even when accurate measurements are obtained. The mechanisms whereby obesity causes hypertension are uncertain, but peripheral vascular resistance is usually normal, while blood volume is increased. Weight loss leads to significant reductions in systemic blood pressure independent of changes in sodium balance.

Hypoventilation syndrome (Pickwickian syndrome) The obesity-hypoventilation syndrome is a heterogeneous group of disorders with differing clinical manifestations. The hypersomnolence that can occur in obesity is a manifestation of nighttime sleep apnea. In these individuals, once sleep begins, upper airway obstruction leads to hypoxemia and hypercapnia, causing arousal with return of normal respiration. Many such episodes occur each night, leading to chronic sleep deprivation and daytime somnolence. The combination of the obese habitus plus sleep-induced relaxation of the pharyngeal musculature is believed to be the cause of the intermittent upper airway obstruction. Occasionally such episodes are life-threatening (causing serious cardiac arrhythmias) and require long-term tracheostomy therapy. Chronic daytime hypoventilation is common but usually is not as severe as that occurring during sleep. Abnormalities of the respiratory control centers may also be important. Patients with hypoventilation display blunted ventilatory responses to hypercapnia and hypoxia and often develop hypercapnia and hypoxemia due to decreased basal ventilation; in addition, ventilation/perfusion mismatch due to mechanical factors may be present. In severe cases polycythemia, pulmonary hypertension, and cor pulmonale can result. Weight reduction will reverse these abnormalities if instituted before permanent cardiac damage develops. Some obese patients with sleep apnea and hypersomnolence do not have daytime hypoventilation and have normal ventilatory responses to hypoxia and hypercapnia. Progestational agents have been used therapeutically in the obesity-hypoventilation syndrome since they stimulate the ventilatory response to hypercarbia and hypoxia in normal subjects. Medroxyprogesterone increases ventilation and improves heart failure and erythrocytosis in these patients, although obstructive sleep apnea continues.

Adrenal function Although Cushing's disease can usually be distinguished from simple obesity on purely clinical grounds, laboratory testing is occasionally necessary. This can lead to confusion since 24-h urinary 17-hydroxycorticoid excretion is often elevated in obesity. Less commonly, plasma cortisol levels are also increased. Corticosteroid levels are usually suppressible with dexamethasone in obesity, but occasionally suppression is incomplete, rendering the diagnosis difficult.

Growth hormone Secretory responses of growth hormone to a variety of stimuli such as hypoglycemia, exercise, and arginine infusion are reduced. Furthermore, the starvation-induced rise in plasma growth hormone levels is attenuated.

Obesity as a risk factor   Obesity is a serious risk factor for the development of coronary artery disease and stroke. Most of the risk imparted by obesity is mediated through the associated hypertension, hyperlipoproteinemia, and diabetes. Nevertheless, even when these abnormalities are factored out, a residual, albeit much smaller, risk can be ascribed to obesity per se.

TREATMENT   Amelioration of hyperinsulinemia, insulin resistance, diabetes, hypertension, and hyperlipidemia can occur following weight loss. These changes are significant and enduring provided the weight loss is maintained. During weight loss all adipose tissue depots diminish proportionately. This generalized loss produces unattractive cosmetic effects. Many techniques, exercises, and other maneuvers have been proposed to effect selective adipose tissue reduction over particular regions of the body, but none is effective.

Methods of weight reduction   In cases where obesity is secondary, the appropriate therapy is to treat the underlying disease. Most of the time the difficult problem of primary weight reduction must be undertaken.

Diet   Caloric restriction is the cornerstone of any weight reduction program. From both the patient's and the physician's standpoint this is a frustrating and demanding undertaking. The basic principles of caloric restriction are simple. If caloric intake is less than caloric expenditure, stored calories, predominantly in the form of fat, will be consumed. In general, a deficit of 7700 kcal leads to loss of about 1 kg fat. By estimating the patient's daily caloric needs (approximately 33 kcal/kg), one can calculate the daily deficit necessary to achieve a given rate of weight loss.

Dietary restriction can range from total starvation to mild caloric deprivation, and these approaches will be discussed separately. Dietary recommendations are most effective when they are specific and geared to the patient's life-style. A dietitian or a similarly trained health professional should interview each patient and estimate his average daily caloric intake, food preferences, and eating patterns. The amount of calories the patient is to consume on the restricted diet should then be carefully explained in terms of quantities of specific foodstuffs. Frequently, the therapist must balance the degree of restriction against potential patient noncompliance. The more restrictive the diet, the more rapid the weight loss, but also the more likely the noncompliance. It is preferable to design a diet with which the patient is happy and comfortable and that produces a modest but steady weight loss.

The process of weight reduction has become a multimillion dollar business in the United States, and there are almost as many diets as there are therapists. Each proponent claims that the presence or absence of certain foodstuffs is desirable for more effective weight loss. However, little evidence exists to support the claim that calorie for calorie one hypocaloric diet will lead to a greater weight loss than another. The relationship between the patient and the therapist, plus patient education and encouragement, are more important to success than are the specific dietary constituents. The major virtue of "fad" diets is that patients are usually motivated to try them, at least initially, and patient cooperation is often better. Provided a particular diet is not harmful, probably the best course for the therapist is to maintain flexibility in the treatment program. Nevertheless, diets markedly deficient in any major class of foodstuff are to be avoided. For example, whole-food diets that are exceedingly low in carbohydrate are by nature high in fat and, depending on the type and quantity of fat ingested, may lead to hypercholesterolemia. The major virtue of a low-carbohydrate diet is the attendant increase in ketosis. (Ketone bod-

ies have a central anorexant effect.) This provides part of the rationale for the widely touted liquid or powdered protein diets. These diets have been dubbed "protein-sparing modified fasts," and claims have been made that they allow drastic long-term caloric restriction without inducing negative nitrogen balance. These claims have not been substantiated, nor has it been shown that the diets lead to a greater degree of tissue weight loss than mixed hypocaloric diets of equal caloric value. Furthermore, a number of deaths have been reported in otherwise healthy individuals participating in such long-term dietary programs, even under medical supervision. Consequently, caution is required when treating obese patients with these approaches. Basically a calorie is a calorie whether it comes from protein, carbohydrate, or fat.

Prior to therapy it is wise to forewarn patients that when caloric restriction is started there is usually a marked initial weight loss, in large part due to fluid loss. The patient should be told that such rapid rates of loss will not persist. Likewise, positive shifts in fluid balance can sometimes mask real loss of adipose mass, a fact that can sometimes be demonstrated to the patient's satisfaction by keeping a record of skin fold thickness at monthly intervals.

Total starvation diets have been advocated for the treatment of obesity; provided underlying diseases such as gout, renal insufficiency, and ketosis-prone diabetes are not present, short-term fasts are usually well tolerated. Ketonemia and hyperuricemia regularly develop during starvation but rarely lead to acidosis or gout. Because of these potential complications, total fasting should be carried out only under medical supervision. Probably the major usefulness of total fasting is as a motivational aid at the beginning of a dietary program or when weight loss has stopped. Even though much of the weight loss during short-term fasting represents fluid, this weight loss can be encouraging to frustrated patients and motivate them to increase their compliance with the long-term weight reduction program.

The major problem in the treatment of obesity is not weight reduction but maintenance of the reduced weight. Provided the therapist works hard and long enough, most motivated patients can eventually lose weight. Unfortunately, only the rare patient maintains the weight loss permanently. Obesity is an eating disorder, and the underlying mechanisms are not reversed by limiting food intake.

Behavior modification   In recognition of the problems involved, the techniques of behavior modification are being used increasingly to treat abnormal patterns of eating behavior. Many studies demonstrate that obese individuals respond less well than normal individuals to internal cues which regulate eating behavior such as gastric contractions, fear, and previous food ingestion. Conversely, obese subjects overrespond to external cues such as taste, smell, food attractiveness, abundance, and the amount of work involved in obtaining food. Given the fact that the obese individual is unusually susceptible to external stimuli, food intake may be altered by changing the pattern and nature of these external cues, and this is the major premise underlying the behavior modification approach to weight reduction.

Behavior modification begins with a detailed individual history of the patient's eating episodes with respect to time of day, length of eating period, place of ingestion (restaurant, dining table, standing in front of refrigerator), simultaneous activities (watching television, reading, idleness), emotional state, companions (relatives, friends, or alone), and finally the kinds and quantities of foods ingested. Once this detailed record is obtained, the therapist and patient can design specific behavioral changes aimed at disrupting or aborting recurring behavior patterns which initiate or prolong abnormal eating activity. As examples: if a patient eats in response to certain emotional states, then other activities can be consciously substituted when the patient perceives such a state; if the patient snacks frequently from readily available food storage areas (refrigerators, cookie jars, etc.), then he is encouraged to eat only while sitting down at a table with a fixed place setting; if eating frequently occurs while watching television alone, then efforts to avoid this activity can be initiated. Obviously, many other examples of specific and general interventions could be given. Results with behavior modification techniques have been encouraging and indicate that patients can maintain long-term weight reduction providing the new behavior patterns are truly "learned."

Exercise In any weight reduction program exercise has its place. However, the importance of exercise in terms of caloric balance must be clearly understood. Table 76-1 shows that even moderate daily exercise would not lead to a large enough increase in caloric expenditure to alter significantly the initial rate of weight reduction. This does not mean exercise is unimportant in weight reduction, since even modest increases in caloric expenditure can lead to large long-term differences in caloric balance, provided exercise is performed on a regular basis. For example, a daily increase in caloric expenditure of 300 cal over a period of 4 months could lead to a 4.5-kg weight loss. More importantly, there is evidence that incorporation of regular exercise into the overall weight reduction program improves the chances that the patient will maintain his weight loss.

Drugs Two classes of drugs are frequently used in the treatment of obesity: anorexants and thyroid hormone supplements. The addition of L-thyroxine or triiodothyronine to a weight reduction program is of no benefit. These drugs are ineffective in promoting adipose tissue loss and, if anything, accentuate lean tissue loss causing negative nitrogen balance. In susceptible individuals, cardiotoxicity may occur. Thus, unless clear-cut hypothyroidism is present, thyroid supplementation has no role in the treatment of obesity.

The major anorexants are amphetamine-like agents, and these drugs presumably exert their effect at the level of the hypothalamus. It is probable that they have a modest effect in promoting short-term weight loss in certain individuals. However, they are effective for a period of only a few weeks, and problems of habituation, addiction, and generalized drug abuse limit their usefulness. Two newer anorexants, diethylpropion and fenfluramine, may be less addictive and, therefore, somewhat more useful. However, none of these agents treats the underlying eating disorder, and they are, therefore, of little use in maintenance of weight reduction.

Injections of human chorionic gonadotropin (HCG) have been popularized as an adjunct to weight reduction, but no evidence exists to indicate a beneficial effect. The primary effectiveness of the HCG-diet program is due to the calorically restricted diet, frequent physician contact, and placebo effects. Comparable weight loss is achieved if saline injections are substituted for HCG.

Jejunoileal shunt Small-bowel bypass is an effective means of achieving weight reduction in morbidly obese patients. However, it is an experimental procedure and should be attempted only in institutions where a trained team is committed to regular, systematic, and long-term follow-up.

The most common operative procedures involve end-to-end or end-to-side anastomosis of about 38 cm of proximal jejunum to 10 cm of terminal ileum. Weight loss is initially rapid, reaching a plateau at 18 to 24 months. While all patients lose weight, few return to ideal weight. In several series the mean weight loss was 30 to 50 percent of initial excess weight, leaving patients still about 50 percent overweight once a steady state was reached. Although some degree of malabsorption occurs, the major portion of the weight loss is due to decreased food intake.

TABLE 76-1
Energy equivalents of food calories expressed in minutes of activity

Food	Calories	Activity				
		Walking*	Riding bicycle†	Swimming‡	Running§	Reclining¶
Apple, large	101	19	12	9	5	78
Bacon, 2 strips	96	18	12	9	5	74
Beer, 1 glass	114	22	14	10	6	88
Bread and butter	78	15	10	7	4	60
Carbonated beverage, 1 glass	106	20	13	9	5	82
Carrot, raw	42	8	5	4	2	32
Cheese, cottage, 1 tbsp	27	5	3	2	1	21
Chicken, fried, ½ breast	232	45	28	21	12	178
Cookie, chocolate chip	51	10	6	5	3	39
Egg, fried	110	21	13	10	6	85
Ham, 2 slices	167	32	20	15	9	128
Ice cream, ⅙ qt	193	37	24	17	10	148
Mayonnaise, 1 tbsp	92	18	11	8	5	71
Milk, skim, 1 glass	81	16	10	7	4	62
Milk shake	421	81	51	38	22	324
Orange, medium	68	13	8	6	4	52
Pancake with syrup	124	24	15	11	6	95
Peas, green, ½ cup	56	11	7	5	3	43
Pizza, cheese, ⅛	180	35	22	16	9	138
Potato chips, 1 serving	108	21	13	10	6	83
Sandwiches:						
Hamburger	350	67	43	31	18	269
Tuna fish salad	278	53	34	25	14	214
Sherbet, ⅙ qt	177	34	22	16	9	136

* *Energy cost of walking for 70-kg individual = 5.2 cal/min at 3.5 mi/h.*
† *Energy cost of riding bicycle = 8.2 cal/min.*
‡ *Energy cost of swimming = 11.2 cal/min.*
§ *Energy cost of running = 19.4 cal/min.*
¶ *Energy cost of reclining = 1.3 cal/min.*

Most teams performing this surgery select patients who are at least 100 lb overweight and in whom adequate attempts at medical management have failed repeatedly. Because of postoperative morbidity, older patients (> 50 years) and psychologically unstable individuals are usually excluded.

Complications of jejunoileal surgery are common. The overall surgical mortality ranges from 0.5 to 7.8 percent with an average of 3.9 percent. Mortality is inversely related to the experience of the surgical team. The major postoperative morbidity is related to wound infection and thromboembolism. The common serious medical complications are cirrhosis and hepatic failure, nephrolithiasis, electrolyte imbalances, cholelithiasis, and arthritis (Table 76-2). Severe liver disease probably occurs in only 5 percent of patients, but milder degrees of hepatic dysfunction are more common. The long-range implications of mild hepatic abnormalities are unknown. Possible causes of liver damage following small-bowel bypass include (1) protein and particularly essential amino acid deficiency, (2) accumulation of hepatotoxic, secondary bile salts, and (3) release of unknown toxic substances from the excluded bowel. Hypokalemia is most likely secondary to diarrhea. Persistent calcium and magnesium deficiency can result from malabsorption and must be treated with appropriate replacement. Transient depression of plasma 25-hydroxyvitamin D levels may also contribute to abnormal mineral metabolism. Nephrolithiasis can occur in up to 30 percent of patients and is due to hyperoxaluria secondary to calcium malabsorption (see Chap. 292). It can be treated by calcium supplements and a low oxalate intake. Migratory polyarthritis has been found in up to 6 percent of patients and may be due to circulating immune complexes.

Gastric surgery Gastroplasty establishes a small upper gastric remnant connected to a larger lower gastric pouch by a narrow 1- to 1.5-cm channel. Gastric bypass excludes the lower 90 percent of the stomach pouch and maintains intestinal continuity of the upper 10 percent via a retrocolic gastrojejunostomy. Both of these procedures cause patients to limit food intake by delaying gastric emptying and providing a small gastric reservoir so that fullness is experienced after a small meal. Weight loss with these procedures has been comparable with that achieved with small-bowel bypass operations but without the complications related to malabsorption, diarrhea, and hepatic dysfunction.

SUMMARY For most patients obesity is an eating disorder, and a major hope for effective long-term treatment of this disease lies in understanding the causes of overeating. Clearly no single etiology explains all cases, and different causes exist for different individuals. At present a variety of techniques, gimmicks, and maneuvers are available to effect initial weight loss. Unfortunately, initial weight loss is not the real therapeutic problem. Rather, the problem is that almost all obese patients eventually regain their weight. An effective means to sustain weight loss is the major challenge in the treatment of obesity today. The technique of behavioral modification, when professionally and rigorously applied, is the best tool for this task. As information develops concerning the hypothalamic "set point," or *adipostat*, and the factors that regulate it, pharmacological and perhaps physiological methods may emerge that will effect long-term correction of abnormal eating patterns.

REFERENCES

Assimacopoulos-Jeannet F, Jeanrenaud B: The hormonal and metabolic basis of experimental obesity. Clin Endocrinol Metab 5:337, 1976

Bray GA: Current status of intestinal bypass surgery in the treatment of obesity. Diabetes 26:1072, 1977

Hashim SA, Porikos K: Food intake behavior in man: Implications for treatment of obesity. Clin Endocrinol Metab 5:503, 1976

Hirsch J, Batchelor B: Adipose tissue cellularity in human obesity. Clin Endocrinol Metab 5:299, 1976

Mann GV: The influence of obesity on health. N Engl J Med 291:178, 226, 1974

Olefsky JM: The insulin receptor: Its role in insulin resistance in obesity and diabetes. Diabetes 25:1154, 1976

Printen KJ, Mason EE: Gastric surgery for relief of morbid obesity. Arch Surg 106:428, 1973

Sims EAH: Experimental obesity, dietary induced thermogenesis, and their clinical implications. Clin Endocrinol Metab 5:377, 1976

TABLE 76-2
Complications of bypass surgery

Complication	Percentage
EARLY	
Perioperative mortality	2–6
Thromboembolic disease	1–5
Wound infection	2–5
Renal failure	3
Severe nausea vomiting	3
Wound dehiscence	1–3
LATE	
Urinary calculi	3–10
Severe electrolyte imbalance	5–8
Acute cholecystitis	0–5
Progressive liver disease	2–4
Intestinal obstruction	2
Peptic ulcer	1–2
Osteoporosis	?
Tuberculosis	1
MINOR	
Diarrhea	100
Weakness	80
Hypokalemia	80
Hypoproteinemia	50
Vomiting	50
Thirst	50
Hypocalcemia	30
Arthralgias	15
Incisional hernias	3
Hyperuricemia	<10
Anemias (Fe, vitamin B_{12}, folate)	<10

77
ANOREXIA NERVOSA

ROBERT M. BOYAR

Anorexia nervosa is a disorder of previously healthy adolescent girls who become emaciated as a result of voluntary starvation. The population at risk consists largely of white girls from middle- to upper-class backgrounds. The disorder rarely occurs in black or oriental women and is almost never seen in men. Primary anorexia nervosa should be distinguished from eating disorders associated with psychiatric diseases such as schizophrenia, depression, obsessive-compulsive states, and hysteria.

CLINICAL PICTURE The anorexia syndrome usually begins before or shortly after puberty but may appear earlier or later (rarely above the middle twenties). Patients frequently communicate a history of having been overweight in childhood. Sometimes a precipitating stressful event can be identified, such as

TABLE 77-1
Criteria for the diagnosis of anorexia nervosa

I Onset prior to age 25
II Anorexia with weight loss of at least 25 percent of original body weight
III Distorted attitude toward eating, food, or weight that overrides hunger, admonitions, reassurances, and threats
IV No known medical illness that could account for the weight loss
V No other known psychiatric disorder
VI At least two of the following manifestations:
  A Amenorrhea
  B Lanugo hair
  C Bradycardia (persistent resting pulse of 60 beats per minute or less)
  D Periods of overactivity
  E Episodes of bulimia
  F Vomiting (may be self-induced)

leaving home for the first time. The characteristic clinical finding is emaciation equivalent to that seen in the concentration camps of World War II. Despite this emaciation the patients deny hunger, thinness, and fatigue. They are often physically active, and ritualized exercise programs are common. If social circumstances require them to eat, they frequently induce vomiting as soon as they can reach a bathroom. Amenorrhea is present almost invariably.

In advanced cases physical examination shows absent body fat. Body hair is often increased. Usually this is of fine, lanugo quality, but frank hirsutism may occur. Interestingly, breast tissue is often preserved. Parotid glands may be enlarged as in other forms of starvation. Edema is common. Because of edema in the legs and parotid gland enlargement, which gives a fullness to the face, the patient's true state of emaciation may be masked when she is fully dressed. The skin tends to be dry. Body temperature is often in the hypothermic range. Blood pressure is low, and the pulse is slow.

Laboratory abnormalities that may be present include anemia and leukopenia with hypocellularity of the bone marrow, hypokalemia, and hypoalbuminemia. Serum β-carotene levels tend to be elevated with a concomitant decrease in vitamin A concentration. The serum cholesterol concentration is sometimes increased. Glucose tolerance is abnormal, as would be expected in any starving subject. Other laboratory tests are usually normal. The endocrine changes of anorexia nervosa will be considered separately below.

A summary of the diagnostic criteria for anorexia nervosa is given in Table 77-1.

PSYCHOLOGICAL ASPECTS While all investigators agree that anorexia nervosa is associated with profound psychological dysfunction, there is disagreement about its nature. One interpretation is that the primary drive is the need to break away from a restrictive family environment. Often there is a history of a strong mother who has imposed eating demands on the child from an early age. The timing of the illness around puberty suggests that developing sexuality and the necessity of accommodating to a widening social circle play significant roles. Poor self-esteem and a sense of ineffectiveness have been commonly noted. Analytically oriented psychiatrists assume that the denial of hunger, the refusal to eat, the self-induced vomiting, and the ritualized exercise are symbolic expressions of the patient's need to take control over her own body. A fear of fatness also seems to play a role, particularly when one or both parents are overweight. A second school believes that the primary problem in anorexia nervosa is depression. Those holding to this view point out that loss of appetite, lack of self-esteem, disinterest in personal appearance, and self-destructive thoughts are common manifestations of depression. Some studies have shown that up to 80 percent of anorexia patients exhibit symptoms of depression. In support of this hypothesis,

a high percentage of first-degree relatives of such subjects have been reported to have a history of manic-depressive or depressive illness. A third theory, held by some biologically oriented psychiatrists, is that an abnormality exists in the satiety center of the hypothalamus in patients with anorexia nervosa. The evidence for this interpretation is not persuasive.

To summarize, while the psychiatric manifestations of anorexia nervosa are well understood at the descriptive level, the mechanisms by which they are produced remain uncertain.

ENDOCRINOLOGIC ASPECTS A number of endocrinologic abnormalities accompany anorexia nervosa. Most are probably the consequence of starvation and malnutrition.

Amenorrhea The onset of amenorrhea is usually associated with significant weight loss, but menses may cease prior to any decrease in body mass. Studies of the 24-h circadian pattern of luteinizing hormone (LH) in patients with anorexia show regression of the maturational stage of LH secretion to a pattern characteristic of prepubertal or early pubertal girls; i.e., episodic LH release is missing or occurs only during sleep (see Fig. 77-1). Administration of clomiphene citrate fails to result in a rise in plasma LH and follicle-stimulating hormone (FSH) concentrations. Normal LH secretory patterns return, and response to clomiphene reverts to normal following weight gain. It is now accepted that menarche usually does not appear (despite spontaneous gonadotropin release activity) until the percentage of body fat reaches 17 percent. Interestingly, return of menses in patients with secondary amenorrhea due to starvation does not occur until body fat reaches 27 percent, a figure some 10 percent higher than the value required for menarche.

FIGURE 77-1

Plasma LH concentration every 20 min for 24 h during acute exacerbation of anorexia nervosa (upper panel) and after clinical remission with return of body weight to normal (lower panel). (From Boyar et al, 1974. Used by permission.)

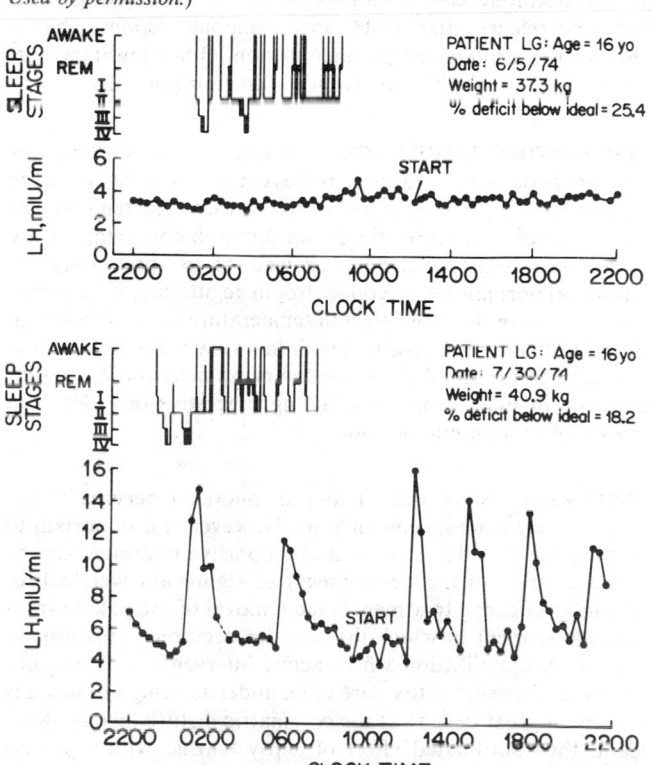

The mechanism for secondary amenorrhea occurring prior to weight loss in patients who subsequently develop anorexia nervosa is unknown. It is possible that amenorrhea with or without weight loss is due to abnormalities in the hypothalamus since injections of gonadotropin-releasing hormone in these subjects results in LH and FSH release. While the initial LH response is blunted, repeated injections are followed by normalization of the LH response. Ovulation has been induced by such treatment.

If anorexia begins before the expected onset of puberty, primary amenorrhea may be the complaint bringing the patient to the physician.

Adrenal function Patients with anorexia nervosa have reduced urinary excretion of 17-hydroxysteroids but normal or elevated plasma cortisol concentrations. Cortisol production rates are normal or slightly elevated, while metabolic clearance is decreased. Plasma half-life of cortisol is prolonged. Some patients, particularly those with agitation or depression, show hyperresponsiveness to adrenocorticotropic hormone (ACTH) and a failure to suppress normally after dexamethasone. Urinary 17-ketosteroids are low, reflecting a decreased production of dehydroepiandrosterone sulfate, dehydroepiandrosterone, and androstenedione.

Thyroid function Thyroid hormone levels of plasma are altered by anorexia nervosa. Both thyroxine (T_4) and 3,3′,5-triiodothyronine (T_3) concentrations are decreased, while levels of the physiologically inactive 3,3′,5′-triiodothyronine (reverse T_3, rT_3) are increased. The latter change is thought to be the consequence of decreased conversion of rT_3 to diiodothyronine. Plasma thyrotropin (TSH) concentrations are normal, and response to thyrotropin-releasing hormone (TRH) is intact. These changes are characteristic of starvation and wasting diseases; they cannot be considered specific for anorexia nervosa.

Pituitary function Patients with anorexia nervosa have normal growth-hormone concentrations but show increased growth-hormone release after TRH, an anomalous response that is also seen in protein-energy malnutrition. Other pituitary hormones, including prolactin, seem to function normally.

TEMPERATURE REGULATION Subjects with moderately severe anorexia nervosa appear to have a defect in temperature regulation. They fail to shiver or to increase core temperature following cold exposure and do not diminish core temperature in response to external heat. In view of the previously described abnormalities in gonadotropin regulation, it is attractive to suppose that the defect in temperature control resides in the hypothalamus. Consistent with this view is the observation that concentration of the urine following dehydration is submaximal in these subjects, a finding suggestive of a defect in release of antidiuretic hormone.

TREATMENT Since the etiology of anorexia nervosa is unknown, there is no specific therapy. However, it is important to identify the disorder early so that supportive treatment can be initiated prior to the development of significant weight loss. The most effective treatment is the removal of the patient from the environment in which the disorder occurred. This usually requires hospitalization where active intervention can be undertaken. The supportive care of an understanding physician is usually of great benefit. If the psychiatric disturbance is significant, the coordinated effort of a psychiatrist with a special interest in the adolescent is often helpful. Antidepressant drugs are occasionally useful. The long-term prognosis is generally good when treatment is initiated early; however, mortality in most series ranges between 2 and 5 percent. Until more is learned about etiology and pathogenesis of the disorder, treatment will be largely supportive in nature. In those instances in which starvation is extreme, parenteral nutrition may be indicated as described in Chap. 78.

REFERENCES

BOYAR RM et al: Anorexia nervosa: Immaturity of the 24 hour luteinizing hormone secretory pattern. N Engl J Med 291:861, 1974

———: Cortisol secretion and metabolism in anorexia nervosa. N Engl J Med 296:190, 1977

BRUCH H: Eating disorders: Obesity, anorexia nervosa, and the person within. New York, Basic Books, 1973

FEIGHNER JP et al: Diagnostic criteria for use in psychiatric research. Arch Gen Psychiatry 26:57, 1972

FRISCH FE, MCARTHUR JW: Menstrual cycles: Fatness as a determinant of minimum weight for height necessary for their maintenance or onset. Science 185:949, 1974

HALMI KA: Anorexia nervosa: Recent investigations. Annu Rev Med 29:137, 1978

MECKLENBURG RS et al: Hypothalamic dysfunction in patients with anorexia nervosa. Medicine 53:147, 1974

MOSHANG T JR et al: Low serum triiodothyronine in patients with anorexia nervosa. J Clin Endocrinol Metab 40:470, 1975

VIGERSKY R (ed): Anorexia Nervosa. New York, Raven Press, 1977

——— et al: Hypothalamic dysfunction in secondary amenorrhea associated with simple weight loss. N Engl J Med 297:1141, 1977

78
DIETARY THERAPY AND PARENTERAL NUTRITION

KHURSHEED N. JEEJEEBHOY

Regular intake of a variety of foods, necessary for survival and growth in normal humans, may be affected by a number of diseases which alter the ability to eat, absorb, or metabolize food. These diseases require dietary therapy. Diabetes mellitus, obesity, malabsorptive states, hyperlipoproteinemia, uremia, and congestive heart failure are obvious examples of illnesses where dietary manipulation plays a major role in treatment and where noncompliance with a dietary prescription may impair or even block the effectiveness of other therapeutic measures. Diets required in these and other conditions are described under the chapters devoted to each illness elsewhere in this book. Details of individual diets, including the foods required and proscribed, are readily available from dietary manuals and will not be described here. If available, a professional dietician should be utilized in initiating dietary therapy. In this chapter, after a brief review of dietary principles, emphasis will be placed on tube feeding and parenteral nutrition. Significant advances have been made in this area, and total parenteral nutrition is now recommended for growing numbers of patients in a wide variety of clinical situations. It is imperative, therefore, that the general internist be familiar with these techniques.

DIETARY THERAPY

In normal humans orally ingested nutrients provide the substrates necessary to meet energy requirements for physical and metabolic activity. Ordinarily intake matches utilization such that body composition remains relatively constant. This homeostasis may be altered by disease in several ways: (1) Intake and absorption of energy may be insufficient to meet body demands. (2) Food intake may be normal or increased but inadequate to meet increased requirements produced by the disease state. In both these situations weight loss and/or malnutrition will result if the illness is prolonged. (3) The intake of nutrients may exceed needs, causing weight gain and obesity. (4) Caloric intake may be appropriate, but specific nutrients may be deficient or present in excess.

In the planning of dietary therapy, the first step is the assessment of the operative pathophysiology, then a decision regarding the alteration of diet that will be required. For example, once the diagnosis of congestive heart failure is made, the need to restrict salt in the diet becomes obvious. Similarly, sprue requires gluten restriction; obesity, caloric limitation; diabetes, elimination of refined sugars; hepatic and renal failure, low protein intake; hypercholesterolemia, increased unsaturated fat; and phenylketonuria, a phenylalanine-free diet. Many other examples could be given. After the proper diet has been selected, other decisions become necessary. A common problem involves the degree of restriction to be prescribed. If limitation of salt is needed, should daily intake be 200 mg or 2 g? Such decisions demand more than a simple assessment of the state of the patient's disease. Also entering the equation is the likelihood of compliance by the patient and his ability to obtain the proper foods. The physician might prefer, for medical reasons, a 200-mg sodium diet but actually prescribe a 2-g sodium intake coupled with diuretic therapy because the patient does not have the economic resources to buy salt-free foods or distilled water to drink. An identical decision might be reached for a person of unlimited economic means who for psychological reasons will not eat a diet with maximum sodium restriction. Similarly the physician caring for a teen-ager with diabetes mellitus might modify the diabetic diet to allow the ingestion of a small amount of dessert on special occasions, despite its ordinary proscription, in order to keep the young person from feeling "different" from his or her peers. The patient with hypercholesterolemia might be allowed to eat eggs or steak once or twice a month in an attempt to enhance compliance with the diet on a day-to-day basis. Both of these are examples of the "treat" technique of dietary therapy. The point to be made is that diets must be prescribed realistically and not simply in accord with an abstract or theoretical ideal.

In most cases diets can be administered orally. In a number of situations, however, this is not possible. Two general problems exist. In the *first*, food cannot be swallowed normally. Examples are the comatose patient and subjects with an impairment of the swallowing mechanism. Cerebral vascular accidents are the most common cause clinically, but other neuromuscular diseases such as myasthenia gravis might act similarly. Obstruction to passage of food by esophageal cancer or scleroderma can preclude normal oral feeding. In these and similar illnesses tube feeding of defined formula diets or administration of such diets via a feeding jejunostomy may be the therapeutic avenue of choice. The *second* general category includes diseases where absorption of food in the intestinal tract is blocked or therapy demands bowel rest to allow healing of the primary pathological process. Regional ileitis and ulcerative colitis are classic examples of the latter. In these situations total parenteral nutrition by intravenous administration is required.

DEFINED FORMULA DIETS AND TUBE FEEDING

Patients unable to eat a normal diet can be nourished without resort to the parenteral route provided the diet can be modified to allow tube feeding without detrimental side effects. Such diets have now become commercially available and are composed of mixtures of precisely defined nutrients capable of being given through a fine silicone rubber feeding tube. They are called *defined formula diets* (DFD). While blenderized foods can also be used in some situations, they require a large-bore nasogastric tube for administration with attendant discomfort, risk of esophagitis, and aspiration.

COMPOSITION OF DEFINED FORMULA DIETS A selection from a vast number of available diets is given in Table 78-1. These diets can be grouped into (1) moderate-residue, lactose-containing diets, (2) low-residue, lactose-free diets with intact protein, and (3) amino acid–based lactose-free diets.

Defined formula diets differ in osmolality, palatability, absorbability, and lactose content. Diets listed in columns A and B (intact protein diets) in Table 78-1 are low in osmolality and are palatable. Amino acid–glucose–fatty acid based diets (Table 78-1, columns C) do not require digestion and hence may be absorbed in the presence of severe malabsorption. Diets in columns A can be given only to patients who do not have

TABLE 78-1
Complete nutritional preparations per 1000 kcal*

Name (Manufacturer):	A			B			C	
	Formula 2 (Cutter)	Compleat B (Doyle)	Sustacal Liquid (Mead Johnson)	Ensure (Ross)	Isocal (Mead Johnson)	Precision Isotonic (Doyle)	Flexical (Mead Johnson)	Vivonex (Eaton)
Protein, g	37.5	40.0	60.3	35.5	32.5	30.0	22.4	20.4
Protein source	Nonfat milk, beef	Nonfat milk, beef	Milk, soy protein	Milk, soy protein	Milk, soy protein	Egg white	Hydrolysed casein	Crystalline amino acids
Fat, g	40.0	40.0	23.0	35.0	42.0	31.3	34.0	1.4
Carbohydrate, g	122.5	120.0	137.8	136.7	125.0	150	154.0	226.3
Lactose, g	37.5	24.4	16.7	0	0	0	0	0
mosmol/kg	435–510	490	625	450	350	300	723	500
Volume needed to meet usual daily requirements, ml	2000	1600	1080	1920	1910	1560	2000	1800

* *Composition is given only in terms of protein and energy, but these diets contain vitamins, minerals, and trace elements to meet requirements. For details see source.*
SOURCE: *After Shils et al.*

lactose intolerance. All diets in columns A and B can be taken orally as well as by tube and are useful in some ambulatory patients with chronic obstructive or inflammatory bowel disease. They are more palatable than those of columns C. The latter are amino acid–glucose based and in theory should be easily absorbed. However, they cause diarrhea in patients with short-bowel syndromes, a side effect which limits their usefulness. They may also cause bloating, nausea, gastric dilatation, and hyperglycemia. Diets in columns A and B have fewer side effects. Even though they utilize intact protein instead of free amino acids, their slower intestinal transit time usually offsets any disadvantage resulting from the requirement for digestion of protein prior to absorption.

MODE OF ADMINISTRATION Diets grouped under columns A and B in Table 78-1 can be fed orally in small quantities at frequent intervals. They are preferably served ice cold. Diets under columns C must be given as a slow intragastric or intraintestinal drip. Intragastric drip should be used in all patients with marked "intestinal hurry," malabsorption, and diarrhea in order to provide a uniform slow input of the formula. The preferred method of administration is an infusion given at the rate of 20 to 30 ml/h via a 2- to 3-mm silicone rubber nasogastric tube. The stomach is aspirated after 4 h, and if the residual volume exceeds 50 ml, the infusion is stopped temporarily. If the volume is less than 50 ml, the rate of infusion is gradually increased to 125 ml/h over a 3- to 4-day period. Blood glucose, blood urea nitrogen (BUN), electrolytes, phosphate, calcium, and magnesium should be monitored three times a week until stabilized. If diarrhea occurs, loperamide or diphenoxylate with atropine may be given. Caution is required with these drugs because of the danger of developing gastric dilatation and vomiting.

INDICATIONS Defined formula diets given orally or by tube feeding are indicated in three general situations. The first consists of conditions where an oral diet cannot be eaten. Examples include unconsciousness, oropharyngeal abnormalities, partial esophageal obstruction, and severe anorexia. A second indication is disease characterized by discomfort after ingestion of normal food, e.g., partial bowel obstruction due to Crohn's disease or adhesions, infiltrative disease of the intestine, and chronic pancreatitis. The third category includes malabsorptive diseases, gastrointestinal fistulas, and short-bowel syndromes. Diets listed in columns C of Table 78-1 are helpful in this group of diseases.

PARENTERAL NUTRITION

This section is mainly concerned with techniques for providing nutrients in circumstances where, owing to disorders of the gastrointestinal tract, patients cannot eat a normal diet, do not absorb an oral diet efficiently, or deteriorate clinically on oral feeding. Such patients need partial or complete nourishment via the parenteral route for varying lengths of time ranging from days to years. The particular combination of nutrients and the route of infusion vary with the needs of the patient and the duration of infusion. Discussed below are the indications for parenteral nutrition and the principles and techniques necessary for rational parenteral therapy.

INDICATIONS FOR TOTAL PARENTERAL NUTRITION The indications for total parenteral nutrition (TPN), are fairly easily recognized. They include the following situations:

1 Malnourished patients who are unable to eat or to absorb an oral diet. In such patients the diagnosis of malnutrition should be based on a number of factors including previous dietary history, evidence of muscle wasting, hypoalbuminemia, edema, reduced skin fold thickness, and body weight. Weight alone is not sufficient to make the diagnosis of malnutrition because edema or previous obesity may mask the degree of nitrogen depletion actually present.

2 For bowel rest in patients with Crohn's disease, intestinal fistulas, and pancreatitis. In these patients food ingestion often results in exacerbation of symptoms with increased inflammation and high output through fistulas, preventing healing. When they are given nothing by mouth and receive TPN, they appear to improve rapidly, heal fistulas without surgery, and maintain nutritional status.

3 For well-nourished patients entering the hospital who will be unable to eat temporarily. In these cases a judgment has to be made about the probable length of time that oral diet will not be available. If the period is likely to exceed 10 to 14 days, then total parenteral nutrition should be administered to avoid undue wasting and malnutrition during the period of starvation. This is especially important if sepsis and trauma complicate the clinical picture since both accelerate catabolism and tissue wasting.

4 Prolonged coma when tube feeding is not possible.

5 Nutritional support in patients with marked hypercatabolism, such as those with severe trauma and burns, even if some oral intake is possible.

6 Nutritional support during therapy for malignant disease. In many patients with malignant tumors weight loss is a prominent feature and is accentuated by surgery, radiation, or chemotherapy. Chemotherapy is particularly prone to cause anorexia and mucosal inflammation that may severely limit oral intake. TPN given prior to and with chemotherapy results in an improved nutritional status in these patients.

NUTRIENT REQUIREMENTS DURING TPN **Energy and fluid requirements** Afebrile patients without septicemia require about 32 kcal per kilogram of ideal body weight daily for weight maintenance and 40 to 45 kcal/kg for weight gain when malnourished. The energy requirement increases to 60 kcal/kg per day with a body temperature of 40°C. While elective surgery does not increase these requirements significantly, septicemia does increase them by 50 percent; in burns exceeding 40 percent of the surface area, the requirements may increase by about 100 percent.

Basal fluid intake should be about 1 to 1.2 ml/kcal infused. To this amount should be added a volume equivalent to losses from diarrhea, stomal output, nasogastric suction, and fistula drainage. In oliguric renal failure a basal intake of 750 to 1000 ml should be given plus a volume equal to that of urine and other losses. In patients with cardiac failure about 40 ml/kg can be infused provided that the sodium intake is restricted to between 20 and 50 meq per day.

Amino acid requirements The efficient functioning of the body requires maintenance of the integrity of the musculoskeletal system and viscera together with normal levels of enzymes, hormones, and plasma proteins. All are dependent on new protein synthesis to meet the demands of normal turnover, and this protein synthesis in turn requires that amino acids be available. A major objective of parenteral nutrition is to provide an adequate supply of amino acids for protein synthesis. The amount required is influenced by several factors. Severe injury, sepsis, and burns dramatically increase nitrogen losses as already mentioned, requiring that larger amounts of amino acids be infused in their presence. The pattern of amino acids infused is important since unbalanced mixtures will not support protein synthesis. Finally, requirements are much larger if amino acids are given as the sole energy source than they are if caloric demands are met by fat or carbohydrate.

In pure dietary starvation the infusion of 100 g glucose per day reduces urinary nitrogen loss but will not produce positive nitrogen balance. Infusion of amino acids also reduces net nitrogen deficits and in large amounts can induce a slight positive nitrogen balance. During starvation a fall in plasma insulin coupled with a rise in glucagon, cortisol, and catecholamines shifts body metabolism toward a fat economy by elevating plasma free fatty acid concentrations and increasing ketone body production. Certain experimental evidence suggests that this elevation of plasma ketones may have a role in minimizing breakdown of muscle protein (and hence the negative nitrogen balance of prolonged starvation). On the basis of these experiments it was postulated by some investigators that the infusion of glucose together with amino acids would be detrimental since a glucose-induced rise in insulin secretion would lower plasma free fatty acids and diminish plasma ketone concentrations, with the result that protein breakdown in muscle would be accelerated. While this area remains controversial, the author believes the evidence to be persuasive that when amino acids are infused with glucose sufficient to meet caloric requirements, they are more efficiently used than when given alone. Significantly positive nitrogen balance is achieved in most malnourished patients (not suffering abnormal losses) by infusing only 0.5 to 1.0 g amino acids per kilogram of ideal body weight per day if nonprotein calories are optimal. Abnormal losses, such as protein-rich exudates in burns, or upper gastrointestinal tract contents rich in pancreatic secretions increase requirements to between 1.5 and 2.0 g/kg per day. As the input of nonprotein energy is increased, there is a concurrent augmentation of nitrogen retention at all levels of amino acid intake until the input of nonprotein energy reaches 55 to 60 kcal per kilogram of ideal body weight. Beyond this point additional calories do not seem to improve nitrogen retention significantly in adults.

Relation of nitrogen retention to the source of nonprotein energy

Both carbohydrates and lipids can be infused with amino acids to provide sufficient nonprotein energy to meet metabolic requirements of the patient. The question then arises whether glucose and lipid are comparable in improving the utilization of amino acids above the level seen in hypocaloric states. The answer, obtained from carefully controlled crossover studies, is that the two types of substrate are equal in efficacy after an initial 3- to 4-day period for adaptation to the source of the energy. Hence the source of nonprotein energy chosen for use in a patient depends on factors other than its effect on nitrogen retention.

The first factor of importance is osmotic pressure. Concentrated glucose solutions are hyperosmolar and cause thrombosis when administered by peripheral vein. TPN regimens using glucose as the primary energy source thus require placement of a catheter in the superior vena cava where rapid blood flow quickly dilutes the hypertonic infusion. A second major consideration is the metabolic state of the patient. Glucose requires insulin for utilization, and hypertonic glucose solutions are probably not ideal in diabetic subjects. Conversely triglyceride emulsions might be contraindicated in hyperlipoproteinemic states.

Glucose infusion mixtures are quite simple and consist of 25 percent dextrose containing 2 percent amino acids together with necessary vitamins and minerals. Lipid emulsions are mixtures of triglyceride, phospholipid (as an emulsifying agent), and glycerol or sorbitol which is added to maintain isotonicity. Lipid can be infused with amino acid–dextrose mixtures using a Y connector to provide 50 to 80 percent of nonprotein calories. These concentrations can be given by peripheral vein without fear of thrombosis. Insulin is not required for metabolism of the fat; indeed, insulin concentrations are low, and free fatty acids and ketones are high during

the administration of lipid when this is providing the major part of nonprotein calories. A valuable additional benefit is that lipid solutions can be discontinued abruptly without danger of hypoglycemia because insulin levels are not elevated. This aspect is particularly important in critically ill patients who may require repeated and unpredictable alterations in their infusions, especially when surgery has to be carried out upon short notice. Finally, lipid infusions meet essential fatty acid requirements since linoleic acid is present in sufficient quantities if as little as 500 ml Intralipid (the commercially available triglyceride emulsion) is given daily. While essential fatty acid deficiency is rare in adults, biochemical signs of deficiency may appear in as little as 1 week with TPN in the absence of lipid, and abnormalities of liver function and skin rash may follow.

It is also possible to carry out TPN with a 1:1 mixture of glucose and lipid calories. Substrate and hormone profiles in the blood following infusion of such a mixture are similar to those seen in the postprandial state.

Recommendations regarding source (type) of nonprotein energy

In North America, in contrast to Europe and the United Kingdom, lipid-free systems were used almost exclusively in the past because triglyceride emulsions had not been approved for nonexperimental use. At the present time lipid-free systems are required only in patients with hyperchylomicronemia. The author believes that most patients should receive lipid as a part of the regimen for total parenteral nutrition. The 80 percent lipid system can be given by peripheral vein, minimizing the threat of catheter sepsis and other catheter-related complications. The 1:1 lipid-glucose solution, given through a central venous line, simulates closely the normal diet and causes neither hyperinsulinemia nor hyperglycemia, thus almost eliminating the need for exogenous insulin.

Other requirements VITAMINS Vitamin requirements are given in Table 78-2. Amounts of vitamins sufficient to meet these needs must be added to the basic parenteral feeding solutions. It is important to avoid infusing excessive amounts of fat-soluble vitamins, in particular vitamins A and D, because of the danger of hypercalcemia and other toxic effects. A combination of 5 ml MVI with 10 ml Soluzyme plus vitamin C on alternate days will meet the requirements for vitamins A and D and will meet or exceed the need for most water-soluble vitamins. These solutions should be supplemented with vitamin K (5 mg) and vitamin B_{12} (200 μg) initially and at intervals of 3 weeks. Folate (5 mg) is given weekly.

ELECTROLYTES Electrolytes are an essential component of the fluids infused during total parenteral nutrition. Potassium, magnesium, and phosphorus are necessary for optimal nitrogen retention and tissue formation. In addition sodium and chloride should be infused to maintain osmolality and acid-base balance. Calcium is required to maintain calcium balance and prevent demineralization of bone. Recommended ranges of intake are given in Table 78-3.

TRACE ELEMENTS The need for trace elements, in particular zinc, copper, and chromium, is becoming increasingly recognized in courses of parenteral nutrition that exceed 1 to 2 weeks.

Zinc is essential for wound healing, for defense against infection, and for the activity of a number of enzymes. In its absence ageusia, loss of hair, night blindness, and a skin rash

TABLE 78-2
Vitamin input and blood or plasma vitamin levels in six patients on long-term TPN

| | Input* provided by: | | | | Plasma/blood vitamin level | |
Vitamin	MVI, per 5 ml	Soluzyme + vitamin C, per 10 ml	Consequent average daily input	Daily (oral) recommended requirement	Average level observed in six patients	Normal range
A	5000 IU		2500 IU	5000 IU	41.6	25–70 μg/100 ml
D	500 IU		250 IU	400 IU	34.4	28–42 ng/ml
E	5 mg		27.5 mg†	30 mg	0.65	0.8–1.2 ng/100 ml
B₁	22 mg	10 mg	16.0 mg	1.5 mg	226	10–64 ng/ml
B₂	5 mg	10 mg	7.5 mg	2.0 mg		
Niacinamide	50 mg	250 mg	150 mg	20.0 mg	16	3–6 μg/ml
Pantothenate	12 mg	45 mg	28 mg	10.0 mg	689	150–400 ng/ml
Pyridoxine	6 mg	5 mg	5.5 mg	2.5 mg	40	30–80 ng/ml
Ascorbic acid	500 mg	500 mg	500 mg	75 mg	2.0	0.4–1 mg/100 ml
Folic acid		5 mg	2.5 mg	0.15 mg	48	4–20 ng/100 ml
B₁₂		25 μg	12.5 μg	1.0 μg	872	100–900 pg/ml
Biotin				300 μg	63	200–500 pg/ml

* Given on alternate days.
† Twenty-five milligrams of the average of 27.5 mg vitamin E per day is provided by infusing 500 ml Intralipid per day.
SOURCE: After KN Jeejeebhoy, Ann Coll Physicians Surg Can 9:287, 1976.

occur. The skin rash is often associated with superficial infection due to staphylococci and yeasts and responds only to zinc supplementation. Zinc deficiency has also been shown to interfere with delayed hypersensitivity. In the absence of excessive gastrointestinal losses, 3 mg zinc per day is sufficient to meet needs. For each liter of intestinal fluids lost through fistulas, stomal output, suction, or diarrhea in patients with extensive resection of the small bowel, an additional 12 mg should be added. If the small bowel is intact, zinc losses are greater and about 17 mg zinc is required per liter of intestinal fluids lost per day.

Deficiency of copper causes anemia and neutropenia. The daily requirement is estimated to be between 0.8 and 1.6 mg with the larger intake to be given patients with major losses of gastrointestinal fluid. Copper should not be given to patients with obstructive jaundice.

The estimated requirement for manganese is about 0.8 mg per day. This element also should not be given if obstructive jaundice is present.

Deficiency of chromium is associated with glucose intolerance and neuropathy. The daily requirement of chromium is about 20 μg.

ROUTES OF ADMINISTRATION   Central venous catheterization

This route allows infusion of fluids irrespective of osmolality and is comfortable for patients since repeated venipuncture is avoided. On the other hand, there is a significant risk of septicemia and thrombosis, especially if the catheter is not properly inserted and cared for during administration of the parenteral nutrition.

TABLE 78-3
Recommended electrolyte intake per day (milliosmoles)

	Na	K	Ca	Mg	P
Basal*	100–120	80–100	10–15	10–12	12–16
Cardiac failure	20–50	80–100	10–15	10–12	12–16
Renal failure	20	†	†	†	†

* To this basal intake, amounts of Na, K, Cl, and HCO₃ are added to meet losses from fistulas, nasogastric tube drainage, diarrhea, and stomal output.
† These ions are added as needed, on the basis of initial and continuing measurements of their circulating level and the clinical state of the patient.

Basic principles of catheter insertion and care are as follows:

1 Catheters should always be placed, and subsequently handled, using completely aseptic technique. Face mask and sterile gloves are required.
2 The catheter should be demonstrated radiologically to be positioned in the superior vena cava prior to commencing total parenteral nutrition with hypertonic fluids. If the tip has entered another central vein (e.g., the internal jugular), thrombosis may occur.
3 Catheters should always be introduced via puncture of a large central vein and not a peripheral vein.
4 The catheter used for TPN should not be used to withdraw blood or measure central venous pressure.
5 The skin puncture site should be cleansed weekly with a detergent, painted with a povidone iodine solution, and occluded with a dressing. A transparent plastic dressing is recommended since it is occlusive and easy to apply and allows for easy inspection of the insertion site for infection, drainage, bleeding, etc.
6 Barium-impregnated silicone rubber catheters (e.g., Silastic, made by Extracorporeal Medical Specialties, Inc., King of Prussia, Pennsylvania) should be used since they do not traumatize the central veins and are less likely to be surrounded with a fibrin clot.

Peripheral venous infusion   This route is safe and not as likely to be a source of septic or thrombotic complications. However the infused fluids must be isotonic or only mildly hypertonic. In order to achieve these conditions, nonprotein energy must be given mainly as lipid. A representative protocol is discussed below.

REPRESENTATIVE PROTOCOLS FOR ADMINISTRATION OF TOTAL PARENTERAL NUTRITION

The three sample protocols given in Table 78-4 are designed for a 60-kg individual. They are intended to be administered throughout 24 h and provide 1 g amino acids and 40 nonprotein calories per kilogram of body weight. Proportionate modifications can be made for larger or smaller persons. Nonprotein energy is provided as (1) glucose, (2) 50 percent glucose and 50 percent lipid, or (3) 85 percent lipid and 15 percent glucose. The latter is suitable for peripheral venous administration. Preparation of the infusion materi-

TABLE 78-4

Representative protocols for the administration of total parenteral nutrition (see text)

100% GLUCOSE

8 A.M. to 8 P.M.:	
2% amino acids with 25% dextrose	1500 ml
Electrolyte additives, as needed[a]	30 ml (approx)
MVI[b] *or*	5 ml
Soluzyme plus vitamin C[c]	10 ml
8 P.M. to 8 A.M.:	
2% amino acids with 25% dextrose	1500 ml
Electrolyte additives, as needed[a]	30 ml (approx)
Trace element mix (1) to (4)[d]	1 ml (each)
Nutrient composition of above regimen:	
Amino acids (60 g)	240 kcal
Glucose monohydrate (750 g)	2550 kcal
Lipid	
Total nonprotein energy	2550 kcal
Total volume	3000 ml (approx)
Electrolytes:[a]	
Na	130 meq
K	80 meq
Ca	10 meq
Mg	11 meq
P	14 meq

50% GLUCOSE AND 50% LIPID

8 A.M. to 8 P.M.:	
4% amino acids with 25% dextrose[e]	750 ml
Electrolyte additives, as needed[a]	30 ml (approx)
MVI[b] *or*	5 ml
Soluzyme plus vitamin C[c]	10 ml
Intralipid 10%[e,f]	500 ml
8 P.M. to 8 A.M.:	
4% amino acids with 25% dextrose[e]	750 ml
Electrolyte additives, as needed[a]	30 ml (approx)
Trace element mix (1) to (4)[d]	1 ml (each)
Intralipid 10%[e,f]	500 ml
Nutrient composition of above regimen:	
Amino acids (60 g)	240 kcal
Glucose monohydrate (375 g)	1275 kcal
Lipid (100 g)	1100 kcal
Total nonprotein energy	2375 kcal
Total volume	2600 ml (approx)
Electrolyte composition: same as for	
100% glucose protocol	

85% LIPID AND 15% GLUCOSE — *Peripheral administration*

8 A.M. to 8 P.M.:	
6% amino acids with 12% dextrose[g]	500 ml
Electrolyte additives, as needed[a]	30 ml (approx)
MVI[b] *or*	5 ml
Soluzyme plus vitamin C[c]	10 ml
Intralipid 10%[f,g]	1000 ml
8 P.M. to 8 A.M.:	
6% amino acids with 12% dextrose[g]	500 ml
Electrolyte additives, as needed[a]	30 ml (approx)
Trace element mix (1) to (4)[d]	1 ml (each)
Intralipid 10%[f,g]	1000 ml
Nutrient composition of above mixture:	
Amino acids (60 g)	240 kcal
Glucose monohydrate (120 g)	408 kcal
Lipid (200 g)	2200 kcal
Total nonprotein energy	2608 kcal
Total volume	3100 ml (approx)
Electrolyte composition: same as for	
100% glucose protocol	

[a] *Total electrolytes have been calculated on the assumption that the amino acid mixture used is electrolyte-free. If another amino acid source is used, the values will be different. The total input of electrolytes given in this table has been found to be capable of maintaining balance in patients without abnormal losses of gastrointestinal secretions. However in patients with such losses appropriate replacement has to be made.*
[b] *MVI injection (USV Pharmaceutical Corp).*
[c] *Soluzyme plus vitamin C (Upjohn).*
[d] *Trace element mix: 1 ml each of (1) 1.6 mg/ml elemental Cu as cupric chloride $(CuCl_2 \cdot 2H_2O)$, 20 μg/ml elemental Cr as chromic nitrate $[Cr(NO_3)_3]$, and 120 μg/ml elemental Se as selenious acid, (H_2SeO_3); (2), 120 μg/ml elemental I as potassium iodide (KI); (3) 3 mg/ml elemental Zn as zinc sulfate $(ZnSO_4 \cdot 7H_2O)$; and (4) 0.7 mg/ml elemental Mn as manganous chloride $(MnCl_3 \cdot 4H_2O)$.*
[e] *The triglyceride emulsion and dextrose–amino acid mixture are infused concurrently through a central venous line using a Y connector for continuous mixing.*
[f] *Intralipid 10% (Cutter Laboratories).*
[g] *It is very important in this system that the amino acid–dextrose solution and Intralipid be infused in correct proportions through the Y connector so that the concentration of the former is diluted adequately by constant mixing with the Intralipid to make the dextrose noninjurious to the peripheral vein. An infusion pump is advisable.*

als must be carried out with great care. In most medical centers such preparation is done exclusively by one or more specially trained pharmacists.

HOME PARENTERAL NUTRITION (HPN) It is now possible to administer parenteral nutrition at home in patients requiring prolonged nutritional support. A permanent silicone rubber catheter is placed in the superior vena cava via a subclavian or jugular vein and led to the outside through a subcutaneous tunnel. These catheters may be left in place for years without need for replacement. The patient receives monthly supplies of prepackaged nutrients ready for infusion. The nutrients are infused during the night while the patient is sleeping. A simple pneumatic cuff placed around the plastic bags containing the prepackaged infusion fluids is safe, cheap, and less cumbersome than mechanical-electrical delivery systems. The system is disconnected in the morning after a 10-h overnight infusion, and the catheter is capped and filled with a heparin solution. The patient is then free to carry out normal social activities or work during the day. This method has revolutionized the life of persons who otherwise would be nutritional cripples because of prolonged hospitalization for TPN.

PARTIAL PARENTERAL NUTRITION Whether amino acids should replace glucose and electrolyte solutions in the management of patients unable to eat for short periods (up to 1 week) following surgery, strokes, or other acute illnesses is debatable. In 7 days a patient has (on average) a net negative nitrogen balance of 100 to 110 g when receiving only glucose replacement. If amino acids are given at a level of 1 g/kg per day, the nitrogen loss is cut to 35 to 45 g. This difference is equal to only about 3 percent of the total nitrogen content in a 60-kg man. Since there is no evidence that such a small deficit makes any difference in clinical outcome (the nitrogen loss is quickly repleted when food intake is restored) and since amino acid solutions are expensive, amino acid infusion is not recommended for fasts of up to 1 week. Beyond 1 week, full TPN should probably be given.

In some patients oral intake is possible but the amounts ingested are inadequate for full nutrition. In such cases an estimate is made of the amount taken orally, and the deficiency is made up by parenteral means. When there is a question about how much of the ingested diet is absorbed (e.g., after bowel resection or with intestinal fistulas), the amount of nutrition given parenterally will have to be determined by trial and error, with evaluation of weight gain and other signs of clinical improvement.

REFERENCES

ANDERSON GH et al: Design and evaluation by nitrogen balance and blood aminograms of an amino acid mixture for total parenteral nutrition of adults with gastrointestinal disease. J Clin Invest 53:904, 1974

——— et al: Dose-response relationships between amino acid intake and blood levels in newborn infants. Am J Clin Nutr 30:1110, 1977

BATSTONE GF et al: Metabolic studies in subjects following thermal injury. Intermediary metabolites, hormones and tissue oxygenation. Burns 2:207, 1976

BLACKBURN GL et al: Protein sparing therapy during periods of starvation with sepsis or trauma. Ann Surg 177:588, 1973

CAHILL GF JR et al: Starvation in man. N Engl J Med 282:668, 1970

CRAIG RP et al: Intravenous glucose, amino acids and fat in the postoperative period. Lancet 2:8, 1977

GREENBERG GR et al: Protein-sparing therapy in postoperative patients. Effects of added hypocaloric glucose or lipid. N Engl J Med 294:1411, 1976

JEEJEEBHOY KN: Protein sparing effect of amino acids, in *Clinical Nutrition Update: Amino Acids,* HL Greene et al (eds). Chicago, American Medical Association, 1977

————: Role of measuring albumin synthesis as a way of measuring protein body repletion, ibid.

———— et al: Metabolic studies in total parenteral nutrition with lipid in man: Comparison with glucose. J Clin Invest 57:125, 1976

———— et al: Total parenteral nutrition at home: Studies in patients surviving 4 months to 5 years. Gastroenterology 71:943, 1976

MENG HC, WILMORE DW (eds): *Fat Emulsions in Parenteral Nutrition.* Chicago, American Medical Association, 1976

MUNRO HN: General aspects of the regulation of protein metabolism by diet and by hormones, in *Mammalian Protein Metabolism,* HN Munro, JB Allison (eds). New York, Academic, 1964, vol I

RUDMAN D et al: Elemental balances during intravenous hyperalimentation of underweight adult subjects. J Clin Invest 55:94, 1975

SHILS ME et al: Liquid formulas for oral and tube feeding. Clin Bull 6:151, 1976

79
DEFICIENCY OF NIACIN (PELLAGRA)

JEAN D. WILSON
LEONARD L. MADISON

NORMAL PHYSIOLOGY OF NIACIN **Biochemistry** Niacin is the accepted generic description for nicotinic acid (pyridine-3-carboxylic acid) and derivatives exhibiting the nutritional activity of nicotinic acid. In one sense niacin is not a vitamin since it can be formed from the essential amino acid tryptophan. Studies in humans indicate that an average of about 1 mg niacin is formed from 60 mg dietary tryptophan. Accordingly, estimates of the adequacy of dietary intake must take into account the tryptophan content of the diet as well as the content of niacin. It should also be recognized that many foodstuffs, especially cereals, contain bound forms of niacin from which the vitamin is not nutritionally available.

The absorption, tissue distribution, and metabolism of the vitamin are poorly understood. In most species approximately a fifth of the vitamin is decarboxylated, and the remainder is excreted in the urine as methylated products, largely *n*-methylnicotinamide and its derivatives.

Mechanism of action Niacin is an essential component of nicotinamide adenine dinucleotide (NAD) and nicotinamide adenine dinucleotide phosphate (NADP), coenzymes for a multitude of important oxidation-reduction reactions in metabolism. Nicotinic acid is transaminated to nicotinamide which subsequently reacts with phosphoribosyl pyrophosphate to form nicotinamide mononucleotide; the latter then reacts with adenosine triphosphate (ATP) to form NAD, and the reaction with a second molecule of ATP results in the formation of NADP.

Requirements The requirements and recommended daily allowances for niacin and tryptophan are listed in Tables 73-1 and 73-2. In contrast to most vitamins there is no clear evidence that requirement is increased during pregnancy. As discussed below, the principal factor that influences requirements may be the amino acid composition of the diet.

EXPERIMENTAL DEPLETION Following the administration of a diet deficient in niacin and tryptophan, the urinary excretion of the metabolites of niacin decreases rapidly, reaching minimal values (< 1.5 mg per day) after 30 to 60 days and remaining constant thereafter. In most instances the first clinical evidence of deficiency is noted within a short period of time after excretion becomes stable at a low level. The symptoms and signs of niacin deficiency include dermatitis, glossitis, stomatitis, diarrhea, proctitis, mental depression, heartburn, abdominal pain, vaginitis, dysphagia, and amenorrhea, findings similar to those in pellagra.

CLINICAL DEFICIENCY **Frequency and clinical context** Pellagra was previously an endemic disease in the American South and in many other parts of the world. Endemic pellagra is usually associated with a high intake of maize (or sorghum) and can be cured by the administration of niacin. However, our understanding of the pathogenesis of pellagra has changed over the years from that of a pure vitamin deficiency to that of a mixed deficiency of tryptophan and available niacin in the diet to that of a vitamin and amino acid deficiency associated with an imbalance in dietary amino acids. This conclusion is based on the following facts: (1) the niacin content of maize is low, and a significant portion appears to be "bound" and unavailable for absorption; (2) however, the niacin equivalent of maize (available niacin and tryptophan) is no lower than in some cereals that are unassociated with endemic pellagra; and (3) the leucine content of common varieties of maize is high. A hybrid strain of maize, opaque 2, has recently been described which differs from the ordinary grain in having lower leucine but similar tryptophan and niacin content. Dogs fed a diet rich in conventional maize or a diet rich in opaque 2 maize supplemented with leucine develop experimental pellagra (black tongue), whereas dogs fed the opaque 2 maize alone do not. This finding presumably explains why pellagra occurs in Indians who ingest a diet rich in sorghum (jowar), which has a leucine content similar to that of maize but a niacin and tryptophan content (and availability) equivalent to that of rice. Leucine is believed to inhibit the synthesis of nicotinic acid mononucleotide and consequently the synthesis of NAD and NADP. Thus, in pathogenic terms, the development of symptoms of niacin "deficiency" depends on the amino acid content of the diet as well as upon the intake of the vitamin and its precursors.

Whatever the exact cause, endemic pellagra disappeared in the United States coincident with the improvement in nutritional education and with the institution of widespread supplementation of grain cereal products with niacin. However, pellagra is an occasional secondary manifestation of two disorders that profoundly affect tryptophan metabolism, the carcinoid syndrome in which up to 60 percent of tryptophan is catabolized by what is ordinarily a minor pathway of metabolism (see Chap. 91) and Hartnup disease, an autosomal recessive disorder in which several amino acids including tryptophan are absorbed poorly from the diet. In both disorders the symptoms of pellagra appear to be the consequence of diminished availability of effective niacin equivalents, and in both the symptoms and signs of pellagra can be cured by the administration of large amounts of the vitamin.

Manifestations The typical presentation of pellagra is that of a chronic wasting disease associated with dermatitis, dementia, and diarrhea. The dermatitis is characteristic; it is bilateral, symmetrical, seen on those parts exposed to sunlight, and due to photosensitivity. The mental changes are less discrete; fatigue, insomnia, and apathy may precede the development of an encephalopathy characterized by confusion, disorientation, hallucination, and loss of memory. Eventually, frank organic psychoses may develop. Paresthesias and polyneuritis seen in pellagra may actually be the result of other coexisting vitamin deficiencies. The diarrhea, when it occurs, is a portion of a widespread inflammation of the mucous surfaces; other manifestations include achlorhydria, glossitis, stomatitis, and vaginitis. After the development of symptoms the course is slowly progressive over a period of several years before death supervenes, usually due to secondary complications.

The exact relation between the known coenzyme functions of NAD and NADP and these various symptoms has never been defined. Levels of NAD and NADP in erythrocytes are lower in patients with pellagra than in normal persons, but the coenzymes are essential to so many reactions in intermediary metabolism that profound deficiency is incompatible with life. Some evidence suggests that the mental changes in pellagra may be associated with diminished conversion of tryptophan to serotonin.

Diagnosis Suspicion and response to replacement therapy must be the basis of diagnosis. No biochemical test is of diagnostic value. As would be predicted, the urinary excretion of the metabolites of nicotinic acid and tryptophan is lower than average but not lower than in patients with generalized malnutrition (Table 74-4). Plasma tryptophan and erythrocyte NAD and NADP levels may be low. Histopathology of the skin is characterized by hyperkeratosis, hyperpigmentation, and desquamation.

Management The administration of small amounts of niacin (10 mg per day) in the face of limiting amounts of dietary tryptophan may be sufficient to cure endemic pellagra. Large doses (40 to 200 mg per day) may be required in Hartnup disease.

REFERENCES

DARBY WJ et al: Niacin. Nutr Rev 33:289, 1977

DE LANGE DJ, JOUBERT CP: Assessment of nicotinic acid status of population groups. Am J Clin Nutr 15:169, 1964

GOLDSMITH GA: Experimental niacin deficiency. J Am Diet Assoc 32:312, 1956

GOPALAN C, RAO KSJ: Pellagra and amino acid imbalance, in *Vitamins and Hormones*, PL Munson et al (eds). New York, Academic, 1975, pp 505–528

JEPSON JB: Hartnup disease, in *The Metabolic Basis of Inherited Disease,* 4th ed, JB Stanbury et al (eds). New York, McGraw-Hill, 1978, pp 1563–1577

80

DEFICIENCY OF THIAMINE (BERIBERI), PYRIDOXINE, AND RIBOFLAVIN

JEAN D. WILSON
LEONARD L. MADISON

THIAMINE

NORMAL PHYSIOLOGY OF THIAMINE Biochemistry Thiamine consists of a pyrimidine ring and a thiazole moiety linked by a methylene bridge (Fig. 80-1). The vitamin is synthesized by a variety of plants and microorganisms but not ordinarily by animal tissues. However, rats and pigeons fed a thiamine-free diet can be protected from developing symptoms of deficiency by being given large quantities of the pyrimidine and thiazole moieties, suggesting that animal tissues have a small capacity to couple the two subunits. Limited amounts may also be synthesized by microorganisms in the gastrointestinal tract. Thiamine is absorbed from the diet by both an active transport process and passive diffusion. The capacity to absorb

the vitamin in the human intestine is limited to about 5 mg per day. In the normal individual approximately 25 to 30 mg is stored in the body, 80 percent as thiamine diphosphate (pyrophosphate), 10 percent as thiamine triphosphate, and the remainder as free thiamine and thiamine monophosphate. Large amounts are found in skeletal muscles (about half of body stores), heart, liver, kidneys, and brain. Three distinct enzymes are known to participate in the formation of thiamine phosphate esters—a pyrophosphate kinase that catalyzes the formation of thiamine diphosphate from adenosine triphosphate (ATP) and thiamine, a phosphoryl transferase that catalyzes the formation of thiamine triphosphate from ATP and the diphosphate, and a pyrophosphatase that hydrolyzes thiamine triphosphate to thiamine monophosphate. Several metabolites of thiamine are excreted in the urine, principally thiamine itself (which is secreted by the renal tubules), an acetylated derivative, and two major end products of thiamine catabolism, thiazole-acetate and pyrimidine carboxylic acid. Indeed, a number of enzymes called *thiaminases* inactivate thiamine by splitting the vitamin into its two component parts.

Mechanism of action The role of thiamine diphosphate as a coenzyme is well established. In mammals thiamine diphosphate is required for a variety of reactions that have in common the cleavage of carbon-carbon bonds—the oxidative decarboxylation of α-keto acids (pyruvate and α-ketoglutarate) and keto analogues of leucine, isoleucine, and valine and the transketolase reaction in the pentose phosphate pathway. (In bacteria thiamine diphosphate also acts as a coenzyme for certain phosphoketolase enzymes.) Thiamine triphosphate, which has no carboxylase function itself, is important in the binding of thiamine diphosphate to its various apoenzymes. Pioneering work by Sir Rudolph Peters and his associates suggested that the entire spectrum of changes in thiamine deficiency could be explained by the inhibition of these key enzymatic reactions and, in some instances, the accumulation of the proximal metabolites. However, in recent years circumstantial evidence has accrued to suggest that thiamine may have a specific role in the process of neural conduction independent of its coenzymatic function in general metabolism. It is of particular interest in this regard that thiamine and its esters are located in axonal membranes of nerves and that electrical stimulation of nerves results in the hydrolysis and release of both thiamine diphosphate and triphosphate.

Requirements The requirements and recommended daily allowances for thiamine are listed in Tables 73-1 and 73-2. The vitamin has a widespread distribution in food and is entirely absent only from oils, fats, cassava, and refined sugar. A large portion of the vitamin in vegetable products is in the form of thiamine itself. In cereal grains the vitamin is especially rich in the outer layers of the grain; hence machine-milled rice is a poor source. In animal tissues it is present largely in the form of phosphate esters. The ester is dephosphorylated by phos-

FIGURE 80-1
Thiamine pyrophosphate.

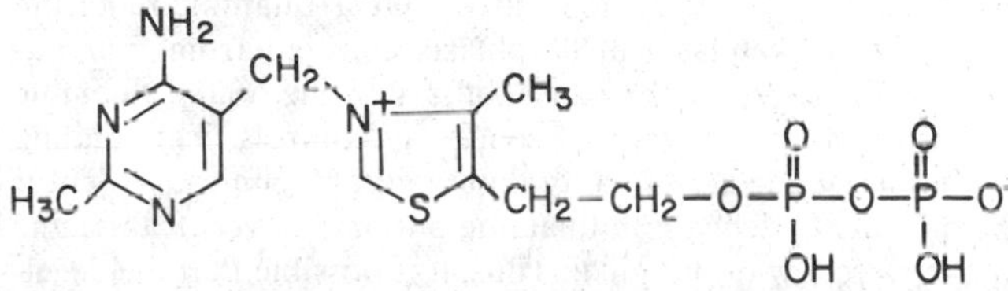

phatases present in the intestine, and only the free vitamin is absorbed. A substantial loss of the vitamin takes place during cooking above 100°C.

Several factors influence the absorption and metabolism of the vitamin (and hence alter daily requirements). One is the presence of thiaminases in foods including fresh fish, clams, shrimp, mussels, and some raw animal tissues. Some microorganisms in the colon may also contain thiaminases. Another factor that influences the requirement is the carbohydrate and caloric intake. Daily needs are reduced when fat forms a large part of the diet and are increased as carbohydrate intake increases. As is true for many vitamins, requirements are increased in pregnancy, during lactation, in thyrotoxicosis, and by fever. Accelerated loss of thiamine from the body may occur as the result of diuretic therapy, hemodialysis, peritoneal dialysis, and diarrhea. Defective intestinal absorption can occur in malabsorption states, alcoholism, chronic malnutrition, and folate deficiency.

EXPERIMENTAL DEPLETION OF THIAMINE Following the institution of a thiamine-free diet in control subjects, thiamine excretion in the urine decreases to 5 percent of the control value by the sixth day and becomes undetectable by day 18. However, the excretion of the pyrimidine and thiazole catabolites of thiamine does not change significantly for as long as 33 days on a deficient diet (about 0.8 mg per day), indicating that the body pool is slowly utilized during a period of deficient intake.

Within 9 days after the institution of a deficient diet, subjects develop a resting tachycardia, followed by the onset of muscle weakness, a decrease in the deep tendon reflexes, and (in some) the appearance of a sensory neuropathy. Subjective symptoms include generalized malaise, headache, nausea, and generalized aching of the muscles. The development of these symptoms is paralleled by a fall in the level of red blood cell transketolase activity. Within a week of thiamine repletion (2 mg per day) all abnormal physical findings disappear; the subjective symptoms clear after 2 weeks. (Experimental depletion in humans has never been carried to the point of development of severe cerebral or cardiovascular symptoms.)

CLINICAL DEFICIENCY Frequency and clinical context In most developed nations thiamine deficiency develops in alcoholics or in the context of special clinical situations, including refeeding after starvation, peritoneal dialysis or hemodialysis, or the administration of glucose to asymptomatic but thiamine-depleted patients. In underdeveloped countries where beriberi may be a common nutritional disease, the causes derive mainly from the consumption of milled rice and foods containing thiaminases and (possibly) other antithiamine factors.

Several factors are involved in the etiology of thiamine deficiency in chronic alcoholics including a low thiamine intake, impaired thiamine absorption, varying rates of destruction of the cofactor, and varying degrees of energy expenditure. However, clinical manifestations of thiamine deficiency develop in only a small fraction of alcoholics and other chronically malnourished persons. Studies by Blass and Gibson suggest that genetic factors are involved in the pathogenesis of clinical manifestations; they demonstrated that a thiamine-requiring enzyme (transketolase) in fibroblasts cultured from four patients with the Wernicke-Korsakoff syndrome bound thiamine diphosphate only a tenth as avidly as controls. This finding implies a genetic abnormality that would be clinically silent if the diet were adequate in thiamine but made overt if thiamine intake were low or marginal. Thus, it is possible that the development of beriberi commonly depends on the presence of an inborn error of metabolism.

Manifestations The two major syndromes of thiamine deficiency involve the cardiovascular (wet beriberi) and nervous systems (dry beriberi and the Wernicke-Korsakoff syndromes). The typical patient has mixed symptoms involving both the cardiovascular and nervous systems, but pure cardiovascular, pure polyneuritic, and pure cerebral forms also occur. The factors that determine the relative preponderance of these manifestations are poorly understood but are related at least in part to the duration and severity of the deficiency, the degree of physical exertion, and the caloric intake. Thus, severe physical exertion, high carbohydrate intake, and a moderate degree of chronic deficiency favor wet beriberi with little or no peripheral neuritis, whereas an equal deficiency with caloric restriction and relative inactivity favors the development of dry (polyneuritic) beriberi.

CARDIOVASCULAR SYSTEM Beriberi heart disease comprises three major physiologic derangements: (1) a state of peripheral vasodilatation leading to a high-output state, (2) a state of biventricular myocardial failure, and (3) retention of sodium and water leading to edema.

In the chronic form, the peripheral vasodilatation leads to increased arteriovenous shunting of blood, rapid circulation time, tachycardia, increased cardiac output, and a venous congestive state characterized by elevated peripheral venous pressure, elevated right ventricular end-diastolic pressure, decreased arteriovenous extraction of oxygen, sodium retention, and edema. Disordered flow of blood to the organs (decreased cerebral and renal blood flow and greatly increased flow to the muscles) is common. It is striking that cardiac output increases to such an extent that, notwithstanding the lowered peripheral vascular resistance, ventricular work, arterial blood pressure, and pulmonary wedge pressure tend to be elevated. Also of interest is the fact that temporary worsening of hypertension occurs during thiamine repletion, presumably due to closing of arteriovenous shunts.

In acute fulminant cardiovascular beriberi, the myocardial lesion appears to be the central feature in a course in which acute cardiovascular collapse develops with death in hours to days. The patient complains of severe dyspnea, intense thirst, restlessness, and anxiety. Physical findings include "stocking-glove" cyanosis, extreme tachycardia, marked cardiomegaly, hepatomegaly, arterial bruits, and neck vein distention. The venous pressure is high, and the circulation time is rapid. Because of the fulminant course little or no edema may be present.

Administration of thiamine rapidly restores peripheral vascular resistance, but improvement in the myocardial abnormality may be delayed so that a low-output failure may supervene during treatment.

NERVOUS SYSTEM Three types of nervous system involvement occur: peripheral neuropathy, Wernicke's encephalopathy (cerebral beriberi), and the Korsakoff syndrome. The neuropathy is characterized by a symmetrical impairment or loss of sensory, motor, and reflex function affecting the distal segments of limbs more severely than the proximal ones. It may or may not be painful. The essential lesion is a noninflammatory, degenerative change affecting the myelin sheaths primarily. No meaningful distinction can be made between this disorder and so-called "alcoholic neuropathy" on the basis of either clinical course or neurologic grounds.

The symptoms of cerebral beriberi ordinarily develop in an orderly progression and consist of vomiting, nystagmus (horizontal more commonly than vertical), palsies of the external recti leading to unilateral or bilateral ophthalmoplegia (and decrease in the nystagmus), fever, ataxia of gait, and progressive mental deterioration that eventuates in a global confusional state and may progress to coma and death. Improvement occurs after the institution of therapy, although symptoms of Korsakoff's syndrome may supervene. Thus, when thiamine therapy is instituted, the eye palsies are corrected, the nystagmus improves in half the patients, the ataxia improves or disappears in two-thirds, and the global confusion state disappears to be replaced by Korsakoff's syndrome. The latter consists of retrograde amnesia, impaired ability to learn, and confabulation (not always present). The patient is usually alert and responsive and exhibits no serious defect in social behavior. Once the Korsakoff disorder supervenes, recovery (complete or partial) can be expected in only half the patients.

In summary, the Wernicke's encephalopathy and the amnesic psychosis of the Korsakoff syndrome are not separate clinical events; instead, the changing ocular and ataxic signs, the transformation of the global confusional state into the amnesic-confabulatory syndrome, and the subsequent development of a nonconfabulatory amnesic state are successive stages in the recovery from a single disease process. The clinical spectrum, differential diagnosis, course, and pathology of cerebral beriberi are discussed in greater detail in Chap. 372.

Diagnosis Various biochemical tests based on thiamine metabolism or the biochemical functions of thiamine diphosphate have been developed to detect thiamine deficiency in humans. These include the measurement of blood thiamine, pyruvate, α-ketoglutarate, lactate, and glyoxylate; the urinary excretion of thiamine and thiamine metabolites; a thiamine-loading test; and measurement of urinary methylglyoxal content. At present the most reliable method is the measurement of whole blood or erythrocyte transketolase activity. Any enhancement in enzymatic activity resulting from added thiamine diphosphate (TPP) is referred to as the *TPP effect* (expressed in percent). If the activity of the enzyme is increased more than 15 percent by the added thiamine diphosphate, then a deficiency state is probably present (Table 74-4). Owing to wide variations in transketolase activity, absolute levels are not very useful, but an increase in activity after treatment coupled with a significant stimulation in vitro by added thiamine diphosphate suggests the presence of thiamine deficiency. Recent work in experimental animals indicates that leukocyte transketolase activity may be a more sensitive index of thiamine nutriture than the red blood cell test.

Another criterion for the diagnosis of thiamine deficiency is the assessment of clinical response to thiamine administration. Clinical improvement may be dramatic in cardiovascular beriberi; an increase in blood pressure and decrease in heart rate may be seen within 12 h after start of therapy. Diuresis and reduction in heart size may be apparent by 24 to 48 h.

Management Prompt administration of thiamine is indicated when beriberi is diagnosed or suspected. Fifty milligrams per day should be given intramuscularly for several days, after which 2.5 to 5 mg per day can be administered by mouth. Larger amounts are usually not absorbed. All patients should also receive other water-soluble vitamins in therapeutic quantities.

THIAMINE-RESPONSIVE INBORN ERRORS OF METABOLISM
A number of thiamine-responsive inborn errors of metabolism have been described in which patients respond to pharmacological doses of thiamine. These include thiamine-responsive megaloblastic anemia, for which the mechanism is unknown; thiamine-responsive lactic acidosis, which is due to low activity of pyruvate carboxylase in liver; thiamine-responsive branched-chain ketoaciduria, which is due to low activity of a ketoacid dehydrogenase; and intermittent cerebellar ataxia

which may result from an abnormal pyruvate dehydrogenase. In addition, it is possible that the autosomal recessive disorder known as *subacute necrotizing encephalomyelopathy* (Leigh's disease) may be related to a diminished amount of thiamine triphosphate in neural tissue; a factor has been isolated from urine of such patients which inhibits the enzyme that synthesizes thiamine triphosphate. The clinical response of patients with Leigh's disease to pharmacological doses of the vitamin appears to be minor, however.

PYRIDOXINE (VITAMIN B$_6$)

NORMAL PHYSIOLOGY OF PYRIDOXINE Biochemistry The biological activity of the vitamin B$_6$ group is displayed by pyridoxine, pyridoxal, and pyridoxamine and their 5-phosphate esters. The coenzyme form is pyridoxal 5-phosphate, and the other compounds owe their enzymatic activity to conversion by tissues to pyridoxal 5-phosphate. Animal tissues contain an oxidase that converts pyridoxine to pyridoxal and a potent pyridoxal kinase that synthesizes pyridoxal phosphate from pyridoxal and ATP. The vitamin is widely and uniformly distributed in all foods; muscle meats, liver, vegetables, and whole-grain cereals are among the best sources.

Mechanism of action Pyridoxal phosphate acts as a cofactor for an exceptionally large number of enzymes involved in amino acid metabolism, including transaminases, synthetases, and hydroxylases. It is of particular importance in humans in the metabolism of tryptophan, glycine, serine, glutamate, and the sulfur-containing amino acids. Pyridoxal phosphate is also required for the synthesis of the heme precursor δ aminolevulinic acid. A large share of body pyridoxine is found in muscle phosphorylase, where it may function not catalytically but to stabilize the enzyme. It also plays a vital (but poorly understood role) in neuronal excitability, possibly as a result of its function in transulfuration reactions or γ-aminobutyric acid metabolism.

Requirements The requirements and recommended daily allowances for the vitamin are described in Tables 73-1 and 73-2. Even more than for most vitamins, the requirement is increased in pregnancy and by the ingestion of estrogenic drugs. In both conditions abnormal tryptophan metabolites are excreted in urine, and this can be prevented by supplementation with pyridoxine. Estrogenic steroids appear to inhibit selectively the pyridoxal phosphate function in tryptophan metabolism. In addition, pyridoxine requirement may be increased by high protein intake. The ingestion of ethanol interferes with the metabolism of pyridoxal phosphate, the ethanol metabolite acetaldehyde displacing the coenzyme from proteins and thus enhancing its degradation.

EXPERIMENTAL DEPLETION OF PYRIDOXINE The feeding to experimental subjects of diets deficient in pyridoxine leads to chemical evidence of deficiency (increased xanthurenic acid and decreased pyridoxine in urine) within a week. Electroencephalographic abnormalities appear within 3 weeks in subjects with previously normal EEGs, and some subjects subsequently have grand mal seizures. Deficiency induced with the pyridoxine antagonist desoxypyridoxine causes, in addition, seborrheic dermatitis, cheilosis, glossitis, and severe systemic symptoms such as nausea, vomiting, weakness, and dizziness.

CLINICAL DEFICIENCY Frequency and clinical context The widespread occurrence of the vitamin in food is probably the reason that a naturally occurring pure pyridoxine deficiency has never been recognized except when the pyridoxine content of food is destroyed during processing, as has occurred in some processed infant formulas. Thus, it is a paradox that at present pyridoxine deficiency is frequent in the United States. This happens because many commonly used drugs act as pyridoxine antagonists. Hydrazines such as isoniazid induce peripheral neuritis that can be prevented by vitamin B_6 supplementation; these drugs appear to combine with pyridoxal or pyridoxal phosphate to form hydrazones. The hydrazones may be excreted in the urine (causing pyridoxal deficiency) but may also inhibit enzymes directly (for example, pyridoxal kinase). The hydrazones may in addition act directly as convulsants. Cycloserine, an antituberculous drug, causes an increase in the excretion of the vitamin in the urine and produces profound neurological effects; it is thought that the drug forms a complex with pyridoxal phosphate which competes with the cofactor for apoenzymes. Penicillamine acts as an antagonist by forming a thiazolidine derivative with pyridoxal phosphate; abnormal tryptophan metabolism and convulsions can be prevented by supplementation with the vitamin.

Diagnosis Estimates of vitamin deficiency have been based upon the cure of clinical signs of deficiency, the excretion of tryptophan metabolites after tryptophan-loading tests, measurement of various amino acid transferase activities in blood, and excretion of pyridoxine or its metabolites or of oxalate in the urine (Table 74-3). Because of the relative ease with which it can be done, the most common index is the measurement of tryptophan metabolites, particularly xanthurenic acid, following tryptophan loading. Alternatively cystathionine can be assayed after a methionine load. It is possible that measurement of red blood cell glutamic pyruvic transaminase in vitro in the presence and absence of pyridoxal phosphate is superior to both loading tests.

Management The appropriate management is prevention of deficiency. Supplementation of the diet with 30 mg pyridoxine normalizes tryptophan metabolism in pregnancy, in contraceptive users, and in patients taking isoniazid. Doses as high as 100 mg per day may be required in subjects taking penicillamine.

PYRIDOXINE-RESPONSIVE DISEASES There are a large number of genetic conditions in which abnormalities in vitamin B_6 metabolism occur. One group, if not provided with large daily supplements of pyridoxine during infancy, develops convulsions and brain damage and dies; these children have an apoenzyme for glutamic acid decarboxylase that has a decreased binding affinity for pyridoxal phosphate. Consequently they do not form γ-aminobutyric acid, a putative physiological inhibitor of neurological activity in the brain, at a normal rate. Another group has pyridoxine-responsive chronic anemia; although pyridoxine supplementation results in prompt hematologic remission, it does not correct the morphological abnormality in the erythrocytes.

The synthesis of cystathionine from homocystine and serine and its cleavage to cysteine and homoserine are catalyzed by two pyridoxal phosphate enzymes. The biochemical changes which occur in deficiency of these two enzymes and in xanthurenic aciduria due to kynureninase deficiency have been reviewed by Mudd. Some patients with vitamin B_6–responsive xanthurenic aciduria or cystathioninuria have a mutant apoenzyme that interacts abnormally with pyridoxal phosphate in a manner which can be largely overcome by elevated concentrations of the cofactor. In contrast, the vitamin B_6 response in patients with homocystinuria due to cystathionine synthetase

deficiency is not due to restoration of the affected enzyme to normal levels but to an enhancement of the activity of the small amount of normal enzyme present.

RIBOFLAVIN

Riboflavin is essential for all oxidation-reduction reactions involving the coenzymes flavin mononucleotide (FMN) and flavin adenine dinucleotide (FAD). In addition, covalently attached flavins are essential to the structure of such enzymes as succinate dehydrogenase and monoamine oxidase. The vitamin is absorbed from the gastrointestinal tract either as free riboflavin or the 5′-phosphate by a specific transport process. The requirements and recommended daily allowances are listed in Tables 73-1 and 73-2. Covalently linked vitamin accounts for less than a tenth of the tissue pool. The vitamin is excreted in urine predominantly in the free form, although a small fraction of the daily turnover is catabolized by microorganisms in the gastrointestinal tract.

Clinical riboflavin deficiency can be induced in human subjects either by feeding a riboflavin-deficient diet and/or by administering riboflavin antagonists such as galactoflavin. The deficiency syndrome is characterized by sore throat, hyperemia and edema of the pharyngeal and oral mucous membranes, cheilosis, angular stomatitis, glossitis, seborrheic dermatitis, and normochromic, normocytic anemia associated with pure red blood cell hypoplasia of the bone marrow. All these features can be rapidly and completely reversed after riboflavin administration.

Riboflavin deficiency almost invariably occurs in combination with other vitamin deficiencies. Certain features of the syndrome such as glossitis and dermatitis may be seen with other vitamin deficiencies as well.

REFERENCES

Pyridoxine

FRIMPTER GW et al: Vitamin B_6-dependency syndromes: New horizons in nutrition. Am J Clin Nutr 22:794, 1969

GERSHOFF SN: Vitamin B_6, in *Nutrition Reviews' Present Knowledge in Nutrition*, 4th ed, DM Hegsted et al (eds). Washington, DC, The Nutrition Foundation, 1976, p 149

HARRIS JW, HORRIGAN DL: Pyridoxine-responsive anemia-prototype and variations on a theme, in *Vitamins and Hormones: Advances in Research and Applications*, RS Harris et al (eds). New York, Academic, 1964, vol 22, pp 721–753

JAFFE IA: The antivitamin B_6 effect of pencillamine: Clinical and immunological implications, in *Advances in Biochemical Psychopharmacology*, vol 4, MS Ebodi, E Costa (eds). New York, Raven Press, 1972

LUHBY AL et al: Vitamin B_6 metabolism in users of oral contraceptive agents. I: Abnormal urinary xanthurenic acid excretion and its correction by pyridoxine. Am J Clin Nutr 24:684, 1971

LUMENG L: The role of acetaldehyde in mediating the deleterious effects of ethanol on pyridoxal 5′-phosphate metabolism. J Clin Invest 62:286, 1978

MUDD SH: Pyridoxine-responsive genetic disease. Fed Proc 30:970, 1971

SAUBERLICH HE et al: Biochemical assessment of the nutritional status of vitamin B_6 in the human. Am J Clin Nutr 25:629, 1972

Riboflavin

LANE M et al: The rapid induction of human riboflavin deficiency with galactoflavin. J Clin Invest 43:357, 1964

RIVLIN RS: Riboflavin metabolism. N Engl J Metab 283:463, 1970

Thiamine

AKBARIAN M et al: Hemodynamic studies in beriberi heart disease. Am J Med 41:197, 1966

BLASS JP, GIBSON GE: Abnormality of a thiamine-requiring enzyme in patients with Wernicke-Korsakoff syndrome. N Engl J Med 297:1367, 1977

BROWN GM: Biogenesis and metabolism of thiamine, in *Metabolic Pathways,* 3d ed, DM Greenberg (ed). Academic, New York, 1970, pp 369–381

KOZAM RL et al: Cardiovascular beriberi. Am J Cardiol 30:418, 1972

PINCUS JH et al: Thiamine derivatives in subacute necrotizing encephalomyelopathy. Pediatrics 51:716, 1973

SCRIVER CR: Vitamin-responsive inborn errors of metabolism. Metabolism 22:1319, 1973

TANPHAICHITR V et al: Clinical and biochemical studies of adult beriberi. Am J Clin Nutr 23:1017, 1970

VICTOR M et al: *The Wernicke-Korsakoff Syndrome.* Philadelphia, Davis, 1971

ZIPORIN ZZ et al: Excretion of thiamine and its metabolites in the urine of young adult males receiving restricted intakes of the vitamin. J Nutr 85:287, 1965

81
DEFICIENCY OF VITAMIN C (SCURVY)

JEAN D. WILSON

NORMAL PHYSIOLOGY OF VITAMIN C **Biochemistry** In most animals vitamin C can be readily synthesized from glucose. Indeed, humans, other primates, and the guinea pig are the only mammals known to be unable to synthesize L-ascorbic acid and consequently to require vitamin C in the diet to prevent scurvy. These three species can perform all the various reactions required for the biosynthesis of the vitamin from *d*-glucose except for one step, the conversion of L-glucono-γ-lactone to L-ascorbic acid. The enzyme that catalyzes this reaction (L-gluconolactone oxidase) is missing because of a mutation that has occurred in these species; thus the need for vitamin C in the diet is the result of a defect in carbohydrate metabolism.

Mechanism of action L-Ascorbic acid readily undergoes reversible oxidation and reduction as follows:

$$\text{L-Ascorbic acid} \rightleftharpoons \text{dehydro-L-ascorbic acid} + 2H^+ + 2e$$

This property of the vitamin is of paramount importance in understanding its physiological role. Indeed, several systems have been characterized in animal tissues in which L-ascorbic acid is coupled with other redox agents. However, there is no direct evidence that the vitamin acts as a conventional cofactor since its requirement can usually be replaced by other compounds with similar redox properties. The most clearly established functional role of the vitamin is in the synthesis of collagen; absence of the vitamin in vitro leads to impairment of peptidyl hydroxylation of procollagen and a reduction in collagen formation and excretion by the connective tissue cell. Nonhydroxylated collagen is unstable and cannot form the triple helix required for normal structures. Many of the clinical findings in scurvy result from this impaired collagen synthesis, including the capillary fragility that underlies the hemorrhagic features, the poor healing of wounds, and (in part) the bony abnormalities of children. Collagens which ordinarily have the highest content of hydroxyproline are most affected, accounting for the disruption of blood vessel adventitia, media, and basal laminae that is characteristic of the disease. Ascorbic acid also acts to prevent oxidation of tetrahydrofolate and thus protect the active folic acid pool. In addition it functions in some manner to regulate iron distribution and storage, probably by influencing the valence of stored iron and thus maintaining a normal ratio of ferritin to hemosiderin. Scorbutic patients also excrete incompletely oxidized products of tyrosine metabolism, but the clinical significance of these metabolites is not clear.

Requirements The requirements and recommended daily allowances for vitamin C are given in Tables 73-1 and 73-2. The vitamin is absent in many common foods but is present in milk and some meats (kidney, liver, fish) and is widely distributed in a variety of fruits and vegetables. A portion of the vitamin is lost after prolonged storage of unprocessed fruits and vegetables (for example, potatoes), but it is partially preserved (half or greater) by most means of food processing (boiling, steaming, pressure cooking, preserving jams and jellies, freezing, dehydration, and canning). As a consequence, fulfilling the recommended daily allowances is easy with even a modest intake of fruits or vegetables. Many factors increase vitamin C requirements including pregnancy, lactation, and thyrotoxicosis which increase utilization, and diarrheal states and achlorhydria which decrease absorption.

EXPERIMENTAL DEPLETION OF VITAMIN C Metabolism of vitamin C has been studied extensively in adults fed diets deficient only in vitamin C and then during repletion in the same subjects. The total body pool varies from 1.5 to 3 g, and when a deficient diet is instituted, the pool is depleted at a constant rate of decay (first order), which varies among individuals (rates as high as 4 percent per day occurring in some). Recent studies in monkeys indicate that the major catabolic pathway involves oxidation of the alcohol at carbon 6 to an aldehyde and then to an acid. Because of differences in initial pool size and rates of turnover, variability in the completeness of deficiency in experimental diets, and variability at the cellular or enzymatic level as well, the time required for the appearance of symptoms ranges from 1 to 3 months in different studies. Symptoms of deficiency correlate better with the total pool size than with plasma or blood levels. In most patients the first symptoms (petechial hemorrhages and ecchymoses) usually do not begin to appear until the pool size is less than 0.5 g; with further depletion (pool size 0.1 to 0.5 g) additional changes appear including gum abnormalities, hyperkeratosis, congested hair follicles, arthralgias, the sicca syndrome, coiled hairs, and joint effusions. When depletion becomes extreme (pool size <0.1 g), dyspnea, edema, oliguria, and neuropathy supervene. After the onset of symptoms, clinical progress of the disease may be rapid.

Symptoms do not improve until the pool size is repleted, and the larger the therapeutic dose, the more rapid the repletion. However, with doses as small as 6.5 mg per day repletion of the body pool and amelioration of symptoms eventually occur in some individuals.

CLINICAL DEFICIENCY **Frequency and clinical background** Clinical scurvy is an unusual disease in the United States and in most of the world today. It occurs for the most part in areas of urban poverty, and from time to time patients are admitted with it to the wards of most municipal hospitals. A peak of incidence occurs at 6 to 12 months of age in infants whose processed milk formulas are unsupplemented with citrus fruit or vegetables as the result of maternal error or neglect. Another peak occurs in middle and old age; edentulous *men* who live alone and cook for themselves are particularly prone to develop the disease. Clinical scurvy is more severe than the experimental disease, doubtlessly because affected individuals usually have deficiencies of other dietary constituents as well and because the groups at risk (infants and the elderly) are especially vulnerable. The disorder has different clinical features in adults and children.

Manifestations In adults the characteristic features include perifollicular hyperkeratotic papules in which hairs become fragmented and buried, perifollicular hemorrhages, purpura beginning on the backs of the lower extremities coalescing to become ecchymoses (Fig. 81-1), hemorrhage into the muscles of the arms and legs with secondary phlebothromboses, hemorrhages into joints, splinter hemorrhages into the nail beds, gum involvement (only in people with teeth) that includes swelling, friability, bleeding, secondary infection, and loosening of the teeth, poor healing of wounds and breakdown of recently healed wounds, petechial hemorrhages in the viscera, and emotional changes. The development of symptoms resembling those of the sicca syndrome has been noted. Terminally, icterus, edema, and fever are common, and convulsions, shock, and death may occur suddenly.

In infancy and childhood, hemorrhage into the periosteum of long bones causes painful swellings and may result in epiphyseal separation (x-ray changes may in fact be diagnostic). The sternum may sink inwardly, leaving a sharp elevation at the rib margins (scorbutic rosary). Skin purpura and ecchymoses may also occur, and gum lesions occur only if the teeth have erupted. Retrobulbar, subarachnoid, and intracerebral hemorrhages may lead to rapidly progressive illness culminating in death if treatment is delayed.

FIGURE 81-1
Hemorrhages and ecchymoses in a patient with scurvy. (Courtesy of LL Madison.)

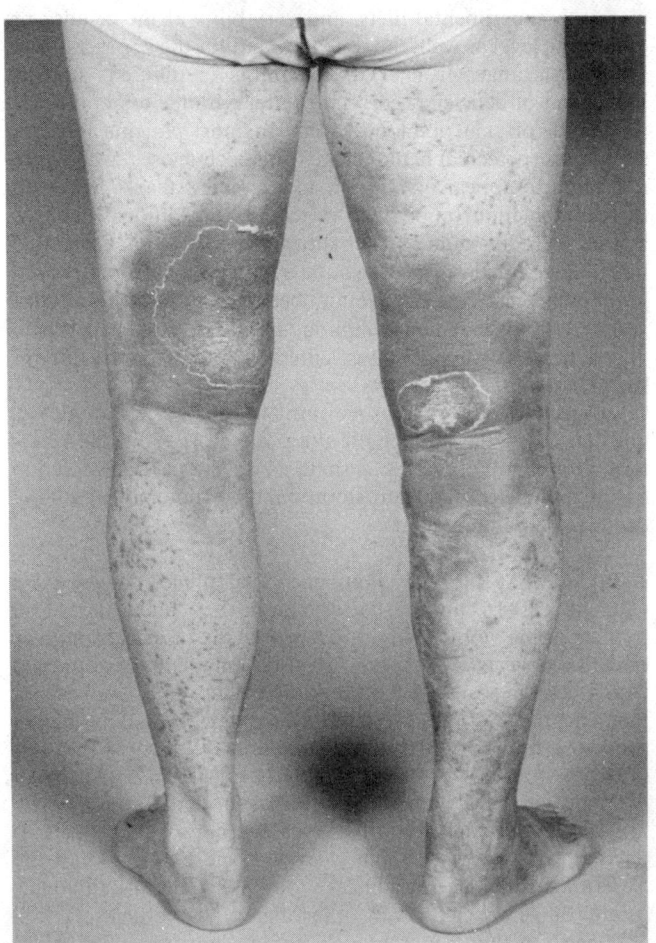

Severe to moderate anemia is a common feature in children and adults and is usually normochromic and normocytic, the result of the bleeding into tissues. On occasion, it may be macrocytic and/or megaloblastic. Many foods which contain vitamin C also contain folate, and a diet that causes scurvy may also cause folate deficiency. However, folate metabolism is also altered in scurvy; ascorbic acid deficiency permits an increased irreversible oxidation of formyl tetrahydrofolic acid to inactive folate metabolites and may thus cause a decrease in the active metabolic pool of the vitamin. Whether changes in iron distribution and storage are involved in the pathogenesis of the anemia is unclear. Whatever the mechanism the anemia is corrected with refeeding and replenishment of vitamin C and the institution of a balanced diet.

Diagnosis In some hospitals platelet ascorbic acid levels are useful in diagnosing scurvy and are usually less than a fourth of the normal value (52 ± 22 μg per 10^{10} platelets). Plasma levels of the vitamin correlate less well with the clinical state (Table 74-3). In infants x-ray changes of the bones may be diagnostic. Indirect bilirubin is frequently elevated. Anemia is usually normochromic, normocytic but may (4 out of 21 patients in one series) be megaloblastic. Capillary fragility is abnormal. The remainder of the laboratory tests are nondiagnostic.

Management If scurvy is suspected, samples of blood should be obtained, and ascorbic acid should be administered promptly. Scurvy is potentially fatal, and treatment should never be delayed. The usual dose of the vitamin in adult patients is 100 mg three to five times a day by mouth until 4 g has been administered, then 100 mg per day. In infants and children 10 to 25 mg three times a day is adequate. A diet rich in vitamin C should be initiated in all patients. Generally, spontaneous bleeding ceases within 24 h, muscle and bone pain subsides quickly, and within 2 to 3 days the gums begin to heal. Even large ecchymoses and hematomas are resolved in 10 to 12 days, although pigmentary changes in areas of extensive hemorrhage may persist for months. Serum bilirubin becomes normal within 3 to 5 days, and the anemia ordinarily is completely corrected within 2 to 4 weeks.

THE MEGAVITAMIN QUESTION Considerable controversy has risen over the claim that large doses of vitamin C (1 g or more per day) are effective in preventing or minimizing the symptoms of the common cold. However, in adequately controlled studies, no significant differences in occurrence, severity, or duration have been demonstrated in subjects treated with a placebo as compared with the vitamin. The long-term toxicity of ascorbic acid in these doses is not known, but large doses can interfere with the absorption of vitamin B_{12}, and by enhancing the development of metabolizing enzymes in the fetus may cause development of scurvy in the offspring of mothers who have ingested large amounts of the vitamin during pregnancy. It must be concluded that common use of the vitamin in this way is both unwarranted and unwise. However, ordinary pharmacological doses (200 mg daily) may correct leucocyte abnormalities in patients with the Chediak-Higashi syndrome (Chap. 56).

REFERENCES

BAKER EM et al: Ascorbic acid metabolism in man. Am J Clin Nutr 19:371, 1966

BARNES MJ, KODICEK E: Biological hydroxylations and ascorbic acid with special regard to collagen metabolism. Vitam Horm 30:1, 1972

BARNESS LA: Nutritional aspects of vegetarianism, health foods and fad diets. Nutr 59:153, 1977

BOXEN LA et al: Correction of leucocyte function in Chediak-Higashi syndrome by ascorbate. N Engl J Med 295:1041, 1976

BURNS JJ: Biosynthesis of L-ascorbic acid; basic defect in scurvy. Am J Med 26:740, 1959

CHALMERS TC: Effects of ascorbic acid on the common cold. Am J Med 58:532, 1975

HODGES RE et al: Clinical manifestations of ascorbic acid deficiency in man. Am J Clin Nutr 24:432, 1971

TOLBERT, BM et al: New information on synthesis and metabolism of ascorbic acid. Nutr Rev 35:22, 1977

VILTER RW: Effects of ascorbic acid deficiency in man, in The Vitamins, WH Sebrell Jr, RS Harris (eds). New York, Academic, 1967, vol 1, p 457

WALLERSTEIN RO, WALLERSTEIN RO JR: Scurvy. Semin Hematol 13:211, 1976

82
DEFICIENCY OF VITAMINS A AND K AND HYPERVITAMINOSIS A

JEAN D. WILSON

VITAMIN A

NORMAL PHYSIOLOGY **Chemistry and metabolism** Vitamin A can be either ingested or synthesized within the body from dietary carotenoids. Preformed vitamin A is found almost exclusively in animals, and the best sources are liver, milk, and kidney, where it is found largely in the form of esters of fatty acids. It is hydrolyzed during the process of digestion, absorbed in the free form, resterified with fatty acids within the intestinal mucosa, and transported in association with lymph chylomicrons. The major substrates for the synthesis of vitamin A are plant carotenoids, mainly β-carotenes, that are widely distributed. β-Carotene can be either absorbed intact or cleaved at the central double bond by a dioxygenase enzyme in the intestinal mucosa (or lumen) to form two molecules of retinaldehyde. Subsequently retinaldehyde is reduced by an aldehyde reductase to retinol. Retinol from whatever source is stored as retinyl esters in the parenchymal cells of the liver. The body pool size in normal subjects varies from 300 to 900 mg.

Prior to release from the liver, the retinyl esters are hydrolyzed, and the free alcohol is mobilized bound to a specific transport protein, retinol-binding protein (RBP). This is the form in which vitamin A is transported to peripheral tissues. In vitamin A deficiency the release of RBP from the liver is inhibited, and the protein accumulates in liver; with repletion rapid release of the protein from preformed stores occurs. The mechanism(s) by which retinol is catabolized and/or excreted has not been defined; approximately equal amounts are excreted in the bile and urine.

Mechanism of action The only physiological function of vitamin A that has been clearly defined in biochemical terms is its role in vision; in the retina vitamin A forms a series of carotenoid proteins that provide the molecular basis for visual excitation. Beyond its role in the visual cycles, vitamin A is known to be required for growth, reproduction, and the maintenance of life. The recent discovery of retinol-phosphate-mannose glycolipid suggests that the vitamin may play a primary role in the synthesis of certain glycoproteins. This process may be one of several functions of the vitamin, but the importance of glycoprotein to every epithelial function implies that this may be a major function of the vitamin.

Requirements The recommended daily allowances for vitamin A are listed in Tables 73-1 and 73-2. The assumed utilization efficiency for the conversion of β-carotene to vitamin A in the human is one-sixth (0.167). Other carotenoids with provitamin activity have, on the average, half the activity of β-carotene. Pregnancy and disease states in which there is impaired absorption or storage, excessive utilization, or increased excretion of vitamin A may lead to increased requirements.

EXPERIMENTAL DEPLETION OF VITAMIN A When experimental subjects are fed a diet deficient in both retinol and carotene, plasma levels fall progressively to less than 10 μg per 100 ml in three-fourths of subjects. The body pool simultaneously shrinks to less than half the control value. A true or manifest deficiency develops in all subjects. Follicular hyperkeratosis, impaired dark adaptation, and abnormalities of the electroretinogram are consistent findings. All these changes are corrected after supplementation with 150 μg retinol or 300 μg β-carotene per day.

VITAMIN A DEFICIENCY **Clinical occurrence and context** Endemic deficiency results from inadequate amounts of the vitamin and the carotene provitamins in the diet and probably never occurs except in conjunction with deficiency of other nutrients or complicating infectious diseases. In many underdeveloped countries vitamin A deficiency is a major cause of blindness in the young; failure to incorporate green leafy vegetables and other rich sources of the provitamin or vitamin into the child's diet is the root of the problem. Vitamin A deficiency may also accompany protein calorie malnutrition, and here the deficiency is due to the defective release mechanism from the liver secondary to inadequate retinol binding protein. In most developed nations, including the United States, vitamin A deficiency is almost always due to either intestinal malabsorption (sprue), abnormal storage (liver disease), or enhanced destruction or excretion of the vitamin (renal disease).

Clinical findings Night blindness is the earliest symptom of deficiency, followed by degenerative changes in the retina. The bulbar conjunctiva becomes dry (xerosis), and small, grey plaques with foamy surfaces develop (Bitot's spots). These lesions are reversible with vitamin A. The more serious effect of vitamin A deficiency is keratomalacia and involves the cornea with ulceration and necrosis, leading to perforation, prolapse, and endophthalmitis. The end result is impairment of vision. Patients may have associated dryness and hyperkeratosis of the skin.

Diagnosis Measurements of dark adaptation, rod scotometry, and electroretinography all suffer the disadvantages of requiring trained personnel and expensive equipment. Vitamin A levels in plasma are not reliable for the assessment of stores in individual cases. The diagnosis ultimately must rest upon a high index of suspicion in every malnourished child.

Treatment Night blindness and the milder conjunctival changes respond well to 30,000 IU vitamin A for a few days. Corneal damage constitutes a therapeutic emergency, and the usual treatment is 20,000 IU per kilogram of body weight per day for 5 days.

OVERDOSAGE **Carotenemia** Hypercarotenemia results from excessive intake of carotene-containing foods, principally carrots. Excess carotene does not appear to be injurious apart from the cosmetic effect; the fact that it never leads to hypervitaminosis A indicates that some step(s) in the conversion of carotene to vitamin A must be regulated. Carotenemia is characterized by yellowing of the skin with greatest intensity on the palms and soles and with a corresponding yellowness of serum. The yellowing of the skin can be distinguished from jaundice in that the scleras remain white. The omission of carrots from the diet always leads to the rapid disappearance of the pigmentation. Yellowness of the skin can also result on occasion from the consumption of excessive amounts of other colored fruits and vegetables. Hypothyroid patients appear to be particularly susceptible.

Vitamin A toxicity Hypervitaminosis A can result from accidental overingestion by hunters or explorers (polar bear liver), as the result of food faddism (usually caused by oversolicitous parents), or as a side effect of inappropriate therapy. It may be either acute or chronic. Acute toxicity from a single massive dose consists of abdominal pain, nausea, vomiting, severe headaches, dizziness, sluggishness, and irritability followed within a few days by generalized desquamation of the skin and recovery. Chronic toxicity occurs in people who take 40,000 units or more daily for protracted periods and is characterized by bone and joint pain, hair loss, dryness and fissures of the lips, anorexia, benign intracranial hypertension, weight loss, and hepatomegaly. The only diagnostic laboratory finding is elevation of the vitamin in serum, chiefly in the form of retinyl esters. The concentration of retinol-binding protein is normal, and the excess vitamin A circulates in association with lipoprotein. Relief is prompt on withdrawal of the vitamin from the diet.

VITAMIN K

Vitamin K occurs in nature in two major forms: vitamin K_1 (phylloquinone) which is present in most edible vegetables, particularly in green leaves, and vitamin K_2 which is produced by intestinal bacteria. All the many compounds with vitamin K activity are structurally related to the simpler compound, 2-methyl-1,4-naphthoquinone (menadione). Menadione may be formed in the gut by the action of intestinal bacteria on vitamins K_1 and K_2. After absorption, menadione is converted in the body to the active menaquinone. Vitamin K is required by humans and other animals to maintain prothrombin and clotting factors VII, IX, X, and possibly V. The vitamin is a component of a specialized microsomal electron transport system coupled to a carbon dioxide fixalin that effects the γ-carboxylation of glutamic acid in several proteins of the plasma, bone, kidney, and urine, including the precursor proteins for the above clotting factors. It is presumed that in deficiency states death from hemorrhage ensues before other abnormalities become manifest.

Under ordinary circumstances about 80 percent of vitamin K is absorbed in the small bowel into the intestinal lymph. Because the naturally occurring forms of vitamin K are fat-soluble and are poorly stored in the body, a conditioned deficiency can occur in association with diseases that interfere with fat absorption. In addition, long-term treatment with certain antimicrobial drugs may temporarily eliminate intestinal bacteria as a vitamin K source. The coumarin anticoagulant drugs appear to induce hypoprothrombinemia by inhibiting the γ carboxylation of the precursor protein.

Newborn infants tend to be deficient in vitamin K, exhibiting low plasma levels of several coagulation factors in the prothrombin complex. Such deficiencies result from minimal stores of vitamin K at birth, lack of an established intestinal flora, and a very limited dietary intake of the vitamin.

Routine determination of prothrombin should be performed before all surgical procedures and deliveries. Patients with values below 70 percent of normal should receive therapy with vitamin K; administration of 75 mg menadione is satisfactory by any route and may be repeated until body stores of vitamin K are repleted. Hypoprothrombinemia secondary to hepatic dysfunction and excessive use of anticoagulants requires multiple dosage of vitamin K_1 for optimal results.

REFERENCES

Doisy EA Jr, Matschiner JT: Biochemistry of vitamin K, in *Fat-Soluble Vitamins*, RA Morton (ed). New York, Pergamon, 1970, vol 9, p 293

Lombaert A, Carton H: Benign intracranial hypertension due to A-hypervitaminosis in adults and adolescents. Eur Neurol 14:340, 1976

Olson RE, Suttie JW: Vitamin K and γ-carboxyglutamate biosynthesis, in *Vitamins and Hormones*, PL Munson et al (eds). New York, Academic, 1977, vol 35, p 59

Sauberlich HE et al: Vitamin A metabolism and requirements in the human studied with the use of labeled retinol, in *Vitamins and Hormones: Advances in Research and Applications*, RS Harris et al (eds). New York, Academic, 1974, vol 32

Shearer MJ et al: Studies on the absorption and metabolism of phylloquinone (vitamin K) in man, in *Vitamins and Hormones: Advances in Research and Applications*, RS Harris et al (eds). Academic, 1974, vol 32, p 513

Smith FR, Goodman DS: Vitamin A transport in human vitamin A toxicity. N Engl J Med 294:805, 1976

Smith JE, Goodman DS: Vitamin A metabolism and transport, in *Present Knowledge in Nutrition*, 4th ed, DM Hegsted et al (eds), Washington, DC, The Nutrition Foundation, 1976

Srikantia SG: Human vitamin A deficiency, in *World Review of Nutrition and Dietetics*, GH Bourne (ed). Basel, Karger, 1975, vol 20, p 185

Wald G: Molecular basis of visual excitation. Science 162:230, 1968

83

DISTURBANCES IN TRACE ELEMENT METABOLISM

DAVID D. ULMER

Inorganic ions are crucial to virtually all biochemical and physiologic processes. Some, present in tissues only in minute quantity, micrograms to picograms per gram of wet organ, are arbitrarily designated *trace elements*. Of these, iron, iodine, cobalt, copper, manganese, molybdenum, selenium, chromium, fluorine, silicon, nickel, zinc, tin, and vanadium are now thought to be essential for animal life.

The functions of trace elements have been defined at levels of biologic complexity ranging from isolated enzymes to intact animals. Thus, many metals participate in enzymic catalysis through substrate binding, activation of the enzyme-substrate complex, or by formation of a tight coordination complex with the enzyme such that the two are isolated together as a unit, i.e., *metalloenzyme*. Metals appear to play a role in the synthesis of both proteins and nucleic acids. Trace elements are also involved in the function of organized subcellular systems, such as mitochondria, in regulation of intracellular heme concentrations, and in membrane transport, nerve conduction, and muscle contraction. Critical biologic functions in animals are disrupted by deprivation of essential metals resulting in discrete deficiency states. Toxic manifestations owing to grossly excessive exposure to metals are also well recognized. The biologic effects of metals, both essential and toxic, are often conditioned by *metal-ion antagonism;* i.e., one metal induces a biologic effect by altering the requirement for another, usually through competition for the same biochemical sites. As a consequence, such metal-ion *imbalances* are likely among the most common and certainly the most elusive sources of either metal-deficiency or intoxication states. This phenomenon complicates investigative efforts and helps to account for the fact that proved manifestations of trace-element deficiency in human beings, except for those due to iron and iodine, are rare despite extensive documentation of deficiency syndromes in many animal species.

ZINC The average adult human body contains 1.4 to 2.3 g zinc; highest concentrations are found in liver, voluntary muscle, bone, prostate, and eye. The minimum daily requirement (about 15 mg) is easily attained in most diets since the element is widely distributed in food, particularly meat, shellfish, liver, gelatin, bread, cereals, lentils, peas, beans, and rice. However, *phytic acid* in the diet binds zinc tightly, limits its absorption, and operates as a conditioning factor to induce zinc deficiency. Zinc is crucial to growth, development, and normal function of all living forms. It is an essential component of many enzymes in the liver, pancreas, and other organs, and its importance for protein synthesis may be surmised from recent evidence that both DNA and RNA polymerases are zinc metalloenzymes. While marked changes in the zinc content of tissues, blood, and urine accompany many different human diseases, the relationship of such alterations to the underlying conditions are, for the most part, poorly understood.

Spontaneous or experimental zinc deficiency in animals results in anorexia, retarded growth, gonadal atrophy, hyperkeratotic dermatitis, loss of hair, parakeratosis of tongue and esophagus, and diarrhea. Two human syndromes exhibit features observed in zinc-deficient animals. Hypogonadal dwarfism, sometimes accompanied by hepatosplenomegaly, anemia, and geophagia, has been described in rural Iranian and Egyptian boys subsisting on diets consisting largely of bread and beans and nearly devoid of animal protein. The youths have decreased zinc concentrations in plasma, red cells, and hair and decreased activity of serum alkaline phosphatase, a zinc-dependent enzyme. Oral zinc supplements enhance growth and sexual maturation beyond that observed with administration of an adequate diet alone. However, the anemia is improved only by correction of concomitant iron deficiency. Delayed growth and sexual maturation accompanied by moderate decreases in serum zinc concentration have also been observed in this country in youths afflicted with chronic illnesses such as intestinal malabsorption and sickle-cell anemia. It is postulated that such patients may have an incomplete form of the hypogonadal dwarf syndrome.

In recent years, *acrodermatitis enteropathica* has been characterized as the first inherited human zinc-deficiency disease. This autosomal recessive disorder is manifested by severe chronic diarrhea, wasting, alopecia, and roughened, thickened, and ulcerated skin about body orifices and on the extremities. Patients exhibit a profound decrease in zinc concentrations in serum and hair, and defective leukocyte chemotaxis. They improve quickly upon administration of zinc. Whether the zinc deficiency results from an intestinal absorptive defect, excessive losses, or other factors is not yet clear. Acrodermatitis enteropathica owing to acquired zinc deficiency has also been observed in adults maintained on long-term parenteral nutrition. The response to zinc administration is equally dramatic.

Demonstration of the value of zinc replacement in patients with acrodermatitis enteropathica has prompted renewed interest in the role of this element in promoting healing of surgical wounds and chronic skin ulcers. Several investigations suggest that wound healing is delayed in patients with zinc deficiency and is restored to normal by oral administration of zinc. However, controlled studies indicate that zinc has no effect in wound-healing in normal persons.

Zinc has been postulated to play a role in the maintenance of normal taste and patients with decreased taste acuity (hypogeusia) may improve with oral administration of zinc sulfate.

Zinc toxicity may result from excessive ingestion of the element in food or drink, although the margin of safety is large. Nausea, vomiting, colic, and diarrhea are predominant manifestations. Toxicity also results from inhalation of high concentrations of zinc oxide fumes, leading to *metal-fume fever* or *brass chills*. Once a fairly common industrial hazard, this self-limited, acute illness is accompanied by fever, shaking chills, excessive salivation, headache, cough, malaise, and pronounced leukocytosis.

COPPER Copper is an essential nutrient for animals and is critical to such diverse activities as heme synthesis, connective tissue metabolism, bone development, and nerve function. Experimental copper deficiency is manifested by severe anemia, abnormalities of hair and skin pigmentation, defective elastic tissue in great vessels resulting in arterial rupture, faulty development of bone and nervous tissue, and decreased concentrations of plasma copper and the serum copper protein, *ceruloplasmin (ferroxidase)*. Ceruloplasmin catalyzes oxidation of ferrous to ferric ions and is postulated to control the rate of iron uptake by transferrin—hence, availability to reticulocytes of iron for heme synthesis. Copper is also a component of a number of other critical metalloenzymes, e.g., cytochrome oxidase, lysine oxidase, polyphenol oxidases, amine oxidases, and the cupreins—cuprozinc proteins in liver, red cells, and brain which appear to function as superoxide dismutases and may also serve in quenching highly reactive singlet oxygen in cells. Copper is important to mitochondrial function and is found frequently as a component of ribonucleic acid.

The copper concentration in adult human beings averages 1.5 to 2.4 μg per gram of fat-free tissue; the metal concentrates in liver, heart, brain, kidneys, and hair; for example, to 18 to 45 μg per gram of dry weight in liver. Balance is maintained on an average intake of 2 to 5 mg copper daily, obtained readily from meats, particularly liver and kidney, shellfish, raisins, whole-grain cereals, dried legumes, and nuts. Bile constitutes a major route of excretion.

Elevated concentrations of copper in serum are observed in a large number of acute and chronic diseases and appear to be a manifestation of response to stress. Hypocupremia is a more specific finding and is associated primarily with hepatolenticular degeneration (Wilson's disease), certain dysproteinemias of infancy, the nephrotic syndrome (secondary to renal loss of copper proteins), intestinal malabsorption, and kwashiorkor. Acute poisoning owing to ingestion of metallic copper manifests as nausea, vomiting, hematemesis, and melena, and may be accompanied by centrilobular liver necrosis. Rapid absorption of copper sulfate through the skin, as employed for therapy of burns, or through use of copper-containing dialysis equipment, has resulted in acute hemolytic anemia. Increased copper accumulation is observed in Wilson's disease (Chap. 95), primary biliary cirrhosis (Chap. 304), and prolonged extrahepatic biliary tract obstruction (Chap. 307).

Frank copper deficiency is rare in human beings, but has been reported in severely malnourished infants, premature infants, and in children and adults receiving prolonged intravenous hyperalimentation (Chap. 78). Anemia, leukopenia, and neutropenia are observed, and the bone marrow is megaloblastoid, contains increased sideroblasts, and shows a predominance of early granulocytes and cytoplasmic vacuolization of erythroid and myeloid elements (maturation arrest). The hematologic abnormalities are reversed by oral copper therapy.

An abnormality in copper transport by intestinal cells has been described in *Menkes's kinky hair disease,* a rare X-chromosome-linked inherited syndrome manifested by rapid central nervous system and arterial degeneration, bony abnormalities, and hypothermia in male infants. As is also observed in copper-deficient animals, the hair of affected patients has less crimp and has a steely texture (pili torti), presumably owing to impaired disulfide bond formation. Concentrations of serum copper and ceruloplasmin are markedly decreased and can be restored to normal by intravenous but not oral administration of copper. Thus far, however, therapeutic efforts to replace copper and prevent early death have failed.

COBALT Although colbalt deficiency occurs in ruminants, the physiologic significance of cobalt to most other animals and humans is limited to its participation in reactions of vitamin B_{12}, of which it is a component (Chap. 311). Acute cobalt poisoning in humans is manifested by nausea, vomiting, diarrhea, tinnitus, and loss of hearing, while chronic administration of cobalt induces polycythemia and, by blocking iodine uptake, may produce goiter, especially in children. During the last decade, cobalt added to beer as an antifoaming agent produced several localized epidemics of an extraordinary cardiomyopathy, often accompanied by pericardial effusion, frequently with fatal outcome.

SELENIUM Selenium deficiency has not yet been verified in humans; however, in animals deficiency results in liver necrosis, striking pallor, and degeneration of skeletal muscle, *white-muscle disease,* occasionally involving the heart. It has been recognized for many years that these alterations resemble certain of the manifestations of vitamin E deficiency in animals and can be ameliorated by dietary supplementation with sulfur-containing amino acids. The nature of these interrelationships has been partially clarified recently by findings that selenium is a component of glutathione peroxidase in red blood cells and likely other tissues. Hence, selenium, like vitamin E, appears to help protect against damage from complex intracellular peroxides.

MANGANESE Manganese activates a host of critical intracellular enzymes; among these, mitochondrial pyruvate carboxylase and superoxide dismutase from chicken liver have recently been identified as manganese metalloenzymes. The metal appears to play a role in such important metabolic functions as oxidative phosphorylation, fatty acid metabolism, and the synthesis of proteins, mucopolysaccharides, and cholesterol. Experimental manganese deficiency has been described in animals, but not as yet in humans.

NICKEL Nickel has been found to be firmly bound to RNA from several tissues and may act to stabilize nucleic acid structure. The metal is also postulated to play a general role in the maintenance of membrane structure and function. A nickel-containing α_2-macroglobulin, nickeloplasmin, has been isolated from both human and rabbit serum, but its significance is uncertain at present. Nickel carbonyl, formed from nickel and carbon monoxide, is exceedingly dangerous and produces severe lung inflammation and liver necrosis. Chronic excess industrial exposure to nickel is associated with an increased incidence of lung and nasal carcinoma.

SILICON (AND SILICA) Silicon is a component of many mucopolysaccharides and may contribute to connective tissue structure by bridging polysaccharide chains or linking polysaccharides to proteins. Inhalation of fine particles of free crystalline silica (SiO_2) produces a pulmonary inflammatory response, granuloma formation, and chronic fibrosis (silicosis).

FLUORINE In pharmacologic doses, fluorine exerts anticariogenic effects, promotes stabilization of newly synthesized bone matrix, and inhibits bone resorption, providing a rationale for its use in treatment of osteoporosis. Chronic ingestion of fluorides in moderate amounts produces mottling of dental enamel (fluorosis); in larger amounts, e.g., from ingestion of insect poisons, fluorides cause nausea, vomiting, abdominal pain, diarrhea, and tetany often resulting in death from cardiovascular collapse.

CHROMIUM Chromium, in the form of a low-molecular-weight organic complex, *glucose tolerance factor,* present in brewer's yeast, animal meats, and grains, is required for normal glucose metabolism in several animal species. The ability of mammals to synthesize glucose tolerance factor appears to be limited, and, in humans, marginal chromium deficiency may possibly accompany protein-caloric malnutrition, pregnancy, and old age. While diabetics often exhibit altered chromium metabolism, the precise relation of this metal to diabetes remains uncertain.

REFERENCES

BURCH RE, SULLIVAN JF (eds): Symposium on trace elements. Med Clin North Am 60:653, 1976

DANKS DM et al: Menkes's kinky hair syndrome: An inherited defect in copper absorption with widespread effects. Pediatrics 50:188, 1972

HALSTED JA et al: Zinc deficiency in man: The Shiraz experiment. Am J Med 53:277, 1972

HOESTRA WG et al (eds): *Trace Element Metabolism in Animals.* Baltimore, University Park Press, 1974

NELDER KH, HAMBRIDGE KM: Zinc therapy of acrodermatitis enteropathica. N Engl J Med 292:879, 1975

SCHWARTZ K: Recent dietary trace element research, exemplified by tin, fluorine, and silicon. Fed Proc 33:1748, 1974

TUCKER SB et al: Acquired zinc deficiency: Cutaneous manifestations typical of acrodermatitis enteropathica. JAMA 235:2399, 1976

ULMER DD: Trace elements. N Engl J Med 297:318, 1977

VILTER RW et al: Manifestations of copper deficiency in a patient with systemic sclerosis on intravenous hyperalimentation. N Engl J Med 291:188, 1974

84

FLUIDS AND ELECTROLYTES

NORMAN G. LEVINSKY

SODIUM AND WATER

PHYSIOLOGIC CONSIDERATIONS Both physiologically and clinically, sodium and water metabolism are closely interrelated. The sodium content of the body depends on the balance between dietary intake and renal excretion of sodium. In health, extrarenal losses of sodium are negligible. Renal sodium excretion is closely regulated to match dietary content. Within 2 to 4 days after sodium intake stops, urinary excretion decreases to 5 meq per day or less. If dietary sodium is abruptly increased, sodium excretion promptly rises. About one-half of the surfeit is excreted within the first 24 h and the remainder over the next few days. Thus, the sodium content of the body remains quite constant despite wide variations in sodium intake; over the range of 0 to 400 meq per day, total body sodium varies only by about 10 percent.

Although detailed knowledge of the mechanism of this renal response is limited, certain general points deserve emphasis because of their clinical relevance. Sodium loads tend to increase glomerular filtration and to depress proximal tubular reabsorption of sodium, while sodium deficits have the opposite effects. Thus, delivery of sodium to the distal segments of the nephron tends to vary in parallel with extracellular sodium. Reabsorption in the loop of Henle and distal convolutions appears to change proportionately with the rate of sodium delivery. This modulates variations in the amount of sodium entering the collecting ducts, where final adjustments are made. Multiple regulatory factors control these tubular adjustments. Of these, only the role of aldosterone is well established; its principal action is to stimulate sodium transport in the distal nephron. There is some evidence for a "natriuretic hormone" which inhibits sodium reabsorption, perhaps at a distal tubular site such as the collecting duct. Changes in proximal tubular reabsorption in response to altered sodium balance appear to be mediated, at least in part, by changes in hemodynamic factors in the peritubular microcirculation. Undoubtedly, other regulatory mechanisms remain to be defined. The multiplicity of control mechanisms prevents abnormalities of any single mechanism from grossly distorting the regulation of sodium excretion. For example, increased aldosterone secretion leads only to limited and transient sodium retention, because the initial accumulation of sodium stimulates opposing natriuretic factors such as increased glomerular filtration and decreased proximal tubular reabsorption.

All but 2 to 5 percent of the sodium in the body is located in the extracellular fluids. (Approximately 40 percent of total body sodium is located in bone, but this fraction does not participate significantly in most physiologic processes and will not be considered further.) Except for minor differences in concentration due to the Gibbs-Donnan effect of plasma proteins, the electrolyte compositions of plasma and interstitial fluid are essentially equal. For practical purposes, plasma composition can be considered representative of the entire extracellular compartment. Total extracellular volume approximates 20 per-

cent of body weight. Of this, 5 percent represents plasma volume and 15 percent the volume of interstitial fluids. Thus, in a 70-kg individual with plasma sodium concentration of 140 meq per liter, extracellular sodium content will approximate 2000 meq. The volume of intracellular fluid is approximately twice as great as that of extracellular fluid, i.e., about 40 percent of body weight. However, since intracellular sodium concentration is less than 5 meq per liter, total intracellular sodium content is only about 100 to 150 meq. The asymmetric distribution of sodium across cell membranes is maintained by expenditure of a large fraction of the energy derived from cell metabolism, which is required constantly to pump sodium out of cells against its electrochemical grandient. All the principal electrolytes are asymmetrically distributed across cell membranes. The principal electrolytes of the extracellular fluids are sodium, chloride, and bicarbonate. The major electrolytes of the intracellular fluids are potassium, magnesium, calcium, and organic anions, including proteins.

Since sodium salts account for more than 90 percent of the total osmolality of the extracellular fluid, variations in plasma sodium concentration are almost always reflected in equivalent changes in plasma osmolality. Exceptions due to accumulation of other solutes in plasma are discussed later. Although the electrolyte compositions of intracellular and extracellular fluids differ markedly, they are always in osmotic equilibrium, since water moves rapidly across cellular membranes to dissipate osmotic gradients. Therefore, although sodium is largely confined to extracellular fluids, plasma sodium concentration is an index of not only the relative proportions of sodium and water in those fluids but also the relation between total body solute and total body water. An example is the effect of shift of sodium from extracellular to intracellular fluid without a change in total body solute. Movement of sodium into cells would not cause hyponatremia, since water would shift into cells with the sodium. On the other hand, a primary decrease in the concentration of osmotically active solute within cells would decrease total body solute; although there would be no change in total body sodium or water, hyponatremia would result from the shift of intracellular water into the extracellular compartment.

A very effective mechanism involving the hypothalamus, the neurohypophysis, and the kidney regulates plasma osmolality. Changes of 2 percent or less in plasma osmolality can be detected by osmoreceptors in the hypothalamus. Small increases in osmolality stimulate the secretion of antidiuretic hormone (ADH) from the neurohypophysis, while small decreases suppress secretion of the hormone. Normal plasma osmolality is approximately 280 to 300 mosmol per kilogram of water; the exact level is determined by the "set" of the hypothalamic osmoreceptors in a given individual. When ADH secretion is maximal, urine volume will be about 500 ml per day, and urine osmolality will be 800 to 1400 mosmol/kg. In the absence of ADH, minimal urine osmolality is 40 to 80 mosmol/kg, and maximum water diuresis can reach 15 to 20 liters per day or more. The capacity of this receptor-effector system is sufficient to maintain plasma osmolality within narrow limits despite large variations in the volume and concentration of dietary fluids.

The total sodium *content* of the body is determined by the

renal sodium regulatory mechanisms described earlier. However, the principal determinant of plasma sodium *concentration* is water metabolism rather than total body sodium content. If excess sodium were to be ingested and retained, hypernatremia would be only transient. Water intake would increase because of thirst, and the fluid ingested would be retained because hypernatremia (hyperosmolality) would stimulate ADH secretion. Expanded extracellular volume, not hypernatremia, would be the end result. Conversely, if the osmoregulatory system is functioning normally, loss of sodium without water would not result in permanent reduction of plasma sodium concentration. The initial reduction would shut off secretion of ADH, and a water diuresis would ensue. The final outcome would be contraction of extracellular volume, while plasma sodium concentration would be restored to normal. It should be apparent that changes in total sodium content tend to cause changes in extracellular volume. In this sense, the sodium content of the extracellular fluid determines extracellular volume. On the other hand, changes in plasma sodium concentration reflect altered regulation of water excretion, not changes in total body sodium content alone. Clinically, plasma sodium concentration per se gives no information about the amount of sodium present in the body. Total body sodium content is determined by the volume of extracellular fluids as well as by the concentration of sodium in these fluids. Extracellular volume is usually the dominant factor since changes in volume tend to be greater than changes in sodium concentration. Plasma sodium concentration reflects merely the relative proportions of sodium and water (or, more exactly, of total body solute and water), not the absolute amount of sodium in the body. Either hyponatremia or hypernatremia may occur when total body sodium content is decreased, normal, or increased.

CLINICAL DISORDERS   Deficits and excesses of sodium and water occur in a great variety of clinical circumstances. The manifestations of the underlying illness may overshadow the clinical features of the fluid and electrolyte disorder. Theoretically, disturbances of sodium and water metabolism can be classified into four categories, reflecting a primary excess or deficit of water or sodium. Practically, such isolated disturbances are uncommon. A primary excess of sodium leads to edema; it is not ordinarily considered as an electrolyte disorder but as a feature of underlying disease, such as congestive heart failure, hepatic cirrhosis, or nephrotic syndrome. Primary sodium deficits are nearly always accompanied by water depletion, leading to the clinical syndrome of extracellular volume depletion. Pure or disproportionate water excess leads to hyponatremia, relative or absolute water depletion to hypernatremia. A practical clinical classification of disorders of sodium and water metabolism is given in Table 84-1.

VOLUME DEPLETION   Combined sodium and water deficits are far more frequent than isolated deficits of either constituent. Although the term *dehydration* is often used for combined deficits, this usage is confusing. Dehydration should be used to describe relatively pure water depletion leading to hypernatremia; *volume depletion* or some similar term should be used for combined deficits.

Pathogenesis   As noted earlier, elimination of sodium from the diet will not by itself lead to sodium depletion, since urinary sodium excretion will quickly fall to very low levels. Therefore, sodium depletion is always due either to extrarenal losses or to abnormal renal losses.

GASTROINTESTINAL   The most common cause of volume depletion is loss of a significant fraction of the 8 to 10 liters of gastrointestinal fluids normally secreted daily. Since the principal secretions contain potassium and hydrogen ion or bicarbonate in large amounts, volume depletion due to gastrointestinal losses is often combined with potassium depletion and acidosis or alkalosis.

Significant volume depletion may be caused by sequestration of secretions within an obstructed gastrointestinal tract or within the peritoneal cavity in peritonitis. Rapid reaccumulation of ascites after paracentesis may cause contraction of the effective circulating blood volume.

SKIN   The sodium concentration of sweat varies from 5 to 50 meq per liter; sodium concentration increases with higher rates of sweating and in adrenal insufficiency. Because sweat is always a hypotonic solution, sweating leads to water deficits out of proportion to sodium losses. In burns, capillary damage may lead to sequestration of large amounts of sodium and water in the injured skin.

RENAL   Abnormal losses of sodium in the urine may occur in both acute and chronic renal diseases. Early in the recovery (diuretic) phase of *acute renal failure,* urinary sodium concentration tends to be high (50 to 100 meq per liter), and substantial deficits may ensue. With rare exceptions, severe sodium wasting does not persist beyond the first few days. It is important to discriminate between increased sodium excretion which represents elimination of excess salt retained during the oliguric period and true tubular sodium wasting which depletes normal extracellular sodium. Only the latter requires replacement. Acute salt wasting due to tubular damage may also occur immediately after relief of prolonged *obstruction* of the urinary tract. Although such a postobstructive diuresis may be severe, it rarely persists for more than several days as a clinically important phenomenon.

Patients with *chronic renal failure* have limited ability to decrease sodium excretion in response to decreased intake. They will become progressively volume-depleted if their intake is restricted by the anorexia, nausea, and vomiting characteris-

TABLE 84-1
Disorders of sodium and water metabolism

I Combined sodium and water depletion (volume depletion)
  A Extrarenal losses
    1 Gastrointestinal (vomiting, diarrhea, gastrointestinal suction, fistulas)
    2 Abdominal sequestration (peritonitis, rapid reaccumulation of ascites)
    3 Skin (sweating, burns)
  B Renal losses
    1 Renal disease (chronic renal failure, salt-wasting tubular disease, diuretic phase of acute renal failure)
    2 Osmotic diuresis (diabetic glycosuria)
    3 Adrenal insufficiency (Addison's disease)
II Hyponatremia
  A Associated with sodium and water depletion (volume depletion)
  B Associated with sodium retention and edema
  C Primary dilutional
  D Adrenal insufficiency
  E Syndrome of inappropriate secretion of antidiuretic hormone
    1 Spontaneous
    2 Drug-induced
  F Essential ("sick-cell syndrome")
  G Osmotic (hyperglycemia, mannitol)
  H Artifactual (hyperlipemia, hyperproteinemia, laboratory error)
III Hypernatremia
  A Extrarenal water loss
    1 Skin (insensible losses, burns, sweat)
    2 Lungs (insensible)
  B Renal water loss
    1 Diabetes insipidus (pituitary, nephrogenic)
    2 Osmotic diuresis (glycosuria, urea diuresis)
  C Primary excess of sodium (excessive salt administration without access to water)
  D Adrenal hyperfunction (Cushing's disease, primary hyperaldosteronism)

tic of uremia or because of their physician's instructions. Large deficits may develop insidiously over many days or weeks. A "vicious circle" may result, in that volume depletion will tend further to compromise renal function. Sodium-wasting renal disease, i.e., negative sodium balance when dietary sodium is normal, is very rare. It occurs in occasional patients with tubulointerstitial diseases of the kidney, especially medullary cystic disease.

Renal sodium wasting in the presence of normal intrinsic renal function occurs in three clinical circumstances. Perhaps the most common is sodium depletion due to continued administration of potent *diuretics* after edema has been relieved or to patients whose edema is sequestered and cannot be mobilized. For example, attempted treatment of cirrhotics with ascites may result in depletion of overall extracellular volume rather than mobilization of ascitic fluid. An obligatory *osmotic diuresis* may also cause renal sodium wasting despite normal renal function. Marked glycosuria in uncontrolled diabetes mellitus is the most frequent clinical example. Administration of osmotic diuretics such as mannitol and urea is a common iatrogenic cause. Volume depletion in patients receiving high-protein tube feedings may be due to an osmotic diuresis of urea formed by protein metabolism. Finally, renal sodium wasting despite normal intrinsic function occurs in *adrenal insufficiency* due to a deficiency of mineralocorticoids.

Clinical features and diagnosis The cause of volume depletion can usually be suspected from a history of inadequate salt and water intake together with vomiting, diarrhea, or excessive sweating; the symptoms of poorly controlled diabetes mellitus or of renal or adrenal disease may be elicited. The key findings on physical examination are those of plasma and extracellular volume depletion. Decreased skin turgor is usually present in patients with significant volume contraction. It can be estimated clinically by noting the slow rate of return of skin to its original position when it is raised between the examiner's fingers. An area of skin normally free of wrinkles and not subject to wide variations in the thickness of subcutaneous tissue, such as that over the sternum, should be selected for this maneuver. With moderate volume depletion, blood pressure is usually normal when the patient is recumbent, although resting tachycardia may be present. Postural hypotension, i.e., a drop of 5 to 10 mmHg in the sitting or standing position, is often present. With greater degrees of volume depletion, even recumbent blood pressure is reduced, and frank shock may occur. The patient with moderate or severe degrees of volume contraction is often lethargic, weak, confused, or obtunded. Such patients are usually oliguric, even when recumbent blood pressure is normal.

LABORATORY FINDINGS The hematocrit and plasma protein concentration are increased, but values within the normal range are interpretable only if prior values are known. Plasma sodium concentration may be decreased, normal, or increased, depending upon the proportion between deficits of sodium and of water. Plasma creatinine and urea nitrogen are usually increased, since the glomerular filtration rate is decreased ("prerenal azotemia"). Urinary sodium concentration may be of value in differentiating extrarenal and renal sources of sodium loss if the probable cause is not clear from the history. With extrarenal losses, urinary sodium concentration will be less than 10 meq per liter; the concentration will usually exceed 20 meq per liter if renal or adrenal disorders are at fault. However urinary sodium may ultimately fall below this level even in patients with renal salt wasting if sodium depletion becomes very severe.

Treatment The principal clinical manifestations of extracellular volume depletion are due to reduction of plasma and interstitial fluid volume. Since there is no convenient clinical method for assessing these volumes, the effect of treatment must be determined by following the clinical response through evaluation of changes in parameters such as blood pressure, urine output, and skin turgor. Modest deficits of sodium and water can often be corrected by increased oral intake in patients not suffering from gastrointestinal disorders. Severe depletion requires therapy with intravenous solutions. Isotonic saline (0.85%) is the infusion of choice in patients whose serum sodium concentration is approximately normal. The amount to be infused can be estimated from the history of prior losses and from the severity of the physical findings of extracellular volume contraction. Patients with clinically moderate volume contraction usually require replacement with 2 to 3 liters of saline, while patients with severe depletion may require much larger volumes. The need for correction of other concurrent electrolyte abnormalities may alter the composition of the required infusion; e.g., some of the sodium may be given as bicarbonate to patients with volume contraction and metabolic acidosis, or potassium may be added in patients with concurrent potassium depletion. In estimating the total amount to be infused, allowance for ongoing losses must be included. Since the amount to be infused cannot be calculated precisely, patients should be monitored carefully to avoid fluid overload and congestive failure.

HYPONATREMIA **Pathophysiology** Hyponatremia indicates that the body fluids are diluted by an excess of water relative to total solute. Hyponatremia is not equivalent to sodium depletion, which is only one of a number of clinical states in which it may occur (see Table 84-1). Most types of hyponatremia can be considered to result from defective urinary dilution. The normal response to dilution of body fluids is a water diuresis, which corrects the hypoosmotic state. Normal water diuresis requires three factors: (1) Secretion of ADH must be suppressed. (2) Sufficient sodium and water must reach the diluting sites of the nephron, in the ascending limb of Henle's loop and the distal convoluted tubule. (3) These nephron segments must function normally, reabsorbing sodium while remaining impermeable to water.

Three general types of mechanisms may cause defective water diuresis in patients with hyponatremia. (1) Secretion of ADH may continue "inappropriately" despite hypotonicity of extracellular fluid, which normally shuts off secretion of the hormone. (2) Insufficient sodium may reach the diluting segments to permit the formation of an adequate amount of dilute urine. Inadequate delivery of tubular fluid to distal sites may be due to reduced glomerular filtration and/or enhanced proximal tubular reabsorption. Even in the absence of ADH, distal tubular segments are not absolutely impermeable to water; small amounts of water continue to leak from the hypotonic tubular fluid into the isotonic cortical and slightly hypertonic medullary interstitial fluid. The amount of water leaking back in this manner becomes an increasingly large fraction of the volume of dilute urine formed, as the diluting process is progressively limited by decreasing delivery. Hence, urine osmolality rises progressively. In some instances, this mechanism may even result in excretion of a urine hypertonic to plasma, despite the absence of ADH. (3) Sodium transport in the diluting segments may be defective or water permeability may be excessive at these sites even in the absence of ADH. One of these three factors can account for most types of hyponatremia. However, it must be recognized that information about actual disease states is incomplete.

Paradoxically, hyponatremia in *volume depletion* and in

edematous states appears to result from similar mechanisms. Delivery of sodium and water to the diluting segments of the nephron is reduced because of decreased gomerular filtration, increased proximal tubular reabsorption, or both. Volume-mediated secretion of ADH may also be a factor in these conditions. Contraction of plasma or extracellular volume is the stimulus to these changes in renal function and hormone secretion during salt depletion. These volumes appear to be normal or increased in most edematous patients. However, it is believed that the "effective" volume is reduced by decreased cardiac output or sequestration of fluid beyond the central circulation. Essential hyponatremia may be an additional mechanism in some edematous patients (see below).

The normal kidney can excrete 15 to 20 liters of dilute urine per day. Normal water intake, regulated by thirst and habit, is a small fraction of this maximum excretory capacity. Hence, *dilutional hyponatremia* usually occurs only when defective water diuresis or water intake unregulated by thirst is present. Oliguric patients may develop dilutional hyponatremia if the volume of oral and intravenous fluids is not limited appropriately. The ability to excrete a normal volume of dilute urine is progressively limited in advancing chronic renal failure. Hyponatremia may be precipitated in patients with advanced renal failure by instructions to force fluids. In the postoperative state, water diuresis is limited by a number of factors, such as secretion of ADH induced by pain or narcotics and extracellular volume contraction. The administration of excessive volumes of hypotonic solutions to such patients is a common cause of hyponatremia. Very rarely, psychogenic polydipsia may be so severe that the rapid ingestion of huge quantities of fluids may overwhelm normal excretory capacity and produce symptomatic dilutional hyponatremia despite normal renal diluting mechanisms.

Multiple factors appear to play a role in limiting water diuresis in patients with *adrenal insufficiency.* Deficient secretion of mineralocorticoid hormones may lead to sodium depletion, with consequent reduction of glomerular filtration and enhancement of proximal tubular sodium reabsorption. Moreover, glucocorticoid deficiency directly reduces filtration. Therefore, adrenal insufficiency will tend to decrease delivery of sodium to diluting sites. In addition, glucocorticoid deficiency directly or indirectly prevents the maintenance of normal water impermeability in distal diluting segments of the nephron. Some evidence suggests a direct effect of glucocorticoid deficiency on water permeability of distal tubular epithelium, but conflicting data indicate that inappropriate secretion of ADH may occur when glucocorticoids are deficient.

Hyponatremia in patients with chronic *inappropriate secretion of antidiuretic hormone* is principally due to water retention, but continued urinary losses of sodium also contribute to producing a mild negative sodium balance. Renal sodium wasting is related to volume expansion, since it can be eliminated by restricting fluid intake. The mechanisms by which extracellular expansion may increase sodium excretion have been discussed above.

A limited number of observations suggest that some patients may be hyponatremic in the absence of a defect in water diuresis. The terms "essential hyponatremia" and "sick-cell syndrome" have been applied to this category. Osmoreceptor cells in the hypothalamus are thought to be "reset" to maintain a decreased level of body fluid osmolality as though it were normal. The genesis of such a syndrome is speculative; it has been suggested that changes in cellular metabolism might lead to a primary reduction in cellular osmolality. Such a reduction in intracellular solute would result in a shift of water out of cells, thereby diluting extracellular fluids and initiating hyponatremia. Once the osmoreceptor was "reset," water and sodium metabolism would behave normally. Urine would become dilute or concentrated if plasma sodium fell or increased slightly from the new "normal" level for that patient.

Hyponatremia due to *accumulation* of *osmotically active solutes* in the plasma is the sole exception to the rule that hyponatremia means decreased plasma osmolality. In this type of hyponatremia, plasma osmolality is increased. Plasma sodium is diluted by movement of water out of cells along the osmotic gradient created by addition to the plasma of the abnormal solute, such as glucose or mannitol. It should be noted that solutes which equilibrate across cell membrances do not induce movement of water from cells. Thus, high plasma urea levels in patients with renal failure do not cause hyponatremia.

Clinical features and diagnosis   In *sodium* (volume) *depletion,* hyponatremia per se is usually of little clinical significance. The major features are those of extracellular volume contraction, described above. Reduction of plasma sodium concentration by more than 10 to 15 meq per liter is rare in the absence of obvious decreases in skin turgor, postural or recumbent hypotension, and some degree of azotemia.

In *edematous states* such as congestive heart failure, cirrhosis, and the nephrotic syndrome, the severity and frequency of hyponatremia correlates to some extent with the magnitude of the edema and the seriousness of the underlying condition. Hyponatremia is usually present in patients with advanced disease unless water intake is restricted. The hyponatremia itself is often of little clinical significance. The principal features are those of the underlying disease. However, symptomatic hyponatremia may occur, most often in connection with vigorous diuretic therapy or excessive oral or parenteral intake of dilute fluids.

The diagnosis of *primary dilutional hyponatremia* is usually evident from the history. This diagnosis should be considered in postoperative patients and in patients with acute or chronic renal failure. Since extracellular fluid volume is expanded by water retention, blood pressure and skin turgor are normal. Plasma creatinine and urea are normal unless preexisting renal disease is present.

The *syndrome* of *chronic inappropriate secretion of antidiuretic hormone* (SIADH) is defined by a unique group of clinical features. (1) Urine osmolality is not maximally dilute even when marked hyponatremia is induced by water loading. In most cases, urine osmolality exceeds plasma osmolality. (The elaboration of hypertonic urine is presumptive evidence of ADH secretion if the glomerular filtration rate is normal.) (2) Plasma creatinine and urea are normal or low, indicating that the glomerular filtration rate is normal or increased. (3) During fluid loading, hyponatremia increases due to water retention and urinary sodium wasting. During restriction of fluid intake, hyponatremia and urinary sodium wasting are corrected. It should be noted that sodium wasting during volume expansion may be minimal or even absent in patients with extreme degrees of hyponatremia. In clinical testing to demonstrate these features, patients with symptomatic hyponatremia or plasma sodium concentrations below 125 meq per liter should first have their fluid intake restricted to 800 to 1000 ml per day or less. Infusion of small volumes of hypertonic saline may be appropriate in symptomatic patients. During restriction of fluid intake, hyponatremia should disappear promptly, and urinary sodium excretion should not exceed intake. Thereafter, plasma and urinary parameters should be evaluated during daily administration of 2 to 3 liters of fluids by mouth or intravenously. Urine osmolality will always exceed 100 mosmol per liter (urine specific gravity greater than 1.003); in the great majority of instances, it will exceed plasma osmolality, despite progressive dilution of body fluids. Urinary sodium excretion will usually exceed sodium intake during this phase of fluid loading. Two to three days of this regimen are ordinarily sufficient to demonstrate the requisite clinical pattern for SIADH without inducing symptomatic hyponatremia.

SIADH has been found frequently in patients with oat-cell carcinoma of the lung but has also been described in patients with a variety of other neoplasms. In some of these patients there is evidence that the tumor is secreting ADH or a substance with analogous biological activity (see also Chap. 334). The syndrome has also been reported in patients with disorders of the central nervous system, including meningitis and encephalitis. It is assumed that ADH in these patients is secreted in response to direct stimulation of the hypothalamic osmoreceptors. SIADH has also been noted in a number of apparently unrelated disorders such as acute porphyria and hypothyroidism. The stimulus to ADH in these patients is unknown.

An ever-increasing list of pharmacological agents has been reported to induce SIADH. The list includes: (1) the oral hypoglycemic agents, chlorpropamide and tolbutamide; (2) antineoplastic and immunosuppressive agents, vincristine and cyclophosphamide; (3) psychoactive drugs, carbamazepine (Tegretol) and amitriptyline (Elavil); and (4) clofibrate. These agents exert their antidiuretic effects either by potentiating the tubular action of small amounts of ADH or by stimulating inappropriate secretion of ADH. In addition, diuretics such as thiazides may induce a syndrome indistinguishable from SIADH, probably by a direct renal action to limit water excretion in patients ingesting moderate to large amounts of dilute fluids.

Since patients with *adrenal insufficiency* may have the combination of defective dilution of the urine and sodium wasting, hyponatremia due to Addison's disease can occasionally be confused with SIADH. Usually, other clinical features of adrenal insufficiency such as hyperkalemia, pigmentation, and hypoglycemia will suggest the correct diagnosis. However, specific tests of adrenal cortical function are indicated whenever the diagnosis is in doubt.

Essential hyponatremia (sick-cell syndrome) may occur in a variety of chronic illnesses, such as pulmonary tuberculosis, congestive heart failure, and hepatic cirrhosis. This type of hyponatremia is asymptomatic; skin turgor, blood pressure, and renal function are normal, unless altered by the primary disease. Definitive diagnosis of essential hyponatremia requires the demonstration of normal urinary dilution in response to water loading, normal urinary concentration during dehydration, and normal renal sodium excretory responses to sodium loading and restriction.

The diagnosis of hyponatremia due to *increased plasma concentrations* of *osmotically active solute* is usually apparent from the history and clinical features of uncontrolled diabetes. Plasma sodium concentration will decrease by about 1.6 meq per liter with every elevation of 100 mg per 100 ml in plasma glucose above normal. This type of hyponatremia should also be considered whenever there is a history of recent administration of mannitol, especially to oliguric patients unable to excrete it promptly. Since plasma osmolality is increased, clinical manifestations of hypotonicity are absent in this type of hyponatremia.

In patients with severe hyperlipemia or, very rarely, with extreme hyperproteinemia, hyponatremia which is clinically *artifactual* may be reported by the laboratory. In severe hyperlipemia part of any unit volume of plasma taken for analysis will be lipid, which is sodium-free. This type of hyponatremia is rarely reported unless the plasma is grossly milky. In patients with extreme hyperproteinemia, proteins occupy more than the normal 7 percent of plasma volume, thereby reducing the proportion of aqueous sodium-containing fluid per unit of plasma taken for analysis. In both cases, hyponatremia will be reported by the laboratory because the sodium concentration will be low in milliequivalents per liter of plasma. However,

sodium concentration per liter of plasma water and plasma osmolality are normal; hence, this type of hyponatremia has no clinical significance.

DIFFERENTIAL DIAGNOSIS   Although the type of hyponatremia can be defined without difficulty in many patients, differentiation among categories may be very difficult. More than one type of hyponatremia may occur in a specific disease entity. For example, hyponatremia in patients with hepatic cirrhosis is usually associated with edema or is due to excessive administration of diuretics, but essential hyponatremia may also occur in this condition. Moreover, current categories may prove artificial or inaccurate when the pathophysiology of hyponatremia is more completely understood and specific diagnostic tests such as a sensitive assay for ADH are readily available. Despite these limitations, the classification outlined above is a useful framework for diagnosis and treatment.

The history is often the most important factor in differential diagnosis. For example, prolonged vomiting, diarrhea, or nasogastric suction will suggest volume depletion. Primary dilutional hyponatremia or hypernatremia associated with sodium losses should be suspected in the postoperative period. Critical information to be derived from the physical examination includes the presence or absence of edema, signs of volume depletion, and evidence of disordered cerebral function. Initial laboratory studies of value include the plasma creatinine and urinary osmolality (specific gravity) and sodium concentration. The combination of high urine specific gravity (above 1.005), increased urinary sodium concentration, and normal or low plasma urea or creatinine in a hyponatremic patient without clinical evidence of volume depletion suggests the diagnosis of SIADH. A maximally dilute urine in a hyponatremic patient suggests psychogenic polydipsia or essential hyponatremia.

CLINICAL MANIFESTATIONS   Neurologic dysfunction is the principal clinical feature of hyponatremia. The severity of symptoms is related to the degree of hyponatremia and the rapidity with which it develops. Patients may be lethargic, confused, stuporous, or comatose. If hyponatremia develops rapidly, signs of hyperexcitability such as muscular twitches, irritability, and convulsions may occur. These are believed due to intracellular movement of water, leading to swelling of brain cells. Hyponatremia rarely causes clinical symptoms when plasma sodium is above 125 meq per liter, although symptoms may occur occasionally at higher levels if the decrease in concentration has been rapid.

Treatment   Hyponatremia itself is often of little clinical significance and requires no specific treatment. When hyponatremia is associated with volume depletion, treatment is directed to correction of the volume deficits. In the occasional patient with sodium depletion whose plasma sodium concentration is less than 125 meq per liter, some of the intravenous sodium replacement fluids should be administered as hypertonic saline. Hyponatremia associated with edema responds to effective treatment of the underlying disease. Moderate, nonprogressive hyponatremia in edematous patients usually does not cause symptoms. Attempts to correct such hyponatremia by restriction of fluid intake induce thirst and discomfort without improving the clinical picture or longevity. Patients with severe or progressive hyponatremia may require some restriction of water intake, especially during vigorous treatment with diuretics. However, moderate limitations to the range of 1000 to 1500 ml per day will often suffice to avoid symptoms or progressive hyponatremia. More severe restriction should be instituted only if specific clinical or laboratory observations warrant. Since edematous subjects have excess total extracellular sodium, hypertonic saline solution should not be administered, except in rare instances in which clinical manifestations of extreme hyponatremia, such as coma or convulsions, justify emergency measures. Dilutional hyponatremia is treated by water restriction. Only if severe symptoms occur is hypertonic saline infusion required. Hyponatremia due to SIADH responds to limitation of fluid intake; restriction to the range of 1000 to 1200 ml per day is ordinarily adequate. Occasional patients with marked hyponatremia due to this syndrome may be symptomatic and require initial therapy with hypertonic saline infusions.

When severe hyponatremia of any type is to be treated intravenously, 5% sodium chloride is the infusion of choice. The amount of sodium to be given should be calculated by multiplying the deficit in plasma sodium concentration (milliequivalents per liter) by total body water (approximately 50 to 60 percent of body weight). Although the administered sodium will remain in the extracellular compartment, the osmotic effect of the hypertonic saline will cause water to shift out of cells. The amount needed to raise plasma sodium concentration to the range of 125 to 130 meq per liter should be calculated and infused over several hours. The patient's symptoms and clinical status, especially with respect to circulatory congestion, should be carefully assessed throughout the infusion. Complete correction of hyponatremia, if clinically indicated, is usually best carried out more slowly, by water restriction or oral sodium supplementation if possible.

HYPERNATREMIA Pathophysiology Hypernatremia is due to a deficit of body water relative to total body solute or sodium content. Without exception, hypernatremia indicates that the body fluids are hypertonic. Since hypertonicity normally stimulates thirst, severe persistent hypernatremia occurs only in patients who cannot respond to thirst by voluntary ingestion of fluid, e.g., infants or mentally obtunded patients. In such individuals, loss of dilute body fluids will progressively elevate body fluid osmolality. Initial losses of water are from the extracellular compartment, but water deficits are rapidly equilibrated throughout total body water. The rise in extracellular fluid tonicity causes intracellular water to shift into the extracellular compartment. In effect, approximately two-thirds of pure water deficits are derived from intracellular fluid. Hence, the clinical findings of extracellular volume depletion occur in patients with relatively pure deficits of water only when such deficits are large. The principal clinical features are attributable to decreased intracellular volume, especially dehydration of cells in the central nervous system. Brain cells appear to adapt to chronic hyperosmolality by accumulating increased intracellular solute. When hyperosmolality is rapidly corrected, the increase in total intracellular solute may promote brain swelling even at normal or slightly elevated plasma osmolality. These mechanisms may account for the clinical observation that rapid correction of hypertonicity sometimes causes deterioration of central nervous function. The identity of the excess brain solute is uncertain; experimental data suggest that electrolyte accumulation accounts only for part of the excess in chronic hypernatremia.

Minimal persistent hypernatremia may be seen in some patients with Cushing's disease and hyperaldosteronism. Presumably stimulation of renal tubular reabsorption by adrenal steroids initiates the hypernatremia. It is not known why the thirst mechanism fails to maintain normal body fluid osmolality.

Pathogenesis The principal causes of hypernatremia are listed in Table 84-1. The most frequent is unreplaced loss of hypotonic fluid from the skin and lungs. Insensible losses of water from these sources may reach several liters per day, especially in patients with fever or increased respirations. Since sweat is hypotonic fluid, hypernatremia will develop if sweating patients are unable to drink. Major losses of insensible water may occur in patients with extensive burns. Renal losses may lead to hypernatremia in two clinical circumstances, diabetes insipidus and solute diuresis. Alert patients with diabetes insipidus ordinarily maintain normal or only slightly hypertonic body fluids despite massive renal water wasting by increasing fluid intake appropriately. However, diabetes insipidus may develop acutely in patients who suffer cerebral trauma or undergo neurosurgical procedures. In such patients, careful attention to replacement of urinary losses is mandatory to avoid severe hypernatremia. In an osmotic diuresis, urinary sodium concentration is less than plasma concentration; therefore, hypernatremia tends to occur. Hypernatremia due to a urea diuresis may develop when patients unable to complain of thirst are placed on a high-protein tube feeding. Examples include patients with severe cerebrovascular accidents who are unable to swallow and postoperative neurosurgical patients. In the syndrome of hyperosmolar nonketotic diabetic coma, severe hyperosmolality of the body fluids is due to a combination of hyperglycemia and relative or absolute hypernatremia. The hypernatremia is a consequence of an intense glucose osmotic diuresis in patients who are unable to ingest fluids. Since hyperglycemia itself causes hyponatremia by inducing a shift of water from cells, the presence of hypernatremia in the face of extreme hyperglycemia indicates that total body water is severely depleted. Hypernatremia due to an osmotic diuresis is usually accompanied by significant extracellular volume depletion, since both sodium and water are lost.

In rare instances, hypernatremia may result from an absolute excess of sodium rather than from water depletion. Examples are hypernatremia caused by accidental substitution of salt for sugar in infant feeding formulas and administration of excessive amounts of hypertonic saline to comatose adults.

Clinical features and diagnosis The principal clinical manifestations of hypernatremia are observed in the central nervous system. Confusion, obtundation, stupor, or coma may develop, depending on the severity of the hyperosmolality. These symptoms appear to be due to dehydration of brain cells; the clinical features are similar whether hyperosmolality is due to hypernatremia or extreme hyperglycemia. In patients with pure water deficits, manifestations of extracellular volume depletion are minimal because only one-third of the deficit is derived from extracellular fluid. As already noted, combined deficits are common, especially in patients who are undergoing an osmotic diuresis; in such individuals, the signs and symptoms of volume depletion may overshadow those due to hypernatremia.

Treatment Water by mouth or intravenous administration of a dilute solution (5% dextrose or 0.45% saline) is the treatment of hypernatremia. Calculation of water requirements must be based on total body water, since water deficits are drawn from both intracellular and extracellular fluid and both must be repleted. Hypernatremia should be corrected slowly; no more than half the water deficit should be replaced in the first few hours. Excessively rapid correction of hypernatremia may cause clinical deterioration of central nervous function.

POTASSIUM

PHYSIOLOGIC CONSIDERATIONS Potassium is the principal intracellular cation. Active transport maintains a cellular concentration of approximately 160 meq per liter, 40 times that in extracellular fluid. All but 2 percent of the 2500 to 3000 meq potassium in the body is within cells. Since potassium is a large fraction of total cellular solute, it is a major determinant of the volume of the cell and the osmolality of the body fluids. Moreover, potassium is an important cofactor in a number of metabolic processes. Extracellular potassium, while a small fraction of the total, greatly influences neuromuscular function. The ratio of intracellular to extracellular potassium concentration is the principal determinant of membrane potential in excitable tissues. Since extracellular potassium concentration is low, small deviations in absolute concentration will produce large variations in this ratio; conversely, only large changes in intracellular potassium will influence the ratio significantly. These relationships have practical consequences. For example, toxic effects of hyperkalemia can be mitigated by inducing movement of potassium from extracellular fluid to cells.

The relation between plasma and cellular potassium is complex and influenced by a number of factors, prominent among them being acid-base balance. Acidosis tends to shift potassium out of cells, and alkalosis favors movement of potassium from extracellular fluid into cells. Thus, a patient with normal total body potassium will tend to be hyperkalemic if acidotic and hypokalemic if alkalotic. During potassium depletion, plasma potassium initially decreases about 1 meq per liter for each 100 to 200 meq lost. However, plasma potassium falls much more slowly after it reaches 2 meq per liter. Thus, a plasma potassium in the range of 2 to 3.5 meq per liter is a reasonably accurate guide to the magnitude of depletion, but plasma potassium concentrations less than 2 meq per liter may reflect a wide range of deficits, from moderate to very severe. Plasma concentration increases about 1 meq per liter after acute administration of 100 to 200 meq potassium. Assuming an extracellular volume of 15 liters, 150 meq would be expected to raise plasma potassium by about 10 meq per liter. Thus, it is evident that the largest fraction of administered potassium rapidly enters cells. Renal excretion also increases promptly. Chronic exposure to high potassium diets enhances both tissue uptake and renal excretion of the ion; the mechanism of these adaptations is uncertain. Sustained hyperkalemia rarely is caused by excess intake, because these mechanisms normally function so efficiently. Impaired renal excretion or cellular transfer are the usual causes of hyperkalemia.

Of the usual potassium intake of 50 to 150 meq per day, all but a few milliequivalents are excreted in the urine. Normally, stool and sweat contain only about 5 meq per day. As already noted, the kidneys respond to acute and chronic changes in potassium intake by corresponding changes in excretion. Excess potassium is excreted promptly; about half of an acute load appears in the urine within 12 h. The renal response to potassium depletion is more sluggish. Excretion does not fall to minimal levels for 7 to 14 days. During this period, a deficit of 200 meq or more may develop in an individual on a potassium-deficient diet. Renal excretory mechanisms for potassium are complex. Potassium in the urine is secreted in the distal convoluted tubule and collecting duct; filtered potassium is nearly quantitatively reabsorbed in more proximal segments. Potassium secretion appears to be determined by the potassium concentration of tubular cells and by an electrochemical gradient favoring diffusion of the ion into tubular fluid. Net excretion is the resultant of secretion and concurrent reabsorption in the distal segments. Among the key influences on this complex system are aldosterone, sodium reabsorption, and acid-base balance. Aldosterone stimulates potassium secretion. Thus, hyperkalemia increases potassium excretion by two mechanisms: it stimulates adrenal secretion of aldosterone, and it directly enhances renal secretion, presumably via increased tubular cell potassium. Sodium reabsorption in the distal tubule creates the electrical gradient which favors potassium secre-

tion. Hence, increased distal sodium reabsorption will favor potassium excretion. For example, administration of diuretics which bring more sodium distally will increase potassium excretion, especially in patients with edema and secondary aldosteronism. Conversely, a low sodium diet decreases potassium excretion even in patients with primary aldosteronism; distal secretion is limited and reabsorption of potassium in collecting ducts is stimulated. Alkalosis enhances and acidosis depresses renal potassium secretion, probably by inducing corresponding changes in cell potassium.

POTASSIUM DEPLETION AND HYPOKALEMIA **Pathogenesis** The principal causes of potassium depletion are listed in Table 84-2. As noted earlier, renal excretion of potassium falls slowly in persons on potassium-deficient diets. During the 10 to 14 days before balance is achieved, significant deficits may occur. Thus, in contrast to sodium, moderate potassium depletion may result from *poor intake* alone. The most frequent cause of potassium deficiency is *gastrointestinal loss*. The potassium concentration of gastric fluid is approximately 5 to 10 meq per liter; significant deficits may result from direct losses of potassium in *vomitus*. The concomitant alkalosis maintains urinary potassium excretion at levels inappropriately high for the degree of potassium depletion. *Diarrhea* may also lead to large potassium deficits, since the potassium concentration of liquid stool is 40 to 60 meq per liter.

The most frequent *renal* cause of potassium depletion is probably administration of *diuretics* without adequate dietary potassium supplementation. All diuretics in common use except spironolactone, triamterene, and amiloride promote potassium excretion, especially in edematous patients with secondary aldosteronism. Potassium excretion is increased during an *osmotic diuresis*. In patients with diabetic ketoacidosis, potassium depletion due to glycosuria may be masked by the shift of potassium out of tissues caused by acidosis. Failure to recognize potassium depletion may lead to serious cardiotoxicity from sudden hypokalemia when the acidosis is corrected with insulin or alkali. A normal plasma potassium concentration in an acidotic patient strongly suggests potassium depletion.

Urinary potassium loss is often due to *excessive mineralocorticoid activity*. Hypokalemia is characteristic of *primary aldosteronism*, but may be minimal in patients with restricted sodium intake. *Secondary aldosteronism* causes renal potassium

TABLE 84-2
Causes of potassium depletion and hypokalemia

I Gastrointestinal
  A Deficient dietary intake
  B Gastrointestinal losses (vomiting, diarrhea, villous adenoma, fistulas, ureterosigmoidostomy)
II Renal
  A Diuretics
  B Osmotic diuresis (glycosuria)
  C Excessive mineralocorticoid effects
    1 Primary aldosteronism
    2 Secondary aldosteronism (including malignant hypertension, Bartter's syndrome, juxtaglomerular cell tumor)
    3 Licorice ingestion
    4 Glucocorticoid excess (Cushing's syndrome, exogenous steroids, ectopic ACTH production)
  D Renal tubular disease
    1 Renal tubular acidosis
    2 Leukemia with lysozymuria
    3 Liddle's syndrome
III Hypokalemia due to shift into cells (no depletion)
  A Hypokalemic periodic paralysis
  B Insulin effect

wasting and hypokalemia in patients with malignant hypertension, Bartter's syndrome, and renin-secreting renal tumors. Bartter's syndrome is most frequent in children and adolescents. *Licorice* contains a compound with mineralocorticoid activity; patients who consume hugh amounts may become hypokalemic. Excessive levels of *glucocorticoids* stimulate secretion of renal potassium (and hydrogen), leading to hypokalemia and alkalosis in patients with *Cushing's syndrome* and those receiving *therapeutic steroids.*

Renal tubular potassium wasting is a feature of *renal tubular acidosis.* Some patients with monocytic or myelomonocytic *leukemia* have developed hypokalemia. Renal potassium wasting in these patients appears to correlate with lysozymuria, and it has been suggested that the enzyme may interfere with tubular function. In *Liddle's syndrome,* a rare familial disorder, renal potassium wasting is an intrinsic tubular abnormality.

Clinical features and diagnosis The most prominent features of hypokalemia and potassium depletion are neuromuscular. Moderate degrees of depletion may be asymptomatic, especially if they develop slowly. Some patients, however, may complain of muscle weakness. With more severe or acute degrees of hypokalemia and potassium deficiency, marked and generalized weakness of skeletal muscles is prominent. Very severe or abrupt development of hypokalemia may lead to virtually total paralysis, including the respiratory muscles. Rhabdomyolysis may occur in patients with potassium depletion. On physical examination, in addition to decreased motor power, the patient may demonstrate decreased or absent tendon reflexes.

Abnormalities in the electrocardiogram are common in patients with hypokalemia and potassium depletion. The characteristic changes include flattening and inversion of the T wave, increased prominence of the U wave, and sagging of the ST segment. These alterations are not well correlated with the severity of the disturbance in potassium metabolism and cannot be relied on as indexes of the clinical significance of a potassium deficit. Although moderate potassium depletion rarely affects cardiac action, severe or rapid reduction in serum potassium may cause cardiac arrest. Potassium deficiency enhances the cardiac toxicity of digitalis preparations.

Renal tubular function is markedly impaired by potassium depletion. The most prominent abnormality is decreased concentrating ability, which may cause polyuria and polydipsia. Glomerular filtration rate is normal or only slightly reduced; moderate reductions may occur in occasional patients with chronic potassium depletion nephropathy. Renal regulation of potassium excretion remains normal. The urinalysis is benign: protein excretion is normal or minimally increased, and the urinary sediment is normal or demonstrates only a slight increase in hyaline or granular casts.

DIAGNOSIS The cause of hypokalemia and potassium depletion is usually evident from the history. However, patients whose potassium deficiency is caused by chronic abuse of laxatives or psychogenic, self-induced vomiting will rarely volunteer an accurate history. Patients with villous adenomas of the rectum sometimes report that their feces are formed; careful questioning will reveal the elimination of the characteristic mucous secretion of the tumor.

When the history is obscure, evaluation of urinary potassium excretion may be helpful in determining the origin of the potassium deficit. If gastrointestinal losses have occurred, urinary excretion will usually be less than 20 to 25 meq per liter. Although renal conservation of potassium is slow, excretion will have fallen to these levels by the time that clinically significant deficits of potassium have accumulated. On the other hand, when renal potassium wasting is the cause, urinary concentration will usually exceed 20 meq per liter. However, lower concentrations may be found in severely depleted patients, in those with excessive mineralocorticoid activity while on low sodium intake, and in patients where diuretics have been stopped at the time of examination.

Treatment When possible, potassium depletion should be corrected by increased dietary intake or supplementation with potassium salts. Potassium chloride is the salt of choice, especially in alkalotic patients. Enteric-coated potassium chloride tablets have been responsible for ulceration of the small bowel, due to release of high concentrations of potassium salts. Organic salts such as gluconate or citrate are adequate in patients who are not severely alkalotic.

Intravenous treatment is required for patients with gastrointestinal disorders or when the potassium deficiency is severe. It must be emphasized that the potassium *concentration* in commonly available intravenous solutions of potassium chloride is 2000 meq per liter. Concentrations in intravenous infusions should not exceed 40 or at the most 60 meq per liter. The rate of infusion should not exceed 20 meq/h or approximately 200 to 250 meq per day, unless the need for more rapid infusion has been demonstrated in the individual patient by evidence of continuing losses large enough to justify more intensive therapy. The results of treatment are best monitored by repeated determinations of plasma potassium and evaluation of clinical symptoms such as muscular weakness or paralysis. Disappearance of electrocardiographic abnormalities correlates only roughly with improvement in total body potassium content. However, during rapid intravenous administration of potassium, the electrocardiogram should be monitored to avoid cardiac toxicity from inadvertent hyperkalemia.

Hypokalemia and hypocalcemia may occur together, for example, in patients with malabsorption syndrome. The neuromuscular effect of each electrolyte abnormality is masked by the other. Treatment of either disorder alone may precipitate symptoms. Thus, treatment of hypokalemia alone may precipitate tetany, and conversely, treatment of hypocalcemia without correcting the hypokalemia may exacerbate the manifestations of potassium deficiency.

HYPERKALEMIA Pathogenesis The causes of hyperkalemia are shown in Table 84-3. *Inadequate renal excretion* is the most frequent cause. When oliguria or anuria is present, as in acute renal failure, progressive hyperkalemia is the rule. Plasma potassium will rise by about 0.5 meq per liter per day if there are no abnormal loads. Chronic renal failure does not cause severe

TABLE 84-3
Causes of hyperkalemia

I Inadequate excretion
   A Renal failure
      1 Acute renal failure
      2 Severe chronic renal failure (especially with marked acidosis or oliguria)
   B Adrenal insufficiency
      1 Hypoaldosteronism
      2 Addison's disease
   C Diuretics which inhibit potassium secretion (spironolactone, triamterene, amiloride)
II Shift of potassium from tissues
   A Tissue damage (muscle crush, hemolysis, internal bleeding)
   B Drugs: succinylcholine, digitalis poisoning
   C Acidosis
   D Hyperkalemic periodic paralysis
III Excessive intake
IV Pseudohyperkalemia
   A Thrombocytosis
   B Leukocytosis
   C Poor venipuncture technique
   D In vitro hemolysis

or progressive hyperkalemia unless oliguria supervenes. Adaptive changes of unknown etiology increase potassium excretion per residual nephron as chronic renal failure progresses. However, patients with chronic renal failure are functioning at the limits of their excretory capacity. Hence, hyperkalemia may develop rapidly if the potassium load is increased or excretory capacity is limited, e.g., by administration of spironolactone.

Hyperkalemia is a cardinal feature of *adrenal insufficiency* (Addison's disease) and of selective *hypoaldosteronism*. In the latter condition, cardiac toxicity (heart block) due to hyperkalemia is the principal clinical manifestation.

A kilogram of tissue such as muscle or erythrocytes contains about 80 meq potassium, and damaged cells release potassium into the plasma. Hence hyperkalemia may be seen when there is *muscle-crushing injury, hemolysis,* or *internal hemorrhage. Acidosis* drives potassium out of cells and leads to hyperkalemia. Severe progressive hyperkalemia is not ordinarily a consequence of increased release of potassium from damaged or acidotic tissues alone. However, acidosis and tissue damage often occur together with acute renal insufficiency; under these circumstances, severe hyperkalemia may develop quickly. In contrast to the increase of 0.5 meq per liter per day typical of uncomplicated anuria, plasma potassium in anuric patients with tissue damage may increase 2 to 4 meq per liter per day. Such rapidly progressive hyperkalemia may be an important cause of death in military casualties. In patients with trauma, burns, or neuromuscular diseases such as paraplegia and multiple sclerosis, the muscle relaxant *succinylcholine* may cause dangerous hyperkalemia. This agent apparently releases potassium from muscle by depolarizing cell membranes. In *hyperkalemic periodic paralysis*, the hyperkalemia is associated with repeated attacks of muscular paralysis. The mechanism of this syndrome is not understood. Ingestion of increased amounts of potassium may precipitate attacks.

Patients with extreme thrombocytosis or, more rarely, extreme leukocytosis in leukemia may demonstrate the phenomenon of pseudohyperkalemia. Platelets or white blood cells release potassium during blood clotting in vitro. While serum potassium may be grossly abnormal, plasma potassium is not increased. Artifactual elevation of plasma potassium may occur if blood is drawn after repeated fist clenching to make veins more prominent during application of a tourniquet. Artifactual hyperkalemia may be suspected when electrocardiographic abnormalities are absent despite apparently marked elevation of serum potassium.

Clinical features and diagnosis The most important toxic effects of hyperkalemia are cardiac arrhythmias. The characteristic sequence of electrocardiographic changes is shown in Fig. 84-1. The earliest manifestation is the development of high peaked T waves, especially prominent in precordial leads. Hyperkalemia does not prolong the QT interval, unlike other disorders which induce peaking of the T waves. Later changes include prolongation of the PR interval, complete heart block, and atrial asystole. As plasma potassium rises further, ventricular complexes may deteriorate. The QRS becomes progressively prolonged and finally tends to merge with the T wave in a sine wave configuration. Terminally, ventricular fibrillation and standstill may occur.

Occasionally moderate or severe hyperkalemia may have striking effects on peripheral muscles. Ascending muscular weakness can occur, progressing to flaccid quadriplegia and respiratory paralysis. Cerebral and cranial nerve function are normal, as is sensation.

Treatment In considering appropriate therapy, it is helpful to classify hyperkalemia according to degree of severity. The seriousness of hyperkalemia is best estimated by considering both the plasma potassium and the electrocardiogram. When the plasma potassium is less than 6.5 meq per liter and electrocardiographic changes are limited to peaking of T waves, hyper-

FIGURE 84-1

Electrocardiographic changes in hyperkalemia. A. Early toxicity in a patient with plasma potassium of 6.8 meq per liter. Note symmetrical peaking of T waves. B. Advanced toxicity in a patient with plasma potassium of 8.6 meq per liter. QRS complexes are abnormally widened, P waves have disappeared, and ventricular rhythm is irregular. (From NG Levinsky, Clinician, 1973.)

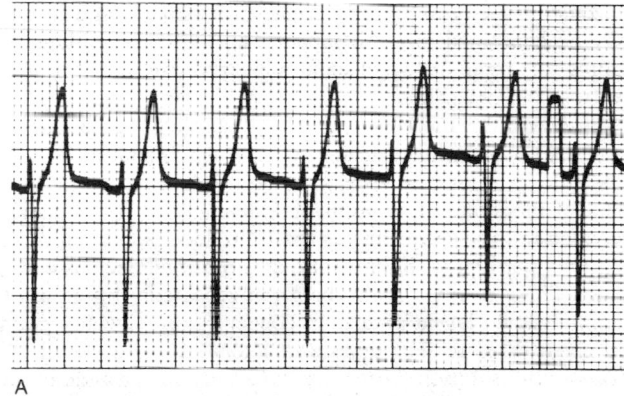

A

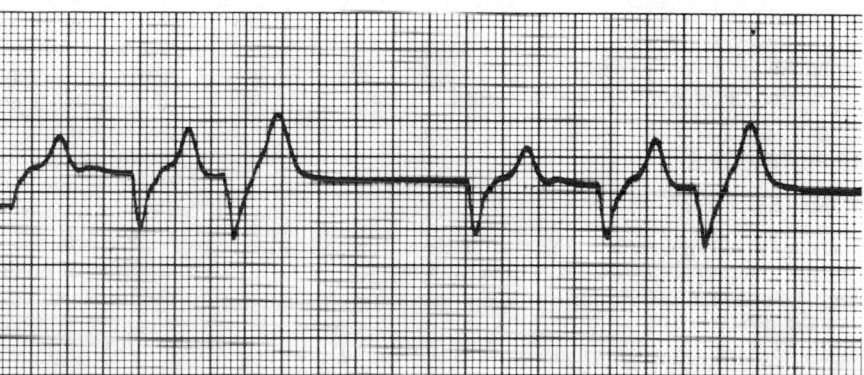

B

kalemia can be considered minimal. When the plasma potassium is 6.5 to 8 meq per liter and T-wave peaking is the only electrocardiographic abnormality, hyperkalemia may be considered moderate. Severe hyperkalemia is present if the plasma potassium exceeds 8 meq per liter or if electrocardiographic abnormalities include absent P waves, widened QRS complexes, or ventricular arrhythmias. Minimal hyperkalemia can usually be treated by elimination of a cause, such as potassium-sparing diuretics, or by treatment of accompanying acidosis. More severe or progressive hyperkalemia requires vigorous therapy. Severe cardiac toxicity responds most rapidly to infusion of calcium; 10 to 30 ml of 10% calcium gluconate may be infused intravenously within a period of 1 to 5 min under constant electrocardiographic monitoring. While calcium infusions do not alter plasma potassium, they counteract the adverse effects of potassium on neuromuscular membranes. The effect of calcium infusions, while almost immediate, is relatively transient if the hyperkalemia is not treated directly.

In moderately severe hyperkalemia, infusion of hypertonic glucose solutions will decrease toxicity by shifting potassium into cells. In the first 30 min, 200 to 500 ml of 10% glucose may be given. An additional 500 to 1000 ml may be infused over the next several hours. Ten units of regular insulin may be given subcutaneously, although this is probably necessary only in insulin-deficient diabetic patients. This treatment may reduce serum potassium by 1 to 2 meq per liter, and effects persist for a number of hours. The infusion of sodium bicarbonate will also help lower serum potassium rapidly by causing potassium to shift into cells; 44 to 132 meq alkali (two to three ampuls) may be added to a liter of glucose. Although this agent is most valuable in acidotic patients, it also is effective in individuals with normal acid-base status. The effect occurs within 1 h and persists for a number of hours thereafter. The infusion of hypertonic sodium solutions may also be effective in reversing cardiac toxicity, especially in hyponatremic or volume-depleted patients. In part the effect depends simply on dilution of plasma potassium, but there may be a direct effect of elevated plasma sodium to antagonize hyperkalemic neuromuscular toxicity as well. Glucose, bicarbonate, and sodium may be combined in a "therapeutic cocktail," formulated by adding an ampul or two of sodium bicarbonate to a liter of 5% dextrose in 0.9% saline.

None of the measures just described removes potassium from the body. Cation exchange resins such as sodium polystyrene sulfonate may be given by retention enema in the treatment of moderate or severe hyperkalemia. Enough potassium may be removed by a single enema to reduce potassium by 0.5 to 2 meq per liter within an hour, and repeated enemas can be given. These resins can also be given repeatedly by mouth to maintain low plasma potassium concentration. Twenty grams are given three or four times a day together with 20 ml of a 70% sorbitol solution, as required to ensure the passage of several loose stools daily. In patients with renal failure, hemodialysis and peritoneal dialysis will effectively control hyperkalemia. However, they are relatively slow techniques, and patients with severe hyperkalemia should be treated first with one of the methods previously discussed.

REFERENCES

Sodium and water

BARTTER FE, SCHWARTZ WB: The syndrome of inappropriate secretion of antidiuretic hormone. Am J Med 42:790, 1967

BERL T et al: Clinical disorders of water metabolism. Kidney Int 10:117, 1976

MILLER M, MOSES AM: Drug-induced states of impaired water excretion. Kidney Int 10:96, 1976

WEINER M, EPSTEIN FH: Signs and symptoms of electrolyte disorders. Yale J Biol Med 43:76, 1970

Potassium

LEVINSKY NG: Management of emergencies: VI. Hyperkalemia. N Engl J Med 274:1076, 1966

MICHELIS MF, MURDAUGH HV: Selective hypoaldosteronism. Am J Med 59:1, 1975

SCHWARTZ WB, RELMAN AS: Effects of electrolyte disorders on renal structure and function. N Engl J Med 276:283, 1967

SURAWICZ B: Relationship between the ECG and electrolytes. Am Heart J 73:814, 1967

WRIGHT FS: Sites and mechanisms of potassium transport along the renal tubule. Kidney Int 11:415, 1977

85
ACIDOSIS AND ALKALOSIS

NORMAN G. LEVINSKY

PHYSIOLOGIC CONSIDERATIONS Normal metabolism continuously produces acids. Despite the addition of some 20,000 mmol carbonic acid and 80 mmol of nonvolatile acids to body fluids daily, the free hydrogen ion concentration of these fluids is fixed within a narrow range. The pH of extracellular fluid is normally between 7.35 and 7.45 (hydrogen ion, 45 to 35 nmol per liter). The pH of intracellular fluids cannot be determined with precision, but most methods suggest a mean intracellular pH in the range of 6.9. It seems likely that hydrogen ion concentration varies among intracellular organelles and cytoplasm even within individual cells. Although the free hydrogen ion concentration of body fluids is exceedingly low, protons are so reactive that even minute changes in concentration significantly influence enzymatic reactions and physiologic processes. Immediate defense against untoward changes in pH is provided by body buffers which can take up or release protons instantaneously in response to changes in acidity of body fluids. Regulation of pH ultimately depends on the lungs and the kidneys.

The principal acid product of metabolism is carbon dioxide, equivalent to potential carbonic acid. The normal concentration of carbon dioxide in body fluids is fixed at 1.2 mmol per liter ($P_{CO_2} = 40$ mmHg) by the lungs; at this concentration, pulmonary excretion equals metabolic production. Although carbon dioxide reacts with water and body buffers during transport from cells to pulmonary alveoli, no net change in body fluid composition results, since the CO_2 excreted by the lungs is directly equivalent to the CO_2 produced by cells. When a nonvolatile acid is produced by metabolism, the protons are removed instantaneously from body fluids by reaction with buffers. In extracellular fluid, bicarbonate is converted to water and carbon dioxide, which is excreted by the lungs. Although this mechanism effectively minimizes changes in acidity, it destroys bicarbonate and uses up cell buffer capacity. The total buffer capacity of the body fluids is about 15 meq per kilogram of body weight. Thus, the normal rate of production of nonvolatile acids would be sufficient to deplete the body buffers completely in 10 to 20 days, were it not for the unique ability of the kidney to eliminate protons from the body by secretion into the urine, thereby regenerating bicarbonate and cell buffer capacity.

The principal source of nonvolatile acid appears to be metabolism of methionine and cystine in dietary proteins, which produces sulfuric acid. Additional sources include the incomplete combustion of carbohydrates and fats, which produces organic acids; the metabolism of nucleoproteins, which produces uric acid; and the metabolism of organic phosphorus compounds, which releases protons and inorganic phosphates. The diet does not normally contain significant amounts of preformed acids or alkalis, but significant amounts of potential acid (e.g., an excess of cationic acids, such as lysine) or alkali (e.g., citrate) may be present.

The principal functions of the kidney in acid-base metabolism can be viewed as retention of existing bicarbonate and generation of new bicarbonate to replace that used to buffer nonvolatile acids. Bicarbonate is reabsorbed in both proximal and distal segments by secretion of protons into tubular fluid. The bicarbonate concentration of extracellular fluid is, in effect, set by this process. If plasma bicarbonate rises so that filtered load exceeds renal reabsorptive capacity, bicarbonate will be excreted rapidly and normal plasma bicarbonate will be restored promptly. New bicarbonate is generated by secretion of protons onto urinary buffers. Normally, one-third is titrated onto phosphate, converting HPO_4^{2-} to $H_2PO_4^-$, the remainder onto ammonia. The amount of free acid which can be excreted in the urine is negligible, even at the minimum urine pH of 4.8. However, acidification of the urine is essential for titration of acid onto phosphate and ammonia. Changes in the pH of body fluids lead to regulatory responses by the kidney. Acidosis stimulates renal hydrogen ion secretion. Ammonia production increases, and more protons can be excreted as ammonium. In extreme acidosis, ammonia production may increase tenfold or more above the normal rate of 40 to 50 meq per day. The rate of bicarbonate reabsorption and hence plasma bicarbonate is determined, in part, by carbon dioxide concentration. Thus, hypercapnia stimulates renal bicarbonate reabsorption and elevates plasma bicarbonate, presumably because the increased concentration of carbonic acid in tubular cells enhances renal hydrogen ion secretion. Hypocapnia has the opposite effects.

The respiratory response to changes in blood pH is almost instantaneous. Acidosis stimulates and alkalosis depresses ventilation. The respiratory center in the medulla appears to respond to a pH intermediate between those of blood and cerebrospinal fluid.

EVALUATION OF ACID-BASE BALANCE In practice, classification of acid-base disorders is based on measurements of changes in the bicarbonate–carbonic acid system, the principal buffer of extracellular fluid. Because intracellular and extracellular buffers are functionally linked, measurement of the plasma bicarbonate system provides useful information about total body buffers. The relationship among the elements of the bicarbonate system is usually described in terms of the Henderson-Hasselbalch equation:

$$pH = pK + \log \frac{[HCO_3^-]}{[H_2CO_3]}$$

(The pK of carbonic acid is 6.1. $[H_2CO_3]$ is calculated as αP_{CO_2}; α, the solubility factor for carbon dioxide in body fluids, is 0.031 mmol per liter per mmHg P_{CO_2}. For a normal P_{CO_2} of 40 mmHg, $[H_2CO_3]$ is calculated to be $40 \times 0.031 = 1.2$ mmol per liter.)

Acidosis is defined as a physiologic disturbance which tends to add acid or remove alkali from body fluids, while *alkalosis* is any physiologic disturbance which tends to remove acid or add base. Since compensatory processes may minimize or prevent a change in the hydrogen ion concentration of the plasma, some authors prefer to use the terms *acidemia* and *alkalemia* to indicate those situations in which the pH of the plasma is measurably altered. *Respiratory* disorders are those in which the primary change is in the concentration of carbon dioxide (carbonic acid). As can be seen from the Henderson-Hasselbalch equation, a fall in carbon dioxide concentration will tend to cause alkalemia, while an increase in carbon dioxide con-

centration will cause acidemia. *Metabolic* disorders are those in which the primary disturbance is in the concentration of bicarbonate. Since bicarbonate appears in the numerator of the buffer salt/acid ratio in the Henderson-Hasselbalch equation, increased bicarbonate concentration causes alkalemia while a decrease in bicarbonate causes acidemia.

A major problem in the clinical assessment of acid-base disorders results from the compensatory responses of the lungs and the kidney. A primary change in carbon dioxide concentration induces a compensatory renal response which alters plasma bicarbonate in the same direction. Conversely, a primary alteration of plasma bicarbonate will induce compensatory changes in plasma carbon dioxide. Consider a patient with chronic respiratory insufficiency who has the following set of acid-base parameters: $P_{CO_2} = 70$ mmHg, $[HCO_3^-] = 33$ mmol per liter, pH = 7.30. The clinician needs to know whether the elevation of plasma bicarbonate is merely the appropriate renal response to the primary hypercapnia or a metabolic acid-base disorder is superimposed. No calculations or a priori reasoning will provide the answer to this key question. Such information can be derived only from in vivo observations in which the usual compensatory response to a given degree of chronic hypercapnia is determined.

Appropriate clinical and experimental observations in humans (and animals) have been made in all common primary acid-base disturbances. They are most readily visualized and used for analysis of clinical acid-base disorders by the "confidence band" technique, as shown in Fig. 85-1. Each band represents the mean ± 2 SD, that is, 95 percent of observations, for the compensatory response to each primary disturbance. In the example under discussion, inspection of the confidence band marked *chronic respiratory acidosis* indicates that 95 percent of individuals with chronic elevation of P_{CO_2} to 70 mmHg would have $[HCO_3^-]$ between 37 and 44 meq per liter, due to renal compensation. Thus, the $[HCO_3^-]$ of 33 meq per liter in

FIGURE 85-1

In vivo nomogram, showing bands for uncomplicated respiratory or metabolic acid-base disturbances. Each "confidence" band represents the mean ± 2 SD for the compensatory response of normal subjects or patients to a given primary disorder. (From Arbus.)

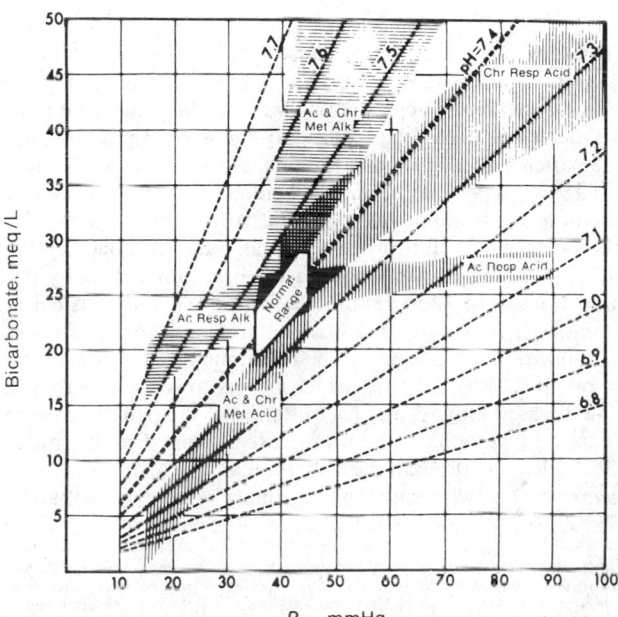

the example cannot be interpreted as solely the result of an appropriate compensatory response to chronic hypercapnia. A second acid-base disorder, presumably metabolic acidosis, must be superimposed. Obviously, the use of this figure is no panacea nor does it obviate the need for commonsense clinical evaluation of alternative possibilities. For example, if the patient under discussion had only recently developed hypercapnia, the $[HCO_3^-]$ of 33 meq per liter would be too high for a purely compensatory response to acute respiratory acidosis and would be interpreted as superimposed metabolic alkalosis. The difference between these two interpretations depends entirely on the clinical recognition of the chronicity of the primary respiratory disorder. The use of Fig. 85-1 in each type of acid-base disturbance is described in the appropriate section of this chapter.[1]

METABOLIC ACIDOSIS

PATHOPHYSIOLOGY Metabolic acidosis is caused by one of three mechanisms: (1) Increased production of nonvolatile acids; (2) decreased acid excretion by the kidney; (3) loss of alkali. In intracellular fluid excess protons replace potassium, which shifts out of cells, tending to elevate plasma levels. Extracellular bicarbonate is reduced by reaction with hydrogen ions or, in patients wasting alkali, by loss of bicarbonate in urine or stool. The decrease in pH stimulates respiration, and P_{CO_2} is lowered. Inspection of the confidence band for metabolic acidosis (Fig. 85-1) indicates that a decrease in P_{CO_2} of roughly 1 mmHg can be expected for each decrement of 1 mmol per liter in plasma bicarbonate. Complete respiratory compensation for primary metabolic acidosis does not occur. Respiratory compensation for acute acidosis tends to be somewhat greater than for chronic metabolic acidosis. The minimum level of P_{CO_2} which can be attained is approximately 10 mmHg; levels below 15 to 20 mmHg are rarely maintained in chronic metabolic acidosis. When kidney function is normal, net acid excretion increases promptly in response to metabolic acidosis. Most of the initial rise is due to increased titration of urinary phosphate as urine pH falls below 5.2. Over several days, ammonia production by the kidney increases and becomes quantitatively by far the most important mechanism for excreting excess protons. Net acid excretion may increase 5 to 10 times above normal, reaching a maximum of several hundred milliequivalents per day.

PATHOGENESIS The major causes of metabolic acidosis are shown in Table 85-1. Renal disease is the most common cause of *chronic* metabolic acidosis. In *chronic renal failure,* the principal defect is decreased ability to excrete ammonium, but some patients also waste bicarbonate, especially at plasma levels of 18 mmol per liter or above. Acidification of the urine and formation of titratable acidity are usually normal. Plasma bicarbonate tends to fall progressively as renal insufficiency becomes increasingly severe, but plasma bicarbonate usually stabilizes at levels of 12 to 18 mmol per liter; it rarely falls below 10 mmol per liter, even in advanced uremia. The mechanisms of stabilization are thought to be (1) stimulation of acid excretion by advancing acidosis, which occurs to some extent even in the diseased kidney, and (2) buffering of the daily metabolic acid load by carbonate and phosphate in bone. Chronic metabolic acidosis is the hallmark of tubular dysfunction in *renal tubular acidosis,* which may be a primary renal disease, part of

TABLE 85-1
Causes of metabolic acidosis

I Renal disease
  A Chronic renal failure
  B Renal tubular acidosis
  C Acute renal failure
II Increased acid production
  A Ketoacidosis
    1 Diabetic acidosis
    2 Associated with alcoholism
    3 Starvation ketosis
  B Lactic acidosis
    1 Secondary to circulatory or respiratory failure
    2 Associated with various disorders
    3 Drugs and toxins
    4 Hereditary forms
  C Poisoning and drug toxicity
    1 High anion gap: salicylates, methanol, ethylene glycol
    2 Normal anion gap: ammonium chloride, lysine and arginine hydrochloride
III Loss of alkali
  A Diarrhea
  B Ureterostomy
  C Carbonic anhydrase inhibitors

the Fanconi syndrome, or associated with a number of non-renal primary disorders (see Chap. 89). In *acute renal failure,* plasma bicarbonate usually decreases by no more than 1 to 2 mmol per liter per day; greater rates of fall suggest the presence of some cause of increased acid production, such as damaged tissue or sepsis.

The most common cause of *acute* metabolic acidosis is increased production of nonvolatile acids. In *diabetic ketoacidosis,* acetoacetic and β-hydroxybutyric acids are produced more rapidly than they can be metabolized. Severe ketoacidosis may occur in *association* with *acute* and *chronic alcoholism.* Typically patients have given a history of prolonged abstention from food, protracted vomiting, and appreciable alcohol intake just before development of the ketoacidosis. β-Hydroxybutyrate, acetoacetate, and lactate accumulate in the plasma. The ketosis may be overlooked because the ratio of β-hydroxybutyrate to acetoacetate tends to be unusually high; the nitroprusside test used for clinical detection of plasma ketones responds only to the latter. Blood sugar is usually normal or mildly elevated in these patients. The mechanism of the syndrome is uncertain. *Starvation* may cause mild ketoacidosis because of increased fat metabolism.

Several types of *lactic acidosis* have been recognized. The most common is *secondary* to severe acute circulatory or respiratory failure, with poor tissue perfusion or arterial oxygen desaturation. The clinical features of shock are usually present. In these patients, lactic acidosis probably is due both to increased production of lactate by hypoxic tissues and to decreased utilization by the liver. Lactic acidosis may also be *associated* with *various disorders* such as acute hepatic necrosis, leukemia, and infections. The biguanide oral hypoglycemic agents, such as phenformin, have been the drugs most often responsible for *drug-induced* lactic acidosis; they recently were removed from general use. Certain sugars used for parenteral alimentation, such as fructose, may cause lactic acidosis. Increased lactic acid production contributes to acidosis in *poisoning* by methanol and salicylates. In infants and children, a variety of congenital defects in enzymes of carbohydrate metabolism have been identified as causes of lactic acidosis. Primary lactic acidosis in patients without an underlying disease has been reported but the existence of such a spontaneous disorder is uncertain. This disorder is discussed in greater detail in Chap. 339.

Poisoning and drug toxicity are causes of acute metabolic acidosis. Among the more common agents are salicylates, ethylene glycol, and methyl alcohol. Each of these intoxicants appears to create a metabolic block, which leads to production of a mixture of endogenous organic acids. The quantities of

---

[1] *Although the confidence band method does not permit automatic identification of simple or complicated acid-base disorders, it is much preferable to other techniques such as "buffer base" or "base excess-deficit" for reasons discussed in detail by Schwartz and Relman. These terms are not used in this chapter.*

acid formed far exceed the amount which can be attributed to acidic properties of the drugs or their metabolites. Salicylates have the additional effect of stimulating the respiratory center directly. Respiratory alkalosis is the earliest derangement in salicylate intoxication and may be the only acid-base disorder in some patients. Several medications may induce hyperchloremic acidosis; these include ammonium chloride, lysine and arginine hydrochloride, and carbonic anhydrase inhibitors (see below).

Loss of *alkali* may be the cause of acute or chronic metabolic acidosis. Severe *diarrhea* or intestinal malabsorption usually causes mild to moderate acidosis due to the loss of bicarbonate in liquid stool, in which concentrations of 40 to 60 mmol per liter may be present. Ureterosigmoidostomy, i.e., transplantation of the ureters into the sigmoid colon, leads to metabolic acidosis both because of exchange of chloride for bicarbonate by intestinal epithelium and because renal disease (obstructive uropathy and pyelonephritis) often develops. Acidosis has virtually been eliminated as a problem by the more modern technique for urinary diversion, in which a bladder is formed from a small isolated loop of ileum. Carbonic anhydrase inhibitors, such as acetazolamide, cause mild to moderate acidosis by increasing bicarbonate loss in the urine.

CLINICAL FEATURES AND DIAGNOSIS There are few specific symptoms or signs of metabolic acidosis; diagnosis depends on recognition of the clinical setting and appropriate laboratory studies. In acute metabolic acidosis, hyperventilation is usually evident and may be extremely intense (Kussmaul respiration). However, it is ordinarily impossible to detect increased respiration by physical examination in patients with chronic metabolic acidosis, despite substantial reduction of P_{CO_2}. Acute, severe acidosis produces a variety of nonspecific symptoms ranging from fatigue through confusion, stupor, and coma; vascular collapse and shock may occur. Chronic metabolic acidosis may produce no symptoms or may be associated with fatigue and anorexia, although it is usually difficult to determine whether these symptoms reflect the acidosis per se or are related to the underlying disease.

The characteristic laboratory features are reduction of plasma bicarbonate and blood pH, together with a compensatory reduction in P_{CO_2} (see Fig. 85-1). Hyperkalemia is often present. In those instances in which the cause of metabolic acidosis is not evident from the history or clinical setting, calculation of unmeasured anions (anion gap) may help in differential diagnosis. Unmeasured anions are calculated by subtracting the sum of plasma bicarbonate and chloride from plasma sodium concentration; the normal value is 4 to 12 mmol per liter. In those instances in which acidosis is due to loss of bicarbonate or to administration of acid with chloride, the anion gap will be normal (hyperchloremic acidosis). This category includes diarrhea, loss of upper intestinal fluid, ureterosigmoidostomy, renal tubular acidosis, and administration of ammonium chloride, lysine, or arginine chloride and acetazolamide. When production of nonvolatile acids is increased or renal failure is present, the anions associated with metabolic acids will accumulate in plasma. An increase in unmeasured anions is typical of renal failure, diabetic and alcoholic ketoacidosis, lactic acidosis, and poisoning by salicylates, ethylene glycol, and methyl alcohol.

TREATMENT The treatment of metabolic acidosis depends on its cause and severity. In *chronic renal failure,* mild or moderate metabolic acidosis does not require treatment. When plasma bicarbonate falls below 15 mmol per liter, it is reasonable to treat patients with oral alkali, such as sodium bicarbonate or sodium citrate. The dose is gradually increased until plasma bicarbonate concentration rises to about 18 to 20 mmol per liter. Some patients appear to benefit symptomatically

from elevation of bicarbonate to this level, and fatigue, anorexia, and malaise tend to be alleviated. Caution must be exerted to avoid excessively rapid alkalinization of the plasma, which may precipitate tetany; excess sodium given with alkali may aggravate hypertension or edema. Acidosis should be corrected as completely as possible in patients with *renal tubular acidosis;* this will avoid hypercalciuria, osteomalacia, nephrocalcinosis, and lithiasis. Patients with *acute renal failure* do not ordinarily require specific therapy for acidosis. Dialysis instituted for management of the renal failure should maintain an adequate plasma bicarbonate.

Diabetic *ketoacidosis* responds to insulin, and most patients do not require treatment with alkali. However, when acidosis is extreme (pH less than 7.1 or $[HCO_3^-]$ less than 6 to 8 meq per liter), intravenous bicarbonate therapy is justified. The ketoacidosis associated with alcoholism responds rapidly to infusions of glucose and saline. Insulin is not required, nor should alkali be given unless acidosis is extreme. The ketoacidosis of starvation is mild and requires no specific treatment.

Lactic acidosis secondary to acute circulatory or respiratory failure is corrected if treatment of the underlying disorder is successful. Since this type of lactic acidosis is usually associated with severe acute circulatory or respiratory failure, the mortality rate is high. Lactic acidosis occurring in other disorders is usually resistant to treatment. Rapid administration of several hundred milliequivalents of alkali may raise plasma bicarbonate in some patients, but in others net production of lactic acid may be so rapid that correction of acidosis is difficult. Since vigorous administration of alkali may lead to circulatory overloading, dialysis may be a useful therapeutic measure. Despite rapid administration of alkali, the mortality rate in these patients is high.

The acidosis associated with *diarrhea* or loss of alkaline upper intestinal secretions is usually associated with other electrolyte abnormalities, including volume depletion and potassium deficiency. Treatment with intravenous infusions appropriate for all these abnormalities may be required.

Some general points about therapy with alkali are worth emphasis. Oral treatment with sodium bicarbonate should usually begin with 1 g three times daily and be increased to maintain the desired plasma bicarbonate level. Some patients find that sodium bicarbonate leads to upper gastrointestinal discomfort; a 10% sodium citrate solution may be more palatable. In treatment of acute metabolic acidosis by intravenous administration of alkali, sodium bicarbonate is the agent of choice. The concentration of bicarbonate to be given depends upon the severity of the acidosis and any associated disorders of serum sodium concentration. Typically, concentrations of bicarbonate between 44 and 132 meq per liter are achieved by adding one to three ampuls of sodium bicarbonate to a liter of dextrose in water. The concentration of bicarbonate in these ampuls is 880 meq per liter (44 meq in 50 ml); they should never be given undiluted in the treatment of acidosis, since rapid infusion may induce serious or even fatal cardiac arrhythmias, especially if given as a bolus through a central venous catheter. The total amount of alkali needed to raise plasma bicarbonate can be estimated from the effects of administration of acid loads. In experiments, approximately equal amounts of acid appear to be buffered by extracellular bicarbonate and by intracellular buffers. (In extremely severe acidosis, a greater fraction of the acid load may be buffered within cells.) Therefore, it is appropriate to calculate the amount of alkali needed by assuming that approximately half will accept protons from intracellular buffers and be destroyed; the other half will elevate plasma bicarbonate concentration. Thus, the calculation would be: millimoles of bicarbonate required equals desired increment in plasma concentration (millimoles per liter) times 40 percent of body weight. The 40 percent figure represents twice the extracellular volume. It is rarely desirable to infuse enough alkali to elevate plasma bicarbonate to normal. Possible untoward effects include hypokalemic cardiac toxicity in patients who are substantially potassium-depleted; tetany in patients with renal failure or hypocalcemia; and congestive failure due to excess sodium. Moreover, alkalosis may supervene. Cerebrospinal fluid bicarbonate does not equilibrate rapidly with plasma. Hence the respiratory center, which responds to acidity both of blood and cerebrospinal fluid, maintains some degree of hyperventilation as plasma bicarbonate is increasing. This type of respiratory alkalosis may sometimes persist for several days after correction of metabolic acidosis. In acute acidosis due to overproduction of metabolic acids, successful treatment of the primary disorder will cause rapid metabolic conversion of lactate and ketone bodies to bicarbonate. Thus, excessive administration of bicarbonate early in therapy also may lead to metabolic alkalosis at a later stage of treatment, when endogenous bicarbonate has been reconstituted by improvement in metabolism.

METABOLIC ALKALOSIS

PATHOPHYSIOLOGY Metabolic alkalosis is usually initiated by increased loss of acid from the stomach or the kidney. However, excretion of bicarbonate at high plasma concentrations is normally so rapid that alkalosis will not be sustained unless bicarbonate reabsorption is enhanced or alkali is continuously generated at a great rate. Clinically, maintenance of metabolic alkalosis is most often due to stimulation of bicarbonate reabsorption by a volume (chloride) deficit. During volume depletion, renal conservation of sodium chloride takes precedence over other homeostatic mechanisms, such as correction of alkalosis. Since in alkalosis a large fraction of plasma sodium is paired with bicarbonate, complete reabsorption of filtered sodium requires reabsorption of bicarbonate as well. Alkalosis is sustained until volume depletion is corrected by administration of sodium chloride. This diminishes tubular avidity for sodium and provides chloride as an alternative anion for reabsorption with sodium; excess bicarbonate can then be excreted with sodium.

The mechanism of metabolic alkalosis in patients with excess mineralocorticoid activity is not fully clarified. Mineralocorticoids stimulate renal hydrogen ion secretion; presumably, elevation of plasma bicarbonate is initiated by increased urinary loss of protons as ammonium and titratable acidity. Stimulation of tubular acid secretion also enhances bicarbonate reabsorption, thereby sustaining the metabolic alkalosis. Patients with excess mineralocorticoid activity are not volume- or chloride-deficient. Hence, this type of metabolic alkalosis does not respond to sodium chloride administration.

The mechanism of alkalosis associated with severe potassium depletion is incompletely understood. To some extent extracellular alkalosis may be initiated by a shift of hydrogen ions into cells as potassium is lost. Renal proton secretion is stimulated by potassium depletion. The older concept that hydrogen and potassium compete for secretion on a transport carrier in the distal nephron has been discarded. Nevertheless, part of the sodium reabsorbed distally does exchange for hydrogen or potassium, although the linkage is now understood to be indirect, in that sodium reabsorption creates a favorable electrical gradient for countermovement of cellular cation into the urine. In potassium depletion cellular potassium concentration falls, and hydrogen ion concentration appears to in-

crease. It seems likely that this change in the intracellular ratio of the two ions in renal epithelial cells promotes hydrogen ion secretion and maintains a high renal threshold for bicarbonate.

Respiratory compensation for metabolic alkalosis is limited. Alveolar ventilation decreases, and P_{CO_2} is elevated. However, since this response is limited by hypoxia, P_{CO_2} rarely rises above 50 to 55 mmHg.

PATHOGENESIS The causes of metabolic alkalosis are outlined in Table 85-2. *Vomiting* and *gastric drainage* usually induce only minimal or moderate alkalosis, but occasional patients, especially those with increased gastric acid secretion, e.g., with acid-peptic disease or the Zollinger-Ellison syndrome, may develop very severe alkalosis.

Alkalosis may be present in patients treated with any *diuretic* except those which specifically inhibit bicarbonate reabsorption, such as acetazolamide, or those which inhibit distal cation secretion, such as spironolactone and triamterene. Alkalosis due to oral treatment with diuretics is usually mild. Acute administration of very potent intravenous diuretics such as ethacrynic acid to patients on low-sodium diets may induce more severe alkalosis due to rapid loss of sodium chloride in the urine. Sudden contraction of extracellular volume elevates plasma bicarbonate; renal excretion of excess bicarbonate is prevented by the mechanism discussed above.

Patients with chronic hypercapnia due to respiratory insufficiency maintain high plasma bicarbonate concentrations (see "Respiratory Acidosis" below). If respiration improves, P_{CO_2} will fall promptly. However, urinary excretion of excess bicarbonate previously generated by renal compensatory mechanisms will take a number of days. In patients on low-salt diets or diuretics who have a volume (chloride) deficiency, *posthypercapnic* alkalosis of this type may persist indefinitely unless sodium or potassium chloride is added to the diet. The mechanism in this condition is the same as that which causes persistent alkalosis in vomiting, described earlier.

Alkalosis is variable in patients with excess mineralocorticoid activity. Minimal or moderate alkalosis is usually present in patients with *Cushing's syndrome* or *primary aldosteronism*. More marked alkalosis may be seen in patients with extreme adrenal hyperfunction associated with ACTH-secreting tumors, such as bronchogenic carcinoma. Moderate alkalosis is typical of patients with *Bartter's syndrome*.

Although alkalosis and *potassium depletion* are often associated, mild or moderate potassium depletion is rarely the sole cause of sustained metabolic alkalosis. However, extreme degrees of potassium depletion (serum potassium usually 2 meq per liter or less) may cause metabolic alkalosis. This type of alkalosis is not corrected by administration of sodium chloride but does respond to administration of potassium.

For reasons noted earlier, alkalosis due to administration of alkali cannot be sustained unless large amounts are given. When renal function is compromised, alkalosis may be sustained by small exogenous loads. This is apparently the mechanism of alkalosis in the milk-alkali syndrome, in which hyper-

TABLE 85-2
Causes of metabolic alkalosis

I Associated with volume (chloride) depletion
  A Vomiting or gastric drainage
  B Diuretic therapy
  C Posthypercapneic alkalosis
II Associated with hyperadrenocorticism
  A Cushing's syndrome
  B Primary aldosteronism
  C Bartter's syndrome
III Severe potassium depletion
IV Excessive alkali intake
  A Acute
  B Milk-alkali syndrome

calcemic nephropathy and alkalosis develop in response to excessive intake of absorbable alkali. The nephropathy limits bicarbonate excretion, thus maintaining the alkalosis.

CLINICAL FEATURES AND DIAGNOSIS There are no specific clinical signs or symptoms. Severe alkalosis may cause apathy, confusion, and stupor. If serum calcium is borderline or low, rapid development of alkalosis may lead to tetany. The diagnosis of metabolic alkalosis depends on recognition of the clinical setting and appropriate laboratory studies. Plasma bicarbonate is increased, and elevation of P_{CO_2} is insufficient to prevent alkalemia (see Fig. 85-1). Plasma potassium concentration is often reduced, and the electrocardiogram may reveal changes in T and U waves typical of hypokalemia; it is uncertain whether these changes are due to alkalosis itself or to associated alterations in potassium metabolism. Despite elevation of plasma bicarbonate, the urine pH is usually less than 7 in patients with sustained metabolic alkalosis. This "paradoxical aciduria" reflects the fact that bicarbonate reabsorption must be increased if metabolic alkalosis is to be sustained.

TREATMENT Mild or moderate metabolic alkalosis rarely requires specific treatment. In patients with gastric alkalosis, infusion of saline solutions is usually sufficient to enhance renal bicarbonate excretion and to correct alkalosis by mechanisms discussed above. Administration of potassium chloride is also helpful in treating or preventing alkalosis in these patients and in treating those with diuretic-induced alkalosis. In patients with adrenal hyperfunction, alkalosis is corrected by specific treatment of the underlying disease. In Bartter's syndrome hypokalemia and potassium wasting may be partly corrected by treatment with prostaglandin synthetase inhibitors such as indomethacin. Whenever alkalosis and potassium depletion occur together, potassium depletion should be treated with potassium chloride, not with an organic salt of potassium.

Rarely, prolonged gastric losses in patients with metabolic alkalosis may be severe enough to require intravenous therapy with acidifying agents. Ammonium chloride or arginine hydrochloride may be given slowly under such circumstances. In most patients the use of potentially toxic acidifying agents can be avoided by appropriate treatment with saline and potassium chloride.

RESPIRATORY ACIDOSIS

PATHOPHYSIOLOGY Failure of ventilation promptly increases P_{CO_2} (carbonic acid) because metabolic production of carbon dioxide is so rapid. Acute respiratory acidosis is modulated to a limited degree by tissue buffers. As can be seen from the curve labeled *acute respiratory acidosis* in Fig. 85-1, immediate tissue buffering is insufficient to elevate plasma bicarbonate more than a few milliequivalents per liter. If hypercapnia is sustained, renal acid excretion is enhanced, and bicarbonate reabsorption stimulated. Over a period of several days, plasma bicarbonate rises approximately 3 meq per liter for each increase of 10 mmHg in P_{CO_2}, thereby minimizing the degree of acidemia. The increment in plasma bicarbonate attributable to renal activity is represented by the difference between the curves marked *chronic respiratory acidosis* and *acute respiratory acidosis*.

PATHOGENESIS *Acute* respiratory acidosis occurs whenever there is a sudden failure of ventilation. Common causes include depression of the respiratory center by cerebral disease or drugs, neuromuscular disorders, and cardiopulmonary arrest. *Chronic* respiratory acidosis occurs in pulmonary diseases such as chronic emphysema and bronchitis, in which ventilation and perfusion are mismatched and effective alveolar ventilation is decreased. Chronic hypercapnia may also result

from primary alveolar hypoventilation or from alveolar hypoventilation related to extreme obesity (Pickwickian syndrome). Acute and chronic diseases characterized principally by interference with alveolar gas exchange, such as chronic pulmonary fibrosis, pneumonia, and pulmonary edema, usually cause hypocapnia rather than hypercapnia. In these conditions, hypoxia stimulates increased ventilation; since carbon dioxide is much more diffusible than oxygen, excretion of carbon dioxide is enhanced despite the barrier to gas exchange. Hypercapnia occurs only with respiratory fatigue or extremely severe disease.

CLINICAL FEATURES AND DIAGNOSIS It is often difficult to separate the manifestations of respiratory acidosis from those of associated hypoxia. Moderate hypercapnia, especially if it develops slowly, probably has no specific clinical features. When P_{CO_2} exceeds 70 mmHg, patients progressively become confused and obtunded. Asterixis may be noted. Papilledema may occur, apparently because intracranial pressure is increased by the cerebral vasodilation characteristic of hypercapnia. Dilatation of conjunctival and superficial facial blood vessels may be noted.

The diagnosis of acute respiratory acidosis is usually evident from the clinical situation, especially if respiration is obviously depressed. Proof requires laboratory confirmation that P_{CO_2} is elevated. Acidemia is always present in patients with acute hypercapnia. Acidosis in acute cardiopulmonary arrest is usually a combination of a metabolic lactic acidosis and acute respiratory acidosis. Patients with chronic hypercapnia are usually acidemic. However, some individuals with minimal or moderate chronic hypercapnia may have normal or even slightly elevated plasma pH, as may be seen from Fig. 85-1. The mechanism of full compensation or of "overcompensation" in such individuals is unknown. However, significant elevation of pH in patients with chronic hypercapnia is almost always due to complicating metabolic alkalosis. Diuretics, low-sodium diets, and posthypercapneic alkalosis are frequent causes of this type of superimposed acid-base disorder.

Because of the differences between plasma bicarbonate in acute hypercapnia and in chronic hypercapnia, proper interpretation of acid-base parameters in respiratory acidosis depends on clinical information. This is discussed in an earlier section of this chapter.

TREATMENT The only worthwhile approach to treatment of respiratory acidosis is correction of the underlying disorder. Rapid infusion of alkali is justified in cardiopulmonary arrest. In other circumstances, attempted treatment of respiratory acidosis with infusions of alkali or with buffers such as THAM is of transient benefit and has no role in practical management.

RESPIRATORY ALKALOSIS

PATHOPHYSIOLOGY Acute reduction in carbon dioxide concentration releases hydrogen ion from tissue buffers, which minimize alkalemia by reducing plasma bicarbonate. Acute alkalosis also enhances glycolysis; increased production of lactic and pyruvic acids lowers serum bicarbonate and raises plasma concentrations of the corresponding anions by a millimole or two. Reduction in P_{CO_2} through its effect on plasma bicarbonate concentration decreases renal bicarbonate reabsorption. In chronic hypocapnia, serum bicarbonate is maintained at a reduced level because of decreased renal reabsorption.

PATHOGENESIS The causes of respiratory alkalosis are shown in Table 85-3.

CLINICAL FEATURES AND DIAGNOSIS Depending on its severity and acuteness, hyperventilation may or may not be clinically apparent. In acute respiratory alkalosis, the clinical picture is rather characteristic: patients complain of paresthesias, numbness, and tingling; of light-headedness; and, if alkalosis is sufficiently severe, of manifestations of tetany. Alkalosis directly enhances neuromuscular excitability; this effect, rather than the modest decrease in ionized plasma calcium induced by alkalosis, is probably the major cause of tetany. Severe respiratory alkalosis may cause confusion or loss of consciousness, perhaps due to cerebral vasospasm induced by hypocapnia.

The diagnosis may be suspected from the clinical setting but must be confirmed by analysis of the plasma bicarbonate system. Hypocapnia together with a variable degree of alkalemia is found; plasma bicarbonate is decreased but is rarely below 15 mmol per liter.

TREATMENT The only successful treatment for respiratory alkalosis is elimination of the underlying disorder. In the acute hyperventilation syndrome, sedation, reassurance, and if symptoms are sufficiently severe, rebreathing into a bag will usually terminate the attack.

REFERENCES

Arbus GS: An in vivo acid-base nomogram for clinical use. Can Med Assoc J 109:291, 1973

Brackett NC Jr et al: Acid-base response to chronic hypercapnia in man. N Engl J Med 280:124, 1969

Cohen RD, Woods HF: *Clinical and Biochemical Aspects of Lactic Acidosis.* Oxford, Blackwell Scientific Publications, 1976

Emmett M, Narins RG: Clinical use of the anion gap. Medicine 56:38, 1977

Levy LH et al: Ketoacidosis associated with alcoholism in non-diabetic subjects. Ann Intern Med 78:213, 1973

Relman AS: Renal acidosis and renal excretion of acid in health and disease. Adv Intern Med 12:295, 1964

Schwartz WB, Relman AS: A critique of the parameters used in the evaluation of acid-base disorders. N Engl J Med 268:1382, 1963

Seldin DW, Rector FC: The generation and maintenance of metabolic alkalosis. Kidney Int 1:306, 1972

86

INTERMEDIARY METABOLISM OF CARBOHYDRATES, LIPIDS, AND PROTEINS

DANIEL W. FOSTER
J. DENIS McGARRY

Fuel metabolism in the human is a complicated and finely regulated process. In this chapter the general principles of the intermediary metabolism of carbohydrates, lipids, and proteins will be briefly reviewed. Emphasis will be placed on the physiology of substrate flow under the influence of the endocrine system rather than on the molecular biochemistry of the various pathways.

It is helpful to consider intermediary metabolism in two phases—*anabolic* and *catabolic*. While each phase will be discussed in some detail, a preliminary overview may be useful. Under ordinary circumstances energy needs of the body are met by exogenous substrate derived from ingested food. In simple terms, oxidation of the constituent molecules of absorbed foodstuffs to carbon dioxide and water is accompanied by the generation of adenosine triphosphate (ATP), the principal high-energy compound of the body (Fig. 86-1). In one sense biological life can be defined as the continued ability to generate ATP (and related high-energy nucleotides) for the preservation of cellular integrity in all its manifestations.

When caloric intake is greater than immediate oxidative needs, as would be the case after the usual meal, excess substrate is stored as fat, structural protein, and glycogen. This stored substrate is readily mobilized for use by the various tissues of the body during fasting or caloric restriction (Fig. 86-2). From conception to adult life net substrate flux is in the anabolic direction (caloric balance is positive) to allow body growth. At maturity anabolic and catabolic cycles ideally balance such that weight is maintained constant. Deviation in a positive direction results in obesity, while prolonged fasting or semistarvation leads to unidirectional flow over the catabolic pathway and weight loss.

Anabolic and catabolic phases of metabolism are hormonally determined, and transition from one to the other is smoothly integrated. Insulin is the primary hormone mediating the anabolic phase, while a rise in plasma glucagon, coupled with a fall in insulin, initiates catabolism. Epinephrine, cortisol, and growth hormone likewise rise during the catabolic phase and doubtless contribute to the metabolic pattern. A summary of the feeding-fasting cycle is given in Table 86-1.

ANABOLIC PHASE

When food is ingested the absorptive process begins through the action of intraluminal and brush border enzymes in the intestine which break down complex carbohydrates, lipids, and proteins to constituent sugars, fatty acids, and amino acids. The normal diet is a mixture of all three components, and absorption and metabolism of carbohydrate, fat, and protein occur simultaneously. For descriptive purposes, however, each will be discussed separately.

CARBOHYDRATE Following a carbohydrate meal, absorbed sugars pass into the portal vein for transport to the liver. In the liver a significant portion of glucose (>60 percent) is retained and utilized primarily for glycogen synthesis. The remainder enters the general circulation as free glucose or, to a much lesser extent, as lactate and pyruvate, products of the hepatic

FIGURE 86-1

Anabolic pathways. Simplified scheme showing a hepatic cell with a mitochondrion. Transport systems and enzymatic details are omitted. Following a meal, a portion of ingested food is used directly to generate energy in the form of ATP while the remainder is available for storage. In the example shown glucose is oxidized via the glycolytic pathway and Krebs cycle, serves as substrate for glycogen synthesis, and is transformed to fat following conversion to citrate in the mitochondrion. Citrate is transported to the cytosol and hydrolyzed to acetyl CoA, the substrate from which malonyl CoA is formed, and oxaloacetate, which then is transported back into the mitochondrion (not shown). Exogenous amino acids and fatty acids are stored as protein and triglyceride in muscle cells and adipocytes, respectively. G-6-P, glucose 6-phosphate, F-6-P, fructose 6-phosphate, F-1,6-P, fructose-1,6-diphosphate; NADH, nicotinamide adenine dinucleotide; ATP, adenosine triphosphate; CoQ, coenzyme Q; Cyto A_3, cytochrome A_3; CoA, coenzyme A.

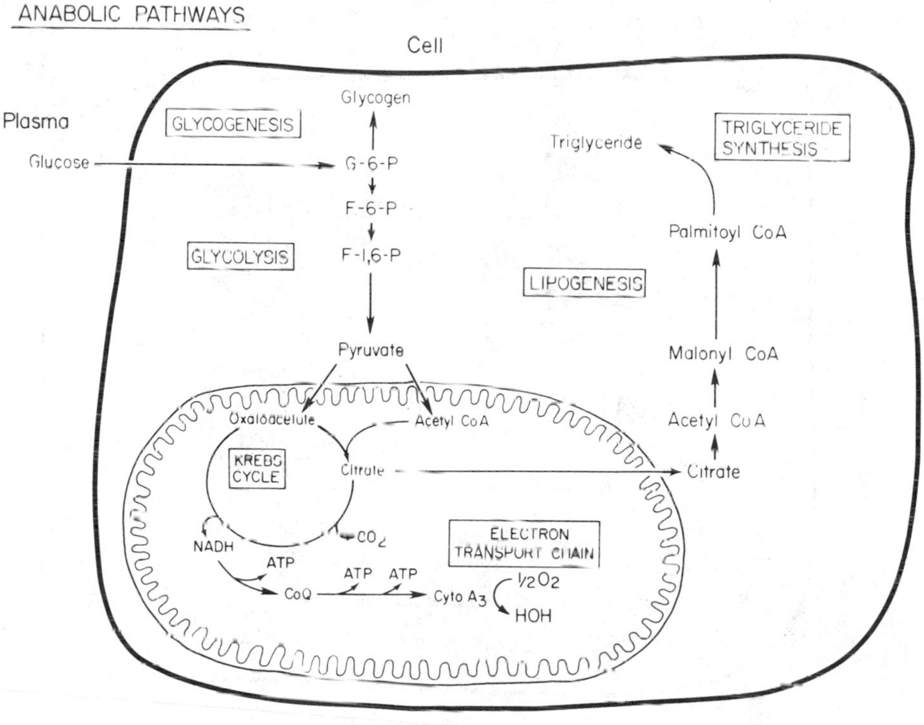

oxidation of glucose. As plasma glucose concentrations rise subsequent to the meal, insulin release from the pancreas is stimulated and glucagon concentrations fall. The magnitude of the insulin response to glucose is increased through the action of other gastrointestinal hormones secreted following food intake. The latter account for the fact that glucose taken by mouth results in much greater insulin release than equivalent amounts given intravenously. Gastric inhibitory polypeptide appears to play a key role in this regard. The newly released insulin, coupled with the fall in glucagon, enhances the capacity of the liver to retain glucose as glycogen and accelerates the disposal of glucose in muscle and adipose tissue. In muscle a portion of the glucose taken up is oxidized while the remainder is stored as glycogen. In adipose tissue glucose is utilized for de novo synthesis of long-chain fatty acids which, in turn, are esterified with glucose-derived glycerol to form triglycerides. A significant amount of triglyceride is also synthesized in liver. It is transported to adipose tissue by very low density lipoprotein molecules.

PROTEIN After a protein-containing meal, absorbed amino acids also pass first to the liver via the portal vein. It is of great interest that the amino acids entering the systemic circulation from the liver do not reflect the makeup of the ingested protein; about 60 percent of the total is accounted for by the branched-chain components valine, isoleucine, and leucine. The precise mechanism whereby selective release of these amino acids is accomplished is unknown. The branched-chain amino acids appear to play a pivotal role in overall protein metabolism in the body. They are markedly responsive to the anabolic effect of insulin in muscle, and one of them—leucine—seems to have a specific stimulatory effect on protein synthesis. It thus is likely that replenishment of protein stores in muscle following a meal is a function of branched-chain amino acid uptake. Muscle also has the capacity (not shared by liver) to oxidize the branched-chain acids for energy purposes. This capacity is important in fasting as will be mentioned below. Amino acids stimulate insulin release from the pancreas but, in contrast to glucose, also cause glucagon secretion. It has been suggested that the role of glucagon is to prevent hypoglycemia when insulin secretion is stimulated by a protein meal under circumstances where dietary carbohydrate is absent or limited.

FAT Fat absorption is much slower than that of carbohydrate or protein and follows a different course. The rate-limiting step

TABLE 86-1
The feeding-fasting cycle

Phase	Primary hormone	Plasma substrates	Substrate flux	Active process
Anabolic*	Insulin	↑ Glucose ↑ Triglycerides ↑ Branched-chain amino acids ↓ Free fatty acids ↓ Ketones	Splanchnic bed → storage and utilization sites	Glycogen storage Protein synthesis Triglyceride formation
Catabolic†	Glucagon	↓ Glucose ↓ Triglycerides ↑ Alanine and glutamine‡ ↑ Free fatty acids ↑ Ketones	Storage sites → liver and utilization sites	Glycogenolysis Gluconeogenesis Proteolysis Lipolysis Ketogenesis

* *Expected findings during the first several hours after ingestion of a mixed meal of fat, carbohydrate, and protein.*
† *The major catabolic phase occurs during the overnight fast, although partial catabolic cycles occur between meals.*
‡ *Arrows indicate plasma concentrations except for alanine and glutamine. While arterial concentrations of these amino acids are relatively constant, uptake by the liver and intestine is increased in the catabolic phase.*

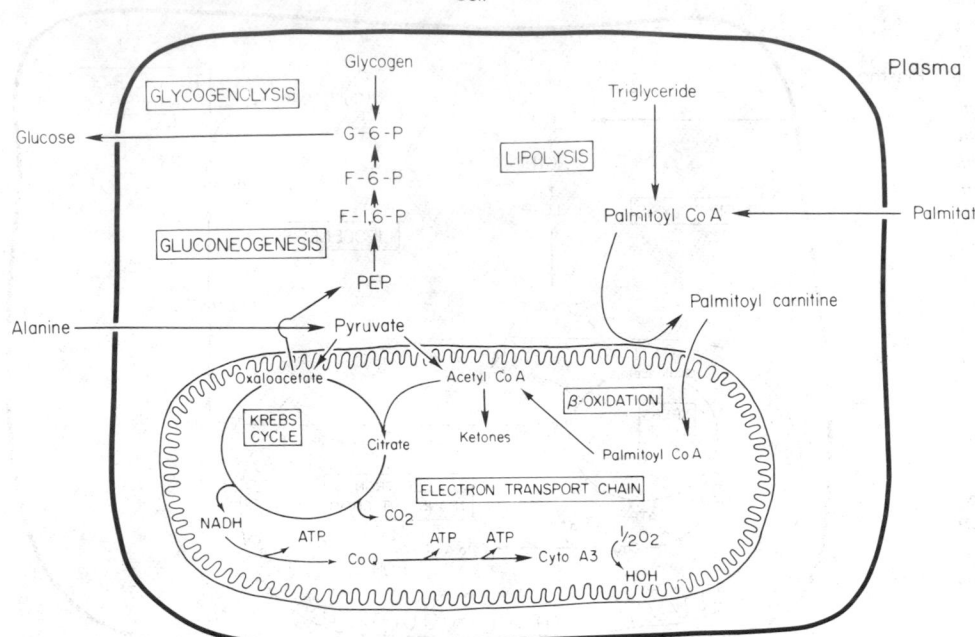

FIGURE 86-2
Catabolic pathways. Simplified scheme showing a hepatic cell with a mitochondrion. Transport systems and enzymatic details are omitted. In the postabsorptive state hepatic glucose production is derived from glycogen breakdown and gluconeogenesis. The latter is largely dependent on amino acids and lactate moving to the liver from the periphery. The energy for gluconeogenesis (ATP) comes primarily from oxidation of long-chain fatty acids released from adipose tissue and from hepatic triglycerides. Fatty acids are also the substrate for ketone body synthesis (see text). PEP, phosphoenolpyruvate; other abbreviations as defined for Fig. 86-1.

is intestinal transport, which may take hours to complete. Following absorption of long-chain fatty acids, triglyceride is reformed inside the intestinal cell and packaged in the form of chylomicrons that then pass into the lymph channels and reach the systemic circulation via the thoracic duct. During transit in both lymph and plasma the apolipoprotein content of the chylomicron is altered by exchange with high-density lipoprotein (HDL). Particularly important is an increase in apoprotein CII, an activator of lipoprotein lipase. In the capillaries of a number of tissues, especially adipose and skeletal tissue and cardiac muscle, the triglycerides of chylomicrons are broken down to free fatty acids and 2-monoglycerides by lipoprotein lipase. Subsequently the monoglyceride is hydrolyzed by a monoglyceridase. The free fatty acids liberated by the two reactions pass into the cell where they may be oxidized for energy purposes or reesterified for storage as triglyceride. The latter pathway predominates in the adipocyte. Most of the triglyceride in the chylomicron is removed in a single passage through the peripheral capillary bed. The cholesterol ester—rich remnant particle then passes to the liver where it serves to regulate hepatic cholesterol synthesis.

The hormonal control of lipid metabolism is slightly more complicated than that of protein and carbohydrate. Pure fat does not stimulate insulin release in humans. However, if carbohydrate is present, triglycerides enhance the insulin response, probably via stimulation of gastric inhibitory polypeptide. Insulin plays an important, if indirect, role in the transport of triglyceride across the plasma membrane of peripheral cells since it is required for synthesis of lipoprotein lipase. Insulin also acts to stimulate fatty acid synthesis and triglyceride formation in the adipocyte and inhibits lipolysis catalyzed by the intracellular hormone-sensitive lipase. In experimental animals triglyceride stimulates secretion of glucagon and enteric glucagon-like material, but this does not appear to be a major response in humans.

SUMMARY The first few hours after a meal are characterized by an anabolic state in which ingested foods pass from the gastrointestinal tract to the liver and peripheral tissues. Under the influence of insulin some substrate is utilized immediately for energy purposes, but significant quantities are stored as

glycogen, structural protein, and fat to be used as needed in the postabsorptive state or during more prolonged fasting.

CATABOLIC PHASE

Postabsorptively[1] a series of metabolic adaptations takes place which ensures adequate fuels for body tissues in the absence of exogenous substrate. Since the brain and other parts of the central nervous system can utilize only glucose or ketone bodies for energy purposes, it is obvious that during a fast plasma glucose concentrations must be sustained in a safe range until acetoacetate and β-hydroxybutyrate concentrations rise to protective levels. Three major processes are involved: (1) The liver is transformed from an organ of glucose uptake to one of net glucose production. Initially the bulk of glucose released comes from glycogen breakdown, while in later stages new glucose production is derived from peripheral precursors via gluconeogenesis. (2) Free fatty acids are mobilized from adipose tissue stores to be utilized directly for oxidative purposes in many tissues of the body and to serve as substrate for ketone body synthesis in the liver. Importantly, free fatty acids also provide the energy required for gluconeogenesis in the liver although they are not themselves substrates for glucose formation. (3) Hepatic ketogenic machinery is activated. As a result of the latter two processes, after only a few days of fasting most tissues of the body utilize free fatty acids and ketones for energy, sparing glucose for the central nervous system. Under these circumstances the enhanced endogenous production of glucose by the liver is adequate to avoid hypoglycemia. In addition the ketone bodies themselves become a major substrate for the brain, sufficient to maintain central nervous system function if for any reason glucose production is impaired. An outline of glucose homeostasis during fasting is given in Table 86-2.

All three of the adaptive processes described above are hormonally induced. In the postabsorptive state there is a fall in insulin release, probably primarily as the consequence of a decline in plasma glucose concentration. Concomitantly there

---

[1] *The term* postabsorptive *is used technically in the literature to indicate an overnight (10- to 12-h) fast. In this discussion it is used to indicate the end of the anabolic phase, which may occur much earlier.*

TABLE 86-2
Maintenance of plasma glucose during fasting

Length of fast	Source of plasma glucose	Mechanism	Tissues using glucose	Primary fuel of brain
3-4 h	Diet	Intestinal absorption	All	Glucose
4-16 h	Liver	Glycogenolysis	All except liver (↓ rates in muscle and adipose tissue)	Glucose
16-48 h	Liver	Gluconeogenesis (± glycogen-olysis)	All except liver (further ↓ rates in muscle and adipose tissue)	Glucose
2-24 days	Liver, kidney	Gluconeogenesis	Brain, RBC, renal medulla	Glucose Ketones
>4 weeks	Liver, kidney	Gluconeogenesis	Brain, RBC, renal medulla (↓ rates)	Ketones Glucose

SOURCE: *After Ruderman et al.*

is a rise in four key counterregulatory hormones: epinephrine, glucagon, cortisol, and growth hormone. If hypoglycemia is rapidly induced, as by insulin injection, epinephrine appears to play the most important role since its release precedes that of glucagon, cortisol, and growth hormone. Moreover, in patients with high spinal cord transection, 2-deoxyglucose administration (which mimics hypoglycemia) is not followed by the appearance of compensatory hyperglycemia as occurs in normal subjects. The quadriplegic patients have a normal rise in glucagon, growth hormone, and cortisol but are unable to release epinephrine, again suggesting a critical role for the catecholamine in activating hepatic glyceogenolysis. When the fall in glucose is more gradual, as in the postabsorptive state, glucagon is thought to be the most important hormone controlling hepatic glucose production. Lipolysis is generally considered to be primarily the consequence of insulin deficiency, while the ketogenic capacity of liver appears to be induced by the rise in plasma glucagon.

GLYCOGENOLYSIS AND GLUCONEOGENESIS Hepatic glucose production in the immediate postabsorptive state is due almost exclusively to breakdown of preformed glycogen. Ordinarily the liver contains sufficient glycogen to maintain the plasma glucose for only 12 to 24 h (depending on activity and caloric demands). Beyond this period gluconeogenesis is required if hypoglycemia is to be avoided. The gluconeogenic substrates are lactate, glycerol, and amino acids. Lactate derived from glucose not completely oxidized in peripheral tissues normally returns to the liver and after an overnight fast accounts for up to 20 percent of hepatic glucose production (Cori cycle). This does not result in net glucose synthesis, however, since the lactate was originally derived from glucose passing to muscle and other tissues. Net glucose synthesis from lactate (as opposed to the recycling sequence) requires its production from stored muscle glycogen. Glycerol utilized for gluconeogenesis comes from triglycerides hydrolyzed in adipose tissue. Its contribution to overall glucose production is relatively minor. Amino acids represent the major substrate for gluconeogenesis, but amino acid metabolism during fasting is complicated. While there is net release of all amino acids, the output of alanine and glutamine is out of proportion to their relative concentrations in muscle protein. Glutamine is preferentially utilized by extrahepatic splanchnic tissues, while alanine uptake by the liver is greater than that of any other amino acid, suggesting a prime role for the latter in the gluconeogenic process. Moreover, alanine extraction by the liver increases during fasting. Glutamine is also taken up by the kidney, serv-

ing as substrate for NH_3 generation and renal gluconeogenesis. While liver is the primary gluconeogenic organ, measurable glucose production occurs in the kidney during prolonged fasting.

It is now thought that the bulk of the alanine released from muscle is derived from transamination of pyruvate which, in turn, is produced from muscle glycogen, glucose from plasma, and possibly directly from amino acids themselves. The source of nitrogen for the transamination of pyruvate is likely the branched-chain amino acids that are released from the breakdown of muscle protein. Following transamination, the α-keto analogues of these acids are oxidized to provide energy for the muscle. The end result is that muscle protein becomes the major source of new glucose formation by the liver, transported to that organ in the form of alanine. Presumably the advantage of alanine resides in its ready ability to enter the hepatocyte and the gluconeogenic pathways.

It is believed that the amino acids utilized in gluconeogensis come from structural protein of muscle rather than from nonfunctional storage pools. As a consequence they represent enzymes, transport molecules, and membrane proteins, all of which are vital to cellular integrity (in contrast to loss of glycogen and triglyceride which are not essential to the cell). For this reason when starvation is extended beyond a few days, limitation of protein loss becomes critical. After several weeks of total starvation (in obese subjects) a definite decrease of nitrogen excretion in the urine has, in fact, been observed. At this stage essentially all tissues of the body are sustained by the oxidation of fat—either as free fatty acids or the ketone bodies. As a result the demand for glucose (and thus the demand for protein as gluconeogenic substrate) markedly diminishes, and the negative nitrogen balance of starvation is blunted. There is suggestive evidence that the ketone bodies somehow signal the muscle to damp amino acid release. Infusion of β-hydroxybutyrate to fasting subjects decreases plasma alanine concentration and acutely lowers urinary nitrogen excretion. Presumably other factors are also involved since massive negative nitrogen balance occurs in diabetic ketoacidosis despite ketone concentrations far higher than maximal levels attained in prolonged starvation. In view of its known anabolic (anticatabolic) effects, insulin may be the required additional factor.

LIPOLYSIS The hydrolysis of adipose tissue triglycerides to free fatty acids and glycerol is mediated by an intracellular, hormone-sensitive lipase which is distinct from the extracellular lipoprotein lipase previously mentioned. This lipase appears susceptible to both positive and negative regulation. Insulin in low concentrations can effectively block lipolysis, while catecholamines activate the process. A number of hormones that increase triglyceride breakdown in rat adipose tissue [e.g., glucagon, growth hormone, adrenocorticotropin (ACTH)] appear to be much less effective in human adipocytes. Activation is thought to involve cyclic adenosine monophosphate (AMP) acting via a protein kinase that phosphorylates the hormone-sensitive lipase. On the negative side both the ketone bodies and adenosine, in addition to insulin, have been suggested to deactivate lipolysis. Free fatty acids rise early in the postabsorptive state and usually reach a maximum of about 1 mM in prolonged fasting.

The importance of lipolysis resides in the fact that body fat represents the organism's primary defense against starvation. This is true because its energy value per gram (about 9 cal) is twice that of protein and carbohydrate (about 4 cal/g) and because its mass is large. Estimates are that the average size person has approximately 140,000 cal stored as fat compared with 24,000 cal as protein and 300 cal as glycogen. If adipose tissue has been depleted (because of disease or famine) or if fatty acids cannot be normally oxidized (see Chap. 340), fatal hypoglycemia or death from protein deficiency may occur.

KETOGENESIS As noted, the ketone bodies play a critical role in the catabolic response to food deprivation. They represent an energy source that can be used by almost every tissue in the body, and they are the only effective alternative substrate for brain metabolism. Interestingly, when total ketones reach concentrations of 4 to 6 mM, hypoglycemia sufficient to cause adrenergic response and mental confusion in a nonketotic individual produces no symptoms. Presumably under these circumstances acetoacetate and β-hydroxybutyrate can meet the metabolic demands of the central nervous system despite inadequate glucose.

Significant ketosis requires changes in both liver and adipose tissue. In the fed state the capacity for fatty acid oxidation in the liver is low. Most of the fatty acid taken up by the hepatocyte is reesterified to triglyceride and either stored or released as a very low density lipoprotein particle. It is now believed that the rate of hepatic fatty acid oxidation is governed by the activity of the carnitine acyltransferase system of enzymes that transports fatty acids into the mitochondria. Present evidence suggests that in the fed state malonyl CoA, a potent inhibitor of carnitine acyltransferase I, keeps the system inactive. This inhibition is removed during fasting through the action of glucagon which lowers the malonyl CoA concentration and simultaneously increases the carnitine content of liver. With these changes the capacity for fatty acid oxidation and ketogenesis in the hepatocyte is maximally activated. (For a more detailed explanation, see Chap. 338.) Once the liver is activated, the rate of ketone body production is determined solely by the rate of delivery of free fatty acids from the periphery; i.e., the higher the free fatty acid concentration in plasma, the greater the hepatic production of acetoacetate and β-hydroxybutyrate until maximal rates are obtained.

Quantitative estimates of substrate flux after a 24-h fast are shown in Table 86-3.

SUMMARY The catabolic changes occurring in the absence of food vary with the duration of the fast. In the first few hours glycogenolysis predominates, while the adaptive response after the first day emphasizes gluconeogenesis and protein breakdown together with acceleration of fat catabolism. If the fast is prolonged, a fat economy is established with diminution of gluconeogenesis and nitrogen wastage. Provided that adipose tissue stores are adequate, prolonged survival can occur in the complete absence of food.

STARVATION AND DIABETIC KETOACIDOSIS

It has long been recognized that diabetic ketoacidosis is a catabolic illness that resembles an accelerated state of starvation. In this situation hepatic gluconeogenesis is markedly increased, plasma-free fatty acids are extremely high (2 to 4

TABLE 86-3
Substrate flux during fasting (per 24 h)*

Amino acids released	75 g
Free fatty acids released:	160 g
Used directly	120 g
Converted to ketones	40 g
Glucose produced	180 g
Ketones produced	60 g

* *Fluxes calculated after 24 h of fasting in a subject with basal energy requirements of 1800 cal.*
SOURCE: *After Cahill.*

TABLE 86-4
Typical laboratory values in fasting and diabetic ketoacidosis

	48-h fast	*Ketoacidosis*
Glucose, mg per 100 ml	65	475
Free fatty acids, mM	0.9	2.1
Acetoacetate, mM	0.8	4.8
β-Hydroxybutyrate, mM	2.2	13.7
Lactate, mM	0.7	4.6
Blood urea nitrogen, mg per 100 ml	16	25
Urinary nitrogen, g per 24 h	12	20
HCO_3^-, mM	22	5
pH	7.35	7.05
Insulin, μU/ml	10	<5
Glucagon, pg/ml	200	400

mM), acetoacetate and β-hydroxybutyrate concentrations are sufficient (18 to 20 mM) to cause frank acidosis, and protein wastage is massive. It seems clear that the quantitative differences between starvation and diabetic coma can be accounted for primarily by the almost complete absence of insulin in ketoacidosis-prone diabetes. As outlined above, normal persons subjected to fasting show a modest fall in plasma glucose which results in diminished insulin release from the pancreatic islets. The fall in insulin concentration, coupled with release of glucagon and other counterregulatory hormones, activates glycogen breakdown, gluconeogenesis, lipolysis, and ketogenesis. Since both ketone bodies and free fatty acids can stimulate insulin release from the beta cell, a protective feedback loop is available during fasting in the normal subject that prevents the occurrence of ketoacidosis; i.e., when total ketones and free fatty acids approach levels sufficient to produce a significant acidosis, insulin release is stimulated (or further fall in insulin is prevented), resulting in modulation of adipose tissue lipolysis and limitation of ketone formation by restriction of fatty acid flow to the liver. In the absence of an adequate insulin feedback loop, as in the juvenile diabetic, lipolysis is unrestrained and ketogenesis becomes maximal, resulting in life-threatening ketoacidosis. Ketoacidosis and the major catabolic responses so characteristic of the uncontrolled insulin-dependent patient do not occur in maturity-onset diabetes. Presumably the difference resides in the fact that insulin deficiency is not as complete in the latter state. A comparison of laboratory values in fasting and diabetic ketoacidosis is shown in Table 86-4.

REFERENCES

BRODOWS RG et al: Neural control of counter-regulatory events during glucopenia in man. J Clin Invest 52:1841, 1973

BUSE MG, REID SS: Leucine. A possible regulator of protein turnover in muscle. J Clin Invest 56:1250, 1975

CAHILL GF JR: Starvation in man. N Engl J Med 282:668, 1970

CROCKETT SE et al: The insulinotropic effect of endogenous gastric inhibitory polypeptide in normal subjects. J Clin Endocrinol Metab 42:1098, 1976

FELIG P: Amino acid and protein metabolism in diabetes mellitus. Arch Intern Med 137:507, 1977

GARBER AJ et al: The role of adrenergic mechanisms in the substrate and hormonal response to insulin-induced hypoglycemia in man. J Clin Invest 58:7, 1976

KHOO JC et al: The mechanism of activation of hormone-sensitive lipase in human adipose tissue. J Clin Invest 53:1124, 1974

McGARRY JD, FOSTER DW: Hormonal control of ketogenesis. Biochemical considerations. Arch Intern Med 137:495, 1977

RUDERMAN NB et al: Gluconeogenesis and its disorders in man, in *Gluconeogenesis: Its Regulation in Mammalian Species*, RW Hanson, MA Mehlman (eds). New York, Wiley, 1976, pp 515–532

SAUDEK CD, FELIG P: The metabolic events of starvation. Am J Med 60:117, 1976

UNGER RH: Diabetes and the alpha cell. Diabetes 25:136, 1976

87

OVERVIEW OF INHERITED METABOLIC DISEASES

LEON E. ROSENBERG

GENE-ENVIRONMENT INTERACTION Metabolism, by definition, comprises all the processes by which living matter is built up (anabolism) or broken down (catabolism). These processes begin with the earliest chemical reactions leading to the formation of the sperm and egg; continue throughout growth, maturation, and senescence; and end inexorably with the death of cell, tissue, organ, and finally the individual. Metabolic processes are controlled by two integrated inputs: the *genes,* which delimit the capacity of any given cell (and pari passu of any organism), and the *environment,* which determines how those genes will be expressed. It follows that all metabolic disorders result from some disturbance in the interaction between genetic and environmental factors, and, in the strictest sense, that no metabolic disorder can be classified as either purely *inherited* or *acquired.* When we have little or no information about the genetic determinants of a disease, as in susceptibility to tuberculosis or to traumatic fractures of bones, we think of the condition as acquired. Conversely, when a metabolic disorder is due to a primary abnormality of a specific protein (and hence to a mutation of a specific gene) and when this abnormality is inherited as a simple mendelian dominant or recessive trait (as in acute intermittent porphyria or phenylketonuria), we consider the metabolic derangement inherited. In fact neither condition might be serious were it not for precipitating and modifying factors in the environment (drugs and hormones in porphyria; dietary phenylalanine in phenylketonuria). Appreciation of this gene-environment continuum is of more than nosologic interest. Thus, identification of genes controlling susceptibility to tuberculosis will, one day, enable us to identify individuals and groups at risk; and additional information about age-related dietary phenylalanine requirements will permit more effective nutritional treatment of phenylketonuria.

CHARACTER OF INBORN ERRORS In the chapters of the section to follow, those metabolic disorders with an "inherited" etiology are emphasized. Literally hundreds of such inherited metabolic diseases or, as they were originally designated by Garrod, "inborn errors of metabolism," are now recognized, and new ones continue to be described at a logarithmic rate. As a group, these conditions affect all phases of metabolism and have contributed enormously to the understanding of normal metabolic pathways (confirming the wisdom of the dictum "treasure your exceptions"). They share only the two common features mentioned earlier: each is inherited as a simple mendelian trait and each has been traced (or is attributed) to a functional abnormality of a specific protein. In other ways the features are diverse. Most are inherited as autosomal recessive traits, implying that a double dose of the mutant gene is required for the disorder to be phenotypically manifest (see Chap. 58); others are inherited as X-linked or autosomal dominant traits. Some have an incidence as high as 1:500 (familial hypercholesterolemia); others have an incidence as low as 1:1,000,000 (alcaptonuria). Some demonstrate prominent racial or ethnic clustering, and others appear to be uniformly distributed in races and groups. Some produce clinical manifestations at birth (or even before), others only in adult life (or not at all). Some are uniformly lethal regardless of treatment; others are compatible with a normal life span and health.

LEVELS OF UNDERSTANDING Since it is generally assumed that the clinical and chemical abnormalities observed in patients with a given inherited metabolic disease reflect the mutational disturbance of a specific gene, it is theoretically possible to understand each inborn error at four levels: the gene, the protein coded for by the gene, the metabolic step at which the protein works, and the clinical or chemical phenotype produced by abnormalities at that step. Of all the genetic disorders, it is only in certain of the hemoglobinopathies that we can approach this level of understanding (see Chap. 315). In hemoglobin S disease (sickle-cell anemia) the specific mutant codon and the precise amino acid substitution in the β globin chain have been identified. Furthermore, physicochemical studies with hemoglobin S have shown why this mutant protein has a tendency to gel in the deoxygenated state and form the tactoids that distort the erythrocyte and lead to the hyperviscosity, sludging, tissue infarction, and hemolysis characteristic of this disorder. Such complete information is possible because hemoglobin is the only human protein that has been studied to date at the level of the gene and messenger RNA. For other loci, understanding stops at the level of the gene product and, even there, in an incomplete way. For example, in one form of galactosemia the activity of galactose 1-phosphate uridyltransferase is deficient; this deficiency leads to accumulation of galactose and galactose 1-phosphate, which results in serious hepatic and central nervous system dysfunction. However, we know little about either the molecular nature of the transferase deficiency or the means by which metabolite accumulation leads to cirrhosis and mental retardation. In other instances, such as Wilson's disease or cystinosis, the particular protein whose function is deranged is unknown, although it is recognized that copper and cystine respectively accumulate in tissues of affected patients. Even more primitive is our understanding of Huntington's disease, which can only be described clinically as an autosomal dominant disease without a known biochemical "handle" with which to grapple with the diagnostic and prognostic dilemmas. Much has been learned about inherited metabolic disorders in the past 25 years, but that quantum of knowledge is trivial compared with the enormity of our ignorance.

PROTEINS AS GENE PRODUCTS

SPECTRUM OF MUTANT PROTEINS Genes and messenger RNAs are polymers of nucleic acids often referred to as "informational macromolecules." Along similar lines proteins and polypeptides can be called "functional macromolecules." These linear polymers of amino acids convert the informational potential of genes and messengers into chemical and physiologic work. Proteins are ubiquitous. They are a vital constituent of the membranes that separate tissues, cells, and organelles from one another. In the blood, lymph, and cerebrospinal fluid they maintain osmotic pressure and selectively bind and transport a large number of small molecules. As enzymes and hormones, whether extracellular or intracellular, they catalyze or regulate reactions that allow anabolic and catabolic pathways to proceed. Proteins display almost limitless variation in size, shape, and function. Molecular weights vary from a few hundred, for the pituitary hormone releasing factors, to more than a million, for gamma macroglobulin. Some are monomeric; others are oligomers of two, three, four, or more like or unlike polypeptide chains. Some are globular while others are helical; still others have both globular and helical regions. Some have metal ions as prosthetic groups or cofactors, while others require organic constituents for activity. Each, however, owes its unique structural features and functional specificity to a single feature—the primary amino acid sequence. Since this primary sequence is dependent on the nucleotide sequence of the gene and messenger RNA that codes for the polypeptide, inherited variations in protein structure or function are the visible expression of gene mutation. Mutations occur in all genes, and hence variation must occur in all proteins. Some variants are detected easily because they lead to obvious chemical or clinical disturbance. Others are detected with great difficulty, either because they produce early lethality or because they are clinically or chemically silent.

In general, mutations responsible for inherited metabolic disorders affect the structural genes that code for the *primary structure* of the protein (see Chap. 58). Single codon changes usually lead to single amino acid substitutions and are referred to as *missense* mutations. Other point mutations (those leading to inappropriately placed terminator codons) as well as deletions and insertions (of codons, segments, or entire genes) produce *nonsense* mutations that result in complete absence of the gene product or one so incomplete or distorted as to be essentially functionless. Alternatively, mutations can modify the *rate* at which a protein is made. Such rate control may be exerted either by modifying control genes or by changing codons in structural genes in a way that leads to accelerated or retarded transcription or translation. Because the messenger RNAs and the genes controlling synthesis of the α and β globin chains of hemoglobin have been purified and characterized, impressive knowledge has been acquired regarding the chemical nature of genetic modifications in this system. Since molecular biological information is lacking for other human loci, inferences about disturbances in gene structure must be drawn from the observed effects of gene-controlled protein functions.

Inborn errors have been described for all types of proteins. In their seminal contributions, Garrod, Beadle, Tatum, and associates stressed enzymatic defects that produce a block in an anabolic or catabolic pathway. More than 100 examples of this type of defect are known (see subsequent chapters), and new enzymatic deficiencies are currently being described at a rate of about ten per year. Although dysfunction of these intracellular catalysts provides the largest body of data concerning the impact of inherited variation on homeostasis, they do not reflect the full scope of functional changes produced by genetic alterations. For example, numerous inherited disorders of cell membrane function have been described. Inborn errors of transport affecting gut and kidney may selectively impair transmembrane movement of sugars, amino acids, phosphate, vitamins, or water (see Chap. 90). Disorders like cystinuria or glycosuria are thought to reflect deficiency of specific membrane carrier proteins required for transepithelial movement of dibasic amino acids or glucose, respectively. Other transport defects lead to abnormal binding of hormones to membrane receptors as in vasopressin-resistant diabetes insipidus or of protein-ligand complexes as in the cell surface receptor defect for low-density lipoprotein in familial hypercholesterolemia (see Chap. 100). Still other mutations alter circulating proteins rather than membrane constituents or intracellular enzymes. Analbuminemia, transcobalamin II deficiency, and abetalipoproteinemia are examples of such deficiencies.

FUNCTIONAL DERANGEMENTS **Increased activity** Simply put, metabolic disorders can be thought of as resulting from too much or too little of a specific protein (or of that protein's activity). Variant forms of G6PD, pseudocholinesterase, and phosphoribosylpyrophosphate synthetase have been described in which enzyme activity is *increased*. In these instances, mutations result in an increase in intracellular enzyme content either because the mutant protein is synthesized more rapidly than normal or is degraded more slowly. In acute intermittent porphyria and familial hypercholesterolemia, rate-controlling enzymes are increased as well (see Chaps. 96 and 100). In the latter disorders, however, enzyme overactivity is a secondary event, reflecting impaired feedback regulation produced by other primary genetic disturbances.

Decreased activity All other inborn errors that have been analyzed in detail are associated with decreased activity (or content) of a protein. The deficiency may be *virtually complete* (as in the classical forms of phenylketonuria and galactosemia) or *partial* (as in the benign variants of those disorders). It should be emphasized that complete loss of enzyme activity cannot be equated with complete absence of a protein. For example, in classic galactosemia, no galactose 1-phosphate uridyltransferase activity can be detected in tissues of affected patients, but immunochemical analyses have shown that such tissues contain a protein that cross-reacts with antibody to the native transferase molecule. Numerous examples of cross-reacting material positive (CRM$^+$) abnormalities are now recognized. They indicate that the mutation has resulted in the synthesis of a protein that has lost catalytic activity but retains antigenic specificity. Other metabolic disorders characterized by complete enzyme deficiency such as muscle phosphorylase deficiency or Von Willebrand disease are CRM$^-$, implying either that no protein is made or that the gene product is so altered that both catalytic and antigenic functions have been lost.

As increasingly sensitive methods of enzyme assay have been developed, it has become apparent that most inborn errors are characterized by partial, rather than complete, loss of activity. Such partial deficiency may result from several different mechanisms. First, it may reflect reduced rate of synthesis of normal or abnormal enzyme molecules. Second, it may result from accelerated destruction of a structurally altered enzyme. Third, reduced activity may reflect reduced affinity of the active enzyme for substrate or cofactor. Fourth, for oligomeric enzymes, reduced activity could result from impaired interaction of identical or nonidentical subunits. Fifth, for those enzymes in which more than a single isoenzyme exists in a tissue, reduced activity could reflect isolated loss of one form of the enzyme. Examples of each of these mechanisms exist among inherited metabolic disorders in humans. Moreover, the same phenotypic manifestations can result from different mechanisms. For example, some G6PD variants exhibit increased lability, others abnormal affinity for substrate, and still others impaired oligomer formation. All these abnormalities result from different structural alterations in a single polypeptide chain.

CONSEQUENCES OF TRANSPORT OR ENZYMATIC DEFECTS

The effect of any given genetic alteration on cellular metabolism and clinical status depends on the role that the mutant protein plays and the severity of the defect. As mentioned earlier, most inborn errors are the result of intracellular enzymatic defects or of membrane transport abnormalities. Since these kinds of mutations are discussed repeatedly in the following chapters, it is appropriate to summarize the possible consequences of inherited transport or enzyme defects. The model reaction sequence shown in Fig. 87-1 is used for illustrative purposes. A, B, C, D, F, and G are substrates or products of a series of enzymatic reactions; T_A, E_{AB}, E_{BC}, and E_{CD} refer to specific transport systems or enzymes catalyzing specific reactions in this sequence. The major pathway involves the conversion of A to D via intermediates B and C. F and G are products of an alternate metabolic pathway. The arrow from D to E_{AB} represents negative feedback control of the first enzyme in the pathway by the final product of the sequence. Wherever possible, examples of specific inborn errors that illustrate specific consequences of transport or enzyme defects will be cited.

PRECURSOR DEFICIENCY If T_A, the receptor or carrier system that transports A into the cell, is defective, the intracellular concentration of A may be so low that E_{AB} will not be saturated with its substrate. This could slow the entire reaction sequence and result in inadequate formation of B, C, and D. In Hartnup disease (see Chap. 90), intestinal transport of tryptophan is defective. This transport defect has important chemical and clinical consequences, since tryptophan is converted to nicotinamide intracellularly. Patients with this disorder may exhibit cerebellar ataxia and temporary or permanent dementia due to nicotinamide deficiency if they do not receive supplements of niacin in the diet. Similarly, patients with inherited defects in intestinal absorption of vitamin B_{12} develop megaloblastic anemia unless the vitamin is supplied parenterally. Precursor or substrate deficiency may also occur if the defect involves a circulating protein that transports substance A in the blood and carries it to the cell surface.

PRECURSOR ACCUMULATION Let us next consider the effect of reduced activity of one of the intracellular enzymes, (E_{AB}, E_{BC}, or E_{CD}). Such a defect might lead to intracellular and extracellular accumulation of the immediate or remote precursors of the reaction. If E_{AB} is defective, only A will accumulate. Such a result is illustrated by the marked increase in lysosomal glucocerebroside content in Gaucher's disease (see Chap. 101) and of blood galactose concentration in galactokinase deficiency (see Chap. 98). Defects of E_{BC} may result in accumulation of A as well as B, and a defect of E_{CD} could lead to the pileup of A, B, and C. In homocystinuria due to cystathionine synthase deficiency, methionine, a remote precursor, accumulates, as does homocystine, the immediate precursor of the blocked reaction (see Chap. 88).

ALTERNATE PATHWAY UTILIZATION If the conversion of A to B is impaired by deficiency of E_{AB}, not only will A accumulate, but the usually minor, alternate pathway to F and G may become prominent. Phenylketonuria represents an excellent example of this phenomenon. The absence of phenylalanine hydroxylase activity leads to gross overproduction and excretion of phenylpyruvic, phenylacetic, and phenyllactic acids, compounds not usually detectable in blood or urine (see Chap. 88). Such alternate pathway augmentation may have important physiologic significance if the products of the alternate pathway interfere with cell processes when present in more than minute concentrations.

PRODUCT DEFICIT If D is the physiologically active product of the hypothetical reaction sequence, a block at any of the steps from A to D results in inadequate synthesis of D. The formation of thyroxine in the thyroid gland proceeds through just such a series of reactions, involving first the transport of iodide into the gland and then its subsequent oxidation and organification. Several enzymatic defects lead to goitrous cretinism due to impaired synthesis of thyroxine. Similarly, in some patients with congenital adrenal hyperplasia due to a defect in hydroxylation at the C_{21} position of the steroid nucleus, aldosterone production is impaired, leading to renal salt wasting and hyponatremic crises. Deficient synthesis of product may cause overproduction of precursors, as in acute intermittent porphyria, because of loss of feedback control (D → E_{AB}).

PRODUCT EXCESS As shown in Fig. 87-1, the end product of the reaction sequence D is presumed to regulate the activity of E_{AB}, the first enzyme in this biosynthetic pathway. The phenomenon of end product inhibition (commonly called feedback inhibition) was first described in microbial systems but is now known to exist for pathways in mammalian cells as well. Several inborn errors demonstrate abnormalities in feedback regulation, but the biochemical events involved are not well understood. In some patients with primary gout urate is overproduced, presumably because the first enzyme in the purine pathway is defective and does not respond to its normal feedback inhibitors, hypoxanthine and adenine. Abnormal feedback control occurs in the congenital adrenal hyperplasias and congenital goitrous cretinism as well, presumably by different chemical mechanisms. In these disorders the formation or release of ACTH and TSH, respectively, is not impeded by their usual "servo" regulators, cortisol and thyroxine, resulting in hyperplasia and functional disturbances in the two target glands.

Faulty feedback control is not the only mechanism capable of producing product excess. In those disorders characterized

FIGURE 87-1

Schematic representation of metabolic pathway including transport system, enzymes, alternate route, and feedback regulation. (From Rosenberg.)

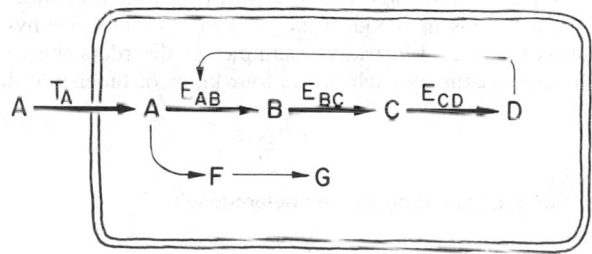

A, B, C, D — Substrate and Products of Major Pathway

F, G — Products of Minor Pathway

T_A — Transport System for A

E_{AB}, E_{BC}, E_{CD} — Enzymes Catalyzing Conversion of A to B, B to C, and C to D

— Cell Membrane

by enzyme excess, such as hyperuricemia resulting from increased PRPP synthetase activity (see Chap. 92), product excess can be explained simply by accelerated conversion of precursor to product.

GENETIC HETEROGENEITY

It is well recognized that a given abnormal phenotype may be produced by more than one genotype. This situation, referred to as genetic heterogeneity, is ubiquitous and important. Clinically, an appreciation of genetic heterogeneity has important diagnostic implications, and since diagnosis defines our approach to treatment and counseling, it is important in these matters as well. Scientifically, elucidation of the mechanisms of heterogeneity is imperative for understanding the ways in which the human genome can be modified and how such genetic manifestations can be expressed phenotypically. As noted in Table 87-1, heterogeneity has been discerned using three general methodologic approaches: clinical, biochemical, and genetic.

CLINICAL EVIDENCE In the absence of independent biochemical or genetic information, it is often impossible to determine whether subtle variations in clinical expression of a given metabolic disorder in any two affected individuals reflect the presence of different mutations or result from modification of an identical mutation by other genetic and environmental influences. However, on the basis of information gleaned from biochemical techniques, such clinical evidence suggesting heterogeneity becomes interpretable. For example, it is likely that patients with juvenile Gaucher's disease have an earlier age of onset and a more rapidly progressive downhill course than do those with adult Gaucher's disease because the mutant glucocerebrosidase in cells from the former group is distinct from and retains less catalytic activity than that in cells from the latter (see Chap. 101). It follows that tissue glucocerebroside content will increase more rapidly if glucocerebrosidase activity is 3 percent of normal than if it is 15 percent of normal. Similarly, the reason that patients with Hunter's disease do not have corneal clouding, whereas patients with the phenotypically similar Hurler's disease do, almost certainly depends on the different enzymatic dysfunctions in the two disorders: iduronate sulfatase deficiency in Hunter's, α-L-iduronidase deficiency in Hurler's.

BIOCHEMICAL TECHNIQUES More often, heterogeneity is first defined through chemical or biochemical assays. Such assays vary greatly in design and complexity—from identification of compounds in blood, urine, or CSF to molecular hybridization analyses. Illustrative examples of disorders shown to be heterogeneous by each of the four kinds of biochemical

TABLE 87-1
Methods of demonstrating genetic heterogeneity

I Clinical analysis
  A Age of onset
  B Severity
  C Specific features
II Biochemical analysis
  A Constituents of blood, urine, and cerebrospinal fluid
  B Enzymatic activity
  C Protein characterization
  D DNA-RNA or DNA-DNA hybridization
III Genetic analysis
  A Chance matings
  B Mode of inheritance
  C Manifestations in heterozygotes
  D Linkage relationships
  E Complementation in mixed cells or heterokaryons

assays noted in Table 87-1 are as follows. First, the "ketotic hyperglycinemia" syndrome, characterized by episodic keto-acidosis, protein intolerance, and hyperglycinemia, was shown by chemical analyses of blood and urine to be a feature of several different disturbances of organic acid metabolism—α-methylacetoacetic acidemia, propionic acidemia, and methylmalonic acidemia. Second, patients with an entity originally called "congenital, nonspherocytic hemolytic anemia" were found to have different deficiencies in glycolytic enzymes when assays were carried out with erythrocyte hemolysates. Third, the nature of the heterogeneity in patients with GM_2 gangliosidosis did not become apparent until the lysosomal hexoseaminidases were subdivided into A and B isozymes whose activities could be measured individually in patients with Tay-Sachs or Sandhoff's disease. The fourth approach is directed at the gene rather than the gene product. Molecular hybridization experiments employing DNA and RNA provided the evidence for two general categories of β thalassemia: β^0, characterized by the apparent absence of β globin mRNA, and β^+, characterized by reduced but clearly detectable amounts of β-globin message. Such hybridization studies were also useful in defining heterogeneity in α thalassemia and in those conditions characterized by hereditary persistence of fetal hemoglobin.

GENETIC METHODS Genetic methods have also been important in demonstrating heterogeneity (Table 87-1). One of the earliest and most convincing evidences of such heterogeneity came from the chance mating of two individuals each affected with autosomal recessively inherited nerve deafness. None of their progeny was deaf, demonstrating conclusively that the mutations that produced deafness in the parents were different and likely nonallelic. In several instances heterogeneity was suggested by different modes of inheritance of phenotypically similar (or identical) disorders. For example, Hunter's and Hurler's diseases were differentiated early because the former is inherited as an X-linked trait, the latter as an autosomal recessive. Similarly, at least three forms of spastic diplegia are now recognized: one inherited as an autosomal dominant, a second as an autosomal recessive, and a third as an X-linked trait. In a few instances heterogeneity was first appreciated by studying obligate heterozygotes for a recessive phenotype. Thus, cystinuria was shown to be heterogeneous by the observation that all obligate heterozygotes in some families excreted increased amounts of cystine and lysine, whereas in other pedigrees urinary findings in obligate heterozygotes could not be distinguished from controls. A fourth genetic tool that has revealed heterogeneity is classical linkage analysis. Through this investigation hereditary elliptocytosis was divided into two forms—one closely linked to the Rh blood group locus, the other not. Finally, heterogeneity has been demonstrated in a number of instances by application of complementation analyses as first worked out in bacteria and neurospora. The general strategy of such studies is simple. Cultured fibroblasts from two affected individuals are cocultivated in the same dish or are fused into heterokaryons with Sendai virus or polyethylene glycol. If the abnormal phenotype expressed in both parental strains remains in the mixed culture, the defect in the two patients is assumed to be identical; if correction occurs in the mixed culture, the defects in the original strains must be different. This approach has been used to define heterogeneity in a wide variety of disorders, including the mucopolysaccharidoses, the GM_2 gangliosidoses, the methylmalonic acidemias, the propionic acidemias, xeroderma pigmentosum, and branched-chain ketoaciduria. Theoretically, positive complementation tests could reflect either of two general mechanisms: intergenic complementation, in which two different loci are involved, or interallelic complementation, in which two different mutations at the same locus are mutually corrective. It seems likely that the vast majority of positive complementation tests reflect the intergenic mechanism.

GENETIC COMPOUNDS One of the important conclusions drawn from these biochemical and genetic demonstrations of heterogeneity is that in some instances individuals with a given metabolic disorder are "genetic compounds" rather than true homozygotes. By genetic compounds we mean individuals who have received a different mutant allele at a given locus from each parent rather than identical mutant alleles. Patients with hemoglobin SC disease were the first compounds identified, having inherited the gene for hemoglobin S from one parent and that for hemoglobin C from the other. These individuals have a double dose of a mutation for β globin chain synthesis and thus make no normal β chains. They are clinically and chemically distinct from true SS or CC homozygotes. More recently, genetic compounds have been identified in patients with cystinuria, iminoglycinuria, galactose 1-phosphate uridyl-transferase deficiency, and L-iduronidase deficiency. Some, but not all, genetic compounds are as severely affected as true homozygotes, depending on the nature of the mutant alleles inherited. Little direct information is available in this area, with the exception of those loci coding for globin chains.

DIAGNOSTIC TECHNIQUES AND TARGETS

PHYSIOLOGIC FLUIDS Most of the early information concerning the mechanisms of the inborn errors and their mode of detection came from chemical studies of blood or urine. Such chemical determinations did more than point out specific biochemical abnormalities; they provided the clues in many instances for the more elegant enzymatic studies that clarified the specific defect involved. They also allowed large populations to be screened for specific disorders, thereby facilitating the detection of affected subjects prior to the onset of overt clinical problems. The use of screening tests in blood and urine has allowed the detection of heterozygous carriers for many conditions. They are also often useful in monitoring the effects of specific dietary, drug, or replacement therapy.

TISSUE ANALYSES During the past 15 to 20 years, enzymatic assays and biochemical studies using human tissue obtained by biopsy made a great impact on the definition and detection of the inborn errors. Analyses of liver, muscle, brain, gut mucosa, kidney, erythrocytes, leukocytes, stratum corneum, and spleen have revealed specific enzymatic defects in more than a hundred metabolic diseases. Membrane transport defects have also been demonstrated in vitro in such disorders as hereditary spherocytosis, cystinuria, and the glucose-galactose malabsorption syndrome by the use of erythrocytes, kidney cortex, and gut mucosa, respectively. These assays have often identified the biochemical and genetic heterogeneity characteristic of the inborn errors, in addition to documenting specific gene product abnormalities. Tissue studies do not lend themselves to population surveys and have the greatest impact when combined with investigations of detectable abnormalities in blood and urine.

CELL CULTURE Within the past decade human fibroblasts grown in tissue culture have yielded important insights into the biochemistry and genetics of numerous inborn metabolic disorders. In some instances (acatalasia, galactosemia, glucose 6-phosphate dehydrogenase deficiency, glycogen storage disease type II, branched-chain ketoaciduria, and orotic aciduria) enzymatic defects initially described in other tissues were confirmed in cultured fibroblasts. In citrullinemia and Refsum's disease, specific enzymatic defects were first demonstrated in fibroblasts, while in the Lesch-Nyhan syndrome defective hy-

poxanthine-guanine phosphoribosyl transferase activity was demonstrated coincidently in erythrocytes, leukocytes, and cultured fibroblasts. Cultured cells are not only of value in defining biochemical abnormalities in affected patients; abnormalities found in cells from heterozygous carriers have also been of significance. For example, the study in obligate heterozygotes of several X-linked traits provided evidence confirming the validity of the Lyon hypothesis.

HETEROZYGOTE DETECTION The detection of heterozygous carriers contributes to the study of inborn errors in two important ways. First, such detection provides the most convincing evidence for a recessive mode of inheritance of a disorder, whether the mutation is autosomal or X-linked. Second, the identification of heterozygous carriers in a single pedigree provides valuable information for counseling family members. Counseling relates to such problems as family planning or the choice of a marriage partner. In those diseases in which clinical manifestations may be observed in the carriers (i.e., in dominantly inherited conditions such as acute intermittent porphyria or familial hypercholesterolemia) heterozygote detection has direct clinical relevance.

Identification of heterozygotes requires many of the same methods employed for the recognition of chemical or enzymatic defects in affected subjects. In a few instances, simple blood or urine screening techniques may be sufficient to detect carriers. Enzymatic assays using blood cells or serum have been helpful in several other conditions. In some disorders blood or urine analyses fail to discriminate between normal subjects and heterozygous carriers, but carriers can be detected after administration of oral or parenteral loads of the metabolic precursor involved in the chemical defect. Thus, heterozygotes for galactosemia and phenylketonuria respond to oral loads of galactose and phenylalanine, respectively, with higher plasma concentrations of these substances than observed in normal subjects.

Finally, carriers for an increasing number of diseases have been detected only by enzymatic assays or phenotypic appearance of cells in biopsy material. These techniques for carrier detection have usually been worked out and utilized in one laboratory or, in some instances, a few centers. Because of their complexity, they have not been employed for carrier detection in large populations.

PRENATAL DETECTION There is now considerable interest in the detection of genetic diseases in utero (see Chap. 58). More than 20 inherited metabolic disorders have been identified by chemical examination of amniotic fluid or enzymatic assays on amniotic fluid cells. The largest group of disorders so detected are those mucopolysaccharide or lipid storage diseases due to deficiency of particular lysosomal hydrolases, but a growing list of disorders of amino acid, organic acid, carbohydrate, and purine metabolism have been identified as well. A few inborn errors have been diagnosed by examination of fetal blood obtained by placental puncture or under fetoscopic control. Sickle-cell anemia, β thalassemia, Duchenne's muscular dystrophy, and hemophilia have been detected in this way.

GENETIC SCREENING

Genetic screening is the search in a population for persons possessing certain genotypes that are known to be associated with or to predispose to disease in the individuals or their descendants. As a research tool, screening can define the incidence of a particular genotype in the population and can be used to search for polymorphism. In the context of this discussion of inherited metabolic diseases, however, screening has two important applications: early identification of at-risk patients with treatable disease prior to onset of clinical symptoms and identification of at-risk couples who may benefit from appropriate genetic counseling. The prototypic example of the former application is neonatal screening for phenylketonuria. The features of this screening application include a relatively common disease (about 1:10,000 in Caucasians) with serious clinical consequences (severe mental retardation); clear evidence that institution of dietary phenylalanine restriction by age 30 days can return blood phenylalanine concentrations to values commensurate with normal or near normal development; and a simple, sensitive, and specific assay that can be performed in the neonatal period. More than 90 percent of neonates in North America and Western Europe are currently being screened for phenylketonuria using the bacterial inhibition assay. The human and monetary savings of this screening program have been enormous and have prompted extension to neonatal detection of other treatable diseases such as galactosemia, hypothyroidism, and homocystinuria. Such "secondary" prevention emphasizes the interaction between environment and heredity, and raises no serious ethical problems.

That statement, however, cannot be made with regard to the other screening application—identification of couples at risk for having offspring with untreatable (or nearly untreatable) disorders. The prototype is Tay-Sachs disease in Ashkenazi Jews. When two Ashkenazim marry, there is a 1:900 chance that both individuals are carriers for the Tay-Sachs gene. Theoretically, if all Ashkenazim were screened before marriage, if all pregnancies in at-risk couples were monitored by prenatal diagnosis and if all affected fetuses were aborted, the incidence of Tay-Sachs disease could be decreased to zero. However, mandatory screening is not a possibility, and compliance for voluntary testing is poor. Education, motivation, and effective follow-up are crucial to the success of such a venture. Similar programs have been mounted in the black community, where 1:100 couples are at risk for having children with sickle-cell anemia. Early results were not only ineffective but indeed counterproductive, owing to inadequate pretesting educational programs, misunderstanding about the difference between sickle trait and sickle-cell disease, and penalties for diagnosis levied by employers and insurance companies. This debacle points out the importance of ethical and social issues in such screening programs.

TREATMENT

A pessimistic approach to the treatment of inherited metabolic disorders is no longer warranted. Effective therapy is available for many of these disorders, particularly those in which the biochemical abnormalities have been defined. As more is learned about the mutational events responsible for specific disorders and about the chemical consequences of the mutations, other inborn errors will surely be controlled or modified by specific therapeutic programs. Two potential levels of treatment exist: the first is directed to means by which the basic genotype of the affected subject can be altered; the second aims to manipulate the environment so as to lessen or eradicate the harmful effect of the mutant phenotype. Successful therapy of the inborn errors has, thus far, been achieved only at the latter level. Although there is great interest in the possibility of genotypic alteration in humans, clinical application remains only a distant hope.

Several prerequisites are necessary for successful therapy. The correct diagnosis must be established. Some inborn errors such as phenylketonuria have harmless phenocopies that produce transient but similar biochemical abnormalities in the newborn. Whereas a low-phenylalanine diet mitigates the central nervous system complications of true phenylketonuria, such a diet may have catastrophic effects on the growth and development of a newborn with transient hyperphenylalaninemia due to delayed maturation of phenylalanine hydroxylase. Next, the physician must be convinced that the disorder is harmful and requires therapy. As stated earlier, some well-defined inborn errors such as pentosuria or iminoglycinuria do not appear to cause any significant clinical pathology and require no treatment. Finally, any therapeutic program must be continually scrutinized for evidence of harmful effects as well as for documentation of beneficial effects of therapy. These may be difficult parameters to dissociate. Penicillamine is an effective drug in Wilson's disease because of its ability to chelate copper; it is also efficacious in solubilizing and preventing the formation of cystine stones in cystinuria. Unfortunately, penicillamine also causes several untoward effects that limit its usefulness and demand careful medical follow-up.

MODALITIES EMPLOYED Phenotypic modification has been approached in many ways, depending on the nature of the defect and the timing of its deleterious effects. Both medical and surgical modalities have been employed, the range and experience with the former far exceeding the latter. Five medical modalities have been used and will be described briefly.

Avoidance For several disorders, clinical consequences can be mitigated or forestalled entirely by avoiding exposure to particular environmental influences. For example, the hemolytic episodes in patients with G6PD deficiency can be modified significantly by avoiding exposure to such drugs as primaquine or sulfa and to such foods as fava beans. Similarly, the prolonged apnea that occurs after succinylcholine administration in individuals deficient in pseudocholinesterase activity will not occur if this anesthetic is not used. Avoiding barbiturates and many other drugs in acute intermittent porphyria and cigarettes and other noxious fumes in α_1-antitrypsin deficiency is another example of this approach.

Restriction There are numerous disorders in which the phenotypic abnormalities result from the accumulation of a specific substrate or its metabolic by-products. Such disorders may respond to restriction of intake of the injurious substrate or its precursors, providing that the substrate is essential in the dietary sense and thus cannot be manufactured by the organism. Phenylketonuria, branched-chain ketoaciduria, homocystinuria, galactosemia, essential fructosuria, and Refsum's disease are examples of inborn errors that have been effectively treated in this way. Similarly, patients with the glucose-galactose malabsorption syndrome who develop profound diarrhea when fed lactose-containing foods do well if their source of dietary carbohydrate is changed. In contrast, dietary restriction is of no value in hyperprolinemia, hydroxyprolinemia, or citrullinemia, because these amino acids are synthesized extensively de novo. Even in those conditions in which dietary restriction is of value, doubt exists about the needed duration of such restriction. The injurious effects of excess phenylalanine, galactose, or branched-chain amino acids or keto acids may be limited to the early years of life when brain development and organization are proceeding at a maximal rate. If this is so, it should be possible to modify or even discontinue dietary restrictions after a given age. There is still considerable uncertainty regarding this matter, however, and more experience is needed before meaningful recommendations can be made.

Replacement Many disorders caused by the failure to make a specific protein or small-molecular-weight product have responded dramatically to replacement therapy. Hemophilia and agammaglobulinemia are examples of inborn errors that respond to parenteral protein replacement. These disorders are amenable to such replacement because the proteins involved normally circulate in abundance. In most instances, however, the missing protein or enzyme is confined to some intracellular organelle and is present in very small amounts. Replacement therapy in these instances may be difficult or impossible for three reasons: first, because large amounts of the protein are difficult to purify or synthesize; second, because parenteral administration of the protein will not increase its entry into the cell where it is required; and third, because the protein may initiate unfavorable immunologic reactions. Despite these drawbacks, attempts along these lines are being made. Pure human glucocerebrosidase has been administered intravenously to a few patients with Gaucher's disease. Tissue glucocerebroside content fell modestly in these patients, suggesting that some enzyme was being taken up by cells and was active intracellularly. More striking success has been reported in combined immunodeficiency due to adenosine deaminase deficit. Administration of frozen, irradiated, normal erythrocytes led to prolonged and dramatic improvement in immune status.

The clinical stigmata of a disorder may be related not to the protein whose synthesis is defective, but rather to the product of the blocked pathway. Cortisol synthesis is blocked in several variants of congenital adrenal hyperplasia, and replacement therapy with this steroid produces dramatic improvement. Similarly, administration of thyroid hormone and uridine reverses the serious clinical disturbances in familial goitrous cretinism and oroticaciduria, respectively.

Supplementation A growing list of metabolic disorders respond clinically and/or chemically to supplementary amounts of specific vitamins. Infants with seizures controlled only by supraphysiologic amounts of pyridoxine provided the first evidence for this phenomenon. Now more than 20 different disorders are known to respond to supplements of a single vitamin. Most of these disorders are caused by primary enzymatic disturbances that result in impaired affinity for cofactor. A growing list, however, are caused by primary abnormalities in the pathway of coenzyme or metabolite synthesis from vitamin precursors. Several disorders responsive to cobalamin (vitamin B_{12}), folate, or vitamin D can now be included in this category. Long-term experience with such vitamin supplements is limited but promising.

Drug administration Clinical disturbances in several inherited metabolic disorders result from deposition of a specific substance in one or more tissues. Successful treatment of these conditions may be achieved by enhancing the excretion of the stored chemical or by preventing its formation. Copper deposition in Wilson's disease can be controlled by drugs such as D-penicillamine, which chelates copper and markedly enhances

its urinary excretion. The excretion of iron in hemochromatosis is augmented by phlebotomy and by the administration of desferrioxamine B. D-Penicillamine is also effective in solubilizing cystine calculi in cystinuria by reacting with cystine to form the more soluble cysteine-penicillamine disulfide. In this instance, the amount of cystine excreted is not changed, but its chemical form is altered in a therapeutically advantageous fashion. Uric acid deposition in gout responds both to drugs that enhance its excretion, such as sulfinpyrazone and probenecid, and to metabolic inhibitors like allopurinol that inhibit uric acid biosynthesis.

Surgical intervention At present, surgery is of limited value in the treatment of the inborn errors. Its use is restricted to a few conditions, such as gout, cystinuria, and oxalosis, in which nephrolithotomy or ureterolithotomy may provide important symptomatic relief while other programs of therapy are initiated. Several reports indicate that tissue transplants may be beneficial in some diseases. Thus, kidney transplants have been undertaken in cystinosis, hyperoxaluria, and Fabry's disease. Here the aim is restoration of renal function in conditions which produce progressive, and ultimately lethal, renal injury. Results have been variable. In hyperoxaluria, the transplanted kidney has been destroyed by oxalate deposition. In cystinosis, this has not occurred. A second, and quite different, goal of transplantation involves restitution of normal function. Thus, in combined immune deficiency, administration of fetal liver cells has produced clinical improvement. Similar beneficial results of bone marrow transplantation have been reported in other immune deficiency diseases. In the future, spleen transplantation may provide lasting benefit to patients with hemophilia or agammaglobulinemia by providing a constant source of antihemophilic globulin or gamma globulin, respectively. It is likewise possible that hepatic homografts may supply specific enzymes in phenylketonuria, branched-chain ketoaciduria, or the glycogen storage diseases and thus prevent the accumulation of toxic substances that lead to clinical abnormalities.

REFERENCES

HARRIS H: *The Principles of Human Biochemical Genetics,* 2d ed. Amsterdam, North-Holland, 1975

ROSENBERG LE: Inborn errors of metabolism, in *Metabolic Control and Disease,* 8th ed, PK Bondy, LE Rosenberg (eds). Philadelphia, Saunders, 1979

STANBURY JB et al: Inherited variation and metabolic abnormality, in *The Metabolic Basis of Inherited Disease,* 4th ed, JB Stanbury et al (eds). New York, McGraw-Hill, 1978

Disorders of amino acid metabolism

88

INHERITED DISORDERS OF AMINO ACID METABOLISM

LEON E. ROSENBERG

All polypeptides and proteins are polymers of 20 different amino acids. Eight of these, referred to as *essential,* cannot be synthesized by humans and must be obtained from dietary sources. The others are formed endogenously by a variety of chemical rearrangements. Although the vast bulk of the body's amino acids are "tied up" in proteins, small but critical pools of *free* amino acids are found intracellularly, and these pools are in equilibrium with extracellular reservoirs in plasma, cerebrospinal fluid, and the lumina of the gut and kidney. Physiologically, amino acids are more than mere "building blocks." Some (glycine, γ-aminobutyric acid) are neurotransmitters. Others (phenylalanine, tyrosine, tryptophan, glycine) are precursors of hormones, coenzymes, pigments, purines, or pyrimidines. Each has a unique and complicated degradative pathway by which its nitrogen and carbon components are used for the synthesis of other amino acids, carbohydrates, and lipids.

Current concepts of inherited metabolic diseases depend to a considerable degree on investigations of amino acid disorders. Three of the conditions analyzed by Garrod in his seminal descriptions of "inborn errors of metabolism" in the first decade of this century involved amino acids (alkaptonuria, albinism, and cystinuria). Although not appreciated at the time, these three conditions contain examples of the two general classes of "aminoacidopathies" now recognized: Enzymatic defects in amino acid catabolism and disorders of transmembrane transport. More than 70 inherited aminoacidopathies are now known, the catabolic defects (approximately 60) discussed in this and the following chapter far outnumbering the transport abnormalities (approximately 10) considered in Chap. 90. Each of these disorders is rare—their incidences range from 1 in 10,000 for phenylketonuria to 1 in 200,000 for alkaptonuria. Collectively, however, they occur in perhaps 1 in 500 to 1 in 1000 live births.

The salient features of inherited disorders of amino acid catabolism, arranged according to structural classes of the respective amino acids, are presented in Table 88-1. In general, these disorders are named for the compound which accumulates to highest concentration in blood (*-emias*) or urine (*-urias*). For many conditions the parent amino acid is found in excess; for others, products in the catabolic pathway accumulate. Which process takes place depends, of course, on the site of the enzymatic block, the reversibility of the reactions proximal to the lesion, and the existence of alternate pathways of metabolic "run-off." For some amino acids, such as the sulfur-containing or branched-chain molecules, defects at nearly each step in the catabolic pathway have been described. For others numerous gaps in our knowledge remain but are being filled rapidly as biochemical screening programs expand and interest in the field grows. Biochemical and genetic heterogeneity

abounds among the aminoacidopathies. At least four distinct forms of hyperphenylalaninemia, three variants of homocystinuria, and five types of methylmalonic acidemia are recognized—variants of both chemical and clinical interest.

The manifestations of these conditions differ widely as noted in Table 88-1. Some, such as sarcosinemia or hyperprolinemia, appear to produce no clinical consequences. At the other extreme, uniform neonatal lethality occurs in the untreated patient with complete deficiency of ornithine transcarbamylase or of branched-chain keto acid dehydrogenase. Central nervous system dysfunction, in the form of developmental retardation, seizures, alterations in sensorium, or behavioral disturbances, occurs in more than half of the disorders. Protein-induced vomiting, neurological dysfunction, and hyperammonemia occur in many disorders of urea cycle intermediates. Metabolic ketoacidosis often accompanied by hyperammonemia is a frequent presenting finding in the disorders of branched-chain amino acid metabolism. Occasional disorders produce focal tissue or organ involvement such as liver disease, renal failure, cutaneous abnormalities, or ocular lesions.

The clinical manifestations in many of these conditions can be prevented or mitigated significantly if diagnosis is achieved early and appropriate treatment (i.e., dietary protein or amino acid restriction or vitamin supplementation) is instituted promptly. For this reason, aminoacidopathies are screened for in mass newborn surveys which analyze blood or urine with an array of chemical and microbiological techniques. Once a presumptive diagnosis is made, confirmation can be provided by direct enzyme assay on extracts of leukocytes, erythrocytes, cultured fibroblasts, or liver. Several (cystinosis, branched-chain ketoaciduria, propionic acidemia, and methylmalonic acidemia) have been diagnosed in utero by chemical analysis on cultured amniotic fluid cells. The remainder of this and the subsequent chapter are focused on selected disorders that illustrate the problems posed by aminoacidopathies.

THE HYPERPHENYLALANINEMIAS

DEFINITION The hyperphenylalaninemias are a group of disorders (Table 88-1), each resulting from impaired conversion of phenylalanine to tyrosine. The most important is phenylketonuria, which in the untreated state is characterized by an increased concentration of phenylalanine in blood, increased concentrations of phenylalanine and its by-products (notably phenylpyruvate, phenylacetate, phenyllactate, and phenylacetylglutamine) in urine, and severe mental retardation.

ETIOLOGY AND PATHOGENESIS Each of the hyperphenylalaninemias results from reduced activity of the enzyme complex called *phenylalanine hydroxylase.* This system is found in appreciable amounts only in liver and kidney. Phenylalanine and molecular oxygen are substrates for the apoenzyme which requires a reduced pteridine, tetrahydrobiopterin, as a cofactor. Tyrosine and dihydrobiopterin are the products of this catalytic system, the latter being reconverted to tetrahydrobiopterin by a second enzyme, dihydropteridine reductase. In classic phenylketonuria activity of the hydroxylase apoenzyme is almost totally deficient. Benign hyperphenylalaninemia results from a less complete deficiency, whereas transient hyperphenylalaninemia (sometimes called transient phenylketonuria) is caused by a delayed maturation of the hydroxylase apoenzyme. In a variant of phenylketonuria, however, persistently impaired hydroxylating activity results not from abnormality in the apohydroxylase but from a lack of tetrahydrobiopterin due to virtually complete deficiency of the dihydropteridine reductase that regenerates it.

As a group the hyperphenylalaninemias occur in about 1 in 10,000 births. Classic phenylketonuria, which accounts for nearly half of these, is inherited as an autosomal recessive trait and is widely distributed among Caucasian ethnic groups and Orientals. It is rare in blacks. Phenylalanine hydroxylase activity in obligate heterozygotes is distinctly less than normal but higher than in homozygotes. Heterozygous carriers are clinically well but usually have slightly increased phenylalanine concentrations in postprandial blood plasma. Each of the other hyperphenylalaninemias also appears to be inherited as an autosomal recessive.

Phenylalanine accumulation in blood and urine and reduced tyrosine formation are direct consequences of the impaired hydroxylation. In untreated phenylketonuria and in dihydropteridine reductase deficiency, plasma concentrations of phenylalanine become sufficiently high (greater than 20 mg per 100 ml) to activate alternate pathways of metabolism and lead to formation of phenylpyruvate, phenylacetate, phenyllactate, and other derivatives that are rapidly cleared by the kidney and excreted in urine. Plasma concentrations of several other amino acids are moderately reduced, probably secondary to inhibition of gastrointestinal absorption or impairment of renal tubular reabsorption by the excess phenylalanine in body fluids. The severe brain damage observed in untreated phenylketonuria appears to be related to several consequences of phenylalanine accumulation: deprivation of other amino acids required for protein synthesis, impaired polyribosome formation or stabilization, reduced myelin synthesis, and inadequate formation of norepinephrine and serotonin. Phenylalanine is a competitive inhibitor of tyrosinase, a key enzyme in the pathway of melanin synthesis. This block plus reduced availability of the melanin precursor, tyrosine, accounts for the hypopigmentation of hair and skin.

CLINICAL MANIFESTATIONS No abnormalities are apparent at birth. Untreated children with classic phenylketonuria fail to attain early developmental milestones and demonstrate progressive impairment of cerebral function with IQ scores usually less than 50. Most require chronic institutionalization within a few years of birth because of the hyperactivity and seizures that accompany the severe mental retardation. Electroencephalogram abnormalities, "mousy" odor of skin, hair, and urine (due to phenylacetate accumulation), and a tendency to hypopigmentation and eczema complete the devastating clinical picture. In contrast, children who are detected at birth and treated promptly show none of these abnormalities. Children with transient hyperphenylalaninemia or with the benign variant are not at risk for any of the clinical consequences seen in untreated classic phenylketonuria. Those few children with dihydropteridine reductase deficiency, however, are the most unfortunate. Seizures appear early, followed by progressive cerebral and basal ganglia dysfunction (rigidity, chorea, spasms, hypotonia). Each has succumbed to secondary infection within a few years despite early diagnosis and standard treatment.

Occasionally, women with untreated classic phenylketonuria have reached adulthood and had children. More than 90 percent of the offspring are markedly retarded, and many have exhibited other congenital anomalies such as microcephaly, growth retardation, and congenital heart defects. Since these children are heterozygous, not homozygous for the phenylketonuria mutation, their clinical manifestations must be attributed to intrauterine damage produced by the elevated maternal concentrations of phenylalanine to which they have been exposed.

DIAGNOSIS Plasma phenylalanine concentrations may be normal at birth in all the hyperphenylalaninemias but rise rapidly after institution of protein feedings and are usually markedly abnormal by day 4. Since diagnosis and initiation of dietary treatment of classic phenylketonuria must be completed before 30 days of age if developmental retardation is to be prevented, most newborns in North America and Europe are screened by determinations of blood phenylalanine concentration using the Guthrie bacterial inhibition assay. Infants with abnormal values are followed up with more quantitative fluorometric or chromatographic assays. In classic phenylketonuria and in dihydropteridine reductase deficiency, values greater than 20 mg per 100 ml are regularly observed. In transient or benign hyperphenylalaninemia concentrations are usually lower but still above control values of less than 1 mg per 100 ml. Distinction of classic phenylketonuria from its benign variants depends on following serial plasma phenylalanine concentrations as a function of age and dietary restriction. In transient hyperphenylalaninemia plasma values return to normal within 3 to 4 months. In benign hyperphenylalaninemia dietary restriction produces a more profound fall in plasma phenylalanine than that observed in classic phenylketonuria. Deficiency of dihydropteridine reductase deficiency must be considered in any child with hyperphenylalaninemia who develops progressive neurological impairment despite prompt diagnosis and dietary treatment. Diagnostic confirmation of this variant can be achieved by enzyme assay on extracts of cultured fibroblasts.

TREATMENT Classic phenylketonuria was the first inherited metabolic disease in which it was demonstrated that mitigating the accumulation of the offending metabolite prevented the clinical abnormalities. This is accomplished by a special diet in which the bulk of protein is replaced by an artificial amino acid mixture low in phenylalanine. By supplementing this formula with a small amount of natural foods, an amount of dietary phenylalanine is provided that is sufficient for normal growth but is insufficient to produce markedly increased quantities of phenylalanine in blood. Ordinarily, plasma phenylalanine concentrations are maintained between 3 and 12 mg per 100 ml.

Until it is determined whether dietary treatment can be terminated safely after 6 to 8 years, dietary restriction in classic phenylketonuria should be continued indefinitely. The transient and benign forms of hyperphenylalaninemia do not require long-term dietary restriction. As mentioned earlier, children with dihydropteridine reductase deficiency deteriorate despite dietary phenylalanine restriction; attempts at pteridine cofactor replacement have been unrewarding.

THE HOMOCYSTINURIAS

The homocystinurias are three biochemically and clinically distinct disorders (Table 88-1), each characterized by increased concentration of the sulfur-containing amino acid, homocystine, in blood and urine. The most common form results from markedly reduced activity of cystathionine β-synthase, an enzyme catalyzing a key step in the transsulfuration pathway by which methionine is converted to cysteine. The two other forms are the result of impaired conversion of homocysteine to methionine, a reaction catalyzed by homocysteine: methyltetrahydrofolate methyltransferase and two essential cofactors methyltetrahydrofolate and methylcobalamin (methyl-vitamin B_{12}). Depending on the underlying disorder, some patients with each of the homocystinurias show chemical and, in some instances, clinical improvement following administration of specific vitamin supplements (pyridoxine, folate, or cobalamin).

CYSTATHIONINE β-SYNTHASE DEFICIENCY Definition Deficiency of this enzyme leads to increased concentrations of methionine and homocystine in body fluids and to decreased concentrations of cysteine and cystine. The clinical hallmark is dislocated optic lenses. Mental retardation, osteoporosis, and thrombotic vascular disease are frequent.

Etiology and pathogenesis The sulfur atom of the essential amino acid methionine is transferred ultimately to cysteine by a series of reactions designated as the transsulfuration pathway. In one of these steps, homocysteine condenses with serine to form cystathionine. This reaction is catalyzed by the pyridoxal phosphate-dependent enzyme, cystathionine β-synthase. Since 1964 more than 200 patients have been described with deficiency of this enzyme. The condition is common in Ireland (1 in 40,000 births) but rare elsewhere (less than 1 in 200,000 births).

Homocysteine and methionine accumulate in cells and body fluids; cysteine synthesis is impaired, resulting in reduced concentrations of this amino acid and its disulfide form, cystine. In approximately half of patients synthase activity in liver, brain, leukocytes, and cultured fibroblasts is absent. In the remaining patients, tissues retain 1 to 5 percent of normal activity. Heterozygous carriers of this autosomal recessive trait show no chemical abnormalities in body fluids but have reduced tissue synthase activity.

Homocysteine interferes with the normal cross-linking of collagen, an effect that likely plays an important role in the ocular, skeletal, and vascular complications.

Altered collagen in the suspensory ligament of the optic lens and in bone matrix may account for the dislocated lenses and osteoporosis. Similarly, interference with normal ground substance metabolism in vascular walls may predispose to the arterial and venous thrombotic diathesis. Recurrent cerebrovascular accidents secondary to thrombotic disease may account for the mental retardation, but direct chemical effects on cerebral cell metabolism have not been excluded.

Clinical manifestations More than 95 percent of patients have dislocated optic lenses. This abnormality usually appears by 3 to 4 years of age and often results in acute glaucoma as well as impaired visual acuity. Mental retardation occurs in less than 50 percent, often accompanied by ill-defined behavioral disturbances. Osteoporosis is a common radiological finding but rarely causes clinical disease. Life-threatening vascular complications, probably initiated by damage to vascular endothelium, are the major cause of morbidity and mortality. Occlusion of coronary, renal, and cerebral arteries with attendant tissue infarction can occur during the first decade of life. Many patients die of vascular disease before age 30. These vascular complications seem to be exacerbated by angiographic procedures.

TABLE 88-1
Inherited disorders of amino acid catabolism

Amino acid(s) affected	Disorder or condition	Enzyme defect
AROMATIC—HETEROCYCLIC		
Phenylalanine	Classic phenylketonuria	Phenylalanine hydroxylase
	Benign hyperphenyl-alaninemia	Phenylalanine hydroxylase
	Transient hyper-phenylalaninemia	Phenylalanine hydroxylase
	Variant phenylketonuria	Dihydropteridine reductase
Tyrosine	Hypertyrosinemia	Tyrosine aminotransferase (cytosol)
	Tyrosinosis	Tyrosine aminotransferase (?)
	Hereditary tyrosinemia	Hydroxyphenylpyruvate oxidase (?)
	Alkaptonuria	Homogentisic acid oxidase
	Albinism (oculocutaneous)	Tyrosinase
	Albinism (ocular)	Unknown
Tryptophan	Tryptophanuria	Tryptophan pyrrolase
	Xanthurenic aciduria	Kynureninase
Histidine	Histidinemia	Histidine-ammonia lyase
	Urocanic aciduria	Urocanase
	Formiminoglutamic aciduria	Formiminotransferase
GLYCINE-IMINO ACIDS		
Glycine	Hyperglycinemia	Glycine cleavage
	Sarcosinemia	Sarcosine dehydrogenase
	Hyperoxaluria (type I)	α-Ketoglutarate: glyoxylate carboligase
	Hyperoxaluria (type II)	D-Glyceric acid dehydrogenase
Imino acids	Hyperprolinemia (type I)	proline oxidase
	Hyperprolinemia (type II)	Δ'-Pyrroline dehydrogenase
	Hyperhydroxyprolinemia	Hydroxyproline reductase
	Iminopeptiduria	Prolidase
SULFUR-CONTAINING		
Methionine	Hypermethioninemia	Methionine adenosyltransferase
Homocystine	Homocystinuria	Cystathione β-synthase
	Homocystinuria	5,10-Methylenetetra-hydrofolate reductase
	Homocystinuria and methylmalonic acidemia (cbl C, D)‡	Cobalamin (vitamin B_{12}) reductase (cytosol) (?)
Cystathionine	Cystathioninuria	Cystathionase
Cystine	Cystinosis	Unknown
S-Sulfo-L-cysteine	S-Sulfo-L-cysteine, sulfite, and thiosulfaturia	Sulfite oxidase
CATIONIC		
Lysine	Hyperlysinemia (type I)	Lysine dehydrogenase
	Hyperlysinemia (type II)	Lysine: α-ketoglutarate reductase
	Saccharopinuria	Saccharopine dehydrogenase
	Hydroxylysinemia	Unknown
	Pipecolic acidemia	Unknown
	α-Ketoadipic aciduria	α-Ketoadipic acid decarboxylase

*Clinical manifestations**

Mental retardation	Neuropsychiatric dysfunction	Protein intolerance	Metabolic ketoacidosis	Ammonia intoxication	Other	Inheritance pattern†
+	+	−	−	−	Hypopigmented skin and hair, eczema	AR
−	−	−	−			AR
−	−	−	−	−		(AR)
+	+	−	−	−		(AR)
+	−	−	−	−	Palmar keratosis, corneal dystrophy	(AR)
−	−	−	−	−	Myasthenia gravis	?
−	−	−	−	−	Cirrhosis, hepatic failure, renal tubular dysfunction	AR
−	−	−	−	−	Ochronosis, arthritis	AR
−	−	−	−	−	Hypopigmentation of hair, skin, and optic fundus	AR
−	−	−	−	−	Hypopigmentation of optic fundus	XL
+	+	−	−	−	Photosensitive skin rash	AR
?	−	−	−	−		?
±	±	−	−	−	Hearing and speech deficit	AR
+	+	−	−	−		?
?	+	−	−	−		(AR)
+	+	−	−	−		AR
−	−	−	−	−		AR
−	−	−	−	−	Renal failure	AR
−	−	−	−	−	Calcium oxalate nephrolithiasis, renal failure	AR
−	−	−	−	−		AR
−	−	−	−	−		AR
−	−	−	−	−		AR
+	−	−	−	−	Crusting, erythematous, ecchymotic dermatitis	AR
−	−	−	−	−		?
±	±	−	−	−	Dislocated lenses, osteoporosis, thrombotic vascular disease	AR
±	±	−	−	−		(AR)
±	±	−	−	−	Megalobastic anemia	(AR)
±	−	−	−	−		AR
−	−	−	−	−	Fanconi syndrome, renal failure, photophobia	AR
+	+	−	−	−	Dislocated lenses	AR
−	+	+	−	+		?
±	±	−	−	−		AR
−	−	−	−	−		?
+	−	−	−	−		(AR)
+	+	−	−	−	Hepatomegaly, dysplastic optic disks	?
±	±	−	−	−		?

Diagnosis The cyanide-nitroprusside test is a simple way of demonstrating increased excretion of sulfhydryl-containing compounds in urine. Since cystine and *S*-sulfocysteine also give a positive test, other disorders of sulfur metabolism must be excluded, but this is usually simple on clinical grounds. Distinction of cystathionine β-synthase deficiency from other causes of homocystinuria can usually be accomplished by measurements of plasma methionine, which tend to be markedly increased in synthase-deficient patients and normal or low in those with impaired methionine formation (see below). Diagnostic confirmation depends on measurements of synthase activity in tissue extracts.

Treatment As with classic phenylketonuria, effective treatment depends on early diagnosis. A few infants diagnosed in the newborn period have been treated successfully with methionine-restricted, cystine-supplemented diets. Their clinical course has, thus far, been benign compared with that of untreated affected siblings. In approximately half of patients, oral supplements of pyridoxine (25 to 500 mg per day) produce a marked fall in plasma and urinary methionine and homocystine and an increase in cystine concentration in body fluids. This effect probably reflects a modest increase in synthase activity in cells of patients in whom the enzymatic defect is characterized by either reduced affinity for cofactor or accelerated degradation of mutant enzyme. Since such vitamin supplementation is simple and apparently harmless, it should be tried in all patients. There are no reports of the effect of pyridoxine supplementation therapy that has been initiated soon after birth.

5,10-METHYLENETETRAHYDROFOLATE REDUCTASE DEFICIENCY
Definition In this form of homocystinuria, methionine concentrations in body fluids are normal or decreased because deficiency of 5,10-methylenetetrahydrofolate reductase leads to impaired synthesis of 5-methyltetrahydrofolate, a cofactor in the enzymatic formation of methionine from homocysteine. Central nervous system dysfunction occurs in most patients.

Etiology and pathogenesis 5-Methyltetrahydrofolate:homocysteine methyltransferase catalyzes the conversion of homocysteine to methionine. The methyl group transferred in this reaction comes from 5-methyltetrahydrofolate, which is converted to tetrahydrofolate in the process. 5-Methyltetrahydrofolate, in turn, is synthesized enzymatically from 5,10-methylenetetrahydrofolate by another folate cycle enzyme, 5,10-methylenetetrahydrofolate reductase. Thus, reductase activity controls both methionine synthesis and tetrahydrofolate generation. This series of reactions is critical to normal DNA and RNA synthesis. A primary defect in the reductase activity results, secondarily, in deficient methyltransferase activity and impaired conversion of homocysteine to methionine. Although the mechanism of the central nervous system dysfunction is unknown, methionine deficiency and impaired nucleic acid synthesis are likely explanations. The disorder appears to be inherited as an autosomal recessive trait.

Clinical manifestations Fewer than 10 children with homocystinuria due to reductase deficiency have been reported. The most severely affected have presented with profound developmental retardation and cerebral atrophy early in life. Others manifested prominent behavioral disturbances (catatonia) during the second decade. In the remainder, mild retardation has

TABLE 88-1 *(continued)*
Inherited disorders of amino acid catabolism

Amino acid(s) affected	Disorder or condition	Enzyme defect
CATIONIC *(continued)*		
	Glutaric aciduria (type I)	Glutaryl CoA dehydrogenase
	Glutaric aciduria (type II)	Medium-chain acyl CoA dehydrogenase (?)
Ornithine	Hyperornithinemia (type I)	Ornithine decarboxylase
	Hyperornithinemia (type II)	Ornithine aminotransferase
UREA CYCLE		
Carbamyl-phosphate	Hyperammonemia (type I)	Carbamylphosphate synthetase I
Ornithine	Hyperammonemia (type II)	Ornithine transcarbamylase
Citrulline	Citrullinemia	Argininosuccinate synthetase
Arginino-succinic acid	Argininosuccinic aciduria	Argininosuccinase
Arginine	Argininemia	Arginase
BRANCHED-CHAIN		
Valine	Hypervalinemia	Valine aminotransferase
Leucine, isoleucine	Hyperleucine-isoleucinemia	Leucine-isoleucine aminotransferase
Valine, leucine, isoleucine	Classic branched-chain ketoaciduria	Branched-chain ketoacid dehydrogenase
	Intermittent branched-chain ketoaciduria	Branched-chain ketoacid dehydrogenase
Leucine	Isovaleric acidemia	Isovaleryl CoA dehydrogenase
	β-Methylcrotonyl glycinuria	β-Methylcrotonyl CoA carboxylase
	β-Hydroxy-β-methylglutaric aciduria	β-Hydroxy-β-methylglutaryl CoA lyase
Isoleucine, valine	α-Methylacetoacetic aciduria	β-Ketothiolase
	Propionic acidemia (pcc A, B, C)‡	Propionyl CoA carboxylase
	Propionic acidemia (bio)‡	Holocarboxylase synthetase (?)
	Methylmalonic acidemia (mut)‡	Methylmalonyl CoA mutase
	Methylmalonic acidemia (cbl A)‡	Cobalamin (vitamin B_{12}) reductase (mitochondrial) (?)
	Methylmalonic acidemia (cbl B)‡	Cobalamin (vitamin B_{12}): ATP adenosyltransferase
DICARBOXYLIC		
Glutamic acid	Glutathionemia	γ-Glutamyl-transpeptidase
	5-Oxoprolinuria	Glutathione synthetase

been observed. Presumably the severity of the clinical manifestations reflects the severity of the reductase deficiency.

Diagnosis and treatment The combination of increased concentrations of homocystine in body fluids with normal or decreased concentrations of methionine should suggest this entity. Serum folate concentrations are low in some patients. Confirmation requires direct reductase assays in tissue extracts (brain, liver, cultured fibroblasts). Although therapeutic experience is limited, one teen-age girl with a catatonic psychosis responded dramatically, both chemically and clinically, to fo-

Clinical manifestations*

Mental retardation	Neuropsychiatric dysfunction	Protein intolerance	Metabolic ketoacidosis	Ammonia intoxication	Other	Inheritance pattern†
−	+	−	−	−		AR
−	+	−	−	−	Hypoglycemia	?
+	+	+	−	+		(AR)
−	−	−	−	−	Gyrate atrophy of choroid and retina	AR
+	+	+	−	+		AR
±	+	+	−	+		XL
+	+	+	−	+		AR
+	+	+	−	+		AR
+	+	+	−	+		AR
+	+	+	−	−		?
+	+	+	−	−		?
+	+	+	+	−	"Maple syrup" odor	AR
±	−	+	+	−		AR
±	±	+	|	−	"Sweaty feet" odor	AR
+	+	−	+	−	"Cat's urine" odor	AR
−	+	+	+	−		?
±	±	+	+	+		AR
±	±	+	+	+		AR
+	±	+	+	−		?
±	±	+	+	+		AR
±	±	+	+	+		AR
±	±	+	+	+		AR
+	−	−	−	−		(?)
±	±	±	+	−		AR

late supplements (5 to 10 mg per day). When the folate was withdrawn, behavior worsened. This observation suggests that early diagnosis followed by folate supplementation may forestall neurological or psychiatric disturbances.

DEFICIENCY OF COBALAMIN (VITAMIN B₁₂) COENZYME SYNTHESIS Definition This form of homocystinuria also reflects impaired conversion of homocysteine to methionine. The primary defect is in the synthesis of methylcobalamin, a cobalamin (vitamin B₁₂) coenzyme required by methyltetrahydrofolate:homocysteine methyltransferase. Methylmalonic acid accumulates in body fluids as well because synthesis of a second coenzyme, adenosylcobalamin, required for isomerization of methylmalonyl coenzyme A (CoA) to succinyl CoA is also impaired.

Etiology and pathogenesis As with 5,10-methylenetetrahydrofolate reductase deficiency, this disorder involves remethylation of homocysteine. The primary defect concerns deficient synthesis of cobalamin coenzymes from precursor vitamin. Since methylcobalamin is required for methyl group transfer from methyltetrahydrofolate to homocysteine, impaired cobalamin metabolism leads to deficient methyltransferase activity. The precise defect responsible for impaired synthesis of meth-

468

ylcobalamin is unknown but involves some early step in lysosomal or cytosolic activation of the vitamin precursor. Somatic cell genetic studies indicate that two distinct lesions underlie deficient coenzyme formation, each of which appears to be inherited as an autosomal recessive trait.

Clinical manifestations The first reported patient died of infection at age 6 weeks following severely arrested development. Clinical manifestations in the other affected children vary: two had megaloblastic anemia and pancytopenia; three had significant spinocerebellar neurological impairment; one exhibited little clinical abnormality.

Diagnosis and treatment Homocystinuria, hypomethioninemia, and methylmalonic aciduria are the chemical hallmarks. These findings may also be present in juvenile or adult onset pernicious anemia in which intestinal cobalamin absorption is impaired. Measurement of serum cobalamin concentrations, low in pernicious anemia and normal in patients with defective conversion of cobalamin vitamin to coenzymes, helps in the differential diagnosis. Definitive diagnosis depends on demonstrating impaired coenzyme synthesis in cultured cells. Treatment of affected children with cobalamin supplements (1 to 2 mg per day) shows promise: Homocystine and methylmalonate excretion fall to near normal values; the hematologic and neurological deficits have also lessened to a more variable degree.

REFERENCES

KNOX WE: Phenylketonuria, in *The Metabolic Basis of Inherited Disease,* 3d ed, JB Stanbury et al (eds). New York, McGraw-Hill, 1972, pp 266–295

KOCH R et al: Phenylalaninemia and phenylketonuria, in *Heritable Disorders of Amino Acid Metabolism,* WL Nyhan (ed). New York, Wiley, 1974, pp 109–140

MCKUSICK VA: Homocystinuria, in *Heritable Disorders of Connective Tissue,* 4th ed. St. Louis, Mosby, 1972, pp 224–281

MUDD SH, LEVY HL: Disorders of transsulfuration, in *The Metabolic Basis of Inherited Disease,* 4th ed, JB Stanbury et al (eds). New York, McGraw-Hill, 1978, pp 458–503

NYHAN WL (ed): *Heritable Disorders of Amino Acid Metabolism.* New York, Wiley, 1974

ROSENBERG LE, SCRIVER CR: Disorders of amino acid metabolism, in *Metabolic Control and Disease,* 8th ed, PK Bondy, LE Rosenberg (eds). Philadelphia, Saunders (in press)

———, TANAKA K: Disorders of amino acid and organic acid metabolism, in *The Year in Metabolism 1977,* N Freinkel (ed). New York, Plenum, 1978, pp 219–246

89
STORAGE DISEASES OF AMINO ACID METABOLISM

LEON E. ROSENBERG

A number of inherited metabolic disorders are characterized by deposition or storage of particular metabolites in tissues. In most, storage reflects impaired degradation of the substance in question; in others, the mechanism is unknown. Many storage diseases involve large molecules such as glycogen, sphingolipids, mucolipids, cholesterol esters, and mucopolysaccharides (see Chaps. 97, 100, and 101); in others, metals such as iron and copper are deposited (see Chaps. 94 and 95). Finally, there is a group of storage diseases in which relatively small organic molecules are deposited. These include gout (see Chap. 92) and a group of disorders of amino acid metabolism.

ALKAPTONURIA

DEFINITION Alkaptonuria is a rare disorder of tyrosine catabolism. Deficiency of the enzyme homogentisic acid oxidase leads to excretion of large amounts of homogentisic acid in urine and to accumulation of oxidized homogentisic acid pigment in connective tissues (ochronosis). After many years ochronosis produces a distinctive form of degenerative arthritis.

ETIOLOGY AND PATHOGENESIS Homogentisic acid is a normal intermediate formed during the catabolism of tyrosine to fumarate and acetoacetate. Activity of homogentisic acid oxidase, the enzyme that catalyzes the opening of the phenolic ring yielding maleylacetoacetic acid, is virtually absent in liver and kidney of patients with alkaptonuria, and homogentisic acid accumulates in cells and body fluids. Patients have minimally increased concentrations of homogentisic acid in blood because it is rapidly cleared by the kidney. As much as 3 to 7 g homogentisic acid may be excreted in the urine per day, but this is of little pathophysiologic significance. However, homogentisic acid and its oxidized polymers bind to collagen, leading to the progressive deposition of a grey to bluish black pigment. The mechanism(s) by which degenerative changes develop in cartilage, intervertebral disk, and other connective tissues is unknown but may involve direct chemical irritation or inhibition of one or more enzyme systems involved in normal connective tissue metabolism.

Alkaptonuria was the first human disease shown to be inherited as an autosomal recessive trait. Affected homozygotes occur with a frequency no greater than 1 in 200,000. Heterozygous carriers are clinically well and excrete no homogentisic acid in urine, even after loading doses of tyrosine.

CLINICAL MANIFESTATIONS Alkaptonuria often goes unrecognized until middle life when degenerative joint disease appears in the majority. Prior to this time the tendency of the patient's urine to darken on standing may go unnoticed, as may slight discoloration of the sclerae and external ears. The latter manifestations of homogentisic acid deposition in tissue are generally the earliest external evidence of the disorder with appearance after age 20 to 30. Foci of grey-brown scleral pigment and generalized darkening of the concha, antihelix, and, finally, helix of the ear are typical. Ear cartilages may feel irregular and thickened. *Ochronotic arthritis* is heralded by pain, stiffness, and some limitation of motion of the hips, knees, and shoulders. Intermittent periods of acute arthritis, which may resemble rheumatoid arthritis, occur, but small joints are usually spared. Limitation of motion and ankylosis of the lumbosacral spine are common late manifestations. Pigmentation of heart valves, larynx, tympanic membranes, and skin occurs, and occasional patients develop pigmented renal or prostatic calculi. An increased incidence of degenerative cardiovascular disease has been reported in older patients, but a clear relationship between these findings and ochronosis has not been established.

DIAGNOSIS A patient whose urine darkens to blackness on standing must be suspected of having alkaptonuria, but because of modern plumbing conditions this finding is not often observed. The diagnosis is usually made from the triad of degenerative arthritis, ochronotic pigmentation, and urine which turns black upon alkalinization. Homogentisic acid in urine may be identified presumptively by other tests: upon addition of ferric chloride, a purple-black color is observed; treatment with Benedict's reagent yields a brown color; and addition of a saturated silver nitrate solution produces an immediate black color. These screening tests can be confirmed by chromatographic, enzymatic, or spectrophotometric determinations of homogentisic acid. X-rays of the lumbar spine are virtually pathognomonic. They show degeneration and dense calcification of the intervertebral disks and narrowing of the intervertebral spaces.

TREATMENT   There is no specific treatment for ochronotic arthritis. It is conceivable that joint manifestations could be mitigated if homogentisic acid accumulation and deposition could be curbed by dietary restriction of phenylalanine and tyrosine, but the long course of the disease has discouraged such therapeutic attempts. Since ascorbic acid impedes oxidation and polymerization of homogentisic acid in vitro, its use has been suggested as a possible means of decreasing pigment formation and deposition. The efficacy of this form of treatment has not been established. Symptomatic treatment is similar to that for osteoarthritis (Chap. 361).

CYSTINOSIS

DEFINITION   Cystinosis is a rare disorder characterized by the intralysosomal accumulation of free cystine in body tissues. This results in the appearance of cystine crystals in the cornea, conjunctiva, bone marrow, lymph nodes, leukocytes, and internal organs. Three clinical forms have been identified: an infantile (nephropathic) form leading to the Fanconi syndrome and renal insufficiency in the first decade; a juvenile (intermediate) form in which renal disease becomes manifest during the second decade; and an adult (benign) form characterized by deposition of cystine in the cornea but not in the kidney.

ETIOLOGY AND PATHOGENESIS   The basic defect has not been identified. Numerous studies of enzymes concerned with cystine metabolism have not yielded any consistent abnormality, nor have investigations of cystine or cysteine transport. The cystine content of tissues in the infantile form may be more than 100 times normal, that in the adult form more than 30 times normal. Intracellular cystine appears to be located only in lysosomes and does not exchange with other intracellular or extracellular pools of this amino acid. Neither plasma nor urinary concentrations of cystine are particularly elevated.

The extent of cystine crystal deposition varies considerably from patient to patient, depending on both the form of the disease and the methods used to prepare pathological specimens. In the kidney cystine accumulation causes renal insufficiency in the infantile and juvenile forms. The kidneys are pale and shrunken, the capsule is adherent, and the corticomedullary junction is obscured. Microscopically, nephron organization is interrupted, glomeruli are hyalinized, connective tissue is increased, and the normal epithelium of the tubules is replaced by cuboidal cells. Narrowing and shortening of the proximal tubule produces the so-called "swan neck deformity" now known not to be specific for cystinosis. Patchy depigmentation of the peripheral retina occurs in the infantile and juvenile forms. This retinal degeneration is to be distinguished from the deposition of cystine crystals in the ocular conjunctiva or uvea.

Each form of cystinosis appears to be inherited as an autosomal recessive trait. Obligate heterozygotes have intracellular cystine contents intermediate between those of normal persons and affected patients but are free of clinical abnormalities.

CLINICAL MANIFESTATIONS   In the infantile form abnormalities are usually apparent by 4 to 6 months of age. Growth retardation, vomiting, fever, vitamin D–resistant rickets, polyuria, dehydration, and metabolic acidosis are prominent. Generalized proximal tubular dysfunction (the Fanconi syndrome)

leads to hyperphosphaturia and hypophosphatemia, renal glycosuria, generalized aminoaciduria, hypouricemia, and often hypokalemia. Pyelonephritis is common and may contribute, along with interstitial fibrosis, to progressive glomerular insufficiency. Death due to uremia or intercurrent infection usually occurs before age 10. Ocular manifestations are also prominent. Photophobia is usually demonstrable within the first few years of life due to cystine deposits in the cornea, and retinal degeneration may appear even earlier.

In contrast, patients with the adult form manifest only ocular abnormalities. Photophobia, headache, and burning or itching of the eyes are major complaints. Glomerular and tubular function and the integrity of the retina are preserved. The findings in the juvenile variant fall between these extremes. These patients have both ocular and renal manifestations, but the latter do not become significant until the second decade. The renal lesion, albeit milder than that seen in the infantile form, eventually leads to renal insufficiency.

DIAGNOSIS   Cystinosis must be considered in any child with vitamin D–resistant rickets, the Fanconi syndrome, or glomerular insufficiency. Hexagonal or rectangular cystine crystals are most easily detected in the cornea (by slit-lamp examination), in unstained preparations of leukocytes from peripheral blood or bone marrow, or in biopsies of rectal mucosa. Diagnosis can be confirmed by quantitative determination of cystine in extracts of peripheral blood leukocytes or cultured fibroblasts. The infantile form of cystinosis has been diagnosed prenatally by the demonstration of vastly increased cystine content in cultured amniotic fluid cells.

TREATMENT   The adult form of cystinosis is benign and requires no treatment. Symptomatic treatment of renal disease in patients with the infantile or juvenile form of cystinosis does not differ from that of other forms of chronic renal insufficiency: maintenance of adequate fluid intake to prevent dehydration; administration of sodium citrate or sodium bicarbonate to correct the metabolic acidosis; and ingestion of supplementary calcium, phosphate, and vitamin D to heal the rickets. Such measures are critical in maintaining growth, development, and well-being in affected children for a time. Two types of more specific therapy have been attempted without much success. Cystine-restricted diets are difficult to prepare and have not prevented progression of renal disease. Likewise, the use of sulfhydryl reagents (D-penicillamine, dimercaprol) and reducing agents (vitamin C) have yielded no long-term benefit.

The most promising form of therapy for nephropathic cystinosis is renal transplantation. More than 20 affected children with end-stage renal disease have been so treated. Those patients who tolerated the procedure and did not develop immunologic problems have shown return of kidney function toward normal. Several patients have been followed for 3 or more years after transplantation. The transplanted kidneys have not developed the functional abnormalities typical of cystinosis (i.e., the Fanconi syndrome or glomerular insufficiency). They may, however, reaccumulate some cystine, apparently owing to migration of interstitial or mesangial cells from the host. This experience justifies offering renal transplantation to patients with terminal renal failure.

PRIMARY HYPEROXALURIA

DEFINITION   Primary hyperoxaluria is the designation for two rare disorders characterized by chronic excessive urinary excretion of oxalic acid and by calcium oxalate nephrolithiasis and nephrocalcinosis. Typically, patients with either form develop renal insufficiency early in life and die of uremia. At postmortem examination, calcium oxalate deposits are generally widespread in renal and extrarenal tissues, a condition referred to as *oxalosis*.

ETIOLOGY AND PATHOGENESIS Since both types of primary hyperoxaluria result from increased oxalate synthesis and since glyoxylate is the only significant precursor of oxalate in humans, the metabolic basis for the primary hyperoxalurias logically involves pathways of glyoxylate metabolism. In type I hyperoxaluria, urinary excretion of oxalate, the oxidized form of glyoxylate, and glycolic acid, the reduced form, is increased. The excessive synthesis of these substances in this condition results from a block in one of the routes of metabolism of glyoxylate. Activity of the cytosolic enzyme α-ketoglutarate:glyoxylate carboligase, which catalyzes the formation of α-hydroxy-β-ketoadipic acid, is markedly reduced in extracts of liver, kidney, and spleen. The resulting expansion of the glyoxylate pool behind this metabolic block leads to oxidation of glyoxylate to oxalate and to reduction of glyoxylate to glycolate. Each of these 2-carbon acids is then excreted in excess in the urine. In type II hyperoxaluria, L-glyceric acid is excreted in excess along with oxalate. In this condition, activity of D-glyceric acid dehydrogenase, an enzyme that catalyzes the reduction of hydroxypyruvate to D-glyceric acid in the catabolic pathway of serine metabolism, is absent in leukocytes (and presumably other tissues). The accumulated hydroxypyruvate is instead reduced by lactic dehydrogenase to the L-isomer of glycerate, which is excreted in the urine. Apparently the reduction of hydroxypyruvate is coupled in some way to the oxidation of glyoxylate to oxalate, thus causing the formation of increased oxalate.

Both disorders appear to be inherited as autosomal recessive traits. Heterozygotes are asymptomatic. Partial enzyme deficiency has been observed in heterozygotes for type II hyperoxaluria, but no studies with type I heterozygotes have been reported.

The pathogenesis of stone formation, nephrocalcinosis, and oxalosis relates directly to the insolubility of calcium oxalate. Extrarenal deposits of oxalate have been most widely reported in the heart, walls of arteries and veins, male urogenital tract, and bone.

CLINICAL MANIFESTATIONS Nephrolithiasis and oxalosis may become manifest during the first year of life. Most patients experience initial symptoms of renal colic or hematuria between ages 2 and 10 and succumb to uremia before age 20. With the onset of uremia, patients may develop severe peripheral arterial spasm and necrosis with resulting vascular insufficiency. In patients with delayed onset of symptoms, survival to age 50 or 60 has been reported, despite recurrent attacks of nephrolithiasis.

DIAGNOSIS Oxalate excretion in normal children or adults is less than 60 mg per 1.73 m² per day. Patients with type I or type II hyperoxaluria generally excrete two to four times this amount. Distinction between the two types of primary hyperoxaluria depends on measurements of the other organic acids that identify them: glycolic acid in type I and L-glyceric acid in type II. Since patients with pyridoxine deficiency or chronic ileal disease may excrete excessive amounts of oxalate, these conditions must be excluded.

TREATMENT There is no satisfactory treatment for primary hyperoxaluria. Urinary oxalate concentration can be reduced

by increasing the urinary flow rate, but success is transient. Large doses of pyridoxine (100 mg per day) may reduce urinary oxalate in some patients, but long-term effects are not dramatic. A diet high in phosphate content seems to reduce the frequency of attacks of renal colic, but oxalate excretion is unaffected. Finally, renal transplantation has been attempted several times, but in each instance renal function was lost because of calcium oxalate deposition in the transplanted kidney.

REFERENCES

Boquist L et al: Primary oxalosis. Am J Med 54:673, 1973

LaDu NB: Alcaptonuria, in *The Metabolic Basis of Inherited Disease*, 4th ed, JB Stanbury et al (eds). New York, McGraw-Hill, 1978, pp 268–282

O'Brien W et al: Biochemical, pathologic and clinical aspects of alcaptonuria, ochronosis and ochronotic arthropathy. Am J Med 34:813, 1963

Schneider JA et al: Cystinosis and the Fanconi syndrome, in *The Metabolic Basis of Inherited Disease*, 4th ed, JB Stanbury et al (eds). New York, McGraw-Hill, 1978, pp 1660–1682

Schulman JD (ed): *Cystinosis*, US Department of Health, Education, and Welfare Publication (NIH) 72–249, 1972

Williams HE, Smith LH Jr: Primary hyperoxaluria, in *The Metabolic Basis of Inherited Disease*, 4th ed, JB Stanbury et al (eds). New York, McGraw-Hill, 1978, pp 182–204

90
INHERITED DEFECTS OF MEMBRANE TRANSPORT

LEON E. ROSENBERG
ELIZABETH M. SHORT

The passage of certain large and small molecules across mammalian plasma cell membranes depends on the existence of specific transport systems that owe their specificity to a variety of membrane receptor and "carrier" proteins. These specific membrane constituents recognize individual substrates or a group of structurally related ones and catalyze their transmembrane movement by mechanisms poorly understood. The disorders considered in this chapter have three features in common: each is characterized by a specific defect in the transport of one or more compounds; each is inherited as a dominant or recessive, implying that a single genetic locus is involved; and each is presumed to reflect a primary alteration in a specific membrane protein. Many of these defects have been well characterized physiologically, but in none has the putative mutant transport protein been isolated.

More than 20 inherited disorders of membrane transport have been described in humans (Table 90-1). Most affect the gut and/or kidney only. Numerous classes of substrates are represented, including amino acids, hexoses, cations, anions, vitamins, and water. Some are discussed elsewhere in this text. Those impairing the transport of amino acids, hexoses, urate, and chloride are discussed here as examples of the range and significance of the abnormalities encountered.

DISORDERS OF AMINO ACID TRANSPORT

As noted in Table 90-1, 10 distinct disorders of amino acid transport have been described. Five of these (cystinuria, dibasicaminoaciduria, Hartnup disease, iminoglycinuria, and dicarboxylicaminoaciduria) show transport abnormalities for groups of structurally related amino acids, thereby implying the existence of group-specific membrane receptors or carriers. With the exception of iminoglycinuria and dicarboxylicaminoaciduria, these defects have important clinical consequences. The remaining five disorders affect the transport of only one amino acid, implying the existence of substrate-specific as well as group-specific transport systems. Each of these conditions affects transport in the kidney, gut, or both; none has been shown to alter transport in other tissues.

CYSTINURIA **Definition** Cystinuria is the most common inborn error of amino acid transport. It is characterized by excessive urinary excretion of the dibasic amino acids: lysine, arginine, ornithine, and cystine. This aminoaciduria results from impaired tubular reabsorption of these amino acids. A similar transport defect exists in the intestinal mucosa. Because cystine is the least soluble of the naturally occurring amino acids, its overexcretion predisposes to the formation of renal, ureteral, and bladder calculi. Such calculi are responsible for the signs and symptoms in affected patients.

Etiology and pathogenesis Massive excretion of cystine and the other dibasic amino acids occurs only in classic cystinuria. The disorder, inherited as an autosomal recessive trait, is believed to result from alterations in a membrane carrier protein essential for transport of this group of amino acids in the apical brush border of proximal renal tubule and small intestinal cells. Renal clearance studies indicate that the putative protein has a greater affinity for ornithine and arginine than for lysine and cystine. Although the endogenous renal clearance of all four amino acids is increased in homozygotes, the presence of some residual transport capacity for these compounds plus the existence of three other disorders marked by selective excretion of members of this group (dibasicaminoaciduria, hypercystinuria, lysinuria) argues for the existence of at least three discrete renal transport systems for these amino acids: one for each amino acid alone; one shared by lysine, arginine, and ornithine; and one for all four amino acids.

Whereas urinary excretion patterns and renal clearance abnormalities in all homozygotes are similar, evidence for three allelic variants has come from studies of intestinal transport in homozygotes and of urinary excretion in obligate heterozygotes. These variants have been designated types I, II, and III. Type I homozygotes lack mediated intestinal transport of cystine, lysine, arginine, and ornithine; their heterozygous relatives have normal urinary amino acid excretion patterns. Type II homozygotes lack mediated lysine transport in the gut but retain some capacity for cystine transport; heterozygotes have moderately increased urinary excretion of each of the four amino acids. Type III homozygotes retain some capacity for mediated intestinal transport of the four involved substrates; heterozygotes have modestly increased urinary lysine and cystine.

Clinical manifestations Cystinuria is among the most common inborn errors, homozygotes occurring with a frequency of 1 in 10,000 to 1 in 15,000 in many ethnic groups. Cystine stones account for 1 to 2 percent of all urinary tract calculi. The maximum solubility of cystine in the physiological urinary pH range of 4.5 to 7.0 is about 300 mg per liter. Since affected homozygotes regularly excrete 600 to 1800 mg per day, crystalluria and calculus formation are a constant threat. Cystine stone formation usually becomes manifest in the second or third decade but has been reported as early as the first year of life. Symptoms and signs are those typical of urolithiasis regardless of etiology: hematuria, flank pain, renal colic, obstructive uropathy, and infection. Recurrent episodes of urolithiasis may lead to progressive renal insufficiency.

Diagnosis The presence of cystine in a urinary tract stone is pathognomonic of cystinuria. However, since 50 percent of the stones excreted by cystinuric subjects are of mixed composition and since as many as 10 percent may contain *no* detectable cystine, a urinary nitroprusside test should be done on all patients with urolithiasis to exclude this diagnosis. The nitroprusside test is also positive (appearance of a cherry red color) in some heterozygotes for cystinuria, in patients with hypercystinuria, homocystinuria, and cysteine β-mercaptolactate disulfiduria, and in the presence of acetone in the urine. When cystine content exceeds 250 mg per liter, cystine crystals may be seen in the sediment of acidified, concentrated, chilled urine. These crystals, in the form of hexagonal plates, are pathognomonic of cystine overexcretion in patients not taking sulfonamides.

Diagnostic confirmation of cystinuria depends upon the demonstration of the characteristic amino acid excretion pattern in the urine. Selective excretion of cystine, lysine, arginine, and ornithine can be demonstrated by paper chromatography or electrophoresis, and quantitative determinations can be made by column chromatography. Quantitation becomes important in differentiating some heterozygotes from homozygotes and in documenting the reduction of free cystine excretion during therapy.

Treatment Medical management of cystinuria is aimed at reducing the concentration of cystine in urine. The single most important aspect of this treatment is maintenance of a large urine volume. Fluid ingestion in excess of 4 liters per day is essential, and 5 to 7 liters per day is optimal. Stones can be prevented and even dissolved by such vigorous hydration. It must be made clear to the cystinuric subject that water is a drug. Solubility of cystine rises sharply in urine above pH 7.5, and various regimens of urinary alkalinization have been used therapeutically. Vigorous administration of sodium bicarbonate, Diamox, and polycitrates is required to maintain a persistently alkaline pH, but this measure introduces the danger of inducing formation of other "alkaline" stones (calcium oxalate, calcium phosphate, magnesium ammonium phosphate) and even of producing nephrocalcinosis.

Another medical approach to treatment involves administration of D-penicillamine (β,β-dimethylcysteine) which undergoes sulfhydryl-disulfide exchange with cystine to form the mixed disulfide of penicillamine and cysteine. Since this disulfide is more than 50 times as soluble as cystine, D-penicillamine (in doses of 1 to 3 g per day) has the capacity to reduce free cystine excretion markedly, thereby preventing new stone formation and promoting dissolution of existing calculi. Unfortunately D-penicillamine is immunogenic, and allergic manifestations include acute serum sickness, agranulocytosis, pancytopenia, immune glomerulitis, and the Goodpasture syndrome. Thus, its use should be reserved for patients who fail to respond to hydration alone or who are in a particularly high-risk category (one remaining kidney, renal insufficiency). When medical management fails, urologic surgery is required. An occasional patient may require renal transplantation because of renal failure.

DIBASICAMINOACIDURIA A number of families have been described in which affected members have a defect in renal tubular reabsorption of lysine, arginine, and ornithine but *not* of cystine. The disorder almost surely reflects mutations in the genes coding for a renal transport protein used by the three dibasic amino acids only. Two clinically distinct variants have been observed, each apparently inherited as an autosomal re-

TABLE 90-1
Genetic disorders of membrane transport

Class of substance and disorder	Individual substrates	Tissues manifesting transport defect	Proposed molecular basis of defect	Major clinical manifestations	Mode of inheritance	Location of discussion
AMINO ACIDS						
Classic cystinuria	Cystine, lysine, arginine, ornithine	Proximal renal tubule, jejunal mucosa	Mutation of shared dibasic-cystine transport protein	Cystine nephrolithiasis	Autosomal recessive	Chap. 90
Dibasicamino-aciduria	Lysine, arginine, ornithine	Proximal renal tubule, jejunal mucosa	Mutation of dibasic transport protein	Type I: Moderate retardation Type II: Protein intolerance, hyperammonemia, retardation	Autosomal recessive	Chap. 90
Hypercystinuria	Cystine	Proximal renal tubule	Mutation of cystine transport protein	Some risk of cystine nephrolithiasis	Autosomal recessive	Chap. 90
Lysinuria	Lysine	Proximal renal tubule, jejunal mucosa	Mutation of lysine transport protein	Seizures, physical and mental retardation	Possible autosomal recessive	Chap. 90
Hartnup disease	Neutral amino acids	Proximal renal tubule, jejunal mucosa	Mutation of neutral amino acid-shared transport protein	Constant neutral aminoaciduria, intermittent symptoms of pellagra	Autosomal recessive	Chap. 90
Tryptophan mal-absorption	Tryptophan	Jejunal mucosa	Mutation of tryptophan transport protein	Indoluria, ?hypercalcemia, ?nephrocalcinosis	Probable autosomal recessive	Chap. 90
Methionine mal-absorption	Methionine	Jejunal mucosa	Mutation of methionine transport protein	α-Hydroxybutyricaciduria, white hair, mental retardation, convulsions, hyperneic attacks, edema	Probable autosomal recessive	Chap. 90
Histidinuria	Histidine	Proximal renal tubule, jejunal mucosa	Mutation of histidine transport protein	Mental retardation	Autosomal recessive	Chap. 90
Iminoglycinuria	Glycine, proline, hydroxyproline	Proximal renal tubule, jejunal mucosa	Mutation of shared glycine-imino acid transport protein	None	Autosomal recessive	Chap. 90
Dicarboxylica-minoaciduria	Glutamic acid, aspartic acid	Proximal renal tubule, jejunal mucosa	Mutation of shared dicarboxylic amino acid transport protein	None	Probable autosomal recessive	Chap. 90
HEXOSES						
Renal glycosuria	D-Glucose	Proximal renal tubule	Mutation of D-glucose transport protein	Glycosuria with normal blood glucose	Autosomal recessive	Chap. 90
Glucose-galactose malabsorption	D-Gluose D-Galactose	Jejunal mucosa, proximal renal tubule	Mutation of shared glucose-galactose transport protein	Watery diarrhea on feeding glucose, lactose, sucrose, or galactose	Autosomal recessive	Chaps. 90, 292
LIPIDS						
Familial hyper-cholesterolemia	Cholesterol	Fibroblasts, lymphoid lines, leukocytes	Mutation of membrane LDL-cholesterol receptor protein	Hypercholesterolemia, tendon xanthomas, arcus corneae, coronary artery atherosclerosis	Autosomal dominant	Chap. 100
URATE						
Hypouricemia	Uric acid	Proximal renal tubule	Mutation of urate transport protein	Hypouricemia, hyperuricosuria, ?hypercalcinuria	Autosomal recessive	Chap. 90
ANIONS						
Familial hypophosphatemic rickets	Inorganic phosphate	Proximal renal tubule, jejunal mucosa	Mutation of inorganic phosphate transport protein	Hypophosphatemia, phosphaturia, phosphatopenic rickets/osteomalacia	X-linked dominant	Chap. 352

TABLE 90-1 (continued)
Genetic disorders of membrane transport

Class of substance and disorder	Individual substrates	Tissues manifesting transport defect	Proposed molecular basis of defect	Major clinical manifestations	Mode of inheritance	Location of discussion
ANIONS (continued)						
Congenital chloridorrhea	Chloride	Ileal and colonic mucosa	Mutation of Cl^-/HCO_3 exchange pump carrier protein	Hydramnios, watery diarrhea, elevated fecal chloride, achloriduria, metabolic alkalosis with volume depletion, hyperaldosteronism	Autosomal recessive	Chaps 90, 292
Familial goiter	Inorganic iodide	Thyroid gland, salivary gland, gastric mucosa	Mutation of iodide transport protein	Congenital hypothyroidism (cretinism), goiter	Probable autosomal recessive	Chap. 335
CATIONS						
Distal renal tubular acidosis (type I— gradient)	Hydrogen ion	Distal renal tubule	Mutation of distal tubule H^+ pump carrier protein	Hyperchloremic acidosis, hypokalemia, acquired nephrocalcinosis, and hypercalcinuria	Autosomal dominant	Chap. 283
Proximal renal tubular acidosis (type II— HCO_3 wasting)	Hydrogen ion	Proximal renal tubule	Mutation of proximal tubule H^+ pump carrier protein	Hyperchloremic acidosis, bicarbonate wasting	Probable autosomal recessive	Chap. 283
Menkes' disease	Copper	Duodenal and jejunal intestinal cells	Possible serosal transport protein or intracellular transport defect	Severe mental retardation, pili torti (kinky hair), typical facies, arterial tortuosity, excess Wormian bones, thermal instability	X-linked recessive	Chap. 83
Hereditary: Spherocytosis Elliptocytosis Ovalocytosis Stomatocytosis	Sodium	Red blood cell (RBC) membranes	Mutation of membrane structure (? lipid or protein) resulting in increased sodium permeability	Increased RBC fragility resulting in variable degrees of hemolytic anemia, splenomegaly, and jaundice; RBC shape respectively spherocytic, elliptocytic, ovalocytic, or stomatocytic (target-shaped)	Each of these diseases of RBC morphology is a separately inherited autosomal dominant	Chap. 314
WATER						
Nephrogenic diabetes insipidus (ADH resistant)	Water	Distal renal tubule	Lack of activation of ADH-responsive luminal membrane adenylate cyclase, possible defect in receptor or enzyme protein	Polyuria, polydipsia, hyposthenuria	X-linked recessive	Chap. 283

cessive trait. Clinical manifestations appear to be related to the significant losses of ornithine, arginine, and perhaps lysine.

In the common form of dibasicaminoaciduria (type II), homozygotes show defective intestinal transport of dibasic amino acids as well as exaggerated renal losses. A defect in hepatic cell uptake of these substances has also been proposed. Affected patients present in childhood with hepatosplenomegaly, protein intolerance, and episodic ammonia intoxication. Plasma concentrations of lysine, arginine, and ornithine are reduced. The clinical findings have been attributed to hyperammonemia resulting from insufficient amounts of arginine

and ornithine to maintain proper function of the Krebs-Henseleit urea cycle. Treatment includes dietary protein restriction and supplementation with arginine and ornithine. Obligate heterozygotes are clinically well and show no excess urinary loss of dibasic amino acids.

Type I dibasicaminoaciduria has been described in only one homozygote. She was moderately mentally retarded but had no clear history of protein intolerance or hyperammonemia. Her urinary losses of dibasic amino acids were not as great as those seen in type II homozygotes. The condition was distinguished from type I by the presence of modest excesses of dibasic amino acids in urine of both asymptomatic parents. Other pedigrees containing asymptomatic heterozygotes have been identified by urinary screening programs.

HARTNUP DISEASE Pellagra-like skin lesions, variable neurological manifestations, and a constant renal aminoaciduria for the monoaminomonocarboxylic amino acids with neutral or aromatic side chains characterize Hartnup disease. Alanine, serine, threonine, valine, leucine, isoleucine, phenylalanine, tyrosine, tryptophan, glutamine, asparagine, and histidine are excreted in urine in quantities from five to ten times normal, and an intestinal transport defect for these same amino acids has been demonstrated. The clinical spectrum appears to relate solely to nutritional deficiency of the essential amino acid tryptophan, caused by the combination of intestinal malabsorption and renal loss. Disease manifestations are episodic, related, at least in part, to metabolic demands for tryptophan.

The major catabolic pathway of tryptophan metabolism leads to the synthesis of niacin and nicotinamide-adenine dinucleotide (NAD). This pathway supplies about 50 percent of daily niacin needs. In patients with Hartnup disease, the renal and intestinal transport defect for neutral and aromatic amino acids, including tryptophan, leads to niacin deficiency. The transport defect likely reflects abnormalities of a group-specific system for neutral amino acids. Renal clearance studies show some residual reabsorptive capacity for each involved amino acid. This suggests that they are transported by other carrier systems as well, a conclusion supported by the subsequent description of patients with substrate-specific transport errors for tryptophan, methionine, and histidine.

Hartnup disease is inherited as an autosomal recessive trait. Homozygotes occur with a frequency of about 1 in 16,000 births. Heterozygotes exhibit no clinical or chemical abnormalities.

Pellagra is the clinical syndrome produced by dietary niacin deficiency, and its clinical features of diarrhea, dementia, and dermatitis are those which characterize Hartnup disease (see Chap. 79). The diagnosis should be suspected in any patient with pellagra without a history of severe dietary niacin deficiency. The neurological and psychiatric manifestations range from attacks of cerebellar ataxia to mild emotional lability to frank delirium and usually accompany exacerbations of the erythematous, eczematoid skin rash. Fever, sunlight, stress, and sulfonamide therapy provoke clinical relapses. Diagnosis is made by detection of the pathological neutral aminoaciduria which does not occur in dietary niacin deficiency. Treatment is directed at niacin repletion and includes a high-protein diet and daily nicotinamide supplementation (50 to 250 mg).

IMINOGLYCINURIA This trait is characterized by excessive urinary excretion of glycine and the imino acids proline and hydroxyproline. Homozygotes for this autosomal recessive disorder occur with a frequency of about 1 in 16,000. The exaggerated renal clearance of glycine, proline, and hydroxyproline reflects a defect in the tubular transport system shared by these three compounds. An intestinal transport defect has been demonstrated in some. This suggests that more than one mutation may lead to persistent iminoglycinuria, a thesis corroborated by studies of urinary amino acid excretion in obligate heterozygotes from different families. No consistent clinical abnormalities have been reported in homozygotes, who are usually detected by urinary amino acid screening programs. Individuals with iminoglycinuria should be reassured as to the benign nature of the disturbance.

DICARBOXYLICAMINOACIDURIA Selective urinary loss and exaggerated endogenous renal clearance of glutamic and as-partic acids have been described in two unrelated children. Intestinal absorption of these dicarboxylic amino acids was impaired in one but not in the other. The former suffered from recurrent hypoglycemia; the latter was asymptomatic. It remains to be determined whether this defect is of clinical significance.

SUBSTRATE-SPECIFIC DEFECTS IN AMINO ACID TRANSPORT Rare pedigrees exist in which individuals have defective renal tubular reabsorption and/or impaired intestinal absorption of a single free amino acid. These disorders, each apparently inherited as an autosomal recessive trait, provide the strongest evidence that transmembrane transport of amino acids is catalyzed by substrate-specific as well as group-specific transport mechanisms.

Hypercystinuria Two siblings exhibited modest cystinuria without excessive urinary excretion of lysine, arginine, or ornithine. Fractional tubular reabsorption of cystine was reduced to about 80 percent of the filtered load, and up to 250 mg per day was excreted in the urine. Neither showed any abnormality in intestinal absorption of cystine. Both were clinically well, although their cystine excretion would appear to place them at some risk for cystine urolithiasis. Urinary cystine excretion by both parents was unremarkable.

Lysinuria Only a single child with selective impairment of renal tubular reabsorption of lysine has been described. Endogenous lysine clearance was increased; intestinal transport was impaired; plasma lysine was reduced. Severe mental and growth retardation and seizures were present. A lysine-supplemented diet appeared to stimulate growth. Urinary excretion of lysine was normal in the parents.

Histidinuria Two siblings, each with moderate mental retardation, exhibited a renal transport defect for histidine only. Urinary loss of histidine approached 40 to 50 percent of the filtered load, and an intestinal transport defect for histidine was also present. The clinically normal parents had normal urinary excretion but a modest defect in intestinal absorption of histidine.

Methionine malabsorption Single children from two pedigrees have shown an intestinal transport defect for methionine. One may have had a renal transport defect as well. This disorder was detected because of urinary excretion of α-hydroxybutyric acid, a distinctive by-product of the intestinal bacterial breakdown of the unabsorbed methionine. This compound, which gives an unusual odor resembling malt or dried celery to the urine, appears to be responsible for the white hair, attacks of hyperpnea, convulsions, edema, and mental retardation. Treatment of one of these children with a methionine-restricted diet was followed by improvement in all clinical manifestations.

Tryptophan malabsorption An isolated defect in intestinal absorption of tryptophan has been described in two siblings. The renal tubular reabsorption of tryptophan was normal. A variety of indoles were excreted in stool and urine. These compounds result from chemical degradation of unabsorbed tryptophan by intestinal bacteria and have been described in patients with Hartnup disease as well. Because of concomitant renal parenchymal disease, hydrolytic enzymes were released into the urine, acted upon the indoles found there, and led to the formation of a blue pigment, indigotin. This sequence of events earned this condition the sobriquet "blue-diaper syndrome." No pellagra-like symptoms were described. The patients' mother also excreted modest excesses of indole compounds, suggesting that she is a carrier of this trait.

DISORDERS OF HEXOSE TRANSPORT

Nondiabetic melituria occurs in a number of conditions. Pentoses, hexoses, heptoses, and disaccharides have been identified in the urine; all except sucrose yield a positive test for reducing substances. Some meliturias result from diffuse renal injury, others from ingestion of nonmetabolizable sugars. In still others the sugars accumulate in blood due to deficient activity of catabolizing enzyme systems and "spill" into the urine. Only among the hexoses have specific inherited disorders of sugar transport been identified. The existence of renal glycosuria and intestinal glucose-galactose malabsorption as heritable, autosomal recessive disorders points to the existence of at least two specific carrier proteins for hexoses in human jejunal and renal brush border membranes: one for glucose and one shared by glucose and galactose.

RENAL GLYCOSURIA   To avoid confusion with diabetes mellitus, Marble's criteria for the diagnosis of renal glycosuria should be followed: (1) glycosuria in the absence of hyperglycemia, (2) constant glycosuria with little fluctuation related to diet, (3) normal (or slightly flat) oral glucose tolerance test, (4) identification of urinary reducing substance as glucose, and (5) normal storage and utilization of carbohydrates. The Fanconi syndrome, in which renal glycosuria occurs as part of generalized proximal tubular dysfunction, should also be excluded. The incidence is less than 1 in 500. The condition is benign, but occasionally glycosuria may be great enough to cause polyuria and polydipsia. Even more rarely, dehydration or ketosis may develop under conditions of stress such as pregnancy or starvation.

In normal persons glucose is present in the glomerular filtrate at a concentration equal to that in plasma water and is actively reabsorbed throughout the proximal renal tubule by a sodium-dependent, phlorizin-inhibitable transport process. Reabsorptive capacity exceeds normal plasma glucose concentration. Thus, glucose does not appear in the urine until the threshold for reabsorption is reached. Titration studies suggest that the plasma concentration at which some filtered glucose begins to escape proximal tubular reabsorption is 200 to 240 mg per 100 ml. Maximal renal reabsorptive capacity is exceeded at a filtered load of 325 ± 36 mg/min per 1.73 m^2, and this value is defined as the tubular maximum for glucose (TmG).

Titration studies in subjects with renal glycosuria have shown two patterns of glycosuria: type A characterized by a reduced tubular maximum reabsorptive capacity and type B showing a reduced threshold for glycosuria, an increased "splay" in the titration curve, and a normal TmG. Marked renal glycosuria occurs in individuals homozygous for either of these recessively inherited mutations of the specific membrane transport process for glucose and in genetic compounds for these presumably allelic mutations. Modest reduction in renal threshold or TmG has been demonstrated in obligate heterozygotes in some pedigrees; modest glycosuria can be expected in such family members when plasma glucose is elevated.

GLUCOSE-GALACTOSE MALABSORPTION   In this condition, infants develop a profuse, watery diarrhea when fed milk or foods containing lactose, sucrose, glucose, or galactose. Fructose or carbohydrate-free formulas are well tolerated. A specific defect in intestinal absorption of glucose and galactose can be demonstrated by oral tolerance tests that produce little or no increase in plasma glucose or galactose. Treatment with a glucose- and galactose-free diet leads to resolution of symptoms in childhood. Although the basic transport defect can be demonstrated throughout life, most patients show an improved tolerance for glucose and galactose as they get older.

Intestinal transport studies performed in vitro on small biopsy specimens of jejunal mucosa have shown a complete absence of active D-glucose and D-galactose transport in affected children and intermediate transport capacity in their parents. These findings confirm the specificity of the mutation for these two sugars and the autosomal recessive inheritance of this transport disorder.

A number of these patients have renal glycosuria at normal plasma glucose concentrations. Renal titration studies generally demonstrate a reduced threshold for glucose reabsorption (type B renal glycosuria) with a normal TmG. Urinary glucose loss is not as severe as in isolated renal glycosuria. This finding suggests the presence of multiple glucose transport proteins in the kidney. One, responsible for the bulk of glucose reabsorption and specific for glucose only, is affected in renal glycosuria; another, shared by glucose and galactose and responsible for transporting less of the filtered load of glucose, is affected in glucose-galactose malabsorption. Either the former is not present in intestinal mucosa or the shared system is more important in that tissue. In both disorders transport of sugars in all other tested tissues is normal, reflecting the multiplicity and tissue specificity of membrane transport proteins.

DEFECTIVE URATE TRANSPORT: HYPOURICEMIA

A small number of pedigrees have been described containing individuals with a selective defect in renal tubular reabsorption of sodium urate. These subjects are identified by the presence of marked hypouricemia. Since little serum urate is bound to plasma proteins, failure to reabsorb filtered urate results in a serum urate ranging from 0.2 to 1.8 mg per 100 ml. No disease is associated with this isolated defect, although the risk of uric acid nephrolithiasis is theoretically present.

Renal urate clearance normally averages 15 percent of glomerular filtration rate, and the excreted urate is composed both of filtered urate that has escaped reabsorption and secreted urate. Subjects with isolated hypouricemia have urate clearances averaging from 33 to 65 percent of the filtration rate; in some, urate clearance exceeds the glomerular filtration rate. Studies with probenecid, which blocks tubular reabsorption of urate, and pyrazinamide, which blocks tubular secretion, suggest that the disorder is due to a partial defect in proximal tubular reabsorption. In two families hypercalcinuria due to enhanced intestinal calcium absorption was also present, but in all others only uricosuria has been demonstrated. The defect is inherited as an autosomal recessive. Urate transport has not been studied in nonrenal tissue or in obligate heterozygotes. The defect is presumed to reflect mutation of a proximal renal tubular membrane protein that selectively transports sodium urate.

DEFECTIVE ANION TRANSPORT: CHLORIDORRHEA

This rare, autosomal recessive disease results from impairment of active transport of chloride in the ileum and colon. Absence of the chloride-bicarbonate ion exchange "pump" causes profound symptoms even before birth (polyhydramnios and absence of meconium). Massive watery diarrhea is apparent from the first days of life. This fluid loss, with its attendant impairment of electrolyte homeostasis, is life-threatening. A hypokalemic, hypochloremic, hyponatremic metabolic alkalosis develops with dehydration and secondary hyperaldosteronism. Fecal fluid contains an excess of chloride ion over the sum of the accompanying cations, sodium and potassium. Fecal chloride concentration always exceeds 90 mmol per liter when volume and serum electrolyte disturbances are corrected, and this chloridorrhea is diagnostic. Renal chloride transport is normal. Decreased urine chloride results from the kidney's attempts to conserve salt and water.

Treatment necessitates adequate, life-long repletion of electrolyte and fluid losses, since no way has yet been found to mitigate the transport disorder. Exact replacement of water, sodium chloride, and potassium chloride can prevent the growth and psychomotor retardation and the development of progressive renal damage. The renal lesion, with hyalinized glomeruli, juxtaglomerular hyperplasia, calcifications, and arteriolar changes, is probably a result of chronic volume depletion.

REFERENCES

ELSAS LJ, ROSENBERG LE: Renal glycosuria, in *Strauss and Welt's Diseases of the Kidney,* 3d ed, LE Earley, CW Gottschalk (eds). Boston, Little, Brown, 1979 (in press)

GORDEN P, LEVITIN H: Congenital alkalosis with diarrhea; a sequel to Darrow's original description. Ann Intern Med 87:876, 1973

HOLMBERG C et al: Congenital chloride diarrhoea. Arch Dis Child 52:255, 1977

KRANE SM: Renal glycosuria, in *The Metabolic Basis of Inherited Disease,* 4th ed, JB Stanbury et al (eds). New York, McGraw-Hill, 1978, pp 1607–1617

ROSENBERG LE: Intestinal hexose transport in familial glucose-galactose malabsorption, in *Membranes and Disease,* L Bolis et al (eds). New York, Raven Press, 1976

———, SCRIVER CR: Disorders of amino acid metabolism, in *Metabolic Control and Disease,* 8th ed, PK Bondy, LE Rosenberg (eds). Philadelphia, Saunders, 1979 (in press)

SHORT EM, ROSENBERG LE: Renal aminoaciduria, in *Strauss and Welt's Diseases of the Kidney,* 3d ed, LE Earley, CW Gottschalk (eds). Boston, Little, Brown, 1979 (in press)

THIER SO, SEGAL S: Cystinuria, in *The Metabolic Basis of Inherited Disease,* 4th ed, JB Stanbury et al (eds). New York, McGraw-Hill, 1978, pp 1578–1592

WYNGAARDEN JB, KELLEY WN: *Gout and Hyperuricemia.* New York, Grune & Stratton, 1976, pp 411–420

91
CARCINOID SYNDROME

JOHN A. OATES

The association of carcinoid tumors with cutaneous flushes, telangiectasia, diarrhea, cardiac valvular lesions, and bronchial constriction eluded recognition until 1953. Once this connection was established by Thorson, Biörk, Björkman, and Waldenström, and independently by Isler and Hedinger, it was clear that the syndrome was mediated by release of one or more biologically active agents by the tumor. Serotonin was the first such agent to be discovered, and overproduction of this amine is the most consistent biochemical indicator of the carcinoid syndrome. Serotonin, however, is not the sole mediator of the clinical syndrome. These tumors vary in their synthesis of indoles and may elaborate chemically unrelated agents such as bradykinin, histamine, and adrenocorticotropic hormone (ACTH). Furthermore, evidence suggests that an additional unidentified substance participates in the production of flushing. Within the broad classification of carcinoid tumors there is great diversity in the production of biologically active substances and in the mechanisms for their storage and release.

Accordingly, there is a varied spectrum of clinical manifestations.

PATHOLOGICAL ANATOMY OF THE TUMOR Carcinoid tumors are slowly growing neoplasms of enterochromaffin cells. The metastatic tumors associated with carcinoid syndrome usually arise from small primary tumors in the ileum. The syndrome is also produced by neoplasms arising from the remainder of the small intestine, from organs derived from the embryonic foregut (e.g., bronchus, stomach, pancreas, and thyroid), and from ovarian or testicular teratomas.

Carcinoid tumors have an unusual proclivity for metastasis to the liver and may involve this organ extensively, with minimal metastatic disease elsewhere. Extrahepatic metastases occur in bone, where they are often osteoblastic, and in lung, pancreas, spleen, ovaries, adrenals, and other organs.

Primary carcinoid tumors of the appendix are common, but they rarely metastasize. Those from the large intestine may metastasize but almost never exhibit endocrine effects.

The usual carcinoid tumor arising from the ileum has the classic histological pattern of dense nests of cells with uniform size and nuclear appearance. Histochemically, they typically exhibit an argentaffin reaction in which the cells convert a silver salt to metallic silver. A positive argentaffin reaction is not required for the diagnosis, however, and carcinoid tumors arising from organs of the embryonic foregut are usually argyrophyllic, containing few if any argentaffin cells. Tumors from these organs also have a broad histological spectrum, which in the lung ranges from typical bronchial carcinoid to a form indistinguishable from oat-cell carcinoma.

Neoplasms of foregut origin with histological features resembling carcinoids may produce excessive amounts of polypeptide hormones such as gastrin, insulin, calcitonin, glucagon, corticotropin, and vasoactive intestinal polypeptide without exhibiting the usual features of carcinoid syndrome. These carcinoid tumors probably share a common embryologic origin with those producing carcinoid syndrome, arising from the neuroectodermal cells of the neural crest.

CLINICAL FEATURES Unlike most metastatic neoplasms, carcinoid tumors have an unusually slow rate of growth; most patients survive for 5 to 10 years after the disease is recognized. For much of the duration of the illness, morbidity may result largely from the endocrine function of the tumor. Death results from cardiac or hepatic failure and from complications associated with tumor growth.

Vasomotor paroxysms The most common clinical feature is cutaneous *flushing.* The typical flush is erythematous and involves the head and neck (blush area). Some patients exhibit vivid color changes from red to violaceous to pallor during its course. Prolonged flushing attacks may be associated with lacrimation and periorbital edema. The systemic effects of the flush are variable. It may be accompanied by tachycardia, and the blood pressure usually falls or does not change. A rise in blood pressure during flushing is rare, and carcinoid syndrome is not a cause of sustained hypertension.

Flushing may be provoked by excitement, exertion, eating, and ethanol ingestion. In addition, the administration of pentagastrin and beta-adrenoceptor agonists such as epinephrine can trigger episodes of vasodilatation; as the hemodynamic changes associated with such pharmacologically induced attacks may be severe, these drugs should be administered with great caution.

Telangiectasia In addition to paroxysms of cutaneous vasodilatation, some patients also develop purple telangiectasia, primarily on the face and neck and most marked in the malar area.

Gastrointestinal symptoms Intestinal hypermotility with borborygmi, cramping, and explosive diarrhea may accompany the episodic flushes. Chronic hypermotility with diarrhea is more common. When this is severe, malabsorption may occur.

Cardiac manifestations There is a unique deposition of fibrous tissue on the endocardium of the valvular cusps and cardiac chambers. It occurs primarily in the right side of the heart, but may involve the left side to a minimal degree. The fibrous deposition does not penetrate the internal elastic membrane. Distortion of the valve cusps, chordae tendineae, and papillary muscles interferes with valvular function in the right side of the heart and may lead to regurgitation, stenosis, or combined functional lesions. There is, however, a tendency for the fibrosing process to produce incompetence at the tricuspid valve and stenosis of the smaller pulmonary orifice, a deleterious hemodynamic combination. A high cardiac output, with its attendant imposition on cardiac function, may be found in some patients with carcinoid syndrome; this is due either to a continuing release of a vasodilator or to excessive flow in the metastatic tumors.

Pulmonary symptoms Bronchoconstriction is a less common feature of the syndrome, but it may be severe. It is usually most pronounced during flushing attacks.

General In addition to the endocrine effects, the tumors themselves may cause intestinal obstruction or bleeding. Necrosis of intestinal or hepatic tumor masses may produce abdominal pain, tenderness, fever, and leukocytosis. Hepatomegaly from the metastatic disease is usually present with the syndrome. Extensive metastatic involvement of the liver by these slowly growing tumors may occur before the liver function test results become abnormal.

ENDOCRINE FUNCTION OF THE TUMORS **Serotonin** The most constant biochemical characteristic of carcinoid tumors is the presence of tryptophan hydroxylase, which catalyzes the formation of 5-hydroxytryptophan (5-HTP) from tryptophan (Fig. 91-1). Most tumors also contain the enzyme aromatic L-amino acid decarboxylase, which catalyzes the formation of 5-hydroxytryptamine (serotonin). Carcinoids from the stomach and from other organs derived from the embryonic foregut, however, are frequently deficient in this decarboxylase and release 5-HTP from the tumor.

Following its release from the tumor, serotonin is inactivated primarily by the enzyme monoamine oxidase; uptake into platelets also contributes to removal of free serotonin from blood. Monoamine oxidase oxidizes serotonin to 5-hydroxyindoleacetaldehyde, which is rapidly converted to 5-hydroxyindoleacetic acid (5-HIAA) by aldehyde dehydrogenase. This acid is rapidly excreted in the urine, and almost all circulating serotonin can be accounted for as urinary 5-HIAA.

Carcinoid tumors vary widely in their capacity to store serotonin, with concentrations of the amine in tumors ranging from a few micrograms per gram to 3 mg/g. The concentration in the tumor appears unrelated to the rate of synthesis of serotonin as reflected by urinary 5-HIAA. Generally, tumors from the ileum have a much higher storage capacity for serotonin than do tumors from organs of the embryonic foregut.

Bradykinin A potent vasodilator peptide, bradykinin is released during flushes in some cases of carcinoid syndrome. In a few of these, excessive amounts continue to be released between flushes. Bradykinin and related kinins are formed by the action of a group of enzymes (kallikreins) which split these peptides from kininogen, a plasma globulin. It is thought that catecholamines and other stimuli initiate bradykinin formation, either by release of kallikrein from the tumor or by initi-

ation of a sequence that leads to activation of the kallikrein normally present in plasma.

Other biologically active substances Some carcinoid tumors, particularly those of gastric origin, produce and release excessive amounts of histamine. This can be detected by an increased excretion of this amine in the urine. In such patients, the release of histamine from the tumors is responsible for the episodic vasodilatation with flushing, tachycardia, and hypotension.

Carcinoid syndrome has been associated with hyperadrenocorticism in a number of instances. This results from ectopic production of an adrenocorticotropic hormone by the tumors, which usually originate from sites other than the ileum (bronchus, pancreas, ovary, and stomach). (See Chap. 347.)

In a few cases, "multiple endocrine adenomas" have been seen in conjunction with carcinoids arising from organs of the embryonic foregut. The associated tumors have included parathyroid adenomas and pancreatic tumors, producing Zollinger-Ellison syndrome. (See Chap. 348.)

FIGURE 91-1
Metabolic pathway of serotonin.

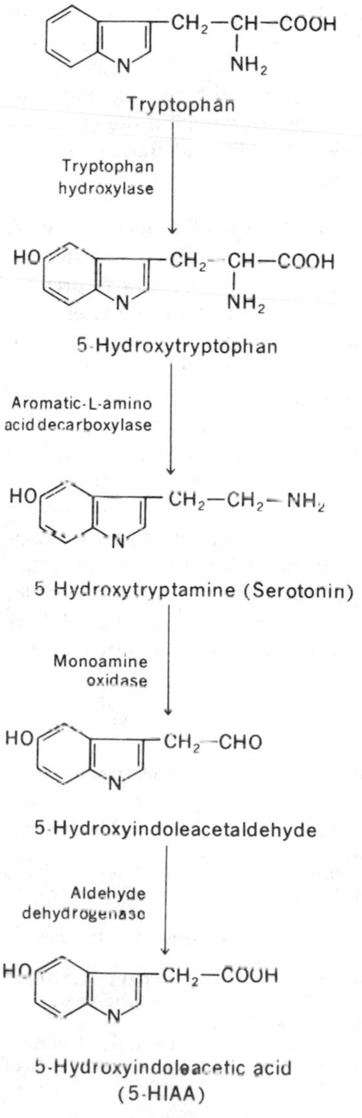

PATHOPHYSIOLOGY Serotonin contributes to those aspects of the syndrome related to intestinal hypermotility, and there is evidence that the fibrous deposits on the endocardium also result from increased levels of circulating serotonin.

A secondary effect of serotonin overproduction occurs when a large fraction of dietary tryptophan is shunted into the hydroxylation pathway, leaving less tryptophan available for the formation of nicotinic acid and protein. When urinary excretion of 5-HIAA exceeds 200 to 300 mg daily, low levels of plasma tryptophan and evidence of nicotinamide deficiency are seen. (See Chap. 79.)

Mechanism of the flush Although the flushes of patients with gastric carcinoids that secrete histamine can be attributed to this amine, the mechanism of the flush in the more typical carcinoid syndrome has not yet been elucidated. Release of the flush-provoking substance(s) can be triggered by the catecholamines, and this probably accounts for the association of flushing with excitement and emotional stimuli. For experimental induction of flushing, injection of isoproterenol in amounts of as little as 0.5 μg may be effective. Pentagastrin in doses of as small as 0.25 μg also can trigger flushing, an action that may explain the provocation of flushes by eating in some patients. Serotonin was originally thought to be the mediator of flushes, but injection of this amine does not produce a mimicking of the carcinoid flush, and patients may exhibit flushes without increased levels of plasma serotonin. Bradykinin is a potent vasodilator, and its injection will simulate one type of carcinoid flush which is characterized by erythema in association with tachycardia and hypotension. Release of this peptide, however, could not be detected in a number of patients during flushing. While bradykinin, serotonin, and histamine may contribute to the varied types of flushes observed in the carcinoid syndrome, there appears to be an additional flush substance which has not yet been identified.

DIAGNOSIS With its full constellation of clinical features, carcinoid syndrome is easily recognized. The diagnosis also must be considered when any one of its features is present.

The diagnostic hallmark of carcinoid syndrome is *overproduction of 5-hydroxyindoles* with *increased urinary excretion of 5-hydroxyindoleacetic acid.* Normally, excretion of 5-HIAA does not exceed 9 mg daily. Ingestion of foods containing serotonin may complicate the biochemical diagnosis of carcinoid syndrome; both walnuts and bananas contain enough serotonin to produce abnormally elevated urinary excretion of 5-HIAA after their ingestion. Some drugs also interfere with the analysis of urinary 5-HIAA; cough syrups containing guaiacolate cause falsely elevated values, and phenothiazines interfere with the colorimetric test. When dietary 5-hydroxyindoles are excluded, a urinary excretion of more than 25 mg 5-HIAA daily is diagnostic of carcinoid. Elevations in the range of 9 to 25 mg may be seen with carcinoid syndrome, nontropical sprue, or acute intestinal obstruction.

Measurement of *serotonin in blood or platelets* is of interest but has less diagnostic value than assay of the major metabolite of serotonin in the urine.

Measurement of an increased concentration of *serotonin in tumor tissue* is a useful and sometimes necessary supplement to histological examination. A portion of suspected tumor should always be frozen for serotonin analysis (see Table 91-1).

VARIANTS OF THE SYNDROME: RELATION TO SITE OF TUMOR ORIGIN The origin of the tumor influences the biologically active substances produced and their storage and release. Carcinoid tumors arising from organs derived from the embryonic foregut (bronchus, stomach, and pancreas) tend to differ from those arising distal to the midduodenum (midgut). The typical carcinoid syndrome usually results from tumors of midgut origin, which almost invariably secrete serotonin with little or no 5-HTP. Tumor serotonin content is likely to be high, and the tumor usually contains dense nests of argentaffin-positive cells. Metastasis to bone and skin is infrequent.

In contrast, tumors arising from the embryonic foregut contain fewer argentaffin cells, have lower serotonin content, and may secrete 5-HTP. Hyperadrenocorticism and multiple endocrine adenomas are more likely to be associated with this group, and metastasis to bone and skin is more frequent.

In addition to the general characteristics of the foregut group, certain clinical and biochemical features have been associated with gastric and bronchial carcinoids. Patients with gastric carcinoids frequently exhibit unique flushing which begins as a bright red patchy erythema with sharply delineated serpentine borders; these patches tend to coalesce as the blush heightens. Food ingestion is especially likely to produce flushes. The tumors usually are deficient in decarboxylase enzyme and secrete 5-HTP; histamine secretion is also common, as is a high incidence of peptic ulceration. Diarrhea and heart lesions are not prominent features in the patients who secrete largely 5-HTP from the tumor without much preformed serotonin.

When the carcinoid tumor arises from the bronchus, attacks of flushing tend to be prolonged and severe and may be associated with periorbital edema, excessive lacrimation and salivation, hypotension, tachycardia, anxiety, and tremulousness. Nausea, vomiting, explosive diarrhea, and bronchoconstriction may progress to a severe degree. This group is therapeutically unique in that the severe flushes often can be prevented by corticosteroids, and chlorpromazine may be helpful in relieving the symptoms.

TREATMENT Recognition of the carcinoid syndrome has led to complete surgical cure of a few patients with tumors arising in ovarian or testicular teratomas or in the bronchus; by releasing their secretions directly into the systemic circulation, tumors from these locations can produce the syndrome before metastatic disease occurs. As the humoral substances released by tumors draining into the portal circulation are largely metabolized by the liver, tumors arising in this location produce the syndrome only after hepatic metastasis. Because of the relatively slow growth of carcinoid tumors, palliative resection of hepatic metastases is beneficial in carefully selected cases. Resection of large isolated hepatic metastases has led to relief of the symptoms of carcinoid syndrome and marked reductions in urinary 5-HIAA excretion for periods of several years. In some cases with multiple metastases, removal of as much as a hepatic lobe may be considered when the metastases are located primarily in the portion of the liver to be resected, as determined by arteriography, scintillation scanning of gamma-emitting colloidal particles taken up by the liver, and inspection of the hepatic surface at surgical exploration.

TABLE 91-1
Outline of diagnostic approach to a patient with suspected carcinoid syndrome

I Quantitative determination of 24-h urinary excretion of 5-HIAA (5-hydroxyindoleacetic acid).
II When elevated 5-HIAA confirms clinical evidence for carcinoid syndrome, curable ovarian, testicular, or bronchial primary tumors should be sought.
III Consideration of possible treatment of the syndrome by surgical resection of hepatic metastases requires:
  A Assessment of the location and character of hepatic metastases with arteriography and scintillation scanning of the liver.
  B Evaluation of hepatic and cardiac function.
  C A search for extrahepatic metastases in bone and other sites.
IV In patients with substantial diarrhea, possible malabsorption of nutrients should be investigated.

Chemotherapy of carcinoid tumors has not yielded the extent or duration of palliation achieved with selective removal of hepatic metastases. Radiation treatment has been effective in some patients.

Pharmacological therapy directed at the humoral mediators of the syndrome is useful in some cases. When the flush is associated with release of histamine, as may be the case with gastric carcinoids, combined treatment with an H_1 antagonist (e.g., diphenhydramine) and an H_2 antagonist (cimetidine) will block the vasodilator action of histamine. Methysergide, a serotonin antagonist, will improve the diarrhea, but prolonged therapy with this agent can produce retroperitoneal fibrosis. Blockade of serotonin synthesis with the tryptophan hydroxylase inhibitor p-chlorophenylalanine also ameliorates the diarrhea. The prevention of severe flushing by corticosteroids and amelioration of the syndrome by phenothiazines are limited largely to patients with tumors arising from the bronchus and other organs derived from the embryonic foregut.

Nicotinamide should be given to those patients who shunt a large fraction of dietary tryptophan into the hydroxyindole pathway.

Hypotensive episodes should not be treated with catecholamines; by stimulating the release of vasoactive substances from the tumor, norepinephrine, epinephrine, and other agents with adrenergic activity can exaggerate and prolong the circulatory disturbance. If hypotension requires therapy, volume expansion or methoxamine infusion is the preferred approach.

REFERENCES

OATES JA, BUTLER TC: Pharmacologic and endocrine aspects of carcinoid syndrome. Adv Pharmacol 5:109, 1967

ROBERTSON JIS et al: The mechanism of facial flushing in the carcinoid syndrome. Q J Med 31:103, 1962

SJOERDSMA A et al: A clinical, physiologic and biochemical study of patients with malignant carcinoid. Am J Med 20:520, 1956

VAN SICKLE DG: Carcinoid tumors; analysis of 61 cases, including 11 cases of carcinoid syndrome. Cleveland Clin Q 39:79, 1972

Disorders of nucleic acid metabolism

92
GOUT AND OTHER DISORDERS OF PURINE METABOLISM

WILLIAM N. KELLEY

Gout is a term representing a heterogeneous group of diseases found exclusively in humans, which in their full development are manifested by (1) an increase in the serum urate concentration; (2) recurrent attacks of a characteristic type of acute arthritis, in which crystals of monosodium urate monohydrate are demonstrable in leukocytes of synovial fluid; (3) aggregated deposits of monosodium urate monohydrate (tophi) chiefly in and around the joints of the extremities and sometimes leading to severe crippling and deformity; (4) renal disease involving interstitial tissues and blood vessels; and (5) uric acid nephrolithiasis. These may occur singly or in combination.

PREVALENCE AND EPIDEMIOLOGY The serum urate value is elevated in an absolute sense when it exceeds the limit of solubility of monosodium urate in serum. At 37°C the saturation value of urate in plasma is about 7.0 mg per 100 ml; a value above this represents supersaturation in a physicochemical sense. The serum urate concentration is relatively elevated when it exceeds the upper limit of an arbitrary normal range, usually defined as the mean serum urate value plus two standard deviations in a healthy population matched for age and sex. In most epidemiological studies the upper limit is about 7.0 mg per 100 ml in men and 6.0 mg per 100 ml in women. In epidemiological terms a serum urate value in excess of 7.0 mg

per 100 ml carries an increased risk of gouty arthritis or renal stones.

Sex and age have an important influence on the serum urate. The serum urate concentration before puberty in both boys and girls averages approximately 3.6 mg per 100 ml. After the onset of puberty levels increase in boys more than in girls. Values in men reach a plateau in the early twenties and are essentially stable thereafter. Values in women are constant from age 20 through 40, but with menopause the values rise and approach or equal those in men. Age and sex differences in the serum urate are thought to be related to differences in the renal clearance of urate, perhaps determined in turn by the levels of estrogens and androgens. Other factors, including warm ambient temperature, obesity, high social status, and achievement or intelligence appear to correlate with a higher serum urate concentration.

Hyperuricemia by one or more of the above definitions is present in 2 to 18 percent of the populations studied. In one hospitalized population, 13 percent of adult men exhibited a serum urate concentration in excess of 7.0 mg per 100 ml.

The prevalence of gout is substantially less than that of hyperuricemia and is widely different around the world. In most of the Western world it ranges from 0.13 to 0.37 percent of the population. Gout is primarily a disease of adult men, and only about 5 percent of cases occur in women; it occurs rarely in the prepubertal child of either sex. The usual form of gout is uncommon before the third decade, and the peak incidence is in the fifth decade.

INHERITANCE In the United States a family history of gout is obtained in 6 to 18 percent of gouty subjects, and figures as high as 75 percent are noted after persistent questioning. A more precise definition of the inheritance of gout is complicated by the numerous environmental factors capable of altering the serum urate concentration. In addition, the identification of several specific genetic causes of gout has established that gout is merely the common clinical manifestation of a heterogeneous group of diseases. Accordingly, study of the inheritance of hyperuricemia and gout in the population or even within families is difficult. Two specific enzymatic causes of gout, hypoxanthine-guanine phosphoribosyltransferase deficiency and 5-phosphoribosyl-1-pyrophosphate (PRPP) synthetase overactivity, are X-linked. Pedigrees have been reported in which the inheritance pattern is consistent with an autosomal dominant mode. More commonly genetic studies suggest multifactorial inheritance patterns.

CLINICAL FEATURES In the full development of its natural history, gout passes through four stages: asymptomatic hyperuricemia, acute gouty arthritis, intercritical gout, and chronic tophaceous gout. Nephrolithiasis may occur in any stage but the first.

Asymptomatic hyperuricemia Asymptomatic hyperuricemia is that stage in which the serum urate level is raised but arthritic symptoms, tophi, or uric acid stones have not yet appeared. In men vulnerable to classic gout hyperuricemia begins at puberty, whereas in women at risk hyperuricemia is usually delayed until menopause. In contrast, patients with certain of the enzyme defects to be described later may be hyperuricemic from birth. While asymptomatic hyperuricemia may last throughout the lifetime with no recognizable consequences, the tendency toward acute gouty arthritis increases as a function of serum urate concentration and the duration of hyperuricemia. The risk of nephrolithiasis also increases as serum urate values increase and correlates with the magnitude of uric acid excretion. While virtually all gouty subjects are hyperuricemic, perhaps no more than 5 percent of hyperuricemics ever develop gout.

The phase of asymptomatic hyperuricemia ends with the first attack of gouty arthritis or nephrolithiasis. In most, gout comes before stone, usually after at least 20 to 30 years of sustained hyperuricemia. However, between 10 and 40 percent of gouty subjects have renal colic prior to the first episode of arthritis.

Acute gouty arthritis The primary manifestation of acute gout is exquisitely painful arthritis, at first usually monoarticular and associated with few constitutional symptoms, but later often polyarticular and accompanied by fever. Attacks last a variable but limited period of time and are separated by intervals of freedom from all symptoms. About 90 percent of first attacks occur in a single joint, and in at least half the initial attack occurs in the first metatarsal phalangeal joint. Ultimately, 90 percent of patients experience an acute attack in the great toe (podagra).

Acute gouty arthritis is predominantly a disease of the lower extremities. The more distal the site of involvement the more typical are the attacks. Following the toe in order of frequency as sites of initial involvement are the insteps, ankles, heels, knees, wrists, fingers, and elbows. While acute attacks may occur in other joints, such as shoulder, hips, spine, sacroiliac, sternoclavicular, and mandibular joints, these sites are rare except in patients with established, severe disease. The patient may report trivial episodes of pain preceding the first dramatic gouty attack. Commonly, the major attack begins at night, is exquisitely painful with inflamed joints, and may be triggered by a specific event such as trauma, alcohol ingestion, certain drugs, dietary excess, or surgery. It is difficult to improve upon Syndenham's classical description:

The victim goes to bed and sleeps in good health. About two o'clock in the morning he is awakened by a severe pain in the great toe; more rarely in the heel, ankle or instep. This pain is like that of a dislocation, and yet the parts feel as if cold water were poured over them. Then follow chills and shivers, and a little fever. The pain, which was at first moderate, becomes more intense. With its intensity the chills and shivers increase. After a time this comes to its height, accommodating itself to the bones and ligaments of the tarsus and metatarsus. Now it is a violent stretching and tearing of the ligaments—now it is a gnawing pain and now a pressure and tightening. So exquisite and lively meanwhile is the feeling of the part affected, that it cannot bear the weight of bedclothes nor the jar of a person walking in the room. The night is passed in torture, sleeplessness, turning of the part affected, and perpetual change of posture; the tossing about of the body being as incessant as the pain of the tortured joint, and being worse as the fit comes on. Hence the vain effort by change of posture, both in the body and the limb affected, to obtain an abatement of the pain.

Intercritical period The attack of gout may last only a day or two or up to several weeks but characteristically subsides spontaneously. An asymptomatic phase termed the *intercritical period* then commences. The patient will be totally free of symptoms during this stage, a feature that is diagnostically important. While approximately 7 percent of patients never have a second attack, most experience a recurrence within 1 year. However, the intercritical period may last up to 10 years. Later attacks tend to be polyarticular, more severe, more prolonged, and associated with fever. In this stage gout may be difficult to differentiate from other types of polyarticular arthritis such as rheumatoid arthritis. While most patients experience the intermittent course just described, rare patients progress directly from the initial acute attack to chronic polyarticular disease with no remissions.

Tophi and chronic gouty arthritis In the untreated patient the urate pool expands and crystal deposits of monosodium urate eventually appear in cartilage, synovial membranes, tendons, and soft tissues. The rate of formation of these tophaceous deposits appears to be a direct function of the degree and duration of hyperuricemia and of the severity of renal disease. The classic location of a tophus is the helix or antihelix of the ear (Fig. 92-1). Tophi also commonly occur along the ulnar surface of the forearm, as saccular distensions of the olecranon bursae (Fig. 92-2), as enlargements of the Achilles tendon, or at other pressure points. Patients with the most severe tophi, interestingly, often have sparing of the helix and antihelix of the ear.

FIGURE 92-1
Tophus of the helix of the ear adjacent to the auricular tubercle.

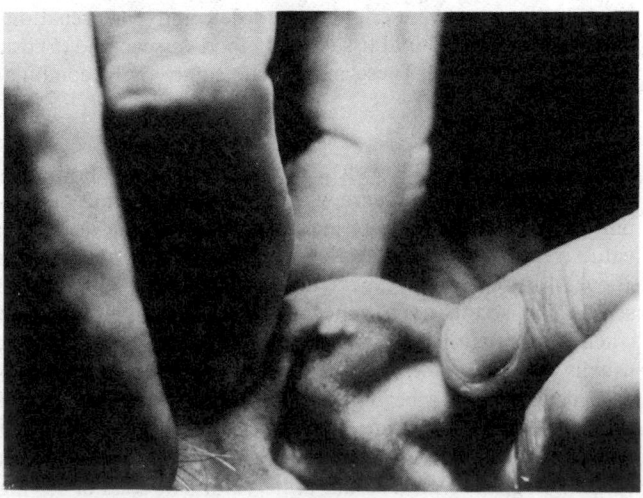

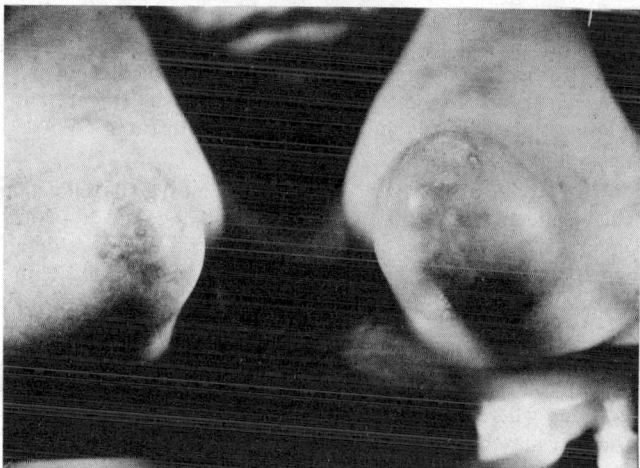

FIGURE 92-2
Effusions of olecranon bursae of patient with gout. Note also the cutaneous deposits of urate and the minimal inflammatory response.

Tophi are difficult to differentiate from rheumatoid nodules and other types of subcutaneous nodules. They may ulcerate and exude chalky or pasty material rich in monosodium urate crystals. In contrast to other subcutaneous nodules, tophi are rarely transient although they may resolve slowly in response to effective treatment of hyperuricemia. For reasons that are unclear, it is rare for a tophus to become infected. Patients with severe tophaceous disease appear to have milder and less frequent attacks of acute gouty arthritis than nontophaceous subjects. Chronic tophaceous gout rarely occurs prior to the onset of gouty arthritis.

Since the advent of effective antihyperuricemic therapy, only a minority of patients develop visible tophi, permanent joint changes, or chronic symptoms. Thus, effective therapy has altered the natural history of the disease.

Nephropathy Some renal dysfunction is present in up to 90 percent of subjects with a history of gouty arthritis. Prior to the advent of chronic hemodialysis, renal failure accounted for 17 to 25 percent of deaths in the gouty population. The initial manifestation of renal involvement may be albuminuria or isosthenuria. If the patient presents in an advanced stage of renal failure it may be difficult to determine whether renal failure is a consequence of hyperuricemia or hyperuricemia is the result of renal disease.

Several types of parenchymal renal damage have been described. The first, urate nephropathy, has been attributed to the deposition of monosodium urate crystals in the renal interstitial tissue. The second, obstructive uropathy, is due to the formation of uric acid crystals in the collecting tubules, renal pelvis, or ureter, with resulting blockage of urine flow.

There is considerable controversy over the pathogenesis of urate nephropathy. While crystals of monosodium urate have been demonstrated in the interstitium of kidneys from gouty subjects, such crystals are not demonstrable in the kidneys of most people with gout. Further, there is a close correlation between the development of renal disease and the presence of hypertension in patients with gout. It is not clear, therefore, whether the hypertension causes the renal disease or the gouty renal disease is the cause of the hypertension.

Acute obstructive uropathy is a severe form of acute renal failure due to the precipitation of uric acid crystals in collecting ducts and ureters. This condition occurs most commonly in (1) patients with profound overproduction of uric acid, particularly subjects with leukemia or lymphoma who are subjected to aggressive chemotherapy, (2) patients with gout and marked hyperuricaciduria, and (3) (possibly) in patients following severe exercise or convulsions. Postmortem studies reveal intraluminal precipitates of uric acid with dilatation of proximal tubules. Therapy designed to decrease the formation of uric acid, accelerate urine flow, and increase the fraction of uric acid present as the more soluble ionized form, monosodium urate, is effective in the reversal of this process.

Nephrolithiasis While the overall prevalence of uric acid stones in the population of the United States is about 0.01 percent, the prevalence in gouty subjects ranges from 10 to 25 percent. The major factor favoring formation of uric acid stones is the increased urinary excretion of uric acid. When the urinary uric acid exceeds 1100 mg per day the incidence reaches 50 percent. There is also correlation with increasing serum urate concentrations, the prevalence reaching approximately 50 percent at a serum urate value of 13 mg per 100 ml or above. Other factors contributing to the formation of uric acid stones include (1) undue acidity of the urine, (2) increased urine concentration, and (3) (perhaps) abnormalities of urinary constituents that affect the solubility of uric acid itself.

Gouty subjects also have an increased frequency of calcium-containing stones, the occurrence in gout is 1 to 3 percent, while that in the general population is about 0.1 percent. While the mechanisms for this association are unclear, there is a high frequency of hyperuricemia and hyperuricaciduria in patients seen because of calcium stones. It is possible that uric acid crystals serve as a nidus for calcium stone formation.

Associated conditions Obesity, hypertriglyceridemia, and hypertension are common. The hypertriglyceridemia of primary gout is strongly associated with obesity or alcohol ingestion and not with hyperuricemia itself. The incidence of hypertension in the nongouty population is correlated with age, sex, and obesity; when these factors are appropriately scored there appears to be little or no direct relationship between hyperuricemia and hypertension. The increased frequency of diabetes is also probably related to factors such as age and obesity and not to hyperuricemia itself. Finally, the increased incidence of atherosclerosis has been attributed to the concomitant obesity, hypertension, diabetes, and hypertriglyceridemia.

Independent analysis of these variables suggests that obesity is most important. Hyperuricemia in the obese subject appears to be related to both increased production and reduced excretion of uric acid.

DIAGNOSIS AND DIFFERENTIAL DIAGNOSIS The diagnosis of acute gouty arthritis can be established by demonstration of monosodium urate crystals in white cells of synovial fluid obtained from the inflamed joint by compensated polarized light microscopy (Fig. 92-3). Such crystals can be identified in synovial fluid from virtually every patient with acute gouty arthritis. Failure to demonstrate urate crystals in synovial fluid after careful search under appropriate conditions makes the diagnosis unlikely.

Demonstration of intracellular urate crystals establishes the diagnosis but does not exclude the possibility that another type of arthropathy is present concurrently.

Synovial fluid analysis may also be helpful in other ways. The total leukocyte count may range from 1000 to more than 70,000 per milliliter. The predominant cell type is the polymorphonuclear leukocyte. As with other inflammatory fluids, the mucin clot is fair to poor. The concentrations of glucose and uric acid are the same as in serum.

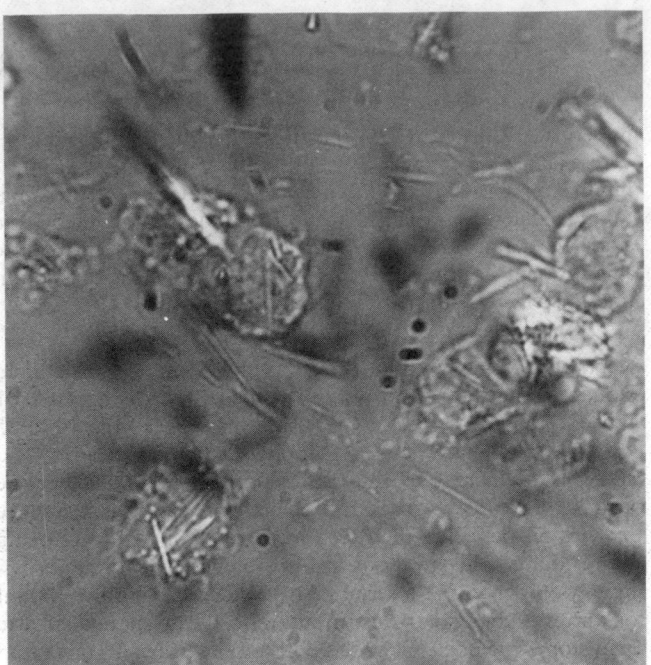

FIGURE 92-3
Crystals of monosodium urate monohydrate in joint aspirate.

In the patient in whom synovial fluid cannot be obtained or in whom intracellular crystals cannot be demonstrated, a presumptive diagnosis of gout can be seriously entertained if the patient has (1) hyperuricemia, (2) the classical clinical features described above, and (3) a dramatic response to colchicine. In the absence of crystals or this highly suggestive triad, the diagnosis of gout should be considered tentative. While a dramatic therapeutic response to colchicine is strongly suggestive of the diagnosis of gouty arthritis, it is not pathognomonic by itself.

Acute gouty arthritis must be differentiated from other conditions in which monoarticular or polyarticular arthritis occurs. The most common initial presentation in the gouty patient is podagra, but many conditions mimic the painful, swollen big toe characteristic of the disease. These include soft tissue infection, inflamed bunions, local trauma, rheumatoid arthritis, degenerative arthritis with acute inflammation, acute sarcoidosis, psoriatic arthritis, pseudogout, acute calcific tendonitis, palindromic rheumatism, Reiter's disease, and sporotrichosis. Rarely, confusion may be caused by cellulitis, gonor-

rhea, fibrosis of the sole and heel, hematoma, and subacute bacterial endocarditis with embolization or suppurative arthritis. Gouty involvement of other joints such as the knee must also be differentiated from acute rheumatic fever, serum sickness, hemarthrosis, and the peripheral joint involvement of ankylosing spondylitis or inflammatory bowel disease.

PATHOPHYSIOLOGY OF HYPERURICEMIA   Classification

The biochemical hallmark and prerequisite of gout is hyperuricemia. The concentration of uric acid in body fluids is determined by the balance between rates of production and elimination. Uric acid is formed by oxidation of purine bases, which may be exogenous or endogenous in origin. About two-thirds of uric acid is excreted into the urine (300 to 600 mg per day), and approximately one-third is excreted into the gastrointestinal tract, where it is ultimately destroyed by bacteria. Hyperuricemia may be due to an excessive rate of uric acid production, a decrease in the renal excretion of uric acid, or a combination of both events.

Hyperuricemia and gout may be classified as primary, secondary, or idiopathic (Table 92-1). In the classification used here *primary* refers to those cases in which gout or hyperuricemia is the central manifestation of the disease, namely, gout that is neither secondary to another acquired disorder nor a subordinate manifestation of an inborn error that leads initially to a major disease unlike gout. While some cases of primary gout have a defined genetic basis, others do not. *Secondary* hyperuricemia or gout refers to those cases which develop in the course of another disease or as a consequence of drugs. Finally, the term *idiopathic* is used to describe those cases in which the underlying defect has not been defined and a more precise classification (overproduction or underexcretion) cannot be made. Further subdivisions within each of the three major categories are based on the identification of overproduction or underexcretion or both as responsible for the hyperuricemia.

Overproduction of uric acid   Overproducers of uric acid by definition excrete in excess of 600 mg per day after a 5-day period of dietary purine restriction; such patients probably represent less than 10 percent of the gouty population. In these patients there is an acceleration in the rate of purine biosynthesis de novo. Overproduction of uric acid can occur either as the result of a specific enzyme defect, as the secondary consequence of a proliferative disorder, or in idiopathic gout. Understanding the basic mechanisms responsible for these abnor-

TABLE 92-1
Classification of hyperuricemia and gout

Type	Metabolic disturbance	Inheritance
Primary:		
Molecular defects undefined:		
Underexcretion (90% of primary gout)	Not established	Polygenic
Overproduction (10% of primary gout)	Not established	Polygenic
Associated with specific enzyme defects:		
P-ribose-PP synthetase variants; increased activity	Overproduction of PP-ribose-P and of uric acid	X-linked
Hypoxanthine-guanine phosphoribosyltransferase deficiency, partial	Overproduction of uric acid; increased purine biosynthesis de novo driven by surplus P-ribose-PP	X-linked
Secondary:		
Associated with increased purine biosynthesis de novo:		
Glucose 6-phosphatase deficiency or absence	Overproduction plus underexcretion of uric acid; glycogen storage disease, type I (von Gierke)	Autosomal recessive
Hypoxanthine-guanine phosphoribosyltransferase deficiency "virtually complete"	Overproduction of uric acid; Lesch-Nyhan syndrome	X-linked
Associated with increased nucleic acid turnover	Overproduction of uric acid	
Associated with decreased renal excretion of uric acid	Decreased filtration of uric acid	
	Inhibited tubular secretion of uric acid, or enhanced tubular reabsorption of uric acid	
Idiopathic		Unknown

SOURCE: *After Wyngaarden and Kelley, 1976.*

malities requires a brief review of purine metabolism (Fig. 92-4).

The purine nucleotides, adenylic acid (AMP), inosinic acid (IMP), and guanylic acid (GMP), are the end products of purine biosynthesis. They can be synthesized in one of two ways: either directly from the purine bases, e.g., guanine to GMP, hypoxanthine to IMP, and adenine to AMP; or they may be synthesized de novo, beginning with nonpurine precursors and progressing through a series of steps to the formation of IMP, which is the common intermediate purine nucleotide. IMP can be converted either to AMP or to GMP. Once the purine nucleotides are formed, they are utilized for the synthesis of nucleic acids, cyclic AMP, cyclic GMP, ATP, and certain cofactors.

The various purine components are degraded to the purine nucleotide monophosphates. GMP is degraded via guanosine, guanine, and xanthine to uric acid. IMP is degraded through inosine, hypoxanthine, and xanthine to uric acid. AMP can be deaminated to IMP and further catabolized through inosine to uric acid, or it may be degraded to inosine by an alternate pathway with the intermediate formation of adenosine.

While the purine pathway is regulated in a complex manner, the intracellular concentration of 5-phosphoribosyl-1-pyrophosphate (PRPP) appears to be a major determinant of the rate of synthesis of uric acid in humans. Generally, when the concentration of PRPP in the cell is elevated, uric acid synthesis is elevated; when the concentration of PRPP is reduced, the synthesis of uric acid is also reduced. Although exceptions are recognized, this concept is applicable to most situations.

From 5 to 10 percent of adult gouty subjects with overproduction of uric acid have a partial deficiency of hypoxanthine-guanine phosphoribosyltransferase, the enzyme that catalyzes the conversion of hypoxanthine to inosinic acid and guanine to guanylic acid (reaction 2, Fig. 92-4). The deficiency of hypoxanthine-guanine phosphoribosyltransferase leads to a decreased consumption and increased accumulation of PRPP, thus accelerating purine biosynthesis and the production of uric acid. These patients typically have the onset of gouty arthritis at a young age (15 to 30 years), a high incidence of uric acid stones (75 percent), and the occasional occurrence of mild neurologic dysfunction characterized by dysarthria, hyperreflexia, incoordination, and/or mental retardation. This disease

is inherited in an X-linked manner so that males are affected through carrier females. A more severe deficiency of the same enzyme leads to the development of the Lesch-Nyhan syndrome.

Several families are described in which there is increased activity of the enzyme PRPP synthetase (reaction 3, Fig. 92-4). The mutant enzymes, of which three different types are recognized, all exhibit increased activity, resulting in increased intracellular concentrations of PRPP, accelerated purine biosynthesis, and elevated excretion of uric acid. The inheritance pattern in this disease is also X-linked. These patients, like those with partial hypoxanthine-guanine phosphoribosyltransferase deficiency, generally develop gout in the second or third decade and have a high incidence of uric acid stones.

These two inborn errors of purine metabolism, hypoxanthine-guanine phosphoribosyltransferase deficiency and PRPP synthetase overactivity, account for less than 15 percent of all patients with what is now considered to be primary hyperuricemia associated with an overproduction of uric acid. The cause of the overproduction in the majority of patients has not been defined (idiopathic).

There are numerous causes of secondary hyperuricemia associated with an increased production of uric acid. In some, the increased excretion of uric acid is related, as it is in primary gout, to an accelerated rate of purine biosynthesis de novo. Patients with glucose 6-phosphatase deficiency (type I glycogen storage disease) uniformly exhibit an increased production of uric acid as well as an accelerated rate of purine biosynthesis de novo (see Chap. 97). It is postulated that patients with this enzyme defect also have an increased concentration of PRPP, which in turn is responsible for the accelerated rate of purine biosynthesis and uric acid overproduction. Patients with the Lesch-Nyhan syndrome, which is due to a virtually complete deficiency of hypoxanthine-guanine phosphoribosyltransferase, also uniformly exhibit a profound overproduction of uric acid and an accelerated rate of purine biosynthesis de novo. In these patients, as in those with gout due to a partial deficiency of hypoxanthine-guanine phosphoribosyltransfer-

FIGURE 92-4

Outline of purine metabolism: (1) amidophosphoribosyltransferase; (2) hypoxanthine guanine phosphoribosyltransferase; (3) PRPP synthetase; (4) adenine phosphoribosyltransferase; (5) adenosine deaminase; (6) purine nucleoside phosphorylase; (7) 5'-nucleotidase; (8) xanthine oxidase.

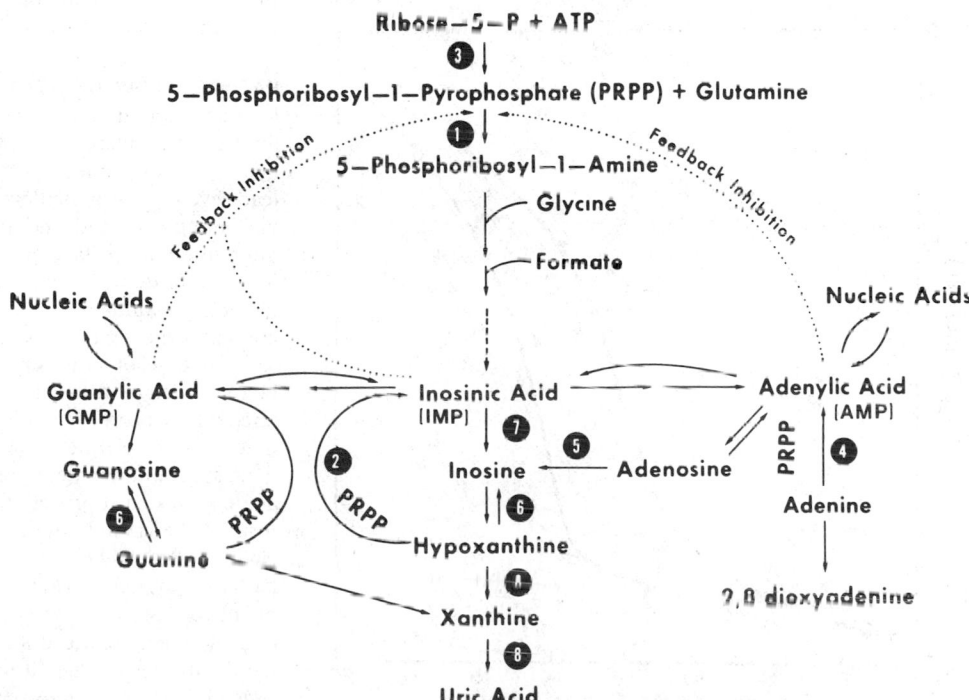

ase, the basic mechanism is thought to be related to a decreased consumption of PRPP.

In the majority of patients with secondary hyperuricemia due to an overproduction of uric acid, the predominant abnormality appears to be an increased turnover of nucleic acids. A number of diseases, including the myeloproliferative and lymphoproliferative disorders, multiple myeloma, secondary polycythemia, pernicious anemia, certain hemoglobinopathies, thalassemia, other hemolytic anemias, infectious mononucleosis, and some carcinomas may be associated with increased marrow activity or increased cell turnover at other sites and an associated increased turnover of nucleic acids. The increased turnover in nucleic acids leads in turn to hyperuricemia, hyperuricaciduria, and a compensatory increase in the rate of purine biosynthesis de novo.

Reduced excretion A large proportion of gouty subjects require a plasma urate value of 1 to 2 mg per 100 ml higher than normal subjects to achieve a given rate of uric acid excretion (Fig. 92-5). This abnormality is most prominent in the gouty subject with a normal production of uric acid and is not present in most subjects with overproduction of uric acid.

The excretion of urate is dependent on glomerular filtration, tubular reabsorption, and tubular secretion. Uric acid appears to be completely filtered at the glomerulus and reabsorbed in the proximal tubule (i.e., presecretory reabsorption). Uric acid secretion then occurs in a subsequent segment of the proximal tubule, and partial reabsorption takes place at a second reabsorptive site in the distal portion of the proximal tubule (i.e., postsecretory reabsorption). While some uric acid reabsorption may also occur in the ascending limb of the loop of Henle and in the collecting duct, these latter two sites are

FIGURE 92-5

Rate of uric acid excretion at various plasma urate levels in nongouty (solid symbols) and gouty (open symbols) subjects. Large symbols represent mean values; small symbols represent individual data of a few mean values selected to illustrate the degree of scatter within groups. Studies were conducted under basal conditions, after RNA feeding, and after infusions of lithium urate. (From Wyngaarden. Reproduced by permission of Academic Press.)

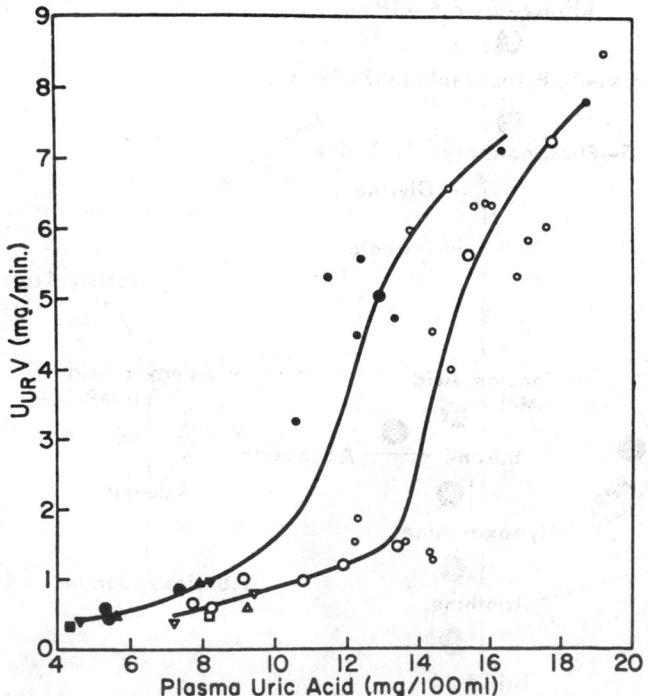

thought to be quantitatively less important. Attempts to define further the location and nature of these latter sites and to quantify their contribution to uric acid transport in normal humans or in various disease states have been largely unrewarding.

Theoretically, the altered renal excretion of uric acid exhibited by most patients with gout could be due to (1) reduced filtration of uric acid, (2) enhanced reabsorption, or (3) decreased secretion. While there are no unequivocal data to establish any one of these three mechanisms as the basic defect, it seems likely that all three types of abnormalities will be found to be operative within the gouty population.

Numerous secondary causes of hyperuricemia and gout can also be attributed to a decrease in the renal excretion of uric acid. A reduction in the glomerular filtration rate leads to a decrease in the filtered load of uric acid and thus to hyperuricemia; patients with renal disease are hyperuricemic on this basis. Other factors, such as decreased secretion of uric acid, have been postulated in patients with some types of renal disease (e.g., polycystic kidney disease and lead nephropathy). Gout is a rare complication of the secondary hyperuricemia due to renal disease.

Diuretic therapy is one of the most important causes of secondary hyperuricemia. Diuretic-induced volume depletion leads to enhanced tubular reabsorption of uric acid as well as decreased uric acid filtration. Decreased secretion of uric acid has also been postulated as a possible mechanism in diuretic-induced hyperuricemia. A number of other drugs lead to hyperuricemia by undefined renal mechanisms; these agents include low-dose aspirin, pyrazinamide, nicotinic acid, ethambutol, and ethanol.

Impaired renal excretion of uric acid is thought to be an important mechanism for the hyperuricemia associated with several disease states. Volume depletion may be important in patients with hyperuricemia associated with adrenal insufficiency and nephrogenic diabetes insipidus. In some situations hyperuricemia has been attributed to competitive inhibition of uric acid secretion by excess organic acids thought to be secreted by the same renal tubular mechanism responsible for uric acid secretion. Examples include starvation (ketosis and free fatty acids), alcoholic ketosis, diabetic ketoacidosis, maple syrup urine disease, and lactic acidosis of any cause. Hyperuricemia in conditions such as hyperparathyroidism, hypoparathyroidism, pseudohypoparathyroidism, and hypothyroidism may also have a renal basis, but the mechanism is unclear.

PATHOGENESIS OF ACUTE GOUTY ARTHRITIS The events leading to the initial crystallization of monosodium urate in a joint after an average of 30 years of asymptomatic hyperuricemia are not completely understood. Sustained hyperuricemia leads eventually to the development of microtophi in the synovial lining cells and perhaps to an accumulation of monosodium urate in cartilage on proteoglycans that have a high affinity for urate. By one of several mechanisms, probably including trauma with disruption of the microtophi and increased turnover of the cartilage proteoglycans, there is an episodic release of urate crystals into the synovial fluid. Other factors, such as a lower temperature in the joint space or an unequal reabsorption of water and urate from the synovial fluid, may accelerate urate precipitation.

A sufficient number of crystals in the joint space triggers the acute attack by a process that appears to include (1) phagocytosis of the crystals by leukocytes with the rapid release of a chemotactic protein from the leukocytes, (2) activation of the kallikrein system, (3) activation of complement with the consequent formation of the chemotactic complement components, and (4) the ultimate urate-mediated disruption of lysosomes within the leukocytes, leading to destruction of white blood cells and release of lysosomal products into the synovial fluid.

While progress in the understanding of acute gouty arthritis has occurred, questions about factors responsible for spontaneous resolution of the acute attack and the effect of colchicine remain to be completely answered.

TREATMENT   The therapeutic aims in gout are (1) to terminate the acute attack as promptly and gently as possible; (2) to prevent recurrences of acute gouty arthritis; (3) to prevent or reverse complications of the disease resulting from deposition of monosodium urate crystals in joints, kidneys, and other sites; (4) to prevent or reverse associated features such as obesity, hypertriglyceridemia, or hypertension; and (5) to prevent formation of uric acid kidney stones.

Treatment of the acute gouty attack   Acute gouty arthritis is treated with an anti-inflammatory agent. Colchicine is the drug most frequently employed. Standard therapy involves administration of 0.5 mg each hour or 1.0 mg every 2 hours by mouth until one of three things occurs: (1) the patient improves, (2) gastrointestinal side effects develop, or (3) a maximum of 6 mg is taken without relief. Colchicine is most effective if therapy is begun shortly after the onset of symptoms. Over 75 percent of patients with gout show major improvement in symptoms within the first 12 h of treatment. However, as many as 80 percent of patients are unable to tolerate an optimal dose because of gastrointestinal side effects, which may precede or coincide with clinical improvement. Intravenous administration of colchicine eliminates the gastrointestinal side effects for the majority and also provides a more rapid response.

Colchicine levels become high in leukocytes, remain constant for 24 h, and are detectable for over 10 days after a single intravenous infusion. As an initial dose 2 mg should be given intravenously, followed by two additional doses of 1 mg at 6-h intervals if needed. Special care must be taken in the intravenous administration of colchicine. The drug is irritative and can lead to severe pain and necrosis if allowed to extravasate to surrounding tissues. It is important to make certain that the intravenous route is secure and that the drug is diluted with 5 to 10 volumes of normal saline and infused over a period of no less than 5 min. Colchicine by either oral or parenteral route may cause bone marrow depression, alopecia, hepatocellular failure, mental depression, seizures, ascending paralysis, respiratory depression, and death. Toxic effects are more likely in patients with significant hepatic, bone marrow, or renal disease and in those subjects on prophylactic maintenance colchicine. The dosage should be reduced for these individuals, and the drug should not be used in neutropenic patients.

Other anti-inflammatory agents, including indomethacin, phenylbutazone, naproxen, and fenoprofen, are also effective in the treatment of acute gouty arthritis. Indomethacin may be given at a dose of 75 mg orally, followed by 50 mg every 6 h and continued at that dose for 24 h after relief is obtained. The drug is then tapered to 50 mg every 8 h for three doses, and then to 25 mg every 8 h for three doses. Side effects of indomethacin include gastrointestinal toxicity, sodium retention, and complaints referable to the central nervous system. While the incidence of side effects may be as high as 60 percent in patients taking the doses described above, the drug is generally better tolerated than colchicine and probably is the treatment of choice in the patient with a well-established diagnosis of acute gouty arthritis. To improve the therapeutic response and thus diminish morbidity of the disease, the patient may be instructed to begin therapy with an anti-inflammatory agent at the first twinge of an acute attack.

Prophylaxis   Once the acute episode has resolved, a number of measures can reduce the likelihood of recurrence. These include (1) the institution of prophylactic daily colchicine or indomethacin, (2) controlled weight reduction for the obese pa-

tient, (3) avoidance of known precipitating factors such as heavy alcohol consumption or a diet rich in purines, and (4) the institution of antihyperuricemic therapy.

The administration of small daily doses of colchicine for prophylaxis against further acute attacks is effective. A program of 1 to 2 mg colchicine a day is completely successful in about three-fourths of patients with gout and fails completely in only about 5 percent. In addition, this program is safe and essentially free of side effects. However, unless serum urate is maintained at normal levels, the patient is spared only acute arthritis and may well proceed to develop other manifestations of gout. Maintenance colchicine therapy is particularly helpful during the first year or two after institution of antihyperuricemic drugs.

Prevention or reversal of the deposition of monosodium urate in tissues   Antihyperuricemic agents are effective in reducing serum urate concentration and should be used in patients with (1) one or more attacks of acute gouty arthritis, (2) one or more tophi, and (3) uric acid nephrolithiasis. The aim of antihyperuricemic therapy is to maintain the serum urate below 7.0 mg per 100 ml, the minimal concentration at which urate saturates the extracellular fluid. Reduction to these levels may be achieved by use of drugs that increase the renal excretion of uric acid or decrease uric acid production. Antihyperuricemic drugs generally do not have anti-inflammatory properties. Uricosuric agents reduce serum urate by enhancing the renal excretion. While a large number of drugs exhibit this property, the most effective agents available in the United States are probenecid and sulfinpyrazone. Probenecid is usually started in doses of 250 mg twice a day; it is increased over a period of several weeks to the dose necessary to achieve effective reversal of the hyperuricemia. A total dose of 1 g per day is appropriate for half of patients; the maximum dose should not exceed 3.0 g per day. Because the half-life is 6 to 12 h, it should be given in two to four evenly spaced doses per day. Hypersensitivity, skin rash, and gastrointestinal complaints are the major side effects. Although serious toxicity is rare, side effects may cause up to a third of the patients to discontinue probenecid.

Sulfinpyrazone is a metabolite of phenylbutazone with no anti-inflammatory activity. The drug is usually started at a dose of 50 mg twice a day and gradually increased to a maintenance level of 300 to 400 mg per day given in three or four divided doses. The maximum effective daily dose is 800 mg. Side effects are similar to those with probenecid, although the incidence of bone marrow toxicity may be higher. Approximately a fourth of patients stop the drug for one reason or another.

Probenecid and sulfinpyrazone are effective in 75 to 80 percent of patients with hyperuricemia and gout. In addition to intolerance, failures can result from poor patient compliance, concomitant salicylate ingestion, or impaired renal function. Aspirin at any dose blocks the uricosuric effect of probenecid and sulfinpyrazone. These agents begin to lose effectiveness as the creatinine clearance falls below 80 ml/min and are completely ineffective when clearance reaches 30 ml/min.

During the negative urate balance that commences upon initiation of uricosuric therapy, the serum urate value drops, and urinary uric acid excretion is elevated above pretreatment levels. With continuation of therapy excess urate is mobilized and eliminated, the serum urate falls, and uric acid excretion returns essentially to pretreatment levels. The transient increase in uric acid excretion, which usually lasts for only a few days, may lead to the development of renal calculi in as many as 9 percent of patients so treated. To avoid this complication uricosuric agents should be started at low doses and gradually increased as described. Maintaining an ample urine flow with adequate hydration and alkalinizing the urine with oral sodium bicarbonate alone or in combination with acetazolamide reduce the likelihood of stone formation. The ideal candidate for uricosuric agents is under 60 years old and has normal renal function (creatinine clearance greater than 80 ml/min), uric acid excretion of less than 700 mg per day on a general diet, and no history of renal stones.

Hyperuricemia may also be controlled by allopurinol, a drug that decreases uric acid synthesis. Allopurinol inhibits xanthine oxidase (reaction 8, Fig. 92-4), the enzyme that catalyzes the oxidation of hypoxanthine to xanthine and xanthine to uric acid. While allopurinol has a half-life in vivo of only 2 to 3 h, it is metabolized largely to oxipurinol, which also is an effective inhibitor of xanthine oxidase and has a half-life ranging from 18 to 30 h. In most patients 300 mg per day represents an effective antihyperuricemic dose. Because of the long half-life of the major metabolite the drug may be administered once a day with no loss of effectiveness. Since oxipurinol is largely excreted in the urine, its half-life is prolonged in patients with renal insufficiency. The dose of allopurinol should, therefore, be reduced by one-half in patients with significant renal dysfunction.

The significant side affects of allopurinol include gastrointestinal distress, skin rashes, fever, toxic epidermal necrolysis, alopecia, bone marrow suppression, hepatitis, jaundice, and vasculitis. The overall incidence of side effects is about 20 percent. Toxic effects appear to be more common in the presence of renal insufficiency. In only 5 percent of patients are the side effects sufficiently distressing to force discontinuation of the medication. Important drug-drug interactions involving allopurinol include prolongation of the half-lives of 6-mercaptopurine and azathioprine and enhancement of the toxicity of cyclophosphamide.

Specific indications for choosing allopurinol over a uricosuric drug include (1) an increased urinary uric acid excretion (greater than 700 mg per day on a general diet), (2) impairment of renal function with a creatinine clearance less than 80 ml/min, (3) tophaceous gout regardless of renal function, (4) uric acid nephrolithiasis, and (5) gout not controlled by uricosuric agents because of ineffectiveness or intolerance. Allopurinol and a uricosuric drug may be used simultaneously in the rare hyperuricemic patient who cannot be controlled by a single medication. The addition of allopurinol to a program that includes a uricosuric drug usually results in further lowering of the serum urate concentration. No modification in the dosage of either agent is required with combination therapy.

Acute gouty arthritis may occur whenever there is a rapid and substantial change in the serum urate concentration. Thus, the initiation of antihyperuricemic therapy with any agent may precipitate an acute attack of gouty arthritis. In addition, recurrent attacks may occur for a year or longer when large tophaceous deposits are present, even if hyperuricemia is controlled. For these reasons, it is prudent to begin prophylactic therapy with colchicine just prior to initiation of antihyperuricemic drugs, and to continue it until the serum urate is controlled for at least a year or until all tophi have resolved. Patients should be warned of the possibility of flare-up during the early phase of therapy. While it is usually not necessary to limit purine intake in most gouty patients, strict dietary purine restriction should be instituted in patients with severe tophaceous gout and/or renal failure.

Prevention and treatment of acute uric acid nephropathy Immediate and vigorous therapy is essential for acute uric acid nephropathy. The first step is to increase urine flow by vigorous hydration coupled with administration of a potent diuretic such as furosemide. The urine should be alkalinized to achieve conversion of uric acid to the more soluble monosodium urate. Alkalinization can be accomplished by the administration of sodium bicarbonate alone or by the simultaneous administration of sodium bicarbonate and acetazolamide. Allopurinol therapy should also be employed to reduce uric acid formation. The initial dose in this setting should be 8 mg/kg per day given as a single daily dose. The dose should be decreased after 3 or 4 days to 100 to 200 mg per day if renal insufficiency persists. Principles of treatment for uric acid kidney stones are similar to those described for acute uric acid nephropathy. In most cases of uric acid nephrolithiasis allopurinol therapy combined only with high fluid intake is effective.

WORKUP OF THE HYPERURICEMIC PATIENT Evaluation of the patient with hyperuricemia is directed toward (1) defining the cause of the hyperuricemia (which may disclose an important disease other than gout), (2) assessing the presence and extent of damage to tissues and organs, and (3) identifying associated abnormalities. From a practical standpoint these inquiries are pursued simultaneously, since decisions about the significance of hyperuricemia and about therapy depend on the answers to all of these.

History Is the hyperuricemia primary or secondary? Is the patient asymptomatic? Has there been hypertension or a history of cardiovascular disease? Is there a family history of hyperuricemia, gout, kidney stones, or renal disease? Is there a history of lead exposure?

Physical examination Are the joints normal? Are tophi present? Is there evidence of atherosclerosis? Are there features suggestive of a secondary cause of hyperuricemia, such as lymphadenopathy, splenomegaly, or hepatomegaly? Is the patient obese?

Initial laboratory test data The most important single test in the hyperuricemic patient is analysis of the urine for uric acid. If a history of stone disease is present, a flat plate of the abdomen and intravenous pyelogram may be indicated. If a renal stone is recovered, analysis for uric acid and other constituents is useful. If joint disease is present, synovial fluid analysis and x-rays of the involved joints are helpful. If there is a history of exposure to lead, measurement of urinary lead excretion after an infusion of calcium EDTA may be useful in documenting the presence of gout due to lead exposure. In cases where the patient appears to be an overproducer, measurement of erythrocyte hypoxanthine-guanine phosphoribosyltransferase and PRPP synthetase levels may be indicated.

Management of asymptomatic hyperuricemia There is considerable controversy about the indications for therapy of the patient with asymptomatic hyperuricemia. Generally, treatment should be withheld unless the patient (1) becomes symptomatic; (2) has a strong family history for gout, nephrolithiasis, or renal failure; or (3) is excreting large quantities of uric acid (greater than 1100 mg per day).

OTHER DISORDERS OF PURINE METABOLISM Lesch-Nyhan syndrome The Lesch-Nyhan syndrome is an X-linked disorder, which was described in 1964. Affected patients have hyperuricemia and a profound overproduction of uric acid. In addition, they have a bizarre neurologic disorder characterized by self-mutilation, choreoathetosis, spasticity, and retardation of growth and mental function. The incidence is estimated at 1:100,000 births. The characteristic biochemical abnormality is a profound deficiency of the enzyme hypoxanthine-guanine phosphoribosyltransferase (reaction 2, Fig. 92-4).

Adenine phosphoribosyltransferase deficiency Adenine phosphoribosyltransferase catalyzes the conversion of adenine to AMP (reaction 4, Fig. 92-4). The first family with a deficiency of adenine phosphoribosyltransferase was discovered in 1968. These subjects were heterozygous for deficiency of the enzyme and had no associated disease. It subsequently became apparent that heterozygosity for this deficiency is common, perhaps as frequent as 1:100. A homozygous deficiency of adenine phosphoribosyltransferase has now been described in three patients with a history of renal stones composed of 2,8-dioxyadenine. Because of chemical similarity, 2,8-dioxyadenine may be confused with uric acid, and in each of these patients an incorrect diagnosis of uric acid nephrolithiasis was made initially.

Adenosine deaminase deficiency and purine nucleoside phosphorylase deficiency Adenosine deaminase catalyzes the deamination of adenosine to inosine (reaction 5, Fig. 92-4). Patients with adenosine deaminase deficiency have severe combined immunodeficiency disease, i.e., a severe abnormality in T-cell function and somewhat milder B-cell dysfunction.

Deficiency of purine nucleoside phosphorylase (reaction 6, Fig. 92-4), the enzyme that catalyzes the conversion of inosine to hypoxanthine and guanosine to guanine also causes combined immunodeficiency disease. These two inborn errors of purine metabolism represent the first enzyme defects to be associated with immune dysfunction.

Xanthine oxidase deficiency Xanthine oxidase catalyzes the oxidation of hypoxanthine to xanthine, xanthine to uric acid, and adenine to 2,8-dioxyadenine (reaction 8, Fig. 92-4). Xanthinuria, the first inborn error of purine metabolism to be defined at the enzyme level, is due to a deficiency of xanthine oxidase. As a result, affected patients with xanthinuria have hypouricemia and hypouricaciduria as well as an increased urinary excretion of the oxypurines, hypoxanthine, and xanthine. Half are asymptomatic and a third have urinary xanthine stones. Several patients have been noted to have a myopathy and one patient with polyarthritis has been reported. Precipitation of xanthine is thought to be the important factor in the development of each of these clinical manifestations.

REFERENCES

GIBLETT ER et al: Adenosine deaminase deficiency in two patients with severely impaired cellular immunity. Lancet 2:1067, 1972

───── et al: Nucleoside-phosphorylase deficiency in a child with severely defective T-cell immunity and normal B-cell immunity. Lancet 1:1010, 1975

KELLEY WN: Crystal-induced arthropathies, in *The Clinics in Rheumatic Diseases*. Philadelphia, Saunders, 1977, vol 3, pp 1–171

───── et al: Hypoxanthine-guanine phosphoribosyltransferase deficiency in gout. Ann Intern Med, 70:155, 1969

SEEGMILLER JE: Diseases of purine and pyrimidine metabolism, in *Duncan's Diseases of Metabolism*, 7th ed, PK Bondy, LE Rosenberg (eds). Philadelphia, Saunders, 1974

TALBOTT JH, YU TF: *Gout and Uric Acid Metabolism*. New York, Stratton, 1976

WYNGAARDEN JB: Gout, in *Advances in Metabolic Disorders*, R Levine, and R Luft (eds). New York, Academic, 1965, vol 2, pp 2–78

─────, Kelley WN: *Gout and Hyperuricemia*. New York, Grune & Stratton, 1976

─────, ─────: Gout, in *The Metabolic Basis of Inherited Diseases*, 4th ed, JB Stanbury et al (eds). New York, McGraw-Hill, 1978, pp 916–1010

93
HEREDITARY OROTIC ACIDURIA

WILLIAM N. KELLEY

Hereditary orotic aciduria is a rare disorder of pyrimidine metabolism usually characterized by retarded growth and development, hypochromic anemia associated with a megaloblastic marrow unresponsive to usual hematinic therapy, and excessive urinary excretion of orotic acid. The first patient with orotic aciduria was recognized and reported by Huguley and coworkers in 1959. Since that time eight additional cases have been described.

PATHOGENESIS The synthesis of pyrimidine nucleotides de novo is outlined in Fig. 93-1. Orotic aciduria occurs when the rate of synthesis of orotic acid exceeds the rate at which it is converted to orotidine 5'-monophosphate in the reaction catalyzed by orotate phosphoribosyltransferase. Patients with hereditary orotic aciduria have a genetically determined deficiency of orotate phosphoribosyltransferase and orotidine 5'-phosphate decarboxylase (type 1) or of orotidine 5'-phosphate decarboxylase alone (type 2). In the former the capacity of the cell to convert orotic acid to orotidine 5'-monophosphate is reduced. In the latter it is assumed that orotidine 5'-phosphate accumulates and thus inhibits orotate phosphoribosyltransferase activity. The two enzymes, orotate phosphoribosyltransferase and orotidine 5'-phosphate decarboxylase, are intimately associated in a complex. In patients with the double enzyme defect, it has been proposed that a mutation affecting the structure of orotate phosphoribosyltransferase destabilizes the complex, leading to the concomitant loss of orotidine 5'-phosphate decarboxylase activity.

Patients with both types of hereditary orotic aciduria excrete 600 to 1500 mg orotic acid in the urine per day, 3000 to 5000 times normal. In addition, patients excrete 15 to 30 mg orotidine per day, 20 to 40 times normal.

The clinical manifestations of hereditary orotic aciduria are due to (1) increased excretion of orotic acid and (2) pyrimidine nucleotide deficiency. Accumulation of orotic acid per se is harmful in that it may crystallize in the urine and obstruct urine flow. Orotidine is more soluble than orotic acid and does not form stones. The remaining clinical features of hereditary orotic aciduria are due to deficiency of nucleic acid precursors.

CLINICAL FEATURES The most specific early finding in patients with hereditary orotic aciduria is severe hypochromic anemia with marked anisocytosis and poikilocytosis, associated with erythroid hyperplasia and atypical megaloblastic changes in the bone marrow. Leukopenia but not thrombocytopenia is also a consistent finding. The megaloblastosis probably results from a selective defect of DNA synthesis which interferes with mitosis. The megaloblasts in hereditary orotic aciduria are not as large as in pernicious anemia or folic acid deficiency, but the cellular abnormalities in orotic aciduria are more pronounced in the more mature red blood cell precursors. The degree of microcytosis and hypochromia in circulating erythrocytes also differentiates this from other megaloblastic anemias. Typically, poor growth and development are evident during the first few months of life with lassitude, pallor, and nonspecific failure to thrive. While no characteristic neurological picture exists, most patients appear to have some mental retardation. Orotic acid crystalluria is uniformly present, and urinary tract obstruction occurs in about half.

GENETICS Orotic aciduria is transmitted as an autosomal recessive disease. Heterozygotes are asymptomatic and excrete only slightly increased amounts of orotic acid in the urine.

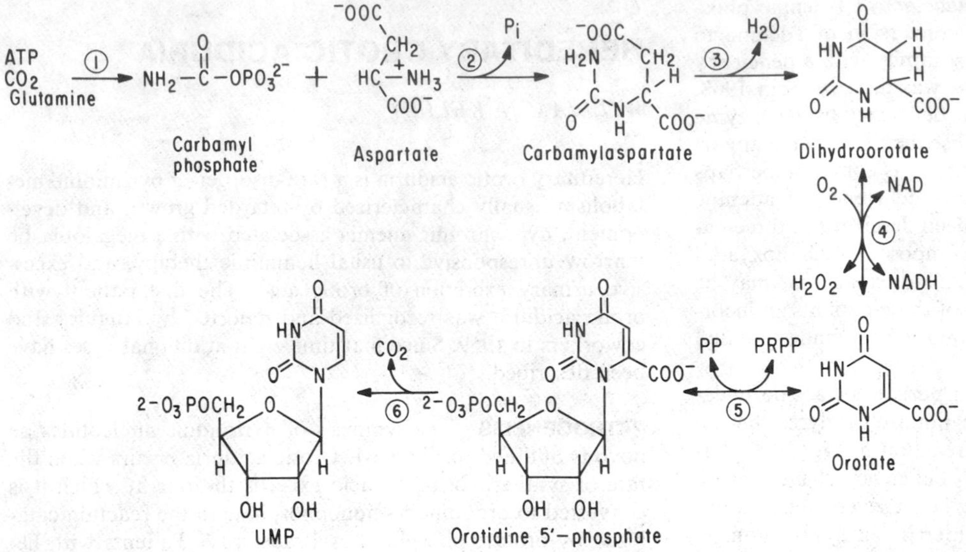

FIGURE 93-1

Pyrimidine biosynthesis de novo. (1) Carbamyl phosphate synthetase, (2) aspartate transcarbamylase, (3) dihydroorotase, (4) dihydroorotic acid dehydrogenase, (5) orotate phosphoribosyltransferase, and (6) orotidine 5'-monophosphate decarboxylase.

TREATMENT The hematologic abnormalities and the retardation of growth and development respond promptly and completely to doses of uridine in the range of 100 to 150 mg/kg per day. Uridine is converted directly to uridine 5'-phosphate in the reaction catalyzed by the enzyme uridine kinase, thus bypassing the enzymatic defect and correcting the pyrimidine nucleotide deficiency and the deficiency in nucleic acid synthesis. Uridine therapy also produces a substantial decrease in the urinary excretion of orotic acid, probably by virtue of the increased levels of pyrimidine nucleotides and the consequent inhibition of pyrimidine biosynthesis de novo. The fatal outcome of untreated hereditary orotic aciduria as well as the residual impairment of mental function that may occur serves to emphasize the importance of early diagnosis and treatment.

Glucocorticoid therapy causes partial hematologic remission without reversal of the megaloblastic changes in the bone marrow. Oral administration of a mixture of yeast nucleotides has also been associated with rapid improvement in the general clinical state with hematologic remission and a decrease in urinary orotic acid. This preparation, however, is not well tolerated because of gastrointestinal side effects.

OTHER CAUSES OF OROTIC ACIDURIA Drugs such as allopurinol, oxipurinol, and azauridine produce modest orotic aciduria and orotidinuria. In each case one or more nucleotide derivatives of the drug are potent inhibitors of orotidine 5'-phosphate decarboxylase. There is no evidence that patients develop a significant deficiency of pyrimidine nucleotides.

5-Phosphoribosyl-1-pyrophosphate (PRPP) is an essential and rate-limiting substrate for the orotate phosphoribosyltransferase reaction. A low intracellular level of PRPP as, for example, in a patient unable to synthesize PRPP due to PRPP synthetase deficiency is also associated with orotic aciduria, megaloblastic anemia, and mental retardation.

Several disorders of the urea cycle, including ornithine transcarbamylase deficiency, argininosuccinic aciduria, and citrullinemia, lead to orotic aciduria. In each of these diseases, carbamyl phosphate utilization in the urea cycle is reduced, and its availability for pyrimidine biosynthesis is enhanced. This shift in carbamyl phosphate utilization to the pyrimidine pathway appears to enhance the rate of pyrimidine biosynthesis de novo up to at least the step of orotic acid formation.

REFERENCES

HUGULEY CM et al: Refractory megaloblastic anemia associated with excretion of orotic acid. Blood 14:615, 1959

KELLEY WN, SMITH LH: Hereditary orotic aciduria, in *The Metabolic Basis of Inherited Diseases,* 4th ed, JB Stanbury et al (eds). New York, McGraw-Hill, 1978, pp 1045–1071

Disorders of metals and metallo proteins

HEPATOMA → 358

94
HEMOCHROMATOSIS

LAWRIE W. POWELL
KURT J. ISSELBACHER

DEFINITION Hemochromatosis (bronze diabetes) is an iron-storage disorder in which an excessive iron absorption and/or parenteral iron loading results in parenchymal deposition of iron with eventual tissue damage and functional insufficiency of the organs involved, especially the liver, pancreas, heart, and pituitary. The increased iron stores may result from one or more different mechanisms (see below). The inherited form of the disease known as *idiopathic hemochromatosis* is now increasingly recognized during its early stages when the iron overload is of lesser degree and organ damage minimal. At this stage the disease is referred to as *latent* or *precirrhotic hemochromatosis.* The first clinical description of the disease was given by Trousseau in 1865; in 1889 von Recklinghausen named the disease *hemochromatosis* and the iron-storage pigment *hemosiderin* because he believed it was derived from the blood.

♂ > ♀   5-10:1

INCIDENCE Hemochromatosis is a rare disease. Estimates of its prevalence have ranged from 1 in 20,000 hospital admissions to 2.5 per 10,000 necropsies and 1 in 10,000 of the white Anglo-Saxon population. It is observed five to ten times more frequently in males than in females. Nearly 70 percent of all patients develop their first symptoms between age 40 and 60. The disease is rarely clinically evident below age 20.

PATHOGENESIS The disease is observed in the following types of patients: (1) those with idiopathic (primary, familial, hereditary) hemochromatosis; (2) those with a defect in hemoglobin synthesis associated with ineffective erythropoiesis (erythropoietic hemochromatosis); (3) those with excessive oral iron intake over many years, usually from an alcoholic beverage, for example, in certain South African Negroes.

Idiopathic hemochromatosis is the consequence of an abnormality in the regulatory mechanism for iron absorption, the nature of which is unknown. The resulting progressive accumulation of iron is reflected in an early increase in the plasma iron and percentage saturation of transferrin. In advanced disease, the tissues contain over 20 g iron; total body iron normally is in the range of 3 to 5 g. The excess iron is deposited mainly in parenchymal cells of the liver, pancreas, and heart. Iron in the liver and pancreas increases 50- to 100-fold; in the heart, 5- to 25-fold; in the spleen, kidney, and skin, about 5-fold. Tissue injury may result from disruption of iron-laden lysosomes. The recent demonstration of an increased incidence of certain histocompatability antigens (viz., HLA-A3, HLA-B14, and HLA-B7) has confirmed the genetic basis for the disease. The mode of inheritance is autosomal recessive although more than one form of the disease may exist. It has been suggested that homozygotes have large iron stores and manifest the disease; heterozygotes tend to have normal or slightly elevated iron stores and develop the disease only when added factors such as alcohol, anemia, or increased oral iron intake contribute to an accumulation of iron in excess of their usual stores.

Erythropoietic hemochromatosis is observed in association with chronic disorders of erythropoiesis, particularly in those with a defect in hemoglobin synthesis and ineffective erythropoiesis. Also in this group of disorders the absorption of iron is increased, and such patients are frequently treated with medicinal iron and transfusions. Erythropoietic hemochromatosis has been observed primarily in patients with sideroblastic anemia and thalassemia. Porphyria cutanea tarda, a disorder characterized by a defect in porphyrin biosynthesis, is also associated with excessive parenchymal iron deposits; however, the magnitude of the iron load is usually insufficient to produce tissue damage.

Alcoholic subjects with chronic liver disease may show evidence of hemochromatosis. Such patients are probably heterozygotes in whom iron accumulation has been accentuated by alcohol. There is evidence that alcohol may enhance iron absorption. Ineffective erythropoiesis in association with folate deficiency or an abnormality in pyridoxal phosphate metabolism may be a complicating factor in some patients. In addition, alcoholic beverages, particularly red wine, may contain appreciable quantities of iron.

Excessive iron ingestion over many years may, in certain circumstances, result in the syndrome of hemochromatosis. This occurs, for example, in certain South African Negroes (Bantu) in whom the intake of excessive iron in an alcoholic beverage results from the practice of brewing fermented beverages in vessels made of iron. There are a few isolated reports of the development of hemochromatosis in normal subjects taking medicinal iron over many years, but it is possible that such subjects have been heterozygous for the inherited trait.

The common denominator in all patients with hemochromatosis is the presence of *excessive amounts of iron in parenchymal tissues* with resultant tissue damage. Parenteral administration of iron in the form of transfusions or iron preparations results in *reticuloendothelial cell* iron overload. Only in patients with an abnormality in erythropoiesis does the parenteral administration of iron result in deposition of iron in parenchymal tissues.

PATHOLOGY At autopsy the enlarged, nodular liver and pancreas present a striking ochre color. Histologically iron is found in increased amounts in many organs, particularly in the liver and pancreas and to a lesser extent in the endocrine glands and the heart. A notable exception is the testis, the iron content of which is relatively low despite the fact that gonadal failure is a characteristic and early feature of the disease. In contrast, the pituitary gland is almost always involved. The epidermis of the skin is thin, and increased *melanin* is found in the cells of the basal layer. Deposits of iron are observed around the synovial lining cells of the joints, and calcium pyrophosphate crystals may be seen to lie within deposits of calcium embedded in the synovial tissue.

As indicated above, iron deposition in the liver of patients with idiopathic hemochromatosis occurs predominantly in the parenchymal cells in the form of hemosiderin. In the early stages, hemosiderin is deposited in the periportal parenchyma being found within lysosomes in the pericanalicular cytoplasm of the hepatocytes. This stage progresses to perilobular fibrosis and deposition of iron in bile duct epithelium, Kupffer cells, and fibrous septa. Inflammatory cells are few in contrast to prominent proliferation of bile ductules. Wedge biopsy specimens show a characteristic pattern of fibrosis with dense fibrous septa surrounding groups of lobules somewhat analogous to the pattern seen in chronic biliary disease. In the advanced stage, an irregular multilobular cirrhosis of postnecrotic type develops.

CLINICAL MANIFESTATIONS The symptoms and signs of hemochromatosis are related to skin pigmentation, diabetes, liver and cardiac impairment, arthropathy, and hypogonadism. The initial symptoms most frequently encountered are weakness, lassitude, weight loss, change in skin color, abdominal pain, loss of libido, and symptoms related to the onset of diabetes. Hepatomegaly, pigmentation, spider angiomas, splenomegaly, arthropathy, ascites, cardiac arrhythmias, congestive heart failure, loss of body hair, testicular atrophy, and jaundice are the most prominent physical signs.

The *liver* is usually the first organ to be damaged, and hepatomegaly is present in more than 95 percent of symptomatic cases. Hepatic enlargement may exist in the absence of symptoms or in the presence of normal liver function tests. Indeed, over half the patients with symptomatic hemochromatosis have little or no laboratory evidence of functional impairment of the liver, in spite of hepatomegaly and fibrosis. Loss of body hair, palmar erythema, testicular atrophy, and gynecomastia are often seen. Manifestations of portal hypertension and esophageal varices may occur but are less commonly observed than in Laennec's cirrhosis. Splenomegaly is present in approximately half the cases. Hepatocellular carcinoma develops in about 35 percent. The incidence of this last complication increases with age and is now the most common cause of death in treated patients.

Excessive *skin pigmentation* is present in about 90 percent of the patients at the time the diagnosis is established. Pigmentation is largely due to *melanin* deposition, and in some instances there may also be some increase in iron. Melanin deposition usually gives rise to bronzing. The characteristic metallic gray hue is believed to result from the presence of increased melanin or both melanin and iron in the dermis. Pigmentation usually is diffuse and generalized, but frequently it is deeper on the face, neck, extensor aspects of the lower forearms, dorsa of the hands, lower legs, genital regions, and in scars. In only 10 to 15 percent of cases is there demonstrable pigmentation of the oral mucosa. Pigmentation of the hard palate and retina has been described.

Diabetes and symptoms therefrom develop in about 65 percent of patients. Diabetes is more likely to develop in patients with a family history of diabetes. The presence of a family history of diabetes, the existence of liver disease, and direct damage to the pancreas by iron deposition may all contribute to the development of diabetes in hemochromatosis. The management of the diabetes is similar to that of diabetes mellitus except for a higher incidence of insulin resistance and of insulin fat atrophy. Late degenerative sequelae are the same as in diabetes mellitus.

Arthropathy, which differs from osteoarthritis and rheumatoid arthritis, develops in 25 to 50 percent of patients. It most commonly occurs after the age of 50 but may occur at any time in the course of the disease, even as a first manifestation or long after therapy. The small joints of the hands, especially the second and third metacarpophalangeal joints, are usually the first joints to be involved. A progressive polyarthritis involving wrists, hips, and knees may ensue. Acute brief attacks of synovitis may occur, associated with deposition of calcium pyrophosphate (chondrocalcinosis or pseudogout), chiefly in the knees. Roentgenologic manifestations consist of cystic changes of sclerosis of the subchondral bones, loss of articular cartilage with narrowing of the joint space, diffuse demineralization, and hypertrophic bone proliferation. The mechanism of these abnormalities and their relationship to iron metabolism is not known.

Cardiac involvement is the presenting manifestation in about 15 percent of patients. The most common cardiac manifestation is congestive heart failure. It is observed not infrequently in young adults, and symptoms of congestive failure may develop suddenly, with rapid progression to death if untreated. The heart is diffusely enlarged, and such cases may be misdiagnosed as idiopathic cardiomyopathy if other overt manifestations are absent. A great variety of cardiac arrhythmias may be present, particularly supraventricular beats and paroxysmal tachyarrhythmias. Atrial flutter, atrial fibrillation, and varying degrees of atrioventricular block have also been described.

Loss of libido and *testicular atrophy* are common in hemochromatosis. The former may antedate the other clinical manifestations of the disease. Testicular atrophy is probably due to the decreased production of gonadotropins associated with impaired hypothalamic pituitary function due to iron deposition. Addison's disease, hypothyroidism, and hypoparathyroidism have been described but are exceedingly rare.

DIAGNOSIS The association of (1) hepatomegaly, (2) skin pigmentation, (3) diabetes mellitus, (4) heart disease, (5) arthritis, and (6) evidence of hypogonadism should suggest the diagnosis of hemochromatosis. However, a parenchymal iron overload of insufficient duration or modest degree may exist without any of these clinical manifestations, or with only some of them. Therefore, the diagnosis should be considered in any patient with unexplained hepatomegaly, idiopathic cardiomyopathy, abnormal skin pigmentation, or loss of libido.

The history should be particularly detailed in regard to disease in other members of the family, alcohol ingestion, and iron intake. The blood should be examined for evidence of anemia and abnormal erythropoiesis to rule out iron loading secondary to a hematologic disorder, such as thalassemia or sideroblastic anemia. Confirmation of the presence of liver, pancreatic, cardiac, and joint disease should be obtained by physical examination, roentgenologic examination, and routine function tests of these organs. It then remains to be demonstrated that there is an increase in total body iron stores and, in particular, an increased parenchymal iron concentration associated with tissue damage.

The methods available for the demonstration of excessive parenchymal iron stores include (1) measurement of serum iron, (2) determination of percent saturation of transferrin, (3) estimation of chelatable iron stores using the agent desferrioxamine, (4) measurement of serum ferritin concentration, and (5) liver biopsy (Table 94-1). Each has its inherent advantages and limitations. The serum iron level and percent saturation of transferrin are elevated early in the course of the disease, but their specificity is reduced by relatively high false-positive and false-negative rates. In particular, an increased serum iron concentration may be present is patients with alcoholic liver disease without iron overload; in this situation, however, the iron-binding capacity is usually not decreased as in hemochromatosis.

There has been considerable focus on the serum ferritin concentration as an estimate of body iron stores. In untreated patients with hemochromatosis, the serum ferritin level is greatly increased (Table 94-1). This test is useful as a noninvasive screening test for the diagnosis of early disease, since it is usually abnormal before there is any morphological evidence of liver damage and the ferritin concentration correlates with the magnitude of body iron stores. It will probably, therefore, replace the more cumbersome screening tests involving urinary iron excretion. However, it should be noted that in patients with infection and hepatocellular necrosis serum ferritin levels may be elevated out of proportion to body iron stores. Also, at least three families have been reported in whom serum ferritin levels in relatives have been normal despite increased iron stores; the reason for the latter finding is unclear but would appear to be an exceptional situation. In clinical practice, the *combined measurements* of the (1) serum iron concentration, (2) percent transferrin saturation, and (3) serum ferritin level provide the simplest and most reliable screening test for hemochromatosis, including the precirrhotic phase of the disease. If any of these tests are abnormal, liver biopsy should be performed since it is the *definitive* test for the diagnosis of hemochromatosis. It permits histochemical estimation of tissue iron, measurement of hepatic iron concentration, and assessment of the extent of tissue damage.

TABLE 94-1
Representative iron values in normal subjects and in patients with idiopathic hemochromatosis

Determination	Normal subjects	Patients with idiopathic hemochromatosis
Plasma iron, μg/100 ml	50–150	180–300
Total iron-binding capacity, μg/100 ml	250–370	200–300
Percent transferrin saturation, μg/100 ml	22–46	80–100
Serum ferritin, ng/ml	10–200	900–6000
Urinary iron,* mg/24 h	0–2	9–23
Liver iron, μg/100 mg dry wt	30–140	600–1800

* *After intramuscular administration of 0.5 g desferrioxamine.*

It is of particular importance to examine family members when the diagnosis of idiopathic hemochromatosis is established. Asymptomatic as well as symptomatic family members with the disease will usually have an increase in plasma iron, a decrease in total iron-binding capacity, an increased saturation of transferrin, and an increased serum ferritin concentration. These changes occur even before the iron stores are greatly increased. A liver biopsy should then be performed, since it is imperative to establish the diagnosis and begin therapy before tissue damage occurs. Preliminary studies suggest that affected relatives usually have an HLA haplotype identical with that of the proband.

The differential diagnosis between parenchymal iron overload and reticuloendothelial iron overload is usually not difficult. Reticuloendothelial iron overload is not associated with tissue damage, the plasma iron is not increased, and the urinary excretion of iron after desferrioxamine administration does not exceed 4 mg. The relative degrees of parenchymal iron overload and reticuloendothelial iron overload can be determined definitively by liver biopsy.

The distinction between idiopathic hemochromatosis and alcoholic cirrhosis associated with iron overload is sometimes difficult. In general, patients with alcoholic cirrhosis of the liver have a lesser degree of iron overload, as determined by the plasma iron concentration, serum ferritin concentration, and urinary iron excretion after desferrioxamine administration. The degree of parenchymal iron deposition in liver biopsy specimens from patients with alcoholic cirrhosis is usually mild in comparison with the degree of fibrosis. Reticuloendothelial (RE) iron deposition is often considerable. In idiopathic hemochromatosis there is very little RE iron, and the amount of parenchymal iron is out of proportion to the degree of fibrosis. Family studies will often resolve the problem, particularly if nonalcoholic relatives are affected and HLA antigen typing may be useful.

TREATMENT The therapy of idiopathic hemochromatosis involves the removal of the excess body iron and supportive treatment of damaged organs.

Iron is best removed from the body by weekly or twice weekly phlebotomy of 500 ml. Although there is an initial modest decline in the volume of packed red blood cells to about 35 ml per 100 ml, the anemia stabilizes after several weeks. The plasma iron concentration remains increased until the available iron stores are depleted. Since one 500-ml unit of blood contains from 200 to 250 mg iron and about 25 g iron must be removed, 2 or 3 years of weekly phlebotomy are usually required. When the plasma iron level becomes normal, phlebotomies are performed at such time intervals as are required to maintain a plasma iron concentration of less than 150 µg per 100 ml. Usually one phlebotomy every 3 months will suffice. The adequacy of the therapy may be evaluated at any time by measuring the plasma iron, the percentage of saturation of transferrin with iron, or the urinary iron excretion after desferrioxamine administration. These measurements become abnormal promptly with iron reaccumulation and precede the increase in serum ferritin concentration.

Chelating agents such as desferrioxamine, when given parenterally, remove 10 to 20 mg iron per day, less than half that mobilized by one weekly phlebotomy. Phlebotomy is not only a more effective but also a less expensive, more convenient, and safer treatment for patients with idiopathic hemochromatosis. Chelating agents may be used as a substitute method for iron removal when anemia or hypoproteinemia is severe enough to preclude phlebotomy.

The management of the hepatic failure, cardiac failure, and diabetes differs little from conventional management of these conditions. Loss of libido and change in secondary sex charac-

teristics are partially relieved by testosterone therapy or gonadotropin therapy.

PROGNOSIS The life expectancy of *untreated* patients with idiopathic hemochromatosis after the disease has become clinically manifest averages 4.4 years, but several instances have been recorded of patients living up to 20 or 30 years. The principal causes of death in *untreated* patients are cardiac failure (30 percent), hepatic coma (15 percent), hematemesis (14 percent), hepatocellular carcinoma (14 percent), and pneumonia (12 percent).

Life expectancy is extended to an average of more than 8 years by removal of the excessive stores of iron and maintenance of these stores at near-normal levels. The 5-year survival rate with therapy is increased from 33 to 89 percent. With removal of iron by repeated phlebotomy, the liver and spleen decrease in size, liver function studies return to normal, pigmentation of skin decreases, and cardiac failure is reversed. Carbohydrate tolerance improves in about 40 percent of cases. The fibrosis in the liver may decrease, but cirrhosis is irreversible. Removal of excess iron has little or no effect on hypogonadism or arthropathy. Hepatocellular carcinoma occurs as a late sequela in about one-third of the patients despite adequate iron removal; the apparent increase in its incidence in treated patients is probably related to their increased life span. This complication does not appear to develop if the disease is treated in the precirrhotic stage. Hence, the importance of family screening and early therapy cannot be emphasized too strongly.

REFERENCES

EDWARDS CQ et al: Hereditary hemochromatosis. N Engl J Med 297:7, 1977

HALLIDAY JW et al: Serum ferritin in the diagnosis of early haemochromatosis: A study of 43 families. Lancet 2:621, 1977

PETERS TJ, SEYMOUR CA: Acid hydrolase activities and lysosomal integrity in liver biopsies from patients with iron overload. Clin Sci Mol Med 50:75, 1976

POWELL LW, KERR JFR: The pathology of liver in hemochromatosis, in *Pathobiology Annual,* H Joacim (ed). New York, Appleton Century Crofts, 1975

SIMON M et al: Idiopathic hemochromatosis and iron overload in alcoholic liver disease: Differentiation by HLA phenotype. Gastroenterology 73:655, 1977

95
WILSON'S DISEASE

I. HERBERT SCHEINBERG

Wilson's disease is an inherited autosomal recessive abnormality in the hepatic excretion of copper that results in toxic accumulations of the metal in liver, brain, and other organs. Deficiency of the plasma copper-protein ceruloplasmin is a characteristic feature.

NATURAL HISTORY Normal babies have low plasma concentrations of ceruloplasmin and high concentrations of hepatic copper. During the first year of life ceruloplasmin values rise, and hepatic copper concentrations fall to normal adult levels.

In contrast, serum ceruloplasmin changes very little in Wilson homozygotes, and the concentration of hepatic copper increases steadily with age. However, clinical manifestations of copper excess are rare before age 6, and half of untreated patients remain asymptomatic to age 16.

Wilson's disease presents with hepatic involvement in somewhat less than half of patients. The toxic effects of copper in the liver may be manifest as acute hepatitis, cirrhosis of the liver, or asymptomatic hepatosplenomegaly. The acute hepatitis is similar to viral hepatitis, can be mistaken for infectious mononucleosis, and may evolve in three different ways. The first is a fulminant, sometimes lethal disease characterized by jaundice, malaise, and at times ascites, hypoalbuminemia, and elevated levels of liver enzymes in plasma. In the acute phase sufficient copper may be released into plasma to cause a hemolytic anemia. The disease may not be diagnosed until autopsy or until the diagnosis in a younger sibling leads to retrospective analysis of preserved tissues. Second, there may be insidious development of parenchymal liver disease resulting in a clinical and histological picture indistinguishable from chronic active hepatitis. Third, patients may apparently recover from the hepatitis. Years or decades may elapse with no sign or symptom of disease. In these patients the past history of an episode of hepatitis can be overlooked unless they are questioned carefully.

More frequently, the copper-induced hepatic disease evolves to cirrhosis without any recognized overt indication of hepatitis. In these patients the initial manifestations are extrahepatic. Neurological or psychiatric disturbances are the first clinical signs in most of this group and are always accompanied by Kayser-Fleischer rings (Plate 8-8). These green or golden deposits of copper in Descemet's membrane of the cornea never interfere with vision but indicate that hepatic copper has been released and caused the brain damage. Rarely Kayser-Fleischer rings may be accompanied by sunflower cataracts. If a patient with frank neurological or psychiatric disease does not have Kayser-Fleischer rings when examined by a trained observer using a slit-lamp, the diagnosis of Wilson's disease can be excluded.

The primary neurological manifestation is that of a movement disorder, particularly resting and intention tremors. Spasticity, rigidity, chorea, drooling, dysphagia, and dysarthria are common. Babinski responses and absent abdominal reflexes are occasionally noted; sensory changes are rare. Psychiatric disturbances, in part due to the toxic effects of copper on the brain and in part to the reactions to a life-threatening disease, are evident in most patients with symptomatic disease. Syndromes indistinguishable from schizophrenia, manic-depressive psychoses, and classic neuroses have been observed, and some bizarre behavioral disturbances defy classification. Improvement in the psychiatric state can occur with pharmacological reduction of the copper excess, but psychotherapy is often also required.

In occasional patients the clinical onset reflects neither a hepatic nor a central nervous system disturbance. For example, primary or secondary amenorrhea may be the first evidence of disease in some young women; in others, repeated spontaneous abortions may result from excess free copper in intrauterine secretions. Routine ophthalmologic examination in patients without symptomatic liver or neurological disease occasionally reveals Kayser-Fleischer rings, leading to the diagnosis. Cirrhosis may be observed incidentally at surgery.

PATHOGENESIS The metabolic defect in Wilson's disease is an inability to maintain a near-zero balance of copper. Excess copper accumulates possibly because hepatic lysosomes lack the normal mechanism to excrete into bile the copper that has been catabolically cleaved from ceruloplasmin. This may cause deficiency of ceruloplasmin since a stoichiometric excess of copper inhibits the formation of ceruloplasmin from apoceruloplasmin and copper. The capacity of hepatocytes to store copper is eventually exceeded, and release into blood and uptake in extrahepatic sites occur (Table 95-1).

Under normal circumstances essentially all tissue copper is present as the prosthetic element of copper proteins such as cytochrome oxidase, tyrosinase, superoxide dismutase, and ceruloplasmin. There is normally little or no free (non-protein-bound) copper. In Wilson's disease more copper is present than can be bound by specific copper proteins; such copper is as toxic as excess iron, zinc, mercury, or lead. Toxicity of these cations is probably effected in large degree by pathological combinations with proteins that ordinarily do not contain metal.

The pathological consequences of the accumulated copper occur first in the liver. Abnormal fat and glycogen deposits are the earliest findings by light microscopy (Fig. 95-1). With electron microscopy mitochondrial abnormalities are observed early and appear to be specific for Wilson's disease (Fig. 95-2). Later, necrosis, inflammation, fibrosis, bile duct proliferation, and cirrhosis are seen. Abnormalities in liver function tests develop later than the histological changes.

Death can occur from copper damage to the central nervous system with little or no evidence of liver dysfunction, but in most subjects significant liver disease becomes apparent sometime during the course. Patients with prolonged survival always show hepatic cirrhosis.

In the brain the excess copper is distributed ubiquitously. Necrosis of neurons with cavitation may be preceded by the appearance of Opalski and Alzheimer type II cells; however neither is specific for Wilson's disease.

Increased copper in the kidney produces little if any structural change and commonly does not alter renal function. He-

TABLE 95-1
Summary of analytical data in patients with Wilson's disease, heterozygous carriers, and control subjects

Group	Serum ceruloplasmin			Hepatic copper concentration		
	No. of patients	Range, mg/100 ml	Mean ± SD, mg/100 ml	No. of patients	Range, µg/g dry weight	Mean ± SD, µg/g dry weight
Wilson's disease:						
Asymptomatic	31	0–19.5	3.6 ± 5.3	36	152–1828	983.5 ± 368
Symptomatic	84	0–43.0	5.9 ± 7.1	33	94–1360	588.3 ± 304
Heterozygous carriers	95*	1–50.1	28.4 ± 8.5	14	39–213	117.0 ± 51
Normal subjects	180	18.5–65.9	30.7 ± 3.5	16	20–45	31.5 ± 6.8

* 71 parents of patients with Wilson's disease and 24 children, each of whom had one parent with Wilson's disease.
SOURCE: Sternlieb and Scheinberg, 1968.

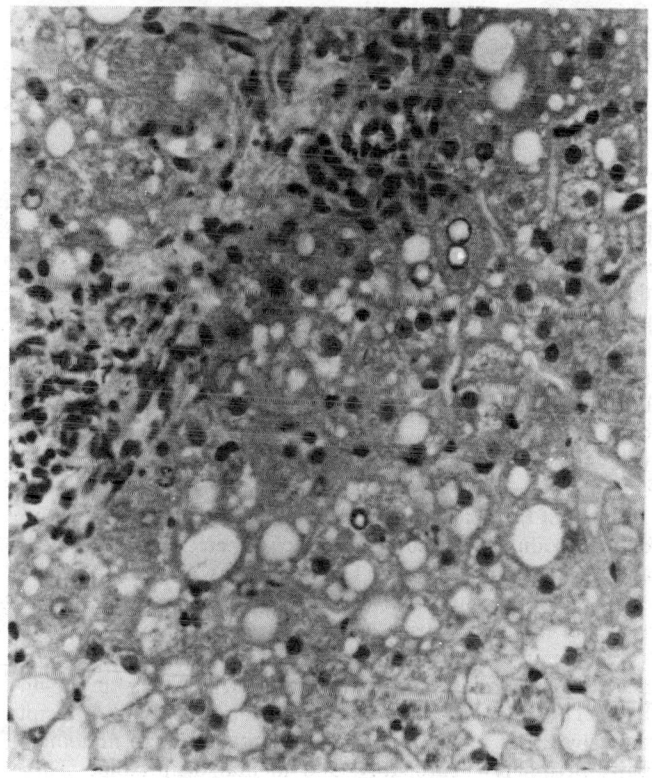

FIGURE 95-1

Fatty changes, glycogen deposits, and cellular infiltrates in a hematoxylin and eosin–stained section of liver from an asymptomatic boy with Wilson's disease.

maturia, proteinuria, the Fanconi syndrome, and renal tubular acidosis occur rarely. Pathological effects in other organs and tissues are minor.

DIAGNOSIS The diagnosis is easy *provided it is suspected.* Wilson's disease should be considered in any patient under the age of 40 with an unexplained disorder of the central nervous system, signs or symptoms of chronic active hepatitis, unexplained persistent elevations of serum transaminase, acquired hemolytic anemia (particularly in the presence of hepatitis), or unexplained cirrhosis, or in any patient who has a relative with Wilson's disease.

The diagnosis is confirmed in suspected cases by the demonstration either of (1) a serum concentration of ceruloplasmin less than 20 mg per 100 ml and Kayser-Fleischer rings, or (2) a serum ceruloplasmin less than 20 mg per 100 ml and a concentration of copper in a liver biopsy sample greater than 250 μg per gram of dry weight. Most patients also excrete more than 100 μg copper per day in urine and exhibit histological abnormalities on liver biopsy.

About 5 percent of patients have a serum concentration of ceruloplasmin greater than 20 mg per 100 ml, and some patients with other hepatic disorders have elevated hepatic copper and Kayser-Fleischer rings. In either circumstance measurement of the ability to incorporate radioactive copper into ceruloplasmin is useful as a discriminating test. Even in the presence of a normal concentration of ceruloplasmin, patients with Wilson's disease incorporate little or no isotope into the protein, while patients with other liver disorders and elevated hepatic copper incorporate the isotope normally.

TREATMENT Treatment consists of removing the deposits of copper as rapidly as possible and should be instituted once the diagnosis is secure whether the patient is ill or asymptomatic.

The drug of choice is D-penicillamine. It is administered orally in an average dose of 1 g daily, usually in divided doses before meals and at bedtime. Since penicillamine has an antipyridoxine effect in animals, 25 mg per day of vitamin B_6 is also given. Effectiveness of therapy should be assayed chemically and clinically. Initially, the patient's 24-h urinary excretion of copper should increase fivefold or more over the pretreatment level, and 1 to 3 mg copper per day may be excreted during the first months of therapy.

White blood cell and platelet counts, urinalysis, and body temperature should be monitored several times weekly for the first month of therapy and at intervals thereafter. Sensitivity to penicillamine usually appears within the first 14 days of treatment and may cause rash, fever, leukopenia, thrombocytopenia, lymphadenopathy, or proteinuria. Discontinuation of treatment is required if sensitivity develops. Therapy can often be resumed if the drug is reinstituted in small and gradually increasing dosage; alternatively, 20 mg prednisone can be given daily for the first 2 weeks of penicillamine treatment and subsequently gradually discontinued. Reactions requiring a desensitizing regimen may recur several times before penicillamine can be administered without a steroid.

Lifelong treatment is required. Inadequate treatment or in-

FIGURE 95-2

Electron micrograph showing portions of two hepatocytes from the liver biopsy of a young asymptomatic woman with Wilson's disease. There are lipid droplets (L) and grossly abnormal mitochondria (M) in the cytoplasm. N, nucleus; P, peroxisome.

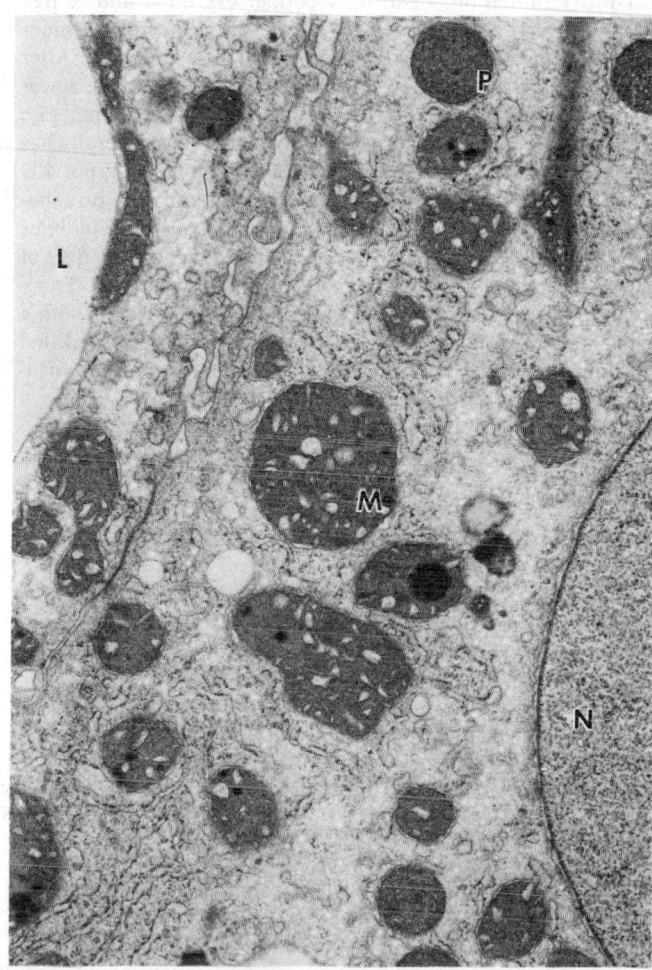

terruption of therapy causes relapse that may be irreversible. Reinstitution of penicillamine after temporary interruption of therapy may be accompanied by the appearance or reappearance of sensitivity reactions. At any time—even after years of uneventful administration—granulocytopenia (or agranulocytosis), thrombocytopenia, the nephrotic syndrome, the Goodpasture syndrome, systemic lupus erythematosus, severe arthralgias, or myasthenia gravis may supervene. Toxicity is sometimes dose-related, and reduction of the dose to a level that is therapeutically effective but nontoxic may be possible. Continued low dosage of steroids may control penicillamine-associated lupus or arthralgias. After temporary interruption of the drug in patients with the nephrotic syndrome, it is sometimes possible to reinstitute therapy without recurrence of proteinuria. However, although irreversible intolerance to D-penicillamine is rare, the toxicity may be such that the drug must be withdrawn permanently. The lifelong administration of dimercaprol by injection is impractical, and the only other alternative mode of therapy is an investigational drug, triethylene tetramine.

After therapy with penicillamine has been successfully instituted, the patient should be seen indefinitely at 1- to 3-month intervals to detect drug toxicity and manage the disease. Physical examination, including relevant neurological assessment and inspection of the corneas with a slit-lamp, together with the patient's own evaluation, provides the best indicator of the efficacy of treatment. Serial determinations of serum transaminase levels, albumin, and bilirubin are useful in following the course of liver function. Lack of clinical improvement or worsening of the disease may be due to irreversible damage present before therapy was begun, to poor patient compliance, or to inadequate dosage of penicillamine. Quantitative determinations of urinary copper excretion and of free copper in serum (total serum copper minus ceruloplasmin-bound copper) can help determine which is the case. After treatment for long periods, urinary copper should be lower than at the onset of therapy and rarely exceeds 1.5 mg per day. Even more helpful, an adequately treated patient generally has a concentration of free serum copper less than 10 μg per 100 ml. After a patient has remained asymptomatic with no laboratory evidence of liver dysfunction for a year and in patients with minimal residual disease that has not changed, the dose of penicillamine may be reduced to 0.75 g per day.

Treatment of more than 100 asymptomatic patients with a confirmed diagnosis over the past 15 years has established that continued administration of D-penicillamine can prevent virtually every manifestation of this disease.

REFERENCES

CARTWRIGHT GE: The diagnosis of treatable Wilson's disease. N Engl J Med 298:1347, 1978

Copper: Report of the Committee on Medical and Biologic Effects of Environmental Pollutants. Washington, DC, National Academy of Sciences, 1977

STERNLIEB I: Evolution of the hepatic lesion in Wilson's disease (hepatolenticular degeneration), in *Progress in Liver Diseases,* vol IV, H Popper et al (eds). New York, Grune & Stratton, 1972

———, SCHEINBERG IH: Prevention of Wilson's disease in asymptomatic patients. N Engl J Med 278:352, 1968

———, ———: Chronic hepatitis as a first manifestation of Wilson's disease. Ann Intern Med 76:59, 1972

WALSHE JM: Wilson's disease (hepatolenticular degeneration), in *Handbook of Clinical Neurology,* vol 27, PJ Vinken et al (eds). New York, American Elsevier, 1976

96
PORPHYRIAS

URS A. MEYER

The porphyrias are a group of clinically heterogeneous diseases associated with inherited or acquired disturbances in heme biosynthesis. Porphyrins are tetrapyrrole pigments that serve as intermediates in this pathway. They are formed from the precursors δ-aminolevulinic acid (ALA) and porphobilinogen. Heme, the ferrous iron complex of protoporphyrin IX, functions as a prosthetic group for hemoproteins such as hemoglobin, microsomal and mitochondrial cytochromes, catalase, tryptophan oxygenase, and others. Disturbances of heme biosynthesis differ from most other metabolic diseases by involving a pathway essential to life and operative in all aerobic cells.

Each of the porphyrias is characterized by a unique pattern of overproduction, accumulation, and excretion of intermediates of heme biosynthesis. These patterns are the metabolic expression of genetically determined deficiencies of specific enzymes of the heme biosynthetic pathway (Table 96-1).

The main clinical manifestations are intermittent attacks of nervous system dysfunction and sensitivity of the skin to sunlight. The *neurological syndrome* is characteristically precipitated by drugs such as barbiturates and results in abdominal pain, peripheral neuropathy, and mental disturbance. These neuropsychiatric symptoms occur only in those porphyrias in which there is great overproduction of the porphyrin precursors ALA and porphobilinogen. The pathogenesis of the neurological lesion is unclear. The *skin photosensitivity* is related directly to increased porphyrin accumulation, although the lesions differ among diseases. The photosensitivity is due to the photodynamic action of porphyrins and is probably mediated through the formation of singlet-oxygen with consequent destructive processes such as the peroxidation of lipids in the membranes of lysosomes. The dominantly inherited human porphyrias exhibit variable expressivity. In many patients only the biochemical or enzymatic abnormalities are apparent. Exacerbations in ordinarily asymptomatic patients can be precipitated by factors such as drugs, hormones, or liver disease. Clinically or chemically latent disease may occur as a phase or persist throughout life.

CLASSIFICATION The porphyrias are usually divided into two main groups, erythropoietic and hepatic, according to the two major sites of heme synthesis where the error of metabolism is expressed (Table 96-1). The only pure erythropoietic form of porphyria is the rare *congenital erythropoietic porphyria* (CEP). In *protoporphyria* (PP) porphyrins accumulate in both erythropoietic and hepatic tissue. In *intermittent acute porphyria* (IAP), *hereditary coproporphyria* (HCP), and *variegate porphyria* (VP), dominantly inherited enzyme deficiencies impair heme biosynthesis predominantly in the liver, apparently without affecting hemoglobin formation. *Porphyria cutanea tarda* (PCT) was previously considered to be an acquired hepatic porphyria. However most if not all patients with this disease have been found to have hereditary deficiency of uroporphyrinogen decarboxylase. Toxic acquired porphyria resembling PCT occurs in individuals accidentally exposed to polychlorinated hydrocarbons and in association with hepatic tumors. Poisoning with lead produces well-recognized abnormalities in porphyrin and heme synthesis (see Chap. 225). Increased urinary excretion of porphyrins or precursors and accumulation of porphyrins in erythrocytes may also occur in numerous clinical conditions; these are secondary phenomena which do not produce symptoms or signs of porphyria.

TABLE 96-1
Characteristics of the porphyrias

| | Erythropoietic porphyria | Hepatic porphyrias | | | | Erythrohepatic porphyria |
	Congenital erythropoietic porphyria (CEP)	Intermittent acute porphyria (IAP)	Hereditary coproporphyria (HCP)	Variegate porphyria (VP)	Porphyria cutanea tarda (PCT)	Protoporphyria (PP)
Enzyme deficiency	Uroporphyrinogen I synthetase and/or uroporphyrinogen III cosynthetase (?)	Uroporphyrinogen I synthetase	Coproporphyrinogen oxidase	Protoporphyrinogen oxidase or ferrochelatase (?)	Uroporphyrinogen decarboxylase	Ferrochelatase
Inheritance	Autosomal recessive	Autosomal dominant	Autosomal dominant	Autosomal dominant	Autosomal dominant	Autosomal dominant
Metabolic expression	Erythroid cells	Liver	Liver	Liver	Liver	Erythroid cells and liver
Signs and symptoms:						
Photosensitive cutaneous lesions	Yes	No	Infrequent	Yes	Yes	Yes
Attacks of abdominal pain, neuropsychiatric syndrome	No	Yes	Yes	Yes	No	No
Laboratory abnormalities:						
Red blood cells:						
Uroporphyrin	+++	N	N	N	N	N
Coproporphyrin	++	N	N	N	N	+
Protoporphyrin	(+)	N	N	N	N	+++
Urine:						
δ-Aminolevulinic acid	N	(+++)	(+++)	(+++)	N	N
Porphobilinogen	N	(+++)	(+++)	(+++)	N	N
Uroporphyrin	+++	++	+	+	+++	N
Coproporphyrin	++	N	++	++	+	(+)
Feces:						
Coproporphyrin	+	N	+++	+	(+)	(+)
Protoporphyrin	+	N	+	+++	N	++

NOTE: N, normal; +, increased levels or excretion; ++, moderately increased; +++, markedly increased; (+), increased in some patients only; (+++), frequently increased only during acute attacks.

BIOCHEMICAL CONSIDERATIONS A schematic outline of heme biosynthesis is presented in Fig. 96-1. The sequence of reactions that leads from the simple substrates glycine and succinyl coenzyme A to ALA, porphobilinogen (PBG), and finally heme is composed of four mitochondrial and four cytosolic enzymes. Differences exist in the regulation of heme biosynthesis among tissues.

In the liver ALA synthetase catalyzes the rate-limiting reaction for heme formation under physiological conditions. The enzymes subsequent to ALA synthetase are present in excess. The principal regulation of ALA synthetase is feedback repression by heme, the end product of the pathway. Increased demands for heme are met by the synthesis of ALA synthetase. Hepatic ALA synthetase can be induced by a large number of lipid-soluble drugs, naturally occurring steroids, and chemicals that are substrates and inducers of cytochrome P_{450}, the terminal oxidase in microsomal drug metabolism. This induction is modulated by multiple genetic, metabolic, and environmental factors. The interdependence of heme synthesis and microsomal drug oxidation is important in some hepatic porphyrias where clinical symptoms are produced by certain drugs.

In the bone marrow ALA synthetase is also rate-limiting in certain cells, but little is known of the role of the enzyme in overall heme synthesis during division, differentiation, and maturation of erythroid cells. With maturation of erythroid cells the nuclei and mitochondria are extruded, and the mitochondrial enzymes of heme synthesis disappear, while the cytosolic enzymes catalyzing the reactions between ALA and coproporphyrinogen persist. Therefore, erythrocytes can be used for the diagnosis and study of porphyrias provided the deficiency is in a cytosolic enzyme.

Bone marrow and liver differ in the role of specific enzymes in control of heme synthesis. The level of ALA synthetase is the major determinant of heme formation in the liver, while heme synthesis in the bone marrow is triggered by the complex process of erythroid differentiation. These considerations probably explain the different phenotypic expression of specific enzyme defects of heme synthesis in erythroid cells and liver.

The porphyrinogens, reduced forms of porphyrins, serve as intermediates between porphobilinogen and protoporphyrin. Porphyrinogens are colorless and nonfluorescent. Porphyrins are by-products that have escaped from the biosynthetic path by irreversible oxidation of the corresponding porphyrinogen. Porphyrins do not possess physiological function but are responsible, through their pigment and fluorescent properties, for the spectacular appearance of urine and erythrocytes in some patients.

The arrangement of two substituent side chains on the pyrrole ring of porphyrins determines the structural isomer types, numbered I to IV. In nature only types I and III have been identified, and only type III serves as substrate for the terminal steps of the pathway leading to protoporphyrin IX and heme. The catabolism of heme does not lead to porphyrins but to noncyclic tetrapyrroles referred to as *bile pigments*.

CONGENITAL ERYTHROPOIETIC PORPHYRIA

DEFINITION Congenital erythropoietic porphyria (CEP; Günther's disease, congenital photosensitive porphyria, erythropoietic uroporphyria) is a rare, recessively inherited defect that causes chronic photosensitivity with severe, mutilating skin lesions and hemolytic anemia.

GENETICS, INCIDENCE, AND PATHOGENESIS Only about 80 cases have been reported. Affected individuals are homozygous

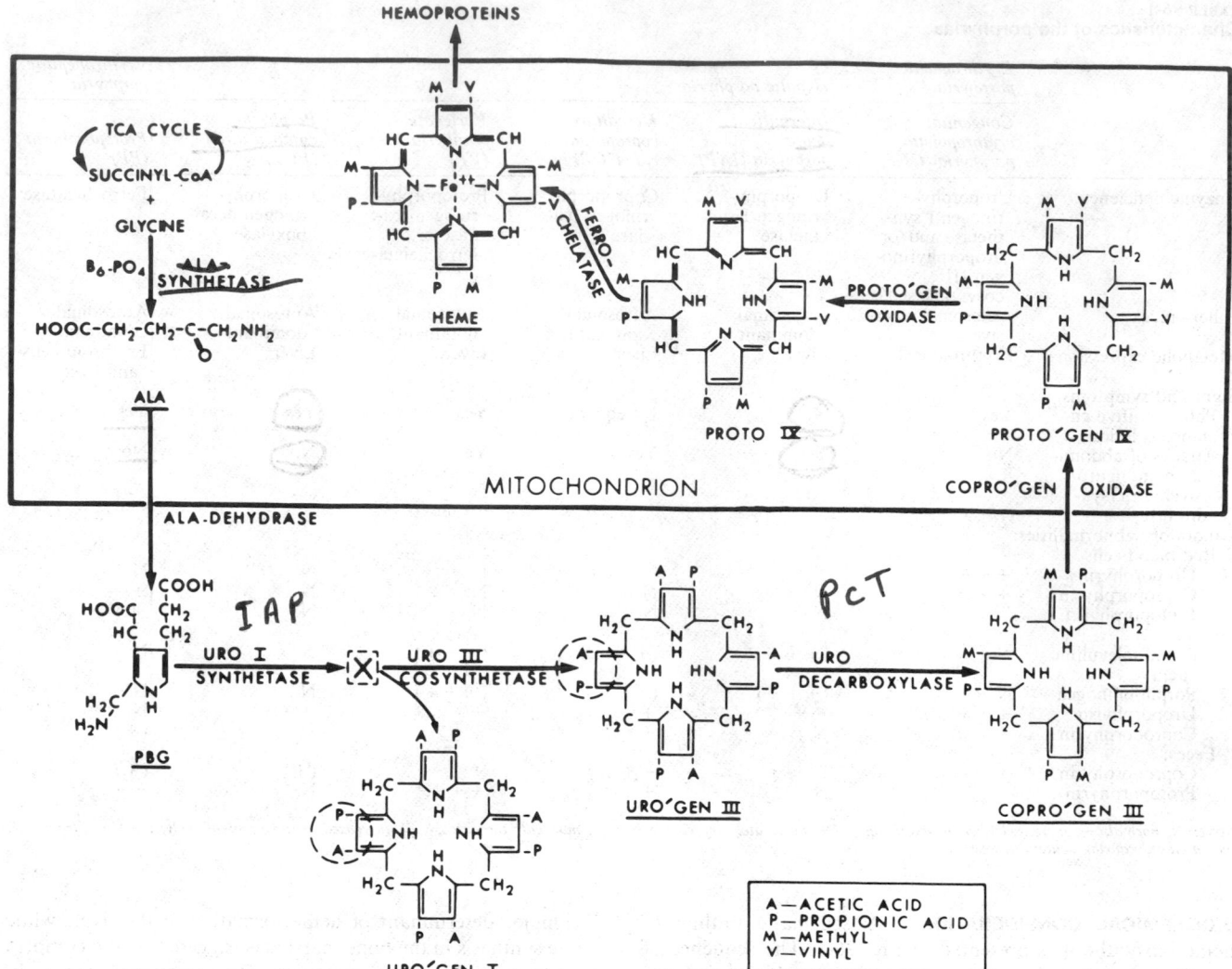

FIGURE 96-1

Outline of heme biosynthesis. (ALA, δ-aminolevulinic acid; PBG, porphobilinogen; URO, uroporphyrin; UROgen, uroporphyrinogen; COPRO-gen, coproporphyrinogen; PROTOgen, protoporphyrinogen; PROTO, protoporphyrin; X, postulated intermediate.)

for an autosomal recessive gene; heterozygotes rarely have demonstrable abnormalities in porphyrin metabolism and appear normal. The underlying enzyme abnormality has not been entirely elucidated, but there appears to be a functional imbalance between the activities of uroporphyrinogen I synthetase and uroporphyrinogen III cosynthetase. The defect is expressed solely in maturing erythroid cells and results in massive overproduction of uroporphyrinogen I while the overall production of uroporphyrinogen III is normal or slightly increased. Uroporphyrinogen I cannot be used for heme synthesis but is converted to coproporphyrinogen I which cannot be metabolized further. Uroporphyrin I, coproporphyrinogen I, and coproporphyrin I accumulate in tissues and are excreted in excess amounts in urine and feces.

CLINICAL PRESENTATION AND DIAGNOSIS Porphyrins accumulate within the body of affected individuals during fetal development. Excretion of pink or red urine usually begins at or shortly after birth, whereas cutaneous photosensitivity, intermittent hemolysis, and splenomegaly may not be detected until later. Hypertrichosis and red discoloration of the teeth and bones are common. Death may occur in childhood. With longer survival, severe scarring and mutilation occur, mostly affecting fingers, nose, and ears. The urine contains high concentrations of uroporphyrin I and increased amounts of coproporphyrin as well as porphyrins with seven, six, five, and three

carboxyl groups, whereas the excretion of ALA and PBG is normal. Large amounts of coproporphyrin I are found in the feces. Normoblasts, reticulocytes, and erythrocytes contain large quantities of uroporphyrin I and lower concentrations of coproporphyrinogen I. Normoblasts and reticulocytes exhibit intense red fluorescence. In accordance with the normal excretion of ALA and PBG, neurological disturbance does not occur in CEP.

TREATMENT Exposure to sunlight should be avoided. In some cases, splenectomy has ameliorated hemolytic anemia, porphyrin excretion, and photosensitivity. The use of hematin infusions and oral beta-carotene remains experimental.

HEPATIC PORPHYRIAS

Three hepatic porphyrias, intermittent acute porphyria (IAP), hereditary coproporphyria (HCP), and variegate porphyria (VP), have many features in common. All are genetically transmitted as autosomal dominants. Acute attacks of a life-threatening neurological syndrome are precipitated by a variety of drugs as well as by hormones and other agents. During acute attacks excessive urinary excretion of the porphyrin precursors ALA and PBG occurs in all, but the patterns of porphyrins excreted in urine and feces differ (Fig. 96-2).

INTERMITTENT ACUTE PORPHYRIA

Definition Intermittent acute porphyria [IAP, acute intermittent porphyria (AIP), pyrroloporphyria] is characterized by recurrent attacks of neurological and psychiatric dysfunction. Photosensitivity does not occur. The primary defect is in uroporphyrinogen I synthetase.

Genetics, incidence, and pathogenesis IAP is inherited as an autosomal dominant trait with variable expressivity. The overall frequency of the abnormal gene is estimated to be between 1 in 10,000 and 1 in 50,000, but in certain regions the incidence may be higher. Homozygous cases of IAP have not been observed. The defect consists of a partial (50 percent) deficiency of uroporphyrinogen I synthetase, the enzyme that converts PBG to uroporphyrinogen I. In the liver this leads to increased activity and/or inducibility of ALA synthetase by drugs and other factors and, consequently, to increased formation and urinary excretion of ALA and PBG. Preformed porphyrins do not accumulate, and, therefore, cutaneous photosensitivity does not occur. Decreased uroporphyrinogen I synthetase activity has been demonstrated in liver, erythrocytes, cultured skin fibroblasts, lymphocytes, and amniotic cells of patients with IAP. Thus, the enzymatic defect of IAP is present, albeit metabolically unexpressed, in tissues other than liver. Deficiency of uroporphyrinogen I synthetase does not necessarily result in clinical manifestations of acute porphyria without additional acquired factors, and families with large numbers of phenotypically normal carriers of the genetic defect have been found (latent porphyria). The relation between the genetic defect and the neurological lesions is unknown.

Clinical presentation and diagnosis Symptoms rarely occur before puberty. Abdominal pain is frequently the initial or most prominent symptom of the porphyric attack. It may be moderate or severe, colicky, localized or generalized; radiation to the back or loins may occur. The pain probably results from autonomic neuropathy causing disturbed gastrointestinal motility with alternate areas of spasm and dilatation. The abdomen is usually soft, and tenderness is not marked. Because it is often accompanied by fever and leukocytosis, the abdominal pain of the acute porphyric attack can mimic any inflammatory abdominal disease. Severe vomiting and persistent constipation are commonly associated. Neurological manifestations and signs of mental disturbance are variable. Peripheral nerves, the autonomic nervous system, brainstem, cranial nerves, or cerebral function may be involved. Sinus tachycardia and labile hypertension with postural hypotension, urinary retention, and excessive sweating are frequent during the acute attack. The pulse rate is a good index of the activity of the disease. Hypertension and tachycardia correlate with increased excretion of catecholamines. Peripheral neuropathy is usually predominantly motor, but sensory components may be present. Deep tendon reflexes are diminished or absent. Neuritic pain in the extremities, areas of hypesthesia and paresthesia, and foot and wrist drop are typical. Paraplegia or complete flaccid quadriplegia may ensue. In the past, complications due to respiratory paralysis were a leading cause of death. Cranial nerve involvement may lead to optic nerve atrophy, ophthalmoplegia, and dysphagia. With more severe CNS involvement, delirium, coma, and seizures occur. Although the neuropathy is reversible to a surprising degree, residual paresis may last for several years following an acute attack. Many patients have a long history of vague nervousness, emotional instability, and functional disturbances. Significant signs of mental disturbance occur in one-third, and an organic brain syndrome with restlessness, disorientation, and visual hallucinations may supervene. During attacks hyponatremia can be severe. Multiple mechanisms (including gastrointestinal loss of sodium, imprudent fluid therapy, and a sodium-losing nephropathy related to a toxic effect of ALA) have been implicated, but the major mechanism appears to be inappropriate release of antidiuretic hormone.

Acute attacks may last from several days to several months and vary considerably in frequency and severity. In periods of remission symptoms may be slight or completely absent. Clinical (and biochemical) manifestations are frequently precipitated by usual therapeutic doses of several drugs including barbiturates, anticonvulsants, estrogens, contraceptives, and alcohol. All these drugs are oxidized by hepatic microsomes and thus involve the hemoproteins of the cytochrome P_{450} system. Impaired hepatic metabolism of some of these drugs has

FIGURE 96-2

Patterns of urinary porphyrin and porphyrin precursor excretion in the hepatic porphyrias in relation to the pathway of heme biosynthesis. Intermediates of the pathway excessively excreted during the acute phase of each of the hepatic porphyrias are within the respective brackets. (ALA, δ-aminolevulinic acid; PBG, porphobilinogen; UROgen, uroporphyrinogen; COPROgen, coproporphyrinogen; PROTOgen, protoporphyrinogen.)

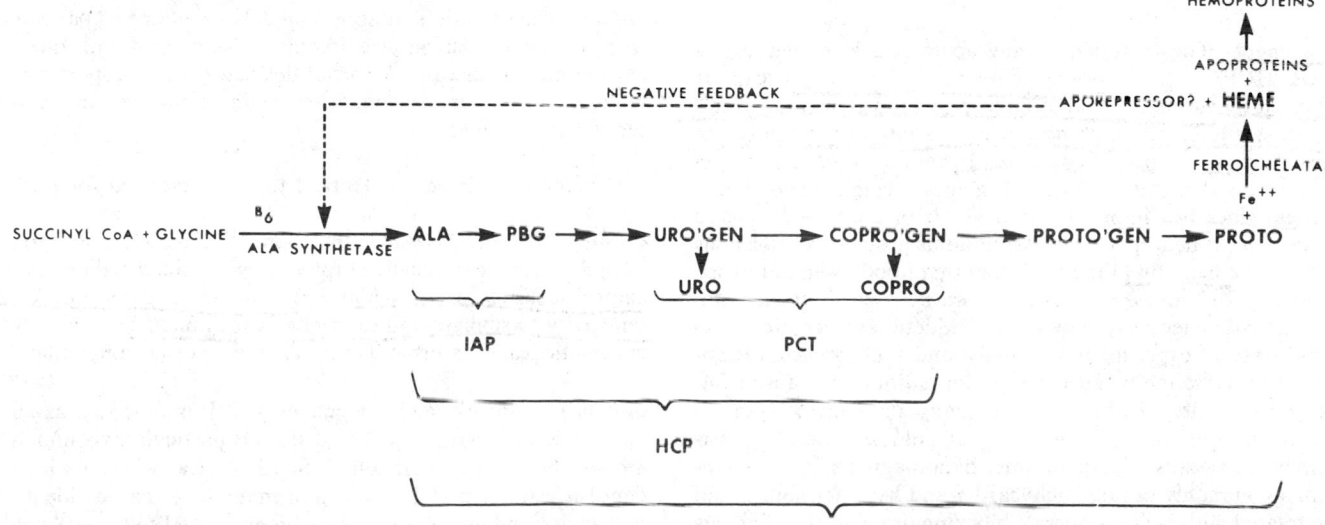

been demonstrated during acute attacks of IAP. In some women, exacerbations are correlated with the menstrual cycle, and latent porphyria may become clinically manifest late in pregnancy or shortly after delivery. Prolonged periods of decreased caloric intake (deliberate fasting) and infections may also provoke attacks.

LABORATORY FINDINGS   Excessive excretion of ALA and PBG in the urine is characteristic during acute attacks. It does not differentiate IAP from HCP and VP, and the levels do not correlate with the severity of the symptoms. The qualitative determination of porphobilinogen in the urine by the Watson-Schwartz or the Hoesch test is a simple and valuable screening aid for the diagnosis of an acute attack in IAP, HCP, and VP. These tests are almost always positive during episodes of neuropsychiatric dysfunction. However, both screening tests become positive only when the concentration of PBG in the urine is three to five times the upper limit of normal; as a consequence, they may be negative in latent cases and in patients in whom urinary excretion of PBG becomes normal following recovery from an acute attack. In these instances urinary ALA and PBG excretion should be measured quantitatively by chromatographic methods. In latent IAP with normal excretion of ALA and PBG, diagnosis is possible only by measuring the activity of uroporphyrinogen I synthetase in erythrocytes, lymphocytes, or cultured skin fibroblasts.

In IAP only the porphyrin precursors ALA and PBG are excreted in increased amounts, consistent with the enzymatic defect. Freshly passed urine is, therefore, colorless and contains little preformed uro- or coproporphyrin. The urine may darken on standing because PBG polymerizes spontaneously to uroporphyrin and porphobilin, a dark brown pigment of unknown structure. The fecal porphyrin concentration in IAP is usually normal. In the other two hepatic porphyrias associated with acute neuropsychiatric attacks, increased amounts of preformed porphyrins are excreted in urine and feces.

Conventional liver function tests are normal except for increased Bromsulphalein (BSP) retention. A moderate reduction in red blood cell mass and blood volume or a transient normochromic, normocytic anemia are the only hematologic disturbances. Numerous metabolic abnormalities may be associated with acute attacks including hypercholesterolemia with increased low-density lipoprotein levels, increased serum thyroxine (without hyperthyroidism), abnormal glucose tolerance, and defective 5α reduction of testosterone in liver. The relationship of these abnormalities to the genetic defect is unknown.

Treatment   The treatment of the acute attack is identical in IAP, HCP, and VP. Some acute attacks seemingly can be aborted by administration of large quantities of carbohydrates (glucose effect), although no objective study of the efficacy of this therapy has been performed. Intravenous administration of glucose at a rate of 10 to 20 g/h is recommended. If the patient does not improve within 48 h of continued glucose infusion or if neuropsychiatric symptoms progress, intravenous infusion of hematin (4 mg per kilogram of body weight infused over 10 to 12 min every 12 h) should be tried. Both hematin and glucose effectively prevent the induction of hepatic ALA-synthetase in experimental animals, and both procedures appear to reverse the biochemical abnormalities and cause clinical improvement within 48 h in many patients. Supportive treatment with careful monitoring of fluid and electrolytes is important because hyponatremia, hypomagnesemia, and azotemia commonly occur. Tachycardia and hypertension should be treated with beta-adrenergic blocking drugs. A list of agents considered to be "safe" or "probably safe" in patients with

TABLE 96-2
Drugs considered to be safe (or probably safe) in patients with intermittent acute porphyria, hereditary coproporphyria, and variegate porphyria

Analgesics:
  Salicylates
  Morphine and related opiates (pethidine)
Antibiotics:
  Penicillins
Psychoactive drugs:
  Phenothiazines (chlorpromazine)
Antihistamines:
  Diphenhydramine
Antihypertensives:
  Guanethidine
  Propranolol
  Reserpine
Miscellaneous:
  Atropine
  Neostigmine
  Propanidid
  Procaine
  Succinylcholine
  Ether
  Nitrous oxide

latent and acute IAP, HCP, and VP is given in Table 96-2. The most important measure in the management is prevention of acute attacks by instructing the carrier of the abnormal gene about the avoidance of provocative factors, namely drugs, steroids, and deliberate fasting. With early recognition of the condition, immediate withdrawal of provocative agents, careful fluid and electrolyte therapy, and the use of glucose and/or hematin infusions most attacks are reversible, and fatalities are rare.

HEREDITARY COPROPORPHYRIA Definition and genetics Hereditary coproporphyria (HCP) is a hepatic porphyria characterized by acute attacks of neuropsychiatric dysfunction identical to those of IAP and VP. In addition, photosensitivity occurs in some. The primary genetic defect is a deficiency of coproporphyrinogen oxidase. The disease is inherited as an autosomal dominant trait. Accurate assessment of the incidence of HCP is difficult since over half of affected individuals remain asymptomatic.

Pathogenesis and clinical picture   Biochemically, HCP is characterized by the excretion of large amounts of coproporphyrin III, mainly in feces but also in urine. Excretion of ALA and PBG is increased during acute attacks (positive Watson-Schwartz or Hoesch test) but usually returns to normal during remission. Acute attacks are indistinguishable from those of IAP and VP and are precipitated by the same factors. Skin photosensitivity occurs in approximately one-third of patients with overt HCP. Its onset is frequently associated with intercurrent hepatic disease. A partial deficiency of coproporphyrinogen oxidase can be demonstrated in leukocytes and cultured skin fibroblasts.

Treatment   Treatment is identical to that described for IAP.

VARIEGATE PORPHYRIA Definition Variegate porphyria (VP; South African genetic porphyria) is characterized by both acute attacks of neuropsychiatric dysfunction and chronic skin sensitivity to sunlight and to mechanical trauma. The primary enzymatic lesion in heme biosynthesis has not been identified.

Genetics, incidence, and pathogenesis   VP is inherited as an autosomal dominant trait. The disease is particularly common among the white population of South Africa, where its incidence is estimated at 1 in 400, and many cases can be identified as descendants of a woman who emigrated to Cape Town from the Netherlands in 1688. Elsewhere the disease is less frequent, but VP has been recognized in many countries. The defect leads to the excretion of large amounts of protoporphyrin in bile and feces (with lesser increases in the fecal excretion of coproporphyrin) and to markedly increased urinary excretion of ALA, PBG, and coproporphyrin during acute attacks. The excretion pattern suggests a deficiency either of protoporphyrinogen oxidase or ferrochelatase, but a defect of these enzymes has not been demonstrated.

Clinical presentation and diagnosis Overt cases with VP usually present in the second or third decade. The clinical picture includes acute attacks of abdominal pain and neuropsychiatric symptoms, coupled with photocutaneous lesions. Neurological and cutaneous manifestations may occur simultaneously or at different times. More than 80 percent of the South African patients have signs of cutaneous involvement, consisting of dermal abrasions, superficial erosions, and blister formation after trivial mechanical trauma. The mechanical fragility usually is limited to light-exposed parts of the skin. The lesions often leave depigmented or pigmented scars. Secondary infection frequently delays healing. Hyperpigmentation of the face and hands is common, and women often have hypertrichosis. The skin lesions are indistinguishable from those of porphyria cutanea tarda (PCT). Severe exacerbations of the cutaneous lesions sometimes are associated with intercurrent hepatic disease, presumably related to diminution of fecal excretion and a concomitant increase in the urinary excretion of porphyrins. Acute attacks of neuropsychiatric dysfunction are indistinguishable from those of IAP and HCP and are precipitated by the same factors. The characteristic chemical finding in VP is the continuous excretion of large amounts of proto- and coproporphyrin, even when clinical manifestations are minimal or absent. The levels of protoporphyrin exceed those of coproporphyrin, the reverse of the situation in HCP. Urinary excretion of ALA, PBG, and porphyrins is either normal or moderately increased in asymptomatic patients or those who have only skin symptoms. During acute attacks the urinary excretion of ALA and PBG is increased (positive Watson-Schwartz or Hoesch test), and there also is increased urinary excretion of coproporphyrin and uroporphyrin. Erythrocyte porphyrins are normal, allowing distinction from protoporphyria.

Treatment Prophylactic measures and treatment of the acute attack with glucose and possibly hematin infusions are the same as for IAP and HCP, although the experience with hematin in VP is limited. Avoidance of exposure to direct sunlight and use of protective clothing (gloves, hats) are advocated.

PORPHYRIA CUTANEA TARDA Definition Porphyria cutanea tarda (PCT; symptomatic cutaneous hepatic porphyria, symptomatic porphyria) is the most common form of porphyria. The disease is characterized by chronic skin lesions, the frequent presence of hepatic disease (and hepatic siderosis), and a distinct pattern of urinary excretion of porphyrins. The disorder is probably caused by an inherited deficiency of hepatic uroporphyrinogen decarboxylase. Neurological manifestations are absent.

Genetics, incidence, and pathogenesis PCT was considered to be an acquired disorder because of its sporadic (and usually nonfamilial) occurrence late in life and its common association (in most series more than 70 percent of patients) with alcoholic liver disease and hepatic siderosis.

The true incidence of the disease has not been evaluated, but PCT is frequent where both alcoholism and iron overload are common, as among the Bantus in South Africa. Recent studies suggest that PCT can be a familial disease, inherited in an autosomal dominant fashion with variable expressivity. The inherited defect consists of a decrease in hepatic and erythrocyte uroporphyrinogen decarboxylase activity; clinically and chemically latent carriers of the defect have been identified. It is not clear whether in some patients PCT also may occur as a consequence of an acquired (or toxic) decrease in hepatic uroporphyrinogen decarboxylase activity. Deficiency (of whatever etiology) in uroporphyrinogen decarboxylase, which catalyzes the conversion of uroporphyrinogen to coproporphyrinogen, leads to a disturbance of hepatic heme synthesis and consequent skin photosensitivity only in the presence of additional factors such as iron overload, usually in association with liver disease. The mechanism by which iron overload causes clinical expression of latent PCT is unknown. In contrast to IAP, HCP, and VP, the enzymatic defect in PCT does not result in altered regulation of the hepatic heme synthetic pathway, and ALA synthetase activity remains normal or only minimally increased even in overt cases. This probably accounts for the absence of acute neuropsychiatric attacks, the usually normal urinary ALA and PBG, and the lack of sensitivity to drugs such as barbiturates.

Clinical presentation and diagnosis Photosensitivity is the only major manifestation of PCT. The skin lesions are indistinguishable from those in VP. Skin symptoms usually begin insidiously, most often in men age 40 to 60, and consist of enhanced facial pigmentation, increased fragility to trauma, erythema, and vesicular and ulcerative lesions. Sclerodermatous changes and increased hair on the forehead, malar region, or forearms are common.

Chemical and histological evidence of liver disease, frequently related to alcohol, is common, and hepatic siderosis is an almost constant finding, although the degree of iron deposition is variable and rarely severe. Spontaneous remission may occur. Occasionally, estrogens (including contraceptive pills) or known hepatotoxic drugs precipitate the clinical disease. The incidence of diabetes mellitus is increased in PCT, and frequent association with systemic lupus erythematosus and other autoimmune syndromes has been noted.

The excretion of uroporphyrin and, to a lesser extent, coproporphyrin in the urine is increased. The urine may be pink or brown. The excretion of ALA and PBG in the urine is usually normal (negative Watson-Schwartz or Hoesch test). Although uroporphyrin is the major porphyrin in the urine, intermediary porphyrins (particularly heptacarboxylic porphyrin) are also found. Increases in fecal porphyrins are less striking and usually restricted to the coproporphyrin fraction. The diagnosis of PCT is established by the combined presence of skin photosensitivity, liver disease, increased urinary uroporphyrin excretion, the lack of an increase in porphyrin precursors (ALA, PBG), and absence of a history of neuropsychiatric attacks.

Toxic acquired porphyria resembling PCT has occurred in individuals accidentally exposed to hexachlorobenzene, polychlorinated biphenyls, tetrachlorodibenzo-p-dioxin (TCDD), and other polychlorinated hydrocarbons. Moreover, several instances of benign or malignant primary tumors of the liver have been observed in association with PCT.

Treatment Abstinence in alcoholic patients usually leads to improvement of PCT. Removal of hepatic iron by repeated phlebotomy is effective and may lead to long-lasting remissions. Alternatively, chelation therapy with desferoxamine may be tried. The administration of small doses of chloroquine apparently removes uroporphyrins from the liver and has been employed successfully in some patients. However, its use is inadvisable because of the risk of hepatic necrosis.

PROTOPORPHYRIA

DEFINITION Protoporphyria (PP; erythropoietic protoporphyria, erythrohepatic protoporphyria) is a genetic disorder in which mild skin photosensitivity is associated with high concentrations of protoporphyrin in erythrocytes. It is due to a deficiency of ferrochelatase. Protoporphyrin also accumulates in the liver in some patients.

GENETICS, INCIDENCE, AND PATHOGENESIS PP is inherited as an autosomal dominant trait with variable expressivity. Several hundred cases have been reported. Deficient activity of ferrochelatase, the mitochondrial enzyme that catalyzes the incorporation of ferrous iron into protoporphyrin, can be demonstrated in bone marrow, peripheral blood, liver, and cultured skin fibroblasts of patients with PP. This generalized enzyme deficiency results in the excessive accumulation of protoporphyrin in late normoblasts, reticulocytes, and young erythrocytes; protoporphyrin leaks into the plasma from erythrocytes as they age. Photosensitivity is mediated by protoporphyrin in plasma and skin and is evoked by visible light (380 to 560 nm). The liver participates in excess porphyrin production in some patients or, alternatively, may take up protoporphyrin from plasma. Many carriers of the genetic defect remain clinically (and chemically) asymptomatic, and detection may be possible only through enzymatic studies. Skin photosensitivity in symptomatic patients shows seasonal variability.

CLINICAL PRESENTATION AND DIAGNOSIS Mild photosensitivity usually begins in childhood. Exposure to sunlight is rapidly followed by pruritus, erythema, and occasional edema (solar urticaria). The lesions subside over hours or days without scarring. In some patients, cutaneous manifestations occur only after prolonged exposure to sunlight; in others the initial skin lesions progress to a chronic eczematous phase (solar eczema). There is no abnormal mechanical fragility or blister formation as is characteristic for VP and PCT. Erythrodontia, hypertrichosis, and hyperpigmentation are absent. Attacks of neuropsychiatric dysfunction do not occur.

PP generally is a benign disease, but a number of patients have been reported who have associated abnormalities of liver, biliary tract, or blood. The incidence of cholelithiasis is increased, and the gallstones contain protoporphyrin. In rare cases, liver disease has developed owing to massive deposition of protoporphyrin; it may progress to fatal cirrhosis. Many patients with overt PP have mild anemia.

PP is diagnosed by the detection of high concentrations of protoporphyrin in erythrocytes. When a smear of blood from a patient is examined under the fluorescent microscope, large numbers of red-fluorescing erythrocytes are seen. Protoporphyrin may also be elevated in plasma and feces, while urinary porphyrins, ALA, and PBG usually are normal.

TREATMENT Topical sunscreens are ineffective. Orally administered β-carotene (usually as a mixture of β-carotene and canthaxanthine) substantially improves the tolerance to sunlight.

REFERENCES

DEAN G: *The Porphyrias,* 2d ed. London, Pitman Medical Publishing Company, 1972

DHAR GJ et al: Effects of hematin in hepatic porphyria. Further studies. Ann Intern Med 83:20, 1975

ELDER GH et al: The porphyrias: A review. J Clin Pathol 25:1013, 1972

MEYER UA, SCHMID R: The porphyrias, in *The Metabolic Basis of Inherited Disease,* 4th ed, JB Stanbury et al (eds). New York, McGraw-Hill, 1978, p 1166

TSCHUDY DP: Porphyrin metabolism and the porphyrias, in *Duncan's Diseases of Metabolism,* 7th ed, PK Bondy, LE Rosenberg (eds). Philadelphia, Saunders, 1974, p 775

Disorders of carbohydrate metabolism

97
DISEASES OF GLYCOGEN METABOLISM

JAMES B. FIELD

The diseases of glycogen metabolism are inherited conditions resulting from deficiencies of specific enzymes involved in glycogen synthesis or degradation. The clinical features and organ involvement depend upon the specific enzymatic defect and its tissue distribution. Although enzymatic defects have been identified in many patients, characteristic clinical features have been described in other subjects whose specific enzymatic defects have not been identified. Such patients complicate attempts at classification based solely on the enzymatic defect and the tissue involved. Furthermore, the same apparent enzymatic deficiency may be associated with different clinical presentations (e.g., the infantile and adult forms of type II, α-1,4-glucosidase deficiency). Although uncommon, the diseases of glycogen metabolism have been of major importance in elucidating pathways of glycogen synthesis and degradation. They were also the first diseases proved to be due to deficiency of a single enzyme. Table 97-1 presents a classification of these diseases. The location of the enzymatic defects in relation to the glycogen metabolism is detailed in Fig. 97-1.

TYPE I GLYCOGENOSIS

Type I glycogenosis (von Gierke's disease) is due to deficient glucose 6-phosphatase activity in the liver, kidney, and intestinal mucosa. While platelets and placenta may also be involved, patients with type 1 glycogenosis have had normal pregnancies. The disease is inherited in autosomal recessive fashion, and heterozygotes have been identified by the demonstration of diminished glucose 6-phosphatase in biopsies of small-bowel mucosa. Type I glycogenosis accounts for about 25 percent of all patients with glycogen storage disease.

PATHOLOGICAL PHYSIOLOGY The absence of hepatic glucose 6-phosphatase causes a profound deficiency in hepatic glucose production from either glycogenolysis or gluconeogenesis, although some glucose may be released from the liver by amylo-1,6-glucosidase (debrancher enzyme). That enzyme hydrolyzes the 6 to 8 percent of the glucose residues in the 1,6 linkage which forms the branch points of the glycogen molecule. Severe hypoglycemia is seen during fasting, with blood glucose values frequently in the range of 10 to 15 mg per 100 ml. Since glucose 6-phosphate cannot be converted to glucose, it traverses the Embden Meyerhof pathway and significantly increases hepatic production of lactic acid. Chronic hypoglycemia is associated with accelerated lipid mobilization and ketonemia. Hypercholesterolemia and hypertriglyceridemia are seen during periods of inadequate carbohydrate intake. Chronic metabolic acidosis may be present due to increased lactic acid and ketone body production. Elevated uric acid levels are characteristic, but clinical gout is usually not a problem until the second decade of life. The hyperuricemia reflects impaired renal excretion secondary to elevated lactic and β-hydroxybutyric acids coupled with increased uric acid production. The mechanism of the latter is not known but might reflect increased production of phosphoribosylpyrophosphate, a precursor of uric acid or increased degradation of adenine nucleotides due to diminished hepatic inorganic phosphate or adenosine triphosphate (ATP) concentrations.

PATHOLOGY The liver is enlarged because of excess glycogen (>5 g per 100 g weight) and fat. Splenomegaly does not occur. Despite hepatomegaly and abnormal histology, liver function is unimpaired except for those parameters involving glycogen metabolism. With increasing age, a significant number of patients develop adenomas of the liver, some of which progress to hepatomas. Renal enlargement is usually not associated with abnormalities of kidney function, although occasional patients may develop Fanconi syndrome. Increased glycogen is present in the renal tubules. Deficient glucose 6-phosphatase in intestinal mucosa seems to be of little clinical consequence although steatorrhea has been reported.

CLINICAL MANIFESTATIONS Although hepatomegaly is usually present at birth, the child with type I glycogen storage disease may not attract medical attention for several months and then present with hypoglycemic seizures, hepatomegaly, or failure to thrive. Respiratory infections, which are common, may precipitate symptomatic hypoglycemia and accentuate the chronic hyperventilation that results from metabolic acidosis. A bleeding diathesis is common and appears to be due to abnormal platelet function. The child may exhibit a typical "doll-like" facies with increased adiposity in the cheeks and buttocks. Eruptive xanthomas on extensor surfaces reflect the hyperlipidemia, and lipemia retinalis is common. The abdomen is greatly enlarged producing a waddling gait. Retarded physical growth, characteristic of this type of glycogen storage disease, may be severe but is not associated with abnormalities in pituitary, thyroid, or adrenal function. It probably reflects hypoglycemia and chronic metabolic acidosis. The latter also causes osteoporosis and negative calcium balance. Adolescent maturation is almost always delayed.

The symptoms usually ameliorate as the patient grows older if death from severe hypoglycemia, overwhelming infections, or metabolic acidosis can be prevented. While brain damage may result from hypoglycemia, the discrepancy between the low blood glucose values and the symptoms of hypoglycemia is noteworthy. Blood sugar values as low as 10 mg per 100 ml appear to be well tolerated, presumably because the brain utilizes the elevated blood ketone bodies as alternative substrate. Symptomatic gout involving both the joints and the kidneys may be a problem in those patients reaching adulthood.

DIAGNOSIS The presence of hypoglycemia, chronic metabolic acidosis, and elevated plasma levels of lactate, free fatty acids, pyruvate, glycerol, triglycerides, phospholipids, cholesterol, ketones, and uric acid suggests the diagnosis of type I glycogen storage disease. Precise diagnosis requires the demonstration of absent glucose 6-phosphatase from properly obtained and processed biopsy material from liver, intestinal mucosa, or kidney. The enzyme assay should include a control for nonspecific phosphatase activity. Histological appearance of the liver is not diagnostic. Open liver biopsy is preferable to a needle biopsy since it provides more tissue for measurement of the structure and content of glycogen and the assay of relevant

TABLE 97-1
Diseases of glycogen metabolism

Type	Enzyme defect	Glycogen		Affected tissues	Alternate names
		Amount	Structure		
I	Glucose 6-phosphatase	Increased	Normal	Liver, kidney, small-bowel mucosa	von Gierke's disease, hepatorenal disease
II	Lysosomal α-1,4-glucosidase	Increased	Normal	Generalized	Pompe's generalized
III	Amylo-1,6-glucosidase (debrancher enzyme)	Increased	Short outer chains (limit dextrin)	Liver, muscle, white blood cells	Cori's limit dextrinosis, Forbes' disease, limit dextrinosis
IV	Amylo-1,4→1,6-transglucosidase (branching enzyme)	Normal or decreased	Long outer chains, few branch points (amylopectin)	Generalized	Andersen's disease, amylopectinosis
V*	Muscle phosphorylase	Increased	Normal	Muscle	McArdle's disease
VI	Liver phosphorylase	Increased	Normal	Liver	Hers' disease
VIa	Liver phosphorylase kinase	Increased	Normal	Liver, white blood cells	
O	Glycogen synthetase	Decreased	Normal	Liver	

* A similar clinical picture results from a deficiency of phosphofructokinase, phosphoglucomutase, or phosphohexoseisomerase in muscle.

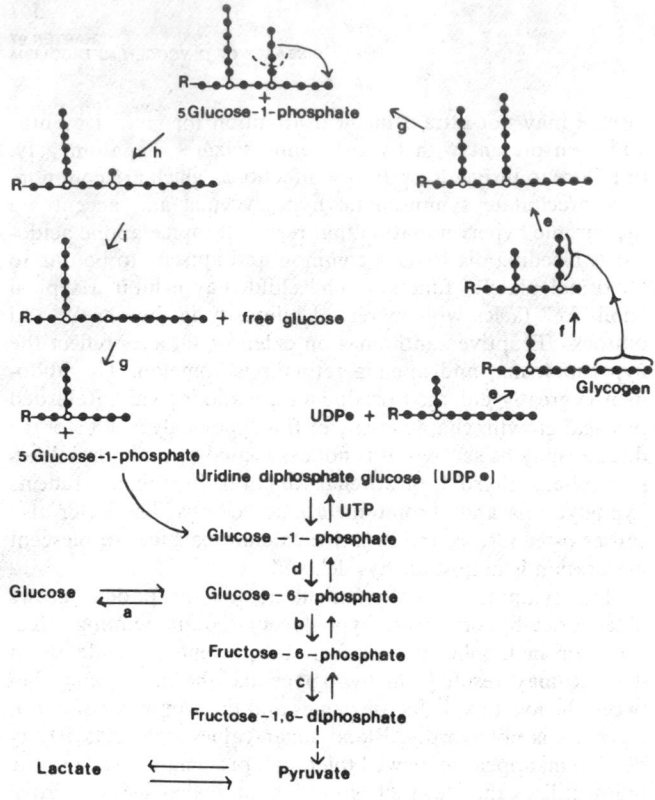

FIGURE 97-1

Pathways of glycogen synthesis and degradation. The pathway of glycogen synthesis involves phosphorylation of glucose to glucose 6-phosphate which is then converted to glucose 1-phosphate. Glucose 1-phosphate plus uridine triphosphate (UTP) reacts to form uridine diphosphate glucose (UDP, •), the donor of glucose residues in glycogen synthesis. The glucose from UDP (•) is transferred to the nonreducing terminal unit of a glycogen molecule in a 1,4 glucosidic linkage (•) by the enzyme, glycogen synthetase (e) to form a glycogen molecule with an additional glucose residue. This is repeated until the chain length contains at least seven glucose residues. A branch point is formed by the enzyme amylo-1,4→1,6-transglucosidase (branching enzyme, f) which transfers a 7-glucose unit from a 1,4 linkage to a 1,6 linkage (○). The repeated action of glycogen synthetase then extends both of these terminal chains until they are the appropriate length to form new branch points.

Glycogen breakdown is initiated by the enzyme phosphorylase (g) which sequentially hydrolyzes terminal glucose residues in 1,4 linkage to form glucose 1-phosphate. Phosphorylase activity continues to within four glucose residues of a branch point. This molecule is known as a phosphorylase limit dextrin. The enzyme oligo-1,4→1,4-glucantransferase (h) then transfers a three-glucose unit from an outer side chain to an outer main chain of the phosphorylase limit dextrin. This then exposes a branch point glucose molecule in 1,6 linkage which is removed as free glucose by the enzyme amylo-1,6-glucosidase (i). These last two enzyme activities have not been separated and are known as the debranching enzyme. After removal of the branch point, the residual glycogen molecule is available to phosphorylase until another branch point is reached. The alternate action of phosphorylase and debranching enzyme is capable of completely degrading glycogen. Glucose 1-phosphate is converted to glucose 6-phosphate by the enzyme phosphoglucomutase (d). Glucose 6-phosphate can be converted to free glucose by glucose 6-phosphatase (a) or to fructose 6-phosphate by phosphohexoseisomerase (b). The latter compound is phosphorylated by phosphofructokinase (c) to form fructose 1,6-diphosphate, which is metabolized by the Embden-Meyerhof pathway to pyruvate and lactate. Another pathway of glycogen degradation involves the lysosomal enzyme acid α-glucosidase which is capable of breaking both 1,4 and 1,6 glucosidic bonds.

enzymes. It also allows adequate hemostasis in patients with a bleeding diathesis. If the appropriate enzyme assays are not available, advance arrangements should be made with a center where they can be done.

Functional tests are helpful in establishing the appropriate diagnosis. Patients with type I glycogenosis do not increase plasma glucose concentrations following administration of epinephrine or glucagon. Since glycogen degradation is normal but free glucose cannot be released, lactate production is augmented by these hormones, thus exaggerating the metabolic acidosis. Administration of fructose, galactose, or glycerol increases plasma lactate but not glucose. Currently the diagnosis of type I glycogen storage disease cannot be made prenatally.

THERAPY Specific therapy for patients with type I glycogenosis is not available. Treatment is aimed at amelioration of hypoglycemia which appears to be responsible for most of, if not all, the clinical abnormalities. Constant nocturnal infusion of a high glucose formula through a small plastic nasogastric tube has been reported to reverse all the metabolic aberrations and increase the growth rate of patients within 4 weeks of initiation. High-starch, low-fat feedings are given every 3 h during the day. This program has been utilized at home by some patients for over a year with good clinical results including reduction of hepatic size. Portacaval transposition and portacaval shunting have also caused improvement in some patients. The results are better when the patients receive hyperalimentation preoperatively. Continuous parenteral nutrition or continuous intragastric infusion is also beneficial during acute intercurrent problems.

TYPE II GLYCOGENOSIS

Type II glycogenosis is associated with deficiency of the lysosomal enzyme α-1,4-glucosidase or acid maltase. (For a discussion of the pathophysiology of lysosomal storage diseases, see Chap. 101.) Increased glycogen concentration has been found in all tissues. The disease occurs in severe infantile and milder adult forms. Different mutant alleles probably exist for α-1,4-glucosidase to account for this clinical heterogeneity. The infantile variety is inherited as an autosomal recessive condition, and the diagnosis can be established before birth by assay of α-1,4-glucosidase in amniotic fluid cells grown in tissue culture. A neutral glucosidase in amniotic fluid precludes its use for this purpose. Type II glycogenosis is present in 1 out of every 150,000 to 400,000 births.

PATHOLOGICAL PHYSIOLOGY Despite the generalized increase in tissue glycogen concentration (especially in lysosomes) the basis for the clinical symptoms and reasons for the differences between infantile and adult forms are not clear. Patients with the infantile form of the disease have no muscle α-1,4-glucosidase, while adult patients may have residual activity. Infantile patients also have decreased neutral maltase activity, whereas this enzyme is normal in the adult variant. Since the enzymes involved in the degradation and synthesis of glycogen are normal, except for the lysosomal α-1,4-glucosidase, hypoglycemia, hyperlipidemia, metabolic acidosis, and other systemic metabolic alterations are not present. Increased lysosomal glycogen concentration can be accounted for by the deficiency of α-1,4-glucosidase, but the explanation for the augmented extralysosomal cytoplasmic glycogen is unknown. In the infantile form, increased glycogen is present in cardiac and skeletal muscle as well as in liver, kidney, and central nervous system. The absent or minimal cardiac involvement in the adult patients may account for their longer survival. Accumulation of glycogen in the lysosomes of cardiac and skeletal muscle may impair their function, but the mechanism is unknown.

CLINICAL MANIFESTATIONS In the infantile form the characteristic clinical features result from myocardial and neuromuscular involvement. Classically symptoms of congestive heart failure with progressive cardiac enlargement begin within a few weeks after birth. Repeated respiratory infections are common. The patients fail to thrive and manifest anorexia, easy fatigability, generalized weakness, drooling, and shortness of breath. The tongue is frequently enlarged. The muscle mass is increased and has a firm, rubbery consistency, but the muscles are weak and hypotonic. The liver is usually firm and moderately enlarged. Neurological abnormalities may be present with retarded motor and intellectual development. The cardiac image is globular and markedly enlarged on chest x-ray. The electrocardiogram demonstrates left axis deviation, short PR interval, QRS complexes of large amplitude, depression of the ST segment, and inversion of the T waves. Death usually occurs within the first year or two of life due to intractable congestive heart failure. About 20 percent of the patients also have endocardial fibroelastosis.

The milder adult form presents with muscle weakness which is greater proximally than distally and involves the pelvic more than the pectoral muscles. Respiratory muscles may also be involved. Symptoms usually become prominent in the third to sixth decade. In the adult form there is no relationship between the clinical picture and the amount of residual α-1,4-glucosidase activity.

DIAGNOSIS Type II glycogen storage disease is diagnosed by demonstrating α-1,4-glucosidase deficiency in white blood cells, cultured skin fibroblasts, or skeletal muscle. The glycogen content of tissue is increased (liver, >5 percent; muscle, >1 percent), but its structure is normal. While the histological localization of increased glycogen in lysosomes is suggestive, the diagnosis should be confirmed by appropriate enzyme assay. It is important to distinguish between neutral and acid α-1,4-glucosidase activity in biopsy specimens.

THERAPY No effective treatment exists for the infantile form. Supportive measures such as digitalis, diuretics, and salt restriction are of little value in the treatment of the congestive heart failure. α-1,4-Glucosidase prepared from both *Aspergillus niger* and human placenta has been administered to infants with type II glycogenosis, but no beneficial effect on the clinical course of the disease was observed.

TYPE III GLYCOGEN STORAGE DISEASE

The enzyme amylo-1,6-glucosidase, the debrancher enzyme, is deficient in this form of glycogen storage disease. The enzyme deficiency in liver and muscle is responsible for the clinical disease, but white and red blood cells also share the defect. Several variants have been described on the basis of tissue distribution of the enzyme deficiency and the method of the enzyme assay. Type III glycogenosis is probably the commonest form of glycogen storage disease and appears to be inherited in autosomal recessive fashion.

PATHOLOGICAL PHYSIOLOGY The absence of amylo-1,6-glucosidase prevents further degradation of glycogen beyond a branch point and results in a molecule with very short outer chains (limit dextrin). Normal glycogen degradation involves removal of glucosyl units in 1,4 linkage in the outer chains by phosphorylase until four such residues remain on either side of the branch point, a glucose molecule which has both a 1,6 and a 1,4 linkage (Fig. 97-1). Three glucose residues on the branched chain are then transferred to the terminal position on the main chain by the enzyme oligo-1,4→1,4-glucantransferase. This enzyme activity has not been separated physically from the amylo-1,6-glucosidase which splits the glucosyl unit

in 1,6 linkage at the branch point to free glucose. Following removal of the branch point, phosphorylase then continues degradation of glycogen until the next branch point is approached. During fasting, the abnormal glycogen (limit dextrin) cannot be further degraded, leading to hypoglycemia. The hypoglycemia is less severe than in patients with type I glycogen storage disease because gluconeogenesis is still intact. Abnormalities in lipid metabolism are also less prominent than in type I glycogen storage disease. Plasma lactate and uric acid concentrations are usually normal. Since amylo-1,6-glucosidase may also be absent in skeletal muscle, the disorder may be associated with hypotonia, muscle weakness, and increased muscle glycogen content.

CLINICAL MANIFESTATIONS The clinical presentation is similar to that of patients with type I glycogenosis but less severe. Hypoglycemia tends to be mild, but growth retardation, hepatomegaly, and splenomegaly may be present. As the patient grows older, the symptoms ameliorate, and hepatomegaly diminishes.

DIAGNOSIS Diagnosis depends upon the demonstration of the enzyme defect in cultured skin fibroblasts or in muscle or liver obtained by biopsy. The finding of increased amounts of glycogen with abnormal structure (short outer-branch chains) is confirmatory. Assay of either white or red blood cells for amylo-1,6-glucosidase and glycogen structure can also be useful in genetic studies. Children with type III glycogenosis frequently have elevations of serum transaminase without other evidence of generalized hepatic dysfunction. Since glycogen cannot be degraded beyond the initial phosphorylase cleavages, administration of glucagon or epinephrine in the fasting state usually does not increase the blood glucose. However, administration of these substances several hours after a meal does cause an elevation in blood glucose since carbohydrate ingestion restores the outer chains of glycogen, rendering them available for degradation by phosphorylase. In contrast to patients with type I glycogen storage disease, glucagon administration does not increase plasma lactate concentration, and administration of fructose, galactose, glycerol, or alanine increases the blood glucose.

THERAPY Hypoglycemia can usually be prevented by frequent feedings, but in some patients the problem is severe enough to warrant portacaval shunting. Generally, constant nocturnal infusion of a high-carbohydrate formula is preferable to surgery, especially since the disease ameliorates with time. In contrast to patients with type I glycogen storage disease, there is no need to restrict the lactose or sucrose content of the diet.

TYPE IV GLYCOGENOSIS

This type of glycogen deposition disease is associated with deficiency of amylo-1,4→1,6-transglucosidase (branching enzyme). This enzyme initiates the branching of glycogen by transferring a 7-glucose unit from a 1,4 linkage to a 1,6 linkage. The enzyme is deficient in multiple tissues including liver, heart, smooth and skeletal muscle, kidney, spleen, central nervous system, and white blood cells. The glycogen content of these tissues may be normal or decreased but is abnormal in structure, resembling amylopectin with decreased branch points and long outer chains. The molecule has a high chromogenicity, and the absorption maximum is shifted. Only 13 cases have been reported, and it appears to be transmitted as an autosomal recessive. Heterozygotes may have diminished branching enzyme in white blood cells, but this has not been found uniformly. Assay of enzyme in amniotic fluid fibroblasts has been used for antenatal diagnosis.

PATHOLOGICAL PHYSIOLOGY This type of glycogenosis is not associated with any abnormality in carbohydrate metabolism since the enzymatic defect does not prevent glycogen degradation by phosphorylase and since gluconeogenesis is unimpaired. However, the disease is associated with progressive development of either cirrhosis or cardiac failure, of unknown mechanism.

CLINICAL MANIFESTATIONS At birth, patients appear normal but fail to thrive in the first few months of life. Hepatomegaly and abnormal liver function usually accompany clinical deterioration, and splenomegaly and ascites develop as the liver failure progresses. The muscles are hypotonic, and congestive heart failure may develop. This disease is uniformly fatal in the first few years of life.

DIAGNOSIS Type IV glycogenosis should be considered in all infants with cirrhosis or congestive heart failure. The diagnosis is established by finding deficient branching-enzyme activity in white blood cells or in tissue obtained by biopsy. The demonstration of glycogen structure resembling amylopectin is indicative of the disease, but the diagnosis should be confirmed by enzyme assay.

THERAPY No specific therapy is available. Cirrhosis and heart failure are treated symptomatically.

TYPE V GLYCOGEN STORAGE DISEASE

Muscle phosphorylase is absent in this form of glycogen storage disease. This enzyme is immunologically and genetically distinct from the liver enzyme. The disease is inherited as an autosomal recessive.

PATHOLOGICAL PHYSIOLOGY Glycogenolysis is an important source of energy for muscle contraction. Phosphorylase deficiency precludes this source of energy and accounts for the difficulty these patients have during sustained muscle activity. Normally during exercise the combination of increased glycogenolysis and inadequate oxygen elevates plasma lactic acid. This normal increase in lactic acid with exercise does not occur in patients with type V glycogenosis.

CLINICAL MANIFESTATIONS For unknown reasons affected patients have very few symptoms during the first or second decade of life. Thereafter, exercise causes weakness and cramping of the involved muscles. Myoglobinuria is common, especially with strenuous exercise, and muscle enzymes are characteristically elevated in the plasma. There are no definitive physical findings, but in later life some muscle atrophy may be present.

DIAGNOSIS The diagnosis is suggested by the lack of increase in plasma lactate after muscular exercise. However, demonstration of absent muscle phosphorylase is necessary to establish the diagnosis since a similar clinical picture with absent lactate elevation has been described in patients with normal phosphorylase activity but other enzyme deficiencies in their muscles. The latter include phosphofructokinase, phosphoglucomutase, and phosphohexoseisomerase, deficiencies of which would impede anaerobic glycolysis in muscle.

THERAPY Ingestion of glucose or fructose prior to and during exercise is frequently associated with improved exercise tolerance. Patients learn their exercise tolerance and avoid symptoms by not exceeding it. Within these limitations, the long-term prognosis is good.

TYPE VI GLYCOGEN STORAGE DISEASE

Abnormalities in the phosphorylase system of the liver are found in patients with type VI glycogen storage disease. A cyclic AMP–dependent protein kinase stimulated by glucagon activates the enzyme phosphorylase kinase which in turn converts inactive phosphorylase to the active enzyme. The product of phosphorylase degradation, glucose 1-phosphate, is then converted to glucose 6-phosphate. While absence of any of the enzymes in this cascade could produce the clinical picture, only deficiencies of phosphorylase kinase and phosphorylase have been adequately documented. The former deficiency is more common. Phosphorylase deficiency, considered as type VI glycogen storage disease, is inherited as an autosomal recessive trait. Type VIa glycogen storage disease is due to deficiency of phosphorylase kinase and exists in two forms. One is inherited as an autosomal recessive and the other as an X-linked recessive trait.

CLINICAL MANIFESTATIONS These patients are similar to those with type III glycogen storage disease and are less symptomatic than patients with the type I disorder. Types VI and VIa glycogen storage diseases are clinically indistinguishable. Hepatic enlargement is prominent during preadolescent years but often disappears with amelioration of symptoms as the child grows older. Fasting hypoglycemia, when present, is usually mild, and hyperlipidemia and metabolic acidosis are usually absent. Frequently the deficiency of phosphorylase is incomplete and, in addition, gluconeogenesis is unimpaired. Patients may have some retardation in physical and motor development initially but almost always ultimately attain normal adult height.

DIAGNOSIS This type of glycogen storage disease should be suspected in patients who present with a picture similar to type III disease. The specific diagnosis can be established by appropriate assay for the enzyme in either liver or leukocytes. Despite the reduction of activity of the phosphorylase system, these patients may have a normal blood glucose response to either epinephrine or glucagon. Several patients have been described who had other defects of the phosphorylase system. One patient with hepatomegaly, truncal ataxia, nystagmus, hypotonia and spasticity had normal total liver phosphorylase, but the enzyme was entirely in the inactive form. An additional patient with defective cyclic AMP–dependent protein kinase in muscle and liver has been reported.

THERAPY Since these patients, for the most part, have mild symptoms that diminish as they grow older, no specific treatment is necessary over and above prevention of hypoglycemia.

PATIENTS WITH MULTIPLE OR NO ENZYMATIC DEFECTS

Several patients with the clinical picture of type I glycogen storage disease have deficiency of another enzyme in addition to glucose 6-phosphatase. The second enzyme is most frequently amylo-1,6-glucosidase, but occasionally it may be phosphorylase. Children in the same family may have different enzymatic defects. It is conceivable that the second enzyme deficiency is an artifact due to inadequate tissue preservation or assay techniques. Patients with the clinical features of glycogen storage diseases have also been reported who have no de-

tectable enzyme defect when the liver biopsy is assayed for all
the enzymes involved in the recognized types of glycogen storage disease.

GLYCOGEN SYNTHETASE DEFICIENCY

This disease is caused by deficiency of hepatic glycogen synthetase, the enzyme responsible for adding glucosyl units to
glycogen. Hypoglycemia is usually the presenting manifestation, although the infant may present because of failure to
thrive. The liver is not enlarged. Fasting ketonuria is present,
and a relationship to ketotic hypoglycemia has been suggested.
Feeding is associated with elevated plasma lactic acid levels,
and glycosuria may occur. Administration of glucagon in the
fed state increases blood glucose somewhat but brings no response during a fast. Plasma alanine levels are low. The diagnosis is established by assay of liver for glycogen synthetase.
Treatment should be aimed at prevention of hypoglycemia by
utilizing a program of constant nocturnal infusion as outlined
for type I glycogen storage disease.

REFERENCES

AYNSLEY-GREEN AW et al: Hepatic glycogen synthetase deficiency.
Definition of syndrome from metabolic and enzyme studies on a 9-
year old girl. Arch Dis Child 52:573, 1977

DRASH A, FIELD JB: The glycogen storage diseases. Dis Mon, October
1971

GREENE HL et al: Continuous nocturnal intragastric feeding for management of type 1 glycogen-storage disease. N Engl J Med 294:423,
1976

HOWELL RR: The glycogen storage diseases, in *The Metabolic Basis of
Inherited Diseases,* 4th ed, JB Stanbury et al (eds). New York,
McGraw-Hill, 1978, p 137

HUG G: Glycogen storage diseases Birth Defects 12:145, 1976

HUIJING F: Glycogen metabolism and glycogen-storage disease. Physiol Rev 55:609, 1975

MAHLER RF: Disorders of glycogen metabolism. Clin Endocrinol Metab 5:579, 1976

SENIOR B, SADEGHI-NEJAD A: The glycogenoses and other inherited
disorders of carbohydrate metabolism. Clin Perinatal 3:79, 1976

98
GALACTOSEMIA

KURT J. ISSELBACHER

DEFINITION Galactosemia refers to an inborn error of metabolism associated with an impairment in the metabolism of
galactose. Two disorders are currently recognized. "Classic"
galactosemia is due to the deficiency of the enzyme galactose
1-phosphate uridyl transferase; it is typically associated with
cataract formation, mental retardation, and cirrhosis. The second disorder, first described in 1965, is due to galactokinase
deficiency and leads primarily to cataract formation.

PATHOGENESIS Lactose, the main carbohydrate in milk, is a
disaccharide containing galactose and glucose; when ingested
it is hydrolyzed by intestinal lactase. Normally the absorbed
galactose is converted in the liver to glucose. The first reaction
in this pathway involves the phosphorylation of galactose to
galactose 1-phosphate by galactokinase:

$$\text{Galactose} + \text{ATP} \xrightarrow{\text{galactokinase}} \text{galactose 1-phosphate}$$

The gene for galactokinase has been assigned to chromosome 17. The next step involves the conversion of galactose 1-
phosphate to glucose 1-phosphate. This involves the participation of uridine diphosphate (UDP) sugars and the enzyme galactose 1-phosphate uridyl transferase as follows:

$$\text{Galactose 1-phosphate} + \text{UDP-glucose} \xrightarrow{\text{transferase}}$$
$$\text{UDP-galactose} + \text{glucose 1-phosphate}$$

The UDP sugars can be reversibly interconverted by an epime-
rase reaction:

$$\text{UDP-galactose} \xrightleftharpoons{\text{epimerase}} \text{UDP-glucose}$$

Several alternate pathways of galactose metabolism appear
to exist. Galactose can be converted (reduced) in the presence
of NADPH (or NADH) to galactitol (dulcitol) by aldose reductase, an enzyme which occurs especially in the lens. Galactose can be oxidized to a limited extent by galactose dehydrogenase leading eventually to the formation of galactonic acid,
xylulose, and CO_2. There is also a pyrophosphorylase reaction
involving the interaction of galactose 1-phosphate with uridine
triphosphate to form UDP-galactose. One or more of these
pathways may account for a limited galactose metabolism in
some patients with galactosemia.

In galactokinase deficiency, galactose accumulates in the
blood and tissues. In the lens galactose is converted by aldose
reductase to galactitol, a sugar to which the lens is impermeable. As a consequence, excessive hydration occurs which, together with a decrease in lenticular glutathione, leads to cataract formation.

In classic galactosemia, transferase deficiency leads to tissue
accumulation of galactose 1-phosphate and galactose. As in
galactokinase deficiency, cataracts develop secondary to galactitol accumulation in the lens. It is assumed but not proved
that the cirrhosis and mental retardation of classic galactosemia are in some manner related to increased amounts of galactose 1-phosphate in these tissues. Elevated blood galactose
levels may lead to a decreased hepatic output of glucose and
hypoglycemia. In the kidney and intestine, accumulation of
galactose and galactose 1-phosphate appears to lead to an inhibition of amino acid transport.

Both galactokinase- and transferase-deficiency galactosemia are transmitted as autosomal recessive traits. Heterozygotes for these disorders have half-normal enzyme levels but
are asymptomatic. Maternal deficiency of galactokinase, together with a significant lactose intake during pregnancy, may
contribute to cataract formation during fetal development.
However, not all persons with half-normal transferase enzymes
in their cells are carriers of galactosemia. Some individuals
homozygous for another gene, called the Duarte variant, normally have only half-normal transferase levels. This group can
be differentiated from galactosemia heterozygotes on the basis
of the electrophoretic properties of the mutant enzyme. In both
types of galactosemia, the disorder is due either to the functional deficiency or absence of the involved enzyme. In the
classic type of galactosemia there is evidence that the disorder
is due to a structural gene mutation and that the enzyme
(transferase) protein is present but structurally altered and not
functioning normally. Several other clinical variants with altered enzyme electrophoretic mobility have been described.

The exact incidence of classic galactosemia is still unclear.
Estimates range from 1 in 18,000 to 1 in 100,000 births. Population studies indicate that 0.8 to 1.3 percent of the population
are heterozygous for the galactosemia gene and about 10 percent carry the Duarte variant.

CLINICAL FEATURES Symptoms of classic galactosemia usually begin within days to several weeks after birth. The infant usually is reluctant to ingest breast milk or milk formulas, develops vomiting, shows poor nutrition, and fails to thrive. Jaundice, hepatomegaly, and evidence of liver disease may then develop. Cataracts are usually not present at birth but occur gradually over a period of weeks to months. Mental retardation may be difficult to detect but becomes evident after 6 or 12 months. Infants with classical galactosemia are subject to bacterial sepsis (especially with *Escherichia coli*), and this may be the primary cause of death in the neonatal period. The only recognized complication of galactokinase deficiency is cataract formation.

DIAGNOSIS Galactokinase deficiency should be suspected in infants or children with cataract formation who have non-glucose-reducing substances in their urine. The diagnosis is made by demonstrating the deficiency of galactokinase in red blood cells.

Classic galactosemia must be considered when one or more of the clinical features described above are found. If the patient is ingesting milk, reducing sugar may be found in the urine, which gives a negative glucose oxidase reaction (i.e., is not glucose) and is identified as galactose by other techniques, such as chromatography. If the child is vomiting, has a poor food intake, or is on intravenous glucose feedings, galactose may not be present in the urine. The definitive diagnosis consists of demonstrating a lack or deficiency of red cell galactose 1-phosphate uridyl transferase. A variety of assay techniques have been described. The disease can also be diagnosed prenatally by enzyme studies on cultured cells obtained by amniocentesis.

In the neonatal period galactosemia needs to be differentiated from primary liver disease. With liver damage, galactose removal from the blood is impaired, and elevated blood galactose levels as well as galactosuria may occur. However, in hepatitis or cirrhosis the transferase levels will be normal.

TREATMENT The treatment of galactosemia consists of the removal of galactose-containing foods from the diet, especially milk. In infants, milk substitutes such as DextriMaltose and Nutramigen are often used. Soybean preparations have also been used in the past, but their polysaccharides contain some galactose and they should be avoided.

The institution of a galactose-free diet usually leads to a dramatic improvement in the patient; in fact, all clinical features except for mental retardation may improve or disappear. In general, patients are kept on galactose-free diets indefinitely or at least until they have reached adequate physical and neurologic development.

REFERENCES

GITZELMANN R et al: Galactose metabolism in a patient with hereditary galactokinase deficiency. Eur J Clin Invest 4:79, 1974

LEVY HL et al: Sepsis due to *Escherichia coli* in neonates with galactosemia. N Engl J Med 297:737, 1975

SEGAL S: Disorders of galactose metabolism, in *The Metabolic Basis of Inherited Disease,* 4th ed, JB Stanbury et al (eds). New York, McGraw-Hill, 1978, p 160

TEDESCO TA et al: The genetic defect in galactosemia. N Engl J Med 292:737, 1975

99

HEREDITARY FRUCTOSE INTOLERANCE

DANIEL W. FOSTER

Hereditary fructose intolerance is an autosomal recessive disorder characterized by vomiting and hypoglycemia following the ingestion of fructose-containing foods. The underlying molecular defect is a deficiency of the enzyme fructose 1-phosphate aldolase.

CLINICAL PICTURE Clinical manifestations of fructose intolerance vary with age, the most severe form occurring in infants. Characteristically the baby is normal when breast fed but develops symptoms once fructose-containing formulas or foods are ingested. The primary response to fructose is severe vomiting and diarrhea with consequent failure to thrive. Hepatic disease is invariable; hepatomegaly is accompanied by hyperbilirubinemia, elevated levels of hepatic enzymes in plasma, hypoalbuminemia, and even ascites. Hemorrhage may be a major problem due to deficiencies of prothrombin, fibrinogen, and other clotting factors. Postprandial hypoglycemia may lead to loss of consciousness or convulsions. Albuminuria and renal tubular acidosis of the proximal type with aminoaciduria and bicarbonate wastage are common. The children are vulnerable to lactic acidosis.

Older children and adults have a less severe syndrome, often because they learn spontaneously to avoid sweets. The usual picture is that of abdominal pain, nausea, bloating, and diarrhea with or without signs of hypoglycemia following the ingestion of foods containing fructose, sucrose, or sorbitol (which is converted to fructose in the body). Hyperuricemia and uricosuria are common, and kidney stones may be present. Dental caries are unusual because of diminished sugar intake. Hepatic disease is less severe in the adult.

If the diagnosis is made early and effective treatment is initiated, all manifestations of the disease disappear; i.e., the renal and hepatic lesions are reversible. Prolonged exposure to fructose in infants may result in permanent liver damage with changes of portal or biliary cirrhosis evident on pathological examination.

PATHOPHYSIOLOGY The disorder is due to deficiency of fructose 1-phosphate aldolase. When fructose is ingested, the first step in its metabolism is the formation of fructose 1-phosphate, a reaction catalyzed by the enzyme fructokinase. Fructose 1-phosphate is then split to form the trioses glyceraldehyde and dihydroxyacetone phosphate by fructose 1-phosphate aldolase. A deficiency of the enzyme results in the accumulation of fructose 1-phosphate in the tissues following ingestion of fructose and sorbitol. This intermediate is presumably directly responsible for hepatic and renal tubular damage. Fructose 1-phosphate also secondarily inhibits other enzymes. Inhibition of fructokinase accounts for fructosemia and fructosuria, while postprandial hypoglycemia is presumably due to inhibition of hepatic glycogen phosphorylase activity, an impairment that also accounts for glucagon unresponsiveness in the syndrome. Fructose 1-phosphate also inhibits fructose 1,6-diphosphate aldolase, thereby blocking gluconeogenesis. While the block in glycogen breakdown is the primary reason for postprandial hypoglycemia, impairment of gluconeogenesis plays a contributing role. Sharp falls in tissue and plasma inorganic phosphate concentrations occur with fructose ingestion and presumably account for the depletion of tissue adenosine triphosphate that characteristically follows. The reason for hyperuricemia is not known but may be related to increased turnover of purine nucleotides.

DIAGNOSIS The diagnosis is usually suggested by history. In infants the differential lies between hereditary fructose intolerance, galactosemia, and tyrosinosis. The latter two syndromes are also associated with postprandial vomiting and failure to thrive and are due to the ingestion of galactose and tyrosine, respectively. If symptoms are immediately relieved by the intravenous infusion of glucose and do not return when a sucrose- and fructose-free diet is consumed, the diagnosis is clear. Confirmation requires testing with fructose. While normal persons develop hypoglycemia with large fructose loads, the administration of small doses of the hexose (0.25 g/kg in adults, 3 g per square meter of body surface area in children) produces symptoms and a fall in plasma glucose and phosphorus concentrations only in subjects with the disease.

TREATMENT Treatment consists of eliminating sucrose, fructose, and sorbitol from the diet.

REFERENCES

FROESCH ER: Essential fructosuria, hereditary fructose intolerance, and fructose-1,6-diphosphatase deficiency, in *The Metabolic Basis of Inherited Disease*, JB Stanbury et al (eds). New York, McGraw Hill, 1978, pp 121–136

ODIÈVRE M et al: Hereditary fructose intolerance in childhood. Am J Dis Child 132.605, 1978

STEINER G et al: Studies of glucose turnover and renal function in an unusual case of hereditary fructose intolerance. Am J Med 62:150, 1977

Disorders of lipid metabolism

100
THE HYPERLIPOPROTEINEMIAS AND OTHER DISORDERS OF LIPID METABOLISM

MICHAEL S. BROWN
JOSEPH L. GOLDSTEIN

The *hyperlipoproteinemias* are disturbances of lipid transport that result from abnormalities in the synthesis or degradation of plasma lipoproteins. The clinical importance of the elevated plasma lipoprotein level derives from the ability of plasma lipoproteins to cause two life-threatening diseases: atherosclerosis and pancreatitis. Some hyperlipoproteinemias are the direct result of *primary* defects in the metabolism of lipoprotein particles. Other hyperlipoproteinemias are *secondary,* that is, the elevated plasma lipoprotein level occurs as part of a constellation of abnormalities caused by an underlying disorder in a related metabolic system, such as thyroid hormone deficiency or insulin deficiency. The primary hyperlipoproteinemias can be divided into two broad categories: (1) *single-gene disorders* that are transmitted by simple dominant or recessive mechanisms and (2) *multifactorial disorders* with complex inheritance patterns in which multiple variant genes interact with environmental factors to produce varying degrees of hyperlipoproteinemia in members of a family.

PHYSIOLOGIC ROLE OF LIPOPROTEINS IN LIPID TRANSPORT
The lipoproteins are globular particles of high molecular weight that transport nonpolar lipids (primarily *triglycerides* and *cholesteryl esters*) through the plasma. A general model for the structure of a lipoprotein particle is shown in Fig. 100-1. Each lipoprotein particle contains a nonpolar *core,* in which many molecules of hydrophobic lipid are packed to form an oil droplet. This hydrophobic core, which accounts for most of the mass of the particle, consists of triglycerides and cholesteryl esters in varying proportions. Surrounding the core is a polar *surface coat* of phospholipids that stabilize the lipoprotein particle so that it can remain in solution in the plasma. In addition to phospholipids, the polar coat contains small amounts of unesterified cholesterol. Each lipoprotein particle also contains specific proteins (termed *apoproteins*) that are partly exposed at the surface. The apoprotein binds to specific enzymes or transport proteins on cell membranes, thus directing the lipoprotein to its sites of metabolism.

Table 100-1 describes the characteristics of the five major classes of lipoproteins that normally circulate in human plasma. These lipoprotein classes differ in the composition of the nonpolar lipids in the core; in the composition of the apoproteins; and in density, size, and electrophoretic mobility.

Lipid transport: the exogenous pathway Figure 100-2 shows the pathways by which lipoproteins transport lipids in plasma. The largest amounts of lipoproteins are involved in the transport of dietary fat, which amounts to more than 100 g triglyceride and about 1 g cholesterol per day. Within intestinal epithelial cells, dietary triglycerides and cholesterol are incorporated into large lipoprotein particles called *chylomicrons.* The chylomicrons are secreted into the intestinal lymph and pass into the general circulation for transport to the capillaries of adipose tissue and skeletal muscle, where they adhere to binding sites on the capillary walls. While bound to these endothelial surfaces, the chylomicrons are exposed to the enzyme *lipoprotein lipase,* which hydrolyzes the triglycerides of the chylomicrons, releasing free fatty acids and monoglycerides. The fatty acids pass through the endothelial cells and enter the underlying adipocytes or muscle cells, where they are either reesterified to triglycerides or oxidized.

After the core triglycerides have been removed, the remainder of the chylomicron dissociates from the capillary endothe-

A. TYPICAL LIPOPROTEIN PARTICLE

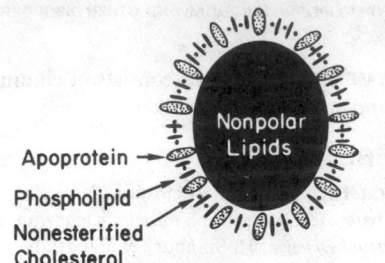

Apoprotein →
Phospholipid →
Nonesterified
Cholesterol →

Nonpolar
Lipids

B. NONPOLAR LIPIDS

Triglyceride

$$CH_2-\overset{\overset{O}{\|}}{C}-(CH_2)_n-CH_3$$
$$CH_2-\overset{\overset{O}{\|}}{C}-(CH_2)_n-CH_3$$
$$CH_2-\overset{\overset{O}{\|}}{C}-(CH_2)_n-CH_3$$

Cholesteryl
Ester

$$CH_3-(CH_2)_n-\overset{\overset{O}{\|}}{C}-O-$$

FIGURE 100-1

A. Diagrammatic representation of the structure of a typical plasma lipoprotein particle. The core of the spherical lipoprotein particle is composed of two nonpolar lipids, triglyceride and cholesteryl ester, which are present in different lipoproteins in varying amounts. The nonpolar core is surrounded by a surface coat composed primarily of phospholipids. Apoproteins are exposed at the surface and extend into the core. Variable amounts of unesterified cholesterol are interdigitated with the phospholip- *ids of the surface coat. The qualitative composition of each of the five major classes of lipoprotein particles in human plasma is summarized in Table 100-1. B. Structures of the two nonpolar lipids, triglyceride and cholesteryl ester. In order for these nonpolar lipids to be assimilated into tissues, the ester bonds between the fatty acids and either glycerol (triglycerides) or cholesterol (cholesteryl esters) must be broken by lipoprotein lipase and the lysosomal cholesterol esterase, respectively.*

lium and reenters the circulation. It has now been transformed into a particle that is relatively poor in triglyceride and enriched in cholesteryl esters. It has also undergone an exchange of apoproteins with other plasma lipoproteins. The net result is the conversion of the chylomicron to a *remnant particle,* enriched in cholesteryl esters and apoproteins B, CIII, and E. This remnant travels to the liver, where it is taken up with great efficiency. The overall result of the chylomicron transport process is to deliver dietary triglyceride to adipose tissue and cholesterol to the liver.

Some of the cholesterol that reaches the liver is converted to bile acids, which are excreted into the intestine to act as detergents and facilitate the absorption of dietary fat. In addition, some cholesterol is excreted into the bile without metabolism to bile acids. The liver also distributes cholesterol to other tissues (discussed below).

Lipid transport: the endogenous pathway Triglyceride synthesis in the liver is enhanced when the diet contains excess carbohydrates. The liver converts the carbohydrate to fatty acids, esterifies the fatty acids with glycerol to form triglycerides, and secretes the triglyceride into the bloodstream in the core of *very low density lipoproteins (VLDL).* The VLDL particles are relatively large, carry five to ten times more triglycerides than cholesteryl esters, and contain apoproteins that are similar to those of chylomicrons (Table 100-1).

The VLDL particles are transported to tissue capillaries, where they interact with the same lipoprotein lipase enzyme that catabolizes chylomicrons. The core triglycerides of the

VLDL are hydrolyzed, and the fatty acids are used for triglyceride synthesis within adipose tissue. The remnants generated from the action of lipoprotein lipase on VLDL are similar to those formed from chylomicrons. However, in contrast to chylomicron remnants, most of the VLDL remnants are not catabolized by the liver in humans. Rather, the VLDL remnants undergo a further transformation in which nearly all the residual triglycerides are removed and replaced with cholesteryl esters. During this conversion, all the apoproteins are removed from the particle with the exception of apoprotein B. The result is the transformation of the VLDL remnant particle into the cholesterol-rich *low-density lipoprotein* (LDL). The core of LDL is composed almost entirely of cholesteryl esters, and the surface coat contains only one apoprotein, apoprotein B. About three-fourths of the total cholesterol in normal human plasma is contained within LDL particles.

The function of LDL is to supply cholesterol to a variety of extrahepatic parenchymal cells, such as adrenal cortical cells, lymphocytes, muscle cells, and renal cells.

These cells have *LDL receptors* localized on the cell surface. LDL that binds to this receptor is taken up and digested by lysosomes within the cells. The cholesteryl esters of LDL are hydrolyzed by a lysosomal cholesteryl esterase (acid lipase), and the liberated cholesterol is used both for membrane synthesis and as a precursor for steroid hormone synthesis. This LDL receptor pathway serves as the major route for the degradation of LDL.

In addition to its degradation by the LDL pathway in extrahepatic parenchymal cells, some of the LDL is degraded by

TABLE 100-1
Characteristics of the major classes of lipoproteins in human plasma

Lipoprotein class	Major core lipids	Major apoproteins	Density, g/ml	Diameter, Å	Electrophoretic mobility
Chylomicrons	Dietary triglycerides	AI, AII, B, CI, CII, CIII	<1.006	800–5000	Remains at origin
VLDL	Endogenous triglycerides	B, CI, CII, CIII, E	<1.006	300–800	Pre-β
Remnants	Cholesteryl esters, triglycerides	B, CIII, E	<1.019	250–350	Slow pre-β
LDL	Cholesteryl esters	B	1.019–1.063	180–280	β
HDL	Cholesteryl esters	AI, AII	1.063–1.210	50–120	α

a scavenger cell system that consists of phagocytic cells in the reticuloendothelial system. In contrast to the receptor-mediated pathway for LDL degradation, the scavenger cell pathway is thought to function solely to degrade LDL when the lipoprotein reaches high concentrations in plasma rather than to supply cholesterol to cells.

As the membranes of parenchymal and scavenger cells undergo turnover and as cells die and are renewed, unesterified cholesterol is released into plasma, where it binds initially to *high-density lipoprotein (HDL)*. This unesterified cholesterol is then coupled to a fatty acid in an esterification reaction catalyzed by the plasma enzyme *lecithin:cholesterol acyltransferase (LCAT)*. The cholesteryl esters that are formed on the surface of HDL are transferred to VLDL and eventually appear in LDL. This establishes a cycle by which LDL delivers cholesterol to extrahepatic cells and by which cholesterol is returned to LDL from extrahepatic cells via HDL. Some of the cholesterol released from extrahepatic tissues is transported to the liver for excretion in the bile. The mechanism by which the liver takes up this cholesterol is unknown, but it is possible that hepatic LDL receptors are involved.

DIAGNOSIS OF HYPERLIPOPROTEINEMIA A variety of diseases cause elevations in the concentrations of one or more lipoprotein classes in plasma. In general, these abnormalities are detected by the finding of an elevated concentration of triglycerides or cholesterol in fasting plasma, a condition called *hyperlipidemia*. The value for plasma cholesterol represents the total cholesterol, which includes both cholesteryl esters and unesterified cholesterol. The absolute and relative values for the plasma cholesterol and triglyceride levels provide information regarding the nature of the lipoprotein particle that is increased. An isolated elevation in plasma triglycerides indicates that the concentrations of chylomicrons, VLDL, and/or remnants are increased. On the other hand, an isolated elevation of plasma cholesterol nearly always indicates that the concentration of LDL is increased. Frequently, both triglycerides and cholesterol are elevated. Such a combined abnormality may be produced by a marked elevation in chylomicrons or VLDL, in which case the ratio of triglyceride to cholesterol in plasma will be greater than 5:1. Alternatively, there may be an elevation of both VLDL and LDL, in which case the triglyceride/cholesterol ratio in plasma is less than 5:1.

The definition of hyperlipoproteinemia is arbitrary because plasma lipid and lipoprotein levels exhibit a bell-shaped distribution in the population, without clear separation between normal and abnormal values. Since lipoprotein concentrations

are influenced by diet and other environmental factors, standards must be established for the population under consideration. What is usually done is to set arbitrary statistical limits of normal concentrations based on the examination of a large number of healthy-appearing subjects of different ages. The cut-off limit that is usually used is the upper 5 to 10 percent of values found in apparently healthy individuals (i.e., the 90th to 95th percentile values). However, a vast amount of epidemiologic data from both industrialized and more agrarian cultures indicate that lipid and lipoprotein concentrations that are "normal" in a statistical sense are not necessarily healthy. As a working rule, clinically significant hyperlipoproteinemia is considered to be present in any individual below the age of 20 whose total plasma cholesterol level exceeds 200 mg per 100 ml or whose triglyceride level exceeds 140 mg per 100 ml. In individuals above the age of 20, significant hyperlipoproteinemia exists whenever the plasma cholesterol level exceeds 240 mg per 100 ml or the triglyceride level exceeds 200 mg per 100 ml.

The various combinations of elevated lipoproteins that occur in disease states have been divided into six lipoprotein types or patterns. These are summarized in Table 100-2. As shown in Table 100-3, most of the lipoprotein types can be caused by several different genetic diseases; conversely, some genetic diseases can produce more than one lipoprotein pattern. In addition, each of the abnormal lipoprotein types can occur as a secondary consequence of another metabolic disease (Table 100-4). Hence, the lipoprotein type is a shorthand notation to describe an abnormal lipoprotein pattern in plasma and not a designation of a specific disease state.

Ordinarily, the simple measurement of plasma lipid levels, coupled with a clinical assessment, is sufficient to classify the type of lipoprotein abnormality present (Table 100-2). Occasionally, paper electrophoresis of the plasma is useful either when an elevation in remnant particles is suspected (type 3 lipoprotein pattern giving a "broad beta" band on electrophoresis) or when chylomicronemia is a possibility (type 1 pattern). Recently, there has been interest in the measurement of HDL levels, since high levels of this lipoprotein class are statistically associated with a decreased risk of myocardial infarction (see Chap. 250). The level of HDL can be estimated in clinical laboratories using standardized lipoprotein separation techniques, but the value of such measurement for predicting

FIGURE 100-2

Model for plasma triglyceride and cholesterol transport in humans. The details of this model are discussed in the text. VLDL denotes very low density lipoprotein, LDL denotes low density lipoprotein, HDL denotes high-density lipoprotein, and LCAT denotes lecithin:cholesterol acyltransferase.

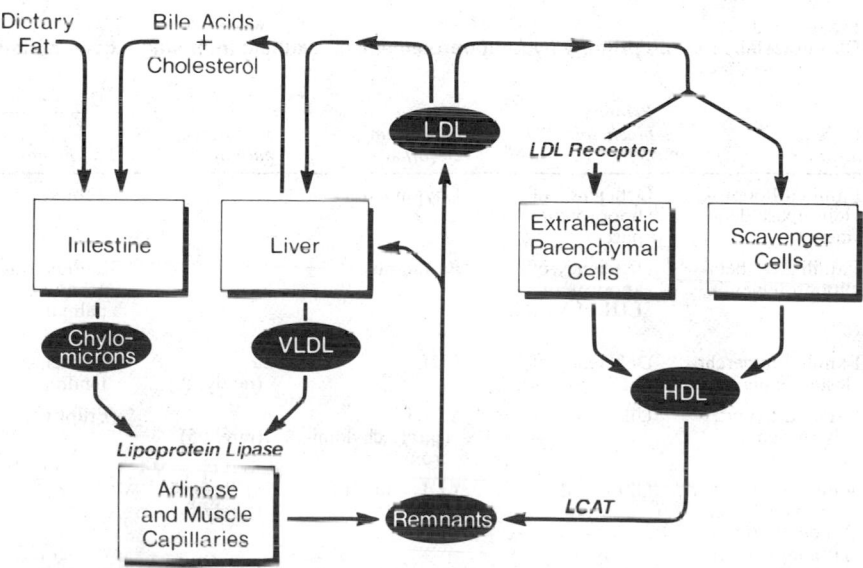

TABLE 100-2
Patterns of lipoprotein elevation in plasma (lipoprotein types)

Lipoprotein pattern	Major elevation in plasma	
	Lipoprotein	Lipid
Type 1	Chylomicrons	Triglycerides
Type 2a	LDL	Cholesterol
Type 2b	LDL and VLDL	Cholesterol and triglycerides
Type 3	Remnants	Triglycerides and cholesterol
Type 4	VLDL	Triglycerides
Type 5	VLDL and chylomicrons	Triglycerides and cholesterol

the occurrence of myocardial infarction in the individual patient has not been established.

PRIMARY HYPERLIPOPROTEINEMIAS RESULTING FROM SINGLE GENE MUTATIONS

FAMILIAL LIPOPROTEIN LIPASE DEFICIENCY This is a rare autosomal recessive disorder due to the absence or marked reduction in the activity of the enzyme lipoprotein lipase. This deficiency leads to a metabolic block in the metabolism of chylomicrons, causing these lipoproteins to accumulate to massive levels in plasma.

Clinical features The disease usually presents in infancy or childhood with recurrent attacks of abdominal pain. The pain is due to pancreatitis occurring as a consequence of the massive elevation of chylomicrons in plasma. Affected individuals intermittently develop eruptive xanthomas, small yellowish papules, frequently surrounded by an erythematous base, that appear predominantly on the buttocks and other pressure-sensitive surfaces. The xanthomas are caused by the deposition of large amounts of chylomicron triglycerides in cutaneous histiocytes. Triglycerides are also deposited at widespread sites in phagocytes of the reticuloendothelial system, producing hepatomegaly, splenomegaly, and foam-cell infiltration of the bone marrow. When the level of chylomicrons in the blood is massively elevated (i.e., plasma triglyceride level greater than 2000 mg per 100 ml), the blood appears pale and creamy and is said to be *lipemic*. When viewed with the ophthalmoscope, the retina appears pale, and the retinal vessels are white, producing the classic appearance of lipemia retinalis. Despite the massive

elevation of triglycerides in the bloodstream, accelerated atherosclerosis does not occur in this disorder.

Pathogenesis Affected individuals are homozygous for a mutation that prevents normal expression of lipoprotein lipase activity. The parents are obligate heterozygotes for this defect, but they are clinically normal. As a result of the deficiency of lipoprotein lipase, chylomicrons cannot be metabolized normally and the level of chylomicrons in the blood rises to high levels after a fat meal. In normal individuals chylomicrons disappear from the blood after a 12-h fast. However, in affected patients high levels of chylomicrons are found in the plasma even after several days of fasting or ingestion of a fat-free diet.

The circulating chylomicrons inflame the pancreas when they pass through its capillaries. Within the capillary lumen in the pancreas, chylomicrons are exposed to small amounts of pancreatic lipase that leaks from the tissue. Partial hydrolysis of the triglycerides and phospholipids of the chylomicron produces toxic products, including fatty acids and lysolecithin, that break down tissue membranes and cause further leakage of lipase from the pancreatic acinar cells. This produces a vicious cycle that eventually causes fulminant pancreatitis.

Diagnosis The diagnosis of familial lipoprotein lipase deficiency is suggested by the finding of lipemic plasma in a young individual who has been fasting for at least 12 h. This lipemic plasma, when collected in the presence of EDTA, has a characteristic appearance after it has incubated overnight in a refrigerator at 4°C. A white layer of cream (which consists of chylomicrons) appears at the top of the tube. The layer beneath the cream is clear. The diagnosis of familial lipoprotein lipase deficiency is supported by the finding of a type 1 pattern on lipoprotein electrophoresis. It is confirmed by the demonstration that lipoprotein lipase levels in plasma fail to increase following the infusion of heparin. In normal individuals, intravenous heparin releases lipoprotein lipase from its binding sites within the capillary endothelium, and increased amounts of enzyme can then be assayed in the plasma.

Treatment All the symptoms and signs of the disease recede when the patient is placed on a fat-free diet. Every attempt should be made to maintain the fasting plasma triglyceride level below 1000 mg per 100 ml to prevent pancreatitis. It has been found empirically that the chronic fat intake in affected adults must be less than 20 g per day to prevent symptomatic

TABLE 100-3
Characteristics of the primary hyperlipoproteinemias resulting from single gene mutations

Genetic disorder	Primary biochemical defect	Plasma lipoprotein elevation	Lipoprotein pattern	Typical clinical findings			Lipoprotein pattern in affected relatives
				Xanthomas	Pancreatitis	Premature atherosclerosis	
Familial lipoprotein lipase deficiency	Deficiency of lipoprotein lipase	Chylomicrons	1	Eruptive	+		1
Familial dysbetalipoproteinemia	Deficiency of apoprotein EIII of VLDL	Remnants	3	Xanthelasma; tuberous; palmar creases		+	3 or 4
Familial hypercholesterolemia	Deficiency of LDL receptor	LDL	2a (rarely 2b)	Xanthelasma; tendon		+	2a (rarely 2b)
Familial hypertriglyceridemia	Unknown	VLDL (rarely chylomicrons)	4 (rarely 5)	(Eruptive)	(+)	+	4 (rarely 5)
Multiple lipoprotein-type hyperlipidemia (familial combined hyperlipidemia)	Unknown	LDL and VLDL	2a, 2b, or 4 (rarely 5)			+	2a, 2b, or 4 (rarely 5)

TABLE 100-4
Clinical disorders associated with secondary hyperlipoproteinemia

Underlying disorder	Plasma lipoprotein elevation				Lipoprotein type	Proposed mechanism for hyperlipoproteinemia	Associated abnormality of carbohydrate metabolism
	Chylomicrons	Remnants	VLDL	LDL			
ENDOCRINE AND METABOLIC							
Diabetes mellitus	+		+ + +		4 (rarely 5)	Increased secretion of VLDL Decreased catabolism of VLDL and chylomicrons due to reduced lipoprotein lipase activity	Insulin deficiency or resistance
von Gierke's disease (glycogenosis, type I)	+		+ + +		4 (rarely 5)	Increased secretion of VLDL Decreased catabolism of VLDL and chylomicrons due to reduced lipoprotein lipase activity	Hypoglycemia with decreased insulin secretion
Lipodystrophies (congenital and acquired forms)			+ +		4	Increased secretion of VLDL	Insulin resistance
Cushing's syndrome			+	+ +	2a or 2b	Increased secretion of VLDL with conversion to LDL	Insulin resistance
Sexual ateliotic dwarfism (isolated growth hormone deficiency)			+ +	+ +	2b	Increased secretion of VLDL with conversion to LDL	Insulin deficiency or resistance
Acromegaly			+		4	Increased secretion of VLDL	Insulin resistance
Hypothyroidism		+		+ + +	2a (rarely 3)	Decreased catabolism of LDL and remnants	
Anorexia nervosa				+ +	2a	Reduced biliary excretion of cholesterol and bile acids	
Werner's syndrome				+ +	2a	Unknown	Insulin resistance
Acute intermittent porphyria				+ +	2a	Unknown	
DRUG-INDUCED							
Alcohol	+		+ + +		4 (rarely 5)	Increased secretion of VLDL in individuals genetically predisposed to hypertriglyceridemia	
Oral contraceptives	+		+ + +		4 (rarely 5)	Increased secretion of VLDL in individuals genetically predisposed to hypertriglyceridemia	Insulin resistance
Glucogenic corticosteroids			+	+ +	2a or 2b	Increased secretion of VLDL with conversion to LDL	Insulin resistance
RENAL							
Uremia			+ + +		4	Decreased catabolism of VLDL due to reduced lipoprotein lipase activity	Insulin resistance
Nephrotic syndrome			+ +	+ + +	2a or 2b	Increased secretion of VLDL Direct secretion of LDL from liver Decreased catabolism of VLDL and LDL	
HEPATIC							
Primary biliary cirrhosis and extrahepatic biliary obstruction					↑ Cholesterol ↑ Phospholipids ↑ Lipoprotein X	Diversion of biliary cholesterol and phospholipids into bloodstream	
Acute hepatitis (nonfulminant)			+ + +		4	Decreased hepatic secretion of lecithin: cholesterol acyltransferase (LCAT)	

TABLE 100-4 *(continued)*
Clinical disorders associated with secondary hyperlipoproteinemia

Underlying disorder	Plasma lipoprotein elevation				Lipoprotein type	Proposed mechanism for hyperlipoproteinemia	Associated abnormality of carbohydrate metabolism
	Chylo-microns	Remnants	VLDL	LDL			
HEPATIC *(continued)*							
Hepatoma				+ +	2a	Lack of feedback inhibition of hepatic cholesterol synthesis by dietary cholesterol	
IMMUNOLOGIC							
Systemic lupus erythematosis	+ +				1	Presence of IgG or IgM that binds heparin, thereby decreasing activity of lipoprotein lipase	
Monoclonal gammopathies (myeloma, macroglobulinemia, lymphoma)		+ +	+ +		3 or 4	Presence of IgG or IgM that forms immune complex with remnants and/or VLDL, thereby decreasing their catabolism	
STRESS-INDUCED							
Emotional stress, acute myocardial infarction, extensive burns, acute gram-negative sepsis			+ +		4	Increased secretion and decreased catabolism of VLDL	

hyperlipemia. Since medium chain triglycerides are not normally incorporated into chylomicrons, they have been employed to help achieve normal caloric intake. The diet should be supplemented with fat-soluble vitamins.

FAMILIAL DYSBETALIPOPROTEINEMIA This is an inherited disorder in which the plasma concentrations of cholesterol and triglycerides are both elevated owing to the accumulation in plasma of remnant-like particles derived from the partial catabolism of VLDL. Also called familial type 3 hyperlipidemia, the disorder is transmitted by a single-gene mechanism, but its expression appears to require the presence of contributory environmental and/or genetic factors (discussed below).

Clinical features Affected individuals characteristically do not manifest hyperlipidemia or any of the other clinical features of the disease until after age 20. A unique clinical feature of the disorder is the occurrence of two types of cutaneous xanthomas. These are xanthoma striata palmaris, which appear as orange or yellow discolorations of the palmar and digital creases, and tuberous or tuberoeruptive xanthomas, which are bulbous cutaneous xanthomas that may vary from pea to lemon size. These tuberous xanthomas are characteristically located over the elbows and knees. Xanthelasmas of the eyelids also occur, but these are not unique to this disorder (see "Familial Hypercholesterolemia," below).

Severe and fulminant atherosclerosis involving the coronary arteries, the internal carotids, and the abdominal aorta and its branches is also a prominent feature. The clinical sequelae include the occurrence of premature myocardial infarctions, strokes, intermittent claudication, and gangrene of the lower extremities. Patients who develop clinical manifestations of dysbetalipoproteinemia often have hypothyroidism, obesity, or diabetes mellitus.

Pathogenesis The hyperlipidemia is caused by the accumulation of relatively large lipoprotein particles that contain both triglycerides and cholesteryl esters. These particles resemble the remnants that are normally produced from the catabolism of VLDL through the action of lipoprotein lipase. In normal

subjects such remnant particles are rapidly taken up by the liver, and hence they are barely detectable in plasma. In patients with familial dysbetalipoproteinemia the uptake of VLDL remnants by the liver is blocked, and these lipoproteins accumulate to high levels in plasma and deposit in tissues, producing xanthomas and atherosclerosis.

The mutation responsible for this disease appears to involve the gene that encodes the structure of apoprotein E, a protein normally found in VLDL and its remnants. This protein is thought to play a role in the uptake of VLDL remnants by the liver. Apoprotein E is actually a family of proteins that can be resolved by isoelectric focusing into three components, designated EI, EII, and EIII. Patients with familial dysbetalipoproteinemia are homozygous for a mutant gene that results in a complete deficiency of EIII in their plasma.

Both parents of an EIII deficient subject and 50 percent of first-degree relatives have half-normal levels of EIII, suggesting that they have one normal allele and one mutant allele at the genetic locus that specifies the EIII apoprotein. Inasmuch as the occurrence of familial dysbetalipoproteinemia requires a complete EIII deficiency, the disease would be expected to behave like a simple autosomal recessive trait. However, several factors make the inheritance pattern atypical for an autosomal recessive disease. First, the frequency of the heterozygous state of EIII deficiency among the general population is high, involving 12 percent of asymptomatic individuals. Moreover, about 1 percent of unselected asymptomatic individuals are homozygous for the EIII deficiency, yet most of these latter subjects have normal lipid levels. Only about 1 in 100 individuals with complete EIII deficiency express the familial dysbetalipoproteinemia syndrome. Thus, all patients with symptomatic familial dysbetalipoproteinemia have homozygous EIII deficiency, but most patients with homozygous EIII deficiency never develop clinical signs of familial dysbetalipoproteinemia. Probably no more than 1 in 10,000 people among the general population show the typical clinical features of familial dysbetalipoproteinemia.

The high frequency of the heterozygous state for EIII deficiency gives rise to pedigrees in which symptomatic familial dysbetalipoproteinemia occurs in several generations of the same family. Such a pseudodominant inheritance pattern is caused by the fact that an individual homozygous for EIII deficiency has a 12 percent chance of marrying a heterozygote. In such a mating half the children have homozygous EIII deficiency, and thus a recessive trait occurs in a parent and a child. In the absence of consanguinity, this situation is rare in typical recessive syndromes where the heterozygous state has a lower frequency in the population.

Some of the factors that produce symptomatic dysbetalipoproteinemia in patients with homozygous EIII deficiency are now known. The disease is exacerbated by hypothyroidism, and many patients with EIII deficiency who develop symptomatic dysbetalipoproteinemia have hypothyroidism. Other factors that predispose to the expression of the disease in an EIII deficient individual include obesity and the independent inheritance of diabetes mellitus or multiple lipoprotein-type hyperlipidemia.

Diagnosis The diagnosis is suggested by the finding of palmar or tuberous xanthomas in a patient with elevated plasma levels of both cholesterol and triglyceride. Approximately 80 percent of symptomatic patients exhibit these xanthomas. The diagnosis is also suggested when a moderate elevation in the plasma concentration of both cholesterol and triglyceride occurs in such a way that the absolute concentrations of cholesterol and triglyceride are nearly equal (e.g., the plasma cholesterol and triglyceride level are both about 300 mg per 100 ml). However, this finding does not always hold true and becomes especially unreliable when the disease is in severe exacerbation, in which case the plasma triglyceride tends to rise higher than cholesterol.

The diagnosis is supported by the finding of a so-called "broad beta" band on lipoprotein electrophoresis (type 3 pattern). This appearance results from the presence of the remnant particles that migrate between β and pre-β lipoproteins and cause a distinctive smear of this region of the electrophoretogram. The diagnosis can be established in specialized laboratories by two procedures. First, the plasma can be subjected to ultracentrifugation, and the chemical composition of the VLDL fraction can be measured. In affected patients, the VLDL fraction contains the abnormal remnant particles and has a relatively high ratio of cholesterol to triglyceride. Second, the diagnosis can be confirmed by the finding of a complete deficiency of apoprotein EIII on isoelectric focusing of the proteins extracted from the remnant particles.

Treatment A vigorous search for occult hypothyroidism should be made, including measurement of plasma thyroid stimulating hormone levels. If hypothyroidism exists, L-thyroxine should be instituted. Patients who have hypothyroidism show a dramatic lowering of lipid levels with treatment. In addition, attempts should be made to control obesity and diabetes mellitus through diet and insulin treatment. If these measures are not successful, patients with familial dysbetalipoproteinemia should be treated with clofibrate. Affected patients usually show a dramatic and sustained reduction in plasma lipid levels when treated with this drug.

FAMILIAL HYPERCHOLESTEROLEMIA This common autosomal dominant disorder affects approximately 1 in 500 persons in the general population. Heterozygotes manifest a two- to three-fold elevation in the concentration of total plasma cholesterol which is attributable to an elevation in the level of LDL. Patients with the homozygous form have six- to eight-fold elevations in plasma LDL cholesterol levels.

Clinical features Heterozygotes with familial hypercholesterolemia can often be diagnosed at birth because their umbilical

cord blood contains a two- to three-fold increase in the concentration of LDL cholesterol. The elevated levels of plasma LDL persist throughout life, but symptoms typically do not develop until the third or fourth decade. The most important clinical feature is the occurrence of premature and accelerated coronary atherosclerosis. Myocardial infarctions begin to occur in affected men in the third decade and show a peak incidence in the fourth and fifth decades. By age 60, approximately 85 percent have experienced a myocardial infarction. In women the incidence of myocardial infarction is also elevated, but the mean age of onset is delayed 10 years as compared with males. Heterozygotes for this disorder constitute about 5 percent of all patients who have a myocardial infarction.

Xanthomas of the tendons constitute the second major clinical manifestation of the heterozygous state. These xanthomas are nodular swellings that typically involve the Achilles and other tendons about the knee, elbow, and dorsum of the hand. They are formed by the deposition of LDL-derived cholesteryl esters in tissue macrophages located in interstitial spaces. The macrophages are swollen with lipid droplets and form foam cells. Cholesterol is also deposited in the soft tissue of the eyelid, producing xanthelasma, and within the cornea, producing arcus corneae. Whereas tendon xanthomas are essentially diagnostic of familial hypercholesterolemia, xanthelasma and arcus corneae are not specific. The latter abnormalities also occur in many adults with normal plasma lipid levels. The incidence of tendon xanthomas in familial hypercholesterolemia increases with age, and up to 75 percent of affected heterozygotes display this sign.

Approximately 1 in 1 million persons in the general population inherits two copies of the familial hypercholesterolemia gene and is a homozygote for the disorder. These individuals have marked elevations in the plasma level of LDL from birth. A unique type of planar cutaneous xanthoma is often present at birth and always develops within the first six years of life. These characteristic xanthomas are raised, yellow, plaque-like lesions that occur at points of cutaneous trauma, such as over the knees, elbows, and buttocks. Xanthomas are almost always present in the interdigital webs of the hands, particularly between the thumb and index finger. Tendon xanthomas, arcus corneae, and xanthelasma are also characteristic. Coronary artery atherosclerosis frequently has its clinical onset in homozygotes before age 10, and myocardial infarction has been reported as early as 18 months of age. In addition to coronary atherosclerosis homozygotes frequently develop cholesterol deposition in the aortic valve, producing symptomatic aortic stenosis. Homozygotes usually succumb to the complications of myocardial infarction before age 20.

In contrast to the disorders causing hypertriglyceridemia, obesity and diabetes mellitus do not occur with increased frequency in familial hypercholesterolemia. A slender body habitus is the rule.

Pathogenesis The primary defect resides in the gene for the LDL receptor. Three types of mutant alleles have been described at this locus. The most common, designated receptor-negative or R^{b0}, specifies a gene product that is nonfunctional. The second most frequent mutant, designated receptor-defective or R^{b-}, produces a receptor that has 1 to 10 percent of normal LDL binding activity. The third type, designated $R^{b+,0}$, produces a receptor that binds LDL normally but is unable to transport the receptor-bound lipoprotein into the cell. This very rare allele produces the so-called "internalization defect."

Phenotypic homozygotes possess two mutant alleles at the

LDL receptor locus, and hence their cells show a total or near-total inability to bind or take up LDL. Heterozygotes have one normal allele and one of the three mutant alleles at the LDL receptor locus, and hence their cells are able to bind and take up LDL at approximately half the normal rate.

Because of the reduction in LDL receptor activity, LDL catabolism is blocked and the level of LDL in plasma rises in a manner that is inversely proportional to the reduction in LDL receptors. In addition to the impaired catabolism of LDL, an increased production of LDL has also been noted in homozygotes. Enhanced production of LDL has been attributed to the lack of an LDL receptor on liver cells such that the liver fails to sense the adequacy of the plasma LDL level. In contrast to normal individuals in whom all plasma LDL appears to be derived from VLDL, in FH homozygotes a large fraction of circulating LDL is secreted directly from the liver into the plasma. This overproduction of LDL, together with its reduced catabolism, accounts for the high concentrations seen in affected patients. The elevated LDL levels cause an increase in the uptake of LDL by scavenger cells, which accumulate at various sites in the body, producing xanthomas.

The accelerated coronary atherosclerosis in familial hypercholesterolemia also results from the high LDL levels, which lead to an enhanced infiltration of LDL into the artery wall following episodes of endothelial damage. The large amounts of LDL that penetrate the artery wall are greater than can be cleared from the interstitial space by the scavenger cells, and atherosclerosis ultimately results. Evidence also indicates that the high LDL levels may act to accelerate platelet aggregation at sites of endothelial injury, thereby enhancing the growth of the atherosclerotic plaque (see Chap. 250).

Diagnosis The diagnosis of heterozygous familial hypercholesterolemia is suggested by the finding of an isolated elevation of plasma cholesterol, with a normal concentration of plasma triglycerides. In nearly all cases, such an isolated elevation in plasma cholesterol is due to an elevation in the plasma concentration of LDL alone (type 2a pattern). However, most individuals in the general population with type 2a hyperlipoproteinemia do not have familial hypercholesterolemia. Rather, they have a form of polygenic hypercholesterolemia that puts them on the upper end of the bell-shaped curve for the general population (see "Polygenic Hypercholesterolemia" below). Type 2a hyperlipoproteinemia is also caused by multiple lipoprotein-type hyperlipidemia (discussed below). In addition, a variety of metabolic disorders, including hypothyroidism and nephrotic syndrome, can cause type 2a hyperlipoproteinemia (Table 100-4).

Among individuals who have a type 2a lipoprotein pattern, those with heterozygous familial hypercholesterolemia can be distinguished from those with polygenic hypercholesterolemia and multiple lipoprotein-type hyperlipidemia on several grounds. (1) In familial hypercholesterolemia the plasma cholesterol level tends to be higher. A plasma cholesterol level in the range of 350 to 400 mg per 100 ml is more suggestive of heterozygous familial hypercholesterolemia than of the other disorders. However, many patients with heterozygous familial hypercholesterolemia have cholesterol levels of 285 to 350 mg per 100 ml, a range in which the other disorders cannot be excluded. (2) The occurrence of tendon xanthomas virtually establishes the diagnosis of familial hypercholesterolemia, since such xanthomas usually do not occur in patients with other forms of hyperlipidemia. (3) In cases in which the diagnosis is in doubt, other family members should be surveyed. In familial hypercholesterolemia the expression of the gene is usually constant with half of first-degree relatives showing an elevated plasma cholesterol level. Hypercholesterolemia is particularly informative when it occurs in children, since elevated levels of cholesterol in childhood are characteristic of familial hypercholesterolemia but not of any of the other aforementioned disorders.

Approximately 10 percent of heterozygotes with familial hypercholesterolemia have concomitant elevation in plasma triglyceride levels (type 2b pattern). In these cases, the disease is difficult to differentiate from multiple lipoprotein-type hyperlipidemia. The finding of a tendon xanthoma or a hypercholesterolemic child in the family favors the diagnosis of familial hypercholesterolemia.

The diagnosis of homozygous familial hypercholesterolemia ordinarily affords no problem, providing the physician is familiar with the clinical picture. Most patients are first seen by dermatologists in childhood because of the cutaneous xanthomas. Occasionally, the presentation is delayed until the onset of angina pectoris or until the child suffers a syncopal episode owing to the xanthomatous aortic stenosis. The finding of a cholesterol level greater than 600 mg per 100 ml with normal triglyceride values in a nonjaundiced child is highly suggestive of the diagnosis. Both parents should have moderately elevated cholesterol levels and other features of heterozygous familial hypercholesterolemia.

In specialized laboratories the diagnosis of both heterozygous and homozygous familial hypercholesterolemia can be made by direct measurement of the number of LDL receptors on cultured skin fibroblasts or freshly isolated blood lymphocytes. Homozygous familial hypercholesterolemia has been diagnosed in utero by the finding of absence of LDL receptors on cultured amniotic fluid cells.

Treatment Inasmuch as the atherosclerosis in this disorder is a consequence of the long-standing elevation in plasma LDL levels, every effort should be made to lower the plasma LDL level into the normal range. Patients should be placed on a diet that is low in cholesterol, low in saturated fats, and high in polyunsaturated fats. This generally means the avoidance of milk, butter, cheese, chocolate, shellfish, and fatty meats and the addition of polyunsaturated cooking oils such as corn oil and safflower oil. With such a diet heterozygotes usually show a 10 to 15 percent drop in plasma cholesterol level.

Bile acid–binding resins, such as cholestyramine, should be added to the regimen when dietary therapy fails to lower the cholesterol levels to the normal range. These resins trap the bile acids excreted by the liver into the intestine and carry them into the feces. Since the body responds to bile acid depletion by converting additional cholesterol into bile acids, the initial result is a dramatic loss of cholesterol from the body. However, affected subjects respond to bile acid depletion by enhancing cholesterol synthesis in the liver, and this compensatory response ultimately limits the long-term success of therapy. With the combination of diet and bile acid–binding resins, the extent of reduction in plasma cholesterol level usually is in the range of 25 percent in heterozygotes. The addition of nicotinic acid may help to block the compensatory increase in hepatic cholesterol synthesis, thus allowing a further lowering of the cholesterol. Major side effects of bile acid–binding resins include gastrointestinal bloating, cramps, and constipation. The major side effect of nicotinic acid is hepatotoxicity; it also produces flushing and headaches in most patients. Probucol has also been used for the treatment of familial hypercholesterolemia, but its efficacy has not been established.

Heterozygotes often show a moderate to marked lowering of plasma cholesterol level in response to the creation of an intestinal anastomosis that bypasses the ileum. This operation has the same functional effect as bile acid–binding resins, i.e., it accelerates the loss of bile acids in the stool. In certain patients in whom drug therapy is not tolerated, the creation of an ileal bypass may be indicated.

Homozygotes tend to be more resistant to treatment. In general, combination therapy consisting of diet, a bile acid–binding resin, and nicotinic acid has little effect. Ileal bypass is uniformly ineffective. Several children have responded to surgical creation of a portacaval anastomosis. However, this procedure is still experimental. The use of a continuous-flow blood cell centrifuge to perform plasma exchanges at monthly intervals is one treatment that will lower the cholesterol in all homozygotes. After each plasma exchange, the plasma cholesterol level drops to about 300 mg per 100 ml and then gradually rises over the ensuing 4 weeks to the pretreatment level. If facilities are available, plasma exchange is the treatment of choice for homozygotes.

FAMILIAL HYPERTRIGLYCERIDEMIA This is a common autosomal dominant disorder in which the concentration of VLDL is elevated in the plasma, causing hypertriglyceridemia.

Clinical features Affected individuals do not usually express hypertriglyceridemia until puberty or early adulthood. Thereafter, the fasting plasma triglyceride level tends to be moderately elevated in the range of 200 to 500 mg per 100 ml (type 4 lipoprotein pattern). The typical affected patient exhibits a clinical triad consisting of obesity, hyperglycemia, and hyperinsulinemia. In addition, hypertension and hyperuricemia are frequent.

The incidence of atherosclerosis is increased. In one study affected patients constituted 6 percent of all individuals with myocardial infarction. However, it has not been established that the hypertriglyceridemia per se causes the increased atherosclerosis. As discussed above, many patients with this disease have diabetes, obesity, and hypertension. Each of these disorders by itself may predispose to atherosclerosis. Xanthomas are not a characteristic feature of familial hypertriglyceridemia.

Affected patients ordinarily have mild to moderate hypertriglyceridemia but can develop a severe exacerbation when exposed to a variety of precipitating factors. These include poorly controlled diabetes mellitus, excessive consumption of alcohol, ingestion of birth control pills containing estrogen, and the development of hypothyroidism. In response to any of these stimuli, the plasma triglyceride level can rise to more than 1000 mg per 100 ml. Under these conditions, large triglyceride-laden particles with the characteristics of chylomicrons appear in plasma. During exacerbations such patients develop *mixed hyperlipemia;* that is, they show an elevation in the concentration of both VLDL and chylomicrons (type 5 lipoprotein pattern). Whenever the concentration of chylomicrons rises to high levels, patients are predisposed to the formation of eruptive xanthomas and the development of pancreatitis. With treatment of the exacerbating condition, the chylomicron-like particles disappear from plasma, and the concentration of triglycerides returns to the moderately elevated basal condition.

In certain families some patients exhibit a severe mixed hyperlipemia, even in the absence of known exacerbating factors. This is the so-called "familial type 5 hyperlipidemia." Other individuals in the same family may have only the mild form of the disease with moderate hypertriglyceridemia and no hyperchylomicronemia (type 4 pattern).

Pathogenesis The disease is transmitted as an autosomal dominant trait, implying a mutation in a single gene. However, the nature of the mutant gene and the mechanism by which it produces hypertriglyceridemia have not been identified. It is likely that the disorder is genetically heterogeneous; that is, the hypertriglyceridemia phenotype in different families may result from different mutations.

Some affected patients have an elevated production rate of VLDL, especially when they ingest diets high in carbohydrate.

However, many of these patients have obesity and diabetes mellitus. Other individuals with obesity and diabetes mellitus, who have normal plasma VLDL levels, also overproduce VLDL. Thus, patients with familial hypertriglyceridemia may have an underlying defect in the ability to catabolize the triglycerides of VLDL. When VLDL production rates become elevated due to obesity or diabetes, they are unable to increase the catabolism of VLDL proportionately and hypertriglyceridemia results. However, lipoprotein lipase activity increases normally in plasma after the administration of heparin, and no abnormalities of lipoprotein structure have been identified.

The increased prevalence of diabetes and obesity in this syndrome is believed to be fortuitous, owing to the fact that both conditions tend to increase VLDL production and hence to exacerbate hypertriglyceridemia. Thus, in family studies, one can find relatives who have diabetes without hypertriglyceridemia and relatives who have hypertriglyceridemia without diabetes, indicating that the two are inherited by independent mechanisms. When an individual inherits both the gene(s) for diabetes and the gene for hypertriglyceridemia, the hypertriglyceridemia is more severe, and such a person is more apt to come to medical attention. Similarly, an individual with familial hypertriglyceridemia who has a normal weight usually has mild hypertriglyceridemia and is less likely to come to medical attention. However, if obesity develops, the hypertriglyceridemia worsens, and a diagnosis is more likely to be made.

Diagnosis The finding of a moderate elevation in plasma triglyceride level, together with a normal cholesterol level, raises the possibility of familial hypertriglyceridemia. In most patients, the plasma is clear to somewhat cloudy on inspection. Chylomicrons typically are not found at the top of the plasma after overnight refrigeration. Electrophoresis of the plasma reveals an increase in the pre-β fraction (type 4 lipoprotein pattern). As mentioned above, an occasional patient exhibits severe hypertriglyceridemia with an elevation in both chylomicrons and VLDL. In this case, a cream layer develops on top (chylomicrons) and a cloudy infranatant (VLDL) is present after overnight storage of plasma in the refrigerator (type 5 lipoprotein pattern).

Given an individual who has an elevation in VLDL levels with or without an elevation in chylomicrons, no simple test exists to determine whether this subject has familial hypertriglyceridemia or hypertriglyceridemia due to some other genetic or acquired cause, such as multiple lipoprotein-type hyperlipidemia or sporadic hypertriglyceridemia. In a typical case of familial hypertriglyceridemia, half of the first-degree relatives have hypertriglyceridemia and no relatives with isolated hypercholesterolemia should be found. Measurement of plasma lipid levels in children is not helpful inasmuch as the disease is typically not manifest until the time of puberty.

Treatment Attempts should be made to control all the exacerbating conditions. Caloric restriction is required in the obese subject. The dietary content of saturated fat should also be limited. Alcohol and oral contraceptives should be avoided. Diabetes mellitus, if present, should be treated vigorously. Thyroid function should be checked, and hypothyroidism treated if found. If the above measures fail, patients respond to the administration of clofibrate, a drug whose mechanism of action is unknown.

MULTIPLE LIPOPROTEIN-TYPE HYPERLIPIDEMIA This common disorder, which is also called familial combined hyperlipidemia, is inherited as an autosomal dominant trait. Affected individuals in a single family characteristically show one of three different lipoprotein patterns: hypercholesterolemia (type 2a), hypertriglyceridemia (type 4), or both hypercholesterolemia and hypertriglyceridemia (type 2b).

Clinical features Hyperlipidemia is not ordinarily present in childhood. Elevations in the plasma cholesterol and/or triglyceride level begin to appear at puberty and continue throughout life. The lipid elevations tend to be mild and vary from time to time so that affected individuals may have a mildly elevated cholesterol level at one examination and/or a mildly elevated triglyceride level at another time. Xanthomas are not a feature. However, premature atherosclerosis occurs, and the incidence of myocardial infarction in middle age is elevated in affected women as well as men.

Patients usually have a strong family history of premature coronary artery disease. This disorder is found in about 10 percent of all patients who have a myocardial infarction. The frequency of obesity, hyperuricemia, and glucose intolerance is increased in affected individuals, especially those with hypertriglyceridemia. However, this association is not as striking as in familial hypertriglyceridemia.

Pathogenesis The disease is transmitted within families as an autosomal dominant trait, implying a mutation in a single gene. Family studies show that about half of the first-degree relatives of an affected individual have hyperlipidemia. However, blood lipid levels are variable among affected individuals in the same family as well as in the same individual at different times. About one-third of hyperlipidemic relatives have hypercholesterolemia (type 2a lipoprotein pattern), one-third hypertriglyceridemia (type 4), and one-third both hypercholesterolemia and hypertriglyceridemia (type 2b). In most affected relatives the plasma lipid levels tend to be just above the 95th percentile for the population and to dip into the normal range intermittently.

While the extent (if any) of the genetic heterogeneity and the nature of the underlying biochemical mechanisms are not known, it has been postulated that affected individuals have an elevated secretion rate of VLDL by the liver. Depending on the interplay of factors governing the efficiency of conversion of VLDL to LDL and the efficiency of catabolism of LDL, this overproduction of VLDL may manifest itself alternatively as an elevation in plasma VLDL levels (hypertriglyceridemia), an elevation in LDL levels (hypercholesterolemia), or both. The hyperlipidemia is worsened by diabetes, alcoholism, and hypothyroidism.

Diagnosis No clinical or laboratory methods exist by which to determine whether an individual with hyperlipidemia has the multiple lipoprotein-type disorder. The 2a, 2b, and 4 lipoprotein patterns can each occur in patients with several other diseases (see Tables 100-3 and 100-4). However, this disorder should be suspected in any individual whose hyperlipoproteinemia is mild and whose lipoprotein type changes with time. The diagnosis is supported by the finding of multiple abnormal lipoprotein types in relatives. The diagnosis can be ruled out by the finding of tendon xanthomas in the patient or his relatives or by the finding of hypercholesterolemia in a relative under the age of 10 years.

Treatment Therapy should be directed at the predominant lipid elevated at the time of examination. General measures such as weight reduction, restriction of dietary saturated fat and cholesterol, and avoidance of alcohol and oral contraceptives are useful. Triglyceride elevations may respond to clofi-

brate. When only the cholesterol level is elevated, a bile acid–binding resin should be given. However, in some individuals the lowering of cholesterol levels with such a drug is accompanied by an increase in triglyceride levels.

PRIMARY HYPERLIPOPROTEINEMIAS OF UNKNOWN ETIOLOGY

POLYGENIC HYPERCHOLESTEROLEMIA By definition, 5 percent of individuals in the general population have LDL-cholesterol levels that exceed the 95th percentile and therefore have hypercholesterolemia (type 2a or type 2b lipoprotein patterns). On the average, among every 20 such hypercholesterolemic persons, one person has the heterozygous form of familial hypercholesterolemia, and two have multiple lipoprotein-type hyperlipidemia. The remaining 17 have a form of hypercholesterolemia, designated polygenic hypercholesterolemia, that owes its origin not to a single mutant gene but rather to a complex interaction of multiple genetic and environmental factors.

Most of the factors that place an individual in the upper part of the bell-shaped curve for cholesterol levels are not known. It is likely that subtle genetic differences exist among people with regard to many processes governing cholesterol metabolism. For example, among normal people there may be genetic polymorphisms in the proteins that govern the rates of intestinal cholesterol absorption, bile acid synthesis, cholesterol synthesis, and LDL synthesis or catabolism. Certain unfavorable combinations of these mildly altered proteins, coupled with an environmental challenge, such as a diet high in cholesterol or saturated fat, may raise the plasma cholesterol level.

Clinically, polygenic hypercholesterolemia can be distinguished from familial hypercholesterolemia and multiple lipoprotein-type hyperlipidemia in two ways: (1) family studies (hyperlipidemia is present in no more than 10 percent of first-degree relatives in polygenic hypercholesterolemia in contrast to 50 percent in the other two disorders) and (2) examination for tendon xanthomas (absent in both polygenic hypercholesterolemia and multiple lipoprotein-type hyperlipidemia but present in about 75 percent of adult heterozygotes with familial hypercholesterolemia).

Certain patients with polygenic hypercholesterolemia respond well to dietary restriction of saturated fat and cholesterol. Other patients require drug therapy to achieve a significant lowering of plasma cholesterol levels. Clofibrate is sometimes effective in this latter group. Cholestyramine may also be used.

SPORADIC HYPERTRIGLYCERIDEMIA In addition to the forms of primary hypertriglyceridemia that show familial aggregation, endogenous hypertriglyceridemia with or without hyperchylomicronemia is sometimes seen in individuals whose relatives do not manifest hyperlipidemia. For purposes of classification, this disorder is called sporadic hypertriglyceridemia. Affected patients comprise a heterogeneous group. Some would undoubtedly be classified under one of the genetic disorders described above if a larger number of relatives were available for lipid measurements. Other than an absence of hyperlipidemic relatives, patients with sporadic hypertriglyceridemia cannot be distinguished clinically from patients with the single-gene forms of primary hypertriglyceridemia. Inasmuch as patients with sporadic hypertriglyceridemia may develop hyperchylomicronemia and pancreatitis, they should be treated with diet and drugs as in the familial disease.

FAMILIAL HYPERALPHALIPOPROTEINEMIA This entity is characterized by elevated plasma levels of HDL, also called alpha lipoprotein. The plasma levels of LDL, VLDL, and triglycerides are normal. The elevated HDL causes a slight elevation in the total plasma cholesterol level. Although a selective elevation in plasma HDL cholesterol can be observed in individuals after exposure to chlorinated hydrocarbon pesticides, in alcoholism and after administration of exogenous estrogen, most cases of hyperalphalipoproteinemia have a genetic basis. In some hyperalphalipoproteinemia is inherited as an autosomal dominant trait, while in others a multifactorial or polygenic basis is suspected.

Individual subjects with familial hyperalphalipoproteinemia show no distinctive clinical features.

Statistical studies suggest that the hyperalphalipoproteinemia is associated with a slightly increased longevity and an apparent protection against myocardial infarction. The mechanism for the increase in plasma HDL levels in this disorder has not been determined.

SECONDARY HYPERLIPOPROTEINEMIAS

A variety of clinical disorders produce secondary hyperlipoproteinemias. These are summarized in Table 100-4 (see references). The most frequently encountered forms of secondary hyperlipoproteinemia occur in association with diabetes mellitus, consumption of alcohol, and ingestion of oral contraceptives.

DIABETES MELLITUS Three distinct patterns of hypertriglyceridemia occur in patients with diabetes mellitus. Classical "diabetic hyperlipemia" consists of a massive elevation in the plasma triglyceride level that occurs in patients who have suffered from insulin deficiency or insulin resistance for many weeks or months. Such insulin-deprived patients develop a progressive increase in concentration of plasma VLDL and eventually of chylomicrons as well. Triglyceride levels as high as 25,000 mg per 100 ml are seen. Eruptive xanthomas, lipemia retinalis, and hepatomegaly can occur. Ketosis is frequently present, but severe acidosis is not characteristic. This form of massive hyperlipemia is only seen in partial insulin deficiency. Patients with this form of diabetic hyperlipemia usually respond to a fat-free diet and to the administration of insulin, although triglyceride levels may not return entirely to normal.

The second type of hypertriglyceridemia in diabetics is associated with acute ketoacidosis. Such patients usually exhibit a mild hyperlipidemia with elevations of VLDL but not chylomicrons. On occasion, however, marked elevations of triglyceride are seen with lipemia retinalis. In this case both VLDL and chylomicrons are present.

The third type of hypertriglyceridemia is a mild to moderate elevation in plasma VLDL that persists even when patients appear to be adequately treated for their diabetes. This chronic triglyceride elevation generally occurs in patients who are obese. Inasmuch as most patients with well-controlled diabetes have normal plasma triglyceride levels, the occasional patient with persistent hypertriglyceridemia is likely to have an underlying familial hyperlipoproteinemic disorder. Indeed, family studies indicate that many of these patients have inherited the trait for familial hypertriglyceridemia in a pattern independent of the inheritance of diabetes mellitus.

The insulin deficiency or insulin resistance of diabetes produces a high VLDL level by two mechanisms. With acute insulin deprivation there is an increase in VLDL secretion from the liver as a secondary response to the increased mobilization of free fatty acids from adipose tissue. As the state of insulin deprivation becomes prolonged, the rate of removal of VLDL and chylomicrons from the circulation declines because lipoprotein lipase activity becomes diminished.

ALCOHOL CONSUMPTION In any individual the daily consumption of large amounts of ethanol can produce a mild, asymptomatic elevation in the plasma triglyceride level due to an elevation of VLDL. However, in a subgroup ethanol ingestion regularly produces massive and clinically significant hyperlipemia with elevations in both VLDL and chylomicrons (type 5 lipoprotein pattern). In most of this group, the VLDL level remains mildly elevated (type 4 lipoprotein pattern), even in the basal state after recovery from the severe alcoholic hyperlipemia. This suggests that these individuals have a form of familial hypertriglyceridemia or multiple lipoprotein-type hyperlipidemia that is exacerbated and converted to a type 5 pattern by the ethanol ingestion.

Ethanol elevates the plasma triglyceride level primarily because it inhibits fatty acid oxidation and enhances fatty acid synthesis in the liver. The excess fatty acids are esterified to triglyceride. Some of this excess triglyceride accumulates in the liver, producing the characteristic enlarged fatty liver of alcoholics. The remainder of the newly formed triglyceride is secreted into plasma, resulting in an increased secretion of VLDL. In those who develop massive alcoholic hyperlipemia, there appears to be a partial defect in the catabolism of these VLDL particles. As the concentration of VLDL increases, the lipoprotein begins to compete with chylomicrons for hydrolysis by lipoprotein lipase, and the plasma concentration of chylomicrons also rises.

In severe alcoholic hyperlipemia, eruptive xanthomas and lipemia retinalis are frequently present. The most serious complication is pancreatitis. Pancreatitis may be difficult to diagnose, since elevated triglyceride levels can interfere with the estimation of serum amylase. There is no solid evidence to indicate that pancreatitis itself can cause hyperlipemia; rather the hyperlipemia is the cause of the pancreatitis.

Plasma from patients with alcoholic hyperlipemia is creamy in appearance. If a blood sample is drawn in EDTA and the plasma placed in the refrigerator at 4°C overnight, the chylomicrons float to the top, and the infranatant layer is turbid, owing to the combined elevation of VLDL and chylomicrons (type 5 pattern).

ORAL CONTRACEPTIVES The ingestion of estrogen-containing birth control pills is regularly associated with an increase in the VLDL secretion rate from the liver. In most women the catabolism of VLDL also increases, so that the overall increase in plasma triglyceride level is only modest. However, in women who have an underlying genetic disorder (such as familial hypertriglyceridemia or multiple lipoprotein-type hyperlipidemia) the plasma VLDL-triglyceride level can increase markedly, and hyperchylomicronemia can develop when estrogen-containing medications are taken. These women generally have mild to moderate hypertriglyceridemia prior to the institution of oral contraceptive therapy, and they presumably are unable to increase VLDL catabolism in response to the stimulation of VLDL production. As the plasma VLDL concentration rises, the elevated VLDL prevents the normal catabolism of chylomicrons by lipoprotein lipase, and secondary hyperchylomicronemia ensues. When the latter develops, severe pancreatitis can occur.

Ingestion of oral contraceptives has also been implicated as a risk factor in promoting thromboembolic disease in young women, especially those with preexisting hypercholesterolemia. Thus, it is important to measure the plasma cholesterol and triglyceride levels prior to the institution of birth control therapy. The finding of hyperlipidemia is a contraindication to the use of these drugs.

TABLE 100-5
Rare autosomal recessive disorders of lipid metabolism

Disorder	Typical age of onset	Plasma lipid abnormality	Major clinical manifestations	Pathogenesis	Treatment
Abetalipoproteinemia	Early childhood	Cholesterol, ~ 50 mg/100 ml; triglycerides, < 10 mg/100 ml	Malabsorption of fat, ataxia, neuropathy, retinitis pigmentosa, acanthocytosis	Defective synthesis of apoprotein B leads to absence of chylomicrons, VLDL, and LDL in plasma	Vitamin E
Tangier disease	Childhood	Cholesterol, 40 to 125 mg/100 ml; triglycerides, normal to slightly elevated	Large orange tonsils, corneal opacities, relapsing polyneuropathy No premature atherosclerosis	Absence of HDL from plasma leads to generation of abnormal chylomicron remnants, which are taken up and stored as cholesteryl esters in phagocytic cells	None
Lecithin:cholesterol acyltransferase (LCAT) deficiency	Young adult	Total plasma cholesterol level variable with marked decrease in esterified cholesterol and increase in unesterified cholesterol; elevated VLDL level Structure of all lipoproteins is abnormal	Hemolytic anemia, renal insufficiency, premature atherosclerosis	Decreased LCAT activity in plasma leads to accumulation of excess unesterified cholesterol in plasma and body tissues	Fat-restricted diet, kidney transplantation
Cerebrotendinous xanthomatosis	Young adult	None	Progressive cerebellar ataxia, dementia and spinal cord paresis, subnormal intelligence, tendon xanthomas, cataracts	Primary defect is unknown Cholesterol and cholestanol accumulate in brain, tendons, and other tissues Defective synthesis of primary bile acids in liver	None
β-sitosterolemia	Adult	Elevated levels of plant sterols in plasma; normal levels of cholesterol and triglycerides	Tendon xanthomas	Increased intestinal absorption of dietary β-sitosterol with accumulation in plasma and tendons	Diet low in plant sterols

RARE DISORDERS OF LIPID METABOLISM

Table 100-5 summarizes the clinical and pathophysiological features of five rare disorders of lipid metabolism, each of which is inherited as an autosomal recessive trait. In two—abetalipoproteinemia and Tangier disease—the major effect of the abnormality is to cause a decrease in lipid levels in plasma. In two—cerebrotendinous xanthomatosis and β-sitosterolemia—the major effect of the inborn error is to cause an accumulation of unusual sterols in tissues. In LCAT deficiency, the underlying mutation produces both an abnormal pattern of lipoproteins in plasma and an accumulation of unesterified cholesterol in tissues.

REFERENCES

EDER HA: Drugs used in the prevention and treatment of atherosclerosis, in *The Pharmacological Basis of Therapeutics,* 5th ed, LS Goodman, A Gilman (eds). New York, Macmillan, 1975, chap 35

FREDRICKSON DS et al: The familial hyperlipoproteinemias, in *The Metabolic Basis of Inherited Disease,* 4th ed, JB Stanbury et al (eds). New York, McGraw-Hill, 1978, chap 30

GOLDSTEIN JL, BROWN MS: The low density lipoprotein pathway and its relation to atherosclerosis. Annu Rev Biochem 46:897, 1977

HAVEL RJ et al: Lipoprotein and lipid transport, in *Diseases of Metabolism,* 8th ed, PK Bondy, LE Rosenberg (eds). Philadelphia, Saunders, 1980, chap 7

JACKSON RL et al: Lipoprotein structure and metabolism. Physiol Rev 56:259, 1976

MOTULSKY AG: The genetic hyperlipidemias. N Engl J Med 294:823, 1976

STANBURY JB et al (eds): *The Metabolic Basis of Inherited Disease,* 4th ed. New York, McGraw-Hill, 1978, chaps 28, 29, 31

UTERMANN G et al: Polymorphism of apolipoprotein E. Clin Genet 15:37, 63, 1979

101
LYSOSOMAL STORAGE DISEASES

ARTHUR L. BEAUDET

GENERAL FEATURES

DEFINITION Lysosomes are cytoplasmic organelles which enclose an acidic environment containing numerous enzymes capable of hydrolyzing most biological macromolecules. Primary lysosomes, the original bodies derived from the Golgi apparatus, may fuse with other membrane-bound vesicles to form secondary lysosomes. Secondary lysosomes contain material derived from outside the cell through endocytosis or material from within the cell through autophagy. The lysosome functions as an efficient recovery system for reutilization of components and disposition of used macromolecules. The continuous remodeling of tissues and turnover of macromolecules underline the importance of this degradative capacity. Recent studies of lipoprotein and vitamin B_{12} metabolism suggest that the lysosome is important not only in the processing of used macromolecules but also in the acquisition of essential compounds from the exterior of the cell through the process of endocytosis and degradation of carrier proteins.

The concept of lysosomal storage diseases arose from the studies of type II (Pompe) glycogen storage disease. The demonstration of lysosomal accumulation of glycogen as the result of α-glucosidase deficiency and data from other disorders led Hers to define an inborn lysosomal disease as one in which (1) a single lysosomal enzyme is deficient and (2) abnormal deposits (of substrate) lie within vacuoles related to lysosomes. This definition can be modified to include single gene defects affecting one or more lysosomal enzymes and thus encompass disorders such as the mucolipidoses and multiple sulfatase deficiency.

The lysosomal storage diseases include most of the lipid storage disorders, the mucopolysaccharidoses, the mucolipidoses, glycoprotein storage diseases, and others, as indicated in Table 101-1. The enzyme deficiencies have an autosomal recessive basis with the exception of Hunter mucopolysaccharidosis II (MPS II), which is X-linked recessive, and Fabry disease, which is X-linked with frequent manifestations in females. The target organs are determined by the usual sites of degradation for a macromolecule. For example, cerebral white matter is affected in patients with defects in degradation of myelin, hepatosplenomegaly develops in those with defects in degradation of glycolipids from red cell stroma, and generalized tissue involvement may occur in patients with defects in the degradation of ubiquitous mucopolysaccharides. The accumulated material often causes visceromegaly or macrocephaly, but secondary atrophy also can occur, particularly in brain or muscle. In simple terms, the symptoms appear to be due to damage from stored material, but exactly how this causes cell death or dysfunction often is unclear. All the disorders are progressive, and many are fatal in childhood or adolescence. Definitive diagnosis is accomplished best by specific enzyme assays on serum, leukocytes, or cultured skin fibroblasts, selecting the appropriate tests on clinical grounds. There is extensive phenotypic variation within disorders with infantile, juvenile, and adult forms of many entities. In addition, varying combinations of visceral, skeletal, and neurological involvement can occur within a single enzyme disorder.

DIAGNOSIS A lysosomal storage disease is usually suspected on the basis of progressive neurological dysfunction, visceromegaly, skeletal dysostosis, or some more specific finding, as outlined in Table 101-1. Progressive or degenerative disease is the hallmark of these disorders. The superimposition of degeneration upon normal childhood development results in a slowing of progress prior to loss of previously acquired abilities. The history should focus on the course of childhood development, neurological symptoms, including seizures and visual or auditory impairment, the course of physical growth, and more specific findings such as coarsening facies, corneal clouding, exaggerated startle response, abdominal distention, joint pain, joint stiffness, and recurrent infection. The family history may reveal similarly affected siblings or consanguinity in autosomal recessive disease or other affected male family members in X-linked disorders. Ethnic background may be helpful since several lipid storage diseases are more frequent in Ashkenazi Jews and since disorders such as mannosidosis and aspartylglucosaminuria may occur with increased frequency in Scandinavian populations.

On physical examination the head circumference may be enlarged. Gigantism occurs early in the course of some MPS disorders and glycoprotein storage diseases, while short stature is a later finding in many disorders. Ophthalmologic examination should include slit-lamp and careful funduscopic examination. Enlargement of the tongue, coarsening of the facies, and hepatosplenomegaly may occur. Skeletal findings may include gibbus deformity, broadening of the long bones, and joint stiffness. Cutaneous findings are rare except in fucosidosis, Fabry disease, and Hunter disease. Careful neurologic examination should attempt to distinguish the extent of involvement of gray matter, white matter, and peripheral nerves. Preliminary diagnostic studies should include examination of the peripheral blood smear for vacuolated or granulated leukocytes, urinary spot test for mucopolysaccharide, and radiological bone survey. The preferred method of diagnosis is to use the above information to select specific enzyme assays in serum, leukocytes, or cultured skin fibroblasts. If a mucopolysaccharide screening test is positive or if clinical findings are suggestive, quantitative mucopolysaccharide analysis can be carried out. If a specific diagnosis is not readily established, biopsy of skin, bone marrow, rectal mucosa, liver, peripheral nerve, or other tissue for light and electron microscopy can be helpful. Electron microscopic findings can direct one toward or away from the general category of lysosomal storage diseases based on the presence or absence of engorged lysosomes. When significant evidence favors a lysosomal storage disease but no enzyme deficiency is demonstrable, chemical analysis of biopsy tissue from liver or brain is an appropriate investigative starting point.

HETEROGENEITY There is extensive clinical and biochemical heterogeneity within the lysosomal storage diseases. The biochemical genetic principles underlying this heterogeneity are reviewed in Chaps. 58 and 87. In general, a structural gene for lysosomal enzyme produces a product which acts to degrade one or more macromolecules. Most or all of the lysosomal enzymes undergo posttranslational modification to become glycoproteins, often resulting in a series of electrophoretic variants or isozymes. These isozymes may hydrolyze one or a variety of substrates, and the substrate specificity of particular isozymes may vary. Differences in substrate specificity also arise from the occurrence of similar but genetically distinct enzymes, for example, the β-galactosidases. Mutations within a gene may totally eliminate or reduce enzyme activity, alter the ability of the enzyme to undergo posttranslational modification, or alter the activity of the enzyme for specific substrates.

Different mutations within the same gene probably account for varying degrees of severity from individual to individual as well as the diverse combinations of visceral, skeletal, neurological, ocular, and other manifestations. The heterogeneity is increased further by the recessive nature of most of the conditions in that each affected individual must have two mutant genes of the same allele. Except in the instance of consanguinity, the exact mutation within each gene may vary so that either one or both may encode some form of residual activity for one or more substrates (so-called "genetic compounds"). An excellent example of a genetic compound is MPS I, to be discussed below. Although it is useful to characterize clinical phenotypes as infantile, juvenile, adult, neuropathic, or nonneuropathic, the existence of different mutant alleles and of genetic compounds provides an explanation for those occasional patients who appear aberrant or intermediate as compared with the usual phenotype. Another type of heterogeneity is illustrated by MPS III A and B, which are virtually indistinguishable clinical disorders caused by different gene defects. Thus these genocopies demonstrate that biochemical heterogeneity can underlie apparent clinical homogeneity.

Further complexity results from the fact that certain enzyme activities are derived from complexes of nonidentical subunits. As a consequence, different mutations can cause deficiency of the same enzyme, as for example, hexosaminidase A deficiency in Tay-Sachs and Sandhoff diseases, and can explain multiple enzyme deficiencies due to a single gene defect as in Sandhoff disease. Genetic disorders involving the post-

TABLE 101-1
Summary of lysosomal storage diseases

Disorder	Heterogeneity (onset)	Enzyme deficiency	Stored material	Neurological
G$_{MI}$ gangliosidosis	Infantile (birth) Juvenile (6-20 mo) Adult	β-Galactosidase	G$_{MI}$ ganglioside Glycoproteins Keratan sulfate	Mental retardation, seizures, blindness; later in juvenile form, variable in adults
Tay-Sachs and variants, G$_{M2}$ gangliosidosis	Infantile (3-6 mo) Juvenile Adult forms	Hexosaminidase A	G$_{M2}$ ganglioside	Mental retardation, seizures, blindness; later in juvenile form
Sandhoff, G$_{M2}$ gangliosidosis	Infantile (3-6 mo)	Hexosaminidase A and B	G$_{M2}$ ganglioside Globoside	Mental retardation, seizures, blindness
Krabbe, galactosylceramide lipidosis	Infantile (2-6 mo) Late onset	Galactosylceramide β-Galactosidase	↑ Galactoscerebroside/sulfatide ratio	Mental retardation, leukodystrophy; variable in late onset
Metachromatic leukodystrophy, sulfatide lipidosis	Late infantile (1-4 yr) Juvenile (4-20 yr) Adult	Arylsulfatase A (cerebroside sulfatase)	Galactosyl sulfatides	Mental retardation, leukodystrophy, psychosis and dementia in adults
Niemann-Pick, sphingomyelin lipidosis	Infantile neuropathic (1-4 mo) Late onset neuropathic Visceral	Sphingomyelinase ? Specific isozymes in some	Sphingomyelin	Mental retardation, ataxia, and seizures in neuropathic forms
Gaucher, glucosylceramide lipidosis	Infantile (1-12 mo) Juvenile (2-6 yr) Adult	β-Glucocerebrosidase	Glucosylceramide	Mental retardation; spastic, later flaccid, ataxia in juvenile; no neurologic symptoms in adult form
Fabry, trihexosyl ceramidosis	Hemizygous males Heterozygous females	α-Galactosidase A	Trihexosylceramide	Painful neuropathy
Acid lipase deficiency	Infantile Wolman disease (0-3 mo) Late onset cholesteryl ester storage disease	Acid lipase	Cholesteryl ester Triglyceride	Mental retardation but mild related to growth failure in Wolman; none in CESD
Farber, ceramide deficiency	Infantile (0-4 mo) Rare juvenile	Ceramidase	Ceramide	Occasional mental retardation, but may be secondary to somatic features
Lactosylceramidosis	May not exist; one report probably represented case of Niemann-Pick disease			
Pompe, glycogen storage type II	Infantile (0-6 mo) Juvenile Adult	Acid maltase (α-1,4- and 1,6-glucosidase)	Glycogen	Probably normal mentally
Acid phosphatase deficiency	Infantile (0-3 mo)	Acid phosphatase	Not characterized	Mental retardation

* *AR = autosomal recessive.*

Liver and/or spleen enlargement	Skeletal dysplasia	Ophthalmic	Hematologic	Genetics	Unique manifestations	References
+ + + + Less in juvenile, variable in adult	+ + + + Variable in juvenile and adult forms	Cherry red spot in 50% of infantile; corneal clouding variable but more in adults	Foam cells Vacuolated lymphocytes	AR*	Coarse facies, edema, macroglossia, mucopolysacchariduria; early blindness in infantile, milder in juvenile; in adults often spondylo-epiphyseal dysplasia +/− mucopolysacchariduria	Hers and Van Hoof, chap 12 Stanbury et al, chap 40 Ho et al
0	0	Cherry red spot in infantile form, rare in juvenile	0	AR	Macrocephaly, hyperaucusis in infantile; increased in Ashkenazi Jews	Hers and Van Hoof, chap 13 Stanbury et al, chap 40 Ho et al
0	0	Cherry red spot	0	AR	Macrocephaly, hyperaucusis, visceral histiocytosis	Hers and Van Hoof, chap 14 Stanbury et al, chap 40 Ho et al
0	0	Optic atrophy	0	AR	Extreme irritability, ↑ CSF protein, fever, globoid cell neuropathology	Hers and Van Hoof, chap 17 Stanbury et al, chap 37 Ho et al
0	0	Optic atrophy, less in juvenile and adult forms	0	AR	↑ CSF protein and early gait abnormalities in late infantile; peripheral neuropathy	Hers and Van Hoof, chap 18 Stanbury et al, chap 38
+ + + + Less prominent in late onset forms	0	Macular degeneration and cherry red spot in neuropathic forms	Distinctive foam cell Vacuolated lymphocytes	AR	Pulmonary infiltrates, brownish skin, infantile neuronopathic form increased in Ashkenazi Jews, sea blue histiocytes	Hers and Van Hoof, chap 19 Stanbury et al, chap 35
+ + + + Hypersplenism common	+ +	Usually normal	Distinctive foam cell	AR	Adult form includes ↑ acid phosphatase, pathologic fractures; Ashkenazi Jewish predilection	Hers and Van Hoof, chap 16 Stanbury et al, chap 36 Ho et al
0	0	Corneal dystrophy, vascular lesions, cataracts	0	X-linked dominant	Cutaneous angiokeratoma, vascular thromboses, hypohidrosis	Hers and Van Hoof, chap 15 Stanbury et al, chap 39 Ho et al
+ + +	0	0	Foam cells Vacuolated lymphocytes	AR	Adrenal calcification, anemia, vomiting and poor growth in Wolman; hepatic fibrosis and ↑ blood cholesterol in CESD	Hers and Van Hoof, chap 20 Stanbury et al, chap 32
+/−	?	Mild macular degeneration	0	AR	Arthropathy—subcutaneous, periarticular and visceral nodules (lipogranulomatosis); ↑ CSF protein	Hers and Van Hoof, chap 24 Stanbury et al, chap 34 Ho et al
Mild hepatomegaly	0	0	0	AR	Lethal skeletal and cardiac myopathy in infantile; primarily skeletal myopathy in adults	See chap 97 Hers and Van Hoof, chap 7 Stanbury et al, chap 7
+ +	0	0	0	AR?	Lethal disorders described in two families	Hers and Van Hoof, chap 21 Hirschhorn and Weissmann

TABLE 101-1 *(continued)*
Summary of lysosomal storage diseases

Disorder	Heterogeneity (onset)	Enzyme deficiency	Stored material	Neurological
Fucosidosis	Infantile (3–12 mo) Juvenile	α-Fucosidase	Glycopeptides Glycolipids Oligosaccharides	Mental retardation
Mannosidosis	Infantile (6–18 mo) Milder form	α-Mannosidase	Oligosaccharides	Mental retardation
Aspartylglucosaminuria	Young adult onset	Aspartylglucosamine amidase	Aspartylglucosamine	Mental retardation
Mucopolysaccharidosis 1H and 1S	Infantile Hurler (6–12 mo) Intermediate Adult Scheie	α-Iduronidase	Dermatan sulfate Heparan sulfate	Mental retardation, absent in Scheie
Hunter, mucopolysaccharidosis II	Severe infantile (6–12 mo) Mild juvenile	Iduronosulfate sulfatase	Dermatan sulfate Heparan sulfate	Mental retardation, less in mild form
Sanfilippo A, mucopolysaccharidosis III A	Late infantile (1–4 yr)	Heparan N-sulfatase (sulfamidase)	Heparan sulfate	Severe mental retardation
Sanfilippo B, mucopolysaccharidosis III B	Late infantile (1–4 yr)	N-Acetyl-α-glucosaminidase	Heparan sulfate	Severe mental retardation
Morquio, mucopolysaccharidosis IV	Some variation	N-Acetylgalactosamine 6-sulfate sulfatase	Keratan sulfate	0
Maroteaux-Lamy, mucopolysaccharidosis VI	Variation in severity and cardiovascular involvement	N-Acetylhexosamine-4-sulfate sulfatase (arylsulfatase B)	Dermatan sulfate	0
β-Glucuronidase deficiency, mucopolysaccharidosis VII	Few patients; infantile to adult forms	β-Glucuronidase	Dermatan sulfate ? Heparan sulfate	Mental retardation ? absent in some adults
Mucopolysaccharidosis VIII	One patient	N-Acetylglucosamine 6-sulfate sulfatase	Heparan sulfate Keratan sulfate	Mental retardation
Multiple sulfatase deficiency	Late infantile (1–4 yr)	Arylsulfatases A, B and C Other sulfatases	Sulfatides Mucopolysaccharides	Mental retardation
Sialidase deficiency	Infantile mucolipidosis I Late myoclonus and cherry red spot	Sialidase (neuraminidase)	Glycoproteins Glycolipids Sialyloligosaccharides	Mental retardation, myoclonus
Mucolipidosis II, I cell disease	Infantile (0–3 mo)	Elevated serum enzymes Primary defect unknown	Glycoproteins Glycolipids	Mental retardation
Mucolipidosis III, pseudo-Hurler polydystrophy	Late infantile (>2 yr)	Elevated serum enzymes Primary defect unknown	Glycoproteins Glycolipids	Mild mental retardation
Mucolipidosis VI	Infantile	Unknown	? Multiple	Mental retardation
Neuronal ceroid lipofuscinoses	Late infantile Juvenile Adult	Unknown	"Ceroid" "Lipofuscin"	Mental retardation, dementia variable in adults, seizures

Liver and/or spleen enlargement	Skeletal dysplasia	Ophthalmic	Hematologic	Genetics	Unique manifestations	References
+ +	+ +	0	Vacuolated lymphocytes Foam cells	AR	Coarse facies, increased sweat electrolytes, nonfunctional gall bladder; angiokeratoma in juvenile	Hers and Van Hoof, chap 11 Ho et al
+ + +	+ +	Cataracts, corneal clouding	Vacuolated lymphocytes Granulated neutrophils	AR	Coarse facies, enlarged tongue	Hers and Van Hoof, chap 11 Hirschhorn and Weissmann
0	+ +	Lens opacities	Vacuolated lymphocytes	AR	Coarse facies, detectable by urine amino acid analysis; Finnish predilection	Hers and Van Hoof, chap 24
+ + +	+ + + +	Corneal clouding	Granulated lymphocytes	AR	Coarse facies, cardiovascular involvement, joint stiffness	Hers and Van Hoof, chaps 8 and 9 Stanbury et al, chap 53 McKusick
+ + +	+ + + +	Retinal degeneration, no significant corneal clouding	Granulated lymphocytes	X-linked	Coarse facies, cardiovascular involvement, joint stiffness	
+	+	0	Granulated lymphocytes	AR	Mild coarsening of facies	
+	+	0	Granulated lymphocytes	AR	Nearly indistinguishable from MPS IIIA	
+	Severe, distinctive	Corneal clouding	Granulated neutrophils	AR	Severe deformity, odontoid hypoplasia, aortic regurgitation	
+ +	+ + + +	Corneal clouding	Granulated neutrophils and lymphocytes	AR	Mild coarsening of facies, joint stiffness, valvular heart disease	
+ + +	+ + +	Corneal clouding	Granulated neutrophils	AR	Coarse facies, ↑ vascular involvement	
+ +	+ +	Normal at age 6	?	? AR	Coarse facies	
+	MPS features	Retinal degeneration	Vacuolated and granulated cells	AR	Icthyosis, combined MPS and metachromatic leukodystrophy phenotype	Hers and Van Hoof, chaps 8 and 18 Stanbury et al, chap 38
+ + Less in late form	+ + Less or absent in late form	Cherry red spot	Vacuolated lymphocytes	AR	ML I patients have MPS phenotype; unclear if all ML I patients have sialidase deficiency	Hers and Van Hoof, chap 8 O'Brien
0/ +	+ + + +	Corneal clouding	Vacuolated and granulated neutrophils	AR	Coarse facies, inclusions in cultured fibroblasts, normal mucopolysacchariduria	Hers and Van Hoof, chap 8 Stanbury et al, chap 38
0	+ + +	Corneal clouding	Vacuolated plasma cells	AR	Coarse facies, inclusions in cultured fibroblasts, joint contractures, valvular heart disease, normal mucopolysacchariduria	
0	0	Corneal clouding, retinal degeneration	0	AR	Diagnosis based on electron microscopy; ? Ashkenazi Jewish predilection	Stanbury et al, chap 38
0	0	Optic atrophy, macular degeneration, retinitis pigmentosa	Vacuolated lymphocytes Granulated neutrophils	AR AR	Electron microscopy helpful, degree of genetic heterogeneity unknown	Hers and Van Hoof, chap 23

translational modification of lysosomal enzymes and general defects in the integrity and function of the lysosome may also cause lysosomal storage diseases. The mucolipidoses II and III appear to represent situations in which a single gene defect alters the ability of a number of lysosomal enzymes to enter or be retained within the lysosome. Thus, mutations outside the structural genes for the enzymes themselves can account for further heterogeneity. Better biochemical understanding of the identity, subunit structure, posttranslational processing, and substrate specificities of lysosomal enzymes should provide further insight into phenotypic and genotypic heterogeneity.

Clinical diagnosis is facilitated but also somewhat complicated by the widespread use of synthetic substrates for measuring lysosomal enzyme activities. These substrates often measure a group of related activities attributable to different enzymes. Thus, the activity of β-galactosidase using an artificial substrate may represent the sum of various β-galactosidases encoded by different structural genes and having different substrate specificities. Clinical reliability generally is achieved by manipulating in vitro conditions to reflect that enzyme activity whose deficiency is characteristic of a clinical disorder. Genetic heterogeneity has, however, resulted in individuals with mutant enzyme that either hydrolyzes the natural substrate and not the artificial substrate, or vice versa. This is exemplified by the normal individuals who have hexosaminidase A deficiency using artificial substrate and by patients with Tay-Sachs disease who have substantial levels of hexosaminidase A activity with artificial substrates. The presence or absence of disease correlates with ability to hydrolyze the natural G_{M2} ganglioside substrate. These phenomena have considerable significance for identification of affected patients, for heterozygote screening and for prenatal diagnosis. They indicate the need to go beyond artificial substrate enzyme assays if normal results occur in the face of overwhelming clinical, electron microscopic, or chemical evidence of a storage disease.

MANAGEMENT AND PREVENTION Specific therapy is not effective in lysosomal storage diseases at present, and care is largely symptomatic. The relentless, progressive course in many instances represents a tragic burden. Transplantation is effective in reversing the renal failure that commonly occurs in Fabry disease, and splenectomy frequently is helpful in adult Gaucher disease. Considerable attention has been focused on enzyme replacement for lysosomal storage diseases using organ or fibroblast transplantation or the infusion of either plasma, leukocytes, purified enzyme itself, or enzyme trapped in erythrocytes or liposomes. Although these approaches offer promise for treatment of manifestations outside the central nervous system, they are not of proved efficacy.

The most distressing aspects of lysosomal storage diseases involve the central nervous system, where the blood-brain barrier and the lack of pinocytotic activity by neurons present additional obstacles to the development of effective enzyme replacement therapy.

Genetic counseling is an important aspect of the management of these disorders. All the lysosomal storage diseases in which the specific enzyme deficiency is known either have been or presumably could be diagnosed in utero, since lysosomal enzyme activities appear to be expressed in cultured amniotic fluid cells as well as in cultured skin fibroblasts. Artificial insemination is an alternative for couples who have children affected with an autosomal recessive disease. Heterozygote detection in close relatives is frequently possible with careful laboratory analysis. This is particularly important in the X-linked Fabry and Hunter disorders, since numerous female members of the family may be at risk for bearing affected children. More effective approaches to prevention require identification of heterozygous couples prior to the birth of an affected offspring. The feasibility of this approach has been demonstrated by heterozygote testing programs for Tay-Sachs disease. Such programs could allow the elimination of these disorders through extensive testing and appropriate reproductive decisions on the part of the rare couples identified as being at risk for having affected offspring; the high frequency of the heterozygous state in Ashkenazi Jews and favorable biochemical aspects of carrier detection for Tay-Sachs disease have facilitated this program. Efficient and extremely accurate heterozygote detection methods are needed to apply this approach to other diseases and to populations with lower heterozygote frequencies. Even under optimal conditions genetic variants might cause false positive or false negative results in any screening process.

SPECIFIC DISORDERS

SPHINGOLIPIDOSES G_{M1} **gangliosidosis** G_{M1} gangliosidosis was recognized in 1965 in infants with features of Tay-Sachs disease and mucopolysaccharidosis and is due to deficiency of β-galactosidase. Prominent features of the infantile form are the presence of abnormalities at or near birth, developmental delay, seizures, coarse facies, edema, hepatosplenomegaly, macroglossia, ocular cherry red spot, and a distinctive mucopolysaccharidosis-like dysostosis multiplex. Death usually occurs in the first or second year of life. The juvenile form is characterized by a later onset, survival to the latter half of the first decade, neurological impairment and seizures, and milder skeletal and ocular findings. In the adult form of spondyloepiphyseal dysplasia similar to MPS IV, corneal clouding and normal intelligence are common. Joint pain and limitation of motion, particularly at the hips, can be disabling in these patients. Prominent spasticity and ataxia with mild bony abnormalities have occurred in other adult patients. A high index of suspicion is necessary to recognize the diverse phenotypes caused by β-galactosidase deficiency in juvenile and adult patients, since almost any combination of skeletal, ocular, neurologic, and visceral findings can occur. Isozymes of β-galactosidase occur, but evidence suggests that these derive from a single gene on chromosome 22. Thus, the diversity of phenotypes is due to different mutations in the structural gene. All forms of G_{M1} gangliosidosis have an autosomal recessive inheritance. There is no ethnic predilection. The frequency of the disease is low, with less than 50 patients reported for any given phenotype.

G_{M2} **gangliosidosis** Tay-Sachs disease, first recognized in 1881, is a relatively common inborn error of metabolism with thousands of documented cases. Although clinically indistinguishable from Sandhoff disease, the two are genetically distinct with deficiency of hexosaminidase A in the former and hexosaminidase A and B in the latter. The presenting features in both are a developmental delay beginning in the third to sixth month with subsequent rapidly progressive neurologic deterioration. Macrocephaly, seizures, retinal cherry-red spot, and an augmented startle response to sound suggest the diagnosis. The diagnosis is confirmed by enzyme assay. Most juvenile onset patients with hexosaminidase deficiency present with dementia, seizures and ocular findings, and some have an atypical spinocerebellar degeneration.

Sandhoff disease is nonallelic with Tay-Sachs disease, but the juvenile forms of hexosaminidase deficiency likely are allelic with Tay-Sachs disease. Tay-Sachs disease is the most frequent form of hexosaminidase deficiency, the risk being about 100-fold in Ashkenazi Jews compared with other ethnic groups. All forms of G_{M2} gangliosidosis are autosomal recessive. There is evidence that hexosaminidase B is composed of β subunits whose structural locus is on chromosome 5, while hexosaminidase A is composed of α and β subunits with the structural locus for the α subunit on chromosome 15.

Although no specific therapy is available, extensive programs for heterozygote detection in the prevention of Tay-Sachs disease have been carried out throughout the world. As of 1976, more than 150,000 people were tested with the identification of more than 6000 heterozygotes and more than 120 couples at risk for Tay-Sachs disease in their offspring. There had been 371 pregnancies monitored by prenatal diagnosis because of a previous affected child and 90 pregnancies monitored based on results of carrier screening.

LEUKODYSTROPHIES Krabbe galactosylceramide lipidosis or globoid cell leukodystrophy is an infantile disease due to deficiency of galactosylceramide β-galactosidase and characterized by onset at 2 to 6 months of age, with irritability, hyperesthesia, hypersensitivity to external stimuli, unexplained fever, optic atrophy, and sometimes seizures. Spinal fluid protein is usually increased. Initially there is hypertonicity and increased deep tendon reflexes with progression to a hypotonic state. Rapid neurologic deterioration, and death occur within 1 to 2 years of onset. Premortem diagnosis is accomplished by enzyme assay. The presence of globoid cells on neuropathologic examination is characteristic and possibly specific for this enzyme deficiency. Galactosylceramide β-galactosidase functions in the degradation of sulfatides derived from myelin. Myelin synthesis is so impaired by tissue damage that the absolute amount of the galactocerebroside substrate is usually not increased in postmortem tissue. Galactosylceramide β-galactosidase is genetically distinct from the β-galactosidase that is deficient in G_{M1} gangliosidosis.

Krabbe disease is relatively rare, with about 150 reported cases and numerous unreported cases. It has an autosomal recessive genetic basis and is present in all ethnic groups with a possible increased frequency in the Scandinavian countries. Although no specific therapy is available, prenatal diagnosis has been accomplished.

Deficiency of arylsulfatase A (cerebroside sulfatase) is the basis of metachromatic leukodystrophy, a lipid storage disease with a frequency of 1 in 40,000. The age of onset is later than that in Tay-Sachs disease or Krabbe disease. Patients develop the ability to walk and frequently present with gait abnormalities in the second to fourth year of life. Initially the patients may be hypotonic with decreased deep tendon reflexes, the latter reflecting peripheral nerve involvement. The disease progresses over the first decade to include ataxia, increased muscle tone, decorticate or decerebrate posturing, and eventual loss of all contact with surroundings. Duration of survival depends on nursing care and support such as nasogastric or gastrostomy feeding.

Diagnosis is accomplished using enzyme assay, originally in urine and more recently in leukocytes or fibroblasts. Changes demonstrable on metachromatic staining of nerve tissue are nonspecific and not an adequate substitute for enzyme assay. Rare patients with a juvenile form of metachromatic leukodystrophy are described with an onset between 4 and 20 years of age and a slower progression. The adult form of this disease deserves special mention as an example of the difficulties presented by subtle, slowly progressive forms of lysosomal storage diseases. The onset is in the second to fifth decade with a slowly progressive dementia. Emotional difficulties, motor dysfunction, and indistinct speech are often present. Even though conduction velocity in peripheral nerves is usually diminished, the deep tendon reflexes are often increased. Typical premortem diagnoses include organic dementia, schizophrenia, and multiple sclerosis; a correct premortem diagnosis has been made in only a minority.

Arylsulfatase A is routinely measured using artificial substrate, and complexities involving low levels of activity in normal individuals and moderate levels of residual activity in symptomatic patients have been described. Heterogencity involving mutations in multiple components of the cerebroside sulfatase activity may exist, but the majority of patients probably have simple allelic disorders on an autosomal recessive basis. Arylsulfatase A deficiency also occurs in multiple sulfatase deficiency discussed below.

NIEMANN-PICK DISEASE Niemann-Pick disease is a lipidosis caused by deficiency of sphingomyelinase which hydrolyzes sphingomyelin ceramide and phosphorylcholine. The most common form is an infantile neuropathic disorder which begins shortly after birth with hepatosplenomegaly, failure to thrive, and neurologic impairment. Retinal cherry red spots occur, but seizures and functional hypersplenism are rare. The diagnosis can be made with considerable confidence by recognition of the distinctive Niemann-Pick cell in the bone marrow, but enzyme assay should be performed. Patients with later onset and slower progression have been described as well as a number of patients with visceral disease and no neurologic involvement. Many patients described with the sea blue histiocyte syndrome may have had sphingomyelinase deficiency; other patients with the sea blue histiocyte syndrome may represent unique disorders not yet biochemically characterized.

GAUCHER DISEASE Gaucher disease is a glucosylceramide lipidosis caused by deficiency of glucosylceramidase. An infantile form is characterized by early onset, marked hepatosplenomegaly, and severe neurological progression to early death. A juvenile form with milder neurologic involvement exists. The adult form of the disease may be the most commonly encountered lysosomal storage disease. Patients with juvenile and adult Gaucher disease have been observed within the same family but not within the same sibships, supporting the hypothesis that these are allelic disorders.

All forms of Gaucher disease have an autosomal recessive genetic basis. The disorder is about 30 times more frequent in Ashkenazi Jews, with an incidence in this ethnic group of about 1 in 2500 births. Although commonly termed "adult Gaucher disease," this variant frequently has its onset in childhood. Absence of neurologic involvement is the criterion for inclusion in this category. Manifestations include hepatosplenomegaly, hypersplenism, bleeding diathesis, bone pain, pathological fractures, and pulmonary involvement with associated pneumonia. Serum acid phosphatase is characteristically elevated. A distinctive storage cell occurs in the bone marrow in all forms of Gaucher disease, but enzyme assay should be performed because the Gaucher cell may also be found in patients with granulocytic leukemia and myeloma.

The clinical course is variable; pulmonary involvement may lead to early death, but in many patients life span is not shortened by the disease. Bleeding secondary to thrombocytopenia frequently responds to splenectomy with considerable benefit. Because of the frequency of the disease and the lack of neurologic involvement, the adult form of Gaucher disease is potentially amenable to enzyme replacement therapy.

FABRY DISEASE Fabry disease involves the accumulation of a trihexoside, galactosylgalactosylglucosylceramide due to deficiency of α-galactosidase A. The disorder is X-linked, and the most severe symptoms are seen in hemizygous males. Onset is in childhood with periodic crises of severe pain in the extremities, cutaneous angiokeratomas, a characteristic corneal dystrophy, hypohidrosis, vascular thromboses, and progressive renal impairment. Death most often results from renal failure, typically in the third to fifth decade. Heterozygous females are affected more mildly. Corneal dystrophy is the most frequent finding, but all other manifestations may also be seen. Life expectancy is greater in women, although fatal complications can rarely occur. Renal failure can be treated by chronic dialysis or transplantation. Enzyme replacement therapy has been attempted in this disease. In addition, patients undergoing transplantation presumably derive normal enzyme from the transplanted kidney. Administration of phenytoin sodium (Dilantin) has been used in treatment of the painful neuropathy.

There is evidence that the α galactosidase A structural gene resides on the X chromosome, although alternative explanations involving regulatory components have been suggested. Clinically the disorder should be considered as an X-linked dominant, since heterozygous females usually manifest the condition.

ACID LIPASE DEFICIENCY Acid lipase deficiency is the basis for two disorders with different phenotypic features. Wolman disease is a severe disorder of early onset, with prominent hepatosplenomegaly, anemia, vomiting, failure to thrive, and characteristic adrenal calcification. Neurologic involvement is minimal compared with the severe somatic handicap. Cholesteryl ester storage disease is a rare disorder with mild phenotypic features by comparison. The most constant features are hepatosplenomegaly and increased plasma cholesterol. Hepatic fibrosis, esophageal varices, and poor growth have occurred. One reported sibship may represent an intermediate phenotype, since two females died at 7 and 9 years of age with unexplained acute hepatic failure, and a third sibling developed adrenal calcification and pulmonary hypertension early in life. Tissues from patients with acid lipase deficiency demonstrate inability to hydrolyze triglycerides as well as cholesteryl esters. Possibly a single enzyme hydrolyzes multiple substrates, but the subunit structure and hydrolytic capacities of various lysosomal lipases are not well studied. Deficiency of acid lipase results in impairment of the LDL pathway as described in Chap. 100 and may be associated with premature atherosclerosis. Both Wolman and cholesteryl ester storage diseases have an autosomal recessive basis.

GLYCOPROTEIN STORAGE DISORDERS Fucosidosis, mannosidosis, and aspartylglucosaminuria are rare, autosomal recessive disorders involving hydrolases that degrade polysaccharide linkages. Glycolipids as well as glycoproteins are accumulated in fucosidosis. All are characterized by mental retardation and varying somatic involvements, as outlined in Table 101-1. Fucosidosis and mannosidosis are most often lethal disorders in childhood, while aspartylglucosaminuria presents as a late-onset lysosomal storage disease with prominent mental retardation and a prolonged course. Abnormal sweat electrolytes and cutaneous angiokeratomas are distinctive in fucosidosis, and an unusual cartwheel-type cataract occurs in mannosidosis. Aspartylglucosaminuria is remarkable in that urinary amino acid analysis is diagnostic with an increase of aspartylglucosamine; it is more frequent in the Finnish population. Each of the disorders can be diagnosed by appropriate enzyme assay.

MUCOPOLYSACCHARIDOSIS (MPS) The mucopolysaccharidoses represent a broad spectrum of disorders due to deficiencies of one of a group of enzymes which degrade three classes of mucopolysaccharides: heparan sulfate, dermatan sulfate, and keratan sulfate. The general MPS phenotype includes coarse facies, corneal clouding, hepatosplenomegaly, joint stiffness, hernias, dysostosis multiplex, mucopolysaccharide excretion in the urine, and metachromatic staining in peripheral leukocytes and bone marrow. Various components of the MPS phenotype are also found in the mucolipidoses, glycoprotein storage disorders, and other lysosomal storage diseases. Detailed clinical and radiologic evaluation and identification of the type of MPS excreted in the urine help to narrow the diagnostic possibilities. Definitive diagnosis requires assay of specific enzymes in various tissues such as cultured skin fibroblasts.

The Hurler or MPS IH disorder is the prototype MPS. Virtually all the components of the phenotype mentioned above are present and expressed in a severe degree. Nasal congestion and grossly visible corneal clouding are early features. Excessive growth during the first year of life is followed by poor growth late in the course. Radiologic features include enlargement of the sella turcica with a distinctive "shoe-shaped" fossa, broadening and shortening of the long bones, and hypoplasia and beaking of the vertebrae in the lumbar area. The vertebral beaking gives rise to an accentuated kyphosis or gibbus deformity. Death occurs within the first decade; postmortem findings include hydrocephalus and cardiovascular disease due to occlusion of the coronary arteries. The biochemical hallmark is α-iduronidase deficiency with accumulation of heparan sulfate and dermatan sulfate.

MPS IS, or Scheie syndrome, is a clinically distinct disorder of adult onset characterized by joint stiffness, corneal clouding, aortic regurgitation, and usually normal intelligence. Surprisingly, this much milder disorder is also the result of α-iduronidase deficiency; it is allelic with the Hurler syndrome, as shown by lack of cross-correction of enzyme activity in cocultures of skin fibroblasts. Phenotypes occur that are clearly intermediate between Hurler and Scheie syndromes. It is believed that patients with an intermediate phenotype represent genetic compounds with one Hurler allele and one Scheie allele. Although genetic compounds must occur, their existence is difficult to distinguish in any one case from still other mutations of intermediate severity.

The Hunter or MPS II syndrome is distinguishable from the Hurler phenotype by the absence of gross corneal clouding and the X-linked recessive inheritance. The infantile form resembles the Hurler phenotype, and a milder form allows survival into adulthood. The severe and mild forms may be allelic, since both are sex-linked and share the same enzyme deficiency (iduronosulfate sulfatase).

The Sanfilippo mucopolysaccharidoses (MPS IIIA and IIIB) are distinguished by the accumulation of heparan sulfate without dermatan or keratan sulfate and by the marked central nervous system involvement with milder somatic involvement. Because the somatic features of this MPS are mild, the condition can be overlooked in the evaluation of an apparently isolated central nervous system problem. Death usually occurs during the second decade. MPS IIIA and MPS IIIB represent hallmark examples of genocopies. That is, two different enzyme deficiencies give rise to a virtually indistinguishable clinical phenotype with the same storage product. The two MPS III disorders can be diagnosed and distinguished by enzyme assay (Table 101-1).

The Morquio or MPS IV syndrome is distinguished by the absence of mental retardation and the presence of a distinctive bony dystrophy which can be classified as a spondyloepiphyseal dysplasia. Marked hypoplasia of the odontoid process can cause cervical dislocation and usually leads to some degree of spinal cord compression. Aortic regurgitation is frequent. The deficiency of N-acetylgalactosamine 6-sulfate sulfatase is the basis for this condition. This enzyme is distinct from an N-acetylglucosamine 6-sulfate sulfatase whose deficiency results in MPS VIII. Bone changes somewhat suggestive of the Morquio syndrome may also occur in MPS VIII, in β-galactosidase deficiency, and in other forms of spondyloepiphyseal dysplasia. The Maroteaux-Lamy or MPS VI disorder is characterized by prominent osseous involvement, corneal clouding, and normal intellect. Allelic forms with variable severity but the same deficiency of arylsulfatase B (*N*-acetylhexosamine 4-sulfate sulfatase) have been described. MPS VII, or β-glucuronidase deficiency has been described in less than 10 patients with a rather complete MPS phenotype. Extreme variability from a lethal infantile form to a mild adult disease has occurred. Two patients with MPS VIII were found to have *N*-acetylglucosamine 6-sulfate sulfatase deficiency with mucopolysacchariduria involving heparan sulfate and keratan sulfate. As might be expected, the patients had a phenotype combining features of MPS III and MPS IV.

MULTIPLE SULFATASE DEFICIENCY Multiple sulfatase deficiency is a unique disorder, which, although autosomal recessive, is characterized by deficiency of five or more cellular sulfatases. Arylsulfatase A, arylsulfatase B, other mucopolysaccharide sulfatases, and a nonlysosomal placental sulfatase are deficient in this condition. The clinical picture combines features of metachromatic leukodystrophy, an MPS phenotype, and ichthyosis. The last feature presumably relates to the placental sulfatase deficiency which also occurs as an isolated X-linked enzyme deficiency characterized by abnormal parturition and ichthyosis. Biochemical studies of this condition should provide further insight into biochemical and clinical genetic heterogeneity.

MUCOLIPIDOSES Mucolipidosis is a general term for lysosomal storage diseases involving some combination of MPS, glycoprotein, oligosaccharide, and glycolipids. Although G_{M1} gangliosidosis, fucosidosis, mannosidosis, and other disorders might qualify as mucolipidoses, these can be considered more specifically since the biochemical basis is understood. Findings in mucolipidosis I include mental retardation, hepatosplenomegaly, an MPS phenotype, and ocular cherry red spot on an autosomal recessive basis. Some or most patients with mucolipidosis I have a deficiency of sialidase (neuraminidase). Another disorder described in the literature, the cherry red spot–myoclonus syndrome, also appears to be due to sialidase deficiency, suggesting that these may be allelic disorders.

Mucolipidosis II, or I-cell disease, is an early onset disorder with mental retardation and an MPS phenotype. The distinctive features are striking inclusions in cultured skin fibroblasts and markedly elevated serum levels of lysosomal enzymes. The disorder has an autosomal recessive basis and is thought to involve a defect in the processes for entry into, or maintenance of, lysosomal enzymes within that organelle. Mucolipidosis III or psuedo-Hurler polydystrophy is a milder disorder with many aspects of the MPS phenotype, particularly dysostosis multiplex. The disorder presents in the first decade with joint stiffness, the diagnosis of rheumatoid arthritis often being considered. The major handicaps are progressive physical disabilities, particularly claw hand deformity and hip dysplasia. Mild mental retardation is common. Aortic and/or mitral valvular disease is routinely present, although often not functionally significant. Survival into adult life with possible stabilization of the condition is characteristic, with greater disability in males than in females. Inclusions in cultured skin fibroblasts and elevation of serum lysosomal enzymes are essentially identical with the findings in mucolipidosis II, suggesting that these may be allelic disorders. Mucolipidosis IV is a disorder with mental retardation, corneal clouding, and retinal degeneration without other somatic features. Diagnosis has been based primarily on electron microscopic findings. A small number of patients, all of Ashkenazi Jewish origin, have been described.

NEURONAL CEROID LIPOFUSCINOSES The neuronal ceroid lipofuscinosis group of disorders includes a wide clinical spectrum with onset in childhood, juvenile, or adult periods. It is unknown whether single or multiple biochemical genetic disorders are present in the patients reported. The clinical features include central nervous system deterioration with cerebral atrophy, usually commensurate with degree of impairment. Seizures, particularly myoclonic jerks, are a prominent feature. Ocular involvement with optic atrophy, retinitis pigmentosa, and macular degeneration is present in the infantile and juvenile disorders but often absent in adult forms. Autosomal recessive inheritance is likely in most instances. The neuropathologic findings form the basis of the descriptive term for the disease. Electron microscopy demonstrates abnormal inclusions within lysosomes throughout a wide variety of tissues, despite the rather isolated neurological clinical involvement. The presence of curvilinear bodies, electron-dense material, and fingerprint profiles on electron microscopy of white blood cells, liver biopsy, or muscle biopsy can be helpful diagnostically.

OTHER LYSOSOMAL STORAGE DISEASES Glycogen storage disease type II (Pompe disease) is the prototype lysosomal storage disease. The predominant clinical features of skeletal and cardiac myopathy are described in Chap. 97. Acid phosphatase deficiency and Farber lipogranulomatosis are included in Table 101-1. Lactosyl ceramidosis appears to represent a variant of Niemann-Pick disease; in vitro hydrolysis of lactosyl ceramide is accomplished by those enzymes that are deficient in G_{M1} gangliosidosis or in Krabbe disease, depending upon the in vitro conditions used. Adrenoleukodystrophy is identifiable as a distinct X-linked disorder with accumulation of long-chain fatty acid cholesteryl esters in tissues, but it is unclear whether this is a lysosomal storage disease. A Sanfilippo C or MPS III C disorder may occur with α-glucosaminidase as its basis. The recognition of females with the Hunter MPS II phenotype and identical enzyme deficiency has raised the possibility of an autosomal recessive form of the Hunter syndrome. Such could occur if the enzyme in question had nonidentical subunits coded for by one autosomal and one X-linked gene, or if regulatory genetic elements were invoked. On the other hand females with phenotypic manifestations could occur, owing to X-chromosome inactivation. One family has been described with G_{M3} gangliosidosis. This is not a lysosomal storage disease but does possibly represent a defect in ganglioside synthesis. The clinical features are similar to those seen in lysosomal storage diseases, but inconsistencies between siblings leave question of whether this is a unique genetic disorder. Other neurodegenerative diseases may eventually become classifiable as lysosomal storage diseases. Disorders such as juvenile dystonic lipidosis, neuroaxonal dystrophy, Hallervorden-Spatz disease, Pelizaeus-Merzbacher disease, and other candidates exist. In addition, it is not unusual to identify patients with distinctive clinical features suggestive of lipidosis, mucolipidosis, or mucopolysaccharidosis, in which none of the present biochemically identifiable disorders can be identified. For these reasons, the number of distinct lysosomal storage diseases is likely to continue to increase.

REFERENCES

Hers HG, Van Hoof F (eds): *Lysosomes and Storage Diseases*. New York, Academic, 1973

Hirschhorn R, Weissmann G: Genetic disorders of lysosomes, in *Progress in Medical Genetics*, AG Steinberg et al, (eds). Philadelphia, Saunders, 1976, vol 1

Ho MW et al: Glycosphingolipid hydrolases: Properties and molecular genetics. Mol Cell Biochem 17:125, 1977

McKusick VA: *Heritable Disorders of Connective Tissue,* 4th ed. St Louis, Mosby, 1972

O'Brien JS: Neuraminidase deficiency in the cherry red spot–myoclonus syndrome. Biochem Biophys Res Comm 79:1136, 1977

Stanbury JB et al (eds): *The Metabolic Basis of Inherited Disease,* 4th ed. New York, McGraw-Hill, 1978

102
RARE DISORDERS OF ADIPOSE TISSUE

Daniel W. Foster

This chapter is concerned with syndromes characterized by abnormalities in adipose tissue. The disorders are rare, the pathophysiology is frequently not clear, and only clinical descriptions can be given.

THE LIPODYSTROPHIES

The lipodystrophies are characterized by generalized or partial loss of body fat and a series of metabolic disorders, including insulin resistance, hyperglycemia, and hypertriglyceridemia.

GENERALIZED LIPODYSTROPHY Generalized lipodystrophy (also called lipoatrophic diabetes) may be either congenital or acquired. The congenital form is transmitted as an autosomal recessive trait. Rates of parental consanguinity are high. Loss of fat is obvious at birth, but the rest of the clinical picture may not develop until later. The acquired disease often develops after some other illness. Infections such as measles, chicken pox, whooping cough, or infectious mononucleosis are common precipitating events, but hypothyroidism, hyperthyroidism, and pregnancy have also been implicated. Some cases begin with the appearance of painful nodular swellings of adipose tissue resembling acute panniculitis (see below). While certain differences exist, the congenital and acquired forms are basically similar in clinical manifestations (Table 102-1).

Fat atrophy Loss of body fat is the characteristic finding. In congenital cases the skin of the face is tightly drawn over the bony structures, and the entire body is devoid of adipose tissue. Rarely, a small amount of breast fat remains. In the acquired form the face may be spared, but all other fat disappears. Microscopically adipose tissue cells can be identified, but they contain no triglyceride stores. Paradoxically the liver is stuffed with fat, and the reticuloendothelial system contains lipid-laden macrophages (foam cells). The cause of the fat atrophy is not known. While many studies have attempted to identify defects in triglyceride transport, triglyceride synthesis, or lipolysis, no uniform abnormality has been found. Small molecular weight fat-mobilizing polypeptides have been reported in the urine of patients with generalized lipodystrophy, but their role in the disease is uncertain. Release of free fatty acids into plasma following norepinephrine infusion is impaired, but this may simply reflect the depleted triglyceride stores. Adipose tissue from a dystrophic site in a patient with partial lipodystrophy accumulates fat when transplanted into a normal region of the body, while fat from an uninvolved region loses its triglyceride on transplantation to a dystrophic area, suggesting a localized (neuropathic?) cause for fat atrophy.

Growth and maturation Linear growth is accelerated in the first few years of life in the congenital disorder and in acquired disease that begins early in childhood. Epiphyses close early, however, so that the final height in most patients is normal. True muscular hypertrophy is present, and patients may have an acromegalic appearance with coarse facial features and large hands and feet. The ears tend to be prominent in the congenital form. Many viscera are enlarged, and generalized lymphadenopathy may be present.

Liver The liver is uniformly enlarged, and as a consequence the abdomen is protuberant. Fatty liver may progress to cirrhosis, especially in the acquired form. Several patients have died from bleeding esophageal varices. Splenomegaly probably does not occur in the absence of portal hypertension.

Kidneys The kidneys are usually enlarged. Subjects with the acquired disorder may have proteinuria and the nephrotic syndrome, although not as frequently as in partial lipodystrophy. Moderate hypertension is common.

Genitalia The external genitalia (penis and testes in males, clitoris in females) are usually hypertrophied in congenital disease. In girls polycystic ovaries are common, resulting in the clinical picture of Stein-Leventhal syndrome.

Skin Acanthosis nigricans is present in most. Hypertrichosis of face, neck, trunk, and limbs is frequent. Scalp hair is usually thick and curly, particularly early in life.

Central nervous system Mental retardation is present in about half the congenital cases. Dilatation of the third ventricle and basal cisterns has been demonstrated by pneumoencephalography. Central nervous system involvement appears to be less marked in the acquired disease, although two patients had astrocytomas arising in the floor of the third ventricle.

Endocrine and metabolic abnormalities Three major disturbances characterize the lipodystrophic patient: (1) Severe insu-

TABLE 102-1
Characteristics of the lipodystrophies

Finding	Congenital general	Acquired general	Acquired partial	Dominant partial
Inheritance	Autosomal recessive	Sporadic	Usually sporadic	Autosomal dominant
Age of onset	Infancy	Childhood to adult	Childhood to adult	Puberty
Sex incidence	Males and females equal	Female preponderance	Female preponderance	Female preponderance
Lipoatrophy	Face, trunk, limbs	Face, trunk, limbs	Face, upper trunk, upper limbs	Trunk and limbs
Liver involvement	+	+ +	Rare	0
Renal disease	+	+	+ +	0
Insulin resistance	+	+	+	+
Hyperglycemia	+	+	+	+
Hypertriglyceridemia	+	+	+	+
Acanthosis nigricans	+	+	Rare	+
Genital hypertrophy	+	+	Rare	+
Bone age	Accelerated	Normal to accelerated	Normal	Normal

lin resistance with hyperglycemia. Diminished affinity of insulin receptors for the hormone has been demonstrated utilizing monocytes from affected patients, and this receptor defect may account for the resistant state. Receptor number is probably normal. Despite insulin resistance, ketoacidosis does not develop, even with severe hyperglycemia. Muscle capillary basement membranes are not thickened, differentiating lipodystrophy from the common forms of diabetes mellitus. (2) Severe hypertriglyceridemia with the accumulation of both chylomicrons and very low density lipoproteins in the blood. The mechanism is not clear. (3) A hypermetabolic state with normal thyroid function. Basal metabolic rates are markedly elevated. Patients do not gain weight with excessive caloric intake, indicating a facile capacity to waste calories as heat. Thyroidectomy in one patient decreased but did not normalize the basal metabolic rate; symptoms and signs of hypothyroidism supervened in this patient, requiring treatment with thyroid hormone despite continued high metabolic rates, thus confirming that hypermetabolism was not due to hyperthyroidism.

ACQUIRED PARTIAL LIPODYSTROPHY This is the most common of the lipodystrophies and usually affects women. Fat atrophy occurs in the upper half of the body, including the face, but spares the lower extremities. Rarely the lower half of the body is affected, leaving the upper torso intact. Occasionally the lesion affects only one side. The other anatomic features of generalized lipodystrophy are usually absent, and liver disease appears to be rare. Proteinuria, with or without the nephrotic syndrome, occurs much more frequently than in other forms. The complement system is abnormal, and C_3 levels tend to be low. C_3 splitting factor ("nephritic factor") is present in the serum. Dermatomyositis and Sjögren's syndrome occur in some patients. Rarely partial lipodystrophy converts or progresses to the generalized form of the disease.

LIPODYSTROPHY WITH DOMINANT TRANSMISSION This syndrome was first described in 1974 and represents a variant characterized by fat atrophy of the limbs and trunk with sparing of the face, which may actually be rounded. The neck may also be exempt. The disease usually begins at puberty but may not appear until middle age. Males are rarely affected. Insulin resistance and hyperglycemia are usual, and severe hypertriglyceridemia with eruptive xanthoma may occur. The vaginal labia are hypertrophied and polycystic ovaries may be seen. Acanthosis nigricans is usually present. Liver and renal disease do not occur.

MULTIPLE SYMMETRIC LIPOMATOSIS

This disease is characterized by the formation of multiple, non-encapsulated lipomas in the nape of the neck, supraclavicular, and deltoid regions to produce an extraordinary bull-necked appearance (sometimes called "Madelung collar"). Lipomas can also appear elsewhere in the body. Expansion of the lipomas with infiltration between fascial planes can cause tracheal, laryngeal, and mediastinal compression. Most cases occur in alcoholics for reasons that are not clear. Hypertriglyceridemia, hyperuricemia, hyperinsulinemia, and renal tubular acidosis have been reported in some subjects.

The etiology is not known. Fat cells in the tumors have been reported to be small, suggesting new formation of adipocytes rather than a defect in triglyceride storage. Catecholamine-induced lipolysis is impaired in tumor tissue, but this may be a result rather than the cause of the lesion.

ADIPOSIS DOLOROSA

Adiposis dolorosa is a rare disease characterized by the presence of painful, circumscribed fatty deposits in the subcutane-

ous tissue of the extremities and occasionally elsewhere in the body. The face is not involved. Pain may occur spontaneously or upon pressure. Involved areas vary in size from 0.5 to 5.0 cm. Affected subjects are usually obese, postmenopausal women who have weakness and asthenia. Epilepsy has been noted in a number of cases, and emotional instability or frank dementia may be present. Most cases probably are sporadic, but familial inheritance in a dominant pattern has been noted. Microscopic examination of involved adipose tissue shows granulomas with giant-cell formation. Fat necrosis is unusual. The only reported biochemical defect is an inability to synthesize 18 carbon fatty acids despite the capacity for normal synthesis of 16 carbon fatty acids. Even if this defect is present, its relation to the clinical picture is uncertain.

Treatment is unsatisfactory, possibly because many of the complaints are functional. Oral analgesics and injection with local anesthetics have been tried. In one patient with extreme pain recalcitrant to all measures, the intravenous infusion of lidocaine (200 to 400 mg) over a 20-min period gave relief for 10 h. After the pain cycle was broken, lidocaine was given as a single infusion every other day. It is not known whether the effects were real or due to a placebo response.

ACUTE (RELAPSING) PANNICULITIS

The appearance of single or multiple crops of tender nodules in subcutaneous fat with a histologic picture of fat cell necrosis, infiltration of inflammatory cells, and development of fat-filled macrophages (foam cells) is the hallmark of panniculitis. The nodules range in size from 0.5 to 10 cm and may be firm or fluctuant. On occasion they drain an oily solution, and suppuration is sometimes seen. Individual lesions last from 1 to 8 weeks before disappearing. Often a pigmented depressed area is left at the involved site. While some patients have only nodular relapsing panniculitis, others develop a syndrome that includes fever, abnormal liver function, involvement of the bone marrow with leukemoid response or bleeding tendencies, nodular pulmonary lesions, evidence of pancreatic disease with elevated plasma amylase and lipase levels, and an unusual prevalence of collagen-vascular disease. This constellation of findings has been called Weber-Christian disease. It now seems clear that painful or nonpainful panniculitis occurs in several conditions and that Weber-Christian disease is not a specific entity. In a series of 34 patients with panniculitis studied at the Mayo Clinic, ultimate diagnoses included erythema nodosum, 15; local skin infections, 6; erythema enduratum, 5; Weber-Christian-like disease, 5; traumatic panniculitis, 2; and vasculitis, 1. Erythema enduratum is probably a localized hypersensitivity vasculitis. It is often found in association with tuberculosis but may develop in the absence of that disease. "Weber-Christian-like" referred to a picture of relapsing, febrile panniculitis with elevation of lipase and amylase activities in the plasma. Some of these patients could, in fact, have had metastatic fat necrosis (see below). Generalized vasculitis as a cause of acute panniculitis may be more common than indicated in the Mayo series, since in 57 autopsied cases presumed to have Weber-Christian disease there were 2 cases of dermatomyositis; 2 of scleroderma; and 6 with either lupus, polyarteritis, or rheumatoid arthritis. A fulminant downhill course in a patient with panniculitis can be assumed to be a collagen-vascular disease or metastatic fat necrosis.

The Weber-Christian notation should probably be abandoned. Patients with histologically proved panniculitis should be diagnosed as having acute (relapsing) panniculitis and a search made for the underlying etiology. Treatment is unsatisfactory, though glucocorticoids are usually tried.

METASTATIC FAT NECROSIS

Metastatic fat necrosis is a syndrome of extensive adipose tissue inflammation and cell death resembling or identical with acute nodular panniculitis. It is accompanied by fever, destructive polyarthritis (which may cause flail joints), lytic bone lesions, pleural and pericardial effusions, ascites, and elevation of lipase and amylase levels in the plasma. Eosinophilia occurs in some patients. Pancreatic disease is invariably present. About two-thirds of patients have pancreatitis, while the remainder have a carcinoma of the pancreas, usually acinar. The cause of the syndrome is unknown. Fat necrosis has been speculated to be due to pancreatic lipase acting at multiple sites in the body, but the entire picture may actually result from an autoimmune phenomenon. Complement levels are low, and involved tissues show immunofluorescent staining for IgG and the third component of complement. Prognosis is poor, and death often occurs within a few months whether or not the underlying cause is cancer.

REFERENCES

Lipodystrophy

DUNNIGAN MG et al: Familial lipoatrophic diabetes with dominant transmission. Q J Med 169:33, 1974

OSEID S et al: Decreased binding of insulin to its receptor in patients with congenital generalized lipodystrophy. N Engl J Med 296:245, 1977

SEIP M: Generalized lipodystrophy. Ergeb Inn Med Kinderheilkd 31:59, 1971

Multiple symmetric lipomatosis

ENZI G et al: Multiple symmetric lipomatosis. A defect in adrenergic-stimulated lipolysis. J Clin Invest 60:1221, 1977

Adiposis dolorosa

BLOMSTRAND R et al: Adiposis dolorosa associated with defects of lipid metabolism. Acta Derm Venereol 51:243, 1971

CANTU JM et al: Autosomal dominant inheritance in adiposis dolorosa (Dercum's disease). Humangenetik 18:89, 1973

Acute (relapsing) panniculitis

FÖRSTRÖM L, RK WINKELMANN: Acute panniculitis. A clinical and histopathologic study of 34 cases. Arch Dermatol 113:909, 1977

MACDONALD A, M FEIWEL: A review of the concept of Weber-Christian panniculitis with a report of five cases. Br J Dermatol 80:355, 1968

Metastatic fat necrosis

GOOD AE et al: Acinar pancreatic tumor with metastatic fat necrosis. Report of a case and review of rheumatic manifestations. Am J Dig Dis 21:978, 1976

POTTS DE et al: Syndrome of pancreatic disease, subcutaneous fat necrosis and polyserositis. Case report and review of literature. Am J Med 58:417, 1975

Genetic disorders affecting multiple organ systems

103
DISORDERS OF CONNECTIVE TISSUE

PHILIP J. FIALKOW

Elastin, collagen, glycoproteins, and proteinpolysaccharides are the major extracellular macromolecules of connective tissue. An inherited abnormality in connective tissue may affect any one of the numerous steps in the biosynthesis and the metabolism of these substances or the processes by which the macromolecules are physically organized and oriented to one another.

Heritable, generalized disorders of connective tissue may be classified as primary or secondary. The former group includes those diseases caused by mutations in genes that directly involve the synthesis or metabolism of elements such as collagen or elastin. In secondary disorders, mutant genes affect metabolism exogenous to connective tissue pathways, resulting in the accumulation of a product that damages connective tissue (e.g., homocystinuria, Chap. 88).

The heritable disorders discussed in this chapter are thought to be primary and to involve collagen or elastic fibers. With some exceptions the basic defects are undefined, and it is not known whether the mutations affect connective tissue primarily or secondarily. In some cases it is not certain whether the abnormalities involve collagen, elastin, or other connective tissue components. All the disorders are genetically heterogeneous, i.e., two or more different mutations produce clinically similar diseases. Diseases primarily affecting mucopolysaccharides are described in Chap. 101.

THE EHLERS-DANLOS SYNDROME

The Ehlers-Danlos syndrome (EDS) constitutes a group of heritable, generalized disorders of connective tissue whose major features include fragile and hyperextensible skin (Fig. 103-1), easy bruising, and loose-jointedness. There are at least seven distinct types that vary in clinical manifestations from mild to severe. The patterns of inheritance include autosomal dominant and recessive and X-linked recessive. The prevalence is uncertain.

The EDS presumably involves collagen fibers. The basic building block of these fibers, the collagen monomer, is a triple helix of three α chains. Several different forms of collagen are known. The ubiquitous molecule (type I) is a triple helix containing two different α chains and is found in skin, tendon, ligament, bone, blood vessels, dentin, and other organs. EDS I,

II, and III are thought to involve this macromolecule. Type II collagen is found primarily in cartilage and consists of three α chains, similar to but not identical with, those found in type I. Type III collagen, the molecule thought to be involved in EDS IV, has three identical α chains which differ from those found in types I and II. It has a similar tissue distribution to type I but is not found in bone or dentin.

EDS I, GRAVIS TYPE   This is the classical EDS, which, because of its severe clinical manifestations, is termed *gravis*.

Clinical manifestations   SKIN   The skin is soft, velvety, and hyperextensible. It can be pulled far away from the underlying structures, but upon release it promptly returns to its original position (Fig. 103-1). With advancing age focal losses of elasticity may cause the skin over some areas such as the palms to become lax. The skin is fragile and easily bruised. Minor trauma often produces a gaping, fish-mouth wound that is hard to suture but does not bleed extensively. Paper-thin scars develop with healing. Minor injury often results in purpura or hematomas which may organize, calcify, and resemble a neoplasm. Another type of pseudotumor develops over pressure points such as the knees and elbows. These smaller, subcutaneous pea-sized "spherules" occur on the extremities, calcify, and are visible on roentgenograms.

MUSCULOSKELETAL SYSTEM   Hyperextensible joints may allow patients to perform unusual contortions (e.g., "India rubber man," "human pretzel"). Because of joint instability, these patients are prone to develop effusions or recurrent dislocations of the hip, patella, shoulder, and other joints. Hemarthroses sometimes occur. Backward curvature of the knees (genu recurvatum), flatfeet, kyphoscoliosis, and looseness of the clavicles at their sternal ends are common. Joint hyperextensibility may decrease somewhat with advancing age. High-arched palate, "pigeon breast," and spondylolisthesis may be seen. Muscle hypotonia, dental abnormalities, and nocturnal leg cramps are frequent.

BLEEDING   This may occur into the skin and joints as described above. Severe gastrointestinal or respiratory tract bleeding occasionally occurs. The gums may bleed with minor trauma (e.g., brushing of the teeth), and bleeding may complicate tooth extraction or tonsillectomy. Weakness of vessel walls or abnormal interactions of platelets with collagen apparently underlies the hemorrhagic diathesis; consistent abnormalities in clotting factors have not been described.

EYES   Blue scleras are common. Epicanthal folds are frequent in younger patients. In older patients the eyes may appear widely spaced.

CARDIOVASCULAR SYSTEM   Mitral valve prolapse occurs in this and other forms of EDS, especially types II and III. Right bundle branch block or other conduction abnormalities are found in some patients with EDS. Aortic valve regurgitation and dissecting aneurysm of the aorta are rare complications.

Congenital cardiac anomalies have also been reported, but their prevalence may not be higher in EDS than in the general population. Vascular complications such as spontaneous rupture of the large arteries and rupture of intracranial aneurysms leading to cerebral vascular accidents are rare and are more likely to be seen in EDS IV. Because the arteries may be friable, cerebral angiography and other diagnostic arterial invasions should be performed cautiously.

OTHER MANIFESTATIONS   Generalized tissue fragility makes surgery and subsequent wound healing difficult and may lead to spontaneous rupture of the bowel or to pneumothorax. Premature birth due to early rupture of the fetal membranes is common. Diaphragmatic and other hernias and gastrointestinal tract diverticula occur with increased frequency.

Inheritance   EDS I is inherited as an autosomal dominant and may itself be genetically heterogeneous.

Pathogenesis   The basic defect in EDS I is unknown. Dermal collagen bundles often appear fragmented, and collagen fibrils are abnormal on electron microscopy. The abnormalities are presumed to involve type I collagen.

EDS II, MITIS TYPE   Clinical manifestations are similar to those of EDS I but are less severe. Hence EDS II is also termed "mitis" type. Skin and joint changes are mild, and hyperextensibility may be limited to joints of the hands and feet. Tissue friability is not a problem, and internal manifestations are uncommon with the exception of mitral valve prolapse. As in EDS I, this form of EDS is inherited as an autosomal dominant and may be genetically heterogeneous. Ultrastructural studies suggest an abnormality in type I collagen.

EDS III, BENIGN HYPERMOBILE TYPE   The striking features are generalized joint hypermobility with joint dislocations and effusions and eventual degenerative arthritis. Cutaneous manifestations are minimal. Mitral valve prolapse may occur. EDS III is transmitted as an autosomal dominant.

EDS IV, ECCHYMOTIC OR ARTERIAL TYPE   In this rare form of EDS, the skin is fragile, thin, and translucent, allowing easy visualization of subcutaneous veins. In contrast to other types of the EDS, the skin is not hyperextensible and may even be tight. Severe bruising occurs easily. Joint hypermobility is usually found only in the digits. Severe complications which may lead to premature death are rupture of hollow viscera or of

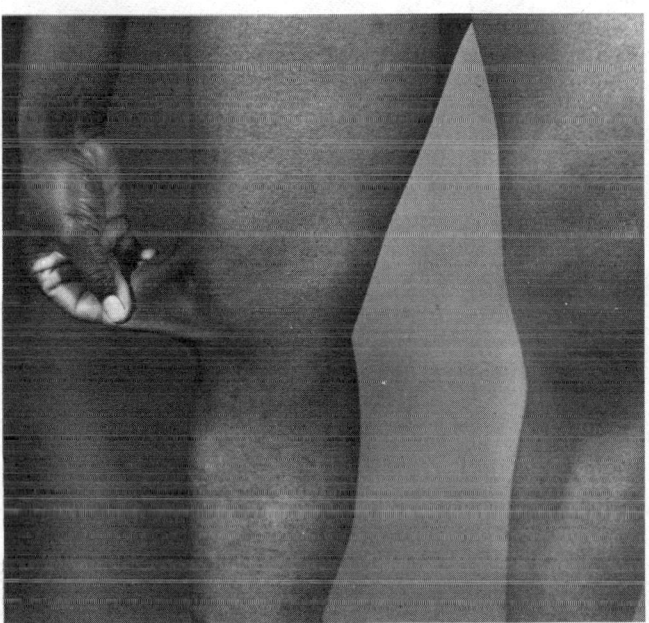

FIGURE 103-1

Hyperextensible skin in a patient with an unclassified form of Ehlers Danlos syndrome.

large arteries. This form of EDS is genetically heterogeneous, and families with autosomal dominant or recessive inheritance have been described. The recessive varieties are more severe and are associated with a decrease in life expectancy. The life expectancy in the dominant variety is only slightly reduced. Normal blood vessels are especially rich in type III collagen, and the tissue content of this type of collagen is decreased in many, if not all, varieties of EDS IV. The precise biochemical defects are unknown.

EDS V, X-LINKED TYPE The most striking feature is hyperextensible skin with moderate fragility, thin scars, and bruising. Joint hypermobility is mild. These features are similar to those of EDS II, and EDS V is distinguished more by its pattern of inheritance (X-linked recessive) than by its clinical manifestations. In some patients with apparently X-linked recessive EDS, short stature, and severe joint hypermobility occur. Such patients may have deficient activity of lysyl oxidase, an enzyme necessary for normal formation of interchain cross-links in collagen (see EDS VI). Deficiency of this enzyme activity is also found in the X-linked recessive form of cutis laxa.

EDS VI, OCULAR TYPE Hyperextensible skin and joints with the ensuing complications are present, but the distinctive features of this type of EDS are the ocular manifestations, severe scoliosis, and mild to moderate arachnodactyly. The cornea may be abnormal in size or shape and, like the sclera, is fragile and prone to rupture from even mild trauma. Glaucoma and retinal detachment also occur.

The primary abnormality in this autosomal recessive disorder is deficient activity of lysyl hydroxylase. The tensile strength of collagen fibrils in tissues depends upon the formation of interchain cross-links, which in large part result from interactions involving lysyl- or hydroxylysyl-derived aldehydes. With deficient lysyl hydroxylase activity, the hydroxylysine residue content of collagen is markedly decreased, hydroxylysine interchain cross-links are diminished, tensile strength is decreased, and the clinical manifestations ensue.

EDS VII, ARTHROCHALASIS MULTIPLEX CONGENITA This rare form of EDS is inherited as an autosomal recessive and is characterized by short stature and marked joint hypermobility with only mild skin hyperextensibility. The primary defect is deficient activity of a protease involved in the formation of collagen from its precursor, procollagen.

DIFFERENTIAL DIAGNOSIS Congenital joint hypermobility occurs as an isolated finding, sometimes in more than one relative, and is probably a distinct entity from the EDS. Loose-jointedness also occurs in the Marfan and Noonan syndromes and in osteogenesis imperfecta. In cutis laxa the skin is not only hyperextensible, but it is also lax, i.e., it has decreased elasticity and may hang in loose folds. Late in the course of EDS the skin in localized areas may resemble that seen in cutis laxa.

TREATMENT AND PROGNOSIS No specific therapy is known. Trauma to skin and joints should be avoided. In moderate and severe forms of the EDS, surgery should be undertaken with caution because of the fragility of skin, arteries, and internal organs. Wound dehiscence is frequent, and sutures should be left in place longer than usual.

Pregnancy may be accompanied by increased bruisability and exacerbation of joint manifestations and carries increased risk for development of abdominal herniae; leg and vulva varicosities; complications of episiotomy and cesarean section; and, in type I EDS, for premature delivery.

Death from arterial rupture is relatively frequent in patients with the severe variety of EDS IV. In other types of EDS death may occasionally occur from internal complications, but the prognosis for normal life expectancy is good. Some patients experience considerable morbidity from cutaneous and joint abnormalities.

MARFAN SYNDROME

The Marfan syndrome is an inherited, generalized disorder of connective tissue with ocular, skeletal, and cardiovascular manifestations. There is wide variability in clinical expression, and some patients have findings in only one or two systems. The prevalence of the disorder has been estimated to be more than 1 in 50,000, perhaps 1 in 10,000 persons.

Clinical manifestations These result from abnormalities in the supporting tissues of the ocular, cardiovascular, and skeletal systems. Although the diagnosis may be apparent during infancy, ordinarily it is not made until the second decade or later.

EYES Weakness and redundancy of the supporting tissues of the lens is the cause of the most characteristic finding in the Marfan syndrome, bilateral subluxation, or dislocation of the lens (ectopia lentis). This occurs in about 80 percent of patients, and its presence may be signaled by tremor of the iris (iridodenesis). The lens dislocation is most frequently upward. Complications of subluxated lens include uveitis, glaucoma, and cataracts. Minor dislocation is frequent and can be excluded only by careful slit-lamp examination. High-grade myopia is also common. Spontaneous retinal detachment may occur, and some patients have blue sclerae.

CARDIOVASCULAR SYSTEM About 90 percent of patients have cardiovascular abnormalities, some of which may be evident only with sensitive diagnostic modalities such as echocardiography. Weakness in the media of the aorta causes the most life-threatening abnormality in the Marfan syndrome, progressive dilatation, and dissecting aneurysm of the proximal portion of the ascending aorta. Clinical manifestations such as diastolic murmur or roentgenographic evidence of aortic dilatation may be detected in infancy or as late as in the fifth or sixth decades. The predilection for involvement of the ascending aorta is not surprising in view of the hemodynamic stresses that occur there.

Although *severe* mitral valve regurgitation is less common than *severe* aortic valve disease, echocardiographic studies in most patients reveal some abnormality of the mitral valve, including mitral valve prolapse (the "click murmur" syndrome, Chap. 242). Echocardiography may also be useful in following patients with aortic root and valve abnormalities. Bacterial endocarditis may involve heart valves with only minor antecedent alterations. Coarctation of the aorta and abnormalities in the conduction system are also found in the Marfan syndrome.

SKELETAL SYSTEM Increased length of the tubular bones is the most conspicuous external feature of the disease (Fig. 102-2). The extremities are long and thin (dolichostenomelia); almost all patients are tall, either absolutely or relatively when their heights are assessed against the background of their families.

Abnormal body proportions are even more specific. The distance from the top of the pubic symphysis to the sole of the foot ("lower segment") is increased in patients with the Marfan syndrome, causing a low ratio of the upper segment (pubic symphysis to crown) to the lower segment of the body. In normal postpubertal whites this ratio is 0.92 ± 0.04, and in normal blacks it is 0.85 ± 0.03. A significant decrease in these values is helpful in establishing the diagnosis of the Marfan syndrome. The arm span may be greater than the height.

Excessively long finger bones (arachnodactyly, "spider fingers") are found in most patients with the Marfan syndrome. When this is subtle, roentgenograms of the hands with calculation of the "metacarpal index" may be helpful. The length of each of the last four metacarpal bones is divided by the width at its midpoint, and the values are averaged. In patients with the Marfan syndrome the index is often greater than 8.4; in normal individuals it is usually less than 8. Sternal displacement upward causes "pigeon breast" (pectus carinatum), and sternal displacement inward causes pectus excavatum. The palate is often high and arched, and the facies, long and narrow.

Weakness and redundancy of the ligaments and other supporting tissues of the joints lead to loose- or "double-jointedness," flatfeet, backward curvature of the knees (genu recurvatum), kyphoscoliosis, and recurrent dislocations, especially of the hip and patella. Inguinal or femoral hernias are frequent.

OTHER MANIFESTATIONS Many patients have sparse subcutaneous fat and muscle hypotonia. Striae may be present, especially in the skin of the pectoral, deltoid, and thigh areas. Lung cysts with spontaneous pneumothorax occasionally occur.

Inheritance The Marfan syndrome is inherited as an autosomal dominant. There is wide variability in clinical expression

FIGURE 103-2

A 16-year-old boy with the Marfan syndrome. Manifestations include dislocated lens, long, thin face, long fingers (arachnodactyly) and extremities (dolichostenomelia), and inward displacement of the sternum (pectus excavatum). (Courtesy of JG Hall.)

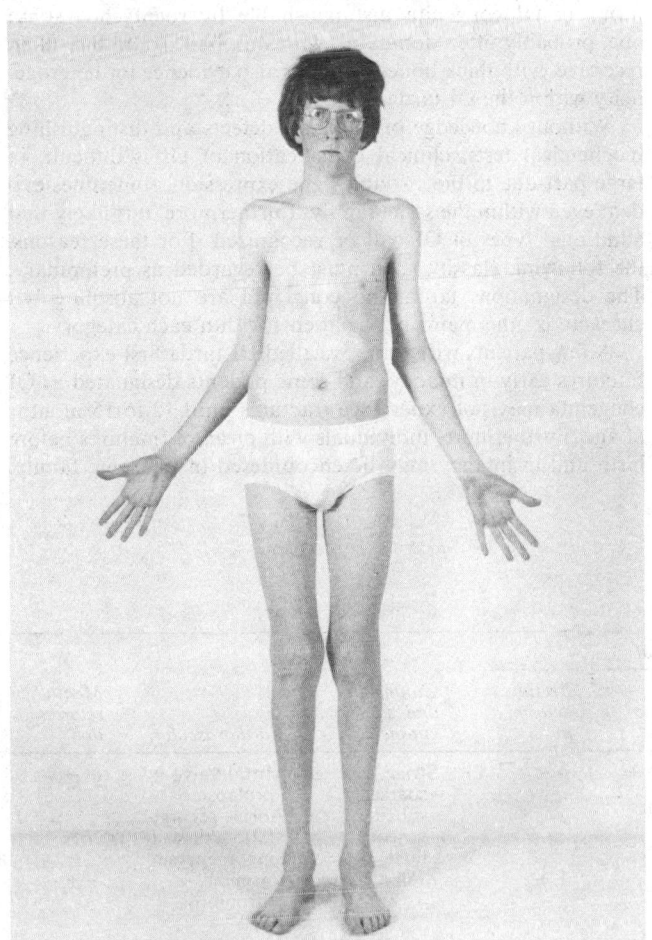

("variable expressivity"), and an affected relative may have only mild manifestations confined to one system (e.g., dislocated lens detected only by slit-lamp examination). Rarely, an individual genetically proved to possess the Marfan gene (e.g., a person with an affected parent and offspring) does not have any detectable expression (lack of "penetrance"). Perhaps 15 percent of cases are sporadic and presumably the result of a fresh mutation in a parental germ cell. Fathers of sporadic cases are, on average, 7 years older than fathers of patients who have inherited the disease from an affected parent. Elevated paternal age is considered a factor in the occurrence of fresh mutations.

Pathology and pathogenesis The basic biochemical abnormality is unknown. Defective collagen cross-linking is possible, but unproved. The early aortic changes are those of cystic medial necrosis (Chap. 252). Later findings are loss of elastic fibers and scarring with irregular whorls of smooth muscle. No histological changes or electron microscopic abnormalities in collagen have been reported in ligaments or tendons.

Differential diagnosis Because the disorder displays wide variability in clinical expression and because there is no specific test for the Marfan syndrome, the diagnosis may be difficult to establish in patients without the classical triad of dislocated lens, aortic dilatation or aneurysm, and excessive length of tubular bones. In such cases careful examination of close relatives and exclusion of disorders resembling the Marfan syndrome can be helpful. It may be impossible to establish the diagnosis definitively in a patient with skeletal or cardiac abnormalities who does not have a dislocated lens or a clearly affected relative.

The homocystinurias, inborn errors of methionine metabolism with secondary effects on connective tissue (Chap. 88), are the principal diseases to be distinguished from the Marfan syndrome. The disorders have dislocated lens and skeletal deformities in common but differ in other clinical manifestations and in their pattern of inheritance (Table 103-1). As its name implies, there is a specific laboratory test for homocystinuria.

A "marfanoid hypermobility" syndrome is characterized by hyperextensible joints and skin changes similar to those seen in Ehlers-Danlos syndrome as well as by arachnodactyly, pectus deformity, and regurgitation of the aortic and mitral valves.

Congenital contractural arachnodactyly, an autosomal dominant disorder associated with severe kyphoscoliosis, generalized osteopenia, and arachnodactyly, is distinguished from the Marfan syndrome by the presence of congenital contractures of the fingers and abnormally shaped ears. It has been suggested that congenital contractural arachnodactyly and the marfanoid hypermobility disorder are forms of, and reflect genetic heterogeneity of, the Marfan syndrome and that the more typical cases of the Marfan syndrome can be subdivided into at least two types: asthenic, mainly in children, and nonasthenic.

Dislocation of the lens is a feature of another genetic disorder of connective tissue, the Weill-Marchesani syndrome, but the skeletal abnormalities in this autosomal recessive disorder are short stature and stiffness of joints.

Treatment and prognosis Estrogen therapy may reduce adult height in girls who are already tall in the prepubertal period and may also partially prevent severe kyphoscoliosis. The potential benefits of estrogens must be weighed against their possible complications, including the psychological and physical effects of inducing precocious puberty. Prophylactic administration of drugs like propranolol which decrease myocardial contractility and diminish the stress on the aorta have thus far not been documented to be beneficial in patients with early aortic changes. The risks of surgery for aortic or valvular disease are high, primarily because the abnormal connective tissue may not hold sutures well. However, therapy is often successful.

The major threats to life, severe cardiovascular complications, may occur anytime from infancy to the seventh decade. These complications include dilatation, dissection, or rupture of the aorta, and severe regurgitation of the aortic or mitral valve. In one series, the mean age at death was 43 for men and 46 for women. Pregnancy may be particularly hazardous for women with aortic disease.

Patients with the Marfan syndrome may be disabled by profound kyphoscoliosis; recurrent joint dislocations; recurrent pneumothorax; or serious visual impairment from myopia, retinal detachment, or the uveitis and glaucoma that result from subluxation of the lens.

OSTEOGENESIS IMPERFECTA

Osteogenesis imperfecta (OI; fragilitas ossium, maladie de Lobstein) is a group of heritable, generalized disorders of connective tissue with clinical manifestations in the skeleton, ear, joints and ligaments, teeth, sclera, and skin. The basic defect is unknown but presumably involves an abnormality in collagen. The frequency of OI has been estimated at more than 1 in every 20,000 births.

Clinical manifestations The cardinal features are blue sclerae, multiple fractures, loose-jointedness, and deafness; clinical expression is variable.

SKELETON Narrow bones with osteoporosis, thin cortices, and excessive fragility underlie the multiple fractures and skeletal deformities characteristic of the common types of OI. The fractures occur with minor trauma and frequently involve the long bones of the legs. Callus formed with healing may be large and on occasion may be mistaken for osteogenic sarcoma. In severe cases multiple fractures in utero allow antenatal diagnosis. Generally, susceptibility to fractures decreases after puberty, but may return later, especially with inactivity, pregnancy, or menopause. The extremities are often short, and associated deformities include saber shins, marked bowing of the legs, and pseudoarthroses. There is often lateral bulging of the calvarium with a characteristic triangular shape of the face. Chest deformities such as sternal displacement inward (pectus excavatum) or outward ("pigeon breast," pectus carinatum) are

frequent. Frequently, dome forehead and overhanging occiput are seen. Roentgenograms of the bones may show osteoporosis, basilar impression of the skull (platybasia), "codfish" or "hourglass" vertebrae, and wormian bones in the skull. This last finding may help establish the diagnosis.

EYES The scleras appear translucent, thin, and usually blue, owing to partial visualization of the underlying choroid. This is the most frequent manifestation of OI.

EARS Progressive hearing impairment from otosclerosis may begin in childhood, but deafness usually does not develop until adulthood. The tympanic membranes may appear blue.

JOINTS Abnormalities in the ligaments and tendons lead to loose-jointedness, which causes in turn the increased frequency of kyphoscoliosis, flatfeet, and recurrent joint dislocations. Tendons may rupture from minor stress.

TEETH Hypoplasia of dentine and pulp causes the characteristically small, misshapen, blue-yellow teeth (dentinogenesis imperfecta).

OTHER MANIFESTATIONS The skin tends to be thin, translucent, and easily bruised. Hernias occur frequently. Cardiovascular disorders, including mitral valve prolapse or aortic regurgitation, may occur.

Inheritance As in the other heritable disorders of connective tissue, clinical and genetic heterogeneity occurs in OI. The subdivision of OI on clinical grounds into congenita (features present at birth) and tarda (onset of fractures afterward) may also have genetic validity. Almost all cases of OI tarda are transmitted as autosomal dominants, but there appear to be two forms of OI congenita distinguishable by roentgenography: one, probably often dominant, with thin bones, and the other, recessive, with thick bones. There is also evidence for heterogeneity within the OI tarda patients.

Without knowledge of the basic defects and distinguishing biochemical tests, clinical classification of OI is difficult, in large part due to the variable gene expression, sometimes evident even within the same family. Furthermore, it is likely that additional types of OI will be recognized. For these reasons, the following classification must be regarded as preliminary. The designations tarda and congenita are not absolute but characterize the majority of patients within each category.

A few patients with what is called OI tarda first experience fractures early in infancy, and some patients designated as OI congenita may not experience fractures until 12 to 15 months of age. Furthermore, individuals with onset of fractures before birth and in infancy may be encountered in the same family.

TABLE 103-1
Comparison of the Marfan syndrome with homocystinuria

Disorder	Mode of inheritance	Basic biochemical defect	Clinical manifestations			Cutaneous and subcutaneous	Cardiovascular	Mental retardation
			Ectopia lentis	Skeletal				
				Arachno-dactyly	Pectus deformities			
Marfan syndrome	Autosomal dominant	Unknown	+++ (usually upward)	++++	+++	Striae; sparse subcutaneous fat	Mitral valve prolapse Aorta: regurgitation/dissecting aneurysm	--
Homocystinuria	Autosomal recessive	Usually decreased cystathionine synthase activity	++++ (usually downward)	++	++	Malar flush	Vascular thrombosis	++

OI TARDA This, the most common variety of OI, is characterized by osteoporosis, frequent fractures, dental abnormalities, blue sclerae, and deafness. Fractures, rare at birth, usually occur by age 3. The course is variable, but skeletal deformities are usually mild. Inheritance is autosomal dominant. There may be two distinct subtypes, one with and the other without dental abnormalities. There may also be a rarer, distinct disorder inherited as an autosomal dominant but without blue sclerae (and perhaps also without deafness). Occasionally, families are encountered in which OI tarda is apparently inherited as an autosomal recessive.

OI CONGENITA I (THIN BONE TYPE) This is a severe disease characterized by osteoporosis, fractures, progressive skeletal deformities with shortness of stature, and thin bones on roentgenograms. The majority of affected infants have fractures at or before birth. The scleras are blue in infancy, but, as in normal children, frequently become white. Deafness may not be an important feature. Live-born infants often survive but may be disabled by multiple fractures and bone deformities, or by complications of intracranial hemorrhage in the perinatal period. The pattern of inheritance is not well defined. Almost all cases occur sporadically. Some patients, however, have an autosomal recessive disease, others an autosomal dominant. The latter presumably result from a fresh mutation in a parental gamete.

OI CONGENITA II (THICK BONE TYPE) This very severe disease is generally lethal in infancy. The bones appear thick and crumpled on roentgenograms. Inheritance is autosomal recessive.

Pathology and pathogenesis The bone cortices and trabeculae are usually thin. Osteoid is diminished and replaced by basophilic, periodic acid-Schiff-staining material. In other tissues mature collagen is not seen. Biochemical studies suggest that the defects in OI involve aberrations in collagen, but the basic abnormalities are unknown.

Differential diagnosis The correct diagnosis is obvious in patients with the classical triad of blue scleras, pathologic fractures, and deafness. However, only 60 percent of affected subjects have clinical bone disease, and some patients manifest only blue scleras or otosclerosis. According to one survey, 60 percent of adult patients with blue scleras have multiple fractures, 60 percent have otosclerosis, and 44 percent have all three manifestations. It is likely that this variability reflects the fact that there are several distinct OI syndromes, i.e., genetic and clinical heterogeneity. However, variability in clinical manifestations can sometimes occur among relatives in the same family.

Without a clear family history, it may be difficult to distinguish OI early in its course from "idiopathic" osteoporosis. The same is true after the menopause in women with OI who have experienced few fractures earlier in life. When the legs are short and the head appears large, OI may resemble achondroplasia. OI congenita must also be distinguished from hypophosphatasia.

Treatment and prognosis No specific therapy is known. Careful orthopedic management is necessary, and immobilization should be avoided. Infants with severe OI congenita are often born dead or die in infancy. OI tarda is a more benign disease, but disability may occur from multiple fractures, skeletal deformities, or deafness. Nonetheless, many patients adjust to their disease and lead normal lives. The frequency of fractures generally decreases after puberty but may again increase later in life. Deafness is present in about 35 percent of patients in the fourth decade and in about 50 percent in the sixth decade.

PSEUDOXANTHOMA ELASTICUM

Pseudoxanthoma elasticum (PXE; Groenblad-Strandberg syndrome) is a genetically determined disorder with protean clinical manifestations most frequently involving the skin, eyes, and arteries. The basic pathogenetic abnormality is unknown but probably involves elastic fibers. Clinical changes usually first appear in the second or third decade and thereafter are progressive. The prevalence of PXE has been estimated at between 1 in 200,000 and 1 in 50,000 adults.

Clinical manifestations SKIN PXE derives its name from the characteristic yellow xanthoma-like papular and reticulated skin lesions. Skin changes are usually evident in the second or third decade and in later life are found in virtually all.

The changes are most notable in the neck and axillae, and the antecubital fossae, periumbilical area, groin, and penis may also be involved. The abnormalities range from a few yellow papules confined to one or two areas (usually the neck, axilla, or both) to confluent yellow papules and plaques that cause redundant folds of lax skin over flexural surfaces. The skin around the mouth, chin, and nasolabial folds may be thickened as well as lax.

The extent of changes detected histologically correlates with the severity of clinical cutaneous lesions, but occasionally changes of PXE may be seen in a biopsy from a patient without obvious clinical alterations.

EYES Angioid streaks are first noted during the second or third decade and found thereafter in all but a very few patients. The streaks are bilateral. They lie beneath the retinal vessels, are flat, are usually three to five times the diameter of retinal veins, and are red, brown, or gray. Angioid streaks are most numerous around the optic disks from which they appear to emanate. Later changes include hemorrhage and chorioretinal scarring; when these alterations are marked, the streaks may be obscured. Visual impairment may result in near blindness.

VASCULAR SYSTEM Most patients with PXE have some combination of peripheral, cardiac, or cerebrovascular abnormalities. Involvement of peripheral arteries results in weak or absent pulses and often in calcification. Easy fatigability of the limbs and intermittent claudication are common. Some patients develop early-onset hypertension or coronary artery disease that usually presents as angina or an altered ECG. Cerebrovascular symptoms are less frequent and may be rare in the absence of hypertension. Hypothyroidism, perhaps from altered thyroid vasculature may occur.

Upper gastrointestinal tract bleeding is frequent, often severe, and occasionally the presenting manifestation. The hemorrhage is probably from arterial disease in the gastrointestinal tract. Sometimes peptic ulcer or hiatus hernia is present, but in many the source of the bleeding is not detected. Uterine bleeding may be severe. Hemorrhage may also occur in the urinary and upper respiratory tracts.

Inheritance PXE is a genetically heterogeneous disorder. In most families it is autosomal recessive, but autosomal dominant inheritance also occurs. There may be at least two varieties of autosomal dominant PXE. Type I is characterized by classic orange-peel-like skin changes, severe vascular manifestations, and choroiditis. Patients with the more frequent type II have a much milder disease. The skin is hyperextensible, and the rash is macular (or focal). Other manifestations such as high-arched palate, blue sclerae, and loose-jointedness may also occur in patients with type II.

Pathology and pathogenesis The basic defect in PXE is unknown, but probably involves, either primarily or secondarily, elastic fibers in the skin, media of arteries, and elsewhere. Angioid streaks in the eyes represent breaks in the Bruch membrane behind the retina. Early skin changes are small patchy areas of swollen, fragmented, and irregularly clumped basophilic elastic fibers in the middermis.

These altered areas have affinity for calcium, and von Kossa staining (for calcium) may be valuable in confirming subtle lesions. Later in the disease all the elastic fibers of the mid and lower dermis are affected. Studies with the electron microscope indicate that the principal alterations are in the elastin moiety of the elastic fibers.

Differential diagnosis Virtually all patients with PXE have characteristic cutaneous changes, and the diagnosis can be confirmed with a skin biopsy. Actinic (or "senile") elastosis may cause confusion in some patients; however, the changes are limited to exposed sites, and the disorder is histologically distinguishable from PXE. Angioid streaks are present in the great majority of patients with PXE, and while their presence is very suggestive of the diagnosis, they are also found in other disorders, including sickle-cell anemia and Paget's disease.

Treatment and prognosis No specific treatment for PXE is known. Skin changes may be a cosmetic problem. Most patients with PXE have some visual impairment, but complete blindness is rare. Early death may occur from hemorrhage, cardiac disease, or cerebrovascular accidents, but some patients have a normal life span.

REFERENCES

BORNSTEIN P, BYERS PH: Disorders of collagen, in *Duncan's Diseases of Metabolism*, 8th ed, P Bondy et al (eds). Philadelphia, Saunders, 1979 (in press)

McKUSICK VA: *Heritable Disorders of Connective Tissue*, 4th ed. St Louis, Mosby, 1972

VITTO J, LICHTENSTEIN JR: Defects in the biochemistry of collagen in diseases of connective tissue. J Invest Dermatol 66:59, 1976

104
OTHER DISORDERS INVOLVING MULTIPLE ORGAN SYSTEMS

PHILIP J. FIALKOW

The pathophysiology of many clinically important genetic diseases is unknown. Most of these disorders are described under the principal organ systems affected. Some others involving multiple organ systems are discussed here.

NOONAN SYNDROME

The Noonan syndrome shows wide phenotypic variability and comprises multiple congenital anomalies of the skin, skeleton, heart, and gonads. Many patients have short stature and intellectual impairment. The prevalence, clinical spectrum, natural history, pathogenesis, and mode of inheritance are poorly delineated. The syndrome probably comprises several distinct

but, as yet, undefined disorders. Furthermore, only within the last 10 to 15 years has it been appreciated that the Noonan syndrome is separable from the Turner syndrome (gonadal dysgenesis), which is due to a partial or complete absence of one sex chromosome. It is likely that most patients previously described as Ullrich, male Turner or female pseudo-Turner syndromes and as Turner, Ullrich, or Bonnevie-Ullrich phenotype with normal chromosomes fall within the spectrum of the Noonan syndrome.

CLINICAL MANIFESTATIONS Since few family studies have been performed, the spectrum and prevalence of individual abnormalities given here cannot be regarded as definitive.

Facies Patients with the Noonan syndrome have a characteristic appearance, including a narrow maxilla and small mandible with triangular-shaped mouth, epicanthic eye folds, hypertelorism, ptosis, downward ("antimongoloid") slant of the eyes, and ears that are prominent, fleshy, low-set and posteriorly rotated (Fig. 104-1). Webbing of the neck and a low posterior hairline are found in about half of patients.

Skin Multiple pigmented nevi and dystrophic nails are frequent. Patients may have congenital lymphangiectatic edema of the hands and feet lasting until age 6 to 9 months or, in some patients, into adulthood. Keloid formation is frequent. The skin may be hyperelastic. Dermatoglyphic patterns may be abnormal but are nonspecific.

Skeletal system Most patients are short. Others have normal stature but are not as tall as would be expected for their genetic background. Skeletal abnormalities are common and include high-arched palate, dental malocclusion, increased car-

FIGURE 104-1
A 14-year-old boy with the Noonan syndrome. Manifestations include downward ("antimongoloid") slant of the eyes, epicanthic eye folds, midface hypoplasia, prominent ears, broad neck, and upturned nose. (Courtesy of JG Hall.)

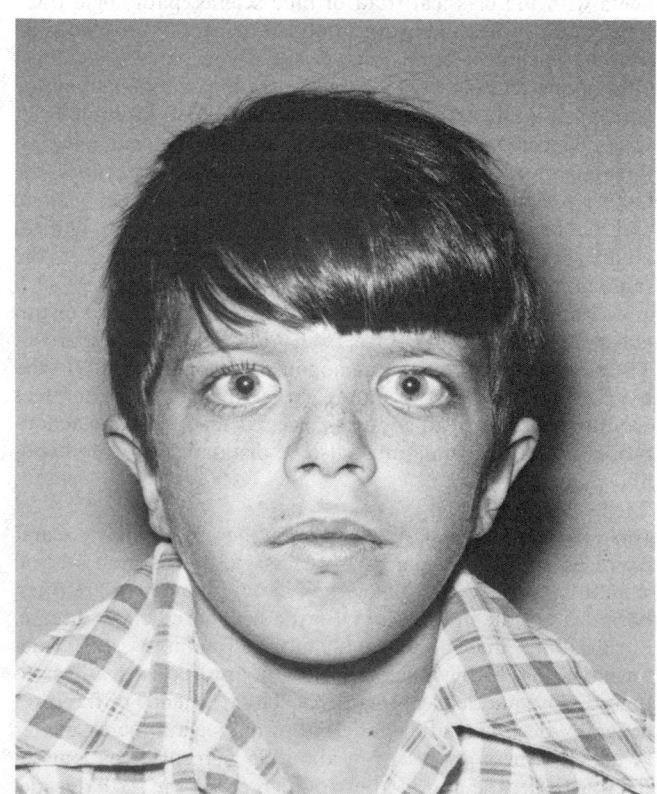

rying angle of the arms (cubitus valgus), shield-shaped chest with wide-spaced nipples, pectus deformities, and kyphoscoliosis. Anomalies of the sternum, vertebrae, limbs, or skull may be seen radiographically. Often the pectus deformity is distinctive in that the upper portion of the sternum is displaced outward and the lower portion is displaced inward; that is, pectus carinatum and excavatum are both present in the same patient. The joints may be hyperextensible.

Intellectual development   Intelligence ranges from superior to profoundly retarded, but most have mild or borderline mental retardation, as compared with nonaffected family members. From 25 to 50 percent of patients have normal intelligence.

Heart   The true prevalence of congenital heart disease is unknown, but may be between 30 and 50 percent. The most frequent finding is valvular pulmonic stenosis, alone or in combination with septal defects (especially atrial), asymmetric septal hypertrophy, or pulmonary artery branch stenosis. The last three abnormalities are less frequent in the absence of valvular pulmonic stenosis. In contrast to the Turner syndrome coarctation of the aorta is rare.

Sexual development   Penile size may be normal or decreased; more than half of the males have cryptorchidism. Fertility is rare in men with the Noonan syndrome. In contrast, most affected females apparently are fertile.

Other manifestations   Hydronephrosis with pyeloureteral obstruction and other renal anomalies occur, but the prevalence is unknown. Other abnormalities include thyroiditis, hypothyroidism, and hepatosplenomegaly in the absence of cardiac failure.

INHERITANCE   Clinical and genetic heterogeneity clearly occurs. There are likely to be several "cardiofacial" syndromes which have in common unusual facies and congenital cardiac abnormalities. Among these is the typical Noonan syndrome.

No chromosomal abnormality has been found in patients with the Noonan syndrome. Autosomal dominant inheritance, described in some families, may be the mode of transmission for most patients. The relatively high proportion of sporadic cases (theoretically representing new mutations) would not be unusual for an autosomal dominant disorder often accompanied by infertility. In some families "unaffected" relatives have mild signs of the disorder.

Genetic counseling should include a discussion not only of disease recurrence risks but also of the wide range of clinical expression, especially as it pertains to cardiac anomalies, intelligence, stature, and fertility. Until the presumed heterogeneity is better defined, prognosis and recurrence risks are difficult to estimate and should be based largely on individual findings in the patient and family. The risk of severe disease in a patient's sibling or child is higher if the patient is severely affected.

DIFFERENTIAL DIAGNOSIS   Noonan syndrome must be distinguished from the Turner syndrome (gonadal dysgenesis) (Chap. 344). Shortness of stature and anomalies of the skeleton, skin, and integument are common in both disorders. Although the characteristic facies is seen to some extent in every Noonan patient, it alone may not be distinctive enough to exclude the Turner syndrome. Clinical features that help identify the Turner syndrome include normal intelligence, infertility, and negative family history for other affected individuals. Pulmonic stenosis is common in the Noonan but infrequent in the Turner syndrome, whereas the reverse is true for coarctation of the aorta. Finally, chromosome studies will usually allow the definitive diagnosis of the Turner syndrome.

The Aarskog syndrome (faciogenital dysplasia) is also associated with shortness of stature and facial anomalies but is further characterized by its X-linked recessive pattern of inheritance and by the fact that the scrotum overhangs the penis ("saddle-bag scrotum"). The fetal alcohol, fetal hydantoin, and Williams syndromes, all characterized by growth retardation, mild to moderate mental retardation and craniofacial abnormalities, must also be distinguished from the Noonan syndrome. In Noonan patients with hyperelastic skin and loose-jointedness, an erroneous diagnosis of Ehlers-Danlos syndrome may be made.

TREATMENT AND PROGNOSIS   Therapy is directed toward correcting debilitating and life-threatening anomalies. Decisions to operate on patients for ptosis and webbing of the neck must be tempered by the reports of increased predilection to keloid formation. Surgical correction of valvular pulmonic stenosis should be performed when indicated, but results may be unsatisfactory because both the valve and contiguous tissue may be dysplastic. Orchiopexy for undescended testes should be attempted but is frequently unsuccessful. Although poorly defined, the life span in the Noonan syndrome, excluding cardiovascular problems and a possible increased frequency of neoplasia, is probably normal.

LAURENCE-MOON-BIEDL SYNDROME

The Laurence-Moon-Biedl (LMB) syndrome (Laurence-Moon-Biedl-Bardet syndrome, Bardet-Biedl syndrome, Biedl-Bardet syndrome) is a heritable disorder characterized by obesity, mental retardation, digital anomalies, hypogonadism, and retinal degeneration with pigmentary changes. The basic defect and the prevalence of the LMB syndrome are unknown. Over 400 cases have been recorded.

CLINICAL MANIFESTATIONS   Obesity   Usually truncal in location, obesity is present in at least 80 percent of patients with the LMB syndrome. It begins in childhood and increases in severity with advancing age.

Eyes   Retinal degeneration occurs in over 90 percent, leading either to typical or atypical retinitis pigmentosa. The electroretinogram may be abnormal before clinical changes are evident. The earliest symptom often is night-blindness. Decreased visual acuity may be discovered at school age and is progressive, culminating in total blindness by age 30. Optic atrophy and congenital tapetoretinal blindness also occur in patients with the LMB syndrome.

Gonads   Hypogonadism is present in at least 75 percent of males and 50 percent of females. In many instances gonadotropin levels are low, but primary gonadal failure also occurs.

Digits   Anomalies are noted in about 80 percent. The most frequent finding is postaxial polydactyly in one or more extremities, but some have only syndactyly or brachydactyly.

Mental retardation   Mild to moderate intellectual impairment is the usual finding. About a tenth of patients have severe retardation and another tenth have normal intelligence.

Kidney   Kidney abnormalities ranging from mesangial tissue proliferation to glomerular sclerosis, interstitial scarring, and cyst formation with death from uremia may occur.

Other manifestations Congenital heart defects may occur. Brachycephaly or other skull anomalies have been described. In contrast to the Alstrom syndrome, diabetes mellitus and nerve deafness are infrequent in the LMB syndrome.

INHERITANCE The LMB syndrome is transmitted as an autosomal recessive disorder. There may be genetic heterogeneity.

DIFFERENTIAL DIAGNOSIS Since there is no specific test for the LMB syndrome, the diagnosis must be established clinically. This can be done with little difficulty in the presence of the five cardinal manifestations (obesity, mental retardation, polydactyly, retinal degeneration, and hypogonadism). However, the limits of the syndrome are poorly defined, and the diagnosis is often extended to patients with only some of these components. Variability in clinical expression occurs even among patients within the same family.

The patients originally described by Laurence and Moon had mental retardation, pigmentary retinal degeneration, hypogenitalism, and spastic paraplegia without obesity or digital anomalies. This is undoubtedly a different disorder from what is now usually called the LMB syndrome. (Thus, in a strict sense the LMB syndrome should be called the Bardet-Biedl syndrome.)

The LMB syndrome must be distinguished from syndromes bearing the eponyms Alstrom, Biemond, and Carpenter. Comparison with the Alstrom syndrome is discussed in the following section. The LMB, Biemond, and Carpenter syndromes are all characterized by hypogonadism, polydactyly, mental retardation, and autosomal recessive inheritance, but only LMB has been associated with retinal degeneration. The Biemond syndrome is distinguished by the presence of iris coloboma, and the Carpenter syndrome is characterized by acrocephalosyndactyly and peculiar facies.

ALSTROM SYNDROME

The Alstrom syndrome is a rare inherited disease with major involvement of the retina, ear, kidney, and endocrine glands. In childhood, the typical patient has obesity, moderately severe nerve deafness, and retinal degeneration with later pigmentary changes ("atypical retinitis pigmentosa") and blindness. In adulthood, carbohydrate intolerance and slowly progressive renal disease develop; obesity may disappear. Males often have an unusual form of primary hypogonadism in which normal secondary sex characteristics occur, despite small testes, low plasma testosterone, and elevated gonadotropin levels. Females lack evidence of hypogonadism, but menses are irregular. Other clinical manifestations include hyperuricemia, hypertriglyceridemia, acanthosis nigricans, baldness, scoliosis, and hyperostosis frontalis. Although signs and symptoms appear early in life, the correct diagnosis is usually not made until the third decade. Before that time cases may be classified as congenital blindness or deafness or the Laurence-Moon-Biedl syndrome.

Although the Alstrom and the Laurence-Moon-Biedl syndromes both have retinal degeneration, childhood obesity, and nephropathy, they can be distinguished clinically. Most noteworthy are the rarity of mental retardation and digital anomalies in the Alstrom syndrome and the rarity of nerve deafness and diabetes mellitus in the Laurence-Moon-Biedl syndrome. Furthermore, total blindness occurs in the Alstrom syndrome at about 7 years and in the Laurence-Moon-Biedl syndrome at about 30 years.

Although the Alstrom syndrome is inherited as an autosomal recessive, suggesting an abnormality in a single enzyme, the primary biochemical defect is unknown. Membrane thickening and hyalinization in the kidney, testes, and skin suggest that the basic abnormality involves an element in membranes common to these organs, the retina, neural apparatus of the ear, and perhaps, adipose tissue. Patients with the Alstrom syndrome are resistant to the action of at least three polypeptide hormones: insulin, vasopressin, and gonadotropins. This resistance may reflect membrane changes or degeneration of cells in the target organs.

REFERENCES

COLLINS E, TURNER G: The Noonan syndrome. J Pediatr 83:941, 1973
GOLDSTEIN J, FIALKOW PJ: The Alstrom syndrome. Medicine 52:53, 1973

|

|

PART FOUR

105
AN APPROACH TO INFECTIOUS DISEASES

ROBERT G. PETERSDORF

INTRODUCTION The vast majority of human and animal diseases of known etiology are produced by biologic agents: viruses, rickettsias, bacteria, mycoplasma, *Chlamydia*, fungi, protozoa, or nematodes. No small part of the past and present importance of infectious diseases in medical practice is attributable to their enormous frequency and the public health implications of their contagiousness. However, developments in sanitary engineering, vector control, immunization, and specific chemotherapy have modified the situation favorably. Although important exceptions remain, infectious diseases as a class are more easily prevented and more easily cured than any other major group of disorders. Despite the virtual elimination of certain infectious diseases such as smallpox and the profound reduction in the morbidity and mortality of many, humans are by no means free of infection. In fact, the total human load of disease produced by microbial parasites has decreased only modestly, primarily through smallpox and malaria control and better health care in developing countries. As certain specific microbial infections have been controlled, others have emerged as troublesome therapeutic and epidemiologic problems. With the introduction of cytotoxic drugs, massive irradiation in the treatment of malignant diseases, and immunosuppressive agents to control the rejection of transplanted organs, the insertion of prosthetic devices into the bloodstream, and the progressive longevity of people with chronic degenerative diseases, infections due to organisms previously considered saprophytic or commensal have increased. These infections have also been termed *opportunistic*. As Dubos has pointed out, microbial infections appear to form an inherent part of human life.

Because of better environmental sanitation and other measures that now prevent contact with many microbial agents, and the development of acquired immunity early in childhood, certain infections have been seen more frequently in adults. For example, as contact with poliomyelitis virus in childhood declined in many countries, paralytic poliomyelitis became more common in young adults. *Hemophilus influenzae* meningitis is being reported more frequently in adults than heretofore, and decreasing infection with the tubercle bacillus raises questions about the status of antituberculous immunity in adults. For reasons that are not clear, hepatitis A is predominantly a disease of young adults, while non-A, non-B hepatitis tends to occur in individuals over 35 years of age.

As antimicrobial agents reduce the mortality associated with certain common infections, other microbes emerge as important causes of human disease. If an infection occurs during or immediately following a course of chemotherapy, it is often caused by a microorganism that is resistant to the drug that was given; such an infection is termed a *superinfection*. While it is relatively unusual nowadays for patients to die of uncomplicated pneumococcal pneumonia, a disease readily handled with available antimicrobials, it is common to see serious disease produced by microorganisms which are much more resistant even though they are often part of the normal microbial flora in humans. These include staphylococci, gram-negative enteric bacilli, and a variety of anaerobes and fungi. One important mechanism by which resistance is conferred on gram-negative enteric bacteria is the action of R factors (Chap. 108).

THE PARASITE AND THE HOST The interaction between microorganism and humans that results in infection and disease is complex. Much has been learned about the way in which microbes enter the body, the ways in which they produce tissue injury, the influence of specific immunity and "nonspecific" resistance of the host, and the mechanisms of recovery. However, it is not yet possible to transfer in any specific way much of the information that has been acquired to the individual patient with an infection. In this and the subsequent chapter, those aspects of the host-parasite relationship that form the basis for diagnostic procedures, that are of importance in deriving therapeutic principles, or that help explain the epidemiology of infection are stressed.

INFECTION AND CLINICAL DISEASE It is well known that microorganisms of different species or different strains of the same species vary widely in their capacity to produce disease and that human beings are not equally susceptible to the disease caused by a given bacterium or virus. Furthermore, while a specific infectious disease will not occur in the absence of the causative organism, the mere presence of the organism in the body does not lead invariably to clinical illness. Indeed, the production of symptoms in humans by many parasites is the exception rather than the rule, and the *subclinical infection* or the "carrier state" is the usual host-parasite relationship. *Dis-*

ease in a clinical sense is not synonymous with the presence of the organism or *infection* in a microbiological sense. In fact, for most organisms the number of subclinical infections far exceeds that of clinical disease.

MECHANISMS OF INJURY It is customary to refer to bacteria or other microorganisms that are capable of producing disease as *pathogenic*. *Virulence,* the *degree* of pathogenicity, should be distinguished from *invasiveness,* the ability to spread and disseminate in the body. For example, *Clostridium tetani* is pathogenic and, by virtue of its exotoxin, highly virulent, but it is almost completely lacking in invasiveness. Moreover, in certain circumstances and in certain anatomic locations, mildly "pathogenic" organisms can produce fatal disease, or highly "pathogenic" species can multiply without producing any harmful effect.

A few parasites produce *toxins* that account for the tissue damage and physiological alterations of infection. *Hypersensitivity* to components of the parasite is demonstrable in several infections to account for the manifestations of disease. For many pathogenic agents, an explanation of their damaging effects upon the host is incomplete or wholly lacking. Generally, therefore, the aim of therapy is to stop multiplication or to kill the parasites with appropriate drugs; in diseases caused by toxin-producing organisms, the use of antiserum (as in tetanus or diphtheria) is the definitive procedure, and chemotherapy is of secondary importance.

The tendency of certain pathogenic organisms to *localize in certain cells or organs* and to produce disease in a specific anatomic site or evoke a combination of symptoms referable to certain organs often suggests the identity of the causative organism. For example, the pneumococcus usually causes infection in the lung but almost never in the kidney, and *H. influenzae* infections are confined almost solely to the respiratory tract and meninges. Similarly, in the presence of disease known to be caused by a given agent, complicating involvement of other tissues can be anticipated or predicted. Examples include the multiple lung abscesses which are so characteristic of hematogenously disseminated staphylococcal disease and the metastatic skin lesions which complicate *Pseudomonas* bacteremia.

Frequently, the proper management of infectious disease involves the use of techniques completely unrelated to microbiology or chemotherapy, in an effort to support the function of damaged organs. Survival in poliomyelitis may depend upon treatment of respiratory failure, the management of heart failure in endocarditis is sometimes a greater problem than the eradication of the causative organism, in cholera the repletion of the volume deficit and in Weil's disease the treatment of acute renal failure with peritoneal or hemodialysis are the important therapeutic objectives.

RESISTANCE AND SUSCEPTIBILITY Many so-called "host factors" are known to influence the likelihood that disease will occur if organisms enter the tissues, or to play a determining role in the outcome once the infection has become established. These include natural or acquired antibodies, interferon, properdin, phagocytic activity, and the level of the general inflammatory response, which is generally manifested by cellular activity such as chemotaxis, phagocytosis, and release of lysozomal enzymes.

In experimental animals, sex, microbial strain, age, route of infection, the presence of specific antibody, other diseases, nutritional state, and the use of such procedures as exposure to ionizing radiation or high environmental temperature or administration of mucin, nitrogen mustard, adrenal steroids, epinephrine, xerosin, and metabolic analogues can be shown to exert a profound effect on infection by bacteria, viruses, and other agents.

In humans, these factors are no less important, although controlled studies are lacking for many. Alcoholism; diabetes; deficiency or absence of immunoglobulins (Chap. 62); defects in cellular immunity (Chap. 65); malnutrition; chronic administration of adrenal hormones; chronic lymphedema; ischemia; the presence of foreign bodies such as bullets, calculi, or bone fragments; obstruction of a bronchus, the urethra, or any hollow tube; agranulocytosis or congenital defects in bactericidal or virucidal activity; various blood dyscrasias, and many other circumstances influence susceptibility to systemic or local infection. Furthermore, in those instances where the extenuating condition is remediable, the probability of recovery is enhanced.

Racial differences in susceptibility, such as the poor resistance of dark-skinned people to tuberculosis and their predilection for developing disseminated coccidioidomycosis, are well established. Resistance to infection may be determined genetically. The relation of sickle-cell trait to malaria is one example. The increased frequency and severity of some infections in children, of others in pregnant women, and still others in the aged are familiar.

Prior contact with an organism or its products, whether by active infection or by artificial immunization, increases resistance to some infections, such as measles, diphtheria, and pertussis by stimulating antibody production, but seems to have little influence on resistance to others, such as gonorrhea.

Knowledge of the factors involved in human resistance and susceptibility is incomplete. Explanations such as changes in physical or chemical activity of phagocytes; antibacterial substances such as lysozyme, phagocytin, or lysozomal enzymes; qualitative or quantitative alterations in serum proteins; disordered metabolism at the cellular level, "products of tissue injury" that influence vascular permeability, and the effects of tissue pressure remain to a considerable extent in the realm of hypothesis.

The profound influence of host factors upon the infectious process makes it clear, however, that their understanding is probably essential for the control of infections in predictable fashion.

PATHOGENESIS OF INFECTION With relatively minor variations, the development of an infectious disease follows a consistent pattern. The parasites enter the body through the skin, nasopharynx, lung, intestine, urethra, or other portal. A number of microorganisms adhere to their site of primary attack through fimbriae, pili, and surface antigens; the adherence of *Bordetella pertussis* to respiratory epithelium, the gonococcus to urethral epithelium, and possibly some gram-negative urinary pathogens to the epithelium of the renal pelvis are some examples. Once established in the host, the organisms can multiply and, in so doing, establish a local or primary lesion. From this site, there may be local spread along fascial planes or tubular structures, such as a bronchus or ureter. The next step may be systemic spread of the microorganisms via the circulating blood. Bacteria can enter the bloodstream by direct invasion of vessels, a relatively unusual occurrence, or more commonly by traversing peripheral lymph nodes to enter the thoracic duct lymph and thence the venous system. In the bloodstream, they spread to other tissues and can produce distant or secondary lesions. In infections such as tetanus and diphtheria, distant lesions are produced by toxins elaborated at the primary site without systemic spread of the parasites. The infectious process may terminate in recovery or death at any stage: the local lesion, systemic spread, or distant lesion.

The apparent inconsistency of this pattern in clinical medicine is attributable to the fact that the infection is recognized as a clinical entity only at the stage when symptoms are most likely to appear. For example, pneumococcal pneumonia is a local lesion, and the distant lesion, pneumococcal meningitis, is referred to clinically as a complication. In meningococcal infections, the local lesion, nasopharyngitis, is rarely symptomatic and has no status as a clinical entity, but the stage of spread, meningococcemia, and the commonest distant lesion, meningitis, are clinical entities. A rarer distant lesion, arthritis, is called a complication. In a patient who has osteomyelitis, a clinical entity, a recent furuncle may be referred to as a predisposing factor. In another patient with extensive furunculosis who develops osteomyelitis, the infection in bone may be regarded as a complication of the superficial infection. The stages mentioned are in no way limited to bacterial diseases; the primary lesion of poliomyelitis is intestinal, viremia may occur without neurological involvement, or a distant lesion manifested by symptomatic involvement of the central nervous system may be established.

Because clinical usage and terminology are based upon the symptomatic illness that leads patients to seek medical aid, the consistency of this general sequence in the pathogenesis of infection is often not recognized. However, the concept is useful and offers some basis for systematizing what may otherwise seem to be a miscellaneous collection of unrelated clinical signs and symptoms.

CLINICAL MANIFESTATIONS OF INFECTIONS So varied are the disorders attributable to infection or infestation of humans by lower organisms that generalizations about them are difficult. The clinical manifestations of infection can duplicate those of diseases of any other etiology. However, certain clinical features are highly suggestive of infection, including abrupt onset, fever, chills, myalgia, photophobia, pharyngitis, acute lymphadenopathy and splenomegaly, gastrointestinal upset, and leukocytosis or leukopenia. It is obvious that the presence of one, several, or all of these features does not constitute proof of the microbial origin of illness in a given patient. Conversely, serious, even fatal, infectious disease may exist in the absence of fever or other signs and symptoms.

Although there is no infallible clinical criterion of infection, it it still possible to recognize accurately many specific infectious diseases from information obtained by *history, physical examination, blood count, and urinalysis*. The importance of interrogation about past illness, predisposing factors such as alcoholism, familial disease, exposure to ill persons, contact with animals or insects, ingestion of contaminated food, type and order of onset of symptoms, and recent or remote residence in endemic areas is discussed in the subsequent chapters that deal with specific diseases and etiologic agents. Cardinal physical signs are also described for each entity.

The mechanisms that produce most of the signs and symptoms of human infection are unknown. The pathogenesis of fever is discussed in Chap. 9. The physiological alterations underlying "malaise," "postinfectious asthenia," "toxicity," and other common complaints are completely mysterious. The factors responsible for leukocytosis or leukopenia are only partially understood (Chap. 56). Why the rash of typhus begins on the trunk while that of another rickettsiosis, Rocky Mountain spotted fever, begins on the extremities is unanswered. Failure to understand these manifestations does not impair their clinical usefulness, although it is probable that understanding them might lead to more accurate diagnosis and better management.

DIAGNOSTIC PROCEDURES The specific procedures for the diagnosis of infectious disease have become sufficiently complex to warrant separate discussion. This is provided in Chap. 106.

Importance of specific diagnosis in infectious diseases The diagnostic procedures employed for infectious diseases are no more absolute than those in other diseases; they cannot be blindly equated with the science of microbiology. The responsibility for interpreting the facts supplied by the bacteriologist, immunologist, and virologist in the total context of a patient's illness remains that of the physician. A positive tuberculin skin test certainly does not indicate that a patient has active tuberculosis. The finding of *Candida albicans* in a stool culture does not necessarily mean that a patient's diarrhea is caused by intestinal candidiasis. The presence of staphylococci in nasal cultures from a patient with headaches does not establish a diagnosis of staphylococcal sinusitis. A throat culture containing group A beta hemolytic streptococci does not rule out diphtheria, nor does such a culture establish that a febrile illness in a patient with mitral stenosis is a recurrence of acute rheumatic fever rather than bacterial endocarditis. A positive serologic test for syphilis may be the first sign of lupus erythematosus.

The etiologic agent From a practical point of view, two important steps are vital to the correct diagnosis of infection: (1) the organ(s) or organ systems involved must be found, and (2) the etiologic agents causing the infections must be identified precisely. Chapter 106 deals with the diagnostic approaches that are available. Most of the remaining chapters in this part take up the specific bacteria, spirochetes, fungi, rickettsias, viruses, *Mycoplasma,* and Protozoa which cause infections. The common syndromes caused by these agents are described either in chapters dealing with specific organisms or in chapters dealing with infections in individual organ systems such as pneumonia (Chap. 260), bacterial endocarditis (Chap. 243), urinary tract infections (Chap. 280), osteomyelitis (Chap. 360), and meningitis (Chap. 368).

When confronted with specific organ involvement, it is important to know the most common pathogens which cause disease in the involved organ. Table 105-1 provides a listing of those pathogens. Used in conjunction with the individual chapters dealing with specific agents and the summary of chemotherapy (Chap. 111), the table should provide a rational guide to treatment which often must be instituted before the results of antimicrobial sensitivity tests are available.

CHEMOTHERAPY The impact of chemotherapy upon mortality and morbidity from infection and upon epidemic disease is a matter of record. These therapeutic agents, however, have in no way lessened the importance of specific diagnosis; indeed, their availability has increased the need for obtaining exact etiologic information. It requires but a moment's reflection to realize that the substitution of a prescription for a broad-spectrum antibiotic or a quick injection of penicillin for the systematic collection of facts and thoughtful consideration of diagnostic possibilities is a fallacious, unwise, and dangerous practice. Numerous antibiotics with overlapping spectra are now available, dosages for different infections vary widely, the drugs themselves are potentially dangerous, and their administration entails considerable expense. They should never be prescribed as placebos, antipyretics, or substitutes for diagnosis. In the vast majority of instances in which this is done, patients recover just as they would if no "therapy" had been given, and the drugs are wasted. More importantly, an inadequate dosage of a drug or the wrong agent may suppress symptoms temporarily without achieving cure and may make isolation of the etiologic agent difficult, delay recognition of the true nature of an illness, and postpone the institution of curative treatment. Furthermore, antibiotics may select out resistant variants or facilitate the transfer of R factors between pathogenic and commensal enterobacteria. Resistant variants can then replace sensitive strains and pose the additional hazard of spread to others. Finally, to expose a patient to the risk of a drug reaction without proper indication is inexcusable, whether the drug is an antibiotic, a sedative, a laxative, or a narcotic.

EPIDEMIOLOGIC AND OTHER CONSIDERATIONS Just as the decision to administer antibiotics to a patient with a febrile illness of presumed infectious etiology must be made on an individual basis, the selection of cases in which extensive cultural and serologic testing is required is a matter of judgment. The majority of common grippe-like illnesses subside spontaneously, and symptomatic treatment is sufficient. However, because of this tendency toward spontaneous recovery and also because the results of serologic tests may not be available until after recovery has taken place, the effort to determine the specific etiology of illness is often considered an impractical, "academic" procedure. Such an attitude fails to recognize that in addition to the individual patient, the welfare of the community must be considered. For example, a clinical diagnosis of "virus pneumonia" may turn out, following serologic tests, to be psittacosis. Although the "index" patient may have recovered completely, others in the community may be at risk until the "pet parakeet" which was the source of the illness has been eliminated.

Pursuing the diagnosis of obscure, often self-limited, illnesses may be academic, but this approach has led to clarification of some important etiologic relations. For example, the syndrome of infectious mononucleosis has been linked with development of antibody to a herpes-like virus, the EB virus (Chap. 195); some cases of erythema multiforme may be due to herpes simplex virus; several patients with encephalitis have been found to have central nervous system infections with myxoviruses. Some congenital anomalies have been related to prenatal viral infections; this relationship is well known for rubella (Chap. 182), but a number of other viruses (CMV, varicella, herpes simplex) have been implicated, although with less certainty. The finding of bacteria-like bodies in the intestinal mucosa of patients with Whipple's disease and the improvement of these patients with tetracycline therapy provides another example of an entity of unknown etiology entering the realm of infectious diseases. Patients with sarcoidosis have been shown to have high titers against herpes-like virus, similar to patients with infectious mononucleosis, Burkitt's lymphoma, and carcinoma of the posterior nasal space. The relation of these viruses to these diseases is not clear; suffice it to say, these associations raise some interesting possibilities concerning the lymphocytic system and virus infections. Along the same vein, the possibility has been raised that the Chédiak-Higashi syndrome, a rare familial disorder characterized by albinism, photophobia, nystagmus, anomalous cellular granules, marked susceptibility to infection, and development of lymphoma, is caused by a virus.

TABLE 105-1
The syndromic approach to treatable infections

Type of infection	Etiologic agents		
	Common	Relatively common	Unusual but important
Skin and subcutaneous tissue	Staphylococcus aureus	Streptococcus pyogenes, Candida, and superficial fungi	Gram-negative bacilli (burns, wounds)
Sinusitis	Streptococcus pneumoniae S. aureus	S. pyogenes, Hemophilus influenzae	Mucorales
Pharyngitis	Respiratory viruses, S. pyogenes	Gonococcus	Corynebacterium diphtheriae
Epiglottitis	H. influenzae		
Otitis, mastoiditis	S. pneumoniae, H. influenzae (children)	S. aureus, S. pyogenes	Pseudomonas, Proteus
Pneumonitis	S. pneumoniae, Mycoplasma pneumoniae, Mycobacterium tuberculosis	S. aureus, Klebsiella-Enterobacter, respiratory viruses, Legionella pneumophilia	S. pyogenes, gram-negative enteric bacilli, psittacosis, systemic fungi, Pneumocystis, H. influenzae, Pasteurella multocida
Empyema and lung abscess	S. aureus, anaerobic streptococcus, Bacteroides, Fusobacterium	Klebsiella (abscess)	
Bacterial endocarditis	Streptococcus viridans, S. aureus, enterococcus	S. pneumoniae, anaerobic streptococci	Pseudomonas, Candida, Staphylococcus epidermidis
Gastroenteritis	Salmonella, Shigella, enteric viruses	S. aureus, Escherichia coli (enterotoxic), clostridia, Giardia	Pseudomonas, Entamoeba histolytica, Vibrio cholerae, V. parahemolyticus
Peritonitis, cholangitis, intraabdominal abscess	E. coli, enterococcus, Bacteroides, anaerobic streptococcus, Fusobacterium	Klebsiella-Enterobacter, Proteus species	Clostridia, S. aureus
Urinary infection (cystitis, pyelonephritis)	E. coli, Klebsiella-Enterobacter, paracolon, Proteus, enterococcus	Pseudomonas	S. aureus
Urethritis	Gonococcus, ?Mycoplasma, Chlamydia, ?Acinetobacter (Mima-herellea)	Treponema pallidum	
Pelvic inflammatory disease	Gonococcus, E. coli Bacteroides, anaerobic streptococci, Chlamydia	Klebsiella-Enterobacter, enterococcus, Fusobacterium	Clostridia, S. aureus
Bones (osteomyelitis)	S. aureus	Salmonella	S. pyogenes
Joints	S. aureus, gonococcus, S. pneumoniae, H. influenzae	S. pyogenes, Neisseria meningitidis	
Meninges	S. pneumoniae, H. influenzae, N. meningitidis	E. coli, Klebsiella-Enterobacter, Proteus, Pseudomonas	S. pyogenes, M. tuberculosis, Cryptococcus, S. aureus, Listeria monocytogenes

This association, among others, relates the field of infection to that of oncogenesis.

Legionnaires' disease (Chap. 138) is the most striking example, demonstrating the importance of identifying the causative organism of an infection definitively. By dint of hard "shoe leather" epidemiology and by application of the most advanced microbiologic techniques available, an important new organism has been identified and steps to contain it have been instituted.

Similar results can be expected from other "academic procedures" which may have little immediate applicability to infection in a particular patient. Yet, just as was the case with Legionnaires' disease, organisms that seem to have little biological significance at present may assume practical importance in the future.

REFERENCES

BURNET M: *Natural History of Infectious Disease*, 4th ed. New York, Cambridge, 1972

CLUFF LE, JOHNSON JE III: *Clinical Concepts of Infectious Diseases*, 2d ed. Baltimore, Williams & Wilkins, 1978

DAVIS BD et al: *Microbiology*, 2d ed. New York, Harper & Row, 1972

DUBOS RJ: *Biochemical Determinants of Microbial Disease*. Cambridge, Harvard, 1954

———: *The Evolution of Microbial Diseases: Bacterial and Mycotic Diseases of Man*, 4th ed. Philadelphia, Lippincott, 1965, p 20

HORSFALL FL, TAMM I: *Viral and Rickettsial Infections of Man*, 4th ed. Philadelphia, Lippincott, 1965

WILSON GA, MILES AA: *Topley and Wilson's Principles of Bacteriology and Immunity*, 6th ed. Baltimore, Williams & Wilkens, 1975

106
THE DIAGNOSIS OF INFECTIOUS DISEASES

JAMES J. PLORDE
ROBERT G. PETERSDORF

The diagnosis of an infectious disease requires the direct or indirect demonstration of a pathogenic microbe on or within the tissues of the afflicted host. This is accomplished in four steps:

1 *Test selection.* The selection of appropriate laboratory tests begins with the performance of a careful history and physical examination. This is followed by the establishment of a provisional etiologic diagnosis based on that examination and consultation with the laboratory concerning the most efficient methods available for confirming the diagnosis.
2 *Specimen collection and transportation.* Detailed written instructions on the appropriate methods for the collection, transportation, and labeling of biological specimens must be available, and these instructions must be followed explicitly by the clinical staff. Failure to do so may result in the contamination of the specimen with normal flora during the process of collection, death of pathogenic microbes during delayed or defective transportation, and/or specimen mix-up during laboratory processing.
3 *Testing.* The clinical microbiology laboratory has a large number of testing procedures available for demonstrating the presence of pathogens within clinical specimens. These include visualization of the organisms by direct microscopic examination of exudates, body fluids, and tissues; cultivation of the organisms in artificial media, tissues, or experimental animals; demonstration of microbial antigens or

their by-products and the demonstration of characteristic host responses to the invading organism such as specific antibody formation or histological reactions.
4 *Data interpretation.* The mere demonstration of a potential pathogen is not prima facie evidence of its etiologic significance. It may represent a member of the patient's normal microbial flora or a contaminant introduced at the time the specimen was collected or processed. Similarly, high titers of specific antibody in the serum may represent a serologic response to resident flora or past exposure to a pathogenic microbe rather than evidence of a current infection.

SPECIMEN COLLECTION

SPECIMEN TYPES The diagnostic value of a culture specimen depends to a large extent on the likelihood that it has been collected free of contamination with either the transient or resident microbial flora. Specimens can be divided into three major categories based on the site from which they are collected.

Deep closed body areas Specimens obtained from closed, normally sterile, body areas are the most satisfactory for bacteriologic examination. Examples include the deep tissues, the vascular and subarachnoid spaces, pleura, peritoneum, and joints. If the specimen is collected by surgical excision or closed needle aspiration following careful disinfection of the overlying skin surface, the likelihood of contamination is small. The recovery of either aerobic or anaerobic organisms under such conditions is strong evidence that they are of pathogenic significance.

Deep communicating body areas As with the areas just mentioned, the lower respiratory tract, bladder, endometrium, and bone are normally devoid of a resident bacterial flora. Usually, however, specimens from these areas are collected only after they have been spontaneously ejected through a communicating pathway such as the oropharynx, urethra, cervix, or a sinus tract. These are invariably heavily contaminated with bacterial flora, including large concentrations of anaerobes. For this reason, these specimens are generally not suitable for anaerobic culture, and even the growth of aerobic or facultative organisms must be interpreted with caution. In many instances the degree of contamination can be lessened by disinfecting the area around the orifice (e.g., periurethra, cervix), cleansing the pathway (e.g., midstream urine), or aspirating through a sterile tube inserted into the pathway. Moreover, true pathogens can, at times, be distinguished from contaminants by their number (e.g., quantitative urine culture) or species (*Staphylococcus aureus* vs. *S. epidermidis*). Nevertheless, areas of confusion cannot be totally eliminated. As a result, cultures from these areas are seldom as reliable as those from deep closed areas unless collection techniques which bypass the colonized pathway, such as transtracheal or suprapubic aspiration, are employed.

Skin and mucous membranes The mouth, throat, gastrointestinal stomata, fissures, and fistulas, and superficial wounds such as decubitus ulcers are heavily contaminated with both transient and permanent organisms. Culture of these areas is unlikely to be helpful unless:

1 There is gross pus.
2 A specific bacterial pathogen that strongly suggests disease is being sought, such as *Salmonella* or *Shigella* from the stool, or *Neisseria gonorrhoeae* from the urethra or vagina.

3 The base of the lesion can be aspirated through normal adjoining skin or biopsied after disinfection of the lesion's surface. The use of swabs is much less satisfactory. The resulting sample size is small, and organisms are exposed to the drying environment of the air. Moreover, the unsaturated fatty acids present in cotton swabs are often toxic to microbes. If swabs are to be used, this inhibitory activity may be minimized by treating the swab with serum or charcoal. Alternatively, the cotton may be replaced with a synthetic fiber such as calcium alginate which is less toxic and is soluble in salt solutions. If the swab is to be used on a dry surface, it should first be moistened in a sterile fluid such as saline or broth. Swab cultures are not satisfactory for recovery of anaerobic bacteria or fungi.

DISINFECTION When specimens from deep closed lesions are collected, the site of percutaneous needle aspiration should be cleansed first by using 70% isopropyl or ethyl alcohol and then disinfected with a 2% tincture of iodine or an appropriate iodophor. The iodine is applied in a concentric fashion beginning at the site of aspiration and allowed to act for 1 to 2 min before the aspiration is performed. The area should not be probed or manipulated unless sterile gloves are worn or the involved fingers have also been disinfected. If the initial attempt at collection fails, subsequent efforts should be carried out with a new needle through a freshly disinfected site. At the completion of the procedure the iodine should be removed with alcohol to avoid the danger of sensitization. If the specimen for culture is drawn through an indwelling cannula, the site of withdrawal must be disinfected in the same fashion.

When specimens are to be collected from the uterus, a draining wound, or sinus tract, the orifice must be thoroughly cleansed and disinfected as described above, a sterile intravenous catheter or multilumen tube is introduced as deeply as possible through the orifice, and the specimen aspirated into a sterile syringe. Culture from an open lesion may be collected by biopsy, aspiration from the margin, or by swabbing the surface. In the first two situations the wound is prepared as for a deep closed lesion. For swab cultures, the wound surface is cleansed only with sterile saline to remove debris and saprophytic flora.

TRANSPORTATION All specimens submitted for microbial culture should be transported to the laboratory as rapidly as possible, preferably within 1 h. Delay beyond this time may result in death of fastidious organisms, overgrowth of contaminants, and/or change in the number of bacteria unless special procedures are employed to overcome these problems. Rapid transportation is particularly important when dealing with blood, body fluid, and exudates which may harbor pathogenic *Neisseria* or anaerobes. The container should be clean, sterile (stool specimens excepted), and appropriately labeled. Respiratory secretions, urine, large pieces of tissue, and large volumes of fluid can be safely transmitted in plastic containers with leakproof lids. Aspirates are conveniently and safely transported in the same syringe used in the collection procedure, providing all air is expressed from the syringe and the needle is capped with a sterile holder. Alternatively, such fluid may be injected into a sealed gassed-out vial suitable for transport of anaerobic specimens. If such vials are used, it is important that the indicator in the vial be checked to ascertain whether it is still colorless. A pink or blue color indicates the presence of oxygen and suggests that the vial is no longer adequate for the transport of specimens for anaerobic culture. Small pieces of tissue (less than 1 cm²) are transported best in sterile rubber-stoppered gassed-out tubes. After the anaerobic indicator is checked, the tube is held upright to minimize the loss of the heavy inert gas, the stopper removed, specimen inserted, and the tube recapped.

Swabs submitted for the culture of group A beta-hemolytic streptococci can be transported in dry sterile test tubes. All other swabs should be submitted in one of several commercially available transport media. These prevent both the desiccation of organisms implanted on the swab and the overgrowth of hardy organisms at the expense of more fastidious ones. Although special anaerobic transport materials are available, use of swab cultures for the recovery of such organisms is not encouraged.

SEROLOGIC STUDIES Although blood is the specimen most commonly examined for the presence of antibody, a variety of other fluids including cerebrospinal, pleural, peritoneal, and joint fluids may be examined under appropriate conditions. Because a rise or fall in antibody titer is more significant than the absolute level, it is usually helpful, and often necessary, to obtain a specimen during both the acute and convalescent phases of illness. The optimum interval between these two specimens averages 10 to 14 days but varies with both the type of antibody being measured and the etiologic agent. The volume should approximate 5 ml whenever possible; much smaller specimens are sufficient for certain types of procedures. The testing laboratory should be consulted for details. Whenever possible the blood should be collected aseptically; if whole blood is required for the test, the specimen should be drawn into a tube containing anticoagulant. When the specimen is to be transported to another institution for testing, a preservative which does not influence the outcome of the serologic test should be added to inhibit bacterial contamination. Alternatively the specimen can be lyophilized or, in some cases, simply dried on filter paper before it is dispatched.

VIROLOGIC SPECIMENS The selection of specimens for the diagnosis of viral illness depends on both the stage of the disease and its clinical presentation. If the patient is seen early in the course of illness, frequently it is possible to demonstrate viral antigen in body tissue or fluids and/or to recover the virus by appropriate culture techniques. If the patient is seen later, during the recovery or convalescent stages, the diagnosis is often best established by serologic means. The type of specimen submitted for culture and the method of specimen transport depend to some extent on the nature of the illness. Throat swabs are helpful in the diagnosis of most viral infections. Because respiratory viruses are extremely labile, the swabs are placed in a buffered, high-protein transport medium containing antibiotic agents. If the specimen is to be transported to another institution, the specimen should be stored at −60°C and shipped on dry ice.

Cerebrospinal fluid from patients presenting with meningitis or encephalitis can also be submitted for culture. As with throat swabs, these specimens should be stored at low temperatures and shipped on dry ice. Stool should be collected in patients with respiratory illnesses, meningitis, or encephalitis, if either adenoviruses or enteroviruses are thought to be involved. Since these organisms are hardy, the feces can be collected in any sterile screw-top bottle and dispatched without refrigeration. Urine cultures are seldom helpful except in the diagnosis of cytomegalovirus infections. Vesicular fluid is a rich source of virus and viral antigen in patients presenting with exanthems. Pericardial fluid may be of help in patients with myocarditis or pericarditis. Viral blood cultures are seldom useful except in the diagnosis of arboviral infections. Isolation techniques for these viruses are highly specialized and are not available in most virus laboratories. Buffy coat cultures for cytomegalovirus and herpesvirus may be of help in immunosuppressed patients. Brain biopsy is the best single method for diagnosing *Herpes simplex* encephalitis (Chap. 193). The biopsy specimen should be placed in a sterile screw-top bottle and stored and dispatched in the frozen state.

LABORATORY PROCEDURES

DIRECT MICROSCOPIC EXAMINATION The direct microscopic examination of body fluids, exudates, and tissues is both the simplest and one of the most helpful laboratory procedures available for the diagnosis of infectious diseases. In many situations the examination allows an accurate, highly specific identification of the causative agent. Examples include the recognition of *Borrelia* or *Plasmodium* species in blood smears taken from patients with relapsing fever or malaria. At times only a tentative identification can be made on the basis of microbial morphology. Nevertheless, this is often sufficiently precise to allow the selection of an appropriate chemotherapeutic agent pending the results of more definitive investigations. A variety of techniques are used in direct microscopy. If the agent being sought is sufficiently large or characteristic, the specimen can be prepared as an unstained wet mount and examined by light-field, dark-field, or phase contrast microscopy. More commonly, a dried smear is made; this allows the application of a variety of stains which assist the visualization and identification of the microbe in question. The smear is prepared in a way that spreads tissue and inflammatory cells evenly in an undamaged monolayer over the glass slide. After drying, the smears are fixed, stained, and examined with a light, fluorescent, or electron microscope.

Wet mounts Dark-field examination of fluid from genital lesions for the spirochete of syphilis is a well-known, but neglected, procedure. More often, wet mounts are used for the diagnosis of fungal and parasitic infections. The examination of hair fragments, skin scrapings, or nail clippings is useful in establishing the presence of superficial mycoses. The specimens are placed in a drop of 10% KOH, a cover slip added, the preparation cleared by heating, and the mount examined under low-power magnification for the presence of hyphae and arthrospores. At times, as for tinea versicolor infections, the fungous elements will be sufficiently characteristic to allow the specific identification of the causative agent. Occasionally a presumptive diagnosis of a systemic fungous infection can also be established with this procedure. Two examples are cryptococcal meningitis by demonstrating the encapsulated organism in an India ink preparation of cerebrospinal fluid, and coccidiodomycosis by finding characteristic spherules in expectorated sputum.

Examination of saline or iodine mounts of stool or duodenal drainage is also the initial first step in establishing the diagnosis of intestinal protozoal infections such as amebiasis and giardiasis. Moreover, it is the definitive procedure diagnosing intestinal helminthic infections including ascariasis, trichuriasis, strongyloidiasis, and hookworm. Finally, filariasis and sleeping sickness can be recognized by demonstrating the characteristic motility of microfilariae and trypanosomes in blood or other body fluids.

Stain-enhanced microscopy Despite many recent technical advances in the field of microbiology, Gram's stain remains, after 90 years of use, the best single technique available for the rapid diagnosis of bacterial infections. It can be applied to virtually all clinical specimens and is of particular value in the examination of exudates, aspirates, body fluids, including cerebrospinal fluid, and urine. Gram's stains should be examined first under the lower-power objective to demonstrate the presence of pink-staining inflammatory cells. The paucity of such cells in the presence of many squamous epithelial cells suggests that the specimen was contaminated during the process of collection and may not be representative of the inflammatory process. After the evaluation under low-power objective, the smear is then examined for the presence of bacteria using the oil immersion lens; bacteria will appear either as dark blue (gram-positive) or pink (gram-negative) bodies. Their color and morphological appearance often make possible a presumptive identification of the genus and occasionally the species with a significant degree of accuracy. The demonstration of pneumococci in the sputum, Enterobacteriaceae in the urine, staphylococci in localized abscesses, gonococci in urethral exudates, clostridia in foul-smelling discharge, and pneumococci, meningococci, or *Hemophilus influenzae* in stained smears of the cerebrospinal fluid permits the initiation of specific chemotherapy with the assurance that the regimen is the proper one. In some immunosuppressed patients *Candida* blastospores and pseudohyphae can be found in blood smears several days before candidemia is demonstrable by culture.

A variety of other stains are available for the demonstration of specific microbes. Mycobacteria have the unique capacity to resist the decolorization by strong mineral acid alcohol solutions once they have been stained with basic carbol-fuchsin or one of the fluorochromes. This allows their immediate recognition in body tissues and fluids. The presence of a large number of acid-fast bacilli in the expectorated sputum establishes the presumptive diagnosis of respiratory tuberculosis and is sufficient evidence for initiating isolation procedures and antituberculosis therapy once additional specimens are collected for culture. Subsequent examination of the sputum with acid-fast stains is an important element in monitoring the success of therapy. The traditional Ziehl-Neelsen and Kinyoun stains are now being supplanted by the fluorochromes which allow a much more rapid scanning of smears using relatively low magnification.

Acid-fast smears can also be used to identify pathogenic strains of *Nocardia* if mineral acid rather than acid-alcohol is used for decolorization. When an even weaker decolorizing agent such as organic acid is used, organisms such as *Actinomyces* may also be visualized.

Both Giemsa's and iodine stains may be used to diagnose chlamydial infections involving the eye, urethra, or cervix. When epithelial cells obtained by scraping these areas are stained with Giemsa's stain, a typical semilunar dense inclusion body composed of many blue- or purplish-staining particles is seen adjoining the nucleus of the cell. Iodine stains reveal a similar reddish brown mass in scrapings from the eye but are not useful in cervical specimens.

A number of stains are available for the definitive identification of parasites. *Pneumocystis carinii* can be recognized in transbronchial brush biopsies using a modified Wright's stain, toluidine blue, or methenamine silver. The latter produces a very distinctive black-stained cyst. Blood and tissue protozoa such as plasmodia and *Leishmania* can be demonstrated best with Romanowsky-type mixtures containing methyline blue and eosin. These render the nuclei red to violet and the cytoplasm blue. The identification of intestinal protozoa, on the other hand, requires the use of stains such as iron hematoxyline or trichome to demonstrate the taxonomically important nuclear detail.

Immune microscopy This method combines the specificity of immunologic procedures with the speed of direct microscopy. In the immunofluorescent technique, smears thought to contain viral, bacterial, fungal, or parasitic organisms are stained with specific antibody preparations labeled with fluorescent compounds and examined with a fluorescent microscope. At present, the most useful application of this technique is the examination of brain tissue for Herpes simplex or rabies virus; lung tissue, pleural fluid, and sputum for the Legionnaires' disease bacillus; and cervical, urethral, and conjunctival scrapings for trachoma-inclusion conjunctivitis agent.

Direct fluorescent antibody staining of nasal epithelial cells may also be used for the rapid diagnosis of influenza, parainfluenza, and respiratory syncytial virus infections.

Finally, the direct immunofluorescence technique for detecting antibody-coated bacteria in the urinary sediment has been useful in distinguishing kidney from bladder infection in females.

Unfortunately, the need for expensive fluorescent microscopes, the poor quality of many of the commercially available conjugated antiserums, and the need for well-trained technologists restrict the routine use of these procedures to reference laboratories.

Enzyme-linked immunoabsorbent assay (ELISA) tests are similar to the immunofluorescence test except that the antiserum is reacted with a peroxidase-labeled antispecies conjugate. After treatment with appropriate reagents, the peroxidase assumes a dark-brown color that can be visualized with the ordinary light microscope, obviating the need for expensive equipment. Its potential application in the diagnosis of a wide variety of infectious diseases is obvious, but its final role in clinical microbiology remains to be established.

Electron microscopy The electron microscopic examination of vesicular fluid or scabs of patients with febrile exanthems allows a very rapid differentiation of varicella-zoster infections from smallpox. This technique also has been useful in the identification of certain viral infections which do not produce cytopathic effects in cell cultures. It has been particularly valuable in the detection of rotaviruses in the stool specimens of infants and small children suffering from gastroenteritis. The large number and characteristic appearance of these virus particles allow specific identification to be made on morphological grounds alone. Electron microscopy has also been used in the diagnosis of the so-called "winter vomiting disease" caused by the Norwalk and Hawaii agents. These agents are morphologically similar to those of the picornavirus group, and specific identification requires aggregation of the virus particles with immune serum. This technique of immune electron microscopy may have wide application in virology and has been used to identify virus-like particles associated with non-A, non-B hepatitis in experimental animals.

CULTURE Despite the time and complexity, the isolation of the etiologic agent by cultivation in artificial media, tissue cultures, or animals is generally the most definitive diagnostic procedure available. When laboratory confirmation of the presence or absence of a specific microorganism such as *Streptococcus pyogenes, Corynebacterium diphtheriae, Salmonella,* or *Shigella* is needed, artificial media specifically designed to recover these organisms are employed. More commonly, however, the laboratory is asked to screen for the presence of any potential bacterial pathogen. In that situation, the specimen is inoculated on a variety of artificial media designed to recover the most commonly encountered pathogens. Differential media, which allow demonstration of certain biochemical characteristics of isolated organisms, and selective media, which inhibit the growth of resident microbes, are commonly included in this initial battery. Special media may be required to recover rare or unusually fastidious microbes, such as *Listeria, Leptospira,* and *Brucella.* The appropriate selection of such media requires close and constant communication between the clinical and laboratory staffs.

For most purposes, the specimen is inoculated onto a small area of solid medium contained in a petri dish and then is distributed over the remainder of the medium's surface with a sterile bacteriologic loop. If this procedure is performed appropriately, the bacterial growth will appear as isolated colonies. These can then be characterized morphologically, subcultured in pure form, identified biochemically, and tested for their sensitivity to antimicrobial agents. In addition, this inoculation procedure allows an estimate to be made of the quantity of organisms present in the original specimen. This is usually recorded in the semiquantitative fashion, but in the case of urine, blood, and occasionally other specimens, the inoculum size can be measured precisely and the total number of colonies enumerated. The clinical significance of bacterial growth must be evaluated both qualitatively and quantitatively. The isolation of certain bacterial pathogens such as *N. gonorrhoeae, Salmonella,* and *Shigella* almost always indicates disease. The isolation of most bacterial pathogens, however, is of questionable significance unless (1) the gross and microscopic appearance of the specimen suggests that it was adequately collected, (2) the bacterial species in question is present in large numbers on both the Gram's stain and culture media, and (3) the organism represents the predominant bacterial species grown.

Although it is often necessary to initiate chemotherapy prior to the availability of culture results, it is mandatory that treatment not be started until the culture specimens have been collected.

There are new developments in identification of a wide variety of viruses in tissue culture, and refinements of these techniques are increasing the value of tissue culture in clinical diagnosis. Many viruses can also be isolated by the inoculation of appropriate animals. This is rarely feasible for ordinary clinical diagnosis, and for several agents it is hazardous. Animal inoculation has also been used for several nonviral infections, including rat-bite fever, certain mycoses, tuberculosis, and some rickettsioses. Although this is a cumbersome procedure for routine use, it may need to be employed with appropriate precautions in selected instances.

DETECTION OF MICROBIAL ANTIGENS AND THEIR BY-PRODUCTS The relative nonspecificity of many direct microscopic methods and the delay inherent in culture procedures have resulted in the introduction of a variety of techniques aimed at the rapid detection of microbial antigens or their by-products.

Counterimmunoelectrophoresis The most widely used of these techniques is counterimmunoelectrophoresis (CIE). In this variation of the agar gel diffusion test, the specimen being tested for antigen is placed in an agar well and specific antiserum in a second apposed well. An electric current is then passed through the agar resulting in rapid confluence of antigen and antibody with the formation of a precipitant within a matter of minutes. CIE has proved most useful for the rapid diagnosis of bacterial meningitis in childhood where the cerebrospinal fluid is checked for the presence of pneumococcal, meningococcal, group B streptococcal, or *H. influenzae* antigens. The technique has approximately the same order of sensitivity as Gram's stain but has the advantage of heightened specificity. CIE has also been used for the detection of the above-mentioned bacterial antigens in serum, pneumococcal capsular antigens in sputum, and the detection of rotavirus and enterovirus in stool.

Latex agglutination This test has been utilized in many of the same situations as CIE. Although greater sensitivity has been claimed for latex agglutination, the test is plagued by false-positive reactions from heat labile serum components and rheumatoid factor. Perhaps its greatest usefulness has been in the detection of cryptococcal antigen in the spinal fluid of patients with chronic meningoencephalitis.

Radioimmunoassay The most spectacular application of this technique is in the detection of hepatitis B surface antigen–associated (HBsAg-associated) infection and in the prevention of such infections by the screening of blood and blood products for the presence of the antigen. This procedure is highly sensitive, and results can be obtained within a few hours with commercially available test kits. In this method HBsAg-labeled ^{125}I competes with antigen in a test serum for a specific antibody in the test mixture. Free and bound antigens are separated by washing. The reactivity of the antigen-antibody complex is then analyzed with a gamma counter.

Gas chromatography This method involves the direct examination of clinical specimens by gas liquid chromatography for the detection of characteristic microbial by-products. It has been thought helpful in differentiating aerobic from anaerobic organisms in pus and blood. It has also been used to differentiate staphylococcal, streptococcal, and gonococcal from traumatic arthritis and to detect *Candida* in the blood of patients with fungemia. Although the role of gas chromatography in the identification of anaerobic bacteria is established, its usefulness in the direct analysis of clinical specimens remains to be determined.

IMMUNOLOGIC METHODS These diagnostic methods are intended to supply evidence of past or present infection by demonstrating antibodies in serum or other body fluids, by indicating changed reactivity of the host (hypersensitivity, allergy) to products of the organism, or, rarely, to detect components of the causative organism in the body.

Serologic tests The finding on a single occasion that a patient's serum contains antibody which reacts with a certain antigen merely indicates that the patient has had previous contact with the antigen or a closely related substance. For this reason, with rare exceptions, the clinical interpretation of serologic tests depends on serial determinations. If the antibody titer is found to *rise or fall significantly,* the response likely is a result of recent contact with the antigen. In subsequent chapters, the need for serologic testing of acute phase and convalescent serum is emphasized repeatedly. *In any patient with a puzzling illness, a sterile specimen of serum should be preserved in a frozen state so that it can, if necessary, be studied and compared with serum collected at a later date.*

Prior contact with an antigen may be the result of past immunization with vaccines; interpretation of serum agglutinin titers for typhoid bacilli is often made difficult by prior immunization. The so-called "anamnestic reaction," a nonspecific stimulation of antibody formation by an acute illness (e.g., a rise in *Brucella* agglutinins in a patient with acute tularemia), occurs only when the two organisms are antigenically related, and rarely presents a serious problem.

The methods employed for detecting antibody rises in various infections have been selected empirically on the basis of the ease with which the test can be performed and careful study to correlate the results of the test with other diagnostic criteria in patients. Therefore, the fact that antibodies against one agent are detected by a precipitin technique, another by agglutination of whole organisms or the production of capsular swelling, another by indirect fluorescent-antibody methods, and still another by complement fixation is a practical matter and bears no necessary relation to the agent, the type of infection, or its pathogenesis. By coating some particulate material, such as erythrocytes or latex, with antigen derived from a cer-

tain organism, antibody can sometimes be demonstrated by an agglutination test rather than by some more complex method.

Particular properties of the causative organism can sometimes be utilized to devise a simplified clinical test for antibody. Two striking instances of this are widely used. The ability of influenza and related viruses to clump erythrocytes makes possible the demonstration of antibody to virus by merely testing the capacity of a patient's serum to prevent the agglutination of red blood cells by suspensions of virus, the so-called "hemagglutination-inhibition" reaction. Similarly, because many microorganisms possess hemolytic components or toxins, the assay of a patient's serum for capacity to prevent lysis of red blood cells is a convenient and simple clinical test for antibody. The antistreptolysin O test in group A *S. pyogenes* infections is an example of this.

In a few infections, predominantly those caused by viruses, the only reliable serologic test is a *neutralization or protection* test, an assay of the protection afforded by the patient's serum against active infection in tissue culture or in experimental animals. This technique is time consuming and is usually performed only in diagnostic virology laboratories.

Some mention of "nonspecific" serologic changes may serve to emphasize again that clinical laboratory tests have come into use *only because they have been found to correlate reasonably well with clinical findings.* In several diseases it has been found, often accidentally, that serum antibody develops which will react with antigens derived from sources other than the etiologic agent (which may actually be unknown). Common examples are heterophil agglutinins in infectious mononucleosis, cold agglutinins in mycoplasma pneumonia, and the agglutination of certain strains of *Proteus* bacilli by serum of patients with rickettsial diseases. The VDRL test for syphilis and related flocculation tests are performed with antigens derived from sources completely unrelated to *Treponema pallidum.*

The results of serologic tests must be interpreted in the light of other information about the patient, including such factors as previous immunizations and illnesses, the possibility of exposure to chemically but etiologically unrelated antigens, and the importance of a changing titer in serial tests as opposed to a single isolated observation.

Skin tests Exposure to antigens of certain types, by various routes, and under circumstances not completely understood often results in the development of immediate (anaphylactic, atopic) hypersensitivity or delayed (bacterial, tuberculin) hypersensitivity.

Active infection with some, but not all, bacteria and viruses results in delayed hypersensitivity to the infecting agent in some, but not all, individuals. Clinically, this allergic state is detected by intradermal injection of the organism or one of its components; in a sensitive individual, induration and erythema will appear at the local site within 24 to 48 h. If an individual is highly "sensitive" or if the amount of antigen injected is excessive, there may be extensive local inflammation with necrosis, vesicle formation, edema, regional lymphadenopathy, and even malaise and fever. Antigens prepared in concentrations unlikely to provoke severe reactions are generally available for intradermal testing for tuberculosis, leprosy, mumps, lymphogranuloma venereum, cat-scratch disease, chancroid, brucellosis, tularemia, glanders, toxoplasmosis, blastomycosis, histoplasmosis, coccidioidomycosis, and many other infections. The immune reaction to vaccination (Chap. 184) is also an example of delayed dermal hypersensitivity.

The reliability, specificity, and usefulness of the individual tests differ and are discussed in the chapters on specific infections. However, certain general principles apply to their use and interpretation:

1 They are highly useful in epidemiologic surveys as indicators of the incidence of infection in a population.
2 In most individuals, dermal reactivity persists for many years or for life. A single positive test means only that at some past time the individual was infected with the organism (or a closely related one). Unless supplementary information in the form of clinical findings, cultural studies, or more specific serologic data bear out the presence of active infection, a diagnosis of the disease is not justified.
3 The appearance of a positive dermal reaction in an individual known to have been nonreactive a short time before is good evidence of recent infection; this is a useful method for detecting tuberculosis.
4 *A negative intradermal test does not rule out past or present infection.* For unknown reasons, patients with measles, Hodgkin's disease, or sarcoidosis often develop a state of *anergy,* or inability to react to intradermally injected antigens. In several diseases, dermal sensitivity develops after weeks or months of infection; an important example is acute histoplasmosis, in which patients can be ill for many weeks without showing a positive skin test. The skin test to coccidiodin is always negative in disseminated coccidioidomycosis; in far-advanced or miliary tuberculosis in elderly patients, failure to react to intradermal tuberculin in the usual amounts employed for testing occurs in as many as 10 to 15 percent of the cases.

Intradermal injection of antigens derived from sources other than microorganisms usually produces an immediate *wheal and erythema* reaction which subsides promptly. The greatest clinical usefulness of this type of reaction is in the detection of allergy to foreign serums, pollens, and animal dander (Chap. 65). The skin tests for demonstrating infestation with helminths (trichinosis, filariasis) produce reactions of the immediate type in allergic individuals, but many of the antigens employed are so nonspecific that they are of little use in diagnosis.

INTERPRETATION AND REPORTING

As the number, cost, and complexity of laboratory procedures increase, so does the need for the clinical laboratory to assist the physician in the selection of tests and in the interpretation of their results. Such consultations can decrease unnecessary testing, avoid inappropriate antimicrobial therapy, and increase the speed and effectiveness of therapy when it is indicated. One important aspect of such consultation is the immediate interpretation of Gram's stain smears because this can be helpful in selecting appropriate antimicrobial agents or in suggesting the need to collect a second more satisfactory specimen prior to the beginning of therapy.

The laboratory should provide the physician with information on the results of all cultures within 24 h and the significance of both positive and negative results for each specimen. Failure of the culture to grow within this time interval may result in recommendations for further testing or occasionally for discontinuation of therapy. Polymicrobial growth on aerobic cultures can also lead to further testing using better collection techniques. Finally, the identification of the organism and its likely susceptibility to antimicrobial agents often can be surmised accurately on the basis of colonial morphology and rapid biochemical testing.

The clinical laboratory may choose not to report certain data if they are likely to be misleading. For example, the laboratory may choose not to report the susceptibility of an organism to a given antimicrobial agent if there is a contraindication to the use of that agent for treatment of the infection in question.

MANAGEMENT OF SPECIFIC SPECIMENS

UPPER RESPIRATORY TRACT Because the throat and nasopharynx are normally heavily colonized by both saprophytic and potentially pathogenic bacteria, culture of this area is seldom useful except when a particular bacterial pathogen is being sought, e.g., *S. pyogenes, Bordetella pertussis, C. diphtheriae,* meningococci, or gonococci.

Throat cultures When throat cultures are submitted to the laboratory without specifying the pathogen being sought, the laboratory will generally report only the presence or absence of *S. pyogenes.* Since a single properly obtained throat swab will detect at least 90 percent of patients with streptococcal pharyngitis, a negative culture is very helpful in excluding the possibility of this disease. Similarly, a heavy or predominant growth of group A beta-hemolytic streptococci in patients presenting with the signs and symptoms of streptococcal pharyngitis is highly predictive of an antibody response to streptococcal antigens and, therefore, presumably disease. It is far more difficult to interpret cultures with a light or nonpredominant growth of *S. pyogenes.* A large proportion of these patients do not mount an appreciable immunologic response, suggesting that bacterial growth represents a carrier state.

Throat cultures may not be indicated in adults presenting with sore throat if they lack fever, cervical lymphadenopathy, or recent exposure to another patient with streptococcal pharyngitis since fewer than 5 percent of this population have positive cultures. Conversely, adults with temperatures of 38°C or higher, tender cervical lymphadenopathy, or pharyngeal exudate are so frequently culture positive that immediate antibiotic therapy is more cost effective than waiting for the result of culture.

Mouth cultures Usually massively mixed flora of aerobic and anaerobic bacteria is present in mouth cultures, and they are not clinically useful except when a careful attempt to avoid contamination with indigenous flora has been made. This is particularly true for the isolation of *Actinomyces israelii.* This organism is part of the normal oropharyngeal flora, and the time and effort required for its isolation is not justified unless an uncontaminated specimen can be provided.

LOWER RESPIRATORY TRACT Although culture of expectorated sputum is the most frequently employed technique for the diagnosis of lower respiratory tract infections, both its sensitivity and specificity are open to question. Studies of patients with bacteremic pneumococcal pneumonia have shown the etiologic agent to be present in the sputum in only 50 to 94 percent of cases. Moreover, expectorated sputum is almost always contaminated with oropharyngeal flora including, in many cases, bacterial species commonly associated with pulmonary infections. Even when a potential pathogen is recovered, its role in the causation of a lower respiratory tract infection is uncertain. Attempts to remove saliva and nasal secretions from the sputum by repeated washing or to differentiate upper and lower tract organisms on the basis of quantitative sputum culture have been ineffective or unacceptably tedious. Some confusion can be avoided if the specimen is collected appropriately and screened carefully for both gross and microscopic characteristics prior to inoculation of the culture. Ideally, sputum specimens should be collected early in the morning under direct supervision of a physician or respiratory therapist. If the patient is unable to produce sputum, coughing may be stimu lated by lowering the head of the patient's bed for a few minutes or exposing the patient to an aerosol of warm hypertonic saline.

Because sputum is rarely homogeneous, it should be examined carefully for bits of pus and blood. These should then be used to prepare a Gram's stain smear which is examined for the presence of squamous epithelial cells (SEC) and leukocytes under the low-power objective (10×) of the microscope. If there are fewer than 10 SEC and greater than 25 leukocytes per field, the results of the culture are more likely to represent lower tract flora. This is particularly true if a single or clearly predominant bacterial type grows, or, in the case of chronic obstructive pulmonary disease, if both pneumococci and *H. influenzae* are isolated. If squamous epithelial cells number more than 10 per low-power field, the specimen can be considered heavily contaminated with oropharyngeal flora and should be discarded. In most cases a second carefully collected expectorated sputum will yield a satisfactory specimen.

Direct endotracheal or endobronchial aspiration may be employed when a satisfactory expectorated sputum cannot be produced. However, such specimens are subject to contamination by oropharyngeal flora which is introduced during the passage of the aspiration instrument. Fiberoptic bronchoscopy, which allows the direct visualization and aspiration of bronchial secretions, is a relatively inocuous procedure and may result in a somewhat better specimen. When possible, however, bronchial brushings or biopsy material should be obtained, because they are less likely to be diluted with topical anesthetics or saliva.

Alternatively, the specimen may be collected by a technique that totally bypasses the oropharynx. The most widely used is transtracheal aspiration. This method entails a definite risk of hemoptysis, subcutaneous and mediastinal emphysema, vagal discharge, or respiratory embarrassment and is contraindicated in the presence of a bleeding diathesis. It should be used only when results from expectorated sputum are unsatisfactory and the infection is severe enough to merit the attendant risks. The technique produces a more reliable sputum specimen than either expectoration or bronchoscopy and is probably the only satisfactory method for collecting specimens for anaerobic culture. However, some 20 percent of specimens from patients without clinical evidence of pneumonia yield potential respiratory pathogens. These "false positive" specimens are primarily from patients who have chronic pulmonary disease, who have recently suffered minor bouts of aspiration, or in whom the tip of the catheter was coughed into the hypopharynx during the collection procedure.

Needle aspiration of a pulmonary infiltrate under fluoroscopic control also produces specimens of excellent quality. The percutaneous method gives both a high yield and accurate results but has at least a 5 percent chance of complications, particularly pneumothorax. The morbidity risk is greater than with transtracheal aspiration biopsy, but the diagnostic yield may be superior.

Whatever technique is used to sample the lower respiratory tract, the physician should always obtain a concomitant blood culture. If a pleural effusion is present, it should also be aspirated and cultured.

In addition to bacterial pathogens, pneumonia can be caused by viruses, *Rickettsia, Chlamydia, Mycoplasma pneumoniae,* and Legionnaires' disease bacillus. Techniques for the recovery of these agents from the sputum are generally not available in a routine clinical microbiology laboratory, and the diagnosis is most frequently made by clinical and/or serologic methods. Legionnaires' disease bacillus can be cultured from lung tissue or empyema fluid. In addition, it can be demonstrated by direct fluorescent antibody staining in both of these specimen types and in transtracheal aspirates. This allows early diagnosis and rapid institution of appropriate therapy. For

discussion of the techniques used for the recovery of mycobacteria and fungi from the lower respiratory tract, the sections devoted to these organisms should be consulted.

URINE CULTURES Voided urine, like expectorated sputum, is usually contaminated with the normal microbial flora, in this case from the urethra and external genitalia. Urine cultures, however, are more reliable than those of expectorated sputum, because the periurethral area can be disinfected and the urethra itself flushed with the first portion of the urine stream before a sample is taken. In addition, quantitation of the bacterial growth is helpful in separating contaminated specimens from true infection. In general, bacterial counts exceeding 100,000 organisms per milliliter of urine indicate true bacteriuria while those less than 10,000 organisms per milliliter reflect contamination with perineal or urethral flora. Before a high bacterial count can be accepted as evidence of infection, however, the following factors need to be considered: (1) the adequacy of the disinfection procedures, (2) the sex of the patient, (3) the interval between specimen collection and plating, and (4) the number of bacterial species isolated. It is important that patients be carefully instructed in the techniques of collecting clean voided specimens or that the collection be supervised by a trained attendant. In brief, the foreskin of males must be retracted completely; in females the labia must be separated widely. The periurethral area is repeatedly cleansed with an appropriate disinfectant and then rinsed with warm sterile water. Following this, the patient voids. After the first 20 to 25 ml is discarded, the specimen is caught directly in a sterile container without interrupting the stream. The cup should be held in a way to avoid contact with the legs or perineal area. When this procedure is followed conscientiously, a single specimen from a male which yields a colony count in excess of 100,000 organisms per milliliter is highly indicative of bacteriuria. In women, the colony count must exceed 100,000 organisms per milliliter in two consecutive urine specimens before infection can be considered to be present. Because urine is a good culture medium, contaminating organisms will multiply to large numbers if the urine is allowed to stand at room temperature for prolonged periods of time. For this reason, specimens which cannot be dispatched to the laboratory within an hour should be refrigerated. They can be held at 4°C for 4 to 6 h without an appreciable change in the bacterial colony count. In most instances, urinary tract infections are caused by a single bacterial species. The isolation of three or more species in a urine culture usually reflects contamination even when the colony count is high. True polymicrobial bacteriuria does occur but is generally restricted to patients with chronic indwelling urethral catheters. In contrast, colony counts of less than 100,000 organisms per milliliter may sometimes represent true bacteriuria. In fact, up to one-third of urinary tract infections are associated with counts in the range of 10,000 to 100,000 organisms per milliliter. This is particularly true of specimens from male patients or patients receiving antimicrobial therapy, and of specimens obtained by ureteral or urethral catheterization and by suprapubic aspiration.

When an adequate clean-voided urine specimen cannot be obtained, or when anaerobic cultures are desired, suprapubic aspiration may be employed. Specimens obtained in this manner are unlikely to be contaminated, and even slight growth may be significant. When an indwelling catheter is in place, a specimen should be collected directly from the catheter by means of a sterile needle and syringe after careful disinfection of the exterior surface. Urine should not be taken from the drainage tube or bag, because these are frequently contaminated. Occasionally Foley catheter tips are submitted to the laboratory for culture when a catheterized patient shows signs or symptoms of urinary tract infection. Statistical analysis has shown this practice to be both futile and potentially misleading.

Examination of a Gram's stain smear of uncentrifuged urine is often helpful in the rapid diagnosis of urinary tract infection. The presence of many squamous epithelial cells and mixed bacterial flora indicates contamination and the need for another specimen. In the absence of the epithelial cells, the presence of one or more bacterial cells per oil immersion field usually indicates true bacteriuria especially when accompanied by one or more leukocytes.

BLOOD CULTURES Because of the peculiar clinical importance of demonstrating bacteria in the bloodstream and because there are varying opinions about optimal timing and sites of sampling for blood cultures, it is of practical importance to understand something about the mechanisms of bacteremia.

Excepting intravascular infections (bacterial endocarditis or endarteritis, mycotic aneurysm, suppurative thrombophlebitis), bacteria usually enter the circulation through the lymphatic system. Consequently, when bacteria multiply at a site of local infection in the tissues, the likelihood of bacteremia parallels the occurrence of local conditions that favor drainage of lymph from the infected area to the thoracic duct and eventually to the venous blood. These factors include the number and anatomic arrangement of local lymph vessels, accumulation of fluid, increase in tissue pressure, and manipulation of the part.

Once bacteria enter the blood, they are removed rapidly by the fixed phagocytes of the reticuloendothelial system in the liver, spleen, and bone marrow and by engulfment in polymorphonuclear leukocytes in capillaries, especially those of the lung.

Clinically, bacteremia can be transient, intermittent, or continuous. Many transient bacteremias result from manipulation of infected or contaminated tissues, common examples being instrumentation of the genitourinary tract, tonsillectomy, dental procedures, and massage or surgical incision of furuncles or abscesses. In the vast majority of instances, the sudden discharge of bacteria into the blood produces no symptoms or, at most, a rigor and brief fever, and the organisms are promptly removed. The great danger of these "man-made" bacteremias is their role in producing bacterial endocarditis in patients with endocardial damage or intracardiac prostheses.

Transient bacteremia accompanies the early phase of many infections. In pneumococcal pneumonia, the typical rigor at the onset is a result of transient bacteremia. In most cases, with localization of the pulmonary lesion, blood cultures rapidly revert to negative. The poor prognosis of patients with pneumonia who continue to have positive blood cultures is not due to the presence of organisms in the blood but reflects spreading infection in the lung itself.

A sudden single influx of microorganisms into the bloodstream may be followed by a shaking chill and fever. However, there is a "lag period" of 30 to 90 min before the febrile response. During this delay, the bacteria are usually promptly removed from the circulation by phagocytosis; consequently, a blood culture taken at the time of the rigor may be negative.

Continuous bacteremia is a feature of the first several days of typhoid fever, of brucellosis, and of intravascular infections such as endocarditis or endarteritis.

Blood cultures should be obtained from all febrile patients who have rigors, are seriously ill, are thought to have endocar-

ditis or intravascular infection, or are immunosuppressed. If viremia, fungemia, brucellosis, tularemia, leptospirosis, or an infection with cell wall–deficient bacteria is suspected, the laboratory should be contacted for special instructions. In general, three blood cultures taken at intervals of no less than 60 min are adequate to document the presence of bacteremia in an adult. In emergent situations, two cultures taken simultaneously from different anatomic sites will usually suffice. In patients who have received antimicrobial agents within the previous 2 weeks or in whom endocarditis is suspected, a total of six cultures taken over a 2-day period may be useful. If the patient is receiving antimicrobial agents, the cultures should be taken immediately prior to the next dose, and the laboratory should be notified to allow the addition of penicillinase and/or extensive dilution of the blood specimen. The collection of specimens over and above the number listed above is seldom helpful in detecting occult bacteremia unless the culture procedures, media, or conditions of incubation are altered to allow detection of fastidious organisms.

Specimens are best collected by percutaneous venipuncture. If possible, aspirations from the femoral vein should be avoided since disinfecting the skin of the groin is often difficult. The increasingly common practice of drawing blood for culture through an indwelling intravascular cannula often results in a higher level of contamination without substantially improving the detection of bacteremia. Similarly there is no evidence that arterial blood cultures possess any advantage over venous cultures. Bone marrow cultures may reveal the etiologic agent when it cannot be obtained by other means in occasional patients with disseminated salmonellosis, tuberculosis, and deep mycoses.

To minimize the chance of contamination with skin flora, the site of aspiration should be carefully disinfected as described in "Management of Specific Specimens" above. Following aspiration, the blood should be inoculated into both aerobic and anaerobic broths immediately. The dilution ratio of blood to broth should be at least 1:10 to minimize the normal bactericidal activity of serum and the activity of any antimicrobial agents that may be present. If direct inoculation into broth is not feasible, the blood may be drawn into a sterile Vacutainer tube containing sodium polyethanol sulfanate (SPS). This anticoagulant is anticomplementary and inactivates leukocytes and certain aminoglycoside and polypeptide antibiotics. Nevertheless, it will not delay bacterial death indefinitely, and Vacutainer specimens should be sent to the laboratory for dilution in broth within 30 min of the time the blood is drawn. If fungemia is suspected, the laboratory should be notified since the standard techniques described above are less satisfactory for the isolation of fungi. The yield can be improved by the use of a large inoculum of blood in a Castaneda-type biphasic medium of brain-heart infusion agar and broth which is incubated for up to 4 weeks.

Gram's stain examination of buffy coat smears is seldom indicated. Although a number of microorganisms, particularly meningococci and staphylococci, can be detected within granulocytes in approximately 4 percent of submitted blood culture specimens, the procedure is time-consuming and seldom of therapeutic value. It may be justified if fungemia is suspected. The toxicity of amphotericin B therapy precludes initiation of treatment without strong evidence of systemic fungal infection. Because these organisms often require 4 to 5 days to grow, a positive buffy coat smear would be of obvious therapeutic importance.

Approximately two-thirds of blood cultures from bacteremic patients are found to be positive within 24 h and 90 percent within 3 days. Despite strict adherence to disinfectant procedures on the ward and sterile technique in the laboratory, contamination occasionally occurs. The following are characteristics of "false-positive" blood cultures: (1) pour plates are seldom positive, (2) repeat cultures are seldom positive for the same organism, (3) bacterial growth in broth generally occurs after 3 days of incubation, and (4) the organisms are often identified as diphtheroids, *Bacillus,* or *S. epidermidis.* However, any of these species can occasionally be responsible for true bacteremia, particularly in immunosuppressed patients.

CEREBROSPINAL FLUID Examination of the CSF from patients suspected of having meningitis represents one of the major emergency procedures faced by the clinical microbiology laboratory. Bacterial meningitis can be rapidly fatal if treatment is delayed or inadequate, and appropriate therapy often requires specific identification of the etiologic agent. Because of the clinical urgency, CSF specimens should be collected as soon as the diagnosis is considered, and the specimen promptly transported to the laboratory. The laboratory should be notified if the specimen has been collected from an abscess within the CNS to ensure that it is cultured both aerobically and anaerobically. If possible, at least 2 ml CSF should be obtained and the specimen sent for glucose, quantitative protein level, and cell count in addition to microbiologic studies. A simultaneous blood sugar also should be drawn for correlation with the CSF glucose level. Fastidious organisms, particularly *N. meningitidis,* may not survive prolonged storage at temperatures below that of the body. If a delay in CSF examination cannot be avoided, specimens should be held at 37°C.

After receipt, the specimen is concentrated by centrifugation or filtration, Gram stained, and cultured aerobically. The inflammatory response in the CSF is helpful in distinguishing acute bacterial meningitis from nonbacterial forms of the disease. In bacterial meningitis, polymorphonuclear leukocytes predominate, while in tuberculous, fungal, or protozoal meningitis, the inflammatory cells usually consist of lymphocytes, and the response is less intense. Although polymorphonuclear leukocytes may dominate early in the course of aseptic meningitis, there is usually a clear shift to mononuclear cells within 8 h. Cytologic changes in the CSF may also be seen in patients with brain abscess. However, smears and cultures are generally negative in these cases unless the abscess ruptures into the subarachnoid space or into the ventricles. The Gram's stain smear of the CSF should be examined carefully for stainable organisms, particularly meningococci, pneumococci, *Enterobacteriaceae, Listeria,* and staphylococci in patients with atrioventricular shunts. Stainable, but nonviable, organisms in the CSF are fairly common and may result in a "false-positive" Gram's stain. In addition, in cases of partially treated bacterial meningitis there is a tendency for gram-positive organisms to stain gram-negative.

When a large number of organisms is present and specific antiserums are available, the etiologic agent can often be rapidly identified by the quellung reaction or a precipitin test. Counterimmunoelectrophoresis is even more sensitive and may be positive when the Gram's stain is not. Moreover, detection of microbial antigens in the CSF by CIE is often the only method of identification of an infectious agent from a patient with partially treated meningitis. In the presence of a significant number of mononuclear cells without stainable bacteria, encapsulated cryptococci or cryptococcal antigen can be identified with the India ink preparation or latex agglutination tests, respectively.

Regardless of the results of these studies, the CSF must be cultured and any resulting growth identified to the species level. Mycobacterial and fungal cultures should be set up on patients who present with chronic meningitis and a mononuclear inflammatory response in the CSF.

Naegleria filaria, the cause of amoebic meningoencephalitis, can often be recognized by its amoeboid movements in wetmount preparations of cerebrospinal fluid. This organism

should be looked for in patients who develop hemorrhagic meningoencephalitis during the summer months (Chap. 199).

GASTROINTESTINAL INFECTIONS Cultures of the mouth, periodontal lesions, or saliva usually yield a mixed flora of aerobic and anaerobic organisms including *A. israelli* and *Candida* spp. The isolation of these organisms is without significance unless the specimen was collected in a way which avoided contamination with indigenous flora. If actinomycosis is suspected, the laboratory should be contacted for special instructions. The diagnosis of oral thrush and Vincent's infection can be made with stained smears from scrapings of the suspected lesion.

Cultures of ileostomy or colostomy stomata, gastrointestinal fistulas, and rectal fissures invariably grow both aerobic and anaerobic intestinal flora. They are seldom helpful, therefore, unless a search is made for specific intestinal pathogens.

Fecal cultures are helpful in determining the etiology of diarrhea and in detecting carrier states. Such specimens are routinely cultured for species of *Salmonella, Shigella,* and *Arizona.* Many laboratories are now also looking for *Vibrio parahemolyticus, Yersinia enterocolitica,* and *Camphylobacter fetus.* There is at present no convenient and reliable method of identifying enterotoxogenic strains of *E. coli* in the clinical laboratory. The physician should indicate whether any of these, or any other unusual infection such as antibiotic-associated pseudomembranous enterocolitis, candidiasis, clostridial food poisoning, or cholera, are suspected.

Although rectal swabs are adequate for the diagnosis of bacterial diarrhea, they are less satisfactory for the detection of carrier states. If swabs are used, they should show obvious soiling and be sent to the laboratory in appropriate transport media. Whole stool should be collected free of urine, placed in clean waxed cardboard cartons, and promptly dispatched to the laboratory. If delivery cannot be made within 1 h, the stool should be preserved in phosphate-buffered glycerol to prevent death of fastidious organisms such as *Shigella* spp. It is seldom necessary to submit more than three consecutive daily specimens. Isolated pathogens should be identified both serologically and biochemically before the final report is issued. It is important, however, that the physician be notified as soon as a potential pathogen has been isolated.

GENITAL TRACT Genital specimens are submitted primarily for the diagnosis of venereal disease including gonorrhea, syphilis, chancroid, trichomoniasis, and chlamydial infections. Instructions for the collection of specimens should be sought in the sections of the text dealing with these specific diseases. In addition to the venereal pathogens, a number of organisms may infect the endometrium, tuboovarian tissues, and vagina. Endometrial cultures must be collected through a double or triple lumen tube inserted through a decontaminated cervical os if contamination with vaginal and cervical flora is to be avoided. The specimens should be delivered to the laboratory in either a gassed-out vial or a sealed syringe to ensure recovery of anaerobic organisms. When a patient presents with vaginitis, a specimen is collected by swabbing the vaginal fornix under direct visualization. If trichomoniasis is suspected, the swab should be placed in a small amount of sterile saline and sent to the laboratory immediately. If the swab is received within 10 to 15 min, the organism can be identified without difficulty by its characteristic motility in a wet-mount preparation. Cultural examination should focus on the recovery of agents thought capable of causing vaginitis such as *H. vaginalis,* group B beta-hemolytic streptococci, and *Candida albicans.*

EXUDATES AND BODY FLUIDS Pus from undrained abscesses as well as pericardial, pleural, peritoneal and synovial fluids is best collected by syringe and needle aspiration through disinfected skin. Prior rinsing of the syringe with a sterile anticoagulant such as heparin or SPS will help prevent formation of clots. Because anaerobic organisms are commonly involved in infection of these areas, the syringe should be sealed and sent immediately to the microbiology laboratory. Alternatively, the aspirate may be injected into a gassed-out anaerobic transport vial. The use of swabs is not encouraged since the sample size is small and fastidious organisms including anaerobes are unusually susceptible to desiccation and oxidation. Deep suppurative lesions which communicate with the surface of the body through fistulas or sinus tracts present a difficult problem in specimen collection. The communicating pathway is generally colonized by a wide variety of bacterial flora which contaminate drainage being ejected through the fistula opening. The degree of contamination can be lessened in many instances by carefully disinfecting the orifice and aspirating material via a sterile plastic catheter inserted deep into the sinus. Even when these precautions are taken, however, sinus tract cultures often fail to correlate well with pathogens isolated from operative specimens. For this reason, a bacteriologic diagnosis of draining suppurative lesions should be based on a culture of currettings or biopsy rather than sinus drainage. If actinomycosis is suspected, the draining sinus tract may be covered with gauze which is left in place until it is thoroughly saturated. The gauze is then submitted to the laboratory where it is carefully examined for the presence of granules which can be picked out and then identified.

SKIN, SOFT TISSUE, AND SUPERFICIAL WOUNDS Specimens collected from these areas are usually heavily contaminated with the normal flora of their respective sites. Swab cultures should be obtained only if gross pus is present or if the physician wishes to confirm the presence or absence of only a single bacterial pathogen, such as *C. diphtheriae;* in this case, the wound should first be cleansed mechanically with saline to remove as much exudate as possible. Material from bullae and areas of cellulitis is best obtained with a syringe. Successful aspiration of an area of cellulitis may require initial injection of a small amount of sterile saline. It is important that this solution not contain a preservative which may affect the viability of some bacteria. Alternatively, a punch biopsy may be obtained of the area after appropriate disinfection. Similarly, cultures from open lesions may be obtained by biopsy or by aspirating from the margins of these lesions using a syringe and needle. Semiquantitative cultures of burn eschars are useful in identifying patients at risk of bacteremia.

Intravenous and intraarterial catheter tips are best collected by disinfecting the area of the skin penetrated by the catheter, carefully withdrawing the catheter, and aseptically cutting off its tip into a sterile container. The tip is then delivered to the microbiology laboratory where semiquantitative cultures are done. In general, catheter tips which are contaminated during removal will have only a few colonies on agar plates, while infected catheter tips will show heavy growth.

REFERENCES

BARRY AL: Clinical specimens for microbiologic examinations, in *Infectious Diseases,* 2d ed, PD Hoeprich (ed). Hagerstown, Md, Harper & Row, 1977

——— et al: Microscopic examinations in infection, in *Infectious Diseases,* 2d ed, PD Hoeprich (ed). Hagerstown, Md, Harper & Row, 1977

BARTLETT RC: Control of cost and medical relevance in clinical microbiology. Am J Clin Path 64:518, 1975

DOLAN CT et al: *Proceedings of the 1975 Aspen Conference on Clinical Relevance in Microbiology.* Chicago, College of American Pathologists, 1977

EISENBERG HD et al: Collection, handling and processing of specimens, in *Manual of Clinical Microbiology,* 2d ed, EH Lennette et al (eds). Washington, DC, American Society for Microbiology, 1974

NEU HC: What should the clinic expect from the microbiology laboratory? Ann Intern Med 89:781, 1978

107
INFECTIONS IN THE COMPROMISED HOST

DAVID C. DALE

DEFINITION An individual who is abnormally susceptible to infections is called a *compromised host.* This heightened susceptibility often is attributable to specific abnormalities in host defense mechanisms (e.g., leukocytes, immunoglobulins, complement, mucosal and epithelial barriers, tissue vascular supply), alterations in normal surface bacteria caused by antibiotics, or the insertion of a foreign body (e.g., endotracheal tube, artificial heart valve, shunt, or catheter) (Table 107-1).

HOST DEFENSE MECHANISMS The skin and mucous membranes are the principal barriers which prevent invasion of the body by microorganisms. A variety of bacteria, including *Staphylococcus epidermidis, Streptococcus pyogenes,* and *Corynebacterium acnes,* inhabit the superficial layers of the normal skin. The mucosal surfaces of the upper respiratory tract, the lower gastrointestinal tract, and lower urinary tract are also in constant contact with bacteria, whereas the lower respiratory and upper urinary tracts are normally free of microorganisms. The subcutaneous tissues are protected from infection by the tough stratum corneum and antimicrobial substances derived from the sweat and sebaceous glands. Mucus in the respiratory and gastrointestinal tracts, together with secretory immunoglobulin (IgA), lysozyme, lactoferrin, α-antitrypsin, and bacteriocins produced by the normal bacterial flora serve to prevent colonization of the mucosal surfaces by new organisms. Bacteria and foreign debris are constantly swept toward the body orifices by the ciliated epithelial cells lining the mucosal surfaces. Normally a constant, low-grade exudation of leukocytes to these surfaces provides added protection.

If an organism penetrates a body surface and enters the tissues, a series of host responses occurs. An inflammatory exudate containing immunoglobulins, complement components, and other plasma proteins quickly appears. If the immunoglobulin is specific for the invading organism, it attaches to the bacterial cell wall, opsonizes the organism, and activates the complement system via the classic pathway. If specific immunoglobulin is lacking, the C3 component of complement will serve to opsonize the organism and facilitate phagocytosis. Complement activation also generates chemotactic factors which attract neutrophils, monocytes, and eosinophils to the inflammatory site (Chap. 56).

Normally within 1 to 3 h, neutrophils have begun to accumulate at a site of inflammation anywhere in the body, and they continue to arrive until the invading microbes are killed and eliminated, or a chronic inflammatory reaction consisting of monocytes, lymphocytes, and macrophages has developed. When infection spreads from the tissues to the blood, the circulating organisms ordinarily are removed by cells of the fixed mononuclear phagocytic system in the lungs, liver, spleen, and bone marrow.

TABLE 107-1
Infections in the compromised host

	Disease	Infection	Etiologic agents
HUMORAL DEFECTS			
Antibody deficiency	Bruton's X-linked agamma-globulinemia, multiple myeloma, chronic lymphocytic leukemia, Waldenstrom's macroglobulinemia, Wiskott-Aldrich syndrome, ataxia telangiectasia, isolated IgA deficiency	Sinusitis, bacterial pneumonia, bacteremia	*S. pneumoniae, H. influenzae, G. lamblia*
Complement deficiency	C3 deficiency, C5 deficiency, other isolated complement factor deficiencies, systemic lupus erythematosus, sickle-cell anemia	Otitis, sinusitis, pneumonia, bacteremia	*S. aureus, E. coli, Pseudomonas, N. gonorrhoeae*
PHAGOCYTIC DEFECTS			
Neutropenia	Agranulocytosis, acute leukemia, aplastic anemia, cyclic neutropenia, cytotoxic drug therapy, Chédiak-Higashi syndrome	Cellulitis, pharyngitis, perirectal abscess, pneumonia, bacteremia	*S. aureus, E. coli, Pseudomonas, Candida, Aspergillus*
Chemotactic defects	Chédiak-Higashi syndrome, diabetes mellitus, rheumatoid arthritis	Cellulitis, abscesses, septic arthritis, skin ulcers	*S. aureus, S. pyogenes*
Phagocytic defects	Acute leukemia	Pharyngitis, perirectal abscess, pneumonia, bacteremia	*E. coli, Pseudomonas, Candida*
Microbicidal defects	Chronic granulomatous disease of childhood, myeloperoxidase deficiency, Chédiak-Higashi syndrome, lysosomal granule deficiency	Recurrent skin abscesses, lymphadenitis, osteomyelitis, liver abscess, lung abscess, pneumonia	*S. aureus, Salmonella, Serratia*
DEFECTS OF CELLULAR IMMUNITY			
T-cell deficit, with intact B cells	Hodgkin's disease, chronic mucocutaneous candidiasis, thymic dysplasia (Nezelof's syndrome), thymic-parathyroid hypoplasia (Di George's syndrome), sarcoidosis, lepromatous leprosy	Superficial skin infections (especially with *Candida*), hepatitis, tuberculosis, fungal pneumonia, chronic meningitis, meningoencephalitis	*Candida, Cryptococcus, M. tuberculosis, Listeria, Toxoplasma, herpes zoster*
Combined B-cell and T-cell defects	Severe combined immunodeficiency (adenosine deaminase deficiency), ataxia telangiectasia, Wiskott-Aldrich syndrome, cartilage-hair hypoplasia, thymoma with immunodeficiency, intestinal lymphangiectasia secondary to Whipple's disease, Crohn's disease, pericarditis, tricuspid regurgitation, chronic lymphocytic leukemia	Disseminated skin infection (especially viral), otitis, sinusitis, bronchitis, pneumonia, bacteremias, abscesses	*Staph. aureus, gram-negative bacilli,* herpes zoster, herpes simplex, *cytomegalovirus*
OTHER DEFECTS			
Impaired tissue perfusion	Diabetes mellitus, nephrotic syndrome, sickle-cell anemia, severe atherosclerosis	Skin ulcers, cellulitis, wet gangrene, osteomyelitis	*S. aureus, E. coli,* and other gram-negative enteric bacilli
Abnormal drainage	Cystic fibrosis, bronchogenic carcinoma, ureteral and urethral obstruction, obstruction tumors at any site	Bronchitis, bronchiectasis, pneumonia with atelectasis, urinary tract infection, ascending cholangitis	*S. aureus, E. coli,* and other gram-negative bacilli
Integumental damage	Burns, eczema, compound fractures	Cellulitis, pneumonia, bacteremia, osteomyelitis	*S. aureus, S. pyogenes, Pseudomonas*
Antibiotics	Superinfection	Pneumonia, bacteremia	*S. aureus,* resistant gram-negative bacilli, especially *Pseudomonas, Serratia, Mima-Herellea, Candida*
Prosthetic devices and foreign bodies		Abscesses, bacteremia, osteomyelitis	*S. aureus, S. epidermidis,* gram-negative enteric bacilli, *Candida*

Certain pathogens, such as mycobacteria, DNA virus, and fungi, which are not readily killed by neutrophils, tend to persist intracellularly; they require a different host response for their containment. This mechanism, commonly referred to as *cellular immunity,* involves the interaction of monocytes and sensitized lymphocytes, the transformation of monocytes to activated macrophages, and the killing of organisms by macrophages and lymphocytes by both intracellular and extracellular mechanisms. The mediators of cellular immunity include migration inhibitory factor, transfer factor, chemotactic factor, and other lymphokines which are produced by T lymphocytes (Chap. 61).

SPECIFIC DEFECTS IN HOST DEFENSES Defects in skin and mucous membranes Burns and extensive trauma which leave patients with raw skin exposed to endogenous and environmental organisms rapidly become infected. *Pseudomonas* infections are frequently encountered in these patients, particularly those who have received antibiotics (Chap. 121). Atherosclerosis and neuropathy commonly predispose diabetic individuals to cutaneous infections of the lower extremities, particularly with staphylococci. Decubitus ulcers which become secondarily infected occur in severely ill patients who are not repositioned regularly. Burns, inhalation of toxic materials, and viral infections, e.g., influenza, can damage the respiratory tract epithelium predisposing to secondary infection by upper respiratory tract flora, especially pneumococci and staphylococci. Obtundation, intubation, and mechanical ventilation also enhance the risk of pneumonia because these factors interfere with the clearance of debris and bacteria from the lower respiratory tract. Urinary tract catheters, intravenous catheters, and other devices which connect the integument to any internal organ provide a route for microbial invasion from the skin. This problem is compounded by the fact that the porous surfaces of these foreign bodies provide crevices where bacteria can grow protected from the host's phagocytic cells.

Defects in the humoral system Immunoglobulin deficiency due to B-lymphocyte deficiency or dysfunction occurs in agammaglobulinemia (Chap. 62), multiple myeloma (Chap. 63), and chronic lymphocytic leukemia (Chap. 326) and with intensive immunosuppressive therapies. It results in decreased bacterial opsonization and inefficient function of the phagocytic system. Patients with these disorders are prone to infections by encapsulated bacteria, particularly pneumococci and *Hemophilus influenzae*. Patients with reduced or absent immunoglobulins and patients with defects of complement components C1, C2, or C4 are able to utilize the alternate complement pathway to activate C3 and the later complement components, i.e., C5 through C9. Patients with early complement component defects have fewer problems with infections than patients with deficiencies of complement components C3 through C9. These complement-related host defense defects are, in general, quite uncommon (Chap. 61).

Defects in the phagocytic system The most frequently encountered problem in phagocytic defenses is neutropenia. Blood neutrophil counts below 500 cells per cubic millimeter, and particularly counts below 100 cells per cubic millimeter, are associated with a greatly increased frequency of fever and infections. This is especially true in idiopathic or drug-induced agranulocytosis, leukemia, and aplastic anemia. Far less commonly, patients are encountered with specific defects in the granulocyte bactericidal mechanisms, e.g., chronic granulomatous disease and the Chédiak-Higashi syndrome (Chap. 56). In some patients with diabetes, uremia, lupus erythematosus, and rheumatoid arthritis, defects in neutrophils have been recognized which are attributed to abnormalities in the environment (excess glucose, uremic toxins, immune complexes) in which the cells function. When these patients' cells are suspended in normal serum or plasma they generally function normally.

Defects in cell-mediated immunity Patients with Hodgkin's disease, sarcoidosis, lepromatous leprosy, chronic mucocutaneous candidiasis, and certain congenital syndromes, e.g., Nezelof's syndrome, Di George's syndrome, Wiskott-Aldrich syndrome, and combined immunodeficiency, have defective lymphocyte-monocyte function most easily identified by reduced or absent cutaneous, delayed hypersensitivity responses

(Chap. 62). Tuberculosis, candidiasis, and disseminated viral infections, particularly herpes zoster infections, seem to occur with increased frequency in these patients.

Splenectomy The magnitude of the risk of overwhelming infection in the splenectomized patient is related to the underlying disease which called for removal of the spleen. However, even splenectomy for trauma in an otherwise normal individual appears to increase the risk of severe bacteremic infections. There is an impressive predominance of pneumococcal infections in splenectomized individuals; other organisms encountered frequently have included *Neisseria meningitidis, Escherichia coli*, and *Pseudomonas*. Malaria and other intracellular parasitic infections such as *Toxoplasma* and *Babesia* also may occur with increased frequency.

Defects induced by drugs *Antibiotics,* particularly when taken orally, regularly alter the normal host bacterial flora and predispose patients to superinfections, i.e., infections occurring specifically as a consequence of antibiotic treatment. Characteristically, these infections are caused by organisms resistant to the antibiotic being administered. These infections occur more commonly when antimicrobials are given in large doses, when several antimicrobials are administered concurrently, or when broad-spectrum agents are used.

It is often difficult to distinguish between superinfections and simple surface colonization by new organisms. Usually superinfections are identified by the occurrence of new symptoms, e.g., fever, cough, dysuria, or diarrhea, and the finding of resistant organisms in an area of new inflammation during the course of treating a defined infection (Chap. 114). Most of the time, antimicrobial therapy does not promote superinfection. However, when the concentration of organisms replacing the normal flora is high and when anatomic conditions are favorable, superinfection is likely. Certain circumstances, such as the tendency for *Pseudomonas* to infect patients treated with the cephalosporins and for *Candida* to infect patients treated with broad-spectrum combinations of antibiotics, are well recognized. Superinfections are also common during treatment of pneumonia in patients with severe, chronic, obstructive pulmonary disease where intubation is necessary, and when urinary tract infections are treated in patients with urinary stones or catheters.

Glucocorticosteroid therapy, particularly when given for long periods and in high doses, is thought to increase the risk of infections in humans. Although this risk is well documented in animal experiments, properly controlled human studies have been difficult to conduct. In the laboratory, steroids decrease mobilization of neutrophils to the sites of inflammation, decrease the killing of microbes by monocytes, and interfere with cell-mediated immune responses, possibly by altering the responsiveness of monocytes and macrophages to lymphokines. Because steroids induce such a broad defect in host defense mechanisms, both common and unusual pathogens must be considered in the steroid-treated patient with a presumed infection.

Immunosuppressive drugs, e.g., cyclophosphamide, chlorambucil, methotrexate, and many others, are now widely used for nonmalignant and malignant diseases. Nearly all of these agents cause neutropenia, lymphopenia, and monocytopenia through suppression of cell production. They also impair the rates of cell renewal in other tissues vital for host defenses including the epithelial cells lining the mucosal surfaces. Most of the infectious complications of these agents occur concomitant with the drug-induced neutropenia. Especially when used with corticosteroids in high doses, patients treated with these agents are severely compromised both in their ability to resist new infections and to handle established ones.

Defects with transplantation Immunosuppressive drugs, antilymphocyte globulin, and corticosteroids are generally used to prolong and to prevent rejection of kidney, heart, and other homografts. Because these agents are used in high doses during periods of impending graft rejection and because cellular resistance to infections may be impaired by the graft rejection process itself, at times these patients are inordinately susceptible to infections, particularly to severe fungal and viral infections (Chap. 69).

Bone marrow transplant patients have marked susceptibility to infection at the time of marrow grafting because of neutropenia and bone marrow ablation. After transplantation and marrow engraftment, despite the rise in their neutrophil counts, their host defenses remain severely compromised for 1 to 3 months because of a persisting impairment in cellular immunity. During this period, they frequently develop catastrophic pulmonary infections due to fungi, viruses, and parasites (Chaps. 69 and 312).

RECOGNIZING THE COMPROMISED HOST Most disease states associated with increased susceptibility to infections are easily identified. Examples include patients with leukemia, lymphoma, or aplastic anemia; therapy with steroids, immunosuppressive drugs, and broad-spectrum antibiotics; and specific anatomic defects such as bronchiectasis, chronic obstructive lung disease, or obstructive uropathy. Not infrequently the occurrence of fever and infection leads to the diagnosis of certain diseases associated with defects in host defenses. For example, a diabetic may be recognized because of recurrent abscesses or candidiasis in the perineal region. A severely granulocytopenic patient may be recognized because of fever, sore throat, or sepsis. Recurrent pneumococcal meningitis may lead to recognition of a small skull fracture with chronic CSF leakage. Recurrent fever and lymphadenitis usually precede recognition of chronic granulomatous disease.

Several reasonably reliable associations of specific organisms and certain host defense defects have been recognized and may be helpful in identifying or caring for the compromised host. These include *Staphylococcus aureus* with foreign bodies; *S. aureus, Serratia,* and *Salmonella* with chronic granulomatous disease; *Streptococcus pneumoniae* with agammaglobulinemia and splenectomy; mucoid *Pseudomonas* strains with cystic fibrosis; *Salmonella* with sickle-cell disease; *Nocardia* with alveolar proteinosis; *Mycobacterium tuberculosis, Cryptococcus,* and herpes zoster with Hodgkin's disease; and *Candida* with hypoparathyroidism.

The evaluation of a patient to identify a defect in host defenses should proceed systematically. After a complete history and physical examination, complete blood cell counts, blood glucose, liver and renal function tests, and chest and other appropriate x-ray examinations are obtained. Serum protein electrophoresis, quantitative immunoglobulins, and isohemagglutinins or selective febrile agglutinins are then measured to evaluate B-lymphocyte function. T-lymphocyte functions are evaluated with a panel of delayed hypersensitivity skin tests, generally including PPD, mumps, *Candida,* trichophytin, and streptokinase-streptodornase. Contact sensitization with dinitrochlorobenzene (DNCB) or keyhole hemocyanin (KLH) may also be performed. Complement defects usually can be recognized by obtaining total hemolytic complement levels (CH_{50}) or C3 assays. The principal screening test for recognizing the various forms of chronic granulomatous disease is the nitroblue tetrazolium (NBT) test. At this point in any patient's evaluation, consultation with an individual engaged in studying host defense defects is usually necessary.

Useful clues for persisting in a patient's evaluation to try to define a specific abnormality are: repetitive episodes of proven bacterial infections with the same organism; infections which do not respond to treatment that is usually considered to be effective or which relapse when therapy is discontinued, and repeated infections caused by unusual organisms.

THERAPEUTIC CONSIDERATIONS Successful treatment of infections in the compromised host depends upon early diagnosis, prompt intervention, and avoidance of certain pitfalls in patient management. Because infections in the compromised host tend to be chronic, long-term care by a concerned physician who understands the patient's host defense deficiency is vitally important. Laboratory facilities for accurate culture and sensitivity testing also are essential. In the febrile compromised host, the clinician must collect blood, body fluids, and exudate for cultures as quickly as possible. When these materials do not yield a diagnosis promptly, aspiration or biopsy of sites of presumed infection is often necessary and should not be delayed.

Often it is necessary to initiate antibiotic treatment before results of cultures and sensitivity tests are available. This is particularly true in patients with shock and presumed bacteremia, patients with fever and severe neutropenia, and those with severe respiratory tract infections where sputum or transtracheal washings are difficult or impossible to obtain. In these instances broad-spectrum coverage with a combination of antibiotics should be used initially (Chap. 111), but the coverage should be narrowed as quickly as possible to avoid superinfections. Often patients with neutropenia, corticosteroid treatment, and certain specific host defense defects fail to mount an inflammatory response as rapidly as normal individuals. Consequently, when these patients have pneumonia, cellulitis, or abscesses, the diagnosis may not be apparent when the patient is first seen. Repeated careful examinations are the only way to establish the diagnosis.

Although sometimes essential, indwelling catheters should be avoided in the compromised host whenever possible (Chap. 108). The prophylactic use of antibiotics in these patients has rarely been successful (Chap. 114). With time, the patients simply become colonized by microbes resistant to the prophylactic agents chosen. Oral nonabsorbable antibiotics can delay infections briefly in the highly susceptible neutropenic host, but patients' acceptance of this form of therapy is poor. Gamma globulin therapy can be helpful in patients with agammaglobulinemia (Chap. 62), but is of no benefit to most patients with multiple myeloma or other hypogammaglobulinemic states in which there is low, but detectable, serum IgG. Active and passive immunization to prevent specific infections and the use of prophylactic granulocyte transfusions are under investigation. Protective isolation with laminar airflow rooms, sterile food, and antibiotic treatment will prevent or delay infection and probably is useful when the duration of maximum susceptibility to the infection is no longer than a few days to a few weeks.

SPECIFIC INFECTIONS Certain organisms are encountered as pathogens almost exclusively in the compromised host, e.g., *Pneumocystis carinii, Phycomyces,* and *Aspergillus.* Others, e.g., *Candida, Histoplasma,* herpes simplex, and cytomegalovirus, are common pathogens for both the normal and compromised host. The following organisms are encountered frequently or present special problems. Separate chapters in the text deal with each of these and their treatment in greater detail.

Staphylococcus In general, staphylococcal infections are not inordinately difficult to manage in the compromised host. Staphylococcal infections related to intravenous catheters present a special problem. Although it is always best to remove the catheter, it may be possible, on occasion, to cure infections caused by antibiotic-sensitive staphylococci at the site of arteriovenous shunts and at the tips of chronic parenteral nutrition catheters (Chap. 116).

Listeria   Bacteremia, peritonitis, and meningitis are encountered particularly in newborns, alcoholics, diabetics, and patients with lymphoreticular malignancies. The diagnosis may be missed initially because relatively few organisms are found in exudate (e.g., peritoneal fluid or cerebrospinal fluid) or the organism is confused with other gram-positive rods, such as diphtheroids, and regarded as a contaminant (Chap. 132).

Corynebacterium   Diphtheroids are among the most common organisms encountered as contaminants of blood cultures. With increasing frequency, however, they are being found as the cause of significant bacteremias, particularly in severely ill patients with intravenous catheters and cerebrospinal fluid reservoirs and shunts.

Gram-negative bacilli   *E. coli, Pseudomonas, Proteus,* and other Enterobacteriaceae remain the major pathogens for patients with compromised host defenses. The portal for entry is generally the gastrointestinal tract. Gram-negative bacteremia, pneumonia, and meningitis are well recognized. *Ecthyma gangrenosum* is an important clue to early recognition of *Pseudomonas* sepsis (Chaps. 120 and 121).

Mycobacterium   With the declining frequency of pulmonary tuberculosis in the United States, an increasing proportion of cases involve patients with compromised host defenses who often present with unusual manifestations of the disease. For this reason it is important to know the tuberculin status of every patient with a chronic debilitating disease which may predispose the patient to infections or which may require treatment with corticosteroids or immunosuppressive drugs. The practice of treating all tuberculin-positive patients receiving steroids with isoniazid is becoming less frequent with recognition of the toxicity of the drug and the relatively small risk of activation of latent disease, at least in certain conditions such as asthma and rheumatoid arthritis. However, this approach necessitates careful follow-up of every tuberculin reactor (Chap. 143).

Candida   This organism has emerged as a major cause for superinfection in the compromised host. *Candida* pharyngitis, laryngitis, esophagitis, pneumonia, and candidemia are common in patients with reduced host defenses who are receiving broad-spectrum antibiotics. The diagnosis of disseminated candidiasis often poses considerable difficulty (Chap. 158).

Histoplasma   Disseminated histoplasmosis is becoming an increasingly important problem, particularly among patients with Hodgkin's disease, chronic lymphocytic leukemia, acute lymphocytic leukemia, and those undergoing intensive immunosuppressive therapy. Both reactivation of latent infections and inordinately severe initial infections have been documented. It is important to establish because the infection responds well to amphotericin in many instances (Chap. 155).

Nocardia   See Chap. 152.

Aspergillus   See Chap. 159.

Phycomyces   See Chap. 160.

Herpes zoster   Disseminated Herpes zoster infections occur with increased frequency in disorders of cellular immunity, especially Hodgkin's disease and chronic lymphocytic leukemia, and in patients receiving corticosteroids and immunosuppressive drugs (Chap. 185).

Herpes simplex   Disseminated infections with diffuse skin lesions, pneumonitis, encephalitis, and hepatitis have been increasing, especially in renal transplant patients and in others receiving intensive immunosuppression (Chap. 193).

Cytomegalovirus   See Chap. 194.

Toxoplasmosis   See Chap. 203.

Pneumocystis   See Chap. 204.

REFERENCES

ALLEN JC: *Infections and the Compromised Host.* Baltimore, Williams & Wilkens, 1976

CLIFT RA et al: Granulocyte transfusions for prevention of infection in patients receiving bone marrow transplants. N Engl J Med 298:1052, 1978

CLINE MJ: *The White Cell.* Cambridge, Mass, Harvard University Press, 1975

CODISH SD, TOBIAS JS: Managing systemic mycoses in the compromised host. JAMA 235:2132, 1976

EDITORIAL: Infective hazards of splenectomy. Lancet 1:1167, 1976

FAUCI AS et al: Glucocorticosteroid therapy: Mechanisms of action and clinical considerations. Ann Intern Med 84:304, 1976

FEIGIN RD, SHEARER WT: Opportunistic infection in children. J Pediatr 87:507, 677, 852, 1975

GREENMAN RL et al: Lung biopsy in the immunocompromised host. Am J Med 59:488, 1975

GURWITH MJ et al: Granulocytopenia in hospitalized patients: I. Prognostic factors and etiology of fever. Am J Med 64:121, 1978

LEVINE AS et al: Hematologic malignancies and other marrow failure states: Progress in management of complicating infections. Semin Hematol 11:141, 1974

NIEMAN PE et al: A prospective analysis of interstitial pneumonia and opportunistic viral infection among recipients of allogeneic bone marrow graft. J Infect Dis 136:754, 1977

RODRIQUEZ V et al: Randomized trial of protected environment–prophylactic antibiotics in 145 adults with acute leukemia. Medicine 57:253, 1978

SCHIMPF SC et al: Three antibiotic regimens in the treatment of infections in febrile granulocytopenic patients with cancer. J Infect Dis 137:14, 1978

SMITH FG, PALMER DL: Alcoholism, infection and altered host defenses: A review of clinical and experimental observations. J Chron Dis 29:35, 1976

VALDIVIESO M et al: Gram-negative bacillary pneumonia in the compromised host. Medicine 56:241, 1977

108
HOSPITAL-ACQUIRED INFECTIONS

PIERCE GARDNER
WILLIAM A. CAUSEY

DEFINITION   Hospital-acquired infections (also called *nosocomial infections*) are significant causes of human morbidity and mortality. They may be defined as clinical infections occurring in patients after admission to the hospital that were neither present nor in a period of incubation at the time of admission. Also included are infections that are contracted in the hospital but do not become clinically evident until after the patient is discharged. Although many of these infections can be prevented, some cannot, and the term *hospital-acquired infection* should not be equated with *iatrogenic infection,* which is usually defined as an infection caused by a diagnostic or therapeutic maneuver such as insertion of an urethral or intravenous catheter. Infections caused by organisms in the patient's own flora are termed *autochthonous infections* and are often unavoidable because they are related to defects in mucosal barriers or other host defenses rather than being preventable environmental risks.

EPIDEMIOLOGY Incidence and cost

Hospital acquired infections occur in from 2 to 15 percent of patients admitted to general hospitals. The highest infection rates are recorded in municipal hospitals and tertiary care centers such as university hospitals, while the prevalence of these infections is much lower in community hospitals. Hospital-acquired infections have a mortality rate of approximately 1 percent and contribute to death in an additional 3 percent of cases. Estimates for the United States indicate that 1.5 million hospital-acquired infections occur annually, cause 15,000 deaths, and contribute to mortality in an additional 45,000 patients. The prolongation in hospital stays and additional diagnostic tests, medications, and physicians' fees contribute significantly to the high cost of hospital care.

ETIOLOGY Causative pathogens

Gram-negative bacilli dominate the list of nosocomial pathogens, although *Staphylococcus aureus,* the scourge of the 1950s and early 1960s, remains an important pathogen in all sites except the urinary tract (Table 108-1). During the past decade antibiotic susceptibility patterns of the gram-positive cocci have remained relatively stable. However, the isolation of strains of pneumococci resistant to penicillins and cephalosporins in South Africa and the possible significance of bacterial tolerance (organisms are inhibited but not killed by bactericidal drugs) among isolates of *S. aureus* to β-lactamase–resistant penicillins suggest that important problems with antimicrobial resistance may lie ahead. The

gram-negative bacilli have tended to develop resistance to many of the antimicrobial agents in common use. In large part, this resistance is due to the acquisition of plasmids called *resistance factors* (R factors). R-factor plasmids consist of extrachromosomal circular deoxyribonucleic acid (DNA) which mediates antibiotic resistance by coding for enzymes that inactivate the drug or by conferring properties altering the permeability of the bacterial cell wall to the drug. Two properties of R factors are of major public health concern: (1) resistance to several antibiotics is often linked on the same R factor, and (2) R-factor transfer can occur across species lines from one gram-negative organism to another. Under the appropriate selective conditions these properties make possible the rapid dissemination of multiple antibiotic resistance among a wide variety of gram-negative pathogens.

Whatever the mechanism, the major reason for the development of antimicrobial-resistant bacteria in the hospital setting is the use of antibiotics. These drugs tend to eliminate susceptible bacteria in the host's own flora, leading to replacement by antibiotic-resistant organisms. Once colonized by these organisms, susceptible individuals may develop clinical infections. The importance of antibiotics as a selective force favoring the emergence of resistant bacteria is emphasized by the observation that a number of hospital epidemics have been aborted by limiting the use of some of these drugs and by interdicting others altogether (Chap. 114).

Opportunistic infections (Chap. 107) may be defined as infections occurring in patients with impaired host defenses which would not ordinarily occur in normal hosts. Commonly they are due to pathogens that do not ordinarily cause disease in healthy persons but colonize and invade individuals whose host defenses are faulty. These infections have become so frequent that *Candida* spp. appears among the list of most com-

TABLE 108-1
Incidence* and relative frequency† of selected pathogens causing nosocomial infections, by site of infection, January to December 1976

	Primary bacteremia	Surgical wound	Lower respiratory	Urinary tract	Cutaneous	Other	All sites
Staphylococcus aureus	2.1 (12.8%)	18.9 (15.5%)	7.4 (10.4%)	2.9 (1.7%)	8.7 (33.7%)	5.8 (12.7%)	45.8 (10.0%)
Staphylococcus epidermidis	1.3 (7.7%)	5.5 (4.5%)	0.4 (0.5%)	5.1 (2.9%)	1.1 (4.3%)	1.6 (3.5%)	15.0 (3.3%)
Streptococcus, group D	1.2 (7.4%)	12.7 (10.3%)	0.9 (1.2%)	24.4 (13.9%)	1.6 (6.1%)	2.7 (5.9%)	43.5 (9.6%)
Escherichia coli	2.4 (14.3%)	19.1 (15.7%)	5.2 (7.2%)	55.3 (31.7%)	2.2 (8.5%)	4.2 (9.2%)	88.4 (19.4%)
Klebsiella spp.	1.8 (10.6%)	6.4 (5.2%)	7.9 (11.1%)	15.3 (8.8%)	1.1 (4.3%)	2.1 (4.6%)	34.6 (7.6%)
Enterobacter spp.	0.9 (5.2%)	4.9 (4.0%)	4.7 (6.5%)	7.2 (4.1%)	0.8 (3.1%)	1.1 (2.4%)	19.6 (4.3%)
Proteus-Providencia spp.	0.6 (3.6%)	8.6 (7.1%)	4.0 (5.6%)	18.2 (10.4%)	1.4 (5.5%)	2.6 (5.7%)	35.4 (7.8%)
Pseudomonas aeruginosa	0.9 (5.2%)	5.0 (4.1%)	5.2 (7.3%)	15.5 (8.9%)	1.2 (4.7%)	2.2 (4.8%)	30.0 (6.6%)
Candida spp.	0.5 (3.3%)	1.0 (0.8%)	2.5 (3.5%)	7.3 (4.2%)	0.7 (2.9%)	3.8 (8.3%)	15.8 (3.5%)
All pathogens	16.6 (100.0%)	121.9 (100.0%)	71.4 (100.0%)	174.6 (100.0%)	25.7 (100.0%)	45.9 (100.0%)	456.1 (100.0%)
Secondary bacteremia	NA	3.8 (3.1%)	3.0 (4.1%)	4.5 (2.6%)	1.3 (5.0%)	3.7 (7.9%)	16.3 (3.7%)

* *Incidence is number of isolates reported per 100,000 discharges; up to four isolates may be reported per infection.*
† *Relative frequency is expressed as percent of all isolates from each site.*
SOURCE: *Center for Disease Control, National Nosocomial Infections Study Report, Annual Summary 1976, Washington, DC, US Government Printing Office, 1978.*

mon nosocomial pathogens. Although surveillance and reporting of opportunistic viral and protozoan infections are variable, cytomegalovirus, *Pneumocystis carinii*, and *Toxoplasma gondii* have gained increased recognition as causes of hospital-acquired infection.

Transmission of nosocomial pathogens Even before the recognition of bacteria as causative agents of disease, Ignaz Semmelweis, by simple epidemiologic methods, identified the contaminated hands of physicians and medical students as the major transmitters of puerperal sepsis, the most significant hospital-acquired infection of his day. Although the major sites and pathogens of hospital-acquired infection have changed during the past century, contact with hospital personnel remains the principal mode of spread of nosocomial pathogens. Usually, transmission occurs via the hands of hospital personnel, but other skin surfaces and respiratory droplets may also be important. Inanimate sources of hospital-associated microorganisms include food and drinking water, sinks and bath water, ventilation systems, contaminated horizontal surfaces, and the catheters and equipment needed for life-support systems and diagnostic procedures.

A *common-source epidemic* occurs when a single contaminating source is responsible for multiple infections. In this situation, patients commonly become colonized with hospital-associated bacteria following exposure to a particular procedure or area of the hospital. The epidemiologic steps in the evaluation of a common-source epidemic include recognition of a clustering of infections in both time and place, use of antibiotic susceptibility patterns or other biologic markers to allow more precise definition of the epidemic strain, and analysis of the geographic distribution and diagnostic experiences which are common to the infected patients but absent in the noninfected patients.

Host factors The age and underlying disease of patients, the integrity of their mucosal and integumentary surfaces, and the status of their immunological defenses are among the major determinants of both the incidence and outcome of hospital-acquired infections (Chap. 107).

COMMON HOSPITAL-ACQUIRED INFECTIONS Urinary tract infections These infections account for approximately 40 percent of hospital-acquired infections and are usually a consequence of instrumentation of the urethra, bladder, or kidneys. The most common predisposing factor is the insertion of an indwelling urethral catheter which permits bacteria to ascend from the external environment to the bladder. Hospital surveys show that 10 to 15 percent of all adult patients have indwelling catheters, a number of which appear to be unnecessary. Because the urinary tract is the most common site of infection resulting in secondary bacteremia, preventive measures involving urethral catheters should be a major focus of efforts to reduce the frequency of gram-negative sepsis in hospitalized patients. Several principles should be followed in managing urethral catheters in hospitalized patients:

1 Indwelling catheters should not be used unless they are required for management of bladder outlet obstruction or for close monitoring of fluid and electrolyte balance in severely ill patients.
2 There should be rigorous adherence to sterile technique during insertion of the catheter.
3 Maintaining a system of closed drainage is essential and can usually keep the urine sterile for 5 to 7 days. After that, the risk of infection increases with time, 5 to 10 percent for each day of catheterization.

4 In catheterized patients, specimens of urine for laboratory tests should be aspirated from the catheter by use of a sterile syringe, and the collecting tubing and bag must be unobstructed and in a dependent position.
5 Daily perineal care including the application of antibacterial ointment at the meatal-catheter junction may also be of benefit.
6 Occasionally, intermittent straight catheterization for patients with anticipated short-term needs for bladder drainage may avoid an indwelling catheter altogether.

Wound infections Most surgical wound infections are due to organisms introduced into the tissues at the time of the operative procedures. Most infecting organisms originate from the resident skin flora of the patient, and airborne bacteria are of little consequence in the etiology of wound infections. The major factors affecting the incidence of wound infection include the type of operation, its duration, the skill of the surgeon, and the basic health of the patient. Operations involving contaminated sites such as the bowel or a previously infected area are more likely to be complicated by infection than sites which are clean prior to surgery. Operations of long duration or in which devitalized tissue, foreign bodies, or hematomas are left behind are associated with a high rate of wound infection. Other factors predisposing to wound infection include advanced age, poor nutritional status, the presence of distant foci of infection, diabetes mellitus, renal failure, and corticosteroid therapy.

Most wound infections appear from 3 to 7 days following surgery. Early postoperative wound infections (those occurring within 24 to 48 h of surgery) are commonly caused by group A *Streptococcus* or *Clostridium* spp. Gram-stained smears of wound exudate, followed by culture, may provide valuable early clues to the bacterial etiology in wound infections. Staphylococcal wound infections characteristically become evident 4 to 6 days after surgery, and those caused by gram-negative bacilli and anaerobic bacteria may not appear for a week or more. If perioperative antibiotics are used, the manifestations of infection may be delayed.

In addition to emphasis on maintaining sterility in the operating room and insistence on operative techniques that minimize tissue trauma and blood loss, increased attention is being given to preventing postoperative wound infections with short prophylactic courses of systemic antibiotics during the perioperative period. The principles that should govern this use of antibiotics include (1) beginning the drug during the immediate preoperative period but not earlier, (2) assuring adequate tissue levels throughout surgery by giving intraoperative doses of antibiotics if necessary, and (3) discontinuing antibiotic prophylaxis within 24 to 48 h of surgery. This use of antibiotics does not appear to significantly alter the flora or promote colonization with resistant strains. Prolonged pre- and postoperative courses are unnecessary, expensive, and potentially harmful because of toxicity or superinfection. Antibiotic prophylaxis administered according to these principles has been reported to reduce infectious morbidity in a variety of orthopedic, gynecologic, and abdominal operations. The antibiotics used for surgical prophylaxis should be aimed at the most likely causative organisms (Chap. 111). Examples are *Escherichia coli* in biliary tree and gynecologic surgery and staphylococci in vascular and cardiac surgery.

Nonsurgical wounds that are common sites of nosocomial infection include burns, injection sites, decubitus ulcers, and cutaneous ulcers resulting from venous or arterial occlusive disease. In general, the offending pathogens are similar to those found in wound infections, with the exception that burn wound infections and soft tissue\infections in neutropenic patients frequently are caused by *Pseudomonas aeruginosa*. Bacteremic *Pseudomonas* infections may result in bacterial arteritis and cutaneous infarction manifested by hemorrhagic bullae (ecthyma gangrenosum, Chap. 121).

Pneumonia Lower respiratory tract infections are the leading cause of mortality among hospital-acquired infections, although they rank third in incidence behind urinary tract infections and wound infections. The major pathogens are the gram-negative bacilli and *S. aureus*, all of which are invasive and characteristically cause a necrotizing bronchopneumonia. These organisms reach the lower respiratory tract by inhalation or aspiration rather than by hematogenous spread. The observation that the pharyngeal flora of seriously ill patients consists predominantly of gram-negative bacilli is consistent with the pathogenesis of this infection. The three settings in which nosocomial pneumonias most commonly occur are (1) in obtunded patients whose gag reflex and cough are ineffective, (2) in patients with underlying pulmonary disease or congestive heart failure whose pulmonary clearance mechanisms are impaired, and (3) in patients who require respiratory tract instrumentation or ventilatory assistance.

Positioning the patient in a swimmer's or Gatch position is the cornerstone of preventing aspiration by obtunded patients. Frequent suctioning of secretions using sterile technique, particularly from intubated or tracheostomized patients, is also an important prophylactic measure. Treatment of congestive failure will improve the effectiveness of the lung's defenses and will also reduce pulmonary edema fluid which serves as an excellent culture medium. Respiratory assistance apparatus must be maintained in the most nearly sterile state possible. Moreover, intermittent positive pressure breathing as part of routine perioperative care is often unnecessary and subjects the patients to the infectious risk inherent in exposure to ventilatory equipment. Finally, regular monitoring of the respiratory flora, particularly in intubated patients, with gram-stained smears and cultures provides useful information in choosing appropriate early therapy for pulmonary superinfections, should they occur.

Hospital transmission of viral respiratory pathogens is common especially on pediatric services but, except for influenza and respiratory syncytial virus (in infants), rarely results in severe disease. When influenza A is widespread in the community, amantadine prophylaxis, as well as immunization, should be considered for unimmunized hospital patients identified as being at high risk for complications of influenza.

Bacteremia Although bacterial invasion of the bloodstream can occur in any nosocomial infection, the infected intravenous cannula is one of the most common and also most remediable causes of hospital-acquired bacteremia. Annually in the United States more than 10 million persons (more than one in four hospitalized patients) receive intravenous therapy, and even a low rate of complications will involve a large number of patients. Intravenous devices account for about 5 percent of all nosocomial infections and 10 percent of all positive blood cultures. The most common isolates from catheter tips are *S. epidermidis, S. aureus,* gram-negative bacilli (especially *Klebsiella, Enterobacter, Serratia*), and enterococci. Although microorganisms can enter at any point, the intravenous system most commonly is contaminated at the site of cannula entry during insertion and subsequent manipulation, and at the connecting points of the intravenous set to the cannula and to the intravenous fluid bag. Intravenous fluids also may become contaminated in the process of manufacture or as a result of addition of medications. The type of intravenous cannula, the choice of intravenous site, the adequacy of skin preparation, and the length of time during which the cannula is in use are important determinants of the risk of septic complications. Steel needles, especially scalp vein needles, are preferable to plastic cannulae which have greater risks of local phlebitis, contamination, and

sepsis. For example, suppurative phlebitis, the most feared complication of cannula-related infections, is virtually unknown with steel needles. Arms are better intravenous sites than legs owing to the lower rate of phlebitis and sepsis. The risk of bacteremia increases with time and is unacceptably high when cannulas are left in place longer than 48 to 72 h. Prolonged use of an intravenous site and failure to remove the cannula at the earliest sign of inflammation or cannula malfunction are common errors. Preventive measures designed to reduce the incidence of intravenous-associated infections are listed in Table 108-2. With meticulous care, catheters used for parenteral hyperalimentation can be maintained free of infection for prolonged periods. However, infectious complications, particularly *Candida* sepsis, are not uncommon in this setting.

Transient bacteremias frequently follow diagnostic or therapeutic manipulations of the mouth or the respiratory, gastrointestinal, or genitourinary tract and are usually well tolerated by the normal host. However, the patient with valvular or congenital heart disease (or a valve prosthesis) may be at risk of developing endocarditis and should receive antibiotic prophylaxis when undergoing procedures associated with significant risk of bacteremia (Chap. 243). These procedures include dental manipulations, urinary tract instrumentation, abdominal surgery, and other surgery involving infected tissue. For patients with prosthetic heart valves, these recommendations have been extended. Detailed programs of prophylaxis are given in the chapter on infective endocarditis (Chap. 243).

Hepatitis B (see also Chap. 302) The risk of hospital-acquired hepatitis B is significant not only for patients, especially those who receive blood products or undergo renal dialysis, but also for hospital personnel who work with patients or handle their blood specimens. The widespread practice of screening blood products for hepatitis B surface antigen (HBsAg) has reduced markedly the incidence of posttransfusion hepatitis B. Currently most posttransfusion hepatitis is caused by unidentified agents (non-A, non-B hepatitis). However, hepatitis B remains an endemic problem on many renal dialysis and oncology services. Moreover, for unknown reasons, infections often are more severe in clinical and laboratory staff than in patients. Meticulous attention to precautions designed to limit spread of pathogens by direct contact is the major focus in the prevention of hepatitis B in dialysis units. Other important control measures include active serologic surveillance of patients and staff, attention to environmental cleanliness, and needle-blood precautions. Hepatitis B immunoglobulin (HBIG) contains high levels of antibodies to hepatitis B (anti-HBs) and is recommended for personnel directly exposed to HBsAg-positive

TABLE 108-2
Guidelines to reduce the incidence of intravenous-associated infections

1 Establish strict indications for use of intravenous fluid therapy.
2 Avoid high-risk sites, such as the leg.
3 Use stainless steel needles in preference to plastic catheters.
4 Adequately disinfect the skin over the intravenous site.
5 Use sterile technique in insertion of cannulas, including careful handwashing, sterile gloves, and, when possible, sterile drapes.
6 Securely anchor cannula to prevent to-and-fro motion.
7 Apply sterile dressing over intravenous site (topical antibiotic ointment optional).
8 Inspect the infusion site daily and remove cannula if inflammation, phlebitis, or cannula malfunction is present.
9 Change the cannula at frequent (~48 h) intervals.

SOURCE: *After Goldmann et al.*

material by accidental needle stick, mucous membrane contact, or oral ingestion.

Standard immunoglobulin (IG) usually contains some anti-HBs and may be effective for pre- and postexposure prophylaxis of hepatitis B. Prophylaxis with HBIG or standard IG for patients and personnel with continuing exposure to hepatitis B virus is not routinely recommended, but may be indicated in epidemic situations.

Considerable concern has been generated about the infectivity of the approximately 1 percent of physicians and dentists who are asymptomatic carriers of HBsAg. Although several instances of physician-to-patient transmission have been identified, the great majority of HBsAg-positive health care personnel do not appear to present a hazard to patients. While they have been encouraged to pay particular attention to handwashing and other measures to prevent contact spread, their patient-related activities need not necessarily be restricted.

CONTROL MEASURES **Infection control team** The goals of those concerned with infection control are (1) to reduce the risk of patients acquiring infections in the hospital, (2) to provide adequate care for patients with a potentially communicable infection, and (3) to minimize risks related to infections to employees, visitors, and community contacts. The functions of the infection control team include (1) development of enforceable policies necessary for appropriate management of patients with communicable infections; (2) development of a surveillance system which identifies patients with communicable infections, quantitates the incidence and prevalence of hospital-acquired infection, and investigates problems that are likely to be remediable; (3) liaison with personnel from nursing, central supply, housekeeping, maintenance, pharmacy, and other services to ensure that appropriate cleaning and sterilization techniques and materials are employed, and to permit evaluation of new germicides and other products as they become available; (4) education of employees in appropriate techniques to prevent spread of infectious agents within the hospital; (5) communication with employee health services to ensure adequate immunizations and to provide whatever care is necessary for susceptible personnel exposed to a communicable disease; and (6) monitoring of antibiotic utilization and the susceptibility patterns of common nosocomial pathogens. Most large hospitals employ full-time nurse(s) and/or physician(s), called *infection control officers*, to lead the multidisciplinary team effort that is necessary to carry out these functions.

Prevention Sir William Osler once remarked, "Soap, water and common sense are the best disinfectants." The basic principles of handwashing between patient contacts, appropriate isolation of patients harboring communicable organisms, and application of epidemiologic methods to identify and correct potential sources of infection remain the cornerstones of preventing nosocomial infections. Specific preventive measures related to particular hazards such as catheters and respirators have been mentioned in preceding sections.

EMPLOYEE HEALTH SERVICE Preventive medicine applies not only to patients but also to hospital personnel, and the employee health service should be encouraged to maintain surveillance for tuberculosis by tuberculin skin tests and/or chest x-rays and to immunize personnel who are susceptible to measles, mumps, poliomyelitis, diphtheria, or tetanus. The availability of improved influenza vaccines makes it rational to recommend annual immunization for all hospital personnel. Premenopausal women should be tested for antibodies to rubella, and rubella immunization should be offered to nonpreg-

nant susceptible women who are practicing effective contraception. Routine smallpox immunization of employees is no longer indicated. Hospital personnel who develop significant infections should be removed from patient contact during the period of communicability. Paronychias and other pustular lesions due to *S. aureus* or group A streptococci are often underrated by staff, and it is commonly forgotten that herpes zoster lesions may cause chickenpox in susceptible contacts.

ADMISSION SCREENING A patient scheduled for elective admission who has, or is thought to be incubating, a communicable disease should be sent home until the period of potential communicability has passed. Admission screening for communicable infections is particularly important for patients being admitted to oncology or dialysis services, which tend to have a high percentage of immunocompromised patients. Infections such as chickenpox and measles can be devastating in such patients, and their spread among them must be avoided at all costs.

CONTAINMENT Microorganisms can be spread from one person to another by several routes, including (1) contact, either directly from person to person or indirectly via contaminated equipment, linens, etc. (including contaminated hands); (2) airborne, via droplet nuclei reaching respiratory tract or wound surfaces; (3) vehicles, such as contaminated food, water, parenteral drugs, or blood; and (4) vectors, such as insects or arthropods.

Each pathogen has its characteristic mode(s) of spread, and, on the basis of this knowledge, isolation precautions can be tailored to fit the situation. Isolation procedures are time-consuming and expensive and can hinder needed patient care if applied too rigidly. They should be used only when necessary and for the shortest period consistent with good practice.

The following are the types of isolation and precautions in common use:

1 *Strict isolation,* where both airborne and contact transmission of an organism are possible, e.g., staphylococcal pneumonia.
2 *Respiratory isolation,* where the infectious agent is contained in airborne droplets of respiratory secretions, e.g., tuberculosis.
3 *Wound and skin isolation,* where direct or indirect contact with skin lesions or dressings may transmit the organism, e.g., a staphylococcal furuncle.
4 *Enteric precautions,* where transmission usually occurs via the fecal-oral route and contact with articles contaminated by feces is to be avoided, e.g., *Salmonella* gastroenteritis.
5 *Protective (reverse) isolation,* where the precautions are designed to protect the patient with impaired host defenses from organisms in the environment or carried by personnel, e.g., patients with total neutropenia or burns.
6 *Blood precautions,* where the transmission is by accidental inoculation or ingestion of blood or blood products, e.g., hepatitis B.

If preventive measures fail and a communicable infection develops in an inpatient, the following principles of containment should be observed:

1 Prevent further transmission of disease by the index case. This is usually accomplished by initiating appropriate isolation procedures or, if the patient's condition allows, arranging discharge home.
2 In cases of contagious disease, identify all contacts of the index case and determine their susceptibility and degree of exposure.
3 Give indicated prophylaxis to exposed susceptibles. The indications for passive immunization, active immunization,

and prophylaxis with antimicrobial agents vary with the pathogen (Chap. 114). The most common nosocomial infections requiring treatment of exposed susceptibles are hepatitis A and B.

4 Design a plan to prevent the spread of the infectious agent from the exposed susceptibles to other patients and personnel. This plan must take cognizance of the epidemiology of the communicable disease, the efficacy and feasibility of various control measures, and the potential consequences of further disease transmission.

The methods commonly employed to limit the tertiary spread of communicable diseases by exposed susceptibles are (1) early discharge of patients when feasible, (2) rearranging personnel assignments to avoid patient contact during the period of communicability, and (3) cohorting—grouping exposed susceptible patients (and personnel) together and treating them as an epidemiologic unit with appropriate precautions during the period of communicability. Cohorting is cumbersome but remains a major control measure for hospital outbreaks of chickenpox and epidemic diarrhea.

PROGNOSIS Most nosocomial infections are diseases of medical progress, and the ever-increasing orientation of modern medicine to technologically sophisticated procedures makes it likely that the risk of patients acquiring infections in the hospital will continue to increase. On the other hand, many of the factors that promote infections in the hospital have been identified, and measures for their control have been developed. Influencing hospital personnel to carry out these control measures, such as handwashing, catheter care, and restraint in the use of antibiotics, remains a major challenge.

REFERENCES

AMERICAN COLLEGE OF SURGEONS: *Manual in Control of Infections in Surgical Patients.* Philadelphia, Lippincott, 1976

BENENSON AS (ed): *Control of Communicable Diseases in Man,* 12th ed. Washington, DC, American Public Health Association, 1975

BENNETT JV, BRACHMAN PS: *Nosocomial Infections.* Boston, Little, Brown, 1978

CAMERON JL, ZUIDEMA GD: Aspiration pneumonia. JAMA 219:1194, 1972

CENTER FOR DISEASE CONTROL: *Isolation Techniques for Use in Hospitals,* 2d ed. Washington, DC, US Government Printing Office, 1975

EVERETT ED, HIRSCHMANN JV: Transient bacteremia and endocarditis prophylaxis. A review. Medicine 56:61, 1977

GARDNER P et al: Hospital isolation and precaution guidelines. Pediatrics 53:663, 1974

————— et al: Hospital management of patients and personnel exposed to communicable diseases. Pediatrics 56:700, 1975

GOLDMANN DA et al: Guidelines for infection control in intravenous therapy. Ann Intern Med 79:848, 1973

JOHANSON WG et al: Nosocomial respiratory infections with gram-negative bacilli. Ann Intern Med 77:701, 1972

SNYDMAN DR et al: Prevention of nosocomial viral hepatitis, type B. Ann Intern Med 83:838, 1975

STAMM WE: Guidelines for prevention of catheter-associated urinary tract infections. Ann Intern Med 82:386, 1975

STEERE AC, MALLISON GF: Handwashing practices for the prevention of nosocomial infections. Ann Intern Med 83:683, 1975

109
GRAM-NEGATIVE BACTEREMIA AND SEPTIC SHOCK

ROBERT G. PETERSDORF
DAVID C. DALE

DEFINITION Septic shock is characterized by inadequate tissue perfusion, usually following bacteremia with gram-negative enteric bacilli. Hypotension, oliguria, tachycardia, tachypnea, and fever are observed in most patients. The circulatory insufficiency is due principally to cell and tissue injury initiated by endotoxin and to the resultant pooling of blood in the microcirculation.

ETIOLOGY Septic shock may be associated with gram-positive infections, notably those due to pneumococci and streptococci, although it is more common following bacteremia with gram-negative bacilli: the Enterobacteriaceae (Chap. 120) and *Pseudomonas* and related organisms (Chap. 121). Gram-negative anaerobic bacteremia with *Bacteroides* species is also a precursor of septic shock, although in this situation the syndrome is less fulminating than with aerobic gram-negative bacilli. The shock syndrome is not due to bloodstream invasion with bacteria per se, but is related to release of endotoxin, the lipopolysaccharide moiety of the organisms' cell walls, into the circulation.

EPIDEMIOLOGY Gram-negative bacteremia and septic shock occur primarily in hospitalized patients who usually have underlying diseases which render them susceptible to bloodstream invasion. Predisposing factors include diabetes mellitus; cirrhosis; leukemia, lymphoma, or disseminated carcinoma; transplantation and its associated immunosuppression; childbirth; and a variety of surgical procedures and antecedent infections in the urinary, biliary, or gastrointestinal tracts. Most adults with gram-negative sepsis are elderly males, but neonates and child-bearing women are also prone to develop this syndrome. There has been an appreciable increase in the prevalence of serious gram-negative infections among hospitalized patients since 1935. The current incidence of gram-negative bacteremic sepsis is about 6 cases per 1000 hospital admissions. In addition to the predisposing factors mentioned above, the widespread use of antibiotics, immunosuppressive and cytotoxic agents, adrenal steroids, intravenous catheters, humidifiers, and other hospital equipment (Chaps. 107 and 108) and the increasing longevity of patients with chronic diseases contribute to this serious problem.

PATHOGENESIS AND PATHOLOGY With the exception of *Pseudomonas* and *Acinetobacter,* which are ubiquitous in the hospital environment, most of the bacteria causing gram-negative sepsis are normal commensals in the gastrointestinal tract. From there they may spread to contiguous structures, as in peritonitis after appendiceal perforation, or they may migrate from the perineum into the urethra or bladder. Gram-negative bacteremia follows infection in a primary focus, usually the genitourinary tract; biliary tree; gastrointestinal tract and adjoining structures or lungs; and, less commonly, the skin, bones, and joints. In patients with leukemia, the skin and subcutaneous tissues or the lungs are often portals of entry, as is also the case in burn patients. In many instances, however, notably in patients with debilitating diseases, cirrhosis, and cancer, no primary focus is apparent. When bacteremia is followed by metastatic lesions in distant sites, classic abscess formation occurs. More often, however, the autopsy findings in gram-negative sepsis reflect primarily the infection at the primary locus and show involvement of target organs: pulmonary edema, hemorrhage and hyaline membrane formation in the lungs; tubular or cortical necrosis in the kidney; patchy necrosis in the myocardium; superficial ulceration in the gastrointestinal tract; and generalized thrombi in the capillaries.

PATHOPHYSIOLOGY **Cellular injury in shock** Exposure of mammalian cells to endotoxin results in cell injury by several mechanisms: (1) direct cell membrane damage by endotoxin, (2) extracellular release of lysosomal enzymes from leukocytes, (3) activation of the complement cascade, and (4) metabolic injury due to tissue anoxia. The toxic component of endotoxin is principally lipid A. When endotoxin is administered to experimental animals, diffuse endothelial cell damage occurs. The cells show vacuolization and other cytoplasmic and nuclear abnormalities. There is diffuse desquamation of the endothelial cells, and the damaged cells often can be seen in the circulating blood. Endotoxin administration also causes an abrupt thrombocytopenia and granulocytopenia; in both instances this is attributed to endotoxin injury to these circulating blood elements. The damaged endothelial cells, leukocytes, and platelets all release substances activating blood coagulation, which leads to fibrin deposition in many tissues. The damaged platelets release the vasoactive substances serotonin and epinephrine. Polymorphonuclear leukocyte injury releases a variety of lysosomal enzymes as well as substances activating the complement system; the complement system is also activated directly by endotoxin, chiefly through the alternate complement pathway (Chap. 61).

Animal studies suggest a number of interactions between the complement system and the changes in platelets and leukocytes. Animals depleted of complement by pretreatment with cobra venom factor, which depletes C3 and later complement components, are less prone to develop thrombocytopenia and granulocytopenia after endotoxin than normal animals. Activation of complement in the circulation by endotoxin, specifically the component C5a, appears to increase granulocyte margination and may enhance the extracellular release of granulocyte enzymes. However, animals depleted of platelets or granulocytes and animals with congenital deficiencies in complement, e.g., C4 deficiency in guinea pigs and C6 deficiency in rabbits, are as susceptible to the lethal effects of endotoxin as normal animals are. These observations suggest that the critical initial event in septic shock is probably direct endothelial cell injury by endotoxin.

Cells in many tissues are also injured by the hypoxia that results from reduced tissue perfusion in endotoxic shock. The tissue injury closely resembles that occurring in hemorrhagic and cardiogenic shock. The result of hypoxia is uncoupling of oxidative phosphorylation and lactic acidosis.

Hemodynamic alterations Endotoxin exerts its major effects on small blood vessels with sympathetic (alpha-receptor) innervation. The toxin causes intense arteriolar and venospasm leading to significant immobilization of blood in the pulmonary, splanchnic, and renal capillaries, and to stagnant anoxia in these tissues. Through the activation of Hageman factor (factor XII), endotoxin activates bradykinin, a potent vasodilator which may be the humoral substance principally responsible for the pooling of blood in the peripheral tissues. It also increases capillary permeability. As a result, blood pools in the capillary bed and plasma proteins leak into the interstitial fluid. This, in turn, results in a sharp decrease in effective circulating blood volume and lowered cardiac output and systemic arterial hypotension, which stimulates the baroreceptors and results in further sympathetic activity, vasoconstriction, and selective reduction of blood flow to visceral organs and skin. If ineffective perfusion of vital organs is permitted to

continue, metabolic acidosis and severe parenchymal damage ensue, and shock is then irreversible. In man, the kidneys and lungs are the organs particularly susceptible to endotoxin; oliguria as well as tachypnea and, in some instances, pulmonary edema develop early. In general, the heart and brain are spared early in shock, and myocardial failure and coma are late and often terminal manifestations of the shock syndrome. There is also experimental evidence that, after the administration of live gram-negative bacteria, significant arteriovenous shunting occurs around the capillary beds of susceptible organs. This intensifies tissue anoxia. Finally, in some instances the cells seem unable to utilize available oxygen. The net result of defective tissue perfusion is a sharp decrease in arteriovenous (AV) oxygen difference and lactic acidemia.

Many of the observations dealing with the pathophysiology of endotoxin shock were made in animals, and the hemodynamic data often varied according to the species studied and the dose of endotoxin administered. The establishment of centers for the study of shock has permitted detailed pathophysiologic studies in man. The results of these studies may vary with the time at which they are performed. For example, early in septic shock, the picture is one primarily of vasodilatation with an increase in cardiac output, a decrease in systemic vascular resistance, a decrease in central venous pressure, and an increase in stroke volume. In contrast, later in septic shock, the predominant picture is one of vasoconstriction with an increase in systemic vascular resistance, a decrease in cardiac output, a decrease in central venous pressure, and a decrease in stroke volume. Despite these differences, certain patterns of septic shock have emerged when large groups of patients have been studied. These may be summarized as follows:

1. Shock characterized by a normal cardiac output, normal blood volume, normal circulation time, normal or high central venous pressure, normal or high pH, and *reduced* peripheral resistance. These patients have warm, dry skin. While hypotension, oliguria, and lactic acidemia are present, the prognosis is generally good. Shock in this group has been attributed to shunting of blood through arteriovenous communications, making it unavailable for perfusion of vital organs.

2. Patients with low blood volume, low central venous pressure, high hematocrit, increased peripheral resistance, low cardiac output, hypotension, oliguria, but only a moderate elevation of blood lactate and normal or slightly high pH. These patients may be hypovolemic before bacteremia, and their prognosis is reasonably good, provided intravascular volume is restored, bacteremia is treated with appropriate antibiotics, septic foci are removed or drained, and vasoactive drugs are given.

3. Shock characterized by normal blood volume, high central venous pressure, normal or high cardiac output, reduced peripheral resistance but *marked metabolic acidosis*, oliguria, and very high blood lactate, indicating ineffective tissue perfusion or impaired oxygen utilization. Despite the presence of warm, dry extremities in these patients, the prognosis is unfavorable.

4. Shock characterized by low blood volume, low central venous pressure, low cardiac output, marked decompensated metabolic acidosis, and severe lactic acidemia. In these patients the extremities are cool and cyanotic. The prognosis is extremely poor.

These observations suggest that there are various stages of septic shock, from hyperventilation, respiratory alkalosis, vasodilatation, and high or normal cardiac output in early shock, to perfusion failure characterized by high-grade lactic acidemia, metabolic acidosis, low cardiac output, and small AV oxygen difference in irreversible, late shock. Moreover, in some patients there is little correlation between the outcome and the hemodynamic abnormalities.

COMPLICATIONS Coagulation defects In most patients with septic shock there is a deficiency in several clotting factors, due to consumption of these factors, a syndrome termed *disseminated intravascular coagulation* (DIC). The pathogenesis of this syndrome involves the activation of the intrinsic clotting system by factor XII (Hageman factor) followed by deposition of fibrin-platelet aggregates on the capillary thrombi that have formed as a result of the generalized Shwartzman reaction. The fibrin-platelet aggregates are typical of DIC, which is characterized by a decrease in factors II, V, and VIII, fibrinogen, and platelets. There may be some degree of fibrinolysis, with appearance of split products. These clotting abnormalities are present to some degree in most patients with septic shock, but usually there is no clinical bleeding, although hemorrhagic phenomena due to thrombocytopenia or deficiency in clotting factors occur occasionally. A more important effect of further disseminated intravascular coagulation is development of capillary thrombi, particularly in the lung. Unless there is bleeding, the coagulopathy requires no therapy and disappears spontaneously as shock is treated.

Respiratory failure Respiratory failure is the most important cause of death in patients with shock, particularly after the hemodynamic aberrations have been corrected. The respiratory lesion has been called the "shock lung," and is characterized by pulmonary edema, hemorrhage, atelectasis, hyaline membrane formation, and formation of capillary thrombi. The severe pulmonary edema may be a consequence of a marked increase in capillary permeability, resulting in a "pulmonary leak." It may occur in the absence of heart failure. Respiratory failure may develop and progress even as other abnormalities return to normal. Pulmonary surfactant decreases, and pulmonary compliance becomes progressively compromised.

Renal failure Oliguria occurs early in shock and is probably due to low intravascular volume and inadequate renal perfusion. If renal perfusion remains inadequate, acute tubular necrosis develops. In an occasional patient, renal cortical necrosis, as occurs in the generalized Shwartzman reaction, is seen.

Cardiac failure Many patients with septic shock develop myocardial failure even though they were free of heart disease before development of shock. On the basis of experimental data, heart failure has been attributed to a product of lysosomal enzyme activity in the ischemic splanchnic region. This product has been termed myocardial depressant factor (MDF). Functionally, there is left ventricular failure as indicated by an increase in left ventricular end-diastolic pressure.

Other organs Superficial ulcerations of the gastrointestinal tract manifested by hemorrhage are common, as are abnormalities in liver function, characterized by hypoprothrombinemia, hypoalbuminemia, and mild jaundice.

CLINICAL MANIFESTATIONS Usually gram-negative bacteremia begins abruptly with chills, fever, nausea, vomiting, diarrhea, and prostration. When septic shock develops, there are, in addition, tachycardia; tachypnea; hypotension; cool, pale extremities, often with peripheral cyanosis; mental obtundation; and oliguria. When present in its full-blown form, gram-negative shock is detected readily, but occasionally the findings are quite subtle, particularly in old, debilitated patients or in infants. Unexplained hypotension, increasing confusion, and disorientation or hyperventilation may be the only clues to septic shock. Some patients are hypothermic, and in the absence of fever the diagnosis is often missed. Jaundice occurs

occasionally and signifies infection in the biliary tree, intravascular hemolysis, or "toxic" hepatitis. As shock progresses, oliguria persists, and heart failure, respiratory insufficiency, and coma supervene. Death usually occurs from pulmonary edema, generalized anoxemia secondary to respiratory insufficiency, cardiac arrhythmias, disseminated intravascular coagulation with bleeding, cerebral anoxia, or a combination of these factors.

LABORATORY FINDINGS The laboratory data in septic shock vary greatly and depend in many instances on the cause of the shock syndrome and on the stage of shock. The hematocrit is often elevated and falls to below normal as the volume deficit is repaired. There usually is *leukocytosis* with a white blood cell count between 15,000 and 30,000 per cubic millimeter with a shift to the left. However, the white blood cell count may be normal, and some patients have leukopenia. The *platelet count* is usually decreased, and the prothrombin time and partial thromboplastin times may be abnormal, reflecting a consumption of *clotting factors.*

The *urinalysis* shows no specific abnormalities. Initially, the specific gravity is high; as oliguria persists, isosthenuria develops. The *blood urea nitrogen* and *creatinine* are elevated, and creatinine clearance is reduced.

Simultaneous measurements of urine and plasma osmolalities are a useful clue to impending renal failure. If the urinary osmolality is greater than 400 mosmol and the ratio of urine to plasma osmolality is greater than 1.5, renal function is preserved and oliguria is probably due to volume depletion. On the other hand, a urine osmolality of less than 400 mosmol and a urine/plasma ratio less than 1.5 signify renal failure. Other useful clues to suggest prerenal azotemia are urine sodium less than 20 meq per liter, a urine creatinine/serum creatinine ratio greater than 40, or a BUN/serum creatinine ratio greater than 20. Electrolyte patterns vary considerably, but there is a tendency to *hyponatremia* and hypochloremia. The serum potassium may be high, low, or normal. The *bicarbonate concentration* is usually low and *blood lactate* is elevated. A high level of blood lactate is the most reliable clue to poor tissue perfusion.

Early in endotoxin shock there is *respiratory alkalosis* manifested by a low P_{CO_2} and high arterial pH, probably because of progressive anoxemia and an attempt to blow off CO_2 to compensate for developing lactic acidemia. As shock progresses, *metabolic acidosis* develops. There often is striking *anoxemia*, and P_{O_2} values below 70 mmHg are common. The *electrocardiogram* generally shows depression of the ST segment, inversion of the T waves, and a variety of arrhythmias, and may mistakenly suggest the diagnosis of myocardial infarction.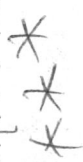

In untreated septic shock, the blood cultures should reveal the causative pathogens, but bacteremia may be intermittent and the blood cultures may be negative. Furthermore, many patients will have received antimicrobial agents when they are first seen, masking the bacteriologic diagnosis. *A negative blood culture does not exclude the diagnosis of septic shock.* Culture of the primary septic focus may aid in the diagnosis, but the bacteriology may have been altered by prior chemotherapy. The ability of endotoxin to coagulate the blood of the horseshoe crab *Limulus* is the basis of a test for endotoxemia, but this test is not widely available and is of limited clinical usefulness.

DIAGNOSIS The diagnosis of septic shock is not difficult in the presence of chills, fever, and an overt focus of infection. However, none of the obvious clues may be present. Elderly, debilitated patients, in particular, may have severe infections in the absence of fever. Unexplained confusion and disorientation and hyperventilation without abnormal chest x-rays should call the diagnosis to mind. Pulmonary embolism, myocardial infarction, cardiac tamponade, aortic dissection, and silent hemorrhage are entities often confused with septic shock.

COURSE The rational treatment of septic shock depends upon careful monitoring of patients. A flow sheet for recording clinical data is very helpful. Specifically four parameters need to be followed at the bedside:

1 The status of the *pulmonary circulation* and, to a lesser extent, of left ventricular function should be monitored by insertion of a Swan-Ganz catheter. A pulmonary wedge pressure in excess of 15 to 18 cmH_2O signifies fluid overload. When a Swan-Ganz catheter is not available, the *central venous pressure* (CVP) should be measured. Insertion of a catheter into the great veins or right atrium provides an accurate index of the relation between right ventricular competence and effective blood volume and should be used as a guide to fluid replacement therapy. When the CVP exceeds 12 to 14 cmH_2O, there is some danger of overloading the circulation and precipitating pulmonary edema. It is important to be sure that the flow through the catheter is free and that the catheter is not in the right ventricle. Either a Swan-Ganz catheter or a CVP line should be placed in every patient with septic shock.

2 The *pulse pressure* serves as an estimate of stroke volume.

3 *Cutaneous vasoconstriction* provides a clue to peripheral resistance, although it does not reflect accurately blood flow to kidney, brain, or gut.

4 Hourly *urine output* should be used to monitor splanchnic blood flow and visceral perfusion. Usually this requires placement of an indwelling urethral catheter.

By means of these four measurements the patient with shock can be followed carefully and managed intelligently. Indirect arterial blood pressure does not provide an accurate picture of the hemodynamic situation, and perfusion of vital organs may be adequate in patients with hypotension; conversely, some patients with normal blood pressures may have marked pooling and inadequate visceral blood flow. Direct measurement of arterial pressure is helpful but usually not necessary.

Where possible, these patients should be treated in intensive care units in hospitals that have laboratories available for measurement of arterial pH, blood gases, blood lactate, renal function, and electrolytes.

TREATMENT **Support of respiration** In many patients with septic shock arterial P_{O_2} is markedly depressed. It is essential to establish an airway at the outset and to administer oxygen nasally or by mask. Tracheal intubation usually suffices; tracheostomy is rarely necessary. However, a positive pressure–volume-cycled respirator should be employed early to achieve proper ventilation and to overcome the severe hypoxia.

Volume replacement With the CVP or pulmonary wedge pressure as a guide, blood volume should be replaced with blood (if anemia is present), plasma, or other colloids, especially human serum albumin, and appropriate electrolyte solutions, primarily dextrose-saline and bicarbonate (which is preferable to lactate for treating the acidosis). Bicarbonate should be given to increase the blood pH to about 7.2 to 7.3 but not higher under most circumstances. The quantity of fluid required may be considerably in excess of "normal" blood volume and may amount to 8 to 12 liters in only a few hours. Large quantities may be required even when the cardiac index

is normal. Oliguria in the presence of hypotension is not a contraindication to continued vigorous fluid therapy. In order to guard against pulmonary edema, diuresis with furosemide should be attempted when the CVP reaches a level of approximately 10 to 12 cmH_2O and the pulmonary artery pressure 16 to 18 cmH_2O.

Antibiotics Blood cultures and cultures of relevant body fluids or exudates should be taken before instituting antimicrobial therapy. Drugs should be given intravenously, and bactericidal agents used when possible. When the results of blood cultures and sensitivities are known, one of the appropriate drugs recommended in the chapters dealing with the specific infections and discussed in Chap. 111 should be given. Usually cultures and sensitivities are not at hand at the onset of shock, and the etiologic diagnosis entails an educated guess based upon culture from the primary focus—urine, bile, pus, or sputum, or on the setting in which the infection occurs. For example, a young woman with dysuria, chills, and flank pain and septic shock is likely to have *Escherichia coli* bacteremia, while gram-negative sepsis in a burn patient is probably caused by *Pseudomonas*. The drugs of choice for gram-negative bacteremia are:

E. coli	Ampicillin or a parenteral cephalosporin
Klebsiella-	Gentamicin
Enterobacter	
Proteus mirabilis	Ampicillin or a parenteral cephalosporin
P. rettgeri,	Gentamicin and/or carbenicillin
morganii, or	
vulgaris	
Acinetobacter	Gentamicin and/or carbenicillin
Pseudomonas	Gentamicin and/or carbenicillin

The dosages and routes of administration for these agents are detailed in Chap. 111. A cephalosporin can be substituted for ampicillin in patients with a history of penicillin allergy. Because of its toxic effect on the vestibular portion of the eighth nerve, gentamicin must be given cautiously to oliguric patients; a single dose of 80 mg achieves blood levels which should suffice throughout the period of oliguria. Similar precautions should be taken with kanamycin, where the loading dose is 1.0 g.

When the cause of septic shock is unknown, therapy should be initiated with both gentamicin and a cephalosporin or a penicillinase-resistant penicillin; many physicians add carbenicillin to this regimen. If *Bacteroides* is suspected, chloramphenicol, 7-chlorlincomycin (clindamycin), or carbenicillin can be added. As soon as culture results become available, the unnecessary drugs can be deleted.

Surgical intervention Many patients with septic shock have an abscess, infarcted or necrotic bowel, inflamed gallbladder, infected uterus, pyonephrosis, or other local situations which lend themselves to surgical drainage or excision. As a rule, successful treatment of shock requires surgical intervention even if the patient is desperately ill. Operations should not be postponed "to get the patient in shape" because these patients' condition will continue to deteriorate unless the septic focus is removed or drained.

Vasoactive drugs Usually, septic shock is accompanied by maximal stimulation of alpha-adrenergic receptors, and pressor agents which act by stimulating these receptors, such as norepinephrine, levarterenol, and metaraminol are generally not indicated. The two groups of drugs which have been of value in septic shock are beta-receptor stimulants (notably isoproterenol and dopamine) and alpha-receptor blocking agents (phenoxybenzamine and phentolamine).

Dopamine hydrochloride is used widely for treatment of

shock. Unlike other vasoactive agents, this drug increases renal blood flow and with it glomerular filtration, sodium excretion, and urine flow. This effect is seen at low doses [1 to 2 (μg/kg)/min]. At a dose of 2 to 10 (μg/kg)/min, the beta receptors in the heart are stimulated with a resulting increase in cardiac output but without increase in heart rate or blood pressure. Between 10 and 20 (μg/kg)/min there is some effect on the alpha receptors with a rise in blood pressure. Above 20 (μg/kg)/min, alpha stimulation predominates, and vasoconstriction may reverse the dopaminergic effects on the renal and splanchnic circulations. Treatment should be started at 2 to 5 (μg/kg)/min and the dose increased until urine flow and blood pressure respond. Most patients respond to doses of 20 (μg/kg)/min or less. Side effects include ectopic rhythms, nausea and vomiting, and occasionally tachyarrhythmias. They usually disappear with reduction in dosage.

Isoproterenol (Isuprel) counteracts arteriolar and venous constriction in the microcirculation by its direct vasodilating effect. In addition, the drug exerts a direct inotropic effect on the heart. Cardiac output is increased by stimulation of the myocardium and by reduction of cardiac work as peripheral resistance decreases. The dose of isoproterenol is 2 to 8 μg/min for the average adult. Ventricular arrhythmias may result from this drug, and shock may be made worse if fluid administration does not keep pace with relieved vasoconstriction.

Phenoxybenzamine (Dibenzyline), an adrenolytic agent, effects a central phlebotomy by reducing resistance and increasing intravascular capacity. Hence there is a redistribution of blood. Blood leaves the lungs, relieving pulmonary edema and enhancing gas exchange. Central venous pressure and left ventricular end-diastolic pressure fall, cardiac output rises, and peripheral venous constriction regresses. The recommended dose is 0.2 to 2.0 mg/kg intravenously. Small doses can be injected instantaneously and large doses over a period of 40 to 60 min. Fluids must be given simultaneously to compensate for the increment in venous capacitance; failure to do so aggravates shock. Dibenzyline is not available for general use, and experience with phentolamine has not been great enough to recommend it.

Chlorpromazine in multiple small doses of 2.5 to 5 mg also relieves vasoconstriction through its direct adrenolytic effect and by ganglionic blockage.

Diuretics and digitalis   It is important to maintain urine flow to try to prevent the development of renal tubular necrosis. Once the volume status of the patient is repaired, a diuretic, preferably furosemide, should be given to keep the hourly urine output up to greater than 30 to 40 ml/h. In patients who remain hypotensive despite an elevated CVP or pulmonary wedge pressure, digitalization with digoxin or Cedilanid may be beneficial. Therapy with digitalis preparations should be undertaken with caution in patients with impaired renal function, elevated serum potassium, and severe acid-base abnormalities.

Glucocorticosteroids   Numerous experimental studies provide a rationale for the use of corticosteroid therapy to ameliorate the effects of endotoxemia and septic shock. Steroids appear to protect cell membranes from endotoxin-mediated injury and to decrease platelet aggregation and the extracellular release of leukocyte enzymes. Some studies suggest that steroids also may have a direct effect on reducing peripheral vascular resistance. Because of the complexity of the clinical circumstances surrounding the patient with endotoxic shock, it has been difficult to prove that steroid therapy is clearly helpful. One controlled study has demonstrated a substantial benefit for treating patients with methylprednisolone (30 mg/kg) or dexamethasone (3 mg/kg) as soon as shock was recognized. Therapy was repeated in 4 h in the most severely ill patients. This study and experience in many shock centers supports the early use of steroids in high doses for relatively brief periods (24 to 48 h). Prolonged steroid therapy substantially increases the problems of hyperglycemia, gastrointestinal bleeding, and other steroid side effects and should be avoided.

Other measures   Hemorrhage must be controlled with whole blood, fresh frozen plasma, cryoprecipitate, or platelet transfusion, depending on the clotting abnormality. Treatment of disseminated intravascular coagulation with heparin remains a controversial and hazardous procedure. Hyperbaric oxygen has been tried in gram-negative bacteremia with indifferent results.

PROGNOSIS   The measures described above usually will resuscitate most patients, at least temporarily. Indicators of a favorable response are:

1 Improved sensorium and general appearance
2 Decreased peripheral cyanosis
3 Warming of the skin over the extremities
4 Urine output of 40 to 50 ml/h
5 Increased pulse pressure
6 Return of CVP and pulmonary artery pressure to normal
7 Increased blood pressure

The ultimate outcome, however, is dependent upon several other factors:

1 Ability to eliminate the source of infection with surgery or antibiotics. The prognosis of urinary tract infections, septic abortions, abdominal abscesses, gastrointestinal or biliary fistulas, and subcutaneous or anorectal abscesses is better than that of primary foci in the skin or lungs. However, extensive abdominal surgery, even if necessary, is associated with a poor prognosis.
2 Previous contact with the organism. Patients with chronic urinary tract infections who develop bacteremia rarely have severe gram-negative shock, perhaps because they have become tolerant to the endotoxin.
3 Underlying disease. Patients with lymphoma or leukemia who develop septic shock while their hematologic disease is out of control rarely recover; conversely, if hematologic remission is achieved, the shock is more likely to respond to therapy. Patients with antecedent heart disease and with diabetes mellitus also have a poor prognosis.
4 Metabolic status. The development of severe metabolic acidosis and lactic acidemia—irrespective of cardiac output—is associated with a poor prognosis.
5 Development of pulmonary insufficiency even after the hemodynamic abnormalities have been corrected is associated with an unfavorable outcome.

The overall mortality rate of septic shock remains 50 percent; however, with better monitoring and more physiologic treatment, the outcome should improve.

PREVENTION   The poor results in the treatment of septic shock are not due to lack of potent antibiotics or vasoactive agents. Rather, failure to institute therapy sufficiently early is a major roadblock to success. Septic shock usually is recognized too late, all too often after irreversible changes have taken place. Because 70 percent of patients who are likely to develop septic shock are in the hospital *before* signs and symptoms of shock appear, it is essential to watch patients who are candidates for development of shock assiduously, to treat their infections vigorously and early, and to perform appropriate surgery before catastrophic complications occur. It is particularly important to watch for infected venous and urinary catheters which may act as portals of entry for the organisms that cause gram-negative sepsis and to remove them from all patients as soon as feasible. There is some preliminary evidence that early therapy of septic shock improves the ultimate outcome. Finally, the protective effect of antiserum in experimental animals may, at some time in the future, be applicable to humans.

REFERENCES

BRYANT RD et al: Factors affecting mortality of gram-negative rod bacteremia. Arch Intern Med 127:120, 1971

CAVANAGH D et al: Septic shock in obstetrics and gynecology. Major Probl Obstet Gynecol 11:1, 1977

CORRIGAN JJ JR et al: Changes in the blood coagulation system associated with septicemia. N Engl J Med 279:851, 1968

FEARON DT et al: Activation of properdin pathway of complement in patients with gram-negative bacteremia. N Engl J Med 292:937, 1975

GOLDBERG LI: Dopamine: Clinical uses of an endogenous catecholamine. N Engl J Med 291:707, 1974

HARDAWAY RM et al: Intensive study and treatment of shock in man. JAMA 199:799, 1967.

JONES LW, WEIL MH: Water, creatinine and sodium excretion following circulatory shock with renal failure. Am J Med 41:314, 1971

MACLEAN LD et al: Patterns of septic shock in man: A detailed study of 56 patients. Ann Surg 166:543, 1967

MCHENRY MC, HANK WA: Bacteremia caused by gram-negative bacilli. Med Clin North Am 58:623, 1974

MILLER RI et al: Biochemical mechanisms of generation of bradykinin by endotoxin. J Infect Dis 128:S144, 1973

NISHIJIMA H et al: Hemodynamic and metabolic studies in shock associated with gram-negative bacteremia. Medicine 42:287, 1973

ROBIN ED et al: Capillary leak syndrome with pulmonary edema. Arch Intern Med 130:66, 1972

ROBINSON JA et al: Endotoxin, prekallikrein, complement and systemic vascular resistance. Am J Med 49:61, 1975

SCHUMER W: Steroids in the treatment of clinical septic shock. Ann Surg 184:333, 1976

TARAZI RC: Sympathomimetic agents in the treatment of shock. Ann Intern Med 81:364, 1974

ULEVITCH RJ et al: Role of complement in lethal bacterial lipopolysaccharide-induced hypotensive and coagulative changes. Infect Immun 19:204, 1978

WINSLOW EJ et al: Hemodynamic studies and results of therapy in 50 patients with bacteremic shock. Am J Med 54:421, 1973

110
LOCALIZED INFECTIONS AND ABSCESSES

ROBERT G. PETERSDORF
JAN V. HIRSCHMANN

GENERAL CONSIDERATIONS

In contrast to many bacterial diseases, which can be conveniently described in terms of their specific etiologic pathogens, there are some in which the clinical picture is determined primarily by their location. Examples of such infections include abscesses, soft-tissue infections, bacterial endocarditis (Chap. 243), pyogenic infections of the central nervous system (Chap. 368), urinary tract infections (Chap. 280), lung abscess (Chap. 260), mediastinitis (Chap. 269), appendicitis and appendiceal abscess (Chap. 296), diverticulitis (Chap. 294), osteomyelitis (Chap. 360), and infections of the pericardium (Chap. 249). Infections in these sites can be caused by many pathogens, and although their bacteriologic identification may be time-consuming, knowledge of the usual flora causing infection in certain anatomic loci should permit institution of therapy before the results of cultures are available. Although treatment of these infections is usually surgical, the internist may be the first one to see these patients and may also be the one to prescribe chemotherapy on the basis of the presumed pathogen.

ETIOLOGY Localized pyogenic infection can develop in any region or organ of the body, and may be initiated by *trauma* and secondary bacterial contamination, by some *alteration in local conditions* that renders a tissue susceptible to infection with organisms already present as part of the "normal flora" to which it is ordinarily resistant, by *contiguous spread* from a nearby lesion, or by *metastatic implantation* of microorganisms carried in blood or lymph.

Under appropriate conditions of lowered tissue resistance, almost any of the common bacteria can initiate an infectious process. Cultures from open lesions such as those of the skin or from intraabdominal foci arising from perforations of the gastrointestinal tract frequently contain several bacterial species; as might be expected, the organisms found most frequently are the "normal flora" of these regions.

Infection in some areas is more likely to be caused by certain organisms, staphylococci in the skin and coliform bacteria in the urinary tract, and special features of the tissue reaction produced by some bacterial species make it possible to recognize infection by them with considerable accuracy. The *staphylococci* produce rapid necrosis and early suppuration with large amounts of creamy yellow pus (Chap. 116). Group A beta-hemolytic streptococcal infections (Chap. 117) tend to spread rapidly through tissues, causing intense edema and erythema but relatively little necrosis and thin, serumlike exudate; anaerobic bacteria (Chap. 142) produce necrosis and profuse, brownish, foul-smelling pus.

The identification of infecting organisms is important in the choice of local or systemic chemotherapy. However, when infection occurs in certain areas, as in paranasal sinuses or cutaneous ulcers, or shows up in sputum, it is unlikely that cultured specimens can ever be rendered sterile. In these locations, serial cultures during antimicrobial administration must be interpreted in this light, and therapy should be guided largely by the clinical response.

PATHOGENESIS Factors predisposing to the initiation and persistence of infection in a tissue include trauma, obstruction of normal drainage (sweat glands, biliary tract, bronchial tree, urinary tract), ischemia (infarction, gangrene), chemical irritation (by gastric contents, bile, or intramuscularly injected drugs), hematoma formation, accumulation of fluid (lymphatic obstruction, cardiac edema), foreign bodies (bullets, splinters, sutures), and others such as the occurrence of stasis or turbulence in the vascular system.

Infection in soft tissue usually begins as a *cellulitis,* a diffuse acute inflammation with hyperemia, edema, and leukocytic infiltration but little or no necrosis and suppuration. With some organisms, this is followed by necrosis, liquefaction, accumulation of leukocytes and debris, suppuration, loculation of the pus, and formation of one or more *abscesses.* Abscess formation is particularly likely to follow infection in a preexisting space or cavity, examples being the fallopian tubes or lung cysts.

The local spread of infection generally follows the path of least resistance along fascial planes; proper surgical treatment is based upon a knowledge of these routes, which will be described for specific infections later in this chapter. Lymphatic spread may lead to lymphangitis, lymphadenitis, or, if the regional nodes suppurate, to the formation of a *bubo*. Involvement of local venules or large veins may lead to infective thrombophlebitis with resulting bacteremia, septic embolization, and systemic dissemination of infection. Staphylococci, streptococci, and *Bacteroides* are notorious for the frequency with which they produce vascular lesions of this type.

Depending upon the infecting organism and the anatomy of the affected region, a small abscess may subside completely; there may be gradual encapsulation of the accumulated pus and persistence of the focus in a quiescent state; or the lesion may "point" and rupture into adjacent tissues or to the outside surface of the body, as usually happens with furuncles. Spontaneous drainage ordinarily leads to subsidence and healing of a superficially situated suppurative focus. However, if the abscess is deeply situated and well encapsulated, there are often persistence of a fistulous tract and the formation of a chronic, draining sinus. *The development of persistent sinuses over an area of suppuration produced by ordinary pyogenic bacteria should always suggest involvement of underlying bone or the presence of a foreign body.* Fistulas that open onto the skin are, of course, soon colonized by microorganisms from the external environment. Ordinary bacterial cultures of drainage fluid almost invariably show a mixed flora and should not be relied upon for the etiologic diagnosis of the underlying disease. This is particularly important in disorders that characteristically lead to persistent sinus formation: tuberculosis, actinomycosis, blastomycosis, melioidosis and glanders, and, rarely, amebic abscess of the liver or cecum. In these situations, superficial organisms about the opening of the sinus tract may mask the true nature of the lesion by obscuring the real pathogen.

MANIFESTATIONS Secondary infection of wounds and cutaneous ulcers is usually recognizable by inspection. Infections of the skin and subcutaneous tissues almost invariably produce the classic manifestations: *redness, tenderness, heat,* and *swelling.* Reddish streaks extending proximally and associated with tender enlargement of regional lymph nodes indicate lymphangitis. Systemic symptoms may be absent or mild, or there may be fever, malaise, prostration, and leukocytosis.

Infection and suppuration in deeper tissues or in body cavities are often manifested by local pain and tenderness, but the task of locating and determining the exact nature of the lesion may be difficult. The palpation of a tender mass is helpful, but muscle spasm and intervening structures often interfere. Abdominal or pelvic examination under anesthesia is sometimes useful in these circumstances.

Auscultation may reveal a friction rub over an abdominal viscus, the pleura, or the pericardium. The rapid development of an effusion in the pericardium, pleura, abdomen, or a joint should suggest infection. Similarly, fluid detected by transillumination of paranasal sinuses or inspection of the tympanic membrane may be the first sign of infection.

Depending on the location of an abscess, symptoms and signs referable to encroachment upon adjacent structures may dominate the picture. Respiratory obstruction may be the first sign of mediastinal abscess; dysphagia often first calls attention to peritonsillar or retropharyngeal abscesses; and tamponade is sometimes the initial clue to pericardial infection. Localizing signs of dysfunction are especially striking and important with brain and spinal cord abscesses, although brain abscesses may be clinically silent (Chap. 368). In some patients local pain and tenderness or signs of dysfunction are mild or equivocal, and fever, prostration, and weight loss dominate the picture. The fever may be low-grade but is often hectic, with repeated rigors and drenching night sweats. Fatigue and anemia are frequent, and weight loss may be so rapid as to result in emaciation within a few weeks. A patient with these symptoms and signs may have chronic subphrenic, perinephric, or other

abscess in the complete absence of any detectable physical sign pointing to the location of a large accumulation of pus. With the advent of antibiotics some deep-seated abscesses present the picture of a chronic illness manifested by no more than malaise, easy fatigability, low-grade fever, mild anemia, and an elevated sedimentation rate because of prior treatment with antimicrobials.

Fluctuation of a mass on palpation is a reliable sign that it contains fluid, perhaps pus, but failure to detect this sign when deeper structures are examined is no guarantee that suppuration is absent and should not be taken by itself to indicate that the mass is noninfectious in origin or that drainage is not required.

LABORATORY FINDINGS Peripheral polymorphonuclear leukocytosis is frequent with abscesses, and significant unexplained elevation of the white blood cell count in any patient should lead to a search for localized suppuration. Depending on the severity and duration of infection, there may be a chronic normocytic, normochromic anemia. The sedimentation rate is almost always rapid. Mild albuminuria, occasionally noted in febrile patients, has no diagnostic import.

Pus or fluid obtained by needle aspiration or incision of a suspected lesion should *always* be stained and examined directly in addition to being cultured aerobically and anaerobically. Pus is a poor metabolic substrate, and bacteria may fail to grow in cultures from an abscess of long standing. In such instances, the findings on microscopic examination may be the only guide in choosing proper chemotherapy. *Failure to examine exudates with Gram's stain is the single greatest deterrent to appropriate antimicrobial therapy;* it is the responsibility of the internist as well as the surgeon to see that this procedure is performed.

Blood cultures are often positive in intravascular infections such as septic thrombophlebitis and endocarditis and in pyogenic infections in which localized abscesses are metastatic, as in staphylococcal, streptococcal, and *Salmonella* bacteremias. Moreover, manipulation, including surgical incision, of any localized infection may be followed by transient bacteremia.

Noninvasive techniques are often helpful in the diagnosis of abscess. X-ray examinations may be of considerable help in detecting localized collections of pus when they show atypical collections of gas, displacement of organs, and tissue densities in abnormal locations. Radionuclide scans may demonstrate abscesses in brain, liver, spleen, and thyroid. The isotope [^{67}Ga] gallium citrate is selectively concentrated in abscesses, but in noninfectious inflammation and neoplasms as well, and many have found gallium scans of limited value in locating abscesses. Of even more potential value is the technique of diagnostic ultrasound, which is not only useful in localizing abscess but also may provide clues to the size of the abscess and to the presence of multiple abscesses or loculation. Angiography is useful in detecting abscesses in highly vascular organs such as the spleen. Computerized tomography (CT scan) may be helpful in demonstrating abscesses, especially in the brain and in areas not easily evaluated by other methods, such as the retroperitoneum.

THERAPEUTIC CONSIDERATIONS Recognition of the striking symptomatic improvement that follows spontaneous evacuation of a suppurative focus led long ago to the adoption of *surgical incision* for the treatment of abscesses. The exact reasons for the amelioration of local and constitutional manifestations that results from drainage of pus are unknown, but, clinically, the benefits of adequate incision and drainage are unequivocal.

Incision of infected tissue before the stage of liquefaction and accumulation of pus is often deleterious and fails to relieve discomfort. Premature incision may even at times facilitate spread of infection. For this reason, it is sometimes necessary to wait until an abscess "ripens," i.e., localizes and "comes to a head." The *application of heat* to an area of inflammation will relieve pain and often speed the subsidence of cellulitis without suppuration. If necrosis of tissue is already under way, hot applications appear to facilitate localization of the process and accumulation of pus, making incision and drainage feasible at an earlier time. Another procedure that aids in reduction of swelling and relief of pain is *elevation of the affected part.*

The availability of specific chemotherapeutic drugs has modified the need for heat, elevation, and incision surprisingly little. The early administration of chemotherapeutics has reduced the incidence of suppurative complications in many disorders, but once suppuration has appeared, antimicrobial drugs become remarkably incapable of eradicating the infecting organisms, although they may mask the classic clinical features of abscess formation.

Some antimicrobials, notably the penicillins, appear to retain their antibacterial activity in the presence of pus, while others, exemplified by the aminoglycosides and the polymyxins, are at least partially inactivated in purulent exudates. However, inability of the drug to penetrate into an area of suppuration is rarely the reason for therapeutic failure. Although this possibility exists in some infections, such as osteomyelitis, it is usually overcome by increasing dosage. Because direct instillation of the antibiotic into an infected area is not, by itself, a curative procedure, other factors are probably more important than faulty diffusion of the agent into the purulent focus.

An established inflammatory exudate is a relatively poor environment for bacterial multiplication. Because the bactericidal action of the penicillins and the cephalosporins is exerted only against multiplying organisms, failure of these antibiotics to eradicate bacteria in an abscess may be related to the organisms' inactive metabolic state. Although the mechanism of their antibacterial action differs from that of the penicillins, bacteriostatic agents such as tetracycline or chloramphenicol also are incapable of eradicating bacteria in the static phase of growth. Furthermore, by definition, these drugs only inhibit multiplication of bacteria and usually exert no direct lethal action; the death of organisms in any infection treated with bacteriostatic agents depends on other mechanisms. For most pyogenic bacteria, phagocytosis is one of the most important of these mechanisms (although there must be others that have not been studied so carefully), and, in the absence of phagocytes or in circumstances which inhibit their activity, bacteriostatic drugs are relatively ineffective. In fluid-filled cavities, particularly in the metabolically unfavorable milieu of an abscess, phagocytosis is greatly reduced. Consequently, despite inhibition of bacterial multiplication, organisms can remain dormant and survive for long periods of time. It is probably a combination of these two circumstances, decreased multiplication of bacteria and decreased phagocytosis, that makes infection in the heart valves, in the kidney, or in the meninges so relatively resistant to antimicrobial therapy. Relatively large doses of bactericidal drugs for long periods are needed to achieve cure.

Antimicrobial drugs may be expected to prevent suppuration if given early or to prevent spread of an existing abscess, but cannot be substituted for surgical drainage. Indeed, their use in the face of a lesion requiring evacuation of pus is one of the most common serious errors in treating pyogenic infections.

In empyema, suppurative pericarditis, or pyarthrosis, excellent therapeutic results are sometimes achieved by aspiration of pus and systemic antimicrobial therapy. The success of this procedure, however, fully depends on the adequacy of drainage as it is upon the instillation of the antibiotic, and if there is loculation or if the exudate becomes too viscid to allow removal, surgical incision and drainage through a large-bore tube become mandatory.

In the presence of infective thrombophlebitis, surgical interruption of the veins by ligation or, in some cases, by total excision of an infected segment is sometimes indicated to prevent seeding of other organs by infected emboli.

CLINICAL FEATURES OF INFECTIONS IN VARIOUS REGIONS

SUPERFICIAL ABSCESSES   Skin and subcutaneous tissues *Impetigo* is a superficial infection caused by group A hemolytic streptococci, sometimes combined with *Staphylococcus aureus.* It is primarily a disease of children, common in warm weather, characterized by multiple erythematous lesions which vesiculate and are intensely pruritic. Local spread occurs through scratching and release of infected vesicle fluid. Serious complications are metastatic abscesses and hemorrhagic nephritis. Treatment consists of local and general cleansing of the skin and appropriate systemic antibiotics.

Deeper infections of the skin are almost invariably staphylococcal in origin and are described in Chap. 116. Erysipelas, a characteristic dermal lesion produced by group A streptococci, is described in Chap. 117.

Lymphadenitis with or without suppuration may complicate any pyogenic skin lesion and is often striking with superficial streptococcal infections. Specific diseases characterized by suppurative regional lymphadenitis include lymphogranuloma venereum (Chap. 174), cat-scratch disease (Chap. 197), tularemia (Chap. 128), and bubonic plague (Chap. 129).

Infections of the hand   These are almost invariably secondary to trauma and are very common. Because of the rapidity with which infection can spread through the complex fascial spaces of the hand, wrist, and forearm, with the production of irreparable functional damage, *any deep infection in this area should receive expert surgical attention immediately.* The importance of such care has in no way been lessened by the availability of antibiotics.

The ordinary *paronychia,* or "run-around," is a superficial infection of the epithelium lateral to a nail, usually a result of tearing a hangnail and most frequently caused by staphylococcus. Hot applications will lead to subsidence of paronychial cellulitis, but often a superficial blister of pus appears. A small incision or simply separation of the nail fold from the nail will promote adequate drainage. If the infection burrows beneath the nail to form a painful *subungual abscess,* incision and drainage with partial or complete removal of the nail are necessary. Recurrence is common, especially in nail biters, and this seemingly trivial infection can cause painful disability. Chronic paronychial inflammation produced by various fungi occurs in diabetics, and a similar lesion is seen in psoriasis and some types of pemphigus.

What appears to be a small furuncle of the webs of the fingers sometimes produces a *collar-button abscess,* consisting of a superficial and deep compartment connected by a narrow tract. Evacuation of the shallow pocket without emptying the deeper abscess can lead to puzzling persistence of infection. Sometimes a foreign-body granuloma forms in the skin of the digital webs. This is most common in barbers, in whom a hair is the core of the foreign-body granuloma, the "barber's inter-digital pilonidal sinus."

Infection of the distal phalanx of a finger, usually acquired by pinprick, thorn prick, etc., may lead to the formation of a *felon,* or *whitlow.* This is a suppurative infection in the tightly enclosed fibrous compartments of the finger pulp, the "anterior closed space," which can compromise the distal blood supply by compression of the digital arteries, with consequent necrosis of bone and the development of osteomyelitis. The manifestations are swelling, extreme pain, and tenderness of the palmar surface of the finger tip. The treatment is immediate incision directly over the lesion, sometimes by the use of a trephine, and cutting all the fibrous septa that radiate from the periosteum to the subcutaneous fascia.

Suppurative tenosynovitis, usually a complication of a puncture wound, is an even more serious infection of the hand from the point of view of functional damage; early diagnosis and treatment are mandatory to prevent permanent disability from destruction of the tendon or its sheath. The three cardinal manifestations of tenosynovitis are (1) exquisite tenderness limited to the course of the sheath, (2) flexion of the fingers, and (3) excruciating pain, most marked at the base of the digit, on extension of the involved finger. *Immediate incision* of the sheath is indicated, not only to prevent damage to the tendon itself but to avoid proximal extension of the process into the major fascial spaces of the hand or forearm. Vigorous antibiotic treatment should accompany surgery. The definitive treatment of any serious infection of the hand is a matter for a skilled surgeon, but the early recognition of the need for surgery often falls to other physicians.

Human bites lead to very important hand infections, which, if neglected, almost invariably produce a highly destructive, necrotizing lesion contaminated by a mixture of aerobic and anaerobic organisms. A deliberately inflicted bite on the hand or elsewhere is usually recognized as dangerously contaminated, but wounds on the knuckles produced by striking an opponent's teeth with the fists may not be recognized as potentially dangerous. In general, bite wounds should be cleaned thoroughly and not sutured. Patients should be given prophylaxis for tetanus and antibiotics, preferably both a penicillinase-resistant penicillin and ampicillin.

Chronic cutaneous ulcers A partial list of the causes of chronic ulcers of the skin includes circulatory disturbances, such as varicose veins and obliterative arterial disease, extensive injury from frostbite or burns, trophic changes accompanying many neurological disorders, bedsores or decubiti, systemic diseases such as sickle-cell disease and myxedema, neoplasms, and various infections. No matter what the underlying disease, secondary infection is very likely to occur and to interfere with healing, complicate grafting or other restorative procedures, or produce extension of the process.

The management of secondary bacterial infection in skin ulcers associated with obliterative arterial disease, a common problem in diabetics, is especially important, because infection is frequently the factor that precipitates spreading gangrene and makes amputation necessary.

Studies of the microflora of chronic cutaneous ulcers have almost invariably shown bacteria of many species, including staphylococci, aerobic and anaerobic streptococci, coliform bacilli, and members of the *Proteus* and *Pseudomonas* groups. Depending on the patient's environment and on systemically or locally administered antimicrobial drugs, the predominating bacterial species show great variation when lesions are cultured serially. Particularly noteworthy is the replacement of sensitive organisms by resistant strains or species during the course of chemotherapy.

Treatment of chronic dermal ulcers should be directed

toward the underlying disorder but should also include *local debridement* and *chemotherapy.* Debridement by surgical excision is often needed, but the local application of wet-to-dry dressings or other forms of "medical debridement" frequently suffice. Intensive systemic administration of antibiotics should be carried out only in conjunction with definitive surgical procedures or when infection can be controlled in no other way. The prevention of infection by "prophylactic" administration of antimicrobial drugs is futile because it results in the development of a flora resistant to the drugs being used. The *local application of antibiotics* is sometimes highly effective, and it is in the management of chronic mixed infections of this type that several potent but toxic antibiotics have great value. An ointment or solution containing neomycin, bacitracin, and polymyxin exerts a bactericidal effect against a wide variety of organisms and will sometimes temporarily sterilize a chronic lesion. Other useful topical medications are furacin and 3 percent acetic acid, which is especially helpful in *Pseudomonas* infections.

Diphtheritic ulcer of the skin is discussed in Chap. 133.

INFECTIONS OF THE HEAD AND NECK Pustules of the nose and upper lip may be particularly dangerous, because they are likely to extend intracranially through the angular vein to the cavernous sinus. These lesions should be treated conservatively, manipulation or incision should be avoided if possible, and systemic antibiotics should be used if local swelling or redness appears.

Suppurative parotitis Typically, suppurative parotitis occurs in elderly and chronically ill patients who have a dry mouth from decreased oral intake, often following general anesthesia and surgery, or from medications with atropine-like effects, such as antihistamines or phenothiazines. In most patients, it is an ascending infection due to *S. aureus,* which normally colonizes the opening to Stensen's duct. Occasionally, there is an obstructing calculus. Its onset, usually sudden, is heralded by unilateral local pain and swelling, frequently with fever and chills. Frank pus can often be expressed from the duct and may show gram-positive cocci in clumps. The gland itself is firm and tender and often shows redness and edema of the overlying skin. Treatment consists of systemic antimicrobial therapy with a penicillinase-resistant penicillin or another agent effective against *S. aureus,* combined with improved hydration and oral hygiene. Massage of the gland and sialagogues, like lemon drops, help promote drainage through the duct. Surgery is usually unnecessary and should be reserved for patients failing to improve after 4 to 5 days of medical management.

Rare complications include fistula formation, facial nerve palsy, or extension of the infection to involve the mediastinum. The mortality rate is about 20 to 30 percent, probably because this infection occurs in severely debilitated patients.

The use of penicillin and other antibiotics has reduced the incidence of many formerly common suppurative complications of streptococcal pharyngitis. However, as a result of streptococcal sore throat, *Bacteroides* infections of the pharynx, or introduction of infection by trauma to the floor of the mouth or the pharyngeal wall, abscesses of the deep cervical structures still occur. *Suppurative cervical adenitis,* once an all-too-common sequel to streptococcal pharyngitis in children, is now rare. *Peritonsillar abscess (quinsy)* is manifested by fever, sore throat, cervical lymphadenopathy, unilateral pain radiating to the ear on swallowing, and enlargement of the tonsil with redness and swelling of the adjacent soft palate. Treatment with penicillin and irrigations of warm saline solution sometimes lead to subsidence of the process, but if digital palpation reveals fluctuation, surgical drainage with or without tonsillectomy is indicated. Organisms associated with peritonsillar abscess include *Streptococcus pyogenes* and oral anaerobic bacteria.

The course of *deep cervical infections* is fully as dependent upon the anatomic arrangement of fascial planes as is that of infections of the hand. Infection in this area is serious and is attended by fever, prostration, and leukocytosis. A tender mass may be palpated, but *surgical evacuation of such an infection should not be delayed because of failure to detect fluctuation,* which is usually absent because of the dense fascial layers.

Infection of the *sublingual* and submandibular spaces, so-called "Ludwig's angina," is characterized by brawny induration of the submaxillary region, edema of the floor of the mouth, and elevation of the tongue. It usually originates from apical abscesses of the second and third mandibular molars. There are severe pain, dysphagia, and, within hours, dyspnea from respiratory obstruction. The causative organisms of this and other neck abscesses are mainly streptococci and oral anaerobes. Mortality was formerly about 50 percent. *Treatment* consists of large doses of penicillin and careful observation. With significant airway obstruction, tracheostomy is necessary. Since the infection is largely a cellulitis, incision and drainage are reserved for evidence of fluctuation.

The retropharyngeal space lies between the muscles anterior to the cervical vertebrae and the pharyngeal mucosa. *Retropharyngeal abscess,* formerly common in children, is manifested by dysphagia, progressive stridor, pain, and fever. The bulging mass is easily seen and can completely occlude the airway within hours. Incision and drainage are mandatory; spontaneous rupture may lead to death by aspiration. Esophageal perforation during endoscopy may result in abscess as a late complication. Tuberculous abscess, secondary to spinal disease, occasionally appears in the retropharyngeal space; it is painless, and relief of obstruction follows surgical incision.

Submastoid abscess, or suppuration in the submastoid space, known as *Bezold's abscess,* is usually secondary to otitis and produces nuchal rigidity, which may lead to a mistaken diagnosis of otogenous meningitis. Infection can extend down the carotid sheath to the mediastinum. A suppurative thrombophlebitis of the jugular vein usually accompanies this infection, and the vessel is easily felt as a tender cord. Bacteremia and systemic spread of infection are common, and the involved venous segment may need to be excised. Spontaneous rupture of the carotid artery with rapid death from exsanguination is a rare complication.

Therapy of head and neck abscesses includes surgical incision and drainage, open treatment of infected wounds, and systemic antibiotics, which should include agents active against anaerobic organisms, particularly if there is foul-smelling pus. Penicillin is usually the drug of choice.

DEEP-SEATED INFECTIONS Hepatic abscess These abscesses are usually amebic (Chap. 199) or bacterial (pyogenic). Bacterial abscesses usually develop by one of five mechanisms: (1) portal vein bacteremia arising from an infected intraabdominal site, such as appendicitis, diverticulitis, or perforated bowel; (2) systemic bacteremia originating from a distant site, in which bacteria reach the liver via the hepatic artery; (3) ascending cholangitis in a biliary tract completely or partially obstructed by stone, malignancy, or stricture; (4) direct extension from a contiguous focus of infection outside the biliary tract, such as a subphrenic abscess; or (5) trauma, either penetrating, with direct introduction of organisms into the liver, or

blunt, causing a hematoma that becomes secondarily infected. In most cases the cause is apparent, but in some the pathogenesis of the abscess is unexplained ("cryptogenic"). Most abscesses are single; multiple abscesses are typically microscopic and associated with systemic bacteremia or complete biliary tract obstruction. In these cases, the onset is acute, and the clinical features of the predisposing disease predominate.

Most other cases of hepatic abscess have a subacute onset, and an illness lasting several weeks is the rule. Fever is nearly always present and is accompanied by such nonspecific symptoms as chills, nausea, vomiting, anorexia, weight loss, and weakness. Right upper quadrant abdominal pain or tenderness is present in about one-half of patients, as is hepatomegaly. Some complain of right pleuritic chest pain. Jaundice is usually evident only when there is biliary tract obstruction.

Laboratory findings in most patients include one or more of the following: anemia, leukocytosis, increased erythrocyte sedimentation rate, increased alkaline phosphatase, decreased serum albumin, and usually mildly increased serum bilirubin. The chest roentgenogram is abnormal in about one-half of patients and shows right-sided basilar atelectasis, pneumonia, pleural effusion, or an elevated hemidiaphragm.

The radionuclide liver scan demonstrates filling defects for most abscesses greater than 2 cm in diameter. Ultrasound scans are usually positive and can distinguish fluid-filled from solid masses, helping to discriminate between infectious and neoplastic lesions. Computerized tomography and hepatic arteriography may also demonstrate the abscesses but generally provide no additional useful information.

The bacteriology of liver abscesses depends upon the cause. With systemic bacteremia staphylococci or streptococci are common. Abscesses originating from an intraabdominal infection, however, usually contain aerobic gram-negative rods, especially *Escherichia coli* and *Klebsiella-Enterobacter;* anaerobic bacteria, especially anaerobic gram-positive cocci, *Fusobacterium nucleatum,* and *B. fragilis;* or a mixture of aerobes and anaerobes. Blood cultures are positive in a substantial minority of patients.

Treatment consists of surgical drainage supplemented by appropriate antibiotic therapy. When the bacteriology is unknown, chloramphenicol or a combination of clindamycin and an aminoglycoside should be effective. Antibiotics are usually continued for several weeks following drainage.

Complications of hepatic abscesses include formation of a subphrenic abscess, bleeding into the abscess, and rupture into the lung, pleural cavity, or peritoneum. In correctly diagnosed and treated patients the mortality rate is about 20 to 40 percent, and is higher in those with multiple rather than single abscesses.

In patients with a clinical picture suggesting a liver abscess and an abnormal hepatic radionuclide or ultrasound scan, it is important to distinguish between a bacterial and an amebic abscess, since the latter usually requires no surgical drainage. Features suggesting an amebic etiology are: age under 50; single rather than multiple abscesses; a history of diarrhea, especially if bloody; the presence of *Entamoeba histolytica* in the stool; and the absence of a condition predisposing to bacterial liver abscess. The most helpful differential point is that nearly all patients with amebic liver abscesses have a positive serology for *E. histolytica.*

Splenic abscess Most splenic abscesses are multiple, small, and clinically silent lesions found incidentally at autopsy and occurring as a terminal manifestation of uncontrolled infection elsewhere. Clinically important splenic abscesses are generally solitary and arise from (1) systemic bacteremia originating in another site, such as endocarditis or salmonellosis; (2) infection, probably by the hematogenous route, of a spleen damaged by bland infarction (as occurs in hemoglobinopathies, especially sickle-cell trait or sickle-cell disease), trauma, penetrating or blunt (with superinfection of a subcapsular hematoma), or other diseases (malaria, hydatid cysts); or (3) extension from a contiguous focus of infection, such as a subphrenic abscess. The most common organisms are staphylococci, streptococci, anaerobes, and aerobic gram-negative rods, including *Salmonella.*

The onset is typically subacute, and the major features are fever and left-sided pain which is often pleuritic and located in the upper abdomen, lower chest, or flank. The pain may radiate to the left shoulder. Left upper quadrant abdominal tenderness and splenomegaly are common, but an audible splenic friction rub is rare. Leukocytosis is usually present.

Radiographic findings may include (1) a left upper quadrant soft-tissue abdominal mass, (2) extraintestinal gas from gas-forming organisms in the abscess, (3) displacement of other organs, including the colon, kidney, and stomach, (4) elevation of the left hemidiaphragm, and (5) left pleural effusion. A liver-spleen radionuclide scan is valuable in detecting abscesses larger than 2 or 3 cm. A combined spleen-lung scan may provide clues to perisplenic (or left subdiaphragmatic) abscesses. An ultrasound scan may be positive for macroscopic splenic abscesses. Arteriography, which may reveal an avascular mass and mycotic aneurysms, or CT scan may be helpful when these other tests fail to demonstrate a suspected lesion.

Treatment consists of appropriate systemic antibiotics and splenectomy. Complications of untreated splenic abscesses include hemorrhage into the abscess cavity or rupture into the peritoneum, bowel, bronchus, or pleural space. Splenic abscesses should be considered a possible, although rare, cause of continued bacteremia in acute endocarditis despite appropriate chemotherapy, and splenectomy may be necessary to achieve final eradication of the infection.

Subphrenic abscess   Peritoneal infections show a striking tendency to localize in the upper part of the abdomen between the transverse colon and the diaphragm. True subphrenic abscesses form between the liver and diaphragm on the left or right, and many so-called "subphrenic infections" are, in fact, subhepatic. Most of these infections are related to perforations in the gastrointestinal or biliary tracts, and over half of them follow operations on the gallbladder, duodenum, or stomach. Subphrenic abscesses following perforated appendicitis occur rarely nowadays. Closed blunt trauma is an important cause. A few abscesses occur without predisposing neighborhood infection. The most common organisms are *E. coli,* non-group A streptococci, staphylococci, *Klebsiella-Enterobacter,* and anaerobes, especially *Bacteroides* spp.; mixed infections are common. About 60 percent of abscesses occur on the right, 25 percent on the left, and 15 percent are bilateral. They are more common in males and elderly patients, who often have a debilitating disease such as cancer. *Any patient with persistent fever and a history of a recent abdominal operation or recent intraabdominal sepsis should be suspected of having a subphrenic abscess.*

Manifestations include fever, upper abdominal pain, and tenderness, usually along the costal margin. Shoulder pain, dyspnea, dullness, and rales at the lung base are more common than abdominal signs and symptoms, and emphasize the location of a true abscess between the liver and the diaphragm. Foul sputum connotes perforation of the abscess into the lung. The localizing signs are by no means striking in all cases, however. The widespread practice of "covering" postoperative patients with antibiotics prophylactically can attenuate subphrenic infection without eradicating it and may result in an insidiously progressive illness with weight loss, malaise, fatigue, and low-grade fever beginning weeks or months after a laparotomy, a syndrome termed *chronic subphrenic abscess.* Roentgenograms may show gas, sometimes with an air-fluid

level beneath the diaphragm. The gas may be from a perforated viscus or the result of bacterial multiplication.

Other radiographic findings include pleural effusion, which is usually sterile, basilar infiltrates, and elevation—but not necessarily fixation—of the diaphragm. Barium meal with the patient in the head-down position may show indentation of the gastric fundus in left subphrenic abscess, a lesion that is often notoriously difficult to localize. Combined lung-liver scintiscan may show a widened subphrenic space. Ultrasound scans are useful in detecting subphrenic abscesses, and CT scan will usually demonstrate extraintestinal gas or fluid.

Treatment includes adequate surgical drainage and appropriate systemic antibiotics. Chloramphenicol or clindamycin and an aminoglycoside are good choices pending culture results. The outlook in subphrenic abscesses is often poor because of delayed diagnosis, the debilitated state of the patient, and failure to attain complete drainage. Even with proper surgery, the mortality rate is about 30 percent.

Retroperitoneal infections   Strictly speaking, all perinephric, most pancreatic, and many subphrenic abscesses are located outside the peritoneum, but the term *retroperitoneal abscess* usually refers to infection in the lumbar and iliac regions. Suppuration in these areas is relatively rare, but the importance of recognizing its existence in patients with fever and pain in the lower part of the back is great. In one series, the average duration of illness in 65 patients before diagnosis was approximately 1 month.

Infection in the retroperitoneal space usually reflects extension from posterior perforations of the appendix, small bowel or colon, pancreatic, renal, or spinal infections, and occasionally suppurative lymphadenitis in the iliac area, usually secondary to streptococcal infections of the lower extremities in children. Sometimes, the infection is apparently spread hematogenously.

Lumbar abscess is characterized by tenderness and spasm of the back muscles on the affected side, and a mass is usually palpable in the lumbar region; or there may be a prominent, tender abdominal mass without lumbar pain or spasm. Infection in the wall of the abdominal aneurysm, often with *Salmonella,* may present as a lumbar abscess. Flexion of the hip (psoas sign) occurs in a few cases but is more often present with infections lower in the retroperitoneal area. *Fever, leukocytosis,* and *lumbar spasm* should suggest the diagnosis. The absence of a palpable mass may lead to protracted observation, and it is in these instances that palpation under anesthesia is often helpful.

Psoas (iliac) abscess is typically attended by abdominal pain in the iliac or inguinal region, and, particularly when the psoas muscle is involved, severe pain may be referred to the hip, thigh, or knee. Careful palpation of the lower part of the abdomen or groin usually reveals a mass, and fullness and tenderness on rectal examination are common. Hip spasm (psoas sign) is often present. Although psoas abscesses characteristically occur in association with tuberculosis of the spine, the acute bacterial form has been reported in perforation or fistula formation of the bowel in appendicitis, diverticulitis, colonic carcinoma, and Crohn's disease (regional enteritis). Roentgenograms may delineate the inflammatory mass; pyelography shows displacement of the kidney or ureter in some cases, scoliosis with concavity on the side of the infection, and blurring of the psoas shadow. Barium studies of the small and large bowel may demonstrate an intestinal site of origin. Computerized tomography may be useful in revealing a suspected abscess when other studies are negative. Treatment consists of surgical drainage and appropriate antibiotic therapy.

Pancreatic abscess   These abscesses usually occur in a site of pancreatic necrosis following acute pancreatitis. Typically, the patient improves after the attack of pancreatitis, but about 10 to 21 days later fever, abdominal pain and tenderness, nausea, vomiting, and sometimes persistent ileus begin; in those cases, persistent fever, leukocytosis, and abdominal findings beyond 7 to 10 days should suggest an abscess. A mass is palpable in about half of cases. The serum amylase is irregularly elevated, but leukocytosis is usually present. The serum alkaline phosphatase may be increased and the albumin decreased.

Chest roentgenograms often show a left pleural effusion, basilar atelectasis or pneumonia, or a raised hemidiaphragm. Plain films of the abdomen or barium studies of the intestinal tract may show extraintestinal gas in the pancreatic area from gas-forming organisms in the abscess or may demonstrate displacement of adjacent structures. Ultrasound is very useful in revealing fluid-filled pancreatic masses. Computerized tomography is also a sensitive test.

Treatment is surgical drainage and appropriate antibiotic therapy. Since the usual organisms are coliforms and anaerobes, chloramphenicol or clindamycin and an aminoglycoside are reasonable choices until culture results return. Complications of undrained abscess include perforation into adjacent structures; erosion of the left gastric, splenic, and gastroduodenal arteries with exsanguination; and the development of further abscesses in the pancreas or peritoneal and retroperitoneal spaces. Even with surgical drainage the mortality rate is about 40 percent, and recurrent abscesses requiring reoperation are common.

Renal abscess   Single or multiple abscesses of the renal *cortex* are almost invariably the result of metastatic implantation of staphylococci from another focus. There is no relationship to previous renal disease; the infection occurs in younger individuals, is usually unilateral, and occurs on the right side oftener than on the left. Many patients give a history of recent skin infection such as furuncle. Although acute pyelonephritis is a diffuse disease with foci of cellular infiltrates in the interstitium of the renal medulla, these inflammatory foci may coalesce to form a distinct abscess cavity in the medulla. This situation probably ensues more frequently than is generally appreciated.

The onset of renal abscess is abrupt, with chills and fever, followed by costovertebral pain and tenderness. If the abscess is cortical, the urine contains *no white blood cells;* medullary abscesses are usually accompanied by pyuria. The stained urinary sediment may show myriads of gram-positive cocci in cortical abscesses and gram-negative organisms in medullary abscesses. Transient gross or microscopic hematuria may occur at the onset. The white blood cell count is usually elevated and may exceed 30,000 cells per cubic millimeter. Physical signs are usually localized to the region of the kidney, but abdominal spasm may lead to confusion with appendicitis, cholecystitis, or pancreatitis. Early in the disease, ureteral calculus or acute hydronephrosis may be considered as possible diagnoses. Sudden onset of *fever, leukocytosis, and renal pain in the absence of pyuria* should suggest the diagnosis of renal abscess, especially in a patient with infection elsewhere. Obstruction of the ureter by pus or cellular debris may also yield a urine sediment sparse in white blood cells and bacteria. Excretory urograms typically reveal an intrarenal mass, and ultrasound scans usually demonstrate the abscess as a fluid-filled defect. *Treatment* consists of appropriate antibiotics, adequate fluids, and relief of pain. An abscess may suddenly discharge into the renal pelvis, with relief of pain and the passage of cloudy urine

containing enormous numbers of leukocytes and bacteria. *Complications* include formation of a thick-walled chronic renal "carbuncle," requiring surgical removal, rupture into the perirenal space, and secondary pyelonephritis, usually produced by coliform bacilli. Recovery is ordinarily prompt, and chronic sequelae are rare. Failure to achieve rapid defervescence following treatment suggests an incorrect diagnosis or the necessity of drainage, either by needle aspiration or by surgery.

Perinephric abscess   Rupture of a renal parenchymal abscess into the perinephric space can cause a perinephric abscess. Such an abscess may be staphylococcal following hematogenous dissemination from another site, usually the skin, but more commonly it arises from pyelonephritis which is usually associated with renal calculus disease. The causative organisms, therefore, are those responsible for acute pyelonephritis: *E. coli, Proteus* sp., and *Klebsiella-Enterobacter.* The main symptoms are fever, chills, and unilateral flank pain. Dysuria is frequently present. Most patients are febrile and have unilateral flank or abdominal tenderness, often with a palpable mass. Leukocytosis, pyuria, and a positive urine culture are typical. Blood cultures are positive in 20 to 40 percent of patients. Perinephric abscess generally can be distinguished clinically from uncomplicated acute pyelonephritis by the longer duration of symptoms before hospitalization (usually more than 5 days) and the failure of patients to become afebrile within 5 days following the institution of antimicrobial therapy.

The chest roentgenograms often show ipsilateral pneumonia or atelectasis, pleural effusion, or a raised hemidiaphragm. An abdominal plain film may reveal the loss of the psoas shadow, a mass, calculi, or extraintestinal gas in the perinephric area secondary to gas-forming organisms. Findings on excretory urogram may include: a nonvisualizing or a poorly visualizing kidney, distorted calyces, anterior displacement of the kidney on lateral views, and unilateral fixation of the kidney that is demonstrated best by fluoroscopy or inspiration-expiration films. Ultrasound scans are very sensitive in detecting perinephric abscesses. Treatment is surgical drainage and relief of any urinary obstruction; occasionally, nephrectomy is necessary. Appropriate systemic antibiotics (not urinary antiseptics) should be administered along with surgical measures.

Rectal abscess   Most of these infections are superficial and involve the perirectal region, and many are associated with fistulas. Infection in the apocrine glands (hidradenitis) or folliculitis in the perianal region, extension of cryptitis or obstructions in the "anal glands" which open into the crypts of Morgagni, and contamination of submucosal hematomas, sclerosed hemorrhoids, or anal fissures may lead to abscess formation. In most patients, the cause of infection is not apparent. These are usually painful, easily palpable, often visible on inspection. Treatment is incision and drainage. Antibiotics may be indicated in some instances.

Difficulties in diagnosis are likely to arise with infections higher in the rectum. Most are in the ischiorectal area, but those above the pelvic diaphragm, the so-called "supralevator abscess," are particularly elusive. Patients with this type of infection often have fever, malaise, and leukocytosis for several days or even weeks before any symptoms referable to the rectum develop. There is vague pelvic discomfort, relieved by defecation, and constipation punctuated by short episodes of diarrhea is common. In males, the inflammation often involves the base of the bladder, and urinary urgency or retention may occur, falsely centering attention on the urinary tract as the source of fever and malaise. Eventually, the abscess produces severe pain, chills, and fever; palpation and instrumentation will reveal the swelling in the rectal ampulla. Such an abscess may surround the rectum and produce narrowing that is differentiated from neoplasm by the fact that the mucosa remains intact. A useful sign of deep rectal abscess is severe pain with pressure in the region between the anus and the coccyx. The supralevator space is continuous with the ischiorectal space, with both the gluteal and obturator regions, and with the retroperitoneal space. In neglected cases, the abscess may drain through the skin of the perineum, the groin, or the buttock or may extend as high as the perirenal areas. Rectal abscesses are not uncommon in patients with preexisting anorectal disease, diabetes, alcoholism, and neurological disease; infections in this area are also peculiarly frequent in patients with acute leukemia, especially when neutropenia is present. Because the clinical picture may be that of "fever of unknown origin" for a long period, it is important that thorough digital and endoscopic examination of the rectum be carried out in patients with unexplained fever. Patients with diabetic ketoacidosis should receive a careful rectal examination because a rectal abscess may be the infection responsible for precipitating the ketoacidosis.

A rectal abscess may be a forerunner of both ulcerative colitis and regional enteritis, and may occur months and even years before other overt manifestations of these diseases. For this reason, proctosigmoidoscopy, colonoscopy, barium enema, and, often, upper gastrointestinal roentgenograms are indicated in nonhealing or recurrent rectal lesions.

Treatment of high rectal abscesses consists of incision and drainage, analgesics, and antibiotics directed at *E. coli, Klebsiella-Enterobacter, Bacteroides,* and a variety of streptococci, which constitute the polymicrobial flora of these lesions.

REFERENCES

BARTLETT JG et al: Anaerobic infections of the head and neck. Otolaryngol Clin North Am 9:655, 1976

CHOW AW et al: Orofacial odontogenic infections. Ann Intern Med 88:392, 1978

CHULAY JD et al: Splenic abscess: Report of 10 cases and review of the literature. Am J Med 61:513, 1976

DOUST BD et al: Ultrasonic diagnosis of abdominal abscess. Am J Dig Dis 21:569, 1976

GOLIGHER JC: *Surgery of the Anus, Rectum, and Colon,* 3d ed. Springfield, Ill, Charles C Thomas, 1975

HARDCASTLE JD: Acute nontuberculous psoas abscess. Report of 10 cases and review of the literature. Br J Surg 57:103, 1970

KONVOLINKA CW et al: Subphrenic abscess. Curr Probl Surg, January 1972

LAZARCHICK J et al: Pyogenic liver abscess. Mayo Clin Proc 48:349, 1973

LINSCHEID RL et al: Common and uncommon infections of the hand. Orthop Clin North Am 6:1063, 1975

RUBIN RH et al: Hepatic abscess: Changes in clinical, bacteriologic and therapeutic aspects. Am J Med 57:601, 1974

SABBAJ J et al: Anaerobic pyogenic liver abscess. Ann Intern Med 77:629, 1972

SPEIRS CF et al: Acute septic parotitis: Incidence, aetiology, and management. Scott Med J 17:62, 1972

THORLEY JD et al: Perinephric abscess. Medicine 53:441, 1974

WARSHAW AL: Inflammatory masses following acute pancreatitis: Phlegmon, pseudocyst, and abscess. Surg Clin North Am 54:621, 1974

111
CHEMOTHERAPY OF INFECTION

WILLIAM M. M. KIRBY

INTRODUCTION From the standpoint of overall reduction in morbidity and mortality rates, the greatest impact of drug therapy has been in the field of infectious diseases. Modern chemotherapy of infectious diseases dates from the mid-1930s when the sulfonamides were introduced. Penicillin G, the first of the antibiotics to be used systemically, came into widespread use in the early 1940s, and since then several dozen chemotherapeutic agents have appeared that are effective in a wide variety of bacterial, rickettsial, fungal, and parasitic infections. The efficacy of antimicrobial agents is due to their action in inhibiting growth of the parasite rather than to an enhancement of defense mechanisms, and it is remarkable that such a large number of substances can interfere effectively with multiplication of invading organisms without seriously damaging the cells of the host. Effective new agents continue to appear in surprising numbers, both from large-scale screening programs in which samples of organic matter are tested for antimicrobial activity and from chemical modifications of the known chemotherapeutic drugs. Specific recommendations for therapy are made in chapters dealing with individual diseases; this section is devoted to general principles of chemotherapy and to a consideration of individual therapeutic agents.

FACTORS INFLUENCING SELECTION OF ANTIMICROBIAL AGENTS AND THE OUTCOME OF THERAPY

SUSCEPTIBILITY OF THE INFECTING MICROORGANISMS No antimicrobial agent is effective against all pathogenic microorganisms; each has its own spectrum of activity against one or a variety of species, within which the majority of strains have been found to be susceptible. There are a few instances, such as the susceptibility of group A streptococci to penicillin G, in which resistant strains occur rarely if at all, and where treatment with penicillin can be given without concern about resistance. With the majority of chemotherapeutic agents, however, a variable percentage of strains of each susceptible species is resistant, i.e., they are not inhibited by concentrations of the drug attainable in the patient's blood and tissues with the usual dosage schedules. It is customary, therefore, in serious infections to determine the susceptibility of most pathogens to a variety of chemotherapeutic agents, and this has become one of the most important functions of clinical microbiology laboratories. *Dilution methods* of susceptibility testing, considered to be the most accurate, involve making serial dilutions of each agent to be tested in agar or broth, adding a standardized inoculum of the infecting organisms, and determining the smallest amount (the minimal inhibitory concentration, MIC) of the drug that inhibits growth after overnight incubation. *Agar dilution tests* are used routinely in some laboratories with sufficient volume to justify them, and mechanized or preprepared *broth dilution methods* are available. Automated methods are also being developed commercially. Although expensive, they are becoming simpler and more accurate, and at least one provides a result within 3 h. For the majority of laboratories, however, the simpler *agar diffusion method,* which is accurate and reliable when properly performed, remains the one usually used. With this technique, zones of inhibition of growth of a standardized inoculum of the infecting organism around filter paper disks impregnated with antibiotics are measured, and the zone sizes are inversely proportional to inhibitory concentrations (MICs) of drug, which are in turn related to the blood levels usually attained. Susceptibility of 8 to 10 chemotherapeutic agents can be tested on a single large agar plate, and a report of *susceptible, intermediate,* or *resistant* can be made. Intermediate sensitivity indicates the organisms' possible susceptibility with increased doses, or in urinary tract infections where high concentrations of drug can be attained in the urine. Disk testing has a number of limitations; it is applicable chiefly to rapidly growing pathogens, and the results are usually not reported until 24 h after the pathogen is isolated.

BACTERICIDAL VERSUS BACTERIOSTATIC AGENTS Although these are relative terms, some chemotherapeutic drugs can be clearly shown to have a killing (bactericidal) action at or near the minimal inhibitory concentration, while others simply inhibit bacterial growth (bacteriostatic), leaving the host to strike the *coup de grâce*. Bactericidal agents include the penicillins, cephalosporins, aminoglycosides, polymyxins, and vancomycin, while examples of bacteriostatic agents are the tetracyclines, sulfonamides, chloramphenicol, erythromycin, and clindamycin. Bactericidal agents give definitely superior results in diseases such as bacterial endocarditis and are more likely to give a favorable response in life-threatening infections, particularly when there is impairment of the host's defense mechanisms. In mild infections in otherwise healthy individuals, on the other hand, there is little to choose between "-cidal" and "-static" agents. In uncomplicated urinary tract infections, due to *Escherichia coli,* for example, the clinical results are as good with sulfonamides as with broad-spectrum penicillins or cephalosporins.

CLINICAL PHARMACOLOGY Knowledge of the clinical pharmacology of antimicrobial agents is helpful in prescribing therapy that is both safe and effective. Important information includes details of absorption and excretion, blood and urine levels with various routes of administration, protein binding, renal clearance, half-lives of drugs, stability in solutions and within the body, and the conversion to metabolic breakdown products. With some agents, such as ampicillin, much higher blood levels are obtained with the same doses given parenterally than orally, whereas with others such as doxycycline, where there is complete absorption from the intestinal tract, the oral and parenteral doses are the same. Because of possible incompatibilities, *it is advisable never to administer more than one agent at a time by the intravenous route.* Absorption from the intestinal tract is impaired by a variety of foods and chemicals, and, in general, antimicrobials should be administered temporally as far removed from food and other drugs, such as antacids, as possible.

Antimicrobials are bound to a varying extent to serum proteins, especially albumin. Although the significance of protein binding is uncertain and controversial, it is clear that the bound antibiotic has no antimicrobial activity, and it is probable that the concentration of free, unbound antibiotic in the tissues, at any one time, is no greater than the peak level of free antibiotic in the blood. All other features being equal, antimicrobials with relatively low binding should be preferable to those with a high degree of binding. In general, this point of view is reflected in the dosages of antimicrobial agents that are commonly recommended.

Renal clearance is one of the most important determinants of antibiotic blood levels and is mainly responsible, for example, for the much higher levels attained with the same dose of cephaloridine than of cephalothin, and of carbenicillin than of ampicillin. Antibiotics with a high renal clearance such as penicillin G and cephalothin have a large component of tubular secretion, and their blood levels are elevated to a greater degree by probenecid than those of ampicillin and cephaloridine, where the tubular contribution is less important. Plasma half-life, the time required for a blood level to fall by one-half,

is also determined primarily by renal clearance mechanisms and is much shorter for those penicillins and cephalosporins that are secreted by the renal tubules than for antibiotics such as the aminoglycosides with little or no tubular component. Protein binding also has an important influence on the half-life of antibiotics, particularly those that are excreted mainly or entirely by glomerular filtration. For example, the plasma half-life of gentamicin, which is not bound by proteins, is 2 h, whereas that of doxycycline, which is over 90 percent protein-bound, is about 16 h. Antibiotics with little or no protein binding have a much larger apparent volume of distribution (AVD) than those with a high degree of binding, i.e., the AVD of gentamicin is 30 percent of body weight compared with 14 percent for cefazolin. Cephalothin has a high plasma clearance with a high rate of nonrenal clearance due to its partial conversion in the body to a less active metabolic breakdown product. These are a few examples of the pharmacologic features of individual antimicrobial agents; others will be mentioned as the individual drugs are considered.

DOSE, ROUTE, AND DURATION OF THERAPY In prescribing dosages of antimicrobial agents, the objective is to deliver a concentration in excess of that needed to inhibit and/or kill the infecting organism at the site of infection. Since it is difficult to measure tissue concentrations, a blood level that exceeds the MIC two- to eightfold is a commonly accepted guideline. This is an arbitrary concentration of drug and obviously does not take into account all the variations in penetration into different tissues, or the role of host defense mechanisms. These variations may be very important because, in many instances, infections have been cured with antibiotics such as the tetracyclines where the concentration of free, active drug in the blood is not much greater than the MIC. The relation between blood levels and MIC does not hold in urinary tract infection, where the concentration of drug cleared by the kidney usually far exceeds the MIC. In this situation, an excess of drug in the urine is obviously important.

The route of administration, as well as the dose, is important in achieving appropriate drug levels. In general, parenteral therapy should usually be given in severe infections to be certain that high, effective blood levels are attained. The *intravenous route* is especially indicated initially in meningitis, endocarditis, and osteomyelitis, where barriers to penetration of the antimicrobial agent can be overcome by high blood levels. Intravenous therapy is also indicated when there is hypotension, and when bleeding diatheses are present. For milder infections, *intramuscular administration* is often an acceptable or preferable alternative, particularly with antibiotics such as procaine penicillin that cause relatively little pain and produce prolonged, effective blood levels. With gentamicin, blood levels are the same with an intramuscular injection as with an intravenous infusion given over a period of 60 min, so that the route can be chosen on the basis of comfort for the patient and the need for other intravenous medications. The *oral route* is used chiefly for mild to moderate infections, and for completion of therapy of severe infections after they have been brought under control with parenteral therapy. Absorption from the intestinal tract is variable even in the fasting state, and all oral antibiotics should be taken at least 1 h before and 3 h after food and other medications. This presents difficulties with drugs such as antacids that need to be taken frequently and that are especially likely to interfere with absorption of antimicrobial agents. Parenteral administration is often the only solution to this problem.

The optimal duration of antimicrobial treatment is unknown for many infections, and there is considerable variation from one medical center to another in the length of time antimicrobial therapy is given. In bacterial endocarditis, for example, the usual course of parenteral therapy may vary from 2 to

8 weeks with an average of about four weeks. For most acute infections a good general rule is to continue therapy for 2 to 3 days after the temperature has returned to normal and all signs of infection have subsided. However, fever can continue for weeks from sterile effusions complicating pneumonia, and cerebrospinal fluid abnormalities can persist for considerable periods in bacterial meningitis, leading to a continuation of chemotherapy for much longer than is necessary. Empiricism needs to be tempered with reason and experience, and in actual practice the guidelines for duration of therapy must be sufficiently flexible to be appropriate for the patient being treated.

ALLERGY AND TOXICITY The patient's allergic history should always be explored before prescribing antimicrobial agents. In addition to allergic manifestations in general, a report of previous drug allergies is of particular importance, and agents that have caused clear-cut reactions should be avoided. Unfortunately, no reliable test is available to determine the presence of allergy to the penicillins, and they may or may not be well tolerated by patients with a history of a previous reaction. The possibility of a severe anaphylactic reaction can be reliably excluded by skin tests containing major and minor determinant mixtures, but only the major mixture is commercially available. When administration of a penicillin is considered essential, one approach is to begin with a very small dose intravenously and increase the amount every few minutes until it is learned whether the patient can tolerate the antibiotic. Specifically, with an intravenous infusion running 1 unit penicillin diluted in 3 to 5 ml saline or glucose solution is injected slowly into the tubing, and 5 min is allowed to elapse to see if an untoward reaction occurs. A solution of epinephrine is available in another syringe to be injected if needed. If no reaction occurs, 2, 5, 10, 25, and 50 units, etc., are injected at 5 min intervals, and within an hour or so it either becomes apparent that the patient can tolerate a full therapeutic dose, or he develops a reaction that is readily controlled by epinephrine. If a reaction occurs, administering another antibiotic is usually best, although in mild reactions, continuing the penicillin along with antihistamines and/or steroids is possible in some instances. Such a program can be quite troublesome as well as risky, requiring frequent adjustments to suppress urticaria and itching. The number of alternative antibiotics available is large enough that switching to another agent is usually the best course to follow.

Drug toxicity related to renal function is of particular importance. Some antimicrobials, such as the penicillins, cephalothin, chloramphenicol, erythromycin, and lincomycin, are relatively safe at normal or only slightly reduced dosage in the presence of impaired renal function. Other agents, such as the aminoglycosides, are potentially quite toxic but can be administered safely at reduced dosage if proper guidelines, based on serial determinations of the serum creatinine, are followed, and particularly if blood levels can be monitored. Certain toxic agents should be avoided if at all possible in the presence of renal insufficiency. These include most of the tetracyclines, streptomycin, cephaloridine, the sulfonamides, the nitrofurans, and nalidixic acid. One of the long-acting tetracyclines, doxycycline, has the same half-life in healthy and uremic subjects, and can be administered to patients with impaired renal function either orally or intravenously. Many patients with chronic renal failure are being maintained on dialysis programs and may require antimicrobials for a variety of infections. Table 111-1 summarizes adult dosage schedules for various antibiotics for patients with renal failure, on or off dialysis.

SITE OF INFECTION Soft-tissue infections in sites with a good blood supply and a minimum of tissue necrosis are, in general,

easily treated. In meningitis and endocarditis, on the other hand, penetration into the site of the infection presents formidable problems and is not infrequently responsible for treatment failures. Penetration across the blood-brain barrier is a complex phenomenon involving protein binding, lipid solubility, and ionization of the drug being administered. In addition, the permeability of this barrier to drugs depends on the degree of inflammation. Because of their low toxicity the penicillins can be administered in doses large enough to provide therapeutic concentrations in the spinal fluid, whereas more toxic drugs such as the aminoglycosides and polymyxins must be injected intrathecally to be effective clinically in meningitis. On the other hand, agents such as the sulfonamides, chloramphenicol, and the tetracyclines appear in the spinal fluid in amounts adequate for the treatment of some types of meningitis when they are given in doses appropriate for the treatment of systemic infections.

Other examples of problems of penetration, and of the influence of localized physiologic conditions, may be cited. The sulfonamides are excreted in the saliva in amounts adequate to eradicate the meningococcal carrier state, whereas most penicillins and tetracyclines are not. However, most of the strains of meningococci encountered at the present time are sulfonamide-resistant. In urinary infections, erythromycin and the aminoglycosides are relatively ineffective at an acid pH, whereas a pH at less than 5.5 is essential for the activity of methenamine mandelate (Mandelamine). The lack of efficacy of sulfonamides in the presence of pus, due to the competition for binding sites by the large amounts of p-aminobenzoic acid present, greatly limits the usefulness of this class of drugs.

Foreign bodies, abscesses, and obstruction to normal pathways of drainage almost always interfere with the response to chemotherapy and usually prevent cure until they are removed, drained, or relieved. Suture materials, prostheses, sequestrations, and calculi are examples of foreign bodies that interfere with drug therapy and usually, but not always, need to be removed. In many abscesses, bacteria tend to be in a metabolically inactive state in which they are not actively synthesizing cell wall and are not susceptible to the damaging effects of some antimicrobial drugs; hence drainage plus chemotherapy is necessary to eradicate the infection. Obstruction to bronchial, biliary, and renal drainage interferes seriously with the response of bacterial infections to antibiotics, and these infections generally cannot be cured with drugs until the obstruction is relieved. A thorough knowledge of the mechanical, metabolic, and physiologic factors is essential in planning therapy that will bring about optimal results in infections located in different parts of the body.

COMBINATION THERAPY, SYNERGISM, ANTAGONISM Once the etiologic agent is known or can be anticipated, most bacterial infections can be treated successfully with a *single* antimicrobial agent. Combination therapy is used frequently, however, to broaden the antibacterial spectrum while awaiting the results of cultures, and also to cover the possibility that a polymicrobial infection might be present. For example, in a hospitalized patient who suddenly becomes ill with presumed sepsis, cephalothin and gentamicin may be given empirically to provide antibacterial activity against a variety of gram-positive and -negative pathogens that might be fatal if therapy were delayed (Chap. 109). Over 100 fixed-dose combinations were once available commercially in the United States for oral or parenteral therapy, but virtually all have been ordered off the market by the Food and Drug Administration on the grounds that it has not been shown in controlled studies that both agents contribute to the claimed therapeutic effects, that the amounts of each agent present were often not appropriate, and that patients were often being exposed to the potential hazards of two drugs when only one was needed. When combination therapy is indicated, it is most rational to prescribe separately the indicated drugs in doses that take into the account the patient's age, weight, and physiologic status.

A clinically significant enhancement of antibacterial activity from exposing microorganisms to two or more drugs is rare. Usually, the drugs have an indifferent effect in vitro; sometimes an additive action is observed, but this is difficult to demonstrate in patients.

True synergism occurs between penicillins and aminoglycosides with a number of gram-positive and gram-negative pathogens. The classic example is enterococcal endocarditis; penicillins (G, V, ampicillin, carbenicillin) disrupt the cell wall, permitting streptomycin to gain access to the ribosomes where their action is lethal. About one-third of enterococci are ribosomally resistant to streptomycin, but few if any strains are resistant to gentamicin and tobramycin, and so these aminoglycosides are replacing streptomycin in treating this disease. Of the penicillinase-resistant penicillins, only nafcillin is synergistic against most strains of enterococci. In contrast, with viridans streptococci streptomycin is synergistic with penicillins against virtually all strains, and it is probable that, in bacterial endocarditis due to viridans streptococci, there are fewer relapses with combined therapy than with penicillin G alone (Chap. 243).

Gentamicin and tobramycin are synergistic with carbenicillin against *Pseudomonas* and some other gram-negative bacilli. Theoretically, it would be possible to reduce doses of the antibiotics, but in severe *Pseudomonas* infections full doses are usually given so as not to risk compromising the therapeutic result.

Trimethoprim-sulfamethoxazole, another synergistic combination, will be described below.

Clinically, significant antagonism between antimicrobial agents is also rare, a prime example being a higher mortality rate in pneumococcal meningitis with penicillin and tetracycline than with penicillin alone. The rate of killing by penicillin

TABLE 111-1
Dosages of antimicrobials in renal failure

Drug	Normal dose	Normal dose interval	Dose interval for degree of renal failure Mild (C_{cr}* 50–80 ml/min)	Moderate (C_{cr}* 10–50 ml/min)	Severe (C_{cr}* 10 ml/min)	Hemodialysis Significant dialysis of drug	Add at end of each dialysis	Peritoneal dialysis Significant dialysis of drug	Add parenterally during dialysis	Alternative, add to dialysate after the regular parenteral loading dose
Ampicillin	0.5–3 g	Every 6 h	6 h	9 h	12–15 h (1 g)	Yes	0.5–1 g	No		50 µg/ml
Amoxicillin	0.25–1 g PO	Every 8 h	8 h	12 h	16 h (0.5 g)	Yes	0.5 g	No		
Penicillin G	0.25–4 million U	4 h	4 h (2 million U)	4 h (1.5 million U)	6 h (1 million U)	No		No		
Methicillin, oxacillin, nafcillin	1–2 g	4 h	4 h	4 h	8–12 h (1 g)	No		No		
Cloxacillin, dicloxacillin	0.5–1 g PO	6 h	6 h	6 h	6 h	No		No		
Carbenicillin	4–5 g	4 h	4 h	6–8 h (2 g)	12 h (2 g)	Yes	1–2 g	No	1 g every 6 h	200 µg/ml
Cephalexin, cephradine	0.25–1 g	4 h	4 h	6 h	Every 6 h (0.25 g)	Yes	0.25–0.5 g	Yes	0.25 g PO every 6 h	
Cephalothin, cephapirin	1–2 g	4 h	4 h	6 h	8–12 h (1 g)	Yes	1 g	Yes	1 g every 6 h	50 µg/ml
Cefazolin	0.5–1 g	8 h	12 h	12 h (0.5 g)	24 h (0.5 g)	No	0.5 g	No		75 µg/ml
Cefamandole, cefoxitin	0.5–2 g	6 h	8 h	12 h (1 g)	12 h (1 g)	No	0.5 g	No		50 µg/ml
Gentamicin,†,‡ tobramycin	1–1.7 mg/kg	8 h	8–12 h	12–24 h	48–72 h	Yes	1.5 mg/kg	No		8 µg/ml
Amikacin,†,‡ kanamycin	7.5 mg/kg	12 h	24 h	24–72 h	72–96 h	Yes	3.5 mg/kg	No		20 µg/ml
Streptomycin	0.5 g	12 h	24 h	24–72 h	72–96 h	Yes	0.25 g	Yes	?	
Chloramphenicol	0.25–1 g	6 h	6 h	8 h	8 h	No		No		
Erythromycin	0.25–1 g	6 h	6 h	8 h	8–12 h	?		?		
Clindamycin	0.3–0.6 g	6–8 h	8 h	8 h	12 h (0.3 g)	No		No		
Vancomycin	0.25–0.5 g	6 h	24 h	48–72 h	7 days	No		No		15 µg/ml
Tetracycline	0.25–0.5 g	6 h	8–12 h	Avoid	Avoid	No		No		
Doxycycline	0.1–0.2 g	12–24 h	12–24 h	24 h	24 h	No		No		
Sulfisoxazole	1 g	6 h	6 h	6 h	8–12 h	Avoid	Yes	?		

* C_{cr} = creatinine clearance rate.
† Frequency of the dose can be estimated more accurately by multiplying the serum creatinine by 8 (for gentamicin and tobramycin) or by 9 (for amikacin and kanamycin).
‡ An alternate method is to give smaller doses at 8- to 12-h intervals by relating the elimination constants of the drugs to the patient's creatinine clearance. A dosing chart applicable to all the aminoglycosides has been described by Sarubbi and Hull.

is slowed by the bacteriostatic agent, tetracycline, and this can alter the outcome when survival depends on rapid killing of the pneumococci.

SUPERINFECTION AND RESISTANCE DURING ANTIMICROBIAL THERAPY A number of microorganisms are genetically resistant to clinically feasible levels of one or more antimicrobials, and they obviously will not be affected by antibiotic therapy. Most antibiotics will alter the host's normal flora by removing those organisms which are sensitive to the drug. In most cases this ecologic change is of little consequence, but occasionally the commensal bacteria of the host set up infection in the same location as the original infection, a state termed *superinfection* (Chap. 107). The superinfecting organism is resistant to the drug being administered, and determining its susceptibility is helpful in selecting the most appropriate antimicrobial drug. Some superinfecting organisms, particularly gram-negatives, acquire resistance to multiple drugs by an episomal transfer mechanism (R factors). For example, multiple-resistant *E. coli* and *Klebsiella-Enterobacter* pose a particular hazard to hospitalized patients.

Comparatively few organisms become resistant to the antibiotic being given during therapy. Some that do develop resistance are *E. coli* to streptomycin and nalidixic acid, occasional strains of staphylococci to erythromycin, and *Pseudomonas* to carbenicillin. In general, however, sensitive organisms are supplanted by resistant ones, rather than acquiring resistance themselves. From a practical point of view, it is important to know which agents are likely to induce resistance, and to look for this phenomenon clinically.

SPECIFIC ANTIMICROBIALS

PENICILLINS Penicillinase-susceptible The prototype, *Penicillin G* (benzyl penicillin), is still widely used, especially parenterally, when high blood levels are desirable as in meningitis and endocarditis. Large doses are necessary either continuously or at 3- to 4-h intervals because of problems of penetration into vegetations and across the blood-brain barrier, and also because of its high renal clearance, which is due chiefly to rapid tubular secretion. Blood levels can be doubled by the concomitant administration of probenecid, 0.5 g every 6 h, but since penicillin G is now quite inexpensive and the optimal blood levels are not known precisely, it is customary in most instances simply to give more penicillin. *Procaine penicillin* is well tolerated intramuscularly and is absorbed quite slowly so that injections need to be given only every 12 h for the treatment of many infections due to susceptible bacteria. In dosage of 300,000 to 600,000 units every 12 h, it is the drug of choice for most patients with pneumococcal pneumonia. *Benzathine penicillin* provides a depot in the muscle that releases penicillin so slowly that low blood levels are present for 2 to 3 weeks. These low levels are adequate for the therapy and prevention of streptococcal pharyngitis, for the treatment of some forms of syphilis, and for the prevention of recurrences of rheumatic fever.

Penicillin G given orally in doses of 250,000 units once or twice daily is also effective in preventing streptococcal sore throats, but less so than benzathine penicillin (Chap. 241). Because of its instability in the presence of acid, however, it is less reliable for therapy than the acid-stable penicillin V (phenoxymethyl penicillin), and attempts to overcome this disadvantage by giving larger amounts of penicillin G are associated with an increased incidence of nausea and diarrhea. This has resulted in the development of a number of penicillin G analogs which continue to have some usefulness because very little resistance has developed to them. An exception are the pneumococci

where a small number of resistant strains have been isolated in various parts of the world.

Broad-spectrum penicillins *Ampicillin* differs from penicillin G only in the presence of an amino group in the side chain, but this minor chemical difference is responsible for some unique features that have led to the widespread use of this antibiotic. Ampicillin is active in low concentrations against a number of gram-negative bacteria causing respiratory (*Hemophilus influenzae*), intestinal (*Shigella*, *Salmonella*), and urinary (*E. coli*, *Proteus mirabilis*) infections. When it is given orally, the peak blood level occurs later (2 to 3 h versus ½ to 1 h) and is lower than with penicillin V, and the ampicillin blood level then declines more slowly. This more prolonged blood level, along with its greater in vitro activity, is probably responsible for the greater efficacy of ampicillin, compared with penicillin V, in the oral therapy of gonococcal urethritis.

When given in an intravenous infusion, blood levels are more than 80 percent higher with ampicillin than with penicillin G chiefly because of the much higher rate of renal clearance of penicillin G (390 versus 210 ml/min per 1.73 m²). When the in vitro activity of the infecting organisms is the same for the two antibiotics, this difference can mean equal efficacy with smaller doses of ampicillin, or higher blood levels with the same dose when maximum serum concentrations are considered necessary. Ampicillin is also more stable in the body, with a serum half-life twice as long as penicillin G, due chiefly to slower breakdown by the liver. Serum protein binding of ampicillin is approximately 20 percent compared with 60 percent for penicillin G and 80 percent for penicillin V; this may mean that with ampicillin there is a higher concentration of free, active antibiotic at the site of infection. All these features contribute to the efficacy and widespread use of ampicillin, and in the United States, competition has led to a marked decrease in the cost in the last few years. Although ampicillin has remained an effective drug against most organisms, increasing resistance has developed among a significant number of strains of *E. coli*, *Salmonella*, *Shigella*, and *H. influenzae*.

Hypersensitivity reactions occur with about the same frequency with ampicillin as with penicillin G and V, and with all three are much more frequent and severe when the drug is given parenterally and topically than by the oral route. About 5 to 10 percent of patients develop skin rashes with oral ampicillin, but the incidence is as high as 90 percent when patients with infectious mononucleosis take this drug. This remarkably high incidence, which does not occur with penicillins G and V, does not represent true penicillin allergy, and its exact nature is not known. Maculopapular (as opposed to urticarial) rashes beginning 4 days or more after initiating treatment with ampicillin do not indicate a need to discontinue therapy, or to avoid subsequent courses of the antibiotic. Although acid-stable, ampicillin is not very well absorbed when taken orally, giving peak blood levels only one-sixth as high as dicloxacillin and cephalexin. *Amoxicillin*, a derivative with a hydroxyl group on the benzene ring, is much better absorbed orally, with blood levels and urinary excretion more than twice as great on the average as ampicillin. Blood levels are roughly equivalent to those of ampicillin given intramuscularly, and amoxicillin has a lower incidence of intestinal side effects when given in half the dose orally. *Bacampicillin*, a rapidly hydrolyzed ester with much better intestinal absorption, provides peak blood levels and urinary excretion of ampicillin more than twice as great as does ampicillin alone. It is not yet available commercially. *Hetacillin*, a penicillin with a complex side chain, is hydrolyzed rapidly in the body to ampicillin, and for practical therapeutic purposes can be regarded as the same as ampicillin.

Carbenicillin is a broad-spectrum penicillin similar chemically to ampicillin, except that the amino group in the side chain is replaced by a carboxyl group. As a result, carbenicillin is active in vitro against *Pseudomonas*, indole-positive *Proteus*, and some strains of *Enterobacter*, in addition to the other gram-negatives that are susceptible to ampicillin. Like ampicillin, it is not active against *Klebsiella*. The MIC for *Pseudomonas* is much higher than that usually considered within the therapeutic range for other antibiotics, i.e., about 75 to 100 µg/ml for most strains and as high as 500 µg/ml for a few. However, extraordinarily high blood levels can be readily attained, in the range of 200 to 400 µg/ml, so that carbenicillin provides the safety and bactericidal activity of a penicillin for some organisms that have been notably refractory to most other antibiotics. The much higher blood levels that can be readily attained with carbenicillin compared to ampicillin are due chiefly to its much lower renal clearance (100 versus 210 ml/min per 1.73 m²). In addition, carbenicillin is much more stable in the body, so that blood levels obtained with 30 g a day in patients with normal renal function can be achieved with only 3 or 4 g a day in patients with no renal function. Since many patients with severe gram-negative infections have considerable renal impairment, reduced doses can be administered with the knowledge that full therapeutic blood levels will be achieved. To give 30 g daily for the therapy of severe *Pseudomonas* infections in patients with normal renal function, it is customary to administer 5 g intravenously every 4 h, diluting each dose in 100 to 200 ml fluid and allowing it to drip into the vein within 1 to 2 h. Except for severe *Pseudomonas* infections, 30 g daily is not necessary, and much smaller doses, 10 or 15 g daily, are adequate for the therapy of other gram-negative infections, including those caused by indole-positive *Proteus* and *Enterobacter*. Urinary concentrations in excess of 1000 µg/ml are attained with 0.5- or 1.0-g doses intramuscularly, so that doses comparable with those used with ampicillin are appropriate for urinary tract infections, including those due to *Pseudomonas*. An oral form of carbenicillin, the indanyl salt of the sodium ester, has become available, and one or two 0.5-g tablets (each equivalent to 382 mg carbenicillin) every 6 h produce urinary concentrations well in excess of MICs for susceptible gram-negative bacilli, including *Pseudomonas*.

An increase in bacterial resistance has been noted in some patients with severe gram-negative infections treated with carbenicillin, but the frequency and extent of the resistance has varied in different reports. The concomitant administration of aminoglycosides has tended to delay the development of resistance to carbenicillin, and in addition a synergistic action has been found to occur with these two antibiotics against many gram-negative bacilli. It has therefore become customary in severe infections to give both these antibiotics, to enhance antibacterial activity, and to delay the emergence of resistance as well. Since there is inactivation of the antibiotics, especially gentamicin, when the two are present in the same solution for several hours, it is preferable to administer them separately, either intramuscularly or intravenously, and under these circumstances the blood levels of each are the same as if they were being given alone. *Ticarcillin*, a newer semisynthetic penicillin, has pharmacokinetic properties very similar to those of carbenicillin but is two to four times as active in vitro against *Pseudomonas*. A daily dose of 18 g is considered equal to 30 g carbenicillin for *Pseudomonas* infections and provides a lower sodium load (both antibiotics contain about 5.5 meq sodium per gram). Disadvantages of the lower dose are that the greater activity of ticarcillin is found only against *Pseudomonas*, and that 18 g ticarcillin is more expensive than 30 g carbenicillin.

Piperacillin, another new penicillin even more active against *Pseudomonas* and other gram-negative organisms, has been quite promising in extensive clinical trials.

Penicillinase-resistant penicillins The advent of these antibiotics in the early 1960s greatly enhanced the ability to cope with severe staphylococcal infections, because at that time over three-fourths of strains causing infections in hospitals were penicillinase producers, and this high incidence has persisted. Furthermore, the number of strains resistant to these new penicillins has remained small, especially in the United States. This is probably due to the low incidence of naturally occurring methicillin-resistant strains, and the fact that only a small proportion of the cells in a "resistant" culture are actually lacking in susceptibility. In contrast, certain European hospitals now report that over 20 percent of strains of *Staphylococcus aureus* are methicillin-resistant; the reason for the difference is unknown.

Five penicillinase-resistant penicillins are currently marketed in the United States: *methicillin, oxacillin, nafcillin, cloxacillin,* and *dicloxacillin*. The first three are available for parenteral administration. Methicillin is less active when tested in broth cultures than are oxacillin and nafcillin, but this is probably offset by its much lower protein binding, 40 percent compared with 90 percent or more for the other two. Clinical studies do not provide convincing evidence of superiority of any of these three penicillins for the parenteral therapy of severe staphylococcal infections. Methicillin is given in the same dose as, or in twice the dose of, the other two because of its lower in vitro activity, i.e., 1 or 2 g every 4 to 6 h in adults. For intravenous administration, each dose is diluted in 50 to 100 ml fluid, and is infused over a period of 30 min to minimize phlebitis. Intramuscular injections are painful and are poorly tolerated for more than a few days. Methicillin nephritis, an uncommon but important allergic reaction, has been reported rarely with oxacillin and nafcillin; it is not known whether this is due simply to the fact that methicillin is more widely used. Nafcillin has been found by many observers to give lower blood levels than equal doses of oxacillin; this appears to be due to sequestration of nafcillin in the liver and possibly in other tissues so that less is available to circulate in the blood. The therapeutic implications of this phenomenon are unknown.

With oral administration, both nafcillin and oxacillin give low blood levels, but cloxacillin gives blood levels twice as high and dicloxacillin four times as high as oxacillin when the same doses are given orally. However, there is also a progressive increase in serum protein binding (92 percent for oxacillin, 94 percent for cloxacillin, and 96 percent for dicloxacillin), so that the differences in free, active antibiotic may offset the blood level differences. In general, cloxacillin or dicloxacillin in doses of 0.25 or 0.5 g four times daily is preferred for oral administration. The efficacy of these antibiotics, either initially in mild to moderate soft-tissue infections, or for completion of therapy following administration of one of the three parenteral preparations described above, is well established.

The chief indication for the penicillinase-resistant penicillins is the therapy of infections caused by penicillinase-producing staphylococci, but they are often administered empirically before the etiologic organism is known. Pneumococci and most streptococci are more susceptible to penicillin G and ampicillin, but blood levels are sufficiently high with the penicillinase-resistant penicillins, especially when given parenterally, so that it is not necessary to give both types of penicillins to provide coverage for these organisms. However, infections caused by enterococci and *Neisseria* cannot be expected to respond to therapy with a penicillinase-resistant penicillin given alone, and if these organisms are suspected, penicillin G or ampicillin should be used.

In addition to the various allergic manifestations mentioned above, reactions to penicillins include myoclonus, seizures, potassium intoxication, hemolysis, leukopenia, thrombocytopenia, and neuropathy, usually with very high blood levels. Mental disturbances occur in a small percentage of patients following large doses of procaine penicillin.

CEPHALOSPORINS The cephalosporins differ from the penicillins in having a six-membered dihydrothiazine ring, instead of a five-membered thiazolidine ring, fused to the beta-lactam ring. As a result of this chemical difference there is no true cross-allergenicity, and most patients who are allergic to penicillins can be treated with cephalosporins without hypersensitivity reactions. The small number in whom this is not possible seem to be highly allergic individuals who react separately to the two groups of antibiotics.

Most bacteria susceptible to the penicillins are also susceptible to the cephalosporins, including group A and viridans streptococci, pneumococci, penicillin G-sensitive and resistant *S. aureus, Neisseria, Clostridia, Actinomyces,* and *Corynebacterium diphtheriae.* Among the gram-negatives most strains of *E. coli, P. mirabilis, Klebsiella* but not *Enterobacter, Shigella, Salmonella,* and most strains of *H. influenzae,* are susceptible. The spectrum has been extended appreciably by the addition of cefamandole and cefoxitin (see below). The cephalosporins act on the cell wall in a manner similar to the penicillins, and are bactericidal. As with the penicillins, there has been little tendency for susceptible species to become resistant despite widespread use of the cephalosporins for more than a decade.

Nine cephalosporins are now marketed in the United States, and at least that many more are under investigation. Orally, *cephalexin* and *cephradine* are very similar and can be considered interchangeable. They are well absorbed, a 0.5 g dose giving an average peak blood level in adults of about 18 μg/ml, six times as high as with the same dose of ampicillin. Serum protein binding is low and comparable with that of ampicillin (about 15 percent), and over 90 percent of these drugs are excreted in the urine, without nephrotoxicity. These two antibiotics are less active in vitro against gram-positive bacteria, especially staphylococci, than the injectable cephalosporins, but, because of the high blood levels, clinical results have been good, particularly after initial parenteral therapy. There is considerable variability in the susceptibility of *H. influenzae,* and twice the usual dose is recommended in the official labeling for otitis media. *Cephaloglycin,* a drug that is poorly absorbed orally and that gives low blood levels, has gradually been abandoned in the treatment of urinary infections because of the superior characteristics of the other two compounds.

Parenteral preparations of seven cephalosporins are commercially available. Both for therapy and prophylaxis *cephalothin* has had the longest and most extensive use. It is usually administered intravenously, 1 or 2 g every 4 or 6 h in at least 50 ml fluid to minimize phlebitis. It is partially converted in the body to a metabolic breakdown product, desacetylcephalothin, which is less active, particularly against gram-negative bacteria. This appears to have no clinical significance because of the large amount of the parent compound present. Cephalothin may cause some nephrotoxicity, especially when given in conjunction with aminoglycosides, but establishing this point clearly has been difficult. *Cephapirin* is very similar to cephalothin in its in vitro activity and pharmacological characteristics and may be interchangeable clinically, although fewer reports of its efficacy are available. *Cephaloridine,* another early cephalosporin, has low serum protein binding and is well tolerated intramuscularly, but clearly causes renal tubular damage in large doses and, because of its potential nephrotoxicity, should not be used. Cephradine is available parenterally as well as orally, but published documentation of efficacy with parenteral administration is not extensive.

Cefazolin has had increasing use parenterally because of its high and prolonged blood levels, which are due to high serum protein binding (85 percent) and low renal clearance. Its serum half-life is 1.8 h compared with 0.5 h for cephalothin. Cefazolin 0.5 g is probably equivalent to 1.0 g cephalothin therapeutically, taking into consideration the differences in blood levels and protein binding. Cefazolin is also well tolerated intramuscularly, whereas cephalothin and cephapirin are not. Also cefazolin is inactivated by large inocula of some strains of *S. aureus* while cephalothin is not; whether the inactivation is of any clinical significance has not been established.

Cefoxitin and *cefamandole* are the latest parenteral cephalosporins that have become available, and their relative usefulness is still being tested. Both agents have similar pharmacological characteristics that are superior to those of cephalothin, and a broader antibacterial spectrum that includes greater activity against indole-positive *Proteus* and *H. influenzae.* Cefamandole also has increased activity against *Enterobacter, Citrobacter,* and *Providencia,* and cefoxitin is active against *Serratia* and *Bacteroides fragilis.* Because of the importance of *B. fragilis* as a pathogen in abdominal and pelvic infections, cefoxitin might replace cephalothin and cefazolin as the antibiotic that is widely used in surgery.

Although cephalosporins penetrate most body fluids quite well, none can be clearly recommended for parenteral therapy of bacterial meningitis. Good results have been observed with cephaloridine in pneumococcal meningitis, but intrathecal therapy has been necessary when the antibiotic is given in recommended doses. Cefamandole has been reported to give a high cure rate in meningococcal meningitis, but, in cases of *H. influenzae* meningitis, the results have been equivocal. Further studies are needed before parenteral therapy can be given routinely, particularly in cases where the causative organism is not known.

Most patients who are thought to be allergic to penicillins can tolerate cephalosporins without adverse reactions. There is probably not true cross-reactivity, but a small number of highly allergic individuals do react to both drugs. In patients with previous penicillin anaphylaxis, or with positive immediate-type skin reactions to penicillin, therapy with cephalosporins should be instituted in small doses that are increased gradually. Rashes, urticaria, and anaphylaxis have been reported with cephalosporins, as have neutropenia, hemolytic anemia, thrombocytopenia, positive Coombs' tests, and transient rise in serum glutamic oxaloacetic transaminase and alkaline phosphatase.

AMINOGLYCOSIDES *Streptomycin,* one of the first antibiotics available for systemic administration, was widely used during the late 1940s and the 1950s. For a number of years it was given almost routinely in conjunction with penicillin in surgical cases for the prophylaxis and treatment of postoperative infections. Because of the tendency for highly resistant organisms to appear within 2 or 3 days, and its potential for causing vestibular damage and deafness, streptomycin has been largely supplanted by kanamycin, gentamicin, tobramycin, and amikacin, although it is still in use for certain specific purposes. Tuberculosis is still treated with streptomycin, particularly when triple drug regimens are used for the first few weeks. Streptomycin is also used in conjunction with penicillin to treat *Strep. viridans* endocarditis and some enterococcal infections and for the treatment of certain less common infections such as brucellosis and tularemia. In addition to vestibular nerve toxicity, other adverse reactions of streptomycin include rashes, fever, contact dermatitis, pancytopenia, anaphylaxis, and renal irritation.

Neomycin, another aminoglycoside that appeared in the 1940s, is no longer used parenterally because of its nephro- and neurotoxicity. Respiratory arrest is a serious adverse reaction that has occurred when neomycin is instilled topically in the peritoneal cavity in anesthetized patients, and deafness has resulted from the topical application of neomycin soaks injudiciously in burns and wounds. Neomycin is useful and relatively safe when given orally in doses of 4 to 6 g daily to "prepare" the bowel preoperatively, and in patients with hepatic insufficiency where inhibition of bacterial growth in the intestine is necessary to reduce the absorption of nitrogenous substances. However, the amount of neomycin absorbed from the intestine is variable, and toxic levels have been demonstrated in some patients. Neomycin is also used as a spray and an ointment to decrease the bacterial count in individuals who are nasal carriers of staphylococci.

Kanamycin is similar in structure to neomycin but less toxic and has been widely used parenterally for infections caused by most commonly encountered gram-negative bacilli except *Pseudomonas. Amikacin,* a semisynthetic derivative of kanamycin, has almost identical characteristics except that it is active against *Pseudomonas.* Both are active in vitro against staphylococci but are not used to treat severe staphylococcal infections because much higher blood levels can be attained safely with penicillins and cephalosporins. These aminoglycosides are not active against common gram-positive pathogens such as streptococci and pneumococci. They should be administered intramuscularly or by slow intravenous infusion in doses not larger than 7.5 mg/kg every 12 h, with the total dose not exceeding 15 g. Excretion is by glomerular filtration, the serum half-life is 2 h, and the drugs are not protein-bound.

Gentamicin and *tobramycin* are widely used aminoglycosides that are very similar except that tobramycin is two to four times more active against most strains of *Pseudomonas.* Smaller doses are used than for amikacin (3 to 5 versus 15 mg/kg per day), giving peak blood levels following intramuscular injections of 4 to 5 μg/ml for gentamicin and tobramycin versus about 20 μg/ml for amikacin. However, minimal inhibitory concentrations are also higher with amikacin, and it has not been shown that the higher blood levels are associated with a better clinical response.

Bacterial resistance, transmitted by plasmids and due to enzymatic transformations, is a potential threat with the aminoglycosides but has been relatively uncommon in most hospitals. Since amikacin has the least potential for resistance by this mechanism, many hospitals have established the policy of holding it in reserve. However, in some hospitals where gentamicin resistance has become a significant problem (25 to 30 percent of resistant strains), amikacin is the drug of choice for seriously ill patients requiring an aminoglycoside.

To minimize ototoxicity and nephrotoxicity, both significant problems with the aminoglycosides, it is important to reduce the dosage in patients with impaired renal function, and this is done in one of two ways. With the first, the full dose is given at an interval determined by multiplying the patient's serum creatinine by 8. This can result in a long interval between doses, when the serum concentration is at a low level. Therefore, the second method, giving a reduced dose at 8- or 12-h intervals, is used more widely. The serum creatinine, or preferably the creatinine clearance, is applied to a nomogram, and blood levels are monitored. The peak level is determined 30 min after an intramuscular, or 5 to 10 min after an intravenous, dose, and is more important than the trough. Serum concentrations can be determined by bioassay or radioimmunoassay within 2 to 4 h. The latter method is more expensive unless at least six or eight specimens are run every day.

With the ever-increasing occurrence of infections due to gram-negative bacteria the aminoglycosides are among the most widely used antibiotics in hospitals. Tobramycin and gentamicin have, to a great extent, replaced kanamycin, because of the adverse effects and bacterial resistance associated with its use. The role of amikacin remains in flux because its relative efficacy, toxicity, and potential for resistance have not been determined with certainty, particularly in relation to gentamicin and tobramycin. *Sisomicin* and *netilmicin* are new aminoglycosides that are being tested clinically and may have some advantages over drugs presently available.

TETRACYCLINES   Since they first appeared in the late 1940s, the tetracycline antibiotics have been used widely because of their broad spectrum of activity against many gram-positive and gram-negative bacteria, and also other microorganisms such as *Mycoplasma, Rickettsia,* and *Chlamydia.* They have been effective, although not necessarily the drugs of choice, in the treatment of common venereal diseases including gonorrhea, syphilis, lymphogranuloma venereum, and granuloma inguinale. Their use has become more restricted during the last decade because of the advent of bactericidal antibiotics such as the cephalosporins, the penicillinase-resistant penicillins, and the aminoglycosides, together with an increasing awareness of the limitations of the tetracyclines. These limitations include the appearance of resistant strains among commonly encountered pathogens such as group A streptococci and pneumococci, the primarily bacteriostatic action of the tetracyclines, the occurrence of hepatotoxicity with high blood levels, the relatively high incidence of superinfections, and the common occurrence of side effects such as nausea, diarrhea, and photosensitivity reactions. Despite these limitations, the tetracyclines are still widely used for respiratory, urinary, soft tissue, and venereal infections.

Chlortetracycline (Aureomycin) and *oxytetracycline* (Terramycin), the two original compounds, have been largely replaced by *tetracycline,* which is marketed by a number of companies, and competition has led to a marked reduction in its price. The usual adult dose is 1 to 2 g daily in two to four equally divided doses. Intramuscular preparations are not very satisfactory, but the intravenous form is well-tolerated and gives relatively high blood levels with doses of 0.5 g every 12 h. Excessive blood levels occur with renal insufficiency unless the dose is decreased, and can cause fatty degeneration of the liver which may be fatal. Tetracycline persists in the body for many days when its normal route of excretion through the kidneys is blocked.

Four long-acting tetracyclines are available: *demeclocycline, methacycline, doxycycline,* and *minocycline.* They have high protein binding (over 90 versus 70 percent for tetracycline) and a prolonged plasma half-life, so that blood levels are well maintained when they are administered orally only every 12 to 24 h. However, the half-life of tetracycline is sufficiently prolonged so that blood levels with administration only every 12 h are similar to those of the smaller doses recommended for the long-acting tetracyclines. Unfortunately, the reduction in dose is not matched by a proportional decrease in price. The potential advantages for the long-active tetracyclines, i.e., greater convenience from less frequent administration and decreased cost from lower doses, have not been realized fully. Doxycycline does not give excessive blood levels in the presence of renal insufficiency following either oral or intravenous administration, and this provides a safety feature when the exact status of the patient's renal function is uncertain or unknown. Doxycycline is also active against the majority of strains of *B. fragilis,* and its efficacy in abdominal and pelvic infections has received considerable attention.

Untoward effects of the tetracyclines include staining of the teeth in children under 10, photosensitivity, intestinal irritation, increased urinary nitrogen loss, potential nephrotoxicity especially when given with other nephrotoxic drugs or with outdated supplies, vertigo (with minocycline), fatty hepatic changes in pregnancy, and increased intracranial pressure in children

ERYTHROMYCIN, LINCOMYCIN, CLINDAMYCIN *Erythromycin* is primarily a bacteriostatic antibiotic that is active against the commonly encountered gram-positive bacteria, and is used chiefly for the oral therapy of respiratory and soft-tissue infections, particularly in patients thought to be allergic to penicillin. The susceptibility of *Mycoplasma pneumoniae* to erythromycin enhances its usefulness in respiratory infections. Erythromycin base is absorbed in an erratic manner, but some enteric-coated preparations now available give good and reliable serum concentrations. Erythromycin estolate has been thought to give much higher blood levels than erythromycin stearate, but the difference may be not as great as was once postulated because the estolate needs to be hydrolyzed in the body to the active form, and the hydrolysis is not as complete as during the blood level assay procedure. The estolate salt is associated with a low incidence of cholestatic hepatitis, which is readily reversible and rarely serious. Clinical results with the estolate, stearate, and the newer enteric-coated preparations appear to be comparable. The usual oral dose is 1 or 2 g daily. Intramuscular preparations are irritating, and intravenous administration is not used widely, partly because the preparations are not entirely satisfactory but chiefly because oral therapy is adequate for most infections treated with erythromycin.

Lincomycin and *clindamycin* are similar in antibacterial activity and clinical usefulness to erythromycin. Clindamycin gives higher blood levels, is more potent, and may cause less gastrointestinal side effects than lincomycin. The usual oral dose is 150 to 300 mg every 6 h. An excellent parenteral preparation of both is available, and 300 to 600 mg is given every 6 or 8 h. Clindamycin is considerably more active against *B. fragilis*, and intravenous administration of this antibiotic in abdominal and pelvic infections is widely advocated for this reason. However, pseudomembranous colitis is a fairly frequent and at times serious side effect which has led to recommendations that these antibiotics be used chiefly for hospitalized patients with significant infections, and that they be discontinued at once if diarrhea occurs. The colitis is probably due to toxin-producing strains of clostridia that are resistant to clindamycin.

CHLORAMPHENICOL This antibiotic has a broad spectrum of activity similar to the tetracyclines and during the 1950s was used widely. However, the occurrence of aplastic anemia, even though quite uncommon (about 1 in 25,000 persons exposed) has led to a restriction of chloramphenicol to those serious infections in which it is quite clearly the drug of choice. Typhoid fever is the principal example, and there are occasionally other severe gram-negative infections where the etiologic agent is susceptible only to chloramphenicol. With increasing interest in anaerobic infections, it is now realized that *B. fragilis* is the commonest of the anaerobic pathogens and that over half the strains are resistant to the penicillins and tetracyclines. This has led to an increase in the use of chloramphenicol since almost all *Bacteroides* strains are susceptible to it. However, clindamycin is also very active against *B. fragilis*, and it has partially replaced chloramphenicol for the treatment of patients with proved or presumed *Bacteroides* infections. Clindamycin lacks the broad gram-negative spectrum of chloramphenicol, and for this reason, the latter may be preferred under certain circumstances. In addition, clindamycin's propensity to producing colitis should restrict its use. Chloramphenicol is also used frequently in bacterial meningitis when the causative organism is not clearly recognizable on Gram's stain of the spinal fluid, since a number of strains of *H. influenzae* are now resistant to ampicillin.

Chloramphenicol is well absorbed by the oral route, and the usual adult dose is 0.5 g every 6 h. The parenteral preparation, chloramphenicol succinate, is hydrolyzed in the body to the active form, and this conversion is incomplete so that the blood levels with intravenous administration are not much higher than when the antibiotic is taken by mouth. With intramuscular administration, blood levels are considerably lower than with the oral route, and although the drug was widely used by this route for a number of years, the present labeling does not authorize intramuscular injections.

In addition to aplastic anemia, which may be an allergic or "idiosyncratic" reaction that usually occurs with prolonged and repeated administration, chloramphenicol inhibits protein synthesis, especially with doses larger than 2 g a day, an effect that is reversible. Clinically this is manifested by leukopenia, inadequate erythropoiesis (anemia), and thrombocytopenia as well as absence of reticulocytosis, high serum iron, and full saturation of transferrin. To monitor toxicity, blood counts should be performed at least twice weekly, and treatment with the antibiotic should be discontinued if there is significant hematologic toxicity. The gray syndrome, consisting of pallor, listlessness, and often death, occurs in neonates who have inadequately developed hepatic and renal mechanisms for metabolizing chloramphenicol; this can be prevented by restricting the dose to 25 mg/kg per day.

POLYMYXINS Polymyxin B and E (colistin) are polypeptide antibiotics that are active against most gram-negative bacteria except for the *Proteus* group. They have been of importance chiefly because of their action against *Pseudomonas aeruginosa*. However, their use systemically has decreased markedly since the advent of the aminoglycosides and carbenicillin which are clearly superior.

Polymyxin B is administered intramuscularly every 8 h, or as a continuous intravenous infusion, in doses no larger than 2.0 mg/kg per day. It is effective in treating urinary infections, but its efficacy in systemic infections is uncertain. Polymyxin B is also administered topically for eye and ear infections, and intrathecally for *Pseudomonas* meningitis. Colistin is available as the sodium salt of colistimethate and is administered in doses of 3.0 to 5.0 mg/kg per day intramuscularly or intravenously as described for polymyxin B.

Polymyxin B and colistimethate both cause perioral paresthesias and other neurotoxic manifestations with excessive blood levels; of these, apnea is the most life-threatening. Renal irritation and azotemia, which are usually reversible, may also occur. It is important to monitor renal function and to decrease the dose in the presence of renal insufficiency.

VANCOMYCIN Vancomycin is a relatively toxic but highly effective antibiotic that warrants special consideration because of its usefulness in treating certain specific infections. Vancomycin is bactericidal and is effective against gram-positive bacteria including penicillinase-producing staphylococci and enterococci. It is particularly useful in treating severe staphylococcal infections when penicillins and cephalosporins cannot be given, and in the treatment of *S. viridans* and enterococcal endocarditis under the same circumstances. It can be given only by the intravenous route, and 0.5 g every 6 h for 2 or 3 weeks is the usual dose. Thrombophlebitis is the principal side effect; it can be minimized by diluting each dose in 100 ml fluid and administering it over a period of at least 1 h. Chills, fever, renal irritation, and deafness are other adverse reactions that have been described, and these can be minimized by slow administration and by reduction of the dose if renal function is impaired. Vancomycin has had a considerable revival. One special indication is infections in patients with renal failure requiring dialysis, where a single dose of 1 g every 7 to 10 days gives adequate blood levels.

SULFONAMIDES The sulfonamides have been used clinically since 1937 and were the principal drugs administered for systemic antibacterial chemotherapy before penicillin and the other antibiotics became generally available. Their role has declined steadily, and they now occupy an important although relatively small place in clinical therapy since they are less active than the antibiotics, they are primarily bacteriostatic, resistant organisms occur frequently, and adverse reactions are common. Uncomplicated urinary tract infections due to *E. coli* are the principal indication for sulfonamides because of their efficacy, relative safety, and low cost. In addition, sulfonamides are the drugs of choice for the therapy of nocardiosis. They are no longer the preferred agents for the treatment of bacillary dysentery, meningococcal infections, and *H. influenzae* meningitis. Sulfonamides are still prescribed on a large scale for upper respiratory infections, but their efficacy in these situations is highly questionable since the majority of such infections is caused by viruses.

Sulfadiazine, once widely used as an all-purpose sulfonamide, tends to produce crystalluria and has been largely replaced by the more soluble *sulfisoxazole* (Gantrisin) and its close congener, *sulfamethoxazole* (Gantanol) which is also used widely now in a fixed-dose combination with trimethoprim (see "Miscellaneous Antibacterial Agents" below). Mixtures of three sulfonamides (trisulfapyrimidines) are also widely used because they are associated with a low incidence of crystalluria. The sulfonamides are usually administered orally, although very satisfactory intravenous preparations of the sodium salts are available. Orally, an initial dose of 2 to 4 g is followed by 1 g every 4 to 6 h.

Long-acting sulfonamides have also been used widely, and their only advantage is that they can be administered orally only once or twice daily. Examples are sulfamethoxypyridazine and sulfadimethoxine. The primary clinical indication for these long-acting compounds has been urinary tract infections, in instances where the convenience of taking only one dose a day has been considered important. However, it is undesirable to use a drug that leaves the body slowly, because this may prolong adverse reactions. Moreover, certain severe toxic reactions such as erythema multiforme or myocarditis have been reported to occur more commonly with long-acting sulfonamides. It is probably best not to use this class of compounds at all.

There are also some poorly absorbed sulfonamides, succinylsulfathiazole (Sulfasuxidine) and phthalysulfathiazole (Sulfathalidine), that are used principally to decrease the number of bacteria in the colon prior to certain types of abdominal surgery. These agents are of doubtful value. The drug Azulfidine (Chap. 294) is of value in ulcerative colitis.

Adverse reactions caused by the sulfonamides include erythema multiforme, serum sickness, hemolytic (in patients with glucose 6-phosphate dehydrogenase deficiency) and aplastic anemias, arthralgias, hepatitis, nausea, vertigo, lesions resembling those of polyarteritis nodosa, and kernicterus.

ANTIFUNGAL AGENTS *Amphotericin B* is a highly toxic antibiotic that is effective in the treatment of deep-seated mycotic infections. It produces marked improvement and occasional cures in cryptococcosis, histoplasmosis, blastomycosis, disseminated candidiasis, and coccidioidomycosis, and has a beneficial effect in at least some cases of aspergillosis and mucormycosis. It is administered intravenously in 5% dextrose solution over a period of 5 or 6 h. The safest procedure is to administer 1 mg on the first day, 5 mg on the second, and 10 mg on the third. The dose is then increased by 5 to 10 mg each day until 1 mg/kg is being administered daily. The dose may then be changed to 1.5 mg/kg every other day; treatment is continued for 2 to 4 months, depending on the severity of the infection and upon the patient's response. In patients with severe infections where intensive therapy is considered essential, it may be necessary to assume the risk of administering 15 mg very cautiously as the initial dose, with the addition of antihistamines and/or steroids to help ameliorate the chills and fever, which are quite variable from patient to patient. In some debilitated patients who develop *Candida* infections with oral or esophageal lesions, or bacteremias secondary to intravenous catheters, 10 or 15 mg amphotericin B daily for only 3 or 4 days may be adequate to bring the infection under control.

Some degree of renal impairment invariably occurs when amphotericin B is administered for several weeks; this is manifested during therapy by a rise in the blood urea nitrogen (BUN) and serum creatinine. Renal function may return to normal following therapy if attention is devoted to giving the minimum amount of drug that is compatible with a satisfactory therapeutic response, and if particular care is exercised in lowering the dose and frequency of administration when the creatinine becomes markedly elevated. Many patients have permanent renal damage; this poses special problems when relapses occur and subsequent courses of therapy are needed. Other adverse effects of amphotericin B include anemia, hypokalemia, thrombocytopenia, and hepatitis.

Nystatin (Mycostatin) is another antifungal antibiotic that is less potent than amphotericin B and is too toxic for systemic administration. It is applied topically in ointments, tablets, and suspension. It is used particularly for oral, intestinal, skin, and vaginal lesions due to *Candida,* and the best results are obtained when applications are made several times a day. The individual dose varies from 100,000 to 1 million units, depending on the location of the lesion.

Flucytosine is an oral antifungal agent that is relatively nontoxic and has been used successfully in cryptococcal, *Candida,* and *Torulopsis* infections. The dose is 150 mg/kg per day administered in divided doses at 6-h intervals. Some cases of cryptococcal meningitis and pulmonary disease have seemed to respond as well as to amphotericin B, but flucytosine is, in general, less potent than amphotericin. An appreciable percentage of initial isolates of *Candida* are resistant to the drug, and resistance also occurs during therapy. Adverse effects have consisted chiefly of nausea, vomiting, diarrhea, and rashes, but pancytopenia and abnormal liver function tests have also been reported. The drug is excreted in the urine, and the dose needs to be decreased in uremia in accordance with the package insert.

Flucytosine is not effective in histoplasmosis, blastomycosis, and coccidioidomycosis. It is indicated chiefly in patients with severe cryptococcal, *Candida,* and *Torulopsis* infections who cannot tolerate amphotericin B. It can also be used for *Candida* infections of the bladder and for superficial lesions that do not respond to topical therapy. There is in vitro evidence of synergism between flucytosine and amphotericin B, and clinical results in some severe systemic infections appear to have been improved by administering these two antifungal agents together.

Miconazole, an investigational synthetic imidazole derivative, has been used intravenously in systemic cryptococcal, *Candida,* and coccidioides infections with at least moderate effectiveness. It causes little or no nephrotoxicity. Itching and nausea have been significant side effects.

ANTITUBERCULOSIS DRUGS *Isoniazid* remains the most important single agent for the treatment of tuberculosis. After years of being considered virtually free from adverse reactions, hepatotoxicity has been reported on a number of occasions. Individuals receiving this drug should be monitored with liver function tests (Chap. 143). *Ethambutol* has largely replaced *p*-aminosalicylic acid (PAS) as the usual companion drug for isoniazid because it avoids the necessity of taking large numbers of tablets and also avoids the gastrointestinal side effects associated with PAS. *Rifampin* is another important drug that is comparable to isoniazid in activity against tuberculosis; it should be used in combination with other drugs to prevent the emergence of rifampin-resistant tubercle bacilli. Streptomycin is still used to some extent, particularly for triple drug therapy in seriously ill, hospitalized patients. The secondary drugs, used chiefly in cases that have failed to respond to initial therapy, are cycloserine, pyrazinamide, ethionamide, and viomycin. These drugs are all associated with significant toxic side effects and should be administered and monitored by experts who are familiar with their use. A more detailed consideration of the antituberculosis drugs and the present treatment regimens are given in Chap. 143.

MISCELLANEOUS ANTIBACTERIAL AGENTS *Spectinomycin* is an antibiotic that is effective in single 2- to 4-g doses intramuscularly for the treatment of gonorrhea. Side effects are minimal, and it is useful to have an agent similar in effectiveness to penicillin available for the treatment of patients who are allergic to penicillin or who have failed to be cured by penicillin.

Nitrofurantoin is an antibacterial agent that is effective in treating urinary tract infections although susceptibility of the *Proteus* group is variable and *Pseudomonas* is resistant. It is usually administered orally in doses of 100 mg four times a day. In addition to treating acute uncomplicated urinary tract infections, it is widely used to suppress symptoms of infection in patients with prostatism and other chronic obstructive uropathies. Nausea is sometimes troublesome, and pulmonary hypersensitivity and peripheral neuropathy may occur. The latter is especially likely to occur with renal insufficiency, and nitrofurantoin should be used very cautiously in the presence of uremia.

Nalidixic acid is another drug used orally for urinary tract infections. Its principal defect lies in the rapidity with which bacteria become resistant to it. This means that cultures should be made during, as well as following, therapy to be sure that bacteria are being cleared from the urinary tract. The usual dose is 4 g daily in divided doses for 1 to 2 weeks. Nausea, vomiting, and rashes are the chief adverse reactions.

Co-trimoxazole, a fixed-dose combination of trimethoprim (80 mg) and sulfamethoxazole (400 mg), is synergistic in this ratio against most gram-negatives causing urinary tract infections except for *Pseudomonas*. It is also active in vitro against a variety of other pathogens and is used in other countries for many types of infections. In the United States it is approved so far for urinary infections, otitis media, and pneumonia due to *Pneumocystis carinii*. Its use prophylactically in immunosuppressed patients appears promising for preventing severe *Pneumocystis* infestations. Because of its cost it should be used chiefly when the infecting organisms are not susceptible to other antimicrobials. It may be of particular value, however, in preventing recurrent bouts of bacteriuria.

Troleandomycin (TAO) is an antibiotic similar to, although less active than, the erythromycins. It is an ester and occasionally causes cholestatic jaundice. In general, erythromycin, lincomycin, and clindamycin are preferable to troleandomycin because of their greater antibacterial activity.

DRUGS OF CHOICE

It is quite clear from reading about the pharmacology of individual agents, as well as about their indications and uses in individual diseases, that many agents are available for the treatment of these diseases. Table 111-2 presents a summary of drugs, indications, dosage schedules, routes of administration, and duration of therapy. The table presents only a limited number of drugs, and many equally acceptable regimens are available. Moreover, while these treatment programs are appropriate for the present, changes in them should be expected as new drugs come on the market and as more experience with the newer agents is gathered.

REASONS FOR FAILURE OF CHEMOTHERAPY

This chapter as well as others dealing with specific disease entities has documented that there are few organisms not sensitive to some antibiotic. Despite this seemingly salutary observation, a large number of patients develop infections and many continue to die from them. In these patients antibiotics appear to have failed. Often this failure of chemotherapy is more apparent than real and may be attributed to one of several causes.

FAILURE TO ADJUST THE DOSE OF THE ANTIBIOTIC Different doses of antibiotics are required in different locations. For example, 600,000 units penicillin G is more than adequate to cure pneumococcal pneumonia, but as much as 20 million units may be required to cure pneumococcal meningitis and more than 50 million units to treat pneumococcal endocarditis. The pneumococcus in each of these locations remains exquisitely sensitive to penicillin, nor is the penetration of the drug inadequate. However, the host's environment is such that higher doses are required to cure the infections in different locations. Failure to appreciate this phenomenon may lead to inadequate doses.

TREATMENT OF NONBACTERIAL INFECTIONS Viral infections do not respond to the drugs generally considered as antibiotic agents, and these drugs must not be expected to exact a therapeutic effect in these situations. Similarly, antibiotics do not prevent bacterial complications of viral infections.

FAILURE TO DRAIN PURULENT MATERIAL OR TO REMOVE OBSTRUCTION Antimicrobial drugs work well only in an environment free of obstruction. Infections will not respond optimally unless obstructions such as a plug of mucus or an enlarged prostate, or a foreign body such as a suture or splinter, are removed, or unless purulent material is drained. It is particularly important to drain an abscess cavity because antibiotics do not kill bacteria enmeshed in pus.

SUPERINFECTIONS The role of antibiotics in promoting superinfections is discussed in Chaps. 107 and 108. In 2 to 3 percent of patients seeming failure of antimicrobials is a consequence of superinfection.

DRUG REACTION The development of drug fever without rash or any other manifestation of hypersensitivity may make it appear as if the infection were not responding to therapy, when instead the fever is due to the very drug being given to cure the infection. Drug fever is extremely common with certain antimicrobials, particularly penicillin. The best way to

TABLE 111-2
Conventional antibiotic regimens for adults with normal renal and hepatic function

Organism	Disease	Drug	Dosage	Route	Duration
Pneumococcus	Lung	Penicillin G (procaine)	600,000 U q 12 h	IM	5–10 days[a]
	Meningitis	Penicillin G	20 million U/day	IV	7–10 days
	Joints	Penicillin G (aqueous)	20 million U/day	IV	7–10 days
	Endocarditis	Penicillin G	20 million U/day	IV	4–6 weeks[b]
Group A *Streptococcus*	Pharyngitis	Penicillin G (procaine)	600,000 U/day	IM	10 days[c]
	Erysipelas	Penicillin G	600,000 U/day	IM	10 days[c]
	Other sites	See pneumococcus			
Coagulase-positive *Staphylococcus*[d]	Furunculosis, cellulitis, abscess	Erythromycin	500 mg q 6 h	PO	7–10 days
		or cloxacillin	500 mg q 6 h	PO	7–10 days
		or cephalexin	500 mg q 6 h	PO	7–10 days
	Pneumonia	Methicillin	1.0 g q 4 h	IM, IV	10–14 days
		or cloxacillin	500 mg q 6 h	PO	10–14 days
		or dicloxacillin	250 mg q 6 h	PO	10–14 days
		or cephalothin	1.0 g q 4 h	IV	10–14 days
	Arthritis	Methicillin	1.0 g q 4 h	IV	10–14 days
		or cephalothin	1.0 g q 4 h	IV	10–14 days
	Meningitis, endocarditis	Methicillin	1.0 g q 2 h	IV	4 weeks
		or cephalothin	1.0 g q 2 h	IV	4 weeks
	Enterocolitis	Vancomycin	500 mg q 6 h	PO	Until diarrhea ceases
Streptococcus viridans	Endocarditis	Penicillin G,	6–12 million U/day	IV	14 days
		then penicillin V	500 mg q 4 h	PO	14 days
		Penicillin G	6–12 million U/day	IV	14 days
		plus streptomycin	500 mg q 12 h	IM	14 days
Streptococcus fecalis (enterococcus)	Genitourinary infection	Ampicillin	500 mg q 6 h	PO	10–14 days
		plus gentamicin	3 mg/kg/day	IM, IV	10–14 days
	Surgical wound	Ampicillin	1 g q 6 h	IM or IV	7–10 days
		plus gentamicin	3–5 mg/kg/day	IM, IV	7–10 days
	Endocarditis	Ampicillin	8–12 g/day	IV	4 weeks
		or penicillin G	20 million U/day	IV	4 weeks
		plus gentamicin,	3–5 mg/kg/day	IM, IV	2 weeks
		or kanamycin	7.5 mg/kg q 12 h	IM	2 weeks
		or streptomycin	500 mg q 12 h	IM, IV	2 weeks
Streptococcus bovis	Endocarditis	Penicillin G	6–12 million U/day	IV	14 days
		then penicillin V	500 mg q 4 h	PO	14 days
		Penicillin G	6–12 million U/day	IV	14 days
		plus streptomycin	500 mg q 12 h	IM	14 days
Neisseria meningitidis	Meningitis, meningococcemia	Penicillin G	20 million U/day	IV	7–10 days
		or chloramphenicol	50–100 mg/kg/day (given q 6 h)	IV	7–10 days
N. gonorrheae	Urethritis	Penicillin G	4.8 million U/day	IM	1 dose
		plus probenecid	1 g	PO	1 dose
		or spectinomycin[e]	2 g/day	IM	1 dose
	Arthritis	Penicillin G (aqueous)	6 million U/day	IV	7–10 days
Hemophilus influenzae	Bronchitis and pneumonia	Ampicillin	500 mg q 4 h	PO	5–7 days
		or tetracycline	500 mg q 6 h	PO	5–7 days
	Meningitis	Ampicillin	8–12 g/day	IV	7–10 days
		plus chloramphenicol	50–100 mg/kg/day (given q 6 h)	IV	7–10 days
Brucella	Brucellosis	Tetracycline	500 mg q 6 h	PO	14 days
		and streptomycin	500 mg q 12 h	IM	14 days
Salmonella typhosa	Typhoid fever	Chloramphenicol[f]	1.0 g q 8 h	IV, PO	14 days
		or ampicillin[f]	1.0 g q 6 h	PO, IM, IV	14 days
Salmonella	Abscess, bacteremia	Ampicillin	1.0 g q 4 h	IV	2–4 weeks
Shigella	Shigellosis	Ampicillin	500 mg q 4–6 h	PO, IM, IV	7 days
Klebsiella	Genitourinary infection	Gentamicin	3 mg/kg q 8 h	IM, IV	10–14 days
		or cephalothin	500 mg q 6 h	IM, IV	10–14 days
		or cefazolin	500 mg q 6 h	IM, IV	10–14 days
		or kanamycin	7.5 mg/kg q 12 h	IM	10–14 days
K. pneumoniae	Pneumonia, bacteremia	Cephalothin	1.0 g q 4 h	IV	7 days
		or cefazolin	1.0 g q 4 h	IV	7 days
		or kanamycin	7.5 mg/kg q 12 h	IM	7 days
		or gentamicin	5 mg/kg/day	IM, IV	7 days

[a] *Last 3–4 days can be given orally as penicillin V 2 g/day in many cases.*
[b] *Last 2 weeks can be given as penicillin V 4–6 g/day orally.*
[c] *Penicillin V 1–2 g/day for 10 days, or a single shot of 1.2 × 10⁶ U benzathine penicillin is an acceptable alternate.*
[d] *Appropriate doses (see Pneumococcus and Streptococcus) of penicillin G (parenteral) or penicillin V (oral) if organism is sensitive to penicillin G.*
[e] *For patients allergic to penicillin.*
[f] *Start with parenteral but switch to oral as soon as possible.*

TABLE 111-2 *(continued)*
Conventional antibiotic regimens for adults with normal renal and hepatic function

Organism	Disease	Drug	Dosage	Route	Duration
Pasturella tularensis	Tularemia	Streptomycin	1.0 g q 12 h	IM	10–14 days
Enterobacter aerogenes	Genitourinary infection	Nalidixic acid[g]	1.0 mg q 6 h	PO	10–14 days
		or kanamycin	7.5 mg/kg q 12 h	IM	7 days
		or gentamicin	3 mg/kg/day	IM, IV	7 days
	Bacteremia	Kanamycin	7.5 mg/kg q 12 h	IM	7 days
		or gentamicin	3–5 mg/kg/day	IM, IV	7 days
		and/or carbenicillin	30 g/day	IV	7 days
Escherichia coli	Genitourinary infection	Sulfisoxazole[h]	1 g q 6 h	PO	10–14 days
		or tetracycline	500 mg q 6 h	PO	10–14 days
		or ampicillin	500 mg q 6 h	PO	10–14 days
		or nitrofurantoin	100 mg q 6 h	PO	10–14 days
	Bacteremia, arthritis, peritonitis	Ampicillin	6–12 g/day	IV	7–10 days
		or kanamycin	7.5 mg/kg q 12 h	IM	7–10 days
		or gentamicin	3–5 mg/kg/day	IM, IV	7–10 days
		or cephalothin	1–2 g q 4 h	IV	7–10 days
	Meningitis	Ampicillin	8–12 g q 4 h	IV	7–10 days
		or chloramphenicol	50–100 mg/kg/day (q 6 h)	IV	7–10 days
Proteus mirabilis	Urine	Ampicillin	500 mg q 6 h	PO	10–14 days
		or cephalexin	500 mg q 6 h	PO	10–14 days
	Blood	Ampicillin	6.0 g/day	IV	7–10 days
		or kanamycin	7.5 mg/kg q 12 h	IM	7–10 days
		or cephalothin	6.0 g/day	IV	7–10 days
		or gentamicin	5 mg/kg/day	IM, IV	7–10 days
Indole-positive *Proteus*	Urine	Kanamycin	7.5 mg/kg q 12 h	IM	10–14 days
		or carbenicillin[i]	1 g q 6 h	IV	10–14 days
		or nalidixic acid	1 g q 6 h	PO	10–14 days
		or gentamicin	3–5 mg/kg/day	IM, IV	10–14 days
	Blood	Kanamycin	7.5 mg/kg q 12 h	IM	7–10 days
		or carbenicillin	4 g q 4 h	IV	7–10 days
		or gentamicin	5 mg/kg/day	IM	7–10 days
Pseudomonas	Blood, joint	Gentamicin	5 mg/kg/day	IM, IV	7 days
		plus carbenicillin	5–6 g q 4 h	IV	7 days
	Meningitis, brain abscess	Gentamicin	5 mg/kg/day	IV, IM	7–14 days
		plus carbenicillin	5–6 g q 4 h	IV	7–14 days
		and gentamicin	4 mg q 12–18 h	Intrathecally	7 days
	Urine	Gentamicin	3 mg/kg/day	IM, IV	10–14 days
		or carbenicillin	2 g q 6 h	IM, IV	10–14 days
		or colistin	75 mg q 6 h	IM	10–14 days
		or polymyxin B	30 mg q 6 h	IM, IV	10–14 days
		or oxytetracycline	500 mg q 6 h	PO	10–14 days
Bacteroides	Abscess, bacteremia	Chloramphenicol	0.5 g q 4 h	IV, PO	10–14 days
		or Clindamycin	0.6 g q 6–8 h *then* 0.3 g q 6 h	IV / PO	10–14 days / As long as necessary
Mycoplasma	Sputum	Erythromycin	250–500 mg q 6 h	PO	7 days
		or tetracycline	500 mg q 6 h	PO	7 days

[g] *Early follow-up cultures are essential to be sure resistance has not developed.*
[h] *Uncomplicated infections only.*
[i] *The indanyl ester of carbenicillin 1 g q 6 h may be given orally.*

make the diagnosis is simply to discontinue therapy. If fever disappears, the diagnosis is established. A second challenge with the suspected drug is neither necessary nor safe.

INCORRECT DRUG Only rarely does chemotherapy fail because the incorrect drug has been administered. Most drugs have a sufficiently broad spectrum, and combinations of drugs are administered with sufficient frequency, whether indicated or not, to make it highly unlikely that the patient is not given an agent active against the etiologic pathogen. One of the most common errors, when the patient is not responding, is to add more antimicrobials indiscriminately, when the correct course should be to discontinue therapy and to watch the patient.

DEFECTS IN HOST RESISTANCE The type of patient requiring antimicrobial therapy has changed from a young or middle-aged individual to an elderly one with degenerative and debilitating disease or one whose host defenses have been compromised by neoplastic disease, large doses of antimicrobials, antineoplastic or immunosuppressive drugs, x-ray therapy, major surgical procedures, or transplants. For a variety of rea-

sons, this type of patient does not, and should not be expected to, respond to antimicrobials as does a normal individual. This factor is often ignored in gauging the results of chemotherapy. It does not mean that antibiotics should not be used when indicated; rather, no miraculous results should be expected in patients with severe associated disease of noninfectious origin.

REFERENCES

APPEL GB, NEU HC: The nephrotoxicity of antimicrobial agents. N Engl J Med 296:663, 1977

BENNETT WM et al: A guide to drug therapy in renal failure. JAMA 230:1544, 1974

CLUFF LE, JOHNSON JE (eds): *Clinical Concepts of the Infectious Diseases*, 2d ed. Baltimore, Williams & Wilkins, 1978

Handbook of Antimicrobial Therapy, rev ed. New Rochelle, NY, Medical Letter, 1978

HOEPRICH PD: *Infectious Diseases*, 2d ed. New York, Harper & Row, 1977

KUNIN CM. Audits of antimicrobial usage. JAMA 237:1003, 1134, 1241, 1243, 1366, 1376, 1481, 1482, 1605, 1607, 1723, 1724, 1725, 1859, 1880, 1967, 1968, 1969; 1977

PRATT WB: *Chemotherapy of Infection.* New York, Oxford University Press, 1977

SARUBBI FA, HULL JH: Amikacin serum concentrations. Ann Intern Med 89:612, 1978

Symposium on Amikacin. Am J Med 62:799, 1977

Symposium on Cefamandole. J Infect Dis 137:S1–194, 1978

112
ACUTE INFECTIOUS DIARRHEAL DISEASE AND BACTERIAL FOOD POISONING

CHARLES C. J. CARPENTER

Acute diarrheal illnesses caused by bacterial, viral, or protozoal pathogens vary from slightly annoying bowel dysfunction to fulminant, life-threatening diseases. Until recent years, a specific etiologic agent could not be isolated from most patients with acute diarrhea. During the past decade, however, largely because of the recognition of enterotoxigenic *E. coli* as a major cause of acute diarrheal disease in adults and the identification of rotavirus as a frequent cause in young children, specific etiologic agents have been isolated from 80 to 85 percent of patients with acute diarrheal illnesses. Those illnesses caused by bacterial pathogens are more serious, although numerically fewer than those due to viruses, at least among adults, and for that reason, they will be addressed first. This chapter is aimed at presenting an overview of these diseases and, in most instances, the entities are discussed in more detail in the chapters dealing with the specific etiologic agent.

In considering the bacterial diarrheas, it is useful to divide them into two groups, those caused by invasive and those caused by noninvasive microorganisms. The invasive pathogens, of which *Shigella* (Chap. 124) may be considered the prototype, generally cause abdominal pain, fever, and other systemic symptoms, often including headache and myalgia. Illness caused by the noninvasive pathogens, of which cholera (Chap. 134) is the prototype, is generally characterized by the absence of fever and few systemic symptoms (except those directly related to intestinal fluid loss). The invasive pathogens characteristically destroy gut mucosal cells, typically involving the terminal ileum and colon, so that both leukocytes and erythrocytes are present, to a variable degree, in the stool. Inflammatory cells are generally absent from the stool in acute diarrheal disease caused by noninvasive bacterial pathogens.

NONINVASIVE BACTERIAL PATHOGENS

ENTEROTOXIGENIC *ESCHERICHIA COLI*   Etiology and epidemiology   Enterotoxin-producing *E. coli,* which has the dual capacity to adhere to small-bowel epithelial cells and to produce one or more diarrheagenic toxins, is now recognized as a major cause of acute diarrheal disease in the adult population throughout most of the world. Largely because current techniques for demonstrating toxigenicity remain cumbersome, the epidemiology of *E. coli* diarrhea is poorly understood. It has been demonstrated that enterotoxigenic *E. coli* is responsible for many cases of "traveler's diarrhea" in visitors to Mexico and in Peace Corps volunteers in East Africa, and that it is also the etiologic agent in most cases of acute diarrheal disease in adolescents and adults in rural Bangladesh. *Escherichia coli* plays a far less important role in episodic diarrheal illness in the United States. There is, as yet, no satisfactory explanation for the observation that *E. coli* has been implicated as a major cause of fulminant, cholera-like diarrheal disease in adult patients only in South and Southeast Asia.

Pathogenesis   The ability to cause diarrheal disease is not restricted to any one *E. coli* serotype, but appears to be dependent upon the presence of both a plasmid-mediated colonization factor, which allows the *E. coli* to adhere to small-bowel mucosal cells, and either one or both of two plasmids which code for the production of the two diarrheagenic toxins which may be produced by *E. coli*. The kinetics and mode of action of one of the toxins, which is heat labile (LT) and of relatively high molecular weight ($> 70,000$), are similar to those of cholera enterotoxin (Chap. 134); the diarrheagenic effect results from stimulation of adenylate cyclase in the gut epithelial cells. The other toxin, which is heat stable (ST) and of a lower molecular weight (< 5000), has a more rapid onset of action and probably exerts its effect through stimulation of guanylate cyclase in the gut mucosal cells. Either or both toxins may be produced by enterotoxigenic *E. coli*. Most isolates from patients with diarrheal disease in Bangladesh produce both LT and ST, whereas isolates from patients in other developing nations have shown widely varying capacities for the production of LT, ST, or both. The wide clinical spectrum may be, in part, related to the predominant production of either LT or ST by the culpable microorganisms.

Manifestations   Both clinical observations and volunteer studies indicate that the incubation period is generally between 24 and 72 h. The illness which follows is quite variable, ranging from the fulminant, cholera-like disease often seen on the Indian subcontinent to the much milder Mexican "turista," in which the symptoms of mild, watery diarrhea, abdominal cramps, and occasional low-grade fever are more troublesome than life-threatening. Vomiting occurs in fewer than half the adults with *E. coli* diarrhea and is seldom responsible for major fluid losses.

In fulminant cases, the severe diarrhea seldom lasts longer than 24 to 36 h, and the response to either oral or intravenous electrolyte repletion is predictable and dramatic. With milder disease, the symptoms subside more gradually, occasionally persisting for a week or longer.

Laboratory findings   As with cholera, no erythrocytes and few, if any, polymorphonuclear leukocytes are seen in a stool preparation stained by Loeffler's methylene blue. Because *E. coli* occurs normally among stool flora, and because its ability to produce enterotoxin is not restricted to any specific serotype, there is no rapid and simple means of laboratory diagnosis of enterotoxigenic *E. coli*. Bioassays for LT, based on the ability of *E. coli* isolates to produce fluid in isolated intestinal loops of experimental animals, or to stimulate adenyl cyclase in cells in tissue culture, as well as the suckling mouse bioassay for ST, are reliable but of little practical value.

Treatment   The intestinal fluid losses are qualitatively identical to those in cholera. Therefore, in those patients who develop clinically significant saline depletion, the principles of fluid administration are identical to those described for cholera (Chap. 134). Oral solutions containing electrolytes plus glucose or sucrose are quite effective in correcting the saline depletion. Antimicrobials have not been shown to be effective in the *treatment* of diarrhea due to enterotoxigenic *E. coli,* although tetracyclines like doxycycline, 100 mg per day, may be of significant short-term *prophylactic* value in preventing *E. coli* diarrhea in travelers. Bismuth subsalicylate, 60 ml hourly for 4 doses, provides symptomatic relief (less frequent stools, less severe abdominal cramps) but has no effect on the total stool volume. Antiperistaltic agents such as anticholinergics or Lomotil are of no demonstrable value in enterotoxigenic *E. coli* diarrhea.

Prognosis With even the more fulminant cases of disease caused by enterotoxigenic *E. coli*, the prognosis is excellent with adequate fluid replacement.

Prevention Careful hygienic practices, with special attention to ingestion of clean water and adequately cooked foods when living in a generally unsanitary environment, provide the most certain protection against enterotoxigenic *E. coli*. Antibiotic prophylaxis is detailed above and is likely to be effective.

CHOLERA See Chap. 134.

OTHER ENTEROTOXIGENIC ENTEROBACTERIACEAE Noninvasive strains of *Klebsiella* and *Enterobacter* occasionally have been incriminated in acute diarrheal disease in the developing areas of the world. The culpable microorganisms have been shown to produce both heat labile (LT) and heat stable (ST) enterotoxins; the LT associated with these microorganisms is immunologically related to *E. coli* LT. The clinical illness produced is indistinguishable from the milder cases of diarrhea caused by enterotoxigenic *E. coli,* and treatment is the same.

CLOSTRIDIUM PERFRINGENS (Chap. 141) This organism remains a significant cause of diarrheal disease and was, in 1973, implicated in more cases of acute food poisoning in the United States than any other single microorganism. Both the epidemiologic background and the clinical picture of *C. perfringens* diarrhea differ strikingly from that caused by *E. coli*. *Clostridium perfringens* diarrhea tends to occur in a microepidemic pattern following ingestion of contaminated meat, poultry products, or legumes. The relatively short incubation period of 6 to 12 h is an important diagnostic clue. Typically, two or more patients who have ingested the same meat dish for dinner become ill at roughly the same time during the early morning hours. The production of a specific enterotoxin by the actively sporulating microorganisms in the intestinal tract appears to be responsible for all the symptoms.

The clinical picture of diarrhea caused by *C. perfringens* is different from that caused by enterotoxigenic *E. coli* in one important respect, namely, that moderately severe, cramping abdominal pain, which is usually not prominent with *E. coli*, is a major presenting symptom.

Treatment consists of symptomatic therapy with codeine to alleviate the cramping abdominal pain, and intravenous fluid therapy in the small proportion of patients in whom there is clinical evidence of saline depletion. The illness is self-limited and rarely lasts for more than 24 h. Because of the relatively short natural course of the illness, antimicrobial therapy is of no value. Because *C. perfringens* normally inhibits mammalian and avian intestinal tracts, prevention is dependent upon adequate cooking and handling of meat and poultry products. The practice of allowing cooked meat products to cool slowly toward room temperature over 12 to 24 h permits germination of contaminating clostridial spores; this practice must be avoided.

STAPHYLOCOCCUS AUREUS (Chap. 116) Acute staphylococcal diarrhea, classical "food poisoning," is due entirely to ingestion of preformed enterotoxin, and the causative organisms are often absent from stool during the acute illness. This form of diarrhea often occurs in institutional outbreaks, and is characterized by a short incubation period (1 to 6 h), relatively short duration (usually less less than 10 h), and very high attack rates (often greater than 75 percent of the population at

risk). In addition to its distinctive epidemiologic features, acute staphylococcal diarrhea differs from other noninvasive bacterial diarrheas by the prominence of vomiting. Vomiting is an almost constant feature, and is apparently mediated by a direct effect of the absorbed toxin on the central nervous system.

Treatment is directed toward correction of the saline depletion (intravenous fluids are required in 10 to 20 percent of patients) and, when necessary, toward symptomatic relief of vomiting. Because staphylococcal food poisoning is caused by preformed enterotoxin and is not perpetuated by viable microorganisms, antimicrobials are of no value.

A good example of the explosive nature of staphylococcal food poisoning was provided by an outbreak on a jet liner flying from Anchorage to Copenhagen. In this episode, 57 per cent of 343 passengers developed an acute illness characterized by vomiting, diarrhea, and cramping abdominal pain. Thirty of the 200 affected individuals required intravenous fluids, but none had serious sequelae. The food, contaminated by a pustule on the hand of a food handler, had not been adequately refrigerated aboard the plane, allowing abundant growth of the staphylococcus, with production of enterotoxin. Since staphylococci are ubiquitous, the prevention of massive contamination is dependent largely on control of growth conditions, primarily temperature. *Staphylococcus aureus* can multiply at temperatures from 4 to 46°C and if contaminated food is allowed to remain at ambient temperatures after cooking, these organisms have ample opportunity to multiply, especially in such items as cream pastries, potato salad, and mayonnaise.

BACILLUS CEREUS *Bacillus cereus* is a cause of acute diarrheal disease which, although uncommon, has been identified with increasing frequency in the past decade, especially in Europe. The illness results from gross contamination of food with this gram-positive rod, which is capable of producing at least two discrete enterotoxins, one of which has characteristics similar to those of the labile enterotoxin of *E. coli*, and the other of which has effects similar to that of staphylococcal enterotoxin. *Bacillus cereus* may therefore cause two distinct clinical syndromes, a diarrheal form resulting from the *E. coli* LT type of enterotoxin and an emetic form caused by the staphylococcal type of enterotoxin. The diarrheal syndrome caused by *B. cereus* is generally similar to that caused by enterotoxin-producing *E. coli*, with the exceptions that abdominal cramps are more common (75 percent of cases) and both the incubation period (6 to 14 h) and median duration of illness (20 h) are shorter. The emetic syndrome is clinically indistinguishable from that caused by staphylococcal enterotoxin, with a short incubation period (median 2 h), short duration (median 9 h), and prominent vomiting (100 percent compared with less than 25 percent in the diarrheal syndrome).

Because both syndromes are self-limited and generally mild, no specific therapy is indicated. When *B. cereus* food poisoning is suspected clinically, the diagnosis can be confirmed by demonstration of 10^5 or more *B. cereus* organisms in epidemiologically incriminated food. *Bacillus cereus* grows readily on simple laboratory media, including blood agar, but will not generally be identified as a pathogen unless such identification is specifically requested. Isolation of *B. cereus* from stool alone does not establish it as the etiologic agent. *Bacillus cereus* is frequently found in the fecal flora of normal individuals.

Since *B. cereus* is ubiquitous in soil, as well as in many raw, dried, and processed foods, proper food handling is the only practical means of preventing this form of food poisoning. The emetic form of *B. cereus* food poisoning has almost invariably been associated with ingestion of contaminated fried rice. *Bacillus cereus* is commonly present in uncooked rice, and its spores survive boiling and germinate, with production of the enterotoxin, when boiled rice is left unrefrigerated. Brief rewarming before serving is not adequate to destroy the relatively heat-stable toxin. Prompt refrigeration of boiled rice will prevent transmission of the disease.

INVASIVE ENTERIC PATHOGENS

Shigellae characteristically invade the colon and terminal ileum, destroy segments of intestinal mucosa, cause extensive inflammatory changes in the lamina propria, and are the prototype of the invasive enteric bacterial pathogens. Other important invasive bacterial enteric pathogens include *Salmonella, Yersinia enterocolitica,* invasive *E. coli,* and *Vibrio parahemolyticus,* which may have the capacity both to damage intestinal mucosa and to produce an enterotoxin. As opposed to the noninvasive pathogens, the invasive enteric organisms frequently cause systemic symptoms, including headache, myalgias, chills, and fever. As a general rule, antiperistaltic agents such as opiates, diphenoxylate, and atropine are contraindicated in diarrheal disease caused by invasive enteric pathogens because they clearly worsen the clinical course in human shigellosis, as well as salmonellosis and shigellosis in animal models.

The major therapeutic challenge in invasive bacterial diarrheas is that of distinguishing between (1) shigellosis and yersiniosis, in which antimicrobial therapy is usually indicated because of the severity of diarrhea and the frequency of rectal bleeding, dysentery, and systemic symptoms, (2) infections caused by salmonella, which are characterized primarily by watery diarrhea and few systemic symptoms and in which antimicrobial therapy may cause prolonged excretion of the pathogen, and (3) invasive *E. coli* infections, in which antimicrobials are of no demonstrable value.

SHIGELLOSIS   See Chap. 124.

SALMONELLOSIS   See Chap. 123.

YERSINIA ENTEROCOLITICA   See Chap. 129.

VIBRIO PARAHEMOLYTICUS   See Chap. 134.

INVASIVE *ESCHERICHIA COLI*   Invasive *E. coli*, which are far less common pathogens than enterotoxigenic *E. coli,* may cause a clinical syndrome quite similar to shigellosis with the exceptions that vomiting seldom occurs with the invasive *E. coli* and the illness is of shorter duration. Diarrhea caused by invasive *E. coli* is rare in the United States but has been a significant cause of short-term disability in Southeast Asia and South America. Since the illness caused by invasive *E. coli* is relatively short-lived antimicrobial therapy has not been shown to be helpful.

ACUTE VIRAL DIARRHEAS

Acute viral gastroenteritis is discussed in detail in Chap. 187. These illnesses are both more common and more life-threatening in small children than adults. In the United States, rotaviruses account for a large proportion of diarrheal illnesses during the first 2 years of life and usually occur during the winter. They have seldom been implicated in adult illness. In rural Bangladesh, infection with rotavirus accounts for roughly 60 percent of episodes of diarrhea in children under the age of 2, for about 5 percent in the 2- to 5-year-old age group, and

seldom occurs in adolescents and adults. The illness usually presents gradually with vomiting, watery diarrhea, and low-grade fever with little or no associated abdominal pain. Vomiting is a prominent and almost constant early manifestation of rotavirus enteritis but rarely persists beyond the first 36 h. Diarrhea often persists for 4 to 6 days. Although the illness is generally not life-threatening, many patients require fluid and electrolyte repletion. Following subsidence of vomiting, this can generally be achieved by the oral route, using the same fluids that are effective in the treatment of cholera (Chap. 134).

The diagnosis can be confirmed by a variety of tests including demonstration of the virus in stool by electron microscopy, a rise in complement-fixing antibody titers, radioimmunoassay, etc. The most useful and reliable test for rapid diagnosis under field conditions consists of direct demonstration of the antigen in stool by the enzyme-linked immunosorbent assay (ELISA).

Other viruses (e.g., Norwalk virus, Hawaii virus), although implicated in occasional common-source outbreaks involving adults, usually cause relatively mild, short ($<$ 36 h), and self-limited disease, for which neither fluid nor antimicrobial therapy is necessary (Chap. 187).

ACUTE PROTOZOAL DIARRHEAS

Over the past decade, *Giardia lamblia* has emerged as a major cause of acute diarrheal disease (Chap. 210). Although formerly thought to be a pathogen only in children and later considered to be a significant cause of diarrheal disease only in developing nations, this organism was the pathogen most commonly incriminated in outbreaks of waterborne diarrheal disease in the United States in 1976. In North America, it occurs most commonly in the Rocky Mountain states, and more frequently causes disease in visitors than in the indigenous population. The illness characteristically presents with the sudden onset of watery diarrhea and malabsorption, accompanied by mild to moderate abdominal discomfort, bloating, and flatulence, and may persist unless appropriate antimicrobials are administered. Prolonged disease with malabsorption occurs from time to time in previously normal individuals but is particularly common in patients with IgA deficiency, who tend to have the most severe form of giardiasis.

The attack rate may be quite high ($>$ 50 percent) in individuals exposed to contaminated water sources. In certain groups of North American travelers returning from Leningrad, where the water supply appears to be heavily contaminated with giardia cysts, up to 60 percent of individuals have developed clinical giardiasis. The usual incubation period is 10 to 20 days. The illness, therefore, frequently develops after a traveler returns home, and the travel history is a critical element in suspecting the diagnosis. Occasionally the disease occurs endemically in individuals who have not traveled. The diagnosis can be confirmed in approximately half the cases by examining the stool for cysts; if the stool examination is negative in a patient with characteristic clinical features, duodenal aspirates or biopsies will usually yield the characteristic trophozoites. Treatment with quinacrine, 100 mg tid for 5 to 7 days, is generally curative; metronidazole, 250 mg tid for 7 days, is an acceptable alternative regimen.

REFERENCES

CENTER FOR DISEASE CONTROL: *Foodborne Outbreaks: Annual Summary 1973.* 1974

DUPONT HL et al: Pathogenesis of *Escherichia coli* diarrhea. N Engl J Med 285:1, 1971

——— et al: Symptomatic treatment of diarrhea with bismuth subsalicylate among students attending a Mexican university. Gastroenterology 73:715, 1977

Evans DG et al: Plasmid-controlled colonization factor associated with virulence in *Escherichia coli* enterotoxigenic for humans. Infect Immunol 12:656, 1975

Gorbach SL et al: Traveller's diarrhea and toxigenic *Escherichia coli*. N Engl J Med 292:933, 1975

Guerrant RL et al: Role of toxigenic and invasive bacteria in acute diarrhea of childhood. N Engl J Med 293:576, 1974

Merson MH et al: Traveller's diarrhea in Mexico. A prospective study of physicians and family members attending a Congress. N Engl J Med 294:1299, 1976

Sack RB et al: Enterotoxigenic *Escherichia coli* isolated from patients with severe cholera-like disease. J Infect Dis 123:378, 1971

——— et al: Human diarrheal disease caused by enterotoxigenic *Escherichia coli*. Ann Rev Microbiol 29:333, 1975

———: Prophylactic doxycycline for traveller's diarrhea. N Engl J Med 298:758, 1978

Terranova W et al: Current concepts. *Bacillus cereus* food poisoning. N Engl J Med 298:143, 1978

113
SEXUALLY TRANSMITTED DISEASES

KING K. HOLMES

INTRODUCTION Venereology today encompasses not only the five "venerable" venereal diseases (gonorrhea, syphilis, chancroid, lymphogranuloma venereum, and granuloma inguinale), but also a growing number of other diseases which might be considered the "new generation" of sexually transmitted diseases (STDs). Many of these newer STDs, like gonorrhea, have become epidemic in nearly all countries of the world during the past two decades. With increasing interest in these diseases and improved methods for diagnosis has come awareness of the growing consequences of STD in areas of health and society which extend beyond the traditional sphere of venereology. In particular, major impact of the newer STDs has been noted on maternal and infant morbidity and on human reproduction and infertility.

CLASSIFICATION OF SEXUALLY TRANSMITTED DISEASES
These diseases can be classified on the basis of either their etiology or their clinical manifestations. Table 113-1 gives an etiologic classification of STD. Sexual transmission has been implicated as a major factor in the propagation of each of the pathogens listed in this table although evidence for sexual transmission of some, such as group B streptococcal infection and cytomegalovirus infection, is quite preliminary. There have been sporadic case reports of sexual transmission of many other pathogenic agents. However, the diseases caused by these other agents are not generally considered sexually transmitted diseases, since sexual transmission seems to be a minor factor in their propagation. For each of the agents listed in Table 113-1, there are one or more diseases or syndromes known to be caused by the agent, and others (indicated by a question mark) for which a causal association is suspected but not proved.

APPROACH TO SEXUALLY TRANSMITTED DISEASE It is necessary for the clinician to consider the approach to STD syndromes before an etiologic diagnosis is established. Table 113-2 lists some of the most common clinical syndromes and complications caused by sexually transmitted pathogens. Strategies for the management of the three most common syndromes seen in venereology are outlined below.

MALE URETHRITIS Urethritis in the male is classified as gonococcal or nongonococcal. The incidence of gonococcal urethritis has stabilized in many Western countries, while that

TABLE 113-1
Twenty-one sexually transmitted pathogens and the diseases they cause

Agent	Disease or syndrome
BACTERIAL	
Neisseria gonorrhoeae	Urethritis, cervicitis, proctitis, pharyngitis, conjunctivitis, endometritis, pelvic inflammatory disease, perihepatitis, bartholinitis, amniotic infection syndrome, disseminated gonococcal infection, ?premature rupture of membranes and premature delivery
Chlamydia trachomatis	Nongonococcal urethritis, epididymitis, cervicitis, salpingitis, inclusion conjunctivitis, infant pneumonia, trachoma, and lymphogranuloma venereum, ?perihepatitis, ?bartholinitis, ?proctitis, ?otitis media
Mycoplasma hominis	Postpartum fever, ?salpingitis
Ureaplasma urealyticum	?Nongonococcal urethritis, ?premature rupture of membranes and premature delivery
Treponema pallidum	Syphilis
Hemophilus vaginalis	?Nonspecific vaginitis
Hemophilus ducreyi	Chancroid
Calymmatobacterium granulomatis	Granuloma inguinale
Shigella spp.	Shigellosis in homosexual men
?Group B streptococcus	Neonatal sepsis, neonatal meningitis
VIRAL	
Herpes simplex virus	Initial and recurrent genital herpes, aseptic meningitis, neonatal herpes, ?carcinoma of the uterine cervix
Hepatitis B virus	Acute hepatitis, chronic active hepatitis, persistent (unresolved) hepatitis, polyarteritis nodosa, chronic membranous glomerulonephritis, ?mixed cryoglobulinemia, ?polymyalgia rheumatica, ?hepatoma
?Cytomegalovirus	Heterophile-negative infectious mononucleosis; congenital infection: gross birth defects and infant mortality; cognitive impairment (e.g., mental retardation, sensorineural deafness); ?cervicitis; protean manifestations in the immunosuppressed host
Genital wart virus	Condyloma accuminata, ?laryngeal papilloma in infants
Molluscum contagiosum virus	Genital molluscum contagiosum
PROTOZOAN	
Trichomonas vaginalis	Trichomonal vaginitis
Entamoeba histolytica	Amebiasis in homosexual men
Giardia lamblia	Giardiasis in homosexual men
FUNGAL	
Candida albicans	Vulvovaginitis, balanitis, and balanoposthitis
ECTOPARASITICAL	
Phthirius pubis	Pubic lice infestation
Sarcoptes scabiei	Scabies

of nongonococcal urethritis (NGU) continues to rise, suggesting that current measures for control of NGU are relatively ineffective. In general, gonorrhea and NGU are equally common among men seen in STD clinics in the United States, whereas NGU is approximately three times as common as gonorrhea among men seen by physicians in private practice and 10 times as common as gonorrhea among college students.

About 40 to 50 percent of NGU is caused by *Chlamydia trachomatis*. Herpes simplex virus and trichomonal vaginitis each cause a small additional proportion of NGU cases in the United States, but about 50 percent of cases cannot be attributed to any of these three pathogens. *Ureaplasma urealyticum* has been implicated in case-control studies as a probable cause of most of the *Chlamydia*-negative cases. Since facilities for isolation of *C. trachomatis* are not widely available, and the role of *U. urealyticum* is not certain, the diagnosis of male urethritis usually does not include cultures for *C. trachomatis* or *U. urealyticum*. The following steps should be taken in evaluating sexually active men with symptoms of urethral discharge and/or dysuria.

1 Establish the presence of urethritis. Urethral discharge should be demonstrated. Commonly in NGU, and less often in gonorrhea, discharge can be demonstrated only by milking the urethra after the patient has gone several hours, preferably overnight, without voiding. If no overt discharge is demonstrable, urethral exudate can be demonstrated by inserting a small urethrogenital swab 1 to 2 cm into the urethra and examining the Gram-stained direct smear prepared from

this swab for leukocytes. Five or more leukocytes per 1000× field in areas containing cells suggest urethritis. Patients with symptoms of urethritis who lack objective confirmatory evidence of urethritis may have functional problems and generally do not benefit from repeated courses of antibiotics.

2 Exclude complications or alternative diagnosis. Epididymitis and systemic complications, such as the gonococcal arthritis-dermatitis syndrome, and *Reiter's* syndrome, should be excluded by brief history and examination. Rectal examination for prostatitis is seldom informative in patients with overt urethritis, unless concomitant symptoms such as perineal, suprapubic, or rectal discomfort are present. Bacterial prostatitis and cystitis should, of course, be excluded by appropriate tests in men with dysuria who lack signs of urethritis.

3 Gram's stain examination of urethral exudate. The diagnosis of gonorrhea is confirmed by demonstrating typical gram-negative diplococci within neutrophils. The diagnosis of NGU is warranted if no gram-negative *Neisseria gonorrhoeae* are found in such cases. Smears containing only extracellular or atypical gram-negative diplococci are equivocal and should lead to attempts to isolate *N. gonorrhoeae* by culture. The above approach is illustrated in Fig. 113-1. The treatment of gonorrhea and NGU is discussed in Chaps. 119 and 174, respectively.

LOWER GENITOURINARY INFECTION IN WOMEN Infections of the female urinary tract, vulva, and vagina produce certain overlapping symptoms in women such as burning on urination, vulvar irritation, and dyspareunia. Infections of the cervix and vagina produce other symptoms such as altered quality or increased quantity of vaginal discharge. There is insufficient consensus on clinical or laboratory guidelines for differentiating among these various categories on the basis of symptomatology, and they are often referred to in vague terms such as "nonspecific genital infection." Lack of nosologic precision is attributable not only to overlapping symptomatology, but also to uncertainty about the etiology of the inflammatory conditions of the urinary tract, vulva, vagina, and cervix in women; to the lack of consistent application of available laboratory testing where the etiology is known; and to the difficulty clinicians experience in differentiating true inflammatory conditions from functional, psychosomatic genitourinary complaints.

Although the etiology of certain genitourinary inflammatory conditions in women remains uncertain, some data allow improved diagnostic precision, which in turn should lead to improved management. One estimate of the relative frequency of diagnostic entities that produce lower urogenital symptoms (unusual vaginal discharge, vulvar itching or irritation, dysuria, frequency, etc.) was provided in a study of 821 young women (mean age 24) examined in a primary care clinic. Vaginitis was found to be more than five times as common as cystitis or urethritis (UTI). Two steps are required in the evaluation of lower genitourinary symptoms in women: (1) differentiation among cystitis, urethritis, vaginitis, cervicitis, and cervical ectopy, and (2) exclusion of associated upper tract disease (e.g., pyelonephritis, salpingitis).

Cystitis/urethritis Although dysuria is more common in UTI than in vaginitis, in young women dysuria is attributable to vaginitis more often than UTI, because vaginitis is so much more common than UTI. However, when women were asked to localize the dysuria as "internal" (felt inside the body) or "external" (felt on the vaginal labia when the stream of urine passed), "internal" dysuria correlated with UTI. Among women considered to have UTI without vaginal infection, about half have bacterial cystitis, with 10^5 bacteria per millili-

TABLE 113-2
Selected syndromes and complications with corresponding sexually transmitted etiologic agents*

Syndrome	Agent
Male urethritis	*N. gonorrhoeae, C. trachomatis,* herpes simplex virus, *?U. urealyticum*
Lower genitourinary infection in women	Vulvitis: *C. albicans,* herpes simplex virus
	Vaginitis: *T. vaginalis, C. albicans, H. vaginalis*
	Cervicitis: *N. gonorrhoeae, C. trachomatis,* herpes simplex virus
	Female urethritis: *N. gonorrhoeae, C. trachomatis*
Genital ulceration	Herpes simplex virus, *Treponema pallidum, H. ducreyi, Cal. granulomatis, C. trachomatis* (LGV)
Pelvic inflammatory disease	*N. gonorrhoeae, C. trachomatis*
Proctitis	*N. gonorrhoeae,* herpes simplex virus, *?C. trachomatis*
Acute arthritis with genital infection	*N. gonorrhoeae, ?C. trachomatis*
Neonate and infant: "TORCHES" syndrome	Cytomegalovirus, herpes simplex virus, *T. pallidum*
Other infant and childhood morbidity	Conjunctivitis: *C. trachomatis, N. gonorrhoeae*
	Pneumonia: *C. trachomatis*
	Otitis media: *C. trachomatis*
	Sepsis, death: Group B streptococcus
	Cognitive impairment: Cytomegalovirus, herpes simplex virus, *T. pallidum*
Infertility: Postsalpingitis, postobstetric, postabortion	*N. gonorrhoeae, C. trachomatis, M. hominis*
Spontaneous abortion	Herpes simplex virus, *?N. gonorrhoeae, ?C. trachomatis,* fetal wastage

* For each of the above syndromes and complications, a variable proportion cannot yet be ascribed to any cause and must currently be considered idiopathic.

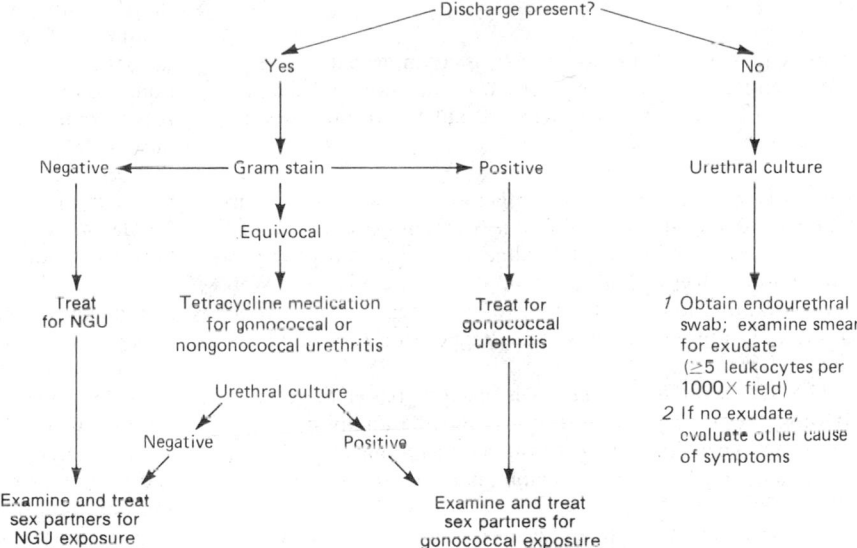

FIGURE 113-1
Diagnosis and management of suspected urethritis in males.

ter of urine, while half have urethritis—often termed the *urethral syndrome*. Both sexual intercourse and oral contraception have been identified as risk factors predisposing to bacterial UTI in women. The role of sexual intercourse in predisposing to the urethral syndrome is uncertain. However, in populations having a high risk of gonorrhea, *N. gonorrhoeae* clearly is a common cause of urethritis among women without significant bacteriuria. *Chlamydia trachomatis* has also been implicated as a cause of urethritis among women (Chap. 174).

DIAGNOSIS AND THERAPY The diagnosis of UTI in young women involves first the differentiation of UTI from vaginitis by history and examination. Among women with suspected UTI, bacterial UTI must then be differentiated from the urethral syndrome. The absence of bacteriuria in women with suspected UTI suggests the diagnosis of the urethral syndrome. Gonorrhea should be excluded by appropriate culture of the cervix and urethra. The value of antimicrobial therapy for the urethral syndrome, if gonorrhea is not present, has not been studied in controlled fashion.

VAGINITIS In self-referred female STD clinic patients, vaginitis is the most common diagnosis. The relative frequency of *Candida albicans, Hemophilus vaginalis,* and *Trichomonas vaginalis* as causes of vaginitis varies, with *T. vaginalis* being relatively more common among those of low socioeconomic status.

Vaginitis, without UTI, is characterized by one or more of the following symptoms: increased volume of discharge; abnormal yellow or green color of discharge, caused by increased concentration of polymorphonuclear leukocytes, which contain myeloperoxidase pigment; vulvar itching, irritation, or burning; introital dyspareunia; and malodor. *Trichomonas vaginalis* produces a profuse, yellow or green purulent discharge which is often malodorous. In contrast, the predominant symptom in *C. albicans* vaginitis is usually vulvar itching, often with signs of vulvitis as well as vaginitis, but without odor. The discharge in *Candida* vaginitis is typically white and may resemble curds of cottage cheese. The vagina occasionally contains adherent thrush-like plaques of matted mycelia, polymorphonuclear leukocytes, and epithelial cells. Nonspecific vaginitis, associated with *H. vaginalis* infection, is associated with moderately increased malodorous vaginal discharge. The discharge is homogeneous, low in viscosity, contains fewer leukocytes than are usually found in *T. vaginalis* or *C. albicans* infection, and is uniformly adherent to the vaginal walls. Colposcopy may show abnormally dilated vessels and/or in-

creased density of vessels on the vaginal or cervical wall in *Candida* and *Trichomonas* vaginitis, but not in nonspecific vaginitis (NSV). While the symptomatology and examination may suggest an etiologic diagnosis, several studies have shown poor correlation between clinical and microbiological findings in determining the etiology of vaginitis. A most important contribution of the clinical evaluation of vaginal discharge is ascertaining by speculum examination whether the discharge emanates from the vagina or cervix, and whether the discharge is, in fact, abnormal. Occasionally, subjective symptoms of vaginitis are not associated with objective signs of vaginitis. Psychological testing is normal in most such cases. The diagnosis and therapy of the three types of vaginitis are summarized in Table 113-3.

***Trichomonas vaginalis* vaginitis** Sexual transmission of *T. vaginalis* is well established, although the age distribution of *T. vaginalis* infection in women is skewed toward the older age group more than for other STDs, suggesting that nonsexual transmission of *T. vaginalis* may be important. Routine sampling indicates that many women and most men with infection are asymptomatic. Among patients with asymptomatic infections, the potential for development of symptoms is high.

TABLE 113-3
Diagnostic features and therapy of infectious vaginitis

Etiology	Diagnostic features	Therapy
Trichomonas vaginalis	Motile trichomonads pH = 5.5–6.0 Amine odor volatilized by adding 10% KOH	Metronidazole 2.0 g single oral dose Metronidazole 250 mg three times daily for 10 days
Candida albicans	Yeast, pseudomycelia pH < 4.5 No odor with 10% KOH Isolation of *C. albicans*	Nystatin vaginal tablet twice daily for 7 days Imidazole (clotrimazole or miconazole) intravaginally once daily for 7 days
Hemophilus vaginalis	Clue cells pH > 4.5 Amine odor with 10% KOH Isolation of *H. vaginalis*	Ampicillin 500 mg four times daily for 7 days Metronidazole 500 mg twice daily for 7 days
Uninfected	Normal vaginal secretions pH < 4.5 No odor with 10% KOH	No medication

Treatment of symptomatic as well as asymptomatic cases is recommended to reduce the reservoir of infection and the possible risk of transmission and to prevent the future development of symptoms.

DIAGNOSIS AND THERAPY The diagnosis in women is confirmed by demonstration of motile trichomonads in vaginal secretions mixed with normal saline and examined promptly under a low-power or high dry (400×) microscopic field. Wet-mount examination is at least 80 to 90 percent as sensitive as culture in symptomatic cases. The diagnosis of T. vaginalis infection in men is difficult.

The pH of vaginal secretions is usually greater than 5.0 in symptomatic T. vaginalis infections, and the addition of 10% potassium hydroxide (KOH) to vaginal secretions may liberate an amine-like fishy odor in trichomonal vaginitis as well as in NSV.

Nitroimidazoles are the only consistently effective drugs for treating trichomoniasis. Several studies show that a single 2.0-g oral dose is as effective as the former higher dosage schedules. Tinidazole, a structurally related 5-nitroimidazole, has a longer half-life than metronidazole (12.5 h vs. 7.3 h after a single oral 2.0-g dose) which might conceivably be of benefit in single-dose therapy, but this drug has not been shown to give better results than metronidazole in single-dose therapy of trichomoniasis.

Several studies have demonstrated T. vaginalis infection in one-third to two-thirds of male sex partners of women with T. vaginalis infections. On the basis of these data, and in view of

FIGURE 113-2

A. Vaginal epithelial "clue cells." Note granular appearance due to adherent H. vaginalis *and indistinct cell margins. 400×. B. Normal vaginal epithelial cells. The cell margins are distinct and lack granularity.*

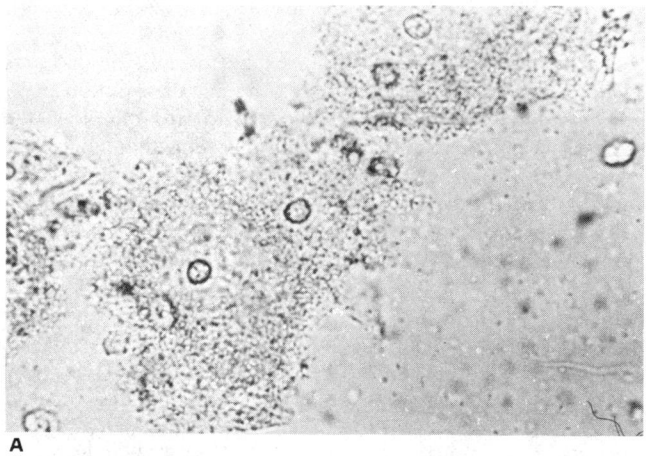

A

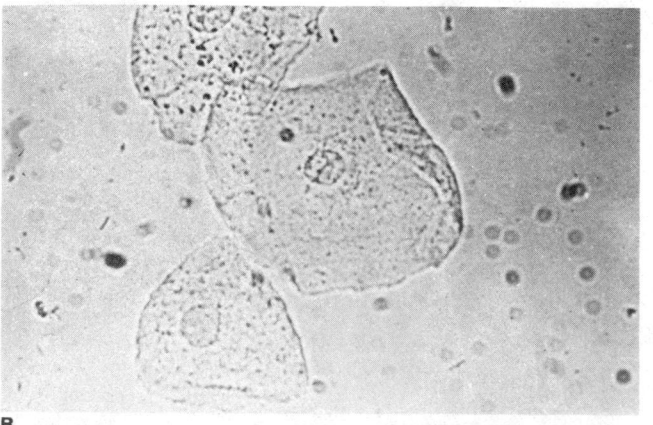

B

the difficulty in demonstrating T. vaginalis in men, routine treatment of sex partners of either sex seems advisable to reduce the risk of reinfection and to reduce the reservoir of infection. However, caution is warranted in using nitroimidazoles. It is recommended that metronidazole not be given to women during the first trimester of pregnancy because of teratogenicity in animals, and that alcohol be avoided for 24 h after treatment because of the Antabuse-like effect of the drug. Metronidazole is also mutagenic, and massive doses cause several types of tumors in rodents.

Nonspecific vaginitis Vaginal discharge not associated with T. vaginalis, C. albicans, or uterine infection is usually attributed to nonspecific vaginitis (NSV). *Hemophilus vaginalis* has been associated with NSV, and although this association has been challenged, it was supported by finding H. vaginalis in vaginal secretions from 17 (96 percent) of 18 women with NSV and only 1 (4 percent) of 18 normal matching women. The concentration of anaerobic bacteria in vaginal washings from women with NSV has also been found to be increased, though no specific anaerobe has been implicated.

The evidence linking H. vaginalis to NSV is somewhat similar to that linking U. urealyticum to Chlamydia-negative NGU. That is, H. vaginalis is recovered more often and in higher quantity from women with NSV than from those with other forms of vaginitis or from normal women, and improvement of clinical signs of NSV correlates with eradication of H. vaginalis. It is clear that H. vaginalis is frequently present in vaginal secretions of asymptomatic women who may or may not have signs of an increased malodorous vaginal discharge. The factors responsible for the presence or absence of symptoms in women infected by H. vaginalis require further study. Evidence for sexual transmission of H. vaginalis is also circumstantial, although recurrence of H. vaginalis–associated NSV after initially successful treatment has been demonstrated after sexual reexposure.

DIAGNOSIS AND TREATMENT In a patient with symptoms and/ or signs of abnormal vaginal discharge the diagnosis of NSV can be made with reasonable certainty by the following:

1 Exclusion of C. albicans, T. vaginalis, cervicitis, and cervical ectopy.
2 Demonstration of the presence of "clue cells" by microscopic examination of vaginal secretions diluted 1:1 in normal saline (wet-mount examination) (Fig. 113-2). Clue cells are vaginal epithelial cells coated with coccobaccillary forms of H. vaginalis, to the extent that the borders of the cells are completely obscured. Several media are available for isolation of H. vaginalis; the addition of colistin and nalidixic acid selectively inhibits other organisms, and addition of 5 percent human blood permits rapid detection of beta-hemolytic colonies of H. vaginalis on primary isolation.
3 Liberation of an amine-like fishy odor immediately after mixing vaginal secretion with 10% KOH (for microscopic identification of yeasts). Vaginal secretions in NSV contain several amines, including putrescine, cadaverine, methylamine, isobutylamine, histamine, tyramine, and phenethylamine. Amines are not produced by H. vaginalis per se. They may also be released from vaginal secretions from women with T. vaginalis infection when KOH is added, but not from secretions from women with Candida vaginitis or from normal women.
4 Demonstration of pH of vaginal secretions greater than 4.5. The elevated pH may be partly due to the presence of amines.

Treatment of H. vaginalis–associated NSV generally has been frustrating. Sulfonamide-containing vaginal creams are ineffective, perhaps because sulfonamides are uniformly inactive against *H. vaginalis* in vitro. Tetracycline therapy is also usually ineffective, partly because many strains of *H. vaginalis* are resistant to tetracyclines in vitro. Ampicillin, 500 mg four times daily for 7 days, has been effective in 33 to 100 percent of cases of NSV. The most consistently effective therapy consists of metronidazole 500 mg twice daily for 7 days, which eradicated *H. vaginalis* and cleared symptoms in 80 of 81 women with NSV. The efficacy of this regimen, which is not approved for use for NSV in the United States, should be weighed against its potential toxicity. Asymptomatic urethral colonization of *H. vaginalis* is demonstrable in most male sex partners of women with NSV and may contribute to reinfection of the female. The need for treatment of male partners of women with NSV and the efficacy of various antimicrobials in men require further study.

Candidal vaginitis *Candida albicans* and *Torulopsis glabrata* were detected in 21 and 4 percent of female STD clinic patients, respectively. Other yeasts were rare. Pruritus and vulvovaginitis were more common among those with *C. albicans* than among those with *T. glabrata*. Other species found with varying frequency in the vagina include *C. tropicalis, C. stellatoidea, C. krusei, C. parakrusei, C. pseudotropicalis, C. parapsilosis,* and *C. guillermondi.* These other species are generally not associated with vaginitis. Sexual transmission from the male and spread of infection from the anus may account for vaginal yeast infection or for reinfection of the vagina following therapy.

DIAGNOSIS AND THERAPY   The diagnosis of *Candida* vaginitis involves demonstration of yeast by microscopic examination of vaginal secretions in saline or 10% KOH, or by Gram's stain. Demonstration of hyphae or pseudohyphae strengthens the diagnosis of *C. albicans* vaginitis. Microscopic examination is less sensitive than culture. The pH of vaginal secretions is less than 4.5 in yeast vaginitis, and the vaginal odor is normal. Vulvitis often accompanies vaginitis and may result in excoriations which must be differentiated from HSV infection. Most clinicians recommend therapy for *C. albicans* vaginal infection only if the patient is symptomatic.

Therapy of yeast vaginitis involves the use of the polyene antifungal agent, nystatin, or one of the imidazoles, clotrimazole or miconazole. Many trials suggest that the imidazoles are more effective than the polyenes. Imidazoles have the apparent additional advantage of requiring only once nightly vaginal application, as opposed to twice daily application currently recommended for nystatin, but imidazoles have the disadvantage of costing more. The recommended duration of therapy for clinical as well as mycologic cure is 7 days for both mycostatin and the imidazoles. The need for simultaneous oral therapy to attempt to eradicate gut infections and for treatment of the male sex partner has not been determined.

MUCOPURULENT CERVICITIS   Cervicitis may accompany vaginitis due to *C. albicans* or *T. vaginalis*. Cervicitis without vaginitis can be caused by *N. gonorrhoeae, C. trachomatis,* or herpes simplex virus. *Neisseria gonorrhoeae* and *C. trachomatis* both produce endocervicitis, with mucopurulent exudate emanating from the cervical os.

Mucopurulent cervicitis requires antimicrobial therapy, and nongonococcal endocervicitis should probably be regarded as being caused by *C. trachomatis* unless infection by that agent can be specifically excluded by culture. The diagnosis of gonococcal cervicitis is made by Gram's stain and culture. If a specimen is properly collected from the endocervical os, after first wiping the cervix clean to remove vaginal flora, then the sensitivity of the Gram's stain showing intracellular gram-negative diplococci, in comparison with culture is about 60 percent, and the specificity approaches 100 percent. The sensitivity of a single endocervical culture is estimated to be 80 to 90 percent.

Chlamydia trachomatis infection of the cervix can be demonstrated reliably only by isolation of the organisms in tissue cell culture, since direct stains and even immunofluorescent stains of exfoliated cervical cells are insensitive. If tissue cell isolate capabilities are lacking, and cultures for *N. gonorrhoeae* are negative, consideration should be given to tetracycline therapy for nongonococcal mucopurulent cervicitis, as is recommended for nongonococcal urethritis in men. The recommended regimen consists of 1 to 2 g tetracycline hydrochloride orally for 1 to 3 weeks. For pregnant women, comparable doses of erythromycin base can be used.

Genital herpes simplex virus (HSV) infection produces ulcerative inflammation of the exocervix, as well as of the endocervix. HSV can be isolated from the cervix in 80 percent of women with an initial attack of genital herpes simplex virus infection, and these patients often have *true* ulcerative erosions of the cervix. In contrast, only 5 percent or less of women with recurrent vulvar HSV infection shed HSV from cervical lesions. If laboratory capabilities for isolation of HSV are not available, HSV can be demonstrated by Papanicolaou smear in about 50 percent of women with HSV cervicitis. In the absence of vaginitis, no infectious cause of cervicitis other than *N. gonorrhoeae, C. trachomatis,* and HSV has been identified.

Cervical ectopy   True cervicitis must be differentiated from cervical ectopy, which is often mislabeled "cervical erosion." Ectopy represents movement of the one-cell thick columnar endocervical epithelium into an exposed visible position on the cervix, where it appears redder than the 20-cell-thick stratified squamous vaginal epithelium. The cervical os contains clear or slightly cloudy mucous in ectopy, but not mucopus. Colposcopy shows that the epithelium is intact and not eroded. The mechanism by which ectopy occurs is uncertain, but oral contraceptive usage favors its development. Ectopy may cause increased vaginal discharge which may be symptomatic but which does not require therapy. The use of traumatic cauterizing procedures to eliminate ectopy is no longer recommended.

ULCERATIVE LESIONS OF THE GENITALIA   Genital skin lesions can be classified as ulcerative or nonulcerative. Patients seen in an STD clinic for nonulcerative genital lesions often have a sexually transmitted infection, such as scabies, genital warts, *Candida* balanoposthitis or vulvitis, and genital molluscum contagiosum, but the differential diagnosis involves a broad spectrum of dermatologic conditions.

The incidence and etiology of ulcerative lesions of the genitalia vary greatly in different areas of the world. In Asia and Africa, genital ulcers are seen as frequently as gonorrhea in some STD clinics, and limited studies suggest chancroid is the commonest form of genital ulceration. In the industrialized Western countries, genital ulcers are considerably less common than urethritis or vaginitis, and genital herpes simplex virus infection is the commonest form of ulceration. Syphilis is less common, chancroid is rare, and lymphogranuloma venereum (LGV) and granuloma inguinale are almost never seen.

Diagnosis and therapy   In industrialized countries, the differential diagnosis of genital ulceration, when trauma and excoriated lesions are excluded, usually rests among genital herpes simplex virus infection, syphilis, and, rarely, chancroid. Epidemiologic factors such as acquisition of infection in a developing country or from a prostitute or homosexual contact,

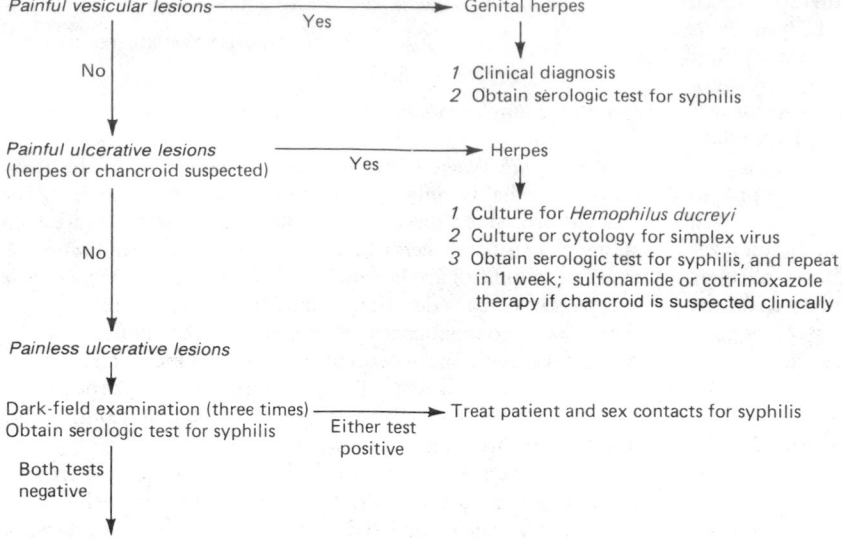

Painful vesicular lesions ───────────────→ Genital herpes
                Yes
                                        1 Clinical diagnosis
No   *2* Obtain serologic test for syphilis

Painful ulcerative lesions ──────────────→ Herpes
(herpes or chancroid suspected)   Yes
                                   1 Culture for *Hemophilus ducreyi*
No   *2* Culture or cytology for simplex virus
                           3 Obtain serologic test for syphilis, and repeat
                              in 1 week; sulfonamide or cotrimoxazole
                              therapy if chancroid is suspected clinically

Painless ulcerative lesions

Dark-field examination (three times) ─────→ Treat patient and sex contacts for syphilis
Obtain serologic test for syphilis Either test
                          positive
Both tests
negative

Repeat syphilis serology at 1 and 6 weeks

FIGURE 113-3
Management of ulcerative genital lesions.

prostitution, or very low socioeconomic status increase the likelihood of chancroid, LGV, or granuloma inguinale. Although the clinical findings are occasionally diagnostic (e.g., presence of herpetic vesicles) and clinical findings plus epidemiologic considerations help dictate the initial therapy pending further studies, most genital ulcerations cannot be diagnosed on clinical grounds. It is axiomatic to exclude syphilis by appropriate serology in all cases. Dark-field examination should also be performed, by experienced technicians when possible, on lesions suggesting primary or secondary syphilis. Chancroid should not be used as a "wastebasket" diagnosis for all ulcerative lesions not attributable to syphilis or genital herpes, since few such lesions are confirmed as chancroid. Newer selective enrichment media for isolation of *H. ducreyi* should be used for the etiologic evaluation of genital ulcers. However, even when all available diagnostic tests are used by an experienced dermatovenereologist, many ulcerative genital lesions are still classified as idiopathic.

The following general guidelines are recommended for management of ulcerative genital lesions (Fig. 113-3):

1 If typical painful herpetic vesicopustules are present: In this case the clinical diagnosis of herpes is warranted, although a reaginic serologic test for syphilis should be performed. The diagnosis can be confirmed by isolation of herpes simplex virus in 90 percent of patients and by cytology (Papanicolaou) smear in about two-thirds.

2 If painful nonvesicular ulcer(s) raise the suspicion of herpes or chancroid: If the lesion(s) or inguinal node(s) are painful or have other features suggestive of herpes or chancroid, attempts to demonstrate herpes simplex virus or *H. ducreyi* are indicated. Cytology for demonstrating herpes virus is slightly less sensitive in the ulcerative stage than in the vesicular stage. Syphilis should be excluded by reaginic serologic testing, which should be repeated 1 to 2 weeks later if negative initially and if other diagnoses cannot be confirmed.

Topical antimicrobial therapy is not indicated for ulcerative genital lesions. In settings where genital herpes is much commoner than chancroid, as in the United States, antimicrobial therapy for painful genital ulcers can generally be deferred, pending the results of initial studies. Initial attacks of genital herpes generally begin to improve spontaneously 10 to 14 days after onset, and recurrent episodes 4 to 7 days after onset. The value of antimicrobial therapy for idiopathic ulcerative lesions of the genitalia is uncertain, but a course

of sulfonamide, cotrimoxazole, or tetracycline therapy, as recommended for chancroid (Chap. 126) seems reasonable for lesions of recent onset that persist or progress during several days of observation and that cannot be attributed to herpes, chancroid, or syphilis. Sulfonamides will not interfere with subsequent dark-field examination and should be given promptly for ulcerative lesions considered "typical" of chancroid, especially if regional lymph node suppuration is present or appears imminent.

3 If painless ulcerative lesions suggest the diagnosis of syphilis: If lesions are at all suggestive of syphilis, or there are reasons to suspect syphilis, such as recent exposure, then dark-field examination and/or a rapid reagin test should be performed for prompt diagnosis. If these are negative, two more dark-field examinations on successive days are recommended, and a serologic test for syphilis should be repeated 1 week and 6 weeks later.

If patients do not improve or worsen during 1 or 2 weeks of observation and the diagnosis remains obscure, attempts to isolate *H. ducreyi* should be made or repeated, and other infectious (e.g., granuloma inguinale) and noninfectious etiologies should be considered.

REFERENCES

CHAPEL TA et al: How reliable is the morphologic diagnosis of penile ulcerations? Sex Trans Dis 4:150, 1977

ESCHENBACH, DA, HOLMES KK: Acute pelvic inflammatory disease: Current concepts of pathogenesis, etiology and management. Clin Obstet Gynecol 18:35, 1975

HART G: *Chancroid, Donovanosis, Lymphogranuloma Venereum,* US Department of Health, Education, and Welfare Publication (CDC) 75-8302

HOLMES KK, KIVIAT MD: Urethritis, in *Campbell's Urology,* HH Harrison et al (eds). Philadelphia, Saunders, 1978, p 538

KAWAMURA N: Metronidazole and tinidazole in a single large dose for treating urogenital infections with *Trichomonas vaginalis* in men. Br J Vener Dis 54:81, 1978

KOMAROFF AL et al: Management strategies for urinary and vaginal infections. Arch Intern Med 138:1069, 1978

ORIEL JD et al: Genital yeast infections. Br Med J 4:761, 1972

PHEIFER TA et al: Nonspecific vaginitis: Role of *Hemophilus vaginalis* and treatment with metronidazole. N Engl J Med 298:1429, 1978

REES E et al: Chlamydia in relation to cervical infection and pelvic inflammatory disease, in *Nongonococcal Urethritis and Related Infections,* D Hobson, KK Holmes (eds). Washington, DC, American Society of Microbiology, 1977, p 67

114

PREVENTION OF INFECTION: IMMUNIZATION AND ANTIMICROBIAL PROPHYLAXIS

LAWRENCE COREY
ROBERT G. PETERSDORF

There are three major ways to prevent infections: (1) by reducing exposure, (2) by acquiring or inducing immunity, and (3) by using antimicrobial agents to prevent colonization and infection. Exposure can be reduced by diminishing the prevalence of the infecting agent, by community-wide vaccination programs, and by cohorting of infected patients. On an individual basis, however, the most reliable way to prevent infectious disease is to provide effective immunization and, less commonly, chemoprophylaxis against the causative agent. This chapter summarizes current immunization practices and principles of antimicrobial prophylaxis. Additional details are provided in the chapters dealing with individual diseases.

IMMUNIZATION

Immunity may be defined as the ability of the individual to resist or overcome infection; it may be innate or acquired. For many infectious diseases, immunity is acquired during recovery from an infection or induced by the administration of vaccines prepared from inactivated or live microorganisms of modified disease-producing potential, or from specific antigen(s) derived from these organisms. The purpose of immunization, therefore, is to provoke a specific immunologic response to a selected microbial agent or its antigens with the expectation that this will result in humoral, and/or secretory, and/or cell mediated immunity. While this protection may diminish over time, future exposures to the same stimulus will result in a rapid return of the immune response because of heightened reactivity of antibody-forming, phagocytic, and other cells that mediate immune mechanisms (Chap. 61).

Certain infectious diseases present special situations that impede the development of vaccines. For example, *Salmonella* organisms and rhinoviruses consist of several hundred antigenically unique strains, making production of a vaccine unfeasible. Secondly, the portal of entry of an organism and the role of local immunity are important in determining whether a vaccine given parenterally will offer protection from either infection or disease. Finally, even when effective immunizing agents are available, difficulties in delivering them to the susceptible population may preclude their use.

GENERAL PRINCIPLES OF IMMUNIZATION Infections can be prevented or controlled by active and/or passive immunization. Active immunization with live attenuated vaccines generally results in subclinical or mild clinical illness which duplicates, to a limited extent, the disease that is marked for prevention; generally, it provides both local and durable humoral immunity. "Killed" or inactivated vaccines, such as influenza, rabies, typhoid, and cholera vaccines, maintain immunogenicity, without infectivity, but have several disadvantages including the large amount of antigen that must be administered by the parenteral route and the greater time period between administration of the antigen and the appearance of a protective effect. Table 114-1 summarizes active immunizing agents.

The use of any biological substance requires balancing its benefits and risks, and each vaccine must be evaluated accordingly. While some immunizations are recommended for all individuals, for example, diphtheria, tetanus, and poliomyelitis, others should be used only in those who have an increased risk of either acquiring the disease or developing complications. Pneumococcal polysaccharide vaccine, influenza vaccine, bacillus Calmette-Guérin (BCG) vaccine, and meningococcal vaccine are some examples.

Inactivated vaccines can be administered simultaneously at separate sites, although vaccines known to be associated with severe side effects should generally be given on separate occasions. Some vaccines contain trace amounts of preservatives or antibiotics to which patients may be sensitive, and, although reactions to them are unusual, reviewing the manufacturers' package insert prior to use of these agents may be helpful. Live virus vaccines prepared by growing viruses in cell culture are usually devoid of potential allergic substances. Many live virus vaccinations can be given simultaneously; measles, mumps, and rubella are some examples. However, when more than one dose of live viral vaccine is required, repeated administration should be separated by at least 1 month.

Contraindications to vaccination Virus replication following administration of live attenuated virus vaccines can be accentuated in immune deficiency diseases and in patients whose immune responses have been suppressed as in leukemia, lymphoma, or generalized malignancy or following therapy with corticosteroids, alkylating drugs, antimetabolites, and radiation. Such patients should not be given live attenuated virus vaccines. Vaccination of persons with severe febrile disease should be deferred to avoid superimposing the adverse effects of the vaccine on the underlying illness. Occasionally, viral interference, as might occur with concurrent enterovirus infection in the gut, may affect the efficacy of vaccines adversely. Because of a theoretical risk to the developing fetus, live attenuated virus vaccines generally should not be given to pregnant women. For some vaccines, particularly live attenuated rubella vaccine, pregnancy is an absolute contraindication to vaccination. Passively acquired antibody can interfere with the response to live attenuated virus vaccines; therefore, administration of live vaccine should be postponed until approximately 3 months after passive immunization.

IMMUNIZATION IN ADULTS Diphtheria The myocardial and peripheral nervous system involvement associated with *Corynebacterium diphtheriae* is due to elaboration of an exotoxin (Chap. 133). Diphtheria toxoid is a cell-free preparation of diphtheria toxin treated with formaldehyde. When administered intramuscularly, it produces a specific immune response to the toxin. While detailed controlled studies have not been undertaken, extensive experience in many countries indicates that the use of diphtheria toxoid has been associated with a steady reduction in the incidence of diphtheria. Moreover, although clinical diphtheria occurs occasionally in immunized individuals, the disease appears milder. Diphtheria toxoid provides protection against only the toxin and not the somatic components of *C. diphtheriae,* and local infection, either in the respiratory tract or skin, occurs occasionally in immune individuals. Nontoxigenic strains also may cause mild, focal infections.

All children less than 7 years of age should receive routine immunization against diphtheria in the form of absorbed diphtheria and tetanus toxoids and pertussis vaccine (DPT). Absorbed toxoids are produced by the addition of aluminum compounds to the formaldehyde-inactivated toxoid and are more antigenic than the fluid (plain) preparation. A preparation without pertussis vaccine is available for primary immunization of children who are unable to tolerate the pertussis vac-

TABLE 114-1
Active immunization in adults

	Type of vaccine	Administration and frequency*	Comments
ALL ADULTS			
Tetanus and diphtheria	Adsorbed toxoid	IM at least every 10 years	Usually administered together as Td vaccine
Poliomyelitis	Live attenuated	Oral polio vaccine (OPV)	Preferred for routine use and during epidemics
	Formalin-inactivated	Inactivated polio vaccine (IPV)	Selective use in unimmunized adults
WOMEN OF CHILD-BEARING AGE			
Rubella vaccine	Live attenuated	SC once	Only to women who are antibody (HI) negative and if pregnancy can be prevented for 3 months post-vaccination
POSTPUBERTAL MALES			
Mumps	Live attenuated	SC once	Prevention of orchitis in susceptible seronegative males
PERSONS AT HIGH RISK OF COMPLICATIONS OF DISEASE (CHRONIC HEART AND PULMONARY DISEASE)			
Influenza vaccine	Inactivated	SC yearly	Directed at reducing morbidity and mortality in those at risk of complications of influenza including those over 65 years
Pneumococcal polysaccharide vaccine	Purified dodecavalent polysaccharide vaccine	SC once	Also useful in patients with functional or surgical asplenia, agammaglobulinemia, cirrhosis, multiple myeloma, and nephrotic syndrome
POPULATIONS EXPOSED TO LOCALIZED OUTBREAKS			
Meningococcal vaccine A, C, AC	Purified capsular polysaccharide	SC once	Control of localized epidemics and adjunct to chemoprophylaxis in household contacts
Measles vaccine	Live attenuated	SC once	Control of outbreaks usually among adolescents or young adults
BCG vaccine	Live attenuated	SC or intradermally, once	Use in groups with excessive risk of new infection with tuberculosis or individuals persistently exposed to sputum-positive tuberculosis
Adenovirus vaccine	Live attenuated bivalent (types 4 and 7)	PO once	Only used for military recruits
Typhoid vaccine	Inactivated bacilli	SC in two doses	Household contact of documented *Salmonella typhi* carrier
Rubella vaccine	Live attenuated	SC once	Control of outbreaks among adolescents and young adults (must screen pubertal females with HI test prior to vaccination)
TRAVELERS TO FOREIGN COUNTRIES			
Smallpox	Live vaccinia virus	Intradermally, every 3-5 years	Presently recommended only for travel to endemic areas
Yellow fever	Live attenuated	SC once per 10 years	Administered at yellow fever vaccination centers
Cholera	Phenol-inactivated suspension of *Vibrio cholerae*	SC approximately every 6 months	Only 50% effective and not effective in decreasing transmission of disease
Typhoid	Inactivated bacilli	SC in half doses 4 weeks apart	70-90% efficacy in "normal" exposure
Typhus	Formaldehyde-inactivated *Rickettsia prowazekii*	SC in two doses 4 weeks apart	Only to persons in close contact to those where disease is indigenous
Plague	Formaldehyde-inactivated *Yersinia pestis*	SC in three injections of 0.5 ml at least 1 week apart, booster approximately every 2 years	Agricultural workers who reside in plague-endemic areas
Poliomyelitis	Oral or inactivated polio vaccine	See text	Most adults already immune
Hepatitis A	Immune serum globulin	IM every 3 months	See "Passive Immunization" in this chapter

* PO, orally; SC, subcutaneously; IM, intramuscularly.

cine (DT). To avoid the febrile reactions that may accompany repeated exposure to diphtheria toxoid among patients with prior exposure to diphtheria antigens, the preparation recommended for use in adults is a combination of tetanus and diphtheria toxoid in which the diphtheria toxoid is reduced to a maximum of two flocculating units per dose. This vaccine (Td) is recommended for primary immunization of adults and children older than 6 years of age and is also routinely used for booster immunization, both for the prevention of tetanus at the time of injury and for diphtheria prophylaxis.

Tetanus (see also Chap. 139) Tetanus toxoid is a formaldehyde-detoxified bacteria-free filtrate of *Clostridium tetani*. The antibody response to toxoid is often variable. However, two doses of the absorbed toxoid or three doses of fluid toxoid generally result in a protective level of antibody, 0.01 units per milliliter tetanus antitoxin toxoid. Tetanus toxoid may be used singly or in combination with diphtheria toxoid (DT or Td), or with both diphtheria toxoid and pertussis vaccine (DPT). When used singly, primary immunization with the fluid toxoid is given in three doses at least 1 month apart with a booster 8 to 12 months later and then at 10-year intervals. The absorbed form should be given in two doses, 1 month apart.

Poliomyelitis (see also Chap. 187) While routine polio vaccination of adults residing in the United States is generally not necessary because most are immune and the risk of exposure is small, susceptible adults at increased risk by virtue of travel or exposure to wild or vaccine polio virus should receive primary immunization with either inactivated or wild attenuated polio vaccines. Both a live attenuated oral polio vaccine (OPV) and an inactivated polio vaccine (IPV) are licensed in the United States. OPV has been favored over IPV because it is easier to administer, orally versus injection, confers more resistance in the alimentary tract to reinfection, and interferes with simultaneous infection by wild polioviruses. These properties are of special value during epidemics of poliomyelitis. Vaccination with OPV results in shedding of virus contained in the vaccine, and spread of virus to unvaccinated persons occurs. Rarely, recipients of oral vaccine or people in contact with them have contracted paralytic polio. Between 1969 and 1976, 132 cases of paralytic poliomyelitis were reported in the United States; 44 were classified as vaccine-associated. The risk of vaccine-associated polio has been estimated to be one case per recipient for every 11.5 million persons vaccinated with OPV, one case in a household contact for every 3.9 million persons vaccinated, and one case in a community contact for every 22.9 million persons vaccinated. The relative risk of paralytic disease is slightly higher in susceptible adults than in children. Such a risk seems acceptable. On the other hand, no serious complications have been reported with IPV. While oral trivalent polio vaccine is the principal vaccine in the United States, use of inactivated polio vaccine may be beneficial in selective circumstances such as primary immunization of susceptible adults.

For infants and children, the primary series of vaccination with OPV consists of three doses. The first two should be given not less than 6 and preferably 8 weeks apart. The third dose should follow 8 to 12 months after the second dose.

A booster dose of trivalent OPV should be given when the child enters kindergarten or first grade. Additional preadolescent immunization (at age 11 to 12) has been recommended by an expert committee of the National Academy of Sciences to provide additional protection during adulthood. The rationale for this recommendation is twofold: (1) vaccine-associated paralytic disease is rare under age 20; and (2) most vaccine-associated cases have occured in young adults following contact with vaccinated infants.

Inactivated polio vaccine should be considered for persons with heightened susceptibility to infection, including immunodeficient children and their siblings, and immunosuppressed persons and adults undergoing initial vaccination when traveling to areas where the incidence of polio is high or whose household contacts are undergoing OPV vaccination. Live attenuated oral polio vaccine is acceptable for adults who have been vaccinated previously or whose circumstances do not allow adequate time for administration of IVP and who are not in a category in which oral vaccine is contraindicated. Primary immunization with IPV consists of four doses: three at 1- to 2-month intervals and a booster 6 to 12 months after the third. Booster doses at 2- to 3-year intervals either with IPV or with one dose of OPV after primary immunization with IPV will sustain long-lasting immunity.

IMMUNIZATION IN WOMEN OF CHILDBEARING AGE Rubella (see also Chap. 182) The purpose of rubella vaccination is to prevent rubella embryopathy in the fetus. The direct approach to this goal would be to immunize all women before they become pregnant. However, the difficulty is being sure that a woman is not pregnant at the time of vaccination, and the increased risk of joint symptoms associated with vaccination in women has rendered this approach impractical. Because children are a major source of spread of rubella to pregnant females, rubella vaccination has been routinely recommended for all children older than 12 months. When given in combination with measles antigen, rubella vaccine should be administered when a child is about 15 months of age to achieve the maximum rate of measles seroconversion.

Since 1969 when rubella vaccine was first licensed, the incidence of rubella has declined steadily, and the lack of a rubella epidemic during the early 1970s suggests that the vaccine is effective in interrupting the 7- to 9-year epidemiologic cycle that has characterized nationwide rubella outbreaks. However, the congenital rubella syndrome still occurs in the United States, and increased emphasis should be placed on vaccinating unimmunized prepubertal girls and susceptible adolescent and adult women who are not pregnant and who agree to prevent pregnancy for 3 months after receiving vaccine. In addition, testing for rubella antibody by hemagglutination inhibition during the perinatal or antepartum period, and vaccination of susceptible women in the immediate postpartum period, are warranted. Routine premarital rubella antibody determinations by either hemagglutination inhibition or enzyme-linked immunoabsorbent assay would enhance effects to identify susceptible females before their first pregnancy. Rubella immunization of medical personnel having frequent contact with pregnant women is also advisable.

Rubella vaccine is prepared in cell cultures and is administered by subcutaneous injection. A single dose induces antibodies in approximately 95 percent of susceptible persons.

Rubella vaccine virus has been demonstrated to cross the placenta and infect the fetus. Infants born to more than 60 susceptible women, who inadvertently received rubella vaccine during early pregnancy and continued their pregnancies to term, did not have any recognizable malformations attributable to rubella. However, fetal infection with vaccine-like rubella virus may produce pathological changes in developing organs. While the risk of teratogenicity is felt to be much lower from the vaccine virus than from the wild virus, if a pregnant woman is inadvertently vaccinated or if she becomes pregnant within 3 months of vaccination, she should be advised of the theoretical risk to the fetus.

VACCINATION OF SUSCEPTIBLE POSTPUBERTAL MALES

Mumps (see also Chap. 188) Mumps is a relatively benign disease of childhood with a low case fatality rate. Meningoencephalitis associated with mumps is usually uncomplicated, self-limited, and, therefore, the stimulus for prevention of mumps by vaccination is due to the occurrence of orchitis in postpubertal males. While this has been documented to occur as frequently as 20 percent of the time in epidemic mumps, the incidence of subsequent sterility is low. Both a live attenuated mumps vaccine (Jeryl-Lynn strain) grown in chick embryo cell cultures and a killed vaccine have been developed, but only live mumps vaccine clearly has demonstrated safety and efficacy. Mumps vaccination is recommended for all children older than 1 year and especially in children approaching puberty, adolescents, and adults, particularly males, who have not had mumps or who have no serologic evidence of mumps immunity. A single dose is given subcutaneously; protective antibodies have been shown to persist for at least 8 years after vaccination. Patients with severe febrile illness or hypersensitivity to egg products, with malignancy who are receiving immunosuppressive therapy, or who are pregnant should not be vaccinated.

VACCINATION OF PERSONS WITH CHRONIC HEART, PULMONARY, AND METABOLIC DISEASE

Influenza (see also Chap. 179) Influenza occurs every year in the United States but with variation in incidence and geographic distribution. Epidemics occur periodically; more are caused by influenza A viruses than by influenza B. More importantly, influenza A epidemics are notable for causing mortality in excess of what is usually expected. In the 1957 to 1958 Asian influenza epidemic, nearly 70,000 excess deaths were reported in the United States during the 12-week epidemic period. Most nationwide influenza epidemics have resulted in 10,000 to 20,000 excess deaths. Repeated observations have indicated that during influenza epidemics deaths occur primarily among children and chronically ill adults, especially those over age 65. These high-risk persons should be vaccinated annually. Vaccination of the entire population has not been considered a reasonable public health policy because protection is of limited duration owing both to the antigenic drift of the virus, as well as the short-lived antibody response to the inactivated vaccine, and the low incidence of serious infections in healthy persons.

Influenza vaccines are inactivated products of the prevalent circulating types of influenza virus. The vaccine is usually bivalent and contains an influenza A as well as an influenza B prototype antigen. Two types of vaccines are available, whole virus vaccines and "split-product" or subunit vaccines. Generally, whole virus vaccines are more immunogenic but have a slightly higher reaction rate than split-product vaccines. Studies with both preparations indicate a 60 to 95 percent protection rate, depending upon the population group studied and the relationship between the "epidemic" strain and the vaccine strain. In adults either form of vaccine can be used, but because of the high frequency of febrile reactions, children under 12 should receive two doses of split-product vaccine at approximately 3 to 6-week intervals. Vaccine is generally administered during the fall of the year and is given subcutaneously. While intradermal vaccination may elicit a good humoral antibody response, the clinical efficacy of this route of administration has not been well documented. Because even the zonally centrifuged inactivated influenza vaccines contain trace amounts of egg protein, patients who are allergic to egg or egg protein should not receive this vaccine. Severe adverse reactions to influenza vaccine are uncommon. The relationship between influenza vaccination and the Landry-Guillain-Barré syndrome is discussed in Chap. 179.

While influenza vaccine is the preferred form of prophylaxis, because of its low cost, greater efficacy, and slight toxicity, amantadine hydrochloride has been effective in preventing influenza infection especially during interepidemic intervals. Patients at risk of developing the complications of influenza who failed to receive their annual influenza vaccination should be placed on 100 mg amantadine hydrochloride twice daily during the period in which influenza A virus is identified in the community.

Pneumococcal vaccine (see also Chap. 115) Despite antibiotic therapy, the morbidity and mortality of pneumococcal disease remains a problem. Bacteremic pneumococcal disease appears to be unusually common in persons with sickle-cell anemia, anatomic or functional asplenia, agammaglobulinemia, multiple myeloma, nephrotic syndrome, cirrhosis, alcoholism, diabetes mellitus, and chronic cardiorespiratory disease; in these situations vaccination is generally indicated. Other situations in which pneumococcal vaccine may be of benefit include closed populations in which systemic pneumococcal disease has been identified as an epidemic or endemic problem, or where an antibiotic-resistant strain of pneumococcus has emerged.

The dodecavalent polysaccharide vaccine licensed for use in the United States is composed of purified capsular material extracted separately from the 14 types of pneumococcal organisms in the vaccine. These 14 types, 1 to 4, 6, 8, 12, 14, 19, 23, 25, 51, and 56, are responsible for at least 80 percent of all bacteremic pneumococcal disease in the United States. One dose of vaccine contains 50 μg of each polysaccharide. The majority of adults and most children over 2 years of age respond with development of measurable humoral antibody. Immunity exists only against the pneumococcal types contained in the vaccine, although theoretically there may be some degree of cross-protection among immunologically similar types. The duration of protection is unknown, but elevated antibody levels appear to persist for at least 2 years after immunization. Booster doses do not seem to increase the levels of antibody, and children under 2 develop lower levels of antibody than adults. Vaccination reduces the likelihood of acquiring the pneumococcal types in the vaccine in the nasopharynx. There has been no evidence of a relative increase in disease caused by other microbial pathogens among vaccine recipients. Vaccination has reduced the incidence of pneumococcal pneumonia and bacteremia due to types in the vaccine by 80 percent. Local erythema and pain at the injection site occur in approximately half the recipients, but serious adverse reactions are rare.

VACCINES USEFUL IN LOCALIZED OUTBREAKS

Meningococcal vaccine (see also Chap. 118) Meningococcal disease is endemic in the United States and throughout the world. In recent years meningococcal disease in civilians has occurred primarily in single isolated cases, usually due to groups B or C or, infrequently, in small localized clusters. Secondary cases occur more frequently in household contacts than in the general population, and appropriate antibiotic prophylaxis has been the principal method of reducing the risk for immediate contacts. Vaccines have been used to curtail recent outbreaks of group A disease in several cities in the Pacific Northwest (Chap. 118) as well as extensive outbreaks in Brazil of groups A and C meningococcal disease. When epidemic meningococcal disease due to groups A or C occurs, the population at risk should be identified and vaccinated. Vaccination also should be considered as an adjunct to antibiotic prophylaxis for household contacts of cases of meningococcal disease. The reason for this is that one-half of the secondary cases in families occurs more than 5 days after the primary case; this is long enough to yield potential benefits from vaccination if antibiotic chemoprophylaxis should not be successful.

Three meningococcal polysaccharide vaccines, monovalent A, monovalent C, and bivalent AC vaccine, are licensed for selective use in the United States. These vaccines are chemically defined antigens consisting of purified capsular polysaccharides and induce specific immunity to the serologic groups. The vaccine is administered parenterally as a single dose. Adverse reactions consist principally of localized erythema lasting 1 to 2 days. The vaccine appears effective in all age groups beyond the first year of life, and there is suggestive evidence of efficacy in children as young as 3 months of age.

Measles (see also Chap. 181) Two categories of live measles vaccine exist: (1) vaccine made from attenuated Edmonston strain and (2) further-attenuated measles vaccine (Schwarz strain) derived from passage of the Edmonston strain in chick cell culture. The further-attenuated vaccines are associated with fewer reactions, can be administered without the concomitant use of gamma globulin, and are the preferable mode of vaccination.

While measles vaccination is highly effective, the number of cases of measles reported in the United States in 1976 and 1977 has increased over that reported in the early 1970s. Much of this increase is due to localized outbreaks among patients 10 to 19 years old, often among populations thought to be highly immunized. It has been suggested that these cases have occurred in children who were vaccinated prior to age 12 months or who received measles vaccine concomitantly with immune serum globulin (ISG). Both of these circumstances may not provide adequate immunity against infection.

Measles vaccination has been recommended for all children older than 12 months. During measles outbreaks, it is recommended that all susceptible children, as well as adolescents and adults at risk, be immunized. Individuals can be defined as susceptible to measles when they lack a certificate of adequate immunization with live measles vaccine at age of at least 12 months or who lack adequate evidence of having had measles. Persons who should not be considered adequately protected and who should be revaccinated include (1) children vaccinated with live vaccine before they were 12 months old (these children should be revaccinated at 15 months of age or older); (2) children who received live vaccine with immune serum globulin, regardless of their age at vaccination; and (3) persons previously vaccinated with killed measles virus vaccine. Repeat vaccination with live measles vaccine poses no increased risk for individuals who have previously had natural measles or who have been vaccinated.

Up to 15 percent of vaccinated children will have fever beginning the sixth day after vaccination and lasting up to 5 days. Local induration and edema at the injection site may occur in persons who previously received killed measles vaccine.

BCG vaccine Efforts to control tuberculosis in the United States are directed toward the early identification and treatment of active cases and preventive therapy with isoniazid. Use of BCG vaccine should be considered for uninfected persons who are exposed repeatedly to infected cases and who cannot or will not obtain or accept treatment. In selected circumstances, where multiple-drug-resistant *Mycobacterium tuberculosis* is the "epidemic" strain, vaccination with BCG may also be useful. In the United States, BCG vaccination should be reserved for persons who are skin test negative to 5 tuberculin units (TU) of tuberculin purified protein derivative (PPD). BCG recipients should have repeat skin tests 2 to 3 months later; if they are negative, vaccination should be repeated. The World Health Organization (WHO) recommends that BCG vaccine be administered by the intradermal route, but vaccine

for percutaneous administration is also available. BCG should not be given to persons with impaired immune responses, and although no harmful effects of BCG on the fetus have been observed, it is best to avoid vaccination during pregnancy.

Adenovirus vaccine The epidemiologic syndrome of epidemic acute respiratory disease due to adenovirus 4 or 7 is almost exclusively a problem of military recruits. While an effective oral attenuated adenovirus vaccine has been manufactured, clinical illness caused by these adenoviruses has not been associated with significant morbidity or mortality in the civilian population, and hence use of this vaccine outside the military is not recommended.

Typhoid vaccine Routine typhoid vaccination is no longer recommended in the United States, but selective immunization is indicated for persons who are household contacts of a documented typhoid carrier. Typhoid vaccine is generally not necessary among persons affected by flooding or other natural disasters or for those utilizing rural summer camps. Typhoid vaccine consists of whole typhoid bacilli that have been killed, concentrated, and preserved by various methods. The vaccine should be given in two doses of 0.5 ml subcutaneously or 0.1 ml intradermally, according to the manufacturers' recommendations. Local reactions such as erythema, induration, and moderate fever for about 24 h are not uncommon. Controlled trials indicate a 70 to 90 percent protection rate, although immunity may be overcome by exposure to high inocula of *Salmonella*.

VACCINATION OF TRAVELERS TO FOREIGN COUNTRIES

There are two objectives for immunization of foreign travelers: (1) to satisfy a country's requirements, as modified by international regulations, regarding prevention of the introduction and spread of disease (e.g., smallpox, yellow fever, and cholera), and (2) to protect the traveler.

Smallpox vaccination (see also Chap. 184) The success of the WHO smallpox eradication program, the concomitant decrease of worldwide smallpox, and the low risk of importation of smallpox make the morbidity of smallpox vaccination greater than the risk of exposure to smallpox itself. For this reason, routine use of smallpox vaccine is no longer recommended in the United States. Only travelers going to endemic areas should be vaccinated before departing the United States. The complications and contraindications to vaccination are outlined in Chap. 184.

Yellow fever vaccine Many countries require a current international certificate of vaccination against yellow fever from persons older than 6 months who have been in the countries reporting yellow fever (South America and the African subcontinent) in the preceding 6 days. Because these requirements change and often vary with the length of stay in the country, all travelers to areas where yellow fever is endemic should seek current information from health departments or international airlines before departing. Yellow fever vaccine must be administered at a designated yellow fever center. Vaccination certificates are valid for a period of 10 years, beginning 10 days after vaccination. The only yellow fever vaccine licensed in the United States is a live attenuated vaccine produced in chick embryos which must be administered subcutaneously in 0.5-ml amounts. Fever and malaise occur in 10 percent of recipients, but major reactions such as encephalitis are fortunately very rare. While pregnant females should generally not be vaccinated with live attenuated virus, the risk to the fetus is felt to be small, and pregnant women who must travel to areas where the risk of yellow fever is high should be vaccinated. Yellow fever virus vaccine should not be given to patients with severe underlying diseases such as leukemia or those receiving immunosuppressive therapy.

Cholera (see also Chap. 134)   Travelers to the Middle East, Asia, and Africa may require evidence of cholera vaccination. Ideally, travelers to these countries should be vaccinated 1 month prior to their departure. A single primary series or booster dose of vaccine is generally sufficient. The risk of cholera for travelers who use ordinary tourist accommodations is very slight, and currently available cholera vaccines are only about 50 percent effective in reducing the incidence of clinical illness for a period of only 3 to 6 months. They do not prevent transmission of disease.

Typhoid   Travelers going to regions where food and water sanitation is poor may wish to receive typhoid vaccine. However, care in selecting food and water is the best protection.

Typhus (see also Chap. 168)   Vaccination against typhus is not required by any country as a condition for entry, and typhus has not occurred in American travelers in recent years. Typhus vaccination is, therefore, suggested only for persons who work in close contact with the organisms in the laboratory or who live in or visit areas where the disease actually occurs and who will be in close contact with the population in such areas. Typhus vaccine is prepared from formaldehyde-inactivated *Rickettsia prowazekii* grown in embryonated eggs. This vaccine provides protection only against louse-borne (epidemic) typhus, not against murine or scrub typhus. Two subcutaneous injections of the vaccine 4 or more weeks apart are recommended. Boosters at yearly intervals may be necessary.

Plague (see also Chap. 129)   Immunization against *Yersinia pestis* is recommended only for laboratory workers and for individuals such as Peace Corps volunteers or agricultural advisors who reside in plague-enzootic or plague-epidemic rural areas where avoidance of rodents and fleas is difficult. Travelers to countries or areas reporting endemic plague do not need to receive vaccine.

UNUSUAL OCCUPATIONAL EXPOSURES   In general, vaccination of personnel such as laboratory or field workers whose vocation or avocation puts them at particular risk of developing an immunizable disease should receive preexposure immunization. For example, laboratory workers involved with rabies, *Y. pestis,* smallpox, *R. prowazekii, R. rickettsii,* yellow fever virus, or Venezuelan or Eastern equine encephalitis viruses, anthrax bacillus, or tularemia should be vaccinated against the appropriate agent. Occupational exposure requiring vaccination includes preexposure immunization against rabies for veterinarians, spelunkers, and other animal handlers exposed to potentially rabid dogs, cats, skunks, foxes, and bats; *Yersinia* vaccination for field workers in endemic areas; and anthrax vaccination for industrial workers who process hides, hair, bone meal, and wool of potentially infected animals.

PASSIVE IMMUNIZATION (See Table 114-2)   Prophylaxis or therapy of infection can also be accomplished in some instances by passive immunization which involves the administration of preformed antibody obtained from humans or other animals who have been actively immunized. Because animal antiserum can induce a hypersensitivity response in the recipient, antiserums from humans are preferable. The duration of immunity provided by passive immunization is brief. Intracellular virus generally is not affected by antibody, and once infection has been initiated, the role of antibody is limited to resisting the spread of the virus.

Hepatitis A (see also Chap. 302)   Immune serum globulin administered before exposure and during the incubation period of hepatitis A is 80 to 90 percent effective in preventing or modifying the disease. The prophylactic effect of ISG is greatest when given early in the incubation period, and the use of ISG more than 2 weeks after exposure or after onset of clinical illness is not indicated. Immune serum globulin is recommended for household contacts of patients with hepatitis A but not for contacts at school, hospital, or work. In institutional settings where periodic epidemics of hepatitis A are common, the administration of ISG to residents and staff may limit the spread of the disease. The dose of ISG for postexposure prophylaxis is 0.02 ml per kilogram of body weight.

The risk of hepatitis A for residents of the United States traveling abroad is small. Travelers to tropical areas or to developing countries who bypass the usual tourist routes should probably be given ISG. In addition, travelers staying in developing countries or in tropical areas longer than 3 months should receive a single injection of ISG, 0.05 ml per kilogram of body weight. This dose should be repeated every 4 to 6 months.

Hepatitis B (see also Chaps. 108 and 302)   Much information remains to be acquired before definite recommendations concerning the passive immunization of hepatitis B can be made. Most studies, however, indicate that either ISG-containing antibody to hepatitis B surface antigen (anti-HBs) or hyperimmune globulin containing a high titer of anti-HBs hepatitis B immunoglobulin (HBI) should be given to susceptible health care personnel who are anti-HBs negative and who have been exposed to needle sticks with blood from documented HBsAg-positive donors. Because of its lower cost, ISG may be used in susceptible persons with needle exposures from unknown sources. The role of passive immunization in the prophylaxis of hepatitis B in dialysis units, or among household contacts, requires further definition. HBI has been partially effective in protecting spouses of patients with acute hepatitis B. However, in endemic environments, like dialysis units, or among persons continuously exposed to chronic HBsAg carriers, passive immunization may only delay the incubation period of the disease. Although data concerning prophylaxis of infants born to mothers with HBsAg-positive hepatitis at the time of delivery are insufficient to form firm recommendations, the information available suggests that administration of either HBI or standard ISG-containing anti-HBs appears warranted.

Zoster serum immune globulin (ZIG)   Within 72 h after exposure, ZIG may prevent or ameliorate varicella-zoster among immunosuppressed susceptible patients. Indications for the use of ZIG are listed in Chap. 185. A list of regional ZIG consultants may be obtained from the Center for Disease Control, Atlanta, Georgia.

Diphtheria antitoxin (see also Chap. 133)   Diphtheria antitoxin may be useful in the prophylaxis of asymptomatic unimmunized household contacts along with (1) chemoprophylaxis with either oral erythromycin or intramuscular benzathine penicillin or (2) immunization with diphtheria toxoid. The risk of diphtheria among household contacts, which was approximately 20 percent before the antibiotic era but is negligible now, versus that of serum sickness from equine antiserum must be weighed before using this product.

TABLE 114-2
Passive immunization

Disease	Preparation	Route and dose*	Comments
Hepatitis A	ISG, human	IM (0.02–0.06 ml/kg)	Household contacts
Hepatitis B	Human, hepatitis B immunoglobulin	IM (0.06 ml/kg; two doses 4 weeks apart)	Prophylaxis of direct parenteral exposure (needle stick) or mucous-membrane contact in susceptibles; both HBIG and ISG with anti-HBs may be useful in preventing nonparenteral transmission of hepatitis B
	ISG, human	IM (0.05 ml/kg; two doses 4 weeks apart)	
Vaccinia immunoglobulin	Human VIG	IM (0.3 ml/kg)	Use in eczema vaccinatum, disseminated vaccinia, vaccinia in pregnancy
Herpes zoster	Human ZIG	IM (1.2 ml/10 kg up to 5 ml)	Prevention and amelioration of varicella in susceptible immunosuppressed patients
Diphtheria	Diphtheria antitoxin, horse	IM or IV (10,000–100,000 units)	Dose dependent on extent of membrane and degree of toxicity; may also be used in unimmunized household contacts
Tetanus	Human tetanus immunoglobulin (TIG)	IM (250 units)	When given with tetanus toxoid, use separate syringes and sites
Rabies	Human rabies immunoglobulin	One half locally and one-half IM (20 IU/kg)	Used for postexposure prophylaxis with 21-dose primary series and two booster doses of duck embryo rabies vaccine
	Equine antirabies globulin	One-half locally and one-half IM (40 IU/kg)	Same as above
Pertussis	Pertussis immunoglobulin, human	IM (1.5 ml, repeat in 5–7 days)	No studies suggest efficacy in susceptible infants
Measles	ISG, human	IM (0.05–0.1 ml/kg)	Susceptible household contacts less than 1 year old, exposed susceptible pregnant females, or immunodeficient persons
Rubella	ISG, human	IM (20–30 ml)	Exposed susceptible pregnant females who will not consider termination
Botulism (Chap. 140)	Horse serum, trivalent AB	One-half IM and one-half IV (8–32 ml)	Use only therapeutically: greatest efficacy in type E
Snake bite (Chap. 215)	Polyvalent crotaline antivenom (pit vipers)	IV (dose function of severity of bite)	See Chap. 215
Spider bite (Chap. 215)	Equine	IM (2.5 ml)	*Latrodectus* (black widow spider) poisoning

* IM, intramuscularly; IV, intravenously.

Tetanus immune globulin (TIG) (see also Chap. 139) The product of choice when contaminated wounds are present in persons whose history of previous tetanus immunization is uncertain or inadequate is TIG. The current recommended prophylactic dose of TIG is 250 to 1000 units given intramuscularly.

Rabies (see also Chap. 189) Postexposure prophylaxis for rabies consists of both passive and active immunization. Although more expensive, human rabies immune globulin is the preferred immunizing agent. The dose is 20 IU per kilogram of body weight given half intramuscularly and half intravenously.

Pertussis (see also Chap. 125) Hyperimmune pertussis globulin does not appear effective in preventing disease among unvaccinated susceptible neonates.

Measles (see also Chap. 181) Immune serum globulin should not be used to control measles outbreaks. Live measles vaccination can usually prevent development of disease if administered within 2 days of exposure. Immune serum globulin should be reserved for susceptible household contacts of measles patients, particularly for those under 1 year of age, exposed pregnant females, or for persons in whom measles vaccine is contraindicated, such as immune deficient hosts. The usual dose is 10 to 20 ml intramuscularly.

Rubella (see also Chap. 182) After exposure to rubella, ISG will not prevent infection or viremia with rubella virus but may modify or suppress symptoms. The routine use of ISG for postexposure prophylaxis of rubella in early pregnancy is not recommended, and infants with congenital rubella have been born to women who were given ISG shortly after exposure.

CHEMOPROPHYLAXIS OF INFECTION

USE OF A SINGLE DRUG Antibiotics have been used prophylactically to (1) prevent the acquisition of an exogenous organism, (2) prevent a resident organism from infecting a normally sterile site, and (3) prevent a dormant pathogenic organism from causing disease. In general, antimicrobial prophylaxis with a single drug, administered over a moderate period of time and directed at a single pathogen, has been successful. Examples of this type of prophylaxis employing low doses of "narrow-spectrum" antimicrobials include the prevention of recurrent episodes of rheumatic fever secondary to group A streptococcal disease with benzathine penicillin, of malaria with chloroquine, and of influenza A with amantadine. Table 114-3 lists some clinical situations where prolonged chemoprophylaxis either to prevent exposure to an exogenous organism or to reactivate a dormant organism in a uniquely susceptible host has been useful.

There are also situations in which the short-term use of antibiotics may prevent bacteremia, as in prophylaxis of bacterial endocarditis in individuals with acquired or congenital heart disease, or may abort localized mucosal infections. Here the use of antibiotics is based on the rationale that brief, low-dose exposure to an antimicrobial, early in the disease before

TABLE 114-3
Drugs that may be administered prophylactically for prolonged exposure or for extended periods of time

Disease/organism	Drug
Group A streptococcus (rheumatic fever)	Penicillin G, sulfonamide
Influenza A infection*	Amantadine
Malaria	Chloroquine
Tuberculosis contacts	Isoniazid
*Pneumocystis carinii** in cancer patients receiving cytotoxic agents	Trimethoprim-sulfamethoxazole
Recurrent urinary tract infection in females	Trimethoprim-sulfamethoxazole, nitrofurantoin

* May require only short courses.

bacterial multiplication has led to established infection, may prevent full-blown disease. Some examples of short-term prophylaxis are given in Table 114-4.

ANTIBIOTIC PROPHYLAXIS IN SURGERY Controlled evaluations of short courses of prophylactic antimicrobials have indicated that the selective use of antibiotics, particularly in operative procedures involving potentially contaminated surgical sites, will lower the rate of postoperative infections. The following principles should be applied in using antimicrobial prophylaxis in surgery (Table 114-5): (1) there must be a high prevalence of postoperative infections that are potentially severe before employing antimicrobial drugs; (2) the prophylactic antimicrobial must be effective against the most frequent postoperative pathogens; (3) the drug should be administered from immediately before and during the operation, and for only a short period thereafter; and (4) where possible, prophylaxis should be carried out with a single drug. This topic is also discussed in Chap. 118. For choice of the appropriate agent, Chap. 111 should be consulted.

TABLE 114-4
Short-term antimicrobial prophylaxis

Disease	Antibiotic
USUALLY EFFECTIVE	
Subacute bacterial endocarditis:	
Streptococcus viridans	Penicillin V, procaine penicillin G plus streptomycin
Enterococcus	Ampicillin or penicillin G plus gentamicin or streptomycin
Neisseria gonorrheae (ophthalmia)	Penicillin, silver nitrate
Neisseria gonorrheae (genital infection)	Tetracycline
Nongonococcal urethritis	Tetracycline
Congenital or incubating syphilis	Penicillin
Toxigenic *Escherichia coli* ("tourista")	Tetracycline
Enteropathogenic *E. coli* diarrhea	Neomycin or kanamycin
Neisseria meningitidis	Sulfonamides (sensitive strains only), rifampin, minocycline
Corynebacterium diphtheriae	Erythromycin, clindamycin, penicillin
SOMETIMES EFFECTIVE	
Shigellosis	Ampicillin, neomycin
Chronic bronchitis*	Ampicillin, tetracycline
Short-term urethral catheterization (<24 h)	Ampicillin, tetracycline, nitrofurantoin, trimethoprim-sulfamethoxazole

* Prophylaxis may require prolonged administration.

TABLE 114-5
Systemic antimicrobial prophylaxis in surgery

PROPHYLAXIS INDICATED

Obstetric-gynecologic surgery:
   Vaginal and abdominal hysterectomy
   Caesarean section after prolonged rupture of membranes
Colorectal surgery
Cardiac surgery
Valvular, noncardiac thoracic surgery
Orthopedic surgery (joint replacement, prosthesis, compound fractures)
Peripheral artery surgery with graft replacement
Contaminated surgical wounds

PROPHYLAXIS OF UNCERTAIN VALUE

Gastroduodenal surgery
Biliary tract surgery
Microsurgical craniotomy
Extensive ear, nose, or throat surgery

PROPHYLAXIS UNLIKELY TO BE OF VALUE

Clean abdominal surgery
Gynecologic surgery (other than mentioned above)
Coronary artery bypass surgery
Prophylaxis of wound infections

ANTIBIOTICS IN SUSCEPTIBLE HOSTS In contrast to short-term antimicrobial prophylaxis with a single drug which, while at times not effective, is unlikely to be deleterious, attempts to prevent infection with multiple drugs administered in high doses for relatively prolonged periods are much more likely to be harmful. Adverse effects of "prolonged" antimicrobial prophylaxis include (1) superinfection (defined as an infection with a resistant organism that has developed during antibiotic therapy), (2) increased incidence of toxic or allergic reactions to drugs, (3) increased cost, and last but not least, (4) a sense of false security on the part of many physicians, resulting in less stringent observation of the patient. However, many of the patients who are given antibiotics prophylactically are precisely the ones who are susceptible to complicating infections, and particular care must be taken to watch assiduously for the development of infection and to treat it promptly when it occurs. Such policy is often superior to the use of antimicrobial prophylaxis.

Prophylactic antibiotics have not been useful in preventing bacterial complications of antecedent viral respiratory illness such as influenza or in preventing colonization of pathogenic organisms in intensive care units. Indeed, in these and many other clinical situations the risk of superinfection with resistant, difficult-to-treat organisms outweighs the unlikely effectiveness of prophylactic antibiotics (Table 114-6).

There are a number of situations in which the use of antimicrobial prophylaxis remains controversial but where these drugs seem to have decreased the frequency of overt infection. One of these is patients with severe neutropenia—less than 200

TABLE 114-6
Antibiotic prophylaxis in susceptible hosts in whom its use is not indicated

OUTPATIENT USE

Viral respiratory disease
Viral exanthems
Preventing acute exacerbations of asthma

HOSPITALIZED PATIENTS

Preventing pneumonia in comatose patients
Preventing tracheal colonization with pathogenic organisms
Preventing infections in patients with congestive heart failure
Prolonged urethral catheterization (>24 h)
Prolonged intravenous catheterization (>48 h)
High-dose steroid therapy
Prematurity
Shock

white blood cells per cubic millimeter in whom fever is often suppressed as long as the patient is receiving antibiotics (Chaps. 107 and 220). The use of antibiotics in burn patients presents the enigma of prophylaxis versus therapy. Most of these patients receive topical antibiotics from the outset and for this and other reasons may have a lower incidence of infection. A textbook of surgery should be consulted for a more detailed treatment of this subject.

REFERENCES

Amman AJ et al: Polyvalent pneumococcal polysaccharide immunization of patients with sickle cell anemia and patients with splenectomy. N Engl J Med 297:897, 1977

Barrett-Conner E: Chemoprophylaxis of malaria for travelers. Ann Intern Med 81:219, 1974

Glasso GJ et al: Overview of clinical trials of influenza vaccines 1976. J Infect Dis S136:S4-25, 1977

Krugman S: Effect of human immune serum globulin on infectivity of hepatitis A virus. J Infect Dis 134:70, 1976

Maynard JE et al: Passive immunization against hepatitis B. A review of recent studies and comment on current aspects of control. Am J Epidemiol 107:77, 1978

Modlin JF et al: Risk of congenital abnormality after inadvertent rubella vaccination of pregnant women. N Engl J Med 294:972, 1976

Nightingale EO: Recommendations for a national policy on poliomyelitis vaccination. N Engl J Med 297:249, 1977

Peltola H et al: Clinical efficacy of meningococcus Group A capsular polysaccharide vaccine in children 3 months to 5 years of age. N Engl J Med 297:686, 1977

Ruben FL: Antitoxin responses in the elderly to tetanus-diphtheria (Td) immunization. Am J Epidemiol 108:145, 1978

Shasby DM et al: Epidemic measles in a highly vaccinated population. N Engl J Med 296:585, 1977

section 2 | Infections caused by gram-positive cocci

115
PNEUMOCOCCAL INFECTIONS

ROBERT AUSTRIAN

ETIOLOGY

The pneumococcus *(Streptococcus pneumoniae)* is a gram-positive encapsulated coccus that usually grows in pairs or short chains. In the diplococcal form, the adjacent margins are rounded and the opposite ends slightly pointed, giving the organisms a lancet shape. In stained preparations of exudate, gram-negative forms are sometimes present. Pneumococcal colonies are surrounded by greenish discoloration on or in blood agar and are confused at times with other alpha-hemolytic streptococci to which they are closely related. Their isolation from respiratory secretions may be facilitated by inclusion of 5 μg gentamicin per milliliter in the medium. Pneumococci can be distinguished by their bile solubility and mouse virulence or by serologic typing. Another method, utilizing inhibition of pneumococci by Optochin-impregnated paper disks, is less cumbersome and very effective, but standard zones of inhibition determined for aerobic cultures cannot be applied to cultures grown in 5% carbon dioxide for the presumptive identification of pneumococcus.

The capsular substances are complex polysaccharides and are the basis for dividing pneumococci into serotypes. Organisms exposed to type-specific antiserum show a positive capsular precipitin reaction, the *Neufeld quellung reaction;* by this means, 84 serotypes have been identified. All are pathogenic for human beings, but types 1, 3, 4, 7, 8, and 12 are encountered most frequently in clinical practice. Types 6, 14, 19, and 23 often cause pneumonia and otitis media in children but are less common in adults.

Specific typing of pneumococci remains of great clinical importance if pneumococcus is to be identified with regularity, but it has largely been abandoned since the introduction of sulfonamides and antibiotics, which are effective against pneumococci of all types. Recognition of pneumococcus has decreased significantly since the abandonment of capsular typing by most clinical laboratories. The detection of pneumococcal capsular polysaccharides in sputum and in other body fluids by counterimmunoelectrophoresis provides an alternative to bacteriologic techniques for the presumptive diagnosis of pneumococcal infection. Because of cross reactions between the polysaccharides of pneumococci and of other bacterial species, immunologic diagnosis is somewhat less specific than bacteriologic diagnosis.

PATHOGENESIS

The mechanism by which pneumococci damage the mammalian host is obscure. It is conceivable that toxic substances may be elaborated, but no such toxin has been shown to play a major pathogenic role in pneumococcal infection. The capsular polysaccharides, though nontoxic, are known to be necessary factors in virulence and to protect the organism to a certain extent from engulfment by phagocytes.

Although "pneumococcal pharyngitis" is a doubtful entity, invasion of the tissue of the nasopharynx may occur in the infant and occasionally in the nonimmune adult and be followed by spread to the circulation via the cervical lymphatics. At times, secondary infection of serous cavities in the absence of demonstrable focal infection of the upper or lower respiratory tract may occur. The organisms multiply readily in vivo and may produce acute inflammation of the lungs, serous cavities, and endocardium.

The normal human respiratory tract is provided with a variety of mechanisms which act to guard the lungs from infection. The lower respiratory tract is protected by the glottis and larynx, and material passing these barriers stimulates the expulsive cough reflex. Removal of small particles impinging on the walls of the trachea and bronchi is facilitated by their mucociliary lining; and growth of bacteria reaching normal alveoli is inhibited by their relative dryness and by the phagocytic activity of alveolar macrophages. Any anatomic or physiologic derangement of these coordinated defenses tends to augment the susceptibility of the lungs to infection. Anesthesia, alcoholic intoxication, convulsions, and disturbed innervation of the larynx depress the cough reflex and may permit aspiration of infected material. Alterations in the tracheobronchial tree leading to anatomic changes in the epithelial lining or to localized obstruction increase the vulnerability of the lungs to infection. Pulmonary edema, local or generalized, resulting from viral infection, inhalation of irritant gases, cardiac failure, or contusion of the chest wall, provides a fluid menstruum in the alveoli for the growth of bacteria and their spread to adjacent areas of the lung. Viral infection of the respiratory epithelium with concomitant disruption of its component cells interferes significantly with the clearance of bacteria from the lungs, an observation in accord with the high incidence of pneumococcal pneumonia during epidemics of viral influenza and its frequent clinical association with sporadic viral respiratory infections.

Pneumonia begins usually in the right lower, right middle, or left lower lobe, those areas to which gravity is most likely to carry upper respiratory secretions aspirated during sleep. Bronchial embolization with infected mucinous secretions during the course of an upper respiratory infection appears to be the initiating factor in many cases of pneumococcal pneumonia. Protected initially from phagocytosis by mucinous material, the bacteria multiply and, in infected alveoli, evoke the outpouring of proteinaceous fluid, which serves both as a nutrient and as a vehicle for spread to adjacent alveoli. Soon thereafter, polymorphonuclear leukocytes migrate from the pulmonary capillaries to phagocytize a part of the pneumococcal population before the appearance of detectable antibody. Delay in the polymorphonuclear leukocytic response occurs during alcoholic intoxication and certain forms of anesthesia, permitting spread of infection. Adrenocortical steroids and their congeners may also interfere with leukocyte migration. Later, as the pneumonic lesion evolves, macrophages appear in the exudate and remove the debris of fibrin and cells. It is probable that antibody to the capsular polysaccharide of the invading pneumococcus makes its appearance locally in the lung before being detectable in the circulation. Such antibody increases the efficiency of phagocytosis approximately twofold and causes agglutination of the organisms and their adherence to alveolar walls, thereby slowing their dissemination in the lung. The outcome of infection depends, therefore, on the rate at which bacteria can multiply in the edema fluid and spread, and on the host's ability to immobilize and destroy them by phagocytosis. Individuals with hypogammaglobulinemia and patients with multiple myeloma incapable of producing anticapsular antibody are liable to recurrent attacks of pneumococcal pneumonia. Repeated infection with the same pneumococcal type should always prompt a search for dysgammaglobulinemia.

Failure of local defense mechanisms in the lung results in lymphatic spread of pneumococci to the hilar lymph nodes. In the sinusoids of these organs, a sequence of events not unlike that in the lung ensues. If infection is not checked in this secondary line of defense, organisms find their way into the thoracic duct and then into the circulation. Although transient bacteremia may occur at the onset of many cases of pneumococcal pneumonia, it is detectable in only 25 to 30 percent of cases. Bacteremia, which reflects the body's inability to localize the pulmonary infection, is a poor prognostic sign and carries with it the danger of metastatic infection. The mortality of treated or untreated bacteremic pneumococcal pneumonia is four times that resulting from comparably managed nonbacteremic infections. Metastatic infection secondary to bacteremia may occur in the meninges, joints, or peritoneum or on the endocardium. Direct spread from the infected lung may give rise to pleural empyema or to pericarditis.

Natural recovery from pneumococcal infection coincides usually, but not invariably, with the appearance of detectable type-specific antibody in the circulation and is often accompanied by a dramatic and abrupt fall in temperature, the so-called "crisis." Antibody aids recovery by increasing the efficiency of phagocytosis and by limiting dissemination of the organisms. Bacteriostatic drugs, such as sulfonamides, facilitate control of the infection by limiting the size of the pneumococcal population, but the host's defense mechanisms are still required for the elimination of the bacteria. Bactericidal agents, such as penicillin, cause the death of pneumococci in the lung and are effective when some of the host's defense mechanisms are compromised. With the arrest of infection, the alveolar exudate undergoes liquefaction, the inflammatory debris is removed by expectoration and via the lymphatic channels, and the lung is restored to its normal state. Necrosis of pulmonary tissue as a result of pneumococcal infection is distinctly uncommon. Primary pneumococcal lung abscess is a rare clinical entity, although the diagnosis is mistakenly made at times when pneumococcal infection complicates lung abscess of other origins.

In addition to causing pneumonia and its metastatic sequelae, pneumococcus can extend from the nasopharynx to its adjacent structures, giving rise to otitis media, mastoiditis, paranasal sinusitis, or conjunctivitis. Soft-tissue abscesses are rare but may occur.

PNEUMOCOCCAL PNEUMONIA

Pneumococcal pneumonia is a disease remarkable for its uniformity, in contrast to other infections such as typhoid fever and tuberculosis. The diseases produced by different pneumococcal serotypes show little variation in severity or in clinical manifestations. The prognosis in type 3 pneumococcal pneumonia is usually regarded as poor, probably because type 3 infections occur frequently in the aged and in patients with other debilitating diseases, such as diabetes and congestive heart failure. The usual lesion in adults is segmental or lobar in distribution, but in children and the aged, bronchopneumonia, characterized by patchy involvement, is frequent.

MANIFESTATIONS Pneumonia is often preceded for a few days by coryza or some other form of common respiratory disease. The onset is usually so abrupt that patients frequently can state the exact hour that illness began. There is a sudden *shaking chill* in more than 80 percent of the cases and a rapid rise in temperature, with corresponding tachycardia and an increase in respiratory rate (tachypnea). Most patients with pneumococcal pneumonia have a single rigor unless antipyretic drugs are administered, and repeated chills should suggest another etiologic agent.

About 75 percent of patients develop severe *pleuritic pain* and *cough,* productive of pinkish or "rusty" mucoid sputum within a few hours. The chest pain is agonizing, and respirations become rapid, shallow, and grunting as the patient tries to splint the affected side. Many patients are mildly cyanotic as a result of hypoxia caused by V/Q abnormality or shunt, which accompanies altered respiration, and show dilatation of the alae nasi when first seen. Patients appear acutely ill; but nausea, headache, and malaise are not prominent, and most individuals are alert. Pleuritic pain and dyspnea are the dominent complaints.

In the untreated disease, there are sustained fever of 102.5 to 105°F, continued pleuritic pain, cough, and expectoration; and *abdominal distention* is frequent. *Herpes labialis* is a common complication. After 7 to 10 days, there are diaphoresis, abrupt defervescence, and dramatic improvement in well-being, the "crisis."

In cases which terminate fatally, there is usually extensive pulmonary involvement, and dyspnea, cyanosis, and tachycardia are prominent. Circulatory collapse or a picture resembling heart failure is common. Death in a few patients is associated with empyema or some other suppurative complication such as meningitis or endocarditis.

Physical examination reveals restricted motion of the affected hemithorax. Tactile fremitus may be decreased during the initial day of illness but is usually increased when consolidation is fully established. Deviation of the trachea away from the affected lung suggests pleural effusion or empyema. The percussion note is dull, and if the lesion is in an upper lobe, impaired motion of the diaphragm can be detected on the affected side. Very early in the course of infection, breath sounds are diminished, but as the lesion evolves, they become tubular or bronchial in quality, and bronchophony and whispered pectoriloquy can be elicited. These findings are accompanied by fine crepitant rales.

EFFECT OF SPECIFIC CHEMOTHERAPY Pneumococcal pneumonia usually improves promptly when an appropriate antimicrobial drug is given. Within 12 to 36 h after initiation of treatment with penicillin, temperature, pulse, and respiration begin to fall and may reach normal values, pleuritic pain subsides, and the spread of the inflammatory process is halted. The temperature of approximately half the patients, however, requires 4 days or longer to become normal, and failure of the patient's temperature to reach normal in 24 to 48 h should not prompt a change in antibacterial therapy in the absence of other indications.

COMPLICATIONS The typical course of pneumococcal pneumonia can be modified by the development of one or more local or distant complications:

In the lung ATELECTASIS Atelectasis of all or part of a lobe may occur during the active stage of pneumonia or after treatment has been instituted. The patient may complain of sudden recurrence of pleuritic pain and show rapid respirations. Small areas of atelectasis are often detected by x-ray in the absence of symptoms. These areas usually clear with coughing and deep breathing, but bronchoscopic aspiration is occasionally necessary. If atelectasis is allowed to persist, the affected area becomes fibrotic and functionless.

DELAYED RESOLUTION Return to normal of physical findings in the lung after pneumococcal pneumonia is usually complete within 2 to 4 weeks. X-ray evidence of residual pulmonary consolidation, however, may persist as long as 8 weeks, and other radiologic manifestations of the infection (volume loss, stranding and pleural disease) may persist for up to 18 weeks. The process of resolution may require a longer time in those over 50 years of age and in those with chronic obstructive airway disease or alcoholism.

ABSCESS Lung abscess is a rare sequel to pneumococcal infection, although pneumococcal pneumonia is a not uncommon complication of lung abscess of other origins. It is manifested by continued fever and profuse expectoration of purulent sputum. X-ray shows one or more cavities. This complication is exceedingly rare in patients who receive penicillin therapy and is most likely to follow infection with pneumococcus type 3.

In adjacent structures PLEURAL EFFUSION Pleural effusion occurs in about 5 percent of patients with pneumococcal pneumonia, even with specific therapy. The amount of fluid is usually not sufficient to cause obvious displacement of mediastinal structures. Usually the effusion is sterile and is reabsorbed spontaneously within a week or two. Sometimes, however, the effusion is large and requires aspiration.

EMPYEMA Before the introduction of effective chemotherapy, empyema occurred in 5 to 8 percent of patients with pneumococcal pneumonia; it is now observed in less than 1 percent of treated cases. It is manifested by persistent fever or pleuritic pain, together with signs of pleural effusion. In the early stages, the gross appearance of infected fluid may not differ from that of a sterile pleural effusion; later, there is a profuse outpouring of polymorphonuclear leukocytes and fibrin, resulting in an exudate of thick greenish pus containing large clots of fibrin. The quantity of exudate may become large enough to displace mediastinal structures. In neglected cases, this process leads to extensive pleural scarring, with limitation of thoracic movement. Rupture and drainage through the chest wall (*empyema necessitatis*) occurs, but is rare. Metastatic *brain abscess* is an occasional complication of chronic empyema.

PERICARDITIS A particularly serious complication is spread of infection to the pericardial sac. This lesion is characterized by pain in the precordial region, a friction rub synchronous with the heartbeat, and distention of cervical veins, although one or all of these findings may be absent. The possibility of coexisting purulent pericarditis should be considered whenever a very ill patient with pneumonia develops empyema.

Metastatic infections *Arthritis* occurs more often in children than in adults. The affected joint is swollen, red, and painful, with a purulent effusion. It usually subsides promptly with systemic administration of penicillin, although aspiration and intraarticular injection of penicillin may be necessary in adults.

Acute bacterial endocarditis complicates pneumococcal pneumonia in fewer than 0.5 percent of cases. Its manifestations and treatment are discussed below. Meningitis, another complication of pneumococcal pneumonia, is also discussed subsequently.

Paralytic ileus Gaseous abdominal distention is commonly present and in severely ill patients may assume such serious proportions that the term *paralytic ileus* is justified. This complication further impairs respiratory movement by elevation of the diaphragm and constitutes a difficult problem in management. A rarer and more serious gastrointestinal complication is acute gastric dilatation.

Impaired liver function Alterations in hepatic function are common during the course of pneumococcal pneumonia, and mild jaundice is not at all rare. The pathogenesis of the jaundice is not entirely clear, although in some patients it appears to be related to glucose 6-phosphate dehydrogenase deficiency.

LABORATORY FINDINGS *Sputum* should be obtained by the physician in his or her presence before the administration of antimicrobial drugs to ensure its quality. Although resort to transtracheal aspiration or lung puncture may be necessary on occasion to establish the cause of pneumonia, routine use of these invasive techniques is not recommended because of their attendant, albeit infrequent, complications. When stained by

Gram's method, the sputum shows polymorphonuclear leukocytes and variable numbers of gram-positive cocci, singly and in pairs. These can be typed directly by the Neufeld quellung or capsular precipitin technique, and this procedure should be followed to facilitate diagnosis whenever possible. The *blood culture* is positive for pneumococci during the first days of untreated illness in 20 to 25 percent of cases. The white blood count usually shows a polymorphonuclear *leukocytosis* ranging from 12,000 to 25,000 cells per cubic millimeter. A normal white count or leukopenia is sometimes observed in patients with overwhelming infection and bacteremia. Occasionally, pneumococci may be seen directly in granulocytes of patients with bacteremia by examining the buffy coat after staining with Wright's stain. These patients often have asplenia. *X-ray of the chest* usually reveals a homogenous density in the affected area of the lung. In well-established cases, the density may occupy one or more entire lobes. Atypical patterns of consolidation may be seen in those with underlying chronic pulmonary disease.

EXTRAPULMONARY PNEUMOCOCCAL INFECTION

PNEUMOCOCCAL MENINGITIS The pneumococcus is second only to the meningococcus as a cause of purulent meningitis in adults; in children, meningitis caused by *Hemophilus influenzae* is also more frequent than pneumococcal infection.

Pneumococcal meningitis can develop as a "primary" disease without preceding signs of infection elsewhere; as a complication of pneumococcal pneumonia; by extension from otitis, mastoiditis, or sinusitis; or following a skull fracture which creates an opening between the subarachnoid space and the nasal cavity or paranasal sinuses. Patients with pneumococcal endocarditis frequently develop meningeal infection. Patients with multiple myeloma and with sickle-cell disease seem to be liable to pneumococcal infection of the meninges, just as they are to pneumonia.

The *manifestations* are of those of any acute pyogenic meningitis (Chap. 368) and include chills, fever, headache, nuchal rigidity, Kernig's and Brudzinski's signs, delirium, and cranial nerve palsies. Evidence of otitis, sinusitis, or pneumonia should be carefully sought by physical and roentgenographic examination in all patients.

The *spinal fluid* is under increased pressure, appears cloudy, often with a greenish tint, and shows a high protein and low glucose content. Stained smears usually reveal gram-positive diplococci and polymorphonuclear leukocytes; in some patients, the number of cells in the spinal fluid is surprisingly small, and much of the cloudiness is produced by the bacterial content. The diagnosis can be established rapidly by identification of pneumococci in the spinal fluid by Gram's stain and by direct typing with the Neufeld quellung reaction.

With appropriate chemotherapy, recovery can be expected in 70 percent of cases; the prognosis is better in children than in infants or in adults. Relapse may occur but is unusual if adequate treatment is carried out. Subarachnoid block, the result of accumulation of large amounts of thick exudate in the meningeal space and at the base of the brain, is now an unusual complication.

PNEUMOCOCCAL ENDOCARDITIS Endocarditis is usually a complication of pneumonia or meningitis. The clinical picture is that of acute bacterial endocarditis (Chap. 243), with remittent fever, splenomegaly, and metastatic infection of the lungs, meninges, joints, eye, and other tissues. Petechiae are uncommon. The infection can attack normal valves and is particularly likely to occur in the aortic valve. The valvular infection is destructive, and loud murmurs and heart failure develop rapidly. Rupture or perforation of cusps or even rupture of the aorta may occur. The blood culture is consistently positive for the pneumococcus in the absence of treatment with antimicrobial drugs; yet at the same time antibodies to the infecting organism may be demonstrable in the blood, a combination of findings seldom observed except in endocarditis or brucellosis. Although the infection is relatively easy to cure with penicillin, damage to valve leaflets, especially to the cusps of the aortic valve, may be followed by rapidly progressive heart failure. Surgical repair or replacement of damaged valvular structures should be carried out early, before heart failure becomes intractable.

PNEUMOCOCCAL PERITONITIS Pneumococcal peritonitis is a rare disease and is probably the sequela to transient pneumococcal bacteremia, although, because of its somewhat greater frequency in young girls, it has been hypothesized that the organism may gain entry to the peritoneum via the vagina and fallopian tubes. Peritonitis was formerly a common complication of the nephrotic syndrome, particularly in children, but it occurs now with a frequency of approximately 2 percent. In adults, the disease is seen in association with cirrhosis or with carcinoma of the liver. The diagnosis is made by examination of the ascitic fluid; blood cultures are often positive, and a polymorphonuclear leukocytosis is the rule.

TREATMENT

SPECIFIC ANTIMICROBIAL THERAPY Although resistance of pneumococci to antimicrobial drugs has not been regarded as a significant problem in the past, some strains have been found to be resistant to one or the other of the following agents: penicillins, cephalosporins, tetracyclines, chloramphenicol, erythromycin, clindamycin, cotrimoxazole, and aminoglycosides. For this reason sensitivity of the infecting organism to the infecting drug should be determined, particularly in extrapulmonary infection. In the absence of resistance or of hypersensitivity to it, penicillin G (benzyl penicillin) is the drug of choice for all manifestations of pneumococcal infection. Strains of pneumococcus manifesting a modest increase in resistance to penicillin have been recovered infrequently from humans; and although the level of such resistance does not preclude treatment with this antibiotic, awareness of the phenomenon is necessary. The minimum curative dose for *pneumonia* caused by strains of usual sensitivity to penicillin G is less than 60,000 units daily, and a total dose of 600,000 units daily provides a good margin of safety for bacteremic and nonbacteremic pulmonary infection in adults in the absence of an extrapulmonary focus. Treatment may be administered at 12-h intervals in doses of 300,000 units aqueous crystalline penicillin G or procaine penicillin. Therapy should be continued until the patient has been afebrile for 48 to 72 h. The response is usually dramatic, and relapse is extremely uncommon. Pneumococcal pneumonia can be treated adequately with oral penicillin, preferably one of the drugs resistant to gastric acid (Chap. 111), in dosage of 1.2 to 2.4 million units daily. *Peritonitis* usually responds within 36 to 48 h to 2 to 4 million units of penicillin daily.

Pneumococcal *meningitis* should be treated with 12 to 20 million units aqueous penicillin G daily intravenously in adults. In many clinics, even larger amounts are used, though care must be taken to avoid neurotoxicity from excessive dosage. Intrathecal administration of penicillin is not necessary. The addition of sulfadiazine to this regimen affords no advantage, and supplementary administration of chlortetracycline (and presumably, of other broad-spectrum drugs) may exert a deleterious effect. In the presence of sinusitis, otitis, or mastoiditis, surgical drainage should be carried out as soon as is feasible. The response of meningitis is usually less dramatic than that of pneumonia; patients often remain febrile and disoriented, and signs of meningeal irritation may persist for several days, but improvement becomes gradually evident with continued treatment.

Large doses are required in pneumococcal endocarditis also—12 to 20 million units daily by intravenous infusion. Rapidly developing heart failure in these patients and the tendency to form myocardial abscess, however, often lead to a fatal outcome despite large doses of antibiotics. Surgical repair or replacement of damaged heart valves should be considered when cardiac failure develops.

Cephalosporins in parenteral doses of 1 to 2 g daily are effective in pneumococcal pneumonia but must be administered with caution to those hypersensitive to penicillin. These drugs should *not* be used to treat pneumococcal meningitis because of their poor ability to penetrate the blood–cerebrospinal fluid barrier. The *tetracyclines* in doses 1 to 2 g daily, *erythromycin* in doses of 1.6 g daily, or *clindamycin* in doses of 1.2 g daily are effective treatment for pneumococcal pneumonia if it is caused by a sensitive strain, but they are recommended only for patients who have had untoward reactions to penicillins or cephalosporins. Despite its efficacy, *chloramphenicol* should not be used to treat pneumococcal infections other than meningitis in patients hypersensitive to penicillin who are infected with a drug-sensitive strain. For patients with illness caused by multiple drug-resistant pneumococci, *vancomycin* in doses of 2 g daily is the drug of choice. Sulfonamides have little place in the present-day treatment of pneumococcal pneumonia and are useless in endocarditis and meningitis. Aminoglycosides, such as gentamicin, tobramycin, and amikacin, should not be employed to treat pneumococcal infection.

Pneumococcal arthritis responds to systemic penicillin, but aspiration and intraarticular instillation of the drug may be necessary.

Empyema should be detected and treated as early as possible. When an effusion is found, the fluid should be examined for organisms; and if they are present, 50,000 to 200,000 units of penicillin G should be injected intrapleurally. In addition the same antibiotic should be administered systemically in doses of 6 to 8 million units a day. Aspiration of fluid and instillation of penicillin should be carried out at 1- to 2-day intervals until cultures are persistently negative and fever disappears. Fluoroscopic guidance may be needed for aspiration of small empyema pockets. If the exudate is especially thick or viscid, streptokinase-streptodornase (Varidase) may facilitate its withdrawal. When definite improvement is not evident in 4 to 6 days or when the empyema is of long duration, a large-lumen intercostal tube should be placed in the pleural cavity to facilitate drainage. Failure to effect prompt cure of empyema may be followed by pleural fibrosis and necessitate subsequent surgical decortication of the lung to restore pulmonary function.

OTHER MEASURES Oxygen administered through a face mask should be used to treat significant cyanosis, cardiac failure, and delirium. Codeine, 32 to 64 mg every 4 h, will usually control pleuritic pain. When pain is severe, it may require intercostal nerve block with 1 to 2 percent procaine for relief.

PROGNOSIS AND PREVENTION

Although the mortality from pneumococcal pneumonia has diminished significantly since the advent of antimicrobial drugs, available evidence indicates that the incidence of the disease has changed little, if at all. The fatality rate in patients over the age of 12 years with bacteremic pneumococcal pneumonia treated with an antibiotic is 18 percent, and in patients over the age of 50 and in those with underlying systemic illness, it is significantly higher.

Signs of poor prognosis in pneumonia include leukopenia, bacteremia, multilobar involvement, any extrapulmonary focus of pneumococcal infection, presence of preexisting systemic disease, circulatory collapse, and occurrence of the infection in the first year of life or after the age of 55. Infection with pneumococcus type 3 has a higher mortality rate than that caused by other pneumococcal types. Death is most likely to occur in individuals sustaining irreversible physiologic damage early in the course which is unaltered by antimicrobial therapy. Until the nature of the injury produced by pneumococcus is understood and ways devised to repair it, vaccination will remain the only means of protecting those at high risk of a fatal outcome.

A tetradecavalent vaccine containing the capsular polysaccharides of pneumococcal types 1, 2, 3, 4, 6, 8, 9, 12, 14, 19, 23, 25, 51, and 56, which are responsible for 80 percent of bacteremic infections in the United States, is available for prevention of pneumococcal infection caused by these types in individuals at high risk of a fatal outcome. Those at higher than average risk are individuals over the age of 55 and patients with a variety of chronic systemic illnesses including heart disease, chronic bronchopulmonary disease, hepatic disease, renal insufficiency, diabetes, and a variety of malignancies. Persons with sicklaemia of all ages have an increased risk of developing pneumococcal infection, and the vaccine is recommended for those with this disorder over the age of 2 years. Since anatomic or functional asplenia is associated with fulminant overwhelming pneumococcal septicemia with disseminated intravascular coagulation, giving rise to a clinical picture resembling the Waterhouse-Friderichsen syndrome, such individuals should also be immunized. It should be recognized, however, that the vaccine contains a limited number of pneumococcal antigens, and that infection caused by other pneumococcal types may occur occasionally in the immunized subject. Reactions to the vaccine are usually absent or mild, although in the occasional individual they may resemble those following immunization with typhoid vaccine: local pain, erythema, and elevation of temperature. The most severe local and systemic reactions to the vaccine appear to be associated with preexisting high levels of antibody to one or more of the antigens in the vaccine. Because of the persistence of pneumococcal antibodies after a single injection of vaccine, reimmunization in less than 3 years after the initial injection is not recommended. The vaccine is 80 to 90 percent effective in adults. The efficacy of the vaccine in infants and in children under 2 years is currently under investigation, and its efficacy in preventing pneumococcal otitis media, pneumonia, and meningitis in individuals in this age group remains to be determined. Further data are needed to assess the efficacy of pneumococcal vaccine in immunosuppressed individuals.

REFERENCES

AMMANN AJ et al: Polyvalent pneumococcal-polysaccharide immunization of patients with sickle-cell anemia and patients with splenectomy. N Engl J Med 297:897, 1977

APPELBAUM PC et al: Multiple-antibiotic resistance of pneumococci South Africa. Morb Mort Week Rep 26:285, 1977

AUSTRIAN R: Pneumococcal endocarditis, meningitis and rupture of the aortic valve. Arch Intern Med 99:539, 1957

————, Gold J: Pneumococcal bacteremia with especial reference to bacteremic pneumococcal pneumonia. Ann Intern Med 60:759, 1964

———— et al: Prevention of pneumococcal pneumonia by vaccination. Trans Assoc Am Phys 89:184, 1976

Gopal V, Bisno AL: Fulminant pneumococcal infections in "normal" asplenic hosts. Arch Intern Med 137:1526, 1977

Heffron R: *Pneumonia with Special Reference to Pneumococcus Lobar Pneumonia.* New York, Commonwealth Fund, 1939

Kauffman CA et al: Purulent pneumococcic pericarditis: Continuing problem in antibiotic era. Am J Med 54:743, 1973

Leach RP, Coonrod JD: Detection of pneumococcal antigens in sputum in pneumococcal pneumonia. Am Rev Respir Dis 116:847, 1977

Lepper MH, Dowling HF: Treatment of pneumococcal meningitis with penicillin compared with penicillin plus aureomycin. Arch Intern Med 88:489, 1951

Merrill CW et al: Rapid identification of pneumococci: Gram stain vs. quellung reaction. N Engl J Med 288:510, 1973

Shulman JA et al: Errors and hazards in the diagnosis and treatment of bacterial pneumonias. Ann Intern Med 62:41, 1965

Stephen JJ et al: The radiographic resolution of *Streptococcus pneumoniae* pneumonia. N Engl J Med 293:798, 1975

Tugwell P, Williams AO: Jaundice associated with lobar pneumonia. Q J Med 46:97, 1977

Wood WB Jr: Studies on the cellular immunology of acute bacterial infections. Harvey Lect 42:72, 1951–1952

Zinneman HW, Hall WH: Recurrent pneumonia in multiple myeloma. Ann Intern Med 41:1152, 1954

116
STAPHYLOCOCCAL INFECTIONS

MARVIN TURCK
WALTER STAMM

INTRODUCTION Staphylococci most commonly produce relatively harmless superficial suppurative infections in human beings. They also produce serious infections of the lungs, pleural space, endocardium, myocardium, long bones, kidneys, and surgical wounds.

The majority of life-threatening staphylococcal infections arise within hospitals, and are among the "diseases of medical progress." Staphylococcal cross infection in hospitals may be less frequent now than it was 10 to 15 years ago, and gram-negative rods are now the most common nosocomial pathogens; nevertheless staphylococci still account for 20 percent of all hospital-acquired infections.

ETIOLOGY Staphylococci are members of the genus *Micrococcus*, which includes many morphologically similar saprophytic microorganisms that do not cause human infection. The parasitic micrococci of primary concern in medicine are grouped in the species *M. pyogenes*. Through established usage these pathogenic micrococci are termed *staphylococci*.

Staphylococci are spherical gram-positive cells. On solid agar media, staphylococcal colonies develop characteristic pigmentation: *M. pyogenes* var. *aureus* (*Staphylococcus aureus*), golden yellow; *M. pyogenes* var. *albus* (*S. albus*), ivory white; and *M. citreus*, lemon yellow. Most human infections are caused by *S. aureus,* and a few are caused by *S. albus* (*S. epidermidis*). The name *staphylococcus* derives from the characteristic grape-like clusters of organisms seen in stained smears prepared from colonies on solid media. In stained smears obtained from pus, smaller clusters, diploids, and short chains

resembling streptococci are seen. In such preparations, staphylococci characteristically retain their uniform round shape, in contrast to the boat-like forms assumed by pneumococci. Staphylococci may be seen within the cytoplasm of polymorphonuclear cells in pus, a rare finding in other gram-positive coccal infections. They can be readily differentiated from streptococci by their positive catalase reaction.

Staphylococci that are coagulase-positive and that ferment mannitol are classified as *S. aureus*. Most laboratories label all coagulase-negative strains as *S. epidermidis,* although other micrococci share this characteristic. Other methods to differentiate *S. aureus* from *S. epidermidis* (pigment production, pattern of hemolysis, and antibiotic susceptibility) are unreliable. In general, *S. aureus* strains possess a broader complement of biochemical activity (production of coagulase, hemolysins, and several toxins) than *S. epidermidis*.

Different strains of *S. aureus* can be recognized by the patterns of lysis produced by staphylococcal bacteriophages. Although it is cumbersome, phage typing has allowed more precise strain characterization and is commonly used in studies of intrahospital disease and epidemics of staphylococcal infection. It provides no information that is useful clinically in treating an individual patient. Methods for subtyping *S. epidermidis* (phage lysis and biotyping) have also been developed.

PATHOGENESIS Little is known of the events which allow staphylococci to invade host tissues. Though strains of staphylococci are common skin and mucous membrane inhabitants, an enormous number of bacteria must be used to establish experimental infections in animals or humans, and more than a million organisms are necessary to produce serious infection in most laboratory animals. The inoculum required to produce infection is greatly reduced in the presence of a foreign body. More than 50 percent of serious staphylococcal infections of deep tissues arise from cutaneous foci, and a smaller number originate in the respiratory or genitourinary tract. Direct inoculation of staphylococci into the bloodstream is also an important route of infection in hospitalized patients with intravenous catheters and in drug addicts. The integument and mucous membranes of heroin addicts and insulin-using diabetics appear to have a unique susceptibility to colonization by *S. aureus*.

Staphylococcal disease is more common in patients with *diabetes, liver disease, renal failure,* and severe *debilitation* and/or *malnutrition*. When skin continuity is broken through *abrasions, wounds, insect bites, burns, exfoliative dermatitis,* or *chronic skin diseases,* the areas affected are commonly infected with staphylococci. *Influenza, measles,* and *mucoviscidosis* appear to predispose to primary staphylococcal invasion of the lung. Patients receiving *broad-spectrum antimicrobial therapy* also appear to have a higher incidence of staphylococcal disease.

Staphylococci often invade the integument via hair follicles and sebaceous glands. When skin continuity has been breached, local microbial multiplication is accompanied by inflammation and tissue necrosis at the site of infection. Polymorphonuclear leukocytes rapidly enter the area and ingest large numbers of staphylococci. Thrombosis of surrounding capillaries occurs; fibrin is deposited about the periphery; and, later, fibroblasts create a relatively avascular wall about the area. The fully developed staphylococcal lesion consists of a central core of dead and dying leukocytes and bacteria which gradually liquefies to form characteristic thick, creamy pus, surrounded by a fibroblastic wall.

When host mechanisms fail to contain the cutaneous or subcutaneous infection, staphylococci may enter the bloodstream. Common sites of metastatic seeding are the diaphyseal ends of long bones in children, lungs, kidneys, endocardium, myocardium, liver, spleen, and brain.

Certain biologic properties of staphylococci appear to contribute to pathogenicity. Many *S. aureus* strains elaborate an *exotoxin* (alpha toxin) capable of causing dermal necrosis in animals. Fever, tachycardia, cyanosis, shock, and death ensue when exotoxin is administered to experimental animals, a picture similar to that seen occasionally in certain fulminating cases of staphylococcal bacteremia in human beings. A delta toxin also has been incriminated in the pathogenesis of severe staphylococcal infection. However, the exact role played by both of these toxins remains uncertain. About 40 percent of *S. aureus* lysed by phages in group II produce an exotoxin that causes intraepidermal cleavage and bulla formation.

The high correlation between *coagulase* production and virulence suggests that this substance is important in the pathogenesis of staphylococcal infections. Coagulase has been said to protect staphylococci from phagocytosis by polymorphonuclear leukocytes, to promote abscess formation in humans and in animal species which have coagulable plasmas, or to protect staphylococci from bacteriostatic substances present in normal serum. However, the precise role of coagulase as a determinant of pathogenicity has not been established.

Some *S. aureus* strains produce a *leukocidin* which destroys human and rabbit leukocytes in vitro. Some strains elaborate *hyaluronidase*. Many staphylococci produce an *enterotoxin* which produces nausea, vomiting, and diarrhea in certain experimental animals and in humans.

In vitro and in vivo studies have indicated that pathogenic staphylococci can survive within human leukocytes, whereas nonpathogenic strains do not. Such intracellular survival may be a means of transporting staphylococci and spreading them to distant tissues. This intracellular survival may also account for the relative refractoriness of staphylococcal infection to antibiotic treatment.

Staphylococcus epidermidis strains appear particularly likely to cause infections in the presence of certain foreign bodies: prosthetic heart valves, CSF shunts, and orthopedic prostheses. The unique ability of some *S. epidermidis* strains to adhere to these foreign surfaces seems to at least partly explain this propensity.

IMMUNITY Some degree of resistance to staphylococcal infections develops with age. For example, primary staphylococcal pneumonia is common in infants but rare in adults. Acute staphylococcal osteomyelitis is almost exclusively a disease of children. Both superficial staphylococcal pyoderma and staphylococcal bacteremia are more frequent in infants, while actual abscess formation occurs more often in adults.

Intact polymorphonuclear leukocytes capable of normal chemotaxis, ingestion, and killing appear to be the major protective mechanism against staphylococcal infections. Persons with inherited or acquired defects in any of these leukocyte functions are particularly susceptible to staphylococcal infections (Chap. 56). Coagulase-positive staphylococci have a characteristic cell wall teichoic acid, which may be antiphagocytic. Certain unusual strains possess a definite mucopolysaccharide capsular structure which impedes phagocytosis, and specific opsonizing antibody is required for the ingestion of these unusual strains. A number of antistaphylococcal antibodies have been shown to pass from mother to fetus, and the incidence of a variety of antibodies rapidly rises with age. Virtually 100 percent of adults possess antibodies to several staphylococcal antigens in their serum. Nevertheless, the role of humoral immunity in modifying or protecting against staphylococcal infection is uncertain. Immunization of animals with alpha toxin, toxoids, coagulase, or whole staphylococci may prolong experimental staphylococcal infection, but does not protect against eventual death. There has been no satisfactory demonstration that human staphylococcal disease is followed by immunity or that infection can be modified significantly by vaccination.

EPIDEMIOLOGY *Staphylococcus aureus* transiently colonizes the nasopharynx of 70 to 90 percent of individuals, and resides relatively permanently in the anterior nares of 20 to 30 percent. Nasal carriage often leads to skin colonization as well. Hospital patients and personnel have significantly higher staphylococcal carrier rates than the general population.

While staphylococci remain viable for long periods in dust, blankets, or clothing, and viable staphylococci are often demonstrable in the environment by air-sampling techniques, the significance of airborne transmission remains uncertain, and the best evidence suggests that direct person-to-person contact is the most important means of transmission of staphylococci. Most often, staphylococci are carried from patient to patient on the hands of hospital workers who neglect handwashing. Patients or hospital employees with active staphylococcal infections are probably a more serious source of cross infection than the simple carrier state. However, in some circumstances asymptomatic nasal carriers have been the source of staphylococcal infections. The factors which cause some staphylococcal carriers to become dangerous disseminators remain poorly understood. Discontinuation of the use of hexachlorophene in hospital nurseries has been associated with an increase in infection in some hospitals, and it is apparent that continued surveillance is necessary to thwart the development of epidemics of staphylococcal infection.

Certain phage types of staphylococci have been associated with intrahospital infections. Some strains, particularly antibiotic-resistant strains in phage group III, appear to have greater "epidemic virulence" than other staphylococci. In specific hospitals, one phage type often emerges and may cause most of the serious intrahospital infections. Such "epidemic strains" have shifted from time to time and vary from hospital to hospital. In other hospitals, multiple phage types cause infection. The high incidence of active staphylococcal disease in carriers of certain strains (e.g., the 80/81 strains) suggests that some staphylococci may possess higher virulence for humans than others. Some of the decrease in the frequency of staphylococcal infection in hospitals has been attributed to the disappearance of 80/81 strains.

ANTIMICROBIAL RESISTANCE In the past, the introduction of new antibiotics active against staphylococci has generally been followed by the appearance of staphylococci specifically resistant to that agent. When penicillin was first introduced, fewer than 10 percent of staphylococcal strains isolated from patients or carriers were resistant. Now 60 to 90 percent of staphylococci isolated from hospitalized patients throughout the Western world are resistant to penicillin G, and the incidence of infection due to penicillinase-producing strains in nonhospitalized individuals is almost as high. The prevalence of resistance to a specific antimicrobial has correlated closely with the frequency of its administration, and the emergence of resistant strains has followed the use of most antibiotics. Vancomycin, first employed in 1958, and the penicillinase-resistant penicillins and the cephalosporins, both introduced in the 1960s, have been exceptions to this rule. In general, these agents have retained a high degree of activity against both penicillin-sensitive and penicillin-resistant staphylococci. However, methicillin-resistant strains have become increasingly common in England and France, and in this country, epidemics of methicillin-resistant staphylococci have occurred in several hospitals and burn treatment centers. Gentamicin-resistant staphylococci have also been isolated with greater frequency in recent years.

Most observations on the prevalence of antimicrobial-resistant strains have been made within hospitals where antimicrobial use is heaviest. It has been shown that drug-susceptible strains carried by patients may be replaced by drug-resistant phage group III staphylococci present in the hospital environment during antimicrobial treatment. These strains are in turn acquired by hospital personnel who serve as reservoirs of potentially pathogenic, antimicrobial-resistant strains. Staphylococci isolated from population groups outside the hospital have shown a slower increase in the percentage of antimicrobial-resistant strains, but in some communities the incidence of extrahospital infections caused by penicillin-resistant strains is similar to that found in hospitalized patients.

MANIFESTATIONS Superficial infections Simple infection of hair follicles manifested by a minute erythematous nodule without involvement of the surrounding skin or deeper tissues is termed *folliculitis*. A more extensive and invasive follicular or sebaceous gland infection with some involvement of subcutaneous tissues is termed a *furuncle,* or *boil.* Itching and mild pain are followed by progressive local swelling and erythema, and the overlying skin becomes exquisitely painful on pressure or motion. Relief of pain occurs promptly after spontaneous or surgical drainage.

Furuncles occur most commonly on the face, neck, axillas, forearms, buttocks, thighs, breast, upper back, and labia. The acne of adolescence is frequently complicated by secondary furunculosis. Staphylococcal infection may involve the sweat glands in the axillas *(hidradenitis suppurativa).* These infections may be deep-seated, slow to localize and drain, and are liable to recurrence and scarring.

Staphylococcal infections within the thick, fibrous, inelastic skin of the back of the neck and upper part of the back lead to formation of a *carbuncle.* The relative thickness and impermeability of the overlying skin lead to lateral extension and loculation, and a large, indurated, painful lesion with multiple ineffective drainage sites results. These extensive lesions appear more frequently among diabetics. Carbuncles produce fever, leukocytosis, extreme pain, and prostration. Bacteremia is common.

Staphylococci frequently colonize impetiginous lesions, but most impetigo in children and adults is due to group A streptococci. However, staphylococcal impetigo does occur, and while it cannot be clearly differentiated from streptococcal impetigo clinically, it tends to produce more localized disease, has a grayish rather than golden yellow crust, and less often produces high fever and lymphadenitis.

One form of impetigo characteristically caused by *S. aureus* is bullous impetigo. This disease represents one of several exfoliative staphylococcal pyodermas. *Staphylococcus aureus* strains lysed by group II phages, usually type 71, cause this group of diseases through production of an exotoxin (exfoliatin), which produces separation of the epidermis at the granular cell layer. Production of this exotoxin is plasmid-mediated.

Several clinical syndromes have been associated with exfoliative toxin-producing strains. Local pyoderma may be followed by a tender, scarlatiniform, finely desquamative rash that can be localized or generalized (staphylococcal scarlet fever). Bullous impetigo is the more severe form of this disease. Characteristically, local pyoderma precedes the sudden onset of generalized erythema, fever, and leukocytosis. Several days later large flaccid bullae form and then burst, resulting in red, denuded skin resembling a burn. The syndrom may be localized or rarely generalized (toxic epidermal necrolysis, Ritter's syndrome, Lyell's disease, or scalded skin syndrome). In the localized form, staphylococci can usually be recovered from the bullous lesions, while in the generalized form they usually cannot be.

Osteomyelitis Staphylococci are responsible for the majority of cases of *acute osteomyelitis.* This infection occurs most commonly in children under the age of 12, but adults also are susceptible to acute osteomyelitis, especially of the spine. There appears to have been a sharp decrease in the incidence of acute osteomyelitis since the introduction of antibiotics. Approximately 50 percent of patients give a history of a furuncle or superficial staphylococcal infection preceding osteomyelitis. Bone involvement follows hematogenous dissemination of bacteria. The frequent localization in the diaphyseal end of long bones is thought to be due to the endarterial circulation of the diaphysis. Many patients give a history of preceding trauma to the involved area. Recently cases of clavicular osteomyelitis secondary to infected subclavian catheters have been reported.

Once established, infection spreads through the newly formed juxtaepiphyseal bone to the periosteum or along the marrow cavity. If the infection reaches the subperiosteal space, the periosteum is lifted, a subperiosteal abscess forms, and rupture with infection of the subcutaneous tissues may occur. Rarely, the joint capsule is penetrated, producing a pyogenic arthritis. There is death of bone, producing a *sequestrum,* followed by new bone formation, the *involucrum.*

Occasionally indolent staphylococcal infections of bone remain localized within dense granulation tissue about a central necrotic cavity. Such a local infection may persist for years as a so-called "Brodie's abscess."

Osteomyelitis in children usually begins abruptly with chills, high fever, nausea, vomiting, and progressive pain at the site of bony involvement. Muscle spasm about the affected bone is a common early sign of osteomyelitis, and the child may refuse to move the affected limb. Leukocytosis is the rule. Blood cultures are positive for staphylococci in 50 to 60 percent of cases early in the disease. The tissues overlying the involved bone become edematous and warm, and the skin become erythematous and shiny. Anemia develops during the course of untreated disease. Roentgenograms are usually normal during the first week, but radionucleide scans may be abnormal. Bony rarefaction, local periosteal elevation, and new bone formation can frequently be seen during the second week.

Staphylococcal spinal infection in the adult differs considerably from acute osteomyelitis in the child. The onset is less abrupt, and there is a greater tendency for bony fusion with obliteration of the disk space (Chap. 360).

DIAGNOSIS Osteomyelitis should be suspected in any child with fever, limb pain, and leukocytosis. Similarly, neck or back pain in an adult, when accompanied by fever, should raise the possibility of acute osteomyelitis or a disk space infection. History of a preceding cutaneous infection, local tenderness over the bone, and the finding of *S. aureus* in blood cultures are confirmatory. In early stages, osteomyelitis must be differentiated from acute rheumatic fever and pyogenic arthritis.

PROGNOSIS Before the advent of antimicrobials, the overall mortality was approximately 25 percent. Death was more common in individuals with demonstrable bacteremia. Chronic osteomyelitis with recurrent activation and metastatic foci in other bones was common. However, acute staphylococcal osteomyelitis is declining in incidence, death is rare, and chronic osteomyelitis is also becoming less frequent.

Staphylococcal pneumonia Staphylococci are the cause of approximately 1 percent of bacterial pneumonias acquired outside hospitals. This disease occurs sporadically except during epidemics of influenza, when staphylococcal pneumonia is more common, although even then it is not as frequent as pneumococcal infection.

Primary staphylococcal pneumonia in infants and young children frequently causes pyopneumothorax, and pneumatoceles occur early and should suggest *S. aureus* infection. In older children and healthy adults staphylococcal pneumonia is generally preceded by an influenza-like respiratory infection (influenza, measles, or other viruses). Onset of staphylococcal involvement is abrupt, with chills, high fever, progressive dyspnea, cyanosis, cough, and pleural pain. Early peripheral vascular collapse is common, and examination frequently reveals a patient who seems sicker than his physical findings would suggest. Sputum in the early phases is not characteristic, but may be bloody or frankly purulent. Admixture with blood may produce a thick, creamy pink sputum.

Staphylococci are one of the causes of pneumonia occurring in hospitalized patients. These infections usually begin insidiously. Increasing fever, tachycardia, and an elevated respiratory rate may be the only indications of infection. Typical pneumonic symptoms may be absent. The disease is also less abrupt when pulmonary involvement occurs during the course of staphylococcal bacteremia, as may be the case in drug addicts or in patients with endocarditis. Staphylococci generally produce patchy, centrally located areas of pneumonia. Pleural involvement and empyema are common. Many of these patients developing nosocomial staphylococcal pneumonia have chronic lung disease, leukemia, mucoviscidosis, or other debilitating diseases.

Because of the central pulmonary involvement, chest findings are variable. Signs of frank consolidation are rare. Scattered fine to coarse rales and rhonchi may be heard over the involved areas. Empyema produces typical signs of pleural fluid. Signs of abscess may appear late in the course of the disease. Bacteremia is not common in primary staphylococcal pneumonia (less than 20 percent of patients), and *its presence should suggest that the pneumonic involvement is metastatic and secondary to foci of infection elsewhere.*

The course of staphylococcal pneumonia may be stormy despite adequate antimicrobial therapy. Gradual defervescence starting 48 to 72 h after the initiation of therapy is the rule. Pulmonary abscesses or empyema cavities may require surgical treatment.

DIAGNOSIS   Staphylococcal pneumonia must be differentiated from other pneumonias. The preceding influenza-like illness, rapid onset of pleural pain, cyanosis, and prostration out of proportion to physical findings should suggest primary staphylococcal pneumonia. The finding of masses of polymorphonuclear leukocytes and gram-positive intraleukocytic cocci strongly suggests the diagnosis. The blood leukocyte count is generally above 15,000 per cubic millimeter. When pneumonia develops suddenly or insidiously, with higher fever, tachycardia, and leukocytosis, in debilitated hospitalized patients receiving antimicrobials staphylococci should be strongly considered as the etiologic agent.

PROGNOSIS   Before 1942, mortality ranged from 50 to 95 percent. The presence of bacteremia was almost invariably associated with a fatal outcome. The prognosis has improved with the use of antimicrobials, but some patients continue to die with staphylococcal pneumonia, especially debilitated individuals acquiring staphylococcal pneumonia in the hospital. Abscess formation and pleural involvement often prolong convalescence.

Staphylococcal bacteremia   Staphylococcal bacteremia may arise from any local staphylococcal infection. Infections of the skin (including infections about inlying venous cutdowns or catheters), respiratory tract, bones, or genitourinary tract precede bacteremia. Trauma to local lesions, such as pinching, or surgical drainage before adequate localization may precipitate bacteremia.

Rarely, patients with bacteremia die in 12 to 24 h, with high fever, tachycardia, cyanosis, gastrointestinal symptoms, and vascular collapse. Commonly, the disease progresses more slowly, with hectic fever and metastatic abscess formation in the skin, bones, kidneys, brain, lungs, myocardium, spleen, or other tissues. *Meningitis* is an occasional complication.

Endocarditis (Chap. 243) may occur in patients with protracted bacteremia. Normal heart valves are frequently involved, the aortic being the most frequent. Typically, staphylococcal endocarditis runs an acute course with high fever, progressive anemia, and metastatic abscesses in the skin and deeper structures. Rupture of the valve leaflets and valve ring abscesses are common. Specific diagnosis of endocardial involvement is difficult; because of its frequency, it should be assumed to be present in patients with staphylococcal bacteremia with demonstrable cutaneous lesions (petechiae or cutaneous pustules) and a significant heart murmur. Echocardiography may facilitate diagnosis if valvular vegetations can be demonstrated. At times, especially among addicts with right-sided valvular lesions, a significant heart murmur may not be demonstrable. In these patients, septic pulmonary emboli often produce chest pain, hemoptysis, and multiple small pulmonary infiltrates. Both coagulase-positive and coagulase-negative staphylococci have been a major cause of endocarditis in patients undergoing cardiac surgical procedures, particularly valve replacement, and both coagulase-positive and coagulase-negative staphylococci occasionally produce a subacute endocarditis indistinguishable from that produced by *Streptococcus viridans*. Persistent *Staphylococcus epidermidis* bacteremia has also been common after ventriculoatriostomy.

Staphylococcal bacteremia is generally accompanied by a polymorphonuclear leukocytosis of 12,000 to 20,000 but a normal leukocyte count or leukopenia is occasionally seen. Diagnosis of bacteremia can be facilitated by doing a Gram's stain of the buffy coat, which may show staphylococci within the cytoplasm of polymorphonuclear cells. Anemia develops rapidly during the course of the illness. Cyanosis and hypoxemia may be seen with staphylococcal bacteremia, even in the absence of significant pulmonary lesions on chest roentgenogram. Demonstration of antibodies to the staphylococcal cell wall component teichoic acid by counterimmunoelectrophoresis has been useful in the diagnosis of culture-negative endocarditis.

PROGNOSIS   Staphylococcal bacteremia is an extremely serious disease. Before the development of antimicrobials, over 80 percent of individuals died, the majority within 10 days of the onset of illness. The development of endocarditis or meningitis during bacteremia was almost invariably fatal. The sulfonamides produced little alteration in this mortality rate. With the administration of effective antibiotics and appropriate surgical treatment of local sites of infection, 50 to 70 percent of patients survive. With left-sided endocarditis, the fatality/case ratio is 30 percent. The prognosis for drug addicts with right-sided endocarditis appears particularly good; only 10 percent die. However, when staphylococcal endocarditis has occurred on a prosthetic cardiac valve, the outcome has been almost invariably fatal unless reconstructive surgery can be performed. Early surgical intervention is indicated in such cases.

Staphylococcal food poisoning   See Chap. 112.

Genitourinary infections *Staphylococcus aureus* rarely causes urinary tract infections by retrograde spread from the bladder. Hence, the isolation of *S. aureus* from a well-collected urine specimen should prompt a search for renal, perinephric, or prostatic abscesses secondary to bacteremic staphylococcal infection elsewhere. Diabetics, drug addicts, and patients with valve protheses are particularly prone to this complication. *Staphylococcus epidermidis* has been increasingly recognized as a cause of acute lower urinary tract infection in young women. Many of these strains have the unique characteristic of being novobiocin and nalidixic acid-resistant and may have a specific species designation *(S. saprophyticus).*

Miscellaneous infections Staphylococci may cause conjunctivitis, otitis, sinusitis, or mastoid infections as well as infection in and around the orbit. Epidemics of staphylococcal pyoderma in newborn infants and maternal breast abscesses are a recurring problem in maternity units.

TREATMENT **Features of staphylococcal infection which influence therapy** While the development of penicillinase-resistant penicillins and cephalosporins has simplified treatment, certain characteristics of staphylococcal disease should be borne in mind in designing therapy.

1 *The host setting in which infection occurs.* Acute staphylococcal infections arising outside the hospital in otherwise healthy adults have a better prognosis than intrahospital infections arising in sick individuals with compromised host defense mechanisms.
2 *The rapid necrosis of tissues produced by staphylococci.* Delays in effective therapy may allow a progressing infection to advance to frank abscess formation. While many antimicrobials reach abscess cavities in adequate concentrations, the physiologic insusceptibility of microorganisms residing in the areas of extensive necrosis or suppuration renders antibiotic therapy quite ineffective in this situation. Surgical drainage of such lesions is often required.
3 *The sluggish response to therapy.* Staphylococci are killed slowly by antimicrobials, and relapses are frequent. Hence antimicrobial therapy must be continued longer than in many bacterial infections.
4 *The problem of antimicrobial resistance.* While treatment must be initiated empirically when serious staphylococcal infection is suspected, rational therapy requires that the antibiotic susceptibility of the infecting strain be known.

Treatment of serious staphylococcal infections The effectiveness of the penicillinase-resistant penicillins has simplified the approach to life-threatening staphylococcal disease. Since nearly all strains of staphylococci are susceptible to penicillinase-resistant penicillins, and because of the high incidence of penicillinase-producing staphylococci as causes of infection, most authorities initiate treatment with methicillin, oxacillin, or nafcillin alone, shifting to aqueous penicillin G if the strain is subsequently proved to be susceptible to that drug. Methicillin is rapidly eliminated from the body, and initial doses of 2 g every 4 h are indicated. Parenteral oxacillin or nafcillin in doses of 1 or 2 g every 4 h can be substituted for methicillin. For penicillin-sensitive strains, adults should be given aqueous penicillin, 20 million units, by continuous infusion.

Despite differences in structure, the major allergenic properties of the penicillins reside in the 6-aminopenicillanic acid molecule. There is significant cross allergenicity between penicillins, and patients who have had well-established allergic reactions to penicillin G should not receive penicillinase-resistant penicillins. Further, there is increasing evidence that a signifi-

cant number of these individuals may react to the cephalosporin derivatives as well. These agents, which are good antistaphylococcal drugs, have a 7-aminocephalosporanic acid nucleus quite similar to that of penicillins and should be used with caution in patients with prior reactions to penicillin.

Several cephalosporins can be given parenterally for treatment of serious staphylococcal infections. Cephalothin is highly active against both penicillin-sensitive and penicillin-resistant strains; intramuscular or intravenous doses of 1 to 2 g every 4 h are recommended. The usual dose of cefazolin for severe staphylococcal infection is 1 g every 6 h intramuscularly or intravenously and the dose and route of administration for cephapirin are similar. Nephrotoxicity and an increased susceptibility to penicillinase limit the usefulness of cephaloridine. Cephalosporins should not be used in the treatment of serious staphylococcal infections caused by methicillin-resistant strains of *S. aureus* or *S. epidermidis.* Such strains are generally resistant to cephalosporins despite disk-diffusion results that may indicate sensitivity.

Vancomycin is uniformly active against coagulase-positive staphylococci regardless of their sensitivity to penicillin. It should be given intravenously in doses of 1 to 1.5 g over a 30- to 40-min period every 12 h.

The development of these new agents has relegated several antibiotics formerly used in treatment to minor or secondary roles. Lincomycin, clindamycin, and erythromycin are still useful in certain circumstances, but are not front-line agents in staphylococcal bacteremia. They are used primarily in patients allergic to penicillin.

Changes in therapy Established staphylococcal infections respond slowly even to the most effective antimicrobial regimens, making it difficult to know when therapy should be considered inadequate. Characteristically, 24 to 48 h elapse before a decline in fever is noted, and recovery is accompanied by slow return of the temperature to normal in 7 to 10 days.

Special therapeutic situations ASYMPTOMATIC NASAL CARRIER STATE The role of asymptomatic carriers in hospital transmission of infection remains controversial. Many hospital personnel carry *S. aureus* in their anterior nares but do not appear to disseminate the strain. However, some persons readily disseminate their strain and are a cause of nosocomial infections. Unfortunately, simple methods for recognition of such "dangerous disseminators" are not available, and they are most often detected when increased numbers of *S. aureus* infections prompt an epidemiologic investigation. It is generally agreed that disseminators must be removed from nursery units, operating theaters, delivery rooms, and surgical floors. Although no method of treatment has been uniformly satisfactory, the following regimens have had limited success in treatment of nasal carriers.

1 Simple removal from the hospital environment for 3 to 4 weeks
2 Frequent baths with vermicidal soaps
3 The use of topical antibiotics of low sensitizing potential in a water-soluble base (i.e., bacitracin, neomycin, gentamicin, or a combination of these agents) four to five times daily for 2 weeks

If the carrier state returns, a second course of treatment is indicated.

SUPERFICIAL INFECTIONS Superficial infections frequently do not require the use of antibiotics. There is no adequate therapy for recurrent furunculosis, but if the disease is severe, antimicrobial treatment may be attempted. Antibiotics to which the strain is susceptible should be administered systemically for a minimum of 10 to 14 days. Cloxacillin (2 g per day divided into four doses) or dicloxacillin (2 g per day divided into four doses) can usually be used. Local moist heat, immobilization of the infected part, and incision and drainage should be utilized. The surrounding skin should be protected with a coating of zinc oxide to prevent maceration. Treatment of the nasal carrier state by the local application of topical antibiotics (see above) may be advisable. Careful daily baths with germicidal soaps, attention to personal and family hygiene, and the passage of time appear to be measures most likely to interrupt the process. Attempts to prevent recurrence by autogenous or other vaccines have not been effective.

EMPYEMA Empyema should be treated by aspiration, generally with a large-bore tube since loculation and thick exudate may prevent adequate needle drainage. Intravenous antibiotics as already outlined for serious infections should be given. Direct instillation of penicillin or methicillin into the pleural space may be beneficial in some instances. Similarly, while the local instillation of proteolytic enzymes may occasionally aid in liquefying the exudate, surgical drainage is generally necessary and should be performed promptly.

OSTEOMYELITIS The initial regimen already outlined for other serious infections is recommended, and treatment should be continued for 14 to 28 days in acute osteomyelitis. Local drainage of abscess cavities in soft tissues or bones should be considered in all patients in whom severe pain persists or when response to antimicrobials is inadequate. If sequestration occurs, devitalized bone should be removed. Lincomycin has been reported to be superior to other agents in the treatment of chronic osteomyelitis, but the evidence for this is not convincing. The optimal duration of treatment in established chronic infection is not known, but frequently several months of antimicrobial therapy are recommended.

BACTEREMIA AND ENDOCARDITIS Most authorities recommend 4 to 6 weeks of parenteral antibiotic therapy in proved or suspected staphylococcal endocarditis. However, shorter courses of therapy may be successful, especially in drug addicts with tricuspid endocarditis. In some centers, gentamicin is given with a penicillinase-resistant penicillin in an attempt to kill staphylococci more rapidly. When staphylococcal bacteremia occurs secondary to a removable focus of localized infection (an abscess or an infected intravenous catheter), 10 to 14 days of parenteral therapy is probably sufficient provided the patient has no clinical evidence of endocarditis and demonstrates prompt clinical improvement.

REFERENCES

EICKHOFF TE: Hospital infections. Dis Mon, September 1972

JANNINI PB, CROSSLEY K: Therapy of S. aureus bacteremia associated with a removable focus of infection. Ann Intern Med 84:558, 1976

JESSEN O et al: Changing staphylococci and staphylococcal infections. N Engl J Med 281:627, 1969

KOENIG MG: Staphylococcal infections: Treatment and control. Dis Mon, April 1968

MUSHER DM, McKENZIE SO: Infections due to Staphylococcus aureus. Medicine 56:383, 1977

NAHMIAS AJ, EICKHOFF TC: Staphylococcal infections in hospitals. N Engl J Med 265:74, 120, 177, 1962

NOLAN CM, BEATY HN: S. Aureus bacteremia: Current clinical patterns. Am J Med 60:495, 1976

WATANAKUNAKORN C et al: Some salient features of Staphylococcus aureus endocarditis. Am J Med 54:473, 1973

WISE RI: Modern management of severe staphylococcal disease. Medicine 52:295, 1973

117

STREPTOCOCCAL INFECTIONS

ALAN L. BISNO

Streptococci are among the commonest bacterial pathogens of humans. They are responsible for a diverse spectrum of diseases including pharyngitis and tonsillitis, scarlet fever, erysipelas, impetigo, lymphangitis, and perinatal infections of mother and child. Certain representatives of this genus are prominent causes of endocarditis and urinary tract infections. In addition to their role in causing acute pyogenic infections, strains of *Streptococcus pyogenes* are capable of giving rise to the delayed nonsuppurative sequels of acute rheumatic fever and acute glomerulonephritis.

ETIOLOGY AND CLASSIFICATION Streptococci are spherical or ovoid bacterial cells which grow in pairs or chains of varying lengths. Most are facultative anaerobes, although some are strict anaerobes. The organisms are gram-positive, usually nonmotile, non-spore-forming, and catalase-negative. No single system of classification suffices to differentiate this heterogeneous group of organisms. Instead, classification depends upon a combination of features, including patterns of hemolysis observed on blood agar plates, antigenic composition, growth characteristics, and biochemical reactions.

When cultivated on blood agar plates, streptococci may produce one of three different patterns of hemolysis. Alpha-hemolytic colonies are surrounded by a zone of partial hemolysis; in addition, such organisms usually produce a greenish discoloration in the medium due to the presence of an unidentified reductant of hemoglobin. This greening reaction gives rise to the term *S. viridans*, which is often applied to alpha-hemolytic strains. Strains of *S. pneumoniae* are alpha-hemolytic, as are many other streptococci which normally inhabit the upper respiratory and gastrointestinal tracts. Beta-hemolytic colonies are surrounded by clear colorless zones within which the red blood cells in the medium have been completely lysed. This pattern of complete hemolysis is exhibited by *S. pyogenes* and many of the other streptococci pathogenic for humans. Gamma streptococci are those which fail to produce hemolysis upon blood agar plates.

Although classification of streptococci on the basis of hemolytic reactions is quite useful in certain clinical situations, more precise identification of beta-hemolytic streptococci is accomplished by differentiation into serogroups, as originally described by Lancefield, on the basis of antigenic differences in cell wall carbohydrates. These antigens are readily extracted from streptococcal cell walls and identified by precipitin reactions using specific antiserums. Groups A to H and K to T are recognized. The vast majority of beta-hemolytic streptococci isolated from human sources belongs to groups A to D, F, and G. Although the Lancefield grouping system was initially devised for identification of beta-hemolytic streptococci, certain alpha-hemolytic and nonhemolytic strains also contain group-specific antigens. The most important of these are the group D streptococci, including the so-called "enterococci," among which many strains fail to show beta hemolysis. There are 21 recognized species of streptococci. Species designation is based upon growth characteristics under varying conditions of temperature, pH, and media composition. Five species do not possess group antigens, and, conversely, a number of serogroups do not encompass any of the recognized species.

Anaerobic and microaerophilic streptococci include members of the family Peptococceae, genus *Peptostreptococcus*; five species are recognized. Hemolytic reactions of these organisms are variable, and no satisfactory method of classifying them has been devised.

GROUP A STREPTOCOCCAL INFECTIONS

Strep pyogenes

Streptococci of Lancefield's group A (*S. pyogenes*) are responsible for the great majority of human streptococcal infections and are uniquely important because of their role as precursors of rheumatic fever and glomerulonephritis.

ETIOLOGY The *group-specific carbohydrate* of group A streptococci is a polymer of rhamnose and *N*-acetylglucosamine. There are more than 60 recognized group A serotypes. The typing system is based upon antigenic differences in a cell wall constituent known as *M protein,* which is the principal virulence factor of group A organisms. Strains rich in M protein are highly resistant to phagocytosis by polymorphonuclear leukocytes in vitro and are capable of initiating disease in humans and experimental animals. Strains lacking M protein are avirulent. Acquired human immunity to streptococcal infection is based upon development of opsonic antibodies directed against the antiphagocytic moiety of M protein. This immunity is type-specific and lasts for many years, perhaps indefinitely. M protein is a macromolecule which contains, in addition to the type-specific determinant, a variety of non-type-specific antigens which are widely shared by strains of differing serotypes. *T protein* serves as the basis of a subsidiary typing system which has been useful in classifying strains not typable by the M systems; unlike M protein, the T antigen plays no role in virulence. *Lipoteichoic acid,* a substance which has a marked affinity for biological membranes, has been found to play a crucial role in colonization by binding group A streptococci to specific receptor sites on human epithelial cells. *Opacity factor,* an α-lipoproteinase closely associated with the M-protein molecule, is produced by certain serotypes only. Strains positive for opacity factor may be somewhat attenuated in their virulence, or at least in their ability to elicit antibody response to type-specific and non-type-specific antigens of M protein. The streptococcal *cell membrane* contains a number of antigenic structures, certain of which have been reported to share determinants with constituents of human heart and with basement membrane of the renal glomerulus. Group A streptococci are enveloped in a slimy *hyaluronic acid capsule* which serves to retard phagocytosis and, therefore, represents an accessory virulence factor. Streptococcal hyaluronate is nonantigenic in humans, presumably because it is identical to that found in human connective tissue.

As streptococci grow in vitro or in vivo, they elaborate a number of extracellular products, a few of which require mention. *Erythrogenic toxin,* which is induced by lysogeny with a temperature bacteriophage, is responsible for the rash of scarlet fever. There are three serologically distinct toxins, the effects of which may be neutralized by antibody. Two distinct hemolysins are elaborated. *Streptolysin O* is reversibly inhibited by oxygen (hence exerting its effect primarily on subsurface colonies) and irreversibly inhibited by cholesterol. It is produced by almost all group A strains as well as by many group C and G organisms. Titration of antistreptolysin O (ASO) antibodies in human serums is the most widely used serologic procedure to detect group A streptococcal infection in clinical practice. Hemolysis on the surface of blood agar plates is due primarily to the action of *streptolysin S.* Although streptolysin S differs from streptolysin O in being oxygen-stable and nonantigenic, both hemolysins possess the capacity to damage membranes of polymorphonuclear leukocytes, platelets, and subcellular organelles. A number of other extracellular products exert effects which might serve to facilitate the organisms' survival in vivo by liquefying pus [streptokinase and deoxyribonucleases (DNases) A to D] or by allowing spread through tissue planes (*hyaluronidase* and *proteinase*).

The role of these substances in streptococcal virulence remains unproved.

The two most frequent types of group A streptococcal infection are pharyngitis and pyoderma. They differ markedly in their epidemiologic, clinical, and bacteriologic characteristics.

STREPTOCOCCAL PHARYNGITIS Epidemiology This is one of the commonest bacterial infections of humans. The incidence is highest in children aged 5 to 15 years; males and females are affected equally. The great majority of such infections are due to group A streptococci, but strains of other serogroups, particularly group C or G, are involved occasionally. The organism is ordinarily transmitted directly from person to person, most likely by droplet spread, and crowding markedly facilitates interpersonal transmission. This may account for the increased incidence of streptococcal pharyngitis in northern latitudes during the colder months of the year, as well as for the explosive outbreaks which occur in military recruit camps and other crowded institutional settings. Common-source epidemics of streptococcal sore throat with high attack rates occasionally occur following contamination of a food item with beta-hemolytic streptococci. Environmental reservoirs of streptococci, such as viable organisms in room dust or on blankets, are not important in spread of disease.

Patients with acute streptococcal pharyngitis harbor large numbers of organisms in the anterior nares and throat. If antibiotics are not administered, the organisms may persist in the upper respiratory tract for weeks to months after symptoms have subsided. However, as the length of the carrier state increases, the organisms decrease in number, disappear from the anterior nasal secretions, and lose detectable M protein. Therefore, convalescent carriers are less likely than acutely ill patients to transmit group A streptococci to exposed individuals. Group A pharyngeal carriage rates vary with geographic location, season of the year, and age group. Among school-aged children, rates of 15 to 20 percent have been reported; the carriage rate among adults is considerably lower.

Symptoms The usual incubation period of streptococcal pharyngitis is between 2 and 4 days. The classic syndrome, as observed in older children and adults, is ushered in by the rather abrupt onset of sore throat, manifested particularly by pain on swallowing. Associated symptoms include headache, malaise, feverishness, and anorexia. Chilliness is a frequent symptom, but true rigors are rare. Nausea, vomiting, and abdominal pain are common in children.

Physical signs The patient appears moderately ill with tachycardia and fever which frequently exceeds 38.3°C (101°F). There is diffuse erythema, edema, and lymphoid hyperplasia of the posterior pharynx. The uvula is edematous. The tonsils, if present, are enlarged, reddened, and covered by a punctate or coalescent exudate which may be yellow, gray, or white. Discrete areas of pinhead-size exudate are frequently present on the posterior pharynx but may be concealed by mucopurulent nasal secretions. The anterior cervical lymph nodes at the angles of the jaw are enlarged and tender. Cough and hoarseness, if present, are mild and, in the absence of the signs and symptoms indicated above, do not in themselves suggest the diagnosis of streptococcal pharyngitis. Laryngeal involvement with loss of voice is not a feature of streptococcal infection.

The full-blown clinical syndrome of acute exudative tonsillopharyngitis is seen frequently during explosive epidemics of streptococcal disease, particularly those occurring in institutional settings such as military recruit camps. In endemically occurring infections among civilian populations, however, the illness is frequently much milder. Indeed, in such circumstances, only about half the children with sore throats and positive cultures for group A streptococci will have tonsillar exudate, and a third or less may have fever greater than 38.3°C (101°F) or marked leukocytosis. Patients who have undergone tonsillectomy tend to experience a milder clinical syndrome. In infants, streptococcal upper respiratory infections tend to be less sharply localized to the lymphoid tissue of the faucial and posterior pharyngeal areas. Infections at this age are characterized by rhinorrhea with excoriation of the nares, low-grade fever, anorexia, and a protracted clinical course. Exudative pharyngitis in children less than 3 years of age is rarely streptococcal in etiology.

Course The course of streptococcal pharyngitis is usually brief and self-limited. Fever abates within a week, usually within 3 to 5 days. Constitutional symptoms and sore throat disappear with defervescence or shortly thereafter. Several weeks may be required, however, for the tonsils and lymph nodes to return to normal size.

Scarlet fever When streptococcal pharyngitis is due to a lysogenic strain producing erythrogenic toxin, and when the host is not immune to the toxin, scarlet fever ensues. The rash usually appears within 2 days after onset of sore throat, involves first the neck, upper chest, and back, then spreads over the remainder of the trunk and the extremities, and spares the palms and soles. The rash may be difficult to appreciate in black patients. It consists of a diffuse erythema, which blanches on pressure, with numerous 1- to 2-mm punctate elevations that impart a "sandpaper" texture to the skin. Discrete lesions are absent from the face, but there is a generalized facial flush which contrasts with the prominent circumoral pallor. The rash is more intense along skin folds, such as those of the antecubital fossae and axillary folds, and in these locations often produces linear striations of confluent petachiae known as *Pastia's lines.* Increased capillary fragility, which contributes to the formation of Pastia's lines, is confirmed by a positive Rumpel-Leede's test.

The exanthem of scarlet fever is accompanied by an enanthem, consisting of punctate erythema and petechiae on the soft palate. Early in the disease, the tongue is covered with a white coat through which hypertrophied papillae protrude as islands of red (strawberry tongue). By the fourth or fifth day the coating is gone and the entire tongue appears beefy red (raspberry tongue). In rare cases, scarlet fever may be complicated by hepatic involvement with jaundice, pleural effusion, and arthralgia. It is unclear how often arthralgia is a manifestation of scarlet fever or how often it presages the development of rheumatic fever.

The rash usually lasts 4 to 5 days and is followed by extensive desquamation which begins as early as a few days or as late as 3 to 4 weeks after onset of the disease and is often a striking feature of the convalescent phase of scarlet fever.

Although scarlet fever usually follows upper respiratory infection due to group A streptococci, rarely other erythrogenic toxins are produced by streptococci of groups C and G and by certain strains of staphylococci. Moreover, scarlet fever may follow streptococcal impetigo or secondary streptococcal infection of superficial wounds. The disease must be differentiated from various of the childhood exanthems, infectious mononucleosis when the latter is associated with rash, and drug eruptions. The management of scarlet fever consists of adequate treatment of the causative infection.

Two tests previously employed in assessment of scarlet fever are no longer in clinical use. The *Dick test* is performed by inoculating erythrogenic toxin intracutaneously. Individuals who are susceptible to the toxin will experience local erythema (positive Dick test), while individuals with antitoxin immunity will have no reaction (negative Dick test). Conversion from a positive to a negative Dick test during the course of a rash illness strongly suggests the diagnosis of scarlet fever. Another test consists of injection of scarlatinal antitoxin into an area of cutaneous rash, which produces blanching if the eruption is due to erythrogenic toxin. This test, previously used for diagnosis of scarlet fever, is known as the Schultz-Charlton reaction.

Complications Streptococcal pharyngitis may give rise to suppurative complications, among which acute otitis media and acute sinusitis are the most frequent. Suppurative cervical lymphadenitis may also occur. Inflammation of the faucial area induced by streptococcal infection may give rise to peritonsillar cellulitis, peritonsillar abscess, or retropharyngeal abscess. The abscesses themselves, however, usually contain a variety of oropharyngeal flora, including anaerobic bacteria, rather than group A streptococci. A variety of other complications, common in the past, are almost never seen in the antibiotic era: (1) extension up the cribriform plate of the ethmoid or via the mastoid, giving rise to meningitis, brain abscess, or thrombosis of cerebral venous sinuses; and (2) bacteremia with metastatic foci of infection such as suppurative arthritis, osteomyelitis, or liver abscess. Much of the intense clinical and investigative interest focused upon streptococcal pharyngitis is due to its association with two delayed nonsuppurative sequels: acute rheumatic fever (ARF) and acute glomerulonephritis (AGN). These are discussed in Chaps. 241 and 278, respectively.

Diagnosis Sore throat due to group A streptococci must be differentiated from that caused by a number of other agents. *Diphtheria* is rare in immunized populations. It is characterized by the presence of an extensive diphtheritic membrane, respiratory embarrassment due to laryngeal involvement, myocarditis, cranial nerve palsies, and positive cultures for *Corynebacterium diphtheriae. Gonococcal* tonsillopharyngitis should be suggested by a history of homosexuality or fellatio. *Vincent's angina* is characterized by sore throat and tonsillopharyngeal exudate. Unlike streptococcal sore throat, however, there is an insidious onset without constitutional symptoms, pharyngeal ulcerations are frequent, and the disease is usually unilateral.

The major differential diagnostic confusion is with viral upper respiratory infections, which occur more frequently than does streptococcal infection. In many cases, the viral etiology may be suspected because of the more prominent catarrhal, "common cold–like" quality of these viral infections. *Adenoviruses* may cause an exudative pharyngitis which is virtually indistinguishable clinically from that due to group A streptococci. *Infectious mononucleosis* also produces severe exudative pharyngitis with fever and toxicity and at times is accompanied by a rash which may be confused with scarlet fever. The generalized lymphadenopathy, splenomegaly, prolonged fever, and presence of abnormal lymphocytes and heterophile antibodies in the peripheral blood serve to differentiate this entity. Pharyngitis due to group A coxsackie viruses (*herpangina*) or to primary infection with *herpes simplex* is characterized by formation of vesicles, which rupture and leave shallow ulcers. *Influenza* virus infections frequently occur in epidemics; they are accompanied by severe myalgias, bronchitis is a frequent clinical feature, and all age groups are affected. *Mycoplasma pneumonia* infections may cause pharyngitis that at times may be exudative. Bullous myringitis, if present, should suggest this diagnosis.

Despite the differential features set forth above, in many instances it is impossible to differentiate streptococcal from nonstreptococcal sore throat on clinical grounds alone. Even experienced observers are able to predict the presence of streptococcal pharyngeal infection in no more than 50 to 75 percent of cases. For this reason, precise diagnosis requires performance of a throat culture. In obtaining the culture, it is important to rub the cotton swab over both tonsils or tonsillar fossae, the oropharynx, and the nasopharynx posterior to the uvula. The swab should be inoculated onto a sheep blood agar plate to allow evaluation of patterns of hemolysis after overnight incubation. If beta-hemolytic streptococci are isolated, they may be presumed to be group A by sensitivity to a low-potency bacitracin disk or may be identified definitively by fluorescent antibody, coagglutination, or precipitin techniques. A number of the positive cultures obtained, particularly those with few organisms on the culture plate, will represent streptococcal carriers rather than cases of acute infection. It is not possible to differentiate cases from carriers confidently on the basis of culture results, but culture does serve to exclude from antimicrobial therapy the bulk of patients with sore throat (approximately 70 percent) who have negative cultures for beta-hemolytic streptococci. Assay of serum antibodies to streptococcal extracellular products (e.g., ASO) provides confirmatory evidence of recent streptococcal infection in patients suspected of having acute rheumatic fever or acute glomerulonephritis, but such tests are of no value in the diagnosis of acute streptococcal infection.

1.2 m∨ BENZATHINE PEN G

Treatment Therapy of streptococcal pharyngitis is directed primarily toward prevention of suppurative sequelae and of ARF. It is unclear whether treatment of the antecedent streptococcal infection will prevent development of AGN. Prevention of ARF depends upon eradication of the infecting organism from the pharynx, and attainment of this objective requires prolonged antibiotic treatment. Penicillin is the drug of choice because it is inexpensive and nontoxic and because all group A streptococci have remained exquisitely sensitive to this agent. A single intramuscular injection of benzathine penicillin G, 600,000 units for children less than 60 lb and 1.2 million units for all others, ensures a prolonged penicillinemia and is the most effective form of therapy. If oral therapy is elected, penicillin G, 250,000 units, or penicillin V, 250 mg, three or four times daily, is the treatment of choice. Penicillin-allergic individuals may be treated with erythromycin, 20 mg/lb per day (not to exceed 1 g per day). Nearly all group A streptococci in the United States have remained susceptible to erythromycin, but extensive resistance has been reported in certain areas of the world such as Japan. On the other hand, tetracycline-resistant strains are encountered with some frequency in the United States, and this drug is not recommended. Sulfonamides are ineffective in eradication of established streptococcal infection, although they are useful prophylactically in preventing new pharyngeal acquisitions of group A streptococci and in preventing recurrences of ARF (Chap. 241). All oral regimens are less effective than intramuscular benzathine penicillin G in eradicating the infecting streptococcus, a fact that is due at least in part to the difficulty of ensuring faithful compliance once the acute symptoms have subsided. It is advisable to reculture the throat within 48 h of completion of oral therapy. If group A streptococci persist, as they may in 15 percent of cases, retreatment, preferably with benzathine penicillin G, is indicated. Multiple repetitive courses of antibiotics are not of further value and should be avoided.

Appropriate antibiotic therapy is effective in preventing ARF, even when initiated as long as 9 days after the onset of acute pharyngitis. Therefore, in the patient seen early after the course of his illness, the delay in initiating therapy occasioned

by obtaining a positive throat culture is not ordinarily a matter of concern. In patients who are severely ill or in whom development of suppurative complications is apparent, therapy may be instituted at the time of the initial visit after a throat culture has been obtained. If oral antibiotic therapy is elected, the throat culture serves as a guide to the necessity of completion of a full 10-day course or, alternatively, of recalling the patient for definitive therapy with an injection of benzathine penicillin G.

Patients with more severe suppurative complications, such as infections involving the mastoid or ethmoids, require larger doses of penicillin than those used for treatment of uncomplicated sore throat. When streptococcal upper respiratory infection is complicated by the development of abscesses associated with suppurative cervical adenitis or in the peritonsillar or retrophyaryngeal soft tissues, incision and drainage are usually required.

The role of tonsillectomy, if any, in the management of patients with frequent recurrences of acute pharyngitis or in the prevention of ARF remains undefined. Clinical episodes of pharyngitis occur less frequently and tend to be milder following tonsillectomy, but this may possibly make detection and appropriate treatment of immunologically significant streptococcal infections more difficult.

Family contacts of patients with streptococcal sore throat frequently develop symptomatic infections or become asymptomatic pharyngeal carriers. Secondary cases in families should, of course, be treated appropriately. Asymptomatic family contacts should also be cultured in high-risk circumstances. These include the presence of a rheumatic subject in the family, known cases of ARF occurring in the general area, and families in a lower socioeconomic group with a large number of children living in crowded circumstances. In situations where the risk is lower, the decision to culture and treat asymptomatic family contacts must be made for each involved individual and should be based upon factors such as the geographic and socioeconomic setting, and the current prevalence of streptococcal disease and its sequels.

STREPTOCOCCAL SKIN INFECTIONS Erysipelas Also known as Saint Anthony's fire, erysipelas is an acute infection of the skin and subcutaneous tissues caused by group A streptococci. Other streptococci, and even staphylococci and pneumococci, have been implicated on rare occasions. The disease most frequently affects infants, young children, and elderly individuals. The commonest site of involvement is the face, where cutaneous infection originates from an upper respiratory source, presumably by way of small or inapparent breaks in the skin. Erysipelas may also result from streptococcal infection of wounds, surgical incisions, or even areas of dermatophytosis, in which case any portion of the body may be involved.

The onset is usually abrupt; initial symptoms include malaise, chilliness, feverishness, headache, and vomiting. The skin lesion may begin with itching and mild discomfort at the site of infection and is followed shortly thereafter by a small area of erythema which enlarges during the ensuing hours. The lesion spreads rapidly, reaching its maximum extent in 3 to 6 days. It is warm, pink to deep red in color, and has an advancing elevated margin which protrudes irregularly into the surrounding areas of normal skin. Vesicles and bullae may appear; these rupture leaving crusts on the surface. While the advancing margin remains inflamed, central clearing may be evident with a return of the skin to normal appearance or with residual pigmentation. The eruption may be less well demarcated in areas where the skin is loose, but edema and erythema are constant features. Facial erysipelas commonly involves the bridge of the nose and one or more cheeks in a "butterfly" distribution (Fig. 117-1).

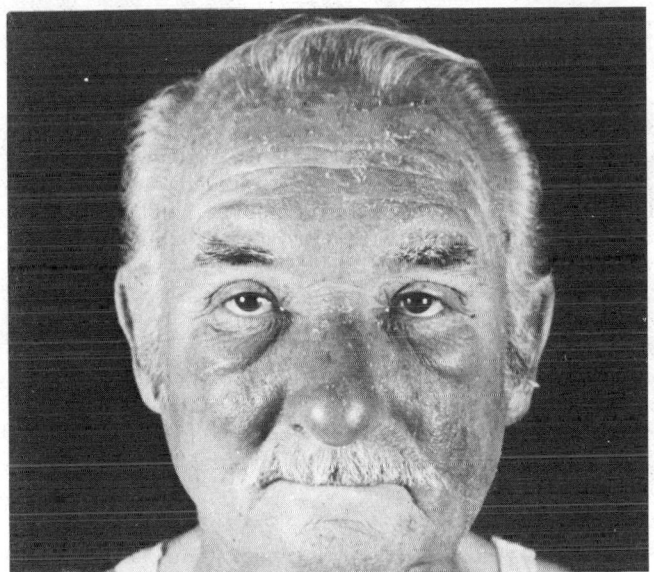

FIGURE 117-1

This patient with facial erysipelas exhibits the characteristic "butterfly" distribution of the lesion. The picture was obtained after 48 h of penicillin therapy when the acute inflammation and systemic toxicity had abated slightly.

The disease process may be accompanied by high fever and bacteremia. Recovery is usually apparent by the end of a week, but this varies with the severity of the infection. The substantial mortality attending bacteremic cases of erysipelas in the preantibiotic era has been markedly reduced by penicillin. Fatalities still occur among children within the first few months of life and elderly, debilitated, immunosuppressed individuals. The disease is noted for its propensity to recur, especially in the areas of chronic lymphatic obstruction.

The diagnosis of erysipelas is primarily clinical. Group A streptococci may at times be isolated from the respiratory tract or the bloodstream. Culture of edema fluid or of saline injected intracutaneously and then withdrawn from the advancing margin may yield streptococci, but this maneuver is rarely successful.

Pyoderma This term is used collectively to denote localized purulent streptococcal skin infections. Some pyoderma lesions represent obvious secondary infections of wounds or burns. For the most part, however, the term is used synonymously with streptococcal impetigo or impetigo contagiosa and refers to discrete purulent lesions which appear to be primary infections of the skin. Streptococcal impetigo differs from streptococcal pharyngitis in a number of particulars (Table 117-1). Epidemiologically, impetigo is more prevalent among underpriviledged children residing in warm, humid climates such as the southeastern United States or the tropics. However, the disease may also occur during the summer in northern settings, such as the American Indian reservations of Minnesota. The peak incidence is in young children (2 to 6 years), and there is no definite sex or racial predisposition.

The mode of spread of streptococcal pyoderma is unknown, but personal contact and insect vectors such as *Hippelates* flies are probably both important. "Skin strains" of group A streptococci (i.e., strains of M and T types usually associated with pyoderma) are capable of contaminating unbroken skin, from where they may be inoculated intradermally by local scratches, abrasions, or insect bites. A number of interesting epidemiologic relationships have been observed; they include secondary streptococcal infection in the lesions of scabies and the co-

existence of *S. pyogenes* and *C. diphtheriae* in impetiginous lesions in Mississippi and Trinidad. Nasal and pharyngeal carriage of skin strains is frequent in children with impetigo, but such carriage does not ordinarily occur until after establishment of cutaneous carriage or overt infection.

The pattern of immunologic responses to streptococcal impetigo differs from that associated with upper respiratory infection. In particular, the ASO response to impetigo is weak, perhaps because streptolysin O is inactivated by lipids present in the skin. Brisk antibody responses to anti-DNAse B and anti-hyaluronidase, as well as to the Streptozyme slide hemagglutination reagent, are observed, however. Type-specific anti-M responses are variable, depending in part upon the antigenicity of the infecting strain, but in general such responses are weaker than in pharyngeal infections. The role of type-specific antibodies in protection against reinfection in pyoderma has not been adequately studied.

Streptococcal impetigo occurs on exposed areas of the body, most frequently on the lower extremities. The lesions remain well-localized but are frequently multiple. They begin as papules but rapidly evolve into vesicles surrounded by an area of erythema. The vesicular lesions are rarely recognized clinically; they give rise to papules which gradually enlarge, then break down over 4 to 6 days to form characteristic thick crusts. The lesions heal slowly, leaving depigmented areas. A deeply ulcerated form of impetigo is known as *echthyma*. Although regional lymphadenitis often occurs, systemic symptoms are not ordinarily present.

In addition to the indolent, impetiginous skin infections of young children, a more severe and extensive form of pyoderma has been observed in combat troops serving in hot, wet environments such as the jungles of Southeast Asia. During the Vietnam conflict, such "jungle sores" became a major medical problem among infantry personnel. In their most common form, they consist of multiple echthymatous ulcers located on the ankle or dorsum of the foot. The ulcers are usually circular, punched-out lesions 0.5 to 3.0 cm in diameter, have borders, and are surrounded by a zone of erythema. They are filled with purulent material and covered with grayish yellow adherent crusts. Secondary cellulitis or lymphadenitis may be present.

TABLE 117-1

Comparative features of pharyngitis and pyoderma due to group A streptococci

	Pharyngitis	*Pyoderma*
Predominant geographic distribution	Temperate	Subtropic-tropic
Season (temperate zone)	Winter-spring	Summer-fall
Peak age group	5-15 years	2-5 years
Mode of spread	Direct contact (droplet)	Unknown (?insects)
Clinical illness	Acute	Indolent
Streptococcal types	Generally lower-numbered M types	Generally higher-numbered M types
ASO responses	Good	Weak
Type-specific antibody responses	Generally good	Variable, often poor
Nonsuppurative sequels	Acute rheumatic fever, acute glomerulonephritis	Acute glomerulonephritis

SOURCE: *After Wannamaker.*

The diagnosis of streptococcal pyoderma is made by bacteriologic culture. Adequate cultures require removal of the surface crusts in order to obtain specimens from the base of the lesions. Although both *S. pyogenes* and *Staphylococcus aureus* may be isolated from the lesions, the former is the major pathogen. Morphologically characteristic lesions respond well to penicillin therapy, even when penicillinase-resistant staphylococci are recovered. These lesions contrast with bullous impetigo, which is ordinarily due to *S. aureus* and not to streptococci. Antibiotic regimens are the same as those for pharyngitis, and benzathine penicillin G, oral penicillin V, or oral erythromycin all result in cure rates in excess of 95 percent. Topical antiseptics and antibiotics are of little, if any, value. Prevention of pyoderma depends primarily upon adherence to good personal hygiene, with special attention to frequent scrubbing with soap and water.

Streptococcal pyoderma does not give rise to ARF. This observation remains unexplained, but may indicate a requirement for infection at the pharyngeal site, with its rich endowment of lymphoid tissue, in order to initiate the immunologic events leading to ARF. On the other hand, studies of populations in which ARF and AGN occur simultaneously indicate that the streptococcal strains responsible for each sequel are distinct and suggest that "pyoderma strains" of group A streptococci may be nonrheumatogenic. When pyoderma is due to a nephritogenic strain of group A streptococcus, AGN may ensue. Indeed, pyoderma is by far the commonest antecedent of poststreptococcal glomerulonephritis in subtropical and tropical regions of the world. Strains of a number of M types (49, 55, 57, and others) have been associated both with sporadic cases and large epidemics of pyoderma-associated nephritis in diverse geographic areas. There are no conclusive data to indicate that treatment of an individual case of pyoderma will prevent the subsequent occurrence of AGN in that patient. Such treatment is important, however, in eradicating nephritogenic streptococci from the environment in epidemiologic settings in which these strains are prevalent.

Cellulitis   Streptococcal cellulitis may occur in areas of tissue damage due to trauma, operative wounds, or stasis ulceration. It is an acute inflammation of the skin and subcutaneous tissues marked by pain, tenderness, erythema, fever, and often regional lymphadenopathy. In contrast to erysipelas, the margins of the lesions are neither elevated nor sharply demarcated from the surrounding uninvolved tissue. Rarely such lesions may progress to frank gangrene. Cellulitis of the perianal area may be manifested by painful defecation or by pruritus; asymptomatic anal colonization has been the source of several outbreaks of hospital-acquired streptococcal infection. Vaginal colonization by group A streptococci has a number of features in common with perianal involvement. In both instances there is a close epidemiologic association with streptococcal upper respiratory infection. Anal and vaginal streptococcal infection may be either symptomatic or asymptomatic. At least one outbreak of nosocomial streptococcal infection has been attributed to an asymptomatic vaginal carrier.

LYMPHANGITIS AND PUERPERAL SEPSIS   Local trauma, whether or not complicated by frank cellulitis, may give rise to *acute lymphangitis*. This entity is characterized by the appearance of red linear streaks extending from the portal of entry to the draining regional lymph nodes, which are enlarged and tender. Systemic symptoms, including chills, fever, malaise, and headache, are prominent, and the process may be accompanied by demonstrable bacteremia. Streptococcal bacteremia, from whatever cause, may give rise to metastatic foci of infection, such as suppurative arthritis, osteomyelitis, peritonitis, endocarditis, meningitis, or visceral abscesses. The clinical course of streptococcal bacteremia may at times be fulminant and lead rapidly to prostration, shock, purpura fulminans, disseminated intravascular coagulation, and death.

Puerperal sepsis follows abortion or childbirth when streptococci invade the endometrium and surrounding structures and then the lymphatics and bloodstream. The pathological process may be further complicated by pelvic cellulitis, septic pelvic thrombophlebitis, peritonitis, or pelvic abscess. The causative organism may be transmitted to the pregnant woman directly by medical personnel or attendants, as was demonstrated by Semmelweiss in the mid-nineteenth century. In recent years, group B streptococci have supplanted other organisms as the most frequent cause of perinatal streptococcal infections of mother and child (see below). Anaerobic streptococci, along with other anaerobic organisms, have also been implicated.

PNEUMONIA AND EMPYEMA   Pneumonia due to group A streptococci is uncommon and usually occurs following viral infections such as influenza, measles, pertussis, or varicella. The illness occurs in epidemic form in military recruit camps and is characterized by abrupt onset of fever, chills, myalgia, dyspnea, cough, pleuritic chest pain, and hemoptysis. Patients are severely ill and often cyanotic. Pathologically and radiologically, this is usually a bronchopneumonia, and lobar consolidation is uncommon. A characteristic feature of streptococcal pneumonia is the early and rapid accumulation of copious amounts of thin, serosanguinous empyema fluid. Bacteremia occurs in 10 to 15 percent of cases. Extension of the pneumonic process to the pericardium may give rise to a purulent pericarditis. Other potential complications include mediastinitis, pneumothorax, and bronchiectasis. Therapy consists of 4 to 6 million units parenteral penicillin in the form of aqueous procaine penicillin G, given every 6 to 12 h intramuscularly, or intravenous aqueous crystalline penicillin G, and adequate drainage of empyema fluid, which usually requires insertion of a chest tube.

GROUP B STREPTOCOCCAL INFECTIONS

Streptococci belonging to serogroup B have long been of interest to veterinarians because of their association with bovine mastitis, an association which led to their species designation as *S. agalactiae*. The organisms are beta-hemolytic and usually, but not uniformly, resistant to bacitracin. In addition to the presence of group B carbohydrate in their cell walls, *S. agalactiae* may be identified by biochemical means, including their production of hippuricase and so-called "cyclic AMP factor." Group B streptococci may be subdivided by means of surface polysaccharides and protein antigens into five serotypes: Ia, Ib, Ic, II, and III.

Human strains of group B streptococci, which appear to be biologically distinct from bovine strains, frequently colonize the female genital tract as well as the throat and rectum. Asymptomatic vaginal carriage rates in postpubertal women generally have ranged between 6 and 25 percent, depending on the bacteriologic methods employed and on the socioeconomic status and geographic residence of the women sampled. The majority of serious group B infections occur as perinatal events. Maternal infections include chorioamnionitis, septic abortion, and puerperal sepsis. *Streptococcus agalactiae* now ranks with *Escherichia coli* as one of the two most frequent causes of neonatal sepsis and meningitis. Neonatal disease takes one of two forms. Early-onset disease, occurring within the first 10 days of life, is usually due to organisms acquired from the maternal genital tract. It involves primarily the lungs, probably as a result of aspiration of infected amniotic fluid, but the organism can be cultured from many sites such as the blood, nasopharynx, skin, and myocardium. Early-onset group B streptococcal infection occurs in approximately two of every thousand live births (the incidence is higher following prolonged or complicated delivery) and is attended by a high mortality rate. Late-onset disease occurs in infants over 10 days old, may be due to nosocomial transmission of group B streptococci, is manifested primarily by meningitis and bacteremia, and has a lower mortality rate than early-onset disease. Although the serotypes involved in early-onset illness are variable, type III organisms predominate as the cause of late-onset meningeal infection. Transplacentally acquired antibodies to type III organisms may protect against late-onset disease: they are reported to be present in serums of most women delivering healthy babies but are usually lacking in serums of mothers whose offspring develop late-onset meningitis due to type III group B streptococci.

Group B streptococci also cause a group of adult infections not associated with the puerperium. These include urinary tract infections in both sexes; the infections in men often occur in elderly individuals, perhaps due to associated prostatism. A second syndrome occurs in patients with adult-onset, insulin-dependent diabetes mellitus, peripheral vascular insufficiency, and suppurative gangrenous lesions, infected with *S. agalactiae*. Bacteremia may accompany this syndrome. Other adult infections due to group B organisms include endocarditis, pneumonia, empyema, meningitis, peritonitis, and terminal bacteremia in patients with malignancy. Although recovered from a small proportion of throat cultures, group B streptococci are rarely, if ever, the cause of clinically significant pharyngitis. All strains are susceptible to penicillin, which is the drug of choice, although group B organisms have slightly higher minimal inhibitory concentrations for penicillin than do group A strains. Only occasional strains are resistant to erythromycin. Tetracyclines should not be used without prior susceptibility testing because resistance to them is quite common.

OTHER STREPTOCOCCAL INFECTIONS

Streptococci of groups C and G are capable of causing exudative pharyngitis, and epidemics of upper respiratory disease due to these organisms have been reported, particularly following ingestion of contaminated food items. Strains of both serogroups produce streptolysin O, and pharyngeal infections with groups C and G elicit rises in ASO titer. However, most reported instances of human disease due to these two serogroups have been skin and wound infections or puerperal infections. Associated bacteremia may result in endocarditis.

Lancefield's group D streptococci consist of enterococcal species (*S. faecalis, S. faecium, S. durans*) and nonenterococci (*S. bovis, S. equinus*). Group D streptococci are frequent causes of urinary tract infection in patients with structural abnormalities of the urinary tract and frequently are associated with bacterial endocarditis. These microorganisms are usually alpha-hemolytic or nonhemolytic but may be beta-hemolytic. The treatment of severe enterococcal infections, particularly bacterial endocarditis, is complicated by the fact that the organisms are frequently resistant to many antibiotics, including the penicillins. In the therapy of enterococcal endocarditis, a combination of intravenous penicillin G or ampicillin in high doses plus an aminoglycoside antibiotic should be used, because this combination exerts a synergistic effect in the killing of enterococci (Chap. 243). While formerly streptomycin was the aminoglycoside of choice, high-level resistance (>2000 µg/ml) to streptomycin and kanamycin has been found in a significant number of enterococcal isolates. This is due to a plasmid which is transferable, by conjugation under laboratory condi-

tions, from resistant to sensitive strains. For this reason, aminoglycosides such as gentamicin or tobramycin should be used along with penicillin or ampicillin in treatment of serious enterococcal infections.

In contrast, nonenterococcal group D streptococci, of which *S. bovis* is the only known pathogen, remain extremely sensitive to penicillin and are amenable to therapy with this agent alone. Laboratory differentiation of *S. bovis* from enterococci is sometimes difficult. Likewise, *S. mutans,* a penicillin-sensitive viridans streptococcus which is normally found in the mouth and occasionally causes endocarditis, may be confused with group D streptococci. A series of precise biochemical tests is required to identify the various species correctly. In particular, enterococci grow in 6.5% sodium chloride broth, while *S. bovis* and *S. mutans* do not. Treatment of life-threatening enterococcal infections in patients who cannot tolerate penicillin is difficult. Cephalothin and clindamycin are of no value, but vancomycin, often in combination with gentamicin, is likely to be effective.

Streptococci of most groups have been isolated at least occasionally from infected heart valves, soft tissues, or visceral abscesses. Such infections may occur as "opportunists" following surgical manipulation or in patients with malignant disease. Danish and Dutch investigators have reported a number of instances of meningitis and bacteremia in humans due to streptococci of serogroup R, a group of organisms well-known as pathogens of swine. In nearly all human cases there had been a history of contact with pigs.

Viridans streptococci are normal inhabitants of the oropharynx and gastrointestinal tract. They remain the most frequent causative agents of subacute bacterial endocarditis (Chap. 243). The taxonomy of these organisms is confused, but one classification scheme recognizes five species (in addition to *S. pneumoniae*): *salivarius, mitior, milleri, sanguis,* and *mutans.* Although viridans streptococci are not usually considered to be highly invasive, *S. milleri* is capable of causing serious pyogenic infections such as liver and brain abscesses, peritonitis, and empyema. Cases of endocarditis due to *S. milleri* are more likely to be complicated by abscess formation in peripheral tissues than are similar infections due to other species of viridans streptococci. *Streptococcus milleri* is usually considered "microaerophilic," and its clinical behavior is similar to that of the anaerobic streptococci. All the viridans species, including *S. milleri,* are susceptible to penicillin. Modest increases in the minimal inhibitory concentrations of oral streptococci to penicillin occur following prolonged oral therapy with this antibiotic.

Anaerobic streptococci (see also Chap. 142) abound in the mouth, intestinal tract, and vagina. They may be found, either alone or in combination with other anaerobic and aerobic microorganisms, in abscess cavities throughout the body. In the head and neck, anaerobic streptococci may be found in infected paranasal sinuses, brain abscess, dental abscess, infections of the retropharyngeal or lateral pharyngeal spaces, and in cases of Ludwig's angina. In the chest, these organisms occur in lung abscesses and empyema fluids. Abscesses of the liver and other intraabdominal viscera, as well as perirectal abscesses and pelvic abscesses in women, may be due in part to peptostreptococci. Finally, these organisms may thrive in dead or devitalized muscle, skin, or subcutaneous tissue. *Streptococcal myositis* is characterized by marked edema, crepitant myositis, pain, and the presence of chains of gram-positive cocci in a seropurulent exudate. *Progressive synergistic gangrene* usually develops about a surgical incision and consists of an ulcerated lesion surrounded by gangrenous skin. The infection is associated particularly with the use of through-and-through sutures after abdominal surgery, and is thought most often to be due to the synergistic action of *S. aureus* and microaerophilic streptococci. *Chronic burrowing ulcer* is a deep soft-tissue infection caused by microaerophilic streptococci which erodes through subcutaneous tissue to emerge as an ulcer at a distant site. Management of anaerobic streptococcal infections consists of drainage of abscesses, debridement of devitalized tissues, and high-dose intravenous penicillin therapy.

REFERENCES

BAKER CJ, DENNIS KL: Immunological investigation of infants with septicemia and meningitis due to group B streptococcus. J Infect Dis 136:598, 1977

BISNO AL et al: Factors influencing serum antibody responses in streptococcal pyoderma. J Lab Clin Med 81:410, 1973

DUMA RJ et al: Streptococcal infections: A bacteriologic and clinical study of streptococcal bacteremia. Medicine 48:87, 1969

KAPLAN EL et al: Diagnosis of streptococcal pharyngitis: Differentiation of active infection from the carrier state in the symptomatic child. J Infect Dis 123:490, 1971

KROGSTAD DJ: Plasmid-mediated resistance to antibiotic synergism to enterococci. J Clin Invest 61:1645, 1978

LERNER PI et al: Group B streptococcus (*S. agalactiae*) bacteremia in adults: Analysis of 32 cases and review of the literature. Medicine 56:457, 1977

MURRAY HW et al: Serious infections caused by *Streptococcus milleri*. Am J Med 64:759, 1978

STOLLERMAN GH: *Rheumatic Fever and Streptococcal Infection*. New York, Grune & Stratton, 1975

WANNAMAKER LW: Differences between streptococcal infections of the throat and the skin. N Engl J Med 282:23, 1970

section 3 | Diseases caused by gram-negative cocci

118
MENINGOCOCCAL INFECTIONS

HARRY N. BEATY

DEFINITION *Neisseria meningitidis* is the causative organism of a variety of infections, notably meningitis and bacteremia.

ETIOLOGY The organism responsible for "cerebrospinal fever" was first described by Weichselbaum in 1887. It was subsequently assigned to the genus *Neisseria*, and is now designated by the binominal *Neisseria meningitidis* and the common name meningococcus. In stained smears, meningococci are gram-negative and characteristically appear as single cocci or diplococci with flattened adjacent sides. They grow well on solid or semisolid media containing blood, serum, or ascitic fluid, and thrive best at temperatures between 35 and 37°C in an atmosphere reduced in oxygen and containing 5 to 10 percent CO_2. The organism is recovered readily from biologic fluids when fresh specimens are inoculated on warm chocolate agar plates which are incubated 18 to 24 h in a candle jar or in a more sophisticated apparatus that provides a suitable environment.

The biochemical reactions of the *Neisseria* are relatively limited, but they contain cytochrome oxidase, which is responsible for the positive "oxidase" test; the clinically significant species usually are differentiated by their ability to produce acid in glucose, maltose, or sucrose. Typically the meningococcus ferments both glucose and maltose, but on occasion maltose-negative strains have been isolated.

Meningococci can be divided into serologic groups on the basis of agglutination reactions with immune serum. The present classification into groups A, B, C, and D was agreed upon in 1950, but since 1960, new groups including X, Y, and Z have been identified. The major groups are remarkably heterogeneous, but subclassification with bacteriocin typing or additional serologic markers has been possible. Subcapsular antigens, some of which are proteins, have provided the basis for serological typing schemes, which have been used to divide strains of groups A, B, C, and Y into distinct types that are independent of their capsular serogroup.

EPIDEMIOLOGY The natural habitat of meningococci is the nasopharynx of humans, and no other reservoir or vector has been recognized. The principal means of spread is through inhalation of droplets of infected nasopharyngeal secretions. It is unlikely that the disease is spread by contact with contaminated fomites. Meningococci cause either epidemic or sporadic disease, and there is a cyclic variation in the prevalence of meningococcal infection with peaks of increased frequency occurring every 8 to 12 years and lasting 4 to 6 years. A minor upward trend in this cycle began in the United States in 1962 and reached a peak in 1965. For the epidemic years 1967 through 1971, the attack rate of meningococcal disease was lower and constant, but subsequently it has declined further. The prevalence of meningococcal infection is also subject to seasonal influences; the lowest attack rate occurs in midsummer and the highest in late winter and early spring. This seasonal variation follows that of other bacterial and viral respiratory infections.

The attack rate of meningococcal disease is highest for children between 6 months and 1 year of age. A second, much lower, peak in incidence occurs among adolescents, and the lowest attack rate occurs in individuals over 25. There is no clear-cut tendency for racial or sexual predominance, but presumably because of an increased opportunity to acquire infection, males develop meningitis and meningococcemia more frequently than females. The attack rate in household contacts of sporadic cases of meningococcal disease is 1000 times the overall endemic rate; in epidemic periods, the attack rate among household contacts may be as much as 15,000 times that of the general population. Experience with recent group A outbreaks in Alaska and the northwestern part of the United States indicates that alcoholics and Alaska natives are at increased risk for infection. Military recruits also are particularly susceptible to meningococcal disease, although outbreaks that appear to be restricted to the military usually parallel less apparent trends in the civilian population.

Since 1915, most epidemics of meningococcal disease have been caused by group A meningococci, and strains of groups B and C have been associated with sporadic, interepidemic infections. However, in the United States outbreaks of 1963 and 1964 a major shift in the pattern of meningococcal infection became apparent as group B meningococci were isolated from the majority of clinical infections in both civilian and military populations. In 1967, over 70 percent of meningococci isolated were group B. However, early in 1968, another shift began, and in the epidemic years 1969 through 1972, the majority of meningococcal strains submitted to the Center for Disease Control were group C. More recently, group B has again become the most prevalent serogroup isolated in the United States, and group Y is increasing in importance. This organism is more likely to cause respiratory disease and pneumonia than meningococcemia and meningitis.

Only a small proportion of the meningococci isolated in this country are group A. However, in Alaska and the Pacific Northwest, group A organisms are isolated from 30 to 60 percent of patients with meningococcal disease.

Studies using a serotyping system have allowed identification of a few strains that possess unique epidemic potential. Isolates from group B, C, and Y outbreaks are almost exclusively representatives of two serotypes, with type CII predominating. These observations may have great significance in future vaccine development, because in the case of group B organisms, it is the type-specific antigen which induces bactericidal antibody formation.

Coincident with these epidemiologic shifts has been a waxing and waning of the proportion of isolates which are resistant to sulfadiazine. When the majority of meningococci causing disease were group B, most strains were resistant to sulfadiazine. Today, approximately 95 percent are sensitive. Similarly, as group C emerged as the predominant serogroup, sulfadiazine resistance was the rule, but in the epidemic year 1974, about one-third of group C isolates were sensitive. Sulfadiazine resistance has been recognized among isolates of all major serogroups, and future major shifts may occur.

The potential for the meningococcus to produce serious outbreaks of disease has been reemphasized by recent events in Brazil and Finland. A large urban epidemic was first recognized in São Paulo in 1971, and it increased in intensity over the next several years. In 1974, the predominant strain of meningococcus producing disease there changed abruptly from group C to group A, and the epidemic spread to other major cities in Brazil. In July and August, 1974, about 13,000 cases of meningococcal disease occurred in São Paulo alone. An epidemic of group A meningococcal disease began in Finland early in 1973. It peaked in 1974 when the incidence of infection rose to 15 per 100,000 population (in the same year, there were 0.6 cases per 100,000 population in the United States). Massive immunization programs apparently have curtailed both of these major epidemics.

Carriers Between epidemics, 2 to 15 percent of the individuals in urban centers harbor meningococci in the nasopharynx. When sporadic cases of meningococcal disease occur, the carrier rate in close contacts may rise to 40 percent, and in closed populations or during epidemics, may approach 100 percent. Although some individuals harbor meningococci for years, nasopharyngeal infection is usually transient, and in 75 percent of carriers the organism disappears within a few weeks to a few months. The relation between the proportion of carriers in a population and the occurrence of meningococcal disease is un-

clear. Case-to-case transmission of infection is documented rarely, and carriers, not patients, are the foci from which disease is spread. It appears that the prevalence of meningococcal disease can be attributed to the prevailing carrier rate only in a general way, and that the occurrence of clinical disease is most dependent on unknown circumstances within the host which lead to spread of infection beyond the nasopharynx.

Immunity The fact that meningococcal meningitis is primarily a disease of childhood has suggested that natural immunity develops in most individuals within the first two decades of life. There is a correlation between susceptibility to meningococcal disease and absence of bactericidal antibody in the serum, and the serum of most adults contains antibodies to pathogenic strains of meningococci. Natural immunization appears to result from asymptomatic carriage of meningococci in the nasopharynx. Not only does the carrier state produce antibodies to the infecting strain, but cross-reacting antibodies may develop, even after colonization with avirulent nongroupable organisms. Nasopharyngeal carriage of a closely related species, *N. lactamica,* also may play a role in the development of natural immunity to meningococcal disease.

The immunity conferred by meningococcal meningitis or meningococcemia is usually group-specific, and second episodes of meningococcal disease have been encountered only infrequently.

PATHOGENESIS The primary focus of meningococcal infection is the nasopharynx. In most instances, this infection is subclinical, but occasionally localized inflammation occurs and mild symptoms develop. Dissemination of meningococci from the nasopharynx occurs via the bloodstream, and generally is followed by clinical manifestations of meningococcal disease. *Purulent meningitis* is the most common form of metastatic infection encountered and is either associated with signs and symptoms of meningococcemia or constitutes the predominant clinical expression of illness. Organisms in the meninges induce an acute inflammatory reaction, and purulent exudate spreads across the surface of the brain. Rarely, a more extensive inflammatory reaction is responsible for an acute diffuse encephalitis.

Although the mechanisms responsible for the pathologic changes associated with meningococcal infection have not been explained entirely, the tissue injury observed in laboratory animals appears to be caused by an endotoxin which is biochemically and biologically similar to endotoxins of enteric bacilli. It may be responsible for hypotension and vascular collapse observed in fulminant meningococcemia and may also play a role in the pathogenesis of the purpura and visceral hemorrhages associated with meningococcal bacteremia. Thrombosis of dermal venules, adrenal sinusoids, and renal glomerular capillaries is most commonly seen in patients who die of fulminant meningococcemia and is strikingly similar to the pathologic changes observed in the experimental Shwartzman reaction. It is postulated that endotoxin either induces a Shwartzman reaction directly or effects the release of clotting factors which initiate intravascular coagulation and produce these characteristic pathologic changes.

CLINICAL MANIFESTATIONS Ninety to ninety-five percent of patients with meningococcal disease have meningococcemia and/or meningitis.

Meningococcemia Thirty to fifty percent of patients who develop overt disease have meningococcemia without meningitis.

The onset of clinical illness may be abrupt, but patients usually have nonspecific prodromal symptoms of cough, headache, and sore throat followed by the sudden development of spiking fever, chills, arthralgia, and muscle pains which may be particularly severe in the lower extremities and back. Patients usually appear acutely ill with an inordinate degree of prostration. In addition to high fever, tachycardia, and tachypnea, mild hypotension may be present. However, clinical shock does not occur unless fulminant meningococcemia supervenes. In the course of meningococcal bacteremia, about three-fourths of the patients develop a characteristic petechial rash. Lesions are frequently sparse, and the axillae, flanks, wrists, and ankles are the most commonly involved sites. Often petechiae are located in the center of lighter-colored macules, and they may become nodular as the disease progresses. The diagnosis of meningococcemia occasionally can be established by demonstrating gram-negative diplococci in scrapings from these nodular lesions. In severe cases, purpuric spots or large ecchymoses develop, and a widespread petechial or purpuric eruption suggests fulminating disease. However, the absence of rash does not necessarily indicate that the illness will be mild.

Fulminant meningococcemia, or the Waterhouse-Friderichsen syndrome, is meningococcemia associated with vasomotor collapse and shock. It occurs in 10 to 20 percent of patients with generalized meningococcal infection, and is associated with a high fatality rate. The onset is abrupt, and profound prostration frequently occurs within a few hours. Petechiae and purpuric lesions enlarge rapidly, and hemorrhage into the skin may be extensive. Early in the preshock stage, there is generalized vasoconstriction; patients are alert and pale, with circumoral cyanosis and cold extremities. Upon entering the shock stage, however, coma develops, the cardiac output decreases, and the blood pressure drops. Unless incipient shock is recognized and appropriate therapy instituted early, death from cardiac and/or respiratory failure almost invariably occurs. Patients who recover may have extensive sloughing of skin lesions and even loss of digits because of gangrene.

Chronic meningococcemia is a rare form of meningococcal infection which lasts for weeks or months and is characterized by fever, rash, and arthritis or arthralgia. Typically, the fever is intermittent, and during afebrile periods, which may last several days, patients appear remarkably well. The usual rash is a maculopapular or polymorphous eruption which waxes and wanes with the fever, but petechial or nodular lesions may be seen. Joint involvement is present in two-thirds of the patients, and splenomegaly is detected in about 20 percent. If the diagnosis is not suspected or treatment is otherwise delayed, complications such as meningitis, carditis, or nephritis may occur.

Meningitis Meningitis is a common form of meningococcal disease which occurs primarily in children over 6 months of age and in adolescents. Fever, vomiting, headache, and confusion or lethargy are the commonest symptoms; in about one-fourth of the patients, symptoms begin abruptly and rapidly increase in severity. The more typical patient, however, has symptoms of an upper respiratory tract infection followed by an illness which progresses over several days. Twenty to forty percent of patients have meningitis without clinical evidence of meningococcemia, and the diagnosis depends upon bacteriologic examination of the cerebrospinal fluid. However, when meningitis occurs in association with a petechial or purpuric rash, a presumptive diagnosis of meningococcal disease is warranted, because this pattern of illness is seen only rarely in other infections.

Barer manifestations The meningococcus is a rare cause of purulent conjunctivitis or sinusitis. Primary pneumonia previously was considered a rare manifestation of meningococcal infection, but increasing numbers of cases are being reported. In one study of military recruits, 68 cases of clinical pneumonia due to group Y meningococci were reported. Bacterial endocarditis, primary pericarditis, and osteomyelitis have also been reported. On rare occasion, meningococci have produced genital infections clinically indistinguishable from gonococcal disease. *Neisseria meningitidis* has been isolated with increasing frequency from the genitourinary tract and anal canal of symptomatic and asymptomatic patients of both sexes.

LABORATORY FINDINGS Aside from bacteriologic data, laboratory studies are of little value in establishing the diagnosis of meningococcal infection. Polymorphonuclear leukocyte counts usually range from 12,000 to 40,000 cells per cubic millimeter, but in meningococcemia, normal or low leukocyte counts may be encountered. Anemia is uncommon, and levels of serum electrolytes and blood urea nitrogen are normal unless shock develops. Patients with prominent hemorrhagic manifestations may have low platelet counts and decreased levels of circulating clotting factors as a result of intravascular coagulation. In meningitis, the cerebrospinal fluid pressure is increased, and the fluid usually contains from 100 to 40,000 polymorphonuclear leukocytes per cubic millimeter. The protein content is increased, and the concentration of glucose is almost always less than 35 mg per 100 ml and often is between 0 and 10 mg per 100 ml.

Meningococci can be recovered readily from cultures of blood or spinal fluid, and, on occasion, material aspirated from skin lesions or joints yields the organism. In addition, gram-negative diplococci may be seen in stains of nodular petechiae or the buffy coat of blood from patients with meningococcemia. In meningococcal meningitis, a smear of the spinal fluid is diagnostic in about half the patients but often shows only a few intracellular bacteria which are located with difficulty.

COMPLICATIONS Herpes labialis occurs in 5 to 20 percent of patients with meningococcal disease. Other complications, which result from neurologic damage or secondary foci of infection, are uncommon following appropriate treatment and are often transient. Seizures or deafness occur in 10 to 20 percent of patients during the acute stages of meningitis, but postmeningitic epilepsy is rare, and the frequency of permanent eighth nerve damage is probably less than 5 percent. Peripheral neuropathy, cranial nerve palsies, and hemiplegia are seen occasionally, but usually clear completely within 2 to 4 months. Hydrocephalus and thrombosis of venous sinuses, once frequent sequelae of meningococcal meningitis, are encountered rarely. A number of patients complain of recurrent headache, emotional lability, insomnia, backache, memory loss, and difficulty in concentrating for months after an episode of meningitis. The organic basis for these symptoms is obscure, but they usually disappear a year or two after the infection.

Arthritis is a common metastatic complication of meningococcemia and occurs in 2 to 10 percent of patients. As a rule, multiple joints are involved, and signs and symptoms may not appear until after treatment of meningitis or meningococcemia has been instituted. Joint fluid usually contains many granulocytes, but meningococci are recovered infrequently. Antibiotic therapy does not appear to influence the course of the arthritis, and permanent joint changes are rare. Other purulent complications have become extremely uncommon since antibiotics have gained widespread use. Pneumonia occurs occasionally, but it is uncertain whether it is caused by the meningococcus or coincident infection with other bacteria. Bacterial endocarditis is quite rare, but *a high proportion of patients who die of meningococcal infection have myocarditis.* The etiology of these myocardial changes is uncertain, but cardiac failure may be an important factor in the pathogenesis of the shock syndrome in meningococcemia. A pericardial friction rub or electrocardiographic change of pericarditis is seen in about 5 percent of patients, and rarely purulent pericarditis may develop.

DIAGNOSIS The diagnosis of meningococcal disease depends upon recovering *N. meningitidis* from cultures of blood, spinal fluid, or petechial scrapings from patients with a typical clinical picture. Where available, counterimmunoelectrophoresis of biological fluids to detect meningococcal antigen may be helpful. Recovery of meningococci from the nasopharynx does not, in itself, establish the diagnosis.

Few diseases need to be considered seriously in the differential diagnosis of meningococcal disease. If meningococcal meningitis is not accompanied by manifestations of bacteremia, it is indistinguishable from meningitis caused by other common pathogens. Occasionally, the common viral exanthems, Rocky Mountain spotted fever (Chap. 164), and vascular purpuras may be confused with meningococcemia, and their differentiation depends upon demonstration of the organism and knowledge of the epidemiology and clinical manifestations of each disease.

TREATMENT Antimicrobial therapy of suspected or documented meningococcal disease should be instituted as early as possible. Penicillin G is the drug of choice, and should be administered intravenously. The dosage for treatment of meningitis in adults is 12 to 24 million units per day, and in the pediatric age group, 16 million units per square meter (day). Meningococcemia can be treated with 5 to 10 million units per day, because it is not necessary to achieve high levels of antibiotic in the spinal fluid. If treatment with these doses is continued for a minimum of 7 days, or 4 to 5 days after the patient becomes afebrile, relapse is extremely rare. Ampicillin in doses of 200 to 400 mg/kg per day is as effective as penicillin G. When bacteriologic confirmation of meningococcal disease is available, however, treatment should be switched to penicillin G because it is less costly. Meningococci are susceptible to other antimicrobial agents such as chloramphenicol and tetracycline, but they should not be used unless a patient is allergic to penicillin. Under these circumstances, chloramphenicol hemisuccinate 4.0 to 6.0 g per day in divided doses (in adults) is an acceptable alternate. Sensitivity tests usually indicate that cephalothin could be a suitable alternative to penicillin, but treatment failures with this drug have been reported. *Because a significant proportion of meningococci isolated are resistant to sulfonamides, these drugs should not be used alone in the treatment of meningococcal infections,* and their use in combination with penicillin offers no advantage.

Patients with meningococcal infections require supportive treatment as well as antimicrobial therapy. Maintenance of fluid and electrolyte balance and prevention of respiratory complications in comatose patients are of primary concern. When shock occurs, visceral perfusion must be improved by maintenance of an adequate intravascular volume, treatment of heart failure, and support of the blood pressure. Vasoactive drugs should be employed according to the pathophysiologic derangement in each individual case. These derangements can be determined best by carefully monitoring the blood pressure, pulse, arterial blood gases, cardiac output, peripheral resistance, pulmonary artery wedge pressures, and arteriovenous oxygen differences. When blood pressure must be raised immediately, norepinephrine may be indicated. However, if improved tissue perfusion is the primary goal, an agent such as dopamine is likely to be more effective. When heart failure is present, diuretics and digitalis should be given. When intravas-

cular coagulation is recognized, treatment with heparin, whole blood, or fibrinogen can be tried, but dramatic results should not be expected. Massive doses of adrenal cortical steroids as used in the treatment of septic shock (Chap. 109) may be helpful, but lower "replacement" doses are of uncertain value.

PREVENTION With the widespread emergence of sulfonamide-resistant meningococci, alternate methods of preventing meningococcal disease in closed populations were sought. High-molecular-weight polysaccharide antigens from organisms of serogroups A and C have been shown to induce a group-specific bactericidal antibody response after subcutaneous injection. Large-scale field trials with the group C vaccine led to a 90 percent reduction in group C disease among vaccinated recruits. Similar results have been observed with group A vaccine in the Brazilian and Finnish epidemics. An effective group B vaccine has not yet been developed.

For intimate contacts of sporadic cases of meningococcal disease, chemoprophylaxis should be administered. If the organism isolated from the patient is sensitive to sulfonamides, these drugs are preferred for prophylaxis. When sensitivities are not known or the organism is resistant to sulfonamides, rifampin in dosage of 600 mg a day for 4 days or minocycline in dosage of 100 mg every 12 h for 5 days can be expected to temporarily eradicate the carrier state and minimize spread of meningococci. Because of some reports of a high incidence of vestibular symptoms with minocycline, rifampin is considered by some to be the drug of choice. However, in large populations, rifampin may not be effective because of rapid appearance of rifampin resistance.

With increased availability of group A and C vaccines, their use as adjuncts to chemoprophylaxis for household or other intimate contacts of sporadic cases of group A or C meningococcal disease has been recommended. The rationale behind this recommendation is sound, and this approach to prevention of secondary cases deserves consideration.

PROGNOSIS Before the introduction of antibiotics, meningococcal meningitis, and meningococcemia were almost invariably fatal. With prompt and appropriate chemotherapy, the mortality rate of meningitis without fulminant meningococcemia has dropped to less than 10 percent in the United States, and neurologic sequelae are rare. The mortality of fulminant infection remains high primarily because patients are often in irreversible shock when treatment is instituted. Most deaths occur within 24 to 48 h of admission, and the capacity of the meningococcus to kill a perfectly healthy individual within a few hours remains one of the most awesome characteristics of this disease.

REFERENCES

DAVIS CE, ARNOLD K: Role of meningococcal endotoxin in meningococcal purpura. J Exp Med 140:158, 1974

JACOBSON JA et al: Trends in meningococcal disease, 1974. J Infect Dis 132:480, 1975

KOPPES, GM et al: Group Y meningococcal disease in United States Air Force recruits. Am J Med 62:661, 1977

MCCORMICK JB, BENNETT JV: Public health considerations in the management of meningococcal disease. Ann Intern Med 83:883, 1975

MENINGOCOCCAL DISEASE SURVEILLANCE GROUP: Analysis of endemic meningococcal disease by serogroup and evaluation of chemoprophylaxis. J Infect Dis 134:201, 1976

PELTOLA H et al: Vaccination against meningococcal group A disease in Finland 1974–75. Scand J Infect Dis 8:169, 1976

———— et al: Clinical efficacy of meningococcus Group A capsular polysaccharide vaccine in children three months to five years of age. N Engl J Med 297:686, 1977

SMILACK JD: Group Y meningococcal disease. Ann Intern Med 81:740, 1974

119
GONOCOCCAL INFECTIONS

KING K. HOLMES

DEFINITION Gonorrhea, an infection of columnar and transitional epithelium caused by *Neisseria gonorrhoeae,* is the most common reportable communicable disease in the United States. Anatomic sites which can be infected directly by the gonococcus include the urethra, anal canal, conjunctivas, pharynx, and endocervix. Local complications include endometritis, salpingitis, peritonitis, and bartholinitis in the female, and periurethral abscess and epididymitis in the male. Systemic manifestations of gonococcemia include arthritis, dermatitis, endocarditis, and meningitis as well as myopericarditis and hepatitis.

ETIOLOGY *Neisseria gonorrhoeae* is a gram-negative diplococcus which forms oxidase-positive colonies and is differentiated from other *Neisseria* by its ability to dissimilate glucose, but not maltose, sucrose, or lactose, or by specific immunofluorescent staining.

At least four morphologically distinct forms of colonies occur when gonococci are passed in vitro. Colony forms T_1 and T_2 retain virulence during repeated selective subculture in vitro and are covered by surface projections called *pili,* which are visible on electron microscopy. Spontaneous transition to colony forms T_3 and T_4 results in some loss of virulence, together with disappearance of pili. Gonococcal strains cannot be differentiated by colonial morphology since each strain gives rise to all colony forms. However, gonococcal strains now can be typed on the basis of nutritional auxotrophic requirements (auxotyping) or surface antigenic variation.

EPIDEMIOLOGY The only natural hosts for *N. gonorrhoeae* are humans. One million cases of gonorrhea were reported in the United States in 1977, and an estimated 2 million cases went unreported. The annual incidence rates quadrupled from 1960 to 1975 and then leveled off. The peak incidence rates occur from ages 20 to 24 (2 cases per 100 population per year); 85 percent of the cases are age 30 or younger. The reported incidence rate in the United States is now three times higher than in England and Wales. The true incidence rate is probably nearly 10 times higher in the United States, since reporting of gonorrhea is far more complete in the United Kingdom, where most patients with gonorrhea are seen in public clinics for sexually transmitted diseases. Suboptimal clinical practice, including use of subcurative therapy and especially failure to trace infected contacts, probably contributes to the higher incidence rate in the United States.

Gonorrhea incidence and prevalence rates are known to be related to age, sex, race, socioeconomic status, and marital status—risk factors which influence sexual behavior, illness behavior, and accessibility of health care. The highest rates occur at ages 18 to 19, in noncaucasians, in the poor, in large cities, and in unmarried persons—particularly those who live alone.

The incidence is perceived as highest in men, while the prevalence is perceived as highest in women. The prevalence rate is so high among women in the United States that endocervical cultures are advocated for gonorrhea case detection in sexually active asymptomatic women age 30 or under. Approximately 2 percent of women tested by private physicians have gonorrhea. Unfortunately, there is now greater reliance in the United States upon routine endocervical culturing than upon contact tracing, which is far more efficient for control of gonorrhea. The single most important axiom about the epidemiology of this disease is that *gonorrhea is usually spread by carriers who have no symptoms or have ignored symptoms.* Symptomatic patients, male or female, have usually been recently infected by such carriers, who must in turn be traced and treated to prevent reinfection. *Men and women with symptomatic gonorrhea should always be interviewed to identify their recent sex contacts, who should be examined and treated if infected.*

There are interesting regional differences in the antibiotic resistance of *N. gonorrhoeae.* Resistance is greatest in Southeast Asia and Africa where prophylactic or low-dose therapy is common; intermediate in the United States and Australia; and least in Scandinavia, the United Kingdom, and Western Europe. Increasing levels of gonococcal resistance to penicillin G and tetracycline were noted during the 1960s in the United States, where subcurative therapy was common and importation of resistant strains occurred during the Vietnam war. From 1970 through 1975, no further increase in resistance to these antibiotics was noted in the United States. However, in 1976, β-lactamase–producing strains of *N. gonorrhoeae,* completely resistant to penicillin and ampicillin, appeared almost simultaneously in two areas of the world: in England, where they had probably been imported from West Africa, and in the United States where they had clearly been imported from the Philippines. Infections with these penicillin-resistant gonococci are not cured by pencillin therapy. The β-lactamase enzymes produced by these strains are coded on small plasmids which have DNA sequences homologous with the β-lactamase plasmid that first appeared in *Hemophilus influenzae* just 4 years earlier. Such plasmids were not present in gonococci prior to 1976. The African and Asian β-lactamase–producing gonococci show intriguing differences. The African plasmid has a molecular weight of 3.2 million Daltons and has been found in only one particular gonococcal auxotype. The Asian plasmid, which can be found in 20 to 50 percent of gonococci isolated in some cities in the Philippine island of Luzon, is slightly larger and has entered several different auxotypes and serotypes of gonococci. This is probably because the Asian β-lactamase frequently coexists with a larger, conjugative plasmid which is capable of transferring the β-lactamase plasmid to other bacterial cells such as other types of gonococci. This type of molecular epidemiology is instructive—both β-lactamase–producing plasmids apparently enter gonococci and persist in gonococci in areas of the world where prostitution is exceptionally common and where access to subcurative antimicrobial therapy is unrestricted. Fortunately, β-lactamase–producing gonococci have not become established in any of the industrialized countries. Although localized outbreaks have occurred in several cities in the United States and England, they have been contained by rapid use of epidemiologic measures (Fig. 119-1).

CLINICAL MANIFESTATIONS The clinical spectrum of gonococcal infections depends upon the site of inoculation, the duration of infection, and the presence or absence of local or systemic spread of the organism.

Gonorrhea in the male The usual incubation period of gonococcal urethritis ("clap") in the male is 2 to 6 days following exposure, although longer intervals are not infrequent, and

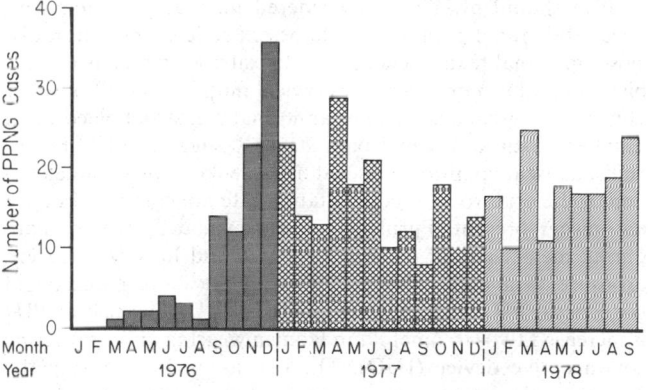

FIGURE 119-1

Penicillinase-producing Neisseria gonorrhoeae (PPNG). The number of cases occurring by month in the United States (including outlying areas) from March 1976 to September 1978. (Courtesy of P Perine.)

some men never develop symptoms. In one study, one fastidious auxotype, which has distinctive nutritional requirements, was associated with 96 percent of asymptomatic infections and only 40 percent of symptomatic infections. Symptoms include a purulent urethral discharge, usually associated with dysuria and frequent urination. Although approximately 90 to 95 percent of men who acquire urethral gonococcal infection develop urethral discharge, most symptomatic men seek treatment and are removed from the infectious pool. The remaining men who never develop symptoms or who ignore their symptoms constitute about two-thirds of the infected men at any point in time, and they serve as the source of spread of infection to women. Before antibiotic treatment became available, symptoms of urethritis persisted for an average of 8 weeks, and unilateral epididymitis occurred in 5 to 10 percent of untreated men. Epididymitis is now an uncommon complication (see below), and gonococcal prostatitis occurs rarely, if at all. Other local complications of gonorrhea which are now unusual include inguinal lymphadenitis, edema of the penis due to dorsal lymphangitis or thrombophlebitis, submucous inflammatory "soft" infiltration of the urethral wall, periurethral abscess or fistula, unilateral inflammation or abscess of Cowper's gland (which lies between the thumb and forefinger when the forefinger is in the anal canal and the thumb is positioned anteriorly on the perineum), abscess of Tyson's gland(s) (which open on either side of the frenulum), and, rarely, seminal vesiculitis.

In homosexual men, anorectal and pharyngeal gonococcal infection are common. Anorectal infection may be asymptomatic from the outset or may produce anorectal burning or pruritus, tenesmus, and a bloody, mucopurulent rectal discharge. Proctoscopy is essential to exclude syphilis, lymphogranuloma venereum, granuloma inguinale, and other conditions which cause similar symptoms. These symptoms may subside without treatment, leaving a chronic asymptomatic carrier state. Pharyngeal gonococcal infection occurs in approximately 20 percent of homosexual men or heterosexual women who engage in fellatio with men who have urethral infection. Pharyngeal infection may produce exudative tonsillitis but frequently is asymptomatic.

Gonorrhea in the female Acute uncomplicated gonorrhea in the female often causes dysuria, frequent urination, increased vaginal discharge due to exudative endocervicitis, abnormal menstrual bleeding, and anorectal discomfort. While dysuria and frequency in young men arouse the suspicion of gonococcal urethritis, the same symptoms in a young woman are often automatically attributed to "cystitis." Actually, only about one-half of young women with these symptoms are found to

have at least 10^5 coliform bacteria per ml of clean voided midstream urine, while many of those without significant bacteriuria have gonococcal infection of the urethra and of Skene's glands. Young women with dysuria should have a pelvic examination and endocervical culture for gonorrhea. Compression of the urethra through the anterior vaginal wall against the symphysis pubis may express urethral exudate which can be examined by Gram's stain and culture. Acute symptoms of gonococcal urethritis in the female may subside spontaneously or following subcurative therapy with sulfonamides or urinary antiseptics. The proportion of women with gonorrhea who never develop symptoms is undefined.

Asymptomatic gonococcal infection in the female involves the endocervix, urethra, anal canal, and pharynx, in decreasing order of frequency. Extension of infection from the endocervix to the fallopian tubes occurs in at least 15 percent of women with gonorrhea. This tends to occur soon after acquisition of infection or during menstruation and results in *acute salpingitis,* the major complication of gonorrhea. Extension of infection to the pelvis may produce signs of pelvic peritonitis, accompanied by nausea and vomiting, and may lead to pelvic abscess. Early antibiotic treatment, before development of adnexal masses, restores normal tubal function and fertility in nearly all cases of salpingitis. However, if prominent adnexal swelling has occurred before treatment is begun, bilateral tubal dysfunction occurs in 15 to 25 percent.

Spread of gonococci into the upper abdomen may cause *gonococcal perihepatitis* (Fitz-Hugh–Curtis syndrome) manifested by right upper quadrant or bilateral upper abdominal pain and tenderness, and occasionally by a hepatic friction rub.

Acute inflammation of Bartholin's gland is usually unilateral and frequently is due to gonococcal infection. The acutely infected duct is surrounded by a red halo and exudes pus at the posterior third of the labium majus. Occlusion of the duct results in formation of a Bartholin's abscess. Chronic Bartholin cysts are rarely caused by active gonococcal infection.

There is suggestive evidence that endocervical gonococcal infection is associated with prematurity and prolonged labor following rupture of membranes, both of which may produce increased perinatal morbidity.

Gonorrhea in children During childbirth, the gonococcus may infect the conjunctivas, pharynx, respiratory tract, or anal canal of the newborn. The risk of contamination increases with prolonged rupture of membranes. Prevention of gonococcal ophthalmia by prophylactic use of 1% silver nitrate eyedrops has led to the emergence of inclusion conjunctivitis caused by *Chlamydia* as a more common form of ophthalmia neonatorum. During the first year of life, infection of the infant usually results from accidental contamination of the eye or vagina by an adult. Between 1 year of age and puberty, most cases of gonorrhea involve vulvovaginitis in females who have been molested by a relative, and medicolegal considerations necessitate a complete bacteriologic diagnosis.

Disseminated gonococcal infection In some areas of the world, from 1 to 3 percent of adults with gonococcal infection develop gonococcemia. Approximately two-thirds of such patients are women. The majority of men and women with gonococcemia do not have symptoms of urogenital, anorectal, or pharyngeal gonococcal infection. Gonococcemia may occur soon after acquisition of new infection or later, during menstruation. There is suggestive evidence that gonococci which cause disseminated infection are uniquely resistant to the complement-mediated bactericidal activity of normal human serum. These organisms tend to be fastidious strains with the same distinctive auxotype that is correlated with asymptomatic urethral infection in men. Patients with deficiency in the sixth, seventh, and eighth components of complement have increased susceptibility to gonococcemia and meningococcemia, but not to other infections. Nine of the first seventeen patients reported to have a deficiency of C6, C7, and C8 had at least one episode of documented bacteremia with *N. gonorrhoeae* or *N. meningitidis*. Serum bactericidal activity, rather than opsonic activity, appears essential for protection against gonococcal bacteremia.

The onset of gonococcemia is characterized by fever, polyarthralgias, and papular, petechial, pustular, hemorrhagic, or necrotic skin lesions. Approximately 3 to 20 such lesions appear, usually on the distal extremities. Gonococci are demonstrable by immunofluorescent staining in about two-thirds of gonococcal skin lesions. The initial joint involvement is characteristically limited to tenosynovitis involving several joints asymmetrically. The wrists, fingers, knees, and ankles are most often involved. Circulating immune complexes have been demonstrated at this stage of infection. Without treatment, the duration of gonococcemia is variable; the systemic manifestations of bacteremia may subside spontaneously within a week. (It is possible that many such cases go undiagnosed and the actual risk of gonococcemia exceeds current estimates.) Alternatively, septic arthritis ensues, often without prior symptoms of bacteremia. Pain and swelling then increase in one or, very occasionally, more joints, with accumulation of purulent synovial fluid, leading to progressive destruction of the joint if treatment is delayed. A continuum exists from the manifestations of bacteremia (polyarthralgias, new skin lesions) to septic arthritis, but the probability of positive blood cultures decreases after 48 h of illness, and the probability of recovery of gonococci from synovial fluid increases with increasing duration of illness. Gonococci are infrequently recovered from early effusions containing less than 20,000 leukocytes per cubic millimeter, but are usually recovered from effusions containing more than 80,000 leukocytes per cubic millimeter. In the individual patient, gonococci are seldom recovered from blood and synovial fluid simultaneously.

Other common manifestations of disseminated gonococcal infection include mild myopericarditis and "toxic" hepatitis. Endocarditis and meningitis are infrequent but severe complications. Endocarditis is suggested by pathological or changing heart murmurs, major embolic phenomena, severe myocarditis, deterioration of renal function, or an unusually large number of skin lesions.

DIFFERENTIAL DIAGNOSIS Gonococcal infection produces several common clinical syndromes which have multiple etiologies or which mimic other conditions. The differential diagnosis of urethritis in men and of vaginitis and cervicitis is discussed in Chap. 113. Three additional complications of gonorrhea are discussed below.

Pelvic inflammatory disease (PID) The incidence of acute, spontaneous PID, unrelated to obstetrical complications or surgery, can be estimated as about a half-million cases per year in the United States. About 50 percent of these are caused by *N. gonorrhoeae*, alone or in combination with cervicovaginal commensal bacteria. Nongonococcal PID is usually caused by cervicovaginal bacteria, including *Bacteroides fragilis* and anaerobic gram-positive cocci. The peak incidence of gonorrhea occurs in the late summer and autumn each year, and the proportion of cases of PID which are associated with gonococcal infection is also highest during these months.

PID should always be considered in young women with lower abdominal pain and tenderness. Pelvic examination discloses maximal tenderness in the adnexal area, which is usually bilateral and is reproduced by cervical motion. Recent onset of abnormal vaginal discharge or abnormal menstrual bleeding in a patient with abdominal pain strongly suggests PID. Fever, chills, nausea, vomiting, adnexal mass, leukocytosis, and elevation of the erythroctye sedimentation rate are common but are *not always* present. Purulent cervical exudate, onset of pain during menstruation, dysuria, proctitis, and history of recent exposure to a male with urethritis all are more common in gonococcal PID than in nongonococcal PID. The risk of PID is increased two- to ninefold in women wearing an intrauterine contraceptive device (IUD). The risk is maximal during the first 2 months after insertion, but persists as long as the device is in place. IUD-associated salpingitis usually is nongonococcal. There is no fever, and the major manifestation is indolent progression of minimally symptomatic adnexal masses.

Gonococcal perihepatitis may mimic acute cholecystitis, with transient nonvisualization of the gallbladder and mild liver function abnormalities. Perihepatitis should be distinguished from the hepatitis which occurs during gonococcemia. Perihepatitis also occurs as a complication of nongonococcal PID, presumably resulting from spread of other bacteria from the pelvis to the upper abdomen. Bacteremia and suppurative pelvic thrombophlebitis are unusual in acute spontaneously occurring PID.

The clinical diagnosis of PID is imprecise, and failure to respond to appropriate antibiotic therapy should always lead to reevaluation of the diagnosis before consideration of a change in antibiotics. Laparoscopy may disclose other diagnoses, such as ectopic pregnancy, acute appendicitis, pelvic endometriosis, corpus luteum hematoma, ovarian tumor, mesenteric lymphadenitis, or occasional complications such as tuboovarian abscess.

Epididymitis Acute epididymitis is almost always unilateral and must be differentiated from testicular torsion, tumor, and trauma. Torsion, a surgical emergency, occurs predominantly in teen-agers and is suggested by the acuteness of the pain, elevation of the testicle within the scrotal sac, and abscess of blood flow on Doppler-flow examination. In men under 35, acute epididymitis is usually caused by *N. gonorrhoeae* or *Chlamydia trachomatis* and is usually, but not always, associated with urethral exudate, demonstrable by milking the urethra. The recommended treatment includes bed rest, scrotal elevation, and antimicrobial therapy. Treatment of gonococcal epididymitis is the same as for gonococcal pelvic inflammatory disease. Optimal treatment for nongonococcal epididymitis (presumably caused by *C. trachomatis* in men under 35) is tetracycline hydrochloride, 500 mg four times daily by mouth for 10 days.

Acute epididymitis in older men is usually caused by urinary pathogens such as *Escherichia coli* or *Pseudomonas aeruginosa*. Urethritis is usually absent, but bacteriuria is present. Treatment should be with the appropriate antibiotics as determined by sensitivity tests.

Acute arthritis The gonococcal arthritis-dermatitis syndrome is probably the commonest form of acute arthritis in young adults, and must be differentiated in particular from Reiter's syndrome, other forms of septic arthritis, acute rheumatoid arthritis, and systemic lupus erythematosus. Gonococcemia may be complicated by myocarditis, which mimics acute rheumatic fever or bacterial endocarditis, and by "toxic" hepatitis, which must be differentiated from hepatitis B viremia. Meningococcemia, *Yersinia* infection, and sarcoidosis are less common causes of acute polyarthritis.

Demonstration of *N. gonorrhoeae* by culture or specific immunofluorescent antibody stain in synovial fluid, blood, cerebrospinal fluid, or skin lesions is diagnostic of acute gonococcal arthritis. Failing this, the diagnosis of gonococcal arthritis is virtually certain if (1) *N. gonorrhoeae* is recovered from the urethra, cervix, pharynx, anal canal, or conjunctiva, or from the patient's sex partner; (2) pustular, hemorrhagic, or necrotic skin lesions are distributed on the extremities; and (3) a therapeutic antibiotic trial produces subjective improvement and normal temperature within 48 h, and loss of all objective signs of arthritis within 2 weeks. Patients with gonococcal arthritis who have highly purulent synovial effusions may, however, have persistent fever and progressive arthritis despite adequate antimicrobial therapy, and may require repeated closed joint irrigations with saline before improvement occurs.

If only two of the above three criteria are met, the diagnosis of gonococcal arthritis remains probable, particularly if other diagnoses listed above are excluded. Conjunctivitis rarely occurs in gonococcal arthritis and suggests the diagnosis of Reiter's syndrome in men with acute arthritis. HLA histocompatibility haplotype B27 is associated with Reiter's syndrome but not with gonococcal arthritis. Gonococcal arthritis has been reported in several women with active lupus erythematosus, in whom hypocomplementemia may predispose to gonococcemia.

LABORATORY DIAGNOSIS The Gram's stain of urethral or endocervical exudate is considered diagnostic of gonorrhea when typical gram-negative diplococci are seen within leukocytes, is equivocal if only extracellular or atypical gram-negative diplococci are seen, and is negative if no gram-negative diplococci are seen. When these criteria are employed by experienced microbiologists, the sensitivity and specificity of Gram's stain of the urethral exudate approach 100 percent. The specificity of Gram's stain of purulent cervical exudate also is high, but the sensitivity is only 60 percent or less. Thayer-Martin (TM) medium, which contains antibiotics to inhibit most other organisms selectively, is most useful for recovering the gonococcus from the endocervix, anal canal, and pharynx, which are colonized by a mixed bacterial flora. After inoculation, the TM medium should be placed in an atmosphere containing 3 to 10 percent carbon dioxide to permit growth of the gonococcus. This can be accomplished in a candle jar, by packaging the TM medium in sealed vials to which carbon dioxide was added before sealing (Transgrow medium), or by generation of carbon dioxide chemically within packets which are sealed after inoculation. Inoculated media should be incubated at 36°C for 48 h, and putative gonococcal colonies should be confirmed by oxidase reaction, Gram's stain, and sugar fermentation tests. The latter are especially important for isolates from the pharynx and anal canal and for cultures obtained from populations which have a low prevalence of gonorrhea, such as prenatal patients. Anal canal cultures are most important as a test of cure in women, since about one-quarter of all treatment failures in women involve only that site.

In men with incubating or chronic asymptomatic urethral infection without exudate, or as a test of cure following treatment, a very thin cotton swab or wire bacteriologic loop should be inserted 2 cm into the anterior urethra and used to inoculate TM medium. Cultures of the pharynx and anal canal should be obtained from all homosexual men with suspected gonorrhea.

The most efficient test for gonorrhea in women is the endocervical culture, which is positive on a single examination in approximately 80 percent of those with gonorrhea. This diagnostic yield can be increased by performing a second endocervical culture on enriched chocolate agar medium which does not contain antibiotics and by performing cultures of the anal canal, urethra, and pharynx.

Standard blood culture broth medium containing 3 to 10 percent carbon dioxide should be used in culturing blood and is also recommended for culturing synovial fluid. In pus from skin lesions, *N. gonorrhoeae* is more often demonstrable by Gram's stain or immunofluorescent staining than by culture. A fourfold or greater rise in gonococcal antibody can be demonstrated in paired serums from many patients with gonococcal arthritis, using complement fixation, immunofluorescent, or gonococcal pili antigen-binding assays, but such tests are not generally available. Techniques designed to detect gonococcal infection by testing of a single serum have been limited thus far by inability to differentiate antibody due to past gonorrhea from antibody due to current infection, and by false-positive tests caused by cross-reactive meningococci in the pharynx.

TREATMENT The preferred drugs for gonococcal infection are penicillin G, ampicillin, or amoxicillin, tetracycline hydrochloride, and spectinomycin. As shown in Table 119-1, the Communicable Disease Center (CDC) recommended treatment schedules now list three regimens as coequal choices for uncomplicated gonorrhea in men and women. Single-dose treatment is preferred in patients who are unlikely to complete the multiple-dose tetracycline regimen. The aqueous procaine penicillin G (APPG) regimen is preferred for men with anorectal infection and for pharyngeal infection in men and women. With parenteral penicillin G, the risk of anaphylaxis in patients who deny previous penicillin allergy has been shown to be 0.04 percent. The risk of procaine reaction due to transient neurotoxic serum concentrations of procaine is probably between 0.1 and 1 percent with the currently recommended dosage. Ampicillin 3.5 g (or amoxicillin 3.0 g) can be given orally with probenecid with nearly equal efficacy and less toxicity. A single intramuscular dose of 2 g spectinomycin is adequate for gonorrhea in both sexes and is recommended for treatment failures, because gonococci which demonstrate increased resistance to penicillin, ampicillin, or tetracycline show no cross-resistance to spectinomycin. Most recurrent infections after treatment with the recommended schedules are due to *reinfection* and indicate a need for improved contact tracing and patient education. Since infection by β-lactamase–producing gonococci is a cause of treatment failure, posttreatment isolates should be tested for β-lactamase production. Spectinomycin is the treatment of choice for β-lactamase producing *N. gonorrhoeae*.

Either spectinomycin or tetracycline can be used for penicillin-allergic patients. Tetracycline is no longer effective for gonorrhea as a single dose. Other tetracyclines are not more effective than tetracycline hydrochloride. Tetracycline has the significant advantage of curing simultaneously acquired *Chlamydia* and *Ureaplasma* infections, thus preventing postgonococcal urethritis (PGU). Usually appearing 2 or 3 weeks after treatment, PGU occurs in from 20 to 50 percent of men treated for gonorrhea with penicillin, ampicillin, or spectinomycin.

About half of the cases of PGU appear to be caused by *Chlamydia trachomatis* which was probably acquired at the same time as gonorrhea but did not become clinically apparent until later because of the longer incubation period of chlamydial infection. When PGU occurs, it can be managed, like nongonococcal urethritis, with tetracycline, 0.5 g four times a day for at least 7 days. Men and women exposed to gonorrhea should be examined, cultured, and treated with one of the recommended treatment schedules.

All patients with gonorrhea should have a serologic test for syphilis at the time of diagnosis. Patients with incubating seronegative syphilis, without clinical signs of syphilis, are likely to be cured by any of the recommended regimens (except spectinomycin) and need not have later follow-up tests for syphilis. However, patients with gonorrhea who also have syphilis or who are established contacts of someone with syphilis should be given additional treatment appropriate to the stage of syphilis. As a test of cure of gonorrhea, follow-up cervical, anal canal, and other appropriate cultures should be obtained from women, and urethral and other appropriate cultures from men,

TABLE 119-1
Recommended treatment for gonococcal infection

Diagnosis	Treatment of choice
Uncomplicated gonococcal infection in men and women	Aqueous procaine penicillin G (APPG), 4.8 million units injected intramuscularly, at two sites with 1.0 g probenecid by mouth *or* tetracycline 0.5 g by mouth four times a day for 5 days (total dosage 10.0 g) *or* ampicillin 3.5 g (or amoxicillin 3.0 g) single oral dose, given with 1.0 g probenecid by mouth
Anorectal infection in men	APPG, 4.8 million units, with 1.0 g probenecid
Pharyngeal infection, either sex	APPG, 4.8 million units, with 1.0 g probenecid
Treatment failures	Spectinomycin, 2.0 g intramuscularly
Penicillinase-producing *N. gonorrhoeae*	Spectinomycin, 2.0 g intramuscularly
Gonorrhea in pregnancy	APPG, 4.8 million units intramuscularly with 1.0 g probenecid by mouth (if pregnant patient is allergic to penicillin, spectinomycin 2.0 g intramuscularly is recommended)
Acute PID, outpatient	Tetracycline 0.5 g orally four times a day for 10 days *or* APPG 4.8 million units intramuscularly plus 1.0 g probenecid orally, followed by ampicillin 0.5 g orally four times a day for 10 days
Acute PID, hospitalized	Aqueous crystalline penicillin G, 20 million units intravenously each day until improvement occurs, followed by ampicillin 0.5 g orally four times a day to complete 10 days of therapy. Since optimal therapy for hospitalized patients has not been established, alternative regimens, such as gentamicin plus clindamycin, or chloramphenicol, are often used for severe PID in hospitalized patients.
Acute epididymitis	Tetracycline 0.5 g orally four times a day for 10 days
Disseminated gonococcal infection	Aqueous crystalline penicillin G, 10 million units intravenously per day until improvement occurs, followed by ampicillin 0.5 g four times daily to complete 7 days of therapy *or* ampicillin 3.5 g orally with probenecid 1.0 g, followed by ampicillin 0.5 g orally four times a day for 7 days *Penicillin allergy:* Tetracycline 0.5 g orally four times daily for 7 days
Pediatric gonococcal infection	See "Gonorrhea—CDC recommended treatment schedules" in References

7 to 14 days after completion of therapy. Because true treatment failure is uncommon with the recommended regimen, some authorities advocate one reexamination approximately 6 weeks after treatment, at which time approximately 15 percent of individuals are again infected, presumably because of reinfection.

Hospitalization is recommended for women with suspected salpingitis if the diagnosis is uncertain and surgical emergencies, such as appendicitis or ectopic pregnancy, must be excluded, if there is suspicion of pelvic abscess, if the patient is pregnant or unable to follow an outpatient regimen of oral medication because of nausea and vomiting, if she is severely ill, or if she is not responding to outpatient therapy. Failure to improve on recommended therapy does not indicate a need for stepwise additional antibiotics but requires clinical reassessment. Most authorities recommend removal of an intrauterine device, if present in a woman with acute PID, although the effect of an IUD on response to therapy and risk of recurrence has not been studied. The treatment schedules recommended in Table 119-1 for PID have given satisfactory short-term results in both gonococcal and nongonococcal PID in limited trials, but additional data are needed. It is clear, however, that the single-dose procaine penicillin G-probenecid regimen recommended for uncomplicated gonorrhea is inadequate for the treatment of PID, even for gonococcal PID. For ambulatory patients with nongonococcal PID, tetracycline is the preferred drug. In severe cases of PID, especially when pelvic abscess is suspected, treatment must be individualized, and alternative antibiotics and surgical drainage may be needed. Adequate treatment of women with acute salpingitis must include examination and appropriate treatment of their sex partners because of their high prevalence of nonsympatomatic urethral infection. Failure to treat sex partners is a major cause of recurrent gonococcal salpingitis.

Treatment of gonococcal arthritis can be accomplished satisfactorily with several regimens. Gonococci recovered from patients with gonococcal arthritis have been significantly less resistant to penicillin or tetracycline than isolates from patients with uncomplicated gonorrhea. However, because of the threat of endocarditis, meningitis, and joint sepsis, all patients with disseminated infection should preferably be hospitalized and treated with aqueous crystalline penicillin G intravenously, 10 million units per day until clinical improvement occurs. Treatment can then be completed on an outpatient basis with ampicillin, 2 g per day orally to complete a 7- to 10-day course of therapy. As summarized in the CDC recommendation, a 3-day course of high-dose intravenous penicillin therapy alone, or treatment with ampicillin, 3.5 g daily orally with 1 g probenecid, followed by 0.5 g four times a day for 7 days, also probably represents adequate therapy for disseminated gonococcal infection. Failure to improve with one of these regimens strongly suggests a diagnosis other than disseminated gonococcal infection. Repeated joint aspiration or closed irrigation of the joint with sterile saline may be required to reduce inflammation in patients with high synovial fluid leukocyte counts. Open drainage is seldom, if ever, required for gonococcal arthritis, except in infants with hip infection. Temporary immobilization of the joint may reduce discomfort for the patient and may be useful during initial ambulation in patients with persistent effusions of the knee or ankle. Antibiotics should not be injected directly into the joint.

Gonococcal conjunctivitis in the adult or newborn should be managed as a medical emergency by irrigation of the conjunctiva with saline, together with penicillin G given intravenously.

PREVENTION AND CONTROL There is probably no more striking illustration than gonorrhea of the failure of a specific treatment alone to eradicate a communicable disease. Vaccination is not available, and there is some doubt as to whether any resistance to reinfection occurs during natural infection, although humoral, local, and cellular immune responses have all been demonstrated during acute or recurrent gonococcal infection. Use of the condom can prevent transmission. Prophylactic antibiotics (e.g., 200 mg minocycline or doxycycline taken soon after sexual exposure) have been shown to be effective but are not recommended for general use or for individuals with known exposure to gonorrhea, who should receive one of the regimens recommended for established gonorrhea. The efficacy of local vaginal antiseptic and spermicidal preparations for prevention of venereal disease requires further study. The most effective additional measure now available for control of gonorrhea is tracing sexual contacts of infected patients. Experienced interviewers are able to identify and bring to treatment an average of one additional case for every patient interviewed.

REFERENCES

BROOKS GF et al: Immunobiology of *Neisseria gonorrhaeae*. Washington, DC, American Society of Microbiology, 1978

CUNNINGHAM FG et al: Evaluation of tetracycline or penicillin-ampicillin for treatment of acute pelvic inflammatory disease. N Engl J Med 296:1380, 1977

ESCHENBACH DA et al: Polymicrobial etiology of acute pelvic inflammatory disease. N Engl J Med 293:166, 1975

FALK V: Treatment of acute nontuberculous salpingitis alone and in combination with glucocorticoids. Acta Obstet Gynecol Scand, vol 44, suppl 6, 1965

Gonorrhea—CDC recommended treatment schedules. Morb Mort Week Rep 28:1, 1978

HANDSFIELD HH et al: Treatment of the gonococcal arthritis-dermatitis syndrome. Ann Intern Med 84:661, 1976

HOLMES KK et al: Disseminated gonococcal infection. Ann Intern Med 74:979, 1971

JACOBSEN L, WESTROM L: Objectivized diagnosis of acute pelvic inflammatory disease. Am J Obstet Gynecol 105:1088, 1969

KARNEY WW et al: Spectinomycin vs tetracycline for the treatment of gonorrhea. N Engl J Med 296:889, 1977

KAUFMAN RE et al: National gonorrhea therapy monitoring study: Treatment results. N Engl J Med 294:1, 1976

ROBERTS M et al: Molecular characterization of two beta-lactamase specifying plasmids isolated from *Neisseria gonorrhoeae*. J Bacteriol 131:557, 1977

———, FALKOW S: Conjugal transfer of R plasmids in *Neisseria gonorrhoeae*. Nature 266:630, 1977

ROBERTS RB: *The Gonococcus*. New York, Wiley, 1977

SCHOOLNIK GK et al: Gonococci causing disseminated gonococcal infection are resistant to the bactericidal action of normal human sera. J Clin Invest 58:1163, 1976

SIEGEL MS et al: Penicillinase producing *Neisseria gonorrhoeae*: Results of surveillance in the United States. J Infect Dis 137:170, 1978

section 4 | Diseases caused by enteric gram-negative bacilli

120
INFECTIONS DUE TO ENTEROBACTERIACEAE

MARVIN TURCK
DENNIS SCHABERG

LActose fermenter

ESCHERICHIA COLI INFECTIONS

ETIOLOGY *Escherichia coli* is a group of gram-negative nonsporing rods which belong to the tribe Enterobacteriaceae. They generally ferment lactose, as opposed to the medically significant non-lactose-fermenting organisms, such as *Salmonella*, *Shigella*, and *Proteus*. The so-called "paracolon" bacilli are organisms which ferment lactose late, irregularly, or not at all, and on more careful biochemical and antigenic testing are found to belong to one or another of the genera of the Enterobacteriaceae, which comprise *Salmonella*, *Arizona*, *Citrobacter*, *Shigella*, *Escherichia*, *Klebsiella*, *Enterobacter*, *Hafnia*, *Serratia*, *Proteus*, and *Providencia*. All these organisms are readily culturable on ordinary media and are aerobic and facultatively anaerobic. All species ferment glucose, reduce nitrates to nitrites, and are oxidase-negative and catalase-positive. They are differentiated among members of their own tribe by biochemical and serologic tests. It is important to make this differentiation, not only taxonomically, but also because of epidemiologic and therapeutic implications.

PATHOGENESIS *Escherichia coli* is regarded generally as a normal commensal in the gastrointestinal tract, from which it may spread to infect contiguous structures if normal anatomic barriers are interrupted, as occurs in appendiceal perforation. It is believed that the urinary tract is infected from without via urethral contamination, but direct hematogenous spread may also account for renal infection. Once infection has occurred in a primary focus, further spread to distant organs may occur via the bloodstream. There is experimental and clinical evidence that *E. coli* tends to settle in avascular or necrotic tissue. In more than 50 percent of *E. coli* infections the urinary tract is the portal of entry; infections of the hepatobiliary tree, peritoneal cavity, skin, and lung are not uncommon. A number of patients with *E. coli* bacteremia have no demonstrable portal of entry; they often have neoplastic and hematologic diseases, and *E. coli* is considered an "opportunistic" invader. There may be other defects in host resistance, including diabetes mellitus, cirrhosis, and sickle-cell anemia, or recent administration of irradiation, cytotoxic drugs, adrenal steroids, or antibiotics. There also is epidemiologic evidence that *E. coli* and other

Enterobacteriaceae tend to colonize the skin and mucous membranes of debilitated patients, possibly accounting for the increased frequency of these infections in patients with advanced illness. Morphologically the lesions produced in various tissues show typical acute inflammation with pus and abscess formation. There is a common misconception that *E. coli* bacterial infections are characterized by a foul-smelling, feculent exudate. Such an odor is caused by anaerobic streptococci or *Bacteroides* species, which are often associated with coliform bacteria in mixed infection. In fact, organisms of the genus *Bacteroides* frequently far outnumber *E. coli* as the most prevalent gram-negative flora in the intestine.

EPIDEMIOLOGY Strains of *E. coli* are characterized by their somatic (O), flagellar (H), and capsular (K or B) antigens, and there are hundreds of different serologic varieties. Any of the strains is capable of causing disease. Clinical and epidemiologic studies have demonstrated that certain specific *E. coli* serotypes are more frequently incriminated in diarrheal disease of the infant and newborn. Strains incriminated in infantile diarrhea probably are disseminated within nurseries by symptomatic or asymptomatic infant carriers, mothers, and nurses. Although fecal contamination is the usual mode of spread, airborne contamination and fomite spread may also occur.

Some epidemiologic studies have suggested that *E. coli* 04, 06, and 075 are responsible for most *E. coli* infections other than infantile diarrhea. It is unclear whether these strains actually are more virulent or merely are more prevalent than other somatic types. In fact, virulence factors may be associated more closely with the K than with the somatic antigen, and may account for the frequency with which certain strains cause parenchymal infection.

MANIFESTATIONS Urinary tract infections *Escherichia coli* accounts for well over 75 percent of urinary tract infections, including cystitis, pyelitis, pyelonephritis, and asymptomatic bacteriuria. Strains cultured from patients with acute, uncomplicated urinary tract infections are almost invariably *E. coli*, whereas other Enterobacteriaceae and strains of *Pseudomonas* become prevalent among patients with chronic infection. Urinary tract infections are discussed in Chap. 280.

Peritoneal and biliary infections *Escherichia coli* can usually be cultured from a perforated or inflamed appendix or from abscesses secondary to perforated diverticula, peptic ulcers, subphrenic or lesser sac abscesses, or mesenteric infarction. Often, other organisms, including anaerobic streptococci, clostridia, and *Bacteroides,* are found along with *E. coli*. Acute cholecystitis with gangrene and perforation is often associated with *E. coli* infection. An air-fluid level associated with stones or a circumferential layer of gas in the wall of the gallbladder may be detectable by x-ray and is characteristic of acute emphysematous cholecystitis. From the gallbladder, infection may ascend via the biliary tree to produce cholangitis and multiple liver abscesses. More rarely *E. coli* infection in the peritoneal cavity may produce a septic thrombophlebitis of the portal vein (pylephlebitis), which in turn is followed by liver abscesses.

Bacteremia Invasion of the bloodstream is the most serious manifestation of *E. coli* infection; it is characterized usually by the sudden onset of fever and chills, but sometimes only by mental confusion, dyspnea, or unexplained hypotension. It is most common in patients with urinary tract infection and biliary or intraperitoneal sepsis, and following abortions or pelvic surgery. In some patients no portal of entry is evident. Most cases occur in elderly males, presumably because of the high incidence of urethral instrumentation and catheterization in this group. Fever ranges between 100 and 106°F and is higher in younger patients. Hyperventilation may be an early sign. Hypotension may be present from the onset but usually occurs within 12 to 16 h after bacteremia; if it is persistent, it is accompanied by oliguria and often by mental confusion, stupor, and coma. The skin is warm and dry initially, but most patients develop some evidence of peripheral vasoconstriction characterized by cold and cyanotic extremities. Fortunately hypotension is transient and self-limited in most patients with *E. coli* bacteremia and is absent altogether in some. However, about 25 percent of patients with bacteremia develop more prolonged hypotension, a syndrome known as *gram-negative* or *endotoxin shock,* which is discussed in Chap. 109.

Occasionally *E. coli* bacteremia develops in patients with cirrhosis without an overt portal of entry. This has been variably attributed to portosystemic shunts both in and around the liver, impaired reticuloendothelial function, and diminution in humoral and cellular defense mechanisms.

Other manifestations *Escherichia coli* may produce abscesses anywhere in the body. Subcutaneous infections are found at the site of insulin administration in diabetics, in extremities with ischemic gangrene, or in surgical wounds. Perirectal phlegmons are not uncommon in patients with leukemia. Subcutaneous abscesses are often characterized by formation of gas in tissue, especially among diabetics, which may be detected by crepitation or by x-ray and which must be differentiated from clostridial infection. From 5 to 10 percent of patients with *E. coli* bacteremia develop metastatic infection in bone, brain, liver, and lung. *Escherichia coli* may cause pneumonia de novo; also, *E. coli* are often cultured from sputum in pulmonary superinfections.

Neonatal infection Neonates, particularly premature infants, often develop *E. coli* bacteremia associated with meningitis and bloodborne pyelonephritis. Fecal soiling and absence of maternal gamma-G globulin (IgM) antibody are two of the factors which render this group particularly susceptible to *E. coli* infections.

Gastroenteritis Children under 2 years of age develop gastroenteritis, typified by nausea, vomiting, and diarrhea. Most outbreaks have occurred in nurseries and have been due to specific strains of enteropathogenic *E. coli* (EPEC). These particular strains produce a toxin similar to the toxin elaborated by *Vibrio cholerae*. Fluorescent antibody techniques have been useful in the rapid identification of organisms with serotypes frequently implicated in this syndrome. Although theoretically any *E. coli* strain might be cultured, since the genetic information coding for toxin production is found on a plasmid and can be transferred between *E. coli* strains, the number of different serotypes involved remains restricted. Although diarrhea is usually mediated through production of enterotoxins, occasionally *E. coli* may be enteroinvasive, involving the mucosa and causing disease akin to *Shigella* dysentery. The rapid dehydration, with its attendant high mortality, demands prompt recognition of this condition, isolation of the infants, and treatment of both patients and contacts with the appropriate antibiotic. *Escherichia coli* is also being recognized as a cause of acute diarrheal disease in adults, especially foreign travelers.

LABORATORY FINDINGS There are no characteristic laboratory abnormalities. The white blood cell count is usually elevated, and there is a preponderance of granulocytes. At times, however, the white count is normal or low. When *E. coli* infection occurs in previously healthy individuals, anemia is absent, but more commonly there is anemia which is usually related to the patient's underlying disease. *Escherichia coli* grows readily in a variety of bacteriologic media and should be cultured from appropriate secretions and blood. In the presence of gram-negative shock, there are often profound metabolic derangements, including azotemia, metabolic acidosis, hypokalemia, and hyperkalemia, as well as variety of coagulation defects (Chap. 109).

DIAGNOSIS *Escherichia coli* cannot be differentiated from most other gram-negative bacteria on Gram's stain, and culture followed by appropriate biochemical characterization is necessary to identify the organism precisely. Fluorescent antibody techniques have been used for identifying EPEC. In addition, serologic typing of *E. coli* may be useful in individual patients with recurrent urinary tract infections in order to help differentiate between relapse and reinfection.

TREATMENT As with other infections, drainage of pus and removal of foreign bodies are essential. If *E. coli* is suspected as the etiologic agent in a particular infection, choice of an appropriate antimicrobial will depend upon the site and type of infection as well as upon its severity. Often the outcome of the infection depends upon the status of the associated disease, rather than on eradication of bacteria. For example, in acute, uncomplicated urinary tract infection in females, the disease is frequently self-limited even without antimicrobial therapy, and there is no evidence that antibiotics are superior to sulfonamides. Conversely, *E. coli* bacteremia in a patient with leukemia may not respond to antimicrobials unless a hematologic remission is achieved simultaneously.

In most situations, antibiotics should be selected, when possible, on the basis of their in vitro sensitivity tests. Although no drug is uniformly active against all strains of *E. coli*, a number of agents are effective against the majority of clinical isolates. If average obtainable plasma concentrations become the criteria for in vitro susceptibility, approximately 75 percent of *E. coli* strains are likely to be sensitive to the tetracyclines, 85 to 90 percent to chloramphenicol or ampicillin, and 90 percent to gentamicin, kanamycin, polymyxin B, or colistin; 50 percent of *E. coli* isolated from hospitalized patients will be inhibited by streptomycin, and 75 to 90 percent by one of the cephalosporin antibiotics. Many strains of *E. coli* are sensitive to high concentrations of penicillin G (50 to 100 μg/ml), and this drug may be used in dosage of 10 to 40 million units intravenously daily, particularly if probenecid is given concomitantly. This regimen has been largely superseded by ampicillin, 2 to 4 g per day intravenously or intramuscularly; for severe infections the dose can be raised to 6 to 12 g per day. The antibacterial spectrum of ampicillin against *E. coli* is probably identical with that achieved with very high concentrations of penicillin G, and with the spectrum covered by the tetracyclines or chloramphenicol. However, the bactericidal properties of ampicillin may be a distinct advantage over these two drugs, particularly in deep-seated infections. Gentamicin has been employed effectively in the initial treatment of severe *E. coli* infections in doses of 5 mg/kg per day in divided doses every 8 h. This drug has superseded kanamycin in the treatment of many patients although kanamycin remains effective against most *E. coli* in doses of 15 mg/kg per day given intramuscularly in divided doses every 8 to 12 h. Cephalosporins in concentration of 25 μg/ml or less are effective against many *E. coli* strains. This serum concentration can be obtained only with 1.5- to 2.0-g dosages at 3- to 4-h intervals with cephalothin. Newer cephalosporins have been developed which give slightly higher peak serum concentrations and in some instances have lower MICs for *E. coli* (Chap. 111). Tetracyclines and chloramphenicol are

still widely used in the treatment of *E. coli* infection, but better drugs are now available. Polymyxin B and colistin are also effective in vitro against the majority of *E. coli*. However, it is difficult to obtain adequate tissue and serum concentrations with these agents, and they should probably not be used for treatment of systemic *E. coli* infections. Although combinations of antimicrobials, i.e., streptomycin and tetracycline or streptomycin and chloramphenicol, have been recommended, there is little need to employ more than one agent in most situations. Nitrofurantoin (400 mg) and nalidixic acid (2 to 4 g) are reserved for treating patients with *E. coli* bacteriuria, and should not be employed when infection is suspected outside the urinary tract. Trimethoprim sulfa is also useful in urinary tract infections (Chap. 280).

PREVENTION Isolation and antimicrobial therapy of infants and contacts are essential to abort epidemic infantile diarrhea. In adults, many *E. coli* infections are hospital-associated, and their incidence can be reduced by limiting use of indwelling urinary and intravenous catheters, by careful surgical aseptic technique, by appropriate isolation of infection-prone patients, and by judicious use of antibiotics, steroids, and cytotoxic agents. There is mounting evidence that the promiscuous use of antibiotics may propagate the transfer of resistance factors among intestinal *E. coli*. These organisms may in turn transmit their resistance to other virulent Enterobacteriaceae, such as *Salmonella*.

KLEBSIELLA-ENTEROBACTER-SERRATIA INFECTIONS

ETIOLOGY Next to *E. coli*, strains of *Klebsiella*, *Enterobacter*, and *Serratia* are the most important enteric organisms infecting man. In many laboratories *Klebsiella* are, in general, more resistant to antibiotics than *E. coli*, and their isolation from blood, purulent exudates, and urine is of more serious epidemiologic and prognostic significance. The Friedländer bacilli *(K. pneumoniae)* are encapsulated gram-negative bacilli, found among the normal flora of the mouth and intestinal tracts. *Klebsiella pneumoniae* has been considered to be a virulent respiratory pathogen since first described by Friedländer in 1882. *Klebsiella* is closely related to the genera *Enterobacter* and *Serratia* and may be differentiated only by certain amino acid decarboxylase tests. In addition to differentiation by these biochemical tests, which group *Klebsiella*, *Enterobacter*, and *Serratia*, strains of *Klebsiella* usually are nonmotile and form large mucoid colonies on solid media, whereas the other species are typically motile. Klebsiellas also are usually sensitive to concentrations of cephalosporin antibiotics, to which *Enterobacter* and *Serratia* are resistant. These characteristics, however, are not invariable enough to differentiate various isolates from clinical sources. Strains of *Klebsiella* can be further distinguished on the basis of type-specific capsular antigens; more than 75 known capsular types have been identified. There is little evidence that certain types are more virulent than others, and the main role of capsular typing of *Klebsiella* is as an epidemiologic tool in nosocomial outbreaks of infection.

Klebsiella rhinoscleromatis is probably the causative agent of rhinoscleroma, and *K. ozenae* has been isolated occasionally from the nose of patients with ozena, a chronic severe rhinitis associated with turbinate atrophy and progressive anosmia.

PATHOGENESIS *Klebsiella*, *Enterobacter*, and *Serratia* are all capable of causing disease in diverse anatomic sites. However, results of clinical and epidemiologic studies suggest that differences in pathogenicity may exist among these genera and that precise taxonomic identification is of value. Although infections of the respiratory tract with *K. pneumoniae* have been emphasized most in the past, the urinary tract presently accounts for the majority of clinical isolates. In this site clinical manifestations and pathogenesis are similar to infections produced by *E. coli,* but klebsiellas are more frequently found in patients with complicated and obstructive urinary tract disease. Infections of the biliary tract, the peritoneal cavity, the middle ear, mastoids, paranasal sinuses, and meninges also are not uncommon. In these locations, *Klebsiella* is more frequent than either *Enterobacter* or *Serratia* and is more likely to produce an illness of greater severity. The apparent increased frequency of infection by *Serratia* represents an increase primarily due to nosocomial spread of this organism.

MANIFESTATIONS Symptoms and signs of common infections caused by *Klebsiella*—namely, those involving the urinary tract, biliary tree, and peritoneal cavity—are indistinguishable from those caused by *E. coli.* These infections commonly occur in diabetics and in the form of superinfections in patients who have received antimicrobials to which these organisms are resistant. *Klebsiella* infection is also an important etiologic factor in septic shock. *Serratia* and *Enterobacter* are almost exclusively nosocomial pathogens. These organisms have been implicated as pathogens in a wide variety of infections, most frequently pneumonia, urinary tract infections and bacteremia.

Pneumonia *Klebsiella* is well recognized as a pulmonary pathogen, but probably accounts for less than 1 percent of all cases of bacterial pneumonia. The disease is most common in men over 40 years of age and is most frequently found in alcoholics. Other factors associated with increased susceptibility include diabetes mellitus and chronic bronchopulmonary disease. Aspiration of oropharyngeal secretions containing *Klebsiella* organisms is the likely inciting factor among alcoholic patients. The clinical manifestations are indistinguishable from those of pneumococcal pneumonia (Chap. 115), with sudden onset of chills, fever, productive cough, and severe pleuritic chest pain. Patients are frequently delirious and prostrated, but this may also occur with pneumococcal infection. A "characteristic" clinical feature, which occurs in only 25 to 50 percent of patients, is the dark-brown or red-currant-jelly sputum which may be so tenacious that the patient has difficulty in expelling it from his mouth and lips. The pulmonary lesion is most frequent in the right upper lobe but often rapidly progresses and, if untreated, may spread from lobe to lobe. Cyanosis and dyspnea develop rapidly, and jaundice, vomiting, and diarrhea may be present. Physical findings consist primarily of signs of consolidation unless pleural effusion or necrotizing pneumonitis with rapid cavitation has intervened. The blood leukocyte count may be elevated but is often low, which probably is merely a reflection of severe infection in an alcoholic patient with poor bone marrow reserve and folate deficiency. Lung abscess and empyema are much more frequent than in pneumococcal pneumonia and are related to the destructive capabilities of this organism. So-called "characteristic" and radiographic features such as bulging fissures and loss of lung volume occur only occasionally, and also may be found in pneumococcal infection, as well as in necrotizing pneumonia caused by other gram-negative species.

Klebsiella, Serratia, and *Enterobacter* are frequently seen in nosocomial pneumonia. Older patients become colonized with gram-negative bacilli in the oropharynx and these organisms can then gain access to the respiratory tract and cause pneumonia or purulent bronchitis. Common-source outbreaks, with contamination of a variety of respiratory therapy devices have been implicated in infections with these pathogens, especially *Serratia.*

Chronic infection of the lung Rarely, infection with *Klebsiella* may progress, often in indolent fashion, to a chronic necrotizing pneumonitis resembling tuberculosis. It may follow acute *Klebsiella* pneumonia but is also seen in patients who give no history of an acute onset. The principal symptoms are productive cough, weakness, and anemia. Hemoptysis, chronic empyema, or sterile serous effusions are also encountered. Cavitation, frequently with thin walls, occurs primarily in the upper lobes.

DIAGNOSIS Diagnosis of community-acquired pneumonia is established by an awareness of the clinical setting in which *Klebsiella* infections occur and by isolation of the organism. A presumptive diagnosis of *Klebsiella* pneumonia should be made on the basis of a Gram stain of the sputum which shows a predominance of short, plump, gram-negative bacilli, frequently surrounded by a clear space because of the capsule. Often these gram-negative organisms occur together with gram-positive cocci, and because the gram-positives are easier to see, the gram-negative bacteria may be ignored and the diagnosis may be missed, which, in turn, may lead to potentially serious delays in instituting therapy. Additional proof of *Klebsiella* infection in the lung is afforded by isolation of the organisms from blood and pleural exudate. In extrapulmonary infections, the organisms are readily seen in, and cultured from, pus or secretions of involved organs.

The diagnosis of nosocomial respiratory infection with these organisms may be more difficult, mainly because colonization has to be distinguished from infection. Careful evaluation of the clinical course is necessary in establishing a diagnosis. Transtracheal aspiration of sputum for culture and Gram's stain may be useful in difficult cases.

TREATMENT *Klebsiella, Enterobacter,* and *Serratia* have variable suceptiblity to antimicrobial drugs, and cultures of these organisms need to be tested in vitro. Frequently, however, antimicrobial therapy needs to be insituted before results of antibiotic susceptibility tests become available. In general, the majority of strains of *Klebsiella* is susceptible to gentamicin, kanamycin, cephalosporins, chloramphenicol, and polymyxin B or colistin. *Klebsiella* isolates do not respond to penicillin and its analogues, although many isolates of *Enterobacter* are inhibited by 25 μg/ml carbenicillin. *Serratia* isolates are frequently resistant to many antimicrobials, and resistance to gentamicin and tobramycin is being encountered with increasing frequency. Amikacin has been used effectively in these drug-resistant infections. The antimicrobial regimen of choice in the treatment of *Klebsiella, Enterobacter,* and *Serratia* infection will vary from one institution to another depending on the resistance patterns as well as upon the degree of clinical severity of infection. In severely ill patients, the combination of an aminoglycoside such as tobramycin or gentamicin (3 to 5 mg/kg per day) or kanamycin (15 mg/kg per day) with cephalothin, cephapirin, or cefazolin (4 to 12 g per day) is usually preferred. Amikacin, a newer aminoglycoside, in a dose of 15 mg/kg per day, may be effective when the organisms are resistant to either gentamicin or tobramycin. Because of the relatively poor blood and tissue levels obtained with the polymyxins, they should not be employed as first-line agents in the treatment of severe *Klebsiella* infections despite apparent in vitro susceptibility. Regardless of the antimicrobial regimen employed, treatment should be continued for a minimum of 10 to 14 days and prolonged if there is extensive cavitation. Pleural effusions must be drained; antibiotic therapy alone is not sufficient treatment for closed-space infections of the pleural cavity. At times, rib resection with open drainage may be necessary, and should be considered if effusions recur.

PROGNOSIS Before the introduction of antimicrobials, the fatality rate from these infections varied from 50 to 80 percent, and death within 48 h was not infrequent. Even with antimicrobial treatment the course of these infections is quite variable and the prognosis must be guarded. For the most part, this prognosis reflects the age group involved and the frequent association of *Klebsiella* infections with alcoholism, malnutrition, and severe underlying disease.

PROTEUS INFECTIONS

ETIOLOGY The genus *Proteus* consists of gram-negative bacilli which do not ferment lactose and are characterized by their active motility and spreading growth on solid media. There are four pathogenic species: *P. mirabilis, P. vulgaris, P. morganii,* and *P. rettgeri. Proteus mirabilis* causes 75 to 90 percent of human infections and is distinguishable from the other three species by its inability to form indole. All four split urea, with production of ammonia. Some strains of *P. vulgaris* share a common antigen with certain rickettsia, accounting for the appearance of antibodies against *Proteus* organisms (Weil-Felix reaction) in typhus, scrub typhus, and Rocky Mountain spotted fever. The *Providence* group of organisms resembles those of the genus *Proteus* closely except that it fails to produce a urease.

EPIDEMIOLOGY AND PATHOGENESIS Members of the genus *Proteus* are normally found in soil, water, and sewage and are part of the normal fecal flora. Occasionally, they have been implicated as a cause of epidemic diarrhea in infants, but the evidence for this is inconclusive. The organism is frequently cultured from superficial wounds, draining ears, and sputum, particularly in patients who have received antibiotics, and replaces the more susceptible flora eradicated by these drugs. *Proteus* organisms often localize in already damaged tissues, where they produce a typical exudative inflammatory reaction.

MANIFESTATIONS *Proteus* organisms are rarely primary invaders but produce disease in locations previously infected by other organisms. These locations include the skin, ears and mastoid, sinuses, eyes, peritoneal cavity, bone, urinary tract, meninges, lung, and bloodstream.

Cutaneous infections *Proteus* organisms are frequently isolated from surgical wounds, particularly following antimicrobial therapy, but they do not interfere with normal wound healing provided that the tissues are viable and foreign bodies are not present. Burns, varicose ulcers, and decubiti may become contaminated with *Proteus* organisms, often in company with other gram-negative organisms or staphylococci.

Infections of the ears and mastoid sinuses Otitis media and mastoiditis in which *Proteus* organisms are present can result in extensive destruction of the middle ear and mastoid sinuses. Fetid otorrhea, cholesteatoma, and granulation tissue constitute a chronic focus of infection in the middle and inner ears and mastoid, and deafness ensues. Paralysis of the facial nerve

is an occasional complication. The great danger of these infections lies in intracranial extension, leading to thrombosis of the lateral sinus, meningitis, brain abscess, and bacteremia.

Ocular infections *Proteus* infection may cause corneal ulcers, usually following trauma to the eye, which occasionally terminate in panophthalmitis and destruction of the eyeball.

Peritonitis Being part of the normal intestinal flora, *Proteus* organisms may be isolated from the peritoneal cavity following perforation of viscera or mesenteric infarction.

Urinary tract infections *Proteus* organisms are a common cause of urinary tract infections, usually in patients with chronic bacteriuria, many of whom have had obstructive uropathy, a history of instrumentation of the bladder, and repeated courses of chemotherapy. The organism is rarely a pathogen in anatomically normal urinary tracts except occasionally in patients with diabetes mellitus. *Proteus* organisms are also often cultured from bacteriuric patients with renal or bladder calculi. This fact may be related to the urease activity of this organism, which renders the urine alkaline and provides a fertile medium for formation of ammonium-magnesium-phosphate stones.

Bacteremia Bloodstream invasion is the most serious manifestation of infection with this organism. In 75 percent of cases, the urinary tract serves as the portal of entry; in the remainder, the biliary tree, gastrointestinal tract, ears and sinuses, and skin are the primary foci. *Proteus* bacteremia is frequently preceded by cystoscopy, urethral catheterization, transurethral prostatic resection, or other operative procedures. Clinically, the signs, symptoms, and laboratory findings of *Proteus* sepsis—high fever, chills, shock, metastatic abscesses, leukocytosis, and rarely thrombocytopenia—are indistinguishable from those of bloodstream infections with other gram-negative bacteria.

DIAGNOSIS The diagnosis of *Proteus* infection depends on culture of the organism from blood, urine, or exudate and its identification by appropriate biochemical tests. It is especially important to separate *P. mirabilis,* the indole-negative species, from *P. morganii, rettgeri,* and *vulgaris,* which are indole-positive, because only *P. mirabilis* is susceptible to the action of penicillin and many other antibiotics. *Proteus* organisms are often present in mixed infections with other pathogens. Particular care should be exercised in the isolation of other organisms growing in the same medium with members of the genus *Proteus* lest they be masked by its spreading growth. The spreading character of this organism may also make antibiotic sensitivity tests difficult to interpret.

TREATMENT Most strains of *P. mirabilis* are sensitive to penicillin in high concentration (10 units per milliliter or greater), ampicillin, carbenicillin, kanamycin, gentamicin or tobramycin, the cephalosporin antibiotics, and chloramphenicol. *Proteus* bacteriuria can be readily eradicated with any of these drugs during treatment; ampicillin in dosage of 0.5 g every 4 to 6 h is highly effective. In severe infection, therapy should be parenteral: 6 to 12 g ampicillin or 20 million units of penicillin G plus kanamycin or gentamicin in divided doses of 15 mg/kg per day and 5 mg/kg per day, respectively, if renal function is adequate. There is good evidence that kanamycin is synergistic with ampicillin and penicillin G in *Proteus* infections, and that chloramphenicol may be ineffective despite the results of in vitro tests. In view of the numerous more effective agents, there is no reason to use chloramphenicol in *Proteus* infections. In general, all strains of *P. mirabilis* are resistant to tetracycline. Most strains other than *P. mirabilis* and *Providence* bacilli are sensitive only to kanamycin, gentamicin, tobramycin or amikacin. Gentamicin, tobramycin and amikacin in particular appear to be effective against indole-positive *Proteus*. In addition, although ampicillin and penicillin G alone are ineffective against indole-positive *Proteus*, a combination of either drug and an aminoglycoside may be synergistic. Carbenicillin and ticarcillin, semisynthetic penicillins, are also effective against the majority of indole-positive *Proteus* species. As with all other gram-negative infections, appropriate attention must be given to drainage of pus, maintenance of fluid and electrolyte status, and treatment of circulatory collapse.

REFERENCES

Enterobacteriaceae: General

PIERCE AK, SANFORD JP: Aerobic gram-negative bacillary pneumonias. Am Rev Respir Dis 110:647, 1974

SCHABERG DR et al: Epidemics of nosocomial urinary tract infection caused by multiply-resistant gram-negative bacilli: Epidemiology and control. J Infect Dis 133:363, 1976

STAMM WE: Guidelines for prevention of catheter-associated urinary tract infections. Ann Intern Med 82:386, 1975

Escherichia coli infections

CONN HO, FESSEL JM: Spontaneous bacterial peritonitis in cirrhosis. Medicine 50:161, 1971

GORBACH SL et al: Travelers' diarrhea and toxigenic *Escherichia coli*. N Engl J Med 292:933, 1975

TILLOTSON JR, LERNER AM: Characteristics of pneumonia caused by *Escherichia coli*. N Engl J Med 277:115, 1967

TULLOCH EF JR et al: Invasive enteropathic *Escherichia coli* dysentery: Outbreak in 28 adults. Ann Intern Med 79:13, 1973

TURCK M et al: Studies on the epidemiology of *Escherichia coli* 1960–1968. J Infect Dis 120:13, 1969

Klebsiella-Enterobacter-Serratia infections

EDMONDSON EG, SANFORD JP: The *Klebsiella-Enterobacter (Aerobacter)-Serratia* group. Medicine 46:323, 1967

MAKI DG et al: Noscomial urinary tract infection with *Serratia marcescens*: An epidemiologic study. J Infect Dis 128:579, 1973

MANFREDI F et al: Clinical observations of acute Friedländer pneumonia. Ann Intern Med 58:642, 1963

MELTZ DJ, GRIECO MH: Characteristics of *Serratia marcescens* pneumonia. Arch Intern Med 132:359, 1973

PRICE DJE, SLEIGH JD: Control of infection due to *Klebsiella* aerogenes in neurosurgical unit by withdrawal of all antibiotics. Lancet 2:213, 1970

Proteus infections

LEWIS J, FEKETY FR: *Proteus* bacteremia. Johns Hopkins Med J 124:151, 1969

MUSHER DM et al: Role of urease in pyelonephritis resulting from urinary tract infection with *Proteus*. J Infect Dis 131:177, 1975

SERIFF NS: Lobar pneumonia due to *Proteus* infection in a previously healthy adult. Am J Med 46:480, 1969

TILLOTSON JR, LERNER AM: Characteristics of pneumonia caused by bacillus *Proteus*. Ann Intern Med 68:287, 1968

TURCK M et al: The role of carbenicillin in treatment of infections of the urinary tract. J Infect Dis 122:529, 1970

121
PSEUDOMONAS, ACINETOBACTER, AND EIKENELLA INFECTIONS

MARVIN TURCK
DENNIS SCHABERG

PSEUDOMONAS INFECTIONS

ETIOLOGY *Pseudomonas aeruginosa* is a gram-negative motile rod which generally is not encapsulated and forms no spores. It grows readily in all ordinary culture media, and on agar it forms irregular, soft, iridescent colonies which usually have a fluorescent yellow-green color because of diffusion into the medium of two pigments, pyocyanin and fluorescin. *Pseudomonas* produces acid but no gas in glucose, and it is proteolytic. It is oxidase-positive and produces ammonia from arginine. A number of different strains have been identified by immunofluorescent techniques or bacteriophage typing. There is no evidence that these strains vary in their virulence for man. Other *Pseudomonas* species (*P. maltophilia, P. cepacia, P. fluorescens, P. testosteroni,* and *P. putida*) also may cause infection in man. For the most part, these organisms have been associated with common-source nosocomial outbreaks; in addition, they have been incriminated in bacteremia, endocarditis, and osteomyelitis in narcotic addicts.

EPIDEMIOLOGY *Pseudomonas* organisms are present on the skin of some normal persons, particularly in the axilla and anogenital regions. They are uncommon in the stools of adults not receiving antibiotics. In the majority of instances, *Pseudomonas* organisms are cultured as avirulent secondary contaminants in superficial wounds, or from the sputum of patients treated with antibiotics. Ordinarily this is of little consequence because the organisms merely fill the bacteriologic vacuum left by the elimination of more sensitive bacteria. Occasionally, however, infections with *Pseudomonas* organisms occur in the ear, lung, skin, or urinary tract of patients, often when a primary pathogen has been eradicated by antibiotics. Serious infections are almost invariably associated with damage to local tissue or with diminished host resistance. Premature infants; children with congenital anomalies and patients with leukemia, usually receiving antibiotics, adrenal steroids, or antineoplastic drugs; patients with burns; and geriatric patients with debilitating diseases are likely to develop *Pseudomonas* infections. Most often these infections occur in the hospital environment and generally are exogenous infections with the organism acquired from sources other than the patient's normal flora. The organisms have been cultured from a variety of sources in hospitals, sharing in common an aqueous environment including such items as sinks, antiseptic solutions, and aqueous medications. The organism is prevalent in urine receptacles and catheters, and on the hands of orderlies, nurses, and physicians; in several outbreaks, *Pseudomonas* urinary tract infections appeared to have been transmitted from patient to patient by human carriers. Similar epidemics have been reported in nurseries among premature infants, and cross infection on burn wards is also common.

PATHOGENESIS The portal of entry of *Pseudomonas* organisms varies with the patient's age and underlying disease. In infancy and childhood, the skin, umbilical cord, and gastrointestinal tract predominate; in old age, the urinary tract is more often the primary focus. Often the infections remain localized in the skin or subcutaneous tissues. In burns the region below the eschar may become massively infiltrated with bacteria and inflammatory cells, and usually serves as the focus for bacteremia, the single most lethal complication. Hematogenous dissemination is characterized by hemorrhagic nodules in many areas, including the skin, heart, lungs, kidneys, and meninges. The histologic picture is one of necrosis and hemorrhage. Typically the walls of arterioles are heavily infiltrated with bacteria, and the vessels are partially or wholly thrombosed.

MANIFESTATIONS *Pseudomonas* infections occur in many locations, including the skin, subcutaneous tissue, bone and joints, eyes, ears, mastoid and paranasal sinuses, meninges, and heart valves. Bacteremia without a detectable primary focus may also occur and should raise the question of contamination of intravenous medications, intravenous solutions, or antiseptics used for preparing the intravenous site, especially when non-*aeruginosa Pseudmonas* species are isolated.

Infections of the skin and subcutaneous tissues *Pseudomonas* organisms are frequently cultured from surgical wounds, varicose and decubitus ulcers, and burns, particularly following antibiotic therapy. Draining tuberculous or osteomyelitic sinuses may become secondarily infected. The mere presence of *Pseudomonas* in these sites is of little significance provided that bacterial multiplication deep in subcutaneous tissues does not occur and bacteremia does not ensue. Cutaneous infections usually heal after removal or slough of devitalized tissue. *Pseudomonas* organisms may be responsible for green nails in persons whose hands are excessively exposed to water, soap, and detergents, who have onychomycosis, or whose hands are subject to mechanical trauma. The organism can usually be cultured from the nail plate.

Osteomyelitis Osteomyelitis is unusual with *Pseudomonas* except as a complication of bacteremia and puncture wounds. If a puncture wound, especially a nail puncture of the foot in children, fails to respond to standard therapy within 3 to 4 days, complicating *Pseudomonas* osteomyelitis must be considered.

Infections of the ear, mastoid, and paranasal sinuses Otitis externa is the most common form of *Pseudomonas* infection which involves the ear. It is particularly troublesome in tropical climates and is characterized by chronic serosanguineous and purulent drainage from the external auditory canal. Otitis media or mastoiditis usually occurs as a superinfection following eradication of pneumococci, streptococci, or staphylococci by antimicrobial agents. Frequently *Pseudomonas* organisms are present in association with other gram-negative or gram-positive organisms.

Infection of the eye Corneal ulceration is the most severe form of ocular *Pseudomonas* infection. It usually follows a traumatic abrasion and may terminate in panophthalmitis and destruction of the globe. Purulent conjuncitivitis occurs as a manifestation of *Pseudomonas* infection in premature infants. Contamination of contact lenses or lens fluid may be an important means of infecting the eyes with *Pseudomonas* organisms.

Urinary tract infections *Pseudomonas* organisms are common pathogens in the urinary tract and are usually found in patients with obstructive uropathy who have been subjected to repeated urethral manipulations or to urologic surgery. At times *Pseudomonas* is one of several pathogenic bacteria in the urine, the others being *Escherichia coli, Klebsiella, Proteus,* and enterococci. *Pseudomonas* bacteriuria is in no way unique and cannot be distinguished from infection with other organisms on clinical grounds.

Gastrointestinal tract *Pseudomonas* organisms have been implicated as a cause of epidemic diarrhea of infancy. In addition, a number of infants dying from neonatal sepsis have the classic necrotic, avascular ulcers of *Pseudomonas* bacteremia in the bowel at autopsy. A "typhoidal" form of *Pseudomonas* infection characterized by fever, myalgia, and diarrhea occurs predominantly in the tropics. This illness, also called 13-day fever or Shanghai fever, is self-limited, and the prognosis is good.

Respiratory tract Primary *Pseudomonas* pneumonia is infrequent, and culture of this organism from the sputum usually is indicative of aspiration of oropharyngeal contents with secondary infection or of superinfection following eradication of a more sensitive flora with antibiotics. The normal oropharyngeal flora of hospitalized patients is frequently replaced by gram-negative rods, including *Pseudomonas,* early in hospitalization. A variety of nosocomial events, most notably administration of sedative medications, endotracheal intubation, and intermittent positive pressure breathing treatments, can predispose to respiratory infection with *Pseudomonas.* Pulmonary infection is often associated with microabscesses. The organism is often isolated from the sputum of patients with bronchiectasis, chronic bronchitis, or cystic fibrosis who have lingering infections punctuated by multiple courses of chemotherapy and is recovered frequently from the stomata of tracheostomy sites. *Pseudomonas* bronchitis and bronchiolitis may be the terminal event in cystic fibrosis and the isolates from these patients often are found to have a characteristic mucoid colonial morphology when cultured on agar.

Meningitis Spontaneous *Pseudomonas* meningitis is most unusual, but the bacilli may be introduced into the subarachnoid space by lumbar puncture, spinal anesthesia, intrathecal medication, or head trauma. Ventriculomastoid or ventriculoatrial shunts performed for hydrocephalus may become contaminated with *Pseudomonas* organisms. Usually revision or removal of the shunt offers the best hope of cure. Meningitis may be a terminal phenomenon in *Pseudomonas* bacteremia and in this instance represents a metastatic infection in the meninges.

Bacteremia Bloodstream invasion tends to occur in debilitated patients, premature infants, children with congenital defects, patients with lymphomas, leukemias, or other malignant tumors, and elderly patients who have undergone surgery or instrumentation of the biliary or urinary tract. *Pseudomonas* bacteremia is an important cause of death in patients with severe burns. In adults, *Pseudomonas* bacteremia is indistinguishable from bloodstream infection with other bacterial species except for two findings: (1) ecthyma gangrenosum, the classic skin lesion, often located in the anogenital or axillary region as a round, indurated, purple-black area about 1 cm in diameter with an ulcerated center and a surrounding zone of erythema; and (2) the passage rarely of green urine, presumably due to the hemoglobin pigment, verdoglobin. Other features of *Pseudomonas* sepsis include hectic fever, shaking chills, hyperventilation, confusion, delirium, and circulatory collapse. Hypothermia, leukopenia, and thrombocytopenia are more common in *Pseudomonas* bacteremia than in other gram-negative bacteremias but are often related to an underlying blood dyscrasia. In addition to ecthyma gangrenosum, other skin lesions consist of hemorrhagic cellulitis and macular lesions on the trunk similar to "rose spots." Organisms usually can be cultured from cutaneous lesions and may provide an early clue to the diagnosis. *Pseudomonas* organisms may be in the bloodstream concomitantly with other organisms, notably Enterobacteriaceae or staphylococci. More often, however, *Pseudomonas* bacteremia follows staphylococcal sepsis in patients with burns.

Bacterial endocarditis A number of cases of *Pseudomonas* subacute bacterial endocarditis have followed open-heart surgery. Usually the organisms become implanted on a silk suture or a synthetic patch employed for closure of septal defects. Reoperation with removal of the vegetation and foreign bodies offers the best hope of cure. *Pseudomonas* endocarditis has been found on normal heart valves in patients with burns or in drug addicts; it has been postulated that staphylococcal endocarditis develops first and that the vegetation is secondarily infected with *Pseudomonas* organisms. Metastatic abscesses in bone, joints, brain, adrenal glands, and lungs are frequent consequences of *Pseudomonas* endocarditis.

TREATMENT Localized *Pseudomonas* infection can be treated by irrigation with 1% acetic acid or topical therapy with colistin or polymyxin B. Debridement and drainage of purulent material is essential when deeper tissues are involved. For deep-seated tissue infections and life-threatening infection, such as pneumonia or bacteremia, parenteral therapy must be employed. The aminoglycoside antibiotics, tobramycin and gentamicin, inhibit most strains of *Pseudomonas*. In patients with normal renal function, 5 mg/kg per day in divided doses will provide inhibitory levels. Amikacin, a newer aminoglycoside, is also active against *Pseudomonas*. It is especially useful against strains which have developed enzyme-mediated drug resistance to tobramycin and gentamicin. It should be given in doses of 15 mg/kg per day in divided doses. Ticarcillin and carbenicillin are also active against many strains of *Pseudomonas* in doses of 24 to 30 g per day for carbenicillin and 16 to 20 g per day for ticarcillin. The combination of an aminoglycoside active against *Pseudomonas* plus carbenicillin or ticarcillin is frequently employed to delay emergence of resistance during therapy and provides some enhanced activity, especially in the granulocytopenic patient with *Pseudomonas* infection. Asymptomatic bacteriuria, particularly when confined to the bladder, should be treated with the least toxic agent, which at times may be a sulfonamide or tetracycline. The antimicrobial susceptiblity of *Pseudomonas*, other than *P. aeruginosa*, is variable and many of these isolates may be sensitive to chloramphenicol and resistant to aminoglycoside antibiotics.

PROPHYLAXIS *Pseudomonas* cross infections in hospitals can be reduced by careful attention to aseptic techniques, particularly in nurseries for premature infants, operating rooms, and urologic wards; avoidance of cold sterilization procedures wherever possible; and scrupulous attention to clean plumbing fixtures, humidifying equipment, etc. Judicious use of antibiotics, steroids, and cytotoxic agents should also diminish the incidence of *Pseudomonas* infections. Systemic antibiotic prophylaxis aimed at preventing colonization and infection with *Pseudomonas* organisms has been notoriously unsuccessful and should be interdicted. A polyvalent vaccine for *Pseudomonas* has been developed as well as hyperimmune λ globulin. The vaccine has proved useful in prophylaxis against *Pseudomonas* infection in patients with thermal injury and may be useful in other selected populations such as those with solid tumors undergoing cancer chemotherapy.

PROGNOSIS The mortality rate in *Pseudomonas* bacteremia is 75 percent and is highest in patients with shock or severe associated disease such as massive third-degree burns, leukemia, or prematurity. When bacteremia originates in the urinary tract and is not accompanied by shock, the prognosis is considerably better. Localized *Pseudomonas* infections do not present a threat to life unless hematogenous dissemination occurs.

ACINETOBACTER INFECTIONS

DEFINITION Organisms of the genus *Acinetobacter* are pleomorphic, gram-negative bacilli which are easily confused with members of the genus *Neisseria*. Severe infections with these organisms, including meningitis, bacterial endocarditis, pneumonia, and bacteremia, have been described with increasing frequency.

ETIOLOGY *Acinetobacter calcoaceticus* var. *lwoffi* was described by DeBord as *Mima polymorpha* in 1939. It is one of two well-characterized varieties of *Acinetobacter*, the other being *Acinetobacter calcoaceticus* var. *anitratus*, formerly called *Herellea vaginicola*. Organisms described as *Bacterium anitratum* and B5W are synonymous with *Acinetobacter*. These organisms are pleomorphic, gram-negative, encapsulated, and nonmotile. They grow well on ordinary media, forming white, convex, smooth colonies. Diplococcal forms predominate in colonies grown on solid media; rods and filamentous forms are more common in liquid media. The species can be differentiated from the Enterobacteriaceae by their negative nitrate reaction and from members of the genus *Neisseria*, which they may resemble morphologically, by their simple growth requirements, their bacillary form in liquid media, and their usually negative oxidase reaction.

EPIDEMIOLOGY AND PATHOGENESIS *Acinetobacter* organisms are ubiquitous and have been cultured from a variety of human sources, including urethral, vaginal, and conjunctival secretions, sputum, pleural fluid, blood, cerebrospinal fluid, feces, cutaneous ulcers, abscesses, chancroid lesions, joint fluid, ascitic fluid, and bone marrow. In addition, these organisms have been found in river water, humidifiers, and oxygen tents. Twenty-five percent of normal subjects are skin carriers of *Acinetobacter*. The striking association of *Acinetobacter* bacteremia with cutdowns or indwelling intravenous catheters favors the skin as a major portal of entry in man. The increasing incidence of *Acinetobacter* pneumonia, both as a primary infection and as a superinfection, also points to the respiratory tract as an important portal of entry. It appears that *Acinetobacter* organisms are normal human commensals of relatively low virulence with colonization much more frequent than infection. Infections seem to occur in patients subjected to the same epidemiologic pressures encountered with nosocomial, gram-negative bacilli producing serious infections under conditions of decreased host resistance, or in the presence of instrumentation and with prior broad-spectrum antimicrobial therapy. The role of these organisms as a cause of conjunctivitis, vaginitis, and urethritis requires further documentation.

MANIFESTATIONS Serious infections caused by *Acinetobacter* include (1) meningitis, (2) subacute and acute bacterial endocarditis, (3) pneumonia, (4) urinary tract infections, and (5) bacteremia. Usually, the signs and symptoms associated with infections in these sites are no different from those produced by other pathogens. For example, subacute bacterial endocarditis has usually been reported in patients with congenital or rheumatic heart disease and pursues an indolent course, while urinary tract infections may be manifested by asymptomatic bacteriuria, cystitis, or pyelonephritis. Pneumonia often occurs in the form of a superinfection in patients who have received antibiotics and who have either a tracheostomy or endotracheal intubation. Bronchopneumonia is the most common roentgenographic finding. Occasionally, *Acinetobacter* may be the cause of a fulminating bacteremia, with high fever, vascular collapse, petechiae, and ecchymoses, indistinguishable from fulminant meningococcemia. More often, however, bacteremia is associated with an overt portal of entry, such as infected cutdowns or indwelling intravenous catheters, surgical wounds, or burns, or it may follow urethral or other surgical instrumentation. These patients usually have severe debilitating disease or have undergone surgery. Many times they have received antibiotics, adrenal cortical hormones, irradiation, or tumor chemotherapy and have had infections with other organisms prior to development of sepsis with *Acinetobacter*. The clinical picture presented by these patients is dominated by endotoxemia, and the prognosis is poor.

DIAGNOSIS The diagnosis of *Acinetobacter* infection can be missed because the clinical bacteriology laboratory is unfamiliar with these organisms and reports them incorrectly or because they are considered contaminant. The confusion attending the taxonomic classification of these organisms has not simplified matters. For practical purposes, isolation of *Acinetobacter* or synonyms (*Mimae herelleae, B. anitratum,* B5W, *Diplococcus mucosus,* or *Neisseria winogradskyi*) from blood, spinal fluid, sputum, urine, or pus should be considered significant unless there is no evidence of infection on clinical grounds. Since *Acinetobacter* isolates are resistant to penicillin and members of the genus *Neisseria* are sensitive, differentiation of these organisms is of obvious importance.

TREATMENT Antibiotic sensitivites of *Acinetobacter* strains vary, but most strains are inhibited by kanamycin, gentamicin, tobramycin, colistin, or polymyxin B. Sensitivity to the tetracyclines is unpredictable, and most strains are resistant to penicillin, ampicillin, cephalothin, erythromycin, and chloramphenicol. For serious systemic infections, the appropriate antibiotic, generally an aminoglycoside, should be administered, and since these organisms may produce localized abscesses, surgical drainage may be necessary.

EIKENELLA INFECTIONS

ETIOLOGY *Eikenella corrodens* is a facultatively anaerobic or capnophilic gram-negative rod which is oxidase-positive. As colonies develop on blood agar, characteristic "pitting" or "corroding" of the agar is seen with many strains and generally requires 48 to 72 h of growth to develop.

EPIDEMIOLOGY *Eikenella corrodens* is an inhabitant of the mouth, upper respiratory tract, and gastrointestinal tract of man. Infections frequently involve bowel or oral contamination. A striking association between *Eikenella* infections and methylphenidate (Ritalin) abuse has been noted, perhaps related to the low redox potential created by "skin popping" of this agent as well as a tendency for needles to become contaminated with oral secretions through needle licking.

MANIFESTATIONS The most common infection caused by *Eikenella* is that of skin or soft tissue. Endocarditis, osteomyelitis, and meningitis are reported but are rare. *Eikenella* infections frequently mimic infections caused by strict anaerobes such as *Bacteroides fragilis* or *Peptostreptococcus*. The infections are indolent, frequently mixed with aerobic gram-positive cocci, and drainage is often foul smelling. Abscess formation is common.

TREATMENT *Eikenella corrodens* is susceptible to penicillin, ampicillin, carbenicillin, and tetracycline. Adequate drainage of purulent material is essential in the management of these infections. Ampicillin or penicillin coupled with surgical drainage generally provides a good response. Of note is the marked resistance of *Eikenella* to clindamycin, making the differentiation of *Eikenella* infections from those caused by mixed anaerobes even more important.

REFERENCES

Acinetobacter infections

GLEW RH et al: Infections with *Acinetobacter calcoaceticus:* Clinical and laboratory studies. Medicine 56:79, 1977

INCLAN AP et al: Organisms of the tribe Mimae: Incidence of isolation and clinical correlation. South Med J 58:1261, 1965

REYNOLDS RC, CLUFF LE: Infections of man with Mimae. Ann Intern Med 58:759, 1963

Eikenella infections

BROOKS GF et al: *Eikenella corrodens,* a recently recognized pathogen. Medicine 53:325, 1974

DORFF GJ et al: Infections with *Eikenella corrodens*. Ann Intern Med 80:305, 1974

Pseudomonas infections

ALEXANDER JW et al: Immunologic control of *Pseudomonas* infection in burn patients: Clinical evaluation. Arch Surg 102:31, 1971

ARTENSTEIN MS, SANFORD JP (eds): Symposium on *Pseudomonas aeruginosa*. J Infect Dis 130:S1, November 1974

BODEY GP: Epidemiologic studies of *Pseudomonas* species in patients with leukemia. Am J Med Sci 260:82, 1970

FLICK MR, CLUFF LE: *Pseudomonas* bacteremia: Review of 108 cases Am J Med 60:501, 1976

PENNINGTON JE et al: *Pseudomonas* pneumonia: A retrospective study of 36 cases. Am J Med 55:155, 1973

PHILLIPS I et al: Control of respirator-associated infection due to *Pseudomonas aeruginosa*. Lancet 2:871, 1974

STONE HH: Review of *Pseudomonas* sepsis in thermal injury. Ann Surg 163:297, 1966

122
MELIOIDOSIS AND GLANDERS

JAY P. SANFORD

MELIOIDOSIS

DEFINITION Melioidosis is a glanders-like infection of human beings and animals with a protean clinical spectrum. Melioidosis, which means "a resemblance to distemper of asses," bears a striking resemblance to glanders both clinically and pathologically, but is epidemiologically dissimilar.

ETIOLOGY Melioidosis is caused by a gram-negative motile bacillus, *Pseudomonas pseudomallei*, which can be differentiated from *Pseudomonas mallei* by bacteriologic and serologic means. *Pseudomonas pseudomallei* (also known as Whitmore's bacillus) is a small, gram-negative, motile, aerobic bacillus. When it is stained with methylene blue, Wayson's, or Wright's stain, marked irregularities with a bipolar "safety pin" pattern are observed. It grows well on standard bacteriologic media, with a characteristic wrinkling of colony surfaces after 48 to 72 h of incubation.

EPIDEMIOLOGY The disease is endemic in Southeast Asia, with the greatest concentration of cases reported from Vietnam, Cambodia, Laos, Thailand, Malaysia, and Burma. Cases in human beings have also been reported from adjacent areas including India, Borneo, the Philippines, Guam, Indonesia, Ceylon, New Guinea, and North Queensland. Cases in humans or animals have been reported from Madagascar, Chad, Central West Africa, and Turkey. Human melioidosis has been described only rarely in the Western Hemisphere (Panama, Ecuador)—a neonatal case in Hawaii and a possible case in Oklahoma. With these exceptions, confirmed melioidosis has occurred in United States or European residents only when they have traveled in endemic areas. As of January 1973, when all American forces had been withdrawn from Vietnam, there had been 343 cases with 36 deaths reported in United States Army personnel who were or had been in Vietnam. The majority of these cases occurred in individuals without intercurrent illness, although patients who sustained burn injuries in Vietnam accounted for a disproportionately high number of the cases.

Pseudomonas pseudomallei is a saprophyte which can be isolated from soil, stagnant streams, ponds, rice paddies, and market produce in endemic areas. Its ubiquitous nature is illustrated by its isolation as a laboratory contaminant. *Pseudomonas pseudomallei* is capable of causing disease in epizootic form among sheep, goats, swine, and horses. Occasional isolates have also been reported from cows, rodents, dogs, and cats. Although animals are susceptible to the disease, they apparently do not represent a reservoir for human disease. Attempts to culture *P. pseudomallei* from the urine and feces of a large variety of healthy animals have been unsuccessful. Arthropod-borne infection does not occur naturally. Human beings contract melioidosis by soil contamination of skin abrasions. Ingestion, nasal instillation, and inhalation are other probable methods of spread. In contrast to glanders, infections have been uncommon in laboratory workers. Person-to-person transmission of melioidosis is rare. Venereal transmission from a patient with chronic prostatitis with *P. pseudomallei* isolated from prostatic secretions to his wife, who had never been in an endemic area and who had a hemagglutination titer of 1:10,240, has been recorded. Also, the development of melioidosis in a 2-day-old newborn in Hawaii and demonstration of a significant antibody titer in a nurse who had never been in an endemic area but who had worked on wards with melioidosis patients raise the question of spread from person-to-person within a hospital.

PATHOLOGY In acute infections, the majority of lesions occur in the lungs, with occasional abscesses in other organs. In subacute infections, lung abscesses tend to be more extensive, and lesions are found throughout the body, in the skin, subcutaneous tissue, meninges, brain, eye, heart, liver, kidney, spleen, bone, prostate, synovial membranes, and lymph nodes. The acute abscesses are characterized by an outer border of hemorrhage, a medial zone heavily infiltrated with polymorphonuclear leukocytes, and an inner core of necrotic debris containing large histiocytes with two or three nuclei that have been termed *giant cells*. A striking histological feature has been the marked karyorrhexis. In chronic infections, the lesion consists of a central area of caseation necrosis, mononuclear and plasma cells, and granulation tissue. Calcification does not occur.

CLINICAL MANIFESTATIONS The clinical manifestations of melioidosis are variable. The illness can present as an acute, subacute, or chronic process. The incubation period has not been defined; however, judging by the lapse of time between injury and the development of infection, it may be as short as 2 days. Following a laboratory accident, an incubation period of 3 days ensued. Clinically inapparent infections may remain latent for a number of years after an individual leaves an endemic area, with an interval of 26 years reported in one patient. Men are more often affected than women, a finding which is thought to represent occupational exposure. Melioidosis may be recognized as inapparent infection, asymptomatic pulmonary infiltration, acute localized suppurative infection, acute pulmonary infection, acute septicemic infection, or chronic suppurative infection.

Inapparent infection In Thailand, Vietnam, and Malaysia, 6 to 8 percent of healthy adult men have significant antibody titers against *P. pseudomallei,* with the prevalence reaching 20 percent in a group of Army recruits from the rice-growing states of Western Malaysia. Only 1 percent of Thai women had positive reactions. None of the serums from a control group from the United States was positive. The prevalence of significant antibody titers has been reported as 2 percent for Europeans living in Vietnam and 1 to 9 percent in unselected patients in United States Army hospitals and in a group of normal uninjured soldiers who had served in Vietnam. Occasionally, asymptomatic infections have been discovered by routine chest x-ray.

Acute localized suppurative infection Infection by inoculation of a break in the skin usually results in a nodule with an area of acute lymphangitis and regional lymphadenitis. There are usually fever and generalized malaise. This form of infection may rapidly progress to the acute septicemic form.

Acute pulmonary infection The most common form of the disease has been pulmonary infection, which may represent a primary pneumonitis or hematogenous spread. The acute pulmonary infection can vary in severity from a mild bronchitis to overwhelming necrotizing pneumonia. The onset may be abrupt without prodromal symptoms or more gradual, with headache, anorexia, and generalized myalgia. Fever occurs in almost all patients, is often in excess of 38.9°C (102°F) and may be associated with rigors. Dull or pleuritic chest pain is common. Cough, with or without sputum, occurs. There may be mild pharyngitis. Tachypnea may be out of proportion to the fever and findings on physical or x-ray examination. Chest findings may be minimal but usually consist of rales in the area of pneumonitis. In the absence of dissemination, the spleen and liver are not palpable. Laboratory findings include total leukocyte counts ranging from normal to 20,000 cells per cubic millimeter. Mild normochromic, normocytic anemia may appear during the illness. The pneumonia usually involves the upper lobes with the radiographic appearance of consolidation. Thin-walled cavities, usually 2 to 7 cm in diameter, frequently occur. Without specific therapy, the temperature may become normal within a few days; however, the upper lobe cavitation persists, resulting in a radiographic appearance of tuberculosis. While uncommon, pleural effusions and a pleural mass have been reported. Progressive pulmonary spread or hematogenous dissemination with the development of septicemic manifestations may ensue.

Acute septicemic infection This is the form originally described primarily among narcotic addicts. Subsequent reports, however, have not shown a predilection for debilitated patients. The onset may be abrupt, with the dominant symptoms depending upon site of major involvement. In individuals with bacteremia complicating pneumonitis, symptoms may include disorientation, extreme dyspnea, severe headache, pharyngitis, watery diarrhea, and development of cutaneous pustular lesions on the head, trunk, or extremities. There is high fever, extreme tachypnea, a flushed skin, and cyanosis. Muscle tenderness may be striking. On examination of the chest, signs may be absent, or rales, rhonchi, and pleural rubs may be heard. The liver and spleen may be palpable. Signs of arthritis or meningitis may appear. Patients with the septicemic form usually have a rapidly progressive fatal course, which in some instances may be too fulminant to be altered by therapy. The leukocyte count may be normal or slightly increased. Chest radiographs most commonly show irregular nodular densities 4 to 10 mm in diameter disseminated throughout the lungs. These enlarge, coalesce, and often undergo cavitation as the disease progresses. Pleural effusion is rare. Other radiographic patterns include unilateral irregular mottled densities which become confluent.

Chronic suppurative infection In some patients secondary abscesses develop which dominate the clinical picture. Organs involved include skin, brain, lung, myocardium, liver, spleen, bones, joints, lymph nodes, and even the eye. These patients may be afebrile.

Recrudescent infection Disease may present as acute localized suppurative, acute pulmonary, acute septicemic, or chronic suppurative infection remote from the probable time of exposure (up to 26 years having been reported). In 11 of 15 reported cases, surgery, trauma, or intercurrent illness appeared to act as triggering events.

DIAGNOSIS Melioidosis should be considered in the differential diagnosis of any febrile illness in an individual who has been in an endemic area, especially if the presenting features are those of fulminant respiratory failure, if multiple pustular or necrotic skin or subcutaneous lesions develop, or if there is a radiographic pattern of tuberculosis in a patient from whom tubercle bacilli cannot be isolated.

Microscopic examination of exudates will reveal poorly staining, small, gram-negative bacilli which show the characteristic staining irregularities and "safety pin" bipolar staining with methylene blue. *Pseudomonas pseudomallei* will grow on most laboratory media, including eosinmethylene blue agar (EMB) or MacConkey's agar, in 24 to 48 h. The organisms can be readily differentiated from *P. mallei* and *P. aeruginosa* by standard bacteriologic procedures. The characteristic wrinkling of the colonies may require 72 h or longer. The hemagglutination, direct agglutination test, and complement fixation test are aids in diagnosis if a fourfold or greater rise in titer is demonstrated in paired serums. Single low titers are difficult to interpret because of nonspecific responses. The complement fixation test is said to be specific with titers above 1:8 during the acute illness, but may cross-react with *P. mallei*. A negative complement fixation test does not exclude disease. The hemagglutination and agglutination tests show more cross-reactions. Titers of 1:40 or more suggest infection.

TREATMENT The treatment regimen should vary with the form of the disease. Individuals with low-titer positive serologic tests but with no clinical evidence of infection do not require therapy. The choice of antibiotics in active infection should be based upon sensitivity studies, and therapy should be given for a minimum of 30 days. *Pseudomonas pseudomallei* is usually sensitive in vitro to the tetracyclines, chloramphenicol, novobiocin, kanamycin, sulfadiazine or sulfisoxazole, and trimethoprimsulfamethoxazole, and in most instances is resistant to penicillin G, ampicillin, carbenicillin, dicloxacillin, streptomycin, gentamicin, tobramycin, cephalosporins, vancomycin, lincomycin, rifampin, nalidixic acid, and colistin. In patients with pneumonitis who are not too ill, effective therapy has included tetracycline, 2 to 3 g daily (40 mg/kg); chloramphenicol, 3 g daily (40 mg/kg); sulfisoxazole, 4 g daily (70 mg/kg); or trimethoprim-sulfamethoxazole (4 mg/kg trimethoprim, 20 mg/kg sulfamethoxazole) for 60 to 150 days. If the patient is severely ill, two of these antimicrobials in combination have been recommended for 30 days followed by another 30 to 120 days of tetracycline alone. The mean interval for sputum cultures to become negative has been 6 weeks. If sputum cultures remain positive for 6 months, surgery with lobectomy should be considered. In patients with extrapulmonary suppurative lesions, therapy should be continued for 6 months to 1 year. The usual principles of surgical drainage should be followed. In desperately ill patients with severe pneumonitis or the septicemic form, multiple antibiotics should be administered by the parenteral route. One such regimen has included the use of chloramphenicol, 12 g per day; novobiocin, 6 g per day; and kanamycin, 4 g per day. In view of the severe potential toxicity of this regimen, its use should be considered only in extremely ill patients, and then only on a short-term basis. Current recommendations for antibiotics in the septicemic form of melioidosis are tetracycline, 4 to 6 g per day (80 mg/kg); chloramphenicol, 4 to 6 g per day (80 mg/kg); and one of the following: trimethoprim-sulfamethoxazole (9 mg/kg trimethoprim, 45 mg/kg sulfamethoxazole), sulfisoxazole (140 mg/kg), kanamycin (30 mg/kg), or novobiocin (60 mg/kg). In vitro studies have revealed antagonism between the following pairs of drugs: chloramphenicol-kanamycin, tetracycline-kanamycin, and sulfadiazine-chloramphenicol. Though the significance of such antagonism in clinical therapy has not been assessed, the data would favor selection of trimethoprim-sulfamethoxazole or novobiocin as the third drug. The dosage should be tapered rapidly as clinical improvement occurs.

PROGNOSIS Prior to antimicrobials, the mortality rate of apparent infection was 95 percent. With better diagnosis and more prolonged appropriate therapy, the mortality rate in all except the septicemic form is low. Even with vigorous appropriate antibiotics and supportive therapy, the mortality rate in patients with melioidosis septicemia is greater than 50 percent. Very few patients have had long-term follow-up, and the incidence of late relapses cannot be predicted.

PREVENTION There is no means of active immunization. In endemic areas, vigorous cleansing of abrasions and lacerations is recommended.

GLANDERS

DEFINITION Glanders is a serious infection of equine animals caused by *P. mallei*, which is transmitted occasionally to other domestic animals and to human beings.

ETIOLOGY *Pseudomonas mallei* is a small, slender, nonmotile, gram-negative bacillus. When it is stained with methylene blue, marked irregularities in staining are observed. Organisms grow on most common meat infusion media but require glycerol for optimum growth.

EPIDEMIOLOGY Glanders was at one time widespread throughout Europe, but owing to the introduction of control measures, its incidence has decreased steadily in most countries. The disease still occurs in Asia, Africa, and South America, but not in the United States. Glanders has never been common in human beings; the occasional infection, however, may be very serious. There have been no naturally acquired infections in the United States since 1938.

Glanders is primarily a disease of horses, mules, and donkeys, although goats, sheep, cats, and dogs sometimes naturally contract the disease. Pigs and cattle are resistant. In horses, the disease may be systemic, with prominent pulmonary involvement (*glanders*) or may be characterized by subcutaneous ulcerative lesions, and lymphatic thickening with nodules (*farcy*). Inhalation, ingestion, and inoculation through breaks in the skin have been suggested as routes of infection in animals. In human beings, the disease occurs primarily in individuals with close contact with horses, mules, or donkeys through inoculation of or a break in the skin or by exposing the nasal mucosa to contaminated discharges. A number of instances of airborne infection have been reported in laboratory workers.

PATHOLOGY The acute lesion is characterized by nodules consisting of polymorphonuclear leukocytes surrounded by a zone of congestion. A characteristic histological feature is a peculiar nuclear degeneration known as *chromatotexis* which occurs early and is extensive. Small foci of deeply staining detritus within the abscess result from this degeneration. In older nodules, the reaction is characterized by epitheloid cells surrounding an area of central necrosis. Giant cells may be present. Virtually any organ may be involved.

CLINICAL MANIFESTATIONS The manifestations which frequently overlap may be categorized as (1) acute localized suppurative infection, (2) acute pulmonary infection, (3) acute septicemic infection, and (4) chronic suppurative infection. Nearly 60 percent of patients have been between the ages of 20 and 40 years. The disease has been rare in women, probably because of less opportunity for contact.

Infection acquired by inoculation through an abrasion in the skin usually results in a nodule with an area of acute lymphangitis. The incubation period is probably 1 to 5 days. In all types of acute glanders, there are usually fever, generalized malaise, and prostration.

Infection of the mucous membranes may result in a mucopurulent discharge involving the eye, nose, or lips followed by extensive ulcerating granulomatous lesions which may or may not be associated with systemic reactions. With systemic invasion, a generalized papular eruption which may become pustular is frequent. This septicemic form of disease is usually fatal in 7 to 10 days.

Infection by inhalation is followed by an incubation period of 10 to 14 days. The more common symptoms include fever, occasionally associated with rigors, generalized myalgia, fatigue, headache, and pleuritic chest pain. Other symptoms consist of photophobia, lacrimation, and diarrhea. Findings on physical examination are usually normal except for fever and occasional lymphadenopathy, especially in the cervical chain, and splenomegaly. Laboratory findings include mild leukocytosis with 60 to 80 percent neutrophilic leukocytes, but leukopenia with relative lymphocytosis has been recorded. In the acute pulmonary form, chest radiographs characteristically reveal circumscribed densities which suggest early lung abscesses. Other findings may include lobar or bronchopneumonia. In the chronic suppurative form of the disease, the most frequent finding consists of multiple subcutaneous and intramuscular abscesses which most often involve the arms or legs. Approximately one-half the patients will have associated fever, lymphadenopathy, and nasal discharge or ulceration. Visceral involvement including pulmonary or pleural, ocular, skeletal, hepatic, splenic, and meningeal or intracranial involvement occurs in some patients.

DIAGNOSIS Microscopic examination of exudates may reveal small gram-negative bacilli which stain irregularly with methylene blue; however, organisms generally are very scanty, and it is often difficult to find them even in acute abscesses. Giemsa or other modifications of the Romanowski stain may be the best way to identify organisms. *Pseudomonas mallei* and *P. pseudomallei* cannot be distinguished morphologically. Culturing is often avoided because of the hazard to laboratory personnel; however, if cultures are made, growth occurs on most meat infusion nutrient media. The material is often contaminated with other microorganisms, and incubation with penicillin G (1000 units per milliliter) prior to culturing may be helpful. Subcutaneous inoculation of material into a guinea pig or hamster affords an alternative means of isolation. Blood cultures are usually negative except in the terminal stages of disease. Serologic tests show a rapidly rising agglutination titer, which reaches levels of 1:640 within 2 weeks. Serum from normal persons has been reported to show agglutination titers in dilutions up to 1:320. The complement fixation test is less sensitive but more specific and usually becomes positive during the third week; it is considered positive in dilutions of 1:20 or greater.

TREATMENT The limited number of recent infections in human beings has precluded evaluation of most of the antibiotic agents. Sulfadiazine has been found to be an effective agent in experimental animals and in humans. The dosage utilized has been approximately 100 mg/kg administered in divided doses. In experimental infections, 3 weeks of therapy gave better results than 1 week. Benzyl penicillin is ineffective in vitro and in experimental infections. Streptomycin is bacteriostatic in vitro but was ineffective in experimental infections in hamsters. Antibiotics such as tetracycline, chloramphenicol, the antipseudomonal aminoglycosides, carbenicillin, the polymyxins, and trimethoprim have not been evaluated. In the absence of clinical experience and pending in vitro susceptibility studies, it would seem most reasonable to utilize the regimens appropriate for patients with various manifestations of melioidosis. In the acute infections, appropriate supportive measures are essential, and in chronic suppurative infections, the usual principles of surgical drainage should be followed.

PROGNOSIS The prognosis depends upon the type of infection. The acute septicemic form has been uniformly fatal. The localized or chronic forms have a much better prognosis.

PREVENTION Next to acquisition from diseased horses, the commonest source of natural disease in human beings has been contact with human glanders. Isolation is indicated.

REFERENCES

EICKHOFF TC et al: *Pseudomonas pseudomallei:* Susceptibility to chemotherapeutic agents. J Infect Dis 121:95, 1970

EVERETT ED, NELSON R: Pulmonary melioidosis, observations in 39 cases. Am Rev Resp Dis 112:331, 1975

HOWE C, MILLER WR: Human glanders: Report of six cases. Ann Intern Med 26:93, 1947

———— et al: The pseudomallei: A review. J Infect Dis 124:598, 1971

JACKSON AE et al: Recrudescent melioidosis associated with diabetic ketoacidosis. Arch Intern Med 130:268, 1972

MAYS EE, RICKETS EA: Melioidosis: Recrudescence associated with bronchogenic carcinoma twenty-six years following initial geographic exposure. Chest 68:261, 1975

MCCORMICK JB et al: Human to human transmission of *Pseudomonas pseudomallei.* Ann Intern Med 83:512, 1975

SANFORD JP: Melioidosis: Another great imitator, in *Infectious Diseases: Current Topics in Diagnosis and Treatment*, DN Gilbert, JP Sanford (eds). New York, Grune & Stratton, 1978

ZAJTCHUK R et al: Surgical treatment of melioidosis. J Thorac Cardiovasc Surg 66:838, 1973

123
SALMONELLA INFECTIONS

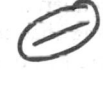

EDWARD W. HOOK
RICHARD L. GUERRANT

INTRODUCTION The genus *Salmonella* consists of three species which include more than 1700 different serologic types. Striking variation in pathogenicity of serotypes occurs, but almost all are pathogenic for animals and humans. Specific host preferences characterize certain serotypes, such as *S. typhi*, which under natural conditions of transmission produces disease only in humans. *Salmonella* infections in humans present a spectrum of clinical syndromes, which sometimes overlap. The syndromes are (1) enteric fever (typhoid or paratyphoid fever), (2) acute gastroenteritis, (3) bacteremia, and (4) localized infection which may occur at almost any site. In addition, *asymptomatic intestinal infections* and *transient convalescent intestinal carrier* states are common. Occasionally, a focus of infection persists in the gallbladder or urinary tract to produce a *chronic carrier* state.

ETIOLOGY Salmonellae are motile gram-negative bacilli that do not ferment lactose or sucrose but ferment glucose. Almost all serotypes produce gas, although *S. typhi* is a notable exception. Salmonellae are divided into three species by biochemical means: *S. typhi, S. cholerae-suis,* and *S. enteritidis.* The species are further subdivided into serotypes, which are identified by highly specific O (somatic) and H (flagellar) antigens. A given serotype will contain a specific combination of multiple O and H antigens. Identification by serotype is accomplished routinely only in large salmonella typing centers, which have the necessary collection of antiserums required for such work. Salmonellae are also divided into groups on the basis of O antigen composition. Most isolates from natural sources fall into five groups, A to E.

The species *S. typhi* and *S. cholerae-suis* consist of only one serotype each (in groups D and C, respectively), whereas the species *S. enteritidis* comprises over 1700 serotypes (in all groups, including C and D). Considerable overlap in antigenic composition is responsible for the cross-reactivity which is commonly seen in serologic tests with salmonellae.

The Salmonella Surveillance Unit of the Center for Disease Control reports 20,000 to 25,000 isolations of salmonellae annually from human beings in the United States. This number has been consistent over the decade from 1967 to 1976. In descending order, the most frequently isolated serotypes in 1976 were *S. typhimurium, S. heidelberg, S. agona, S. newport, S. enteritidis, S. infantis, S. saint-paul, S. typhi, S. oranienburg,* and *S. muenchen.* The 10 most frequently isolated serotypes account for about 70 percent of the total isolates from man over this period. *Salmonella typhimurium* perennially accounts for 25 to 35 percent of the isolates. A significant recent change in serotypes isolated from human sources in the United States is the rapidly increasing rate of isolation each year of *S. agona,* an organism apparently introduced indirectly via animals fed Peruvian fish meal in 1971. Concern has also arisen over the multiple-drug-resistant *S. wein,* which was the most frequent *Salmonella* isolate in France in 1974 and which is now being isolated in the United States; *S. wein* is resistant to chloramphenicol, ampicillin, sulfonamides, and tetracyclines.

In the subsequent section, typhoid fever, the classic example of enteric fever, is considered separately from other *Salmonella* infections because of its historical importance, the host specificity of *S. typhi,* and the extensive clinical experience with the disease.

TYPHOID FEVER

DEFINITION Typhoid fever is an acute systemic disease resulting from infection with *S. typhi.* The disease is unique to humans. It is characterized by malaise, fever, abdominal discomfort, transient rash, splenomegaly, and leukopenia. The most prominent major complications are intestinal hemorrhage and perforation. The disease is the classic example of enteric fever caused by salmonellas. However, enteric fever, similar to typhoid, can also be caused by other *Salmonella* serotypes and is termed *paratyphoid fever.*

EPIDEMIOLOGY *Salmonella typhi* gains access to the body by the oral route in almost all cases as a consequence of the ingestion of contaminated food, water, or milk. Humans are the only true reservoir of *S. typhi* in nature, and persons with typhoid fever or convalescent or chronic carriers always serve as the ultimate source of infection. Infected individuals can excrete millions of viable typhoid bacilli in the feces, which are the usual source of contamination of food or drink. Patients with active disease also occasionally have organisms in respiratory secretions, vomitus, or other body fluids. Flies or other insects can carry organisms from feces or other infected material to food or drink and have been implicated in a few outbreaks. The fact that *S. typhi* may survive freezing or drying enhances the possibility of spread by contaminated ice, dust, foods, and sewage. Oysters or other shellfish are contaminated at times in polluted waters and occasionally serve as sources of typhoid.

The incidence of typhoid fever has steadily decreased in the United States during the past century to the present relatively low level of less than 400 cases per annum. The decrease in incidence has been coincident with improvement in socioeconomic conditions and is specifically related to development of pure water supplies, effective sewage disposal, pasteurization of milk, and methods to detect and control spread of organisms from persons with active disease or from carriers. Typhoid continues to occur on a large scale in countries where sanitation is suboptimal. About 40 percent of the patients with typhoid fever in the United States appear to have acquired the infection in another area of the world.

Typhoid can be eradicated ultimately because the infection is confined to humans and both the disease and the carrier state can be controlled by appropriate therapy. The importance of sewage disposal, a pure water supply, and control of carriers is highlighted repeatedly by the occurrence of outbreaks which develop when defects in sanitation occur during natural disasters such as flood.

The sex distribution of patients with typhoid fever in the United States shows no significant predilection. In recent years, about 75 percent of cases have occurred in persons less than 30 years of age. In contrast, the chronic carrier state is much more common in females than males (the female/male ratio is 3:1) and in older individuals (88 percent over 50 years of age).

There is no seasonal variation in incidence of typhoid fever in the United States. However, in areas of the world where the disease is endemic, the incidence increases in the summer months.

PATHOGENESIS The outcome of the interaction between the typhoid bacillus and humans is determined during the early hours after ingestion of the organisms. Typhoid bacilli reach the small intestine shortly after ingestion and may multiply there. The organisms may then penetrate the mucosa with minimal epithelial destruction and enter intestinal lymphatics, perhaps via the Peyer's patches, to be carried to the bloodstream. This initial early bacteremia apparently occurs within 24 to 72 h after ingestion of organisms and is rarely detected in natural infections because patients are usually asymptomatic at this early stage. The bacteremia is transient and is rapidly terminated as bacilli are phagocytized by cells of the reticuloendothelial system. Nevertheless, viable bacilli are disseminated throughout the body and apparently persist within reticuloendothelial cells. If multiplication at the intracellular site takes place, organisms reenter the bloodstream, producing a continuous bacteremia for days or weeks. The reappearance of bacteremia corresponds with the onset of manifestations of the disease. The intracellular organisms are eventually destroyed as manifestations of disease subside and recovery ensues. Enhanced intracellular killing and recovery appear to be related to the onset of delayed hypersensitivity. Recovery is unrelated to the appearance, even in high titer, of agglutinins against the somatic, flagellar, or Vi antigens of the typhoid bacillus.

The number of organisms ingested is of obvious importance in determining whether typhoid fever results from exposure to *S. typhi.* Studies in volunteers have shown that about 10^7 typhoid bacilli of the Quailes strain must be taken orally to produce typhoid fever in 50 percent of normal volunteers. The number of organisms ingested also influences the incubation period, and short incubation periods, in general, correspond to large doses of organisms. The volunteer studies have also demonstrated that different strains of typhoid bacilli vary considerably in their capacity to produce disease in humans.

The normal flora of the upper intestinal tract is an important protective mechanism against invasion by *S. typhi.* Volunteer studies have demonstrated that antimicrobial therapy a day or so before oral challenge with *S. typhi* markedly decreases the number of viable bacilli required to produce disease. It is possible that certain factors known to be associated with typhoid outbreaks, such as malnutrition, enhance susceptibility to typhoid infection by alterations in the intestinal flora.

During the phase of persistent bacteremia, all organs are repeatedly exposed to typhoid bacilli. Abscess formation may occur but is unusual. However, localization does occur in the gallbladder in almost all cases. Organisms multiply in the bile to high titer, usually without manifestations of cholecystitis, and are excreted with bile into the intestinal tract. Stool cultures, which are usually negative for *S. typhi* during the incubation period and early phases of the disease, become positive in a large proportion of cases during the third or fourth week of the disease, when excretion of organisms multiplying in the bile reaches a peak.

The factors responsible for the fever, leukopenia, and other manifestations of typhoid fever have been inadequately defined. Typhoid bacilli contain biologically active lipopolysaccharides or endotoxins which produce fever, leukopenia, thrombocytopenia, and hyperplasia of reticuloendothelial cells when injected into animals or humans. It has been assumed for years that these materials play an important role in the patho-

genesis of the signs and symptoms of typhoid fever. However, the evidence regarding the role of endotoxin in the genesis of the manifestations of typhoid is inconclusive. For example, tolerance to the pyrogenic effects of endotoxins can be demonstrated during convalescence from typhoid fever, which suggests release of endotoxins during infection. While laboratory evidence for low-grade, subclinical disseminated intravascular coagulation can often be demonstrated in patients with typhoid fever, endotoxemia is usually not detectable. Other studies show that typhoid fever follows a normal course in volunteers rendered tolerant to endotoxins prior to challenge, indicating that more complex mechanisms than endotoxemia alone are responsible for the sustained fever and toxemia.

PATHOLOGY The most prominent microscopic lesion in typhoid fever is proliferation of large mononuclear cells in many different tissues. Mononuclear hyperplasia leads to lymphadenopathy, splenomegaly, and impressive enlargement of lymphoid tissues in the intestines, especially in the terminal ileum (Peyer's patches). Proliferating mononuclear cells may also be observed in bone marrow, liver, and lung. Studies in volunteers using ^{131}I-tagged aggregated albumin have shown increased phagocytic activity of the reticuloendothelial system by the third to fifth days after onset of symptoms. Necrosis in hyperplastic Peyer's patches may be associated with erosion of blood vessels in the lesions in the intestinal tract, which leads to oozing of blood or massive hemorrhage. Lesions may extend deep into the intestinal wall and cause perforation of the bowel, an event which characteristically occurs late in the disease, most often in the third febrile week. The site of perforation is usually in the distal 24 in of the ileum.

The gallbladder and bile ducts are routinely infected during the disease. As a rule, this biliary infection is asymptomatic, although acute cholecystitis may occur occasionally. Biliary infection terminates spontaneously during convalescence in the vast majority of patients within 12 months, but about 3 percent of adults continue to harbor organisms in the gallbladder and become chronic carriers of the typhoid bacillus.

MANIFESTATIONS The incubation period averages about 10 days but may vary from extremes of 3 to 60 days depending on the infecting dose.

The clinical manifestations and duration of illness vary markedly from one patient to another. Mild forms of the disease, characterized primarily by fever, may last only a week, or illness may be prolonged, lasting 8 weeks or more if untreated.

In a typical patient not treated with antimicrobials, the illness lasts about 4 weeks. The onset is insidious with headache, malaise, anorexia, and fever. Headache may be the first manifestation of disease and is usually generalized and severe. Chilly sensations are common, and frank chills may be observed. The fever is remittent, frequently increasing in a step-like manner from day to day as the illness develops. Abdominal discomfort, bloating, and constipation are common during the early phase of illness. A dry cough is observed in about two-thirds of the patients and occasionally may be so prominent as to direct attention away from the generalized nature of the infectious process. Nosebleeds may occur during the early phase of illness.

The temperature gradually increases for 5 to 7 days and then plateaus as a continuous or mildly remittent fever in the range of 39 to 40°C. The temperature may be sustained at these levels with little variation for 2 or 3 weeks. A relative bradycardia occurs in 30 to 40 percent of the patients. The prolonged persistent fever leads to general debility; patients are weak and anorectic. Mental dullness is common and delirium may occur. Abdominal pain and marked distention are usual. Constipation, relatively common during the early phase of illness, may give way to diarrhea later in the course of the disease.

The characteristic rash (rose spots) is most often observed during the second week of the disease. The lesions are small, 2- to 4-mm, erythematous macules which occur in small numbers on the upper abdomen and anterior thorax. The lesions blanch on pressure and last only 2 to 3 days. Some reports describe rose spots in as many as 90 percent of patients, whereas other reports indicate a frequency of only 10 percent or even less. The evasive nature of the rash and the difficulties encountered in detecting lesions in highly pigmented individuals probably account for the marked variation in incidence reported in the literature.

The liver and spleen are frequently enlarged and palpable from the end of the first week of illness. The spleen is palpable in about three-quarters of the patients. The liver may be tender, and occasionally a friction rub is audible over the spleen.

Abdominal tenderness is frequent and distention occurs in the majority of cases. Marked abdominal pain with signs of peritonitis should call attention to the possibility of perforation of the bowel.

After the third week, the symptoms slowly abate, and the temperature returns to normal over a period of days.

Jaundice secondary to extensive mononuclear cell infiltration in the liver and hepatic cell necrosis is a rare complication of typhoid. Acute renal failure also is observed rarely; the pathogenesis of this so-called "typhoid nephritis" has not been adequately defined. Disseminated intravascular coagulation may develop in severe typhoid and lead to additional clinical manifestations secondary to thrombosis or hemorrhage.

Complications   Prior to the introduction of chloramphenicol, the prolonged febrile course of typhoid often led to profound debility, weight loss, and multiple nutritional deficiencies. Intestinal hemorrhage and bowel perforation, the most feared complications, were common causes of death. The frequency of complications in typhoid fever has been reduced since the advent of effective chemotherapy.

INTESTINAL HEMORRHAGE   Erosion of blood vessels in hyperplastic and necrotic Peyer's patches or in other mononuclear cell accumulations in the wall of the intestine leads to bleeding into the intestinal tract. Occult blood in feces is quite common during the course of the disease, occurring in 20 percent or more of patients. Gross blood is present in feces in about 10 percent of patients, and massive hemorrhage occurs occasionally. Major hemorrhage is usually a late complication, occurring most often during the second or third week of disease. A sudden drop in blood pressure or temperature may be the first manifestation of hemorrhage.

INTESTINAL PERFORATION   The pathological process in the lymphoid tissues of the intestine may also involve the muscular and serosal layers of the bowel and lead to perforation. Prior to the advent of chloramphenicol, perforation occurred in about 3 percent of patients with typhoid. The incidence has been reduced by antimicrobial therapy to about 1 percent. Perforation is most common in the distal 24 in of ileum and is observed most frequently during the third week of the disease. The onset of perforation may be quite unexpected during an otherwise uncomplicated convalescence. Pain in the right lower quadrant of the abdomen is the most frequent initial manifestation, but signs of localized or generalized peritonitis develop rapidly.

OTHER COMPLICATIONS   Typhoid bacilli may localize in any tissue in the body with the production of localized suppurative infection. Meningitis, chondritis, periostitis, osteomyelitis, ar-

thritis, and pyelonephritis are examples of localized infections that may be observed occasionally. Pneumonia is not unusual and may be related to the typhoid bacillus or to a secondary bacterial invader, such as the pneumococcus. Severe deep thrombophlebitis may occur during the febrile period. Late complications also include peripheral neuritis, deafness, and alopecia. Hemolytic anemia may be observed, especially in infected individuals deficient in glucose 6-phosphate dehydrogenase.

Relapse   After illness has subsided for a variable period, usually about 2 weeks, all the manifestations which characterized the initial infection may recur. Blood cultures, negative during convalescence, may become positive again. Although relapse may be severe, it is usually milder and of shorter duration than the original illness. The incidence of relapse was about 5 to 10 percent prior to the introduction of effective chemotherapy. Chloramphenicol has not decreased the frequency of relapse; in fact, the relapse rate in chloramphenicol-treated patients is higher than in patients not receiving the drug. Periods of antimicrobial therapy longer than 2 weeks do not seem to alter the incidence of relapse. Relapse cannot be correlated with the titer of agglutinins against the flagellar, somatic, or Vi antigens of the typhoid bacillus.

Chronic carriers   Although the vast majority of patients with typhoid fever eradicate the site of infection in the gallbladder during convalescence, about 3 percent of adults do not, and these individuals become chronic typhoid carriers who continue to excrete organisms in feces for years, usually for life. A chronic carrier is defined as a person documented to have been excreting typhoid bacilli in the stool for a period of at least 1 year. In the United States, almost all chronic carriers have a persistent site of infection in the gallbladder from which organisms reach the intestinal tract in bile. Chronic carriers may be detected by follow-up of patients with typhoid fever, but many carriers give no history of typhoid. In these patients, it is assumed that the initial illness was so mild as to go unrecognized or undiagnosed. Once organisms have been demonstrated in the stools for as long as a year, it is quite unlikely that the focus of infection in the gallbladder will terminate spontaneously. The chronic carrier state is rare in children and occurs more commonly with increasing age and is about three times more common in women than men. It is possible that these age and sex characteristics are related to the greater prevalence of gallbladder disease in older women, a factor which would favor persistence of organisms in the biliary tract.

The chronic biliary carrier is usually asymptomatic. Despite millions of organisms entering the intestine in each milliliter of bile, patients show no systemic manifestations. Gallstones and dysfunction of the gallbladder on cholecystogram can be demonstrated in a large proportion of chronic carriers, and carriers occasionally develop acute cholecystitis.

In areas of the world where *Schistosoma haematobium* infections are common, a chronic urinary carrier state results from localization of typhoid bacilli or other *Salmonella* serotypes in the obstructed urinary tract or adjacent lesions resulting from the schistosomiasis. These chronic urinary carriers not only excrete *Salmonella* in the urine but also may have intermittent bacteremic episodes which are not necessarily accompanied by fever.

LEUKOPENIA ; stool – MONONUCLEAR LEUKOCYTOSIS

LABORATORY FINDINGS   Leukopenia of 3000 to 4000 cells per cubic millimeter is characteristic of the febrile phase of typhoid fever. A sudden increase in leukocyte count to 10,000 cells per cubic millimeter or higher should suggest the possibility of intestinal perforation, hemorrhage, or a pyogenic complication, but these complications may occur in the absence of leukocytosis. A normocytic normochromic anemia develops during the course of the disease and may be aggravated by blood loss from intestinal lesions. Occult blood and a mononuclear leukocytosis in feces is common from the second week of disease. Urine is usually normal except for transient albuminuria during the febrile period.

The most dependable way to establish a definitive diagnosis of typhoid fever is by blood culture. Organisms can be recovered by culture of blood in 70 to 90 percent of patients during the first week of disease. Bacteremia is continuous and prolonged. Positive blood cultures are obtained in as many as 30 or 40 percent of patients during the third week of disease, but the incidence of bacteremia rapidly decreases after this time. Blood cultures frequently are positive during relapse. Recent evidence in partially treated cases suggests that culture of bone marrow may yield the organism when other cultures are negative.

Only about 10 to 15 percent of patients have positive stool cultures during the first week of disease. However, the frequency of positive stool cultures increases as the disease progresses, reaching a maximum of about 75 percent during the third or fourth week of illness. The frequency of positive cultures then begins to decline so that only about 10 percent of patients have positive stool cultures 8 weeks after onset of illness. Most of these patients' cultures become negative over the next several weeks or months, but about 3 percent of adults continue to excrete organisms even after 1 year. Persistent excretion in these chronic carriers is secondary to infection in the gallbladder and biliary tract.

The incidence of positive urine cultures varies markedly during the course of typhoid fever and parallels the frequency of positive stool cultures. At least some of the positive cultures represent contamination of urine with feces harboring typhoid bacilli.

The majority of patients, but by no means all, develop a fourfold or greater rise in agglutinins against the somatic or O antigens of the typhoid bacillus during the course of the disease. A fourfold or greater increase in titer in the absence of recent typhoid immunization is compatible with infection with S. typhi but is by no means specific. All the group D organisms, one of which is S. typhi, as well as organisms in groups A and B, have certain common antigens which can evoke the formation of antibodies reactive with the O antigen used in the Widal test. Agglutinins against flagellar or H antigens also appear, frequently in higher titer than agglutinins against the O antigens. However, the H agglutinins are even more subject to nonspecific variation than O agglutinins and are of no value in diagnosis. Agglutinins begin to appear after about 1 week of illness and reach a peak titer during the fifth or sixth week. Early antimicrobial therapy may dampen the immunologic response in patients with typhoid fever. Relapse bears no relation to agglutinin titer. Rheumatoid factor activity in high titer can be detected in a large proportion of patients with typhoid or paratyphoid fever.

DIFFERENTIAL DIAGNOSIS The clinical features of typhoid fever, while characteristic and suggestive of the diagnosis, are certainly not pathognomonic. Many other diseases give a clinical picture which may be confused with typhoid; these include the rickettsioses, brucellosis, tularemia, leptospirosis, psittacosis, infectious hepatitis, infectious mononucleosis, primary atypical pneumonia, miliary tuberculosis, malaria, lymphoma,

and rheumatic fever. Typhoid should be considered in any patient with unexplained fever, especially if there is a history of recent foreign travel to endemic areas.

TREATMENT Antimicrobial therapy Chloramphenicol is the antibiotic of choice for the treatment of typhoid fever. Despite the fact that a number of antimicrobial agents show excellent in vitro activity against S. typhi, chloramphenicol has consistently been shown to be more effective in terminating the febrile toxic course of the disease in the greatest proportion of patients in the shortest period of time. Nevertheless, the response to chloramphenicol is not dramatic or rapid. Subjective improvement usually occurs within about 48 h after beginning therapy, but the temperature usually does not return to normal for 2 to 5 days after initiating treatment. Bacteremia usually clears within hours after therapy is instituted, but occasionally organisms can be recovered from the blood 24 to 48 h after beginning treatment. The dose of chloramphenicol should be 50 mg per kilogram of body weight per day divided into three or four equal doses given orally at intervals of 6 to 8 h. After the patient has become afebrile, the dose may be reduced to 30 mg/kg per day. Therapy should be continued for 2 weeks. If chloramphenicol cannot be given by the oral route, comparable doses should be given parenterally.

Ampicillin in doses of 80 mg/kg per day or 6 g per day for adults divided into four or six doses given parenterally or a combination of trimethoprim and sulfamethoxazole is effective in the treatment of typhoid, but the response is not as predictable or as prompt as with chloramphenicol. If there is a contraindication to therapy with chloramphenicol, ampicillin, amoxicillin, or trimethoprim-sulfamethoxazole is recommended.

Occasional patients with typhoid without evidence of suppurative complications do not respond clinically even after 4 or 5 days of antimicrobial therapy, even though blood cultures become negative. Delayed responses of this type occur in only about 1 percent of patients treated with chloramphenicol, in contrast to 5 or 10 percent of patients treated with ampicillin.

Chloramphenicol-resistant strains have been reported since 1972 from Mexico, Southeast Asia, and India. Resistance is due to a transferable R factor which also codes for resistance to sulfonamides, tetracycline, and streptomycin. Salmonella typhi resistant to both chloramphenicol and ampicillin have been isolated from a few patients. If chloramphenicol resistance is encountered, then ampicillin, amoxicillin, or trimethoprim and sulfamethoxazole should be used.

Adrenal hormones The administration of prednisone or steroids with similar activity can terminate within a matter of hours the severe febrile toxemic state seen in some patients. Because of the lag in time between institution of antimicrobial therapy and evidence of response, patients with life-threatening toxemia should be treated with a brief course of adrenal corticosteroids in addition to chloramphenicol. An appropriate regimen is 60 mg prednisone the first day; no additional steroid therapy should be administered. Hypothermia and hypotension occasionally occur within hours after initiation of steroids.

Supportive treatment Nursing care and attention to nutritional requirements are important. Laxatives and enemas should be avoided despite constipation because of the danger of precipitating hemorrhage or perforation. Salicylates should not be used, because in addition to their effects on blood platelets and irritating action on the bowel, these compounds can induce wide swings in temperature with very uncomfortable chills and sweats. Hypothermia and hypotension occur in some patients after administration of salicylates.

Hemorrhage and perforation Patients should be observed carefully to detect these complications at an early stage. Typing and cross matching should be carried out at the time of initial diagnosis of typhoid, and transfusion is indicated in the event of significant hemorrhage. Patients with typhoid are poor surgical risks. If perforation is suspected, emphasis should be placed on efforts to combat shock and decompress the bowel. Additional antimicrobials may have to be added to control peritonitis. Small perforations may localize and can be managed without surgical intervention. However, if evidence of localization does not develop, surgical intervention may be required.

Relapse The therapy of relapse is identical to that for the primary episode.

Chronic carriers Chronic carriers should be investigated for the presence of gallstones or a nonfunctioning gallbladder. Carriers without evidence of gallstones or gallbladder disease on cholecystogram usually can be cured with a prolonged course of ampicillin. One program which has been found to be effective consists of 6 g ampicillin divided into four equal oral doses each day with probenecid for a period of 6 weeks. If gallstones or a nonfunctioning gallbladder are demonstrated on cholecystogram, antimicrobial therapy is unlikely to be effective in terminating the carrier state. These patients should have cholecystectomy, which cures the chronic carrier state in about 85 percent of patients. Ampicillin may be used in conjunction with cholecystectomy. Therapy should be started a few days prior to the procedure and continued for 2 or 3 weeks.

PREVENTION AND CONTROL Although immunization with typhoid vaccine affords significant protection against typhoid infection, the degree of immunity is not great and can be readily overcome with a large dose of organisms. Nevertheless, immunization is recommended for individuals living or traveling in areas where the disease is endemic and for persons working with the organism in laboratories. Adults should receive 0.5 ml vaccine on two occasions separated by a period of 1 or 2 weeks. A yearly booster is required to maintain immunity. Immunization with typhoid vaccine causes a transient elevation for several months in titer of agglutinins against typhoid O antigens and a persistently elevated titer for H antigens.

All typhoid patients should be reported to local health authorities, and stool specimens should be cultured during convalescence. Three consecutively negative stool cultures obtained at weekly intervals indicate that a carrier state has not developed.

Caution should be observed to prevent spread of infection from persons with active disease or from carriers. Chronic or convalescent carriers should not be allowed to prepare food until clear documentation shows that at least three or more stool cultures are negative for typhoid bacilli. Carriers should be cautioned regarding routine sanitary techniques.

PROGNOSIS The mortality rate of typhoid fever prior to the introduction of chloramphenicol was about 12 percent. Death was associated with toxemia, inanition, pneumonia, bowel perforation, and intestinal hemorrhage. The mortality rate is still 2 or 3 percent; deaths are observed primarily in infants, the aged, or individuals with malnutrition or other underlying diseases.

OTHER *SALMONELLA* INFECTIONS

DEFINITION Bacteria of the genus *Salmonella* may produce asymptomatic infection of the intestinal tract in humans or

several different clinical syndromes including acute gastroenteritis (or enterocolitis), bacteremia, paratyphoid fever, or localized infections ranging from osteomyelitis to endocarditis. The clinical syndromes resulting from infection with *Salmonella* cannot always be sharply differentiated and sometimes overlap.

Salmonella infections are among the most prevalent communicable diseases caused by bacteria in the United States today. These infections are transmitted in the vast majority of cases from animals to humans and occasionally from person to person and are usually brief, self-limited, and mild.

EPIDEMIOLOGY Salmonellas can be isolated from the intestinal tracts of humans and many lower animals. The prevalence of asymptomatic excretors of these organisms in the general population is about 0.2 percent, but the most important reservoir of salmonellas is in domestic and wild animal species in which infection rates vary from less than 1 to more than 20 percent. An incomplete list of animals from which *Salmonella* species have been isolated includes chickens, turkeys, ducks, pigs, cows, dogs, cats, rats, parakeets, as well as certain cold-blooded animals and insects. Animals sold as pets, especially baby chicks, ducks, and turtles, may also harbor *Salmonella* and serve as sources of infection.

Salmonella infection is almost always acquired by the oral route, usually by ingestion of contaminated food or drink. Any food product is a potential source of human infection. The source of contamination of food or drink may be asymptomatic human carriers or persons with active clinical disease, but the greatest single source of human infection in the United States is the vast reservoir of *Salmonella* in lower animals. The high incidence of infection in domestic animals used as a source of food for humans and present methods of processing foods and food products in bulk result in the availability of foods for human consumption with a potentially high incidence of contamination with *Salmonella*. For example, a significant proportion varying from 1 to more than 50 percent of raw meats purchased in retail markets is contaminated with *Salmonella*. Meat is contaminated by many routes, but the most common are natural infection of the animal used as a source of meat and contamination of the carcass during slaughter and processing. Eggs or egg products, including dried or frozen eggs, are also common sources of *Salmonella* infection. Of the various animal species, domestic fowl, including chickens, turkeys, ducks, and eggs and egg products, constitute the single largest reservoir of infection and the source most often responsible for infection of humans. Adequate cooking of food prior to human consumption serves to decrease the possibility of infection. However, salmonellas may survive cooking at low temperature, or food may be recontaminated after cooking by organisms from kitchen equipment or personnel.

Food or drink may also be contaminated by rats, mice, insects, or other vermin harboring these organisms. Cross infection occurs occasionally by the airborne route from dried foods such as egg whites or dust which contain viable *Salmonella*. *Salmonella* contamination of a large variety of processed foods has also been documented. Some of these foods contain ingredients of animal origin such as eggs, whereas others contain contaminated products of vegetable origin such as coconut or yeast. A variety of pharmaceutical products of animal origin have been shown to be responsible for *Salmonella* infections of humans; these products include carmine dye, pancreatin, bile salts, and extracts of various organs such as thyroid, adrenal, and stomach

Pet turtles may be an important source of *Salmonella* infection in humans, especially in children, accounting for perhaps as many as 10 to 20 percent of reported *Salmonella* infections in certain areas. Turtles are infected on breeding farms and continue to excrete organisms in feces into tank water for long periods of time. Although knowledge of the manner of transmission to humans is incomplete, it is likely that turtle feces or tank water harboring salmonellas contaminate hands of handlers, from which organisms are passed to the mouth or to food or drink.

Salmonella species may also be transmitted directly or via fomites from humans to humans or from animals to humans without the intervention of contaminated food or drink, but this method of spread is not common. However, cross infection of this type has been shown to be responsible for a number of outbreaks of salmonellosis among patients in nurseries and hospitals. Nosocomial salmonellosis poses a particular threat to newborns, immunosuppressed patients, patients in burn units, and those receiving multiple broad-spectrum antibiotics, who may be infected by relatively few organisms. Multiple-drug-resistant salmonellas are often found in this setting. Nursery outbreaks have been traced to newborn infants from mothers with recent *Salmonella* infections.

Fish meal, meat meal, bone meal, and other by-products of the meat-packing industry are often contaminated with *Salmonella* organisms. These products are incorporated in animal and poultry feeds and apparently play an important role in the perpetuation of infection among domestic animals that can be spread to humans.

The true incidence of *Salmonella* infection is difficult to determine. The reported isolations of salmonellas from humans in the United States represent about 10 cases per 100,000 population per annum. However, reported cases represent only a small proportion of the actual number because bacteriologic studies are usually performed only on patients with severe or protracted diarrhea, and many outbreaks are not investigated. Although *Salmonella* infection occurs throughout the year, the Salmonella Surveillance Unit of the National Communicable Disease Center has observed a distinct seasonal pattern with the greatest number of isolations reported from July through October for each year.

A close correlation exists between the *Salmonella* serotypes most often responsible for human infection and those isolated from animals in any specific geographic area. The similarities document the importance of nonhuman reservoirs of *Salmonella* in the epidemiology of *Salmonella* infection in man.

PATHOGENESIS The course of events after salmonellas have gained access to the gastrointestinal tract is determined by the dose, serotype, and invasive potential of the organism, and by the resistance of the host. Different *Salmonella* serotypes show marked variation in invasive potential and capacity to produce disease in man. For example, *S. anatum* characteristically produces asymptomatic intestinal infection and rarely invades the bloodstream. In contrast, *S. cholerae-suis*, the most invasive serotype, frequently produces bacteremia and metastatic infection. Bloodstream invasion may occur as a complication of gastroenteritis but usually develops without preceding intestinal symptoms. Bacteremia with any serotype may be transient or prolonged, and may be accompanied by recurrent chills and fever or manifestations of paratyphoid fever. Bloodborne bacteria may localize at any site and lead to suppuration in bone, joints, meninges, pleura, or other tissues.

Multiplication of ingested organisms in the intestinal tract may be followed by symptoms of gastroenteritis. The intestinal irritation and inflammation are produced by a true infection deep in the mucosa as evidenced by polymorphonuclear leukocytes typically found in the diarrheal stool. However, studies in animals have shown that mucosal invasion alone is not sufficient to account for the intestinal fluid observed in experimental infections. The secretory effects of certain strains of *S. typhimurium* can be abolished in animals by indomethicin without altering the invasive process. This has led to the hypothesis of a possible enterotoxin-like effect on upper intestinal transport. An enterotoxin-like effect has also been shown in animals and tissue culture models used to study *Escherichia coli* and cholera enterotoxins.

Studies in human volunteers indicate that large numbers of viable organisms must be ingested to produce clinically apparent disease. However, a transient carrier state can be produced with doses 10 or 100 times smaller than those required to evoke symptoms of infection. The minimal infectious dose varies markedly among different serotypes.

Many host factors influence the frequency and nature of *Salmonella* infections. The minimal infectious dose varies considerably among different individual hosts and can be reduced by antacids, antimotility drugs, or antimicrobial agents in experimental animals. Some have reported the precipitation of severe systemic disease following antimotility therapy for mild gastroenteritis.

The bacterial flora of the intestine is important in determining the fate of ingested salmonellas. Administration of certain antibiotics by the oral route to mice results in a 10,000-fold increase in susceptibility to infection with *S. enteritidis*. Somewhat similar observations have been made in experimental typhoid fever in volunteers. In these studies the dose of *S. typhi* required to initiate infection by the oral route in humans can be reduced sharply by giving certain antimicrobials orally prior to challenge. Epidemiologic studies have also shown that prior antimicrobial therapy alters the capacity of the human intestinal tract to eradicate *Salmonella* acquired naturally. The effect of antibiotic therapy may be related to a marked diminution in number of *Bacteroides* or other organisms which produce antimicrobial substances such as short-chain fatty acids that are active against *Salmonella*. Alteration in intestinal flora also has been suggested as a mechanism of the increased susceptibility of patients with previous major gastric surgery, especially gastrectomy and gastroenterostomy, to intestinal infection with salmonellas. However, reduced acidity or rapid emptying time consequent to gastric surgery also appear to play a role by increasing the number of viable organisms reaching the small intestine.

Cell-mediated immune mechanisms appear to be important in host resistance to infection with salmonellas. About one-third of patients who are hospitalized because of salmonellosis have some type of major underlying disease, such as leukemia, lymphoma, lupus erythematosus, or aplastic anemia. This may be coincidence but more often reflects a decrease in resistance to bacterial infection in general. In a few diseases there is evidence to indicate an almost specific predisposition to infection by salmonellas that exceeds susceptibility to other bacterial species. Patients with sickle-cell anemia and other hemolytic processes are unusually susceptible to bloodstream invasion by salmonellas. In patients with sickle hemoglobinopathies there is a strong tendency for localization in bone, and salmonellas, not staphylococci, are the most common cause of osteomyelitis in patients with sickle-cell diseases. *Salmonella* bacteremia is also an unusually frequent complication of the acute hemolytic phase of bartonellosis (Chap. 136).

Infants are more susceptible to *Salmonella* infection and remain convalescent carriers for a longer period of time than adults. The mortality rate from the disease is also higher in infants and in the elderly than in young adults.

CLINICAL MANIFESTATIONS Gastroenteritis Although gastroenteritis often occurs in large epidemics among individuals who have eaten the same contaminated food, family outbreaks and sporadic cases are even more common. After an incubation period of 8 to 48 h, there is sudden onset of colicky abdominal pain and loose, watery diarrhea, occasionally with mucus or blood. Nausea and vomiting are frequent but are rarely severe or protracted. Fever of 38 to 39°C is common, and there may be an initial chill. Patients usually have mild to moderate abdominal tenderness on palpation, but severe tenderness, even with rebound, occurs in occasional patients. Peristalsis is usually hyperactive. Abdominal findings may be prominent in some patients and lead to confusion with certain intraabdominal emergencies, such as acute appendicitis or acute cholecystitis. Symptoms usually subside promptly within 2 to 5 days and recovery is uneventful. However, the illness is occasionally more protracted, with persistence of diarrhea and low-grade fever for 10 to 14 days. Fatalities rarely exceed 1 percent of the affected population and are limited almost entirely to infants, the aged, and debilitated patients.

The causative organism can often be isolated from the suspected food and from feces during the acute illness. Stool cultures usually become negative for salmonellas within 1 to 4 weeks, but occasional patients continue to excrete organisms for months. Organisms tend to persist in the stools of infants and young children for longer periods than in older children or adults. The blood leukocyte count is usually normal. The blood culture is usually negative.

Enteric or paratyphoid fever Certain species can produce an illness clinically indistinguishable from typhoid fever, with prolonged fever, rose spots, splenomegaly, leukopenia, gastrointestinal symptoms, and positive blood and stool cultures. The organisms most likely to produce this picture are *S. choleraesuis* and *S. enteritidis,* serotypes *paratyphi A* and *paratyphi B.* Occasionally a typical attack of food poisoning is followed in a few days by manifestations of paratyphoid fever. Generally, paratyphoid fevers tend to be milder than *S. typhi* infections, but differentiation on clinical grounds is not possible in the individual case. Recovery may be followed by continued excretion of the causative organism in the stools for several months, but the chronic carrier state is less frequent than in typhoid fever.

Bacteremia *Salmonella* species may produce a syndrome characterized primarily by prolonged fever and positive blood cultures. Although symptoms of gastroenteritis can precede bacteremia, they are usually lacking, and most cases arise sporadically. In many instances, the only manifestations are prolonged fever, which is usually spiking and is accompanied by repeated rigors, sweats, aching, anorexia, and weight loss. The characteristic features of typhoid and paratyphoid fever, such as rose spots, persistent leukopenia, and sustained fever, are absent. Stool cultures are usually negative. In contrast to the constant bacteremia of typhoid fever, discharge of organisms into the bloodstream is intermittent, and repeated blood cultures may be required to demonstrate the causative organism. At some time in the course of the illness, localizing signs of infection appear in about one-fourth of the cases. Pulmonary infection in the form of bronchopneumonia or abscess, pleurisy, empyema, pericarditis, endocarditis, pyelonephritis, meningitis, osteomyelitis, and arthritis are relatively common. The blood leukocyte count is usually normal, but with the development of focal lesions, polymorphonuclear leukocytosis as high as 20,000 to 25,000 cells per cubic millimeter occurs. *Salmonella* bacteremia can be a very puzzling disorder, especially before localization takes place, and should be considered in cases of fever of unknown origin.

A prolonged febrile illness lasting weeks or months and characterized by weight loss, marked anemia, hepatosplenomegaly, and bacteremia with *Salmonella* has been described in Brazil and other areas of the world in patients with hepatosplenic schistosomiasis due to *Schistosoma mansoni.* Intermittent bacteremia with *Salmonella* also occurs in patients with *Schistosoma haematobium* infection who are also urinary carriers of *Salmonella.*

Local pyogenic infections *Salmonella* organisms can produce abscesses in almost any anatomic site, and these can occur independently of previous symptoms of gastroenteritis or other systemic illness, or as complications of bacteremias. There is nothing characteristic about the suppurative lesions, and the correct etiologic diagnosis is rarely made on the basis of clinical findings alone. There is a strong tendency for salmonellas to localize in tissues that are the site of preexisting disease. Localization has been described in aneurysms, bone adjacent to aortic aneurysms, hematomas, and many different tumors, including hypernephroma, ovarian cyst, and pheochromocytoma. Meningeal localization of infection is common in newborns and infants, and occasional small outbreaks of *Salmonella* infection in nurseries have consisted almost entirely of meningitis. In addition to suppurative joint disease, a chronic aseptic polyarthritis has been described.

DIAGNOSIS Febrile gastroenteritis produced by presumed viral agents and shigellosis can be distinguished from *Salmonella* gastroenteritis only by appropriate stool cultures, especially in sporadic cases. Polymorphonuclear fecal leukocytes are frequently present in *Salmonella* gastroenteritis and in bacillary dysentery (shigellosis), but not in viral, giardial, or enterotoxin-induced gastroenteritis. Staphylococcal food poisoning usually is not associated with fever, and vomiting is a more prominent feature than in most *Salmonella* infections. Systemic manifestations are usually absent in patients with gastroenteritis caused by enterotoxigenic *E. coli* and *Clostridium perfringens.* Many toxic agents and drugs can produce diarrhea, nausea, and abdominal pain, but fever is rarely a feature of these disorders, and the diagnosis depends upon a history of exposure or ingestion. The diagnosis of paratyphoid fever or *Salmonella* bacteremia depends upon isolation of the causative organism. Agglutination tests with acute and convalescent serums as performed in the usual clinical laboratory are not very helpful. The possibility of an underlying disease should be considered in every patient with a severe *Salmonella* infection.

TREATMENT The treatment of *Salmonella* gastroenteritis is supportive. Dehydration should be corrected by parenteral administration of fluids and electrolytes. Abdominal cramps and diarrhea often are much improved if the patient takes nothing by mouth for 8 to 12 h. Antimicrobial therapy, irrespective of type, does not appear to exert a beneficial effect on the clinical course of *Salmonella* gastroenteritis or decrease the duration of excretion of organisms in the stool. In fact, recent studies show that the period of excretion of *Salmonella* in stools during convalescence is actually longer in patients who have been treated with antimicrobial drugs during the acute illness than in patients who received no antimicrobial therapy. Unless there is documented bacteremia or a protracted febrile course suggesting the diagnosis of enteric fever, antibiotics are *not* indicated in uncomplicated *Salmonella* gastroenteritis.

Chloramphenicol in doses of 3 g daily in adults is the antibiotic of choice in systemic infections including *Salmonella* bacteremia, metastatic infection, and paratyphoid fever. The response is characteristically slow, and the temperature rarely returns to normal until 3 to 4 days after beginning therapy. Therapy should be continued for at least 2 weeks, but in certain infections, such as osteomyelitis or meningitis, the duration may have to be extended. Resistance to multiple antibiotics, including chloramphenicol and ampicillin, occurs, particularly in salmonellas acquired outside the United States. Therefore, antibiotic sensitivity of the organism should be tested in cases of bacteremia, metastatic infection, or enteric fever.

Ampicillin is also effective in systemic infections caused by *Salmonella* strains sensitive to the action of this antibiotic. However, a significant proportion of *Salmonella* strains are highly resistant to ampicillin in vitro. For this reason, ampicillin should not be used in therapy of serious infections unless it is known that the causative organism is sensitive. As in cases of typhoid fever, the combination of trimethoprim and sulfamethoxazole may hold promise in the therapy of salmonella infection when the organism is resistant to chloramphenicol and ampicillin. The tetracycline derivatives have sometimes appeared to exert a beneficial effect, but streptomycin, polymyxin, neomycin, kanamycin, and the sulfonamides are generally ineffective. Antimicrobial resistance is usually related to transferable resistance factors.

Antimicrobial therapy is usually not indicated in convalescent or asymptomatic transient carriers of *Salmonella* species. The carrier state will cease spontaneously in 1 to 3 months in the vast majority of individuals.

The chronic carrier state with localization of infection in the gallbladder and positive stool cultures for a period of time exceeding 1 year is rarely caused by *Salmonella* serotypes other than *S. typhi* and *S. paratyphi* A and B. Its treatment has been discussed. Surgically accessible suppurative lesions should be drained.

PREVENTION AND CONTROL Continuous surveillance and careful reporting of all *Salmonella* isolates improve awareness of new strains, common sources, antibiotic resistance, and the carrier state. Because of the great number of specific serotypes, surveillance and serotyping have occasionally brought attention to widespread occurrence of relatively rare serotypes traced to single sources. Central surveillance of all reported serotypes led to the discovery of an international outbreak in 1974 of *S. eastbourne,* an otherwise rare serotype that was traced to Canadian chocolates. Adequate cooking of meat and egg products and careful surveillance of poultry products and persons who handle food have been only moderately successful in controlling salmonellosis. Probably most important, besides food surveillance, is personal hygiene, including handwashing. Transient or permanent carriers should be warned to take these precautions and, as much as possible, to avoid food preparation. Minimizing the time that foods are allowed to stand at room temperature (as between cooking and refrigeration) should reduce the chances of bacterial growth to infectious inocula.

Careful obstetrical histories for any diarrheal illness at the time a woman enters for delivery should always be obtained, and mothers and infants so affected should be isolated until cultures rule out *Salmonella* carriage. Finally, because of the increasing antibiotic resistance and the enhanced susceptibility of patients receiving antibiotics, the indiscriminate use of unnecessary or "prophylactic" antimicrobial agents should be avoided.

REFERENCES

BAINE WB et al: Institutional salmonellosis, J Infect Dis 128:357, 1973

BENNETT IL JR, HOOK EW: Some aspects of salmonellosis. Ann Rev Med 10:1, 1959

BUTLER T et al: Typhoid fever: Studies of blood coagulation, bacteremia and endotoxemia. Arch Intern Med 138:407, 1978

CLARK GM et al: Epidemiology of an international outbreak of *Salmonella agona.* Lancet 2:490, 1973

DINBAR A et al: The treatment of chronic biliary salmonella carriers. Am J Med 47:236, 1969

FELDMAN RE et al: Epidemiology of *Salmonella typhi* infection in a migrant labor camp in Dade County, Florida. J Infect Dis 130:354, 1974

FREITAG JL: Treatment of chronic typhoid carriers by cholecystectomy. Public Health Rept US 79:7, 1964

GIANNELLA RA et al: Pathogenesis of salmonellosis: Studies of fluid secretion, mucosal invasion, and morphologic reaction in the rabbit ileum. J Clin Invest 52:441, 1973

HORNICK RB et al: Typhoid fever: Pathogenesis and immunologic control. N Engl J Med 283:686, 739, 1970

KAYE D et al: Treatment of chronic enteric carriers of Salmonella typhosa with ampicillin. Ann NY Acad Sci 145:429, 1967

MCHUGH GL et al: Salmonella typhimurium resistant to silver nitrate, chloramphenicol, and ampicillin: A new threat to burn units? Lancet 1:235, 1975

OLARTE J, GALINDO E: *Salmonella typhi* resistant to chloramphenicol, ampicillin, and other antimicrobial agents: Strains isolated during an extensive typhoid fever epidemic in Mexico. Antimicrob Agents Chemother 4:597, 1973

REYNOLDS EW et al: Diagnostic specificity of Widal's reaction for typhoid fever. JAMA 214:2192, 1970

RICE PA et al: *Salmonella typhi* infections in the United States, 1967-1972: Increasing importance of international travelers. Am J Epidemiol 106:160, 1977

ROBERTSON RP et al: Chloramphenicol and ampicillin in salmonella enteric fever. N Engl J Med 278:171, 1968

Salmonella surveillance: Annual Summary 1976. Atlanta, Center for Disease Control, 1977

SCHROEDER SA et al: Epidemic salmonellosis in hospitals and institutions: A five-year review. N Engl J Med 279:674, 1968

124
SHIGELLOSIS

HARRY N. BEATY

DEFINITION Shigellosis is an acute, self-limited infection of the intestinal tract of humans which is characterized by diarrhea, fever, and abdominal pain. The disease is frequently called *bacillary dysentery,* but the term *shigellosis* is preferred.

ETIOLOGY The genus *Shigella* of the family Enterobacteriaceae includes a group of closely related species which are nonmotile, nonencapsulated, slender, gram-negative rods. They are aerobes or facultative anaerobes and grow best at 37°C. Nutritional requirements are relatively simple, and the ability of these organisms to grow in the presence of bile salts is used in devising selective media which facilitate their isolation. However, *S. dysenteriae* type 1 may be inhibited by these media, and growth may not be apparent for several days. Fermentation of carbohydrates differs according to species, but all strains produce acid in glucose and either fail to ferment lactose or do so only slowly. The shigellas are classified into subgroups A, B, C, or D on the basis of biochemical and antigenic characteristics. The clinically important species within the respective groups are *S. dysenteriae, S. flexneri, S. boydii,* and *S.*

sonnei. While these shigellas share antigens among themselves and with other enteric bacilli, serologic classification is not difficult, and with the exception of *S. sonnei* a number of serotypes of each species has been recognized.

The somatic antigen of the shigellas is an endotoxin which is chemically and biologically similar to the endotoxins of other gram-negative bacilli. *Shigella dysenteriae* type 1 (Shiga bacillus) also produces an exotoxin(s) which has cytotoxic, neurotoxic, and enterotoxic properties. The role of this exotoxin in the pathogenesis of shigellosis is unknown, but a biologically and antigenically similar toxin is elaborated by certain strains of *S. flexneri* and *S. sonnei,* and there is increasing speculation that toxin may be a virulence factor.

EPIDEMIOLOGY The principal habitat of the shigellas is the gastrointestinal tract of higher primates. Natural disease occurs in humans, gorillas, and some species of monkey. The convalescent or asymptomatic carrier is the only recognized reservoir. In 1972 a family outbreak of the disease was attributed to a pet monkey. Spread of infection from person to person occurs primarily when organisms on hands and inanimate objects contaminated with infected feces are ingested. In the United States, common source outbreaks usually involve food which has been contaminated by careless handlers. Outbreaks associated with drinking water have been reported, and swimming in contaminated rivers or pools can be a cause of infection. In regions where sanitation is poor, flies which have been in contact with infected human feces may serve as an important vector in the transmission of this disease.

Shigellosis is worldwide in distribution, and is particularly common in countries where effective sanitation is lacking. Around 10,000 cases are reported annually in the United States, but many more undoubtedly occur. *Shigella sonnei* is responsible for about three-fourths of the infections encountered in this country; *S. flexneri* is isolated from all but a small percentage of the rest. *Shigella dysenteriae* type 1, which formerly produced disease predominantly in Asia, has been responsible for large outbreaks of diarrhea in Central America. In the United States, infections with this species occur almost exclusively among foreign travelers or their contacts.

Major epidemics of shigellosis are uncommon in this country, but high-risk groups exist in the inner cities, in mental or penal institutions, and on Indian reservations. Poor sanitation, low standards of personal hygiene, crowded conditions, and a high proportion of children in a population favor spread of the infection. Infected persons may excrete organisms intermittently during convalescence, but the carrier state infrequently persists longer than 3 months.

Humoral antibodies to somatic antigens and toxins frequently develop in response to clinical infection, but there is no evidence that they influence the course of the disease or protect against reinfection. Nevertheless, persons living in endemic areas seem to develop immunity to recurrent episodes of clinical disease, and volunteers infected with a specific strain are resistant to rechallenge with that strain for weeks to months. This immunity may be mediated by coproantibody, which has been identified in the stool of patients with shigellosis, or by cellular defense mechanisms in the wall of the bowel. In any event, it has led to the development of live, attenuated vaccines which, given orally, induce the same degree of immunity as natural infection. Parenteral vaccines are of no value.

PATHOGENESIS AND PATHOLOGY The pathogenesis of shigellosis is complex, but reasonably well understood. In order to produce disease, viable organisms must first adhere to the mucosal surface and then penetrate the epithelial cell lining. These virulence properties are genetically controlled by at least

three separate regions of the chromosome; loss of any one through mutation renders a strain avirulent. Unlike members of the genus *Salmonella,* which require a large inoculum to produce infection, as few as 10 to 100 virulent *Shigella* can cause disease.

Once organisms penetrate the mucosal surface, they multiply within epithelial cells and rarely extend beyond the limits of the intestinal mucous membrane. Although superficial, the inflammatory reaction is severe and usually involves the entire colon. A fibrinous exudate often develops, and necrosis of the mucosa produces shallow ulcers that bleed readily. Microscopic examination shows that the submucosa and muscularis mucosa are infiltrated with bacteria and polymorphonuclear leukocytes. Ulcers are sharply demarcated and are not undermined. The question of whether toxins are important in the pathogenesis of shigellosis is unsettled. However, there is mounting evidence that species other than *S. dysenteriae* are toxigenic, and the hypothesis has been proposed that toxin produced in the lumen of the jejunum binds to specific receptors on epithelial cells, leading to activation of adenylate cyclase and production of cholera-like diarrhea in the early stages of shigellosis. It has long been proposed that systemic manifestations of this disease are due to absorbed toxins, because bacteremia is extremely rare except when infection is due to the Shiga bacillus.

CLINICAL MANIFESTATIONS *Shigella* infections are characterized by fever, abdominal pain, and diarrhea. However, mild diarrhea alone or asymptomatic infection occurs in a significant proportion of individuals infected. The incubation period is usually 24 to 48 h, and the first symptom is often colicky abdominal pain which is followed within an hour by high fever and diarrhea, often accompanied by tenesmus. Other symptoms include nausea, vomiting, headache, myalgia, and convulsions in children. The stools are liquid, greenish in color, contain shreds of mucus, and in 20 to 30 percent of cases various amounts of gross blood. Depending upon the severity of diarrhea and the height of fever, patients may become profoundly dehydrated, and circulatory collapse can occur. Lower abdominal tenderness and hyperactive bowel sounds are common, but there is no peritoneal irritation. Splenomegaly has been reported, but is rare. Sigmoidoscopic examination reveals diffuse mucosal inflammation, often with multiple ulcerations.

LABORATORY FINDINGS Blood leukocyte counts usually range between 5000 and 15,000 per cubic millimeter, but a leukemoid reaction with counts in the range of 30,000 to 50,000 per cubic millimeter is seen occasionally with *S. dysenteriae* infections. Anemia is uncommon. Microscopic examination of stool reveals shreds of mucus and erythrocytes. A methylene blue wet mount preparation shows many polymorphonuclear leukocytes, which helps to distinguish diarrhea caused by *Shigella* from that caused by *Salmonella typhosa* or nonbacterial infections. Stool cultures usually are positive, but blood cultures rarely are. Electrolyte abnormalities depend on the degree of vomiting and diarrhea.

COURSE Shigellosis is generally a self-limited disease, and patients usually become afebrile in about 4 days. Diarrhea and abdominal cramps may continue a few days longer, but within a week most patients have recovered. However, a significant proportion of untreated patients continue to shed organisms in the stool for 2 or more weeks. In about 10 percent of cases a clinical or bacteriologic relapse occurs unless antibiotics are given. In the United States, the overall mortality rate associated with shigellosis is less than 0.1 percent. However, among young children and elderly patients, the illness is often more severe and the prognosis poorer. *Shigella dysenteriae* type 1 produces particularly severe infections, and mortality rates of 25 to 50 percent have been recorded in epidemics produced by this species.

Complications of *Shigella* infections are encountered infrequently. An uncommon but significant problem is perforation of the colon. Hematogenous dissemination of the shigellas is also rare, but these organisms have been encountered in metastatic foci of infection such as abscesses and meningitis. In some series, bacteremia due to other gram-negative bacilli has been seen in association with shigellosis. Reiter's syndrome has been reported following shigellosis and is particularly likely to occur in patients who have the histocompatibility antigen B27. Likewise, the hemolytic-uremic syndrome has been recognized as an infrequent complication of shigellosis. Conjunctivitis, iritis, and peripheral neuropathy accompany shigellosis on rare occasions.

DIAGNOSIS A definitive diagnosis can be established when pathogenic members of the genus *Shigella* are isolated from cultures. Stool cultures are positive in over 90 percent of cases if they are obtained in the first 3 days of illness; but only about 75 percent are positive if they are obtained more than 1 week after the onset of diarrhea. The organisms survive for only a short time in feces, and fresh stool specimens or rectal swabs should be cultured promptly. Recovery of the shigellas is facilitated if saline suspensions of stool are streaked directly onto selective media such as SS agar or desoxycholate citrate agar. Antibodies can be detected in the serum of the majority of patients with positive cultures and may occasionally be of value in establishing the diagnosis of shigellosis. Immunofluorescent techniques which allow rapid detection of organisms in the stool have been developed.

Shigellosis infection should be considered in every febrile illness associated with diarrhea. Occasionally, children with infections such as tonsillitis or otitis have diarrhea, but the major differential diagnosis of shigellosis includes acute ulcerative colitis, viral enteritis, amebic dysentery, salmonellosis, and clostridial or staphylococcal food poisoning. Shigellosis can closely mimic acute ulcerative colitis, and should be excluded with cultures in patients thought to have this disease. In viral infections, fever is uncommon, and the stool usually does not contain gross blood or pus. The onset of amebic colitis is gradual, and the diarrhea is relatively mild. Staphylococcal food poisoning is associated with more nausea and vomiting, and usually is not associated with fever. *Salmonella* infections can be differentiated with certainty only by bacteriologic studies.

TREATMENT The treatment of shigellosis is primarily supportive, and the major goal is correction of fluid and electrolyte abnormalities. Antibiotics are of secondary importance, and are used chiefly to shorten the duration of illness and to prevent relapse. Sulfonamides formerly were effective in the treatment of bacillary dysentery, but almost 90 percent of *S. sonnei* isolated in the United States are resistant to these drugs. More significantly, since 1955 epidemics of shigellosis in various parts of the world, including the United States, have been caused by organisms resistant to multiple antibiotics. The molecular basis for multiple drug resistance involves the episomal transfer (R factor) of drug-resistant determinants between enteric bacilli.

Currently, increasing numbers of isolates in the United States are resistant to a number of antimicrobials. Ampicillin and tetracycline were the drugs of choice for shigellosis, but widespread resistance to these agents makes it advisable to determine the antibiotic susceptibility of all *Shigella* isolates before chemotherapy with these drugs is instituted. Cotrimoxazole, which has proven to be as effective as ampicillin, is preferred by many for the treatment of these infections. The decision whether to treat patients with antimicrobials should be based on several factors such as the nature of the organism (e.g., *S. dysenteriae* infections should be treated), the severity of the illness, the availability of safe and effective drugs, and the patient's social and physical environment.

Lomotil and antispasmodics such as paregoric should not be used in individuals with shigellosis, because these agents have an adverse effect on the course of infection caused by invasive pathogens.

PREVENTION The most important prophylactic measures are the maintenance of proper sanitation and adequate sewage disposal. The detection and elimination of carriers are difficult and rarely practical. Methods for increasing resistance with oral vaccines may be useful in preventing outbreaks among susceptible populations.

REFERENCES

DuPont HL, Hornick RB: Clinical approach to infectious diarrheas. Medicine 52:265, 1973

Gemski P Jr, Formal SB: Shigellosis: An invasive infection of the gastrointestinal tract, in *Microbiology 1975,* D Schlessinger (ed). Washington, DC, American Society for Microbiology, 1975, p 165

Keusch GT, Jacewicz M: Pathogenesis of *Shigella* diarrhea: VII. Evidence for a cell membrane toxin receptor involving β-1,4 linked *N*-acetyl-*d*-glucosamine oligomers. J Exp Med 146:535, 1977

Nelson JD et al: Trimethoprim-sulfamethoxazole therapy for shigellosis. JAMA 235:1239, 1976

125
HEMOPHILUS INFECTIONS

DAVID W. SMITH

Hemophilus influenzae was isolated by Pfeiffer in 1892 from the sputum of individuals afflicted during an influenza pandemic. The requirement of blood for in vitro growth and its presumptive role in the pandemic prompted the designation of this genus. Other species have since been classified as members of the *Hemophilus* genus on the basis of morphology and physiology: small, pleomorphic, facultatively aerobic, nonmotile, nonspore-forming, gram-negative bacilli that require enriched media containing blood or certain derivatives and that are strict parasites of humans. Certain of these species are closely related genetically.

Hemophilus influenzae and *H. pertussis* are the most important cause of human disease among this genus; other pathogenic species include *H. aegyptius, H. aphrophilus, H. ducreyi, H. parapertussis,* and *H. vaginalis. Hemophilus hemolyticus, H. parainfluenzae,* and *H. bronchiseptica* infect the upper respiratory tract but rarely cause disease.

HEMOPHILUS INFLUENZAE

ETIOLOGY *Hemophilus influenzae* is distinguished by its growth requirement of a heat-labile V factor and a heat-stable

X factor found in erythrocytes and by its inability to hemolyze erythrocytes during growth. V factor can be replaced by coenzyme I (DPN), coenzyme II (TPN), or nicotinamide nucleoside, and X factor by hematin. X factor is not required for anaerobic growth. Fermentation reactions and tests of other metabolic activities are not useful in identification but may help in "biotyping" individual isolates.

Hemophilus influenzae will grow in any enriched supplemented medium, but optimal growth occurs on media in which erythrocytes are disrupted to release the growth factors, e.g., chocolate or Levinthal agar. "Satellitism" around colonies of hemolytic *Staphylococcus aureus* growing on solid blood agar is often used to identify *H. influenzae*. Some strains grow best in 5 to 10 percent carbon dioxide; many laboratories therefore incubate specimens suspected of containing *H. influenzae* in a candle jar or an incubator purged with carbon dioxide. Since viability of this bacterium is lost rapidly on drying or heating, clinical specimens should be inoculated without delay.

The organism exists with or without a polysaccharide capsule. Colonies of nonencapsulated isolates are usually 0.5 to 1.5 mm in diameter and appear granular after overnight incubation on solid agar; those of encapsulated isolates are usually 3 to 4 mm in diameter and initially appear mucoid or glistening. *Hemophilus influenzae* grown on enriched media appear microscopically as relatively uniform, small coccobacilli (1 by 0.3 μm); under less than optimal growth conditions, long filaments or short chains are common. The morphology of *H. influenzae* in clinical specimens is generally variable. Moreover, the organism does not always react optimally with safranin dye. *Hemophilus influenzae* is, therefore, not infrequently misdiagnosed in gram-stained smears of infected material.

The outer membrane of *H. influenzae*, like that of other gram-negative bacilli, is composed of a lipopolysaccharide (endotoxin)-containing cell wall and a number of immunogenic proteins. The antigenic composition of *H. influenzae* endotoxin and the outer-membrane proteins is poorly defined. Only a small percentage of isolates recovered from the respiratory tract are encapsulated. Six antigenically distinguishable capsular types, designated a to f, have been identified. Each is a complex carbohydrate. Type a, b, and c capsules share antigenic determinants with certain pneumococci, while that of type b, polyribose ribitol phosphate (PRP), cross-reacts immunologically with the capsules or cell walls of several species of gram-positive cocci and rods, and with enteric bacilli.

Strains with decreased or absent capsular antigen arise spontaneously from encapsulated strains. This variation most likely proceeds from M (fully encapsulated) → S (partially encapsulated) → R (nonencapsulated). The genetic basis of this variation and the natural existence of its converse, that is, R→S→M, are not well described. Alexander demonstrated that DNA purified from an M strain could transform an R strain to the serotype of the donor M strain. Transformation of *H. influenzae* in the host has not been studied, but the demonstration of pneumococcal transformation in experimentally infected mice supports that possibility. Transformations between *H. aegyptius* and *H. influenzae* and between *H. influenzae* and *H. parainfluenzae* demonstrate the close genetic relation of these species.

Hemophilus influenzae type b releases its capsular antigen (PRP) during growth in vitro and in vivo. PRP can be identified immunologically by countercurrent immunoelectrophoresis or agglutination of latex particles to which antibody is absorbed.

Hemophilus influenzae was previously susceptible to many antibiotics, but resistance to tetracycline has been increasing, and up to 10 percent of type b and a higher percentage of nonencapsulated strains isolated in the United States are now resistant to ampicillin. Chloramphenicol-resistant and multiply resistant (chloramphenicol, tetracycline, and/or ampicillin) strains have been isolated in Europe. Resistant strains are widely but variably distributed and are as pathogenic and transmissible as antibiotic-sensitive strains.

EPIDEMIOLOGY *Hemophilus influenzae* infects only humans, primarily their upper respiratory tracts. It can be recovered from the nasopharynx of up to 80 percent of healthy individuals, with the frequency of infection related inversely to age, being greatest with young persons. Asymptomatic nasopharyngeal infection lasts days to a few months, is not eradicated by systemic antibody, and often is not eliminated by antibiotic therapy adequate to cure type b meningitis. Of the isolated strains, up to 25 percent are encapsulated, one-half of which are type b.

Hemophilus influenzae diseases occur worldwide and for the most part are endemic. Unusually high attack rates of systemic type b diseases occur in certain communities and within closed populations of susceptible persons. A 10-year review of patients with systemic type b disease revealed multiple cases in 3 percent of affected families. Systemic *H. influenzae* b diseases occur more commonly among impoverished and rural populations and blacks. Persons with sickle-cell disease, splenectomy, agammaglobulinemia, and treated Hodgkin's disease are unusually susceptible. Alcoholic adults appear to be at increased risk of *H. influenzae* pneumonia. Systemic *H. influenzae* diseases have a marked age relationship: newborns, older children, and adults are uncommonly affected. In temperate climates, these diseases occur most commonly during the winter months.

The incidence of systemic *H. influenzae* b diseases seems to have increased during the past 30 to 40 years, and more adults are being affected. The basis for this increased attack rate is not understood. Improved diagnostic laboratories and diminution in the prevalence of protective antibody due to excessive use of antibiotics have been implicated. The possibility that the organism has changed its antigenic composition and/or virulence also deserves evaluation.

PATHOGENICITY The relatively common asymptomatic nasopharyngeal infection occasionally develops into symptomatic disease which may spread contiguously to involve the sinuses, middle ear, or bronchi. Nonencapsulated strains produce luminal diseases. Encapsulated strains may invade local tissues, causing epiglottitis, pneumonia, pericarditis, or facial cellulitis, or they may enter the bloodstream and produce metastatic disease in the meninges or joints.

Virtually all *H. influenzae* causing systemic disease are encapsulated, and at least 90 percent are type b. The pathogenicity of invasive strains is related directly to the inhibition of phagocytosis produced by the capsule. The basis for the disproportionate virulence of type b strains is unknown. The role of outer membrane proteins and other constitutents in pathogenicity is also ill-defined. Synergy between *H. influenzae* and certain respiratory viruses has been demonstrated in studies of human disease and in experimental models.

IMMUNITY Susceptibility to *H. influenzae* b meningitis was always correlated inversely to the presence of anticapsular antibody. The role of anti-PRP has been questioned recently, however, because of its apparent variable distribution among adults who have no increased incidence of *H. influenzae* b disease. The interpretation of these data remain in question because of the lack of standard methods in performing the classic bactericidal assay for antibody. Moreover, the limits of sensitivity of the bactericidal assay (about 200 ng antibody per milliliter) exceed by tenfold the antibody concentration needed to protect animals from lethal, experimental disease. Radioimmunoassays which detect 10 ng anti-PRP per milliliter should provide important insights into this question.

Although recent evidence suggests that immunity to *H. influenzae* is mediated by antibody of multiple specificity, anti-PRP antibody is a potent resistance factor. It promotes phagocytosis and bacteriolysis in vitro, protects animals from a lethal concentration of *H. influenzae,* and was responsible for the beneficial effects of rabbit anti-*H. influenzae* serum in human disease. Moreover, recent field trials with a purified PRP vaccine have demonstrated protection of young children from systemic diseases when an antibody response is mounted.

Antibody to PRP can be stimulated by infection with bacteria bearing cross-reactive surface antigens. Such antibody is bacteriolytic in vitro and protective in experimental disease. Antibody to *H. influenzae* outer membrane (OM) antigens also promotes phagocytosis and bacteriolysis in vitro and protects experimentally infected animals. Antibody to OM antigens has been found in high titers in certain adults and older children clinically resistant to *H. influenzae* but deficient in anti-PRP antibody. This observation suggests that natural resistance to this pathogen appears to result from a composite of antibody activities stimulated by each of several antigens.

Studies of patients recovering from systemic *H. influenzae* b disease and of those immunized with PRP have revealed a marked age relation to anti-PRP antibody: infants respond infrequently and poorly; younger children have intermediate reactivity; all older children and adults develop marked, nonboostable responses. The level of detectable antibody activity following disease is further complicated by antigenemia, which may last days to weeks, and which is more common and prolonged in infants. A few children have failed to produce anti-PRP antibody (measured by radioimmunoassay) following systemic disease and subsequently developed a second distinct episode of type b invasive disease. Although these children appear to have been "immunologically nonreactive" for periods up to months, all those studied to date have subsequently raised anti-PRP antibody activity. These observations indicate the need for further study and close follow-up of young children recuperating from invasive *H. influenzae* b disease. Likewise, survivors of intensive radio- and/or chemotherapy for Hodgkin's disease, many of whom have also had a splenectomy, are incapable of an appropriate anti-PRP antibody response, even following systemic disease.

Children recuperating from certain *H. influenzae* b diseases were found in one study to have lower anti-PRP titers and significant differences in the composition of certain erythrocyte and/or lymphocyte antigens compared with healthy blood donors. These data support the concept of a genetic basis for the production of anti-PRP antibody and/or development of certain *H. influenzae* b diseases, and deserve further evaluation.

CLINICAL MANIFESTATIONS *Hemophilus influenzae* can cause local respiratory tract or invasive diseases. A 1-year survey of children hospitalized in Denver, Colorado, revealed that *H. influenzae* b was the most common cause of bacteremic disease and that 54 percent of children with *H. influenzae* disease had meningitis; 14 percent, pneumonia (4 percent with pericarditis); 11 percent, bacteremia without a primary focus; 11 percent, facial cellulitis; 10 percent, epiglottitis; and 1 percent, pyarthrosis. Adults may develop *H. influenzae* bacteremia, meningitis, and, less commonly, epiglottitis; however, in them bronchitis, due to nonencapsulated strains, and pneumonia are more common.

Hemophilus influenzae diseases are generally acute with symptoms reflecting the pyogenic process; however, the clinical course of certain of these diseases may be surprisingly prolonged and subacute.

Meningitis (see also Chap. 368) *Hemophilus influenzae* is the most common cause of bacterial meningitis, primarily affecting children 9 months to 4 years of age. The signs and symptoms depend on the patient's age and the time in the course of the disease when medical care is sought. Young children and those early in the disease generally have a nonspecific clinical picture: preceding upper respiratory tract symptoms, fever, anorexia, lethargy, vomiting, and, in older children and adults, headache. A history of stiff neck or back may be elicited. Confusion, paresis of one or another cranial nerve, coma, convulsions, opisthotonus, and shock occur with more prolonged and serious disease. The clinical findings are indistinguishable from other bacterial meningitides. Age and certain concurrent manifestations, such as cellulitis, pyarthrosis, or epiglottitis, suggest *H. influenzae,* but the diagnosis depends on bacteriologic studies.

Pneumonia *Hemophilus influenzae* may cause either a broncho- or lobar pneumonia. Approximately one-half of the children with lobar pneumonia have an associated empyema. The pneumonic disease sometimes spreads to produce a purulent pericarditis. Lobar disease, particularly with pleural involvement, is most often confused with pneumococcal or *S. aureus* pneumonia, but the course may be prolonged enough to suggest tuberculosis. Elderly adults, particularly those with chronic obstructive lung disease and/or alcoholism, are being affected increasingly with *H. influenzae* pneumonia (Chap. 260).

Bacteremia without local disease Children, particularly those between 6 months and 3 years of age, may develop bacteremia without evidence of local disease. The diagnosis is made most often in those with a temperature greater than 38.9°C (102°F) and an elevated circulating neutrophil count. Persons with sickle-cell disease, previous splenectomy, and chemotherapy for Hodgkin's disease are at increased risk of bacteremia without local disease. Although pneumococci are the most common cause of this syndrome, *H. influenzae* b is the second most common etiologic agent. Fever, chills, anxiety, anorexia, and lethargy dominate the clinical picture. Among highly susceptible hosts, the disease may be fulminating with rapid progress to shock and death within a few hours.

Cellulitis *Hemophilus influenzae* causes a cellulitis, particularly among children 6 to 24 months of age, which is characterized as a raised, warm, tender area with a distinctive reddish blue hue, usually located on one cheek or, less commonly, in the periorbital area. The child is moderately febrile and has a history of preceding rhinorrhea, fever, and, at times, ipsilateral otitis media. The cellulitis develops and spreads within a few hours. *Hemophilus influenzae* cellulitis involving the limbs and hands is seen rarely, usually in older children. The distinctive color, location, and clinical course suggest the etiology. A significant percentage of the involved infants develops sepsis and metastatic disease, notably meningitis.

Epiglottitis *Hemophilus influenzae* b is the leading cause of this potentially lethal, septic disease with a dramatically rapid course that primarily affects preschool-age children. Acute onset of high fever, dysphagia, and an aura of not feeling well are followed by puddling of oropharyngeal secretions and tachypnea with inspiratory retractions. Increasing airway obstruction is accompanied by increasing hypoxia and anxiety. Over one-half of these patients require hospitalization and airway intubation within 12 h after the onset of initial symptoms. The diagnostic examination can provoke further edema of the markedly swollen, inflamed epiglottis and should, therefore, be conducted only in a locale in which an airway can be inserted.

Pyarthrosis *Hemophilus influenzae* b joint disease occurs during a septic invasion with or without other systemic disease. Although an uncommon manifestation of *H. influenzae* sepsis, pyarthrosis in children under 2 years of age is most commonly caused by *H. influenzae*. Single, large weight-bearing joints are usually involved without osteomyelitis (Chap. 360). Response to systemic antibiotics without surgical drainage is dramatic and curative, but long-term follow-up reveals some joint dysfunction in a significant percentage of children

Pericarditis *Hemophilus influenzae* b causes purulent pericarditis usually as a part of a bout of pneumonia. The clinical signs and symptoms are similar to those of pyogenic pericarditis of other etiology, although the course is often less acute (Chap. 249).

Other respiratory tract diseases *Hemophilus influenzae* is the second leading cause of childhood otitis media and often causes sinusitis. Nearly all the etiologic strains are nonencapsulated. These diseases cannot be distinguished clinically from those produced by other microbial agents (Chap. 267), nor can the disease caused by encapsulated or nonencapsulated *H. influenzae* be differentiated clinically. Fever, local pain, irritability, and, in sinusitis, foul breath, postnasal drip, and cough predominate. Chronic bronchitis, particularly among adults and those with agamma- or hypogammaglobulinemia, is often caused by nonencapsulated *H. influenzae* or mixed bacterial species among which *H. influenzae* predominates. Cough productive of purulent sputum, dyspnea with prolonged expiration, and anorexia dominate this process which is aggravated by smoking and other respiratory pollutants.

Other diseases *Hemophilus influenzae* can cause endocarditis and brain abscess, but such cases are very rare and are usually associated with a primary underlying disease. *Hemophilus influenzae* endophthalmitis, renal disease, and osteomyelitis have been reported. Pharyngitis is only rarely caused by *H. influenzae*, and the role of this organism in bronchiolitis has been dismissed.

DIAGNOSIS The etiology of many *H. influenzae* diseases, i.e., pyarthrosis in a child under 2 years, facial cellulitis, and epiglottitis, can generally be suspected on the basis of the history and clinical findings. Chemical analysis of infected fluids is consistent with any pyogenic etiology. A leukocytosis is common, and children often have a significant anemia. Gram's stains of infected body fluids, e.g., spinal fluid, correlate with culture results in 70 percent of cases. Of the rest of culture-positive specimens, 15 percent have negative smears, while another 15 percent have misinterpreted smears. Staining such specimens with methylene blue generally does not improve these results. Quellung reactions are usually even less accurate.

PRP can be detected by countercurrent electrophoresis in the serum, CSF, or concentrated urine of 90 percent of children with meningitis. Despite the apparent widespread distribution of immunologically cross-reactive antigens among bacteria in nature, false-positive reactions are unusual. False-positive reactions due to antibodies to serum constituents may occur in some acutely infected patients. PRP is generally detected in infected pericardial fluid or joint fluid but is found infrequently in the serum of children with epiglottitis, presumably because the fulminant course of this disease does not entail the time required for antigen to be released from the invasive bacteria. Detection of antigen in the supernatant of liquid cultures can expedite the laboratory diagnosis. Antigen, and nonviable bacteria, often persist in serum and other body fluids following antibiotic therapy. This makes antigen detection very helpful in the diagnosis of patients with *H. influenzae* meningitis who have received prior antibiotics.

Positive nasopharyngeal cultures are not meaningful because of the high carriage rate of *H. influenzae* by healthy individuals. Needle aspiration of the edge of the site of cellulitis or of diseased lung markedly increases the rate of bacterial isolation and may be necessary, particularly in sick patients. Cultures of empyema, pericardial, and joint fluid and an inflamed epiglottis are usually diagnostic. Blood cultures are positive in up to 80 percent of patients with *H. influenzae* septic arthritis, facial cellulitis, epiglottitis, and meningitis prior to the onset of antibiotic therapy. Even if antibiotic therapy has been initiated, the yield is sufficiently great to recommend that blood cultures be taken. It has been suggested that *H. influenzae* pneumonia, in which 30 percent of persons have a positive blood culture, is underdiagnosed. The role of antigen detection in the diagnosis of this disease deserves further evaluation.

TREATMENT Without treatment, systemic *H. influenzae* disease, particularly meningitis and epiglottitis, has a very high, if not uniform, mortality. Therapy with intrathecal streptomycin and a systemic sulfonamide was one of the earliest therapeutic regimens for meningitis. It produced reasonably satisfactory results but is no longer advocated. Chloramphenicol yields very high concentrations of antibiotic in the joint and cerebrospinal fluids relative to serum and produces excellent clinical results. However, the potential toxicity of chloramphenicol and the highly satisfactory results obtained with ampicillin for many years made ampicillin the antibiotic of choice for *H. influenzae* diseases. The current prevalence of ampicillin-resistant strains requires that all systemic diseases potentially due to *H. influenzae* be treated with chloramphenicol, 100 mg/kg per day for children, or 4 g per day for adults, given intravenously at 6-h intervals until the etiologic agent is proved to be sensitive to ampicillin. Some, including the American Academy of Pediatrics, also recommend that ampicillin be used along with chloramphenicol. If the etiologic strain is sensitive, ampicillin is given intravenously in dosage of 200 to 400 mg/kg per day for children and 4 g per day for adults divided into six infusions given at 4-h intervals. Other antibiotics are also useful in *H. influenzae* infections. Carbenicillin is thought to be particularly sensitive to the β-lactamase of *H. influenzae*, and high concentrations of bacteria, as found in clinical disease, are resistant to carbenicillin. Moreover, carbenicillin is no more effective than ampicillin in therapy of experimental *H. influenzae* b meningitis caused by ampicillin-resistant strains. Amoxicillin is useful in ambulatory therapy of ampicillin-sensitive *H. influenzae* infections. Tetracycline can be used to treat bronchitis and other respiratory diseases caused by sensitive strains. Cephamandole appears promising in the therapy of non-life-threatening ampicillin-sensitive or resistant *H. influenzae* diseases. Trimethoprim-sulfa therapy has recently been approved for *H. influenzae* upper respiratory tract disease.

The duration of chemotherapy for *H. influenzae* disease depends on the disease and the status of the individual patient. All systemic diseases are treated intravenously at least until cultures of the infected area are sterile and the patient is afebrile and without clinical and laboratory evidence of active infection for 3 to 5 days. Patients with meningitis are usually treated for 10 to 14 days. Occasionally, ampicillin does not clear the bacteria from the CSF, and clinical relapses follow the cessation of therapy. Such therapeutic failures have often been associated with antibiotic courses that were too brief, dosages too low, or administration of the drug by a route other than the intravenous one. In a few instances, treatment failures could be attributed to loculated disease that was not completely eradicated by acceptable therapy. Treatment failures require retreatment with ampicillin or chloramphenicol.

Children with endocarditis or pericarditis should receive 6 weeks of intravenous therapy. Ampicillin or chloramphenicol diffuse well into inflamed joint spaces, and there is no indication for local instillation of antibiotics in septic arthritis. Children with otitis media may be treated orally with amoxicillin in dosage of 50 mg/kg per day, adults with 2 g per day, in four divided doses until their symptoms are alleviated or for a total course of 7 to 10 days. Sinusitis requires therapy for 3 or more weeks; therapy of bronchitis may be prolonged even further, depending upon the symptoms.

Only a few H. influenzae isolates resistant to chloramphenicol have been recovered in the United States, but their isolation in European centers strongly suggests the need to test invasive organisms for chloramphenicol sensitivity routinely, particularly when the results of chloramphenicol therapy are disappointing.

Antibiotic therapy is only one facet of the management of the patient with a systemic H. influenzae disease. Careful evaluation of the airway, consideration of oxygen therapy and transfusion, vigorous treatment of shock and defects in coagulation, conservative fluid replacement, anticonvulsant therapy, and medical management of cerebral edema are often critical. Repeated aspirations of an infected joint or an empyema or placements of a pericardial "window" for drainage may be needed.

PREVENTION Although secondary cases of invasive H. influenzae diseases occur at significantly increased rates among young, close contacts of primary cases, no successful antibiotic prophylactic regimen currently exists. The increased attack rate, constant mortality (5 to 10 percent), and significant neurological morbidity during the past two decades for H. influenzae meningitis in children and the prevalence of ampicillin-resistant strains has promoted attempts to produce a vaccine to prevent H. influenzae diseases. Because of the primacy of the type b capsule in pathogenicity and the efficacy of anticapsular serum, attention was focused initially on a vaccine composed of purified capsular PRP. Such a vaccine has been prepared and found nontoxic and immunogenic for older children and adults. Recent data indicate that a single dose of this vaccine protects children older than 18 months from meningitis and sepsis for at least 2 years; however, the vaccine is not immunogenic or protective for younger children. New approaches have, therefore, been initiated to develop an effective agent for younger children.

A less purified, systemically administered vaccine in which the native outer membrane complex of lipopolysaccharide-protein-PRP of H. influenzae b is conserved is currently being evaluated. Protective antibiotics directed to PRP and to the OM proteins are generated in adults and children; the efficacy of this vaccine in infants is under study.

HEMOPHILUS AEGYPTIUS

Often known as the Koch-Weeks bacillus, H. aegyptius causes conjunctivitis in humans. Morphologically and biochemically, this organism closely resembles an unencapsulated H. influ-

enzae. Moreover, H. aegyptius and H. influenzae share certain antigens, and each can be transformed by DNA of the other species.

The conjunctivitis primarily affects children and occurs throughout the world often in epidemics and, in some areas, seasonally. This organism must be distinguished from trachoma-inclusion conjunctivitis (TRIC) agents, adenoviruses, and other bacterial agents, e.g., pneumococcus, Staphylococcus aureus, Neisseria gonorroheae. Therapy consists of local instillation of antibiotic drops or ointment, sulfonamide, polymyxin B, or gentamicin five or six times daily and moist soaks to keep the eyelids clean.

HEMOPHILUS APHROPHILUS

Hemophilus aphrophilus is an uncommon cause of bacteremia, bacterial endocarditis, acute and chronic sinusitis, pneumonia, and deep tissue abscesses, such as brain abscess. This organism requires X but not V factor and extra carbon dioxide for aerobic growth; it grows anaerobically without X factor. Most strains are sensitive to most families of antibiotics: penicillin, cephalosporins, aminoglycosides, and chloramphenicol.

HEMOPHILUS DUCREYI

See Chap. 126.

HEMOPHILUS PARAINFLUENZAE

This species differs from H. influenzae by requiring V but not X factor for growth. Since H. influenzae does not require X factor for anaerobic growth, diagnostic confusion can arise, particularly in stabbed cultures. This phenomenon may have played a role in certain instances of systemic disease allegedly caused by H. parainfluenzae which, on further testing, were found to be caused by H. influenzae.

Acute upper respiratory disease, including otitis media, and less commonly meningitis, pneumonia, endocarditis, and brain abscess have been ascribed to H. parainfluenzae. A small but significant percentage of H. parainfluenzae carry plasmids mediating β-lactamase production and ampicillin resistance.

HEMOPHILUS VAGINALIS (See Chap. 113)

Hemophilus vaginalis (sometimes called Corynebacterium vaginale) appears to cause vaginitis, and less commonly septic abortion and puerperal fever, and asymptomatic urethal infection in men. The growth requirements are not precisely defined but include factor V and probably X; incubation in increased carbon dioxide is important.

The pathogenic role of H. vaginalis is disputed because of its recovery from asymptomatic persons. However, recent data have revealed a significant correlation between isolation of H. vaginalis and nonspecific vaginitis. The results of therapy support the causal relationship. The clinical diagnosis is suggested by the presence of "clue" cells—vaginal epithelial cells to which multiple gram-negative bacilli are attached—in a vaginal discharge with a pH $\geq$ 5.0 which releases an amine-like odor upon alkalinization. Hemophilus vaginalis is not eradicated by oral tetracycline, ampicillin, or sulfonamide vaginal cream. Oral metronidazole is effective, but its use must be weighed against the drug's potential toxicity and the high potential of reinfection from sexual partners.

HEMOPHILUS PERTUSSIS

This bacterium causes an acute bronchitis, primarily in infants and young children, that is characterized by a repetitious, paroxysmal cough and prolonged, inspiratory stridor, "whooping cough."

ETIOLOGY *Hemophilus pertussis* is a minute, aerobic nonmotile, gram-negative coccobacillus that grows slowly and, as a primary isolate, only on a complex medium. The classic Bordet-Gengou medium, which contains blood, is used for primary culture. Charcoal, ion-exchange resin, or starch can be substituted for the blood which apparently binds toxic lipids rather than providing essential growth factors. The absence of an antigenic relationship and inability to transform *H. pertussis* with *H. influenzae* DNA, or vice versa, also suggest that these species are not closely related. *Hemophilus pertussis* is closely related to *H. parapertussis,* which can cause a milder, similar disease in humans, and *H. bronchiseptica,* which causes such a disease in animals but rarely in humans.

Primary isolates, phase I cells, change morphology and antigenic content and lose pathogenicity on in vitro culture; this conversion to phase IV cells is a type of S→R conversion. Killed phase I cells provoke several physiological changes when injected into experimental animals: increased sensitivity to histamine and serotonin, increased susceptibility to experimental allergic encephalomyelitis, a heightened antibody response to heterologous antigens, and lymphocytosis. Factors responsible for these phemonena as well as human pathogenicity of *H. pertussis* are subjects of considerable study and include O antigen (endotoxin), six different K antigens (agglutinogens), which are probably outer-membrane proteins, a heat-labile and a heat-stabile toxin, a hemagglutinin, and a histamine-sensitizing factor. Recent studies suggest that the pilus of *H. pertussis* is identical to the previously identified lymphocytosis-promoting factor. This protein can apparently attach to certain lymphocytes and inhibit their sequestration in lymphoid tissues. The characteristic lymphocytosis in *H. pertussis* disease may result from the prolonged circulation of these lymphocytes. The presence of a capsule on *H. pertussis* is reported only irregularly. The surface antigen content, including the K antigens, can shift phenotypically and genotypically. Such shifts are reflected in changes of vaccine potency. This plethora of antigens also has provoked the development of multiple serologic methods.

EPIDEMIOLOGY *Hemophilus pertussis* exists worldwide and in nature affects only humans; however, primates and mice can be experimentally infected. Pertussis is one of the most contagious of infectious diseases because it is transmitted by aerosolized droplets. The infectivity of respiratory secretions and contact transmission has not been well studied. Up to 90 percent of exposed, susceptible persons develop disease. Asymptomatic infection is rare. Although pertussis may occur endemically, it produces epidemics in a susceptible population. The incidence is greater in the winter in temperate climates. Although adults were earlier thought resistant, recent studies have revealed that neither disease nor active immunization provides life-long immunity. Hospital personnel are at increased risk, as evidenced by reports of epidemics involving hospital staff and patients. The level of maternal immunity and the lack of transplacental transfer of bacteriolytic antibody (which is an IgM globulin) leave the infant particularly susceptible; not surprisingly, more than 50 percent of *H. pertussis* disease occurs in infants.

About 3000 cases of pertussis are officially reported each year in the United States. Most observers think this number is falsely low owing to the difficulty in bacteriologic confirmation. Pertussis remains a very significant health problem in developing countries, particularly in areas of poor nutrition and immunization. The recent decline (1978) in the rate of immunization to pertussis in Great Britain to 30 percent of children has been accompanied by an epidemic affecting as many persons as in the prevaccine era. Certain adenoviruses can cause an identical clinical picture, but there is little doubt that *H. pertussis* can be a primary pathogen.

PATHOGENICITY Inhaled *H. pertussis* attaches to the respiratory epithelium by a specialized pilus; the organisms multiply on the surface of the airway lumen but do not invade the lung or the bloodstream. Acute inflammation results; epithelial cell ciliary action is inhibited, and mucous secretion is stimulated. The subsequent necrosis results in patchy ulceration of the epithelium. The bronchi and bronchioles are primarily affected; the trachea, larynx, and nasophyarynx may be involved, but less severely. The mucopurulent exudate can compromise the diminutive airway of the infant or small child. Focal atelectasis and emphysema are common; peribronchial infiltration by inflammatory cells, particularly lymphocytes, occurs, but the alveoli are spared. The basis for the neurological symptoms—whether from the primary action of a bacterial neurotoxin or secondary hypoxia—remains undefined.

CLINICAL MANIFESTATIONS Following an incubation period of 7 to 10 days, sneezing, mild fever, rhinorrhea, anorexia, and a mild cough become evident (catarrhal period). After 1 to 2 weeks the cough increases in frequency and intensity. Paroxysms are followed, particularly in infants, by a prolonged, often distressing gasp (the whoop). The cough occurs at variable intervals, often every few minutes, for 2 to 3 weeks (paroxysmal period). The disease is much more severe in the infant. The cough inhibits oral intake, and swallowed mucus provokes vomiting. Dehydration and weight loss can be significant. The cough can provoke venous congestion with hemoptysis, epistaxis, and hemorrhage from small blood vessels. Hypoxia may be more common and severe than is commonly appreciated. Apprehension is a major symptom in infants; convulsions and cerebral dysfunction are very rare. Adults and older children are less ill but have the symptoms of a severe, prolonged bronchitis. A recovery period of 1 to 6 weeks follows. During this period the cough decreases, but spasms can be provoked, particularly by smoke or irritating inhalants.

Death results primarily from dehydration and electrolyte imbalance, cerebral anoxia or hemorrhage, or secondary bacterial pneumonia. Mortality is now less than 5 percent among children hospitalized in the United States, but it is significant in developing countries. Up to 90 percent of deaths occur in children under 1 year of age, up to 70 percent in those of 6 months or younger. Among survivors, transient atelectasis is frequent, but bronchiectasis, reported commonly a few decades ago, is now uncommon. Permanent cerebral dysfunction is also unusual among children provided with optimal therapy.

DIAGNOSIS Pertussis is exceedingly difficult to diagnose clinically in the catarrhal state without a history of contact but should be considered in any nonimmune person with a repetitious cough. The differential diagnosis includes viral tracheobronchitis, *Mycoplasma pneumoniae* pneumonia, particularly in adults, and, in infants, *Chlamydia* infection (Chap. 174).

A marked absolute and relative lymphocytosis is characteristic. The organism is isolated from a deep nasopharyngeal (NP) culture; the recovery rate on "cough plates" is too low to recommend this technique. NP swabs must be plated immediately because *H. pertussis* loses viability rapidly with drying. Optimal results occur with fresh medium that contains an antibiotic, such as penicillin, to prevent the growth of NP flora. *Hemophilus pertussis* can be isolated from as many as 90 percent of patients during the catarrhal stage of the disease, but from no greater than 50 percent during the paroxysmal stage. Fluorescent-labeled antibody can detect *H. pertussis* in NP smears; the positive identification rate is generally up to twice that of NP cultures, but false-positive results may be 30 to 40 percent. Serologic studies are of little value. Blood cultures are sterile and should not be done; a chest x-ray, which may show peribronchial thickening, is not diagnostic. Dual infection with adenoviruses occurs, and positive viral cultures do not exclude *H. pertussis* as an etiologic agent.

TREATMENT General supportive care is critical: careful nursing, avoidance of stimuli that provoke paroxysms, oxygen, suctioning of respiratory secretions, and attention to caloric needs and fluid and electrolyte balance. A recent single controlled study reported beneficial effects of steroids for severely ill infants.

Hemophilus pertussis is sensitive to many antibiotics in vitro. Antibiotics can eliminate infection and, if given in the catarrhal phase, prevent disease. Since the pathological process is well developed by the time paroxysms occur, antibiotic therapy given thereafter does not affect the clinical course. Erythromycin is the preferred drug and should be used to prevent interpersonal transmission. Tetracycline and chloramphenicol are nearly as effective but are not recommended because of potential toxicity, particularly for infants. Ampicillin appears to be relatively ineffective in eradicating nasopharyngeal infection. Hyperimmune, antibacterial rabbit serum has no proved effect on bacterial shedding or clinical manifestations and is not recommended.

PREVENTION Patients suspected of having pertussis should be isolated until the diagnosis is disproved or infection eradicated by antibiotics. Exposed susceptibles should be vaccinated to prevent disease (see below) and treated with erythromycin to prevent infection and retransmission.

Prior to the availability of a vaccine, pertussis caused as many deaths in the United States as all other contagious diseases of children *combined!* In order to prevent the disease, a vaccine composed of a chemical extract of bacterial cells was developed. Because of the risk of pertussis to infants, start of immunization as early in life as possible was proposed. Unfortunately, pertussis immunization at 7 days of age produces a limited antibody response in only a small percentage of infants, and it results in reduced booster responses at 1 year. This vaccine is now mixed with diphtheria and tetanus toxoids, for convenience and because pertussis enhances the antibody responses to the toxoids, and is given five times through the first 6 years of life, with three doses being given at 2-month intervals starting at 8 weeks of age.

Although the vaccine was 70 to 80 percent effective in preventing disease among intimately exposed children, its effectiveness and toxicity have been questioned. Completely immunized children may develop pertussis, although the disease is milder than among the unimmunized. Furthermore, the protection provided by the vaccine is transient with only minimal resistance being evident a decade following the last immunization. Indeed, improved housing, hygiene, and nutrition are cited by some as responsible for the dramatic decline in pertussis during the past several decades. However, available data indicate that the degree of decline in the attack rate of pertussis in the United States has been positively affected by the vaccine. The association of an epidemic of pertussis in Great Britain, with a decline in pertussis immunization, also strongly supports the efficacy of the vaccine.

Pertussis vaccine provokes local reactions in up to 50 percent of recipients; neurological complications, including uncontrollable screaming fits, convulsions, and encephalopathy, are a rare but real risk. Neurological complications of pertussis vaccine are more common in families with neurological disease, such as epilepsy. Unfortunately, pertussis vaccine preparations are not uniform in composition, and the risk of any given inoculation is hard to calculate. Any neurological response to pertussis vaccine precludes reimmunization. Vaccine is rarely recommended for persons older than 6 years because of the potential neurotoxicity and decreased risk of pertussis as a life-threatening disease. However, pertussis vaccine (not diphtheria-pertussis-tetanus vaccine) has been used in reduced dosages successfully and without complications among hospital personnel involved in an epidemic. Patients with active pertussis or convalescent from it may have a very severe reaction to the vaccine and should not be immunized.

REFERENCES

Hemophilus aphrophilus

ELSTER SK et al: *Hemophilus aphrophilus* endocarditis: A review of 23 cases. Am J Cardiol 35:72, 1975

SUTTER VL, FINEGOLD SM: *Hemophilus aphrophilus* infections: Clinical and bacteriologic studies. Ann NY Acad Sci 174:468, 1970

Hemophilus influenzae

ALEXANDER HE: Treatment of type b *Hemophilus influenzae* meningitis. J Pediatr 25:517, 1975

AMERICAN ACADEMY OF PEDIATRICS COMMITTEE ON INFECTIOUS DISEASES: Ampicillin-resistant strains of *Hemophilus influenzae* type b. Pediatrics 55:145, 1975

BRADSHAW MW et al: Bacterial antigens cross-reactive with the capsular polysaccharide of *Hemophilus influenzae* b. Lancet 1:1095, 1971

FOTHERGILL LD, WRIGHT J: Influenzal meningitis: Relation of age incidence to bactericidal power of blood against causal organism. J Immunol 24:273, 1933

JACOBSEN JA et al: Epidemiologic characteristics of infections caused by ampicillin-resistant *Hemophilus influenzae*. Pediatrics 58:388, 1976

LEVIN DC et al: Bacteremic *Hemophilus influenzae* pneumonia in adults: Report of 24 cases and review of the literature. Am J Med 62:219, 1977

PELTDA H et al: *Haemophilus influenzae* type b capsular polysaccharide vaccine in children: A double-blind field study of 100,000 vaccines 3 months to 5 years of age in Finland. Pediatrics 60:730, 1977

ROBBINS JB et al: *Haemophilus influenzae* type b: Disease and immunity in humans. Ann Intern Med 78:259, 1973

SMITH DH et al: Responses of children immunized with the capsular polysaccharide of *Hemophilus influenzae* type b. Pediatrics 52:637, 1973

SMITH EWP JR, HAYNES RE: Changing incidence of *Hemophilus influenzae* meningitis. Pediatrics 50:723, 1972

TODD JK, BRUHN FW: Severe *Haemophilus influenzae* infections. Am J Dis Child 129:607, 1975

VANKLINGEREN B et al: Plasmid-mediated chloramphenicol resistance in *Haemophilus influenzae*. Antimicrob Agents Chemother 11:383, 1977

Hemophilus parainfluenzae

CHUNN CJ et al: *Haemophilus parainfluenzae* infective endocarditis. Medicine 56:99, 1977

HABLE KA et al: Three *Hemophilus* species. Am J Dis Child 121:35, 1971

Hemophilus pertussis

BASSILI WR, STEWART GT: Epidemiological evaluation of immunisation and other factors in the control of whooping cough. Lancet 1:471, 1976

BRADFORD WL, SLAVIN B: Nasopharyngeal cultures in pertussis. Proc Soc Exp Biol Med 43:590, 1940

BYERS RK, MOLL FC: Encephalopathies following prophylactic pertussis vaccine. Pediatrics 1:437, 1948

DONALDSON P, WHITACKER J: Diagnoses of pertussis by fluorescent antibody staining of nasopharyngeal smears. Am J Dis Child 99:423, 1960

KURT TL et al: Spread of pertussis by hospital staff. JAMA 221:264, 1972

LAMBERT HJ: Epidemiology of a small pertussis outbreak in Kent County, Michigan. Public Health Rep 80:365, 1965

MEDICAL RESEARCH COUNCIL INVESTIGATION: The prevention of whooping cough by vaccination. Br Med J 1:1463, 1951

OLSON LC: Pertussis. Medicine 54:427, 1975

Report of the Committee on Infectious Diseases, 17th ed. Evanston, Ill, American Academy of Pediatrics, 1974

Hemophilus vaginalis

GARDNER HL, DUKES CD: Haemophilus vaginalis vaginitis: A newly defined specific infection previously classified "non-specific vaginitis." Am J Obstet Gynecol 69:962, 1955

PHEIFER TA et al: Non-specific vaginitis. Role of Haemophilus vaginitis and treatment with metroindazole. N Engl J Med 298:1429, 1978

REGAMEY C, SCHOENKNECHT FD: Puerperal fever with Haemophilus vaginalis septicemia. JAMA 225:1621, 1973

126
CHANCROID

KING K. HOLMES
ALAN R. RONALD

DEFINITION Chancroid, or soft chancre, is an acute, sexually transmitted infection characterized by painful genital ulcerations usually associated with inflammatory, inguinal adenopathy which often progresses to suppuration. A presumptive diagnosis is supported by exclusion of syphilis, genital herpes, and other specific causes of genital ulceration, together with improvement following sulfonamide therapy. A specific diagnosis is proved only when *Hemophilus ducreyi* is isolated from the lesion or suppurative node.

ETIOLOGY The specific microbial etiology of chancroid has repeatedly been supported by isolation of Ducrey's bacterium, *H. ducreyi*, in mixed culture from chancroidal ulcers and rarely in pure culture from buboes. However, *Bacteroides fragilis, B. melaninogenicus,* and gram-positive cocci are often present in genital ulcers, and anaerobic spirochetes which can be confused with *Treponema pallidum* are occasionally seen as well. The role of such organisms as synergistic or independent pathogens remains undefined. The reported frequency of recovery of *H. ducreyi* from typical chancroid ulcers ranges from 15 to 90 percent. *Hemophilus ducreyi* is a poorly characterized gram-negative aerobe which requires hemin (X factor) but not nicotinamide adenine dinucleotide (V factor) for growth. No unique colonial, biochemical, or immunologic characterizations have been demonstrated, and isolates are identified principally by their streptobacillary "chaining" appearance on Gram's stain.

EPIDEMIOLOGY The incidence of chancroid is unknown, since bacteriologic diagnosis is difficult, clinical diagnosis inaccurate, and reporting incomplete. However, chancroid on a worldwide basis is estimated to be more prevalent than syphilis. Chancroid is most common in Southeast Asia, Africa, and South and Central America but is rare in developed countries. Less than 1000 cases of chancroid are reported annually in the United States. Localized outbreaks of disease do occur. The sex ratio of reported cases in the United States is five males to one female. Uncircumcised men are more susceptible to chancroid than circumcised men. Prostitution plays a significant role in transmission, and among merchant seamen and military troops whose sexual contacts are prostitutes, chancroid appears to be far more common than syphilis. The extent of the organism's reservoir and the role of carriers in the spread of chancroid are undetermined. Commonly female contacts of infected males will not have genital ulcers. It is presumed that they are carriers of *H. ducreyi*, and organisms resembling *H. ducreyi* have been recovered from smegma of normal men and the vagina of normal women.

CLINICAL MANIFESTATIONS After an incubation period of 3 to 5 days, a small inflammatory papule appears, which becomes pustular or occasionally vesiculopustular and ulcerative within 2 to 3 days. The classic chancroid (Fig. 126-1) is superficial and shallow, ranging from a few millimeters to 2 cm in diameter. The edge usually appears ragged or scalloped and is surrounded by an inflammatory red halo. The base is covered by a necrotic exudate and bleeds easily when the exudate is removed. In contrast with syphilitic chancre, the chancroidal ulcer is extremely painful and tender and is not indurated. In men, the most frequent locations are the preputial orifice or internal surface of the prepuce and the frenulum; in women, the labia, fourchette, and perianal region. The lesions in females tend to be more superficial and less painful. Multiple ulcers are more common than single ulcers. Extragenital ulcers can occur but are rare.

FIGURE 126-1
The classic chancroid.

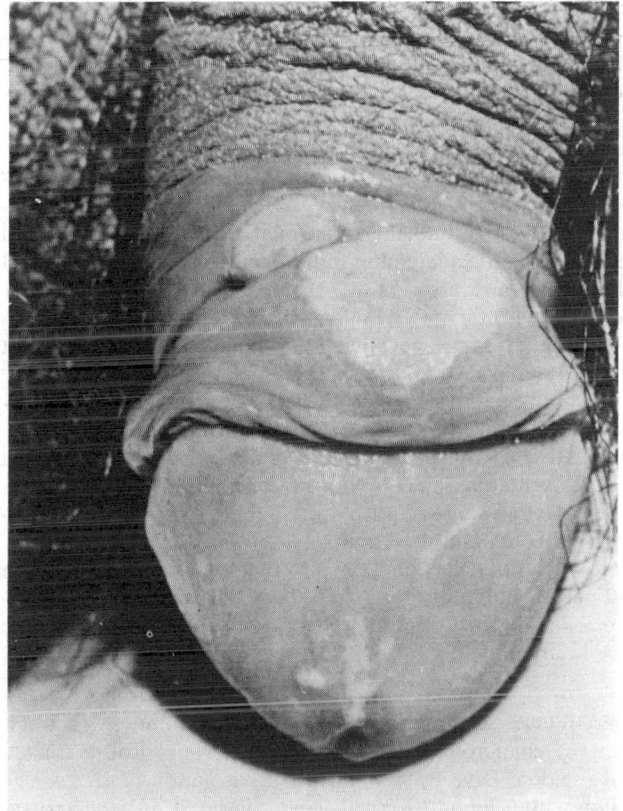

Acute, painful, tender, inflammatory inguinal adenopathy accompanies over 50 percent of cases and is unilateral in about two-thirds. In untreated patients, the involved nodes become matted, forming a unilocular suppurative bubo. The overlying skin becomes erythematous, tense, and thinned and finally ruptures, forming a single ulcer.

DIAGNOSIS Other diseases which may be confused with chancroid in decreasing order of frequency are genital herpes, primary syphilis, and lymphogranuloma venereum (LGV). One United States study of 100 consecutive men with penile ulceration disclosed genital herpes in 22, syphilis in 17, and traumatic lesions in 8. Classic chancroid ulcers were noted in 12, only 2 of which yielded *H. ducreyi* on culture. Most of the remaining ulcers were of uncertain etiology. The morphological diagnosis of genital lesions is fraught with error, and the majority of lesions diagnosed as chancroid in clinical practice probably are actually genital herpes, syphilis, or traumatic lesions. Careful repeated dark-field search for *T. pallidum* are serial serology for syphilis should be carried out even in patients with clinical features of chancroid.

Primary genital infection with herpes simplex virus produces tender inguinal adenopathy in approximately 50 percent of cases, but primary genital herpes can usually be readily distinguished by the history of onset with vesicular lesions. Primary genital herpes often produces dysuria and symptoms suggestive of viremia, such as fever, myalgia, and arthralgia, whereas chancroid rarely causes systemic symptoms. Over 80 percent of women with primary herpes have transient cervical ulcerations. A localized cluster of vesicles and a past history of similar lesions characterize recurrent genital herpes.

If viral isolation cannot be attempted, a simple means for diagnosing genital herpes is by cytology (Papanicolaou) smear obtained from the base of the genital lesion. Multinucleated cells and/or intranuclear inclusions can be seen in about two-thirds of vesicular or pustular herpetic lesions and about 50 percent of ulcerative lesions. In primary syphilis, the chancre is indurated, and the associated adenopathy is bilateral, nontender, and nonsuppurative. However, at least three dark-field examinations should be performed on separate days together with monthly serologic tests for syphilis for 3 months, to exclude syphilis.

The inguinal adenopathy of LGV differs from that of chancroid. The adenopathy of LGV develops after the genital lesion is healed, is indolent, often bilateral and nontender, and develops multilocular suppuration and fistulas. Chancroidal adenopathy appears rapidly, nearly always before the ulcer has healed, is more often unilateral, is more painful, and develops suppuration. A negative LGV complement fixation test provides evidence against LGV.

The only reliable method for laboratory diagnosis of chancroid consists of isolation of *H. ducreyi* from the ulcer or bubo. Inoculation of pus into rabbit blood has been the standard culture technique. Overgrowth of concomitant flora has usually precluded successful isolation. Direct plating onto chocolate agar containing 1% Isovitalex plus 3 μg/ml vancomycin is more likely to yield the organism. Incubation in 5% CO_2 with 100 percent humidity for 3 to 5 days is necessary for discernible colonial growth. Immunodiagnostic tests for chancroid are needed urgently.

TREATMENT Comparisons of various antibiotics for treatment of chancroid have been inconclusive, because treated cases seldom have been confirmed by isolation of *H. ducreyi*. Small genital lesions, treated only with good hygiene and saline soaks, may heal in 2 to 4 weeks without antibacterial ther-apy. Genital herpes usually begins to improve spontaneously about 10 days after onset of primary lesions and 4 days after onset of recurrent lesions, while primary syphilis usually heals 4 to 6 weeks after onset. Sulfonamides are considered more effective than tetracycline or streptomycin for chancroid. Also sulfonamide therapy will not interfere with dark-field examination for *T. pallidum* or with development of a positive serologic test for syphilis. If initial dark-field examination of a chancroidal lesion is negative, sulfonamide therapy can be started, and the dark-field examination can be repeated on subsequent days. Sulfisoxazole (Gantrisin) is usually effective in a dose of 4 g daily and should be continued until the lesion and adenopathy have healed, which usually requires about 2 weeks. Fluctuant lymph nodes should be aspirated to prevent rupture, since suppuration may progress despite therapy. Buboes larger than 5 cm in diameter almost always require drainage. After three successive dark-field examinations have been negative, if the response to sulfisoxazole is unsatisfactory, tetracycline hydrochloride should be added in a dose of 2 g daily. *Hemophilus ducreyi* is susceptible to a number of antibiotics including streptomycin, chloramphenicol, erythromycin, and usually penicillin. Plasmid-mediated resistance to one or multiple antibiotics is present in some strains.

REFERENCES

CHAPEL T et al: The microbiological flora of penile ulcerations. J Infect Dis 137:50, 1978

HAMMOND GW et al: Antimicrobial susceptibility of *Haemophilus ducreyi*. Antimicrob Agents Chemother 13:608, 1978

———— et al: Comparison of specimen collection and laboratory techniques for isolation of *Haemophilus ducreyi*. J Clin Microbiol 7:39, 1978

———— et al: Determination of the hemin requirement of *Haemophilus ducreyi:* Evaluation of the porphyrin test and media used in the satellite growth test. J. Clin Microbiol 7:243, 1978

KERFER RE et al: Treatment of chancroid. A comparison of tetracycline and sulfisoxazole. Arch Dermatol 100:604, 1979

SULLIVAN M: Chancroid. Am J Syph Gonorrhea Vener Dis 24:482, 1940

127
BRUCELLOSIS

WESLEY W. SPINK

DEFINITION Brucellosis (undulant fever) is caused by microorganisms belonging to the genus *Brucella* and is transmitted to human beings from lower animals. The acute illness is frequently characterized by fever without localized findings, while the chronic form consists of fever, weakness, and vague complaints, which may persist for months and years.

HISTORY The first clear-cut picture of the disease was presented in 1863 by Marston, and the etiologic agent (*Brucella melitensis*) was discovered by Bruce in 1886. In 1897, Bang reported that *B. abortus* was the cause of contagious abortion in cattle in Denmark. Traum first identified *Brucella* organisms (*B. suis*) from aborting sows in 1914. New species include *B. canis,* which causes abortions in dogs, especially the beagle breed, and *B. ovis,* which causes epidemics that result in sterility in rams.

ETIOLOGY Human brucellosis is primarily due to one of three species: *B. melitensis* (goats), *B. suis* (hogs), and *B. abortus* (cattle). Several subtypes have been described under each of these three main categories. *Brucella suis*, subtype II (*B. rangiferi tarandi*), is a serious disease of reindeer in Alaska and Siberia, and a common cause of human illness. *Brucella canis* has caused illness in few humans, and no human disease has been ascribed to *B. ovis*. Brucellae are small, nonmotile, non-spore-forming, gram-negative rods. Growth is best at 37°C in trypticase soy broth or tryptose phosphate broth having a pH of 6.6 to 6.8, under conditions in which 10 percent of the air is displaced by carbon dioxide. The differentiation of the three species is dependent upon biochemical and serologic reaction. Strain 19, *B. abortus,* is a viable attenuated strain used widely for vaccinating cattle. Accidental injection through the skin in veterinarians causes an acute febrile illness, which should be treated with tetracycline.

EPIDEMIOLOGY

The natural reservoir of brucellosis is in domestic animals, particularly cattle, swine, goats, and sheep. The disease is very rarely transmitted from person to person.

Studies in the United States and elsewhere indicate that the majority of cases are acquired through contact, and fewer cases are caused by the ingestion of milk or milk products. This trend is due to the enactment of local and state ordinances requiring all milk sold for human consumption to be pasteurized. There is some evidence that brucellosis may be airborne, the disease resulting from the inhalation of *Brucella*. Infections caused by *B. abortus* are spread through cow's milk or through dermal contact with *Brucella*. Contact with infected porcine tissue is a common cause of infections due to *B. suis*. Thus, brucellosis is primarily an occupational disease of rural areas, involving primarily meat-packing plant employees, farmers, veterinarians, and livestock producers. Disease due to *B. melitensis* is the most common type of brucellosis on a worldwide basis. It occurs in local areas in the United States and is due to the ingestion of goat's milk cheese.

PATHOGENESIS

Following invasion of the body by brucellae through the oropharynx or through the skin, the organisms tend to localize in tissues of the reticuloendothelial system, such as the bone marrow, lymph nodes, liver, spleen, and also the kidneys. A characteristic but nonspecific reaction of these tissues to the brucellae is the appearance of epithelioid cells, giant cells of the foreign body and Langhans' types, and lymphocytes and plasma cells. Necrosis and caseation rarely occur in these granulomatous areas. When caseation is encountered, it is usually caused by *B. suis*. The granulomas are similar to those of sarcoidosis and tuberculosis. Other, less frequent, sites of localization of *Brucella* organisms are the bones (especially the spine), the endocardium, and the testes. Although the central nervous system and peripheral nerves are commonly affected deleteriously by brucellae, the mechanism whereby this takes place is not known. Like other blood-borne bacilli, brucellae may on occasion localize in any tissue or organ in the body. Though brucellosis is a common cause of abortions in cattle, swine, and goats, authentic human abortions occur no more frequently with this disease than with other bacteremias. Orchitis in the male is rarely the cause of subsequent sterility.

MANIFESTATIONS

The incubation period varies between 5 and 21 days, though many months may elapse between the time of infection and the first appearance of symptoms. The onset in many instances may be insidious; patients have a low-grade fever with no localized findings and complain of headache, weakness, insomnia, sweats, anorexia, constipation, pain over the spine, and generalized aches and pains. Less frequently, the disease may be ushered in by chills, high fever, and prostration, but, again, localizing abnormal physical findings may be absent. An enlarged and tender spleen is usually associated with the more severe cases. Pain on pressure over

the vertebrae occurs occasionally, and pain along the course of peripheral nerves, particularly the sciatic nerve, is encountered. Orchitis appears after several days of illness and, like the orchitis of mumps, is ushered in with a chill or chilliness, high fever, and tender and enlarged testes. Painful and swollen joints are seen occasionally, but persistent and deforming arthritis is rare. Signs and symptoms referable to the lungs and pleurae are uncommon. A rare but serious complication is subacute bacterial endocarditis. Ocular disorders are associated with the more chronic forms of the disease.

The initial febrile stage of the illness may last from a few days up to several weeks. The persistence of fever and symptoms is definitely related to physical activity. Rest in bed during the acute illness is frequently associated with prompt improvement. The natural course of the disease in the majority of patients is marked by a permanent remission of fever and symptoms within 3 to 6 months or sooner. A small number of patients with bacteriologically proved cases may have an illness that persists for a year or more.

The status of *chronic brucellosis* is extremely difficult to assess. There is no doubt that the infection may persist in a relatively small number of individuals for months and years. Such patients are in a state of ill health manifested by weakness, fatigue, mental depression, vague aches and pains, and no abnormal physical findings. Intermittent fever may occur. Of considerable importance in the suspected chronic case is the investigation of possible sites of chronic suppuration manifested by calcified caseating areas in the liver and spleen that can be detected by careful x-ray films of the abdomen or by liver or spleen scan. Abacteriuric pyuria should suggest, among other causes, renal suppuration due to brucellae.

LABORATORY FINDINGS

A precise diagnosis of brucellosis is dependent upon the results of laboratory procedures.

Blood The total leukocyte count is usually normal, or slightly reduced, but is rarely over 10,000 cells per cubic millimeter. The differential count reveals a relative lymphocytosis. The erythrocyte sedimentation rate is of no specific diagnostic aid, being normal or accelerated.

The most practical method for screening suspected cases of brucellosis is the agglutination reaction. Agglutinins usually appear during the second or third week of illness. If proper techniques and antigens are employed, agglutinins are demonstrated in the vast majority of bacteriologically proved cases. Active brucellosis is usually associated with titers of 1:100 or above. On rare occasions, the titer may be depressed by "blocking antibodies" in chronic illness. Only very rarely are agglutinins absent in patients with bacteriologically proved disease. Agglutinins for brucellosis are not always specific, since cross reactions occur with the cholera vibrio and with *Pasteurella tularensis*. Agglutinins may persist in the blood long after the patient has recovered. One of the most critical diagnostic problems in the sporadic case of brucellosis is the interpretation of an agglutination titer of 1 to 100 or lower in the absence of definitive bacteriologic data and localizing signs. *Brucella*-agglutinating immunoglobulins in serum consist of both 7S and 19S globulins, but only 7S globulins have been associated with active disease in acute and chronic cases, providing a stimulating dose of antigen (skin test) has not been given before obtaining blood from the patient. The absence of 7S agglutinating antibody in the serum of a suspected case of brucellosis strongly militates against the presence of active disease as the cause of illness.

At least one, and preferably more, cultures of blood should be carried out in every suspected case of brucellosis and kept for 6 weeks before being discarded as negative. Brucellae have been isolated from aspirated sternal bone marrow when simultaneous blood cultures were sterile. It is too impractical for routine purposes to attempt to isolate brucellae from the urine, bile, or feces.

Intradermal tests A positive reaction to *Brucella* antigen has no more significance than that obtained with tuberculin in suspected cases of tuberculosis. A positive reaction indicates previous invasion of the body by brucellae and does not mean that active disease is present. When agglutinins are absent and cultures remain sterile, considerable caution must be exercised before making a diagnosis of brucellosis, even though the skin test is positive.

DIFFERENTIAL DIAGNOSIS Brucellosis must be differentiated from other acute febrile illnesses such as influenza and other upper respiratory diseases of doubtful etiology. Other diseases from which it must be differentiated include malaria and typhoid fever. Brucellosis may be confused with infectious mononucleosis.

Chronic brucellosis simulates psychoneurosis, anxiety states, and chronic nervous exhaustion. Indeed, a patient with brucellosis may also have these nervous disorders.

TREATMENT Patients with acute brucellosis should be reassured that a large majority of those with the disease recover spontaneously. Rest and psychotherapy are important during the febrile illness.

The course of acute brucellosis can be shortened and complications prevented by the prompt use of tetracycline, in dosage of 0.5 g four times daily orally for at least 3 weeks. In case of a relapse, this dose schedule can be repeated. Except in rare instances there is no advantage in more than two courses of tetracycline therapy. For more seriously ill patients streptomycin in dosage of 0.5 g twice daily may be used in addition to tetracycline. Tetracycline therapy, with and without streptomycin, is also effective in proved chronic brucellosis.

Febrile patients with either acute or chronic brucellosis sometimes have severe anorexia, depression, and generalized debilitation. Such individuals should receive an adrenocorticoid steroid preparation in addition to antibiotic therapy. Prednisone in oral dosage of 20 mg can be given twice daily for 72 to 96 h, or 100 mg hydrocortisone can be administered intravenously, followed by 50 mg orally twice daily.

The therapeutic use of brucella vaccine in chronic brucellosis is of questionable value and is not recommended.

For the relief of headache and the generalized aches and pains, salicylates may be prescribed; the occasional use of barbiturates is desirable for the insomnia which is so commonly a part of the disease.

PROGNOSIS Although brucellosis may be a chronic and disabling disease, the overall mortality rate is low. Even without the aid of effective drug therapy, only 15 percent of patients have an illness exceeding 3 months.

Cases of bacteriologically proved brucellosis in which the disease has continued for up to 25 years have been studied at the University of Minnesota Hospitals, but such cases are rare. So-called "chronic brucellosis" is diagnosed all too often on the basis of procedures of doubtful value, especially the intradermal test with *Brucella* antigen.

Relapses occur in some chronic cases of brucellosis. These recurrences are not common and are manifested by fever, mental and physical disability, and generalized aches and pains. Too little attention has been given to the problem of reinfections. Clinical observations in meat-packing plant employees have confirmed studies made in experimentally infected animals, showing that the immunity induced by one attack of brucellosis is only relative and that second and third infections do take place. In individuals who continue to be exposed to the disease, it may be quite difficult to differentiate between relapses and reinfections. Furthermore, patients who have recovered from brucellosis have an acquired *Brucella* hypersensitivity that may render them extremely susceptible to the effects of contact with *Brucella* antigen. This is particularly applicable to veterinarians who have accidentally injected viable *Brucella* antigen into their skin while immunizing animals. Violent local and systemic febrile reactions follow such an incident within a few hours.

PREVENTION As long as a reservoir of brucellosis persists in domestic animals, human brucellosis will occur. The only practical means of eliminating the disease in human beings is to eradicate the disease from cattle, hogs, sheep, and goats. Control measures in animals have been worked out in the United States, especially for cattle, and considerable progress is being made in eliminating *B. suis* from herds of swine. Since human brucellosis may be contracted through the ingestion of contaminated milk and milk products, it is essential that only properly pasteurized milk be utilized for human consumption. Brucellosis is an occupational disease involving farmers, livestock workers, veterinarians, and those working in meat-packing plants, and there is no entirely safe means for immunizing these groups against the disease.

REFERENCES

BUCHANAN TM et al: Brucellosis in the United States, 1960–1972. An abattoir-associated disease. Medicine 53:403, 1974

CENTER FOR DISEASE CONTROL: *Brucellosis Surveillance: Annual Summary 1976.* October 1977

MEYER ME: Advances in research on brucellosis, 1957–1972, in *Advances in Veterinary Science and Comparative Medicine,* vol 18, CA Brandly, CE Cornelius (eds). New York, Academic, 1974, pp 231–249

SAEGUSA J et al: A survey of *Brucella canis* infection in dogs from Tokyo area. Jpn J Vet Sci 40:75, 1978

SPINK WW: *The Nature of Brucellosis.* Minneapolis, University of Minnesota Press, 1956

———: The significance of bacterial hypersensitivity in human brucellosis: Studies on infections due to strain 19, *Brucella abortus.* Ann Intern Med 47:861, 1957.

128
TULAREMIA

LEIGHTON E. CLUFF

DEFINITION Tularemia (rabbit fever, deer-fly fever, Ohara's disease) is an infectious disease of animals transmitted to human beings by direct contact or by insect vectors. A cutaneous or mucous membrane lesion at the site of inoculation and regional lymph node enlargement are the characteristic manifestations of the disease in humans. Pneumonia or fever without regional manifestations also is a feature of tularemia.

HISTORY The microorganism responsible for tularemia was identified by McCoy and Chapin in 1912 among infected ground squirrels in Tulare County, California. The first description of tularemia in man was by Wherry and Lamb in 1914.

ETIOLOGY *Francisella (Pasteurella) tularensis* is a pleomorphic, nonsporulating, gram-negative bacillus. It can be cultured only on media containing glucose, cystine, and serum. Thorough cooking renders meat from infected animals safe for eating, but tularemia can develop in persons handling carcasses that have been frozen for many days. *Francisella tularensis* is related antigenically to the causative organisms of brucellosis and plague and possesses an endotoxin similar to those of many other gram-negative bacteria.

EPIDEMIOLOGY AND PATHOGENESIS Contact with infected animals is the commonest source of tularemia in humans, but the disease also may be acquired from insects or by exposure to the organism in the laboratory. A variety of rodents, carnivores, ungulates, birds, and arthropods are naturally infected by *F. tularensis,* including rabbits, squirrels, woodchucks, muskrats, skunks, coyotes, foxes, cats, opossums, mice, rats, quail, chickens, pheasants, snakes, ticks, and flies. The Rocky Mountain tick, western wood tick, eastern dog tick, and the Lone Star tick (*Dermacentor andersoni, D. variabilis, D. occidentalis,* and *Amblyomma americanum*) may act as reservoirs of infection. One species of deerfly (*Chrysops discalis*) and, in Sweden, a mosquito (*Aedes cinereus*) can transmit tularemia to humans. Ticks are an important reservoir of the disease because the microorganism is transferred transovarially from the female to her progeny. Sporadic episodes and epidemic tularemia have occurred among humans after contact with water and fish contaminated by infected animal carcasses. However, human-to-human transmission of infection does not occur. Wild cottontail rabbits are the principal source of tularemia in the United States. A large-scale epidemic, presumably transmitted by infected muskrats, occurred in Vermont in 1968. A case of human infection has been reported after a cat bite.

Human beings are highly susceptible to tularemia; the organism usually invades through the skin, mucous membrane, gastrointestinal tract, or respiratory tract. Hunters, butchers, and housewives are most often affected.

PATHOLOGY Microscopically, the primary cutaneous lesion shows neutrophilic infiltration, granulomatous reaction, and necrosis. The regional lymph nodes develop similar changes and often suppurate. The granulomatous reaction in tularemia resembles tubercles in liver, spleen, lung, and kidney *Francisella tularensis* has been recovered from lymph nodes many days after apparent subsidence of the disease.

MANIFESTATIONS The incubation period is 3 to 7 days. The typical lesion of skin or mucous membranes begins as a reddened papule that may be pruritic and soon ulcerates. The primary lesion in this *ulceroglandular* form of the disease is rarely very painful, is usually present before onset of systemic symptoms, and may not heal until convalescence is well under way. Frequently it is overlooked, or its relation to severe systemic symptoms is not recognized. Regional lymph node enlargement is usually more prominent than that accompanying infections of similar severity produced by other microorganisms. The involved nodes are often exquisitely tender, fluctuant, hot, and reddened. Drainage can occur spontaneously. Generalized lymphadenopathy is present in some cases, but the regional nodes are most prominently involved. There is considerable variation in the intensity of the systemic symptoms of ulceroglandular tularemia; the patient may be almost asymptomatic or severely ill. Clinical and roentgenographic evidence of pneumonitis may accompany this form of the disease, illustrating its disseminated character, but bacteremia is rarely demonstrable.

Localized lymph node enlargement without a detectable skin lesion is referred to as *glandular* tularemia. The patho-

genesis of this form of the disease is probably identical with that of ulceroglandular tularemia, and the features of the illness are also the same.

Rarely, the portal of entry of the organism is the conjunctiva, where there develops an ulcer, with edema, congestion, lacrimation, photophobia, and pain. In this *oculoglandular* type of tularemia the preauricular, submaxillary, and anterior cervical lymph nodes may enlarge. Corneal ulceration and scarring or perforation of the globe may occur.

Ingestion of contaminated meat or water may result in primary lesions in the *gastrointestinal tract.* This rare form of the disease produces diarrhea, abdominal pain, nausea, vomiting, melena, and hematemesis, but otherwise differs little from tularemia introduced through other portals. Ulcerative lesions are often found in the buccal mucosa, pharynx, or intestine, and the mesenteric or cervical lymph nodes are involved early in the disease.

Tularemia without obvious primary ulcer or localized lymphadenitis is referred to as *typhoidal.* Constitutional symptoms in typhoidal tularemia differ in no way from those in other types of the disease, although there is usually more prostration. In the absence of localized manifestations, the diagnosis of tularemia is more difficult and depends on serologic tests, isolation of the organism, or a strong epidemiologic history.

Pneumonia may accompany tularemia. Involvement of the lung is secondary to hematogenous dissemination, even when infection is acquired by inhalation of the organism (as in bacteriology laboratories). Pneumonitis in tularemia may cause cough, mucoid sputum, hemoptysis, pleuritic pain, dyspnea, and cyanosis; but extensive x-ray evidence of pneumonitis is sometimes present in the absence of any symptoms of pulmonary disease. Physical findings often correlate poorly with the roentgenologic changes, which consist of diffuse patchy or lobar infiltrations and inconstant hilar adenopathy. Pleural effusion may occur, but lung abscess is rare.

Rarely *F. tularensis* causes endocarditis, pericarditis, peritonitis, appendicitis, osteomyelitis, or meningitis.

Fever in tularemia develops abruptly, often with rigors, and in untreated patients may persist with temperatures of 104 to 106°F for as long as 4 weeks. The fever is sustained or mildly remittent, and defervescence is by lysis.

Splenomegaly is detectable in many patients. An evanescent macular or papular rash is sometimes present on the trunk and extremities early in the disease.

Convalescence in untreated tularemia is prolonged; and fever, lassitude, fatigability, myalgia, irritability, or anorexia may persist or recur for many months. Recovery is usually prompt if acute tularemia is treated with antibiotics. When therapy is delayed, however, patients are more likely to be left with mild debilitation that is unresponsive to further administration of antimicrobial drugs.

Recovery from tularemia is usually followed by immunity to recurrence of disease. However, immunity is not complete, and several instances of second, even third, attacks of tularemia have been recorded. Almost invariably, they have consisted of the development of a local lesion and mild regional adenopathy without systemic symptoms and with little or no fever.

LABORATORY FINDINGS Serum agglutinins for *F. tularensis* are present after the second week of illness. Cross-agglutination may occur with antigens of *Brucella,* but this is not a constant finding. The procedure of choice is a microagglutination method, although the standard tube agglutination test is equally sensitive

Francisella tularensis can be recovered by appropriate cultures or animal inoculation. It is rarely found in blood but can be isolated from the mucocutaneous ulcer or regional lymph nodes with regularity. The organism has been cultured from the sputum and gastric washings, even in patients without roentgenographic evidence of pneumonitis. Accidental infection of personnel in diagnostic laboratories may occur.

The skin test with a diluted suspension of killed *F. tularensis*, or purified antigen, becomes positive during the first week of disease. The cutaneous hypersensitivity response is "delayed" and resembles the tuberculin reaction. The skin test may become positive earlier and may remain so longer than the agglutination test.

The total blood leukocyte count is usually normal. The erythrocyte sedimentation rate is normal in ulceroglandular or mild disease but is frequently elevated in severe typhoidal tularemia.

DIFFERENTIAL DIAGNOSIS Brucellosis, typhoid fever, disseminated tuberculosis, the early stage of several rickettsial diseases, and infectious mononucleosis may closely resemble typhoidal tularemia. History of possible contacts is important, and appropriate serologic and cultural studies are usually successful in differentiating these infections. Pneumonic tularemia must be distinguished from viral, mycotic, and other bacterial infections of the lung. The differential diagnosis of pneumonia is discussed in Chap. 260. Oculoglandular syndromes likely to be confused with tularemia are described in Chap. 197.

Ulceroglandular tularemia must be distinguished from a variety of infections in which a *local cutaneous ulcer with regional lymphadenopathy* may occur. Besides pyoderma caused by streptococci or staphylococci, these infections include lymphogranuloma venereum, cat-scratch fever, rat-bite fever, bubonic plague, anthrax, glanders, several rickettsioses of which the important one in this country is rickettsialpox, several viral infections of the skin such as orf and cowpox, and inoculation syphilis or tuberculosis. In all these, with the exception of lymphogranuloma venereum and cat-scratch fever, the regional lymph node involvement is usually proportional to the size of the cutaneous ulcer. Extragenital lymphogranuloma is rare; fever and systemic symptoms in cat-scratch fever are rarely severe for more than a few days.

TREATMENT Streptomycin is the antibiotic of choice for tularemia. The dosage is 0.5 to 1 g every 12 h for 10 days. *Francisella tularensis* cannot be recovered from lymph nodes or skin lesions after 24 to 48 h of therapy. However, the regional lymph nodes may continue to enlarge and suppurate for several days. Pulmonary lesions usually subside rapidly, although the evolution of the cutaneous lesion is not interrupted. The tetracycline antibiotics and chloramphenicol also are effective, although fever and other manifestations may recur 7 to 14 days after cessation of therapy. Recrudescent illness, however, responds rapidly to readministration of the antibiotic. Aspiration of pus from suppurating nodes rarely is necessary; but if fistulas persist, total surgical removal of the involved tissue can be carried out. Surgery may be followed by transient recurrence of fever despite failure to demonstrate the organism in excised tissues.

PROPHYLAXIS A killed bacterial vaccine developed by Foshay has been shown to stimulate serum agglutinins and induces positive skin reactions to the bacterial antigens, but it produces little immunity to infection with *F. tularensis*. An attenuated live bacterial vaccine has been developed, however, and is effective in inducing protection against infection, particularly the typhoidal form.

Antibiotic prophylaxis with streptomycin after exposure to tularemia will protect against infection. Chloramphenicol and tetracycline, however, only prolong the incubation period of the disease and do not prevent its occurrence.

Avoidance of contact with possible sources of infection is important in prevention, and the incidence of tularemia in several localities has fallen sharply with the introduction of laws prohibiting the sale of wild rabbits by butchers.

PROGNOSIS The mortality rate in untreated tularemia is 6 to 7 percent. With antimicrobial therapy, death is rare.

REFERENCES

BUCHANAN TM et al: The tularemia skin test: 325 skin tests in 210 persons: Serologic correlation and review of the literature. Ann Intern Med 74:336, 1971

BURKE DS: Immunization against tularemia: Analysis of the effectiveness of live *Francisella tularensis* vaccine in the prevention of laboratory-acquired tularemia. J Infect Dis 135:55, 1977

MASSEY ED, MANGIAFICO JA: Microagglutination test for detecting and measuring serum agglutinins of *Francisella tularensis*. Applied Microbiol 27:25, 1974

STUART BM, PULLEN RL: Tularemic pneumonia: Review of American literature and report of fifteen additional cases. Am J Med Sci 210:233, 1945

YOUNG LS et al: Tularemia epidemic: Vermont 1968. Forty-seven cases linked to contact with muskrats. N Engl J Med 280:1253, 1969

129
YERSINIA (PASTEURELLA) INFECTIONS, INCLUDING PLAGUE

JOSEPH E. JOHNSON III

Gram-negative bacilli of the genus *Pasteurella* have been reclassified recently in accordance with increasing knowledge about the characteristics of the bacteria. *Pasteurella pestis* (the plague bacillus) and *P. pseudotuberculosis* are now included in the genus *Yersinia* along with a third closely related organism, *Y. enterocolitica*. *Pasteurella multocida* (formerly *P. septica*) initially included a group of several closely related species producing hemorrhagic septicemia in animals and man. Related species with at least potential pathogenicity for humans include *P. urae*, *P. haemolytica*, and *P. pneumotropica*.

PLAGUE Definition Plague is an infectious disease of animals (principally wild and domestic rodents) which is transmitted to humans through the bite of infected ectoparasites (especially the rat flea). Disease in humans is usually characterized by the abrupt onset of high fever, lymphadenopathy with painful enlargement of regional lymph nodes draining the exposure site, bacteremia, and prostration. This clinical form of the disease is known as *bubonic* plague because of the presence of enlarged lymph nodes, or *buboes*. Secondary pneumonia may occur and lead to direct respiratory transmission by infectious aerosols from person to person. This primary *pneumonic* type of human disease is highly fatal.

History Plague was known and feared in ancient times and has been the subject of dread as well as a source of literary stimulation to authors from Dionysius in the third century to Camus in the present. At least three major pandemics have occurred in which large segments of the population were destroyed. The first authentic pandemic was recorded in the sixth century A.D.; the second great pandemic occurred in the fourteenth century and was known as the "Black Death," and the last major pandemic originated in China in 1894, spread eventually to all continents, and was first recognized in the United States in 1900. It is likely, however, that the disease was present in the wild rodent population (sylvatic plague) in California long before this. The disease is now well established in wild rodents in many parts of the world, including the western United States. It is present on every continent except Australia. Human disease is endemic in parts of Asia, Africa, and South America, and sporadic human cases still occur in the United States.

Etiology The causative agent, *Yersinia pestis*, is a gram-negative, nonmotile, and non-spore-forming bacillus which grows both aerobically and anaerobically. It is pleomorphic in exudate or sputum and may appear bacillary, ovoid, or coccal. When stained with Giemsa's or Wayson's stain, it displays a bipolar "safety pin" structure. *Yersinia pestis* grows readily although somewhat slowly on ordinary culture media, forming small, round, transparent colonies which assume a "beaten-copper" appearance after 48 h. At least two types of toxins have been identified, including a soluble exotoxin-like protein and an insoluble endotoxic lipopolysaccharide. Although readily killed by sunlight, organisms have been shown to survive in sterile soil for 16 months and in nonsterile soil for as long as 7 months, and it is likely that organisms may be present in rodent burrows in the absence of fleas and rats for long periods.

Epidemiology Plague is firmly entrenched as an enzootic among approximately 200 species of rodents in many parts of the world. While the disease in wild rodents (sylvatic plague) is not usually a direct threat to man, it nevertheless serves as a vast reservoir for infection of domestic rats (murine or rat plague) which, along with their ectoparasites, live in close association with man. The endemic reservoir of sylvatic plague includes wild rats, ground squirrels, rock squirrels, mice, marmots, gophers, rabbits, prairie dogs, and chipmunks. Other animal species which are not reservoir hosts are important potential transmitters of the disease. Sick domesticated cats have been implicated in human cases. Dogs are relatively resistant to plague, showing seroconversion following exposure but usually without clinical illness. In the Western Hemisphere the disease is firmly entrenched in the wild rodent population of California, Oregon, Washington, Utah, Idaho, Nevada, New Mexico, Texas, Arizona, Colorado, Montana, Wyoming, and in wide areas in South America. The principal murine hosts are the domestic rats, *Rattus rattus* and *R. norvegicus,* which are found throughout the world. Although ticks, lice, and bedbugs may occasionally serve as vectors, the principal ectoparasite vectors are the oriental rat fleas, *Xenopsylla cheopis* and *Diamanus montanus.*

Between epidemics the infection persists as a chronic disease of wild rodents which is maintained by the insect vector. Although occasionally acquired through contact with wild rodents and their parasites, in major outbreaks of human disease infection has usually resulted from association with domestic rats and occurs in urban areas in the wake of rat epizootics. When the concentration of people and of rats under circumstances of poor sanitation provides opportunity for the migration of fleas from rats to man, an outbreak is likely to occur. Because sylvatic plague appears virtually impossible to eradicate, it will continue to pose a constant threat of extension into urban rat populations and thence to man. Infection of the flea takes place through ingestion of blood of a bacteremic animal. After multiplication in the intestinal tract of the flea, the organisms are regurgitated when the flea attempts to ingest another blood meal. Because rat fleas will attack man if rats are not immediately available, the infection is likely to be transmitted as the rat population decreases and the fleas transfer from dead hosts to human beings. Plague can be acquired by direct contact with the tissues of an infected animal, by its bite, or by scratching of infected material into the skin.

The bubonic form of the disease rarely results in transmission from person to person because bacteremia in human disease is rarely of a level sufficient to allow infection of fleas. The principal mode of spread from person to person is by the pulmonary route, which occurs when a patient with bubonic disease develops secondary plague pneumonia and thereafter excretes large quantities of organisms in the sputum. Airborne infection by droplet nuclei is highly contagious, and primary pneumonic plague is common among those attending such a patient. Although asymptomatic oropharyngeal carriers have been identified among healthy family contacts of bubonic plague patients in Vietnam, the role of these carriers in the transmission of the disease has not been determined.

Pathogenesis In the more common bubonic form of disease, *Y. pestis* gains entry into the human host through the bite of an infected flea. Organisms are carried to the local lymphatics, then to the bloodstream and finally are disseminated. The prominent clinical manifestations are usually in the lymphatic system. In bubonic plague, a hemorrhagic zone of edema surrounds an inflamed and suppurating group of regional lymph nodes. The glands are hyperplastic and show multiple areas of necrosis, in which there are swarms of organisms. Metastatic lesions sometimes develop in other lymphatics or in the viscera. Particularly likely is the occurrence of secondary pneumonia, which constitutes a potential source of pneumonic spread. Hemorrhages are numerous, probably as a result of a toxin produced by *Y. pestis* and it is not unusual for individuals given chemotherapy late in the disease to die of toxemia when plague bacilli can no longer be cultured from any organ. Primary pneumonic spread occurs through the inhalation of infectious aerosols emanating from another case or, rarely, from infected fomites. It is apparent that the tonsils and/or oropharyngeal mucous membranes may occasionally serve as portals of entry resulting in a cervical bubonic-septicemic form of the disease. Rarely a skin papule forms at the site of entry of the bacillus and may develop into a pustule or a carbuncle.

Bacteremia is a constant feature of bubonic and pneumonic plague. The precise mechanisms by which the plague bacillus and its toxic factors produce severe tissue injury are not understood completely.

Manifestations After an incubation period of 1 to 12 days (usually 2 to 4 days), the patient develops an acute and often fulminant illness. In the more common *bubonic* variety, symptoms begin abruptly with chills, a rise in temperature to 38.9 to 40.6°C (102 to 105°F), tachycardia, headache, vomiting, uncertain gait, marked prostration, and delirium. The spleen is sometimes palpable. The fleabite at the portal of entry rarely can be seen; if present, it is marked by a papule or vesicle which ultimately becomes pustular. Pain and tenderness are present in the infected regional lymph nodes. Of the buboes, 60 to 75 percent are in the inguinal or femoral regions because the lower extremities are more commonly the site of the initial fleabite. Less often, especially in children, buboes are found in the axillary or cervical regions. Infection may extend to other superficial or deeply situated groups of glands. The bubo consists of a firm, matted group of glands measuring 2 to 5 cm in diameter and is surrounded by a boggy and frequently hemorrhagic zone of edema. It may occasionally suppurate and drain spontaneously after 1 or 2 weeks, although in some instances there is complete resorption.

There is a marked hemorrhagic tendency, presumably because of the effect of plague toxin on blood vessels, and the development of an intravascular coagulopathy (DIC). Petechiae or ecchymoses occur often. Bleeding may occur into a viscus or a serous cavity, or from the nose and alimentary, respiratory, or urinary tracts.

The course of bubonic plague is marked by an irregular or remittent fever, which often drops at the time of appearance of the bubo, only to rise again. In favorable cases, the temperature falls gradually during the second week concomitant with improvement in the general clinical condition. A rise to hyperpyrexic levels or a precipitous fall to normal or to subnormal frequently heralds approaching death. Most fatalities occur during the first week of illness. Although bubonic plague is usually severe, mild cases called *pestis minor* are sometimes seen during epidemics.

The "primary septicemic" form of plague is actually a variant of bubonic disease. The patient experiences a sudden and overwhelming systemic illness. There is a marked constitutional reaction, with chills, fever, rapid pulse, severe headache, nausea, vomiting, and delirium. Death ensues within a few days, before localizing lesions become clinically apparent. Nevertheless, autopsy usually reveals inflammation in some part of the lymphatic system.

Plague also may take the form of pneumonia. The initial cases appear in patients with bubonic plague, of whom as many as 5 percent develop secondary lesions in the lungs. These individuals may provide the starting point for a person-to-person epidemiologic cycle of airborne primary pneumonic plague. It is a fulminating infection accompanied by great prostration, cough, dyspnea, and, in the later stages, cyanosis. The sputum is abundant, blood-stained, and teeming with *Y. pestis*. Often there are no clear-cut pulmonary signs, though scattered rales or areas of dullness may be found. In the absence of specific therapy, plague pneumonia invariably ends fatally within 1 to 5 days.

Infection may localize in other regions of the body. Subcutaneous abscesses and cutaneous ulcerations sometimes occur, and occasionally the meninges are involved.

Laboratory findings Laboratory confirmation of plague is relatively simple, although the disease is often misdiagnosed in the United States because of its rarity. Consideration of epidemiologic and clinical features provides highly characteristic leads, and once a suspicion of plague is entertained, it can readily be verified by smear, culture, or animal inoculation of appropriate specimens. The technique of staining a suspected specimen with fluorescent specific antiserum provides an elegant method for rapid identification of *Y. pestis*. If a bubo is present, a small quantity of interstitial fluid should be aspirated from its center. Large numbers of morphologically characteristic bacilli are usually seen in a stained smear. Infected sputum likewise contains many organisms. Bacteremia of varying degrees occurs at some time during the course of the disease in nearly all cases, and methylene-blue staining of venous blood may be useful. Pus and sputum should be cultured on blood agar plates, while blood is inoculated into nutrient broth. Organisms are identified by their morphologic and colonial characteristics, by agglutination with specific antiserum, fluorescent antibody staining, and biochemical reactions. The phage lysis test is relatively simple and helpful in distinguishing *Y. pestis* from other *Yersinia*. Caution should be observed in handling infected materials or animals, because of the great danger of infection to laboratory workers.

Specific antibodies appear in the serum of patients convalescing from the disease and can usually be detected early in the second week by complement fixation, agglutination, passive hemagglutination, or immunoelectrophoretic agar-gel precipitation methods. A passive mouse-protective test serves to indicate the immune status of a convalescent or vaccinated individual.

The white blood cell count is elevated to levels often above 20,000 cells per cubic millimeter, and there is a predominance of polymorphonuclear leukocytes. The red blood cell count usually is normal.

Diagnosis Early in the acute phase of illness, before the appearance of localizing signs, plague may be confused with severe systemic illnesses such as typhoid, typhus, or malaria. The presence of buboes may suggest other forms of infectious lymphadenitis, including tularemia, syphilis, and lymphogranuloma venereum, as well as lymphadenitis of staphylococcal or streptococcal origin. Pneumonic plague must be distinguished from tularemic, pneumococcal, and other gram-negative pneumonias as well as from anthrax, psittacosis, and mycoplasma pneumonia. The consideration of epidemiologic factors, plus bacteriologic studies, will aid in the differentiation. Serologic diagnosis is important for retrospective confirmation. When plague is suspected, it is imperative to begin treatment as soon as adequate specimens have been taken for culture because early institution of therapy is essential to ensure recovery. To delay treatment may risk toxemic death in the face of a bacteriologic cure.

Treatment When antibiotic treatment is instituted early in the course of the disease, the response is usually dramatic and complete. Early treatment in pneumonic and septicemic disease is particularly urgent since irreversible progression may occur within 15 h after onset. Streptomycin and tetracycline are the drugs of choice. Streptomycin is given intramuscularly in doses of 0.5 g every 4 h for 48 h followed by 0.5 g every 6 h for a total of 7 to 10 days or until the patient has been afebrile at least 3 days. Kanamycin is also effective and may be particularly useful if streptomycin resistance increases. Tetracyclines are given in initial doses of 2 to 3 g daily intravenously, and the dose is reduced to 2 g daily orally when improvement occurs. Chloramphenicol is also a potent antiplague agent and should be given in initial doses of 6 to 8 g daily intravenously (100 mg/kg) and the dose reduced to 3 g (50 to 75 mg/kg) daily orally for a total dose of 20 to 25 g. Sulfonamides are less effective, especially in pneumonic plague, and should be used only when the other agents are not available. Trimethoprim-sulfamethoxazole (co-trimoxazole) has been used successfully. Buboes are treated with hot, moist applications. Incision and drainage is not indicated unless the lesion becomes clearly fluctuant and the patient has been treated with antibiotics.

Control Prevention of plague must be directed toward elimination of endemic rodent foci, and in endemic urban areas constant vigilance is required in detecting and combating rodent epizootics. Prevention includes eradication of ectoparasite vectors, extermination of rats, and sometimes the immunization of the human population. Rats are attacked by poisoning and trapping, by elimination of harborage areas, and by separating them from their food supplies. Unfortunately, rodent control has proved to be most difficult in the endemic areas because of generally poor living standards. Vector control with DDT has been used with brilliant success in diminishing the flea population infecting both rodents and human beings, but studies in Southeast Asia show a significant incidence of DDT-resistant fleas; however, these may yield to other insecticides such as aldrin, dieldrin, and chlordane. The complete elimination of sylvatic plague appears to be impossible in the foreseeable future, and the control program must be aimed at eradicating foci of wild rodent infection around areas of human habitation. In these peripheral zones, the wild and the domestic rodents live commensally, exchange fleas, and threaten the human community.

Patients must be disinfested and carefully isolated, while other intimately exposed persons should be quarantined. Prophylaxis has been achieved effectively in the past by administering sulfadiazine in a dose of 3 g per day for 1 week. However, there is now significant in vitro resistance to sulfadiazine. Alternatively, prophylaxis with streptomycin in a dose of 1 g per day or with tetracycline is often effective.

Vaccines have been used for many years and apparently provide limited and transitory immunity. Several types of vaccines have been available. A formalin-killed vaccine approved for use in the United States has been advised for all persons traveling to plague-enzootic areas such as Southeast Asia, for those whose vocations bring them into frequent and regular contact with wild rodents in plague enzootic areas, such as Peace Corps volunteers and agricultural workers, and for all laboratory personnel working with *Y. pestis* or with plague-infected rodents. Although the precise effectiveness of this vaccine has not been measured satisfactorily, it appears to reduce the incidence and severity of the disease. A second promising vaccine is a living attenuated strain of the organism which may be particularly suitable for endemic areas in Asia. Studies in the U.S.S.R. indicate that the attenuated vaccine administered by the aerosol route may be especially valuable in prevention of pneumonic plague. A third vaccine consisting of a chemical extract has been effective in experimental laboratory infections. Immunity is relative, and protection is not always conferred by the active disease, since a number of reinfections have been described. Although general vaccination may be worthwhile in an area threatened by an epidemic, the results are too slow for immediate prophylaxis. In such epidemic situations, combined use of all available control measures is indicated.

Prognosis The availability of effective antibiotic therapy has improved the prognosis in this formerly highly fatal disease. In the past the mortality rate of bubonic plague varied from 50 to 90 percent, and the pneumonic, septicemic, and meningitic forms were almost invariably fatal. In treated cases the mortality is 5 to 10 percent, and even the gravest varieties of infection respond to chemotherapy if treated early enough.

OTHER *YERSINIA* INFECTIONS (*Y. PSEUDOTUBERCULOSIS* AND *Y. ENTEROCOLITICA*) Etiology *Yersinia pseudotuberculosis* is a gram-negative, aerobic, facultatively anaerobic, non-spore-forming bacillus, which is coccobacillary when virulent and bacillary when avirulent. It is easily confused with other non-lactose-fermenting Enterobacteriaceae. It is nonmotile at 37°C (98.6°F) but usually motile at 22°C (71.6°F). *Yersinia enterocolitica*, a closely related organism, has similar characteristics but is distinguished on the basis of biochemical reactions.

Manifestations *Yersinia pseudotuberculosis* is a ubiquitous animal pathogen, worldwide in distribution but identified only in the last decade as a potentially significant human pathogen. Several hundred cases of human infection have now been identified in Europe (especially Scandinavia) and increasingly from Canada and the United States. *Yersinia enterocolitica*, isolated less frequently from animals in the United States, has also now been recognized as a potential cause of a variety of human disease syndromes. Both organisms have been associated with diarrheal diseases, both acute and chronic, and also a usually benign and self-limited form of mesenteric adenitis, clinically

simulating appendicitis. Cervical adenitis has also been seen. Rarely, potentially fatal typhoidal and septicemic forms of infection have been described, especially in patients with underlying debilitating diseases. Increasingly, polyarthritis with and without associated erythema nodosum has been associated with *Yersinia* infection.

Reported cases have indicated a 3:1 male predominance especially in older children and young adults infected with *Y. pseudotuberculosis,* while equal sex distribution and a greater incidence in young children and infants has been observed with *Y. enterocolitica.* In addition, *Y. enterocolitica* has been incriminated in institutional and multiple-family outbreaks.

Transmission has usually been traced to contact with infected animals or contaminated food or water, although person-to-person, hand-to-mouth transmission appears also to be a significant possibility.

Diagnosis Diagnosis may be confirmed by culture of lymph nodes, occasionally of stools, or by serologic titers. Cross reactions with *Salmonella, Brucella,* and *Escherichia coli* antigens occur, and serums must be cross-absorbed. With use of both agglutination and hemagglutination methods, titers up to 1:10,240 have been found. Titers lower than 1:160 are not considered significant. The highest antibody titers usually occur during the acute phase of illness, rapidly disappearing by the fourth or fifth month of convalescence, probably reflecting the elicitation of IgM-type antibodies.

Although both species are easily grown on standard laboratory media, identification is more difficult, and routine methods for pathogenic Enterobacteriaceae are inadequate.

The variety of clinical syndromes which have been observed in association with *Y. pseudotuberculosis* and *Y. enterocolitica* may also be confusing. Acute or subacute yersinial enteritis may mimic salmonellosis, shigellosis, and other common enteropathogenic syndromes. Fever, diarrhea, and vomiting are the most common findings in infants and younger children. Fecal leukocytosis has been found in yersinial enteritis indicating ulceration of the intestinal mucosa. Ulcerative colitis may be simulated. Acute septicemic yersiniosis may resemble systemic salmonellosis and other "typhoidal" syndromes. Subacute localizing yersiniosis with hepatic or splenic abscesses may resemble amebic hepatitis. Patients with mesenteric adenitis (usually children) may present the clinical picture of acute appendicitis with mid- or right-lower quadrant abdominal pain, fever, and leukocytosis. At laparotomy the appendix is usually normal, but large inflamed mesenteric lymph nodes are found, sometimes with associated terminal ileitis. Histologic examination of inflamed nodes has revealed reticulogranulocytic infiltration with or without small abscess formation. Polyarthritis of varying severity and duration has been observed and most often mimics rheumatic fever or juvenile rheumatoid arthritis. Reiter's syndrome may also be simulated. Erythema nodosum has also been increasingly identified in patients with agglutinin rises to *Yersinia,* with or without associated arthritis. Common features in adults have been abdominal pain and fever, with or without arthritis or erythema nodosum. Possible associations of *Yersinia* infection with glomerulonephritis, thyroid disease, and pulmonary lesions have been reported but need further clarification.

Treatment Antibiotic treatment is indicated in the more severe cases, especially the septicemic and subacute localizing forms of disease. *Yersinia pseudotuberculosis* is usually susceptible to the aminoglycoside antibiotics (gentamicin, streptomycin, or kanamycin) as well as to tetracycline, chloramphenicol, ampicillin, and the cephalosporins. *Yersinia enterocolitica* is resistant to penicillin G and only variably sensitive to ampicillin and the cephalosporins. In vitro studies indicate a potential role for trimethoprim-sulfamethoxazole.

PASTEURELLA MULTOCIDA INFECTION   Definition   *Pasteurella multocida* (formerly *P. septica*) is a gram-negative nonsporulating bacillus which differs from *Yersinia* organisms in cultural characteristics, antibiotic sensitivity, and pattern of animal parasitism. For example, all strains of *P. multocida* are sensitive to penicillin. *Pasteurella multocida* is frequently identified as a commensal in cattle, horses, swine, sheep, fowl, dogs, cats, and rats, and on occasion causes hemorrhagic septicemia, or chronic pulmonary infiltrates, in these species. Human infection with *P. multocida* is uncommon and usually related to animal contact. Related species which have occasionally been identified as human pathogens include *P. urae*, *P. haemolytica*, and *P. pneumotropica*.

Manifestations   Human disease due to *P. multocida* is usually a consequence of a dog or cat bite and appears as a localized wound infection with cellulitis, suppuration, and adenitis. Osteomyelitis sometimes ensues. Rarely, in patients with bronchiectasis, *P. multocida* is isolated from sputum, and animal handlers are sometimes identified as asymptomatic respiratory carriers. Empyema has occasionally been associated with the organisms. Bacteremia with fever and chills may develop after an animal bite, occasionally without an apparent local lesion. Meningitis, brain abscess, pyogenic arthritis, endocarditis, and pyelonephritis may occasionally complicate the bacteremia.

Not all *P. multocida* infections follow documented animal bites or animal contact.

Diagnosis   Except for the association with animal (especially cat) bites, local infections with *P. multocida* show no unique characteristics, and may resemble cat-scratch fever, tularemia, or staphylococcal or streptococcal infection. Leukocytosis, uncommon in tularemia and cat-scratch fever, is the rule in *P. multocida* infection.

Gram's stain of infected material shows pleomorphic gram-negative bacilli which are usually extracellular. The bacteria may have bipolar staining and may be mistaken for gram-negative diplococci prior to cultural identification.

Treatment   Penicillin in a dosage of 600,000 to 1.2 million units daily is the preferred antibiotic, but a variety of other antibiotics may be effective.

REFERENCES

Plague

CANTEY JR: Plague in Vietnam, clinical observations and treatment with kanamycin. Arch Intern Med 133:280, 1974

GIRARD G: Plague. Annu Rev Microbiol 69:253, 1955

HIRST LF: *The Conquest of Plague: A Study of the Evolution of Epidemiology.* Fair Lawn, NJ, Oxford University Press, 1953

MEYER KF et al: Plague immunization. I. Past and present trends. J Infect Dis 129:S13, 1974

POLAND JD et al: Human bubonic plague from exposure to a naturally infected wild carnivore. Am J Epidemiol 97:332, 1973

POLLITZER R: *Plague.* Geneva, World Health Organization, 1954

REED WB et al: Bubonic plague in the southwestern United States. Medicine 49:465, 1970

RUST JD et al: The role of domestic animals in the epidemiology of plague. I. Experimental infection of dogs and cats. J Infect Dis 124:522, 1971

VON REYN CF et al: Epidemiologic and clinical features of an outbreak of bubonic plague in New Mexico. J Infect Dis 136:489, 1977

WHO EXPERT COMMITTEE ON PLAGUE: Fourth report. Tech Rep Ser 447, Geneva, 1970

P. Multocida

BEARN AG et al: *Pasteurella multocida* septicemia in man. Am J Med 18:167, 1955

MORRIS AJ et al: *Pasteurella multocida* and bronchiectasis. Bull Johns Hopkins Hosp 91:174, 1952

SWARTZ MN, KUNZ LJ: *Pasteurella multocida* infections in man: Report of two cases—meningitis and infected cat bite. N Engl J Med 261:888, 1959

Yersinia

ARVASTON B et al: Clinical symptoms of infection with *Yersinia enterocolitica.* Scand J Infect Dis 3:37, 1971

GUTMAN LT et al: An inter-familial outbreak of *Yersinia entercolitica* enteritis. N Engl J Med 288:1372, 1974

HUBERT WT et al: *Yersinia pseudotuberculosis* infection in the United States: Septicemia, appendicitis and mesenteric lymphadenitis. Am J Trop Med 20:679, 1971

JEPSEN OB et al: *Yersinia enterocolitica* infection in patients with acute surgical abdominal disease: A prospective study. Scand J Infect Dis 8:189, 1976

LEINO R, KALLIOMAKI JL: Yersiniosis as an internal disease. Ann Intern Med 81:458, 1974

RABSON AR et al: Generalized *Yersinia enterocolitica* infection. J Infect Dis 131:447, 1975

SAARI TN, TRIPLETT DA: *Yersinia pseudotuberculosis* mesenteric adenitis. J Pediatr 85:656, 1974

SHENKMAN L, BOTTONE EJ: Antibodies in *Yersinia enterocolitica* in thyroid disease. Ann Intern Med 85:735, 1976

SPIRA TJ, KABINS SA: *Yersinia enterocolitica* septicemia with septic arthritis. Arch Intern Med 136:1305, 1976

130
RAT-BITE FEVER (*STREPTOBACILLUS MONILIFORMIS* AND *SPIRILLUM MINUS* INFECTIONS)

JAN V. HIRSCHMANN

DEFINITION   *Rat-bite fever* refers to infection by either *Streptobacillus moniliformis* or *Spirillum minus*. The latter infection is also known by its Japanese name *sodoku*.

ETIOLOGY AND EPIDEMIOLOGY   *Streptobacillus moniliformis* is an aerobic nonmotile gram-negative bacterium that may grow in chains of fusiform bacilli. In blood cultures the typical puffball colonies generally appear in 2 to 7 days. Stable L forms frequently develop spontaneously.

The nasopharynx of rats is the natural reservoir of *S. moniliformis,* which grows from as many as half those studied. Human infection usually follows bites from wild rats, but bites from laboratory rats and occasionally other rodents have caused disease. Infection may also occur from ingestion of contaminated food. An epidemic in Haverhill, Massachusetts, in 1926 involving 86 people and caused by contaminated milk or ice cream has led to the term *Haverhill fever* when infection is food-borne.

Spirillum minus is a short, thick spiral gram-negative spiral organism 2 to 5 μm with two to five curves and terminal flagellae that increase its total length to 6 to 10 μm. On dark-field microscopy the organism has characteristic spasmodic motions of the body and darting movements of the flagella. Although it may be visible on Wright's stains of blood from infected patients or animals, it does not grow on artificial media and requires animal inoculation for isolation from patients.

Carrier rates in wild rats, the natural reservoir, are as high as 25 percent in some locations. In them it may cause interstitial keratitis and conjunctivitis. Human infections with *S. minus* almost always follow rat bites.

CLINICAL MANIFESTATIONS Although up to 22 days may elapse, the incubation period for *S. moniliformis* infection is generally short, typically less than 10 days, usually 1 to 3 days. The onset is sudden, with fever, chills, headache, and myalgias the initial symptoms. The bite site is usually unimpressive; occasionally swelling, ulceration, and regional lymphadenopathy are present. A macular rash develops in about 75 percent of cases, usually 1 to 3 days after the onset of symptoms, and is most prominent on the extremities, where it may involve palms and soles. Sometimes it may be generalized, petechial, purpuric, or pustular. Arthralgias or arthritis occurs in about half the cases within the first week, usually with multiple, asymmetric large joint involvement. Without treatment the course of disease may be prolonged for several weeks with persistent or recurrent fever and arthritis. Complications of *S. moniliformis* infection include endocarditis and localized abscesses in soft tissues or brain.

In *Spirillum minus* infections the incubation period is typically longer, usually 1 to 4 weeks, with a range of 1 to 36 days. Usually the bite site, after initial prompt healing, becomes swollen, painful, and red at the onset of fever and chills. There is often lymphangitis and regional lymphadenopathy as well. The fever is usually relapsing, with febrile periods of 2 to 4 days alternating with afebrile periods of about the same duration. During the fever, headache, photophobia, nausea, and vomiting may occur. Joint complaints are rare. A rash develops in more than half the patients that is usually macular and reddish brown or purple-red and occurs typically on the extremities. When untreated, this relapsing illness may persist for months. Rarely, bacterial endocarditis occurs.

LABORATORY FINDINGS In *S. moniliformis* infections the leukocyte count is typically elevated, with neutrophilia and increased immature forms. The organism can be isolated from blood, joint fluid, or pus. Serologic response can be demonstrated during the second week by agglutination tests.

In *S. minus* infections the leukocyte count may be normal or elevated. The organism may be visible on Wright's stained smears or dark-field examination of the patient's blood. In suspected cases the blood should be injected into the peritoneum of mice or guinea pigs; 5 to 15 days later the organism will be visible on dark-field examination of the animals' blood or peritoneal fluid. In about one-half of patients there are biological false-positive tests for syphilis.

DIFFERENTIAL DIAGNOSIS With a history of a rat bite, the major clinical features distinguishing *S. moniliformis* from *S. minus* infection are the differences in the incubation period, the condition of the bite site, the nature of the fever, and the presence or absence of joint symptoms.

TREATMENT AND PROGNOSIS Before effective chemotherapy was available, the mortality rate from *S. moniliformis* infections was about 10 percent; for *S. minus* it was about 6 percent. The treatment of choice is the same for both organisms: 7 to 10 days of procaine penicillin, 600,000 units twice daily intramuscularly, or oral penicillin V, 2 g daily in four divided doses. For penicillin-allergic patients oral erythromycin or tetracycline, 2 g daily in four divided doses, are alternatives. Patients with endocarditis should receive a 4-week course of intravenous penicillin G in a daily dose of 12 to 16 million units.

REFERENCES

Cole JS et al: Rat-bite fever. Ann Intern Med 71:979, 1969
McCormack RC et al: Endocarditis due to *Streptobacillus moniliformis.* JAMA 200:77, 1967
Roughgarden JW: Antimicrobial therapy of rat-bite fever: A review. Arch Intern Med 116:39, 1965

section 5 | Other aerobic bacterial infections

131 ANTHRAX

LEIGHTON E. CLUFF

DEFINITION Anthrax (also called malignant pustule, charbon, splenic fever, milzbrand, woolsorter's disease) is a disease of wild and domesticated animals that is transmitted to human beings by contact with infected animals or their products and, rarely, by insect vectors which act as mechanical carriers of the etiologic organism. The characteristic lesion of human anthrax is a necrotic cutaneous ulcer, the *malignant pustule.* The disease also may be associated with disseminated infection and mediastinitis without mucous membrane involvement or cutaneous ulcer.

HISTORY The classic studies of Robert Koch in 1877, showing that *Bacillus anthracis* was the cause of anthrax, serve as the prototype for the establishment of causation of infectious diseases.

ETIOLOGY *Bacillus anthracis* is a large, encapsulated, gram-positive, aerobic, spore-forming microorganism that grows well in most nutrient media. Its pathogenicity for laboratory animals differentiates it from *Bacillus subtilis,* which it closely resembles. The spores are killed by boiling for 10 min, but can survive for many years in soil and animal products, an important factor in the persistence and spread of the disease. The anthrax bacillus possesses a capsule of glutamyl polypeptide, which interferes with phagocytosis of the microorganism. In addition, it contains an anticomplementary substance and elaborates a "protective" antigen and a toxin which is probably of importance in determining virulence.

EPIDEMIOLOGY Anthrax is worldwide; repeated outbreaks have occurred in Southern Europe, Africa, Australia, Asia, and on both American continents.

Cattle, horses, sheep, goats, and swine are most commonly infected. There have been outbreaks of anthrax among animals in the United States, centering mostly in South Dakota, Nebraska, Arkansas, Mississippi, Louisiana, Texas, and California. The disease tends to occur in animals in late summer and early fall. An outbreak of anthrax, acquired from goatskin bongo drum heads and goatskin rugs, occurred in Haiti in 1973, and though importation from Haiti of goatskins or products made in whole or part from them has been restricted since 1974, commercial importation of potentially contaminated raw goatskin for tanning is not restricted in the United States. In 1974, an epidemic of anthrax developed in cattle in Texas, and in the state of Washington in horses infected from contaminated saddle packs containing goat hair imported from Pakistan.

The disease in human beings is acquired by butchering, skinning, or dissecting infected carcasses or by handling contaminated hides, wool, hair, or other materials. It is seen principally in agricultural and industrial employees. The majority of cases of human anthrax involve workers handling imported and unprocessed wool, hair, or hides. The disease usually follows inoculation of bacilli or spores into the skin, often through a wound or abrasion. Intestinal infection has followed ingestion of contaminated meat, and anthrax may develop after inhalation of spores.

PATHOGENESIS The malignant pustule which follows cutaneous inoculation of anthrax organisms is characterized by vesiculation, neutrophilic infiltration, gelatinous edema, and necrosis. Suppuration is rare in the absence of secondary pyogenic infection. Spread of the bacilli to the regional lymph nodes may be followed by systemic dissemination. Examination of tissues from fatal human cases reveals masses of the bacteria in blood vessels, lymph nodes, and the parenchyma of various organs. There is scanty or no cellular exudation at these foci, but hemorrhage and edema are widespread. So-called "anthrax pneumonia" and "anthrax meningitis" are, in all probability, an expression of this generalized hemorrhage and edema.

The blood of fatally infected experimental animals contains a lethal toxin, which can be neutralized by specific antiserum. This toxin has been isolated in vitro and is important in the pathogenesis of some of the manifestations of the disease.

MANIFESTATIONS The malignant pustule of human anthrax begins usually on an exposed body surface, as a painless, pruritic, erythematous papule which vesiculates and ulcerates to form a black eschar. Tiny satellite vesicles are frequent. The ulcer may be surrounded by extensive edematous swelling, which is nontender, nonpitting, and so characteristic of anthrax that it is a valuable diagnostic sign. After about 5 days the ulcer begins to subside, but edema may persist for many days or weeks. Mild tenderness and enlargement of regional lymph nodes are frequently present. Constitutional symptoms are often absent despite extensive local changes, but there may be mild fever, headache, and malaise. In disseminated anthrax, high fever, prostration, and a rapidly fatal course are seen. So-called "woolsorter's disease," a highly fatal disseminated infection, is characterized by cyanosis, dyspnea, mediastinitis, and hemoptysis and is probably dependent on the pulmonary route of inoculation. Human infection may occur from ingestion of poorly cooked meat of infected animals. This form of the disease is called *intestinal anthrax*. Clinically, it resembles an acute abdomen; massive diarrhea similar to cholera may be present. The disease is usually eventually fatal.

LABORATORY FINDINGS The fluid from the cutaneous lesion frequently contains many bacilli, demonstrable by Gram's stain and culture. Bacilli may be found on direct examination or culture of the blood of patients with bacteremia. The blood leukocyte count is normal in mild cases, but there is polymorphonuclear leukocytosis in severe disease. Similarly, the erythrocyte sedimentation rate may be increased. Patients with meningeal involvement show bloody spinal fluid, in which the organisms are easily found by direct examination or culture.

DIAGNOSIS An indirect microhemagglutination test (IMH test) has supplanted the agar-gel precipitation (AGPI) test because it is more sensitive and less time consuming. The IMH test has detected antibodies in 93 percent of patients, 98 percent of vaccinees, and none of the controls. It is useful in confirming the diagnosis, which can, of course, also be established by isolation of the organism in culture. A history of occupational exposure and characteristic eschar and edema should suggest the proper diagnosis. Pyogenic infections of the skin are usually painful; the malignant pustule is not. In addition, cutaneous anthrax is rarely purulent. The differential diagnosis of other diseases characterized by local ulceration at the portal of entry is discussed in Chap. 128.

TREATMENT AND PROPHYLAXIS Many antibiotics are effective in the treatment of human anthrax, including penicillin, chloramphenicol, tetracycline, erythromycin, and streptomycin. A dose of 600,000 units penicillin should be given twice daily until the local edema subsides. The eschar goes through its natural evolution in spite of treatment, and lymph node enlargement may persist for several days. *Bacillus anthracis* cannot be recovered from the skin lesion after 24 to 48 h of penicillin therapy, but it may persist for a longer period when chloramphenicol or tetracycline is used.

Infection of personnel in industrial plants where contaminated animal products are handled still occurs. An outbreak of inhalation anthrax with a high mortality rate was reported in a goat hair processing mill in the United States in the late 1950s. Sterilization of all raw wool, mohair, etc., would probably remove the hazard but has had only limited use. A vaccine prepared from the "protective" antigen of *B. anthracis* is available and is effective in reducing the incidence of infection in an exposed population. Spore vaccines of various types are used with good effect in domestic animals in endemic areas but are not suitable for use in human beings.

Transmission of anthrax from one human being to another has never been recognized. The cutaneous disease was fatal in 20 to 30 percent of cases before antimicrobial drugs were available. The mortality rate now is less than 1 percent with proper treatment.

REFERENCES

BRACHMAN PS: Anthrax, in *Tice's Practice of Medicine,* vol 3. Hagerstown, Md, Harper & Row, 1970

BUCHANAN TM et al: Anthrax indirect microagglutination test. J Immunol 107:1631, 1971

CENTER FOR DISEASE CONTROL: Morb Mort Week Rep, February 4, 1977

GOLD H: Anthrax: Report of 117 cases. Arch Intern Med 96:387, 1955

NALIN DR et al: Survival of a patient with intestinal anthrax. Am J Med 62:130, 1977

132

INFECTIONS CAUSED BY *LISTERIA MONOCYTOGENES* AND *ERYSIPELOTHRIX RHUSIOPATHIAE*

PAUL D. HOEPRICH

LISTERIA MONOCYTOGENES INFECTIONS

DEFINITION Listeriosis, a disease caused by *L. monocytogenes,* consists of many clinical syndromes. Perinatal infection, acquired either transplacentally or during parturition, is the most nearly unique form of listeriosis.

ETIOLOGY *Listeria monocytogenes* are gram-positive, non-acid-fast, microaerophilic, motile bacilli that form smooth colonies, but do not produce either capsules or spores. Several serotypes have been defined on the basis of O and H antigens. The epidemiologically essential aid of typing is available from the Center for Disease Control in Atlanta, Georgia. Types 4b, 1b, and 1a account for most of the cases in the United States. Weakly hemolytic gram-positive bacilli are presumed to be listerias if they are motile (when grown at 20 to 25°C), reduce 2,3,5-triphenyltetrazolium chloride, and display characteristic animal pathogenicity. The Anton test is classical: 3 to 5 days after inoculation into the conjunctival sac of a rabbit or a guinea pig, *L. monocytogenes* causes a keratoconjunctivitis. Also, general listeriosis in the rabbit typically provokes a monocytosis, and focal hepatic necrosis is usual in lethal murine listeriosis.

EPIDEMIOLOGY AND PATHOGENESIS Found on every continent save the Antarctic, *L. monocytogenes* may be primarily saprophytic on decaying organic matter in nature. They are distinct from the nonhemolytic, nonpathogenic, nonmonocytogenic, and serologically different bacilli (found mainly in soil, decaying matter, and feces) which have been variously assigned either to the genus *Listeria* or to a new genus *Murrayi.* Although typical *L. monocytogenes* have been isolated from silage, other vegetative sources, and 1 to 5 percent of specimens of human feces, listeriosis is uncommon and occurs sporadically; moreover, listeriosis is actually more common in urban than rural dwellers, occurring most frequently in July and August (Northern Hemisphere). The reservoir from which human beings become infected is frequently occult and the mode of transmission often obscure. Direct transmission from an infected nonhuman animal via contaminated secretions has been documented only rarely. On the other hand, transmission from the infected pregnant female to her offspring is well established as a route of infection.

Transplacental perinatal infection results in disseminated fetal listeriosis. The fetus is usually stillborn or is prematurely ejected, virtually always with lethal listeriosis. Fetal listeriosis acquired during delivery is typically not clinically evident for 1 or 2 weeks postpartum and usually presents as a meningitis.

Listeriosis is preponderantly a disease of persons under 1 month (about 27 percent) and over 40 years (about 56 percent) in age.

Persons in apparent good health may develop listeriosis. However, other diseases, particularly those with diminished cell-mediated immunity (listerias are cytophilic), facilitate the occurrence of listeriosis: for example, neoplasias (especially of the lymphoreticular system) and any conditions requiring treatment with pharmacologic doses of glucosteroids, irradiation, or cytotoxic agents; alcoholism; cardiovascular disease; diabetes mellitus; and tuberculosis.

MANIFESTATIONS *Meningitis* accounts for about three-fourths of the cases verified by culture and is the predominant clinical form of listeriosis in the United States. Clinically, meningitis caused by *L. monocytogenes* cannot be distinguished from meningitis caused by other kinds of bacteria.

Listeriosis of the newborn, the most nearly unique clinical form of listeriosis, ranges from meningitis that is clinically apparent within 1 month postpartum to diffuse disseminated disease in aborted, premature, stillborn infants, and neonates, who die within minutes to days after birth. If clinical disease is delayed to 1 to 4 weeks postpartum, it is generally localized to the central nervous system, as is the rule when children 1 month to 6 years of age are afflicted.

Infants born alive with listeriosis may or may not have fever; yet these babies are critically ill, with cardiorespiratory distress, vomiting, and diarrhea. Dark-red skin papules are frequent, particularly on the lower extremities. Hepatosplenomegaly may be present. This form of listeriosis is also known as septic or miliary granulomatosis, granulomatosis infantiseptica, argentophil-rod infection, or pseudotuberculosis. The findings at postmortem examination are characteristic and mimic those seen in listeriosis of rodents: widely disseminated abscesses varying in size from grossly visible to microscopic, involving, in order of decreasing frequency, liver, spleen, adrenal glands, lungs, pharynx, gastrointestinal tract, central nervous system, and skin. Typically, the lesions are abscesses, but classic granulomas may be seen, depending principally on the duration of infection before death. Microscopic examination of a Gram's stained smear of meconium from the normal newborn infant does not disclose bacteria; fetal listeriosis results in meconium laden with gram-positive bacilli. For this reason, examination of meconium by Gram's stain and by culture should be carried out whenever there is gross soiling of the amniotic liquid with meconium, prematurity, or unexplained fever in the mother before or at the onset of labor. This is particularly important because listeriosis in the pregnant woman may be asymptomatic or may cause a nonspecific illness. Thus, a week to a month prepartum, there may have been malaise, a chill, diarrhea, pain in the back or flanks, and itching. Even when symptomatic, the disease is benign and self-limited in the mother; however, as symptoms subside, a decrease or cessation of fetal movement may be noted. Infection of the fetus may occur as early as the fifth month of gestation. Following delivery of infants with proved fetal listeriosis, cervical cultures are, or soon become, negative for *L. monocytogenes;* subsequent conception, gestation, and delivery of normal offspring are usual.

Oculoglandular listeriosis is the rare human analog of the illness initiated in the rabbit by conjunctival inoculation of *L. monocytogenes.* There is a purulent conjunctivitis, which may lead to corneal ulceration. Regional-node involvement usually limits the spread from the eye. However, listerial meningitis has been reported as a complication of oculoglandular listeriosis.

Other rare syndromes caused by *L. monocytogenes* include general illness with bacteremia and high fever, endocarditis, polyserositis, and cutaneous infection.

LABORATORY FINDINGS Although *L. monocytogenes* bacilli grow well on the usual culture media, etiologic diagnosis by isolation and identification may be hampered by failure of differentiation from *Corynebacterium* spp. *Erysipelothrix rhusiopathiae*, and *Streptococcus* spp. Recognition of listerial colonies in a mixed culture, as may result with vaginal or cervical specimens, is difficult and may be aided by using selective media and/or enrichment procedures.

Serodiagnosis by assay for agglutinins has not been useful because of the common finding of so-called "natural antibodies." Such nonspecific reactions may reflect the known antigenic relationship between *Staphylococcus aureus* and several listerial serotypes. The humoral antibody response to listeriosis in humans is almost exclusively IgM throughout the disease, whereas staphylococci elicit IgG as well as IgM; i.e., treatment of serums with 2-mercaptoethanol may not eliminate nonspecific reactivity.

Monocytosis is not common in human listeriosis. Leukocytosis with neutrophilia, as in any acute bacterial infection, is seen in listerial meningitis, oculoglandular infection, bacteremia, and endocarditis. The cerebrospinal fluid in meningitis is compatible with that in other purulent meningitides.

DIFFERENTIAL DIAGNOSIS Abortion, premature delivery, stillbirth, and neonatal death are more often due to causes other than listeriosis: Rh incompatibility, syphilis, or toxoplasmosis.

In patients with leptomeningitis, conjunctivitis, endocarditis, bacteremia, or polyserositis, reports of isolation of "diphtheroids" or "nonpathogens" must always be challenged. A statement that *L. monocytogenes* has been excluded should be required.

TREATMENT *Listeria monocytogenes* are susceptible to several antimicrobals in vitro, including penicillin G, tetracyclines, and erythromycin. Dosage and duration of therapy should vary according to the kind of listerial infection under treatment.

In fetal listeriosis, therapy must be rapidly effective and should be bactericidal. Penicillin G [100 to 150 mg (160,000 to 240,000 units) per kilogram of body weight per day given intravenously in six equal portions, one every 4 h] along with either gentamicin (4 to 5 mg/kg per day given intravenously in four equal portions, one every 6 h) or erythromycin (25 to 30 mg/kg per day given intravenously in four equal portions, one every 6 h) should be given.

Listerial meningitis will usually respond to treatment with penicillin G in a dose of 150 mg (240,000 units) per kilogram of body weight per day, given intravenously in six equal portions, one every 4 h. Cephalothin is not an acceptable alternative. Erythromycin as the gluceptate or lactobionate can be given in a dose of 60 to 75 mg/kg per day in four equal portions given intravenously, one every 6 h. Tetracycline is effective—15 mg/kg per day in four equal portions given intravenously, one every 6 h. Treatment should be continued in full dosage by intravenous injection for 7 days after defervescence.

Listeriosis in the pregnant female and oculoglandular listeriosis can be treated with a 2-week course of erythromycin (25 to 30 mg/kg per day given as four equal portions, one every 6 h by mouth).

Endocarditis and bacteremia from an unknown site require vigorous therapy: penicillin G 150 mg (240,000 units) per kilogram of body weight per day by continuous intravenous injection. The addition of erythromycin or gentamicin (doses as given for meningitis) should be evaluated by assay of serum bactericidal activity against the patient's isolate.

PROGNOSIS Prompt, vigorous antimicrobial treatment of the acute forms of listeriosis, excepting fetal listeriosis, is usually curative. On the basis of agglutinin titers, specific antibody disappears during the months following cure. However, reinfection has not been reported.

ERYSIPELOTHRIX RHUSIOPATHIAE INFECTIONS

DEFINITION Erysipeloid is the commonest and most nearly unique form of infection in humans caused by *Erysipelothrix rhusiopathiae*. Infective endocarditis and arthritis are rare forms of erysipelothricosis in human beings.

ETIOLOGY As gram-positive, microaerophilic bacilli, *E. rhusiopathiae* may be confused with nontoxinogenic *Corynebacterium* spp. and *Listeria monocytogenes*. However, *E. rhusiopathiae* is nonmotile and fails to grow on media selective for *Corynebacterium* spp. Also, unlike *L. monocytogenes*, *E. rhusiopathiae* only rarely causes conjunctivitis, following conjunctival inoculation, or monocytosis, after intravenous inoculation, in the rabbit. Because alpha hemolysis is commonly evident after 48 h of incubation of *E. rhusiopathiae*, confusion with streptococci may also occur. Isolates of *E. rhusiopathiae* appear to be serologically homogeneous. Although serodifferentiation from other gram-positive bacilli is possible, few laboratories are capable of definitive serodiagnosis.

EPIDEMIOLOGY AND PATHOGENESIS Primarily a saprophyte, *E. rhusiopathiae* is worldwide in distribution. Human beings are virtually always infected by traumatic dermal inoculation; erysipeloid is the usual result. The disease is almost wholly restricted to persons who in their occupations handle edible or nonedible dead animal products. If the bacilli are not successfully confined to the skin, bacteremia may result and may lead to infective endocarditis; in about half the reported cases, there was no evidence of preexisting valvular heart disease.

The seasonal incidence of erysipeloid parallels that of swine erysipelas, being highest in summer and early fall. Yet persons who tend pigs, even pigs ill with porcine erysipelas, do not commonly develop erysipeloid.

MANIFESTATIONS Erysipeloid begins 2 to 7 days after injury, often after the initial lesion has healed. An itching, burning, painful irritation may precede and always accompanies the appearance of the maculopapular, nonvesiculated, sharply defined, raised, purplish red zone surrounding the site of entry. There is local swelling, and when, as is usual, a finger or the hand is involved, nearby joints may become stiff and painful. Centrifugal spread from the site of inoculation is apparent in a day or so. Movement is slow, 1 to 2 cm per 24 h maximally, and more rapid proximally than distally; involvement of the terminal phalanx of a finger is rare, while spread to other fingers and the hand below the wrist is common. With extension, the original center subsides without desquamation or suppuration. There are usually no systemic signs or symptoms; regional lymphangitis and lymphadenitis are rare. Untreated, the disease heals within 3 weeks in most patients, although relapse has been observed.

The manifestations of erysipelothrical endocarditis may be either acute or chronic, depending on the virulence of the infecting strain and on the state of resistance of the host. Usually, there are no classic erysipeloid skin lesions to suggest the disease at the time that endocarditis is clinically evident. However, a history of recent erysipeloid may be helpful.

Erysipelothrical arthritis is not clinically characteristic but usually can be related to erysipeloid or erysipelothrical bacteremia. Isolation of *E. rhusiopathiae* from synovial fluid has not been reported.

LABORATORY FINDINGS The usual culture media are adequate for the growth of *E. rhusiopathiae.* However, differentiation from diphtheroids, listerias, and streptococci depends primarily on the clinician's alerting the laboratory to the possibility of erysipelothricosis.

In erysipeloid, *E. rhusiopathiae* are best recovered by incubating, in broth containing glucose, a full-thickness biopsy of skin removed from the advancing edge of a lesion. Culture of an aspirate obtained after injection of sterile, bacteriostat-free 0.9% NaCl solution into the periphery of a lesion is less likely to yield *E. rhusiopathiae.*

With endocarditis and arthritis, the findings are in keeping with the respective clinical syndromes and are in no way characteristic for *E. rhusiopathiae.*

DIFFERENTIAL DIAGNOSIS The appearance and location of erysipeloid, its slow and limited spread, the lack of constitutional reaction, the history of occupation and injury, all serve to identify this disease. The afflicted skin in *erysipelas* is very erythematous, and the face and scalp are affected; there are regional lymphangitis and lymphadenitis, leukocytosis, fever, and malaise. Eczematous lesions may itch, but they display vesicles and little abnormal color. The various erythemas have a different location and do not usually itch or burn; they are more apt to be chronic and nonmigratory.

TREATMENT The penicillins, the cephalosporins, erythromycin, clindamycin, the tetracyclines, and chloramphenicol inhibit *E. rhusiopathiae* in vitro at concentrations practical in therapy. Penicillin G is the agent of choice. Erysipeloid is adequately treated by injection of 1.2 million units of benzathine penicillin G. Erythromycin (15 mg/kg per day in four equal portions taken orally for 5 to 7 days) is an alternative. Cure of erysipelothrical endocarditis has been effected by the daily injection of 2 to 20 million units of penicillin per day for 4 to 6 weeks; the dose should be monitored by determination of the bactericidal activity of serum from the patient against his infecting strain. Intractable cardiac failure may oblige surgical excision of an infected valve and insertion of a prosthesis.

PROGNOSIS Penicillin therapy is highly effective in curing erysipelothrical infections. As with infective endocarditis from any cause, the prognosis is primarily a function of the severity of the valvular damage. Of reported cases, approximately half have been fatal; earlier diagnosis, and, perhaps, earlier resort to surgical excision and replacement of infected valves, may improve the outcome.

REFERENCES

BOISEN-MOLLER J: Human listeriosis. Diagnostic, epidemiological and clinical studies. Acta Pathol Microbiol Scand B 229:13, 1972

HOEPRICH PD: Listeriosis, in *Infectious Diseases,* 2d ed, PD Hoeprich (ed). New York, Harper & Row, 1977, chap 48

————: Erysipeloid, in *Infectious Diseases,* 2d ed, PD Hoeprich (ed). New York, Harper & Row, 1977, chap 99

MOORE RM, ZEHMER RB: Listeriosis in the United States—1971. J Infect Dis 127:610, 1973

NELSON E: Five hundred cases of erysipeloid. Rocky Mt Med J 52:40, 1955

SEELIGER HPR: *Listeriosis.* Basel, Karger, 1961

WIGGINS GL et al: Antibiotic susceptibility of clinical isolates *Listeria monocytogenes.* Antimicrob Agents Chemother 13:854, 1978

133

DIPHTHERIA

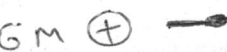 GM ⊕ —

JAMES P. HARNISCH

DEFINITION Diphtheria is an acute infectious disease produced by *Corynebacterium diphtheriae.* It is characterized by a local inflammatory lesion, usually in the upper part of the respiratory tract, and by remote effects resulting from toxin, which affects particularly the heart and peripheral nerves.

ETIOLOGY *Corynebacterium diphtheriae* is a gram-positive, nonsporulating, nonmotile rod. There is a characteristic swelling at one end of the bacillus, which gives it a club shape. A Chinese letter configuration is usually seen in stained smears owing to the alignment of the bacilli at sharp angles with each other. Diphtheria bacilli have been classified into *mitis, gravis,* and *intermedius* groups on the basis of colonial morphology, appearance on tellurite medium, fermentation reactions, and ability to produce hemolysis. European workers have suggested that there is a significant difference in the clinical manifestations and in the severity of disease related to the strain; gravis and intermedius infections are thought to be accompanied by more severe toxic manifestations and a higher death rate. In the United States, the gravis strain is comparatively uncommon, and less significance is attached to the relationship of the type of organism and the clinical form of the disease.

Corynebacterium diphtheriae produces a protein exotoxin which is responsible for many of the clinical manifestations; as little as 0.0001 mg is lethal for guinea pigs. Strains of diphtheria bacilli which elaborate exotoxin are lysogenic. Absence of lysogeny generally is associated with lack of toxin formation and virulence. However, symptomatic diphtheria may also follow invasion by strains of *C. diphtheriae* that cannot be shown to produce toxin.

EPIDEMIOLOGY Diphtheria occurs primarily in the Temperate Zone and is still very common in some parts of the world. Since 1966, there has been an irregular increase in the number of cases of diphtheria in the United States. Two outbreaks in Texas early in this decade accounted for most of the cases. However, since 1973, more than 75 percent of the cases were reported from the Pacific Northwest and the Southwest. The western provinces of Canada experienced a similar increase in diphtheria. Until this geographic trend was recognized, the highest frequency had been in children between 1 and 9 years of age. The attack rate for unimmunized children was 70 times higher than the rate for children who had received primary immunization. In the Pacific Northwest, 77 percent of isolates have been obtained from adults with symptomatic skin lesions. Another striking change has been a decrease in the incidence of laryngeal involvement. In general, diphtheria is acquired by droplet transmission from active cases or carriers, but fomites may play a role in the spread of cutaneous infection. Each diphtheria infection must be classified as either a case or a carrier. A *case* is an individual who is colonized in the respiratory tract with *C. diphtheriae* and is symptomatic. The concomitant presence of other organisms, such as beta-hemolytic streptococci, does not change the definition or prognosis of a diphtheria case. A *carrier* is colonized with *C. diphtheriae* but lacks symptoms. No attempt should be made to classify an instance of cutaneous diphtheria as a case or a carrier.

PATHOGENESIS AND PATHOLOGY The commonest portal of entry for the diphtheria bacillus is the upper respiratory tract. The skin, genitalia, eye, and middle ear may also be sites of invasion. Growth of the organism is superficial in most cases, and there is little tendency to invade the lymphatics or bloodstream except in the terminal stages. The exotoxin elaborated in the local lesion is absorbed and carried by the blood to all parts of the body. The intensity of the toxic effects is greatest when the primary lesion is in the pharynx, less when it is in the larynx, and least when it is on the nasal mucosa or skin. Simultaneous involvement of the pharynx, larynx, trachea, and bronchial tree is associated with most severe intoxication.

The *membrane,* the primary lesion of diphtheria, is thick, leathery, and blue-white and is composed of bacteria, necrotic epithelium, phagocytes, and fibrin. It is surrounded by a narrow zone of inflammation and is firmly adherent to the underlying tissues; bleeding follows its forcible removal. Ulceration is not a regular feature. Regional lymphadenitis is frequent.

The *toxic manifestations* involve primarily the heart, kidneys, and peripheral nerves. The brain is rarely affected. Cardiac enlargement is frequent; this appears to be related to myocarditis rather than hypertrophy. The kidneys may be enlarged and reveal cloudy swelling and interstitial changes. Bronchopneumonia due to *C. diphtheriae* or to secondary invading organisms occurs in some patients, especially those with laryngeal involvement. Membrane is present throughout the bronchial tree when the diphtheria bacillus is responsible for the pulmonary infection. The peripheral nerves may reveal fatty degeneration, disintegration of the medullary sheaths, and involvement of the axis cylinder. Both motor and sensory fibers are affected, but the main impact is on motor innervation. The anterior horn cells and the posterior columns of the spinal cord may be damaged. Other central nervous system involvement includes cerebral hemorrhage, meningitis, and encephalitis. Petechial and purpuric lesions are occasionally present in the kidneys, skin, or adrenals. Endocarditis due to *C. diphtheriae* is rare.

Death results from respiratory obstruction by membrane or edema, or from the effects of toxin on the heart, nervous system, or other organs.

IMMUNITY Susceptibility to the complications of diphtheria is related to the presence or absence of circulating antibody to exotoxin. The Schick test yields a rough estimate of the quantity of antitoxin in the circulation. This test is carried out in the following manner: 0.1 ml purified diphtheria toxin (one-fiftieth the minimum lethal dose) dissolved in buffered human serum albumin is injected intradermally on the volar surface of the forearm; 0.1 ml purified diphtheria toxoid is injected into the other arm as a control. These areas are examined at 24 and 48 h and between the fourth and seventh days and interpreted in the following way:

1 *Positive reaction:* The site of injection of toxin begins to redden in 24 h; the reddening increases and reaches a maximum in about a week, at which time the lesion may be as large as 3 cm in diameter and moderately swollen and tender. There is usually a small (1 to 1.5 cm) dark red central zone which gradually turns brown, desquamates, and leaves a pigmented area. The area of toxoid injection shows no reaction. A positive test indicates little or no circulating antitoxin and no immunity.
2 *Negative reaction:* There is no reaction at the site of injection of either toxoid or toxin. This is consistent with a blood antitoxin level of 1/30 to 1/100 unit and immunity to ordinary exposure.
3 *Pseudoreaction:* Inflammation at both sites of injection within 12 to 14 h, which reaches a maximum in 48 to 72 h and then fades. This usually indicates immunity plus hypersensitivity to the toxin or other materials in the solution.

4 *Combined reaction:* This begins like the pseudoreaction, but the inflammatory response at the toxin site persists after that in the area of toxoid injection has faded. It indicates delayed sensitivity to toxin or other proteins and either low levels or no antitoxin. The incidence of combined reactions increases with age and is highest in unimmunized groups living in areas where diphtheria is prevalent.

Individuals with negative Schick tests occasionally contract diphtheria, and some persons with positive Schick reactions do not develop the disease after exposure. In some parts of the United States fewer than 50 percent of adults have "protective" levels of circulating antitoxin. The Schick test is not used routinely in the United States, and the lack of ability to perform it should not delay the treatment of asymptomatic contacts of diphtheria.

Second attacks of respiratory diphtheria are rare despite the fact that about 10 percent of patients who have had the disease remain Schick-positive. This suggests that factors other than antitoxin may play a role in protection against infection. In general, immunized patients have a milder illness than unimmunized ones when the initial clinical picture and level of circulating antitoxin are the same. Early therapy of diphtheria with antibiotics may lead to recurrence of the disease if exposure to fresh infections occurs shortly after discontinuation of treatment, suggesting that the development of antitoxic immunity is suppressed in these cases. Full immunization with diphtheria toxoid does not prevent nasopharyngeal carriage of the organism but significantly reduces the case fatality ratio. It also ameliorates the symptoms of active disease.

CLINICAL MANIFESTATIONS The incubation period of diphtheria is 1 to 7 days. The local symptoms vary with the site of the primary lesion. A membrane is not always present. The constitutional reaction usually is of only minor to moderate severity in uncomplicated disease. Fever is usually low [37.8 to 38.3°C (100 to 101°F)], unless infection with another organism (often group A *Streptococcus pyogenes*) supervenes. When toxic manifestations are absent, patients feel well except for a varying degree of discomfort at the site of the local lesion. Pallor, listlessness, tachycardia, and weakness are common in more severe cases. Nausea or vomiting is more frequent in young children. Peripheral vascular collapse often develops in the terminal stages of the disease.

Nasal diphtheria Diphtheria is occasionally restricted to the nasal mucosa. It is usually localized to the septum or turbinates in the anterior portion of one side of the nose, does not extend, and may persist for a long time. A foreign body is frequently present. A unilateral serosanguineous discharge is characteristic. When the disease is located in the posterior nasal areas, it commonly extends to the pharynx, from which toxin is absorbed.

Pharyngeal diphtheria The early diphtheritic membrane in the pharynx consists of small areas of soft exudate which wipe off easily and leave no bleeding points. As the disease progresses, the discrete exudate coalesces to form an easily removable thin sheet which spreads to cover tonsils or pharynx, or both. Later, it becomes thicker, bluish white, gray, or black, depending on the degree of hemorrhage, and is so firmly attached to the underlying tissues that attempts to remove it result in bleeding. If infection with group A *Streptococcus pyogenes* is superimposed, the pharynx is diffusely red and edematous. Sore throat is the most common complaint. Pain on swallowing may occur in over 25 percent of the cases and in some patients may be severe. There is a moderate leukocytosis with 15,000 or fewer white blood cells per cubic millimeter.

Local spread of the pharyngeal membrane may occur, and the throat, tonsils, and soft and hard palates become completely covered. Patients with severe disease may develop so-called "malignant" diphtheria, characterized by marked edema of the submandibular areas and the anterior neck, giving the characteristic "bullneck" appearance. Respiration is noisy, the tongue protrudes, the breath is foul, and the speech thick. The pharyngeal tissues are red and edematous, and the cervical lymph nodes are enlarged. The skin is pale and cool. The patient complains of overwhelming weakness. Purpuric eruptions of the skin, particularly on the neck and anterior chest wall, may appear occasionally. Drowsiness and delirium are common.

Laryngeal diphtheria Involvement of the larynx is usually the result of extension of the diphtheritic membrane from the pharynx. The infection may rarely be limited to the larynx or trachea. This possibility must be considered in the differential diagnosis of all cases of "croup"; it can be ruled out only by direct examination of the airway. The clinical features of this type of disease are described below.

Cutaneous diphtheria Until recently, diphtheria of the skin was a problem primarily in tropical areas where it is responsible for some cases of "jungle sore." However, since 1972, there has been a significant increase in skin diphtheria in the Pacific Northwest and the Southwest. A high attack rate has occurred in native Americans and in indigent males living in "skid row" areas where crowding and poor personal and community hygiene abound. *Corynebacterium diphtheriae,* being unable to penetrate unbroken skin, invades wounds, burns, or abrasions. Any break in the skin may be colonized with *C. diphtheriae.* Coagulase-positive *Staphylococcus aureus* and/or beta-hemolytic streptococci frequently are recovered concomitantly. Although the lesions develop most often on the extremities, they may appear at any site including the perianal area. In tropical zones, the typical lesion appears as a round, deep "punched-out" ulcer, 0.5 cm to several centimeters in diameter. In the early stages, it is covered by a gray-yellow or gray-brown membrane which strips off easily to reveal a clean hemorrhagic base that dries quickly and becomes covered by a thin, leathery, dark-brown or black, adherent membrane. In the untreated case, this separates spontaneously 1 to 3 weeks after infection. The margin of the fully developed ulcer is usually slightly undermined, purple, rolled, and sharply defined. When lesions are infected with a toxigenic strain, anesthesia over the lesion develops within a few weeks. In temperate climates, the lesions are not sufficiently specific to permit visual diagnosis. Cutaneous diphtheria should be suspected in any adult with skin lesions, particularly in the proper epidemiologic setting. Antibiotic therapy will change the character of the skin lesions. Twenty percent of patients with cutaneous diphtheria also have infections in the nasopharynx with the same biotype. Myocarditis or neuropathy occurs in about 3 to 5 percent of patients with cutaneous diphtheria. The Landry-Guillain-Barré syndrome develops occasionally.

Diphtheritic lesions in other areas Diphtheria may involve the uterine cervix, vagina, vulva, bladder, urethra, or penis (after circumcision). Toxic manifestations are common. The tongue, buccal mucous membrane, gums, and esophagus may also be affected. Infection of the conjunctiva occurs rarely. Otitis media may occur as an isolated syndrome or secondary to diphtheria in the upper part of the respiratory tract; the aural infection may become chronic; virulent organisms may be isolated from the discharge for many months.

COMPLICATIONS OF DIPHTHERIA The complications of diphtheria are of two types: (1) those that result from spread of the membrane in the respiratory tract, and (2) those due to the effects of the toxin.

Extension and spread of membrane The membrane of diphtheria may spread from the fauces over the posterior pharyngeal wall into the larynx, trachea, and, uncommonly, the bronchial tree, leading to severe illness and a high incidence of toxic manifestations. Occlusion of the airway is manifested by tachypnea and, as obstruction increases, restlessness, use of accessory muscles of respiration, cyanosis, and finally death. In some cases, the membrane extends diffusely into the bronchial tree and produces clinical manifestations of pneumonia. Hoarseness and a croup-like cough are seen with laryngeal involvement. Bronchopulmonary diphtheria is very serious, not only because of obstruction but also because of the large surface from which toxin can be absorbed; the death rate is very high. When the pulmonary lesion regresses, pieces of membrane may break off and produce sudden occlusion of the airway; a cast of the bronchial tree may be coughed up. Occasionally, pharyngeal membrane has extended into the esophagus and cardia of the stomach.

Toxic complications of diphtheria Diphtheria toxin is produced only by isolates of *C. diphtheriae* lysogenic for corynephages that carry the tox structural gene. Nontoxigenic strains can be converted to toxin-producing organisms through transference of this phage. The bacterial host regulates expression of the tox structural gene. The toxin is a single polypeptide chain composed of two fragments. Fragment B recognizes specific surface receptors on sensitive cell membranes, and fragment A crosses the plasma membrane. In the cytoplasm, protein synthesis is inhibited by fragment A through the inactivation of the eukaryotic translocating enzyme, elongation factor 2. A cofactor, nicotinamideadenine dinucleotide, is required for activity of the toxin. The effects of the toxin on the myocardium are thought to result from its ability to decrease the rate of oxidation of long-chain fatty acids by interfering with the metabolism of carnitine. Because of this action, triglycerides accumulate in the myocardium and cause fatty degeneration of muscle.

Myocarditis develops in about two-thirds of patients with diphtheria. However, it is clinically evident in only about 10 percent of cases; alterations in the intensity of the heart sounds, systolic murmurs, bundle branch block, incomplete or complete heart block, atrial fibrillation, and ventricular premature beats or tachycardia, or both, are common. Ventricular fibrillation is a constant threat and is frequently responsible for sudden death. Ninety percent of patients with atrial fibrillation, ventricular tachycardia, or complete heart block die. Overt congestive cardiac failure is uncommon. Evidence of decompensation of the right side of the heart usually develops first; the most common symptom is pain in the right upper quadrant of the abdomen due to rapid engorgement of the liver. Failure of the left side of the heart may appear later. Diphtheritic heart disease is not necessarily "benign" in survivors of the disease; permanent cardiac damage may occur. Fibrosis of the myocardium has been observed in patients who have expired several weeks after "mild" myocarditis was detected electrocardiographically. The degree and extent of fibrotic change have often been greater than could have been predicted on the basis of the type of abnormality present in the ECG.

Peripheral neuritis may occur in the course of diphtheria. Paralysis of the soft palate and posterior pharyngeal wall occasionally appears very early in the disease (2 to 3 days). A more common neuritis (10 percent of cases) usually develops 2 to 6 weeks after onset of the disease. It is characterized by cranial nerve dysfunction; the third, sixth, seventh, ninth, and tenth nerves are most commonly involved. Loss of accommodation, nasal voice, and difficulty in swallowing are the most frequent manifestations. However, any of the peripheral nerves may be affected, with resulting paralysis of the extremities, diaphragm, or intercostal muscles; death may occur from failure of respiration. The peripheral neuritides which appear in the second to the sixth week of the disease are characterized primarily by motor loss; sensory changes are uncommon and, when present, are minor. Peripheral neuritis may not appear until 2 to 3 months after the onset of diphtheria. In these cases, the clinical picture and course resemble infectious polyneuritis. The outstanding findings are loss of sensation in the "glove-and-stocking" distribution and albuminocytological dissociation in the cerebrospinal fluid identical with that observed in the Landry-Guillain-Barré syndrome. Motor weakness and areflexia may develop with progression of involvement. Facial diplegia may accompany the other neurological manifestations. A fatal, rapidly ascending paralysis of the Landry type may develop rarely. Complete recovery is the rule in this late peripheral neuritis, although it may require as long as a year. Encephalitis is a rare toxic complication of diphtheria.

Shock, which develops suddenly and without warning, is an occasional cause of sudden death in this disease. In some instances, this may be a consequence of myocarditis; in others, no cause can be discovered.

Other complications Cerebral infarction with hemiplegia occurs rarely; it is probably due to embolization from atrial thrombi in patients with myocarditis and cardiac dilatation. Superinfection of the lungs is a risk in all patients with diphtheria who are given antimicrobial agents. Purpuric skin eruptions may be seen in severe, malignant cases; thrombocytopenia occurs rarely. A mild morbilliform rash may be present during the early stage of diphtheria. Secondary invasion of the pharynx by group A *S. pyogenes* may take place in patients who have not received an antibiotic. Serum sickness occasionally follows the use of antitoxin. Relapses of diphtheria may occur when patients given antimicrobial agents are exposed to fresh cases soon after therapy has been discontinued. Bacteremia, endocarditis, and meningitis are rare complications.

COURSE AND PROGNOSIS The diphtheritic membrane may be present for only 3 to 4 days in mild cases, even when no antitoxin is given; it usually lasts for about a week in cases of moderate severity. Commonly, the pharyngeal lesion increases in extent and thickness during the first 24 h after the administration of antitoxin. As the disease begins to recede, the exudate softens, wipes off easily, leaving no bleeding areas, becomes patchy so that it resembles the picture of "follicular" tonsillitis, and finally disappears, leaving normal underlying mucous membrane.

The fatality rate of diphtheria prior to the use of specific antitoxin was about 35 percent in average cases and 90 percent in those with laryngeal involvement. Since specific serotherapy has been employed, this rate has been reduced to a range of 3.5 to 22 percent, but it is still highest when the larynx is affected. The overall death rate in the United States is about 10 percent. Death is most frequent in the very young and the old. Immunization is a factor of great importance in prognosis. The fatality rate in immunized individuals is one-tenth that in the unimmunized population. Paralysis is five times and "malignant" disease 15 times less common in immune than in nonimmune

individuals. As a rule, the longer the delay in the administration of antitoxin, the greater the incidence of complications and death. However, antitoxin is ineffective in reducing risks of complications and death if it is given much later than 48 h after diphtheria begins.

A white blood cell count higher than 25,000 per cubic millimeter is associated with a higher risk of complications and death.

DIAGNOSIS The clinical features of the fully developed diphtheritic membrane, especially in the pharynx, are sufficiently characteristic to suggest the possibility of the disease in most instances. However, the appearance of the pharyngeal exudate alone does not clinch the diagnosis. There are a number of other infections in which pseudomembranes resembling those of diphtheria are present; among those are infectious mononucleosis, streptococcal pharyngitis, viral exudative pharyngitis, fusospirochetal infection, and acute pharyngeal candidiasis.

The specific diagnosis of diphtheria depends completely on demonstration of the organism in stained smears and their recovery by culture. Methylene blue–stained preparations are positive, in experienced hands, in 75 to 85 percent of cases. Diphtheria bacilli can be recovered by culture on Loeffler's medium in 8 to 12 h if patients have not been receiving antimicrobial agents. *Corynebacterium diphtheriae* also multiplies, but more slowly, on ordinary blood agar. If an antibiotic, especially penicillin or erythromycin, has been administered prior to obtaining cultures, the organisms may not grow for as long as 5 days or may fail to grow at all.

Staining of suspected material with fluorescein-labeled diphtheria antitoxin may allow rapid diagnosis. Toxigenicity of *C. diphtheriae* isolates should be determined by passive agar diffusion (Elek plate method), guinea pig inoculation, or counterimmunoelectrophoresis.

TREATMENT Patients with diphtheria should be isolated and kept at strict bed rest; physical effort should be reduced during the early convalescent stages. Local therapy of the diphtheritic pharyngeal lesion is useless. The only specific treatment for diphtheria is antitoxin. Antiserum must never be given until the patient's sensitivity to horse serum, using the eye and skin tests, has been determined. There are several regimens for the administration of antitoxin, and the amount given is often based on an empiric decision. In general, the more severe the disease or the more extensive the membrane formation, the greater is the amount of antitoxin required. Mildly symptomatic cases may be treated with 10,000 to 20,000 units. Moderately severe cases, such as those with a pharyngeal membrane, should be given 20,000 to 40,000 units. Severe diphtheria, as with laryngeal involvement, requires 50,000 to 100,000 units. The total dose should be given at one time rather than in split doses over a long period. For doses less than 20,000 units, the intramuscular route is convenient. When this method is used, only one-half the dose should be given intramuscularly and the remainder intravenously in order to expedite delivery of the antitoxin. Alternatively, after appropriate testing for sensitivity, the entire amount of antitoxin may be given intravenously in 100 to 200 ml isotonic saline over a 30-min period. Desensitization should be attempted if the initial skin or eye test is positive. A rare patient may be sensitive to such a high degree that the antiserum cannot be administered without the risk of death.

Antitoxin should be given as early in the course of diphtheria as possible. It is capable of binding or inactivating only the toxin present in blood or extracellular fluid. Once the toxin has entered the cell, the effect cannot be reversed or prevented. Antitoxin must be given when diphtheria is suspected clinically; laboratory confirmation prior to administration of the antitoxin is not necessary. Since mortality increases directly with delay in use of antitoxin, it is better to treat clinically suspect but culture-negative cases than to withhold specific therapy.

The history of military service is not reliable proof of adequate immunization. From World War II until 1956, immunization for diphtheria in the United States military was inconsistent. Since 1957, all branches of the Armed Forces have routinely immunized their personnel. When the immunization history is not clear, it is best to provide antitoxin promptly. Antimicrobial agents do not alter the course, incidence of complications, or outcome of diphtheria.

Patients with laryngeal obstruction should be watched very carefully. In mild cases, inhalation of warm or cool steam may be beneficial. If advancing signs of airway obstruction develop, intubation or tracheostomy is indicated. These procedures must never be delayed until cyanosis appears, because, at this point, stimulation of the pharynx or trachea may produce cardiac standstill and death. Sedative or hypnotic agents should never be given because they may obscure increasing respiratory difficulty.

The pulse and blood pressure should be measured frequently. Little can be done to alter the course of the myocarditis. Quinidine has been tried to prevent and treat arrhythmias but appears to be of no value; there is some suspicion that it may produce deleterious effects. The use of procainamide when ventricular premature beats or tachycardia supervene has been suggested, but no documented observations of its effect have been recorded. The administration of digitalis for cardiac failure in diphtheria is controversial. Some consider this drug to be completely contraindicated; others feel, however, that, used carefully, digitalis may be given safely and with beneficial effects. Shock should be treated according to its etiology (Chaps. 30 and 109). There is no evidence that corticosteroids or corticotropin are of any value in the treatment of diphtheria or any of its complications. Antibiotics should be used to treat symptomatic cases only after antitoxin is administered. Circulating exotoxin is not affected by antibiotics, and their prompt use may give false assurance to the clinician. Patients with diphtheria should be quarantined until two successive cultures of the nose, throat, or other infected areas, taken at 24-h intervals, are negative. If antibiotics have been given, cultural studies should not be initiated until at least 24 h after cessation of therapy.

Treatment of carriers *Corynebacterium diphtheriae* usually disappears from the upper part of the respiratory tract after 2 to 4 weeks in patients who do not receive antimicrobial drugs; in a small number of individuals the organism may persist for a long time or be present permanently. The most effective treatment of the acute and chronic carrier state is erythromycin. A dose of 2 g per day orally in divided doses for 7 days appears to be adequate. Alternative antimicrobials include procaine penicillin G, 600,000 units intramuscularly every 12 h for 10 days; clindamycin, 150 mg four times a day orally for 7 days; and rifampin, 600 mg as a single oral dose for 7 days. Tetracyclines, semisynthetic penicillins, aminoglycosides, and oral cephalosporins are inadequate for the eradication of *C. diphtheriae*. Parenteral cephalosporins such as cephalothin or cephamandole are effective. In some areas of the United States endemic for cutaneous diphtheria, resistance of *C. diphtheriae* to erythromycin has been recognized. Retreatment is indicated for carriers whose organisms do not disappear on the first trial. This is preferable to tonsillectomy, which may be considered as a last resort should the carrier state persist despite repeated courses of antibiotic. Persistence of the organism after appropriate antimicrobial therapy may represent a lack of compliance rather than drug resistance.

PREVENTION Diphtheria is, for the most part, a preventable disease. Immunization at the age of 3 months should be routine. Diphtheria toxoid is best given together with tetanus toxoid and pertussis vaccine (DPT), because antibody titers are higher with combined immunization than with either agent alone. Booster doses should be administered at the age of 1 year and again just before a child goes to school. Although it has been suggested that Schick testing is not necessary in those who have been immunized, many physicians still carry this out to determine the status of antitoxic immunity. A Schick test acts as a booster. A negative reaction does not indicate absolute protection. The development of highly purified toxoid has made it possible to protect adults with little or no risk of untoward sequelae. In this situation, a combination of adult tetanus-diphtheria (Td) toxoid containing 1 to 2 flocculation (Lf) units per milliliter should be used. With this preparation, severe reactions can be avoided. The Moloney test need not be carried out. Adults should receive booster doses at least every 10 years.

Treatment of unimmunized persons exposed to an active case of diphtheria remains controversial. One approach has been to administer 3000 units of antitoxin intramuscularly, after appropriate skin and eye tests. Alternatively, cultures for *C. diphtheriae* can be taken, and a primary series of immunizations initiated. The exposed individual then can be observed closely for signs of active disease. If symptoms occur, antitoxin can be given immediately. In those who have been previously immunized, a booster dose of toxoid is usually sufficient. Cultures from the nasopharynx or open wounds should be obtained from close contacts or family members of a diphtheria case or carrier.

REFERENCES

BELSEY MA, LeBLANC DR: Skin infections and the epidemiology of diphtheria: Acquisition and persistence of *C. diphtheriae* infections. Am J Epidemiol 102:179, 1975

BROOKS GR et al: Diphtheria in the United States 1959–1970. J Infect Dis 129:172, 1974

GOOD I: Myocardial changes in fatal diphtheria: A summary of observations in 221 cases. Am J Med Sci 219:257, 1948

GOOR RS, PAPPENHEIMER AM JR: Studies on the mode of action of diphtheria toxin. J Exp Med 126:899, 913, 923, 1967

IPSEN J: Circulating antitoxin at the onset of diphtheria in 425 patients. J Immunol 54:325, 1946

———: Immunization of adults against diphtheria and tetanus. N Engl J Med 251:459, 1954

LIVINGOOD CS et al: Cutaneous diphtheria: A report of 140 cases. J Invest Dermatol 7:341, 1946

McCLOSKEY RV et al: The 1970 epidemic of diphtheria in San Antonio. Ann Intern Med 75:495, 1971

NAIDITCH MJ, BOWER AG: Diphtheria: A study of 1,433 cases observed during a ten-year period at the Los Angeles County Hospital. Am J Med 17:229, 1954

PAPPENHEIMER AM JR: Diphtheria toxin. Annu Rev Biochem 46:69, 1977

SCHEID W: Diphtherial paralysis: An analysis of 2,292 cases of diphtheria in adults which include 174 cases of polyneuritis. J Nerv Ment Dis 116:1095, 1952

THOMPSON NL, ELLNER PD: Rapid determination of *Corynebacterium diphtheriae* toxigenicity by counterimmunoelectrophoresis. J Clin Microbiol 7:493, 1978

WITTELS B, BRESSLER R: Biochemical lesion of diphtheria toxin on the heart. J Clin Invest 43:630, 1964

134

CHOLERA AND *VIBRIO PARAHEMOLYTICUS* INFECTIONS

CHARLES C. J. CARPENTER

CHOLERA

DEFINITION Cholera is an acute illness which results from colonization of the small intestine by *Vibrio cholerae*. The disease is characterized by its epidemic occurrence and the production in the more severe cases of massive diarrhea with rapid depletion of extracellular fluid and electrolytes.

ETIOLOGY AND EPIDEMIOLOGY *Vibrio cholerae* is a curved, aerobic, gram-negative bacillus with a single polar flagellum. It is rapidly motile and possesses both O and H antigens. Serologic identification is based on differences in the polysaccharide O antigens.

Cholera has been endemic for a century and a half in the Gangetic Delta of West Bengal and Bangladesh and is often epidemic throughout South and Southeast Asia. The seventh and most recent pandemic spread of this disease, from 1961 to 1975, extended from the Celebes northward to Korea and westward to the whole of Africa and Southern Europe. The last major epidemic of cholera in the Western Hemisphere occurred during 1866 to 1867. However, in August and September 1978, at least 11 persons developed cholera, serotype Inaba, after ingestion of inadequately cooked crabs caught in lakes or coastal waters of Louisiana.

The majority of major epidemics have clearly been waterborne, but direct contamination of food by infected feces probably contributes to spread during major outbreaks. Poor sanitation appears to be primarily responsible for the continuing presence of cholera, but host factors, such as relative or absolute achlorhydria, also play an important role in the susceptibility of the individual to infection. In endemic areas, cholera is predominantly a disease of children; in rural Bangladesh attack rates are 10 times greater in the 1- to 5-year-old age group than in those above 14 years of age. However, when the disease spreads to previously uninvolved areas, the attack rates are initially at least as high in adults as in children.

A chronic gallbladder carrier state has been observed in a small percentage of elderly convalescent cholera patients. These chronic *V. cholerae* carriers may provide a vehicle for spread outside of endemic areas. The basis for the annual cholera epidemics throughout the Gangetic Delta, for the periodic outbreaks throughout the remainder of South and Southeast Asia, and for the occasional global pandemics has, however, not been clearly delineated.

PATHOGENESIS *Vibrio cholerae* produces a protein enterotoxin which appears to be responsible for all known pathophysiologic aberrations in cholera. This enterotoxin, which has a molecular weight of 84,000, stimulates adenyl cyclase in the intestine epithelial cells, and the resultant increase in intracellular cyclic adenosine 3′,5′-monophosphate leads to secretion of isotonic fluid by all segments of the small intestine. The enterotoxin-induced electrolyte secretion occurs in the absence of any demonstrable histologic damage to intestine epithelial cells or to the capillary endothelial cells of the lamina propria. Precise studies have demonstrated that the stool of the adult cholera patient is nearly isotonic, with sodium and chloride concentrations slightly less than those of plasma, a bicarbonate concentration approximately twice that of plasma, and a potassium concentration three to five times that of plasma. Disease caused by all known strains of *V. cholerae* results in the same stool electrolyte pattern. The pathophysiologic defect in cholera is extracellular fluid depletion with resultant hypovolemic shock, base-deficit acidosis, and progressive potassium depletion. There is no evidence that the cholera *Vibrio* invades any tissue, nor has the enterotoxin been shown, in human disease, to have any direct effect on any organ other than the small intestine.

MANIFESTATIONS The incubation period is generally from 6 to 48 h. This is followed by the abrupt onset of watery, generally painless diarrhea. In the more severe cases, the initial diarrheal stool may be in excess of 1000 ml, and several liters of isotonic fluid may be lost within hours, leading rapidly to profound shock. Vomiting generally follows, but occasionally precedes, the onset of diarrhea; the vomiting is characteristically effortless and not preceded by nausea. As saline depletion progresses, severe muscle cramps, commonly involving the calves, occur.

When first seen, the typical severely ill cholera patient is cyanotic, with pinched facies, scaphoid abdomen, poor skin turgor, and thready or absent peripheral pulses. The voice is faint, high-pitched, and often inaudible, and there are tachycardia, hypotension, and varying degrees of tachypnea. In all epidemics there are many subclinical or mild cases in which gastrointestinal fluid loss is not severe enough to require hospitalization. With the *el tor* strain of *V. cholerae,* which has been responsible for the most recent pandemic, the ratio of subclinical infections to clinical cholera cases is greater than 10:1.

The disease runs its course in 2 to 7 days, and subsequent manifestations depend on the adequacy of electrolyte repletion therapy. With prompt fluid and electrolyte repletion, physiologic recovery is remarkably rapid, and mortality exceptionally rare. The important causes of death, in inadequately treated patients, are hypovolemic shock, metabolic acidosis, and uremia resulting from acute tubular necrosis.

LABORATORY FINDINGS In epidemics or in endemic areas, the clinical picture should arouse strong suspicion immediately. The most reliable technique for identification of *V. cholerae* consists of direct plating of a sample of cholera stool on bile salt, gelatin-tellurite-taurocholate (GTT), or thiosulfate-citrate-bile salt-sucrose (TCBS) agar. On bile salt or GTT agar the organisms appear as typical translucent colonies within 24 h. On TCBS agar, *V. cholerae* appear at 24 h as distinct, large, yellow colonies. Further classification requires agglutination with type-specific antiserums. In mild or convalescent cases, recovery of vibrios may be enhanced by initial enrichment for 6 h in alkaline peptone water followed by subculture on bile salt, GTT, or TCBS agar. Rapid diagnosis is possible either by directly observing immobilization of vibrios by type-specific antiserums, using dark-field or phase microscopy, or identifying the organisms by immunofluorescent methods.

TREATMENT Successful therapy requires only prompt and adequate replacement of gastrointestinal losses of saline and alkali. A uniformly satisfactory solution for intravenous fluid therapy can be simply prepared by the addition of 5 g sodium chloride, 4 g sodium bicarbonate, and 1 g potassium chloride to 1 liter of pyrogen-free distilled water. If commercially prepared fluids are available, a combination of isotonic sodium bicarbonate (or acetate or lactate) and isotonic sodium chloride, infused in a 2:1 ratio, may be employed. The intravenous fluids are initially infused at 50 to 100 ml/min, until a strong pulse has been restored. The same fluids should subsequently be infused in quantities equal to the gastrointestinal losses. If losses cannot be measured accurately, intravenous fluids should be given at a rate sufficient to maintain a normal radial pulse and normal skin turgor. Overhydration can be avoided by careful observation of neck venous filling and auscultation of the lungs. Close observation is mandatory during the acute phase of the illness, because the cholera patient can lose as much as 1 liter of isotonic fluid per hour during the first 24 h of the disease. Inadequate or delayed restoration of fecal fluid losses may result in a high incidence of acute renal failure. Serious hypokalemic symptoms are rare in adults, and potassium repletion can be carried out orally if potassium-containing intravenous fluids are not available. Hypokalemia contributes significantly, however, to the morbidity in inadequately treated pediatric cholera, and potassium, 10 to 13 meq per liter, should be included in the intravenous fluids administered to pediatric patients.

Although adequate intravenous saline and alkali repletion alone results in rapid recovery of virtually all cholera patients, a dramatic reduction in the duration and volume of the diarrhea and early eradication of vibrios from the stool may be effected by antibiotic therapy. Oral tetracycline, 500 mg every 6 h for the first 48 h of treatment, has been most successful. Other antibiotics, including chloramphenicol and furazolidone, are also of value, but both appear to be slightly less effective than tetracycline.

Oral therapy Since the cholera enterotoxin does not alter glucose-facilitated sodium absorption, fluid repletion can be effected by the oral administration of glucose-containing electrolyte solutions. Since the limiting factor in treatment of cholera in both epidemic and endemic situations is often the lack of adequate quantities of intravenous fluids, the availability of an oral treatment regimen has greatly reduced the mortality from cholera outbreaks during the most recent pandemic spread of this disease. A solution containing glucose 20 g per liter (or sucrose 40 g per liter), sodium bicarbonate 2.5 g per liter, sodium chloride 3.5 g per liter, and potassium chloride 15 g per liter can be readily prepared and should be satisfactory for treatment of all age groups. This solution, administered orally at a rate equal to the stool losses, can be given to patients with milder cholera throughout the course of illness and is satisfactory in the more severe cases, once the hypovolemic shock has been corrected by intravenous fluid therapy. Oral therapy does not decrease the rate of intestinal fluid loss but provides an electrolyte solution which can be absorbed at a rate sufficient, in most cases, to counterbalance the continuing fluid losses. Therefore, successful management of the cholera patient with oral therapy requires just as close supervision, with careful monitoring of pulse volume, skin turgor, and neck veins, as does management with intravenous solutions. Supplemental intravenous fluids must be administered whenever clinical signs of saline depletion recur.

PROGNOSIS Under ideal conditions and with prompt and adequate fluid replacement, mortality approaches zero, and significant sequelae are rare. Unfortunately, death rates as high as 60 percent still occur, especially during the initial phases of certain outbreaks. This high mortality reflects lack of pyrogen-free intravenous fluids in remote areas, the difficulties of initiating treatment promptly when large numbers of cases are occurring in poverty-stricken populations, and the compromises which may have to be made under emergency conditions.

PREVENTION Immunization by standard commercial vaccine, containing 10 billion killed organisms per milliliter, provides only limited (40 to 60 percent) protection for a relatively short (4- to 6-month) period. Vaccination, therefore, is not recommended for Americans who are traveling abroad. Careful hygiene provides the only sure protection against cholera.

VIBRIO PARAHEMOLYTICUS INFECTION

ETIOLOGY AND EPIDEMIOLOGY *Vibrio parahemolyticus* is a curved, aerobic, nonmotile, gram-negative bacillus. Although present in coastal waters throughout the temperate zone, it has most commonly been associated with acute diarrheal illness in Japan, presumably because of the frequency of ingestion of raw seafood. It has been implicated in several outbreaks of acute diarrheal disease in the coastal United States, always as a common-source outbreak related to ingestion of inadequately cooked seafood, usually shrimp. Secondary cases caused by person-to-person transmission occur rarely, if at all. Several epidemics of *V. parahemolyticus* infections on cruise ships have been reported.

PATHOGENESIS Although *V. parahemolyticus* produces a toxin capable of causing intestinal fluid accumulation in the experimental animal, the role of this toxin in human disease is less clear-cut than is that of the cholera enterotoxin. The volume of fluid lost with *V. parahemolyticus* infection is relatively small, and intravenous fluids are seldom required. Unlike *V. cholerae*, *V. parahemolyticus* causes an inflammatory response in the intestinal mucosa: stools usually contain numerous polymorphonuclear leukocytes and are occasionally grossly bloody. The illness is almost always self-limited, with a median duration of just under 24 h.

MANIFESTATIONS Within 6 to 48 h after ingestion of raw or inadequately cooked seafood, the patient develops an acute diarrheal illness. The volume of fluid lost is generally not great, moderately severe abdominal cramps may be a prominent feature, and chills and fever are observed in roughly half the cases. Vomiting is generally not a prominent feature and occurs in no more than one-third of patients. The illness is almost invariably self-limited, and no deaths have been reported in outbreaks involving over a thousand patients in the United States.

LABORATORY FINDINGS When a common-source outbreak of acute diarrheal disease occurs in a group exposed to fresh or frozen seafood, the index of suspicion should be high and the diagnosis should be confirmed by plating a rectal swab on thiosulfate–citrate–bile salt–sucrose (TCBS) agar, on which typical colonies of *V. parahemolyticus* appear at 24 h. (This organism grows poorly and is therefore easily overlooked on deoxycholate culture plates). The stool generally has numerous polymorphonuclear leukocytes and smaller numbers of erythrocytes, but these findings are generally less prominent than in shigellosis.

TREATMENT No therapy is required by the large majority of patients. The disease is self-limited, and antimicrobial therapy shortens neither the course nor the duration of pathogen excretion. Antiperistaltic agents are not of clear-cut benefit. An occasional patient may lose sufficient quantities of intestinal fluid to require oral or intravenous therapy, guided by the same principles employed in the treatment of cholera.

PROGNOSIS The outcome is almost always good. Fatal cases, occasionally reported from Japan, appear to have occurred in rare instances in patients with serious underlying disease.

PREVENTION Since *V. parahemolyticus* is widely distributed in coastal waters, the only effective preventive measure is avoidance of ingestion of inadequately cooked shellfish.

REFERENCES

Cholera

CARPENTER CCJ et al: Clinical studies in Asiatic cholera, I-VI. Bull Johns Hopkins Hosp 118:165, 1966

GANGAROSA EF et al: The nature of the gastrointestinal lesion in Asiatic cholera and its relation to pathogenesis: A biopsy study. Am J Trop Med Hyg 9:125, 1960

HIRSCHHORN N et al: The treatment of cholera, in *Cholera*, D Barua, W Burrows (eds). Philadelphia, Saunders, 1974, p 235

MAHALANOBIS D et al: Oral fluid therapy of cholera among Bangladesh refugees, Johns Hopkins Med J 132:197, 1973

WALLACE CK et al: Optimal antibiotic therapy in cholera. Bull WHO 39:239, 1968

WATTEN RH et al: Water and electrolyte studies in cholera. J Clin Invest 38:1879, 1959

Vibrio parahemolyticus

BARKER WH JR et al: *Vibrio parahemolyticus* outbreak in Covington, Louisiana in August, 1972. Am J Epidemiol 100:316, 1974

THATCHER FS, CLARK DS (eds): *Microorganisms in Foods: Their Significance and Methods of Enumeration*. Toronto, University of Toronto Press, 1968, p 14

ZEN-YOJI H et al: Epidemiology, enteropathogenicity and classification of *Vibrio parahemolyticus*. J Infect Dis 115:436, 1965

135
CAMPYLOBACTER FETUS AND NONCHOLERAIC VIBRIO INFECTIONS

MARVIN TURCK
DENNIS SCHABERG

CAMPYLOBACTER FETUS INFECTIONS

DEFINITION *Campylobacter fetus* (formerly *Vibrio fetus*) infection is economically the most important cause of infectious abortion in cattle. In human beings, this organism may be associated with obscure febrile illnesses, subacute bacterial endocarditis, meningoencephalitis, and perhaps abortion.

ETIOLOGY *Campylobacter fetus* is a motile, comma-shaped or spirillar, gram-negative rod with a single unipolar flagellum. It is best identified by its appearance in smears made from cultured material. The organism is slow-growing and microaerophilic, and grows best in liquid media incubated under increased CO_2 tension. Several serotypes have been isolated by agglutination with antiserums from human and bovine strains. Cross-agglutination reactions occur with other bacterial species, particularly *Brucella abortus*.

EPIDEMIOLOGY AND PATHOGENESIS *Campylobacter* causes a venereal infection of cattle, sheep, and goats; when transmitted to gravid heifers or ewes, it results in abortion. The male acts as an asymptomatic carrier of the infection, and the organism has been isolated from the genitalia and semen of bulls. Although *Campylobacter* infection has been thought to occur only rarely in humans, reports of this disease are appearing with increasing frequency. *Campylobacter* infection in human beings may result from direct contact with the organism,

as happens in laboratory-acquired infection, or from direct contact with infected cattle. Food and water have been implicated, without convincing evidence, as vehicles for infection. The mouth has been postulated as a portal of entry because cases of *C. fetus* endocarditis have followed dental extractions. Because *C. fetus* has been isolated from several aborted fetuses and has been the cause of neonatal meningitis, a venereal route of infection has been postulated. It is presumed that, as in cattle, the male acts as an asymptomatic carrier who transmits the infection to a pregnant partner. The relation of *C. fetus* to prematurity, abortion, and neonatal meningitis requires further documentation. In most instances of *Campylobacter* infection, the portal of entry is not known.

MANIFESTATIONS Fever is the only characteristic sign of *Campylobacter* infection in adults, and may be relapsing in character. Thrombophlebitis involving both arms and legs is not uncommon. The disease may also present as classic subacute bacterial endocarditis; septic arthritis or osteomyelitis; chronic, indolent meningoencephalitis; and fever and abortion in pregnant women. A number of patients have had coexisting disease, including cirrhosis, cardiac amyloidosis, and chronic lymphatic leukemia, or antecedent gastric surgery. Several neonates with fulminating, lethal meningoencephalitis have been reported. It has been postulated that infection was transmitted to these infants via the placenta. *Campylobacter* has also been implicated in the etiology of outbreaks of acute gastroenteritis.

DIAGNOSIS Lack of awareness of *Campylobacter* infection by both the bacteriologist and the clinician has resulted in mistaken diagnosis in most instances. The organisms have been erroneously described as "fastidious strains of *Hemophilus*." Recovery of spirillar organisms in blood cultures should suggest the diagnosis because other spirochetes causing relapsing fever usually do not grow in artificial media. Failure to incubate blood cultures under increased CO_2 tensions may delay growth. Identification of the organisms in smears of cultures is the only definitive method of making the diagnosis, which should then be confirmed by agglutinating the vibrios with specific antiserums. Complement-fixing antibody may be present in high titers in the active phase of the disease. Clinically, *Campylobacter* infection should be suspected in obscure febrile illnesses associated with thrombophlebitis or abortion and premature delivery in pregnant women.

TREATMENT There are few reports of antibiotic sensitivity of the organisms, and various antibiotics, alone or in combination, have been used. A 10-day course of tetracycline or chloramphenicol in dosage of 2 g per day, alone or coupled with streptomycin, 1 g per day, should eradicate the organisms in most instances. In cases of endocarditis, antimicrobial therapy should be extended to 6 weeks. Kanamycin and erythromycin have also been effective in vitro. Penicillin, novobiocin, vancomycin, and polymyxin B are ineffective.

NONCHOLERAIC VIBRIO INFECTIONS

DEFINITION *Vibrio parahemolyticus*, *V. alginolyticus*, and an unnamed lactose-positive *Vibrio* species are halophilic marine vibrios associated with wound infections, septicemia and, in the case of *V. parahemolyticus*, food-borne gastroenteritis (Chaps. 112 and 134). Nonagglutinating *V. cholerae* is biochemically identical with, but serologically distinct from, true *V. cholerae* and has been implicated in gastroenteritis as well as sepsis and wound infection.

EPIDEMIOLOGY AND PATHOGENESIS These marine vibrios are ubiquitous organisms found in oceans worldwide. Infection appears to result from direct contact of wounds with seawater or from handling or ingesting seafood. In the United States the majority of infections are acquired in the coastal states. Acquisition of the organism also occurs in travelers outside the United States.

MANIFESTATIONS Illness can begin as a wound infection or can present as a systemic illness without antecedent wound infection. Rapidly developing swelling, erythema, and bullae formation at the site of a wound exposed to seawater should raise the possibility of *Vibrio* infection. Secondary bloodstream invasion can develop.

Presentation as a systemic illness typically involves fever and chills. Hypotension and leukopenia are not uncommon findings. A history of recent seafood ingestion, especially raw oysters, is often obtained in those patients who have preexisting hepatic disease. Progression to a full-blown syndrome of gram-negative sepsis with shock, disseminated intravascular coagulation, and mortality has been noted in up to one-third of cases.

DIAGNOSIS Clinically, noncholeraic *Vibrio* infection should be suspected when patients present with wound infection and seawater exposure or present with a systemic febrile illness, preexisting hepatic disease, and a history of seafood ingestion. These marine vibrios grow well in artificial media, although when *Vibrio* infection is suspected, the use of thiosulfate–citrate–bile salts–sucrose (TCBS) agar may facilitate isolation. Cultures of wound drainage and blood will yield the causative agent within 24 to 48 h of incubation.

TREATMENT A wide variety of antimicrobial agents has been used in the therapy of noncholeraic *Vibrio* infections. Limited clinical experience and in vitro studies would suggest that tetracycline or chloramphenicol in doses of 2 g per day should be effective. In vitro studies also show that cephalothin or aminoglycoside antibiotics should be effective, but clinical experience with these agents is lacking.

REFERENCES

Campylobacter infections

FRANKLIN B et al: Human infection with *Vibrio fetus*. West J Med 120:200, 1974

LAWRENCE GD et al: Infection caused by *Vibrio fetus*. Arch Intern Med 120:459, 1967

SKIRROW MB: *Campylobacter* enteritis: A "new" disease. Br Med J 2:9, 1977

Noncholeraic *Vibrio* infections

BLAKE PA et al: Disease caused by a marine *Vibrio*: Clinical characteristics and epidemiology. N Engl J Med 300:1, 1979

HOLLIS DG et al: Halophilic *Vibrio* species isolated from blood cultures. J Clin Microbiol 3:425, 1976

HUGHES JM et al: Non-cholera *Vibrio* infections in the United States: Clinical, epidemiologic, and laboratory features. Ann Intern Med 88:602, 1978

136
BARTONELLOSIS

JAMES J. PLORDE

DEFINITION Bartonellosis (Carrión's disease) is an infection with *Bartonella bacilliformis*. Two well-defined clinical stages occur: an acute febrile anemia of rapid onset and high mortal-

ity, designated *Oroya fever*, and a benign eruptive form with chronic cutaneous lesions, called *verruga peruana*. Either of these types may be mild, and asymptomatic cases constitute the greatest epidemiologic hazard.

ETIOLOGY *Bartonella bacilliformis* is a small, motile, aerobic, pleomorphic, gram-negative bacillus which stains reddish violet with Giemsa's stain. It can be cultured on enriched media and does not produce a hemolysin. The organisms are sensitive to several antibiotics in vitro.

EPIDEMIOLOGY The disease is limited to certain valleys in the Andes Mountains comprising parts of Peru, Ecuador, and Colombia. It occurs in regions between the altitudes of 2400 and 8000 ft where the sandfly vector, *Phlebotomus*, propagates. Although only *P. verrucarum* has been shown to transmit the disease, other species are undoubtedly involved. Asymptomatic cases and convalescent carriers are the only known reservoir of infection. A low-grade bacteremia may persist for years following resolution of symptoms, and *B. bacilliformis* can be recovered from the blood of 5 to 10 percent of the apparently normal population in an endemic area. Epidemics often coincide with immigration of workers from uninfected areas.

PATHOLOGY AND PATHOGENESIS The manifestations of the disease are thought to reflect the immune status of the host. In nonimmune individuals Oroya fever develops. Large numbers of the *Bartonella* bacteria enter the bloodstream, adhere to erythrocytes, and invade the endothelial cells of the capillaries and lymphatics. The presence of the organisms on the surface of the red blood cell results in their phagocytosis and destruction by the liver and spleen. The red blood cell life span is greatly shortened, and anemia develops. This is accentuated by a defective erythropoietic response early in the course of infection. The pathogenesis of the hemolytic anemia remains unknown. Agglutinins and hemolysins have not been found, and tests for mechanical fragility of red blood cells have given variable results. Invasion and swelling of capillary endothelial cells may lead to vascular occlusion and tissue infarcts. It is possible that an impairment of reticuloendothelial function secondary to massive phagocytosis of red blood cells is responsible for the frequency with which *Salmonella* and other coliform bacteremias are seen in Oroya fever.

With developing immunity, the bacteria nearly disappear from the peripheral blood and capillary endothelium. After a latent period they reappear in the skin and subcutaneous tissue where they are apparently responsible for the development of the hemangioid lesions of verruga peruana. Second attacks of Carrión's disease are unusual. When they occur, they almost invariably present as verruga.

CLINICAL MANIFESTATIONS The incubation period is approximately 3 weeks but may be longer. The initial symptoms are fever and pains in the bones, joints, and muscles. At this point the disease often resembles influenza or malaria, but blood cultures are positive. After these prodromes, the patient usually develops one of the two classic forms of the infection.

Oroya fever This form is characterized by sudden onset of high fever, extreme pallor, weakness, and a precipitous drop in the number of red blood cells. The count may fall from normal to 1 million per cubic millimeter within 4 or 5 days. The anemia is characterized by normochromic macrocytes in the peripheral blood, striking polychromasia and polychromatophilia, nucleated red blood cells, Howell-Jolly bodies, Cabot rings, and basophilic stippling. There may also be a mild leukocytosis with a shift to the left. Organisms are numerous in the blood, and stained smears may show 90 percent of the erythrocytes heavily invaded. Salmonellosis, malaria, amebiasis, tuberculosis, and other intercurrent infections may occur and are an important factor in fatal cases.

Muscle and joint pain and headache are severe, and insomnia, delirium, and coma are the terminal manifestations. In untreated patients, the mortality rate may exceed 50 percent; death occurs within 10 days to 4 weeks. With treatment, or sometimes spontaneously, recovery results if the organisms decrease and fever abates. The red blood cell count stabilizes and approaches normal values in about 6 weeks, when convalescence begins.

Verruga peruana This form of the disease, characterized by a profuse skin eruption, may follow the anemic form or may occur in patients without previous symptoms. The verrugas vary in color from red to purple. They may be miliary, nodular, or eroding, and they range in size from 2 to 10 mm up to 3 or 4 cm in diameter. The three types of verruga may occur together; since eruption takes place in successive crops, verrugas of all types and in all stages of development may be found on the same patient. The chief sites involved are the limbs and face, and less frequently the genitalia, scalp, and mucosa of the mouth and pharynx. They may persist for 1 month to 2 years. The eruption is accompanied by pain, fever, and moderate anemia. Bartonellas may be demonstrated in the lesions and cultured from the blood.

DIAGNOSIS A clinical diagnosis can be made with accuracy in endemic areas. During Oroya fever the organism is easily seen on peripheral blood smears. It may be recovered from blood cultures in all stages of the disease.

TREATMENT Oroya fever responds dramatically to a number of antibiotics including tetracycline and chloramphenicol. The latter in a dose of 2 g per day for 7 days is often preferred because of the frequency with which *Salmonella* infections complicate this disease. Fever disappears within 48 h, and the patient recovers rapidly. Transfusions may be required when the anemia is severe. Antibiotic therapy of the verrugal stage may hasten the involution of these lesions. The use of DDT in both the interior and exterior of human dwellings is highly effective in controlling the night-biting sandflies. Insect repellents and bed netting afford personal protection.

REFERENCES

Caudra MC: Salmonellosis complication in human bartonellosis. Tex Rep Biol Med 14:97, 1956

Kaye D et al: Factors influencing host resistance to *Salmonella* infections: The effects of hemolysis and erythrophagocytosis. Am J Med Sci 254:205, 1967

Ricketts WE: Clinical manifestations of Carrión's disease. AMA Arch Intern Med 84:751, 1949

Schultz MG: Daniel Carrión's experiment. N Engl J Med 278:1323, 1968

Ureteaga OB, Payne EH: Treatment of the acute febrile phase of Carrión's disease with chloramphenicol. Am J Trop Med 4:507, 1955

Weinman D: The bartonella group, in *Bacterial and Mycotic Infections of Man*, 4th ed, RJ Dubos, JG Hirsch (eds). Philadelphia, Lippincott, 1965, p 775

137
GRANULOMA INGUINALE

KING K. HOLMES

DEFINITION Granuloma inguinale is a mildly contagious, chronic, indolent, progressive, autoinoculable, ulcerative disease involving the skin and lymphatics of the genital or perianal areas. The disease may be sexually transmitted and is associated with the presence in affected tissues of an intracellular microorganism, identified morphologically as the Donovan body.

ETIOLOGY Granuloma inguinale was described by McLeod in India in 1882, and in 1905 Donovan described the intracellular bodies which are thought to cause the disease. Granuloma inguinale has been reproduced in humans by inoculation of pus containing Donovan bodies. Similar attempts to reproduce the disease in experimental animals have been unsuccessful. Encapsulated bacteria resembling Donovan bodies have been recovered from lesions and pseudobuboes of granuloma inguinale by inoculation of chick embryo yolk sacs or yolk-agar medium. These bacteria, which are known as *Calymmatobacterium granulomatis,* are antigenically related to *Klebsiella* species but do not reproduce the disease when inoculated intradermally in humans. It is uncertain whether these isolates are responsible for the disease. Similar bacteria have been isolated from feces. Electron microscopic studies of Donovan bodies confirm their morphological resemblance to gram-negative bacteria.

EPIDEMIOLOGY Granuloma inguinale is endemic in the tropics, particularly in New Guinea and among Hindus in India. In the United States the disease is rare. Most cases occur in the southeastern states and involve male homosexuals. In reported cases the sex ratio of males to females is nearly 10:1. The disease is uncommon in Caucasians. The reported frequency of granuloma inguinale in conjugal partners of chronically infected patients ranges from 1 to 64 percent. Evidence for sexual transmission includes the age-specific incidence, which corresponds to that of other sexually transmitted diseases, the frequent concomitant presence of syphilis, and the predilection for genital involvement in heterosexuals and for anorectal infection in male homosexuals.

CLINICAL MANIFESTATIONS The incubation period ranges from 8 days to 12 weeks, but most lesions appear within 30 days after sexual exposure.

Granuloma inguinale begins as a papule, which ulcerates and develops into a painless elevated zone of clean, beefy-red, friable granulation tissue. The edges are irregular and spread by continuity or by autoinoculation of approximated skin surfaces. Secondary anaerobic infection may produce pain and a foul-smelling exudate. Less common complications of the disease include deep ulcerations, chronic cicatricial lesions, and exuberant epithelial proliferation which grossly resembles carcinoma. In men, the lesions are usually located on the glans, prepuce, or shaft of the penis (Fig. 137-1*A*) or the perianal area, while infection of the labia is most common in women. Lesions in women often arise at the fourchette and progress anteriorly in a V shape along the vulva. Extragenital lesions may occur, involving the face, neck, mouth, and other sites. The chronicity of the disease is of diagnostic importance, since several months often elapse before patients seek treatment. Extension to the inguinal region by autoinoculation or via the

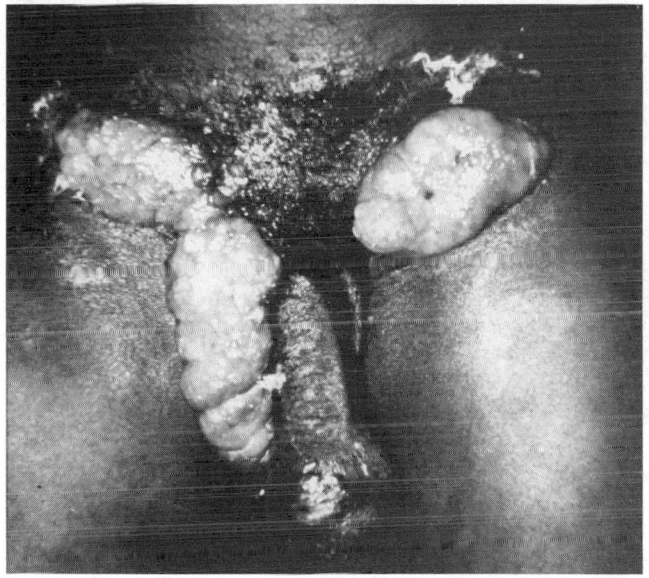

A

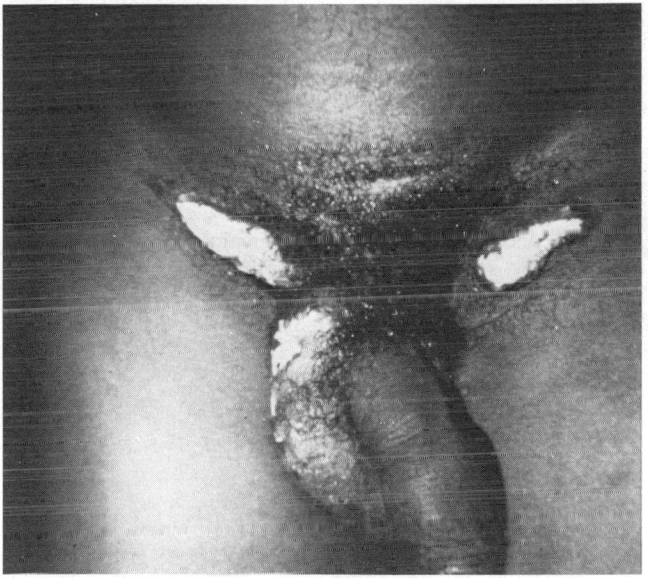

B

FIGURE 137-1

A. Extensive granuloma inguinale, extending along the scrotum and involving both inguinal areas, with elevated, clean, exuberant granulation tissue. B. Same patient, following treatment. (Courtesy of A Brathwaite.)

lymphatics results in diffuse intradermal and subcutaneous swelling or suppuration, known as "pseudobubo," because involvement of the underlying lymph nodes is minimal. Locally destructive lesions and secondary infection may produce severe morbidity or death. Fatal disseminated disease, involving the bones or joints, has been reported after several years of chronic local infection. The relationship of granuloma inguinale to subsequent carcinoma of the genitalia is uncertain.

DIAGNOSIS Early granuloma inguinale may be mistaken for the primary chancre or condyloma latum of syphilis. Epithelial proliferation resembling neoplasia in the genital or perianal region in a young subject should always raise the suspicion of granuloma inguinale if unnecessary destructive surgery is to be avoided. Chronic ulcerative or cicatricial changes may resemble lymphogranuloma venereum. Histological studies in granuloma inguinale reveal marked acanthosis and pseudoepitheli-

omatous hyperplasia. Because Donovan bodies are seldom detectable in sections stained with hematoxylin and eosin, these changes may lead to an erroneous diagnosis of carcinoma and to unnecessary, destructive surgery. Although silver impregnation techniques are useful for demonstration of Donovan bodies in sections, the diagnosis is best made by examination of impression smears prepared from specimens obtained by punch biopsy from the periphery of a lesion; the deep portion of the specimen is removed, crushed between two slides which are air-dried and fixed in methanol, and stained with Wright-Giemsa stain. With this method, Donovan bodies appear as very rounded coccobacilli, 1 by 2 μm in size, which lie within cystic spaces in the cytoplasm of large mononuclear

FIGURE 137-2

Biopsy from granuloma inguinale ulcer, showing mononuclear cells containing Donovan bodies. Wright-Giemsa stain.

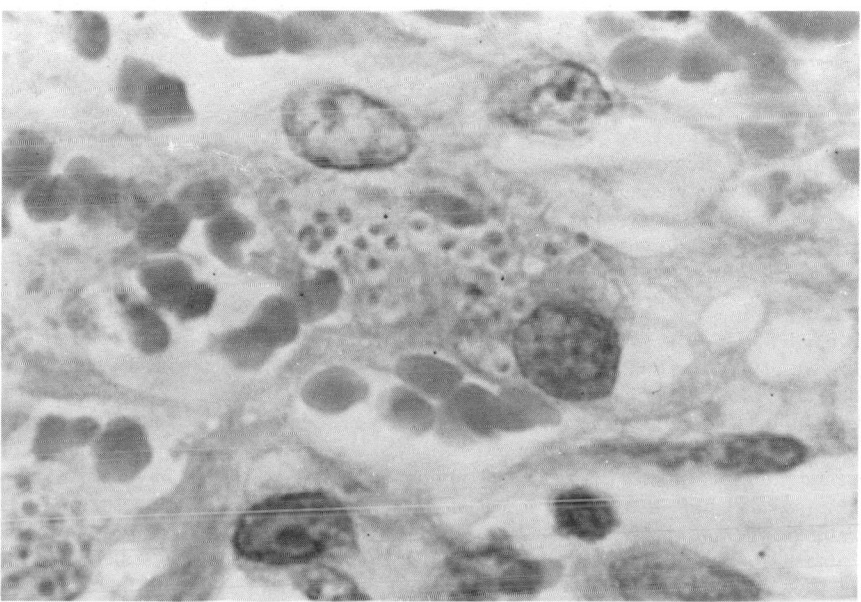

cells (Fig. 137-2). The capsule stains as a dense acidophilic zone surrounding the bipolar basophilic bacterium, which resembles a closed safety pin. The pathognomonic mononuclear cell is 25 to 90 μm in diameter and has many cystic areas containing Donovan bodies.

Perianal granuloma inguinale may resemble condylomata lata of secondary syphilis. Other venereal diseases, particularly syphilis, very frequently coexist with granuloma inguinale. Repeated dark-field examinations of lesions before treatment and a serologic test for syphilis should therefore be performed.

TREATMENT The treatment of choice is tetracycline, 2 g daily, continued for at least 10 days. The risk of relapse is reduced if treatment is continued until healing is complete. Healing is usually apparent within 3 weeks, as the lesions become pale, flatter, and develop peripheral reepithelialization (Fig. 137-1*B*). Donovan bodies disappear from lesions within a few days after onset of therapy. If tetracycline cannot be given, streptomycin may be used in a dose of 1 g intramuscularly every 12 h for 10 to 15 days. In New Guinea, chloramphenicol or gentamicin is used for cases which appear resistant to tetracycline.

REFERENCES

BEERMAN H, SONCK CE: The epithelial changes in granuloma inguinale. Am J Syph Gonorrhea Vener Dis 36:501, 1952

DAVIS CM: Granuloma inguinale. A clinical, histological, and ultrastructural study. JAMA 211:632, 1970

GOLDBERG J: Studies on granuloma inguinale. Br J Vener Dis 40:140, 1964

LAL S: Continued efficacy of streptomycin in the treatment of granuloma inguinale. Br J Vener Dis 47:454, 1971

——, NICHOLAS C: Epidemiological and clinical features in 165 cases of granuloma inguinale. Br J Vener Dis 46:461, 1970

Management of chancroid, granuloma inguinale, lymphogranuloma verereum in general practice. US Public Health Serv Publ 255:15, 1964

RIBEIRO J: Granuloma inguinale. Practitioner 209:628, 1972

138
LEGIONNAIRES' DISEASE   GRAM ⊖ BACILLUS

HARRY N. BEATY   Lgionella PNEumophilia

DEFINITION Legionnaires' disease is an acute respiratory infection caused by a newly recognized, distinctive gram-negative bacterium that was first isolated from fatal cases of pneumonia among individuals attending an American Legion Convention in Philadelphia.

HISTORY In July of 1976, an explosive outbreak of severe respiratory illness occurred in Philadelphia—chiefly among delegates of an American Legion Convention. Initial investigation failed to document a familiar infective or toxic etiology, and so a comprehensive, coordinated effort was undertaken to define the epidemiology and cause of the outbreak. As the ensuing saga unfolded, it became apparent that at least 182 cases of pneumonia—29 of which were fatal—resulted from a common source of airborne infection that was present for several days inside and in the immediate vicinity outside one of the convention hotels. The infective agent was proved to be a previously unknown gram-negative bacterium.

Using serologic techniques, it has been shown that the same organism, or antigenically related species, has caused at least eight other outbreaks of respiratory illness. The earliest of these occurred in 1965 when 80 patients in a psychiatric hospital in Washington, D.C., developed an unexplained pneumonic illness; 12 of these patients died. Other clusters of cases with additional deaths have occurred in Spain (1973) and England (1977). One outbreak of particular significance involved visitors and employees in an office of the county health department in Pontiac, Michigan (1968). Pneumonia was not seen among the 144 persons who developed an influenza-like illness, and there were no deaths. The agent responsible for Legionnaires' disease has been directly linked to this outbreak, because it has been isolated from environmental samples and tissues of experimental animals, which were stored in the frozen state after they were studied unsuccessfully during the initial investigation.

ETIOLOGY The bacterium responsible for Legionnaires' disease was first isolated by inoculating suspensions of lung tissue from four of the fatal Philadelphia cases intraperitoneally into guinea pigs. Suspensions of spleen and other organs from animals with a progressive febrile illness produced infection in embryonated eggs. From infected eggs, the organism was isolated in pure culture on an artificial medium. An inoculum from this medium was used to induce infection in guinea pigs, fulfilling Koch's postulate.

The bacterium is a gram-negative bacillus which is 0.3 to 0.4 μm in width and usually 2 to 3 μm long. However, bacilli from 10 to 50 μm have been seen. Pleomorphism is affected by the medium on which the organism is grown; in tissue, the filamentous forms are not encountered. Electron microscopy reveals a structure typical of gram-negative rods, but gas-liquid chromatography shows a distinctive branched-chain fatty acid profile that is more characteristic of gram-positive bacteria.

With the use of the direct fluorescent-antibody technique, no antigenic cross-reactivity was found with 374 strains including 25 bacterial genera and 59 species. One strain each of *Pseudomonas fluorescens* and *P. alcaligenes* has shown some reaction with anti-Legionnaires' agent conjugate, but numerous other strains of the same species have been tested without additional evidence of cross-reactivity. Studies of DNA relatedness also have failed to show that the bacterium responsible for Legionnaires' disease is related to any other organism. As a consequence of all of these studies, the organism has been named *Legionella pneumophilia* to establish it as the first isolate of a previously unrecognized genus and species.

Legionella pneumophilia is fastidious, and either does not grow or grows rather poorly on most artificial media. For this reason it is infrequently isolated directly from patients. Mueller-Hinton agar containing 1 percent hemoglobin and 1 percent IsoVitale X was the medium used in early studies, but more recently a yeast extract agar containing activated charcoal has produced better growth of the organisms. Inoculated plates should be incubated at 35°C in 5% CO_2 or in candle jars. On clear media, a soluble brown pigment that fluoresces under a Wood's lamp can be seen. The organism is catalase-positive and causes a weakly positive oxidase reaction.

Several distinct serogroups of *L. pneumophilia* have been identified; some were isolated from patients with Legionnaires' disease and others from soil and/or water. Serologic cross-reactions between groups may be absent or weak, which necessitates the use of multiple diagnostic conjugates to detect all strains of *L. pneumophila.*

EPIDEMIOLOGY Knowledge of the distribution of *L. pneumophilia* in nature is incomplete, but it has been isolated from soil and water. Several outbreaks of Legionnaires' disease have been linked to contaminated condensates from air-conditioning cooling towers, and prolonged survival in drinking water has been documented experimentally. The possibility that organisms in soil became airborne during excavation was raised as a possible cause of disease early in the epidemiologic studies of the Philadelphia outbreak.

Infection appears to be acquired by the respiratory route with a usual incubation period of 2 to 10 days. By use of the direct fluorescent-antibody technique, organisms have been identified in the sputum of patients with Legionnaires' disease, but person-to-person spread has not been documented. Common-source outbreaks have received the greatest public attention, but hundreds of sporadic cases of Legionnaires' disease occur each year. Incidence may increase in the summer and early fall, but the disease occurs year-round.

Although this infection has been reported in children, most patients are middle-aged or older. Cigarette smokers and individuals with serious underlying diseases such as chronic renal failure, malignancy, and immunosuppression have increased susceptibility to infection. The mortality rate of Legionnaires' pneumonia that is serious enough to require hospitalization is around 15 percent; among immunocompromised patients it may exceed 50 percent.

Serologic surveys using the indirect fluorescent-antibody technique have shown that less than 5 percent of healthy individuals from around the United States have reciprocal antibody titers to *L. pneumophilia* of 128 or higher. However, some more geographically restricted surveys have shown that 15 to 25 percent of the population have similar serologic evidence of significant exposure to *L. pneumophilia* or antigenically related organisms. This suggests that the infection may be endemic in some regions.

Most cases of Legionnaires' disease are diagnosed by demonstration of at least a fourfold rise in serum antibody titer to *L. pneumophilia*. A significant proportion of patients maintain high titers for years. It is not known whether these individuals are immune to reinfection with the same or closely related organisms.

PATHOLOGY AND PATHOGENESIS Pathologic features of Legionnaires' disease are limited to the lungs. Apparent lobar involvement almost always represents confluent bronchopneumonia. Prominent microscopic features include extensive exudation of proteinaceous fluid and inflammatory cells into alveoli. In most cases, the cellular component of the exudate is a mixture of polymorphonuclear neutrophils and macrophages. Extensive lysis of inflammatory cells, with accumulations of nuclear debris and fibrin, is a distinctive feature of this pneumonia. Alveolar septa usually are edematous and infiltrated with inflammatory cells; hyalin membranes are seen in about half the cases. Terminal bronchioles are routinely involved, but larger bronchioles and bronchi are unaffected. None of these changes is unique to Legionnaires' pneumonia, but the histopathologic alterations are sufficiently distinctive to suggest the diagnosis.

Bacteria usually can be demonstrated in the inflammatory exudate with the Dieterle stain or by direct fluorescent-antibody techniques. Other stains are less reliable. Many bacilli appear to be intracellular, and an increase in the number of organisms is associated with lysis of inflammatory cells.

Little is known about the pathogenesis of Legionnaires' pneumonia. The fact that cigarette smokers are more susceptible to infection than nonsmokers suggests that the defective alveolar macrophage function plays a role in development of disease. The extensive lysis of inflammatory cells and the edema of the interstitium raise the possibility that a toxin is produced by the Legionnaires' disease bacterium. Such a toxin might be responsible for some of the clinical features seen with this infection.

CLINICAL MANIFESTATIONS The total spectrum of clinical manifestations of Legionnaires' disease is not known. Mild respiratory illness has been recognized, and asymptomatic infection has not been excluded as a possible explanation for elevated antibody titers among healthy individuals. The outbreak in Pontiac, Michigan, was characterized by the acute onset and short duration of a moderately severe influenza-like syndrome of fever, myalgia, and headache.

The more typical patient with Legionnaires' disease has pneumonia. In the Philadelphia outbreak over 80 percent of the recognized cases were severe enough to require hospitalization. Some patients have a constellation of symptoms that strongly suggest the diagnosis, particularly in a setting of known Legionnaires' disease activity. These patients have malaise and a slight headache, which precedes a rapidly rising fever by less than a day. Within 24 to 48 h, temperatures reach 40°C in about half the patients, and shaking chills are common. A modest, nonproductive cough frequently is present early; it progresses in severity over the first few days of illness and usually becomes productive of variable amounts of mucoid to mucopurulent sputum. Minimal hemoptysis is seen in about 20 percent of patients. Additional symptoms that occur less frequently include dyspnea, pleuritic chest pain, and myalgia. About 25 percent of patients have various combinations of gastrointestinal symptoms which include nausea and vomiting, diarrhea, and abdominal pain. In a few patients, these manifestations predominate despite the presence of pneumonia. In some individuals, the onset of Legionnaires' disease is more protracted and the clinical expression less distinctive. These cases are likely to be missed unless the epidemiologic setting or subtle clinical clues stimulate physicians to suspect the diagnosis. The findings on physical examination are not specific for Legionnaires' disease, and they are affected by patients' associated diseases. High fever, tachypnea, and tachycardia are common. Patients frequently are flushed, mildly diaphoretic, and appear moderately to severely prostrated. Examination of the chest shows moist rales, but signs of consolidation usually are absent. Chest roentgenograms characteristically show more involvement of the lungs than is suspected on clinical grounds.

During the first 4 to 6 days, the disease becomes progressively worse. An additional 4 to 5 days may pass before definite clinical improvement begins. The average duration of fever in one large series was 13 days. Clearing of pulmonary infiltrates lags significantly behind improvement of other manifestations of infection, and minor residual scarring is not uncommon. Many patients experience weakness and easy fatigability for weeks after the acute stages of the illness.

The major complication of Legionnaires' disease is respiratory failure. Twenty to thirty percent of patients sick enough to require hospitalization have hyperventilation and hypoxemia. In about half of these patients, progression of disease leads to intubation and mechanical ventilation. The mortality rate among patients with respiratory failure is high. Hypotension and shock, with secondary acute renal failure, are additional complications that may be encountered. Whether these are caused by undetected bacteremia or toxemia has not been determined.

684

LABORATORY FINDINGS Most patients have a modest granulocytosis, but about 20 percent have leukocyte counts in excess of 20,000 per cubic millimeter. The erythrocyte sedimentation rate is elevated, and there is moderate proteinuria. Transient renal insufficiency and mild changes in liver function have been reported, but it is not always possible to attribute these abnormalities to the infection.

Chest roentgenograms show unilateral pulmonary parenchymal infiltrates in about 65 percent of cases early in the illness. By the time of maximal involvement, the pneumonia has progressed to involve both sides in most cases. Nonspecific poorly marginated rounded opacities or diffuse patchy lobar shadows predominate. Small pleural effusions are seen in about a third of cases.

Routine bacteriologic studies including blood and sputum cultures are negative. Lower respiratory tract secretions obtained by transtracheal aspiration or other suitable techniques show many granulocytes and alveolar macrophages but are sterile on Gram's stain and currently available culture media.

DIAGNOSIS The diagnosis of Legionnaires' disease has been made in a very few instances by isolation of the causative organism from lung tissue or pleural field. As bacteriologic techniques improve, this may become more common. For the moment, the diagnosis depends on demonstration of a significant rise in antibody in paired serum specimens or by identifying organisms in fresh or Formalin-fixed lung tissue by the direct fluorescent-antibody technique. Serum antibody can be measured in a number of ways, but the indirect fluorescent-antibody method is the most specific and sensitive one available. Because antibody titers rise slowly in some patients, the first serum specimen should be obtained during the first week of illness, and the second at least 21 days after the onset of symptoms.

In some cases, *L. pneumophilia* has been demonstrated in sputum by the direct fluorescent-antibody technique. When this is accomplished in a patient with pneumonia and a single reciprocal antibody titer of 256 or greater, a presumptive diagnosis of Legionnaires' disease can be made. Because antibody titers are known to remain elevated for years in some patients, simple demonstration of a high titer without supporting evidence does not establish the diagnosis with certainty.

Legionnaires' disease may be difficult to differentiate from "atypical" pneumonias. When patients have a constellation of findings which include temperature elevations to 40°C, granulocytosis, and sterile lower respiratory tract secretions that contain many granulocytes and alveolar macrophages, Legionnaires' disease should be suspected. In immunocompromised patients, *Pneumocystis* or fungal infection enters into the differential diagnosis. Rarely, pulmonary embolism can be confused with early Legionnaires' disease.

TREATMENT Although in vitro sensitivity tests indicate that a number of antibiotics might be effective in the treatment of Legionnaires' disease, clinical experience has shown that the lowest case-fatality ratio is achieved with erythromycin in a dose of 0.5 to 1 g every 6 h for adults and 15 mg/kg every 6 h for children. Erythromycin also has been shown to be highly efficacious in treatment of experimental infections in embryonated eggs and guinea pigs. Tetracycline is less effective in all these settings. Rifampin has shown promise in laboratory testing, but its propensity to induce resistance may limit its potential usefulness.

Although the case-fatality ratio of patients treated with erythromycin is low, response to treatment frequently is not dramatic. If therapy is continued for at least 14 days, relapses are uncommon. When they occur, they usually respond to a second course of erythromycin. Because Legionnaires' disease can cause pneumonia in patients not sick enough to be hospitalized and who are assumed to have either *Mycoplasma* infection or early pneumococcal infection, erythromycin should be considered the drug of choice for the treatment of pneumonia in an ambulatory care setting.

There is more to treatment of Legionnaires' disease than administration of antibiotics. High fever, diaphoresis, and tachypnea produce excessive fluid loss, and volume replacement with intravenous fluids may be needed. Hypoxic patients should receive supplemental oxygen.

PROGNOSIS The overall mortality rate of Legionnaires' disease is unknown. Among patients with pneumonia who are sick enough to require hospitalization, the mortality rate is around 15 percent. The presence of complicating associated illnesses may raise that figure two- or threefold. Individuals who recover from Legionnaires' pneumonia usually have no significant residua of their infection. It is not known whether they are immune to reinfection with the same or related organisms.

REFERENCES

Beaty HN et al: Legionnaires' disease in Vermont, May to October 1977. JAMA 240:127, 1978

Fraser DW et al: Legionnaires' disease—description of an epidemic of pneumonia. N Engl J Med 297:1189, 1977

Kirby, BD et al: Legionnaires' disease: Clinical features of 24 cases. Ann Intern Med 89:297, 1978

McDade JE et al: Legionnaires' disease—isolation of a bacterium and demonstration of its role in other respiratory disease. N Engl J Med 297:1197, 1977

Winn WC et al: The pathology of Legionnaires' disease—fourteen fatal cases from the 1977 outbreak in Vermont. Arch Pathol Lab Med 102:344, 1978 *[handwritten margin notes: Antiserum (Tetanus immunoglobulin TIG) Diazepam (Valium) PENG → But no evidence it alters course of Disease ~ Trach]*

139

TETANUS

[handwritten: Anaerobe, Clostridia tetani, clubbed shaped, Gram ⊕ Rod]

HARRY N. BEATY

DEFINITION Tetanus is an acute, often fatal, disease caused by an exotoxin produced in a wound by *Clostridium tetani.* It is characterized by generalized increased rigidity and convulsive spasms of skeletal muscles.

ETIOLOGY *Clostridium tetani* is a strictly anaerobic, gram-positive rod which is motile and readily forms endospores. In stained preparations, organisms may occur singly, in pairs, or in long chains. Spore-bearing bacilli usually contain a single, spheric, terminal endospore which swells the end of the organism and produces a characteristic "clubbed" appearance.

The organism grows well on blood agar at 37°C under anaerobic conditions. Slight hemolysis is usually apparent, but isolated colonies are rare because the organism tends to swarm. *Clostridium tetani* is relatively inert biochemically, with no proteolytic activity and no fermentation of carbohydrates. Vegetative forms of the tetanus bacillus are no more resistant to adverse conditions than other bacteria are, but spores are highly resistant to antiseptics and moderately resistant to heat.

Ten distinct types of *C. tetani* can be distinguished on the basis of flagellar antigens. All these types have one or more common somatic antigens, and are capable of producing at least two exotoxins. One, a hemolysin, is relatively unimportant clinically. The other, tetanospasmin, generally referred to as tetanus toxin, is a protein with a molecular weight of approximately 145,000 in its dimer form, and is responsible for the clinical manifestations of tetanus. The tetanospasmins produced by the various types of *C. tetani* are nearly identical antigenically, and only one antitoxin is needed to neutralize the tetanus toxins produced by all strains.

EPIDEMIOLOGY The tetanus bacillus is found in the superficial layers of soil and as a saprophyte in the intestinal tract of man and certain animals. It is most frequently encountered in densely populated regions in hot, damp climates and in soil rich in organic matter. This explains, in part, why the disease is rare in the polar regions and relatively uncommon in the U.S.S.R., North America, and most of Europe. Urbanization, mechanization of agriculture, and socioeconomic factors such as poverty and lack of availability of health services also significantly influence the occurrence of this disease.

Worldwide, there are probably 300,000 to 500,000 cases of tetanus each year, with a mortality rate of roughly 45 percent. There is no racial predilection, but the male-to-female ratio is 2.5:1, even among neonates, in which the opportunity for infection is presumably equal. In the United States, there are less than 200 reported cases each year, and these occur almost exclusively in nonimmunized or only partially immunized individuals. The highest incidence of disease is among nonwhites in the southern states. However, spores of *C. tetani* are distributed widely throughout urban centers and rural areas of the entire country, and are found commonly on clothing and in house dust, placing the nonimmune individual at risk after relatively minor household injuries. Tetanus has been known to follow surgery and innocuous procedures such as skin testing or intramuscular injection of medication. The disease is inordinately common in narcotic addicts, perhaps because heroin is frequently "cut" with quinine, which drastically lowers the redox potential at the site of injection and favors the growth of *C. tetani.*

Tetanus neonatorum is a major cause of infant mortality in developing countries and is directly related to poor obstetric conditions and lack of maternal immunization programs.

PATHOGENESIS AND PATHOLOGY *Clostridium tetani* is a noninvasive organism. Therefore, tetanus can occur only after spore or vegetative bacteria gain access to tissues and produce toxin locally. The usual mode of entry is through a puncture wound or laceration on the hand, foot, or leg. However, tetanus may follow elective surgery, burn wounds, otitis media, dental infection, abortion, and pregnancy. Neonatal tetanus usually follows infection of the umbilical stump. The disease not infrequently follows injuries too trivial to be seen by a physician, and in 20 to 40 percent of cases there is neither a history of injury nor a detectable lesion.

Wounds are undoubtedly contaminated frequently with spores of *C. tetani*, but tetanus develops rarely because germination of spores occurs only when the oxygen tension is much lower than that of normal tissue. Spores may survive in the body for months to years and finally produce disease at some later date after minor trauma which alters local conditions. Toxin production in wounds is favored by necrotic tissue, foreign bodies, calcium salts, and associated infections which establish low oxidation-reduction potentials. Infection caused by the tetanus bacillus remains strictly localized, but the toxin produced is transported to the central nervous system via neural pathways. Toxin entering the circulation persists for days, and probably must enter peripheral nerves to spread centrally and cause disease.

The typical clinical manifestations of tetanus are caused by the effect of tetanospasmin on the central nervous system. The toxin attacks synaptic functions to produce disinhibition of both the alpha and gamma motor systems. Generalized muscle rigidity arises from uninhibited afferent stimuli entering the central nervous system from the periphery. When the stimuli become more vigorous, spasms occur. Emotional and, to a lesser extent, visual stimuli can also cause muscle spasm. Tetanus toxin also has other effects. Peripherally it produces neuromuscular blockade similar to that of botulinum toxin, and it acts directly on muscle to produce contraction which is unaccompanied by an action potential in nerves. Certain clinical observations have raised the possibility that tetanus toxin also has an effect on the sympathetic nervous system.

All the effects of tetanus toxin appear to be self-limited and completely reversible, because patients who recover from the disease have no residual defect. Although there are no distinguishable pathologic changes which are characteristic of tetanus, brainstem lesions have been reported in patients dying from tetanus, and toxic myocarditis has been recognized.

CLINICAL MANIFESTATIONS The *incubation period* of tetanus, i.e., the time between injury and the appearance of unmistakable symptoms, ranges from 2 to 56 days. However, over 80 percent of patients become symptomatic within 14 days. A short incubation period indicates severe disease, and when symptoms occur within 2 or 3 days of injury, the mortality rate approaches 100 percent.

Nonspecific premonitory symptoms such as restlessness, irritability, and headache are encountered occasionally, but the commonest presenting complaints are pain and stiffness in the jaw, abdomen, or back and difficulty in swallowing. As the disease progresses, stiffness gives way to rigidity, and patients often complain of difficulty in opening their mouths. In fact, trismus is the commonest manifestation of tetanus and is responsible for the familiar descriptive name of *lockjaw*. As more muscles are involved, rigidity becomes generalized, and sustained contractions of facial muscles produce a characteristic expression called *risus sardonicus*. The intensity and sequence of muscle involvement is quite variable. In a small proportion of patients, only local signs and symptoms develop in the region of the injury. In the vast majority, however, most muscles are involved to some degree, and the signs and symptoms encountered depend upon the major muscle groups affected.

Reflex spasms usually occur within 24 to 72 h of the first symptoms, an interval referred to as the *onset time*. As in the case of the incubation period, a short onset time is associated with a poor prognosis. Spasms are caused by sudden intensification of afferent stimuli arising in the periphery, which increases rigidity and causes simultaneous and excessive contraction of muscles and their antagonists. Spasms may be both painful and dangerous. As the disease progresses, minimal or inapparent stimuli produce more intense and longer-lasting spasms with increasing frequency. Respiration may be impaired by laryngospasm or tonic contraction of respiratory muscles which prevents adequate ventilation. Hypoxia may then lead to irreversible central nervous system damage and death.

Patients are almost invariably conscious and mentally alert at the time of admission. Low-grade fever, profuse sweating, and tachycardia are common. Deep tendon reflexes are hyperactive, and there may be labile hypertension. The physical examination should be undertaken with care, because reflex convulsive spasms may be precipitated easily. The wound through which *C. tetani* was introduced should be evaluated, and the examination should determine the extent of rigidity; the severity of trismus; the presence or absence of dysphagia and respiratory embarrassment; the frequency, intensity, and duration of convulsive spasms; and the presence of complications such as respiratory infection.

Characteristically, the manifestations of tetanus increase in severity for about 3 days after the first sign, and then remain stable for the next 5 to 7 days. After about 10 days, spasms begin to occur less frequently, and by the end of 2 weeks, they disappear altogether. Although residual stiffness may persist for a prolonged period, most survivors recover completely in 4 weeks.

Tetanus neonatorum is a severe form of the disease which usually occurs within 10 days of birth. Early signs include difficulty in sucking, irritability, and excessive crying, associated with peculiar grimacing. Intense rigidity characteristically produces opisthotonus, flexion of the arms, clenched fists, extension of the legs, and plantar flexion of the toes. Typical spasms occur with minimal stimuli.

Complications Complications contribute significantly to the morbidity and mortality of tetanus. Some result from overly vigorous therapy and prolonged bed rest, while others are attributed to the action of tetanus toxin. Inadequate ventilation, either from laryngospasm or spasm of respiratory muscles, is a constant threat. In addition to hypoxia, atelectasis is a common consequence of impaired respiration. Difficulty in swallowing leads to aspiration of secretions, which may also cause atelectasis and initiate pulmonary infection. Thrombophlebitis is occasionally encountered, but bland venous thrombosis is more common and may lead to pulmonary embolization. Cardiovascular complications thought to be due to hyperactivity of the sympathetic nervous system include vasomotor instability, hypertension, tachycardia, arrhythmias, and severe vasoconstriction. Pulmonary edema and hypotension may occur as a consequence of myocarditis. High fever usually signifies secondary infection. Pneumonia is a common late complication of tetanus, and is found in 50 to 70 percent of autopsied cases. Other frequent sites of secondary infections include the original wound, decubitus ulcers, and the urinary tract of patients with indwelling bladder catheters. Fractures of midthoracic vertebrae are probably due to severe spasms, and are particularly common among children and adolescents. Gastrointestinal complications include acute peptic ulceration, paralytic ileus, and constipation. Hemolysis is seen in a small proportion of patients.

Pneumonia is a major cause of death. Other autopsy findings in early deaths include intense congestion of viscera and, occasionally, intracranial hemorrhage or thrombosis. In about 20 percent of cases, no obvious pathology is identified, and death is attributed to the direct effects of tetanus toxin.

LABORATORY FINDINGS There are no laboratory findings characteristic of tetanus. Granulocytosis is seen in about one-third of patients, but anemia is rare. Blood chemistries are almost always normal initially, but various fluid and electrolyte disturbances may arise in the course of the disease. The electrocardiogram usually shows only sinus tachycardia, but occasionally T-wave inversion is seen. Roentgenograms are not helpful except in the evaluation of complications.

The diagnosis of tetanus is entirely clinical and does not depend upon bacteriologic confirmation. *Clostridium tetani* is recovered from the wound in only 30 percent of cases, and not infrequently it is isolated from patients who do not have tetanus. Laboratory identification depends on cultural and morphologic characteristics, absence of fermentative activity, and, most importantly, demonstration of toxin production in mice.

DIFFERENTIAL DIAGNOSIS No disease resembles fully developed tetanus. However, strychnine poisoning and dystonic reactions due to phenothiazines and metoclopramide produce a syndrome that has been referred to as pseudotetanus. These rare reactions usually follow brief exposure to drugs, and subside 24 to 48 h after their administration is discontinued. Early in the course of true tetanus, exclusion of local causes of jaw pain may be difficult, and the combination of neck stiffness and fever may suggest meningitis. However, this can be excluded by lumbar puncture, because in tetanus the spinal fluid is normal. When there is doubt about the diagnosis, clinical observation usually settles the issue within a matter of hours.

TREATMENT In order to formulate a rational plan of therapy, it is useful to assess the severity of tetanus. *Mild tetanus* is characterized by an incubation period of at least 14 days and an onset time of more than 6 days. Trismus is usually present, but dysphagia is absent, and generalized spasms are brief and mild. *Moderately severe tetanus* has a somewhat shorter incubation period and onset time; trismus is marked, dysphagia and generalized rigidity are present, but ventilation remains adequate even during spasms. The criteria for *severe tetanus* include a short incubation time, an onset time of 72 h or less, severe trismus, dysphagia and rigidity, and frequent, prolonged, generalized convulsive spasms. Because of the poor prognosis of tetanus in older individuals, the disease should be considered moderate to severe in all patients over 50.

General measures Patients should be hospitalized in an intensive care unit. After initial evaluation, necrotic tissue and foreign bodies should be removed from the infected wound, and abscesses should be drained. Patients should be placed in a quiet room and observed closely for development of complications or unexpected changes in the course of the disease. While it is a good general principle to disturb patients as little as possible, vital signs must be monitored and aspiration must be averted by positioning the patient carefully and by aspirating nasopharyngeal secretions frequently. Care must be taken to prevent development of decubitus ulcers or contractures, but many routine nursing procedures should be omitted because they may precipitate uncomfortable or dangerous spasms. Initially, nutrition is not a major consideration, and fluid and electrolyte balance should be maintained over the first several days by administration of appropriate solutions intravenously, accompanied by careful recording of intake and output. Patients with severe tetanus are in an intense catabolic state, and may have tremendous fluid losses. Early consideration should be given to intravenous hyperalimentation as a means of meeting the nutritional requirements of these patients.

Antiserum Antiserum does not neutralize tetanus toxin fixed in the central nervous system, and does little to ameliorate symptoms already present at the time of admission. However, the case/fatality ratio in mild to moderately severe disease is reduced significantly when antiserum is administered early. Human tetanus immune globulin (TIG) is generally available in the United States, and is far superior to equine antiserum. Because its half-life is about 25 days, only one dose of 3000 to 10,000 units intramuscularly is recommended, even though as little as 500 units may be equally effective. Local infiltration at the site of the wound is of no proved value, but intrathecal injections may prove to be effective after more careful study. Hypersensitivity reactions do not occur with TIG, obviating the need for pretreatment testing.

If human antitoxin is not available, a single dose of equine antiserum should be given after the patient has been tested for hypersensitivity to horse serum. Although the dosage of heterologous antitoxin often recommended for adults is 100,000 to 200,000 units, 10,000 units is probably optimal. Anaphylaxis can occur despite negative sensitivity tests, and patients must be observed carefully to institute treatment at the first sign of an anaphylactic reaction. Up to 25 percent of patients develop delayed reactions including serum sickness after equine antitoxin. Occasionally, serious neurologic complications accompany other manifestations of serum sickness.

Active immunization of patients with tetanus is necessary, because the disease does not confer natural immunity. However, there is no need to begin primary immunization until the patient has recovered.

Management of muscle spasms Muscle relaxation is the key to therapy, but mild sedation is desirable also because it reduces the effect of sensory stimuli. Ideally, this should be accomplished without significantly affecting respiration. Although a variety of agents have been used in the treatment of tetanus, none has achieved universal acceptance. Among the barbiturates, phenobarbital, in adult doses of 50 to 100 mg every 3 to 6 h, produces adequate sedation which may suffice in the management of mild tetanus. When rapid action is required, amylbarbital or pentobarbital, 50 to 200 mg intravenously, may be used. Frequent and severe spasms cannot be managed with barbiturates alone, because the dosage required

for control leads to unconsciousness and suppressed respiration. For this reason, muscle relaxants usually are used, either alone or in combination with barbiturates, in the treatment of moderate or severe tetanus. Electromyographic studies have shown that the phenothiazines effectively produce relaxation while sparing the sensorium and respirations. Chlorpromazine, in doses of 200 to 300 mg a day, minimizes rigidity and decreases the frequency of spasms. Diazepam, in adult doses of 40 to 120 mg a day, is very effective in the treatment of tetanus; it acts quickly, relieves rigidity, and has significant sedative effect without depressing respiration. Given alone to patients with moderately severe disease, diazepam has been shown to lower oxygen consumption from levels that are three to five times normal to near normal. In combination with other drugs, diazepam may significantly reduce mortality in nonneonates with severe tetanus. Other drugs which have been employed extensively include mephenesin, meprobamate, paraldehyde, and chloral hydrate.

Another approach to the management of muscle spasms involves the use of neuromuscular blocking agents such as tubocurare or pancuronium. This method can be used only where facilities and personnel are available to provide controlled mechanical ventilation for the paralyzed patient. It should be reserved for treatment of severe tetanus that is not adequately controlled by other measures. In centers with a team experienced in handling these patients, this approach, in conjunction with meticulous attention to other details of care, has produced encouraging results.

Tracheostomy Tracheostomy has an important role in the management of tetanus. It protects against suffocation due to laryngospasm, reduces the risk of aspiration, and facilitates mechanical assistance of ventilation. While most patients with mild tetanus and some with more severe disease can be managed without it, all patients should be considered candidates for tracheostomy, and the necessary equipment should be at the bedside. Where secretions are copious or respiration has been compromised, the need for tracheostomy should be recognized early, and whenever possible it should be performed electively rather than as an emergency.

Other measures Although antibiotics are frequently prescribed to treat the infected wound and prevent toxin production, there is no indication that they influence the disease favorably. If antibiotics are used, penicillin G is the drug of choice because it is highly effective against the tetanus bacillus, and its limited spectrum is less likely to predispose patients to superinfections. Appropriate cultures to detect complicating infections should be obtained periodically throughout the course of the disease, and specific antibiotics prescribed when indicated. Adrenocortical steroids have been used empirically in the treatment of tetanus, but there is no experimental or clinical evidence to support their effectiveness. Likewise, beneficial results have been claimed for hyperbaric oxygen, but insufficient information is available to evaluate its potential.

PREVENTION *Clostridium tetani* is so ubiquitous in nature that the only hope for prevention of tetanus lies in massive immunization programs. Effective active immunization is possible, and if applied universally, according to recommendations, tetanus could be virtually eliminated. Even tetanus neonatorum could be prevented, because infants are protected by antibody which passes the placental barrier. Two types of tetanus toxoids are available for immunization, a fluid and an adsorbed form. The adsorbed toxoid is preferred because it pro duces higher antitoxin titers and longer-lasting immunity. Immunization failures are exceedingly rare.

According to current recommendations, children 2 months to 6 years of age should be immunized with diphtheria and tetanus toxoids and pertussis vaccine (DPT). Ideally, the first dose should be administered within 2 or 3 months of birth, the second and third should follow at 4- to 6-week intervals, and the fourth dose should be given 1 year after the third. Schoolchildren and adults should be immunized with three doses of adult-type tetanus and diphtheria toxoids (Td). The second dose should be given 4 to 6 weeks after the first, and the third 6 months to 1 year after the second. A booster of DPT is recommended for children at the time of entrance into kindergarten or elementary school. Thereafter and for everyone else who has received a primary immunization series, routine boosters of Td should be given every 10 years. Side effects are uncommon after the primary series, but occur more frequently in persons who have received an excessive number of booster injections. Reactions usually take the form of local swelling, erythema, lymphadenopathy, and fever, but on rare occasions more severe hypersensitivity reactions occur.

In the management of wounds, the question of prophylaxis against tetanus frequently arises. Because active immunization is so effective, a reliable immunization history can greatly simplify the problem. If a patient has received three or more doses of toxoid, antiserum need not be given, and a toxoid booster is required only if more than 5 to 10 years has elapsed since the last dose. The shorter interval pertains for all but clean, minor wounds. In all other instances, the decision must be made on an individual basis, taking into consideration the characteristics of the wound, the conditions under which it was incurred, its age, and the patient's previous active immunization against tetanus. Table 139-1 provides guidelines which may be useful in making appropriate decisions about tetanus prophylaxis. For patients who have received fewer than two doses of toxoid, the primary immunization series should be completed in the succeeding weeks to months.

When passive immunization is contemplated, TIG is preferred to horse serum because it offers longer protection and freedom from serious reactions. The currently recommended prophylactic dose for adults is 250 units intramuscularly, which ensures a protective level of antitoxin in the plasma (> 0.01 unit per milliliter) for as long as 4 weeks. If TIG is not available, equine antitoxin in doses of 3000 to 6000 units should be administered after careful screening for sensitivity to horse serum. When both toxoid and antitoxin are indicated, they can be given simultaneously, but separate syringes and separate injection sites should be used.

Prompt and adequate care of wounds is also important in preventing tetanus. They should be cleaned carefully, and foreign bodies or necrotic, devitalized tissue should be removed. Administration of tetracycline or penicillin is advocated by some to prevent multiplication of *C. tetani*, but tetanus may

occur in spite of prophylactic antibiotics, and their role in the prevention of tetanus has not been established. However, severe wounds should be examined regularly and treated promptly with antimicrobials if infection develops.

PROGNOSIS The overall case/fatality ratio of tetanus is variable, but in the United States it ranges between 40 and 60 percent. This reflects the fact that the incidence of tetanus is eight to ten times greater among people over 60 compared with people 10 to 20 years of age, and the mortality rate is 25 to 50 times greater in the elderly. Neonatal tetanus is uncommon in this country but is fatal in more than 60 percent of cases. The shorter the incubation period and onset time, the poorer the prognosis in tetanus. Three-fourths of the deaths occur within the first week, primarily from pulmonary infection, aspiration, or pulmonary embolization. Survivors recover completely, but remain susceptible to the disease unless actively immunized with tetanus toxoid.

REFERENCES

BLAKE PA et al: Serologic therapy of tetanus in the United States. JAMA 235:42, 1976

COCHLIN DL: Dystonic reactions due to metoclopramide and phenothiazines resembling tetanus. Br J Clin Pract 28:201, 1974

FURSTE W: Four keys to 100 percent success in tetanus prophylaxis. Am J Surg 128:616, 1974

———, WHEELER W: Tetanus: A team disease, in *Current Problems in Surgery*. Chicago, Year Book, 1972

TSUEDA K et al: Cardiovascular manifestations of tetanus. Anesthesiology 40:588, 1974

140
BOTULISM

HARRY N. BEATY
ROBERT W. GRAEBNER

DEFINITION Botulism is an acute form of poisoning which results from ingestion of a toxin produced by *Clostridium botulinum*. The illness is characterized by progressive descending muscle paralysis, and is often fatal.

HISTORY AND EPIDEMIOLOGY The disease was first recognized over 200 years ago by South German physicians who adopted the term *botulismus* for the often fatal syndrome which sometimes followed the consumption of spoiled sausage (*botulus* is Latin for sausage). Botulism was rare in the United States before World War I. The growth of commercial and home canning at this time led to a great increase in cases. A series of studies by K. F. Meyer and his associates in the early 1920s defined the habitat of *C. botulinum*, the foods often incriminated, and the conditions necessary for the destruction of *C. botulinum* spores. This knowledge led to the virtual elimination of botulism from the commercial canning industry, and most cases of clinical botulism now follow consumption of improperly canned, home-preserved foods. However, the need for constant surveillance is emphasized by periodic outbreaks of botulism caused by commercially processed foods. For example, in 1977, 59 people developed botulism after eating home-canned peppers in a restaurant in Pontiac, Michigan; and in 1978, 32 people manifested the disease after dining at a country club in Clovis, New Mexico. These are the largest outbreaks ever reported in the United States, and contrast sharply with the usual situation in which fewer than three individuals are affected after eating home-canned foods.

TABLE 139-1
Guidelines for tetanus prophylaxis

Active immunization	Toxoid	Antitoxin	
		Minor wound*	Other wounds
Uncertain	Yes	No	Yes
None	Yes	No	Yes
< 3 doses	Yes	No	Yes‡
≥ 3 doses	No†	No	No

* *Fresh, clean, minor wounds incurred in a setting unlikely to cause tetanus.*
† *Unless more than 10 years since last dose.*
‡ *Except in patients who have received at least two previous doses of toxoid and have fresh non-tetanus-prone wounds.*

ETIOLOGY *Clostridium botulinum* is a strictly anaerobic, spore-forming, gram-positive rod which elaborates a potent exotoxin during growth and autolysis. Morphologically and culturally similar strains are differentiated into types A, B, C, D, E, or F on the basis of antigenic characteristics of the toxin each produces. Type A, B, and E toxins have been implicated most frequently in human disease in the United States. Only two outbreaks of type F botulism have been reported. Types C and D produce disease almost exclusively in animals, including wild waterfowl, cattle, horses, and mink.

Type A and B spores are widely distributed in soil throughout the world. Type A spores are most common in the United States, especially along the Pacific Coast and the Rocky Mountain states. Type B spores have been found more frequently in the Eastern states and in Europe. Type E spores have been demonstrated in lakeshore mud, coastal sand, and sea-bottom silt in northern latitudes. Fish apparently contaminate their intestinal tracts with these spores, which accounts for the high incidence of type E strains in fish-borne botulism. Type F spores have been found in marine sediments collected off the coast of California and Oregon and in salmon taken from the Columbia River.

Botulinus toxins are the most potent poisons known. Types A through F have been purified and identified as simple proteins. Although they differ in terms of antigenicity, molecular size, electrophoretic mobility, and amino acid content, they appear to have a similar effect on neuromuscular transmission. Pharmacologic differences are manifested by the variable susceptibility of specific animal species to the different toxins.

Spores of *C. botulinum* can withstand 100°C for several hours. Moist heat at 120°C for 30 min will destroy spores of all types, but the toxins are considerably more heat-labile. All varieties of toxin are destroyed by boiling for 10 min, or by temperatures of 80°C for 30 min.

PATHOGENESIS Most human botulism follows the ingestion of foodstuffs contaminated with preformed botulinus toxin. Rarely, wounds infected with *C. botulinum* have been the portal of entry of the toxin. Until recently, there was convincing evidence that the botulinus bacillus produces toxin in the human gastrointestinal tract. That is still the case in adults, but the newly recognized syndrome of infant botulism results from ingestion of *C. botulinum* followed by sporulation and toxin production. Symptoms are slowly progressive because toxin is absorbed as it is produced rather than all at once, which is the case when toxin is ingested in contaminated food. Clinical botulism can occur when the following conditions are met: (1) a food product is contaminated with viable *C. botulinum* bacilli or spores; (2) proper conditions for germination of the spores exist; (3) time and conditions permit production of toxin before eating; (4) the food is not heated or is heated insufficiently to destroy botulinus toxin; and (5) the toxin-containing food is ingested by a susceptible host (Table 140-1). Though a relatively anaerobic environment and temperatures above 30°C (86°F) are optimal for toxin production, strict anaerobic conditions are not necessary and toxin production by some type E strains has been observed at temperatures as low as 6°C (42.8°F).

Although a variety of home-processed foods have been sources of botulism in the United States, certain foods seem to be safer than others. This may be because low pH (acidity) inhibits germination of spores and, therefore, toxin production. Commercially processed smoked fish, tuna, peppers, and soup (vichyssoise) have been implicated in outbreaks of botulism. Contaminated foods may appear putrefied, but frequently look and taste perfectly normal, regardless of toxin type. Honey has been proved to be the source of *C. botulinum* in a number of cases of infant botulism. This and the finding of botulinal organisms in a number of random samples of honey tested have led to the recommendation that honey not be fed to children less than 1 year old. None of the samples tested contained botulinus toxin, so honey remains a safe food for older children and adults.

Botulinus toxins are absorbed primarily in the stomach and upper part of the small intestine. The toxins are large protein molecules which are absorbed after they have been reduced in size by proteolytic enzymes which do not destroy activity. In fact, the toxicity of type E toxin may be enhanced by tryptic digestion. Either absorption is incomplete or toxins are inactivated partially by digestion, because the amount of toxin which appears in the bloodstream is variable, and in animals the lethal dose orally is 1000 times greater than the lethal dose intravenously. Toxin which reaches the lower part of the small intestine and colon may be absorbed slowly, which probably accounts for the delayed onset and the prolonged symptoms observed in many patients.

Botulinus toxins exert their major effect by blocking neuromuscular transmission in cholinergic nerve fibers. They either inhibit the release of acetylcholine or bind with it at or near its site of release within presynaptic clefts. Muscle reactivity to acetylcholine applied directly to the motor end plate is unimpaired. Central nervous system cholinergic pathways do not appear to be affected significantly in human beings.

CLINICAL MANIFESTATIONS Botulism may vary from a mild illness for which patients seek no medical advice to a fulminant disease which ends in death within 24 h. Symptoms usually begin 12 to 36 h after ingestion of toxin, although the extremes of 3 h to 14 days are recorded. In general, the earlier the symptoms appear, the more serious the disease.

The commonest symptoms are ocular; diplopia, blurred vision, and photophobia are frequently the first to appear. Bulbar weakness is manifested by dysphonia, dysarthria, dysphagia, and weakness of the tongue. Symmetric paralysis of the extremities appears, and may progress rapidly in a descending or ascending manner. Weakness of the respiratory muscles may occur early, but this is often asymptomatic until function is moderately impaired.

Impairment of cholinergic autonomic transmission may result in constipation, urinary retention, and reduced salivation and lacrimation. Nausea and vomiting are early symptoms in half the patients, but the absence of these symptoms does not rule out botulism. Gastrointestinal symptoms are more common in type B and E disease than in type A. Some patients with type B disease may have minimal weakness but marked constipation and decreased secretions.

TABLE 140-1
Important factors in the pathogenesis of botulism

SPORES

1 Survive at 6°C (42.8°F) for several months
2 Can withstand boiling for several hours
3 Destroyed at 120°C (248°F) after 30 min

TOXIN PRODUCTION

1 Strict anaerobic conditions not always required
2 Can occur at 6°C (42.8°F)
3 Optimal temperature 30°C (86°F)
4 Reduced at low pH

TOXIN

1 Destroyed at 80°C (176°F) after 30 min or 100°C for 10 min
2 Unstable at high pH
3 Type E toxin activated by trypsin

On examination patients are usually alert, oriented, and afebrile, even with severe disease. Ocular signs include ptosis, weakness of extraocular motion, and in some patients failure of accommodation. The pupils are normal in many patients, but in some cases may react sluggishly or may be dilated and unreactive to light. Widespread neuromuscular block results in symmetric flaccid weakness of the palate, tongue, larynx, respiratory muscles, and extremities. Severe paralytic ileus and bladder distention may be present. Deep-tendon reflexes are intact in milder cases, but if significant paralysis is present they are reduced or absent. No pathologic reflexes are detectable. Findings on sensory examination are always entirely normal. Some patients have apparent gait disturbances and incoordination, but this is due to generalized weakness.

Once symptoms are noted, the disease may progress rapidly over several days, with significant changes in status occurring at hourly intervals. A period of stabilization is then followed by gradual recovery over a period of days to months, depending on the severity of intoxication. The mechanism of recovery is not well understood. In wound botulism the patient may be febrile, but the clinical manifestations are otherwise similar. A 10- to 14-day incubation period is common from the time of infection to the onset of toxic symptoms. In the infant form of botulism, constipation is usually the first manifestation; slowly progressive weakness of skeletal muscles, poor feeding, and "floppiness" follow.

LABORATORY FINDINGS Routine laboratory studies do not aid in diagnosing botulism. When botulism is suspected, public health authorities should be consulted to assist in special studies to confirm the diagnosis. Specimens of blood, feces, and gastric contents, as well as suspected foods and their containers, should be obtained. Because of the extreme potency of botulinus toxin, careful collection and laboratory precautions should be used. The food, stool, and serum should be studied for the presence of toxin by injecting extracts intraperitoneally into mice. If toxin is present, the animals will develop botulism and die within 24 h. Mice protected by specific antiserum will survive. The food and stool should be submitted for special anaerobic culture. This battery of tests will result in an overall case recognition rate of about 85 percent. Immunofluorescent techniques are useful for the early recognition of the organisms. If wound botulism is suspected, the exudate should be submitted for culture and toxin analysis.

The spinal fluid is always normal. Electrocardiographic abnormalities, including minor disturbances in conduction, nonspecific T-wave and ST-segment changes, and various disorders of rhythm, have been described. Electrodiagnostic studies have been shown to be of value in differentiating botulism from other paralytic diseases. The evoked motor action potential may be of low voltage, but will facilitate with tetanic stimulation in a manner similar to the myasthenic syndrome (Eaton-Lambert syndrome). Electromyography may show small, short-duration, overly abundant motor units. In severe cases, denervation can occur, resulting in fibrillation activity after several weeks.

DIFFERENTIAL DIAGNOSIS Botulism must be differentiated from other conditions that produce generalized paralysis. In the Guillain-Barré syndrome, mild sensory abnormalities are nearly always present, and the spinal fluid protein is often elevated. The variant of the Guillain-Barré syndrome with ophthalmoplegia, areflexia, and ataxia (Fisher's syndrome) may prove particularly confusing. The course of myasthenia gravis is seldom so acute, and the deep tendon reflexes and pupils are normal. Some patients with botulism may show mild improvement after injection of edrophonium (Tensilon), but this im-

provement is not of the magnitude seen in myasthenia gravis. In tick paralysis the weakness is generally of an ascending pattern, patients may have paresthesias, and a tick is found. In diphtheria, palatal weakness is frequently the first symptom, and a history of prior pharyngitis may be obtained. Cutaneous diphtheria can be differentiated from wound botulism by appropriate cultures. In poliomyelitis the spinal fluid is abnormal and the weakness is often asymmetric and spares the ocular muscles. Vascular accidents of the brainstem can be recognized by associated neurologic signs. Belladonna poisoning presents with markedly dilated pupils and delirium. In organophosphate poisoning the pupils are markedly miotic. Shellfish poisoning, aminoglycoside antibiotic paralysis, and familial periodic paralysis might also prove confusing.

Patients with marked dry mouth may develop a picture simulating pharyngitis. Patients with gastrointestinal complaints and ileus may appear to have other forms of food poisoning or intestinal obstruction.

TREATMENT The most immediate threat to the survival of patients with botulism is respiratory failure. Patients with symptoms or known exposure should be hospitalized. Close observation is essential, and vital capacity should be measured frequently. If respiratory insufficiency develops, the patient may require assisted ventilation with a respirator. Respiratory difficulties may develop rapidly; elective tracheostomy should be performed before onset of respiratory failure, and may be needed to manage secretions even if ventilation is otherwise adequate. Some milder cases may be managed with endotracheal intubation.

If there is no ileus, cathartics and enemas should be given to remove unabsorbed toxin from the intestine, but magnesium citrate and magnesium sulfate should not be given, as the magnesium may potentiate the neuromuscular block produced by botulinus toxin. Nasogastric suction and intravenous hyperalimentation may be needed if ileus is severe. If the bladder is atonic a catheter will be required. Meticulous nursing care and physical therapy are essential to prevent complications.

As soon as the diagnosis of botulism is suspected, the patient should be tested for hypersensitivity to horse serum and treated with trivalent ABE antitoxin (Connaught), which is available from public health authorities. Type-specific antitoxin has been shown to be of benefit in several outbreaks of type E intoxication, but the value in type A and B outbreaks is less certain, particularly when paralysis has already occurred. Nonfatal hypersensitivity reactions occur in 15 to 20 percent of patients receiving the equine antitoxin, and those that react to a test dose must be desensitized prior to further treatment.

Because there is little evidence that *C. botulinum* can multiply in the gastrointestinal tract of adults, antibiotics should be reserved for specific infectious complications. In infant botulism, where multiplication of ingested organisms may be a factor, antibiotics have been ineffective in eradicating the organism, though this eventually may occur spontaneously. The value of antibiotic therapy in wound botulism has not been determined. It is essential that public health officials be notified so that toxin-containing foods can be confiscated and so that those with possible exposure can be notified.

A number of reports have appeared since 1967 describing the use of guanidine hydrochloride in the treatment of botulism. This drug presumably acts by enhancing the release of acetylcholine from terminal nerve fibers. About two-thirds of the reported cases have shown some improvement with oral doses of 15 to 50 mg/kg per day, but the drug seems ineffective in those patients with severe respiratory impairment, and probably has no effect on mortality rate. Dose-related side effects include gastrointestinal upset, paresthesias, and fasciculations. Idiosyncratic reactions include cardiac arrhythmias and blood dycrasias.

PROGNOSIS The current mortality rate of botulism in the United States is about 10 percent, with type A outbreaks having somewhat higher mortality than types B and E. Death is due to complications such as respiratory failure and pneumonia. With rapid diagnosis and aggressive supportive care, even severely involved patients can recover fully. Some patients may have mild residual weakness due to denervation atrophy. Artificial respiratory support may be required for many months, and clinical weakness and autonomic symptoms may be noted for as long as 1 year after the onset of disease.

REFERENCES

ARNON SS et al: Infant botulism: Epidemiological, clinical, and laboratory aspects. JAMA 237:1946, 1977

BLACK RE, ARNON SS: Botulism in the United States, 1976. J Infect Dis 135:829, 1977

CENTER FOR DISEASE CONTROL: *Botulism in the United States, 1899–1973. Handbook for Epidemiologists, Clinicians, and Laboratory Workers.* June 1974

CHERINGTON M: Botulism: Ten-year experience. Arch Neurol 30:432, 1974

DOWELL VR et al: Coproexamination for botulinal toxin and *Clostridium botulinum:* A new procedure for laboratory diagnosis of botulism. JAMA 238:1829, 1977

FAICH GA et al: Failure of guanidine therapy in botulism A. N Engl J Med 285:773, 1971

KOENIG MC et al: Type B botulism in man. Am J Med 42:208, 1967

MERSON MH, DOWELL VR: Epidemiologic, clinical and laboratory aspects of wound botulism. N Engl J Med 289:1005, 1973

WERNER SB, CHIN J: Botulism—diagnosis, management and public health considerations. Calif Med 118:84, 1973

141
OTHER CLOSTRIDIAL INFECTIONS

EDWARD W. HOOK
MERLE A. SANDE

INTRODUCTION Bacteria of the genus *Clostridium* are normal inhabitants of soil and the gastrointestinal tracts of humans and animals. Most of the species that have been described are saprophytic, but some are pathogenic for humans and animals, usually under conditions of lowered host and tissue resistance. Infections with these organisms are often associated with profound systemic manifestations, and all pathogenic clostridia, except *C. tetani* and *C. botulinum,* are capable of causing extensive tissue destruction. Diseases caused by these other clostridia are gas gangrene, cellulitis, postabortal and puerperal sepsis, and, on occasion, pneumonia, empyema, peritonitis, meningitis, endocarditis, osteomyelitis, and arthritis. Ingestion of food contaminated with *C. perfringens* type A is a common cause of enterocolitis, and *C. difficile* has recently been implicated in antibiotic-induced (clindamycin) pseudomembranous colitis.

ETIOLOGY Wounds complicated by gas gangrene usually contain a mixture of pathogenic and saprophytic clostridia, often including *C. tetani,* as well as a variety of other bacteria. *Clostridium perfringens,* the most common, *C. novyi,* or *C. septicum* can be cultured from most cases of gas gangrene and clostridial cellulitis, and *C. perfringens* causes virtually all clostridial infections of the uterus. *Clostridium bifermentans, C. histolyticum,* and *C. fallax* are less virulent organisms that occasionally cause gas gangrene but are more commonly associated with localized cellulitis. Proliferation of *C. botulinum* in

wounds occasionally leads to clinical manifestations of botulism (Chap. 140).

The clostridia of gas gangrene and related infections are anaerobic or microaerophilic gram-positive bacilli that produce abundant gas in artificial media and form subterminal endospores. *Clostridium perfringens* is encapsulated and nonmotile, rarely sporulates in artificial media, and produces spores that can usually be destroyed by boiling.

Clostridium difficile has been isolated in large numbers from stools of patients with antibiotic-associated pseudomembranous colitis. This organism produces a toxin that is destructive to the intestinal mucosa and is usually resistant to clindamycin, the antibiotic most commonly implicated in enterocolitis.

EPIDEMIOLOGY AND PATHOGENESIS Clostridia can be cultured from one-third to two-thirds of severe traumatic wounds, but gas gangrene develops in only an occasional case. The most important prerequisite for the conversion of clostridial contamination of a wound to a progressive infection is an environment with low oxidation-reduction potential, which permits spore germination and anaerobic growth. Local oxidation-reduction potential can be reduced by failure of the blood supply to a contaminated area, by the presence of foreign bodies such as clothing, soil, or fragments of metal or wood, or by the multiplication of other bacteria in the wound. Once multiplication and toxin production are established, rapid invasion and destruction of healthy tissue follow.

The pathogenicity of clostridia is related to the capacity of these organisms to form exotoxins which destroy tissue cells. The nature and amount of toxins vary considerably for different species and strains. For example, at least 12 different extracellular *toxins* are produced by *C. perfringens.* Alpha toxin, a lecithinase, is clearly the most important and is the principal tissue-destroying, hemolytic, and lethal toxin. Other *C. perfringens* products include collagenase, hyaluronidase, hemolytic theta toxin, leukocidin, deoxyribonuclease, and fibrinolysin.

Gas gangrene is characterized by marked systemic symptoms and a local reaction with extensive necrotizing myositis, edema, thrombosis of small vessels, interstitial gas bubbles, and minimal infiltration by leukocytes. The local reaction in infected tissue can be explained by the action of clostridial toxins, especially alpha toxin, but the factors responsible for the systemic reaction are unknown. Alpha toxin, or other clostridial toxins, have not been demonstrated in circulating blood during the course of severe clostridial myonecrosis.

The toxin responsible for antibiotic-associated pseudomembranous colitis has not been completely characterized. It is found in high titer in cell-free filtrates of feces from patients with this disease. The toxin is produced by *C. difficile* which is usually resistant to clindamycin and proliferates in the colon when the antibiotic-sensitive flora is suppressed. The toxin is heat-labile and cytopathic for certain cells in culture, and it produces an increase in vascular permeability and hemorrhage after injection intradermally in rabbits. Pseudomembranous colitis can be produced by introducing the toxin or the organism into the cecum of hamsters or by treating hamsters with clindamycin. The toxic effects can be blocked by either gas-gangrene equine antitoxin or *C. sordellii* antitoxin; the latter has been shown to cross-react with toxin produced by *C. difficile.*

CLINICAL MANIFESTATIONS **Clostridial myonecrosis (gas gangrene, clostridial myositis)** Gas gangrene develops in anoxic devitalized tissues in which the arterial circulation has been compromised by trauma, constricting tourniquets or casts, or obliterative arterial disease. Infection is most frequent after extensive injury to skeletal muscle, particularly of the thigh and buttock, and is more common in wounds complicated by compound fractures or lodgment of foreign bodies. It may also follow surgical procedures, especially those involving the large bowel and rectum; amputation of ischemic limbs; and reconstructive surgery of the hip. Gas gangrene has also been described following intramuscular injection, especially injection of epinephrine. Minor trauma also occasionally activates clostridial spores dormant in scar tissue and leads to development of myonecrosis years after original injury. Once infection is established, it rapidly spreads to involve healthy muscle undamaged by previous trauma or ischemia.

The incubation period is usually 1 to 4 days but may vary from 3 h to 6 weeks or longer. The earliest symptom is sudden, severe pain in the injured part which may develop an intense "woody hard" edema. The distal portion of an involved limb becomes cold and edematous within a few hours, and eventually pulseless and gangrenous. The wound drains a watery, brown, or hemorrhagic material which may have a peculiar sweet odor. The appearance of the wound is usually not that of a pyogenic inflammatory lesion. Depending on the duration of the process, the surrounding skin may be normal, white, and tense, or dusky brown and reddish. Vesicles or hemorrhagic bullae may develop, particularly in *C. septicum* infections. Gas is usually not detectable in the tissues by palpation except in advanced lesions, although it may be visible easily by x-ray. Occasionally, tiny bubbles may be seen in the discharge from the wound; rarely, crepitation can be detected at an early stage by auscultation. The involved muscle appears dark red or black, may herniate through the wound, and is noncontractile when stimulated.

Systemic manifestations developing shortly after onset of severe pain and swelling of an injured extremity strongly suggest gas gangrene. The patient is prostrated, pale, and motionless but is usually well oriented, alert, and extremely apprehensive. The temperature usually does not exceed 38.3°C (101°F) and may be normal. As the illness progresses, there may be anorexia, vomiting, profuse watery or bloody diarrhea, and eventually circulatory collapse. The pulse rate usually exceeds 120 beats per minute and is elevated out of proportion to the temperature. Massive intravascular hemolysis is rare in patients with clostridial myositis. Pericardial effusion is sometimes noted. Delirium and coma may precede death, but more commonly the patient dies suddenly several days after onset of illness, often during surgery or anesthesia. Acute renal failure is occasionally a late complication.

Gas gangrene must be differentiated from nonclostridial infections of gangrenous limbs caused by anaerobic streptococci, aerobic gas-forming coliform bacilli (most commonly *Escherichia coli*), *Bacteroides* species, and group A streptococci.

Clostridial cellulitis　This is a relatively benign infection of skin and subcutaneous tissues that occurs in a small proportion of wounds contaminated with pathogenic clostridia. The disease is characterized by spreading necrosis of superficial tissues and a profuse, foul-smelling, brown, seropurulent exudate. Gas, which crepitates on palpation, invariably forms in the subcutaneous tissues and may involve an entire limb or form a localized gas pocket. In clostridial cellulitis, the underlying skeletal muscle is not involved, pain is not severe, and the only systemic manifestations are slight fever and moderate tachycardia. It can usually be differentiated from group A streptococcal cellulitis by the presence of subcutaneous gas and the absence of erythema.

Postabortal and puerperal sepsis　Uterine infections with *C. perfringens* usually occur after incomplete abortions induced under unsterile conditions and occasionally after spontaneous abortions, prolonged labor at term, ruptured membranes, or operative interference with pregnancy. The organisms presumably invade the damaged endometrium through the retained products of conception. The earliest symptoms may be related to instrumentation and consist of metrorrhagia, suprapubic and back pain, chills, and fever. Fever of 37.8 to 39.4°C (100 to 103°F), often with chills, usually recurs several days after abortion, but the incubation period can be as short as 6 h. Vaginal bleeding is almost invariably present, and there is often a brown, foul-smelling, vaginal discharge containing necrotic tissue. The cervix is soft and patulous, and the uterus and adnexae are usually very tender. The lower abdominal wall is often tense, or signs of generalized peritonitis may be present, secondary to perforation of the uterus or parametrial extension of infection. Nausea, vomiting, and profuse diarrhea are often prominent.

Systemic manifestations may appear with dramatic suddenness. Massive intravascular hemolysis, accompanied by hemoglobinemia, hemoglobinuria, and jaundice, may be the most striking feature of the disease. Icterus may appear within hours after onset of illness. As in gas gangrene, the clinical picture may be dominated by circulatory collapse with hypotension, extreme tachycardia, cyanosis, hyperpnea, and pulmonary edema. Despite severe prostration, the patient is frequently well oriented, alert, and apprehensive. The mortality rate in postabortal or puerperal sepsis caused by *C. perfringens* and associated with intense hemolysis is 40 to 70 percent. Death may occur a few hours after onset or may be delayed for days. Acute renal failure secondary to shock, dehydration, or hemolysis occurs frequently.

Unusual local complications of uterine infection are gas gangrene of the vagina and rectum and clostridial cellulitis of the anterior abdominal wall following cesarean section or hysterectomy. At times, the infectious process is confined to the endometrium and myometrium with intrauterine gas formation (physometra).

Septic abortion with *C. perfringens* bacteremia without overt hemolysis is a more common occurrence than bacteremia with gross hemolysis, as described above. Death is unusual in the absence of hemolysis.

Diseases to be considered in the *differential diagnosis* include perforated uterus, ruptured ectopic pregnancy, ingestion of toxic abortifacients, septic endometritis caused by aerobic or anaerobic streptococci, enteric bacilli or other microorganisms, pelvic thrombophlebitis with septic pulmonary emboli, acute hepatic necrosis of pregnancy, and sickle-cell crisis.

***Clostridium perfringens* food poisoning**　Meat and meat products contaminated with *C. perfringens* type A are frequently responsible for outbreaks of acute gastroenteritis. In 1976 in the United States, *C. perfringens* accounted for 14.2 percent of cases in reported foodborne outbreaks.

Most outbreaks of *C. perfringens* food poisoning have been associated with the ingestion of meat or poultry dishes. Most market meats and poultry are heavily contaminated, and the organism can be isolated with ease from soil, water, air, and human or animal feces. The usual story is that the food has been prepared and cooked 24 h or more before consumption, allowed to cool slowly at room temperature, and then served either cold or warmed. During this period of incubation, contaminating spores which have survived cooking germinate, and clostridia grow to large numbers sufficient to constitute an infectious inoculum. *Clostridium perfringens* food poisoning can be reproduced experimentally in humans by feeding the actively growing organisms which apparently multiply and sporulate in the small intestine. Sporulation is associated with the production of an enterotoxin in situ.

Typical symptoms of diarrhea with abdominal pain and cramps develop 6 to 24 h after ingestion of meat (especially beef and poultry), stew, or soup which has been stored at a warm temperature for several hours after cooking. Nausea occurs occasionally, but vomiting is rare. Systemic manifestations are usually absent, and recovery is uneventful after 12 to 24 h.

A severe form of clostridial infection termed *enteritis necrotans* was observed in Germany after World War II. This disease was characterized by hemorrhagic necrosis of the small intestine, bloody diarrhea, severe dehydration, shock, and death. A similar infection termed *necrotizing jejunitis* has been described in natives of New Guinea who had eaten inadequately cooked pork.

Antibiotic-associated colitis Diarrhea has been reported in up to 20 percent of patients receiving clindamycin. In one study up to one-half of these patients were found to have evidence of pseudomembranous colitis on proctoscopic examination although the usual rate is much less. *Clostridium difficile* has been implicated as the etiologic agent, but whether this organism accounts for all or only a portion of the cases has not been established. Symptoms of cramping, lower abdominal pain, fever, and diarrhea are common. Fever and cramps precede or coincide with the onset of diarrhea which usually develops between the fourth and ninth days of clindamycin therapy. In some cases, colitis develops within 5 days after discontinuation of the drug. The diarrhea is usually watery but rarely bloody. The symptoms usually subside within a week after administration of clindamycin is discontinued; however, the diarrhea may become protracted, lasting up to 2 to 4 weeks especially if administration of the drug is continued. In patients with severe protracted diarrhea, electrolyte imbalance, protein loss, and death may occur, especially in patients with significant underlying disease. Patients with pseudomembranous colitis occasionally will have associated abdominal tenderness with rebound and leukocytosis. Toxic megacolon is a rare complication. Although clindamycin has received the most attention, other antibiotics such as lincomycin, ampicillin, cephalexin, tetracyclines, and chloramphenicol also produce diarrhea and have been implicated as a cause of pseudomembranous colitis. The role of clostridia in diarrheal disease associated with these agents has not been completely defined, although the *C. difficile* toxin has been found in ampicillin-associated colitis.

Miscellaneous clostridial infections Clostridia can be isolated from bile obtained at elective cholecystectomy in patients without symptoms of clostridial infection. Clostridial cellulitis or myonecrosis may occasionally follow surgical procedures, particularly surgery on the gastrointestinal tract or gallbladder. Pathogenic clostridia are occasionally introduced into the abdomen, thoracic cavity, or cranium through penetrating wounds. Primary pneumonia in the absence of a penetrating wound or distant focus has been described. Clostridial pleurisy may involve the underlying lung but is usually an indolent localized infection with minimal systemic manifestations. Meningitis is usually secondary to a puncture wound of the skull and is often associated with a necrotizing cerebritis. Clostridial peritonitis may occur spontaneously but usually follows perforation of the gallbladder, appendix, or other viscus and is usually rapidly fatal.

Clostridial septicemia also develops occasionally in patients with aplastic anemia or far-advanced neoplastic disease, including leukemias, lymphomas, and metastatic solid tumors. Over two-thirds of these patients have been receiving antineo-

plastic chemotherapy or radiation therapy. The primary site of invasion is usually the gastrointestinal tract which is frequently extensively involved by the neoplastic process. Abdominal surgical procedures, endoscopy, small-bowel series, and paracentesis have been reported to predispose to sepsis in these patients. The course of the disease is rapid, death often occurring within 24 h after onset of recognizable infection. Hypotension, hyperpyrexia, and dyspnea are the most common clinical manifestations. Jaundice and hemolysis occur occasionally. Cellulitis, with or without crepitation, may appear in the flanks and should suggest the diagnosis, especially in patients with leukemia or lymphoma.

Cystitis with pneumaturia, gaseous cholecystitis, endocarditis, osteomyelitis, arthritis, and bursitis after needle aspiration are other examples of rare clostridial infections.

LABORATORY FINDINGS The diagnosis of gas gangrene, clostridial cellulitis, postabortal sepsis, or other clostridial infections is based primarily on clinical criteria. Smears of wound exudate, uterine scrapings, or cervical discharge may show abundant large gram-positive rods, as well as other organisms. Spores are rarely observed in smears of exudates. Thioglycollate broth, deep meat broth, and blood-agar plates incubated in an anaerobic jar should be inoculated for definitive identification of specific clostridia. However, interpretation of positive wound cultures is difficult because clostridia are frequent contaminants. *Clostridium perfringens* bacteremia is common in postabortal infections but rare in gas gangrene.

Polymorphonuclear leukocytosis occurs frequently in gas gangrene and invariably in postabortal sepsis; total blood leukocyte counts range from 15,000 to 40,000 cells per cubic millimeter and occasionally exceed 60,000 cells per cubic millimeter. Marked thrombocytopenia develops in about 50 percent of patients with clostridial sepsis. The urine frequently contains protein and casts. Renal insufficiency may lead to severe uremia.

X-ray examination sometimes provides the first clue leading to the correct diagnosis by revealing the presence of gas in muscle, subcutaneous tissue, or uterus; however, demonstration of gas in tissues is not diagnostic of clostridial infection. Other bacteria, especially *Enterobacter* and *Escherichia*, may be responsible for gas production, and occasionally air is sucked into a wound at the time of penetrating injury.

Profound alterations of circulating erythrocytes are common in postabortal sepsis but are much less frequent in other clostridial infection. Hemolytic anemia may develop with almost unbelievable rapidity; the red blood cell count occasionally decreases by 2 million cells per cubic millimeter in less than 24 h and is associated with hemoglobinemia, hemoglobinuria, and elevated levels of serum bilirubin. Spherocytosis, increased osmotic and mechanical red blood cell fragility, erythrophagocytosis, and methemoglobinemia have also been described. Abnormalities of the clotting mechanism characteristic of intravascular coagulation may be observed in patients with severe clostridial infections.

The diagnosis of antibiotic-associated pseudomembranous colitis is established by proctoscopy, which shows raised yellow-whitish plaques that cover an erythematous edematous base. The membrane is composed of mucus, fibrin, desquamated epithelial cells, and polymorphonuclear leukocytes. The radiographic findings on plain films of the abdomen are of thickened and distorted haustra, generalized thickening of the colonic wall, "thumbprinting," small marginal irregularities (representing the pseudomembranous plaque), and total colonic involvement. The small bowel is usually not involved. Barium enema is not recommended in patients suspected to have colitis because of the possible association with toxic megacolon.

TREATMENT The traditional therapeutic approach to serious clostridial infection, such as diffuse, spreading myositis, is immediate surgical intervention with wide radical debridement followed by open drainage without closure or open amputation when necessary. Early surgery not only aids diagnosis, but permits decompression of fascial compartments and excision of devitalized muscle and may obviate amputation. A number of authorities feel that hyperbaric oxygen therapy has modified this traditional approach to gas gangrene by assuming priority over radical surgical debridement. Proponents report that hyperbaric oxygenation produces impressive, almost immediate improvement in patients with gas gangrene, with rapid disappearance of systemic toxicity and prompt arrest of local spread of the gangrenous infection. Opinions differ about whether conservative debridement should be carried out before or after hyperbaric oxygen therapy. Advocates emphasize that a single 90-min compression treatment frequently results in a clear-cut demarcation between healthy and devitalized tissue and aids in the surgical debridement. Hyperbaric oxygen alone is not adequate therapy for gas gangrene. Oxygen toxicity consequent to hyperbaric oxygenation has lead to convulsions in some patients.

Curettage of the uterus should be performed for diagnosis and treatment of postabortal clostridial infections. In the absence of hemolysis, standard therapy for septic abortion with antibiotics and uterine curettage usually produces rapid improvement, even in patients with bacteremia. The mortality rate in patients with abortion, *C. perfringens* bacteremia, and intense hemolysis is high irrespective of the therapeutic approach. The role of hysterectomy is controversial and ill-defined; some surgeons strongly advocate hysterectomy, whereas others feel that the potential benefits of the procedure do not outweigh the risks. Heparinization, exchange transfusion, and hyperbaric oxygen have been utilized but are not of established benefit.

Simple excision and adequate drainage usually suffice for treating clostridial cellulitis.

Penicillin is the antibiotic of choice for most clostridial infections and should be administered in doses of 20 million units a day by continuous intravenous infusion. Cephalosporins and chloramphenicol are also active against most strains of *Clostridium*, and either may be used as an alternative to penicillin in patients with hypersensitivity. Clostridial myonecrosis has developed while patients were receiving cephalothin (2 to 6 g intravenously daily) for prophylaxis, and only high doses (8 to 12 g intravenously daily) are recommended for treatment. Clostridia are also generally, but not universally, susceptible in vitro to carbenicillin, clindamycin, doxycycline, minocycline, and tetracycline.

The efficacy of polyvalent gas gangrene antitoxin is controversial. Most centers have discontinued the use of antitoxin in the management of patients with suspected gas gangrene or clostridial postabortal sepsis because of questionable efficacy and the risk of hypersensitivity reactions. At the present time this antitoxin is not being produced in the United States.

Intravenous infusions of blood, plasma volume expanders, fluids, and electrolytes are required to combat shock, anemia, and dehydration. Renal insufficiency should be treated in the same manner as acute tubular necrosis from other causes.

The most reliable protection against gas gangrene is early and adequate wound debridement. Antitoxin is ineffective as a

prophylactic agent. The use of clostridial toxoids for prophylactic immunization of individuals in hazardous occupations awaits evaluation.

Therapy of antibiotic-associated pseudomembranous colitis includes immediate discontinuation of the antibiotic, and intravenous fluid to maintain an adequate intravascular volume and electrolyte balance. Vancomycin by the oral route has been effective in eradicating the experimental infection in hamsters. Treatment with vancomycin 500 mg orally every 6 h also appears to be beneficial in stopping the diarrhea in humans.

REFERENCES

Bartlett JG et al: Antibiotic-associated pseudomembranous colitis due to toxin-producing clostridia. N Engl J Med 298:531, 1978

Darke SG et al: Gas gangrene and related infection. Br J Surg 64:104, 1977

Holland JA et al: Experimental and clinical experience with hyperbaric oxygen in the treatment of clostridial myonecrosis. Surgery 77:75, 1975

MacLennan JD: The histotoxic clostridial infections of man. Bacteriol Rev 26:177, 1962

Mahn E, Dantuono LM: Postabortal septicotoxemia due to *Clostridium welchii:* Seventy-five cases from the maternity hospital, Santiago, Chile. 1948–1952. Am J Obstet Gynecol 70:604, 1955

Murrel TGC et al: Pig-bel: Enteritis necroticans: A study in diagnosis and management. Lancet 1:217, 1966

Nakamura M, Schulze JA: *Clostridium perfringens* food poisoning. Annu Rev Microbiol 24:359, 1970

Pritchard JA, Whalley PJ: Abortion complicated by *Clostridium perfringens* infection. Am J Obstet Gynecol 111:484, 1971

Rifkin GD et al: Antibiotic-induced colitis: Implication of a toxin neutralized by *Clostridium sordellii* antitoxin. Lancet 2:1103, 1977

Tedesco RJ: Clindamycin and colitis: A review. J Infect Dis 135S:S95, 1977

Weinstein L, Barza MA: Gas gangrene. N Engl J Med 289:1129, 1973

Wyne JW, Armstrong D: Clostridial septicemia. Cancer 29:215, 1972

142
INFECTIONS DUE TO MIXED ANAEROBIC ORGANISMS

LAWRENCE L. PELLETIER, JR.

Anaerobic bacteria require conditions of reduced oxygen tension and low redox potential for growth. Anaerobes constitute the predominant normal flora on the skin and mucous membranes of humans and outnumber aerobic bacteria 1000 to 1 in the colon and 10 to 1 on the skin, mouth, and vagina. On body surfaces, anaerobic bacteria often coexist with other anaerobic species and aerobic and facultative organisms in poorly understood symbiotic relationships. Any site in the body is susceptible to infection by these endogenous organisms when skin and mucous membrane barriers are compromised by surgery, trauma, or tumor, and when local tissue redox potentials are reduced by ischemia, necrosis, or infection. Multiple species of anaerobic, facultative, or aerobic organisms are often present in infection, and their synergistic interaction is required for pathogenicity. Mixed anaerobic infections frequently cause dental abscess, chronic otitis media and sinusitis, brain abscess, subdural empyema, otogenic meningitis, necrotizing gingivitis, Ludwig's angina, aspiration pneumonia, lung abscess, thoracic empyema, liver abscess, pylephlebitis, peritonitis, intraabdominal abscesses, endometritis, tuboovarian abscess, pelvic cellulitis, gangrene, postsurgical wound infection, perirectal abscess, and human bite infections.

Botulism (Chap. 140), tetanus (Chap. 139), clostridial myonecrosis (Chap. 141), and actinomycosis (Chap. 151) are discussed elsewhere.

ETIOLOGY Because most mixed anaerobic infections develop from normal host flora associated with adjacent mucosal membranes, knowledge of the predominant bacteria at different sites and the pathogenicity of these organisms may permit the selection of appropriate therapy before the results of cultures are available. Advances in culture techniques and methods of microbial identification have clarified the taxonomic classification of anaerobic organisms and the relative pathogenicity of some species in mixed anaerobic infection, but the relative importance of many organisms that participate in mixed infections needs to be established. Certain organisms such as *Vibrio* spp., spirochetes, anaerobic gram-negative cocci, or very oxygen-labile anaerobes that may be seen in stains of clinical material or isolated from culture are not virulent in experimental infections. Formerly, many mixed anaerobic infections of the pharynx, lung, and genital tract were classified as fusospirochetal infections because fusobacteria and spirochetes were seen on stains of material from the lesions. Since spirochetes are not pathogenic and many other species of anaerobes and aerobes have been isolated from infected sites, it is more appropriate to term these infections as mixed anaerobic infections.

Lest normal flora be discounted as undesirable, it should be recognized that normal anaerobic flora play critical roles in protecting against both colonization and infection with pathogenic microorganisms and overgrowth of potentially pathogenic endogenous organisms. Administration of clindamycin or other antimicrobials that suppress the majority of anaerobic colon bacteria may be complicated by the overgrowth of clindamycin-resistant *Clostridia difficile*, which produces toxins that may damage colonic mucosa and cause pseudomembranous colitis (Chap. 141). Likewise, antibiotic suppression of normal flora may predispose to oropharyngeal or perianal symptomatic *Candida* spp. infection (thrush) (Chap. 158) or prolonged carriage of *Salmonella* spp. in the gut.

The functions of anaerobic gastrointestinal flora in health and disease are poorly understood, but it is known that vitamin K synthesis by *Escherichia coli* and *Bacteroides fragilis* in the gut represent important sources of this essential vitamin. *Bacteroides fragilis* and other organisms deconjugate bile acids in the intestine, permitting their reabsorption in the distal ileum and maintaining the bile acid pool. Alterations in the microbial flora in relation to diet may predispose to the development of carcinoma of the colon and to altered metabolism of dietary chemicals and orally administered drugs. Because of both the complexity of the flora and problems in sampling it, knowledge of this area of normal bacterial physiology is scanty, and it is a fertile area for future investigation.

The major anaerobic pathogens from clinical material include (1) gram-negative bacilli (*B. fragilis, B. melaninogenicus, Fusobacterium nucleatum, F. varium, F. necrophorum,* and *F. mortiferum*), (2) gram-positive cocci (*Peptostreptococcus* spp., *Peptococcus* spp., microaerophilic cocci, and streptococci), (3) gram-positive spore-forming bacilli (*Clostridia* spp.), and (4) gram-positive nonsporulating bacilli (*Actinomyces* spp., *Arachina* spp., *Eubacterium* spp., and *Bifidobacterium eriksonii*).

Anaerobic gram-negative bacilli and anaerobic gram-positive cocci are the most commonly isolated anaerobes from clinical infections; *B. fragilis* is the most frequently isolated species. Microaerophilic cocci and streptococci that require reduced oxygen tension and the presence of carbon dioxide for

growth are facultative rather than true anaerobic bacteria. *Clostridia* spp. or *Actinomyces* spp. may produce disease as single pathogens or as one organism among many in mixed infections. Anaerobes should be considered significant pathogens when isolated from body fluids or tissues that are normally sterile, or from infected sites where they are repeatedly isolated in high concentrations when measures have been taken to reduce or eliminate contamination by normal flora.

Table 142-1 lists aerobic and anaerobic organisms constituting normal skin and mucosal flora that are potential pathogens. Normal skin flora include anaerobic *Propionibacterium acnes,* a common blood culture contaminant that produces significant infections only in association with a foreign body such as a prosthetic heart valve or cerebral spinal fluid shunts. Anaerobic gram-negative bacilli, e.g., *C. perfringens,* and other anaerobes may be transient skin flora of the perineum and lower extremities and may cause mixed anaerobic infection of decubitus, ischemic, or diabetic ulcers.

Organisms in the oropharynx may play a role in local disease or be involved in pleuropulmonary infections following aspiration of oropharyngeal secretions. Hospitalized patients have a higher frequency of colonization with aerobic coliform bacilli or *S. aureus,* and anaerobes play a greater role in aspiration pneumonias occurring outside the hospital.

Multiple aerobic and anaerobic pathogens are encountered in infections of the abdomen and female genital tract. All potential pathogens isolated from abdominal and genital tract infections should be considered significant with the possible exception of enterococci encountered in abscesses and soft tissue infections.

EPIDEMIOLOGY Mixed anaerobic infections are frequently encountered in hospitals with active surgical, trauma, and obstetrics and gynecologic services. No reliable data are available to establish the true incidence and prevalence of mixed anaer-

TABLE 142-1
Potential pathogens that constitute normal flora at different body sites

	Anaerobes	Aerobes
Skin	Gram-positive cocci Eubacterium spp.	S. epidermidis S. aureus C. albicans S. pyogenes
Pharynx	B. melaninogenicus Fusobacterium spp. Gram-positive cocci Actinomyces spp. Bifidobacterium spp. Eubacterium spp.	Pneumococcus S. aureus S. pyogenes H. influenzae S. viridans K. pneumoniae Meningococcus Gram-negative coliform bacilli C. albicans
Colon	B. fragilis B. melaninogenicus Gram-positive cocci Clostridium spp. Bifidobacterium spp. Eubacterium spp. Fusobacterium spp.	Gram-negative coliform bacilli Achromobacter spp. Enterococcus P. aeruginosa S. viridans S. aureus
Vagina	B. fragilis B. melaninogenicus Gram-positive cocci Bifidobacterium spp. Clostridium spp. Eubacterium spp. Fusobacterium spp.	Gram-negative coliform bacilli Enterococcus spp. C. vaginalis Mycoplasma spp. C. albicans S. viridans

obic infections. The lack of appropriate cultures, the submission of cultures contaminated by anaerobes from normal flora, and the lack, until recently, of reliable culture techniques have made accurate sampling of infectious anaerobes impossible. Anaerobic bacteria, predominately *B. fragilis* and anaerobic cocci, constitute 8 to 11 percent of blood culture isolates in many centers, and anaerobes have been isolated from 10 to 54 percent of clinical cultures.

PATHOGENESIS Anaerobes generally are not highly invasive; infection is usually secondary to an underlying disease, surgical procedure, or therapy which impairs the normal defenses of the host. These organisms utilize substances other than oxygen as the final electron acceptor in reactions which generate energy, and will grow only in an environment with a low redox potential. Healthy, well-vascularized tissue has a relatively high redox potential and will not support growth of anaerobes. Conditions that significantly lower redox potential, such as impairment of blood supply, tissue necrosis, or growth of aerobic bacteria, are necessary to create an environment conducive to proliferation of anaerobes. Infections, therefore, frequently occur secondary to vascular disease, trauma, surgery, a perforated viscus, shock, aspiration, intramuscular epinephrine injections, or malignancy.

Obligate anaerobes generally do not possess catalase or superoxide dismutase enzymes to protect them from peroxides that form in oxygenated surroundings. However, if the redox potential is low, many species can exist in sites that are well oxygenated, such as the mouth. Pathogenic anaerobic species tend to be more resistant to oxygen exposure than nonpathogenic strains.

Anaerobes involved in local infections originating from mucosal surfaces in the mouth, intestinal tract, or vagina may form pseudomembranes on mucosal surfaces. spreading gangrene from a site of trauma or a localized abscess. The characteristic foul odor of anaerobic lesions is caused by certain metabolic end products of bacterial origin, primarily short-chain fatty acids and volatile amines. Many species of anaerobes produce collagenases and proteinases that account for the propensity for abscess formation. Some bacteroides species produce a heparinase which may frequently lead to localized septic thrombophlebitis seen adjacent to areas of infection. Many bacteroides species also possess a capsule that may interfere with phagocytosis by granulocytes. Infection characteristically remains localized, but bloodstream invasion or direct extension to other areas may occur. Localization of bloodborne organisms at distant sites is not unusual and may result in abscess formation in brain, lung, liver, joints, kidneys, or other organs.

CLINICAL MANIFESTATIONS Anaerobic infection should be suspected when a foul odor emanates from lesions or pus; when infection is situated near a mucosal surface; when necrotic tissue or neoplasm is present; when a spreading gangrene involves skin, subcutaneous tissue, fascia, or muscle; when pseudomembranes or abscesses are formed; when gas in tissues is indicated by roentgenogram or crepitance; when septic thrombophlebitis or pulmonary embolus occurs following intraabdominal or pelvic infections; or when infection progresses despite aminoglycoside therapy.

Dental–periodontal infections Root canal infection caused by mixed anaerobic and aerobic oral flora may result from dental caries and produce dental pulp necrosis with periapical destruction of bone. Without drainage of the root canal, mandibular osteomyelitis or extension of the infection into the maxil-

lary sinus, buccal tissues, and submandibular or submental spaces may occur depending upon the teeth involved. Periodontitis with purulent gingival pockets or abscesses may result in spreading anaerobic infection that involves adjacent bone or soft tissues. Secondary pulmonary anaerobic infection may occur from aspiration of purulent material. Mandibular osteomyelitis may also result from infection complicating tooth extraction, from open fractures, or in association with debilitation, diabetes mellitus, radiation therapy, and malnutrition.

Acute necrotizing ulcerative gingivitis (trench mouth, Vincent's stomatitis) The onset of disease is usually sudden and is associated with tender, bleeding gums, fetid breath, and a bad taste. The gingival mucosa, especially the papillae between the teeth, becomes ulcerated and may be covered by a gray exudate which is removable with gentle pressure. Although involvement of the gums is usually patchy, the process may extend to most of the gingival tissue. If the ulceration is extensive, fever, cervical lymphadenopathy, and leukocytosis are present. The disease may spread to involve other tissues of the oropharynx; it may become less severe and chronic; or it may subside spontaneously. Recurrent ulceration has been described. Most patients who develop ulcerative gingivitis are young adults with poor oral hygiene. Tartar deposits and eruption or extraction of teeth may damage the gums and allow bacterial invasion. Edentulous persons develop the disease infrequently. Ulcerative gingivitis is prevalent in wartime when nutritional deficiency, crowding, and emotional upsets are common. The role of these factors in pathogenesis is not known.

Acute necrotizing ulcerative mucositis (cancrum oris, noma) Occasionally, ulcerative gingivitis spreads to the buccal mucosa, the cheek, and the mandible or maxilla, resulting in widespread destruction of bone and soft tissue. The first indication of cancrum oris is usually slight inflammation of the skin of the cheek. The destruction of tissue proceeds very rapidly. The teeth may fall out, and large areas of bone, even the whole mandible, may be sloughed. A strong, putrid odor is present. The lesions are not usually painful. The gangrenous lesions eventually heal, but large disfiguring defects are left. Cancrum oris is seen most commonly following a debilitating illness in severely malnourished children in underdeveloped areas of the world. Cancrum oris may complicate acute leukemia or develop in individuals with a genetic deficiency of catalase.

Gangrenous pharyngitis (Vincent's angina) Necrotizing infections of the pharynx may occur alone or in association with ulcerative gingivitis. The main complaints are an extremely sore throat, foul breath, bad taste in the mouth, sensation of choking, and fever. The pharynx in the area of the tonsillar pillars is swollen, red, and ulcerated and is covered with a grayish membrane that peels easily. Lymphadenopathy and leukocytosis are common. The disease may last for only a few days or may persist for weeks if not treated. The lesion begins unilaterally but may spread to the other side of the pharynx or to the larynx. Aspiration of infected material may result in lung abscess.

Sinusitis Acute sinusitis is seldom caused by anaerobic organisms unless it is associated with a dental abscess. However, gram-positive anaerobic cocci and bacteroides are isolated from about one-half of patients undergoing surgery for chronic or recurrent maxillary sinusitis. Anaerobic organisms are also associated with chronic otitis media and mastoiditis. Chronic anaerobic sinusitis, otitis, or mastoiditis may lead to subdural or extradural empyemas, brain abscess, or anaerobic meningitis (Chap. 368).

Ludwig's angina Mandibular dental or periodontal infections, particularly of the third molar, may produce submandibular cellulitis that results in marked local swelling of tissues with pain, trismus, and superior-posterior displacement of the tongue. Submandibular swelling of the neck also develops. Inability to swallow and respiratory obstruction may result; tracheostomy may be lifesaving. Anaerobes and aerobes originating from oral flora have been implicated in this dramatic clinical syndrome.

Brain abscess Anaerobic bacteria, particularly bacteroides and anaerobic streptococci, have been isolated from 30 to 80 percent of brain abscesses in adults. In one study, 16 of 18 nontraumatic brain abscesses contained anaerobes, and half of these were bacteroides, including both *B. fragilis* and *B. melaninogenicus*. These lesions may result from either direct extension of suppurative infection involving the sinuses, middle ear, or mastoids, or from hematogenous dissemination from infections elsewhere, particularly the lungs. There is an increased incidence of brain abscess in patients with cyanotic heart disease. Signs and symptoms are mainly those of a space-occupying intracranial lesion with headache followed by changes in mentation, focal neurologic signs, and papilledema. The course may be indolent, and fever is frequently absent. Cerebrospinal fluid findings are variable but may mimic those of purulent or aseptic meningitis. Focal defects are usually present on computerized tomographic or radionucleotide scans of the brain and may need to be differentiated from neoplasms by cerebral angiography.

Pleuropulmonary infection Aspiration of oral secretions leads to production of mixed anaerobic infection of the lungs and pleura. The likelihood of anaerobic pulmonary infection is increased in the presence of poor dental hygiene, periodontal disease, and gingivitis. Bacteroides, fusobacteria, and anaerobic streptococci are isolated alone or in combination in a majority of cases of lung abscess and necrotizing pneumonia. Pneumonitis without necrosis or abscess formation may also occur. These anaerobes are second only to the pneumococcus as a cause of acute bacterial infection of the lungs. Although *B. melaninogenicus* is the most frequent *Bacteroides* species isolated in anaerobic pulmonary infections, *B. fragilis* can be found in 15 to 25 percent of cases. These infections occur primarily in patients with conditions that predispose to aspiration, such as oral surgical procedures, esophageal dysfunction, and altered consciousness due to alcoholism, major motor seizure disorders, general anesthesia, and drug abuse. Anaerobes may also produce infection distal to obstructive lesions of the bronchus. These infections are characterized by tissue necrosis, abscess formation, and the production of foul-smelling and foul-tasting sputum. Empyema is not an unusual complication of lung abscess or necrotizing pneumonia. Empyema with anaerobes may also occur as an extension from subdiaphragmatic infection. Septic pulmonary emboli may originate from abdominal or female genital tract infections. The bacterial flora of bronchiectatic cavities frequently includes bacteroides and other anaerobes.

Abdominal infection Intraabdominal abscesses and generalized peritonitis almost always contain anaerobes, especially when they are secondary to perforation or leakage from the gastrointestinal tract. These infections are uniformly polymicrobial, with an average of five anaerobic and aerobic pathogens that originate from bowel flora. Symptoms include fever with chills, localized or generalized abdominal pain with peritoneal signs, nausea, and vomiting. The abscess cavity will rarely be large enough to be palpable on abdominal or pelvic examination. *Bacteroides fragilis* is isolated from approximately 50 percent of abdominal surgical wounds after trauma involving perforation of the gut and in greater than 50 percent of wound infections following elective colon resection. Anaerobic wound infections may occur following appendectomy or may follow surgery on the small bowel, stomach, gallbladder, and biliary tract. Polymicrobial bacteremia may complicate local infection and frequently is due to facultative gram-negative bacilli or *B. fragilis*. Abdominal ultrasound, combined liver-spleen scans, and gallium scans may be helpful in localizing intraabdominal abscesses, but often surgical exploration may be necessary to establish the site of intraabdominal infection.

Intrahepatic infection Anaerobic bacteria have rarely been implicated in infections of the gallbladder, but they may produce ascending cholangitis and are isolated from 20 to 45 percent of pyogenic intrahepatic abscesses. Bacteroides account for approximately half the bacterial isolates from liver abscess. They may reach the intrahepatic tissue by direct extension from an ascending infection or by embolization from septic portal vein thrombosis. In most cases, the disease is manifested by fever, chills, abdominal pain particularly in the right upper quadrant—hepatomegaly, and liver tenderness. The presence of jaundice and marked elevation of serum alkaline phosphatase usually indicates multiple abscesses. Hepatic abscesses may be detected by hepatic ultrasound or radionucleotide scanning of the liver.

Pelvic infection The predominant organisms isolated in greater than 75 percent of nongonococcal gynecologic infections are anaerobic species found in normal vaginal flora. Anaerobic species are the major cause of Bartholin's abscess, endometritis, parametritis, parametrial abscess, pelvic peritonitis, and nongonococcal tuboovarial abscesses. These infections often complicate malignancy or recent surgery and commonly develop within necrotic tissue or products of conception. They are characterized by drainage of foul-smelling pus or blood from the uterus, generalized uterine or localized pelvic tenderness, and continued fever and chills. Suppurative thrombophlebitis of the pelvic veins may complicate these infections and lead to repeated episodes of small septic pulmonary emboli.

Nonclostridial anaerobes, principally bacteroides and anaerobic streptococci, are also the major invasive pathogens in septic abortions. Bacteremia is often transient, frequently polymicrobic, and can be demonstrated in 50 to 60 percent of these patients.

Cutaneous infections Following operation or injury associated with contamination of the subcutaneous tissues, an *anaerobic cellulitis* may develop consisting of a spreading necrosis of skin and subcutaneous tissues with associated subcutaneous gas. This infection is frequently due to a mixed infection from which clostridia, anaerobic gram-positive cocci and gram-negative bacilli, and facultative coliform bacilli, streptococci, and staphylococci may be isolated. The onset of anaerobic cellulitis is usually gradual, with erythema, tenderness, and edema of involved tissues followed by the development of necrosis, crepitation, pus, and foul odor over a 2- to 5-day period. Local pain is not marked, and the deep fascia and muscle are spared. Once established, the infection may be associated with high fever, toxemia, and positive blood cultures. In diabetics, an identical syndrome may be produced by gas forming facultative coliform bacilli or *Staphylococcus aureus*. On occasion, intraabdominal abscesses may present as an anaerobic cellulitis or abscess of the thigh. Areas of involvement should be opened surgically with debridement of necrotic tissue and drainage of pus and gas. At surgery, the status of the underlying fascia and muscle should be ascertained.

Necrotizing fascitis caused mainly by group A streptococci, *S. aureus,* or facultative gram-negative rods is associated with separation of the skin from necrotic fascia. A surgical probe may be passed without obstruction in a plane superficial to the deep fascia into areas of undermined skin. Gas gangrene caused by clostridia is usually associated with a more rapid onset and progression than anaerobic cellulitis, with severe pain in the involved areas, tense white overlying skin, and severe systemic toxicity. At surgical exploration, the involved muscle is nonviable.

Bacterial synergistic gangrene occurs 1 to 2 weeks after abdominal or thoracic surgery and is caused by microaerophilic or anaerobic streptococci combined with *S. aureus* or aerobic coliform bacilli. The margin of the surgical wound becomes red, swollen, and tender; central necrosis of skin and subcutaneous tissues occurs; and the margin slowly expands to involve adjacent skin. Systemic toxicity is usually minimal, and treatment consists of local debridement and systemic antibiotics. *Meleney's chronic undermining ulcer* is also a slowly progressive gangrene that occurs following surgery without marked systemic toxicity. It differs from bacterial synergistic gangrene because cutaneous fissures and sinus tracts form and are separated from the leading margin of the ulcer by undermined but intact skin. Anaerobic and microaerophilic streptococci are the usual causative organisms.

Fournier's gangrene is an anaerobic cellulitis involving the scrotum, perineum, and anterior abdominal wall in which mixed anaerobic organisms spread along deep external fascial planes and cause extensive loss of skin. Diabetics are susceptible to a necrotizing infection of skin and subcutaneous tissues that also may involve fascia and muscle. These infections have a foul discharge, marked local pain, gas in tissues, and severe systemic toxemia; they are caused by mixed anaerobic and aerobic organisms, and are associated with bacteremia in one-third of patients.

Mixed anaerobic infection may complicate decubitus ulcers, diabetic ulcers, pilonidal cysts, hidradenitis suppurativa, and vascular gangrene.

Other local infections Anaerobic urinary tract infections are rare and are usually the result of invasion from adjacent foci of infection or from bacteremia. Usually, osteomyelitis also results from adjacent ischemic or diabetic ulcers or abscess, but an increasing number of hematogenous bone and joint infections are being reported. Gangrenous lesions resulting from human bites commonly contain mixed oral anaerobic flora. Gangrenous balanitis and ulcers and gangrene of the vulva have been associated with a mixed anaerobic flora.

Bacteremia Invasion of the bloodstream by anaerobes is usually secondary to local infection, particularly those involving the abdominal cavity and pelvis. The initial manifestations are determined by the portal of entry and may be those of endometritis, appendicitis, intraabdominal abscess, or others. When bloodstream invasion occurs, the patient may become extremely ill with chills and hectic fevers ranging from 101 to 106°F. Shock and disseminated intravascular coagulation may develop. The clinical picture may be quite similar to that seen in sepsis with gram-negative bacilli (Chap. 109), except for the occasional association of thrombophlebitis. When bacteremia complicates facial or oral infection, the internal jugular vein may be the site of suppurative thrombophlebitis; and in pelvic infections, the iliac and femoral veins may be involved. Palpation along the course of the involved veins may disclose a firm, tender cord, indicating the presence of a thrombus. Emboli may be dislodged from peripheral sites of thrombophlebitis, resulting in multiple septic pulmonary infarcts. The pulmonary abscesses or empyema then become the main focus of clinical attention rather than the initial site of infection.

Transient anaerobic bacteremias may occur following dental manipulation, extraction, peridontal procedures, nasotracheal intubation, percutaneous liver biopsy, barium enema, gastrointestinal surgery, and urinary tract catheterization but usually are not symptomatic. From 8 to 11 percent of clinically significant bacteremias are caused by anaerobes, most commonly by *B. fragilis* originating in abdominal or female genital tract infections. Anaerobic streptococcal bacteremias usually originate from the female genital tract, and fusobacteria from the oropharynx. Anaerobes cause less than 10 percent of infective endocarditis and are predominately microaerophilic or anaerobic streptococci. *Bacteroides fragilis* is a rare cause of endocarditis. Routine anaerobic cultures should be performed in all cases of suspected bacteremia.

DIAGNOSIS Correct specimen collection and transport are critical for the isolation of anaerobic organisms. Even brief exposure to oxygen may kill the pathogens in clinical specimens. Abscess cavities should be aspirated directly with a syringe, the air expelled, and the needle capped with a sterile rubber stopper. The specimen can then be injected into a carrier bottle containing a reduced environment or transported immediately for direct culture on anaerobic media. Such a technique is preferred over the use of cotton swabs. If swabs must be used, then a swab from a gassed-out container should be placed in a reduced semisolid carrying medium before transport to the laboratory. Delays in transport may lead to failure to isolate anaerobes due to exposure to oxygen or overgrowth with facultative organisms which may eliminate or obscure the anaerobes that are present.

Only certain specimens should be cultured for anaerobic bacteria. Since all mucosal surfaces contain anaerobes, culturing them is of no value, and in fact, may lead to erroneous labeling of culture specimens as "contaminated" with mucosal bacteria, such as occurs in expectorated sputum, nasotracheal aspirates, bronchoscopic aspirates, feces, voided urine, vaginal secretions, or secretions from mucosal surfaces which normally harbor anaerobes. Acceptable materials for culture include blood, pleural fluid, transtracheal aspirates, pus obtained by direct aspiration from abscess cavity, culdocentesis, suprapubic bladder aspirates, and other tissues or fluids that are sterile under normal conditions.

All clinical specimens from suspected anaerobic infections should be Gram stained and examined diligently for organisms with characteristic morphology. Organisms may be seen on Gram's stain that are not isolated in culture. Purulent materials that are "sterile" or that demonstrate organisms on Gram's stain but do not grow on culture should be viewed with suspicion, and the method of collection, transport, and handling in the laboratory reviewed to assure that all reasonable precautions have been taken to permit isolation of fastidious anaerobes. Repeat cultures with immediate inoculation of freshly prepared media and prolonged anaerobic incubation may be required in special circumstances. Promising new techniques for rapid anaerobic diagnosis include fluorescent antibody staining of clinical materials with species specific antisera and direct gas-liquid chromatographic analysis of clinical specimens. However, definitive diagnosis depends upon the isolation and identification of pathogenic organisms.

TREATMENT Due to the association of anaerobic infections with abscess formation, tissue necrosis, and compression, appropriate surgical management is often essential for the control and elimination of infection. Drainage of abscess cavities should be carried out as soon as fluctuation and localization occur; perforations must be closed promptly; devitalized tissues or foreign bodies removed; closed space infections drained; tissue compartments decompressed; and an adequate blood supply established. Drainage of local suppurative lesions may be all that is required for cure in many cases. However, antimicrobial therapy is indicated in infections involving vital organs; to check the spread of infection into healthy tissues; or when bacteremia or systemic manifestations are present. Surgery also may be indicated to obtain appropriate material for culture by biopsy or excision. Thrombophlebitis not controlled by anticoagulation or recurrent septic pulmonary emboli may require surgical removal of thrombi or vein ligation.

It is often necessary to begin antimicrobial treatment of anaerobic infections before culture and susceptibility data are available. The type and location of infection combined with Gram's stain findings should suggest the likelihood of certain bacterial species and serve as a guide to antibiotic therapy. Chloramphenicol is the preferred drug for seriously ill patients with suspected anaerobic infection before susceptibility data are available. Generally, anaerobic infections above the diaphragm caused by oral or upper respiratory tract flora are susceptible to penicillin G. However, if *B. fragilis* is isolated, treatment with clindamycin or chloramphenicol is usually indicated. Mixed abdominal or pelvic infections necessitate multiple drug therapy due to the likelihood of penicillin-resistant strains of *B. fragilis* and facultative or aerobic gram-negative rods. A regimen for serious intraabdominal infection includes penicillin G, 24 to 30 million units a day, combined with chloramphenicol, 4 g per day, or combined with clindamycin, 300 to 600 mg every 6 h, and gentamicin, 1.6 to 2.0 mg/kg every 8 h. Chloramphenicol is the drug of choice for central nervous system anaerobic infections as well, although penicillin G and metronidazole also pass the blood-brain barrier. Bactericidal agents such as penicillin G, ampicillin, carbenicillin, and metronidazole have a definite advantage over bacteriostatic agents only in the presence of endocarditis or in patients with profound neutropenia.

Penicillin G and ampicillin have a wide range of activity against anaerobic bacteria. However, over 90 percent of *B. fragilis* strains, and some strains of fusobacteria, non-*C. perfringens* clostridia, and *B. melaninogenicus*, are resistant. Carbenicillin (25 to 30 g per day) or ticarcillin combine the antimicrobial spectrum of penicillin G with activity against 95 percent of *B. fragilis* strains and may be selected for mixed infections associated with resistant aerobic or facultative gram-negative rods such as *Pseudomonas aeruginosa* or *Proteus* organisms. Semisynthetic penicillinase-resistant penicillins are not active against anaerobes. Many anaerobes are susceptible to cephalothin or cephapirin, but *B. fragilis* is resistant to the cephalosporins. However, cefoxitin possesses activity against *B. fragilis.*

Chloramphenicol or clindamycin remain the drugs of choice for *B. fragilis* infections. Both drugs should be reserved for serious infections and should be administered intravenously. Chloramphenicol produces fatal aplastic anemia in 1 of 40,000 to 100,000 patients who receive the drug. The development of aplastic anemia is independent of a dose-related bone marrow suppression that is common with prolonged high dose regimens. Clindamycin produces pseudomembranous colitis in 0.1 to 10 percent of patients and diarrhea in as many as 20 percent of patients. Since diarrhea may precede pseudo-

membranous colitis, the administration of drug should be stopped if diarrhea develops during therapy. Resistance to chloramphenicol is rare, but clindamycin resistance is common for *F. varium* and for clostridia other than *C. perfringens;* rarely *B. fragilis* or peptococci are resistant.

Metronidazole has bactericidal activity against many anaerobes and is clinically effective in *B. fragilis* infections. However, actinomyces, eubacteria, and microaerophilic streptococci are resistant to this agent. Metronidazole has not been approved by the Food and Drug Administration for use in anaerobic infections, and a parenteral form is not yet available.

Tetracycline is not reliable due to widespread resistance among anaerobes. The role of doxycycline and minocycline, newer tetracycline derivatives with increased activity against anaerobes, is unclear. Erythromycin may be used in minor soft tissue infections above the diaphragm or in bowel preparation for colon surgery, but is less effective than clindamycin. Anaerobes are almost uniformly resistant to the aminoglycosides. Vancomycin is active against most gram-positive anaerobes and is administered orally to treat clostridia induced pseudomembranous colitis.

Anaerobic lesions that fail to respond to treatment or relapse after responding initially should be recultured, and the need for surgical drainage or debridement should be reassessed. Superinfection with resistant gram-negative facultative or aerobic bacteria may necessitate changes in antimicrobial therapy. During treatment with broad-spectrum antibiotics, superinfection with *Candida* or *Torulopsis* may lead to systemic fungemia.

Additional supportive measures in the management of anaerobic infections include careful attention to fluid and electrolyte balance since extensive local edema formation may lead to hypovolemia; immobilization of infected extremities; therapy for septic shock (Chap. 109); maintenance of adequate nutrition during chronic infections by central or peripheral intravenous hyperalimentation if oral intake is inadequate; relief of pain; and anticoagulation with heparin for thrombophlebitis. Hyperbaric oxygen therapy is of unproven value.

OUTCOME Mortality rates may be substantial for serious anaerobic infections and approach 50 percent for brain abscess, 30 percent for necrotizing pneumonia, 25 percent for liver abscess, and 16 to 43 percent for *B. fragilis* sepsis.

PREVENTION Preventive measures include proper therapy of localized infection to prevent metastatic disease; effective debridement, cleansing, removal of foreign bodies, reestablishment of circulation, and early antimicrobial therapy of open traumatic wounds; early exploration and antibiotic therapy for penetrating abdominal wounds associated with bowel perforation; good dental and periodontal hygiene; prophylactic antibiotics for amputation of ischemic lower extremities, vaginal hysterectomy, radical pelvic surgery, and cesarean section with ruptured membranes; measures to prevent pulmonary aspiration; and possibly neomycin-erythromycin bowel preparation for colon surgery.

REFERENCES

BALOWS A et al: *Anaerobic Bacteria: Role in Disease.* Springfield, Thomas, 1974

BARTLETT JG, FINEGOLD SM: Anaerobic pleuropulmonary infections. Medicine 51:413, 1972

———— et al: Percutaneous transtracheal aspiration in the diagnosis of anaerobic pulmonary infection. Ann Intern Med 79:535, 1973

Busch DF et al: Activity of combinations of antimicrobial agents against *Bacteroides fragilis.* J Infect Dis 133:321, 1976

Chow AW et al: Orofacial odontogenic infections. Ann Intern Med 88:392, 1978

————, Guze LB: Bacteroidaceae bacteremia: Clinical experience with 112 patients. Medicine 53:93, 1974

Finegold SM: *Anaerobic Bacteria in Human Disease.* New York, Academic, 1977

Gorbach SL, Bartlett JG: Anaerobic infections. N Engl J Med 290:1177, 1237, 1289, 1974

Ledger WJ: *Infection in the Female.* Philadelphia, Lea & Febiger, 1977

Lennette EH et al: *Manual of Clinical Microbiology,* 2d ed. Washington, DC, American Society for Microbiology, 1974

Raff MJ, Melo JC: Anaerobic osteomyelitis, Medicine 57:83, 1978

Salaki JS et al: *Bacteroides fragilis* resistant to the administration of clindamycin. Am J Med 60:426, 1976

Smith LDS: *The Pathogenic Anaerobic Bacteria.* Springfield, Thomas, 1974

Sutter VL et al: *Wadsworth Anaerobic Bacteriology Manual,* 2d ed. Los Angeles, UCLA Press, 1975

section 7 | Mycobacterial diseases

143 TUBERCULOSIS

WILLIAM W. STEAD
JOSEPH H. BATES

DEFINITION

Tuberculosis is a necrotizing bacterial infection with protean manifestations and wide distribution. The lungs are most commonly affected, but lesions may occur also in the kidneys, bones, lymph nodes, or meninges or be disseminated throughout the body. The infection may cause clinical disease either (1) shortly after inoculation (sometimes called "primary" tuberculosis) or (2) after a period of months or decades of dormancy (still sometimes erroneously referred to as "reinfection" tuberculosis). In the Western world where bovine tuberculosis has been controlled, the portal of entry in humans is almost exclusively the lung.

HISTORY

Some human races (Caucasian, Mongolian) have lived with tubercle bacilli throughout much of their history, and in them the infection produces a more chronic disease, only rarely being fulminant. On the other hand, African, American Indian, and Eskimo peoples have had contact with tuberculosis over a much shorter period, and in them the infection is more prone to produce fulminant disease. Tuberculosis was named to indicate its formation of firm nodules, or *tubercles.* For many years the chronic form (then often called *phthisis* or *consumption*) was considered a degenerative or hereditary disease, quite unrelated to the tuberculosis of childhood which was obviously infectious. Laennec (1819) was the first to recognize the chronic form as merely a later development in the same infection. Koch (1882) identified the causative organism. There has been a great drop in prevalence of tuberculosis in the economically developed countries. The death rate from tuberculosis had already begun to fall by 1900, coincident with improvement in nutrition and standard of living. For the person with clinical tuberculosis, however, the most important development occurred in 1944 with the discovery of streptomycin. With the introduction of *p*-aminosalicylic acid (PAS) in 1947, isoniazid (INH) in 1952, ethambutol in 1967, and rifampin in 1971, specific therapy became progressively better and easier to administer.

ETIOLOGY

Mycobacterium tuberculosis is a rod 2 to 4 μm in length and 0.3 μm in thickness. Its distinguishing staining property, i.e., resistance to decolorization by acid alcohol when stained with basic fuchsin, is related to the waxy component of the cell wall. This "acid fastness" is dependent in some way upon the structural integrity of the bacillus; it is lost when the organisms are damaged by grinding but is not affected by prolonged extraction with fat solvents.

Tubercle bacilli are strict aerobes and thrive best at a P_{O_2} of about 140 mmHg. The organs most commonly affected by tuberculosis are those with relatively high oxygen tension; metastatic foci are most common in the apexes of the lungs where the P_{O_2} is in the range of 120 to 130 mmHg in the upright position, followed by the kidney and the growing ends of bones, where P_{O_2} approaches 100 mmHg. The liver and spleen, where the P_{O_2} is quite low, are rarely affected, except in overwhelming disseminated infection.

Two species of tubercle bacilli affect humans: *M. tuberculosis* and *M. bovis.* By far the greatest number of cases in the United States are caused by the former strain. Programs for eradication of bovine tuberculosis have been so effective that the disease now appears only sporadically in this country.

Several other species of mycobacteria have been noted to cause chronic pulmonary infection (Chap. 145). The most common are *M. avium-intracellulare* and *M. kansasii.* Clinical infection due to other atypical mycobacteria is rare. These mycobacteria appear not to be transmissible, and the epidemiology of the infections they cause remains obscure. They tend to infect lungs that have been damaged by silicosis or chronic obstructive lung disease. *Mycobacterium kansasii* responds well to antituberculous drugs in high dosage, but *M. avium-intracellulare* is resistant to nearly all drugs presently in use, and a favorable clinical response is less common.

TRANSMISSION

Most cases of communicable tuberculosis among adults develop because of a late recrudescence of dormant infection with no history of recent exposure. The liquid caseum from a cavity in such a case abounds in tubercle bacilli which are excreted in aerosolized droplets during coughing, sneezing, and speaking. When inhaled, droplets larger than 10 μm are usually caught on the mucociliary blanket and cleared from the lung without harm, but droplets of smaller size may reach the respiratory bronchiole and deposit bacilli beyond the protective mucous blanket. There, in a susceptible host, the organisms may invade tissue and establish an infection. Persons who have been infected previously are largely protected from reinfection by specific immunity, which is mediated by T lymphocytes. Teachers, school bus drivers, and nursery workers with infectious tuberculosis are of particular epidemiologic significance because of the great susceptibility of children.

Infection in a susceptible host is caused by inhalation of tubercle bacilli in *fresh* droplet nuclei expelled by a person with cavitary tuberculosis. Transmission can be blocked effectively by irradiation of the upper air of the room with ultraviolet light and adequate ventilation and by chemotherapy of the infectious case. Even though tubercle bacilli can be cultured from dust in a room of a tuberculous person, they constitute no hazard to others in this state because the irregular shape and electrostatic charge of the attached dust particles prevent them from being carried beyond the mucociliary protective mechanism. Early in the course of tuberculous infection, persons are rarely infectious because they expel very few organisms. Tuberculosis cannot be spread on hands, dishes, glasses, utensils, or fomites.

Patients who are on an effective regimen of chemotherapy lose their ability to transmit infection within a short time (probably 2 weeks or less), despite the continued presence of tubercle bacilli on smear and culture of the sputum.

PREVALENCE AND INCIDENCE

There has been a great fall in prevalence of tuberculosis in the United States since 1900. Early in this century over 80 percent of the population was infected *before* the age of 20 years. In an autopsy study in 1946, there was evidence of tuberculosis in 80 percent of the persons over the age of 50. In 1978, only 2 to 5 percent of young adults reacted to tuberculin (except in some urban areas), whereas about 25 percent of persons over the age of 50 reacted. The decline in incidence of the infection is most apparent among children and young adults and is due to a reduction in the number of infectious cases, which in turn is attributable to an improved standard of living, reduced risk of late progression of infection, and more prompt recognition and treatment of infectious cases.

The great majority of persons who harbor tubercle bacilli have latent or dormant ("healed") tuberculosis. Apical scars containing viable organisms may remain dormant for many years and then reactivate and produce clinical tuberculosis. Other sites in which tubercle bacilli may lie dormant for years and then recrudesce include the kidney (from which bacilli may spread to the genital tract in the male), spine, long bones, fallopian tubes, brain, and lymph nodes in the hilum and in the neck.

In 1976 there were about 32,000 new cases of clinical tuberculosis in the United States, an incidence of 15 per 100,000, down from 24 in 1966 and 53 in 1953. There were about 15 million tuberculin reactors, indicating a prevalence of infection of 7000 per 100,000. Of these, 60,000 were under therapy for tuberculosis and 500,000 had healed or dormant tuberculosis. The remainder had never developed clinical tuberculosis but simply harbored foci of latent infection. It is toward the latter group that programs of prophylactic therapy with INH are directed.

Of new tuberculous infections revealed by conversion of tuberculin reaction from negative to positive, 5 to 15 percent progress to serious disease within 5 years if left untreated. The risk of direct progression varies with age: it is greatest when infection begins in the first years of life and next greatest in young adults and adolescents. Among those remaining well for 5 years, a further 3 to 5 percent may develop late recrudescence at some time during life. Thus, the total morbidity rate in persons infected with *M. tuberculosis* is 8 to 20 percent. Both the early and late appearance of tuberculosis can be prevented in 80 percent of individuals if prompt treatment with INH is given when tuberculin "conversion" is discovered.

Mortality has fallen steadily over the past 70 years. Tuberculosis has ceased being the leading cause of death, with over 200 deaths per 100,000 in 1906 but only 1.5 per 100,000 in 1976. This figure may be somewhat low, because residual pulmonary scarring may lead to cor pulmonale and cause death secondarily.

IMMUNITY

NATURAL RESISTANCE The Caucasian and Mongolian races have a distinct natural resistance to tuberculosis consisting of an ability to develop an immune response to the infection which permits spontaneous recovery from initial infection. However, late recrudescence may result in chronic disease characterized by cavitation and scarring. Africans, American Indians, and Eskimos were generally spared tuberculous infection until extensive contact began with personnel of European heritage. The former group shows a decreased ability to develop an effective immune response to new infection, and in them the infection tends to be more rapidly progressive.

SPECIFIC (ACQUIRED) IMMUNITY Immunity to tuberculosis is mediated largely by T lymphocytes, which, in response to specific antigenic stimulation, liberate several lymphokines which facilitate the killing of mycobacteria and may actually block the effect of sensitized T lymphocytes. The role of immunoglobulins in the process is less clear, although IgA is often increased in patients with active tuberculosis and drops as the infection is controlled by therapy.

The mechanism by which latent infection recrudesces is not completely understood. From the fact that it occurs more commonly in old age and during other forms of illness, recrudescence appears likely to be due to reduced immunologic surveillance by T lymphocytes.

TUBERCULIN HYPERSENSITIVITY The most readily obtained evidence of a past or present infection with tubercle bacilli is the finding of hypersensitivity to tuberculin, a protein derivative of the broth in which tubercle bacilli have been grown. Epidemiologic evidence strongly suggests that tuberculin hypersensitivity indicates the presence of living tubercle bacilli. The larger the skin reaction, the greater the chance that the infection is of clinical significance.

PATHOGENESIS AND PATHOLOGIC ANATOMY

INITIAL INFECTION ("PRIMARY" TUBERCULOSIS) In the nonimmune subject tubercle bacilli can gain entrance to the body by several routes: lung, gastrointestinal tract, and direct cutaneous or percutaneous inoculation (as in an accident at the autopsy table). For practical purposes, the only route that is of importance in the United States is the lung. The majority of lesions in the early phase of infection are in the lower two-thirds of the lungs, where ventilation is best and deposition of droplet nuclei more likely. Because they produce no toxins and no tissue reaction, tubercle bacilli initially are free to multiply without deterrence. After phagocytosis in the nonimmune host, they remain viable within macrophages for an extended period. Prolonged intracellular survival, which is the key to virulence and persistence, is associated with failure of the bacilli-containing phagosomes to fuse with lysosomes. This defect of fusion protects the bacilli from the killing effect of the digestive enzymes. The organisms reach regional (hilar) nodes and even the bloodstream before their progress is inhibited by the gradual development of specific immunity over a period of several weeks. At this time, the characteristic tissue reaction develops, with epithelioid cell granulomas and caseation necrosis in the pulmonary lesion, regional lymph nodes, and any site to which the bacilli have spread. The number of bacilli drops drastically with the appearance of caseation necrosis, indicating that caseation is associated with the release of lymphokines from T lymphocytes which, in turn, release lysosomal enzymes from macrophages and destroy host tissues as well as tubercle bacilli. Thereafter, the infection in the primary site usually heals by a combination of resolution, fibrosis, and calcification. Occasionally defenses fail, and the infection may overwhelm the host or proceed directly to a chronic stage.

SILENT DISSEMINATION   Early in the course of a new infection tubercle bacilli reach the general circulation in varying numbers. This event is marked only by fever and mild symptoms and is recognized as tuberculosis only when a patient is being observed closely because of recent exposure to tuberculosis. This stage is important in the pathogenesis of tuberculosis, because it is the time when bacilli reach distant sites to establish metastatic foci of infection that are the seeds from which clinical tuberculosis may develop much later.

While bacilli presumably reach all organs during this silent bacillemia, they establish lesions with frequency in only a limited number of sites, which have one feature in common: high tissue oxygen tension. Despite a paucity of ventilation, the apexes of the lungs in the upright position have the highest oxygen tension in the body (130 mmHg) due to a high ventilation-perfusion ratio. Probably for this reason they are the most frequent sites in which viable bacilli persist in a dormant state in metastatic (Simon's) foci and produce clinical disease at a later time.

LATENT (DORMANT) INFECTION   When a tuberculous lesion regresses and heals, the infection enters a latent phase in which it may persist without producing illness. Though the infection may remain dormant for life, it may develop into clinical tuberculosis at any time if the persisting intracellular organisms begin to multiply rapidly.

CLINICAL TUBERCULOSIS   Fibrocaseous tuberculosis may develop from either direct progression of the initial infection or recrudescence of a dormant lesion, most commonly in the apical portion of the lung. An old caseous hilar lymph node occasionally liquefies and spills its contents into a bronchus, to produce a segmental or lobar tuberculous pneumonia. Massive bloodstream invasion (miliary tuberculosis) may also occur at any stage. Tuberculosis is characterized by localized nodular infiltrations, fibrosis, and cavitation.

MANIFESTATIONS

RECENT INFECTION   Uncomplicated initial tuberculous infection often produces no significant clinical illness. It is usually diagnosed only when contacts of an infectious case are examined or when it progresses to a serious form of disease. The incubation period is 4 to 8 weeks from inoculation to appearance of mild fever, malaise, and tuberculin hypersensitivity. Symptoms usually subside without specific therapy because of the appearance of adequate specific immunity. Occasionally, however, the infection progresses, either in the lung or by dissemination through the bloodstream. This turn of events is extremely serious unless detected promptly and treated adequately.

Massive hematogenous dissemination is most likely to occur in a recently infected child of 3 years or younger. In older children infection only rarely progresses to a fatal form and often passes completely unnoticed. The principal danger arises later during adolescence or early adulthood when the infection may undergo late progression.

Initial tuberculous infection occasionally produces pleurisy with effusion, cervical lymphadenitis, miliary tuberculosis, or meningitis. In addition, allergic manifestations occasionally develop, e.g., erythema nodosum and phlyctenular conjunctivitis.

In the United States, 90 to 98 percent of young adults have never been infected with tuberculosis. There have been several "epidemics" of tuberculosis among such susceptible young persons. For example, when infectious tuberculosis develops aboard ship or in prison, many persons may be infected and some secondary cases may develop. Persons working in the Peace Corps, Armed Forces, or State Department who are assigned to countries where the prevalence of tuberculosis is high may be heavily exposed to the disease. As in children, recent tuberculous infection usually produces only mild and nonspecific symptoms, but in the young adult it has a greater tendency to progress to clinical disease. There may be an area of pneumonitis in any portion of the lung, but obvious hilar adenopathy is not common. When a young adult has a pleural effusion or a parenchymal infiltrate in the lung, a tuberculin test should be performed. If the skin test is positive, the possibility of tuberculosis should be considered strongly. The source of infection is usually an adult with cavitary tuberculosis.

PULMONARY TUBERCULOSIS   Pulmonary tuberculosis may follow the initial infection directly or after a short or long period of dormancy. Progressive disease has been observed to develop after 60 years of clinical dormancy. The most striking features of late recrudescent tuberculosis are (1) absence of recent exposure to tuberculosis, (2) tendency to chronicity and cavitation, and (3) production of fibrous tissue of repair. The last two phenomena are characteristic of the responses in persons sensitized to tubercle bacilli. While the solid caseation necrosis of the initial stage contains few bacilli, the *liquid* caseum in a tuberculous cavity contains abundant bacilli and may spread infection via bronchi to other portions of the lungs and into the environment.

Symptoms   In most instances, the onset of pulmonary tuberculosis is insidious, and the patient may be entirely asymptomatic. Many cases are discovered because a routine roentgenogram is taken upon admission of an elderly person to a hospital for some other illness.

The earliest symptoms are constitutional and probably result chiefly from liberation of lymphokines stimulated by absorption of tuberculoprotein from numerous bacilli in a hypersensitive host. Abdominal symptoms may dominate the clinical picture. It is common for a patient with tuberculosis to be unaware of a fever as high as 40°C. General malaise may be present, but often there is nothing more than irritability, depression, and excessive fatigue at the end of the day. Defervescence during sleep gives rise to profuse sweating which may soak the patient's pajamas (night sweat).

Weight loss may precede symptoms but is often passed off as being due to overwork or to voluntary caloric restriction. Often weight is well maintained until late in the course of the illness. When abdominal symptoms predominate, loss of weight may be rapid.

Headache may be noted occasionally, especially in the evening. Palpitation may occur during mild exertion. Menstruation is usually not disturbed until the disease is advanced, when amenorrhea may develop.

Cough is frequent but not invariable and is often passed off as a "cigarette cough." When sputum is produced, it is usually odorless, green or yellow in color, and raised principally upon arising in the morning. Hemoptysis may accompany the cough and usually consists of streaking of the sputum with small amounts of blood. In some patients the onset of pulmonary tuberculosis is relatively sudden, with fever, productive cough, or pleuritic pain suggestive of bacterial pneumonia.

Physical and roentgen examinations Early asymptomatic infiltrations due to tuberculosis are usually undetectable by physical examination, even though obvious by x-ray. Crepitant rales may be present, especially when inspiration is preceded by full expiration and a small cough (posttussive rales).

Long-standing tuberculosis with extensive fibrosis causes contraction and distortion of pulmonary tissue and of bronchi. In such instances, a wide variety of physical signs may be present, such as apical dullness and bronchial breath sounds, coarse rales, deviation of the trachea, and diminished mobility of one hemithorax.

Because findings on examination of the lungs in the early stages are so frequently unremarkable, the importance of the chest roentgenogram in the diagnosis of tuberculosis cannot be overemphasized. Of particular importance is the comparison of the x-ray film with one made months or years earlier, so that subtle changes can be detected in clinically dormant lesions. Because fibrous tissue does not change appreciably with time, any change in the lesions on serial films must be interpreted as indicating pathologic activity of some disease. Among 90 patients over the age of 50 with recently developed pulmonary tuberculosis, over 70 percent showed evidence of preexisting tuberculous scars. Comparison of abnormal films with those taken in previous examinations makes it possible to detect and treat tuberculosis before liquefaction has occurred with spread of bacilli to other portions of the lungs or to other persons.

Complications of pulmonary tuberculosis CAVITATION When defense mechanisms fail, tuberculosis produces liquefaction necrosis and cavitation. The liquid material abounds with tubercle bacilli, making the disease highly infectious.

HEMOPTYSIS In the majority of instances of bleeding from the lungs in tuberculosis, the blood arises from ulceration of the bronchial mucosa and presents as streaks of bright red blood on the sputum. Bleeding usually subsides spontaneously if the patient lies quietly. Bleeding from the pulmonary artery is much more serious. While the branches of the pulmonary artery within a tuberculous lesion usually thrombose, occasionally one may remain open, may be eroded by the liquefaction, and form a mycotic (Rasmussen's) aneurysm. This may rupture and cause death from exsanguination or obstruction of airways. The blood expectorated is copious and dark because of deoxygenated hemoglobin in the pulmonary artery.

PLEURISY WITH EFFUSION A superficial tuberculous lesion may involve the overlying pleura and give rise to "dry" pleurisy, attended by localized pleuritic pain on deep inspiration. Or a small caseous pulmonary focus may actually erode through the visceral pleura and extrude a small amount of

liquid caseum. The immune response to such pleural contamination is a vigorous inflammatory reaction with formation of considerable pleural exudate. Although a pleural effusion may develop at any stage of tuberculosis, it is most common within a few months of the initial infection, particularly in young adults (age 15 to 35 years). The fluid is usually clear and light yellow. Its exudative nature is identified by a high protein content (> 3 g per 100 ml), an elevated lactic dehydrogenase (LDH) level, a lymphocytic-cell response, and pH < 7.20.

The importance of recognizing the tuberculous nature of such a pleural exudate in a young adult is reinforced by the finding that 65 percent of untreated patients sooner or later develop active tuberculosis. The diagnosis must often be clinical, because smears of the pleural fluid rarely reveal tubercle bacilli, and even the culture is positive in only 20 to 25 percent of cases. Percutaneous needle biopsy may reveal granulomatous pleuritis, but organisms are often not demonstrable. In most instances, proof of tuberculosis is lacking at the time the antituberculous treatment must be given if development of manifest tuberculosis is to be prevented. Fortunately, the intermediate tuberculin skin test is so regularly negative in healthy young adults that a positive reaction in a patient with a lymphocytic pleural exudate constitutes adequate evidence of tuberculous etiology to warrant initiation of two-drug therapy. However, it is not uncommon for the intermediate-strength purified protein derivative (PPD) test to be negative in patients with large tuberculous effusions, perhaps because the circulating tuberculin-specific T lymphocytes are rendered inactive by suppressor-adherent cells. A second-strength PPD will almost always be positive if the effusion is of tuberculous etiology.

TUBERCULOUS PNEUMONIA The onset of tuberculosis occasionally is quite acute, resembling that of bacterial pneumonia. This picture is seen most often in blacks, persons with diabetes, children with overwhelming infection, and elderly persons whose lungs are flooded with bacilli discharged from an area of liquid necrosis in the lung or hilar nodes. Chills, fever, productive cough, pleuritic chest pain, and leukocytosis may be noted. A stained smear of the sputum usually reveals numerous tubercle bacilli.

BRONCHOPLEURAL FISTULA AND EMPYEMA Though minimal pleural contamination from a small superficial caseous focus produces only a clear exudate, massive contamination from rupture of a large caseous lesion produces pneumothorax (bronchopleural fistula) and tuberculous empyema. This is one of the most dreaded complications of pulmonary tuberculosis. Tubercle bacilli are usually easily found in the purulent exudate. Management is largely surgical and consists of establishing adequate drainage, in combination with the administration of effective antituberculosis drugs.

TUBERCULOSIS OF BRONCHI, TRACHEA, AND LARYNX These organs are all protected from implantation of *M. tuberculosis* by a covering of secreted mucus but may become involved in advanced cavitary pulmonary tuberculosis with excretion of numerous tubercle bacilli. Bronchial ulceration may result in hemoptysis and a localized wheeze during respiration. The bronchial lumen also may be compromised by pressure of enlarged hilar lymph nodes early in the course of infection.

In a patient with cavitary pulmonary tuberculosis, hoarseness and pain in the throat accentuated by swallowing suggest tuberculous laryngitis. The diagnosis can be confirmed by indirect laryngoscopy. It is important to exclude cavitary tuberculosis before a laryngectomy is performed for carcinoma of

704

the larynx, because tuberculous laryngitis is occasionally mistaken for carcinoma, even on histologic examination. Antituberculous chemotherapy is highly effective for tuberculosis of the mucous membranes.

Bronchi which lie within tuberculous lesions are regularly weakened by the inflammatory process and dilated by contraction of fibrous tissue in healing. In the upper lobes this is rarely clinically significant, but in portions of the lung which are dependent when the patient is upright, it may lead to secondary infection, producing chronic productive cough and sporadic hemoptysis (see "Bronchiectasis," below).

GASTROINTESTINAL TUBERCULOSIS The normal gastrointestinal tract is resistant to penetration by tubercle bacilli, but in cavitary pulmonary tuberculosis associated with excretion of large numbers of bacilli, the mucosa may be penetrated in the ileocecal region. The symptoms consist chiefly of intermittent abdominal pain, cramping, and diarrhea. Occasionally the infection spreads through the wall of the intestine, to produce tuberculous peritonitis (see "Peritoneum," below).

Differential diagnosis The clinical picture presented by pulmonary tuberculosis varies widely and may simulate a great number of other diseases.

CARCINOMA OF THE LUNG (Chap. 268) Tuberculosis is commonly confused with carcinoma of the lung because the highest incidence of both diseases is in the upper lobes and in older men. Both cause loss of weight, chronic cough, blood-streaked sputum, and mild fever. In addition to bacteriologic studies for tubercle bacilli, sputum cytology, bronchial brushing, and bronchoscopy should be employed to aid in the differentiation. Comparison of prior roentgenograms may be of considerable help, but in many instances nothing short of a diagnostic thoracotomy will serve to make the distinction. When tuberculosis is considered among the diagnostic possibilities, therapy with two antituberculous drugs should be instituted a few days before thoracotomy in order to minimize complications in the event the lesion is tuberculous.

MYCOTIC INFECTIONS (Chaps. 151 to 161) When tubercle bacilli cannot be isolated from a patient suspected of having tuberculosis, appropriate tests should be made for the various fungus infections, which may present with a clinical picture indistinguishable from pulmonary tuberculosis. Helpful skin and serologic tests are available for coccidioidomycosis, histoplasmosis and aspergillosis, but blastomycosis, mucormycosis, cryptococcosis, and sporotrichosis can be diagnosed only by demonstrating the organisms in a biopsy specimen or on culture.

ACTINOMYCOSIS AND NOCARDIOSIS Although usually referred to as fungus diseases, these infections are actually caused by bacteria. Diagnosis is made by culture.

SARCOIDOSIS (Chap. 216) The typical patient with sarcoidosis is afebrile and has a negative tuberculin test and a roentgen picture of diffuse pulmonary infiltrations and hilar adenopathy, but the disease is protean in its manifestations and may mimic tuberculosis. Mediastinoscopy with biopsy of lymph nodes or lung biopsy is of greatest value in establishing this diagnosis. The Kveim test may be helpful when the antigen can be obtained.

ASPIRATION PNEUMONIA, LUNG ABSCESS (Chap. 260) Pulmonary infection which is introduced by the drainage of contaminated saliva during sleep from a focus of pyorrhea occurs predominantly in the upper and midposterior portions of the lung and can mimic tuberculosis. The distinction can usually be made eventually, but much valuable time may be lost while the patient is treated for the wrong disease. The presence of putrid sputum, hemoptysis, fever, and leukocytosis in a patient who has pyorrhea and has recently undergone surgery or who drinks alcohol to excess strongly suggests a pyogenic abscess. If the differentiation cannot be made readily, it may be advisable to treat with antimicrobials in addition to antituberculosis medications.

OTHER FORMS OF PNEUMONIA Bacterial or mycoplasma infection (Chap. 172) may present with clinical and roentgen appearances which at first may be indistinguishable from pulmonary tuberculosis. Cultures, cold agglutinins, precipitin, and complement fixation tests often establish the correct diagnosis. Cavitation is rare, and sputum examination does not yield tubercle bacilli. Early in the course of infection, tuberculosis may present with a localized infiltrate in the lung and slowly subside spontaneously or coincidentally with tetracycline therapy, similar to mycoplasma pneumonia. If clearing is incomplete, tuberculosis should be strongly considered. A tuberculin skin test should be performed in all patients with "viral pneumonia," particularly if a significant pleural effusion is present, since this is rare in viral pneumonia. A positive tuberculin skin test in an adolescent or young adult with pneumonitis strongly suggests tuberculosis because of the rarity of dormant infection in this age group.

PNEUMOCONIOSIS Pulmonary infiltrations associated with exposure to silicon dioxide, asbestos, ferrous oxide, and beryllium as well as hypersensitivity reactions to various organic inhalants may present a roentgenographic appearance suggestive of tuberculosis (Chap. 258). Silicosis may present great difficulty in diagnosis because it may produce conglomerate masses and even cavitation that mimic tuberculosis. Silicosis impairs the pulmonary defense against tubercle bacilli. When the tuberculin skin test is positive in a patient with silicosis, smoldering tuberculosis is so likely that two-drug therapy is indicated if activity is suggested by x-ray, and prophylaxis with isoniazid is justified if there is no evidence of activity.

BRONCHIECTASIS (Chap. 261) A productive cough due to chronic infection in dilated bronchi occurs much less frequently than formerly because of more effective antibiotic therapy for necrotizing pneumonias of childhood and the reduction in the number of children whose bronchi have been damaged by tuberculosis. The lower and middle lobes (or lingula on the left) are most often involved, and a bronchogram effectively demonstrates the pathologic condition. If the tuberculin skin test is positive, isoniazid should be administered prophylactically to prevent late progression of tuberculosis from coexistent foci in apexes, whether or not they are visible radiographically.

CONFUSION CAUSED BY SYSTEMIC EFFECTS OF TUBERCULOUS INFECTION Because of the insidious nature of tuberculosis, the clinical picture may be mistaken for that produced by several other disorders. Malaise, easy fatigability, inability to concentrate, anorexia, and loss of weight may be mistaken for psychoneurosis. The symptoms may suggest hyperthyroidism or diabetes mellitus, but with a little care the distinction can be made. Tuberculosis should always be considered in the differential diagnosis of fever of unknown origin (Chap. 10). If the roentgenogram reveals a pulmonary infiltrate, the possibility of tuberculosis is increased, but in cases of disseminated or extrapulmonary tuberculosis, the chest roentgenogram may be normal. In these cases biopsy of an enlarged lymph node, bone marrow, or liver may be of help. Formerly, tuberculosis was overdiagnosed in patients presenting with general systemic symptoms. Today, however, because of a lessening awareness of tuberculosis, the principal danger is that tuberculosis will be overlooked. Furthermore, tuberculosis may appear by recrudescence without recent reexposure, in anyone who has ever been infected in the past.

TUBERCULOSIS OF OTHER ORGANS Localized tuberculous infection may occur in a number of other organs, notably, the lymph nodes, kidney, long bones, genital tract, brain, and meninges. Organisms reach these sites during the silent bacillemia which often occurs early in the infection.

Lymph nodes The most common involvement of lymph nodes occurs in the hilus draining the pulmonary site of initial infection. The enlargement is usually modest but may be massive and give rise to obstruction and even ulceration of a major bronchus. The prognosis is good with proper chemotherapy, but the nodes may continue to enlarge for a few weeks after therapy is started and then resolve slowly.

Cervical adenitis (scrofula) This disease has become uncommon in the United States as a result of the elimination of tuberculous cattle and pasteurization of milk, but it occasionally occurs early in the course of infection. Cervical lymphadenitis may also appear as a late manifestation, especially in blacks. The nodes may be large (several centimeters in diameter) and matted together in a mass with an area of soft fluctuation. Signs of acute inflammation are rarely present. Swelling begins insidiously without systemic symptoms. Spontaneous rupture may occur, with drainage of caseous material. In some cases the offending organism is *M. scrofulaceum* or *M. kansasii*, and for this reason culture of the pus is necessary for accurate diagnosis.

Kidney Second to the upper lobes of the lungs, the kidney is the most common site for the late appearance of localized tuberculous infection. The mechanism of implantation is the same as that in the pulmonary apexes, namely, by hematogenous spread early in the infection. The oxygen tension in the cortical portion of the kidney approaches that in arterial blood, which enhances the growth and persistence of tubercle bacilli. As in the lungs, foci of tuberculosis may remain dormant for many years and produce clinical disease late in life. The pathologic process is the same as in the lung: inflammation, followed by caseation, liquefaction, and discharge of contaminated material into the collecting system and down the ureter to the bladder and, in men, to the genital tract.

Symptoms of renal tuberculosis are usually insidious and may be overlooked completely until the appearance of cystitis or epididymitis. Gross or microscopic hematuria and pyuria with a "sterile" urine on culture for bacteria should always call tuberculosis to mind and lead to the performance of a tuberculin skin test and culture of urine for tubercle bacilli. Intravenous pyelography may reveal a cortical cavity communicating with the calyceal system. Symptoms usually subside promptly with chemotherapy. Resection of residual areas of destruction is only rarely necessary.

Male genitals Infection of the genital tract in the male is secondary to renal tuberculosis. Bacilli discharged from a caseous lesion in the kidney may reach the seminal vesicles, prostate gland, and epididymis through their connections with the excretory tract. Symptoms begin insidiously, most commonly with scrotal pain due to inflammation of the epididymis and vas deferens. Tenderness and swelling may be found in the vas, seminal vesicles, and/or the prostate gland.

Female genitals When tuberculosis infection occurs after puberty, tuberculosis occasionally spreads hematogenously to the highly vascular fallopian tube. Infection may then spread into the uterus and give rise to endometritis. Symptoms are usually mild and of insidious onset, with abdominal pain, white vaginal discharge, metromenorrhagia, and dyspareunia. Systemic symptoms and signs are uncommon, probably because the infection is indolent and localized. The most common manifestation is sterility, but tubal scarring may cause pregnancy to be ectopic. Tuberculosis of the fallopian tube may also spread to the peritoneum and produce either a tuberculous pelvic abscess or generalized peritonitis.

Osseous tuberculosis Hematogenous spread of tuberculosis to the long bones and vertebrae is most common when infection occurs in childhood, because of the high P_{O_2} associated with the vascularity at the epiphyseal plates during active bone growth. It usually occurs within 3 years of infection, but dormant lesions may be reactivated by trauma years later. Infection begins in the ends of the long bones but becomes obvious when it involves the adjacent joint: hip, knee, elbow, or wrist. Tenosynovitis is most common at the wrist.

Tuberculous spondylitis (Pott's disease) This disease may result from hematogenous seeding or from spread of infection from paravertebral lymph nodes draining a tuberculous pleurisy. Spondylitis may develop in childhood or be delayed until later in life. Localized pain in the back may be present for months before x-rays reveal an abnormality. Though infection begins in the body of a vertebra, the first radiographic sign is usually destruction and narrowing of an intervertebral disk. A paravertebral abscess may be seen as a fusiform density extending the length of several vertebrae and occasionally dissects downward to the inguinal area. Therapy with two bactericidal drugs is the keystone of management, although some patients may require surgical drainage. Extensive orthopedic procedures are no longer necessary.

Peritoneum The peritoneum may be implanted with tubercle bacilli when they spread by any of at least four routes: (1) through the wall of infected intestine, (2) from a mesenteric lymph node, (3) from an infected fallopian tube, or (4) from hematogenous seeding in the course of disseminated tuberculosis. Symptoms are insidious, with increasing abdominal girth, but ultimately the patient has fever, night sweats, weakness, diarrhea, and abdominal pain. As with other forms of tuberculosis, there is an increased frequency among alcoholics. Tuberculosis should be strongly considered whenever ascitic fluid contains protein in excess of 3 g per 100 ml, when LDH is elevated, and when the white blood cells are mostly lymphocytes. Diagnosis may be made by open or percutaneous needle biopsy.

Pericardium Tuberculous infection may spread from the mediastinal lymph nodes or contiguous segments of lung to the pericardium in the same manner as to the pleura. The pathologic process is the same as in tuberculous pleurisy, with outpouring of a clear exudate, formation of granulomas, and subsequent fibrosis. The clinical picture may be that of chronic pericardial tamponade, with hepatomegaly, edema, friction rub, and enlargement of the cardiac shadow during the active phase, and constriction during the phase of fibrosis. When such an illness is accompanied by afternoon fever or night sweats and a positive tuberculin reaction, tuberculosis should be strongly considered. The diagnosis is made best by open pericardial biopsy. A tuberculous pericardial effusion contains more than 3 g protein per 100 ml, an elevated LDH, and lymphocytes. Early in the disease, multiple-drug chemotherapy accompanied by corticosteroids is usually sufficient, but surgical resection of the pericardium is occasionally necessary when the process is well established before therapy is begun.

If tuberculous pericarditis has undergone spontaneous healing, the patient may present years later with the picture of constrictive pericarditis (Chap. 249). Pericardiectomy at this stage may improve cardiac function but may be technically difficult because of extensive calcification extending into the myocardium. The procedure may be complicated by marked impairment of cardiac output postoperatively due to cardiac dilatation and myocardial atrophy.

Adrenals Occasionally hematogenous tuberculosis localizes in the adrenal glands and may result in their total destruction, giving rise to adrenal cortical insufficiency (Addison's disease, Chap. 336). This must be differentiated from adrenal cortical atrophy, which is more common, and from other causes of adrenal destruction, such as histoplasmosis. Therapy consists of prolonged administration of antituberculosis agents plus physiologic doses of adrenal steroids.

TRYPTOPHAN IN CSF

Meninges Tuberculosis may involve the meninges, either as a part of miliary tuberculosis or as extension of infection from a focus within the brain. In areas with a high incidence of tuberculosis, tuberculous meningitis is seen most commonly in young children during the first year of infection. In areas of low incidence such as the United States, meningitis is more common among older adults as a result of late reactivation of dormant infection. Pathologically, the meninges contain small tubercles and a fibrinous exudate over the base of the brain.

Symptoms consist of headache, restlessness, and irritability, usually accompanied by fever, malaise, night sweats, and loss of weight. Nausea and vomiting may be prominent. Stiffness of the neck and Brudzinski's sign are usually present. Spinal puncture usually reveals increased pressure, clear fluid containing an increased amount of protein, reduced glucose (less than half the blood glucose), and 100 to 1000 white blood cells per milliliter, 80 to 95 percent of which are lymphocytes. Demonstration of tryptophan in the spinal fluid provides a presumptive diagnosis of tuberculous meningitis upon which to institute chemotherapy.

The differential diagnosis includes partially treated pyogenic meningitis, fungal meningitis, carcinomatosis or sarcoidosis of the meninges, and subarachnoid hemorrhage. There is considerable urgency in establishing the correct diagnosis because specific therapy is most effective when instituted early in the course of the illness. Irreversible brain damage may result from waiting 6 to 8 weeks for cultural proof of diagnosis. For this reason it is frequently necessary to begin therapy for tuberculosis on the basis of a presumptive clinical diagnosis while awaiting results of bacteriologic studies. Therapy should include isoniazid and rifampin, both of which cross the blood-brain barrier. Steroids are indicated only when there is an impending subarachnoid block or cerebral edema. Intrathecal therapy is not indicated.

Inappropriate secretion of antidiuretic hormone (ADH) Older persons with tuberculous meningitis or overwhelming pulmonary tuberculosis occasionally present with somnolence or coma associated with a very low serum sodium concentration (110 to 125 meq per liter), because of inappropriate secretion of ADH. This must be distinguished from adrenal insufficiency, in which the sodium serum concentration is also depressed in concert with an elevated serum potassium level. In addition to antituberculosis agents, adequate sodium chloride should be administered and water intake restricted.

DISSEMINATED TUBERCULOSIS Silent bacillemia Hematogenous dissemination of a small number of tubercle bacilli is common early in the course of infection but usually produces little clinical illness. The principal importance of the event is the seeding of bacilli in sites far removed from the pulmonary site of inoculation.

Massive dissemination (miliary tuberculosis) When a liquid caseous focus empties its contents into a vein, there is a massive dissemination of tubercle bacilli throughout the body. Defense mechanisms are overwhelmed, and tubercles become established in all organs of the body. Without specific therapy, death is almost a certainty.

Miliary tuberculosis is the most dreaded manifestation of tuberculosis. It may arise shortly after infection or from recrudescence of a dormant focus years or decades later. Because the resistance of the body is overwhelmed, lesions are not limited to those organs with an elevated P_{O_2} but are often found in the liver, spleen, bone marrow, and meninges. The best way to make the diagnosis of miliary tuberculosis is to perform a biopsy of the liver, lymph node, or bone marrow in search of caseating granulomas and tubercle bacilli.

Symptoms are usually nonspecific and consist of weight loss, weakness, gastrointestinal disturbance, fever, and sweats. The patient has usually had a course of penicillin or broad-spectrum antibiotics without control of the fever before the diagnosis comes to mind. Cough is not a prominent feature, but dyspnea may be. The correct diagnosis is often not suspected until the typical "miliary" pattern is noted on the chest roentgenogram. The white cell count may be normal or low, or may show a leukemoid pattern suggesting leukemia. There may be a monocytosis. An identical clinical picture can be presented by histoplasmosis, coccidioidomycosis, blastomycosis, cryptococcosis, and other chronic infections. Therefore, it is imperative to obtain any material possible by biopsy or aspiration to establish a correct diagnosis on which to base therapy.

Subacute and chronic dissemination Instead of a single massive invasion of the bloodstream, smaller numbers of tubercle bacilli may escape into the circulation intermittently and give rise to a variety of clinical manifestations, including myelophthisic anemia, low-grade fever, lymphadenopathy, effusion into pleural and peritoneal cavities, and plenomegaly. There may be destructive lesions of bones, kidneys, subcutaneous tissue, or skin. Such a clinical picture is most common in elderly persons with recrudescent infection.

The protean manifestations and bizarre clinical picture caused by subacute and chronic forms of hematogenous tuberculosis provide a tremendous diagnostic challenge. To add to the confusion, the tuberculin reaction is often suppressed in persons with overwhelming infection. The intermediate-strength tuberculin test is often negative, and the PPD no. 2 (see "Diagnosis," below) occasionally so. The solution to the clinical problem most commonly comes when the possibility of tuberculosis is belatedly considered. Confirmation must be sought from appropriate histologic and bacteriologic studies. The prognosis is uniformly bad without treatment but good with appropriate chemotherapy.

DIAGNOSIS

TUBERCULIN SKIN TEST Tuberculin is a protein fraction of tubercle bacilli. When introduced into the skin of a person with tuberculous infection, whether clinically apparent or dormant, it triggers release of several lymphokines which over the next 24 to 72 h cause a localized thickening of the skin due to edema and accumulation of sensitized lymphocytes. Although there are several methods for testing healthy populations with tuberculin for evidence of unsuspected infection, the method preferred in clinical practice is to inject 0.1 ml of a solution containing 5 tuberculin units (TU) of purified protein derivative stabilized with Tween 80 (5 TU of PPD-T) into the skin of the volar aspect of the forearm with a small needle—an "intermediate-strength tuberculin test." The test is read 48 to 72 h later and is considered positive if the diameter of skin thickening measures 10 mm or more, doubtful if it is 5 to 10 mm, and negative if it is less than 5 mm.

Intermediate-strength PPD produces a positive reaction in the majority of persons infected with tubercle bacilli. However, it is a biologic test which is dependent upon the presence of an adequate number of circulating sensitized T lymphocytes. False-negative results may occur in 15 to 20 percent of persons with clinical tuberculosis if sensitized T lymphocytes are temporarily nonfunctional, as in persons who are clinically ill, febrile, or have a large pleural effusion. If the intermediate PPD is negative in a patient in whom tuberculosis is suspected, the test should be repeated using "second-strength" PPD (100 or 250 TU). If this is also negative, tuberculosis can be dismissed with considerable certainty, although persons who are moribund from tuberculosis may fail to react even to PPD no. 2.

A positive reaction to intermediate-strength PPD indicates the presence of a tuberculous infection but does not help in distinguishing clinical from dormant infection. This distinction must be made on clinical, bacteriologic, and radiographic grounds. A positive reaction which is elicited only by PPD no. 2 in a patient who is clinically ill means that active tuberculosis cannot be dismissed as a diagnostic possibility. In healthy persons, however, it usually signifies only healed tuberculosis or infection with mycobacteria other than *M. tuberculosis*.

RADIOGRAPHY   While never providing an etiologic diagnosis, x-rays of the chest provide extremely valuable information. The abnormality which is most suggestive of tuberculosis is a multinodular infiltrate with cavitation in one or both of the upper lobes of the lung. Because of the propensity of tuberculosis to spread via bronchi to other parts of the lungs, the basilar areas may also be involved. Occasionally, especially in the elderly, the lesions are limited to the lower lobe(s). Multiple infiltrates, especially if bilateral, are most suggestive of tuberculosis, because pyogenic pneumonia and primary carcinoma are much more likely to produce single lesions. Carcinoma usually produces a solid lesion, in contrast to the multinodular infiltrate of tuberculosis. Planigrams (laminagrams) are particularly valuable in making such distinctions and in detecting cavitation. Lateral, lordotic, and oblique films are also of value in defining the location and character of lesions. Initially tuberculous infection is not usually apical in location but may involve any other segment of the lungs. Hilar adenopathy is common early in the course of infection in children, but may not be obvious by x-ray in adults. Large pleural effusions are easily detected, but for small or infrapulmonary effusion it may be necessary to place the patient on the *involved* side to permit the fluid to be seen along the lateral chest wall (lateral decubitus film).

BACTERIOLOGIC DIAGNOSIS   The only absolute proof of active tuberculosis is the cultural identification of *M. tuberculosis* from tissue or body fluid: sputum, gastric washing, urine, cerebrospinal fluid (CSF), serous effusion, or pus from an abscess or sinus. A useful preliminary examination, however, is to make a smear of the material and stain it for standard microscopy or to apply auromine-rhodamine stain for easier detection by fluorescence microscopy. The smear is not a very sensitive method, but it has the virtue of quickly identifying the patient who is discharging great numbers of organisms into the environment. For positive identification, cultures must be

made either on solid egg medium (Löwenstein-Jensen) or Middlebrook 7H-11 medium using 20 to 40 mmHg CO_2 in the incubator.

The most commonly examined material is sputum. When it can be produced spontaneously (usually in the early morning), it makes the most satisfactory material for both smear and culture. If none can be produced spontaneously, the patient may be asked to inhale aerosolized heated saline to stimulate production of bronchial secretions. Bacteriologic specimens may also be collected by bronchial washing, bronchial brushing, or tracheal aspiration. Sputum should never be collected over a 24-h period because this increases the frequency of contamination.

When no sputum can be collected, as in young children or senile or psychotic persons, fasting morning gastric contents may be aspirated and cultured. Diagnosis by smear of this material is less reliable than examination of sputum because of the frequency of saprophytic acid-fast bacteria in the stomach, but the presence of large numbers of acid-fast bacilli strongly suggests that they are significant.

Multiple specimens may be needed before the organisms are recovered. This is particularly true early in the course of tuberculous infection, tuberculous pleurisy with effusion, and when the pulmonary lesions are small and noncavitary. Patients with old chronic tuberculous lesions may shed organisms only intermittently.

HEMATOLOGY   The white blood cell count is usually not significantly elevated, except in tuberculous pneumonia (when it may suggest a pyogenic infection) and in miliary tuberculosis (when a leukemoid reaction may be mistaken for leukemia). Hemoglobin and hematocrit are usually normal unless a prolonged period of illness has produced anemia of infection.

URINALYSIS   There are no specific changes except when a urinary tract lesion is present. Renal tuberculosis is not rare in older persons; it most often presents with microscopic hematuria and pyuria with negative cultures for pyogens. Two or three early morning specimens should be submitted for culture. About 10 percent of persons with pulmonary tuberculosis excrete bacilli in their urine, even without detectable urinary tract lesions.

OTHER TESTS   Despite great efforts to develop one, there is no specific serologic test to distinguish clinical from dormant tuberculosis. Biopsy of the liver, bone marrow, or lymph node can be of great aid in reaching a presumptive diagnosis of disseminated tuberculosis by revealing caseating granulomas containing acid-fast bacilli. Such a finding may be lifesaving by permitting initiation of specific therapy without allowing the disease to progress while awaiting culture confirmation.

TREATMENT   Treatment of tuberculosis is based upon intensive and prolonged exposure of the organisms to bacterial antagonists. With proper management tuberculosis can be cured in 95 percent of patients, even though return to health may be limited by an associated disease. Heretofore conventional therapy has required 18 to 24 months, but by using a regimen of two bactericidal drugs treatment can now be completed in 9 months. Either form of therapy can be accomplished while the patient is ambulatory and even at work.

PRINCIPLES OF CHEMOTHERAPY   To be effective in therapy, a drug must interfere with a vital function of the tubercle bacillus without harming the host. The choice of therapy should be guided by several well-established principles:

1 Drugs should be chosen to which the bacilli are likely to be susceptible. Fortunately, in the United States this presents little difficulty in most newly discovered cases because most strains are susceptible to the major drugs. If a patient has been treated previously or contracted the infection in an area where drug resistance is common (e.g., Southeast Asia, Phillippines, Mexico), it must be assumed that the bacilli will be resistant to isoniazid (INH) and the regimen should include at least two other drugs until the results of susceptibility studies are known.

2 Even in a generally susceptible population of bacilli, a naturally resistant mutant occurs about once in 10^5 to 10^6 organisms. For this reason at least two effective drugs should always be given to patients with clinical tuberculosis to avoid multiplication of drug-resistant mutants.

3 Bactericidal drugs are always preferred. Both rifampin and isoniazid are bactericidal for both extra- and intracellular bacilli. For this reason these two drugs are effective both for immediate reduction in the large extracellular population of bacilli and for ultimate eradication of the smaller intracellular population.

4 When treatment appears to be failing (bacteriology fails to become negative within 3 to 4 months), the addition of a single drug is an invitation to disaster. Therapy should always be changed to an entirely new regimen of at least two new drugs, and great care should be taken to ensure that the patient takes the medication regularly.

5 Therapy must be continued long enough to eradicate the bacilli from the body. When two bactericidal drugs are used, this can be accomplished in 9 months, but when one of the drugs is bacteriostatic, a treatment period of 18 to 24 months is required.

6 All medications should be given before breakfast and in a single dose, if possible, in order to achieve a single combined peak concentration for maximum effect on the bacilli.

MAJOR DRUGS   **Isoniazid (INH)**   Isoniazid interferes with DNA synthesis and intermediary metabolism of the tubercle bacillus. It is the keystone of antituberculous chemotherapy. It is acetylated in the liver and excreted by the kidney.

DOSE.   The usual dose for adults is 5 mg/kg per day, usually 300 mg, given in a single dose. In children the dosage is higher because of more rapid excretion: 10 to 15 mg/kg per day. It is a safe drug for use in pregnancy, although elective chemoprophylaxis should be deferred until after delivery. Although some persons acetylate INH more rapidly than others, this has proved to be of little clinical significance unless the interval between doses is 5 days or more. When used in "pulse" therapy, the dose is about 15 mg/kg given twice weekly or 10 mg/kg given three times per week. A matrix form of INH for slower release is under investigation as a means of reducing the frequency of doses. In renal failure, the standard dose is usually tolerated well.

TOXICITY.   Although not common, three types of toxicity from INH occur: (1) Direct toxicity consists of peripheral neuropathy and anemia due to competition of INH with pyridoxine. Pyridoxine in a dose of 30 to 50 mg per day effectively combats this problem, which is most common when a large dose is used and in alcoholics whose nutrition is impaired. (2) Allergic reactions consist of skin rash, swelling of the tongue, arthralgia, and fever and may require withdrawal of the drug. (3) Hepatocellular toxicity is the most serious toxic effect of INH. Contrary to earlier thought, hepatitis is not due to allergy but may be due to a reaction to a metabolic product of INH degradation in the liver. Symptoms consist of malaise and anorexia followed by nausea, vomiting, fever, and finally, jaundice. The best way to detect INH hepatitis is to acquaint each patient with the symptoms for which to be alert (anorexia, nausea, vomiting) with the request that they be reported without delay. No more than a 1-month supply of INH should be given, and inquiry about symptoms should be made each time the patient is seen. A suspected reaction must be confirmed by the following procedure: discontinue INH at once and draw blood for determination of SGOT, alkaline phosphatase, and serum bilirubin. If these tests are normal or SGOT is only mildly elevated, INH therapy may be reinstituted cautiously. If any of the tests show a threefold elevation, INH hepatitis is very likely and the drug should not be given. For minor elevations, one should repeat the studies; if they are normal, restart treatment with INH, beginning with 50 mg (one-sixth of a 300-mg tablet), and recheck the laboratory results. If symptoms recur and the SGOT shows a sharp rise, INH toxicity exists and the drug should be discontinued. The only therapy required is the withdrawal of the drug, but if INH is continued in the face of symptoms of hepatitis, it may prove fatal.

Rifampin (RIF)   Rifampin acts by inhibition of RNA polymerase of both extra- and intracellular bacilli. The dose is about 10 mg/kg per day, or 450 to 600 mg per day, for adults and about 15 mg/kg per day for children. Although RIF has not been cleared for use during pregnancy, wide experience has produced no evidence of teratogenicity. Toxicity consists of jaundice (about 1 percent), gastrointestinal symptoms, and fever. Hypersensitivity reactions such as "flu syndrome," renal failure, and thrombocytopenia may occur when a large dose (900 to 1200 mg) is administered intermittently, but are uncommon when smaller doses (450 to 600 mg) are administered two or three times per week. Hypersensitivity reactions may occur when RIF is resumed after a longer interruption. While there is some laboratory evidence of suppression of immunity, there appears to be no clinical effect.

Streptomycin (SM) and capreomycin (CM)   These drugs inhibit protein synthesis and are bactericidal for extracellular bacilli. They do not penetrate the cell walls of macrophages to reach the intracellular organisms. Dosage for each is 1 g per day for adults, reduced to 0.5 g per day in persons over age 60, of small stature, or with renal impairment. Dosage in children is 20 mg/kg per day. Actually, daily medication can be given 5 days per week with no apparent loss of effectiveness, which facilitates administration of medication by visiting nurses. Toxicity may be allergic in type with fever, rash, malaise, etc., or related to the eighth cranial nerve or the renal tubule. The latter two are total-dose related; therefore, medication is best given daily (five times per week) for only about 2 months and then two or three times per week for an additional 4 to 6 weeks to minimize the total amount of the drug used. Streptomycin is safe during pregnancy, although it may exert a toxic effect upon the eighth cranial nerve of the fetus in late pregnancy. Slight dizziness and circumoral paresthesias are common immediately after injections, but are generally harmless.

Pyrazinamide (PZA)   A very effective drug whose mode of action remains obscure, PZA penetrates the cell wall of the macrophage and is bactericidal in the acid intracellular milieu. When used with SM or CM, a very effective bactericidal combination results against organisms in both locations. Dosage is 30 mg/kg per day given in a single daily dose. PZA can also be given twice a week in a dose of 50 mg/kg. It regularly causes a striking increase in serum uric acid, due to interference with renal excretion of uric acid, but this is harmless except in persons with gout. Toxicity consists of jaundice (rare), fever, or rash.

Ethambutol (EMB) *optic neuritis* Ethambutol inhibits RNA synthesis and is bacteriostatic against extracellular tubercle bacilli. Its principal value is inhibition of the growth of mutants which are resistant to INH or RIF. It was the second most commonly used drug in the United States until it was realized that the combination of RIF and INH makes it possible to administer two bactericidal drugs and thus reduce the total duration of therapy. Its principal use now is as a substitute drug used when toxicity precludes the use of a more effective one. EMB is well tolerated in a dose of 15 mg/kg per day with only rare instances of ocular toxicity (optic neuritis). In the more effective dose of 25 mg/kg per day which is necessary as a substitute drug, the incidence of optic neuritis approaches 1 percent and requires careful surveillance. It is not recommended in pregnancy or in children too young to cooperate in the testing of vision. In addition to periodic examination of visual acuity, color vision, and visual fields, patients should be asked to report any reduction in acuity noted in reading newsprint with their usual glasses. This drug can be used in supervised twice weekly treatment for which the dosage is 50 mg/kg.

OTHER DRUGS Ethionamide (ETA) Ethionamide inhibits protein synthesis and is of value in re-treatment of patients who harbor organisms that show multiple drug resistance. Dosage is 750 to 1000 mg per day for adults. Because gastric irritation is so common, this drug must be given in divided doses after meals.

Cycloserine (CS) This drug inhibits cell wall synthesis and is of use in re-treatment cases. Dosage is 750 to 1500 mg per day for adults, divided into two doses, each accompanied by pyridoxine, 100 mg. CS should not be used in epileptics or persons with a history of psychosis.

p-Aminosalicylic acid (PAS) *p*-Aminosalicylic acid interferes with intermediary metabolism and is bacteriostatic for the tubercle bacillus. Because of a high incidence of gastrointestinal intolerance, it is infrequently used today. It should not be used with RIF because PAS interferes with its absorption. Dosage is 200 mg/kg per day in divided doses.

Kanamycin An aminoglycoside, kanamycin interferes with protein synthesis and can be used in selected re-treatment of resistant cases. Eighth nerve toxicity is so common and severe that it greatly limits its usefulness.

Thiacetazone and isoxyl These are inexpensive drugs in common use in developing countries. They are not available for clinical use in the United States, however, because of a high incidence of toxic side effects.

Viomycin This drug is no longer manufactured in the United States.

CHOICE OF THERAPY FOR CLINICAL TUBERCULOSIS The immediate goal of chemotherapy is to kill the organisms without permitting the selection of resistant mutants. It is very important to adhere to the principles of therapy outlined above in choosing and carrying out a therapeutic regimen. Chemo-

therapy of tuberculosis is so effective that such modalities as bed rest, collapse therapy, surgical resection, etc., need no longer be discussed.

Initial treatment It is now apparent that therapy for tuberculosis, regardless of the organ involved, can be completed in 9 months *provided two bactericidal drugs are given together for the full period.* If the regimen consists of only one bactericidal drug and one bacteriostatic drug, therapy must be given for 18 to 24 months to achieve comparable success.

Preferred regimens When there is no reason to suspect resistance to INH (see the first principle of therapy), the regimen should consist of INH and RIF from the start and usually no other drug is needed. Where the possibility of INH and/or SM resistance is recognized, additional drugs should be given to ensure that at least two effective agents are included pending the report of drug susceptibilities.

Several safe and effective short-course regimens of therapy for tuberculosis have been described. INH 300 mg and RIF 600 mg daily for 9 months is curative in 95 percent of cases with a relapse rate of less than 2 percent. A 9-month regimen has been in use in Arkansas for over 3 years that has been equally effective and requires only one-third as much RIF. In the Arkansas regimen, INH and RIF are given daily for 4 to 6 weeks. At that time RIF is given in the same dose of 600 mg, but the INH dose is increased to 15 mg/kg (usually 900 mg for adults) twice a week (e.g., on Tuesdays and Fridays) for the remainder of the 9 months. We have had no serious allergic reactions in giving RIF in this manner to over 600 patients, many of whom were quite elderly. Another advantage of this regimen is that it lends itself to total supervision of drug ingestion when necessary to ensure compliance.

The regimen used in Great Britain consists of RIF 450 to 600 mg and INH 300 mg for 9 months with the addition of either SM 0.75 g or EMB 25 mg/kg daily for the first 2 months. The third drug adds little if the organisms are sensitive to INH, but can be good insurance against failure if the organisms should be resistant to INH.

In recent studies four bactericidal drugs have been given at the outset to reduce the population of organisms as quickly as possible in an effort to shorten therapy still further. For the moment, however, this appears to have little advantage to offset the disadvantage of increased drug toxicity, except when drug resistance is known or suspected.

About 4 to 6 percent of patients are unable to take RIF and INH because of toxicity, forcing the discontinuance of the offending drug(s) and substitution of others (e.g., SM, PZA, EMB). Hepatic toxicity is uncommon, i.e., less than 2 percent in our experience. Whenever the advantage of giving two bactericidal drugs together is lost, therapy then must be prolonged to 18 to 24 months to achieve success.

Prior to the introduction of the bactericidal therapy described above, the most widely used regimen was a combination of INH 300 mg per day combined with EMB in a dose of 15 to 25 mg/kg per day. When a large population of organisms was indicated by a positive sputum smear, it was common practice to add SM 1 g per day for the first 2 months in order to reduce further the risk of selection of INH-resistant mutants. The total period of therapy with this regimen must be 18 to 24 months in order to ensure lasting success. This form of therapy is now used principally when toxicity secondary to a bactericidal drug forces substitution of a bacteriostatic one.

With the bactericidal combination of RIF and INH, conversion of cultures to negative is quite prompt, i.e., 89 percent in 2 months and 96 percent in 3 months. This is appreciably better than what could be achieved with earlier regimens. Relapse after successful therapy with RIF and INH has been less than 2 percent, largely within the first 6 months following completion of 9 months of therapy. If the full course of 18 to 24 months of the formerly used regimen is followed, relapses should be uncommon (about 3 to 4 percent), but this is often difficult to achieve. When relapse occurs following treatment with RIF and INH, the organisms almost always remain sensitive to both drugs and further treatment with the same regimen given for a longer period of time is usually successful. When relapse occurs following other forms of therapy, the chance of INH-resistant organisms is greater and a multiple-drug retreatment regimen is often necessary to achieve ultimate success.

The two most important tasks during treatment are (1) careful bacteriologic monitoring to be certain of the effectiveness of the medications and to provide samples of the bacilli to test for susceptibility in the event of failure and (2) careful monitoring for the toxic side effects of the drugs being given. To achieve both these ends, the patient should be seen no less frequently than every week or two at the outset and then at monthly intervals when the patient appears stable and recovery is going smoothly. To detect the occasional relapse, sputum specimens should be collected at monthly intervals for the first 6 months after completion of therapy and then every 3 months for an additional year.

When the patient's clinical condition requires hospitalization, it should be brief. Effective chemotherapy reduces infectiousness promptly even while the sputum smear is still positive for tubercle bacilli. For home therapy to be successful, the patient must comprehend enough of the nature of the disease and chemotherapy to ensure cooperation. Irregularity of medication or premature discontinuation are the major causes of failure and relapse. The booklet *Understanding Tuberculosis Today* by W. W. Stead (Central Press, Milwaukee, 1979) is available from many local affiliates of the American Lung Association. It explains tuberculosis and its therapy in terms most patients can comprehend and is helpful in achieving compliance.

Re-treatment of "resistant cases"   Need for a regimen for re-treatment may arise from inadequate use of drugs at the outset, from premature discontinuation of medication, or from relapse after apparently successful therapy. The skill required to manage a re-treatment case is greater than for initial therapy, and advice should be sought from a physician experienced in this field. Re-treatment must always involve a completely *new regimen of drugs*. When the patient has received several drugs in the past, it is usually desirable to await results of susceptibility tests before selecting therapy. When INH resistance is suspected but not yet proved, an excellent regimen is SM, PZA, RIF, and INH. The drugs should be given daily for 6 to 8 weeks or until drug susceptibilities are known. CM may be substituted if SM resistance is suspected. If the bacilli are later found to be susceptible to RIF and INH, daily or twice weekly therapy with only these medications for another 7 months is adequate. If INH resistance is confirmed, RIF, SM, and PZA should be continued either daily or twice weekly for a total of 9 months. For poorly compliant patients whose ingestion of medication must be supervised, the twice weekly regimen is preferable. When EMB must be substituted for any of the drugs, therapy must be continued for at least 12 to 15 months *after conversion* of sputum to negative.

Corticosteroids   The use of cortisone and its derivatives has been shown to increase the chance of recrudescence of dormant tuberculosis. Despite this, in patients who are very seriously ill with tuberculosis, these agents may be lifesaving. They should be used only when there is an immediate threat to life, such as hypotension, debilitating fever, dyspnea, or an impending blockage of the subarachnoid space in tuberculous meningitis. Prednisone may be used in a dosage of 40 mg per day for 1 to 2 weeks, then 20 mg for another 8 weeks, and then gradually withdrawn over a period of 3 to 4 weeks in order to prevent a "steroid rebound." The effect upon the temperature and the general well-being of the patient may be dramatic, but there is no decrease in residual fibrosis. In general, the frequency of side effects makes the routine use of steroids in conjunction with chemotherapy unwise.

PREVENTION

Chemoprophylaxis   Clinically inapparent tuberculous infection can be prevented from developing into tuberculosis by judicious use of isoniazid therapy both in recently infected persons and in those with a dormant infection.

Recently infected persons   Close contacts of an infectious case of tuberculosis should be tested with tuberculin. Hospital and nursing home personnel should be tested at the time of employment and then annually. Any reactor with detectable disease or symptoms should be examined bacteriologically and given treatment with two drugs as outlined earlier. Newly infected persons with normal chest x-rays should be given preventive treatment with isoniazid. The risk of development of clinical tuberculosis in such persons is appreciable (see "Prevalence and Incidence," above) and greatly exceeds the risk of toxicity from isoniazid.

Close contacts of an infectious case who are under the age of 4 years are at special risk and should be started on therapy even though the tuberculin test is negative and they appear well. If in 3 months the skin test is still negative, therapy may be discontinued; if positive, treatment should be given for a full year.

Persons with dormant infections   Dormant tuberculous infection may be prevented from developing into clinical disease by treatment with isoniazid. Treatment is generally recommended for reactors under the age of 35 years and especially for those under 25. Over the age of 35 the risk of hepatitis from isoniazid increases somewhat, and preventive therapy is recommended for reactors of unknown duration only if one of the following factors that increases the risk of tuberculosis is present: (1) radiographically detectable apical scars (Simon's foci) suggestive of healed tuberculosis, (2) diabetes mellitus, (3) prolonged steroid therapy, (4) history of gastrectomy, (5) silicosis, or (6) any chronic malignancy, such as Hodgkin's disease.

Preventive therapy consists of isoniazid, 300 mg for adults and 5 to 10 mg/kg for children given in a single daily dose for 9 to 12 months. Preventive therapy reduces the risk of clinical tuberculosis by about 80 percent, and protection appears to be lasting. When the apparent source case excretes tubercle bacilli which are resistant to isoniazid, rifampin should be given for a year as prophylaxis.

Toxic reactions to isoniazid are uncommon below age 35, but thereafter may be as high as 2 to 3 percent. They need not be serious if early symptoms are heeded and the medication stopped promptly, as outlined earlier. The booklet *Understanding Tuberculosis Today*, mentioned above, can help patients understand the risk of tuberculosis and the rationale for prophylactic chemotherapy.

BIOLOGIC PROPHYLAXIS BCG vaccine BCG, or bacillus Calmette-Guerin, is a live, attenuated strain of bovine tubercle bacilli which has been used widely in many countries to induce specific immunity against tuberculosis. Although it does not reduce the chance of natural infection, it does prevent the development of serious forms of tuberculosis when natural infection occurs. There has been controversy on the effectiveness of BCG, but most authorities agree that it affords about 80 percent protection against the development of clinical tuberculosis. Its greatest value is in infants in countries with high prevalence where exposure of children is common. In the United States vaccination is indicated only for nonreactors who cannot avoid exposure, as when assigned to countries of high prevalence in the Peace Corps, State Department, Armed Forces, etc.

ERADICATION OF TUBERCULOSIS The decline in mortality rates from tuberculosis early in the century led some to predict the eradication of the disease in the United States by 1945. This prediction was based on the idea that infection with tubercle bacilli was harmless and that only reinfections were dangerous. It was reasoned that tuberculosis would disappear when reinfections could be prevented by isolating all infectious cases. It is now clear, however, that clinical tuberculosis developed largely from reactivation of dormant infections and that eradication must await the natural disappearance of tubercle bacilli from the population. It is hoped that this process can be accelerated by the judicious use of INH as prophylactic therapy, but clinical tuberculosis will continue to occur for many years.

IMPLICATIONS OF A POSITIVE TUBERCULIN REACTION In the United States, the chance of a tuberculin reactor developing clinical tuberculosis from a dormant infection is greater than that of a nonreactor acquiring an infection. Therefore, it is preferable to be tuberculin-negative, unless the positive reaction is induced by vaccination. On the other hand, living in a country of high prevalence a nonreactor would be more likely to become infected than a healthy reactor. Under these circumstances, it would be preferable to be tuberculin-positive and to have the immunologic protection against acquiring a new infection.

REFERENCES

BATES JH: Treatment of tuberculosis. Adv Intern Med 20:1, 1975

————, STEAD WW: Effect of chemotherapy on infectiousness of tuberculosis. N Engl J Med 290:459, 1974

DUTT AK, STEAD WW: Short-course chemotherapy for tuberculosis with largely twice-weekly isoniazid-rifampin: Results up to 30 months. Chest 75:441, 1979

FOX W, MITCHISON DA: State of the art "short-course chemotherapy for pulmonary tuberculosis." Am Rev Respir Dis 111:325, 1975

JOHNSTON RF, WILDRICK KH: The impact of chemotherapy on the care of patients with tuberculosis. Am Rev Respir Dis 109:636, 1974

STEAD WW: Pathogenesis of the sporadic case of tuberculosis. N Engl J Med 277:1008, 1967

————, BATES JH: Evidence of "silent" bacillemia in primary tuberculosis. Ann Intern Med 74:559, 1971

————, TEXTER EC: Isoniazid hepatitis. A backlash of progress. Ann Intern Med 79:125, 1973

———— et al: The clinical spectrum of primary tuberculosis in adults: Confusion with reinfection in the pathogenesis of chronic tuberculosis. Ann Intern Med 68:731, 1968

YOUMANS GP: Relationship between delayed hypersensitivity and immunity in tuberculosis. Am Rev Respir Dis 111:109, 1975

144

LEPROSY

CHARLES C. SHEPARD

DEFINITION Leprosy (Hansen's disease) is a chronic granulomatous infection of man, which, in its various clinical forms, attacks superficial tissues, especially the skin, peripheral nerves, and nasal mucosa. The two major clinical types are *lepromatous* and *tuberculoid;* when the disease has features of both these types, it is called *borderline*. In addition, an early indeterminate form is seen, which may later develop into one of the three types mentioned.

ETIOLOGY *Mycobacterium leprae,* or Hansen's bacillus, is the causal agent of leprosy. It is an acid-fast rod, found in enormous numbers in lepromatous lesions. Although it has not been cultivated in artificial media, nor convincingly in tissue cultures, it can be propagated in cooler tissues of small rodents, very consistently in the foot pads of mice. The bacillus will also produce heavy systemic infections in a proportion of nine-banded armadillos; armadillos have a lower body temperature. The bacillus multiplies very slowly, so mouse experiments take 6 to 12 months and armadillo experiments take several years. The mouse model has been used much for the study of antileprosy drugs, and the high bacterial yield from armadillos is making many immunologic studies possible. Estimates of bacillary viability can be made microscopically by determination of the "solid ratio" or "morphologic index"; only viable bacilli are thought to stain solidly.

Lepromin is a suspension of killed *M. leprae* prepared from the tissues of lepromatous patients. Intradermal injection elicits, somewhat irregularly, a tuberculin-like reaction at 48 h (Fernandez' reaction) and more consistently, a papular reaction at 4 weeks (Mitsuda's reaction). The Mitsuda reaction is usually positive in tuberculoid patients and negative in lepromatous patients and is therefore an aid in clinical classification. However, because it is also positive in nearly all normal adults, it has no diagnostic value.

EPIDEMIOLOGY At present, there are probably 10 to 20 million persons affected with leprosy in the world. The disease is more common in tropical countries, in many of which 1 to 2 percent or more of the population is affected. It is also common in certain regions with cooler climates, such as Korea, China, and central Mexico. In the United States the chief leprosy areas are Texas, California, Hawaii, Louisiana, Florida, and New York. Some of the cases are acquired domestically, some are acquired abroad.

Leprosy is frequently a family infection. Many patients give a history of prolonged exposure, and in close family contacts (spouse-spouse) of untreated lepromatous patients the attack rate is 5 to 10 percent. Among young children of untreated lepromatous parents, 30 to 50 percent develop a mild, single-lesion type of leprosy which heals spontaneously. After the index case is under treatment, spread within the family does not occur. Transmission from patients with tuberculoid leprosy is uncommon. The portal of entry is a matter of conjecture, but is probably either the skin or the nasal mucosa. The chief portal of exit is thought to be the nasal mucosa of lepromatous patients.

The incubation period is frequently 3 to 5 years, but it has been reported to range from 6 months to several decades.

CLINICOPATHOLOGIC CLASSIFICATION As is true of other chronic infections, such as syphilis and tuberculosis, the manifestations of leprosy are many and variable. The classification now in general use is based on clinical findings, histopathologic changes, and the lepromin test.

Lepromatous leprosy is one of the polar forms. The involvement is extensive, diffuse, and bilaterally symmetrical. Histologically, there is a diffuse granulomatous reaction with macrophages, large foam (Virchow's) cells, and many intracellular bacilli, frequently in spheroidal masses (globi). The lepromin reaction is negative.

Tuberculoid leprosy is the other polar type. Skin lesions are single or few and are sharply demarcated. Neurologic involvement is relatively pronounced and may be severe. The histologic picture consists of lymphocytes, epithelioid cells, and perhaps giant cells; bacilli are few and sometimes difficult to demonstrate. The lepromin reaction is usually positive.

Borderline, or *dimorphous,* leprosy is a form in which the clinical features and histologic changes are a combination of the two polar types. The disease may shift toward the lepromatous form in the untreated patient or toward the tuberculoid form in the treated patient. Change of either polar type to the other is exceedingly rare.

In all forms of leprosy peripheral nerve involvement is a constant feature. In any histologic section involvement of nerves will tend to be more severe than involvement of other tissues, and in some sections the nerves may be the only tissues involved.

PATHOGENESIS *Mycobacterium leprae* probably enters the body through the skin or nasal mucosa. The early stages of infection have not been described accurately. In lepromatous leprosy bacillemia is frequent and often so profuse that the organisms can be seen in stained smears of peripheral blood. Even in the most advanced lepromatous cases, destructive lesions are limited to the skin, peripheral nerves, anterior portion of the eye, upper respiratory passages above the larynx, testes, and structures of the hands and feet. The probable reason for the predilection of the disease for these tissues is that they are all usually several degrees cooler than 37°C. Two sites of preferential involvement are the ulnar nerves near the elbow and the peroneal nerves where they pass around the head of the fibula; above and below these levels where these nerves take deeper courses, they are much less severely involved. In mice that have been experimentally infected in the foot pads, bacillary multiplication is maximal when the mice are kept at air temperatures at which the foot pad tissues are about 30°C; this is also the usual temperature of the most severely involved tissues of human beings. In patients with lepromatous leprosy, collections of bacilli are also found in the liver, spleen, and bone marrow, but these are probably scavenged from the blood.

A profound lack of cellular immunity for *M. leprae* in lepromatous leprosy is indicated by the histology and by the negative lepromin reaction. Further evidence comes from observations that lepromatous patients' lymphocytes fail to react in vitro to *M. leprae* antigens either with a mitogenic response or by the formation of migration inhibitory factor (MIF). Under the same in vitro conditions the lymphocytes of tuberculoid patients react positively. Moreover, many normal persons exposed to leprosy give positive reactions, indicating the presence of subclinical infections. In addition to this depressed specific cellular immunity for *M. leprae,* lepromatous patients frequently have a partial depression of cellular immunity in general. They have been shown to be deficient in the ability to develop delayed hypersensitivity, their lymphocyte transformation response to plant mitogen may be weak, and the paracortical areas of their lymph nodes are deficient in lymphocytes. Furthermore, mice that have been rendered T-cell deficient by thymectomy and irradiation followed by bone marrow replacement respond to inoculations of *M. leprae* by developing heavier infections. For these reasons, lepromatous leprosy is thought to be the result of a poor immune response, and tuberculoid leprosy the result of a stronger immune response, but whether these differences in immune state precede the infection or are caused by it is not clear.

CLINICAL MANIFESTATIONS Early leprosy The first signs of leprosy are usually cutaneous. One or more hypopigmented or hyperpigmented macules or plaques may be seen. Often an anesthetic or paresthetic patch is the first symptom noted by the patient, but on careful examination skin involvement can also be found. When contacts are being examined, a single skin lesion is often noted, especially in children; usually, this is a hypesthetic macule that may clear in a year or two without treatment, but specific treatment is usually recommended.

Tuberculoid leprosy Early tuberculoid leprosy is frequently manifested by a hypopigmented macule, sharply demarcated and hypesthetic. Later the lesions are larger, and the margins are elevated and circinate or gyrate. There is peripheral spread and central healing. The lesions appear singly or are few in number and are not symmetrical. Nerve involvement occurs early, and the nerves leading from the lesions may be enlarged. The larger peripheral nerves may be palpably and visibly enlarged, especially the ulnar, peroneal, and greater auricular nerves. There may be severe neuritic pain. Neural involvement leads to muscle atrophy, especially of the small muscles of the hand. Contractures of the hand and foot are frequent. Trauma, especially from burns and splinters from excessive pressure, leads to secondary infection of the hands and to plantar ulcers. Later, resorption and loss of phalanges is frequent. When the facial nerves are involved, there may be lagophthalmos, exposure keratitis, and corneal ulceration leading to blindness.

Lepromatous leprosy The skin lesions are macules, nodules, or papules. The macules are often hypopigmented. The borders of the lesions are not sharp, and the centers of raised lesions are convex (rather than concave as in tuberculoid disease). There is also diffuse infiltration between the lesions. The sites of predilection are the face (cheeks, nose, brows), ears, wrists, elbows, buttocks, and knees. Involvement with infiltration and little or no nodulation may progress so subtly that the disease goes unnoticed. Loss of the eyebrows, especially the lateral portions, is common. Much later the skin of the face and forehead becomes thickened and corrugated (leonine facies), and the earlobes become pendulous.

Nasal symptoms (nasal "stuffiness," epistaxis, and obstructed breathing) are common early symptoms. Complete nasal obstruction, then laryngitis and hoarseness, are also frequent. Septal perforation and nasal collapse lead to saddlenose.

In adult males infiltration and scarring of the testes lead to sterility. Gynecomastia is common. Invasion of the anterior portion of the eye leads to keratitis and iridocyclitis. Painless inguinal and axillary lymphadenopathy occurs.

Neurologic involvement, of the same type as that seen in tuberculoid disease, is less prominent in the lepromatous form. A diffuse hypesthesia involving the peripheral portions of the extremities is common in advanced lepromatous disease.

Reactional states The general course of leprosy is indolent, but it may be interrupted by two types of reaction, which tend to complicate chemotherapy.

Erythema nodosum leprosum (ENL) occurs in lepromatous patients, most frequently toward the end of the first year of treatment. Tender, inflamed subcutaneous nodules develop, usually in crops. Each nodule lasts a week or two, but more develop. ENL may last only a week or two, or it may continue for long periods. Low-grade fever accompanies severe ENL, and lymphadenopathy and arthralgias may appear. Even in untreated patients with ENL the bacilli have greatly reduced viability, as indicated by low infectivity for mice and by low "solid ratios." Histologically, ENL is characterized by polymorphonuclear infiltration and deposits of IgG and complement; hence, it resembles an Arthus reaction.

Borderline reaction is seen in borderline patients, more often during treatment. Existing skin lesions develop erythema and swelling, and new lesions may appear. An early influx of lymphocytes is followed by edema and a shift toward tuberculoid histology. Cellular immunity increases. Borderline reactions can be differentiated from frank progression, such as occurs when drug-resistant bacilli appear, by mouse inoculations to test bacillary viability and by histologic studies.

The *Lucio phenomenon* is limited to patients with a diffuse nonnodular lepromatous disease; it is seen more often in Mexico and Central America. Arteritis leads to ulceration of the skin, in a characteristic angular shape, and subsequently to angular thin scars.

COMPLICATIONS The crippling that follows involvement of the peripheral nerves has been mentioned. Leprosy is probably the most frequent cause of crippling of the hand in the world. Blindness also is common.

Amyloidosis is a complication of severe lepromatous disease in the United States but is less common in many other countries.

Patients with leprosy are said to be likely to develop other chronic infections. Tuberculosis is the chief cause of death in many leprosariums.

DIAGNOSIS The demonstration of acid-fast bacilli in the skin smears made by the scraped-incision method is strong evidence for leprosy, but in tuberculoid disease bacilli may be too few for demonstration. Wherever possible, a skin biopsy specimen confined to the affected area should be sent to a pathologist knowledgeable in leprosy. The histologic involvement of peripheral nerves is pathognomonic.

The lepromin reaction has no diagnostic value. No diagnostic blood changes occur. Lepromatous patients frequently have mild anemia, elevated erythrocyte sedimentation rate, and hyperglobulinemia. From 10 to 40 percent of lepromatous patients have false-positive serologic tests for syphilis.

The combination of a chronic skin disease and peripheral nerve involvement should always lead to the consideration of leprosy.

The differential diagnosis includes conditions such as lupus erythematosus, lupus vulgaris, sarcoidosis, yaws, dermal leishmaniasis, and a host of banal skin diseases. The skin lesions of leprosy, especially of tuberculoid disease, are characterized by hyperesthesia, however, and peripheral nerve involvement can always be demonstrated. Peripheral neuropathy from other causes and syringomyelia may be confused with leprosy.

TREATMENT The treatment of leprosy is largely in the hands of specialists, and hospitalization is advantageous for the first few months while the treatment is being established.

Specific chemotherapy Dapsone (4,4'-diaminodiphenylsulfone, DDS, diaphenylsulfone) is the principal drug. The daily dosage is 50 to 100 mg in adults, often raised gradually to that level during the first few weeks. In a few months in lepromatous disease enough bacilli are killed to render mouse inoculations negative. However, in this form of the disease nonviable

bacilli disappear only slowly and may be found in the tissues for 5 to 10 years. Moreover, a few viable bacilli (persisters) may persist in the tissues for many years and may cause a relapse if treatment is discontinued. Consequently in lepromatous disease, treatment should be continued at least 6 to 10 years after bacilli are no longer demonstrable in skin smears, or perhaps for life.

Sulfone resistance occurs in some patients. After 5 to 20 or more years, during which the response is favorable, such a patient will develop clinical and bacteriologic relapse in spite of regular therapy, and sulfone resistance can be proved on isolates in mice. The frequency of this secondary resistance has been 2 to 8 percent in different countries, depending on the sulfone used and regularity of administration. Recently, primary resistance in previously untreated patients has been described.

Because of the problems of drug-resistant bacilli and of persister bacilli, multiple-drug therapy is now recommended for lepromatous disease. The additional drugs most commonly used are clofazimine (B663) and rifampin (rifampicin). Because clofazimine results in cutaneous pigmentation, light-skinned patients often object to the drug. It is also moderately expensive. As rifampin is even more expensive, regimens combining two or three of these drugs in various schedules are under study. In infections with dapsone-resistant *M. leprae*, clofazimine and rifampin are given in combination. Rifampin-resistant *M. leprae* has been demonstrated in patients relapsing after treatment with this drug alone. Other drugs such as prothionamide, ethionamide, thiambutosine, and thiacetazone, thought to be unsuitable for single-drug therapy, are now being studied in combination with dapsone.

Other sulfones, such as sulfoxone or Sulphetrone, are not used much. Acedapsone (DADDS), a repository sulfone, which releases dapsone slowly and is given only five times a year, is under extensive study; in lepromatous leprosy, it has been found necessary to add a 90-day course of rifampin to the continued acedapsone.

In tuberculoid and indeterminate leprosy, persistent and drug-resistant bacilli have not been a problem, and treatment with dapsone or acedapsone alone has been sufficient. Treatment is continued until all signs of activity have been absent for 3 years. The treatment of borderline leprosy depends upon the severity of the disease.

The clinical response to adequate therapy may be confused by the reactional conditions, but the disease stops progressing and the skin lesions gradually improve. Recovery from neurological impairment is limited.

Treatment of reactional states Moderate ENL is managed by antipyretics and analgesics. If severe, it can be treated with corticosteroids; the dosage is adjusted to alleviate severe distress but not to eliminate all signs of reaction. Sulfone therapy should be continued, if necessary, in reduced dosage. In the past some leprologists have discontinued sulfone therapy at the first signs of ENL, but most now feel that such action is not warranted because it allows bacillary multiplication. Corticosteroid therapy promotes the viability of *M. leprae* in mice not given antileprosy drugs. Thalidomide is the most effective drug and in appropriate dosage can completely suppress ENL. Because of its teratogenicity, however, its use is severely restricted, and it can be used only when its administration can be strictly controlled.

Borderline reactions, if severe, can be controlled with corticosteroids. They do not respond to thalidomide.

Other measures Many of the deformities and disabilities of leprosy are preventable through proper attention from the beginning of treatment. Plantar ulcers, which are very common, may be prevented by rigid-soled footwear or walking plaster casts and contractures of the hand may be prevented by physical therapy and application of casts. Reconstructive surgery is sometimes helpful. Nerve and tendon transplants and release of contractures can give patients more functional ability. Vocational retraining is often necessary for those with permanent disability. Plastic repair of facial deformities assists acceptance of patients in society. The psychologic trauma which results from prolonged segregation is now minimized by permitting patients to continue therapy at home as soon as possible.

CONTROL Early detection and treatment of the disease, which prevent the further development of deformities and simplify sulfone therapy, can be aided by education of physicians and laity in endemic areas. Because the disease is best treated by specialists, the establishment of clinics is helpful. Regular and complete skin examination of family contacts is essential. Field trials of BCG vaccination in endemic areas have shown contradictory results. Chemoprophylaxis with low dosages of dapsone or with acedapsone injections should be considered for family contacts and groups with high attack rates. Removal of patients from their families and normal environment is not necessary, unless the patient fails to cooperate with his therapeutic program.

REFERENCES

Cochrane RG, Davey TF (eds): *Leprosy in Theory and Practice*, 2d ed. Baltimore, Williams & Wilkins, 1964

Fasal P: A primer in leprosy. Cutis 7:525, 1971

Immunological problems in leprosy research. 1. Bull WHO 48:345, 483, 1973

Leprosy—United States, Puerto Rico. Morb Mort Week Rep, May 28, 1976

Ridley DS: Histological classification and the immunolgical spectrum in leprosy. Bull WHO 51:451, 1974

Shepard CC: The first decade in experimental leprosy. Bull WHO 44:821, 1971

WHO Expert Committee on Leprosy: Fifth Report. WHO Technical Report Series 607, 1977

145
OTHER MYCOBACTERIAL INFECTIONS

CHARLES C. SHEPARD

The two most important human mycobacterial pathogens are *Mycobacterium tuberculosis* and *M. leprae,* but morphologically similar acid-fast bacteria are widely distributed in nature as saprophytes and as pathogens of lower animals. In addition, a number of other mycobacteria are known to cause human disease, chiefly chronic cutaneous disease, pulmonary disease, or lymphadenitis. Sometimes in the past, these other human mycobacterial pathogens have been called "atypical mycobacteria" or other confusing terms. An early, tentative classification by Runyon was an important step. In it the slowly growing cultures were placed in three groups: group I, photochromogens; group II, scotochromogens; and group III, nonchromogens. Rapidly growing cultures formed a group IV.

As numerical taxonomic studies have now allowed identification of the several pathogenic and nonpathogenic species contained in the groups, the species names should be used. As is the case with other microbial pathogens, individual species cause particular diseases and sometimes several species cause very similar diseases (Table 145-1).

SKIN INFECTIONS *Mycobacterium marinum (M. balnei,* **"swimming pool" or "fishtank" bacillus)** This acid-fast organism inhabits swimming pools, aquaria (saltwater and freshwater), and natural bodies of water that are usually brackish or saline. From contaminated swimming pools, it gains entry through human epidermis through cutaneous abrasions from rough concrete; from aquaria, through cuts; and from fish, through cuts and wounds. A few weeks later nodules develop at the site; they may become verrucous, or they may ulcerate and enlarge to form superficial granulation tissue. The involved area is usually not extensive. In another form, new lesions form centrally from the initial site. The lesions usually remain minor and regress after a year or two, but they may last for years. *Mycobacterium marinum* grows optimally at 25 to 35°C and poorly, if at all, at 37°C. This temperature range probably accounts for the lack of systemic spread; regional lymph nodes remain uninvolved unless secondary pyogenic infection occurs.

The diagnosis is made by culturing the organism, usually from biopsy material, at appropriate temperatures. Although it grows slowly on primary isolation, on transfer it grows more rapidly. Histologically, a chronic granuloma with epithelioid and giant cells and sometimes with caseous necrosis is seen. Acid-fast bacteria may be difficult to observe. Many, but not all, patients become tuberculin-positive.

If chemotherapy is needed, ethambutol and rifampin are indicated. Tests for antibiotic sensitivity are helpful.

Prevention of swimming pool outbreaks requires disinfection of the pool. The pool may need to be reconstructed to eliminate rough concrete surfaces.

Mycobacterium ulcerans The ulcers caused by the organism are known by several local names, such as Bairnsdale, Kaferiku, and Buruli, but they are best designated by the name of the organism, since local differences are trivial. The characteristic disease is extensive granulomatous ulceration that destroys subcutaneous tissue down to the muscle or fascia and extends peripherally under an undermined edge. The extensor surfaces of arms or legs are most often affected, but the trunk may be involved. Histologically, necrosis is prominent, and epithelialization extends under the overhanging margins. Systemic invasion does not occur, although new lesions may develop at distant sites. In its natural course, the lesion starts as a local swelling which then ulcerates; it may heal spontaneously or persist for many years with extensive ulceration and contractures. Originally observed in Southern Australia, the disease has since been described in Central Africa, Southeast Asia, and tropical America. Recently, large outbreaks have been described near swamps in Uganda. While a soil habitat is the suspected source, the organism has not been isolated from soil.

Mycobacterium ulcerans grows optimally at 30 to 33°C and poorly, if at all, at 37°C. It grows very slowly even at optimal temperature, and colonies require 7 weeks to grow. Inoculation of mouse foot pads may be helpful in isolation.

Treatment is best carried out with surgical extirpation of necrotic tissue and overlapping margins of the ulcer, followed by skin grafting. Although experimental results indicate that clofazimine and rifampin are active against the organism, chemotherapy seems not to be beneficial in human disease.

Other mycobacteria Mycobacterial skin infection caused by an unidentified mycobacterium occurs in a geographically limited area centered on Minnesota and southern Manitoba. A single red raised area enlarges over a period of weeks to a papule, which often breaks down in 1 to 2 months with some drainage. Most patients have enlarged regional lymph nodes. Recovery is prompt after surgery or chemotherapy. Most infections occur in fall or winter and involve people of all ages. Only a few cases have been described in adult males.

Mycobacterium avium-intracellulare, *M. scrofulaceum*, *M. kansasii*, and *M. fortuitum* occasionally cause infections that involve skin.

PULMONARY INFECTIONS Several mycobacterial species other than *M. tuberculosis* can cause chronic progressive pulmonary disease with cavitation and fibrosis closely resembling pulmonary tuberculosis.

Etiology The species are listed in Table 145-1. *Mycobacterium avium* and *M. intracellulare* are closely related organisms, sometimes difficult to differentiate, and best spoken of as a complex. Cultures have been isolated from soil and from animals, especially chickens, but the source of infection is not established. Cultures of *M. kansasii* have been isolated from the environment. *Mycobacterium xenopi* was first isolated from a toad. *Mycobacterium szulgai* is the most recently recognized species, and all cultures have originated from human disease. *Mycobacterium scrofulaceum* needs to be differentiated from *M. gordonae*, also scotochromogenic and commonly found in soil and water. The *M. fortuitum-chelonei* complex includes *M. abscessus* as a subspecies of *M. chelonei*.

Since similar species may be isolated from normal sputum and the identification of the several species is often carried out in reference laboratories, the etiologic diagnosis may be delayed. However, isolation of the suspect culture from repeated specimens and the presence of multiple (more than 10) colonies in the primary cultures are strong evidence that the organism has an etiologic role.

Epidemiology The mode of transmission of all these pulmonary infections is unsettled. There is cross-sensitization between antigens of the tubercle bacillus and other mycobacteria, but sensitization to the etiologic organism is greater. Comparative tests with antigens from *M. avium-intracellulare* and the tuberculin indicate that many healthy individuals in the southeastern United States have been infected by organisms of this group, and in this area, chronic pulmonary disease that is not caused by *M. tuberculosis* is often caused by *M. avium-intracellulare*. In Texas, Oklahoma, and Chicago *M. kansasii* is a more frequent causative agent than *M. avium-intracellulare*. The proportion of new cases caused by myco-

bacteria other than *M. tuberculosis* varies from 2 to 15 percent and is expected to increase as the number of infections due to *M. tuberculosis* decreases. In contrast to tuberculosis, multiple cases in the same family are very rare, and isolation of the patient is not necessary. In terms of frequency *M. avium-intracellulare* and *M. kansasii* are much the most important, followed by *M. scrofulaceum*. Infections with other species are rare.

Manifestations The symptoms and signs are those of pulmonary tuberculosis (Chap. 143), although there is some tendency for most of the infections to be more indolent. Infections with *M. avium-intracellulare* are more frequent in older adults and in men. Underlying chronic obstructive pulmonary disease is often present in infections due to *M. avium-intracellulare*, *M. scrofulaceum*, and *M. fortuitum-chelonei*, and is sometimes present with the other mycobacteria. Extrapulmonary lesions are rare.

Treatment Rational chemotherapy depends upon identification of the etiologic mycobacterium and determination of its drug sensitivity. *Mycobacterium kansasii* infections usually respond well to intensive triple-drug therapy with rifampin and a pair selected from isoniazid, ethambutol, and streptomycin. *Mycobacterium avium-intracellulare* infections are often resistant to chemotherapy. Treatment with four drugs chosen from isoniazid, rifampin, ethambutol, ethionamide, and streptomycin (or capreomycin or kanamycin) is recommended, along with appropriate surgery for unclosed cavities. Infections with *M. scrofulaceum* also are often resistant to drugs, and therapy is the same as for *M. avium-intracellulare*. Infections with *M. szulgai* have responded well to chemotherapy, but the others have been difficult to treat.

OTHER INFECTIONS *Mycobacterium avium-intracellulare* and *M. scrofulaceum* cause lymphadenitis in children, especially of the nodes draining the buccal mucous membrane. Excision of the node before it has ruptured or drained is the treatment of choice. The *M. fortuitum* and *M. chelonei* cause local abscesses, particularly from injections given with contaminated needles or syringes; cervical lymphadenitis and cellulitis also occur, with the site of entry probably the mouth. *Mycobacterium chelonei* has caused two recent outbreaks of infection of sternal incisions after cardiac surgery (coronary bypass and valve replacement). The source of the organism could not be determined. In addition, contamination of porcine cardiac valve prostheses by *M. chelonei* has occasionally been detected, but

TABLE 145-1
Human mycobacterial pathogens other than *M. tuberculosis* and *M. leprae*

Mycobacterium	Pigmentation of culture*	Usual site of disease	Usual source of infection	Response to drugs
M. marinum	P	Skin	Swimming pools, aquaria, fish	Good
M. ulcerans	N	Skin	Tropical environment	Variable
M. avium-intracellulare	N	Lungs	Environment, animals?	Poor
M. kansasii	P	Lungs	Environment?	Good
M. xenopi	S	Lungs	Water, animals?	Variable
M. szulgai	S†	Lungs	?	Good
M. scrofulaceum	S	Lungs, lymph nodes	Water, soil	Poor
M. fortuitum	N	Skin (abscesses), lungs	Soil, dirt	Poor
M. chelonei	N	Skin (abscesses), lungs	Soil, dirt	Poor

* P = photochromogenic (develops yellow-orange pigment only when exposed to light). N = nonpigmented. S = scotochromogenic (develops yellow-orange pigment in dark light).
† Scotochromogenic at 37°C, photochromogenic at 25°C.

infection following the implantation of the contaminated valves has been rare. *Mycobacterium kansasii* and *M. scrofulaceum* can cause disease of bones and joints. Widely disseminated, usually fatal infections with any of these mycobacteria can occur, especially in immunosuppressed patients.

REFERENCES

BARKER DJP: Epidemiology of *Mycobacterium ulcerans* infections. Trans R Soc Trop Med Hyg 67:43, 1973

FELDMAN RA, HERSHFIELD E: Mycobacterial skin infection by an unidentified species. A report of 29 patients. Ann Intern Med 80:445, 1974

JOLLY HW JR, SEABURY JH: Infections with *Mycobacterium marinum.* Arch Dermatol 106:32, 1972

KUBICA GP: Differential identification of mycobacteria. VII. Key features for identification of clinically significant mycobacteria. Am Rev Respir Dis 107:9, 1973

LINCOLN EM, GILBERT LA: Disease in children due to mycobacteria other than *Mycobacterium tuberculosis.* Am Rev Respir Dis 105:683, 1972

WOLINSKY E: Nontuberculous mycobacterial infections of man. Med Clin North Am 58:639, 1974

section 8 | Spirochetal diseases

146
SYPHILIS

KING K. HOLMES

The great ailment of modern syphilological practice is a lack of comprehension of the why and wherefore, rather than the what to do.

J. H. Stokes

DEFINITION Syphilis is a chronic systemic infection caused by *Treponema pallidum*, is usually sexually transmitted, and is characterized by an incubation period averaging 3 weeks, followed by a primary lesion associated with regional lymphadenopathy; a secondary bacteremic stage associated with generalized mucocutaneous lesions and generalized lymphadenopathy; a latent period of subclinical infection lasting many years; and, in about one-third of untreated cases, a tertiary stage characterized by progressive destructive mucocutaneous musculoskeletal or parenchymal lesions, aortitis, or central nervous system disease.

ETIOLOGY The discovery of *Treponema pallidum* in syphilitic material was made by Schaudinn and Hoffman in 1905. *Treponema pallidum* is one of the many spiral-shaped microorganisms which propel themselves by spinning around their longitudinal axis. The spiral organisms of medical significance, the Treponemataceae, include three groups which are pathogenic for humans and for a variety of other animals: the *Leptospira*, which cause human leptospirosis; the *Borrelia*, including *B. recurrentis* and *B. vincentii*, which cause relapsing fever and Vincent's angina, respectively; and the *Treponema*, responsible for the diseases known as treponematoses. The *Treponema* include *T. pallidum; T. pertenue*, and *T. carateum*, the organisms which cause yaws and pinta (Chap. 147); and *T. cuniculi*, the cause of rabbit syphilis. Other treponema include nonpathogenic species found in the human mouth and several species of anaerobic saprophytic genital treponemes of low pathogenicity which often coexist with anaerobic gram-negative rods in ulcerative genital lesions (so-called "fusospirochetal" infections). These can also be confused with *T. pallidum* on dark-field examination by inexperienced individuals.

Treponema pallidum is a thin, delicate organism with 6 to 14 spirals and tapered ends, measuring 6 to 15 μm in total length and 0.2 μm in width. The cytoplasm is surrounded by a trilaminar cytoplasmic membrane, which in turn is surrounded by a delicate inner mucopeptide layer, the periplast, thought to be composed of alternating molecules of N-acetyl glucosamine and N-acetyl muramic acid, and which provides some structural rigidity, while an outer lipoprotein membrane is selectively permeable and osmotically sensitive. The unique spiral structure of *T. pallidum* is maintained by six fibrils, three arising at each end of the organism, which wind around the cell body in a groove between the inner cell wall and the outer cell membrane, and may be the contractile elements responsible for motility. None of the four pathogenic treponemes has yet been cultured in vitro, and no convincing morphological, serologic, or metabolic differences between them have been discerned. They are distinguished primarily according to the clinical syndrome they produce. Limited animal inoculation studies also indicate some differences in host range and virulence, even among different strains of *T. pallidum*. The only known natural host for *T. pallidum* is the human being. Most mammals can be infected with *T. pallidum*, but only humans, higher apes, and a few laboratory animals regularly develop syphilitic lesions. Virulent strains of *T. pallidum* are maintained in rabbits.

HISTORY The first clear descriptions of syphilis were recorded at the end of the fifteenth century, when a pandemic known as the great pox, as distinguished from smallpox, swept over Europe and Asia. Severe morbidity or death often occurred during the secondary stage, indicating an unexplained virulence then which is almost unknown today, except in congenital syphilis. The source of the European pandemic 500 years ago is controversial. The sudden appearance and high morbidity of syphilis in 1494 led to the theory of the importation of a highly virulent strain of *Treponema pallidum* from America. However, many historians discern earlier references to syphilis in various writings dating from Hippocrates.

The sexual mode of transmission of syphilis was recognized early during the European pandemic, and description of the primary and secondary stages of the disease followed. The major cardiovascular and neurological complications of late syphilis were recognized during the eighteenth and nineteenth centuries. However, the erroneous concept that gonorrhea, chancroid, and syphilis were the same disease was strengthened by John Hunter, who developed syphilis following self-inoculation with gonorrheal pus in 1767. These three diseases were finally distinguished by Ricord and his students in the mid-1800s, although their etiologies were not established until the turn of this century. Gummas were not recognized as being syphilitic in origin until this century.

A rapid series of important advances began in 1903 with the successful inoculation of syphilis into primates by Metchnikoff and Rowe. The discovery of *Treponema pallidum* in serum from secondary lesions was made by Schaudinn in 1905 and was confirmed by Landsteiner by dark-field microscopy in 1906. In 1910, Wasserman introduced the complement fixation test for the diagnosis of syphilis, and in the same year, Ehrlich and Hata introduced an arsenic derivative, arsphenamine (Compound 606, Salvarsan), which was effective in treatment. More importantly, arsphenamine was the first specific antimicrobial drug.

EPIDEMIOLOGY Nearly all cases of syphilis are now acquired by sexual contact with infectious lesions (i.e., the chancre, mucous patch, or condyloma latum). Uncommon modes of transmission include nonsexual personal contact, contact with contaminated fomites, or infection in utero or following blood transfusions.

In the United States, infant deaths due to syphilis, and new admissions of patients with syphilitic psychoses, have fallen by 99 percent since 1940. The total reported number of cases of late and late latent syphilis has fallen almost every year since 1943. The 10.4 cases per 100,000 population reported in 1977 represent a decrease of 91 percent since 1943. Only 463 cases of congenital syphilis were reported in 1977, a decrease of 97 percent since 1941. The number of new cases of infectious syphilis reached a peak in 1947, then fell steadily to about 6000 in 1957, but then began to increase again.

Although the reported incidence of syphilis appears higher in nonwhites than in whites, and is higher in urban than in rural areas, these differences partly reflect the fact that indigent urban racial groups are treated at public clinics, where case reporting is complete. The case rates of early syphilis are highest in the South and Southwest, and in those states with large urban populations. The peak incidence of syphilis occurs in the age group 20 to 24. In the United States, the male/female ratio of reported early cases (<1 year) has increased from 0.8:1 in 1950 to over 2:1 in 1977. In England the ratio is 6:1.

Of all men with primary, secondary, or early latent syphilis interviewed in the United States during 1977–1978, one-half were homosexual or bisexual. Primary syphilis is usually not diagnosed in women or in homosexual men. For example, during 1974 in the United States, 42 percent of cases of early syphilis in heterosexual men were detected in the primary stage, whereas only 23 percent of early cases in homosexual men and 11 percent of early cases in women were detected in the primary stage. Anorectal chancres make up over 50 percent of primary syphilis among homosexuals examined in venereology clinics in the United Kingdom, but only 15 percent of primary syphilis among homosexuals examined in the United States. This remarkable difference suggests either a greater reticence of physicians in the United States to examine the anal canal or failure to consider syphilis in the evaluation of anal lesions in men.

In 1977, there were 20,362 cases of primary and secondary syphilis and 21,297 cases of early latent syphilis reported, and the number of unreported cases was estimated to be two to three times greater. Comparison of reported case rates of primary and secondary syphilis in the United States with those in England for 1975 shows that the rates per 100,000 persons between ages 20 and 24 were 3.6 times higher for males and 6.1 times higher for females in the United States than in England. The actual difference in case rates between the United States and England is undoubtedly greater, because most cases of syphilis in England are treated by venereologists and reported, whereas most cases in the United States are seen by physicians in private practice and many are not reported. The higher case rates in the United States may be partly attributable to inadequate tracing of sexual contacts of unreported cases.

Interviews of patients with early syphilis disclose an average of 2.8 sexual contacts at risk per patient, and "cluster" tracing of additional associates of the patient or his or her contacts discloses an average of 0.7 others who are also at risk. Approximately one of two individuals named as contacts of infectious syphilis becomes infected. Many contacts will have already developed manifestations of syphilis when they are first seen, and about 30 percent of apparently uninfected contacts of infectious syphilis who are examined within 30 days of exposure will actually be in the incubation stage and will themselves develop infectious syphilis if not treated. Because of this, the identification and "epidemiologic" treatment of all recently exposed contacts has become an important aspect of syphilis control. Also important is the identification of syphilitics by serologic testing of pregnant women, hospital admissions, military inductees, and persons undergoing examination in physicians' offices. Of 43 million blood specimens examined during 1977 in the United States, 1.5 million tests were reactive, representing untreated syphilis, previously treated syphilis, or false-positive tests. Over one-half of all reported early syphilis cases of less than 1 year's duration were detected as a direct result of either contact tracing or serologic testing. More controversial are laws and regulations requiring routine premarital serologic testing for syphilis. This program, which drains approximately 10 percent of all public funds for control of sexually transmitted diseases, yields very few cases of early syphilis. Syphilis is under control in some states in which new cases are limited to sporadic outbreaks which tend to involve homosexual men and are contained by aggressive contact tracing.

NATURAL COURSE AND PATHOGENESIS OF UNTREATED SYPHILIS *Treponema pallidum* can rapidly penetrate intact mucous membranes or abraded skin and within a few hours enters the lymphatics and blood to produce systemic infection and metastatic foci long before and after the appearance of a primary lesion. Thus, blood from a patient with incubating syphilis is infectious. The generation time of *T. pallidum* in humans is 30 to 33 h, and the incubation period of syphilis is inversely proportional to the number of organisms inoculated. The concentration of treponemes generally reaches at least 10^7 per gram of tissue before the appearance of a clinical lesion. In experimental infection in rabbits or humans, a single treponeme can initiate infection which leads to a discernible lesion only after 6 weeks, although histopathologic changes are evident earlier, while intradermal injection of 10^7 organisms usually produces a lesion within 72 h. The median incubation period in humans is about 21 days. Although the incubation period is traditionally stated as ranging from 9 to 90 days, experimental inoculations of humans and rabbits show that the period from inoculation until the primary lesion is discernible rarely exceeds 6 weeks. Subcurative therapy during the incubation period may delay the onset of the primary lesion but does not seem to prevent ultimate development of symptomatic disease.

The primary lesion appears at the site of inoculation, persists for 2 to 6 weeks, and then heals spontaneously. Histopathology of primary lesions shows perivascular infiltration, chiefly by plasma cells and histiocytes, capillary proliferation, and eventually obliteration of small blood vessels. At this time

T. pallidum is demonstrable in the chancre in spaces between epithelial cells as well as within invaginations or phagosomes of epithelial cells, fibroblasts, plasma cells, and the endothelial cells of small capillaries, within lymphatic channels, and in the regional lymph nodes. Macrophages and polymorphonuclear leukocytes can be seen taking up treponemes into phagocytic vacuoles where the organisms are destroyed.

The generalized parenchymal, constitutional, and mucocutaneous manifestations of secondary syphilis usually appear about 6 weeks after healing of the chancre, although secondary lesions may appear while the chancre is still present, or only after several months have passed. Secondary maculopapular skin lesions show histopathologic features of hyperkeratosis of the epidermis, capillary proliferation with endothelial swelling in the superficial corium, and dermal papillae with transmigration of polymorphonuclear leukocytes, and in the deeper corium, perivascular infiltration by plasma cells. Treponemes are found in many tissues including the aqueous humor of the eye and the cerebrospinal fluid. Cerebrospinal fluid abnormalities are detected in as many as 17 to 33 percent of patients during the secondary stage. Immune complex–induced glomerulonephritis occurs. Generalized lymphadenopathy is present and is characterized by marked follicular hyperplasia, with histiocytic infiltration and lymphocyte depletion of the paracortical areas, where treponema are present in greatest numbers. The reason for the paradoxical appearance of secondary manifestations in the face of high titers of humoral antibody (including immobilizing antibody) to *T. pallidum* is unknown. The secondary lesions subside within 2 to 6 weeks, and the patient enters the latent stage, which is detectable only by serologic testing. Approximately 25 percent of untreated patients experience one or more subsequent generalized or localized mucocutaneous relapses at some time during the first 2 to 4 years after infection. Since 90 percent of such infectious relapses occur during the first year, identification and examination of sexual contacts are most important for patients with syphilis of less than 1 year's duration. However, in the International Classification of Diseases, latent syphilis is arbitrarily divided into early latent (less than 2 years' duration) and late latent (over 2 years' duration) stages. About one-third of patients with untreated latent syphilis develop clinically apparent tertiary disease. In the past, the most common type of tertiary disease was the gumma, a usually benign granulomatous lesion. Today, gummas are very uncommon, perhaps because they respond to very low doses of antitreponemal drugs. The remaining tertiary lesions are caused by obliterative small-vessel endarteritis which usually involves the vasa vasorum of the ascending aorta and less often the central nervous system. Factors which determine development of tertiary disease are unknown, except that trauma may predispose to gumma.

The course of untreated syphilis has been studied retrospectively in a group of nearly 2000 patients with primary or secondary syphilis diagnosed clinically, before the dark-field and Wasserman tests came into use (the *Oslo Study,* 1891–1951); prospectively in 431 Negro men with seropositive latent syphilis of 3 or more years' duration (the *Tuskegee Study,* 1932–1972); and retrospectively in a review of 198 autopsies of patients with untreated syphilis.

In the Oslo Study, 24 percent of the patients developed relapsing secondary lesions within 4 years, and 28 percent eventually developed one or more manifestations of late syphilis. Cardiovascular syphilis, including aortitis, was detected in 10.4 percent, with no cases occurring in those infected before age 15; symptomatic neurosyphilis occurred in 6.5 percent, and 16 percent developed benign tertiary syphilis (gumma of the skin, mucous membranes, and skeleton). Syphilis was the

primary cause of death in 15.1 percent of males and 8.3 percent of the females. However, many patients alive when the Oslo Study was completed remained at risk for developing complications, while tuberculosis and other infections prematurely eliminated others before complications of syphilis occurred, so the Oslo figures probably represent minimum estimates of the risk of late complications. Cardiovascular syphilis was found in 35 percent of men and 22 percent of women who eventually underwent autopsy. In general, serious late complications were nearly twice as common in men as in women.

The Tuskegee Study showed that the death rate of syphilitic Negro men, 25 to 50 years of age, was 17 percent greater than in nonsyphilitics, and 30 percent of all deaths were attributable to cardiovascular or central nervous system syphilis. By far the most important factor in increased mortality was cardiovascular syphilis. Anatomic evidence of aortitis was found in 40 to 60 percent of autopsied syphilitics (versus 15 percent of controls), while central nervous system lues was found in only 4 percent. Hypertension was also increased in the syphilitics. Thus, the incidence of cardiovascular syphilis was higher and central nervous system syphilis lower in the prospective Tuskegee Study, as compared with the Oslo Study. These studies each show that about one-third of patients with untreated syphilis develop clinical or pathological evidence of tertiary syphilis; about one-fourth die as a direct result of tertiary syphilis; and additional excess mortality not directly attributable to tertiary syphilis is also seen. Untreated syphilis may make people more susceptible to other diseases, or individuals who get syphilis coincidentally may be more susceptible to other diseases, perhaps because of socioeconomic factors.

MANIFESTATIONS Primary syphilis The typical primary chancre usually begins as a single painless papule which rapidly becomes eroded and usually, but not always, is indurated, with a characteristic cartilaginous consistency on palpation of the edge and base of the ulcer. Histological examination of the ulcer shows mononuclear and histiocytic infiltrates with obliterative endarteritis and periarteritis of small vessels. *Treponema pallidum* is seen by electron microscopy to lie in interstitial perivascular spaces and within invaginations or phagosomes of neutrophils, macrophages, endothelial cells, and plasma cells.

In heterosexual men, the chancre is usually located on the penis. In homosexual men, the chancre is often found in the anal canal, usually within view if the buttocks are spread, within the mouth, or on the external genitalia. It may occur on any site of the body. In women, primary sites which are commonly overlooked include the cervix and labia. Regional lymphadenopathy accompanies the primary lesion, appearing within 1 week of the onset of the lesion. The nodes are firm, nonsuppurative, and painless. Inguinal lymphadenopathy is bilateral. The chancre heals within 4 to 6 weeks (range 2 to 12 weeks), but the lymphadenopathy may persist for months.

Atypical primary lesions are common. The clinical appearance depends upon the number of treponemes inoculated and upon the preinfection immune status of the patient. A large inoculum produces a dark-field positive ulcerative lesion in nonimmune human volunteers, but in individuals with a previous history of syphilis produces either a small dark-field negative papule, an asymptomatic but seropositive latent infection, or no response at all. A small inoculum usually produces only a papular lesion, even in nonimmune humans. Thus, syphilis should be considered even in the evaluation of trivial or atypical, dark-field negative, genital lesions. The most common genital lesions which must be differentiated from primary syphilis include traumatic, superinfected lesions, genital herpes simplex virus infection (Chap. 193), and chancroid (Chap. 126). *Primary genital herpes* may produce inguinal adenopathy but is initially characterized by multiple painful vesicles which later ulcerate, and with systemic symptoms including fever; *recurrent genital herpes* typically begins with a cluster of painful vesicles without associated adenopathy. *Chancroid* produces painful, superficial exudative, nonindurated, usually multiple ulcers; adenopathy is either unilateral or bilateral, tender, and may suppurate.

Secondary syphilis   The manifestations of the secondary stage are protean but usually include localized or diffuse symmetric mucocutaneous lesions and generalized nontender lymphadenopathy. The remnant of the healing primary chancre is still present in many cases. The skin rash consists of macular, papular, papulosquamous, and occasionally pustular syphilides, often with one or more forms present simultaneously. Initial lesions are bilaterally symmetric, pale red or pink, nonpruritic, discrete, round macules, 5 to 10 mm in diameter, distributed on the trunk and proximal extremities. After 1 to 2 months, red, papular lesions 3 to 10 mm in diameter also appear. These may progress to necrotic (pustular) lesions in association with increasing endarteritis and perivascular mononuclear infiltration. These lesions are distributed widely and may occur on the palms, soles, face, and scalp. Tiny papular *follicular syphilides* involving hair follicles may result in patchy alopecia and loss of eyebrows or beard. Progressive endarteritis obliterans and ischemia result in superficial scaling of papules (*papulosquamous syphilides*) and eventually may lead to central necrosis (*pustular syphilide*). In warm, moist, intertriginous areas, including the perianal area, vulva, scrotum, and inner thighs, axillas, and the skin under pendulous breasts, papules enlarge and become eroded, to produce broad, moist, pink or gray-white highly infectious lesions called *condyloma lata.* Superficial mucosal erosions, called *mucous patches,* occur in about a third of patients and may involve lips, oral mucosa, tongue, palate, pharynx, vulva and vagina, glans penis, or inner prepuce. The typical mucous patch is a silver-gray erosion surrounded by a red periphery and is usually painless.

During relapses of secondary syphilis, condyloma lata are particularly common, and skin lesions tend to be asymmetrically distributed and more infiltrated, resembling skin lesions of late syphilis, perhaps reflecting increasing cellular immunity.

Constitutional symptoms which may accompany secondary syphilis include fever, weight loss, malaise, and anorexia. Headache and meningismus are common. Acute meningitis occurs in only 1 to 2 percent of patients, but increased cells and protein have been found in the cerebrospinal fluid in 30 percent or more of patients. *Treponema pallidum* has also been recovered by rabbit inoculation from cerebrospinal fluid during secondary syphilis even in the absence of other cerebrospinal fluid abnormalities.

Other less common complications described in secondary syphilis include hepatitis, nephropathy, arthritis and periostitis, and iridocyclitis. It is uncertain whether the association between secondary syphilis and hepatitis is causal or coincidental. *Syphilitic hepatitis* is distinguished by an unusually high serum alkaline phosphatase and by a nonspecific histological appearance which is unlike viral hepatitis and includes moderate inflammation with polymorphonuclear leukocytes and lymphocytes, some hepatocellular damage, and no cholestasis. The *renal involvement* is associated with proteinuria, an acute nephrotic syndrome, or rarely with hemorrhagic glomerulonephritis, and which is characterized by subepithelial electron-dense deposits and glomerular immune complexes, suggesting that this complication is a form of immune complex glomerulonephritis. Anterior uveitis has been reported in 5 to 10 percent of patients with secondary syphilis, and *T. pallidum* can be demonstrated in the aqueous humor in such cases. Posterior uveitis occurs rarely.

Latent syphilis   A diagnosis of latent syphilis is established by the finding of a positive specific treponemal antibody test for syphilis, together with a normal cerebrospinal fluid examination, the absence of clinical manifestations of syphilis on physical examination and chest films, and a history of primary or secondary lesions, history of exposure to syphilis, or delivery of an infant with congenital syphilis. *Early latent* syphilis encompasses the first 2 years after infection, during which relapse of mucocutaneous lesions may occur, while *late latent* syphilis, beginning 2 years after infection, in the untreated patient, is associated with immunity to infectious relapse and with resistance to reinfection. *Treponema pallidum* may still intermittently seed the bloodstream during this stage, pregnant women with latent syphilis may infect the fetus in utero, and transfusion syphilis has been transmitted from patients with latent syphilis of many years' duration. Until recently it was thought that untreated late latent syphilis had three possible outcomes: (1) it could persist throughout the life of the infected individual; (2) it could end in development of late syphilis; or (3) it could end with spontaneous cure of infection, with reversion of serologic tests to negative. It is now apparent, however, that the more sensitive treponemal antibody tests rarely if ever become negative. Thus, 50 to 70 percent of untreated patients with latent syphilis never develop clinically evident late syphilis, but the occurrence of spontaneous cure is in doubt.

Late syphilis   The onset of slowly progressive inflammatory disease of the aorta or central nervous system begins early during latent syphilis. Pathogenic studies have shown evidence of early syphilitic aortitis soon after the secondary lesions subside, while asymptomatic neurosyphilis can be detected readily during life by cerebrospinal fluid (CSF) examination.

ASYMPTOMATIC NEUROSYPHILIS   In patients with untreated latent syphilis, if the CSF is normal 2 years or more after infection, there is probably no future risk of subsequent development of neurosyphilis, except for the purely vascular type. The diagnosis of asymptomatic neurosyphilis is made in patients with no clinical manifestations of neurosyphilis who have cerebrospinal fluid abnormalities, including pleocytosis, elevated protein, or positive cerebrospinal fluid Wasserman or Venereal Disease Research Laboratory (VDRL) test. One or more of these findings are present in 20 to 30 percent of patients with untreated syphilis after 2 years. The risk of progression to symptomatic neurosyphilis is two or three times greater in Caucasians than in Negroes and is twice as common in men as in women. The risk of parenchymal neurosyphilis (tabes dorsalis or general paresis) is five times greater in men than in women, supposedly because pregnancy after the initial infection somehow protects women from parenchymal neurosyphilis. In patients with untreated asymptomatic neurosyphilis, the overall cumulative probability of progression to clinical neurosyphilis is about 20 percent in the first 10 years, but increases with passing time, and is highest in those who show the greatest degree of pleocytosis or protein elevation. The fluorescent treponemal antibody (FTA) test on undiluted cerebrospinal fluid has been found to be reactive far more often than the VDRL test in cases of latent syphilis. The prognosis of patients with a positive CSF-FTA test without other cerebrospinal fluid abnormalities is not known, but very likely this finding merely represents passive transfer of serum antibody into the CSF, not asymptomatic neurosyphilis. Similarly, the finding of a positive CSF-FTA test without other cerebrospinal fluid abnormalities in patients with a positive serum FTA-ABS (fluorescent treponemal antibody-absorption) associated with nonspecific neurological findings does not necessarily prove a diagnosis of "atypical" neurosyphilis. However, a therapeutic trial of penicillin in doses adequate for neurosyphilis is warranted in any patient with a positive serum treponemal antibody test who also has unexplained neurological findings.

SYMPTOMATIC NEUROSYPHILIS   The risk of neurosyphilis is two or three times greater in Caucasians than in Negroes, and is twice as common in men as in women. Although mixed features are common, the major clinical categories of symptomatic neurosyphilis include meningovascular and parenchymatous syphilis. The latter category includes general paresis and tabes dorsalis. The average interval from infection to onset of symptoms is 5 to 10 years for meningovascular syphilis, 20 years for general paresis, and 25 to 30 years for tabes dorsalis. However, many patients with symptomatic neurosyphilis do not present a classic picture, but have mixed or incomplete syndromes. *Meningovascular syphilis* is associated with inflammation of the pia and arachnoid, together with evidence of focal or widespread cerebrovascular disease or often only with pupillary or reflex changes. The manifestations of *general paresis* reflect widespread parenchymal damage and include abnormalities corresponding to the mnemonic *paresis* [*p*ersonality, *a*ffect, *r*eflexes (hyperactive), *e*ye (e.g., Argyll Robertson pupils), *s*ensorium (illusions, delusions, hallucinations), *i*ntellect (decreased recent memory orientation, calculations, judgment, insight), and *s*peech]. *Tabes dorsalis* presents symptoms and signs of demyelinization of the posterior columns, dorsal roots, and dorsal root ganglia. Symptoms include ataxic, wide-based gait and footslap, paresthesias, bladder disturbances, impotence, and signs including areflexia, loss of position, deep pain, and temperature sensation. Trophic joint degeneration (Charcot's joints) and perforating ulceration of the feet may result from loss of pain sensation. The Argyll Robertson pupil, seen in both tabes dorsalis and paresis, is a small, irregular pupil which reacts to accommodation but not to light. *Optic atrophy* also occurs frequently in association with tabes.

CARDIOVASCULAR SYPHILIS   Cardiovascular manifestations are limited to the large vessels in which the blood supply is provided by vasa vasorum. Endarteritis obliterans of the vasa vasorum produces medial necrosis with destruction of elastic tissue, particularly in the ascending and transverse segments of the aortic arch, resulting in uncomplicated aortitis, aortic regurgitation, saccular aneurysm, or coronary ostial stenosis. Until recently, these complications had not been described following congenital syphilis or syphilis acquired before age 14, suggesting some unexplained resistance of the large blood vessels in youth to invasion by *T. pallidum*. The onset of symptoms occurs from 10 to 40 years after infection. Cardiovascular complications are commoner and occur at an earlier age in men than in women, and in Negroes than in Caucasians. The incidence of symptomatic cardiovascular complications in late untreated syphilis is approximately 10 percent, with aortic regurgitation being two to four times as common as aneurysm. However, syphilitic aortitis can be demonstrated at autopsy in about one-half of Negro males with untreated syphilis.

Asymptomatic syphilitic aortitis may be suspected in life if linear calcification of the ascending aorta is demonstrated on chest x-ray films, since arteriosclerotic disease seldom produces this sign. Aortic dilatation and a tambour quality of the sound of aortic closure are unreliable signs of aortitis. Syphilitic aneurysms are usually saccular, occasionally fusiform, and do not lead to dissection. Approximately 1 in 10 aortic aneurysms of syphilitic origin may involve the abdominal aorta, but tend to occur above the renal arteries, whereas arteriosclerotic abdominal aneurysms usually are found below the renal arteries. With increasing age, the nervous system is also affected in up to 40 percent of patients with cardiovascular syphilis.

LATE LESIONS OF THE EYES   Iritis associated with pain, photophobia, and dimness of vision or chorioretinitis occurs not only during secondary syphilis, but also as a relatively common manifestation of late syphilis. Adhesions of the iris to the anterior lens may produce a fixed pupil, not to be confused with Argyll Robertson pupil.

LATE BENIGN SYPHILIS (GUMMA)   Gummas may be multiple or diffuse, but are usually solitary lesions which range from microscopic size to several centimeters in diameter, and histologically consist of nonspecific granulomatous inflammation with central necrosis surrounded by mononuclear, epithelioid, and fibroblastic cells, occasional giant cells, and perivasculitis. Although *T. pallidum* cannot be demonstrated microscopically, it can be recovered from the lesions by rabbit inoculation. The most commonly involved sites are the skin and skeletal systems, mouth and upper respiratory tract, larynx, liver, and stomach. Virtually any organ may be involved. Gummas of skin produce painless nodular, papulosquamous, or ulcerative lesions, which are indurated, and form characteristic circles or arcs, with peripheral hyperpigmentation. The lesions are usually indolent, and may heal spontaneously with scarring, but may also be explosive in onset and are often destructive. These lesions may resemble many other chronic granulomatous conditions, including *tuberculosis* and *sarcoidosis* of skin, leprosy, and *deep fungal infections*. Skeletal gummas involve long bones of the legs with greatest frequency, although any bone may be affected. Trauma may predispose to involvement of a specific site. Presenting symptoms usually include focal pain and tenderness. When sufficiently advanced to produce radiographic abnormalities, the findings may include periostitis or destructive or sclerosing osteitis. Gummas of the upper respiratory tract can lead to perforation of the nasal septum or palate. Gummatous hepatitis may produce epigastric pain and tenderness and low-grade fever, and may be associated with splenomegaly and anemia.

The histopathology and extensive tissue necrosis associated with gummas suggest that delayed hypersensitivity to *T. pallidum* produces these lesions. Certain individuals appear to develop an exaggerated delayed hypersensitivity response to *T. pallidum*, presumably mediated by sensitized T lymphocytes and macrophages. In areas where syphilis is endemic in childhood, reinfection may result in gummas; when one member of a household acquires a fresh infection, other members of the household who then become reinfected develop gummas. Experimental inoculation of *T. pallidum* into individuals with latent or late syphilis also sometimes results in gumma formation at the site of inoculation.

Since the histological changes may be suggestive but are nonspecific, the diagnosis of late benign syphilis is confirmed by serologic testing and by therapeutic trial. Treatment with penicillin results in rapid healing of active gummatous lesions.

Congenital syphilis   Transmission of *T. pallidum* from a syphilitic mother to her fetus across the placenta may occur at any stage of pregnancy, but the lesions of congenital syphilis develop only after the fourth month of gestation, when immunologic competence begins to develop. This suggests that the pathogenesis of congenital syphilis may depend upon the immune response of the host rather than upon a direct toxic effect of *T. pallidum*. The risk of infection of the fetus during untreated early maternal syphilis is estimated to be 80 to 95 percent, decreases to about 70 percent at 4 years, and is still lower during late latent maternal syphilis. Adequate treatment of the mother before the sixteenth week of pregnancy should prevent fetal damage. During the past decade, the number of reported cases of congenital syphilis in the United States has remained steady at about 5 cases per 100 reported cases of primary and secondary syphilis in women. A study of cases reported in 1972 showed that 37 percent of the mothers of infected children had not sought prenatal examination, while 44 percent had had a nonreactive serologic test during the first trimester, presumably due either to false-negative first trimester tests or to acquisition of syphilis during pregnancy. Syphilis acquired during pregnancy is likely to remain subclinical in the mother while nearly always causing serious fetal infection. Untreated early maternal infection may result in up to 40 percent fetal loss (stillbirth is more common than abortion, because of the late onset of fetal infection), prematurity, neonatal death, or nonfatal congenital syphilis. Therefore, routine serologic testing in early pregnancy as well as at delivery and repeat serologic testing of "high risk" pregnant women in the third trimester are fully justified.

Only fulminant cases of congenital syphilis are clinically apparent in live infants at birth, and these babies have a very poor prognosis. The most common clinical problem is the healthy appearing baby born to a mother who has a positive serologic test.

The manifestations of congenital syphilis can be divided into (1) early manifestations, which appear within the first 2 years of life, often between 2 and 10 weeks of age, are infectious, and resemble severe secondary syphilis in the adult; (2) late manifestations, which appear after 2 years, and are noninfectious; and (3) the residual stigmata of congenital syphilis. Only about 25 percent of cases of congenital syphilis are diagnosed during the first year of life.

The earliest sign of congenital syphilis is usually rhinitis ("snuffles") soon followed by other mucocutaneous lesions. These may include bullae (syphilitic pemphigus), vesicles, superficial desquamation, petechial, and later, papulosquamous lesions, mucous patches, and condyloma latum. The most common early manifestations are osteochondritis and osteitis, particularly involving the metaphyses of long bones, progressing in severity during the first 6 months of life, then spontaneously subsiding; and periostitis, which continues to progress after the first 6 months. Hepatosplenomegaly, lymphadenopathy, anemia, jaundice, thrombocytopenia, and leukocytosis are common. The anemia is usually hypoproliferative but may be hemolytic (paroxysmal cold hemoglobinuria). The nephrotic syndrome in early congenital syphilis, as in adult secondary syphilis, represents an immune complex-induced glomerulonephritis.

Neonatal congenital syphilis must be differentiated from other generalized congenital infections, including rubella, cytomegalovirus infection, and toxoplasmosis, and also from erythroblastosis fetalis. Neonatal death is usually due to pulmonary hemorrhage, secondary bacterial infection, or severe hepatitis. Pathological findings include interstitial and perivascular inflammation followed by variable fibroblastic proliferation, involving skin, bones, liver, kidneys, pancreas, spleen, lungs, and intestines, and extramedullary hematopoiesis.

Late congenital syphilis is defined as congenital syphilis which remains untreated after 2 years of age. In perhaps 60 percent of cases, the infection remains latent, while the clinical spectrum in the remainder differs in certain respects from that of acquired late syphilis in the adult. For example, cardiovascular syphilis rarely develops in late congenital syphilis, whereas interstitial keratitis is much more common and occurs between ages 5 and 25. The onset is acute with photophobia, pain, and circumcorneal injection, followed by superficial and deep vascularization of the cornea, which progresses despite antibiotic therapy, and eventually becomes bilateral. The symptoms and signs may be suppressed with corticosteroid therapy. Although treponemes have occasionally been demonstrated in aqueous humor in interstitial keratitis, the pathogenesis is obscure and is ascribed to "hypersensitivity." Other manifestations associated with interstitial keratitis are eighth-nerve deafness and recurrent arthropathy. Bilateral knee effusions are known as *Clutton's joints*. Examination of CSF discloses asymptomatic neurosyphilis in about one-third of untreated patients without other late clinical manifestations, and clinical neurosyphilis occurs in a quarter of untreated individuals with congenital syphilis over 6 years of age. The clinical manifestations of congenital neurosyphilis correspond to those seen in adult neurosyphilis. Gummatous periostitis occurs between ages 5 and 20 and, as in endemic nonvenereal childhood syphilis, tends to cause destructive lesions of the palate and nasal septum.

Characteristic stigmata include Hutchinson's teeth, the centrally notched, widely spaced, peg-shaped upper central incisors, and "mulberry" molars, sixth-year molars which have multiple, poorly developed cusps, rather than the usual four. The abnormal facies, which includes frontal bossing, saddle-nose, and poorly developed maxilla, may also be seen in congenital ectodermal dysplasia. Saber shins, or anterior tibial bowing, are rare but were probably more common in the past when syphilitic periostitis of the anterior tibia was associated with vitamin D deficiency. *Rhagades* are linear scars at the angles of the mouth and nose caused by secondary bacterial infection of the early facial eruption. Other stigmata include unexplained nerve deafness, old chorioretinitis, optic atrophy, and corneal opacities due to past interstitial keratitis.

LABORATORY EXAMINATIONS   Dark-field examination technique   Dark-field examination is essential in evaluating cutaneous lesions, such as the chancre of primary syphilis, or condyloma lata of secondary syphilis. Although it is difficult to demonstrate *T. pallidum* in dry maculopapular lesions in secondary syphilis by dark-field examination, the organism may be demonstrated by saline aspiration of lymph nodes during this stage. The surface of the suspected ulcerated lesion should be cleaned with saline and gauze, then gently abraded further with dry gauze, without production of bleeding. The lesion is then squeezed to express a serous transudate, and a drop of the transudate is picked up on the surface of a glass slide. A drop of saline (without bacteriostatic additives) may be mixed with the transudate if necessary, and this is then covered with a coverslip and examined immediately for *T. pallidum* with a dark field or phase contrast microscope by an experienced individual. A single negative examination does not exclude syphilis, since at least 10^4 treponemes per milliliter transudate must be present to be detected, and prior use of topical antiseptic or cleansing by the patient may obfuscate the examination. Cleansing or use of topical medication should, therefore, be avoided, and the dark-field examination should be repeated on three successive days before being considered negative.

Serologic tests for syphilis   The profusion of serologic tests for syphilis causes much unnecessary confusion. Syphilitic infection produces two types of antibodies, the *nonspecific reaginic antibody* and *specific antitreponemal* antibody.

The term *reagin* is unfortunate, since the unrelated gamma-E globulin (IgE) antibody involved in certain allergic phenomena is also known as *reagin*. The nontreponemal reaginic antibodies produced in syphilis contain both IgG and IgM immunoglobulins directed against a lipoidal antigen that results from the interaction of *T. pallidum* with host tissues, and possibly against a lipoidal antigen of *T. pallidum* itself. The cardiolipin antigens initially used in the detection of reaginic antibody are relatively crude extracts of beef heart, and it is not surprising that false-positive reactions were extremely common in many conditions other than syphilis. The cardiolipin-cholesterol-lecithin antigen now in use in a variety of tests for reaginic antibody (Table 146-1) is more purified and gives fewer false-positive reactions than did earlier antigens. The tests for treponemal antibody employ antigens derived from *T. pallidum*, rather than from tissues, and detect antibody related only to past or present treponemal infections.

The most widely used reagin antibody tests are the sensitive rapid plasma reagin (RPR) tests, which can be automated and are used to screen large numbers of serums, and the VDRL slide flocculation test, which is used to determine quantitatively the exact titer of serum reagin antibody. The reagin titer reflects the activity of the disease: false-positive VDRL titers usually do not exceed 1:8; a fourfold or greater rise in titer may be seen during the evolution of primary syphilis; VDRL titers usually reach 1:32 or higher in secondary syphilis; a persistent fall in titer following treatment of early syphilis provides essential evidence of an adequate response to therapy.

The standard antitreponemal antibody test is the FTA-ABS test. The patient's serum is first absorbed with a nonpathogenic treponemal antigen (sorbent) to remove group-specific antibody which may be produced against saprophytic oral and genital treponemes. The patient's absorbed serum is then placed on a slide which contains dried *T. pallidum*. If specific antibody to *T. pallidum* remains in the patient's serum after the absorption step, it is fixed to the dried treponemes, and then is detected by the addition of fluorescein-labeled antihuman gamma-globulin and subsequent examination of the slide by fluorescence microscopy. The *T. pallidum* immobilization (TPI) test, in which immobilization of live *T. pallidum* is produced by immune serum plus complement, is more laborious and in the United States is available only in research laboratories. The *T. pallidum* hemagglutination tests (MHA-TP and TPHA) are convenient tests for treponemal antibody but less sensitive than the FTA-ABS test for detection of early primary syphilis. Both the MHA-TP and FTA-ABS tests are very specific when used for confirmation of positive reaginic antibody tests but give false-positive rates as high as 1 to 2 percent when used for screening normal populations. The relative sensitivities of the VDRL, FTA-ABS, TPI, and MHA-TP tests in the various stages of syphilis are shown in Table 146-2.

The VDRL is negative in nearly one-third of patients with primary or late syphilis. Obtaining a reagin antibody test alone is not sufficient in evaluating late symptomatic syphilis; the more sensitive FTA-ABS test should be routinely obtained in suspected late syphilis. In early primary syphilis, the detection of antibody can be maximized either by performing an FTA-ABS test or simply by repeating a VDRL test after 1 to 2 weeks if the initial VDRL was negative. However, both tests are always positive during secondary syphilis, and a negative VDRL or FTA-ABS virtually excludes syphilis in a patient with otherwise compatible mucocutaneous lesions. (An estimated 1 percent of patients with secondary syphilis have a negative VDRL test with undiluted serum which becomes positive in higher dilutions—the *prozone* phenomenon.)

False-positive serologic tests for syphilis An estimated 20 to 40 percent of all positive reagin tests are false-positive tests, but the percentages vary widely depending upon the population being examined. False-positive reagin tests are classified as acute if they become negative within 6 months. Acute false-positive reagin tests occur during mycoplasma pneumonia, malaria, and various acute bacterial or viral infections, and following smallpox vaccinations. Chronic reactions, which persist 6 months or longer, occur in addiction, autoimmune diseases, and aging. False-positive reagin tests occur in 25 percent of narcotics addicts, and in 10 to 20 percent of patients with active systemic lupus erythematosus. Other antibodies which have been found with great frequency in serums from chronic false-positive reactors include antinuclear, antithyroid, and antimitochondrial antibodies, as well as rheumatoid factor and cryoglobulins. The Donath-Landsteiner antibody responsible for paroxysmal cold hemoglobinuria is a hemolysin which appears in syphilis. The autoimmune nature of the false-positive reagin test is further suggested by the occurrence of systemic lupus erythematosus or other connective tissue diseases in 15 to 45 percent of chronic false-positive reactors. The prevalence of false-positive reagin tests increases with advancing age, and 10 percent of people over 70 years of age have false-positive reactions. Other diseases associated with hyperglobulinemia, such as leprosy, may also produce chronic false-positive reactions.

In the patient with a false-positive reagin test, syphilis is excluded by obtaining a negative FTA-ABS or MHA-TP test. The results of the FTA-ABS test are reported as negative, borderline, or positive. *Borderline* results are more common in patients who are pregnant or have diseases associated with abnormal or increased globulins, and are frequently not associated with either clinical, historical, or other serologic evidence of syphilis. Borderline results should, therefore, always be repeated in questionable cases and interpreted with caution. A typical "positive" FTA-ABS occurs infrequently in conditions other than syphilis. Although false-positive FTA-ABS tests have been reported in 15 percent of patients with active systemic lupus erythematosus, the fluorescent staining is "borderline" or has an atypical "beaded" appearance in most cases (thought to be due to attachment of antinuclear antibody to treponemal DNA or nucleoprotein leaked through breaks in the outer treponemal membranes). However, because of the occasional occurrence of false-positive FTA-ABS tests, only a positive TPI provides conclusive proof of past or present treponemal infection. Both the FTA-ABS and TPI tests are positive in patients who have had yaws or pinta.

For practical purposes, most clinicians need to be familiar with the three uses of serologic tests for syphilis: (1) for screen-

TABLE 146-1
Common serologic tests for syphilis

NONSPECIFIC (REAGIN) ANTIBODY TESTS

Flocculation: VDRL
Complement fixation: Kolmer
Agglutination: rapid plasma reagin (RPR)

SPECIFIC TREPONEMAL ANTIBODY TESTS

Immunofluorescence: fluorescent treponemal antibody-absorption (FTA-ABS)
Immobilization: *Treponema pallidum* immobilization (TPI)
Hemagglutination: *T. pallidum* hemagglutination assay (MHA-TP, TPHA)

TABLE 146-2
Reactivity of serodiagnostic tests in untreated syphilis

Test	Stage of disease,* % positive			
	Primary	*Secondary*	*Latent*	*Tertiary*
VDRL	72	100	73	77
FTA-ABS	91	100	97	100
TPI	46	98	95	95
MHA-TP	69	100	98	100

* *Percentage figures provided should not be interpreted as absolute values because there are small numbers in certain categories and test results vary from study to study.*
SOURCE: *Data compiled by the Center for Disease Control.*

ing large numbers of serums for reaginic antibody (e.g., RPR); (2) for quantitative measurement of reaginic antibody titer in order to assess the clinical activity of syphilis, and to follow the reagin titer in response to therapy (e.g., VDRL); and (3) to confirm the diagnosis of syphilis in a patient with a positive reagin antibody test or with a suspected clinical diagnosis of syphilis (e.g., FTA-ABS).

IgM-FTA-ABS test for active congenital syphilis in the newborn
All newborn infants of mothers with reactive VDRL or FTA-ABS tests will themselves have reactive tests whether or not they have become infected, because of passive transplacental transfer of maternal IgG immunoglobulins which are reactive in these tests. However, if IgM antitreponemal antibody is present in the infant's serum, it reflects fetal antibody production in response to intrauterine infection, particularly if there is a rise in titer, since maternal IgM antibody does not cross the intact placental barrier. Neonatal IgM antibody is detected in cord or neonatal serums in a modified FTA-ABS test, employing fluorescein-labeled antihuman IgM to detect antitreponemal IgM antibody. Similar tests have been developed for detection of congenital toxoplasmosis, rubella, and cytomegalovirus infections. The IgM-FTA-ABS test is sensitive and is positive in infants with active congenital syphilis. When the mother and fetus become infected very late during pregnancy, this test may be negative in the neonatal period. However, the specificity of this test is in doubt because of evidence that infants with a variety of congenital infections may produce IgM antibody to maternal allotypes of IgG. Thus, IgM antibody detected in the IgM-FTA-ABS test may be directed against maternal IgG antibody bound specifically to *T. pallidum*, rather than against *T. pallidum* itself.

TREATMENT AND FOLLOW-UP MANAGEMENT   Penicillin G is the drug of choice for all stages of syphilis. *Treponema pallidum* is killed by very low concentrations of penicillin G, although a long period of exposure to penicillin is required for treatment because of the unusually slow rate of multiplication of the organism. The efficacy of penicillin for syphilis remains undiminished after 30 years of use. Other antibiotics which are effective in syphilis include the tetracyclines, erythromycin,

and the cephalosporins. Streptomycin inhibits *T. pallidum* only in very large doses, and the sulfonamides are inactive. The optimal dose and duration of therapy have not been established for any antimicrobial for any stage of syphilis. The United States Public Health Service recommendations are based on limited therapeutic trials and should be interpreted in light of the considerations noted below.

Recurrence rates for a given regimen increase as infection progresses from incubating syphilis to seronegative primary to seropositive primary to secondary to late syphilis. Therefore it is probable, but unproved, that a longer duration of therapy is required to effect cure as the lesion progresses. For these reasons some authorities use more prolonged penicillin therapy than that recommended by the United States Public Health Service when treating secondary, latent, or late syphilis.

The optimal dose and duration of therapy have not been carefully evaluated in well-controlled studies. A variety of data suggest that it is necessary to achieve serum levels of penicillin G of 0.03 μg/ml or more for at least 7 days to effect cure of early syphilis. Other tentative conclusions which can be gleaned from published studies include the following: (1) extending therapy with aqueous procaine penicillin G beyond 2 weeks does not improve cure rates for primary or secondary syphilis; (2) studies of experimental syphilis show that *T. pallidum* begins to regenerate if penicillinemia is allowed to fall to subinhibitory levels for periods of 18 to 24 h; (3) in humans, increases in the dosage of crystalline penicillin G administered over 9 h from 0.03 to 0.6 mg/kg progressively increased the rate of disappearance of *T. pallidum* from chancres, but further increases in dosage did not further speed the disappearance of treponemes; and (4) the serum concentration of penicillin G achieved after one injection of 2.4 million units of benzathine penicillin G probably does not kill *T. pallidum* at the maximum rate.

The treatment regimens currently recommended for syphilis by the Center for Disease Control are summarized in Table 146-3 and described below.

TABLE 146-3
Recommended therapy for syphilis

Stage of syphilis	Patients without penicillin allergy	Patients with penicillin allergy
Primary, secondary, or early latent	Benzathine penicillin G, 2.4 million units single dose (1.2 million units in each hip) *or* aqueous procaine penicillin G, 600,000 units daily for 8 days	Erythromycin base, stearate, or ethyl succinate, 2 g daily for 15 days *or* tetracycline hydrochloride, 2 g daily for 15 days
Late latent or latent or uncertain duration	*CSF normal:* Treat as primary *CSF abnormal:* Treat as neurosyphilis	Lumbar puncture *CSF normal:* Treat as primary *CSF abnormal:* Treat as neurosyphilis
Late neurosyphilis* (asymptomatic or symptomatic)	Aqueous procaine penicillin G, 600,000 units daily for 14 days *or* aqueous penicillin G, 12 to 24 million units per day intravenously for at least 10 days	Erythromycin base, stearate, or ethyl succinate, 2 g daily for 30 days *or* tetracycline hydrochloride, 2 g daily for 30 days
Late cardiovascular or benign tertiary	Benzathine penicillin G, 2.4 million units weekly for 3 weeks *or* aqueous procaine penicillin G, 600,000 units weekly for 10 days	Treat as for neurosyphilis
Congenital (treat *all* neonates with either proved *or* suspected congenital syphilis)	Aqueous penicillin G, 50,000 units/kg per day for at least 10 days *or* aqueous penicillin G, 50,000 units/kg per day in two divided daily doses for at least 10 days *or, only if CSF normal:* Benzathine penicillin G, 50,000 units/kg in a single dose	Antibiotics other than penicillin should not be used

* *Benzathine penicillin G has given inferior results for treatment of symptomatic neurosyphilis. Although only erythromycin or tetracycline was recommended by the CDC Syphilis Therapy Advisory Committee for CNS Syphilis, chloramphenicol may be theoretically preferable, since it reaches higher concentrations in the CSF.*
SOURCE: *From CDC recommendations, revised 1976.*

Early syphilis In very early incubating syphilis, treatment of concurrently acquired gonorrhea with 4.8 million units of procaine penicillin G (plus 1.0 g probenecid) aborts the syphilis. The ampicillin-probenecid and tetracycline regimens recommended for gonorrhea are probably also effective against incubating syphilis, although proof is not available. Follow-up serologic testing for syphilis is considered unnecessary in patients treated for gonorrhea with the recommended dose of procaine penicillin G, ampicillin, or tetracycline. Preventive (abortive, "epidemiologic") treatment is recommended for seronegative individuals without signs of syphilis who were exposed to syphilis when the contact was infectious and the exposure occurred within the previous 6 weeks. Before treatment is given, every effort should be made to establish a diagnosis by examination and serologic testing. The regimens recommended for preventive treatment are the same as those recommended for early syphilis.

Benzathine penicillin G is the most widely used form of treatment for early syphilis, although it is more painful on injection than procaine penicillin G. A single dose of 2.4 million units cures over 95 percent of cases of primary syphilis. Because efficacy for secondary syphilis may be slightly lower, some physicians administer a second dose of 2.4 million units 1 week after the initial dose for secondary syphilis.

Pregnant patients with early syphilis should receive penicillin in the same doses used for nonpregnant patients. If they have well-documented penicillin allergy, no satisfactory alternative is available. Erythromycin, the leading alternative in penicillin-allergic nonpregnant patients, crosses the placenta poorly, with total blood levels varying from 0 to 20 percent of maternal levels. Erythromycin estolate is associated with frequent liver toxicity in pregnancy. Doxycycline 100 mg twice daily for 15 days, or a cephalosporin, may be preferable alternatives, although doxycycline has potential toxicity in pregnancy and cephalosporins may be cross-allergenic in penicillin-allergic patients. After treatment, a quantitative reagin test should be repeated monthly throughout pregnancy, and if a fourfold rise in titer occurs, treatment should be repeated.

If adequate treatment of the mother is accomplished during pregnancy, the risk of congenital syphilis in the newborn is minimal; the child should then be examined monthly after delivery until his or her reaginic antibody test becomes negative. However, if the seropositive mother received inadequate penicillin treatment or treatment other than penicillin, or her treatment status is unknown, or if the infant may be difficult to follow, treatment should be given promptly. It is unwise to require proof of diagnosis before treatment in such cases. Similarly, every infant with suspected or proved congenital syphilis should be treated promptly. The CSF should be examined as a base line before treatment of such infants. The calculation of penicillin dosage for treatment of late congenital syphilis is the same as for that used in the infant, until dosage based upon body weight reaches that used for adult neurosyphilis.

The response of early syphilis to treatment should be determined by following the quantitative VDRL titer 1, 3, 6, and 12 months after treatment. Because the FTA-ABS and TPHA tests remain positive after 2 years in nearly all patients treated for seropositive early syphilis, this test is not useful in following the response to therapy. However, IgM antibody detected in the FTA-ABS test is uniformly present in untreated syphilis in all stages, but disappears over a period of several months after successful treatment. After successful treatment of seropositive primary or secondary syphilis, the VDRL titer progressively declines, becoming negative within 3 to 12 months in about 75 percent of seropositive primary cases and 40 percent of second-

ary cases. After 2 years, nearly all patients with primary syphilis have a negative VDRL, although 25 percent of secondary cases and a higher proportion of those treated for early latent syphilis still maintain low titers of reagin. If the VDRL becomes negative or reaches a fixed low titer within 1 or 2 years, performing a lumbar puncture is unnecessary at that time, since the spinal fluid examination is invariably normal and there is no risk of subsequent neurosyphilis. However, if a VDRL titer of 1:8 or more fails to fall at least fourfold within 12 months, the VDRL titer rises fourfold, or clinical symptoms persist or recur, re-treatment is indicated. Every effort should be made to differentiate treatment failure from reinfection. If signs of secondary syphilis recur, the CSF should be examined. Suspected treatment failures, especially those with abnormal CSF, should be treated as described for neurosyphilis. If the patient remains seropositive but asymptomatic after such re-treatment, no further therapy is necessary.

Asymptomatic neurosyphilis The activity of asymptomatic neurosyphilis correlates best with the degree of cerebrospinal fluid pleocytosis. Changes in the cerebrospinal fluid cell count, and to a lesser extent, in cerebrospinal fluid protein concentration, provide the most sensitive index of response to treatment. Spinal fluid examination should be performed every 3 to 6 months for 3 years after treatment of asymptomatic neurosyphilis. An elevated cerebrospinal fluid cell count falls to 10 or less per cubic millimeter within 3 to 12 months in 95 percent of adequately treated cases, and becomes normal in all cases within 2 to 4 years. Elevated levels of cerebrospinal fluid protein fall more slowly, and the cerebrospinal fluid reagin titer declines slowly over a period of several years. Since benzathine penicillin G given in single doses of 2.4 million units to adults or 50,000 units per kilogram to infants does not produce detectable concentrations of penicillin G in cerebrospinal fluid, this form of penicillin is unreliable for the treatment of neurosyphilis in the adult, or for congenital syphilis, and asymptomatic neurosyphilis has been found to relapse in up to one-quarter of patients treated with 2.4 million units of benzathine penicillin. Symptomatic neurosyphilis has rarely, if ever, occurred in patients who received a total dose of 6 million units or more of other forms of penicillin G for asymptomatic neurosyphilis.

Late syphilis Lumbar puncture should be performed even in the evaluation of late complications other than symptomatic neurosyphilis, since asymptomatic neurosyphilis may coexist with other late complications, and abnormal cerebrospinal fluid findings can then be followed serially as a guide to therapy. No studies of benzathine penicillin G for cardiovascular syphilis have ever been reported, and the efficacy of penicillin therapy in any form for cardiovascular syphilis has not been proved. The response of cardiovascular syphilis to penicillin is seldom dramatic because aortic aneurysm and aortic regurgitation cannot be reversed by antibiotic treatment, although further progression of these lesions may be arrested by treatment.

In contrast, the response of benign tertiary syphilis and of meningovascular syphilis to penicillin G is usually impressive. The response of parenchymal neurosyphilis has been variable. In a cooperative study of the treatment of 1086 general paretics with penicillin, the frequency of clinical improvement or termination of progression ranged from 38 percent of those with severe involvement to 81 percent of those with mild involvement. All patients who relapsed following initial improvement in cerebrospinal fluid pleocytosis had received less than 6 million units of penicillin, and all improved with subsequent therapy. Tabes dorsalis or optic atrophy responds less often. In general, treatment of inactive neurosyphilis in which permanent neurological damage has already occurred may not produce any clinical change, and re-treatment of such cases is not warranted. However, persistence of cerebrospinal fluid pleocytosis, or recurrence following initial response to treatment, indicates continuing active infection, which should respond to additional treatment. The optimal dose and duration of penicillin for neurosyphilis has not been determined, but administration of 600,000 to 900,000 units of procaine penicillin G daily for 10 days has been about 90 percent effective. Some physicians advocate administration of intravenous penicillin G in doses of 12 million units per day or more for 10 days or longer, to ensure maximally treponemacidal concentrations of penicillin G in cerebrospinal fluid. Such therapy has occasionally cured patients who failed to respond to conventional therapy. There are no data to support the use of antibiotics other than penicillin G for the treatment of neurosyphilis. Therefore follow-up for at least 3 years, with reexamination of spinal fluid every 3 to 6 months, is especially important if antibiotics other than penicillin were used.

Jarish-Herxheimer reaction   A dramatic reaction consisting of fever (average temperature elevation, 1.5°C), chills, myalgias, headache, tachycardia, increased respiratory rate, increased circulating neutrophil count (average total white blood cell count, 12,500 per cubic millimeter), and vasodilatation with mild hypotension, may occur following initiation of treatment of syphilis. This reaction occurs in approximately 50 percent of patients with primary syphilis, 90 percent with secondary, and 25 percent with early latent syphilis. The onset occurs within 2 h of treatment, the peak temperature occurs at about 7 h, and defervescence takes place within 12 to 24 h. In patients with secondary syphilis, an increase in erythema and edema of the mucocutaneous lesions occurs; occasionally subclinical or early mucocutaneous lesions may first become apparent during the reaction. The pathogenesis of this reaction may involve release of endotoxin in tissues. Patients should be warned to expect such symptoms, which can be managed by bed rest and aspirin. The Jarisch-Herxheimer reaction in neurosyphilis or cardiovascular syphilis has, on very rare occasions, been associated with acute progression of irreversible organ damage.

Persistence of treponemal forms   The persistence of *T. pallidum* in the aqueous humor, cerebrospinal fluid, lymph nodes, brain, inflamed temporal arteries, and other tissues following "adequate" penicillin treatment of latent or late syphilis has been suggested by dark-field microscopy and by immunofluorescent antibody and silver staining techniques. Treponemal forms have also been demonstrated in patients with various clinical findings suggestive of syphilis, but in whom serologic tests, including the FTA-ABS test, were negative. Although many of these findings could be explained by artifact or by the coincidental presence of nonpathogenic treponemes, in a few cases the persistence of pathogenic *T. pallidum* after antibiotic treatment was proved by rabbit inoculation experiments. The question has been raised as to whether the lifelong persistence of antitreponemal antibody measured in the TPI and FTA-ABS tests following treatment of latent or late syphilis represents prolonged immunologic memory or continued antigenic stimulation by persisting treponemes in lymph nodes and other tissues.

It is not surprising that *T. pallidum* might persist in the aqueous humor or cerebrospinal fluid despite penicillin treatment, because of poor penetration of the antibiotic, but persistence in lymph nodes and other sites remains unexplained. Limited evidence indicates no increase in resistance to penicillin of such persistent treponemes. Since the data on persisting

treponemes are scanty, no modification of the treatment recommendations for latent or late syphilis seems warranted.

IMMUNITY AND PREVENTION OF SYPHILIS   Only about 50 percent of the named contacts of primary and secondary syphilis become infected. The actual risk of infection from a single exposure is probably much lower. The relative importance of variations in sexual and hygienic practices, inoculum size, body and environmental temperature, and other local and systemic factors affecting transmissibility of syphilis remains undefined. There is some interest in the possible efficacy of intravaginal contraceptive gels as prophylactics against venereal diseases including syphilis, since many available preparations have bacteriostatic as well as spermicidal properties.

Humans have no natural resistance to infection by pathogenic treponemes. The rate of development of acquired resistance to *T. pallidum* following natural or experimental infection is quantitatively related to the amount of the antigenic stimulus, which depends upon both the size of the infecting inoculum and the duration of infection prior to treatment.

Resistance to reinfection or superinfection by challenge inoculation develops about three months after the primary (immunizing) infection in animals with experimental syphilis. Resistance of human beings to reinfection by intradermal inoculation of *T. pallidum* was studied in volunteers. Those who had previously been treated for *early* syphilis developed a primary lesion and a serologic response, while the majority of those who had previously been treated for *late latent* syphilis and all those with *untreated latent* syphilis developed neither primary lesions nor serologic response following inoculation. Two patients treated for late latent or late congenital syphilis developed gummas at the site of inoculation.

The role of serum antibody in conferring immunity to syphilis remains controversial. Reagin antibody is not protective, and the evidence is equivocal that antibody directed against specific treponemal antigens confers immunity. Nonetheless, passive transfer of serum antibody from rabbits recovering from experimental syphilis partially protects antibody-recipient rabbits from experimental infection with *T. pallidum*. Delayed hypersensitivity to *T. pallidum* has been demonstrated by skin test in late syphilis, and lymphocytes from patients with syphilis have been demonstrated to undergo blast transformation when exposed to treponemal or cardiolipin antigen. The histopathology of gummas suggests that the cellular immune response is somehow involved in the pathogenesis of these lesions.

Inability to cultivate pathogenic treponemes in vitro has hindered analysis, purification, and concentration of treponemal antigens, and attempts to induce immunity to syphilis by vaccination have shown limited promise. Injection of rabbits with motile strains irradiated with x-rays or with strains of *T. pallidum* inactivated during cold storage has conferred limited immunity, but many injections over long periods of time were required. Attempts to provide cross-resistance by immunization of rabbits with cultivated nonpathogenic treponemas have been unsuccessful. Experiments in humans have shown that varying degrees of cross-immunity exist in patients infected with *T. pallidum*, *T. pertenue*, and *T. carateum*, but chimpanzees with experimental pinta have not developed cross-resistance to syphilis. These findings indicate that the prospects for a syphilis vaccine remain remote, and that the prevention of syphilis depends upon use of mechanical or antiseptic prophylactic agents, and upon detection and treatment of infectious cases.

REFERENCES

CLARK EG, DANBOLT N: The Oslo study of the natural course of untreated syphilis. Med Clin North Am 48:613, 1964

IDSOE O et al: Penicillin in the treatment of syphilis. Bull WHO 47(suppl):1, 1972

JAFFE HW: The laboratory diagnosis of syphilis: New concepts. Ann Intern Med 83:846, 1975

JOHNSON RC (ed): *The Biology of the Parasitic Spirochetes.* New York, Academic, 1976

MAGNUSON HG et al: Inoculation syphilis in human volunteers. Medicine 35:33, 1956

MERRITT HH et al (eds): *Neurosyphilis.* New York, Oxford, 1946

O'NEILL P, NICOL CS: IgM class antitreponemal antibody in treated and untreated syphilis. Br J Vener Dis 48:460, 1972

REIMER CB et al: The specificity of fetal IgM: Antibody or anti-antibody? NY Acad Sci 254:77, 1975

ROSAHN PD: *Autopsy Studies in Syphilis,* CDC Publication no 433. US Department of Health, Education, and Welfare, 1960

SCHROETER AL et al: Treatment for early syphilis and reactivity of serologic tests. JAMA 221:471, 1972

Sexually Transmitted Disease (STD) Statistical Letter, CDC Publication no 127. US Department of Health, Education, and Welfare, 1978

SHERLOCK S: The liver in secondary (early) syphilis. N Engl J Med 284:1437, 1971

SHORT DH et al: Neurosyphilis, the search for adequate treatment: A review and report of a study using benzathine penicillin G. Arch Dermatol 93:87, 1966

Syphilotherapy 1976. Position paper for the current USPHS recommendations. J Am Vener Dis Assoc 3:98, 1976

TURNER TB: *Syphilis and the Treponematoses, Infectious Agents and Host Reaction,* S Mudd (ed). Philadelphia, Saunders, 1970, p 346

WORLD HEALTH ORGANIZATION: Treponematosis research: Report of a WHO scientific group. WHO Tech Rep Ser 455, 1970

147

NONVENEREAL TREPONEMATOSES: YAWS, PINTA, AND ENDEMIC SYPHILIS

KING K. HOLMES
PETER L. PERINE

GENERAL CONSIDERATIONS Nonvenereal treponematoses occur in remote, impoverished areas of the world. Yaws, pinta, and endemic syphilis are distinguished from venereal syphilis solely by clinical and epidemiologic features. Yaws and pinta are caused by treponemes which are conventionally designated as unique species (*Treponema pertenue* causes yaws, and *T. carateum* pinta), but no convincing morphologic or antigenic differences have yet been demonstrated among *T. pertenue, T. carateum,* and *T. pallidum.* The etiologic agent of endemic syphilis is generally held to be identical with *T. pallidum* and is sometimes designated as *T. pallidum endemicum.* Pinta involves the skin alone; yaws affects skin and bones; and endemic syphilis involves the skin, bone, and mucous membranes. Congenital infections and cardiovascular and central nervous system involvement occur rarely if ever in the nonvenereal treponematoses but are common in syphilis. It remains unclear whether the clinical and epidemiologic differences among yaws, pinta, endemic syphilis, and venereal syphilis are solely determined by environmental and host factors or are attributable to undefined biological differences among the causal treponemes. The relationship of the treponematoses is summarized in Table 147-1.

EPIDEMIOLOGY Treponemal antibodies are demonstrable in a high proportion of nonhuman primates in regions of Africa where human yaws and endemic syphilis are common, and pathogenic treponemes have been found in skin lesions and lymph nodes of seropositive animals. These treponemes have produced yaws-like lesions in susceptible monkeys and hamsters. Treponemes related to or identical with *T. pertenue* thus may antedate *Homo sapiens.*

Yaws and endemic syphilis are diseases of young children. Yaws occurs throughout the world between the Tropics of Cancer and Capricorn, in humid, warm environments. Transmission of yaws among children is favored by scanty clothing, poor hygiene, and frequent skin trauma. Spread occurs by direct contact with infected lesions and perhaps by passive transfer of treponemes by insects. Endemic syphilis occurs in arid subtropical or temperate climates in Africa, the eastern Mediterranean, the Arabian Peninsula, Central Asia, and Australia. It is not observed in the Western Hemisphere. Skin-to-skin transmission is less important than in yaws; instead, infection of mucous membranes results from direct mouth-to-mouth contact or from contaminated fomites, such as shared drinking or eating utensils. Household outbreaks of endemic childhood syphilis still occur in modern cities when crowding and poverty favor childhood transmission of *T. pallidum.*

Although cutaneous pigmentary changes resembling pinta occur in yaws or endemic syphilis, most authorities believe pinta is a separate, more benign disease which occurs only in the Western Hemisphere. The onset is typically later than in yaws or endemic syphilis, usually when the person is between 10 and 20 years of age. The method of transmission is not well defined.

The WHO/UNICEF-assisted mass campaign for eradication of endemic nonvenereal treponematosis from 1948 to 1965 was an unusually successful public health campaign. Over 160 million people were examined in 46 countries, and approximately 50 million cases, contacts, and latent infections were treated. The impact of this program was remarkable. The prevalence of active yaws lesions was reduced from over 20 percent to less than 1 percent in many rural areas. In Bosnia, Yugoslavia, endemic syphilis was eradicated—the only example of eradication of endemic treponematosis.

Unfortunately, relaxation of active surveillance activities after the mass campaigns has led to a resurgence of yaws, particularly in Africa. Yaws has not been eradicated in any large area. For example, in Ghana reported cases of yaws increased fivefold from 1970 to 1974, and recrudescences have been reported in Senegal, the Congo, and the Ivory Coast. Among pygmies in Cameroon and Zaire surveyed from 1969 to 1978, the prevalence of clinical yaws was 10 percent, and the prevalence of FTA-ABS antibody ranged from 75 percent for children under 5 years to 90 percent or more for those over 20. Similarly, WHO surveys during the early 1970s showed that the prevalence of active endemic syphilis, though lower than before the eradication program, ranged from 1 to 5 percent in remote poor populations of Senegal, Mauritania, Mali, Chad, Niger, Upper Volta, Kenya, Ethiopia, and Somalia.

Antitreponemal and reaginic seroreactivity has been detected in a small percentage of children without clinical disease born after the mass campaigns in some areas (e.g., Nigeria, New Guinea, and Bosnia). This may represent asymptomatic infection or may simply reflect the decreased predictive value of serologic tests (probability that disease is present if the test is positive) when the prevalence of disease is sharply reduced.

In the Americas, the major residual foci of yaws are Haiti; Dominica, St. Lucia, and St. Vincent; Peru, Colombia, and Ecuador; a few areas of Brazil; and possibly Guyana and Surinam. Pinta is confined to Central America and Northern South America, where it appears to have regressed to remote Indian villages.

TABLE 147-1
Etiology, epidemiology, and clinical manifestations of the treponematoses

	Venereal syphilis	Endemic syphilis	Yaws	Pinta
Organism	Treponema pallidum	T. pallidum endemicum	T. pertenue	T. carateum
Transmission	Sexual, transplacental*	Household contacts: mouth-to-mouth or via drinking, eating utensils	Skin-to-skin ? Insect vector	Skin-to-skin ? Insect vector
Usual age	Adult	Early childhood	Early childhood	Adolescent
Primary lesion	Cutaneous ulcer (chancre)	Rarely seen	Framboise (raspberry), or "mother yaw"	Nonulcerating papule with satellites
Secondary lesion	Mucocutaneous; occasional periostitis	Florid mucocutaneous lesions (mucous patch, split papule, condyloma latum); osteoperiostitis	Cutaneous papulosquamous lesions	Pintides
Tertiary	Gumma, cardiovascular, and CNS lues	Destructive cutaneous osteoarticular gummas	Destructive cutaneous osteoarticular gummas	Dyschromic, achromic macules

* Since the nonvenereal treponematoses are usually acquired in childhood and treponemal bacteremia ceases with time, only in adult-onset venereal syphilis is there any likelihood of a mother giving birth to an infected child.

BIOLOGICAL RELATIONSHIPS Specific humoral antibodies to *T. pallidum* are produced in individuals with yaws, pinta, or endemic syphilis, but the time of appearance of antibodies after onset of infections is variable. The fluorescent treponemal antibody absorption (FTA-ABS) test, the *T. pallidum* hemagglutination test (TPHA), and the *T. pallidum* immobilization (TPI) test cannot differentiate among the treponematoses.

In addition to the clinical and epidemiologic differences among the treponematoses in humans, the range of susceptible animal hosts and some manifestations of experimental infection are also different. In particular, *T. carateum* has produced an infection in chimpanzees which resembles pinta, but attempts to infect other experimental animals have usually been unsuccessful. Turner and Hollander reported differences between *T. pallidum* and *T. pertenue* in infections produced in the rabbit and golden hamster, and also found that experimental rabbit infection with one species conferred greater immunity to reinfection with the homologous species than with the heterologous species. However, these interspecies differences in superinfection immunity are no greater than intraspecies differences which exist among different strains of *T. pallidum*. Individuals who have had yaws or pinta are considered relatively immune to syphilis, and the extensive studies of Medina in Caracas show that persons with active pinta or syphilis cannot be superinfected with *T. pertenue* by experimental inoculation.

CLINICAL MANIFESTATIONS Yaws Also known as pian, framboesia, buba, or bouba, yaws is a chronic infectious disease of childhood caused by *T. pertenue*. The disease is characterized by an initial skin lesion followed by relapsing, nondestructive, secondary lesions of skin and bone. In the late stages, destructive lesions of skin, bone, and joints occur.

The incubation period following experimental inoculation of susceptible human beings is 3 to 4 weeks. Disruption of the skin by insect bites, abrasions, or injuries promotes acquisition of natural infection from infected contacts. The initial early lesion is a single papule which is usually located on a leg. The lesion enlarges and becomes papillomatous. This lesion is known as a framboise (raspberry) or "mother yaw." It becomes superficially eroded and covered by a thin yellow crust of serous exudate containing *T. pertenue*. Erythema and induration are not common. The lesion is pruritic, and regional lymphadenopathy occurs. The initial lesion usually heals in 6 months. As a result of treponemal bacteremia, a generalized secondary eruption of similar lesions appears either before or after the initial lesion has healed and is most extensive on the exposed surfaces of the body. These early cutaneous lesions of yaws have a variety of forms including desquamative macular

and papular as well as papillomatous types. Painful papules on the soles of the feet result in a crab-like gait referred to as *crab yaws*. Early lesions are infectious and heal slowly; they may result in scarring, hyperpigmentation, or depigmentation, resembling the pigmentary changes seen in pinta. Histological findings are mononuclear-cell infiltration, acanthosis, hyperkeratosis, and the presence of many treponemes. Other manifestations of early yaws include lymphadenopathy and nocturnal bone pain and polydactylitis due to periostitis. Fever and other constitutional symptoms may occur. Infectious cutaneous relapses may occur any time during the first 5 years after infection. Late yaws lesions occur 5 years or more after infection and differ histologically from early lesions in showing endarteritis. Late lesions include gummas of the skin and long bones, particularly of the legs, hyperkeratoses of the soles and palms, osteitis, periostitis, juxtaarticular fibromatous nodes, and hydrarthrosis.

Late lesions of yaws are characteristically extensive and usually destructive. Destruction of the nose, maxilla, palate, and pharynx, termed *gangosa*, or *rhinopharyngitis mutilans*, occurs in late yaws, as well as in leprosy and leishmaniasis. Hypertrophic paranasal maxillary osteitis produces distinctive facies known as *goundou*.

The clinical features of yaws have become less reliable for diagnosis as the prevalence of yaws has decreased, necessitating the use of easily performed serologic tests, such as the rapid plasma reagin (RPR) card test, by paramedical field workers engaged in the consolidation phase of yaws surveillance.

Treponema pertenue can be demonstrated by dark-field examination in early cutaneous lesions but should not be confused with other spirochetes found in tropical ulcers. The serum reagin antibody tests become positive after 1 month, and the FTA-ABS test is also positive.

Endemic syphilis Synonyms for endemic syphilis are Bejel, Siti, Dichuchwa, Njovera, Belesh, and Skerljevo. It is a chronic nonvenereal, treponemal infection of childhood characterized by early mucous membrane or mucocutaneous lesions, a latent period of indeterminate duration, and late complications including gummas of bone and skin. The causative organism is indistinguishable from *T. pallidum*. Endemic syphilis differs from congenital syphilis in that dental changes, interstitial keratitis, and neurosyphilis rarely occur. Cardiovascular complications are considered rare in both endemic and congenital syphilis.

Primary cutaneous lesions are infrequent and when present are extragenital. The earliest manifestation of endemic syphilis is usually an intraoral mucous patch or mucocutaneous lesion resembling the split papules or condylomata of secondary syphilis. Periostitis is common. Regional lymphadenopathy occurs, but generalized lymphadenopathy is unusual. Treponemes are abundant in the moist early lesions and in aspirates from regional lymph nodes. After a variable latent period, late lesions may develop and are the most frequent clinical manifestations. These resemble the lesions of late benign syphilis and include osseous or cutaneous gummas. Destructive gummas, osteitis, and periostitis of nasopharyngeal structures are more common than in late yaws. Gummas occur on the nipples of mothers who have themselves previously had endemic syphilis who breastfeed infants with oral lesions. Both early and late forms of endemic syphilis thus may coexist in the same family. The tertiary lesions of endemic syphilis sometimes may be a consequence of repeated reexposure of a previously sensitized host to reinfection.

Pinta   Also known as mal del pinto, carate, azul, or purupuru, pinta is an infectious disease of the skin caused by *T. carateum*. This disease has three cutaneous stages characterized by marked changes in the skin color, does not involve the viscera, and causes no disability other than that associated with cosmetic disfigurement.

The initial lesion is a small papule which appears 7 to 30 days after exposure and is located most often on the extremities, face, neck, or buttocks. It increases in size slowly by peripheral extension and by coalescing with smaller satellite papules. Regional lymphadenopathy occurs. A secondary eruption not associated with generalized lymphadenopathy appears 1 month to 1 year after the appearance of the initial lesion. The secondary lesions are termed *pintides*, may be numerous, and evolve into a psoriatic or circinate configuration. Pintides are initially red but become deeply pigmented, reaching a slate-blue color after a period of time which is related to exposure to sun. Pigmentation occurs most rapidly on the exposed parts of the body. These pigmented lesions are known as dyschromic macules and contain treponemes which are located principally in the epidermis in older lesions. Histologically there is deposition of pigment in the dermis with decreased melanin pigment in the basal-cell layer. Within 3 months to a year, most of the pintides show varying degrees of depigmentation, becoming brown and finally white and giving the skin a mottled appearance. The porcelain-white achromic lesions represent the "late" stage of the disease in which the epidermis is atrophic and melanocytes and melanin are absent. *Treponema carateum* can be demonstrated in transudates from initial, early secondary, or dyschromic lesions. Serologic reaginic and antitreponemal antibody tests are positive, but may take four times longer to become positive in pinta than in venereal syphilis.

TREATMENT   Treatment is similar for all the treponematoses. Intramuscular injection of 2.4 million units of benzathine penicillin G in adults and half this dose in children results in rapid resolution of lesions and prevents recurrence. Procaine penicillin G in oil and 2% aluminum monostearate (PAM) has been used extensively. In persons who are allergic to penicillin, tetracycline hydrochloride in a dose similar to that used for infectious syphilis (Chap. 146) is effective. In areas where less than 5 percent of the population has active disease, cases are managed on an individual basis, and all contacts of infected persons are treated with antibiotics.

PREVENTION   Although the nonvenereal treponematoses are less amenable to eradication than smallpox, the resurgence of yaws has led some authorities to suggest that the application of *selective epidemiologic control* as used in smallpox eradication be applied to yaws control. This strategy would emphasize ongoing active surveillance, investigation of outbreaks, and treatment of active cases and their contacts rather than mass treatment.

REFERENCES

Bibliography on Yaws 1905–1962. Geneva, WHO, 1963

FURTADO T: Some problems of late yaws. Int J Dermatol 12:123, 1973

GRIN EI, GUTHE T: Evaluation of a previous mass campaign against endemic syphilis in Bosnia and Herzogovina. Br J Vener Dis 49:1, 1973

GUTHE T: Clinical, serological and epidemiological features of framboesia tropica (yaws) and its control in rural communities. Acta Derm Venereol 49:343, 1969

HACKETT CJ: An international nomenclature of yaws lesions. Geneva, WHO, 1957

HOPKINS DR: After smallpox eradication: Yaws? Am J Trop Med Hyg 25:860, 1976

————: Yaws in the Americas, 1950–1975. J Infect Dis 136:548, 1977

HUDSON EH: *Nonvenereal Syphilis*. Edinburgh, E and S Livingstone, 1958

MARQUEZ F et al: Mal del pinto in Mexico. Bull WHO 13:299, 1955

PAMPIGLIONE S, WILKINSON AE: A study of yaws among pygmies in Cameroon and Zaire. Br J Vener Dis 51:165, 1975

TANEJA BL: Yaws: Clinical manifestations and criteria for diagnosis. Indian J Med Res 56:100, 1968

Treponematoses Research: Report of a WHO Scientific Group, WHO Technical Report Series 455, 1970

TURNER TB, HOLLANDER DH: *Biology of the Treponematoses*, WHO Monograph Series 35, 1957

WILLCOX RR: Changing patterns of treponemal disease. Br J Vener Dis 50:169, 1974

148
LEPTOSPIROSIS

JAY P. SANFORD

DEFINITION   *Leptospirosis* is a term applied to disease caused by all leptospiras regardless of specific serotype. Correlation of clinical syndromes with infection by differing serotypes leads to the conclusion that a single serotype of *Leptospira* may be responsible for a variety of clinical features; conversely, a single syndrome, e.g., aseptic meningitis, may be caused by multiple serotypes. Hence there is a preference for the general term leptospirosis rather than the synonyms such as Weil's disease and canicola fever.

ETIOLOGY   The genus *Leptospira* contains only one species, *L. interrogans*, which may be subdivided into two complexes, interrogans and biflexa. The interrogans complex includes the pathogenic strains, while the biflexa complex includes saprophytic strains. Within each complex the organisms show antigenic variations that are stable and allow them to be classed as serotypes (serovars). Serotypes with common antigens are arranged in serogroups. Despite contrary common usage, an example of the correct designation of *Leptospira* is as follows: Pomona serogroup of *L. interrogans* or *L. interrogans* serovar pomona, not *L. pomona*. The interrogans complex now contains about 130 serotypes arranged in 16 serogroups (the number in parentheses refers to number of serotypes within the serogroup): Icterohemorrhagiae (13), Hebdomadis (28), Autumnalis (13), Canicola (11), Australis (10), Tarassovi or Hyos (10), Pyrogenes (9), Bataviae (8), Javanica (6), Pomona (6), Ballum (3), Cynopteri (3), Celledoni (2), Grippotyphosa (2), Panama (2), and Shermani (1). At least 22 serotypes of *Leptospira* occur naturally in the United States.

EPIDEMIOLOGY Although leptospirosis is not a common disease, it has been reported from all regions of the United States. Between 1964 and 1976, approximately 50 to 150 cases were reported annually. Occasional upswings in number of cases have been the result of common-source outbreaks. Infection in human beings is an incidental occurrence and is not essential to the maintenance of leptospirosis. The disease occurs in a wide range of domestic and wild animal hosts. In many species, such as opossums, skunks, raccoons, and foxes, infectivity ratios in the range of 10 to 50 percent are not unusual. Interspecies spread of specific serotypes of leptospiras between animal hosts is frequent, e.g., Pomona, a serotype principally associated with livestock, has been demonstrated in dogs. Infection in animals may vary from inapparent illness to severe fatal disease. The carrier state, in which the host may shed leptospiras in its urine for months to years, may develop in many animals. Immunization of dogs may not prevent the carrier, or shedder, state.

Survival of pathogenic leptospiras in nature is governed by factors including pH of the urine of the host, pH of soil or water into which they are shed, and ambient temperature. Acid urine permits only limited survival; however, if the urine is neutral or alkaline and is shed into a similar moist environment which has low salinity, is not badly polluted with microorganisms or detergents, and has a temperature above 22°C, leptospiras may survive for several weeks. Human infections can occur either by direct contact with urine or tissue of an infected animal or indirectly through contaminated water, soil, or vegetation. The usual portals of entry in humans are abraded skin, particularly about the feet, and exposed conjunctival, nasal, and oral mucous membranes. The previously held concept that organisms could penetrate intact skin has been questioned. While leptospiras have been isolated from ticks, these arthropods appear to be unimportant in transmission.

With the ubiquitous infection of animals, leptospirosis in human beings can occur in all age groups, at all seasons, and in both sexes. However, it is primarily a disease of teen-age children and young adults (about one-half of patients are between the ages of 10 and 39), occurs predominantly in males (80 percent), and develops most frequently in hot weather (in the United States one-half of infections occur from July to October). The wide spectrum of animal hosts results in both urban and rural human disease. Leptospirosis has been considered an occupational disease; however, improved methods of rat control and better standards of hygiene have reduced the incidence among occupational groups such as coal miners and people who work in sewers. Currently less than 20 percent of patients have direct contact with animals; they are mostly farmers, trappers, or abattoir workers. In the majority of patients exposure is incidental; two-thirds of cases occur in children, students, or housewives. Swimming or partial immersion in contaminated water, e.g., riding motorcycles through contaminated pools of water, has been implicated in one-fifth of patients and has accounted for most of the recognized common-source outbreaks.

PATHOLOGY In patients who have died with either hepatic involvement (Weil's syndrome), renal involvement, or both, the significant gross changes include hemorrhages and bile staining of tissues. The hemorrhages, which vary from petechial to ecchymotic, are widespread and are most prominent in skeletal muscle, kidneys, adrenals, liver, stomach, spleen, and lungs.

In skeletal muscle, focal, necrotic, and necrobiotic changes thought to be typical of leptospirosis occur. Biopsies early in the illness demonstrate swelling and vacuolation. Leptospiral antigen has been demonstrated in these lesions by the fluorescent antibody technique. Healing ensues by the formation of new myofibrils with minimal fibrosis. The renal lesions in the acute phase involve predominantly the tubules and vary from simple dilatation of distal convoluted tubules to degeneration, necrosis, and basement membrane rupture. Interstitial edema and cellular infiltrates consisting of lymphocytes, neutrophilic leukocytes, histiocytes, and plasma cells are uniformly present. Glomerular lesions either are absent or consist of mesangial hyperplasia and focal foot process fusion which are interpreted as representing nonspecific changes associated with acute inflammation and protein filtration. Microscopic alterations in the liver are not diagnostic and correlate poorly with the degree of functional impairment. The changes include cloudy swelling of parenchymal cells, disruption of liver cords, enlargement of Kupffer cells, and bile stasis in biliary canaliculi. The changes in the brain and meninges are also minimal and are not diagnostic. Microscopic evidence of myocarditis has been recorded. Pulmonary findings consist of a patchy, localized hemorrhagic pneumonitis. Special staining techniques utilizing silver impregnation methods have demonstrated organisms in the lumina of renal tubules but rarely in other organs.

CLINICAL MANIFESTATIONS General features The incubation period following immersion or accidental laboratory exposure has shown extremes of 2 to 26 days, the usual range being 7 to 13 days and the average 10 days.

Leptospirosis is a typically biphasic illness. *During the leptospiremic* or *first phase*, leptospiras are present in the blood and cerebrospinal fluid. The onset is typically abrupt, and initial symptoms include headache, which is usually frontal, less often retroorbital, but occasionally may be bitemporal or occipital. Severe muscle aching occurs in most patients, the muscles of the thighs and lumbar areas being most prominently involved, and often is accompanied by severe pain on palpation. The myalgia may be accompanied by extreme cutaneous hyperesthesia (causalgia). Chills followed by a rapidly rising temperature are prominent. Following the abrupt onset, the leptospiremic phase typically lasts 4 to 9 days. Features during this interval include recurrent chills, high spiking temperatures [usually 38.9°C (102°F) or greater], headache, and continued severe myalgia. Anorexia, nausea, and vomiting are encountered in one-half or more of the patients. Occasional patients have diarrhea. Pulmonary manifestations, usually either cough or chest pain, have varied in frequency of occurrence from less than 25 percent to 86 percent. Hemoptysis occurs but is rare. Examination during this phase reveals an acutely ill, febrile patient, with a relative bradycardia and normal blood pressure, although European authors comment on early hypotension. Disturbances in sensorium may be encountered in up to 25 percent of patients. The most characteristic physical sign is conjunctival suffusion, which usually first appears on the third or fourth day. It may be lacking in some patients but more often is overlooked. This may be associated with photophobia, but serous or purulent secretion is unusual. Less common findings may include pharyngeal injection, cutaneous hemorrhages, and skin rashes that are usually macular, maculopapular, or urticarial and usually occur on the trunk. Uncommon findings are splenomegaly, hepatomegaly, lymphadenopathy, or jaundice. The first phase terminates after 4 to 9 days, usually with defervescence and improvement in symptoms. This coincides with the disappearance of leptospiras from the blood and cerebrospinal fluid.

The second phase has been characterized as the "immune" phase and correlates with the appearance of circulating IgM antibodies. The concentration of C3 in serum has remained within normal range during this phase. The clinical manifestations of this phase show greater variability than those during the first phase. After a relatively asymptomatic period of 1 to 3 days, the fever and earlier symptoms recur and meningismus may develop. The fever rarely exceeds 38.9°C (102°F) and is usually of 1 to 3 days' duration. It is not uncommon for fever to be absent or quite transient. Even when symptoms or signs of meningeal irritation are absent, routine examination of cerebrospinal fluid after the seventh day has revealed pleocytosis in 50 to 90 percent of patients. Less common features include iridocyclitis, optic neuritis, and other nervous system manifestations, including encephalitis, myelitis, and peripheral neuropathy.

Some clinicians recognize a third or convalescent phase, usually between the second and fourth weeks, when both fever and aching may recur. The pathogenesis of this stage is not understood.

Leptospirosis during pregnancy may be associated with an increased risk of fetal loss.

Specific features WEIL'S SYNDROME Weil's syndrome, which may be due to serotypes other than Icterohemorrhagiae, is defined as severe leptospirosis with jaundice, usually accompanied by azotemia, hemorrhages, anemia, disturbances in consciousness, and continued fever. There is uncertainty as to the pathogenesis of the syndrome, i.e., whether it represents direct toxic damage due to leptospiras or whether it is the consequence of immune response to leptospiral antigens. The consensus favors toxic damage.

The onset and first stage are identical with the less severe forms of leptospirosis. The distinctive features of Weil's syndrome appear from the third to the sixth days but do not reach their peak until well into the second stage. As in milder forms of leptospirosis, there is a tendency for defervescence about the seventh day; however, with recurrence, fever is marked and may persist for several weeks. Either renal or hepatic manifestations may predominate. Hepatic disturbances include tenderness in the right upper quadrant and hepatic enlargement, both of which are common when jaundice is present. Serum glutamic oxaloacetic transaminase (SGOT) values are rarely increased more than fivefold regardless of the degree of hyperbilirubinemia, which is predominantly conjugated (direct): e.g., serum bilirubin, 40 mg per 100 ml; SGOT, 170 IU. The predominant mechanism appears to be an intracellular block to bilirubin excretion.

Renal manifestations consist primarily of proteinuria, pyuria, hematuria, and azotemia. Dysuria is rare. Serious renal damage usually occurs in the form of acute tubular necrosis associated with oliguria. The peak elevation of blood urea nitrogen usually is seen on the fifth to seventh day. Hemorrhagic manifestations are most prevalent in this group of patients and include epistaxis, hemoptysis, gastrointestinal bleeding, hemorrhage into the adrenal glands, hemorrhagic pneumonitis, and subarachnoid hemorrhage. These have been explained on the basis of diffuse vasculitis with capillary injury. In addition, in some patients hypoprothrombinemia and thrombocytopenia have been observed.

ASEPTIC MENINGITIS A leptospiral etiology has been incriminated in 5 to 13 percent of sporadic cases of aseptic meningitis. The pleocytosis is not present before the immune phase, when it develops rapidly. There are usually tens to hundreds of leukocytes, occasionally 1000, per cubic milliliter, among which neutrophils or mononuclear cells may predominate. The cerebrospinal fluid glucose concentration is almost always normal, but occasional instances of lowered glucose levels (hypoglycorrhachia) have been recorded. In contrast to the observations with many viral causes of aseptic meningitis, with leptospirosis

the cerebrospinal fluid protein may exceed 100 mg per 100 ml early in the course. Xanthochromic cerebrospinal fluid has been observed in the presence of jaundice. Each of the serotypes of leptospiras that are pathogenic for human beings is probably capable of causing aseptic meningitis. The most prevalent serotypes have been Canicola, Icterohemorrhagiae, and Pomona.

PRETIBIAL (FORT BRAGG) FEVER An illness was observed in the summer of 1942 that had an onset identical with that of the first phase of leptospirosis. The most distinctive feature was the development on about the fourth day of a rash, characterized by 2- to 5-cm, slightly raised, erythematous lesions that were usually symmetrically distributed over the pretibial areas. In contrast to other leptospiral syndromes, splenomegaly occurred in 95 percent of these patients. This outbreak was shown to be due to the Autumnalis serogroup. Subsequently, Pomona has been observed in association with rashes, which are usually truncal but which have also been pretibial.

MYOCARDITIS Cardiac arrhythmias including paroxysmal atrial fibrillation, atrial flutter, ventricular tachycardia, and premature ventricular contractions have been described but are usually of little clinical significance. However, on rare occasions definite cardiac dilatation with acute left ventricular failure has been observed. Associated manifestations have included jaundice, pulmonary infiltrates, arthritis, and skin rashes. The serotypes thus far incriminated have included Icterohemorrhagiae, Pomona, and Grippotyphosa.

CHILDREN Several clinical features occur in children which are not seen or are very rare in adults: hypertension, acalculous cholecystitis (five of nine children in one series), pancreatitis, abdominal causalgia, and peripheral desquamation of a rash which may be associated with gangrene and cardiopulmonary arrest. The features of desquamation, myocardial involvement, and hydrops of the gallbladder suggest mucocutaneous lymph node syndrome (Chap. 180).

LABORATORY FEATURES Leukocyte counts vary from leukopenic levels to mild elevations in the anicteric patients. In patients with jaundice, leukocytosis as high as 70,000 cells per cubic millimeter may be present. However, regardless of the total leukocyte count, neutrophilia of greater than 70 percent is very frequently encountered during the first stage.

Hemolytic substances have been demonstrated in cultures of pathogenic leptospiras. In contrast to many hemolysins of bacterial origin which are not hemolytic in vivo, the leptospiral hemolysins appear to be active in vivo. In patients with jaundice, anemia may be severe and is most characteristically due to intravascular hemolysis. Other mechanisms of anemia include azotemia and blood loss secondary to hemorrhage. Anemia due to leptospirosis is unusual in anicteric patients.

Rarely thrombocytopenia sufficient to be associated with bleeding is encountered. Additional hematologic abnormalities include elevation of the erythrocyte sedimentation rate in over one-half of patients, but it is usually less than 50 mm/h.

Urinalysis during the leptospiremic phase reveals mild proteinuria, casts, and an increase in cellular elements. In anicteric infections, these abnormalities rapidly disappear after the first week. Proteinuria and abnormalities in the urine sediment usually are not associated with elevations in blood urea nitrogen. Since the anicteric form of the disease often has gone undiagnosed, estimates of the frequency of azotemia and jaundice are probably high. Azotemia has been reported in approximately one-fourth of patients. In three-fourths of these patients, the blood urea nitrogen is less than 100 mg per 100 ml. Azotemia is usually associated with jaundice. The serum bilirubin levels may reach 65 mg per 100 ml; however, in two-thirds of patients the levels are less than 20 mg per 100 ml. During the first phase, one-half of the patients have increased serum creatine phosphokinase (CPK) levels, with mean values of five times normal. Such increases are not seen in viral hepatitis, and a slight increase in transaminase with a definite increase in CPK suggests leptospirosis rather than viral hepatitis.

DIAGNOSIS Diagnosis is based upon culture of the organism or serologic proof of its existence. The most common initial diagnostic impressions in patients with leptospirosis are meningitis, hepatitis, nephritis, fever of undetermined origin (FUO), and influenza. Leptospiras may be isolated quite readily during the first phase from blood and cerebrospinal fluid or during the second phase from the urine. Leptospiras may be excreted in the urine for up to 11 months after the onset of illness and may persist despite antimicrobial therapy. Whole blood should be inoculated immediately into tubes containing semisolid medium, such as Fletcher's medium. If culture medium is not available, leptospiras reportedly will remain viable up to 11 days in blood to which anticoagulants, preferably sodium oxalate, have been added. Animal inoculation (preferably either suckling hamsters or guinea pigs) may be used and is of particular value if specimens are contaminated. Direct examination of blood or urine by dark-field methods has been employed; *however, this method so frequently results in failure or misdiagnosis that it should not be employed.* Serologic methods are applicable during the second phase; antibodies appear from the sixth to the twelfth days of illness. Two serologic methods are commonly used: a macroscopic or slide agglutination test which is easy to perform but lacks specificity and sensitivity, and hence is suitable for screening only, and the microscopic agglutination test which is more complicated but also more specific. Serologic criteria for diagnosis include a fourfold or greater rise in titer during the course of illness. Cross-agglutination reactions between various serotypes commonly occur so that the infection serotype often cannot be determined with certainty without isolation of leptospiras.

PROGNOSIS The prognosis is dependent upon both the virulence of the organism and the general condition of the patient. In 1976, there were six deaths (7 percent) in the 81 patients reported in the United States. Age is the most significant host factor related to increased mortality. In a representative series, the mortality rose from 10 percent in men less than 50 years of age to 56 percent in those over 51 years of age. The virulence of the infecting leptospiras correlates best with the development of jaundice. In anicteric patients, mortality does not occur, but with the development of jaundice, mortality in various series has ranged from 15 to 40 percent. The long-term prognosis following the acute renal lesion of leptospirosis is good. Glomerular filtration rates have returned to normal; however, a few patients show residual tubular dysfunction such as a defect in renal concentrating capacity.

TREATMENT A variety of antimicrobial drugs, including penicillin, streptomycin, the tetracycline congeners, chloramphenicol, and erythromycin, have been effective in vitro and in experimental leptospiral infections. Data concerning the efficacy of antibiotics in human beings are conflicting. If antimicrobial drugs are to have any beneficial effect, they must be administered within 4 days, and preferably within 2 days, of the onset of illness. Large doses of penicillin G (usually 600,000 units intramuscularly every 4 h) are considered the preferred treatment, although the tetracyclines are also effective. Within 4 to 6 h after initiation of penicillin G therapy, a Jarisch-Herxheimer type of reaction, which suggests antileptospiral activity, may occur. There is general agreement that antimicrobials administered after the fifth day of illness have no beneficial effect. There exists the clinical impression that early bedrest may minimize subsequent morbidity. Azotemia and jaundice require meticulous attention to fluid and electrolyte therapy. Since the renal damage is reversible, patients with azotemia should be considered for peritoneal dialysis or hemodialysis. From case reports exchange transfusion has been suggested to be beneficial in the management of patients with extreme hyperbilirubinemia.

REFERENCES

ALSTON JM, BROOM JC: *Leptospirosis in Man and Animals.* Edinburgh, E & S Livingstone, 1958

CENTER FOR DISEASE CONTROL: *Leptospirosis Surveillance: Annual Summary 1976.* April 1978

EDWARDS GA, DOMM M: Human leptospirosis. Medicine 39:117, 1960

FEIGIN RD, ANDERSON DC: Human leptospirosis. CRC Crit Rev Clin Lab Sci 5:413, 1975

HEATH CW JR, ALEXANDER AD: Leptospirosis in the United States: Analysis of 483 cases in man, 1949-1961. N Engl J Med 273:857, 915, 1965

JOHNSON ND JR et al: Serum creatine phosphokinase in leptospirosis. JAMA 233:981, 1975

JOHNSON RC: *The Biology of Parasitic Spirochetes.* New York, Academic, 1976

TURNER LH: Leptospirosis. Br Med J 1:537, 1973

WONG ML et al: Leptospirosis: A childhood disease. J Pediatr 90:532, 1977

149
RELAPSING FEVER

JAMES J. PLORDE

DEFINITION Relapsing fever refers to a group of acute infectious diseases that are characterized clinically by cyclic periods of fever and apyrexia. They are caused by spirochetes of the genus *Borrelia* and occur in two epidemiologic varieties, louse-borne and tick-borne.

ETIOLOGY Borreliae are slender helical organisms which measure 10 to 20 μm in length. They have 3 to 10 irregular coils, move in a corkscrew fashion, and divide by transverse fission. Unlike other spirochetes, they readily stain with aniline dyes. *Borrelia recurrentis* is the causative agent of louse-borne relapsing fever. Many strains of *Borrelia* have been found in tick-borne disease; *B. turicatae, B. parkeri,* and *B. hermsii* are responsible for the disease seen in this country. The organisms grow poorly on artificial media and readily in developing chick embryos.

EPIDEMIOLOGY Louse-borne relapsing fever is transmitted from person to person by the human body louse. Spirochetes that are ingested by the vector during feeding penetrate the wall of the intestine and multiply in the body cavity. Human infection occurs when the louse is crushed against an abrasion or wound. There is no known animal reservoir. The disease persists in endemic focuses in Ethiopia, the Sudan, South America, and the Far East. Like typhus, it occurs in epidemic form during war and famine. Major epidemics involving millions of people occurred in Europe and Africa after both the

First and Second World Wars. A third, much smaller, outbreak was seen at the time of the Korean conflict. An occasional case of louse-borne relapsing fever has been imported into the United States.

The tick vectors of relapsing fever belong to several species of the genus *Ornithodoros*. These soft ticks are reclusive night feeders whose bites are quick and painless. They then detach themselves, leaving their host with a 2- to 3-mm pruritic eschar. Like lice, they ingest the borreliae during feeding. The organisms may remain viable in the ticks for several years and can be passed transovarily to the next generation, making the tick a major reservoir of the disease. It is likely that rodents and other small animals act as vertebrate reservoirs in some locales. Human beings are involved when they come into contact with an infected tick in its natural habitat. Transmission occurs if the tick's saliva or coxal fluid contaminates the feeding site. The tick-borne disease is found in localized areas throughout the world. In the United States it occurs primarily in Western mountain states, from Texas in the South to Washington, Montana, and Idaho in the Northwest. Outbreaks have occurred among Boy Scouts in northeastern Washington and tourists visiting the north rim of the Grand Canyon. In both outbreaks, the patients contracted the disease while sleeping overnight in tick-infested cabins. The disease has also been carried to other parts of the country, where it usually does not occur, by western travelers.

PATHOGENESIS AND PATHOLOGY After inoculation into a human being, the borreliae reach the bloodstream, producing spirochetemia and a febrile illness. After several days, immobilizing and borrelicidal antibodies appear, the organisms are cleared from the peripheral blood, and the fever resolves. Following a latent period of approximately 1 week, during which the spirochetes are sequestered in the body, a new antigenic variant of the organism arises. There is reinvasion of the bloodstream, causing a second paroxysm of fever and eventually, with the formation of specific antibodies, a second defervescence by crisis. The continued sequential production of new antigenic variants and specific antibodies results in the characteristic relapsing febrile course. Endotoxin has been detected in the blood of febrile patients with louse-borne disease. Whether the toxin is released by dying spirochetes or is liberated from anoxic gutwall is not known. However, decreased blood levels of Hageman factors and prekaillekrein as well as hypocomplementemia all suggest a role for endotoxin in the pathogenesis of this disease (Chap. 109).

At autopsy follicular splenic abscesses, histiocytic interstitial myocarditis, intracranial hemorrhage, and hepatitis with focal necrosis may be seen. Spontaneous splenic rupture and hemorrhagic gastrointestinal lesions have been noted occasionally. Borreliae have been recovered from the brain, heart, spleen, liver, and skin.

MANIFESTATIONS Clinical manifestations vary from outbreak to outbreak and between the tick- and louse-borne varieties of the disease. Generally, patients with louse-borne relapsing fever are more seriously ill but have fewer relapses than those with tick-borne illnesses. After an incubation period of 4 to 18 days, the disease begins abruptly with rigors, headache, anorexia, nausea, vomiting, photophobia, and pain in the muscles and joints. The temperature rises rapidly, reaching 39 to 40°C (102.2 to 104°F), where it remains until the time of the crisis. The patient appears dull, apathetic, and is uncomplaining. He may have conjunctival suffusion and a macular or petechial rash. Cough, tachypnea, and rhonchi are common. A gallop rhythm and premature ventricular beats may occur in the louse-borne variety. Cardiac enlargement and heart failure are more uncommon. Upper abdominal tenderness is frequent. The liver and spleen are palpable and tender in 20 to 80 percent of cases, and may enlarge 6 to 10 cm during the course of fever. Jaundice secondary to hepatocellular destruction is present in 7 to 36 percent of patients. It is usually seen in louse-borne disease, occurs relatively late in the illness, and if severe, is often associated with purpura.

Bleeding is common in louse-borne relapsing fever. Petechiae develop in the skin and serous membranes, apparently as a result of damage to the capillary endothelium by clumps of spirochetes. Mild epistaxes and microscopic hematuria are present in many patients early in the disease. Later, with the development of liver disease, severe prolonged epistaxes and widespread ecchymoses occur. Infrequently, there may be massive gastrointestinal, urinary, or intracranial hemorrhage. Disseminated intravascular coagulation has been described. Neck stiffness, confusion, and transient focal neurologic signs may be seen even without intracranial bleeding. Patients with tick-borne disease with repeated relapses may develop iritis or iridocyclitis with permanent visual impairment. Pregnant women with relapsing fever often abort.

Three to six days after the onset of illness, the attack ends in a crisis. Clinically this is characterized by a chill and an abrupt but transient rise in temperature, heart rate, respiratory rate, and arterial blood pressure. As the spirochetes disappear, the patient becomes flushed, diaphoretic, and hypotensive. Occasionally, cardiovascular collapse and death may occur at this point. More frequently the blood pressure and temperature return to normal over several hours, leaving the patient comfortable but exhausted. After 7 to 10 afebrile days, a relapse occurs which mimics the original illness. In the louse-borne disease there is usually only a single relapse, but in tick-borne relapsing fever there may be several, each somewhat briefer and milder than the preceding one.

LABORATORY FINDINGS A moderate anemia is common. The leukocyte count is usually normal or slightly elevated. During the crisis, a marked leukopenia occurs which may be followed by a transient rebound leukocytosis. A consumptive thrombocytopenia is seen in most cases, and the prothrombin and partial thromboplastin times may be prolonged. Fibrinogen levels are increased. Liver function tests reveal disturbed hepatocellular function. In severe cases, the total serum bilirubin level may reach 16 mg per 100 ml. Azotemia unrelated to extracellular fluid depletion is common among jaundiced patients. Electrocardiogram abnormalities, including a prolonged QTc interval and ST-T wave changes, may occur. Reagin tests for syphilis are positive in 5 to 10 percent of cases, and experimental data suggest that false-positive FTA-ABS tests may also occur. Patients with louse-borne relapsing fever frequently develop agglutinins to *Proteus* OXK antigens.

The definitive diagnosis is made by demonstrating borreliae in the peripheral blood during a febrile episode. This is most easily accomplished by examining thick and thin films stained with Giemsa's and Wright's stains. Repeated examinations may be required, especially in tick-borne disease. Blood spun in a microhematocrit tube and examined microscopically may reveal organisms when thin and thick smears are negative. Spirochetes may also be seen in wet mounts with phase-contrast microscopy. When the direct methods are negative, blood may be injected into mice or rats and their blood examined frequently for the presence of borreliae.

DIFFERENTIAL DIAGNOSIS Many acute febrile illnesses, including malaria, salmonellosis, typhus, dengue, rat-bite fever, and Weil's disease, must be considered. Practically, there is seldom confusion if blood films are examined carefully.

TREATMENT　The peripheral blood is quickly cleared of spirochetes by a variety of drugs, including penicillin, tetracycline, and chloramphenicol. Treatment with these antimicrobial agents, however, is accompanied by a Jarisch-Herxheimer-like reaction which contributes to the morbidity, and perhaps mortality, of the disease. The reaction appears both clinically and pathophysiologically to be an exaggeration of the spontaneously occurring crisis. Its mechanism is unknown, but it may be related to an accelerated release of endotoxin liberated during destruction of spirochetes. It is certainly related temporally to disappearance of spirochetes from the blood, and its severity appears to depend upon the speed with which they are removed.

In louse-borne relapsing fever, where the spirochetemia is often intense and the Jarisch-Herxheimer reaction severe, the drug of choice is a repository penicillin such as penicillin aluminum monostearate (PAM). Unlike tetracycline, this drug achieves a very gradual clearing of the spirochetes and a correspondingly mild reaction. The drug is given intramuscularly in a dose of 600,000 units. If the shorter-acting procaine penicillin is used, the dose should be repeated in 12 to 24 h to prevent relapse. In epidemics, a single 0.5-g oral dose of tetracycline, erythromycin, or chloramphenicol can be used with good results.

In tick-borne disease where penicillin is not effective in terminating relapses, tetracycline is most rapidly borrelicidal. This drug should be given in a dose of 0.5 g four times a day for 5 to 10 days. Doxycycline, 100 mg twice daily, is also effective. The Jarisch-Herxheimer reaction tends to be less severe in this form of the disease.

PROGNOSIS　When epidemics strike a nonimmune population, the high mortality rate due to the louse-borne disease shows the potential menace of this disease. Most patients, however, recover quickly and completely; relapses do not occur if antibiotic therapy is adequate. Adverse signs are deep jaundice, uncontrolled bleeding, and a grossly prolonged QTc interval.

Typhus and enteric fever may occur simultaneously with louse-borne relapsing fever, and they probably contribute to the mortality rate, particularly during epidemics.

REFERENCES

BOYER KM et al: Tick-borne relapsing fever: An interstate outbreak originating at Grand Canyon National Park. Am J Epidemiol 105:469, 1977

BRYCESON ADM et al: Louse-borne relapsing fever: A clinical and laboratory study of 62 cases in Ethiopia and a reconsideration of the literature. Q J Med 39:139, 1970

BUTLER T et al: *Borrelia recurrentis* infection: Single dose antibiotic regimens and management of the Jarisch-Herxheimer reaction. J Infect Dis 137:573, 1978

GALLOWAY RE et al: Activation of protein mediators of inflammation and evidence of endotoxemia in *Borrelia recurrentis* infection. Am J Med 63:933, 1977

JOHNSON RC: The spirochetes. Annu Rev Microbiol 31:89, 1977

JUDGE DM et al: Louse-borne relapsing fever in man. Arch Pathol 97:136, 1974

SOUTHERN PM JR, SANFORD JP: Relapsing fever. Medicine 48:129, 1969

section 9 | Infections caused by higher bacteria and fungi

150
GENERAL CONSIDERATIONS

JOHN F BENNETT

Actinomycetes and fungi are being considered together in this section, but this should not obscure profound differences between these two groups of organisms. The agents of actinomycosis, nocardiosis, and actinomycetoma are actinomycetes. These organisms are gram-positive higher bacteria which branch but have the diameter, antibiotic susceptibility, and ability to induce a neutrophilic inflammatory response in common with other bacteria. Actinomycetes resemble fungi in causing infections which may be extremely chronic and which are poorly transmissible from person to person. *Actinomyces israelii* and *Candida albicans* colonize the gastrointestinal tract early in life, presumably by person-to-person spread. Infection results in later life when specialized conditions permit entry of normal flora into deeper tissue. The largest number of actinomycetes and fungi enter the body from a source in nature, where the microbe grows as a saprophyte. The two major means of entry into the body are by inhalation into the lungs (histoplasmosis, coccidioidomycosis, blastomycosis, cryptococcosis, nocardiosis, mucormycosis, aspergillosis, paracoccidioidomycosis) and by cutaneous inoculation (sporotrichosis, mycetoma, chromomycosis, dermatophytosis).

Certain problems with names of actinomycetes and fungi need to be recognized. The taxonomy of agents causing actinomycetoma and chromomycosis has been unstable, resulting in a disconcerting number of name changes. The discovery of a perfect state for several fungi has created an additional name for these species. *Perfect state* or *sexual state* refers to a part of the fungal life cycle in which meiosis occurs. This part of the life cycle usually is not encountered in a routine diagnostic laboratory so the report ordinarily should give the name of the species in the imperfect state, generally a more familiar name.

Several facts common to the diagnosis and treatment of many mycoses are most economically dealt with in this section. Fungi are not detected reliably in histological sections stained with hematoxylin and eosin. Gomori methenamine silver stain with a homogeneous counterstain is the most sensitive procedure. Periodic acid–Schiff will stain many fungi, but the lesser contrast makes a small number of organisms more difficult to detect.

Therapy with intravenous amphotericin B is best initiated with a test dose of 1 mg. Patients with profound febrile reactions to this dose will require gradual increments in dose. Patients with fulminant mycoses should have their doses advanced rapidly to at least 0.3 mg/kg per day. Hydrocortisone hemisuccinate added to the infusion may help control febrile reactions. Double-dose alternate-day therapy has the same toxicity and efficacy as single-dose daily therapy, with the following exceptions. Alternate-day double-dose therapy causes more fever, but the patient has fewer infusions and therefore less phlebitis. Appetite and ambulation may be improved on the days-off therapy. The final dose will depend on nephrotoxicity and the specific mycosis. Intrathecal amphotericin B is used in coccidioidal and sometimes other mycotic meningitides. In experienced hands, intracisternal injections are preferable. Triweekly doses are increased from 0.05 to 0.5 mg over six doses. Addition of hydrocortisone 15 mg to the intrathecal injection decreases side effects. As the meningitis is controlled, the frequency of injection can be decreased to once or twice a week. The same schedule may be used for lumbar hyperbaric intrathecal injections or for intraventricular injections via a subcutaneous reservoir. These routes encounter more complications.

REFERENCES

AL-DOORY Y (ed): *The Epidemiology of Human Mycotic Diseases.* Springfield, Ill, Charles C Thomas, 1975

BAKER RD (ed): *Human Infections with Fungi, Actinomycetes and Algae.* New York, Springer-Verlag, 1971

BENNETT JE: Chemotherapy of systemic mycoses. New Engl J Med 290:30, 320, 1974

BUECHNER HA (ed): *Management of Fungus Diseases of the Lungs.* Springfield, Ill, Charles C Thomas, 1971

EMMONS CW: *Medical Mycology.* Philadelphia, Lea & Febiger, 1977

FETTER BF et al: *Mycoses of the Central Nervous System.* Baltimore, Williams & Wilkins, 1967

RIPPON JW: *Medical Mycology.* Philadelphia, Saunders, 1974

151
ACTINOMYCOSIS

JOHN E. BENNETT

DEFINITION Actinomycosis is an indolent suppurative infection caused by certain anaerobic actinomycetes. The microorganisms grow within the tissue as grossly visible tightly knit clusters, called *grains.*

ETIOLOGY *Actinomyces israelii* is the usual causative agent but *A. naeslundi* and *Arachnia propionica* are occasional causes. These gram-positive branching, anaerobic or microaerophilic organisms are the same width as bacteria. When they are cultured on blood agar, small colonies appear after 2 to 4 days of incubation at 37°C under anaerobic conditions. Catalase and other biochemical tests distinguish these organisms from the common skin contaminant *Propionibacterium acnes.* Final identification is best left to a reference laboratory.

PATHOLOGY AND PATHOGENESIS All agents of actinomycosis are commensals in the mouth and gastrointestinal tract of humans. The portal of entry appears to be either a break in the integrity of the mucosa or aspiration into the lung. Poor dental hygiene and dental abscess predispose to oral lesions. Within the gastrointestinal tract, the appendiceal area is the most common site. Infection presents as a chronic suppurative inflammation, usually in the cervicofacial, thoracic, or abdominal area. In histopathologic section, each grain is typically surrounded by polymorphonuclear neutrophils. Adjacent tissue shows subacute or chronic inflammation with extensive fibrosis and formation of sinus tracts. Giant cells are infrequent. The grain stains variably with hematoxylin and eosin. Grains may have an eosinophilic coating composed of human proteins. Hyphal filaments cannot be seen on hematoxylin and eosin stain but may be demonstrated in the periphery of the grain by tissue Gram's stain (such as Brown and Brenn) or by a heavily stained Gomori methenamine silver. These stains may be useful if there is chance for confusion with the grains of eumycetoma or staphylococcal botryomycosis. Grains are a few millimeters in diameter, making them difficult to miss if they are present in the histological section being examined. Several sections may have to be searched to find a grain. Grains may be observed grossly in pus or on bandages covering draining sinuses. These pale yellow, cheese-like particles can be crushed on a microscope slide, and the gram-positive branching filaments demonstrated on Gram's stain.

Infection spreads by direct extension and hematogenously. Direct extension through the skin causes one or more chronic draining sinuses to appear in the abdomen, chest, or cervicofacial area. Hematogenous foci may appear in bone, brain, liver, or other organs.

CLINICAL MANIFESTATIONS Cervicofacial actinomycosis presents as a red or purplish firmly indurated subcutaneous mass, typically in the submandibular area or in the anterior cervical triangle near the angle of the mandible. One or more draining sinuses may be present. Tenderness is slight or absent. Lethargy, weight loss, variable low-grade fever, anemia, and leukocytosis are infrequent in cervicofacial actinomycosis but common in thoracic and abdominal actinomycosis. Localizing findings in the latter forms include draining sinuses and, in thoracic actinomycosis, cough and purulent sputum. Pain or a palpable mass may appear in abdominal actinomycosis. Pelvic actinomycosis, once rare, is now being seen in women with an implanted intrauterine device for contraception. The indolent onset, variable low-grade fever, abdominal pain, and adnexal mass may lead to an erroneous diagnosis of pelvic inflammatory disease or tumor. In all forms of actinomycosis, disease typically has been present for weeks or months at time of diagnosis.

Chest x-ray may reveal an area of dense pneumonitis. Fibrosis, empyema, or cavitation may be seen. Periappendiceal abscess may appear as an extrinsic mass on barium enema.

DIAGNOSIS Laboratory tests other than culture or histological section are not helpful. Blood cultures are rarely positive. Isolation of *Actinomyces* or *Arachnia* species from the mouth, sputum, stool, or feculent draining sinuses is not diagnostic. Demonstration of a grain in pus or deep tissue is diagnostic, if botryomycosis and mycetoma can be excluded. Nocardiosis can be distinguished by the absence of grains, identification of the organism in culture, and, usually, by the weak acid-fast staining of *Nocardia.*

TREATMENT Milder cases of actinomycosis, including most cervicofacial infections, respond well to oral tetracycline or penicillin V, an adult dose being 500 mg qid of either drug. Oral erythromycin would be second choice. More severe cases, including many thoracic and abdominal infections, should receive parenteral penicillin G for roughly 6 weeks (adults receive 2 to 5 million units per day) followed by prolonged therapy with oral penicillin V or tetracycline. The likelihood of relapse is reduced if the total duration of therapy is 2 to 4 months in mild cases and up to 6 to 12 months in severe forms. Drug resistance has not been encountered in relapsed cases. Curettage of bone lesions and surgical drainage of empyema, brain abscess, or other large collections of pus appear to facilitate recovery but are usually not curative by themselves.

It is common in actinomycosis to isolate microbes other than actinomycetes from pus. In general, the antibiotic susceptibility of these secondary organisms does not have to be considered in the selection of therapeutic agents.

REFERENCES

Davies M, Keddie NC: Abdominal actinomycosis. Br J Surg 60:18, 1973

Eastridge CE et al: Actinomycosis. A 24 year experience. South Med J 65:839, 1972

Fradis M et al: Actinomycosis of the face and neck. Arch Otolaryngol 102:87, 1976

Seabury J: Actinomycosis and nocardiosis, in *Management of Fungus Disease of the Lungs,* HA Buechner (ed). Springfield, Ill, Charles C Thomas, 1971, pp 197–211

Seligman P et al: Tubo-ovarian actinomycosis. NY State J Med 76:278, 1976

Slade PR et al: Thoracic actinomycosis. Thorax 28:73, 1973

152
NOCARDIOSIS

JOHN E. BENNETT

DEFINITION Nocardiosis is an acute, subacute, or chronic infection, most often beginning in the lung.

ETIOLOGY *Nocardia asteroides, N. brasiliensis,* and *N. caviae* are the etiologic agents of two different diseases, nocardiosis and mycetoma. In the latter infection, the organism enters the skin by trauma, forms grains within tissue, and spreads slowly to contiguous tissue (see Chap. 161). In nocardiosis, the organism usually enters via the lung, does not form grains, and is prone to hematogenous spread. Even though the etiologic agents of these diseases do overlap, *N. asteroides* causes most cases of nocardiosis and *N. brasiliensis* is the species usually isolated from mycetoma. *Nocardia caviae* is a rare cause of either disease. *Nocardia brasiliensis* can also cause a lymphocutaneous disease closely resembling sporotrichosis; this infection differs from mycetoma by its lymphangitic spread and by the absence of grains.

Nocardia species are aerobic actinomycetes with branching hyphae the same width as bacteria. Hyphae are weakly gram-positive and weakly acid-fast. Growth appears in 2 to 5 days on blood agar, Sabouraud's agar, or other simple media. Incorporation of antibiotics into the media to inhibit bacterial growth usually inhibits *Nocardia* as well. Colonies become rough and chalky with an orange or yellow hue. Identification of *Nocardia* species, including distinction between *Streptomyces, Actinomadura,* and *Nocardia,* is difficult and best assigned to a reference laboratory.

PATHOGENESIS AND PATHOLOGY *Nocardia* is a soil saprophyte widely distributed throughout the world. Infection is acquired from sites in nature, never from infected persons or animals. Males are infected two to three times more commonly than females. No age or exposure is known to predispose to nocardiosis. Many patients have serious preexisting conditions, such as adrenal corticosteroid therapy, cancer, pulmonary alveolar proteinosis, or chronic granulomatous disease of childhood.

Lesions of nocardiosis show suppuration, necrosis, and abscess formation. Neutrophils are the predominant inflammatory cell. Hyphae are scattered throughout the lesion without formation of grains. Tissue Gram's stain or overstained methenamine silver best demonstrate the hyphae. A modified Fite-Faraco stain of histological sections can be used to demonstrate acid-fastness, but this property is not always demonstrable.

CLINICAL MANIFESTATIONS *Nocardia* pneumonia presents with fever and productive cough of several days' or up to several months' duration. The initial illness may resemble a bacterial pneumonia, but slow radiologic progression continues despite antibiotic therapy often with cavitation of radiodense central areas. Hematogenous dissemination to brain and subcutaneous tissue is frequent in nocardiosis. A pulmonary portal is usually but not always detectable clinically. Brain lesions are typically multiple thin-walled abscesses. Purulent meningitis may result from rupture of an abscess into the ventricle. The subcutaneous lesion typically consists of one or a few indolent abscesses. Hematogenous dissemination to other organs occurs but is rarely detectable clinically.

DIAGNOSIS *Nocardia* is difficult enough to detect in sputum culture, Gram's stain, or histological section so that the diagnosis is readily missed. A progressive pneumonia with purulent sputum should suggest the diagnosis, particularly if cavitation or spread to brain or subcutaneous tissue occurs. Sputum, pus, bronchial brushing, or bronchial washing specimens should be examined by Gram's stain and modified acid-fast stain. On Gram's stain the hyphae are usually branching, beaded, and refractile. They are not strongly gram-positive but take the red counterstain even less well. Conventional acid-fast staining procedures such as Ziehl-Neelsen or a fluorochrome do not stain *Nocardia.* Identification of branching, weakly acid-fast organisms in histological section or smear of pus or sputum is sufficient to establish the diagnosis of nocardiosis. Cultural confirmation is highly desirable, but isolation of *Nocardia* from heavily contaminated specimens is difficult. Isolation of *Nocardia* from otherwise sterile pus is readily accomplished. *Nocardia* is rarely isolated from blood, but diphasic culture media are said to facilitate isolation.

When *Nocardia* is isolated from sputum, the diagnosis of nocardiosis should be suspected, but occasionally no disease can be detected. Rarely, *Nocardia* is an airborne contaminant.

TREATMENT Surgical drainage of empyema and abscesses in brain or subcutaneous tissue is helpful but not sufficient therapy. Virtually all patients should receive prolonged chemotherapy. The treatment of choice is a sulfonamide, given in sufficient dose to maintain a blood concentration of 10 to 15 mg per 100 ml. Sulfadiazine is preferred because of its penetration into the cerebrospinal fluid and other tissues. Also, more experience is available with sulfadiazine than other sulfonamides. The danger of crystalluria and oliguria requires copious fluid intake and urine alkalinization during high-dose sulfadiazine. A reasonable starting regimen is sulfadiazine 100 mg/kg per day and sodium bicarbonate 50 mg/kg per day, both in four divided doses. Patients who show progressive improvement may be changed to sulfisoxazole or trisulfapyrimidines,

60 mg/kg per day after 4 to 6 weeks. Therapy is continued for a total of 12 to 18 months.

Sulfisoxazole is a reasonable starting drug when fluid loading and urine alkalinization are difficult. Trimethoprim-sulfamethoxazole has been used successfully in a few cases, but the contribution of trimethoprim is unclear. Addition of other antibiotics to sulfa drugs may be indicated in patients who show continued deterioration. Ampicillin 150 mg/kg per day is preferred. High doses of minocycline or erythromycin also have been advocated. Parsimonious use of other drugs during sulfa therapy of nocardiosis minimizes the probability that a drug allergy will necessitate discontinuance of sulfa. Antimicrobial susceptibility tests are used to guide therapy of patients with serious allergic reactions to sulfa drugs, but such regimens are not of proved efficacy.

Pulmonary nocardiosis in a previously normal host has a 50 to 60 percent chance of cure with appropriate therapy, and cerebral nocardiosis a 13 percent chance. Continued use of immunosuppressive therapy seems to impair therapeutic response in nocardiosis.

REFERENCES

FRAZIER AR et al: Nocardiosis. A review of 25 cases occurring during 24 months. Mayo Clin Proc 50:657, 1975

KRICK JA et al: Nocardia infection in heart transplant patients. Ann Intern Med 82:18, 1975

PADRON S et al: Lymphocutaneous *Nocardia brasiliensis* infection mimicking sporotrichosis. South Med J 66:609, 1973

PALMER DL et al: Diagnostic and therapeutic considerations in *Nocardia asteroides* infection. Medicine 53:391, 1974

153
CRYPTOCOCCOSIS

JOHN E. BENNETT

DEFINITION Cryptococcosis is an infection caused by the yeast-like fungus *Cryptococcus neoformans*. The most common presentation is as a subacute or chronic meningoencephalitis.

ETIOLOGY *Cryptococcus neoformans* should be divided into two different species, one of which would retain the name *C. neoformans* and the other species would be called *C. bacillisporus*. Mating of compatible strains within these two species yields a perfect state called *Filobasidiella neoformans* and *Filobasidiella bacillispora*. There are biochemical, epidemiological, and serotypic differences between *C. neoformans* and *C. bacillisporus,* but the clinical disease and response to therapy appear to be the same. Therefore, the remainder of this chapter will follow the older practice of calling the two species simply *C. neoformans.*

Cryptococcus neoformans reproduces by budding and forms round, yeast-like cells 4 to 6 μm in diameter. Within the host and on certain culture media, a large polysaccharide capsule surrounds each yeast cell. The fungus grows well as smooth, creamy white colonies on Sabouraud's or other simple media at 20 to 37°C. Certain culture media for ringworm contain cycloheximide, which inhibits *C. neoformans*. Identification is based on gross and microscopic appearance, biochemical tests, and growth at 37°C.

PATHOGENESIS AND PATHOLOGY Infection is thought to be acquired by inhalation of fungus into the lungs. Pulmonary infection has a tendency toward spontaneous resolution and is frequently asymptomatic. Silent hematogenous spread to the brain leads to clusters of cryptococci in the perivascular areas of cortical gray matter, basal ganglia, and, to a lesser extent, other areas of the central nervous system. Inflammatory response around these foci is usually scant. In the more chronic cases, a dense basilar arachnoiditis occurs. Lung lesions exhibit an intense granulomatous inflammation. Cryptococci are best seen in tissue by staining with methenamine silver or periodic acid–Schiff. A strongly positive mucicarmine stain of the organism in tissue is diagnostic, but staining varies from intense to absent.

Cryptococcus neoformans has been isolated from several sites in nature, particularly weathered pigeon droppings. Patients are usually unaware of any unusual exposure to pigeon droppings. No significant case clustering, highly endemic areas, or racial or occupational predisposition is known. Infection before puberty is uncommon. The male/female ratio is about 2:1. Approximately half the patients have a predisposing condition, such as lymphoma, sarcoidosis, or supraphysiological doses of adrenal corticosteroids. Cryptococcosis occurs in animals, especially the cat family. Transmission from animals to humans or from person to person has never been documented.

CLINICAL MANIFESTATIONS The majority of patients has meningoencephalitis at time of diagnosis. This form of the infection is invariably fatal without appropriate therapy, and death occurs anywhere from 2 weeks to several years from onset of symptoms. Early manifestations include headache, nausea, staggering gait, dementia, irritability, confusion, and blurred vision. Both fever and nuchal rigidity are usually mild or absent. Papilledema is present in one-third of the patients at time of diagnosis. Cranial nerve palsies, typically asymmetric, occur in about one-fourth of the patients. Other lateralizing signs are rare. With progression of the infection, deepening coma and signs of brainstem compression appear. Autopsy often reveals cerebral edema in the more acute cases or hydrocephalus in more chronic cases.

Pulmonary cryptococcosis is asymptomatic or associated with dry cough or mild, dull chest ache. Chest x-ray shows one or more dense infiltrates, which are often well circumscribed. Cavitation, pleural effusions, or hilar adenopathy are infrequent. Calcification is not present, and fibrotic stranding is rarely noticeable.

Skin lesions are present in 10 percent of patients with cryptococcosis. These appear to be hematogenously disseminated because the vast majority of patients will be found to have disseminated infection. One or a few asymptomatic tiny papular lesions appear, slowly enlarge, and tend to show central softening leading to ulceration. Osteolytic bone lesions occur in 4 percent of patients and usually present as a cold abscess. Rare manifestations of cryptococcosis include prostatitis, endophthalmitis, hepatitis, pericarditis, endocarditis, and renal abscess.

DIAGNOSIS Cryptococcal meningoencephalitis must be distinguished from tuberculosis, neoplasm, coccidioidomycosis, histoplasmosis, candidiasis, viral aseptic meningitis, and sarcoidosis. Focal lesions are virtually never demonstrable in cryptococcosis by technetium brain scan, cerebral angiography, or electroencephalogram. Computerized tomography (CT) scan will occasionally show one or two sharply demarcated radiodense masses with a central area of lesser density. Lumbar puncture is the single most useful test. An India ink smear of centrifuged spinal fluid sediment reveals encapsulated yeast in one-half the cases, but artifacts resembling cryptococci may cause confusion. Cerebrospinal fluid glucose is reduced in half the cases, protein concentration is usually increased, and

20 to 600 leukocytes per cubic millimeter are typically present and consist predominantly of lymphocytes. Approximately 90 percent of patients with cryptococcal meningoencephalitis, including all those with a positive cerebrospinal fluid smear, will have capsular antigen detectable in cerebrospinal fluid or serum by latex agglutination. False-positive tests occur occasionally, making culture the definitive diagnostic test. *Cryptococcus neoformans* is often present in urine in patients with meningoencephalitis. Fungemia occurs in only 10 percent of patients and portends a lethal outcome.

Pulmonary cryptococcosis mimics malignancy by x-ray and symptoms. Sputum culture is positive in only 10 percent, and serum antigen tests are positive in only a third. Occasionally, *C. neoformans* appears in one or multiple sputum specimens as an endobronchial saprophyte. Biopsy is usually required for diagnosis of pulmonary cryptococcosis. Cutaneous cryptococcosis may be mistaken for a comedone, basal-cell carcinoma, or sarcoidosis. Biopsy reveals a myriad of cyptococci. Osseous cryptococcosis resembles tuberculosis.

TREATMENT Patients with meningoencephalitis and previously normal kidney and bone marrow function should be treated with oral flucytosine 150 mg/kg per day in four divided doses and intravenous amphotericin B 0.3 mg/kg per day. Flucytosine toxicity may be minimized by careful observation for leukopenia, thrombocytopenia, and enterocolitis, as well as appropriate reduction in dose if azotemia is present. As a rough guide, the total daily dose should be:

$$\text{Total daily dose (mg/kg)} = \frac{150}{\text{serum creatinine}}$$

Flucytosine in patients with unstable, moderate, or severe azotemia is hazardous without frequent serum flucytosine assays. Intravenous amphotericin B used alone in dosage of 0.5 to 0.6 mg/kg once daily or 1.0 to 1.2 mg/kg every other day cures 50 to 70 percent of patients with cryptococcal meningoencephalitis and has the advantage that azotemia and hemodialysis do not alter drug clearance. Treatment with either regimen is continued for at least 6 weeks and until at least four weekly cultures of 2 to 4 ml cerebrospinal fluid are sterile. Intrathecal amphotericin B is usually reserved for treatment of severely azotemic patients not receiving dialysis or for patients who have relapsed. Permanent sequelae include dementia, personality change, hydrocephalus, and blindness.

Patients with extraneural cryptococcosis most often require intravenous amphotericin B, with or without flucytosine. Observation or excision of lesions may suffice for some patients who are previously normal, who have a single focus in lung, skin, or bone, and who have no cryptococci in the cerebrospinal fluid, urine, or blood. All too often, however, patients who present with a presumed single focus of extracranial cryptococcosis are discovered to have early asymptomatic meningoencephalitis or dissemination to other organs.

REFERENCES

Bennett JE: Flucytosine. Ann Intern Med 86:319, 1977

Diamond RD, Bennett JE: Prognostic factors in cryptococcal meningitis. Ann Intern Med 80:176, 1974

Gordonson J et al: Pulmonary cryptococcosis. Radiology 112:557, 1974

Littman ML, Zimmerman LE: *Cryptococcosis.* New York, Grune & Stratton, 1956

Schupbach CW et al: Cutaneous manifestations of disseminated cryptococcosis. Arch Dermatol 112:1734, 1976

Tunes B et al: Variant forms of pulmonary cryptococcosis. Ann Intern Med 69:1117, 1968

154
BLASTOMYCOSIS

JOHN E. BENNETT

DEFINITION Blastomycosis (North American blastomycosis) is the infection caused by the fungus *Blastomyces dermatitidis.* Illness most often presents as a chronic pneumonia, chronic skin lesions, or both.

ETIOLOGY *Blastomyces dermatitidis* is a dimorphic fungus, growing at room temperature as a white or tan mold but growing within the host or at 37°C as budding, round yeast-like cells. The fungus is identified by its appearance, its dimorphism, and by the appearance of small spores borne on hyphae of the mold form. When isolates of the two opposite mating types are grown closely together on specialized culture media, sporulating structures appear which characterize the perfect form, *Ajellomyces dermatitidis.*

PATHOGENESIS AND PATHOLOGY The infection is restricted by geography and age. Blastomycosis is uncommon in any locality, but the majority of cases have occurred in the Southeast, Central and Midatlantic areas of the United States, with occasional cases in other localities in the United States and Canada. Cases have also been encountered in Africa, Mexico, Central America, and, rarely, South America. Infection is most common between the ages of 25 and 65 years. The male/female ratio is about 10:1. There is no occupational predisposition.

Infection appears to be acquired by inhalation of the fungus from nature, but the reservoir remains unknown. To date, the fungus has been isolated only from infected humans or animals. No carrier state or transmission from animal to human or from person to person has been observed. Patients presenting with infection in other sites but no detectable lung lesion appear to represent the self-healing that is seen, albeit rarely, in documented lung lesions. Infection has a marked propensity to spread to skin, subcutaneous tissue, and bone, but infection of mucous membranes, genitourinary tract, central nervous system, liver, and spleen is not rare. The inflammatory response includes lymphocytes, giant cells, and neutrophils. Pseudoepitheliomatous hyperplasia may be striking and lead to a mistaken diagnosis of squamous-cell carcinoma.

CLINICAL MANIFESTATIONS One-third of patients present with detectable infection in only one organ, usually the lung or skin. In multiorgan disease, the lung and skin remain the two most common sites so that, overall, about two-thirds of patients have lung disease and an equal portion skin disease. Pulmonary blastomycosis may present subacutely with pulmonary consolidation resembling bacterial pneumonia on chest x-ray. More commonly, the onset is indolent and the infiltrate on chest x-ray is more likely to be fibronodular, contracted, and, in about one-fourth of patients, cavitary. Calcification, hilar adenopathy, and large pleural effusions are rare. Skin lesions may be single or multiple from the head and extremities and enlarge over weeks or months. Each lesion tends to be painless, well circumscribed, and verrucous or ulcerated. A dark eschar may cover the ulcer. Large chronic lesions may show central healing with scarring and contracture. Mucous membrane lesions in the mouth, nose, and larynx resemble squamous-cell carcinoma. Subcutaneous lesions form draining abscesses. Blastomycosis of bone, joint, prostate, and epididymis resembles tuberculosis. Fatal cases show lesions in many viscera. In contrast to paracoccidioidomycosis (South American blastomycosis), gastrointestinal lesions are very rare. If all forms of blastomycosis are considered together, the most prominent symptoms are cough, weight loss, malaise, skin or subcutaneous lesions, chest pain, and fever.

DIAGNOSIS The diagnosis is made best by demonstrating the fungus in culture of sputum, pus, or urine. In experienced hands, diagnosis by appearance of the organism in wet smear or histopathologic section is adequate. Skin tests and serologic tests lack sufficient sensitivity and specificity to be useful.

TREATMENT A few patients have been observed with transitory lung lesions, but no guidelines are known to distinguish these patients from those who will progress locally or disseminate. Therefore, every patient should receive intravenous amphotericin B. Skin and noncavitary lung lesions should be treated for about 8 to 10 weeks. Cavitary lung disease or infection beyond the lung and skin should be treated for about 10 to 12 weeks. Hydroxystilbamidine is less effective and rarely indicated. Iodide therapy is ineffective. The mortality rate in appropriately treated cases is 15 percent or less.

REFERENCES

BLASTOMYCOSIS COOPERATIVE STUDY OF THE VETERANS ADMINISTRATION: Blastomycosis. I. A review of 198 collected cases in Veterans Administration Hospitals. Am Rev Resp Dis 89:659, 1964

BUSEY JF: Blastomycosis. III. A cooperative study of 2-hydroxystilbamidine and amphotericin B therapy. Am Rev Resp Dis 105:812, 1972

CUSH R et al: Clinical and roentgenographic manifestations of acute and chronic blastomycosis. Chest 69:345, 1976

WITORSCH P, UTZ JP: North American blastomycosis: A study of 40 patients. Medicine 47:169, 1968

155
HISTOPLASMOSIS

JOHN E. BENNETT

DEFINITION Histoplasmosis is the mycosis acquired by inhalation of spores from *Histoplasma capsulatum*.

ETIOLOGY *Histoplasma capsulatum* is a dimorphic fungus that grows in nature or on Sabouraud's agar at room temperature as a mold. Hyphae bear both large and small spores that are used for identification. *Histoplasma capsulatum* grows as a small budding yeast in host tissue and on enriched agar, such as blood cysteine glucose, at 37°C. Despite the name, the fungus is unencapsulated. When two isolates of the opposite mating type, both in mold form, are grown closely together on an appropriate culture medium, specialized spore-bearing structures are formed which characterize the perfect state, *Emmonsiella capsulata*.

PATHOGENESIS AND PATHOLOGY Infection with *H. capsulatum* has been encountered in many areas of the world but is much more frequent in certain areas. Within the United States infection is more common in the Southeastern, Midatlantic, and Central states than in other areas. Endemic areas are probably determined by the availability of proper conditions in nature for growth of the fungus. *Histoplasma capsulatum* prefers moist surface soil, particularly when it is enriched by droppings of certain birds and bats. The fungus has not only been isolated repeatedly from such sites but many case clusters have occurred 5 to 18 days after groups were exposed to such dust, for example, by raking, cleaning dirt floored chicken coops, bulldozing, or cave exploring. In many endemic areas, 80 percent or more of residents over age 16 have been exposed, judging by skin test reactivity.

Microconidia, or small spores, of *H. capsulatum* are small enough to reach the alveoli on inhalation and are transformed to budding forms. With time, an intense granulomatous reaction occurs. Caseation necrosis or calcification may mimic tuberculosis. The primary infection in children usually heals completely but may leave spotty calcification in the hilar nodes or lung. Transient dissemination may leave calcified granulomas in the spleen. In adults, a rounded mass of scar tissue, with or without central calcification, may remain in the lung. This has been called a *histoplasmoma*. Previous exposure is thought to confer some protection against reinfection, but infection of persons with prior positive skin tests clearly has occurred.

In a small proportion of patients, histoplasmosis becomes a progressive, potentially fatal infection. The disease occurs either as chronic fibrocavitary pneumonia or, less commonly, as disseminated infection. Patients with either form lack a history of acute primary pulmonary histoplasmosis. Chronic pulmonary infection favors otherwise healthy males over the age of 40 years. A history of cigarette use seems unusually common. An acute, rapidly fatal course is most likely to be encountered in young children and immunosuppressed patients. A more chronic but equally lethal disseminated infection is more common in previously healthy adults.

CLINICAL MANIFESTATIONS The vast majority of infections are either asymptomatic or mild, and the diagnosis is elusive. Cough, fever, malaise, and chest x-ray findings of hilar adenopathy with or without one or more areas of pneumonitis occur. Erythema nodosum and erythema multiforme have been reported in a few outbreaks. Hilar adenopathy may cause temporary compression of the right middle lobe bronchus in children and young adults. Subacute pericarditis may occur, probably by extension from contiguous lymph nodes. Rarely, many hilar nodes undergo a caseous, granulomatous reaction with perinodal fibrosis. Mediastinal structures become encased by progressive fibrosis, and, over many years, compression of the pulmonary veins, superior vena cava, pulmonary arteries, and esophagus may occur. Late in mediastinal disease only rare nonviable histoplasma can be found in caseous residua of lymph nodes.

Patients with chronic pulmonary histoplasmosis have a gradual onset over weeks or months of increasing productive cough, weight loss, and sometimes nightsweats. Chest x-ray reveals uni- or bilateral fibronodular apical infiltrates. Approximately one-third of cases will stabilize or improve spontaneously early in the course. The remainder have insidious progression. Retraction and cavitation of the upper lobes occur with spread to the apex of the lower lobes and other areas of the lung. Emphysema and bullae formation further compromise pulmonary function. Death from cor pulmonale, bacterial pneumonia, or histoplasmosis occurs after months or years.

Acute disseminated histoplasmosis may be mistaken for miliary tuberculosis. Common findings include fever, emaciation, hepatosplenomegaly, lymphadenopathy, jaundice, anemia, leukopenia, and thrombocytopenia. All these features may occur in chronic dissemination, but the disease tends to be more localized. Indurated ulcers of the mouth, tongue, nose, or larynx occur in about a fourth of patients. Other focal findings include granulomatous hepatitis, Addison's disease, gastrointestinal ulceration, endocarditis, and chronic meningitis. Chest x-ray abnormalities occur in half the cases and show discrete nodules or a miliary pattern.

The presumed ocular histoplasmosis syndrome is a distinct clinical form of uveitis. Although a positive histoplasmin skin test is a requisite for diagnosis, none of these patients has had active histoplasmosis, despite the frequent use of adrenal corticosteroid therapy.

DIAGNOSIS Histoplasmosis may be suspected by serologic tests and clinical manifestations, but definitive diagnosis requires demonstration of the organism by culture or histology. Serologic tests are performed with either histoplasmin, a culture filtrate, or whole yeast form cells. The results are interchangeable. Complement fixation is quantifiable and is the best test. Agar gel diffusion with histoplasmin is a useful but not quantifiable test. Frequent false negatives and false positives limit all current serologic tests. Serologic conversion is helpful but occurs rarely except in acute pulmonary histoplasmosis. Higher complement fixation titers, such as 1:32 or greater, are most suggestive of the diagnosis, but no titer is diagnostic. Cross-reactions with serologic tests for blastomycosis are very common. A 5-mm or more diameter area of induration 24 to 48 h after skin testing with histoplasmin has been very helpful in identifying prior exposure to histoplasma, but false negatives and false positives are so frequent that skin testing has little value in the study of ill patients. Further, approximately one-fourth of normal volunteers with a positive skin test will convert their histoplasmin serology from negative to positive after skin testing.

Culture of *H. capsulatum* from sputum is difficult but is the procedure of choice in chronic pulmonary histoplasmosis. Digestion by proteolytic enzymes and centrifugation of sputum are helpful. In disseminated histoplasmosis, cultures of bone marrow, blood, centrifuged urine, and biopsy specimens are most often positive. Cultures should be performed on agar surfaces of enriched media at room temperature. Growth occurs in 2 to 6 weeks. Histological sections of bone marrow, liver, lymph node, lung, and mucosal lesions may yield the diagnosis.

TREATMENT Acute pulmonary histoplasmosis requires no therapy. Mediastinal fibrosis may benefit by surgery, but the ultimate progress is poor. All patients with disseminated or chronic fibronodular pulmonary histoplasmosis should receive intravenous amphotericin B. Rapid culture conversion and a cure rate in excess of 50 percent can be achieved in both forms, but a formidable relapse rate after short courses has led to use of a 10- to 12-week course of 0.4 to 0.6 mg/kg per day. In chronic pulmonary histoplasmosis, chest x-ray abnormalities improve somewhat, but pulmonary function improves very little. Successful therapy prevents progression. Addisonian crisis is a preventable cause of death in disseminated histoplasmosis.

AFRICAN HISTOPLASMOSIS Patients have been encountered in Africa who seem to be infected with *H. capsulatum* except that the yeast form is larger. Clinical manifestations resemble blastomycosis more than histoplasmosis, because skin and bone lesions are very common.

REFERENCES

GOODWIN RA et al: Mediastinal fibrosis complicating healed primary histoplasmosis and tuberculosis. Medicine 51:227, 1972

PARKER JD et al: Treatment of chronic pulmonary histoplasmosis. N Engl J Med 283:225, 1970

SAROSI GA et al: Disseminated histoplasmosis: Results of long term follow-up. Ann Intern Med 75:511, 1971

SMITH JW, UTZ JP: Progressive disseminated histoplasmosis. Ann Intern Med 76:557, 1972

SUTLIFF WD: Histoplasmosis cooperative study. V. Amphotericin B dosage for chronic pulmonary histoplasmosis. Am Rev Resp Dis 105:60, 1972

COCCIDIOIDOMYCOSIS

JOHN E. BENNETT

DEFINITION Coccidioidomycosis is the mycosis acquired by inhalation of *Coccidioides immitis*.

ETIOLOGY *Coccidioides immitis* is a dimorphic fungus, growing as a white fluffy mold on most culture media but as a nonbudding spherical form, a spherule, in host tissue or under specialized conditions. Reproduction in the host tissue is by formation of small endospores within mature spherules. After rupture of the spherule, the released endospores enlarge, become spherules, and repeat the cycle. The fungus is identified by its appearance and by formation of thick-walled, barrel-shaped spores, called *arthrospores,* in the hyphae of the mold form.

PATHOGENESIS AND PATHOLOGY *Coccidioides immitis* is a soil saprophyte in certain arid regions of the United States, Mexico, Central America, and South America. Within the United States, most cases are acquired in California, Arizona, West Texas, and New Mexico. A few cases are acquired in bordering areas and by exposure to fomites from endemic areas, such as cotton bales.

Infection in humans and animals results from inhalation of windborne arthrospores arising from soil sites. This primary pulmonary infection is symptomatic in only 40 percent of individuals, with symptoms ranging from a mild, influenza-like illness to severe pneumonia. Mild, self-limited infections may come to medical attention because of case clusters or hypersensitivity reactions: erythema nodosum, erythema multiforme, toxic erythema, arthralgia, arthritis, conjunctivitis, or episcleritis. Case clusters occur 10 to 14 days after a group of susceptible individuals is exposed to dust in an endemic area through such activities as unearthing Indian relics, rock hunting, military maneuvers, or construction. The usual course of primary pulmonary infection is complete healing, though an area of pneumonitis on x-ray may heal by forming a coin-like lesion, or coccidioidoma. Less commonly, a single thin-walled cavity remains as a chronic sequela in the area of consolidation. Also, the consolidation may persist as a chronic pneumonia or progress to fibronodular, cavitary disease.

Pleural effusion may be the only manifestation of primary infection. Self-healing of this form is common.

An uncommon but dreaded complication of coccidioidomycosis is dissemination beyond the lung and hilar lymph nodes. Dissemination is more frequent in blacks, Filipinos, native Americans, Mexican-Americans, and pregnant or immunosuppressed patients.

Coccidioides immitis incites a chronic granulomatous reaction in host tissue, often with caseation necrosis. Lung and hilar node lesions may show calcification. Both IgM and IgG antibodies against *C. immitis* are induced by infection but neither appears protective. The amount of specific IgG antibody is a rough measure of the antigenic mass, i.e., of the amount of infection, making a high titer a poor prognostic sign. Appearance of delayed hypersensitivity to antigens of *C. immitis* is most common in those clinical forms of disease with a good prognosis, such as self-limited primary pulmonary disease. Negative skin tests to *Coccidioides* antigens in roughly half the patients with disseminated disease has led to therapeutic trials of "transfer factor." Conversion of skin tests and in vitro tests correlating with delayed hypersensitivity has been achieved with transfer factor, but whether the infection has improved remains unclear.

CLINICAL MANIFESTATIONS Symptomatic primary pulmonary infection is manifested by fever, cough, chest pain, malaise, and sometimes hypersensitivity reactions. Chest x-ray may show an infiltrate, hilar adenopathy, or pleural effusion. Peripheral blood may show a mild eosinophilia. Spontaneous improvement begins after several days to 2 weeks of illness and usually culminates in complete recovery.

The symptoms of a chronic thin-walled cavity include cough or hemoptysis in half the cases; the other patients are asymptomatic. Chronic progressive pulmonary coccidioidomycosis produces cough, sputum, variable degrees of fever, and weight loss. The first indications of dissemination usually appear during the primary infection. Reactivation with dissemination in later years occurs occasionally, especially if Hodgkin's disease, non-Hodgkin's lymphoma, renal transplantation, or other immunosuppression has supervened. Dissemination should be suspected when fever, malaise, hilar or paratracheal lymphadenopathy, and elevated sedimentation rate show abnormal persistence in patients with primary pulmonary coccidioidomycosis. High complement fixation titers support this concern. With time, lesions appear in the bone, skin, subcutaneous tissue, meninges, joints, and other sites. Without therapy, dissemination may progress rapidly to death or wax and wane for years.

DIAGNOSIS When coccidioidomycosis is suspected, sputum, urine, and pus should be examined for *C. immitis* by wet smear and culture. The laboratory request should indicate clearly that coccidioidomycosis is suspected because the mold form must be handled with extreme care to prevent infection of laboratory personnel. On biopsy, smaller spherules must be distinguished from nonbudding forms of *Blastomyces* and *Cryptococcus,* but appearance of the mature spherule is diagnostic.

Serologic tests are very helpful in coccidioidomycosis. Latex agglutination and agar gel diffusion tests are useful in screening serums for antibody to coccidioides. The complement fixation test is used on cerebrospinal fluid and to confirm and quantitate serum antibody detected by screening tests. The number of cases with a positive complement fixation test will depend upon the severity of disease and upon the laboratory performing the test. Positive tests are least common in patients with solitary pulmonary cavities or primary pulmonary infection, while serums from patients with multiorgan disseminated disease are nearly all positive. Seroconversion is helpful in primary pulmonary coccidioidomycosis but may not occur for up to 8 weeks after onset. A positive complement fixation test in unconcentrated cerebrospinal fluid is diagnostic of meningitis.

Conversion of skin test from negative to positive ($\geq$ 5 mm induration at 24 or 48 h) with either coccidioidin or spherulin, the two commercially available antigens, may be observed between the third and twenty-first days of symptoms in primary pulmonary coccidioidomycosis. Skin testing can also be helpful in epidemiologic studies, such as investigation of case clusters or definition of endemic areas. The utility of skin testing as a diagnostic tool is limited by the presence of persistent positive tests resulting from remote exposures to coccidioides and by the frequency of negative skin tests in many patients with either thin-walled cavities or disseminated coccidioidomycosis.

TREATMENT Primary pulmonary coccidioidomycosis usually resolves spontaneously. Some physicians give a few weeks of intravenous amphotericin B when patients show an unusually severe or protracted primary infection, hoping to abort disseminated or chronic pulmonary disease. There is no solid evidence to support this practice, but the stronger the suspicion of dissemination becomes in any given patient, the more logical this approach appears. Once evidence for dissemination becomes incontrovertible, amphotericin B may be palliative rather than curative. Nevertheless, every patient with disseminated coccidioidomycosis should receive sufficient amphotericin B to attempt cure, usually 0.5 to 0.7 mg/kg per day or a double dose every other day for 10 to 12 weeks. Surgical curettage of bone lesions, drainage of abscesses, and resection of lung lesions contribute to cure. Unfortunately, intravenous amphotericin B is not curative in coccidioidal meningitis, and all such patients should receive prolonged therapy with intrathecal amphotericin B. In all forms of disseminated coccidioidomycosis, relapse after months or years of therapy is frequent. Intravenous miconazole has resulted in improvement of disseminated coccidioidomycosis, but its efficacy compared with amphotericin B is unknown.

Patients with a thin-walled solitary pulmonary cavity will close the cavity spontaneously in 25 to 50 percent of cases. Lobectomy with perioperative amphotericin B may be indicated for hemoptysis, superinfection, or progressive enlargement of such cavities.

REFERENCES

DERESINSKI SC, STEVENS DA: Coccidioidomycosis in compromised hosts. Medicine 54:377, 1974

DRUTZ DJ, CATANZARO A: Coccidioidomycosis. Am Rev Resp Dis 117:559, 727, 1978

FIESE MJ: *Coccidioidomycosis.* Springfield, Ill, Charles C Thomas, 1958

LONKY SA et al: Acute coccidioidal pleural effusion. Am Rev Resp Dis 114:681, 1976

WERIN WA: A long term study of 300 patients with cavitary-abscess lesions of the lung of coccidioidal origin. Dis Chest 54 (suppl 1):12, 1968

157
SPOROTRICHOSIS

JOHN E. BENNETT

DEFINITION Sporotrichosis is the mycosis caused by *Sporothrix schenckii.*

ETIOLOGY *Sporothrix schenckii* lives as a saprophyte on plants in many areas of the world. In nature and on culture at room temperature the fungus grows as a mold, but within host tissue or at 37°C on enriched media it grows as a budding yeast. Identification is by appearance of the fungus in mold and yeast forms. Small spores with a hair-like attachment to hyphae give the fungus the name, *Sporothrix.*

PATHOGENESIS AND PATHOLOGY Infection results when minor trauma inoculates the fungus into subcutaneous tissue. Nursery workers, florists, and gardeners acquire the illness from roses, sphagnum moss, and other plants. Infection may be limited to the site of inoculation (plaque sporotrichosis) or extend along proximal lymphatic channels (lymphangitic sporotrichosis). Spread on an extremity, the usual site, even as far as inguinal or axillary nodes is rare, and hematogenous dissemination from the skin remains unproved. The portal for osteoarticular, pulmonary, and other extracutaneous forms of sporotrichosis is unknown but is likely the lung.

Untreated sporotrichosis shows little evidence of self-healing and is capable of extreme chronicity. The inflammatory response contains both clusters of neutrophils and a marked granulomatous response with epithelioid cells and giant cells.

CLINICAL MANIFESTATIONS Lymphangitic sporotrichosis, by far the most common manifestation, forms a nearly painless red papule at the site of inoculation. Over the next several weeks, similar nodules form along proximal lymphatic channels. Nodules intermittently discharge small amounts of pus. Ulceration may occur. The proximal extension of these lesions, often with skip areas, is quite distinctive but may be mimicked by lesions of *Nocardia brasiliensis, Mycobacterium marinum,* or, on rare occasions, by *Leishmania brasiliensis* or *M. kansasii.*

Plaque sporotrichosis is a nontender red maculopapular granuloma confined to the site of inoculation. Osteoarticular sporotrichosis presents as mono- or polyarticular arthritis of indolent onset and progression over months or years, involving the elbows, knees, wrists, ankles, and, rarely, smaller joints of the extremities. Periarticular bone gradually appears "motheaten," and draining sinuses may appear over joints and bursas. Hematogenous spread to the skin may be observed during polyarticular disease, but none of the skin lesions shows lymphangitic spread. Immunosuppression predisposes to such spread. Pulmonary sporotrichosis usually presents as a single chronic cavitary upper-lobe lung lesion.

DIAGNOSIS Culture of pus, joint fluid, sputum, or skin biopsy specimen is the preferred method of diagnosis. Appearance of *S. schenckii* in tissue is quite variable. In skin lesions, organisms are hard to find.

TREATMENT Cutaneous sporotrichosis can be cured with oral administration of a saturated solution of potassium iodide, given in increasing divided daily doses up to 9 to 12 ml per day for adults. Gastrointestinal disturbance or acneform rash over the cape area and face are common, but therapy should be continued for 1 month after resolution of all lesions. Patients with serious allergic reactions to iodides may respond to local heat, particularly when plaque sporotrichosis is the only form of disease. Extracutaneous sporotrichosis does not respond to iodides, but cures have been obtained in over half such patients with prolonged courses of intravenous amphotericin B.

REFERENCES

CROUT JE et al: Sporotrichosis arthritis. Clinical features of seven patients. Ann Intern Med 86:294, 1977

LYNCH PJ et al: Systemic sporotrichosis. Ann Intern Med 73:23, 1970

ORR ER, RILEY HD: Sporotrichosis in childhood, report of ten cases. J Pediatr 78:951, 1971

WILSON DE et al: Clinical features of extracutaneous sporotrichosis. Medicine 46:265, 1967

158 CANDIDIASIS

JOHN E. BENNETT

DEFINITION Candidiasis (moniliasis, candidosis) is infection caused by any of several species of the yeast-like fungus, *Candida.* Candidiasis of mucous membranes is also called *thrush.*

ETIOLOGY *Candida albicans* is the most common cause of candidiasis, but *C. tropicalis, C. parapsilosis, C. guilliermondii, C. krusei,* and a few other species can cause candidiasis and may even be fatal. *Candida parapsilosis* is particularly notable for its ability to cause endocarditis. All *Candida* species pathogenic for humans are also encountered as commensals of humans, particularly in the mouth, stool, and vagina. These species grow rapidly at 25 to 37°C on simple media as oval budding cells. In specialized agar media, hyphae or elongated branching structures called pseudohyphae are formed. *Candida albicans* can be identified presumptively by its ability to form germ tubes in serum or by the formation of thick-walled large spores, called *chlamydospores.* Final identification of all species requires biochemical tests.

PATHOGENESIS AND PATHOLOGY Either local or systemic factors may lead to tissue invasion by *Candida.* Chronic maceration predisposes to cutaneous candidiasis, as in diaper rash, intertrigo in obese patients, or paronychia in bartenders or cannery workers. Age is important because neonatal colonization often leads to oral thrush. Women in the third trimester of pregnancy are prone to vulvovaginal thrush. Patients with diabetes mellitus or hematologic malignancy, or who are receiving broad-spectrum antibiotics or supraphysiologic doses of adrenal corticosteroids, are especially susceptible to candidiasis. Breaks in the integrity of the skin or mucous membranes may provide access to deeper tissues. Examples include: perforation of the gastrointestinal tract by trauma, surgery, and peptic ulceration; indwelling catheters for intravenous alimentation, peritoneal dialysis, and urinary tract drainage; severe burns and intravenous drug abuse.

Candida grows within tissues in both yeast and pseudohyphal forms. Rarely, only one form is present. Visceral lesions are characterized by necrosis and a neutrophilic inflammatory response. Neutrophils kill *Candida* yeast cells and damage segments of pseudohyphae in vitro, suggesting a major role for the neutrophil in host defense against this fungus. Visceral lesions show a preference for kidney, brain, spleen, heart, and liver.

CLINICAL MANIFESTATIONS Oral thrush presents as discrete and confluent adherent white plaques on the oral and pharyngeal mucosa, particularly in the mouth and tongue. These lesions are usually painless, but fissuring at the corners of the mouth can be painful. Cutaneous candidiasis presents as red, macerated intertriginous areas, paronychia, balanitis, or pruritus ani. Candidiasis of the perineal and scrotal skin may be accompanied by discrete pustular lesions on the inner aspects of the thighs. Chronic mucocutaneous candidiasis or *Candida* granuloma typically presents as circumscribed hyperkeratotic skin lesions, crumbling dystrophic nails, partial alopecia in areas of scalp lesions, and both oral and vaginal thrush. Systemic infection is very rare, but disfigurement of the face and hands can be severe. Other findings may include chronic epidermophytosis, dental dysplasia, and hypofunction of the parathyroid, adrenal, or thyroid glands. A variety of defects in T-cell function have been described in these patients. Vulvovaginal thrush causes pruritus, discharge, and sometimes pain on intercourse or urination. Speculum examination reveals an inflamed mucosa and a thin exudate, often with white curds.

From one to multiple small shallow ulcerations due to *Candida* may appear in the esophagus or gastrointestinal tract. Esophageal lesions favor the distal third and may cause dysphagia or substernal pain. Other such lesions tend to be asymptomatic but assume importance in the leukemic patient as a portal for disseminated candidiasis. Within the urinary tract, the most common lesions are either hematogenously disseminated renal abscesses, which can cause azotemia, or bladder thrush. Bladder invasion usually follows catheterization or instrumentation of a patient with diabetes mellitus or who is receiving broad-spectrum antibiotics. This lesion generally is asymptomatic and benign. Rarely, retrograde invasion of the renal pelvis leads to renal papillary necrosis.

Hematogenous dissemination of *Candida* presents with fever and toxicity but with few localizing findings. One or more retinal abscesses may appear and extend slowly into the vitreous humor. The patient may note orbital pain, blurred vision, scotoma, or opacities floating across the visual field. Pulmonary candidiasis is almost always hematogenous and is visible on chest x-ray only when the abscesses are numerous enough to cause a diffuse, vaguely nodular infiltrate. Candidiasis of the endocardium or around intracardiac prostheses resembles bacterial infection of these sites. Chronic *Candida* meningitis or arthritis may occur, from either disseminated disease or insertion of a plastic prosthesis in the case of arthritis. Rare focal manifestations of disseminated disease include osteomyelitis, pustular skin lesions, myositis, and brain abscess.

DIAGNOSIS Demonstration of pseudohyphae on wet smear with confirmation by culture is the procedure of choice for diagnosing superficial candidiasis. Scrapings for the smear may be obtained from skin, nails, and oral and vaginal mucosa. Culture alone is not diagnostic.

Deeper lesions of *Candida* may be diagnosed by histological section of biopsy specimens or by culture of cerebrospinal fluid, blood, joint fluid, or surgical specimens. Blood culture in vented bottles is very useful in *Candida* endocarditis but is positive less often in other forms of disseminated disease. The utility of serodiagnosis remains controversial.

TREATMENT Cutaneous candidiasis of macerated areas responds to measures which reduce moisture and chafing plus a topically applied antifungal agent in a nonocclusive base. Nystatin, clotrimazole, miconazole, and amphotericin B appear roughly equivalent. The first three of these are available also for vaginal application. Oral candidiasis should be treated with nystatin suspension. Swallowing nystatin suspension or sucking on the tablets compounded for vaginal use may improve symptoms of esophageal candidiasis. When esophageal symptoms are pronounced, a 5- to 10-day course of intravenous amphotericin B, 0.3 mg/kg per day, may be beneficial. Bladder thrush responds to bladder irrigations with amphotericin B, 50 μg/ml for 5 days. In all forms of skin and mucosal candidiasis, relapse after successful treatment is common.

Intravenous amphotericin B is the drug of choice in disseminated candidiasis. The drug is usually given as 0.4 to 0.5 mg/kg every day or as a double dose on alternate days for several weeks. In patients with no contraindication to the use of flucytosine, administration of that drug in dosage of 100 to 150 mg/kg per day plus amphotericin B, 0.3 mg/kg per day, is an effective alternative. *Candida* isolated from a properly obtained blood culture should be considered significant, for true false positives are rare. Whether a patient with candidiasis should receive antifungal therapy will depend on the degree of illness and the likelihood of spontaneous recovery. For example, a febrile, severely immunosuppressed patient with one positive blood culture should receive prompt therapy because a rapidly fatal course is common. A nonimmunosuppressed patient acquiring candidiasis from an indwelling intravenous plastic catheter may recover spontaneously if the catheter is removed promptly. The species of *Candida* is irrelevant to this decision. Patients with candidiasis in whom antifungal therapy is withheld should be observed carefully for the development of endophthalmitis, endocarditis, arthritis, osteomyelitis, or other visceral lesions that require therapy.

REFERENCES

EDWARDS JE et al: Ocular manifestations of Candida septicemia. Review of 76 cases of haematogenous candida endophthalmitis. Medicine 53:47, 1974

ERAS P et al: Candida infection of the gastrointestinal tract. Medicine 51:367, 1972

GAINES JD, REMINGTON JS: Disseminated candidiasis in the surgical patient. Surgery 72:730, 1972

ROSE HD, SHETH NK: Pulmonary candidiasis. A clinical and pathological correlation. Arch Intern Med 138:964, 1978

YOUNG RC et al: Fungemia with compromised host resistance. Ann Intern Med 80:605, 1974

159
ASPERGILLOSIS

JOHN E. BENNETT

DEFINITION The name *aspergillosis* embraces a variety of widely differing diseases having in common only some pathogenetic relationship to the fungus *Aspergillus*. In these diseases the fungus either elicits an allergic reaction, invades tissue, or grows within air spaces, such as a bronchus, pulmonary cavity, or paranasal sinus.

ETIOLOGY *Aspergillus fumigatus* is the most common pathogen, but *A. flavus, A. niger,* and several other species can cause disease. *Aspergillus* is a mold with septate hyphae about 4 μm in diameter. Sporulating structures, called *conidial heads,* may be seen when the fungus is growing in nature, on an artificial medium, or within air-containing spaces of the body. The appearance of the colonies and of conidial heads is used for identification.

PATHOGENESIS AND PATHOLOGY All the common species of *Aspergillus* which cause disease in humans are ubiquitous in the environment, growing on dead leaves, stored grain, compost piles, hay, and other decaying vegetation. Inhalation of *Aspergillus* spores must be extremely common, but disease is rare. Invasion of lung tissue is almost entirely confined to immunosuppressed patients. Roughly 90 percent will have two of these three conditions: less than 500 granulocytes per cubic millimeter of peripheral blood, supraphysiological doses of adrenal corticosteroids, and a history of taking cytotoxic drugs such as azathioprine. Infection in such patients is characterized by hyphal invasion of blood vessels, thrombosis, necrosis, and hemorrhagic infarction. Chronic granulomatous disease of childhood also predisposes to invasive pulmonary aspergillosis, but here the inflammatory response is granulomatous. Blood vessel invasion is rare.

Massive inhalation of *Aspergillus* spores by normal persons can lead to an acute, diffuse, self-limited pneumonitis. Epithelioid granulomas with giant cells and central pyogenic areas containing hyphae are seen. Spontaneous recovery taking several weeks is the usual course.

Aspergillus can colonize the damaged bronchial tree, pulmonary cysts, or cavities of patients with underlying lung disease. Balls of hyphae within cysts or cavities may reach several centimeters in diameter and be visible on chest x-ray. Tissue invasion does not occur. The term *allergic bronchial aspergillosis* denotes the condition of patients with preexisting asthma who have eosinophilia, IgE antibody to *Aspergillus,* and fleeting pulmonary infiltrates from bronchial plugging. Some of these asthmatic patients also have endobronchial colonization with *Aspergillus*. It is not clear what role *Aspergillus* plays in noninvasive lung disease. Plugs of hyphae may obstruct bronchi. Perhaps allergic or toxic reactions to *Aspergillus* antigens cause bronchial constriction and damage.

CLINICAL MANIFESTATIONS Endobronchial pulmonary aspergillosis presents as chronic productive cough and often hemoptysis in a patient with prior chronic lung disease, such as tuberculosis, sarcoidosis, bronchiectasis, or histoplasmosis. *Aspergilloma* refers to a ball of hyphae within a lung cyst or cavity, usually in the upper lobe. *Aspergillus* may be spread from its endocavitary or endobronchial site to the pleura during the course of bacterial lung abscess or surgery.

Invasive aspergillosis in the immunosuppressed host presents as an acute pneumonia. Infection progresses by hematogenous spread as well as extension to surrounding lung and other contiguous structures. Occasionally the portal of infection in the immunosuppressed host is the paranasal sinus, gastrointestinal tract, skin, palate, or epiglottis.

Aspergillus sinusitis in nonimmunosuppressed patients may take two forms. A ball of hyphae may form in a chronically obstructed paranasal sinus, without tissue invasion. A chronic, fibrosing granulomatous inflammation with scanty *Aspergillus* hyphae within tissue may begin in the sinus and spread slowly to the orbit and brain.

Growth of *Aspergillus* on cerumen and detritus within the external auditory canal is termed *otomycosis*. Trauma to the cornea may cause chronic *Aspergillus* keratitis. Endophthalmitis follows introduction of *Aspergillus* into the globe by trauma or surgery. *Aspergillus* may infect intracardiac or intravascular prostheses.

DIAGNOSIS Culture of *Aspergillus* from sputum usually has no diagnostic significance. Repeated isolation of *Aspergillus* from sputum or demonstration of hyphae in the sputum smear suggests endobronchial colonization. Fungus ball of the lung is usually detectable by chest x-ray. Antibody of the IgG class to *Aspergillus* antigens is demonstrable in the serum of many colonized patients and of virtually all patients with fungus ball.

Biopsy is usually required to diagnose invasive aspergillosis of the lung, paranasal sinus, or sites of dissemination. Blood cultures are rarely positive, even in patients with infected cardiac prosthetic valves. *Aspergillus* hyphae can be identified presumptively by histology, but culture is required for confirmation and determination of species. Serologic and skin tests have not proved helpful in invasive aspergillosis.

TREATMENT Patients with severe hemoptysis due to fungus ball of the lung may benefit by lobectomy. Poor pulmonary function in residual lung and dense pleural adhesions around the lesion can complicate the resection. Systemic chemotherapy is of no value in endobronchial or endocavitary aspergillosis.

Intravenous amphotericin B has resulted in arrest or cure of invasive aspergillosis when immunosuppression is not severe. Combined flucytosine–amphotericin B may be useful in non-neutropenic patients with invasive aspergillosis, but current information to evaluate this regimen is inadequate.

REFERENCES

AISNER J et al: Treatment of invasive aspergillosis: Relation of early diagnosis and treatment to response. Ann Intern Med 86:539, 1977

GREEN WF et al: Aspergillosis of the orbit. Arch Ophthalmol 82:302, 1969

KILMAN JW et al: Surgery for pulmonary aspergillosis. J Thorac Cardiovasc Surg 57:642, 1969

MEYER RD et al: Aspergillosis complicating neoplastic disease. Am J Med 54:6, 1973

YOUNG RC et al: Aspergillosis: Spectrum of the disease in 98 patients. Medicine 49:149, 1970

MUCORMYCOSIS

JOHN E. BENNETT

DEFINITION Mucormycosis is an acute infection caused by fungi of the order Mucorales. *Zygomycosis* and *phycomycosis* are synonymous terms which encompass mucormycosis and several entirely different diseases.

ETIOLOGY *Rhizopus* and *Mucor* species are the principal pathogens. These molds have broad, rarely septate hyphae of uneven diameter, ranging from 6 to 50 μm. The fungus is inexplicably difficult to grow from infected tissue. When it occurs, growth is rapid and profuse on most media at room temperature. Identification is based upon gross and microscopic appearance of the mold.

PATHOGENESIS AND PATHOLOGY *Rhizopus* and *Mucor* species are ubiquitous, appearing on decaying vegetation, dung, and foods of high sugar content. Infection is uncommon and largely confined to patients with serious preexisting diseases. Mucormycosis originating in the paranasal sinuses and nose occurs predominantly in patients with poorly controlled diabetes mellitus. Mucormycosis in patients with hematologic malignancy or organ transplantation more often originates in the lung than in the nose and paranasal sinuses. Gastrointestinal mucormycosis occurs in a variety of conditions, including uremia, severe malnutrition, and diarrheal diseases. Infection is acquired from nature, with no person-to-person spread.

In all forms of mucormycosis, vascular invasion by hyphae is prominent. Ischemic or hemorrhagic necrosis is the predominant histological finding.

CLINICAL MANIFESTATIONS Mucormycosis originating in the nose and paranasal sinuses produces a characteristic clinical picture. Low-grade fever, dull sinus pain, and sometimes nasal congestion or a thin, bloody nasal discharge are followed in a few days by double vision, increasing fever and obtundation. Examination reveals a unilateral generalized reduction of ocular motion, chemosis, and proptosis. The nasal turbinates on the involved side may be dusky red or necrotic. A sharply delineated area of necrosis, strictly respecting the midline, may appear in the hard palate. The skin of the cheek may become inflamed. Fungal invasion of the globe or ophthalmic artery leads to blindness. Opacification of one or more sinuses is found on x-ray. Carotid arteriogram may show invasion or obstruction of the carotid siphon. Coma is due to direct invasion of the frontal lobe. Early symptoms mimic bacterial sinusitis. Clouding of the sensorium may be attributed to diabetic acidosis. Cavernous sinus thrombosis may be considered when orbital invasion occurs. Without treatment, death may occur in a few days to a few weeks.

Pulmonary mucormycosis is a progressive severe pneumonia, accompanied by high fever and toxicity. The necrotic center of large infiltrates may cavitate. Hematogenous spread to other areas of the lung, as well as to brain and other organs is common. Survival beyond 2 weeks is unusual. Gastrointestinal invasion presents as one or more ulcers which tend to perforate. Hematogenous dissemination can originate from the gastrointestinal tract, lung, or paranasal sinuses. Sometimes no portal of entry can be found.

DIAGNOSIS Lesions of the lung and craniofacial structures are best diagnosed by biopsy and histological section. Cultural confirmation should be attempted. Wet smear of crushed tissue can provide rapid diagnosis. Cultures of blood and cerebrospinal fluid are negative. Smear and culture of sputum may be positive during cavitation of a lung lesion. Serologic tests are under investigation but are unlikely to aid diagnosis of rapidly fatal cases.

TREATMENT Regulation of diabetes mellitus and decreasing immunosuppressive drugs aid in the treatment. Extensive debridement of craniofacial lesions appears to be very important. Orbital exenteration may be required. Intravenous amphotericin B is clearly of value in craniofacial mucormycosis and should be employed in the other forms of mucormycosis as well. Maximum tolerated doses are given until progression is halted. The drug is continued for a total of 10 to 12 weeks. Appropriate management results in cure of about half of the craniofacial infections. Survival of patients with pulmonary, gastrointestinal, or disseminated mucormycosis is rare.

REFERENCES

ADDLESTONE RB, BAYLIN CJ: Rhinocerebral mucormycosis. Radiology 115:113, 1975

BARTRUM RJ et al: Roentgenographic findings in pulmonary mucormycosis. Am J Roentgenol 117:810, 1973

LOWE JT, HUDSON WR: Rhinocerebral phycomycosis and internal carotid artery thrombosis. Arch Otolaryngol 101:100, 1975

MEYER RD, ARMSTRONG D: Mucormycosis—changing status. CRC Crit Rev Clin Lab Sci 4:421, 1973

161
OTHER DEEP MYCOSES
Paracoccidioidomycosis, petriellidiosis, torulopsosis, mycetoma, and chromomycosis

JOHN E. BENNETT

PARACOCCIDIOIDOMYCOSIS

DEFINITION Paracoccidioidomycosis, formerly called *South American blastomycosis,* is the mycosis caused by *Paracoccidioides brasiliensis.*

ETIOLOGY A dimorphic fungus, *P. brasiliensis* grows as a budding yeast but may be grown as either yeast or mold on a culture medium. Identification is by gross and microscopic appearance. A superficial resemblance to *Blastomyces dermatitidis* may cause misdiagnosis.

PATHOGENESIS AND PATHOLOGY Infection is thought to be acquired by inhalation of spores from environmental sources, but the reservoir in nature remains obscure. Pulmonary infection produces few symptoms initially. Hematogenous spread to the mucous membranes of the mouth and nose, the lymph nodes, and other sites brings the patient to medical attention. Fatal cases show spread to the adrenal, the gastrointestinal tract, and many other viscera.

CLINICAL MANIFESTATIONS Common symptoms include indurated ulcers of the mouth, oropharynx, larynx, and nose, enlarged and draining lymph nodes, lesions of the skin and genitalia, productive cough, weight loss, dyspnea, and sometimes fever. Acquisition of infection is restricted to South America, Central America, and Mexico, but the extreme indolence of this infection may lead to recognition many years after the patient has left the endemic area. Chest x-ray most often shows a bilateral patchy pneumonia.

DIAGNOSIS Cultures of sputum, pus, and mucosal lesions are often diagnostic. The diagnosis can be made by smear or histological section, though confirmation by culture is preferable. Serologic tests are useful in suggesting the diagnosis and monitoring therapy.

TREATMENT Milder cases may be cured by several years of treatment with oral sulfonamide therapy. More advanced cases are given intravenous amphotericin B, followed by prolonged oral sulfa drugs.

PETRIELLIDIOSIS

DEFINITION Petriellidiosis refers to all mycoses caused by *Petriellidium boydii* other than mycetoma.

ETIOLOGY Also called *Allescheria boydii, P. boydii* is a mold frequently found in soil. When the fungus is isolated in the imperfect state, it is called *Monosporium apiospermum.*

PATHOGENESIS AND PATHOLOGY Wind-borne spores of *P. boydii,* arising in soil, are the presumed source of infection. The fungus grows as a mold within tissue, causing necrosis and abscess formation.

CLINICAL MANIFESTATIONS *Petriellidium boydii* resembles *Aspergillus* in its ability to colonize the endobronchial tree, to form fungus balls in the lung or paranasal sinuses, to invade the cornea or globe following trauma or surgery, and by its propensity to invade the immunosuppressed host. Hyphae of *P. boydii* in tissue may be difficult to distinguish from *Aspergillus.* Infection with *P. boydii* is much less common than with *Aspergillus. Petriellidium boydii* is the single most common cause in the United States of mycetoma. Intravascular hyphae, a hallmark of invasive aspergillosis, are less prominent in petriellidiosis. Occasional normal patients have developed necrotizing pneumonia or abscesses in brain or other organs due to *P. boydii.*

DIAGNOSIS Demonstration of hyphae in tissue and culture confirmation are required for diagnosis.

TREATMENT Intravenous miconazole has been recommended, but therapeutic response to all drugs has been poor.

TORULOPSOSIS

DEFINITION Torulopsosis is the infection caused by *Torulopsis glabrata.*

ETIOLOGY *Torulopsis glabrata* is a small yeast-like fungus, the same size as the yeast form of *Histoplasma capsulatum. Torulopsis glabrata* does not form hyphae or pseudohyphae. Identification is by biochemical tests.

PATHOGENESIS AND PATHOLOGY *Torulopsis glabrata* is a normal inhabitant of the human gastrointestinal tract and vagina. Within tissue, *T. glabrata* causes abscess formation with a neutrophilic inflammatory response. In immunosuppressed patients, a scanty or mononuclear inflammatory response may be seen.

CLINICAL MANIFESTATIONS Torulopsosis mimics many of the manifestations of candidiasis, but infection is less common and often less severe. Clinical entities include intravenous catheter–induced sepsis or endocarditis, gastrointestinal and disseminated infection in immunosuppressed patients, and retrograde infection of the urinary tract.

DIAGNOSIS Torulopsis may be difficult to distinguish from yeast cells of *Candida* in histological section. Culture is the most reliable diagnostic tool.

TREATMENT Therapeutic measures used in candidiasis appear appropriate for torulopsosis.

MYCETOMA

DEFINITION *Mycetoma* is a chronic suppurative infection originating in subcutaneous tissue and characterized by the presence of grains, which are tightly clumped colonies of the causative agent.

ETIOLOGY *Actinomycetoma* refers to infection by actinomycetes of the genus *Nocardia, Streptomyces,* and *Actinomadura. Eumycetoma* is caused by true fungi of many different genera. The most common agent varies with the locality.

PATHOGENESIS AND PATHOLOGY The pathogens live in the soil and enter the skin through minor trauma. The most common site of infection is the foot. Infection runs a relentless course over many years, with destruction of contiguous bone and fascia. Grains are found in purulent foci, surrounded by fibrosis and a mononuclear cell inflammatory response.

CLINICAL MANIFESTATIONS The infected site shows painless swelling, woody induration, and sinus tracts which discharge pus intermittently. Systemic symptoms and spread to distant sites in the body are not seen.

DIAGNOSIS The clinical picture is characteristic, but confusion with chronic osteomyelitis or botryomycosis may occur. The diagnosis requires demonstration of grains in pus from the draining sinus or in biopsy sections. Many histological sections may need to be examined to locate a grain.

TREATMENT Actinomycetoma may respond to prolonged therapy with sulfonamides, trimethoprim-sulfamethoxazole, or other antibacterial agents. Eumycetoma does not respond reliably to any drug. Amputation may be required.

CHROMOMYCOSIS

DEFINITION *Chromomycosis* is a clinical syndrome characterized by chronic verrucoid, ulcerated, or crusted skin lesions.

ETIOLOGY The five species of fungi currently recognized as causing this syndrome have received a bewildering number of different names. Using Emmons' classification, these fungi are called *Phialophora verrucosa, P. pedrosoi, P. compacta, P. dermatitidis,* and *Cladosporium carrionii.*

PATHOGENESIS AND PATHOLOGY Infection occurs in tropical and subtropical areas where workers acquire many small puncture wounds from thorns or splinters. Histopathologic section of the skin lesion shows pseudoepitheliomatous hyperplasia and a granulomatous dermal infiltrate. Microabscesses with neutrophils also occur. Clumps of the pathogenic organism are found in these abscesses or elsewhere in the dermis as rounded, thick-walled brown cells. The epidermis and superficial crusts may contain branching brown hyphae.

CLINICAL MANIFESTATIONS The site of the lesion depends upon the area of trauma but is usually the foot or leg. The lesion begins as a pimple, pustule, or ulcer with slow progression over many years. Lesions may remain flat or become pedunculated. Pain is minimal, but itching is common. Infection usually remains confined to the same extremity, but a few cases have spread hematogenously to cause brain abscess.

DIAGNOSIS Demonstration of the characteristic organisms in histological sections of skin biopsy is the best diagnostic method. Positive cultures are obtained readily, but accurate identification may require the service of a reference laboratory.

TREATMENT Prolonged therapy with oral flucytosine appears to be the regimen of choice. Relapse with secondary drug resistance has been encountered, but no reliable alternative treatment is known.

REFERENCES

Chromomycosis

MAUCERI AA et al: Flucytosine. An effective oral treatment for chromomycosis. Arch Dermatol 109:873, 1974

Mycetoma

GREEN WO, ADAMS TE: Mycetoma in the United States. Am J Clin Pathol 42:75, 1964
MAHGOUB ES, MURRAY IG: *Mycetoma.* London, Heinemann, 1973, pp 1–97

Paracoccidioidomycosis

LONDERO AT, RAMOS CD: Paracoccidioidomycosis. A clinical and mycologic study of forty-one cases observed in Santa Maria, RS, Brazil. Am J Med 52:771, 1972
MURRAY HW et al: Disseminated paracoccidioidomycosis (South American blastomycosis) in the United States. Am J Med 56:209, 1974
RESTREPO A et al: Paracoccidioidomycosis (South American blastomycosis). A study of 39 cases observed in Medellin, Columbia. Am J Trop Med Hyg 19:68, 1970

Petriellidiosis

ARNETT JC, HATCH HB: Pulmonary allescheriasis. Report of a case and review of the literature. Arch Intern Med 135:1250, 1975
LUTWICK LI et al: Visceral fungal infections due to *Petrillidium boydii (Allescheria boydii).* Am J Med 61:632, 1976
WINSTON DJ et al: *Allescheria boydii* infections in the immunosuppressed host. Am J Med 63:830, 1977

Torulopsosis

KAUFFMAN CA, TAN JS: *Torulopsis glabrata* renal infection. Am J Med 57:217, 1974
PANKEY GA, DALOVISO JR: Fungemia caused by *Torulopsis glabrata.* Medicine 52:395, 1973
VALDIVIESO M et al: Fungemia due to *Torulopsis glabrata* in the compromised host. Cancer 38:1750, 1976

162
DERMATOPHYTOSIS

JOHN E. BENNETT

DEFINITION Dermatophytosis, also known as ringworm or tinea, is a chronic fungal infection of the skin, hair, or nails.

ETIOLOGY Species of *Trichophyton, Microsporum,* and *Epidermophyton* are called *dermatophytes.* They grow in and remain confined to the keratinous structures of the body. Other mycoses can show fungal invasion of keratinous structures, such as candidiasis, pityriasis versicolor, and tinea nigra, but are traditionally not termed *dermatophytoses*.

PATHOLOGY AND PATHOGENESIS Dermatophyte species are called anthropophilic, zoophilic, or geophilic, depending on whether their usual reservoir within nature appears to be humans, animals, or soil. Infectivity of all those sources is low and group outbreaks are largely confined to an occasional case clustering of scalp infections in children. Acquisition of a dermatophytosis appears to be favored by minor trauma, maceration, and poor hygiene of the skin. Infection does not seem to confer solid immunity. Repeated infection with the same species is commonplace, particularly with anthropophilic species. Infrequency of scalp infection in adults has been attributed to local factors rather than immunity.

Invasion of the stratum corneum by dermatophytes may cause little inflammation, or, particularly with zoophilic fungi, inflammation can be intense. Shedding of the stratum corneum is increased by inflammation. To the extent that fungal growth cannot keep up with shedding, inflammation may help terminate infection. Conversely, infection is probably favored when shedding is reduced by corticosteroids and cytotoxic drugs. Antifungal drugs interfere with the ability of fungal growth to keep up with shedding.

CLINICAL MANIFESTATIONS The disease varies with the site of infection and fungal species. Foot infection (athlete's foot, tinea pedis) may present as fissuring of the toe webs, scaling of the plantar surfaces, or vesicles around the toe webs and soles. Interdigital lesions may be pruritic or, when bacterial superinfection occurs, may be painful. Hand infection is less common but resembles foot infection. Scalp dermatophytosis (tinea capitis) is characterized by areas of alopecia and scaling. In so-

called "endothrix infection," the hair shaft breaks off at the skin surface, leaving the hairs visible as black dots in the scalp. With some forms of scalp infection an intense boggy suppuration occurs, called a *kerion*. Dermatophytosis of the glabrious skin (tinea corporis) presents as circumscribed lesions with a wide variety of appearances. Scales, vesicles, or pustules may appear. Inflammation may be minimal or intense. Central healing of less inflamed lesions may be seen. The serpiginous border of inflammation is the source of the name *ringworm*. Dermatophytosis of the bearded area (tinea barbae) appears as a pustular folliculitis. Onychomycosis (tinea unguium) presents as white discolored nails or thickened, chalky crumbling nails. Peeling and fissuring of the perinychia or keratotic debris under the nail edge may also be seen.

DIAGNOSIS Discolored hairs, scales, and keratotic debris under infected nails should be collected for KOH smear and culture. In the scraping of skin lesions, a drop of water on the skin site may keep the removed scales from flying off and aid in their collection. Culture is important in distinguishing dermatophytes from *Candida* and fungal saprophytes growing in keratinaceous debris.

TREATMENT Skin lesions should be treated topically if the lesions are few and small or located on the feet. Miconazole or clotrimazole cream should be applied twice daily until the lesion disappears and smears are negative. Undecylenic acid, haloprogin, or tolnaftate can also be used. Extensive skin lesions and infection of hair or nails should be treated with oral griseofulvin. The recommended dose for adults is 500 mg bid. Treatment must be continued until all infected keratin is gone. Cutting of infected hair, epilating nails, and cleansing interdigital webs can expedite cure. Secondary bacterial infection of the foot may require soaks or antibacterial agents. Relapse of dermatophyte foot infections may be decreased by measures to keep the feet clean and dry.

section 10 | The rickettsioses

163
GENERAL CONSIDERATIONS

THEODORE E. WOODWARD

The rickettsial diseases of humans consist of a variety of clinical entities caused by microorganisms of the family Rickettsiaceae. The rickettsias are obligate intracellular parasites about the size of bacteria and are usually seen microscopically as pleomorphic coccobacilli. Each of the rickettsias pathogenic for human beings is capable of multiplying in one or more species of arthropod as well as in animals and humans. Indeed, the majority of the rickettsias are maintained in nature by a cycle which involves an insect vector and an animal reservoir, and infection of humans is unimportant in the cycle. Epidemic typhus presents a number of points of dissimilarity to most of the other rickettsioses, because the natural cycle of the infection involves only humans and the louse.

A compendium of information of the rickettsial diseases is given in Table 163-1. Because each of the rickettsioses responds therapeutically to tetracyclines or chloramphenicol, the table mentions no therapy. Procedures for diagnostic isolation of the rickettsias are omitted because they generally are less useful than serologic methods, and the techniques which they require are highly specialized and hazardous. Information on isolation may be found in textbooks devoted to viral and rickettsial diseases.

HISTORY OF THE RICKETTSIAL DISEASES Of all the afflictions of the human race the rickettsial diseases, particularly epidemic typhus, rank among the foremost as a cause of suffering and death.

The record of deaths from epidemic typhus in this century in the Balkan countries and in Poland and Russia reached astounding figures. Typhus ravaged Russia and eastern Poland from 1915 to 1922, infecting 30 million of the inhabitants and causing an estimated 3 million deaths.

The past two decades have seen the development of excellent methods for the prevention and treatment of rickettsioses. In fact, these measures have been so successful that the rickettsioses have become of minor importance in the United States and in many other countries. Although conquered, the rickettsioses have not been eliminated, and they could again become rampant if the will to control them, the present high standards of sanitation, and the necessary industrial capacities for production of effective insecticides and therapeutic agents should be decreased through war or disaster.

Gerhard in 1836 differentiated typhoid fever from louse-borne typhus fever. In 1899, Maxcy described the clinical manifestations of Rocky Mountain spotted fever. In a series of studies from 1906 to 1909, Ricketts, for whom the rickettsial microorganisms are named, successfully transmitted this disease to guinea pigs, incriminated the wood tick as a vector, and observed rickettsias in smears prepared from tick tissues.

Nicolle in 1909 reproduced typhus fever in monkeys and demonstrated transmission by the body louse. Von Prowazek in 1914 and Da Rocha-Lima in 1916 demonstrated small microorganisms in the tissues of lice taken from typhus patients.

Brill in 1910 recognized a febrile disease in patients in New York City as an example of mild epidemic typhus unassociated with lousiness. Zinsser in 1934 postulated that this disease was a recurrent form of typhus occurring in patients during periods of stress or waning immunity. Subsequent studies have confirmed Zinsser's hypothesis. This entity is now called Brill-Zinsser disease.

Weil and Felix, working with typhus patients in Poland in 1915, recognized that agglutinins for certain *Proteus* organisms appeared in the serum of convalescent patients. The Weil-Felix reaction, although nonspecific, affords a simple and valuable screening method for several rickettsioses.

In 1926, Maxcy, on purely epidemiologic evidence, surmised that typhus in the United States had its reservoir in rodents and was transmitted to humans by ticks or fleas. Confirmation of Maxcy's hypothesis was obtained in Baltimore in 1930 by Dyer and others when they isolated rickettsias from

TABLE 163-1
Rickettsial diseases

Disease Type	Agent	Geographic distribution	Natural cycle Arthropod	Mammal	Principal means of transmission to humans	Weil-Felix reaction	CF, MA, and IFA reactions*
SPOTTED FEVER GROUP							
Rocky Mountain spotted fever	R. rickettsii	Western Hemisphere	Ticks	Wild rodents; dogs	Tick bite	Positive OX-19 OX-2	Positive group- and type-specific
Boutonneuse fever	R. conorii	Africa, Europe, Middle East, India					
Queensland tick typhus	R. australis	Australia		Marsupials, wild rodents			
North Asian tick-borne rickettsiosis	R. sibirica	Siberia, Mongolia		Wild rodents			
Rickettsial-pox	R. akari	United States, Russia, Africa(?)	Blood-sucking mite	House mouse, other rodents	Mite bite	Negative	
TYPHUS GROUP							
Endemic (murine)	R. mooseri	Worldwide	Flea	Small rodents	Infected flea feces into broken skin	Positive OX-19	Positive group- and type-specific
Epidemic	R. prowazekii	Worldwide	Body louse	Humans	Infected louse feces into broken skin	Positive OX-19	
	R. Canada	North America	Ticks	?Flying squirrels		Positive OX-19	
Brill-Zinsser disease	R. prowazekii	Worldwide	Recurrence years after original attack of epidemic typhus			Usually negative	
Scrub	R. tsutsugamushi	Asia, Australia, Pacific islands	Trombiculid mites	Wild rodents	Mite bite	Positive OX-K	Positive in about 50% of patients
OTHER RICKETTSIAL DISEASES							
Q fever	R. burnetii	Worldwide	Ticks	Small mammals, cattle, sheep, goats	Inhalation of dried infected material	Negative	Positive
Trench fever	R. quintana†	Europe, Africa, North America	Body louse	Humans	Infected louse feces into broken skin	Negative	None available

* *CF = complement fixation; MA = microscopic agglutination; IFA = immunofluorescent antibody.*
† *Some authorities no longer place the agent in the genus Rickettsia because it can be cultured on artificial media.*

the brains of rats and shortly thereafter incriminated the flea as a vector. This disease, caused by *Rickettsia mooseri* and now designated endemic or murine typhus, is distinct from epidemic typhus and Brill-Zinsser disease. There is increasing evidence of the presence of *R. prowazekii* in flying squirrels as well as infection of its ectoparasites. This poses a potential human threat. *Rickettsia canada* is a member of the typhus group of rickettsias isolated from *Haemphysalis leporis-palustris* ticks in Canada in 1967. Human infections resemble mild Rocky Mountain spotted fever.

The development of suitable vaccines and specific diagnostic antigens was impeded until it was possible to prepare appreciable quantities of highly infectious rickettsial material in the laboratory. The most important steps were (1) the Weigl vaccine (1930), a phenolized suspension of gut tissue obtained from body lice which had been injected intrarectally with the rickettsias of epidemic typhus; (2) the killed murine typhus prepared by Casteneda (1939) from lung tissues of rats, injected intranasally; and (3) the inactivated Rocky Mountain spotted fever vaccine obtained by Cox (1941) from infected yolk sacs of embryonated hen eggs. The low cost and relative simplicity of the egg techniques have led to their general use for preparation of vaccines and diagnostic antigens. A new formalin-inactivated vaccine prepared by sucrose density-gradient centrifugation of *R. rickettsii* grown in chick embryo cell tissue is under development.

The years of World War II saw many strides in the conquest of the rickettsioses; perhaps greatest among these were the highly successful attacks on the arthropod vectors. The lousicide DDT proved to be ideal for control when dusted on the clothes of infested persons. The epidemic at Naples during the winter of 1943 to 1944 established a milestone, because it was the first to be suppressed by the use of insecticides. Scrub typhus (mite-borne typhus) was creating a major problem in the Pacific area. Here, too, the major contributions to successful control were concerned with application of miticidal chemicals to persons and their clothes.

The advent of broad-spectrum antibiotics—first chloramphenicol, then chlortetracycline, and later oxytetracycline—provided dramatic therapeutic results in each of the rickettsioses.

PATHOGENESIS Rickettsial diseases develop after infection through the skin or the respiratory track. Agents of the typhus and spotted fever group are introduced through the bite of the infected arthropod vector. Ticks and mites, which transmit the agents of spotted fever and scrub typhus, inoculate the rickettsias directly into the dermis during feeding. The louse and flea, which transmit epidemic and murine typhus, respectively, deposit infected feces on the skin; infection occurs when organisms are rubbed into the puncture wound made by the arthropod. The rickettsias of Q fever gain entry through the respiratory tract when infected dust is inhaled; moreover, the respiratory route is occasionally implicated in epidemic typhus when infection results from inhalation of dried infected louse feces.

Although organisms probably multiply at the original site of entry in all instances, local lesions appear with regularity only in certain diseases, namely, the initial cutaneous lesions of scrub typhus, rickettsialpox, and boutonneuse fever, and the pneumonitis which develops in about half the persons infected with Q fever.

Volunteers infected with either scrub typhus or Q fever develop rickettsemia late in the incubation period, often some hours before the onset of fever. Similar events probably occur in all the rickettsial diseases; circulating rickettsias can be detected during the early febrile period in practically all patients.

Little is known about the pathogenesis of infection during the midportion of the incubation period. However, it is reasonable to assume that during this time, in patients with typhus or spotted fever, a transient low-grade rickettsemia results from release of organisms multiplying at the initial site of infection and that this seeds infection in the endothelial cells of the vascular tree. Vascular lesions developing at such sites account for the pathologic changes, including the rash.

Rickettsias apparently invade and proliferate in the endothelial cells of small blood vessels. Endothelial cell destruction occurs from the proliferation of organisms and eventual disruption. Rickettsias may exert a cytotoxic effect on endothelial cells; in mice the rickettsial toxin causes remarkable increase in capillary permeability, independent of proliferation. Later manifestations in rickettsial diseases may result from immunopathologic mechanisms, since humoral antibodies are present during the second febrile week, when increases in capillary permeability and vascular thrombosis and ecchymoses are greatest. Also, a delayed type of hypersensitivity occurs during infection.

The underlying cause of the toxic-febrile state which characterizes the rickettsial diseases remains unknown. Several rickettsial species contain type-specific toxins which are lethal for mice; these may play a role.

PATHOLOGIC PHYSIOLOGY Peripheral vascular collapse results in death in fulminating cases during the first week, with capillary dilatation and pooling of blood without increased capillary permeability or loss of fluid into extravascular spaces. As proliferative and thrombotic lesions develop in small vessels, anoxia occurs in the areas supplied, resulting in necrosis and increased capillary permeability, with loss of water, electrolytes, proteins, and erythrocytes. This in turn results in a decrease in blood volume, together with an increase in extravascular space and clinical edema. Edema, anoxia of the myocardium, and histologic evidence of myocarditis are disclosed by electrocardiographic abnormalities, including serious arrhythmias. Liver function is impaired. The azotemia which develops in seriously ill patients appears to be prerenal. Clinical manifestations resulting from the peripheral vascular collapse are oliguria and anuria, azotemia, anemia, hypoproteinemia, hyponatremia, edema, and coma. In spotted fever and typhus patients with hemorrhagic skin lesions, consumptive coagulopathy is present. All these alterations are absent or minimal in mild cases or in those who are given specific treatment early.

PATHOLOGY The basic changes in the spotted and typhus fever groups are vascular, with resultant widespread lesions in adjacent parenchymatous tissues throughout the body. They are most common in the skin, muscles, heart, lung, and brain. The most conspicuous and diverse are found in Rocky Mountain spotted fever. Here swelling, proliferation, and degeneration of the endothelial cells occur, frequently with thrombus formation which partially or completely occludes the lumen. The muscle cells of the arterioles undergo swelling and fibrinoid changes. The adventitial tissues are infiltrated with mononuclear leukocytes, lymphocytes, and plasma cells. The vascular damage is scattered along the arteries, veins and capillaries, with normal architecture prevailing throughout most of the vascular bed. The changes in murine, epidemic, and scrub typhus fevers resemble those in Rocky Mountain spotted fever, but thrombosis is uncommon and involvement of the musculature is rare.

Interstitial myocarditis occurs in each of these diseases but is usually most extensive in Rocky Mountain spotted fever and in scrub typhus. In the brain glial nodules are found in all members of the group, but microinfarcts in the brain tissue or in the myocardium are most often observed in spotted fever.

A rickettsial pneumonitis occurs, at least to some extent, in many patients with spotted or typhus fever and is the characteristic pathologic change in patients with Q fever. The process is patchy and consists microscopically of areas of congestion and edema. Within the consolidated areas the alveoli are filled with compact fibrinocellular exudate containing lymphocytes, plasma cells, large mononuclear cells, and erythrocytes but few, if any, polymorphonuclear leukocytes.

Rickettsias can occasionally be observed microscopically in sections of tissue. Failure to demonstrate them is of no diagnostic significance.

LABORATORY DIAGNOSIS Diagnostic procedures which depend on isolation of the etiologic agent from blood or other clinical material are expensive, time-consuming, and hazardous to laboratory personnel. Primary isolation of rickettsias by inoculation in the yolk sac of the chick embryo or tissue cells usually fails because of the small number of organisms in the patient's blood. Rickettsias have been identified in stained cultured monocytes of infected monkeys and by direct or indirect immunofluorescence of tissues of animals infected with *R. rickettsii*. Except in unusual circumstances, however, currently available serologic tests are adequate for laboratory confirmation of the clinical diagnosis in each of the rickettsial diseases. The demonstration of a rise in titer of specific antibody during convalescence is of prime importance in establishing the laboratory confirmation. Table 163-2 summarizes the serologic results usually encountered in persons who have rickettsial diseases in the United States. The Weil-Felix test employing *Proteus* strains OX-19 and OX-2 gives positive results in patients with spotted fever and murine typhus and negative results in those with rickettsialpox and Q fever. It is useful as a screening procedure but cannot be relied upon to differentiate spotted fever from murine typhus. In patients with Brill-Zinsser disease the *Proteus* OX-19 reaction is usually negative or low in titer.

Serologic tests employing group-specific rickettsial antigens provide data which clearly differentiate the most common infections, i.e., murine typhus, Rocky Mountain spotted fever, and Q fever. Moreover, if type-specific rickettsial antigens are employed, it is generally possible to distinguish rickettsialpox from spotted fever and Brill-Zinsser disease from murine typhus.

Antibodies during response to a primary infection of epidemic typhus or Rocky Mountain spotted fever are usually 19S globulins. In patients with Brill-Zinsser disease, which is a recrudescence, antibodies occur more quickly (within several days after onset of illness), rise to a higher titer, and are 7S globulins.

Utilizing better antigens, other serologic procedures for rickettsial diseases not only distinguish between specific rickettsioses but help to determine the type of immunoglobulin in acute (IgM) and late or recurrent (IgG) illness, such as in recrudescent typhus (Brill-Zinsser disease). The Weil-Felix and complement fixation tests are useful for routine diagnosis; microscopic agglutination, immunofluorescent antibody, and hemagglutination reactions are valuable for specific identification.

Specific antibiotic therapy has little effect on the time of appearance of antibodies or on their ultimate titer, provided treatment is instituted some days after onset of the illness. However, if the illness is cut short by early and vigorous treatment, antibody production may be delayed for a week or so, and also the maximal titers attained may be below those illustrated in Table 163-2. Under these circumstances a sample of blood taken 4 to 6 weeks after onset of illness should also be tested.

The immunofluorescent antibody test is a very useful procedure for detecting rickettsia in the tissues of patients with the typhus group of rickettsioses, the spotted fevers, and Q fever. Identifiable rickettsias have been visualized in skin lesions of patients with Rocky Mountain spotted fever as early as the fourth day of illness and as late as the tenth day. The technique also visualizes rickettsias in ticks and the tissues of animals.

Normochromic anemia occurs in patients severely ill with rickettsial diseases. The white blood cell count in Rocky Mountain spotted fever, rickettsialpox, murine and epidemic typhus, Brill-Zinsser disease, Q fever, and other rickettsial diseases is usually within the normal range; 6000 to 10,000 cells per cubic millimeter. Leukopenia is occasionally observed, and in the presence of complications, such as superimposed infections and extensive vascular lesions, moderate leukocytosis occurs. The differential blood cell count is usually normal.

Thrombocytopenia occurs in severely ill spotted and scrub typhus fever patients with extensive vascular lesions; hypofibrinogenemia, prolonged prothrombin and partial thromboplastin times, and other clotting abnormalties occur. In primates showing peripheral gangrenous ecchymoses caused by *R. rickettsii* there are decreases in complement fractions C2 and C3.

REFERENCES

See Chap. 171.

TABLE 163-2
Serologic diagnosis of rickettsial diseases of the United States

| | | | Weil-Felix reaction | | | Complement fixation tests with type-specific antigen | | | | |
| | | | Illustrative titer | | | | Illustrative titer | | | |
Group	Disease	Proteus	10th day	20th day	Cases with diagnostic titer	Rickettsial antigen	10th day	20th day	30th day	Cases with diagnostic titer
Spotted fever	Rocky Mountain spotted fever	OX-19	40	320	Most	R. rickettsii	20	160	80	Most
		OX-2	20	160						
	Rickettsialpox	OX-19	0	0	None	R. akari	0	64	128	Most
		OX-2	0	0						
Typhus	Murine typhus	OX-19	160	640	Most	R. mooseri	0	160	160	Most
		OX-2	10	40						
	Brill-Zinsser disease	OX-19	160	20	Infrequent	R. prowazekii	1280	640	320	Most
		OX-2	0	0						
	Q fever	OX-19	0	0	None	R. burnetii	10	80	160	Most
		OX-2	0	0						

164

ROCKY MOUNTAIN SPOTTED FEVER

THEODORE E. WOODWARD

[handwritten: TETRACYCLENE, CHLORO   RASH ~100%   STARTS IN EXTREMITIES, MOVES CENTRALLY   ↑ SPLEEN 50%]

DEFINITION Rocky Mountain spotted fever is an acute febrile illness caused by *Rickettsia rickettsii*. It is transmitted to humans by ticks. The disease is characterized by sudden onset with headache and chills and by fever which persists for 2 to 3 weeks. A characteristic exanthem appears on the extremities and trunk about the fourth day of illness. Delerium, shock, and renal failure occur in the severely ill.

ETIOLOGY AND EPIDEMIOLOGY The causative microbe *R. rickettsii* is the prototype for the rickettsial group of agents. The minute organisms are purple when stained by Giemsa's method or red by Macchiavello's technique; most of them are gram-negative. These organisms often occur in pairs and possess a cell wall similar in structure and chemical composition to that of gram-negative bacteria; one finds a cell membrane, cytoplasmic granules corresponding to ribosomes, and prokaryotic organization of nuclear material. The cell membrane is selectively permeable; the cell wall is the focus of important antigens and an endotoxin-like substance.

The rickettsias grow in the nucleus and the cytoplasm of infected cells of ticks, mammals, and embryonated eggs; the intranuclear situation of the organisms is shared by the other members of the spotted fever group, but not by rickettsias of the typhus group. *Rickettsia rickettsii* is readily distinguishable from the agents of the typhus fevers by cross-immunity tests in guinea pigs and by complement fixation tests employing antigens prepared from infected yolk sac tissues. The differentiation of *R. rickettsii* from closely related members of the spotted fever group frequently requires elaborate procedures. Strains of the agent of Rocky Mountain spotted fever vary considerably in their virulence for humans and animals.

The first reports of spotted fever in Idaho and Montana during the final decade of the last century led to the name Rocky Mountain spotted fever. However, the disease has been reported from almost all states, as well as from Canada, Mexico, Colombia, and Brazil. Although related diseases are found on other continents, this particular infection is limited to the Western Hemisphere. In the years 1976 and 1977, 937 and 1115 cases respectively were reported. The mortality rate was about 20 percent in the days before specific therapy but has decreased to about 7 percent. More than half the cases occur in the South Atlantic and South Central states, with the greatest number of these in North Carolina, Virginia, Georgia, Maryland, Tennessee, and Oklahoma.

A number of species of ticks are found infected with *R. rickettsii* in nature, but only two are important in transmitting spotted fever to humans. These are *Dermacentor andersoni,* the wood tick, which is the principal vector in the West, and *D. variabilis,* the dog tick, which assumes this role in the East. Infected female ticks transmit the agent transovarially to at least some of their offspring. Ticks which become infected, either through the egg or at one of the stages during their development cycle by feeding on an infected mammal, harbor the rickettsias throughout their lifetime, which may be several years. Thus, the tick serves as a reservoir in addition to being a vector. Small wild mammals are suspected of playing an important role in spreading the rickettsias in nature by infecting ticks which feed on them during rickettsemia.

Disease in humans is generally acquired from the bite of an infected tick. Transmission is unlikely unless the tick remains attached for a number of hours. Infection may also be acquired through abrasions in the skin which become contaminated with infected tick feces or tissue juices; hence, the hazard associated with crushing ticks between the fingers when removing them from persons or animals. The agent of Rocky Mountain spotted fever has been transmitted accidentally to humans by transfusion of blood taken from a donor just before onset of illness.

There are seasonal variations in the incidence of cases of spotted fever, as well as differences in age and sex distribution of cases. In each instance these differences are related to exposure to ticks. Most cases are seen during the period of maximal tick activity, i.e., late spring and early summer, and 60 percent of cases occur in individuals under 20 years of age. This age distribution is undoubtedly influenced by propinquity to the wood and dog ticks, respectively. The mortality rate increases with the age of the patient.

Rocky Mountain spotted fever has been acquired by laboratory workers via aerosol transmission, and special precautions are necessary when the agent is handled in the laboratory.

CLINICAL MANIFESTATIONS Incubation period and prodromata A history of tick bite is elicited in approximately 80 percent of patients. The incubation period varies between 3 and 12 days with a mean of 7 days. A short incubation period usually indicates a more serious infection.

Onset In nonvaccinated persons, the onset is usually abrupt, with severe headache, a sudden shaking rigor, prostration, generalized myalgia, especially in the back and leg muscles, nausea with occasional vomiting, and fever which reaches 103 to 104°F within the first 2 days. Pain in the abdominal muscles may be severe, and arthralgia is not uncommon. Deep muscle palpation often elicits tenderness. Occasionally the debut of illness in children and adults is mild, accompanied by lethargy, anorexia, headache, and low-grade fever. These symptoms are similar to those of many acute infectious diseases, making specific diagnosis difficult during the first few days.

Pyrexia Fever continues for approximately 15 to 20 days in untreated cases. The febrile course in children may be shorter. Hyperthermia of 105°F or greater is of unfavorable prognostic significance, although fatalities may occur when the patient is hypothermic, with concurrent vasomotor collapse. Fever generally terminates by lysis over a period of several days, but rarely does so by crisis. Recurrent fever is uncommon except in the presence of secondary pyogenic complications.

The *headache* is generalized and excruciating, and frequently more intense over the frontal area. It persists throughout the first and second weeks of illness in untreated cases. Occasionally headache is mild. Malaise continues for the first week; irritability is notable, and the patient shuns distractions such as questioning and examination.

Cutaneous manifestations The rash which is present in practically all cases is the most characteristic and helpful diagnostic sign. It usually appears on the fourth febrile day; the range is 2 to 6 days. The initial lesions are on the wrists, ankles, palms, soles, and forearms. The first lesions are macular, nonfixed, pink, irregularly defined, and measure 2 to 6 mm. A warm compress applied to the extremity accentuates the rash in the early stages. The exanthem is most prominent when the temperature is elevated. After 6 to 12 h, the rash extends centripetally to the axilla, buttocks, trunk, neck, and face. (This is in contrast to the eruption of typhus fever, which begins on the trunk and spreads centrifugally, rarely involving the face, palms, or soles.) The rash becomes maculopapular after 2 to 3 days (it may be felt by light palpation) and assumes a deeper red hue. By about the fourth day it is petechial and fails to fade on pressure. Not uncommonly, the hemorrhagic lesions coalesce to form large ecchymotic blemishes; these lesions tend to form over bony prominences and may ultimately slough to form indolent, slow-healing ulcers. Patients who have had the typical rash show brownish discolorations at the site for several weeks during convalescence. In milder cases, the rash does not become purpuric and may disappear within a few days. Antibiotic therapy may abort the early exanthem; the later fixed lesion fades less rapidly with specific therapy. Occasionally, a rash does not occur or is unnoticed, particularly in dark-skinned patients.

The application of tourniquets for several minutes, or the occasional taking of the blood pressure may provoke additional petechiae (Rumpel-Leede phenomenon), further evidence of capillary abnormalities.

Cardiovascular and respiratory features During the early stages, the pulse is full and regular but accelerated in proportion to the height of the temperature, and the blood pressure is well sustained. During the peak of illness in seriously ill patients, the pulse is rapid and feeble, and hypotension of 90 mmHg is common. If circulatory failure is sustained, the resultant hypoxia and shock lead to agitation and delirium and contribute to the formation of ecchymoses and gangrene of fingers, toes, genitalia, buttocks, earlobes, and nose. Cyanosis of the peripheral parts of the body is common. Venous pressure determinations show no elevation. A reduction of the total blood volume is occasionally found, as is myocardial impairment as shown by low voltage of ventricular complexes, minor ST-segment deflections, and occasionally delay in atrioventricular conduction on the electrocardiogram. These changes are transient and nonspecific. Severely ill patients have a puffy appearance of the face, hands, ankles, feet, and lower parts of the sacrum.

Respirations are either normal or slightly accelerated. Cough may be harassing and nonproductive, and localized pneumonitis may occur, but pulmonary consolidation is extremely rare. Pulmonary edema may develop after injudicious use of intravenous fluids.

Hepatic and renal manifestations In the majority of patients, there is little alteration in renal or hepatic function. The liver may be enlarged, but jaundice is unusual. Oliguria commonly occurs in the seriously ill, and anuria may mark the critically ill patient. Azotemia is common; when marked, it is a very unfavorable sign. Abnormalities in liver function are probably responsible for the hypoproteinemia, with reduction in the albumin fraction.

Neurologic manifestations The principal neurologic manifestations are headache, restlessness, and varying degrees of insomnia. Stiffness of the back is common. The cerebrospinal fluid is clear, with normal dynamics and normal chemical constituents. Coma and muscular rigidity may occur. Athetoid movements, convulsive seizures, and hemiplegia are grave manifestations. Deafness during the active stages of the disease is not uncommon. As a rule, all neurologic signs abate without residua. Findings based upon follow-up examinations and electroencephalograms may be interpreted as indicative of minor residual brain damage for a year or more following recovery of certain patients from Rocky Mountain spotted fever.

Other physical manifestations Patients become dehydrated, with extreme dryness of lips, gums, tongue, and pharynx. The skin is hot and dry, the conjunctivas are frequently injected, and the eyes suffused. Photophobia is common in the early stages of illness. Petechial hemorrhages may be noted in the conjunctivas or in the retina. The spleen is enlarged in approximately one-half the cases and is firm and nontender. Abdominal distention is frequent, and occasionally some degree of intestinal ileus is observed. Constipation is usual.

COURSE In patients with mild and moderately severe cases who are given no specific antibiotic therapy, the disease abates within 2 weeks, and convalescence is rapid. In fatal cases death usually occurs during the latter part of the second week as a result of toxemia, vasomotor weakness, and shock or renal failure. In a few patients, the course is fulminant with death occurring as early as the sixth day of illness.

In vaccinated individuals who contract the disease, the illness is mild, with a short febrile course and an atypical rash.

COMPLICATIONS AND PROGNOSIS If the serious manifestations of spotted fever mentioned above are regarded as intrinsic parts of the disease, then complications are uncommon and consist mainly of secondary bacterial infections, namely, bronchopneumonia, otitis media, and parotitis. Thrombosis of major blood vessels may result in gangrene of a portion of an extremity. Hemiplegia and peripheral neuritis are rare sequelae.

The overall mortality rate for spotted fever was formerly about 20 percent. Death occurred in more than half of persons over 40 years of age, but the mortality rate was much lower in children and young adults. Since the introduction of the broad-spectrum antibiotics and the development of more precise knowledge regarding correction of the physiologic abnormalities which develop during the disease, fewer deaths occur from this infection. Some of the fatalities can be attributed to failure to consider spotted fever in the differential diagnosis.

DIFFERENTIAL DIAGNOSIS During the early stages of infection before the rash has appeared, differentiation from other acute infections is difficult. History of tick bite while living or traveling in a highly endemic area is helpful. The rash of meningococcemia (Chap. 118) resembles Rocky Mountain spotted fever in certain aspects, because it is macular, maculopapular, or petechial in the chronic form, and petechial, confluent, or ecchymotic in the fulminant type. The meningococcal skin lesion is tender and develops with extreme rapidity in the fulminant form, whereas the rickettsial rash occurs on about the fourth day of disease and gradually becomes petechial. *Spotted fever is often confused with measles.* The exanthem of rubeola rapidly becomes confluent, while that of rubella *usually remains discrete.*

Murine typhus is a milder disease than Rocky Mountain spotted fever; the rash is less extensive, nonpurpuric, and nonconfluent, and renal and vascular complications are uncommon. Not infrequently differentiation of these two rickettsial infections must await the results of specific serologic tests. Epidemic typhus fever is capable of causing all the pronounced clinical, physiologic, and anatomic alterations seen in patients with Rocky Mountain spotted fever, i.e., hypotension, peripheral vascular collapse, cyanosis, skin necrosis and gangrene of digits, renal failure and azotemia, and neurologic manifestations. However, the rash of classical typhus is noted initially in the axillary folds of the trunk and later extends peripherally, rarely involving the palms, soles, or face. The serologic patterns in these two diseases are distinctive when specific rickettsial antigens are employed. Moreover, louse-borne typhus is not recognized in the United States except in the form of Brill-Zinsser disease (recurrent typhus fever). Rickettsialpox, although caused by a member of the spotted fever group of organisms, is usually readily differentiated from Rocky Mountain spotted fever by the initial lesion, the relative mildness of the illness, and the early vesiculation of the maculopapular rash. The Weil-Felix reaction is positive in Rocky Mountain spotted fever and in murine and epidemic typhus, but is negative in rickettsialpox. Agglutinins against *Proteus* OX-19 and OX-2 appear in the serum of patients with spotted fever, but only those against OX-19 are generally found in murine and epidemic typhus.

THERAPY Certain physiochemical changes occurring in the patient seriously ill with one of the diseases of the typhus-spotted fever group should be understood before a therapeutic regimen is outlined. These changes are circulatory collapse, coma, oliguria and anuria, azotemia, anemia, hypoproteinemia, hypochloremia and hyponatremia, and edema. These alterations are often absent in the mildly ill, and in them management is much less complicated. The therapeutic principles necessary for treatment of all rickettsioses are (1) specific chemotherapy and (2) supportive care. Attention to both is mandatory for the seriously ill patient first recognized late in the disease. During the first week in the moderately ill patient, supportive therapy may be less energetic, because specific chemotherapy usually suffices. The early mild case may be successfully treated at home; later in the course of the disease patients should receive hospital care.

Therapeutic measures advisable for the management of Rocky Mountain spotted fever will be described in detail. Variations of this regimen which apply to the other rickettsioses are described in subsections dealing with other diseases of the typhus-spotted fever group and Q fever.

Specific therapy Specific therapy is most effective when initiated during the early stages of disease coincident with the appearance of the rash. When therapy is delayed until the rash has become hemorrhagic and widespread, the response is less dramatic. The antibiotics of choice are chloramphenicol and the tetracyclines, which are effective because of their rickettsiostatic properties. They are not rickettsiocidal.

The following antibiotic regimen is considered optimal: for chloramphenicol, an initial dose of 50 mg per kilogram of body weight, and for tetracycline, 25 mg/kg. Subsequent daily doses are the same as the initial loading dose, with the requirement divided equally and given at 6- to 8-h intervals. Antibiotic treatment is continued until the patient has improved and has been afebrile approximately 24 h. In patients too ill to take oral medication, an intravenous preparation of one of the antimicrobials should be employed.

Adrenal cortical hormones may need to be utilized for their antitoxemic effects, in patients first observed late in the course of severe illness. Large doses for brief periods of about 3 to 5 days, in combination with specific antibiotics, are recommended in critically ill patients.

Therapy with antibiotics is continued until the toxemia has abated, the general condition has markedly improved, and the temperature has remained at normal levels for 24 h. In uncomplicated cases of spotted fever, there is symptomatic improvement within 24 h and the temperature becomes normal in 60 to 72 h.

Supportive care Frequent turning of the patient relieves pressure from prominent bony parts and also militates against the development of aspiration pneumonia. Proper mouth care, with frequent swabbing of the oral cavity, may avert the development of parotitis and gingivitis. Sucking of the juice of a lemon or the oral use of glycerin or mineral oil is helpful.

A generous intake of protein should be provided by frequent feedings as soon as the disease is suspected, in order to avoid subsequent protein deficiency. Usually food is well tolerated by patients with rickettsial disease, and the daily diet should provide 3 to 5 g protein per kilogram of normal body weight, with adequate carbohydrate and fat to make it palatable. When the patient is uncooperative, the diet may be supplemented by hourly liquid protein feedings via stomach tube, provided that there is no abdominal distention.

At the critical stage, when hypoproteinemia is present and changes in capillary permeability lead to edema and vascular embarrassment, careful attention must be given to parenteral hyperalimentation with high concentration of glucose and amino acids. When indicated by hematologic studies, whole-blood transfusions given slowly are helpful. The judicious administration of one of the plasma expanders at this stage may have a definite favorable effect upon impending circulatory collapse. If the patient is anuric and azotemia is pronounced, overloading the circulation with fluids should be governed by clinical judgment and very careful laboratory studies. Frequent determinations of hemoglobin, hematocrit, electrolytes, and protein, sometimes at intervals of a few hours during crucial periods are necessary in order to ascertain abnormalities and to permit institution of corrective measures. Dialysis is indicated when there is clear-cut evidence of acute tubular necrosis (Chap. 275).

Complications *Pyogenic complications,* including otitis media and parotitis, are encountered in patients severely ill with Rocky Mountain spotted fever and other rickettsioses. These localized infections respond to therapy with appropriate antibiotics combined with surgical measures.

Pneumonitis usually develops as a result of specific rickettsial action. The sputum is scant but should be examined to determine whether superimposed bacterial infection is present. Specific therapy is guided by the results of these laboratory studies. The pneumonitis generally responds to the antibiotic therapy the patient is receiving, but if staphylococcal pneumonia is suspected, a penicillinase-resistant penicillin should be added to the broad-spectrum drug.

Circulatory failure of peripheral or central origin is combated by careful administration of plasma expanders and fluids. Heart failure may develop from the disease or as a result of overzealous intravenous therapy and is recognized by rapid pulse, gallop rhythm, and increase in venous pressure. When the clinical signs reveal unmistakable evidence of cardiac failure, digitalis should be employed. Oxygen therapy improves the cardiac and circulatory status and is helpful in hypoxemic patients with involvement of the central nervous system.

PREVENTION Prevention is attained primarily by avoidance of tick-infested areas. When this is impractical, prophylactic measures include (1) spraying the ground with dieldrin or chlordane for area control of ticks (though there are environmental objections to the use of residual insecticides in area control of ticks, under special conditions, such procedures may be warranted); (2) application of repellents such as diethyltoluamide or dimethylphthalate to clothing and exposed parts of the body, or in very heavily infested areas the wearing of clothing which interferes with the attachment of ticks, i.e., boots and a one-piece outer garment, preferably impregnated with repellent; and (3) daily inspection of the entire body, including the hairy parts, to detect and remove attached ticks. In removing attached ticks great care should be taken to avoid crushing the arthropod with resultant contamination of the bite wound; touching the tick with gasoline or whisky encourages detachment but gentle traction with tweezers applied close to the mouth parts may be necessary; the skin area should be disinfected with soap and water or other antiseptics. Similarly, precautions should be employed in removing engorged ticks from dogs and other animals, because infection through minor abrasions on the hands is possible. Improved vaccines containing inactivated *R. rickettsii* are under development and should be available commercially for those at great risk, namely, persons frequenting highly endemic areas and laboratory workers exposed to the agent. Because the broad-spectrum antibiotics are such excellent therapeutic agents in spotted fever, there has been less impetus for vaccination of persons who run only a minor risk of infection.

After tick bite in a known endemic area an exposed person should be observed for signs of fever, headache, prostration and rash; therapy is very effective at the early stage of illness.

REFERENCES

See Chap. 171.

165
OTHER TICK-BORNE RICKETTSIAL DISEASES

THEODORE E. WOODWARD

DEFINITION Boutonneuse fever, North Asian tick-borne rickettsiosis, and Queensland tick typhus, three diseases occurring in the Eastern Hemisphere, are caused by rickettsias closely related to one another and to the agent of Rocky Mountain spotted fever. Each is transmitted by the bite of an ixodid tick. These mild to moderately severe illnesses are characterized by an initial lesion (called *tache noire* in boutonneuse fever), a fever of several days to 2 weeks, and a generalized maculopapular erythematous rash which appears on about the fifth day and usually involves the palms and soles. Specific complement-fixing antibodies appear in the patients' serums during convalescence, but agglutinins to *Proteus* OX-19 (Weil-Felix reaction) are frequently found only in low titer.

ETIOLOGY AND EPIDEMIOLOGY The etiologic agents of these three diseases are all members of the spotted fever group of rickettsias. Together with *Rickettsia rickettsii* and *R. akari* they possess common group antigens which are readily demonstrated by agglutination, complement fixation, microscopic agglutination, and immunofluorescent antibody reactions.

Boutonneuse fever, which may be regarded as the prototype of the three, is caused by *R. conorii*. Modern serologic methods employing specific rickettsial antigens have shown this rickettsia to be the causative agent for a single widely disseminated disease known by various local names. Information on the distribution and etiology of the various tick-borne rickettsial diseases is contained in Table 163-1.

In general, the epidemiology of these tick-borne rickettsioses resembles that of spotted fever in the Western Hemisphere. Ixodid ticks and small wild animals maintain the rickettsias in nature; if humans intrude accidentally into the cycle, they become a dead end in the transmission chain. In certain areas, the cycle of boutonneuse fever involves domiciliary environments, with the brown dog tick *Rhipicephalus sanguineus* as the dominant vector.

CLINICAL MANIFESTATIONS These three tick-borne rickettsioses, which occur in different parts of the Eastern Hemisphere, resemble one another closely. The clinical course is usually milder than that of spotted fever, with a shorter febrile period and fewer severe complications; fatalities are rare and generally limited to the aged and debilitated. The initial lesion, which is present in most cases at the onset of fever, heals slowly; the regional lymph nodes are enlarged. The rash usually remains papular and only in severe cases becomes hemorrhagic.

The clinical picture (including the primary lesion), the geographic location, and epidemiologic considerations are helpful in establishing the diagnosis. The typhus fevers, meningococcal infections, and measles must be considered in the differential diagnosis; the serologic reactions, i.e., Weil-Felix and complement fixation tests, are of value here.

TREATMENT AND PREVENTION Chloramphenicol and the tetracyclines are effective therapeutic agents for boutonneuse fever. Patients generally become afebrile after 2 to 3 days of treatment, and recovery is rapid. The therapeutic procedures are comparable to those used in spotted fever. Presumably these measures are also applicable to North Asian tick-borne rickettsiosis and Queensland tick typhus.

The major effective methods of control are concerned with avoidance of tick bites; these include application of new repellents and prompt removal of attached ticks. Effective vaccines are not available commercially.

REFERENCES

See Chap. 171.

166
RICKETTSIALPOX

THEODORE E. WOODWARD

DEFINITION Rickettsialpox is a mild, nonfatal self-limited, febrile illness caused by *Rickettsia akari*, which is transmitted from mouse to humans by mites. It is characterized by an initial skin lesion at the site of the mite bite, a week's febrile course, and a papulovesicular rash.

ETIOLOGY AND EPIDEMIOLOGY Rickettsialpox was first recognized in New York City in 1946, and about 180 cases were reported annually for several years thereafter. It has been diagnosed in several other areas of the United States, and outbreaks have been reported in European Russia. The vector is a small, colorless mite, *Allodermanyssus sanguineus* (Hirst), which infests small mice and rodents. House mice serve as the reservoir of infection.

Rickettsia akari is morphologically and biologically similar to other rickettsias and is antigenically related to, but distinct from, *R. rickettsii*, the cause of Rocky Mountain spotted fever. Mice, guinea pigs, and fertile hen eggs are susceptible to experimental infection. Diagnostic antigens prepared from infected yolk sacs and tissue culture cells are used in serologic reactions.

CLINICAL MANIFESTATIONS The initial skin lesion appears about 7 to 10 days after the mite bite as a firm red papule 1 to 1.5 cm in diameter. In a few days, the center vesiculates, and the papule is surrounded by an area of erythema. The regional lymph glands are moderately enlarged. The primary lesion, which is never painful, becomes covered with a black scab; it heals slowly, and a small scar is visible on separation of the crust.

The febrile phase begins 3 to 7 days after the initial lesion, and exanthem may accompany the fever or begin several days later. The onset of fever is sudden, with chilly sensations or frank chills, headache, sweats, myalgia, anorexia, and photophobia. The pyrexia ranges from 103 to 104°F and continues for about a week, occasionally with morning remisssions.

The exanthem is maculopapular-vesicular, generalized in distribution, and may be abundant or scant. The lesions may involve the oral cavity but not the palms or soles. In a week, the vesicles dry and form scabs which eventually scale but leave no scar.

The constitutional symptoms are generally mild, and the course of illness is uncomplicated. No fatal cases have been reported.

The disease may be confused with chickenpox, which is different because it occurs usually in childhood and has no initial lesion and the papular cutaneous lesion is entirely transformed into a vesicle. Variola (smallpox) is accompanied by a more severe constitutional reaction, and the vesicles become pustules. The skin lesions of the other rickettsioses differ in their lack of vesiculation. The Weil-Felix reaction is usually negative in this rickettsial disease but specific complement fixation, microscopic agglutination, and immunofluorescent antibody reactions are useful diagnostic aids even though there is considerable crossing with materials from Rocky Mountain spotted fever.

TREATMENT AND PREVENTION Chloramphenicol and the tetracycline antibiotics are all effective for treating patients with rickettsialpox. The temperature reaches normal levels in about 2 days, and recovery is rapid.

Control measures should be directed toward elimination of house mice and the vector mites responsible for transmitting the disease.

REFERENCES

See Chap. 171.

167
MURINE (ENDEMIC) TYPHUS FEVER

THEODORE E. WOODWARD

DEFINITION Murine typhus fever is an acute febrile disease caused by *Rickettsia mooseri* and transmitted to humans by fleas. The clinical illness is characterized by fever of 9 to 14 days, headache, a maculopapular rash appearing on the third to fifth day, and myalgia.

ETIOLOGY AND EPIDEMIOLOGY *Rickettsia mooseri* resembles other rickettsias in morphologic properties, staining characteristics, and intracellular parasitism. Under the electron microscope *R. mooseri* is seen to contain dense masses of nuclear material in a less dense homogeneous protoplasmic substance, the whole of which is surrounded by a limiting membrane. It differs from *R. rickettsii* in that it always multiplies within the cytoplasm of cells, in contrast to the intranuclear and cytoplasmic positions of spotted fever rickettsias.

Invasion of the body by *R. mooseri* provokes specific and nonspecific immunologic responses. Utilizing highly purified antigens, specific antibodies may be demonstrated readily by complement fixation, microscopic agglutination, and immuno-

fluorescent antibody reactions. The positive Weil-Felix reaction which occurs in this disease is nonspecific, because it is attributable to the presence of a common carbohydrate antigen in *Proteus* OX-19 and *R. mooseri* and because the reaction is also positive in epidemic typhus and spotted fever. Group-specific rickettsial antigens are common to both *R. mooseri and R. prowazekii*. Furthermore, both murine and epidemic rickettsias possess toxic factors which are lethal to mice and rats and can be neutralized by convalescent serum from humans or lower animals.

The common vector of *R. mooseri* for rats and humans is the rat flea (*Xenopsylla cheopis*). In nature, the rat louse (*Polypax spinulosis*) may transmit the agent among rodents. Customarily, rat fleas become infected on ingestion of blood from diseased rats; the rickettsias multiply within the intestinal cells of the arthropod and are excreted in the feces. Infection in humans occurs after the flea bite and contamination of the broken skin by rickettsia-laden feces. Dried flea feces may also infect via the conjuntivas or the upper part of the respiratory tract.

Rats and mice are naturally infected with murine typhus, and although the rodent disease is nonfatal, viable rickettsias persist in the brain for variable periods.

Murine typhus is one of the most benign and widespread of the rickettsioses in the United States. Prevalent in the Southeastern and Gulf Coast states, it has been identified in most of the other states and in harbor centers throughout the world wherever rats and fleas abound. Through control of rats and their fleas a sharp decline in incidence has occurred since 1951, particularly in the Southern United States. In urban areas the disease is more prevalent during the summer and fall months and occurs predominantly among persons working in proximity to granaries or food depots. There has been an extension to certain rural areas when changing agricultural practices have provided rats with ready access to adequate food supplies. Three cases of endemic typhus were reported in laboratory workers in 1978. This emphasizes the importance of taking special precautions when working with rickettsial organisms in the laboratory.

CLINICAL MANIFESTATIONS **Incubation period and prodromata** The incubation period ranges from 8 to 16 days, with a mean of 10. Common prodromata are headache, backache, arthralgia, and chilly sensations. Nausea, malaise, and transient temperature rises may precede the true onset of disease.

Onset and general symptoms A frank shaking chill and repeated rigors are present at the onset, associated with a severe frontal headache and fever. This triad of headache, chill, and pyrexia is usually followed within a few hours by nausea and vomiting. Prostration, malaise, and weakness are sufficient to enforce cessation of activity in adults, in contrast to children, whose illness is less severe. Occasionally, mild symptoms make it difficult to define the actual onset.

Pyrexia The usual febrile course in murine typhus lasts for about 12 days in adults; the temperature ranges from 102 to 104°F but may reach 105 to 106°F in children. The temperature may reach high levels abruptly after onset or ascend in a stepwise manner during the first few days. With the appearance of the rash, fever is usually sustained, with partial daily remissions which occasionally reach normal levels in the morning. Defervescence is generally by lysis over several days but sometimes occurs by crisis. Transient mild fever of 100°F is not uncommon during early convalescence. A few patients experience only low-grade fever throughout, but this does not necessarily connote a mild illness.

Cutaneous manifestations The early lesions, which are sparse and discrete, are hidden in the axillae and inner surface of the arm. Most patients then develop with surprising suddenness a generalized, dull red macular rash of the upper part of the abdomen, shoulders, chest, arms, and thighs. The individual lesions are discrete and pea size, with an ill-defined border, and fade on pressure during the first 24 h. They later become maculopapular, in contrast to the exanthem of epidemic typhus, which is persistently macular. The distribution over the trunk with sparse involvement of the extremities, palms, soles, and face differs from the peripheral distribution and facial involvement of Rocky Mountain spotted fever. The murine rash generally appears initially on the fifth febrile day, but rarely it is seen concurrently with the onset of fever or develops as late as the seventh day.

Eighty percent of patients develop a rash which persists for 4 to 8 days and fades before defervescence. The cutaneous manifestations vary greatly in intensity and duration and may be fleeting. They are readily overlooked in dark-skinned patients, in whom they should be sought by light palpation and indirect lighting.

Cardiovascular and respiratory features An irritating, nonproductive cough is frequent and is occasionally associated with moderate hemoptysis. Early in the second week, rales may be detected in the basilar lung areas. These changes are generally rickettsial rather than bacterial in origin and respond to the broad-spectrum antibiotics. Pulmonary congestion occurs in extremely ill and elderly patients.

Accelerated pulse, hypotension, and general circulatory weakness occur in this disease, although less frequently than in patients with epidemic typhus or Rocky Mountain spotted fever.

Neurologic manifestations Headache is the most common neurologic manifestation of murine typhus and may dominate the clinical picture. It is frontal and continues into the second week of illness. Stupor and prostration may occur in the second week, and in severe cases, there may be muttering delirium, extreme agitation, or coma. Coma in elderly patients after 2 weeks of illness presages death. Nuchal rigidity and general spasticity often suggest meningitis, although the spinal fluid is normal except for slight increases in pressure and lymphocytes (5 to 30 per cubic millimeter). Transient partial deafness occurs occasionally, but rarely is there localized neuritis or hemiplegia. Neurologic sequelae are unusual. Children experience minimal neurologic changes.

Other physical manifestations During the first 2 days of illness the patient may be nauseated and vomit, but vomiting later in the illness should arouse suspicion of an intercurrent complication. Abdominal pain is bothersome; when associated with diarrhea it responds to intravenous alimentation. Hepatomegaly and jaundice are unusual. There is splenomegaly in approximately 25 percent of patients.

Photophobia, retroocular pain, suffusion of the eyes, and congestion of the conjunctivas are common but are less severe than in the other typhus and spotted fevers.

Renal function is usually unaltered except in elderly patients with prolonged hypotension. Under these circumstances, azotemia may develop to the degree observed in epidemic typhus. In severe murine typhus, as in the epidemic typhus, hyponatremia and hypoalbuminemia are encountered.

COURSE After defervescence, murine typhus patients recover rapidly. Fatalities occur between the ninth and twelfth days in elderly or debilitated patients, usually as a result of circulatory and renal failure or intercurrent bacterial infection.

PROGNOSIS The mortality rate in murine typhus was low even before the introduction of modern specific therapy. Only 1 death occurred in 114 cases studied by Maxcy and none in the 180 reported by Stuart and Pullen.

DIFFERENTIAL DIAGNOSIS Because murine typhus and Rocky Mountain spotted fever occur in many of the same states, the problem of differential diagnosis often arises. Flea-borne murine typhus, which is predominantly an urban disease, is more likely to occur in late summer and autumn. In contrast, spotted fever is a rural and suburban disease in which exposure to ticks is important. Most cases occur in the spring and summer.

TREATMENT AND PREVENTION The therapeutic procedures are comparable to those used in spotted fever. Both chloramphenicol and the tetracycline antibiotics have controlled the disease.

Prevention of murine typhus in humans is attained by reducing the natural reservoir and vector by applying measures for eliminating rodents and employing appropriate insecticides in rat-infested areas to control fleas. Spraying of rat burrows with DDT effectively reduces the population of the vector.

REFERENCES

See Chap. 171.

168
EPIDEMIC TYPHUS FEVER AND BRILL-ZINSSER DISEASE

THEODORE E. WOODWARD

EPIDEMIC (LOUSE-BORNE) TYPHUS FEVER

DEFINITION The classical epidemic form of typhus is a severe, febrile disease caused by *Rickettsia prowazekii* and transmitted to humans by the body louse. Intense headache, continuous pyrexia of about 2 weeks, a macular skin eruption appearing on about the fifth febrile day, malaise, and vascular and neurologic disturbances represent the principal clinical features. Confirmation of the diagnosis is made by demonstration of *Proteus* OX-19 agglutinins and of specific complement-fixing antibodies in convalescence. The broad-spectrum antibiotics are specific therapeutic agents.

ETIOLOGY AND EPIDEMIOLOGY The causative microbe, *R. prowazekii*, is closely related to *R. mooseri*, which causes murine typhus; indeed, the two have a number of common antigens.

Human beings generally are infected when rickettsia-laden louse feces are rubbed into the broken skin; scratching the louse bite facilitates this process. *Pediculus humanus corporis*, which is peculiarly adapted to humans, is the only important vector of epidemic typhus. It dies of its infection and fails to transmit rickettsias to its offspring. *Rickettsia prowazekii* has been isolated from flying squirrels, and the organism probably infests their ectoparasites. Generally, however, the organism is maintained by a cycle involving human-louse-human. New epidemics apparently originate from patients with Brill-Zinsser disease (recurrent epidemic typhus). Pathogenic rickettsias reside for long periods in patients with epidemic typhus as well as Rocky Mountain spotted fever and scrub typhus. Lice readily become infected when fed on patients with recurrent typhus. Inhalation of dust containing dried louse feces may cause infection. An established nonhuman reservoir would pose a serious threat.

Epidemic typhus, if uncontrolled, behaves as a cyclic disease in a susceptible population, extending over a 3-year period. During the first year there is a gradual seeding of cases throughout the group; during the second there is epidemic spread; and during the third the epidemic tapers off, because the majority of persons have become immune. Outbreaks of epidemic typhus last occurred in the United States in the nineteenth century, and its presence is now recognized only in the form of Brill-Zinsser disease.

CLINICAL MANIFESTATIONS Epidemic typhus resembles murine typhus but is more severe. After an incubation period of about 7 days an abrupt onset of headache, chill, and rapidly mounting fever ushers in the illness. Headache, malaise, and prostration continue unabated until the rash appears on the fifth febrile day. It is initially macular in the axillary folds but ultimately invades the trunk and extremities as a pink, irregular macular lesion, which becomes fixed, petechial, and confluent in the later stages.

Neurologic features range from headache and general spasticity to extreme agitation, stupor, and coma. Circulatory disturbances consisting of tachycardia, hypotension, and cyanosis are more profound than those observed in murine typhus and are almost as severe as in Rocky Mountain spotted fever. Ultimately, in untreated cases azotemia often reaches high levels as a result of vascular and renal failure, and death occurs late in the second week of illness. Furthermore, thrombosis of major blood vessels and cutaneous gangrene develop in a manner similar to that seen in the virulent form of Rocky Mountain spotted fever.

The complications and sequelae of epidemic typhus are more severe than those in murine typhus, but not as severe as those in Rocky Mountain spotted fever. However, during certain outbreaks, epidemic typhus was fatal in 60 percent of those infected, and convalescence in survivors was prolonged. Broad-spectrum antibiotics have almost eradicated mortality in this dread disease, provided therapy is instituted before irreversible changes have been established in the tissues.

DIFFERENTIAL DIAGNOSIS Differentiation of epidemic typhus from the various rickettsioses and other diseases with which it may be confused is described in Chap. 164. The disease in epidemic form never occurs in the absence of lousiness in the general population. Under the conditions in which typhus epidemics are likely to occur, other diseases which may cause confusion include malaria, relapsing fever, pneumonia, and tuberculosis. Classic typhus contracted by a previously vaccinated person is usually mild and may be clinically indistinguishable from murine typhus except by serologic methods. An illness simulating Rocky Mountain spotted fever is caused by *R. Canada,* a member of the typhus group.

TREATMENT AND PREVENTION Both chloramphenicol and the tetracycline antibiotics have been found to be highly efficient therapeutic agents in epidemic typhus. Usually the patient becomes afebrile after 2 days of treatment. The therapeutic procedures are comparable to those used in spotted fever. Under field conditions, 100 mg doxycycline in a single oral dose resulted in abatement of clinical manifestations and defervescence in epidemic typhus.

The most effective measures for controlling epidemic typhus are those which eliminate lousiness. DDT or lindane powder when dusted into clothing is suitable for this purpose. If resistant lice are found, malathion or carbaryl may prove effective.

A commercially available vaccine prepared from formalin-treated suspensions of infected yolk sac tissue is an effective immunizing agent. A viable vaccine utilizing an attenuated strain of *R. prowazekii* is under development.

BRILL-ZINSSER DISEASE (RECRUDESCENT TYPHUS)

DEFINITION Brill-Zinsser disease is a recrudescent episode of epidemic typhus fever which occurs years after the initial attack, in persons who had recovered from the epidemic disease acquired while residing in countries where it was prevalent. *Rickettsia prowazekii* have been isolated from lice fed on patients during the active stages of illness.

CLINICAL MANIFESTATIONS The clinical entity, not always mild, resembles epidemic typhus in the character of the rash, circulatory disturbances, and hepatic, renal, and nervous system changes. Recovery is the rule. The Weil-Felix reaction with the various *Proteus* antigens is usually negative, or positive in very low titer. The specific complement fixation, microscopic agglutination, and immunofluorescent antibody reactions are valuable in establishing the diagnosis. In Brill-Zinsser disease the specific complement-fixing antibodies appear as early as the fourth day after the onset of illness; the peak response is attained by the eighth to tenth days. Specific antibody titers in the primary attack of epidemic typhus begin later, about the eighth to twelfth day, with maximum titers on about the sixteenth day after onset. Antibodies in Brill-Zinsser disease and the primary attack are associated with 7S and 19S globulins, respectively. Therapy is like that used in spotted fever.

REFERENCES

See Chap. 171.

169
SCRUB TYPHUS

THEODORE E. WOODWARD

DEFINITION Scrub typhus is limited to eastern and southeastern Asia, India, northern Australia, and the adjacent islands. It is caused by *Rickettsia tsutsugamushi* and characterized by a primary lesion at the site of the bite of an infected mite, a fever of about 2 weeks' duration, a cutaneous rash which develops about the fifth day, and the appearance late in the second week of agglutinins against the OX-K strain of *Proteus* bacillus. The broad-spectrum antibiotics are specific therapeutic agents.

ETIOLOGY The agent of scrub typhus resembles other rickettsias in its physical properties but differs from them in antigenic structure, vector, and reservoir. The disease is transmitted by larvae of several species of mites, especially

Leptotrobidium (*Trombicula*) *akamushi* and *L. deliense*. These tiny chiggers attach themselves to the skin and during the process of obtaining a meal of tissue juice may acquire infection from the host or transmit rickettsias to the vertebrate. The infection is maintained in nature by a cycle involving mites and small rodents and by transovarial transmission in mites; human infection represents an accident attributable to propinquity.

CLINICAL MANIFESTATIONS About 10 to 12 days after infection, illness begins abruptly with chilliness, severe headache, fever, conjunctival injection, and moderate generalized lymphadenopathy, which is most prominent in the nodes draining the area of the primary lesion. The initial lesion at the beginning of fever is evidenced by an erythematous indurated area 1 cm in diameter, surmounted by a multiloculated vesicle; within a few days the vesicle ulcerates and becomes covered with a black crust.

Fever increases progressively during the first week, generally reaching 104 to 105°F, but the pulse remains relatively slow, 70 to 100 beats per minute. The red macular rash, which begins on the trunk about the fifth day and spreads to the extremities, sometimes becomes maculopapular but usually fades in a few days. The course of the disease and the complications resemble those of endemic and epidemic typhus; however, interstitial myocarditis is more prominent than in the other typhus fevers.

PROGNOSIS Before the introduction of the broad-spectrum antibiotics the mortality rate varied from 1 to 60 percent, depending on the geographic area and the virulence of the local strains of *R. tsutsugamushi,* and convalescence was prolonged. With modern therapeutic methods, deaths are rare and convalescence is short.

DIFFERENTIAL DIAGNOSIS Scrub typhus is to be differentiated from the other members of the typhus and the spotted fever group of diseases as well as from measles, typhoid fever, and the meningococcal infections. The geographic localization of scrub typhus, the primary lesion, and the occurrence of OX-K agglutinins are especially useful in establishing the diagnosis.

TREATMENT AND PREVENTION Chloramphenicol and the tetracycline antibiotics are valuable specific therapeutic agents in scrub typhus. The therapeutic procedures are comparable to those used in spotted fever. In fact, scrub typhus is more amenable to drugs than are the other rickettsial infections, and patients with this disease regularly become afebrile and are decidedly improved within 24 to 36 h after beginning treatment, irrespective of the stage of disease. Antibiotic treatment may be discontinued after several afebrile days.

Relapse of clinical illness is unusual unless specific treatment is initiated early, such as before the fifth febrile day. Under these circumstances, recrudescence is obviated by giving the antibiotic for several days and resuming treatment about 5 days after cessation of the initial course of therapy.

Prevention of disease in the individual is accomplished by the application of miticidal chemicals (dibutyl phthalate, benzyl benzoate, diethyltoluamide, and others) to clothing and the skin. There is no satisfactory vaccine.

REFERENCES

See Chap. 171.

170

Q FEVER

THEODORE E. WOODWARD

DEFINITION Q fever is an acute infectious disease caused by *Coxiella burnetii* and characterized by a sudden onset of fever, malaise, headache, weakness, anorexia, and interstitial pneumonitis. Rickettsemia occurs during the febrile period, and specific complement-fixing antibodies are present during convalescence. In contrast to the other rickettsioses, the disease is not associated with a cutaneous exanthem or agglutinins for the *Proteus* bacteria (Weil-Felix reaction).

ETIOLOGY AND EPIDEMIOLOGY *Coxiella burnetii* possesses the general properties of other rickettsias but is somewhat more resistant to inactivation in unfavorable environments and more pleomorphic than the others. Its infectivity after drying under natural conditions is of importance in the spread of infection to humans. *Coxiella burnetii* has a wide host range in nature, but guinea pigs and embryonated eggs are the common laboratory hosts employed for its propagation.

Human cases of Q fever are contracted by inhalation of infected dusts, by handling infected materials, possibly by drinking milk contaminated with *C. burnetii* and, in one instance, by blood transfusion. The disease in Australia is enzootic in animals, especially bandicoots, and is transmitted in nature by ticks. Rickettsia-laden tick feces may contaminate cattle hides, and inhalation of this material has caused infection in humans. In the United States, a number of species of ticks are naturally infected, among them *Dermacentor andersoni* and *Amblyomma americanum,* and in North Africa transovarial transmission of the agent in indigenous ticks has been demonstrated. Sheep, goats, and cows have been found to be naturally infected in North America and in Europe, and *C. burnetii* has been recovered from the milk of such animals. Milk, as well as infected excretions from livestock, probably accounts for certain outbreaks of human disease following inhalation by cows of infected dust from barns and pens. The airborne route of dried contaminated material is the most likely method of spread. A number of epidemics have occurred among laboratory workers engaged in studies on *C. burnetii.* The disease is not transmitted between humans.

CLINICAL MANIFESTATIONS After incubation of approximately 19 days (the range is 14 to 26 days), the disease begins with headache, chilly sensations, fever, malaise, myalgia, and anorexia. For several days, the temperature ranges from 101 to 104°F; the entire course rarely exceeds 2 weeks and usually ranges from 3 to 6 days. There may be wide fluctuations in the fever. Respiratory and gastrointestinal symptoms are not conspicuous in the early stages. Headache and fever predominate. A dry cough and chest pain occur after about 5 days, when rales are usually audible. Roentgenographic findings indistinguishable from those of primary atypical pneumonia are present usually by the third to fourth day of disease, first as patchy areas of consolidation involving a portion of one lobe, giving a homogeneous ground-glass appearance. These manifestations persist beyond the febrile period and may appear in patients who are unaware of pulmonary involvement. Complications are rare, and coincident with defervescence the appetite begins to return. Convalescence progresses slowly for several weeks, during which time the principal disability is weakness. It is not uncommon for patients to lose 15 to 20 lb during the active stages of disease. The disease may be protracted in approximately 20 percent of cases, with fever persisting for longer than

4 weeks, particularly in elderly patients. Occasionally relapse occurs, especially in patients treated with antibiotics during the first several days of disease.

Hepatitis, with the development of clinically detectable icterus, occurs in approximately one-third of patients with the protracted form. This form of Q fever is characterized by fever, malaise, absence of headache or respiratory signs, and hepatomegaly with right upper quadrant pain. Liver biopsy specimens show diffuse granulomatous changes with multinucleated giant cells and scattered infiltrations of polymorphonuclear leukocytes, lymphocytes, and macrophages. *Coxiella burnetii* may be demonstrated in such specimens with the fluorescent antibody technique. Therefore, Q fever must be included in the differential diagnosis of liver granulomas such as tuberculosis, sarcoidosis, histoplasmosis, brucellosis, tularemia, syphilis, and others.

Endocarditis also has been reported, and *C. burnetii* has been identified by smear and isolation in vegetations on the heart valves obtained at operation or autopsy. The aortic valve is most commonly involved, often with large vegetations. It is important, therefore, to suspect the possibility of Q fever in cases of apparent subacute bacterial endocarditis with persistently negative blood cultures. Operative intervention with replacement of damaged valves is usually necessary for recovery because the available antibiotics are not rickettsicidal.

A high complement-fixing antibody titer to phase I antigen is present in patients with endocarditis and granulomatous hepatitis.

PROGNOSIS Few fatalities have been recorded and, except for the patient with protracted illness and hepatic involvement or endocarditis, the course of disease is generally uncomplicated and benign.

TREATMENT AND CONTROL The tetracycline antibiotics and chloramphenicol are effective in the treatment of patients with Q fever. Most patients, when treated early in the course of disease, respond promptly and recover without relapses. The therapeutic procedures are comparable to those used in spotted fever.

Control of Q fever depends primarily on immunization of susceptible persons with specific vaccines. Vaccines made from phase I rickettsias are potent and afford considerable protection to slaughterhouse and dairy workers, herders, rendering-plant workers, woolsorters, tanners, laboratory workers, and others at risk. Measures should be taken to avoid exposure to infected aerosols; milk from infected domestic livestock must be pasteurized or boiled.

REFERENCES

See Chap. 171.

171
TRENCH FEVER

THEODORE E. WOODWARD

DEFINITION Trench fever is a febrile disease transmitted between humans by the body louse, *Pediculus humanus corporis.* It is characterized by a sudden onset with headache and severe pain in the muscles, bones, and joints. In most cases, the fever and other symptoms assume a relapsing character. Fatalities are rare. The disease is also known as shin bone fever, Volhynia fever, His-Werner disease, and Quintan fever.

ETIOLOGY AND EPIDEMIOLOGY *Rickettsia quintana,* the etiologic agent, grows extracellularly in the louse gut, in contrast to other pathogenic rickettsias which can multiply only within cells. A European strain of *R. quintana* has been cultivated on blood agar, and typical trench fever has been induced in volunteers.

Humans are the only known reservoir of infection. The louse does not transmit the organism transovarially but acquires its infection by ingesting the blood of a person with rickettsemia. The organisms multiply extracellularly in the louse gut, without injury to this host, and are excreted in large numbers with the feces. Humans become infected by the inoculation of the contaminated feces into abraded skin or conjunctivas. *Rickettsia quintana* may be recovered periodically from human blood for several years after convalescence from an acute attack. Trench fever is known to exist in Mexico, Tunisia, Eritrea, Poland, the U.S.S.R., and possibly China, and there is serologic evidence for its occurrence in Bolivia, Burundi, and Ethiopia.

PATHOLOGY Since there have been no recorded fatalities, histologic examination has been confined to excised macules of the skin, which have shown nonspecific perivascular infiltrates without the involvement of the vessel walls that is seen in typhus fever.

CLINICAL MANIFESTATIONS A variety of clinical manifestations is displayed in trench fever, ranging from a mild afebrile disease to a debilitating illness with a protracted clinical course involving numerous relapses. Following an incubation period of 10 to 30 days the onset may be insidious or dramatically abrupt. The acute disease is characterized by malaise, headache, fever, and bone and body pain, especially severe in the shins. In some cases only one fever peak occurs; in others the fever continues for 5 to 7 days; and in others there is an initial febrile episode lasting 1 to 3 days followed by relapses which characteristically occur at 4- to 5-day intervals. In some cases the fever and symptoms are continuous for 2 or 3 weeks. Enlargement of the spleen and a red macular rash occur in 70 to 80 percent of the cases. Pain and soreness in the muscles usually recur with each febrile relapse.

The disease is marked by a persistent rickettsemia, which is present during the initial attack and which continues during the relapses, throughout the asymptomatic periods between relapses, and for months or even years after cessation of physical symptoms. A relapse has been reported 10 years after the original attack.

PROGNOSIS The disease causes no known deaths, but its duration is variable. About 85 percent of patients are able to return to work within 2 months of onset, but about 5 percent of all cases become chronic. Recovery is even more delayed in the aged and debilitated.

DIFFERENTIAL DIAGNOSIS During epidemics, typical cases are easily diagnosed on the basis of symptoms. The disease may be differentiated from influenza, typhoid, typhus, dengue, and relapsing fever by the specific laboratory tests available for the diagnosis of each of these diseases.

TREATMENT AND PREVENTION *Rickettsia quintana* is highly sensitive in vitro to the broad-spectrum antibiotics but no reliable information has been obtained about the value of these drugs in treating trench fever. The treatment is symptomatic. Aspirin is used to control pain and discomfort, but codeine may be necessary. The patient should remain in bed for a week or more after complete cessation of subjective and objective evidence of infection. He should be kept under observation for several months and returned to bed at the first sign of relapse.

The methods employed to control epidemic typhus should be equally efficacious in controlling trench fever. These are based on the elimination of lousiness and the improvement of living conditons with provision for frequent bathing and washing of clothing. DDT or lindane powder should be applied by hand or power duster at appropriate intervals to clothes and persons of populations living under conditions favoring lousiness. If resistant lice are found, malathion or other effective lousicides may be substituted as a dusting powder.

REFERENCES

ANDREW R et al: Tick typhus in North Queensland. Med J Aust 2:253, 1946

BOZEMAN FM et al: Serologic evidence of *Rickettsia canada* infection in man. J Infect Dis 121:367, 1970

—— et al: Epidemic typhus rickettsiae isolated from flying squirrels. Nature 255:545, 1975

DERRICK EH: The epidemiology of Q fever: A review. Med J Aust 1:245, 1953

DESHAZO RD et al: Early diagnosis of Rocky Mountain spotted fever. Use of primary monocyte culture technique. JAMA 235:1353, 1976

FERGUSON IC et al: Clinical, virological and pathological findings in a fatal case of Q fever endocarditis. Br J Clin Pathol 15:235, 1962

GAMBRILL MR, WISSEMAN CL JR: Mechanisms of immunity in typhus infections. Infect Immun 8:519, 1973

HARRELL GT: Rickettsial involvement of the nervous system. Med Clin North Am 37:395, 1953

HATTWICK MAW et al: Rocky Mountain spotted fever: Epidemiology of an increasing problem. Ann Intern Med 84:732, 1976

HAZARD GW et al: Rocky Mountain spotted fever in the Eastern United States. N Engl J Med 280:57, 1969

MARMION BP, STOKER MGP: The epidemiology of Q fever in Great Britian: An analysis of the findings and some conclusions. Br Med J 2:809, 1958

MCKIEL JA et al: *Rickettsia canada:* A new member of the typhus group of rickettsiae isolated from *Haemaphysalis leporis-palustris* ticks in Canada. J Microbiol 12:503, 1967

MOHR CO, SMITH WW: Eradication of murine typhus fever in a rural area. Bull WHO 16:255, 1957

MOULTON FR (ed): *The Rickettsial Diseases of Man.* Washington, DC, American Association for the Advancement of Science, 1948

MURRAY ES et al: Brill's disease: I. Clinical and laboratory diagnosis. JAMA 142:1059, 1950

——, SNYDER JC: Brill's disease: II. Etiology. Am J Hyg 53:22, 1951

ORMSBEE RA et al: The influence of phase on the protective potency of Q fever vaccine. J Immunol 92:404, 1964

—— et al: Serologic diagnosis of epidemic typhus fever. Am J Epidemiol 105:261, 1977

OSTER CN et al: Laboratory acquired Rocky Mountain spotted fever: The hazard of aerosol transmission. N Engl J Med 297:859, 1977

PEDERSEN CE et al: Demonstration of *Rickettsia rickettsii* in Rhesus monkeys by immune fluorescence microscopy. J Clin Microbiol 2:121, 1975

PHILIP RN et al: A comparison of serologic methods for diagnosis of Rocky Mountain spotted fever. Am J Epidemiol 105:56, 1977

PRATT HD: The changing picture of murine typhus in the United States. Ann NY Acad Sci 70:516, 1958

ROSE HM: The clinical manifestations and laboratory diagnosis of rickettsialpox. Ann Intern Med 31:871, 1949

SCHACHTER J et al: Potential danger of Q fever in a university hospital environment. J Infect Dis 123:301, 1971

SCHAFFNER W, KOENIG MG: Thrombocytopenic Rocky Mountain spotted fever. Arch Intern Med 116:857, 1965

SMADEL JE: Influence of antibiotics on immunologic responses in scrub typhus. Am J Med 17:246, 1954

—— (ed): *Symposium on Q Fever,* Medical Science Publication 6. Washington, DC, Walter Reed Army Institute of Research, 1959

——, JACKSON EB: Rickettsial infections, in *Diagnostic Procedures of Viral and Rickettsial Diseases,* 3d ed. New York, American Public Health Association, 1964, p 743

SOMENSHINE DE et al: Epizootiology of epidemic typhus (*Rickettsia prowazekii*) in flying squirrels. Am J Trop Med Hyg 27:339, 1978

VINSON JW: Etiology of trench fever in Mexico, in *Industry and Tropical Health,* vol V. Boston, Harvard School of Public Health, 1964, p 109

WOODWARD TE: Rickettsial diseases in the United States. Med Clin North Am 43:1507, 1959

——: A historical account of the rickettsial diseases with a discussion of unsolved problems. The First Maxwell Finland Lecture. J Infect Dis 127:583, 1973

——: Identification of *Rickettsia* in skin tissues. J Infect Dis 134:297, 1976

section 11 | Mycoplasmal diseases

172
RESPIRATORY INFECTION WITH *MYCOPLASMA PNEUMONIAE*

VERNON KNIGHT

INTRODUCTION The mycoplasmas, formerly called pleuropneumonia-like organisms (PPLO) after the organism that caused a highly contagious form of bovine pneumonia and pleurisy in Europe in the eighteenth century, are now designated class Mollicutes, family Mycoplasmataceae, genus *My-*

coplasma. There are 37 species, 8 of which have been isolated from human beings (Table 172-1).

The only mycoplasma of importance in respiratory disease is *M. pneumoniae. Mycoplasma pneumoniae* grows on peptone-enriched beef-heart infusion broth as small round colonies partially buried in the agar without the "fried egg" periphery characteristic of growth of other mycoplasmas. *Mycoplasma pneumoniae* grows aerobically and anaerobically.

Mycoplasma pneumoniae is resistant to penicillin and antibiotics known to interfere with polymerization of cell wall precursors, and it does not retain the dye-iodine complex of Gram's stain. It is inhibited by tetracyclines, erythromycin, chloramphenicol, and some other antibiotics. Like bacteria, it

TABLE 172-1
The human mycoplasmas

Species	Usual site of occurrence
M. pneumoniae	Respiratory tract
M. salivarium	Oropharynx
M. orale 1	Oropharynx
M. orale 2	Oropharynx
M. orale 3	Oropharynx
M. fermentans	Oropharynx and genital tract (rarely detected)
M. hominis	Genital tract
T-strain mycoplasmas (ureaplasma urealyticum)	

grows outside the cell, possesses ribonucleic and deoxyribonucleic acids, reproduces by fission, and generates metabolic energy.

PNEUMONIA AND RESPIRATORY TRACT DISEASE CAUSED BY MYCOPLASMA PNEUMONIAE
Synonyms are primary atypical pneumonia, Eaton's agent pneumonia, cold agglutinin-positive pneumonia, and "virus" pneumonia.

Definition Pneumonia caused by *M. pneumoniae* is characterized by fever, pharyngitis, cough, and pulmonary infiltration, often multilobular, in which roentgenographic signs are more extensive than indicated by physical examination. This organism also causes upper respiratory illness without pneumonia and asymptomatic infection.

Etiology *Mycoplasma pneumoniae* is distinguished from other mycoplasmas by rapid hemolysis of guinea pig erythrocytes and utilization of glucose and other sugars. It also hemolyzes human and rat erythrocytes. It may also be distinguished from other mycoplasmas by fluorescent antibody, complement fixation, growth inhibition, and indirect hemagglutination tests, all of which are useful for serologic diagnosis of human infection. In addition to growing on agar, the organism grows on the surface of cells of embryonated eggs and monkey kidney cell culture with little evidence of cytopathic effect. In human cell cultures, however, there is intracellular growth with cytopathic effects.

Epidemiology In the general population *M. pneumoniae* infection is characterized by intrafamily spread. In most cases the infection is introduced into the family by a schoolchild. Once it is introduced, most family members become infected. In family outbreaks, pneumonia occurs with greatest frequency among school-age children, with a predominance in males. The disease is rare above age forty. *Mycoplasma pneumoniae* pneumonia occurs throughout the year, although prolonged wintertime outbreaks may occur in college groups or communities. The total incidence of *M. pneumoniae* pneumonia in a study in Seattle was 1.3 per 1000 per year, which constituted about 15 to 20 percent of pneumonia from all causes. At intervals of several years, epidemics of *M. pneumoniae* pneumonia may occur with about double the usual incidence of disease.

In the military, *M. pneumoniae* infections account for a small proportion of upper respiratory illness in recruits—in one study, 6.3 percent. However, it accounted for almost one-half of cases of pneumonia in the same military population. No more than 10 percent of infected military personnel develop pneumonia; the rest are asymptomatic. The disease appears to be endemic at military bases.

Mycoplasma pneumoniae is probably spread by means of infected respiratory secretions. The organisms can be cultured from sputum of naturally occurring cases and from volunteers inoculated artificially. Primary atypical pneumonia has been induced in volunteers both by nasopharyngeal inoculation and by inhalation of a small-particle aerosol containing the agent. In volunteers naturally acquired antibody is associated with a high degree of resistance to infection.

Clinical manifestations The incubation period is from 9 to 12 days, but the interval between cases in families is approximately 3 weeks. Illness usually begins with symptoms of upper respiratory infection, which in some patients progresses to bronchitis and pneumonia. Four syndromes of respiratory disease have been identified: pneumonia, tracheobronchitis, pharyngitis, and bullous myringitis. About one-third of cases in family members will develop pneumonia, up to one-half will have tracheobronchitis, 10 percent exhibit only pharyngitis, and 10 percent will be asymptomatic. Children 5 to 10 years old, especially boys, have the greatest incidence of disease. Ear involvement consisting of congestion of the tympanic membrane and of bullous and, rarely, hemorrhagic myringitis may occur in as many as 10 percent of cases of pneumonia, most often in children. Cough is almost universal in pneumonia and is frequent in cases without pulmonary involvement. Blood-flecked sputum may occur in the more severe cases, but gross hemoptysis is rare. A variety of other respiratory and systemic complaints may occur. Fever, nasal congestion, and sore throat are common. In pneumonia, harsh or diminished sounds are frequent but bronchial breathing is uncommon. Fine inspiratory rales are found in most patients but are not impressive. Pleural rubs and pleural effusion are infrequent. Studies on the distribution of pneumonia in one large series showed that more than one-half of cases were multilobular and slightly less than one-half were bilateral. Lower-lobe pneumonia was appreciably more frequent than upper-lobe pneumonia. Pulmonary infiltrates may occur as an isolated area in the lung periphery but more often spread from the hilum.

The disease is variable in severity, but high fever may persist for 1 to 2 weeks in untreated cases. X-ray changes last for as long as 3 weeks in untreated cases, but for 7 to 10 days in treated cases. Even in untreated cases, complications are rare and consist of occasional purulent sinusitis, persistent cough, and, rarely, pleurisy. Prolonged weakness and malaise follow the untreated illness in adults.

Rare complications include meningoencephalitis, polyneuritis, monoarticular arthritis, Stevens-Johnson syndrome, pericarditis, myocarditis, hepatitis, diffuse intravascular coagulation, and hemolytic anemia. Stevens-Johnson syndrome and other mucocutaneous reactions occur in patients with *M. pneumoniae* pneumonia in the absence of treatment, but the frequency is greatly increased in patients who have received antimicrobial drugs.

Laboratory findings During acute illness leukocytosis in the range of 10,000 to 15,000 leukocytes per cubic millimeter occurs in about 25 percent of cases. Increase in sedimentation rate above 40 mm/h occurs in at least two-thirds of cases. Urinalysis, electrocardiograms, and fluid and electrolyte and liver function studies show no characteristic changes. The complement fixation, fluorescent antibody, indirect hemagglutination, and growth inhibition tests all yield highly specific diagnostic information. The simplicity of the complement fixation text recommends it for general use. Fourfold rises in titer often occur within 2 weeks, and maximum rise is achieved in 4 weeks. A nonspecific test for *M. pneumoniae* infection in use for many years is the detection of cold agglutinins. The end point is the dilution of the patient's serum, which agglutinates human type O red blood cells at 4°C. The test depends on the presence of a macroglobulin antibody to phase I antigen of red blood cells. In *M. pneumoniae* infection, cold agglutinins appear at the end of the first week of illness and disappear in a week or so. The test is positive in a majority of patients, more commonly in those who are severely ill. The cold agglutinin reaction is nonspecific, however, and occurs with other red blood cell antigens in infectious mononucleosis, lymphoproliferative diseases and in several respiratory infections, particularly in children.

Differential diagnosis Pneumonia due to *M. pneumoniae* needs to be distinguished from pneumonia of all other types. It is usually less severe, is associated with less dense pulmonary infiltration than pneumococcal and other bacterial pneumonias, and occurs throughout the year. Pulmonary infiltrate in the absence of symptoms or physical signs may initially suggest acute pulmonary tuberculosis. In military populations adenoviral pneumonia must be excluded. Pneumonic involvement as a direct result of influenza viral infection or its complication by pneumococcal, streptococcal, staphylococcal, or *H. influenzae* infection may cause difficulty in diagnosis. Q fever, psittacosis, and tularemia are less frequent causes of pneumonia that may be difficult to distinguish from *M. pneumoniae* infection. In children, especially young infants, pneumonia due to respiratory syncytial, parainfluenza, adenovirus, and influenza viruses may resemble *M. pneumoniae* infection. Legionnaires' disease (Chap. 138) resembles severe cases of *M. pneumoniae* pneumonia.

Treatment Tetracycline derivatives and erythromycin are effective in treatment of pneumonia due to *M. pneumoniae*. Demethylchlortetracycline may be given to adults in daily doses of 0.9 g; tetracycline, 1.5 g; erythromycin stearate, 1.5 g. Response to treatment is characterized by prompt defervescence, rapid clearing of x-ray signs of pneumonia, and disappearance of malaise and weakness. Persistent cough, despite treatment, is a relatively common finding, especially in women.

Treatment temporarily reduces the frequency of positive cultures from the respiratory tract, but shedding may continue for several weeks after treatment, a finding similar to that in psittacosis pneumonia. Relapse of *M. pneumoniae* pneumonia occurs occasionally, but such cases respond to re-treatment. In cases in which there is doubt between the diagnosis of *M. pneumoniae* and pneumococcal infection, erythromycin should be used in preference to a tetracycline.

Prevention Although antibody is apparently highly protective, effective vaccines are not available. Acutely ill patients should be isolated from very young children and persons in whom a complicating respiratory illness would constitute a special hazard.

REFERENCES

CHERRY JD et al: *Mycoplasma pneumoniae* infections and exanthems. J Pediatr 87:369, 1975

COUCH RB: *Mycoplasma pneumoniae*, in *Viral and Mycoplasmal Infections of the Respiratory Tract*, V Knight (ed). Philadelphia, Lea & Febiger, 1973

FOY HM et al: Viral and mycoplasmal pneumonia in a prepaid medical care group during an eight year period. Am J Epidemiol 97:93, 1973

MCDADE JE et al: Legionnaires' disease. Isolation of a bacterium and demonstration of its role in other respiratory disease. N Engl J Med 297:1197, 1978

section 12 | Chlamydial infections

173
GENERAL CONSIDERATIONS

J. THOMAS GRAYSTON
KING K. HOLMES

The genus *Chlamydia* has two species, *C. trachomatis* and *C. psittaci*. The *C. trachomatis* species includes the two important exclusively human pathogens causing trachoma and lymphogranuloma venereum (LGV). The finding that the trachoma organisms are a major cause of venereal disease has led to a broadening of interest in these organisms in the past decade. The *C. psittaci* species contains a number of strains whose primary hosts are animals and birds. They infect humans as accidental hosts. All organisms in the *Chlamydia* genus have a common heat-stable lipopolysaccharide antigen. The species can be differentiated by inclusion type. The *C. trachomatis* inclusions stain with iodine and are compact, while the *C. psittaci* inclusions fail to stain with iodine and are diffuse. *Chlamydia trachomatis* is sensitive to sulfanomides, while *C. psittaci* is not.

NOMENCLATURE In the past the *Chlamydia* organisms have been known by a variety of names: *Miyagawanella*, *Bedsonia*, and psittacosis-LGV-trachoma (PLT). The trachoma organisms of *C. trachomatis* have also been referred to as *TRIC* (trachoma-inclusion conjunctivitis) *agents*. This terminology is being discarded because of confusion with *Trichomonas*. It is the non-LGV, *C. trachomatis* organisms that cause classic trachoma, nonendemic trachoma, and paratrachoma, inclusion conjunctivitis of both the newborn and the adult, nongonococcal urethritis (NGU), epididymitis, various diseases of the female genital tract (Chap. 174), and a distinctive pneumonia syndrome in infants.

MICROBIOLOGY Until recent years, the *Chlamydia* were considered large viruses because they are obligate, intracellular parasites. While remaining a unique group of microorganisms, they are now considered to be bacterial. They have a discrete cell wall quite similar to those of the gram-negative bacteria, contain both RNA and DNA, multiply by binary fission, and are susceptible to a variety of antimicrobials. Their intracellular parasitism is due to their inability to synthesize adenosine triphosphate (ATP), making them energy parasites.

The complex development cycle of the *Chlamydia* is not fully understood. There are two forms of the organisms: the reticulate (initial) body which is a metabolically active intracellular growth form and the elementary body which is the infectious extracellular form. The elementary body attaches to the surface of the host cell and is actively ingested by endocytosis. *Chlamydia* appears to induce its own phagocytosis. Within 6 to 8 h the elementary body is reorganized into the metabolically active reticulate body which divides continuously by binary fission within the phagosome for 18 to 24 h after infection, after which reticulate bodies reorganize into elementary bodies. The mature intracellular inclusion of *C. trachomatis* is shown in Fig. 173-1, just prior to rupture and dissemination of elementary bodies extracellularly.

IMMUNOTYPES The *C. trachomatis* strains of human origin have been classified immunologically. A total of 15 immunotypes have been identified, using a microimmunofluorescence (micro-IF) test. There are 12 types of trachoma organisms—A, B, Ba, C, D, E, F, G, H, I, J, and K—and three types of LGV organisms—L_1, L_2, and L_3. The three LGV types are closely related to the trachoma types. L_1 and L_2 to B, E, and D, and L_3 to K. Other relationships have been shown among the 15 serotypes. By use of the analogy of senior-junior relationship among influenza viruses, existence of similar associations can be shown among the *C. trachomatis* organisms. The LGV strains are all junior, while the types most often associated with endemic trachoma (B and C) are senior.

BIOLOGICAL CHARACTERISTICS OF LGV VERSUS TRACHOMA
Despite the close immunologic relationship of LGV to trachoma organisms, the former have clearly different biological characteristics. They are lethal when inoculated into mice intracerebrally, while the trachoma agents are not. The LGV agents will grow by cell-to-cell serial transmission in tissue culture, while the trachoma agents require mechanical assistance for good growth.

FIGURE 173-1

Giemsa-stained human conjunctival cells. Three cells have cytoplasmic inclusions of trachoma organisms. Each inclusion is in the late stage of development prior to release of elementary bodies (1000×).

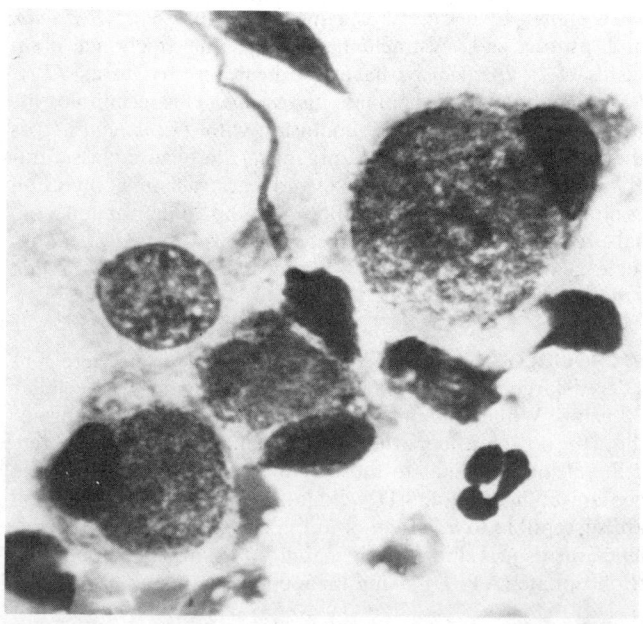

LATENCY OF CHLAMYDIA Latency has been recognized as an important part of the pathogenesis of chlamydial infection in both humans and animals. Psittacosis, LGV, and trachoma are all known to be capable of causing relapsing disease many years after the original infection. Because the organisms are obligate intracellular parasites, they do not simply persist in the body in some nonreplicating form; rather, they remain viable through low levels of multiplication which are held in check by the host's defense mechanisms. An example of this phenomenon is the ability of cortisone eye ointment to precipitate acute trachoma disease in patients with long-dormant eye infection.

PATHOGENESIS Trachoma organisms grow primarily in the columnar epithelium of the conjunctiva, urethra, and cervix. The role of serum and local antibody in *C. trachomatis* infections is uncertain. Similarly, the role of cellular immunity in limiting chlamydial infections or in contributing to its immunopathology remains undefined. The first eye infection with *C. trachomatis* organisms usually results in a self-limited acute papillary and follicular conjunctivitis. The chronic eye pathology of trachoma is thought to be related to an immunopathological response to reinfection. Primates are the only laboratory animals susceptible to eye infection with trachoma organisms.

DIAGNOSIS All diseases caused by *C. trachomatis*, except classic trachoma, require laboratory confirmation for diagnosis. The laboratory procedures include direct microscopic examination for typical intracytoplasmic inclusions or specific antigen, isolation of the organism, and detection of antibody in the serum or in local secretions. Direct microscopic examination of Giemsa- or iodine-stained cell scrapings is inefficient and has a low yield except in neonatal inclusion conjunctivitis. Nevertheless, it may be the only laboratory method available in many areas of the world. Unfortunately, false-positive interpretations by inexperienced observers are common. Direct fluorescent antibody staining of cell smears is more sensitive but is also inefficient and requires as much sophistication as cell culture isolation and serology. Cell culture techniques have replaced the yolk sac of embryonated eggs for isolation of *C. trachomatis*. The cell cultures are much more convenient and are more sensitive, particularly for strains from the genital tract. While LGV strains grow well in many cell lines, the trachoma strains are much more difficult to culture. The most common cell lines used are McCoy cells and HeLa 229 cells. Both cell lines require special pretreatment and centrifugation of the inoculum onto the monolayer for efficient isolation of trachoma strains. Positive cultures are determined by identifying typical intracytoplasmic inclusions stained by Giemsa's, iodine, or immunofluorescent techniques. Isolates may be immunotyped in the micro-IF test.

A complement fixation (CF) test with the heat-stable group-reactive antigen has been used for a long time to diagnose psittacosis and LGV with limited success. It is too insensitive to be useful with non-LGV *C. trachomatis* (trachoma organisms) infections. The micro-IF test with *C. trachomatis* antigens is sensitive and strain-specific. While it has been greatly simplified for diagnostic purposes, it remains available only in research laboratories. The test measures antibodies by immunotype specificity and by immunoglobulin class (IgM, IgG, IgA, secretory IgA) in both serum and local secretions.

ANTIBIOTIC SUSCEPTIBILITY *Chlamydia*, like other bacteria, is susceptible to certain antibiotics. In laboratory tests, death of inoculated mice and chick embryos, as well as growth in cell cultures, is prevented or inhibited by tetracyclines, erythromycin, rosarimicin, choramphenicol, and rifampin; sulfonamides and cycloserine are active against *C. trachomatis* but not *C. psittaci;* bacitracin and polymyxin B are less effective; penicillin and ampicillin suppress *Chlamydia* multiplication but do not eradicate the organisms in vitro. Streptomycin, gentamicin, neomycin, kanamycin, vancomycin, ristocetin, spectinomycin, and nystatin are not effective at concentrations inhibitory for most bacteria and fungi. For treatment of human infection, the tetracyclines and erythromycin are the most useful. The sulfonamides are also effective clinically against *C. trachomatis.*

REFERENCES

GRAYSTON JT, WANG SP: New knowledge of *Chlamydiae* and the diseases they cause. J Infect Dis 132:87, 1975

SCHACHTER J: Medical progress. Chlamydial infections. N Engl J Med 298:428, 490, 540, 1973

174

DISEASES DUE TO *CHLAMYDIA TRACHOMATIS*

KING K. HOLMES
J. THOMAS GRAYSTON
CHANDLER R. DAWSON
PETER L. PERINE

TRACHOMA AND INCLUSION CONJUNCTIVITIS

DEFINITION Trachoma is a chronic conjunctivitis. It is still the most important cause of preventable visual loss, having produced an estimated 20 million cases of blindness throughout the world. Inclusion conjunctivitis is an acute ocular inflammation caused by sexually transmitted chlamydial agents in adults exposed to infected genital secretions and in their newborn offspring.

EPIDEMIOLOGY Epidemiologically, two types of eye disease are caused by the trachoma organisms of the *Chlamydia trachomatis* species. In trachoma-endemic areas where the classic eye disease is seen, transmission is from eye to eye, via hands, towels, flies, etc. In nonendemic areas, the organisms are transmitted from the genital tract to the eye, usually causing only the inclusion conjunctivitis syndrome with or without keratitis. Rarely the eye disease progresses with the development of pannus and scars similar to endemic trachoma. These cases are referred to as *paratrachoma* to differentiate them from eye-to-eye transmitted endemic trachoma.

The worldwide incidence and severity of trachoma have decreased dramatically during the past 30 years in areas with improving hygienic and economic conditions. Endemic trachoma is still the major cause of preventable blindness in North Africa, sub-Saharan Africa, the Middle East, Australia, and parts of Asia. Transmission of the endemic disease occurs primarily through close personal contact, particularly among young children in the affected rural communities. In endemic areas, trachoma is usually associated with repeated exposure, but the infection can also be latent. In the United States a mild form of endemic trachoma still occurs in American Indians and in Mexican Americans as well as in immigrants from areas where trachoma is endemic. Acute relapse of old trachoma may be seen occasionally following treatment with cortisone eye ointment or in very old persons exposed in their youth.

Chlamydia trachomatis eye infection in nonendemic areas is a complication of what is now recognized as one of the most common venereal infections (see "Nongonococcal Urethritis" below). Adult inclusion conjunctivitis and paratrachoma are uncommon complications of genital infections, usually in sexually promiscuous young adults. These sporadic, infrequent eye infections occur following transfer of infected genital discharges to the eye, either on the fingers or by orogenital sexual activities. Newborns become infected by exposure in the infected birth canal of their mothers during delivery.

CLINICAL MANIFESTATIONS Both endemic trachoma and adult inclusion conjunctivitis present initially as a conjunctivitis characterized by small lymphoid follicles in the conjunctiva. In regions with hyperendemic classic blinding trachoma, the disease usually starts insidiously before the age of 2 years. Reinfection is common. The cornea becomes involved with inflammatory leukocytic infiltration and superficial vascularization (pannus formation). As the inflammation continues, there is conjunctival scarring that eventually distorts the eyelids, causing them to turn inward so that the inturned lashes constantly abrade the eyeball (trichiasis and entropion); eventually the corneal epithelium is abraded and may then develop a bacterial corneal ulcer with subsequent corneal scarring and blindness. Destruction of the conjunctival goblet cells, lacrimal ducts, and lacrimal gland may produce a "dry-eye" syndrome with resultant corneal opacity due to drying (xerosis) or secondary bacterial corneal ulcers. Communities with blinding trachoma often experience seasonal epidemics of bacterial conjunctivitis with *Hemophilus influenza* (biotype III or the Koch-Weeks bacillus) and rarely with *Neisseria gonorrhoeae,* which contribute to the intensity of the inflammatory process. In such areas the active infectious process usually resolves spontaneously in affected persons between 10 and 15 years of age, but the conjunctival scars continue to shrink, producing trichiasis and entropion and subsequent corneal scarring in adult life. In areas with milder and less prevalent disease the process may be much slower, with active disease continuing into adulthood; blindness is rare in these cases.

Eye infection with genital *C. trachomatis* strains, usually in sexually active young adults, presents with acute onset of unilateral follicular conjunctivitis and preauricular lymphadenopathy similar to acute adenovirus or herpes virus conjunctivitis. If untreated, the disease may persist for 6 weeks to 2 years. It is frequently associated with corneal inflammation in the form of discrete opacities ("infiltrates"), punctate epithelial erosions, and minor degrees of superficial corneal vascularization. Very rarely conjunctival scarring and eyelid distortion occur, particularly in patients treated for many months with topical corticosteroids. Recurrent eye infections occur most often in patients whose sexual consorts are not treated with antibiotics.

DIAGNOSIS The clinical diagnosis of classic trachoma can be made if two of the following signs are present:

1 Lymphoid follicles on the upper tarsal conjunctiva
2 Typical conjunctival scarring
3 Vascular pannus
4 Limbal follicles or their sequelae, Herbert's pits

For public health purposes, it is necessary to determine whether a substantial proportion of the population has these minimal signs. Public health intervention will depend on the intensity of active inflammatory disease and on the prevalence of blinding or potentially blinding sequelae. In endemic trachoma, laboratory tests to support the clinical diagnosis should be obtained from children with more marked degrees of inflammation. Intracytoplasmic chlamydial inclusions occur in 10 to 60 percent of Giemsa-stained conjunctival smears in such populations, but isolation in cell cultures is more sensitive. Follicular conjunctivitis in adult Europeans or Americans living in trachomatous regions is rarely trachoma, although their children may acquire mild, nonblinding trachoma.

Sporadic cases of adult inclusion conjunctivitis must be differentiated from adenovirus and herpes simplex virus keratoconjunctivitis during the first 15 days after onset, and later from other forms of chronic follicular conjunctivitis. Laboratory demonstration of chlamydial infection by Giemsa- or immunofluorescent-stained smears or by isolation in cell cultures constitutes definitive evidence of infection, but only a few laboratories carry out these procedures. Serologic demonstration of antibody in serum cannot be taken as evidence of eye infection with chlamydial agents, since so many sexually active young adults have serum antibody titers. A practical diagnostic procedure in cases with chronic follicular conjunctivitis is treatment for 6 days with an oral tetracycline or erythromycin; a marked symptomatic response within 3 to 4 days is highly suggestive of inclusion conjunctivitis, and treatment should be continued for at least 3 weeks.

DIFFERENTIAL DIAGNOSIS Several viral eye infections should be considered in the differential diagnosis of trachoma and inclusion conjunctivitis. The eye and its adnexa may be infected during the course of many cutaneous and systemic viral diseases. Sometimes these ocular infections produce minor manifestations, such as the transient loss of accommodation of dengue and the milder forms of conjunctivitis in systemic adenovirus infections. Other virus infections, however, such as herpes simplex (Chap. 193), herpes zoster (Chap. 185), measles (Chap. 181), and vaccinia or smallpox (Chap. 184), occasionally produce serious and permanent visual loss. In addition, congenital viral infections are an important cause of blindness, particularly rubella, which leads to cataracts, microphthalmus, and cytomegalic inclusion disease with retinal involvement.

Among the viral infections limited to the outer eye and manifested as a follicular conjunctivitis are epidemic keratoconjunctivitis, herpes simplex keratoconjunctivitis, Newcastle disease virus (NDV) conjunctivitis, and acute hemorrhagic conjunctivitis.

Epidemic keratoconjunctivitis (EKC) Adenovirus types 8 and 19 are the usual cause of epidemics of EKC, although milder cases may be associated with other adenovirus types. The most common method for transmission of EKC is through manipulation of the eye by medical personnel, e.g., for foreign-body removal in industrial dispensaries (thus the name "shipyard eye") or during an ophthalmologic examination. The virus, which is unusually resistant to inactivation, is transmitted on the fingers, by instruments, or in solutions. Medical personnel not infrequently contract the disease and may act as a source of infection for patients.

Following an incubation period of 5 to 12 days, EKC presents a moderate to very severe follicular conjunctivitis with preauricular lymphadenopathy that is usually unilateral at onset. Severe cases may have subconjunctival hemorrhages and conjunctival membrane formation with subsequent conjunctival scarring. In adults, the associated systemic manifestations are minimal with little if any fever, headache, or malaise, but in children adenovirus type 8 infections may present as febrile upper respiratory disease, or otitis media, with only a minor conjunctivitis; such children may be a source of infection for adults. In EKC, the usual onset of focal corneal involvement is 7 days after onset of conjunctivitis when there is a severe foreign-body sensation, photophobia, and lacrimation. As the conjunctivitis subsides during the second week of the disease,

subepithelial corneal opacities 1 to 2 mm in diameter appear, and these opacities may persist for 2 years or longer.

There is no specific treatment for the acute stage of EKC, but the late opacities can be suppressed temporarily with topical corticosteroids if vision is impaired. Explosive epidemics in industrial dispensaries and ophthalmologists' offices can be prevented or controlled by scrupulous hand washing, adequate cleansing of instruments, and replacement of eye drops to break the chain of infection. Medical personnel with conjunctivitis should not come into contact with patients.

Herpes simplex virus (HSV) keratoconjunctivitis Occasionally HSV produces an acute follicular conjunctivitis that is usually accompanied by one or multiple herpetic skin vesicles on the eyelids. In children this may be the primary herpetic infection, but in adults the conjunctivitis is often a recurrent herpetic infection at a new site. The skin lesions may be inconspicuous, misdiagnosed as a sty, or even not present, so that the disease is indistinguishable from early EKC. The cornea may have focal epithelial lesions, a typical linear, branching (dendritic) ulcer, or no involvement at all. The conjunctivitis usually resolves in 2 weeks. If definite herpetic lid lesions are present or if HSV is isolated, treatment with a topical antiviral (idoxuridine, adenine arabinoside, or trifluorothymidine) should be given three to four times daily to prevent corneal involvement. Overt dendritic ulcerations or other corneal involvement should be treated more vigorously as described in Chap. 193. Topical corticosteroids should not be used in acute HSV infections of the eye except in rare instances and then under frequent supervision by an ophthalmologist.

Newcastle disease virus conjunctivitis Human infection with this avian virus, which is related to influenza, occurs mainly in poultry workers, veterinarians, and virologists. In humans, accidental introduction of contaminated material from naturally infected animals or from live virus (e.g., vaccines) is followed in 24 to 72 h by conjunctivitis, edema of the lids, and tearing. Systemic symptoms occur very rarely, and recovery is complete in 10 to 14 days. The diagnosis may be confirmed by virus isolation in embryonated eggs.

Acute hemorrhagic conjunctivitis (AHC) This disease was first described in 1969 in epidemics in Africa and Asia. It presents as an acute conjunctivitis with numerous punctate hemorrhages on the bulbar conjunctiva which become confluent within 24 h. There is also minor involvement of the cornea. The inflammation subsides in 4 to 5 days, but the hemorrhages do not resolve for 7 to 10 days. The only reported complication has been the rare occurrence of lumbar radiculomyelitis with resultant flaccid paralysis like poliomyelitis. Enterovirus 70 (a member of the picornavirus group) has been identified as the etiologic agent in most epidemics, but some outbreaks have been caused by coxsackievirus A24, another picornavirus. Epidemics of AHC have occurred in the crowded urban populations of developing countries, affecting all age groups and social classes. Occasional outbreaks in Europe have been centered around eye clinics. The disease has not been reported in the Western Hemisphere.

TREATMENT *Chlamydia trachomatis* strains are susceptible to the sulfonamides, tetracyclines, and erythromycin. Public health control programs for endemic trachoma consist of the mass application of tetracycline or erythromycin ointment to the eyes of all children in affected communities for 21 to 60 days or on an intermittent schedule. These programs also include surgical correction of inturned eyelids by a mobile surgical team that visits each locality. At one time systemic sulfonamides for 3 weeks were utilized, but the rate of untoward reactions was unacceptably high. Oral erythromycin, but not oral tetracyclines, offers a useful alternative method of mass antibiotic treatment for trachoma of young children and pregnant women.

Adult inclusion conjunctivitis responds well to treatment with full doses of systemic tetracycline or erythromycin for 3 weeks. Treating all sexual consorts of the patient simultaneously is also necessary to prevent ocular reinfection and to avoid the genital diseases due to chlamydial infection. Topical antibiotic treatment is not required in patients treated with systemic antibiotics.

PREVENTION Efforts to develop a practical trachoma vaccine have not been successful. General hygienic measures associated with improved living standards are effective in the elimination of trachoma. Adequate water supply for personal cleanliness may be a key factor. In some areas the reduction of flies in the household is important. In order to prevent spread of trachoma to uninfected family members, treatment of healthy contacts with antibiotic ointment may be effective.

NONGONOCOCCAL URETHRITIS AND OTHER GENITAL INFECTIONS

SPECTRUM OF *C. TRACHOMATIS* GENITAL INFECTIONS In adults the newly defined clinical spectrum of sexually transmitted *C. trachomatis* infections is easily understood because it parallels exactly the spectrum of gonococcal infections (Table 174-1). Although the causal role of *C. trachomatis* is not firmly established, both agents have been associated with urethritis, epididymitis, mucopurulent cervicitis, acute salpingitis, bartholinitis, and the Fitz-Hugh–Curtis syndrome (perihepatitis), and both can be associated with systemic complications, particularly with arthritis. The etiologic significance of *C. trachomatis* infection in certain of these syndromes, such as the Fitz-Hugh–Curtis syndrome and Reiter's syndrome, requires further study. The possible role of *C. trachomatis* in idiopathic proctitis in homosexual men and in women remains to be defined.

EPIDEMIOLOGY Genital infections other than LGV are caused by *C. trachomatis* immunotypes D through K. Although data are lacking, the incidence of genital *C. trachomatis* infection is probably increasing, since the incidence of nongonococcal urethritis (NGU) has risen dramatically over the last two decades, and *C. trachomatis* has consistently been isolated from 30 to 50 percent of men with NGU. The peak age incidence of genital *C. trachomatis* infections is in the late teens and early twenties, resembling other sexually transmitted infections. Further evidence for sexual transmission is the rising prevalence of serum antibody to *C. trachomatis* in proportion to an increasing number of sex partners of infected individuals. In the United States, the prevalence of *C. trachomatis* in the cervix of pregnant women is five to ten times higher than that of *N. gonorrhoeae*. The prevalence of genital infection with either agent is highest in individuals who are indigent, nonwhite, unmarried, and between ages 18 and 24. The ratio of chlamydial to gonococcal urethritis is highest for heterosexual men and those with high socioeconomic status, and lowest for homosexual men and indigent populations. The ratio of symptomatic to asymptomatic infections appears to be lower for *C. trachomatis* than for *N. gonorrhoeae*, as does the clinical severity of symptomatic infections. However, because the total number of *C. trachomatis* infections exceeds that of *N. gonorrhoeae* infections in industrialized countries, the total morbidity caused by *C. trachomatis* genital infections is comparable with that caused by *N. gonorrhoeae*. The prevalence of *C. trachomatis* is higher than that of *N. gonorrhoeae* in industrialized countries, in part because measures such as treatment of sex partners and routine cultures for case detection in asympto-

matic individuals are being applied much more effectively for gonorrhea control than for control of *C. trachomatis* infection.

Nongonococcal and postgonococcal urethritis Nongonococcal urethritis is a diagnosis of exclusion that is applied to men with symptoms and/or signs of urethritis who do not have gonorrhea. Postgonococcal urethritis (PGU) refers to nongonococcal urethritis which develops 2 to 3 weeks after treatment of gonococcal urethritis in men. *Chlamydia trachomatis* causes 30 to 50 percent of the cases of NGU and PGU. The cause of the remainder is uncertain, although considerable evidence suggests that *Ureaplasma urealyticum* causes an additional 30 to 40 percent.

DIAGNOSIS The most suitable method for diagnosis of *C. trachomatis* urethritis is isolation of the agent in tissue cell culture. It is necessary to insert an endourethral swab 1 to 2 cm into the urethra to obtain an adequate specimen, since cultures of expressed exudate lack sensitivity, as do direct Giemsa-stained or immunofluorescent smears. Serologic techniques are as difficult to perform as culture, and serologic diagnosis by microimmunofluorescence (micro-IF) testing of serum requires demonstration of IgM antibody (lacking in the many patients who have previously experienced infection with the same immunotype) or a fourfold rise in antibody titer in paired serums. Because *C. trachomatis* infections are often mild, many patients do not seek therapy until it is too late to demonstrate a rise in antibody titer. Serologic techniques, therefore, often cannot differentiate current from past infections.

Where culture is not available, current practice is to diagnose NGU by documentation of a leukocytic urethral exudate and by exclusion of gonorrhea by Gram's stain or culture, rather than to pursue a specific etiologic diagnosis of NGU. *Chlamydia trachomatis* urethritis is generally less severe than gonococcal urethritis, although in an individual patient these two forms of urethritis cannot be differentiated solely on clinical grounds. Symptoms include urethral discharge, dysuria, and urethral itching, and there are meatal erythema and tenderness and a urethral exudate which is often demonstrable only by stripping the urethra in the morning before voiding. A substantial proportion of men with *C. trachomatis* urethral infection have no demonstrable signs and may or may not have symptoms of urethritis. An estimated 5 to 10 percent of male STD clinic patients have asymptomatic *C. trachomatis* urethral infection. Such patients frequently have first glass pyuria (15 leukocytes per 400× microscopic field in the sediment of first-

TABLE 174-1
Similarity of clinical manifestations of sexually transmitted infections caused by *Neisseria gonorrhoeae* and *Chlamydia trachomatis*

Site of infection	N. gonorrhoeae	C. trachomatis
MALE		
Urethra	Urethritis	Urethritis
Epididymis	Epididymitis	Epididymitis
Systemic	Disseminated gonococcal infection	Reiter's syndrome
FEMALE		
Cervix	Cervicitis	Cervicitis
Salpinx	Salpingitis	Salpingitis
Urethra	Urethritis	Urethral syndrome
Bartholin's gland	Bartholin's gland abscess	Bartholin's gland abscess

voided early morning urine) or an increased number of leukocytes on gram-stained smear prepared from a urogenital swab inserted 1 to 2 cm into the anterior urethra. The smear is first scanned at low power to identify areas of the slide containing the highest concentrations of leukocytes. These areas are then examined under oil immersion (1000×). An average of four leukocytes in five 1000× (oil immersion) fields is indicative of urethritis and correlates with recovery of *C. trachomatis*. To differentiate between true urethritis and functional symptoms among symptomatic patients, or to make a presumptive diagnosis of *C. trachomatis* infection in asymptomatic men [e.g., male patients in sexually transmitted disease (STD) clinics, sex partners of women with nongonococcal salpingitis or mucopurulent cervicitis, fathers of children with inclusion conjunctivitis], the examination of an endourethral specimen for increased leukocytes is useful.

Epididymitis *Chlamydia trachomatis* is also a cause of epididymitis in sexually active males. In one study, *C. trachomatis* infection was found by cultures of the urethra, urine, semen, or epididymal aspirate or by serology in 11 of 13 men under 35, but in 1 of 10 over 35 who presented with epididymitis. Coliform bacteria and *Pseudomonas aeruginosa* are the most common causes of epididymitis in men over 35. The presence of a urethral discharge in association with epididymitis suggests the diagnosis of chlamydial or gonococcal epididymitis, whereas the presence of midstream pyuria and bacteriuria in an older patient without urethral discharge suggests coliform or *Pseudomonas* infection.

Reiter's syndrome In recent studies, *C. trachomatis* has been recovered from the urethra from up to 70 percent of men with untreated Reiter's syndrome who have associated urethritis. This striking association is unexplained.

Genital *C. trachomatis* infection in women As with gonococcal infection, in recent studies *C. trachomatis* has been isolated from the cervix of 30 to 60 percent of women with gonorrhea, or contact with gonorrhea, from 10 to 20 percent of women attending sexually transmitted disease clinics who do not have a history of contact with a partner with urethritis, and from about 5 percent of United States college students, or young women attending gynecology clinics or prenatal clinics.

CERVICITIS Although many women with *C. trachomatis* cervical infection have a normal cervix or only nonspecific changes, there is a significant correlation of this infection with endocervicitis, manifested by mucopurulent exudate in the cervical os. A distinctive pattern of hypertrophic (edematous and congested) cervical erythema and increased friability also may be seen. Herpes simplex virus causes inflammation and ulceration of the exocervix, rather than of the endocervix alone, but can be confused with gonococcal or chlamydial cervicitis. The presence of mucopurulent endocervicitis suggests the presence of *C. trachomatis* or *N. gonorrhoeae* infection. If tests for gonorrhea are negative, nongonococcal endocervicitis should be treated with tetracycline, just as nongonococcal urethritis is treated, and male sex partners should be examined for NGU.

SALPINGITIS AND PERIHEPATITIS *Chlamydia trachomatis* has recently been implicated as a cause of acute salpingitis. In one study, it was isolated from the cervix of 19 of 53 women with acute salpingitis verified by laparoscopy, and it was recovered from the fallopian tube in the absence of other pathogens from six of seven who had *C. trachomatis* in the cervix.

A related development is the demonstration of IgM antibody to *C. trachomatis,* suggestive of recent *C. trachomatis* infection, in 7 of 11 women with acute peritonitis and or perihepatitis (Fitz-Hugh–Curtis syndrome).

OTHER MANIFESTATIONS *Chlamydia trachomatis* has also been isolated from the rectum of 10 percent of women with genital chlamydial infection and from pus expressed from Bartholin's gland in association with bartholinitis. Other data suggest that *C. trachomatis* is a cause of some cases of the urethral syndrome in women.

CHLAMYDIA TRACHOMATIS INFECTION IN PREGNANCY *Chlamydia trachomatis* infection in pregnant women entails a risk of transmitting infection to the neonate. *Chlamydia trachomatis* in pregnancy also has been associated with fetal wastage and with a high risk of postpartum endometritis and salpingitis. Whether these complications are attributable to *C. trachomatis* remains to be determined. If so, detection and treatment of *C. trachomatis* in the mother and father early during pregnancy may be particularly important.

THERAPY OF GENITAL *C. TRACHOMATIS* INFECTION Therapy of *C. trachomatis* urethritis is more effective than therapy of other forms of NGU. *Chlamydia trachomatis* is eradicated from the urethra by treatment with tetracycline hydrochloride, 500 mg four times daily for 7 days. Alternative regimens which are also effective include erythromycin, 500 mg four times daily for 14 days, and sulfisoxazole, 500 mg four times daily for 10 days. However, sulfonamides are not effective for *Chlamydia*-negative NGU. Minocycline and doxycycline are more active than tetracycline against *C. trachomatis* in vitro and are effective clinically in a dose of 100 mg daily for 7 days. *Chlamydia trachomatis* is not reliably eradicated by single-dose therapy with any antimicrobial.

Eradication of *C. trachomatis* from the cervix has been demonstrated with similar doses of tetracycline and erythromycin. Erythromycin base, 500 mg four times daily for 7 to 10 days, is the regimen of choice for pregnant women with *C. trachomatis* infection. Tetracycline hydrochloride, 500 mg four times daily for 10 days, produces clinical and microbiological cure of epididymitis or salpingitis associated with *C. trachomatis* infection.

Treatment of sex partners The increase in genital *C. trachomatis* infections is related in part to changes in sexual behavior, but probably is also due to failure of the medical profession to diagnose and treat *C. trachomatis* infections in symptomatic patients or their sexual partners. Cases of NGU,' epididymitis, Reiter's syndrome, and mucopurulent endocervicitis are frequently not treated with antimicrobials, and sex partners are treated even less often. Furthermore, even though 20 percent of men and 30 to 60 percent of women with gonorrhea have concurrent *C. trachomatis* infection, only one of the four treatment regimens recommended by the Center for Disease Control for gonorrhea (tetracycline, but not single-dose procaine penicillin G, ampicillin, or spectinomycin) eradicates *C. trachomatis*. *Chlamydia trachomatis* urethral or cervical infection has been well documented in the sex partners of patients with NGU, epididymitis, Reiter's syndrome, salpingitis, or endocervicitis. This is analogous to the problem of asymptomatic gonococcal infection in sex partners of patients with gonorrhea. In the absence of facilities for specific diagnosis of *C. trachomatis* infection, sex partners of patients with symptoms that are attributable to *C. trachomatis* infection should be examined and counseled. Those partners who themselves have clinical evidence of *C. trachomatis* infection clearly should be treated with an effective antimicrobial. Even those without evidence of clinical disease, who have been recently exposed to possible chlamydial infection (e.g., NGU), should probably also be offered therapy.

NEONATAL INCLUSION CONJUNCTIVITIS AND PNEUMONIA

EPIDEMIOLOGY Several studies in the United States have found *C. trachomatis* infections of the cervix in from 5 to 13 percent of pregnant women. In these studies from 3 to 6 percent of the newborn children showed laboratory evidence of *C. trachomatis* infection. Roughly half of the infants born to mothers with cervical infection developed laboratory evidence of infection, and half of these (or 25 percent of the group exposed) developed clinical inclusion conjunctivitis. In addition to eye infection, the *C. trachomatis* organisms were isolated frequently and persistently from the nasopharynx and even the rectum. Pneumonia and otitis media have also been shown to result from these birth canal infections.

INCLUSION CONJUNCTIVITIS OF THE NEWBORN (INCLUSION BLENNORRHEA)

In the newborn, inclusion conjunctivitis can be differentiated from gonococcal ophthalmia by its longer incubation period (5 to 14 days versus 1 to 3 days). The other common causes of conjunctivitis in newborns include *Staphylococcus aureus*, *Hemophilus influenza*, and herpes simplex virus. Neonatal inclusion conjunctivitis has an acute onset and produces a profuse mucopurulent discharge with membrane formation and occasional scar formation on the conjunctiva. Inclusions within epithelial cells usually can be demonstrated in Giemsa-stained conjunctival smears. Relapses of the eye disease are frequent following treatment with topical tetracycline ophthalmic ointment. The therapy recommended is oral erythromycin (40 to 50 mg per kilogram of body weight) for 2 to 3 weeks. Rarely a trachoma-like eye disease with chlamydial infection occurs in children living in nonendemic areas and probably is the late result of neonatally acquired infection.

INFANT PNEUMONIA There is a distinctive pneumonia syndrome in infants infected with *C. trachomatis*, which appears to occur in two to six cases per 1000 live births. This pneumonia has been found in infants from 1 to 4 months of age. The onset is gradual and the course protracted, but the child is usually afebrile. There is diffuse interstitial involvement of the lungs. Most of the infants have a distinctive cough (a series of closely spaced staccato coughs, each separated by a brief inspiration), tachypnea, rales, hyperinflation, slight eosinophilia, and elevated serum immunoglobulins. Clinical illness lasts several weeks, while inspiratory rales and radiological signs may persist for months. About half of the infants with pneumonia also have conjunctivitis. While many of the pneumonia cases have recovered without therapy, a few have been severe. The diagnosis of *C. trachomatis* pneumonia has been confirmed by isolation of the organisms from lung biopsy. A probable diagnosis can be made by isolation of organisms from the nasopharynx, eye, or rectum, and by demonstration of a rising titer of IgG antibody (passively acquired maternal antibody will decrease) or by the presence of specific IgM antibody. Specific treatment with oral systemic erythromycin should be accompanied by supportive measures. Because *C. trachomatis* causes disease in adults, both parents should be treated with systemic erythromycin (especially nursing mothers) or tetracyclines.

LYMPHOGRANULOMA VENEREUM

DEFINITION Lymphogranuloma venereum (LGV) is a sexually transmitted infection caused by *C. trachomatis*. The acute disease in men is characterized by a transient primary genital lesion followed by multilocular suppurative regional lymphadenopathy. Women, homosexual men, and occasionally, heterosexual men may develop hemorrhagic proctocolitis with regional lymphadenitis. Acute LGV is almost always associated

with nonspecific systemic symptoms, usually with fever and leukocytosis, and rarely with systemic complications such as meningoencephalitis. After a latent period of years, late complications include genital elephantiasis, strictures, and fistulas of the penis, urethra, and rectum.

ETIOLOGY Only three immunotypes of *C. trachomatis*, designated L_1, L_2, and L_3, cause LGV, with L_2 being most common. LGV immunotypes also have other distinguishing biological characteristics: they are more invasive than the other immunotypes of *C. trachomatis*, cause disease primarily in lymphatic tissue, grow more readily in tissue culture, and are pathogenic when inoculated intracerebrally into mice and monkeys.

EPIDEMIOLOGY Lymphogranuloma venereum usually is sexually transmitted, but occasional transmission by nonsexual personal contact, fomites, or laboratory accidents has been documented. The peak incidence corresponds to the age of greatest sexual activity, the second and third decades of life. The worldwide incidence of LGV is falling, for unexplained reasons, but the disease is still endemic and a major cause of morbidity in certain countries of Asia, Africa, and South America. In the United States, only 348 cases were reported during 1977, of which about one-third were from Washington, D.C.

Prevalence studies of LGV are difficult to interpret. Most have employed the Frei skin test or LGV complement fixation (CF) serologic test. Since the antigens used in these tests cross-react with other strains of *C. trachomatis* which are much more widely prevalent in developed countries than the three LGV strains, the specificity of the Frei and LGV CF tests is open to question. For example, 18 percent of patients attending a STD clinic had positive skin tests and 2 percent had high LGV titers, but only 1 percent had signs of LGV. Of the cases reported to the Center for Disease Control in 1977, many were based on the LGV CF test and could not be confirmed by the more specific microimmunofluorescence test.

The frequency of infection following exposure is believed to be much less than that associated with gonorrhea and syphilis. Early manifestations are recognized far more often in men than in women, who usually present with late complications. In the United States, where the reported sex ratio is 3.4 males to 1 female, most cases involve travelers, seamen, and military personnel returning from abroad; male homosexuals; and individuals of low socioeconomic status living in areas of low endemicity in the Southeast. The main reservoir of infection in the United States is presumed to be asymptomatically infected individuals, but attempts to isolate LGV strains from the urethra or cervix of sexually active persons without clinical LGV have been unsuccessful.

CLINICAL MANIFESTATIONS A *primary genital lesion* occurs from 3 days to 3 weeks after exposure. It is a small, painless vesicle or nonindurated ulcer or papule located on the penis in men or on the labia, posterior vagina, or fourchette in women. The primary lesion is noticed by less than one-third of men with LGV and only rarely by women. It heals in a few days without scarring and even when noticed is not recognized as LGV except in retrospect when it is followed by or merges with lymphadenitis. LGV strains of *C. trachomatis* have occasionally been recovered from the male urethra and the endocervix of patients who present with inguinal adenopathy, suggesting that these areas may be the primary site of infection in some cases.

In women and homosexual men, *primary anorectal infection* occurs following rectal intercourse. In women, this may also occur by spread via the pelvic lymphatics, or by direct spread of infection from the genitalia along the perineum to the anal canal. Anorectal colonization also occurs in women with cervical infections and in homosexual men. After an incubation period of unknown length, multiplication within intestinal epithelial cells leads to symptoms which include mucopurulent or bloody anal discharge, tenesmus, and diarrhea. Sigmoidoscopy reveals diffuse proctitis or discrete ulcerations limited to the rectosigmoid colon.

From the site of the primary infection, the organism spreads via the regional lymphatics. Penile, vulvar, and, occasionally, anal infection can lead to inguinal and femoral lymphadenitis. Anorectal infection produces hypogastric and deep iliac lymphadenitis. Upper vaginal or cervical infection results in enlargement of the obturator and iliac nodes. The most common presenting picture in heterosexual men is the *inguinal syndrome.* This also occurs in about 10 percent of men with anorectal infection. It is characterized by painful inguinal lymphadenopathy beginning 2 to 6 weeks after presumed exposure; rarely the onset occurs after a few months. The inguinal adenopathy is unilateral in two-thirds of cases, and palpable enlargement of the iliac and femoral nodes is often present on the same side as the enlarged inguinal nodes. The nodes are initially discrete, but progressive periadenitis results in a matted mass of nodes which become fluctuant and suppurative. The overlying skin becomes fixed, inflamed, and thinned and finally develops multiple draining fistulas. Extensive enlargement of chains of inguinal nodes above and below the inguinal ligament ("the sign of the groove") is characteristic but is present in only a minority of cases (Fig. 174-1). Histological involvement of nodes initially shows characteristic small stellate abscesses surrounded by histiocytes. These abscesses coalesce to cause large, necrotic, suppurative foci. Spontaneous healing usually occurs after several months, leaving inguinal scars or granulomatous masses of varying size which persist for life. Massive pelvic lymphadenopathy in women or homosexual men may lead to exploratory laparotomy.

Constitutional symptoms are common during the state of regional lymphadenopathy and include fever, chills, headache, meningismus, anorexia, myalgias, and arthralgias. These findings in the presence of lymphadenopathy are often mistaken

FIGURE 174-1
Lymphogranuloma venereum. Bilateral inguinal buboes, with the "sign of the groove," caused by adenopathy above and below Poupart's ligament. (Courtesy of A Brathwaite.)

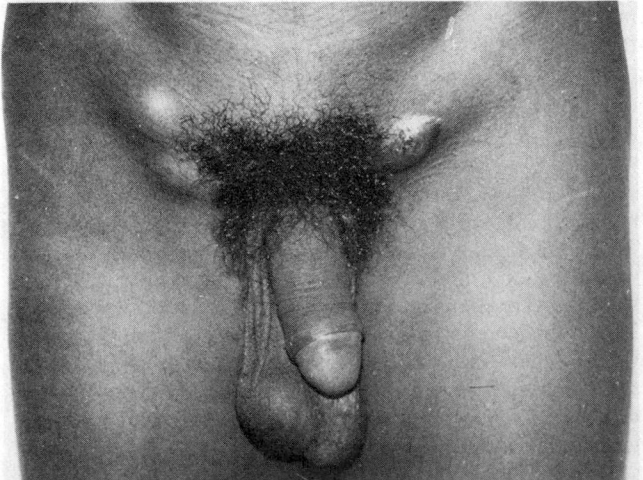

for malignant lymphoma. Other systemic complications are infrequent but include arthritis with sterile effusion, aseptic meningitis, meningoencephalitis, conjunctivitis, hepatitis, and erythema nodosum. Chlamydiae have been recovered from the cerebrospinal fluid, and in one case from the blood in a patient with severe constitutional symptoms, indicating the occurrence of disseminated infection. Associated laboratory findings during the acute stage of infection include leukocytosis and mild elevation of the sedimentation rate. Abnormal liver function tests, hyperglobulinemia, mixed cryoglobulinemia, rheumatoid factor activity, and elevated IgG, IgA, and IgM have been reported in subacute and chronic LGV. False-positive serologic tests for syphilis are rare, and syphilis should be suspected if these tests are positive, as is often the case.

Complications of anorectal infection include perirectal abscess, fistula in ano, and rectovaginal, rectovesical, and ischiorectal fistulas. Secondary bacterial infection probably contributes to these complications. Rectal stricture is a late complication of anorectal infection and usually occurs 2 to 6 cm from the anal orifice, within reach on digital rectal examination. The stricture may extend proximally for several centimeters, leading to a mistaken clinical and radiographic diagnosis of carcinoma.

Approximately 5 percent of cases of LGV in men present with chronic progressive infiltrative, ulcerative, or fistular lesions of the penis, urethra, or scrotum. Urethral stricture may occur and usually involves the posterior urethra, causing incontinence or difficulty with micturition.

An uncommon late complication of LGV is *genital elephantiasis,* a chronic induration and edema of the penis or vulva caused by lymphatic obstruction. Polypoid swelling of the skin and large stellate hyperplastic keloidal scars of the genitalia may be associated with vulvar induration or lymphedema and are difficult to distinguish clinically from granuloma inguinale and genital tuberculosis. Chronic ulcerations of the vulva (esthiomene) and smooth pedunculated perianal growths (lymphorrhoids) also occur. The significance of reports of malignant changes associated with chronic anorectal or genital LGV is uncertain.

DIAGNOSIS Although LGV is uncommon, it frequently enters the differential diagnosis of common conditions such as inguinal lymphadenopathy; vesicular, papular, or ulcerative genital lesions; and perirectal abscess, fistula in ano, or proctocolitis. When methods for culture and serodiagnosis become more available, diagnostic testing for LGV in these conditions should increase.

The most reliable method of diagnosis is isolation of an LGV strain of *Chlamydia* from aspirated bubo pus or from the urethra, endocervix, or infected tissue. Isolation has been possible from bubo pus in about 30 percent of cases with both clinical and serologic evidence of LGV. The methods needed for isolation in tissue cell culture are widely available but seldom used. The most widely used immunodiagnostic tests have been the LGV complement fixation test and the Frei skin tests. The LGV complement fixation test becomes positive (serum titer ≥ 1:32) shortly after the bubo first appears and is positive in 80 to 90 percent of patients with the inguinal syndrome. The titer may not increase in paired serums since most patients have already been infected for several weeks when first seen. The Frei skin test is less sensitive than the LGV complement fixation test. It is performed by intradermal inoculation of 0.1 ml of a crude antigen prepared from infected yolk sac into the flexor surface of the forearm. The test is read at 72 h and is positive (≥ 6 mm induration and erythema at the site of antigen inoculation, with no induration at the site of normal yolk sac control inoculation) in less than 50 percent of patients who present with the inguinal syndrome. The frequency of positive skin tests increases with the duration of untreated infection, and positive tests remain positive for life. *A negative Frei test does not exclude the diagnosis of LGV*. Conversely, a positive LGV complement fixation test or Frei skin test may not be specific for LGV. When other causes of inguinal or pelvic lymphadenopathy are suspected clinically, a positive Frei or LGV CF result should not unduly delay definitive diagnostic testing, which often means lymph node aspiration or excisional biopsy.

However, two serologic tests for LGV have been developed which appear to be both sensitive and specific. Limited experience indicates that the microimmunofluorescent antibody test developed by Wang detects antibody to *C. trachomatis* in nearly all patients with culture-proved LGV. Serum microimmunofluorescent antibody titers from patients with LGV exceed the highest titers that occur in chlamydial NGU and can usually be shown to be directed against immunotypes L_1, L_2, or L_3. A counterimmunoelectrophoresis test has also been developed using the soluble *C. trachomatis*-specific antigen extracted from the LGV strain. This test is positive in over 95 percent of patients whose microimmunofluorescent test shows antibody to LGV strain, but is negative in patients with chlamydial NGU. The histopathology of excised nodes or of rectal biopsy specimens is seldom definitive, but suggestive findings may raise the question of LGV and lead to more specific tests.

TREATMENT LGV chlamydiae are susceptible in vitro to the tetracyclines, sulfonamides, erythromycin, rifampin, and chloramphenicol and are slightly sensitive to the penicillins. They are resistant to the aminoglycosides such as streptomycin, as well as to bacitracin, vancomycin, and the polymyxins. Occasional isolates have been resistant to sulfonamides. Despite their in vitro activity, antibiotics do not have a dramatic effect on the duration and healing of inguinal buboes. However, acute constitutional symptoms are often terminated abruptly. Antibiotics are usually not helpful in improving late complications such as rectal stricture or genital elephantiasis unless secondary infection is also present. Genital elephantiasis and rectal, penile, and urethral strictures and fistulas require surgical correction, although sometimes urethral and even rectal strictures can be managed by repeated mechanical dilation.

The recommended treatment regimen is tetracycline hydrochloride, 0.5 g four times a day for 3 or 4 weeks. A sulfonamide preparation, 4 g per day for 3 or 4 weeks, can also be used, but occasional isolates have been resistant to sulfonamides in vitro. Fluctuant buboes should be aspirated through normal skin with a syringe and 18-gauge needle as often as necessary to prevent spontaneous rupture. It is not unusual for buboes to increase in size or to develop at another site after initiation of treatment. Although these seldom progress to fistula formation, they should be aspirated if fluctuant. A fourfold or greater fall in complement fixation titer occurs in most treated patients, and LGV *Chlamydia* cannot be isolated from lesions after the initiation of antibiotic treatment.

REFERENCES

General

SCHACHTER J, DAWSON CR: *Human Chlamydial Infections.* Littleton, Mass, PSG Medical Books, 1978

Lymphogranuloma venereum

ABRAMS AJ: Lymphogranuloma venereum. JAMA 205:199, 1968

CALDWELL HD, KUO CC: Serologic diagnosis of lymphogranuloma venereum by counterimmunoelectrophoresis with a *Chlamydia trachomatis* antigen. J Immunol 118:442, 1977

GREAVES AB: The frequency of lymphogranuloma venereum in persons with perirectal abscesses, fistula-in-ano, or both. Bull WHO 29:797, 1963

HOPSU-HAVU VK, SONCK CE: Infiltrative, ulcerative, and fistular lesions of the penis due to lymphogranuloma venereum. Br J Vener Dis 49:193, 1972

KING AF et al: Intradermal tests in the diagnosis of lymphogranuloma. Br J Vener Dis 32:208, 1956

SCHACHTER J et al: Lymphogranuloma venereum: I. Comparison of the Frei test, complement fixation test, and isolating the agent. J Infect Dis 120:372, 1969

Neonatal inclusion conjunctivitis and pneumonia

BEEM MO, SAXON EM: Respiratory tract colonization and a distinctive pneumonia syndrome in infants infected with *Chlamydia trachomatis.* N Engl J Med 296:306, 1977

HARRISON JR et al: *Chlamydia trachomatis* infants pneumonitis. N Engl J Med 298:702, 1978

Nongonococcal urethritis

BERGER RE et al: *Chlamydia trachomatis* as a cause of acute "idiopathic" epididymitis. N Engl J Med 298:301, 1978

BOWIE WR et al: Etiology of nongonococcal urethritis: Evidence for *Chlamydia trachomatis* and *Ureaplasma urealyticum.* J Clin Invest 59:735, 1977

HOLMES KK et al: Etiology of nongonococcal urethritis. N Engl J Med 292:1199, 1975

MARDH PA et al: *Chlamydia trachomatis* infection in patients with acute salpingitis. N Engl J Med 296:1377, 1977

REES E et al: Chlamydia in relation to cervical infection and pelvic inflammatory disease, in *Nongonococcal Urethritis and Related Infections,* D Hobson, KK Holmes (eds). Washington, DC, American Society for Microbiology, 1977, pp 67–76

Trachoma and inclusion conjunctivitis

DAWSON CR et al: Infections due to adenovirus type 8 in the United States: III. Epidemiological, clinical and microbiological features of epidemic keratoconjunctivitis. Am J Ophthalmol 69:473, 1970

——— et al: Blinding and nonblinding trachoma. Bull WHO 52(3):279, 1975

———, TOGNI B: Herpes simplex eye infections: Clinical manifestations, pathogenesis and management. Surv Ophthalmol 21:121, 1976

GRAYSTON JT et al: Epidemic keratoconjunctivitis on Taiwan. Am J Trop Med 13:492, 1964

HALES RH, OSTLER HB: Newcastle disease conjunctivitis with subepithelial infiltrates. Br J Ophthalmol 57(9):694, 1973

MORDHORST CH et al: Childhood trachoma in a nonendemic area. JAMA 283:1765, 1978

O'DAY DM et al: Clinical and laboratory evaluation of epidemic keratoconjunctivitis due to adenovirus types 8 and 19. Am J Ophthalmol 81(2):207, 1976

WHITCHE JP et al: Acute hemorrhagic conjunctivitis in Tunisia: Report of viral isolations. Arch Ophthalmol, January 1976

175

PSITTACOSIS

VERNON KNIGHT

DEFINITION Psittacosis is an infectious disease of birds caused by an organism that has a number of properties in common with gram-negative bacteria. Transmission of infection from birds to humans results in a febrile illness characterized by pneumonitis and systemic manifestations. Inapparent infections or mild influenza-like illnesses may also occur. The term *ornithosis* is sometimes applied to infections contracted from birds other than parrots or parakeets, but *psittacosis* is the preferred generic term for all forms of the disease.

ETIOLOGY The causative agent *Chlamydia psittaci* is a gram-negative obligate intracellular parasite, formerly classified as a virus. Now chlamydias, along with the rickettsias, may be considered specialized bacteria. Both synthesize ribonucleic acid (RNA) and deoxyribonucleic acid (DNA), reproduce by binary fission, and are susceptible to antimicrobial drugs. In contrast to rickettsias, the chlamydias are dependent on their hosts for metabolic energy. Slight but definite homology of the DNA of members of the *Chlamydia* genus with the DNA of *Neisseria meningitidis* has been shown. The psittacosis agent is the prototype of a biologically and antigenically homogeneous class of microorganisms that includes the causative agents of lymphogranuloma venereum, trachoma, and 30 or more mammalian parasites which rarely produce human disease.

EPIDEMIOLOGY Psittacosis is widely distributed throughout the world, and almost any avian species can harbor the agent. Psittacine birds are most commonly infected, but human cases have been traced to contact with pigeons, ducks, turkeys, chickens, and many other birds. Psittacosis may be considered an occupational disease of pet-shop owners, poultry raisers, pigeon fanciers, taxidermists, and zoo attendants. The incidence of human infection in the United States rose steadily from 1930, owing in large measure to the increasing popularity of parrots and parakeets as pets and, as subsequently recognized, transmission of infection by barnyard fowl and pigeons. The number of reported cases reached a peak in 1956 and gradually declined thereafter. By 1963, with acceptance of control measures such as incorporation of tetracyclines in poultry feed, the disease had again become relatively uncommon. However, in recent years the disease has increased with cases occurring primarily among employees of poultry processing plants. In 1976 a plant in Nebraska experienced an outbreak involving 28 of 98 employees, whose disease was contracted from turkeys shipped from Texas. Other outbreaks of this type have occurred. In 1975 and 1976, 58 and 80 cases of psittacosis, respectively, were reported to the Center for Disease Control. The disease appears to be more common in England, where budgerigars are common household pets and where restrictions on the importation of these birds have been eased.

The agent is present in nasal secretions, excreta, tissues, and feathers of infected birds. Although the disease can be fatal, infected birds frequently show only minor evidence of illness, such as ruffled feathers, lethargy, and anorexia. Asymptomatic avian carriers are common, and complete recovery may be followed by continued shedding of the organism for many months.

Psittacosis is almost always transmitted to humans by the respiratory route and one-half or more of patients infected in fowl-processing plants may have pneumonia indicative of aerosol transmission of the infection. On rare occasions the disease may be acquired from the bite of a pet bird. Intimate and prolonged contact is not essential for transmission of the disease; a few minutes spent in an environment previously occupied by an infected bird has resulted in human infection. The severity of the disease in humans bears no apparent relationship to closeness or duration of contact, although sick birds are more likely to transmit infection than healthy ones. Transmission of a psittacosis-like agent between humans has occurred among hospital personnel, with severe and sometimes fatal infections. There is evidence that these "human" strains are more virulent than native avian organisms. There is no record of infection acquired by eating poultry products.

PATHOGENESIS The psittacosis agent gains entrance to the body through the upper part of the respiratory tract and eventually localizes in the pulmonary alveoli and in the reticuloendothelial cells of the spleen and liver. Invasion of the lung probably takes place by way of the bloodstream rather than by direct extension from the upper air passages. A lymphocytic inflammatory response occurs on both the interstitial and respiratory surfaces of the alveoli as well as in the perivascular spaces. The alveolar walls and interstitial tissues of the lung are thickened, edematous, necrotic, and occasionally hemorrhagic. Histologically, the affected areas show alveolar spaces filled with fluid, erythrocytes, and lymphocytes. The picture is not pathognomonic of psittacosis unless macrophages containing characteristic cytoplasmic inclusion bodies (LCL bodies) can be identified. The respiratory epithelium of the bronchi and bronchioles usually remains intact.

MANIFESTATIONS The clinical manifestations and course of psittacosis are extremely variable. After an incubation period of 7 to 14 days, or longer, the disease may start abruptly with shaking chills and fever ranging as high as 105°F, but the onset is often gradual with increasing fever over a 3- to 4-day period. Headache is almost always a prominent symptom; it is usually diffuse and excruciating and often the patient's chief complaint.

Many patients present with a dry hacking cough which is usually nonproductive, but small amounts of mucoid or bloody sputum may be raised as the disease progresses. Cough may appear early in the course of the disease or as late as 5 days after the onset of fever. Chest pain, pleurisy with effusion, or a friction rub may all occur but are rare. Pericarditis and myocarditis have been reported. Most patients have a normal or slightly increased respiratory rate; marked dyspnea with cyanosis occurs only in severe psittacosis with extensive pulmonary involvement. In psittacosis, as in most nonbacterial pneumonias, the physical signs of pneumonitis tend to be less prominent than symptoms and x-ray findings would suggest. The initial examination may reveal fine, sibilant rales, or clinical evidence of pneumonia may be completely lacking. Rales usually become audible and more numerous as the illness progresses. Signs of frank pulmonary consolidation are usually absent. Symptoms of upper respiratory tract infection are not prominent, although mild sore throat, pharyngeal infection, and cervical adenopathy are often present; on occasion they may be the only manifestations of illness. Epistaxis is encountered early in the course of nearly one-fourth of the cases. Photophobia is also a common complaint.

There is commonly a complaint of generalized myalgia, and spasm and stiffness of the muscles of the back and neck may lead to an erroneous diagnosis of meningitis. Lethargy, mental depression, agitation, insomnia, and disorientation have been prominent features of the illness in some epidemics, but not in others; delirium and stupor occur near the end of the first week in severe cases. Occasional patients are comatose when first seen, and the diagnosis of psittacosis may be missed. Gastrointestinal complaints such as abdominal pain, nausea, vomiting, or diarrhea are present in some cases; constipation and abdominal distention sometimes occur as late complications. Icterus, the result of severe hepatic involvement, is a rare and ominous finding. A faint, macular rash (Horder's spots) simulating the rose spots of typhoid fever has been described.

Patients without cough or other clinical evidence of respiratory involvement come to the physician with fever of unknown origin. The pulse rate is slow in relation to the fever. When splenomegaly is present in a patient with acute pneumonitis, psittacosis should be considered; the reported incidence of splenomegaly ranges from 10 to 70 percent. Nontender hepatic enlargement also occurs, but jaundice is rare. Thrombophlebitis is not unusual during convalescence; indeed, pulmonary infarction is sometimes a late complication and may be fatal.

In untreated cases of psittacosis, sustained or mildly remittent fever persists for 10 days to 3 weeks, or occasionally as long as 3 months. Defervescence is by lysis and is accompanied by abatement of respiratory manifestations. Psittacosis contracted from parrots or parakeets is more likely to be a severe, prolonged illness than infections acquired from pigeons or barnyard fowl. Relapses occur but are rare. Secondary bacterial infections are uncommon. Immunity to reinfection is probably permanent.

Laboratory findings The x-ray of the lungs in psittacosis mimics that in a great variety of pulmonary diseases. The pneumonic lesions are usually patchy in appearance but can be hazy, diffuse, homogeneous, lobar, atelectatic, wedge-shaped, nodular, or miliary. The white blood cell count is normal or moderately decreased in the acute phase of the disease but may rise in convalescence. The erythrocyte sedimentation rate is frequently not elevated. Transient proteinuria is common. The cerebrospinal fluid sometimes contains a few mononuclear cells but is otherwise normal. Cold agglutinins are rarely present.

The diagnosis can be confirmed only by isolation of the causative microorganism or serologic studies. The agent is present in the blood during the acute phase of the disease and in the bronchial secretions for weeks or sometimes years after infection, but it is difficult to isolate. Psittacosis is most readily diagnosed by the demonstration of a rising titer of complement-fixing antibody in the patient's blood. An acute and convalescent specimen should always be tested. Even a low titer of antibody during the acute febrile phase constitutes presumptive evidence of psittacosis. The prompt initiation of treatment with tetracycline has been shown to delay antibody rise in convalescence for several weeks or months. Interpretation of a single complement fixation test may sometimes be difficult because of the antigenic cross reaction between the agent of psittacosis and that of lymphogranuloma venereum.

Differential diagnosis A history of exposure to birds may be the only clinical basis for differentiating psittacosis from a great variety of infectious and noninfectious febrile disorders. A partial list of pneumonic disease that may be confused with psittacosis includes *Mycoplasma* pneumonia, Q fever, coccidioidomycosis, tuberculosis, carcinoma of the lung with bronchial obstruction, and bacterial pneumonias. In the early stages, before pneumonitis appears, psittacosis may be mistaken for influenza, typhoid fever, miliary tuberculosis, and infectious mononucleosis. A newly described entity, Legionnaires' disease (Chap. 138), caused by a difficult-to-cultivate gram-negative bacillus, causes pneumonia similar to psittacosis.

Treatment The tetracyclines are consistently effective in the treatment of psittacosis. Defervescence and alleviation of symptoms usually occur in 24 to 48 h after instituting therapy with 2 g daily in four divided doses. To avoid relapse, treatment should probably be continued for at least 7 days after defervescence. In severe cases, oxygen and other supportive measures are indicated.

REFERENCES

CENTER FOR DISEASE CONTROL: Morb Mort Week Rep 25:301, October 1, 1976
————: *Psittacosis Annual Summary, 1974,* June 1975.

section 13 | Viral diseases

176
INTRODUCTION TO VIRUS INFECTIONS: CLASSIFICATION, PATHOGENESIS, EPIDEMIOLOGY, DIAGNOSIS, AND CONTROL

A. MARTIN LERNER

Clinical virology has passed from the unitary realm of the research physician. Knowledge of the clinical syndromes associated with specific viruses, understanding of appropriate diagnostic tests, and utilization of available means for prevention and therapy are required of all internists. Common virus infections vary from inapparent to life threatening. Rapid progress continues. Of particular note have been (1) recognition of the causes of viral gastroenteritis, (2) further definitions of immunopathologic mechanisms of hepatitis viruses, and (3) definitive evidence for therapeutic efficacy of intravenous adenine arabinoside (ara-A) in disseminated varicella-zoster and herpes simplex virus encephalitis.

GENERAL PROPERTIES AND CLASSIFICATION OF VIRUSES
Viruses are grouped according to their biophysical characteristics: (1) presence of nucleic acid, (2) size, (3) sensitivity to ether, (4) presence of an envelope, and (5) symmetry (cubic or helical). They contain macromolecular cores of ribonucleic acid (RNA) or deoxyribonucleic acid (DNA), but not both. (On the other hand, chlamydiae, *Mycoplasma,* and Rickettsiae contain both RNA and DNA.) Viruses have marked species and organ specificities, and on the whole, viruses infecting plants, insects, rickettsiae, bacteria, and other animals are distinct from their human counterparts.

Human viruses range in size from 17 nm (picornavirus) to 300 nm (poxvirus). They may be naked and contain only nucleic acid (genome) which is protected by a closed shell or tubing, the capsid. Other viruses have, in addition, a lipid envelope, acquired during maturation as virus evaginates from the nucleus (herpes simplex virus) or cytoplasm (influenza, herpes simplex virus). The lipid coat of these viruses surrounds the capsid. The capsid consists of protein and is composed of repeating subunits, capsomeres. Mature virus particles are called *virions* (Fig. 176-1). Specific antigens of the capsid may penetrate the lipid envelope.

The nucleic acid contains all the genetic material necessary to reproduce itself (transcription) and code for structural proteins and enzymes (translation) important in synthesis and attachment to susceptible cells. The nucleic acid core plus the capsid is known as the *nucleocapsid.* When the virion is stripped of its capsid, nucleic acid may enter a host of foreign

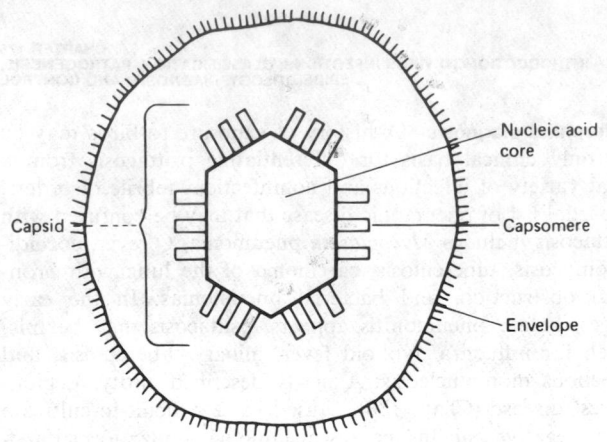

FIGURE 176-1

Components of a complete virus particle (virion).

Labels in figure: Nucleic acid core, Capsomere, Envelope, Capsid

species and produce a single cycle of mature virus (e.g., poliovirus in mouse renal cells). Species and organ specificities of virus-cell union are functions first of complementary physical characteristics and then of covalent union between proteins of the virus and susceptible cell membranes. For instance, molecules of neuraminic acid act as receptors on human red blood cells, allowing hemagglutination by influenza virus. Within several hours after virus adsorption, neuraminidase, one of the proteins of the influenza capsid, digests the neuraminic acid. Elution of influenza virus from red blood cells follows. Cells which allow virus multiplication are termed *permissive,* while those which do not are termed *nonpermissive.* The membrane fit may be HLA dependent and change with aging of the host. Some virus-cell unions may be permissive at one temperature

(37°C) but not at the lower temperatures of the upper respiratory tract (~30°C).

At present, there are seven known groups of RNA viruses (picornavirus, reovirus, arbovirus, myxovirus, rhabdovirus, coronavirus, arenavirus) and four groups of DNA viruses (papovavirus, adenovirus, herpesvirus, poxvirus) (Table 176-1). Nucleic acids of infectious and serum hepatitis viruses have not been absolutely identified. However, the agents of hepatitis A and non-A, non-B resemble RNA-containing enteroviruses, while hepatitis B has a herpesvirus-like lipid coat and contains a DNA genome. Rotaviruses (reovirus-like) and parvoviruses are recently discovered causative agents of viral gastroenteritis.

VIRUS MULTIPLICATION Virus adsorption is a specific physical and then chemical reaction. After absorption, virus enters the cell by pinocytosis and is uncoated; i.e., nucleic acid is stripped from the capsid. With DNA viruses, specific virus DNA strands are transcribed into specific messenger RNA (mRNA) which is then translated to synthesize virus-specific proteins and enzymes necessary for biosynthesis of virus DNA. In the case of virus RNA, single-stranded RNA serves as its own messenger. The mRNA is translated, resulting in the formation of an RNA polymerase. Synthesis of host cell protein and nucleic acid is suppressed to variable degrees. Assembly of protein subunits around virus DNA results in formation of complete virions which may be released by cell lysis or budding from the cytoplasm. Virions of RNA tumor viruses contain an enzyme which is capable of catalyzing synthesis of DNA. The product consists of small fragments of DNA, most of which are complementary in base sequence to 70S RNA of the virion. Thus, information can travel not only from DNA to RNA but also, at least in certain cases, in the reverse direction.

Virus multiplication may lead to a cytolytic infection with release of virus with necrosis of the infected cell, but other infections are persistent or latent and may reactivate at a later

Major groups of viruses infecting human beings

Generic name, nucleic acid, and prototype virus	Size, nm	Ether sensitive	Envelope	Symmetry
Picornavirus (RNA) Coxsackieviruses A and B; echo-, rhino-, and polioviruses	17–30	No	No	Cubic
Reovirus (RNA)	74	No	No	Cubic

Arbovirus (RNA)
  Group A (equine encephalitis, Semliki Forest)
  Group B (Japanese B, Russian tick-borne, yellow fever, dengue)
  Group C (Morituba, Oriboca)
  Ungrouped (Rift Valley, Colorado tick fever, sandfly)
	20–100	Yes	?	

Myxovirus and paramyxovirus (RNA) Influenza A, B, and C: parainfluenza, mumps, rubeola; respiratory syncytial	80–200	Yes	Yes	Helical
Rhabdovirus: rabies (RNA)	65–180	Yes	Yes	
Coronavirus (RNA)		Yes	Yes	

Arenavirus (RNA)
  Togavirus: rubella (most arboviruses of groups A and B)
  Tacaribe-LCM: lymphocytic choriomeningitis, South American hemorrhagic fevers (Lassa, Machupo)
	50
	50–300
		Yes
		Yes
			Yes
			Yes	

Papovavirus (DNA) Warts, simian virus 40	45–55	No	No	Cubic
Adenovirus (DNA)	65–85	No	No	Cubic
Herpesvirus (DNA) Herpes simplex, monkey B, varicella-herpes zoster, cytomegalovirus, Epstein-Barr	120–180	Yes	Yes	Cubic
Poxvirus (DNA) Variola, vaccinia, molluscum contagiosum, orf (milker's nodules)	150–300	Yes or no	Yes	Cubic

Classifications incomplete
  Hepatitis A: "Enterovirus-like"
  Hepatitis, non-A, non-B: "Enterovirus-like"
  Hepatitis B: Nucleic acid is DNA, contains lipid coat
  Rotavirus (arbovirus, duovirus): "Reovirus-like"
  Parvovirus (Norwalk, Hawaii, Montgomery County agents)				

time. In turn, the virus nucleic acid may become incorporated into the genome of the cell leading to malignant transformation. Virus infection may also lead to fusion of cellular membranes (giant cells) or demyelinization.

PATHOGENESIS OF VIRUS INFECTIONS The primary site of virus multiplication depends upon the route of acquisition and the special receptor-site complementarity of the host (Table 176-2). The modes of transmission of human virus infections

TABLE 176-2
Modes of transmission of human viruses

Mode of transmission*	Symptoms/ other	Viruses
Respiratory (droplets or droplet-nuclei in air, bites, salivary transfer, mouth to hand or object)	Local	Adenoviruses (many serotypes) Rhinoviruses (many serotypes) Influenza viruses A, B, C Parainfluenza viruses (several serotypes) Coronaviruses (many serotypes)
	General	Varicella-zoster; Epstein-Barr (EB) virus Variola (smallpox) Rubella Mumps; rubeola (measles) Lymphocytic choriomeningitis; Lassa virus
Alimentary	Local	Adenoviruses (a few serotypes) Enteroviruses (a few serotypes) Parvoviruses (Norwalk agent) Reoviruses (including rotavirus)
	General	Enteroviruses (many serotypes, including polioviruses) Hepatitis viruses A, B, non-A, non-B
Contact (skin)		Papilloma (warts) Herpesviruses [herpes simplex viruses, type 1 (oral) and 2 (genital)]; EB virus Molluscum contagiosum; cowpox; milker's nodes
Arthropod bite	General	California encephalitis virus Western equine encephalitis virus Venezuelan equine encephalitis virus St. Louis encephalitis virus Colorado tick fever virus (reovirus-like orbivirus)
Animal bite	General	B virus Rabies virus
Infection by transfusion	General	Hepatitis B Cytomegalovirus (CMV); EB virus; hepatitis B; hepatitis, non-A, non-B
Transplacental	General	CMV Rubella
Instruments	Tonometer (examination for glaucoma)	Adenoviruses
	Corneal transplants	Jakob-Creutzfeldt "viroid"
	Neurosurgical or ophthalmologic procedures	
	Electrodes (electroencephalograms)	

* Prevention and isolation/control are specifically directed by understanding the mode of transmission.

773

CHAPTER 176
INTRODUCTION TO VIRUS INFECTIONS: CLASSIFICATION, PATHOGENESIS, EPIDEMIOLOGY, DIAGNOSIS, AND CONTROL

are: respiratory, alimentary, contact (mucosal, bite, injection), or transplacental. Respiratory viruses are also exchanged by kissing or by the hands. The hands are also vital in fecal virus transfers.

Virus-specific structures (inclusion bodies) may be present within the cytoplasm (variola), nucleus (herpes simplex virus, varicella-zoster, adenovirus), or both (measles) of infected cells. Viremia may or may not occur. In many virus infections, in distinct contrast to bacteremias, viremia occurs during the incubation period when the patient is well. Viremia is usual with the exanthems of enteroviruses, rubeola, and varicella-zoster. Herpesviruses may multiply within lymphocytes sequestered from antibodies and phagocytes when there is no viremia. During coxsackievirus B3 viremia in mice, virus is present in the plasma, but erythrocytes, polymorphonuclear leukocytes, and platelets do not contain virus. On the third day of this plasma viremia infectious T and B lymphocyte-virus complexes circulate. Secondary sites of infection may be heart, liver, pancreas, kidneys, or brain.

RESPONSES OF THE HOST At sites of virus multiplication extracellular virus often abounds. Macrophages and a few polymorphonuclear leukocytes migrate to the area producing inflammation. Interferon (see below) is produced locally, and B and T lymphocytes appear. Macrophages attach to antigen markedly augmenting the efficiency of virus inactivation by specific neutralizing antibodies or sensitized T lymphocytes. During the first days of many virus infections there is a circulating lymphopenia of both B and T cells. Lymphocytes migrate to sites of infection and to the liver, spleen, or other organs of the mononuclear phagocytic system.

Interferon Viruses, endotoxin, certain parasites, and double-stranded RNA synthetic polyribonucleotide complexes such as polyinosinic polycytidilic ribonucleic acid (poly rI:rC) stimulate interferon, an antiviral protein. Within several hours after onset of virus infection, and days before humoral antibodies can be measured by ordinary methods, interferon is found in tissues where virus is synthesized and in the blood. Interferon is probably most effective as an antiviral substance early in infection when viral titers are low. Later, interferon's effect on virus in tissues is small. Interferon also has an important function as an immunoregulatory substance, either stimulator or depressor, depending upon the time during infection.

A delay in the appearance of interferon in vesicular fluid has been associated with viremic dissemination in herpes zoster. Likewise, decreased in vitro responsiveness of the patient's lymphocytes after stimulation by herpes simplex virus in the production of interferon has been correlated with recurrences of herpes labialis. Severe repetitive and exhausting exercise in mice infected with coxsackievirus B3 results in a delay in the appearance of circulating interferon and, later, in both a delay and a depression in the quantity of type-specific neutralizing antibody in serum. A marked increase in the quantity of myocardial virus and mortality follows. Exercise augmentation of coxsackievirus B3 virulence is also associated with thymic atrophy. Rest may be a very important factor in recovery from virus infections.

Interferons of two classes are produced. The first, a high-molecular-weight protein (8.5×10^4 daltons), is preformed and released within 2 h after infection. At 18 h, the serum contains proteins with biologic activity of interferon with molecular weights of 3 to 4×10^4 daltons. Interferon is acid-stable (pH 2), trypsin-sensitive, nondialyzable, and nonsedimentable by ultracentrifugal forces sufficient to pellet viruses. Most cells tested produce interferon, but those of the reticulo-endothelial system (especially the spleen) and lymphocytes are particularly important.

Interferon has no effect upon extracellular virus. Following entry of virus nucleic acid into a susceptible cell, the cell nucleus is stimulated to produce interferon. Interferon is released through the cytoplasm of the infected cell. Synthesis of virus-directed coat proteins and enzymes is prevented. New virus is not formed.

Interferons are not virus-specific and are active against a wide variety of viruses. However, interferon is an effective antiviral substance only in cells of the same species in which it is produced. For instance, anti-influenza A interferon produced in hamster tissue cultures is effective against influenza in hamsters but not in humans. Likewise, interferon produced in human leukocytes or human tissue cultures is effective in humans.

Viruses vary greatly in their sensitivity to interferon. Myxoviruses are quite sensitive, while herpesviruses are more resistant. The importance of interferon in recovery from virus infection probably varies. With coxsackievirus B3, interferon titers in tissues actually parallel virus titers. In animal models, interferon has been shown to have a prophylactic effect in a number of virus infections, but once the titers of virus are high, interferon is ineffective.

Antibodies Proteins of the virus capsid stimulate B lymphocytes (immunoglobulin-bearing, bone marrow–derived) to synthesize humoral antibodies (IgM, IgG, IgA, IgD) and secretory antibodies (IgA). Cell-associated antibodies (IgE) are also produced. Immunoglobulins are synthesized in local lymph nodes, at body surfaces (saliva, respiratory secretions, colostrum), and in inflammatory exudates within organs (kidney, brain, cervix). During the first 3 to 10 days after an initial exposure to a virus, IgM antibodies predominate. Later, IgG antibodies prevail. Immunoglobulin M is important in clearing viremias remaining within vascular spaces; IgG antibodies also enter interstitial spaces. On surfaces, IgA antibodies contain an added secretory piece, allowing their functional integrity in the presence of hydrolytic enzymes of the secretions. Many molecules of antibody combine with a single virion. Covering a critical number of essential sites on the virion renders an antigen-antibody complex noninfectious. Antigen-antibody complexes attract components of complement which are the mediators for chemotaxis of polymorphonuclear leukocytes. Immune complexes may be fixed in tissues, circulate or precipitate in the glomerulus, in the synovia of joints, or in the skin.

Secretory IgA antibodies in respiratory secretions are vital to the body's defenses against respiratory viruses. During viral respiratory infections viremia does not occur regularly. Humoral antibodies persist only for months. Immunity is transient and reinfections with the same virus occur. On the other hand, after systemic infections, humoral antibodies and immunity persist. After administration of killed virus vaccines immunity is also briefer than that which follows attenuated virus vaccines.

Circulating neutralizing antibody is effective protection against viremia, except possibly against very large inocula or in the presence of low antibody titers. Some viruses multiply and spread from cell to cell even in the presence of neutralizing antibodies. Herpes simplex virus, type 1, and rubeola in nervous tissues are examples. Cell-mediated immunity is the most important means of defense against herpesviruses, while antibody is vital to recovery from enteroviruses. In some cases antibodies or T lymphocytes (cytotoxic "killer" cells) may be

important in continuing the pathogenic process. Cytolytic T cells may be directed against neoantigens induced by, but biochemically different from, any structural component of the virus. This appears to be the pathogenetic mechanism in chronic murine coxsackievirus B3 myocardiopathy.

Antibodies to viruses are measured by neutralization of their cytopathic effects in tissue cultures, or by protection tests using embryonated eggs or animals. Complement fixation, precipitin, indirect hemagglutination, fluorescent antibody, immune hemadsorption, and radioimmunoassay are among the techniques used to measure viral antibodies. Early after infection, certain viruses such as herpes simplex virus, type 1, and cytomegalovirus induce complement-requiring neutralizing antibodies. Myxoviruses, some enteroviruses, and reoviruses hemagglutinate several species of red blood cells. In these cases antibodies can be measured by inhibition of hemagglutination. Virus capsids of nonhemagglutinating viruses may be absorbed to the surface of tanned sheep red blood cells. Antibodies are then assayed by indirect hemagglutination. Kinetics of rises and falls of the several antibodies suggest that different assays may test separate immunoglobulin responses to distinct proteins of the virus capsid.

Cell-mediated immunity Thymic-derived T lymphocytes are responsible for cellular immune functions. In most virus infections, both T and B lymphocytes participate in the containment of virus replication. After a latent period, usually lasting 3 to 4 days, stimulated T lymphocytes transform to lymphoblasts. They release a number of nonspecific, nondialyzable effector molecules which migrate with albumin on electrophoresis. Among these effector molecules are lymphocyte-transforming factor, migration-inhibitory factor, cytotoxin factor, and interferon. Components of complement react with the surface of sensitized lymphocytes, releasing a chemotactic factor to monocytes, which are the important phagocytes in cellular immunity. After stimulation by an antigen, evoking a potent T-lymphocyte response, macrophages are "activated," becoming more efficient phagocytes. This increased phagocytic ability of activated macrophages is not limited to the stimulating virus.

There are at least three subpopulations of T lymphocytes: T_o (cytolytic cells, antigen specific, without receptors for the F_c portion of immunoglobulin molecules); T_m (helper cells with F_c receptors on their surface for IgM); and T_g (suppressor cells with F_c receptors on their surface for IgG). T_m cells are necessary for a sustained IgG response. The elucidation of the functions of these T-cell subpopulations will clarify understanding of the pathogenesis of virus infections.

EPIDEMIOLOGY OF VIRUS INFECTIONS Virus infection occurs with disease, or it may be asymptomatic. Clinical illness is the rule with measles (rubeola virus), but inapparent infection is common with enteroviruses. The severity of disease may also be age-related. In adults, chickenpox and mumps are often severe with complications (varicella pneumonia, mumps orchitis, or encephalitis) which are rare during childhood.

The *incidence* of infection is the number of new cases of a disease occurring in a unit of time, while the *incidence rate* is the number of new cases occurring divided by the number of persons in the total population at risk in the area being studied. The incidence rate is usually calculated as the ratio of the number of new clinical cases divided by the population under surveillance in a given year. Incidence rates may also be calculated by measuring virus excretion or rises in antibody titers using acute and convalescent phase serums.

The *prevalence* is the number of cases of a disease existing at one time, while the *prevalence rate* is the number of cases of a given disease at one time divided by the population at risk. The *point prevalence* or *period prevalence* may be calculated.

775

CHAPTER 176
INTRODUCTION TO VIRUS INFECTIONS: CLASSIFICATION, PATHOGENESIS,
EPIDEMIOLOGY, DIAGNOSIS, AND CONTROL

Unlike most bacterial infections, isolation of virus from an ill patient and even demonstration of a fourfold rise in specific antibodies to that virus in temporally related acute and convalescent serums does not always prove a causative relation to the illness in question. Epidemiologic support is often required for firm etiologic associations. Age-matched, sex-matched, and time- and place-matched controls (compeer groups) must be studied in the same manner as the patients in question. The families of patients are an excellent group to examine. Inapparent simultaneous infection must be sought. Patients within the hospital as well as persons living in the immediate neighborhood of the patient are also often studied. Virus isolation and/or antibody rises in a patient group in significant excess over controls are strong evidence for an etiologic association. In this regard, *serologic epidemiology* is the systematic testing of blood specimens from a defined sample of a healthy population for the presence of antigens, antibodies, or other components.

Virus infections often occur in clusters of cases determined by the presence of the virus in the community and the susceptibility (antibody titers to the virus) of the population. An *epidemic* or outbreak is present when the number of cases is in excess of the expected number at that locality based upon past experience. For instance, an increased incidence of a mix of viral respiratory infections and pneumonias is expected each winter, but influenza epidemics occur over 4- to 6-week intervals only every several years. On the other hand, the occurrence of only a dozen cases of St. Louis encephalitis in Michigan during the late summer would constitute an epidemic.

Influenza A epidemics often affect several continents at the same time. When this occurs, *pandemic* influenza is present. Epidemic influenza B is rarely pandemic.

When an epidemic of echovirus type 9 aseptic meningitis occurs in the summer months, most cases of meningitis (often with rash) during mid- to late summer are due to this agent. However, each case must be studied individually so that discovery of the occasional case of bacterial meningitis or herpes simplex virus encephalitis is certain to be made.

The greater the number of persons immune to a given virus among the population of an area, the less is the likelihood of disease due to that agent among that population at that time. "Population immunity," or *herd immunity,* is usually measured by the presence of neutralizing or other protective antibodies. Susceptibles in the population are protected because of the high number of persons in the group who are immune.

The *incubation period* is the time period from first exposure to first symptom. With short incubation periods of 2 to 4 days (e.g., enteroviruses), multiple cases of illness occur at the same time. With longer incubation periods (e.g., several weeks as with chickenpox), illnesses occur sequentially. If common exposure to several persons occurs, illness may be simultaneous irrespective of the length of the incubation period.

An appropriate environment is necessary for the spread of human disease. Mosquito-borne St. Louis encephalitis ends with effective mosquito control or after the first frost. Respiratory contagion is facilitated by rebreathed air laden with aerosolized virus from coughs, sneezes, or speech. Droplets of water over 10 μm in size containing virus travel short distances through air, while droplet nuclei, minus moisture and less than 10 μm in size, waft over greater distances. Successful primary infection in a susceptible host depends upon (1) the number of virions circulating per cubic foot of air, and (2) the time of exposure which, in turn, determine the total size of the inoculum. For instance, if an aerosol contains four virions per liter of air and 30 virions are required for infection, then persons breathing this air will inspire an infectious dose within a half-hour. The smaller number of respiratory infections during summer may be due to the multiple exchanges of air that result from open windows. In hospitals, walls reaching to the ceilings and closed doors are required for adequate respiratory isolation.

DIAGNOSIS OF VIRUS INFECTIONS   Isolation or recognition of viruses   Materials for virus isolation must be obtained as early during illness as possible. The earlier the specimen is taken, the higher is the titer of virus usually present, and the more likely that the specimen will be positive. Generally, specimens are collected in sterile screw-capped vials containing a balanced salt solution with antibiotics. Depending upon the pathogenesis of the particular infection, throat swab (or sputum), stool (or rectal swab), cerebrospinal fluid (CSF), urine, vesicular fluid, or tissues (biopsy or autopsy) should be obtained for inoculation into susceptible tissue cultures (or mice), prepared for electron microscopy, immunofluorescent radioimmunoassay, or enzyme-linked immunoassay (ELISA). These procedures can recognize viral antigens. If the specimen cannot be processed immediately, it should be frozen promptly to −70°C.

Vesicles should be opened and fluids or scrapings inoculated for virus. Scrapings and impression smears should be stained with Tzanck, Wright, and Gram's stains. Instructions relating to collection of specimens for various clinical syndromes are listed in Table 176-3.

Serologic tests   At the initial visit with a patient suspected of a viral illness a sample of 10 ml blood should be taken and allowed to clot. The serum should be separated to prevent hemolysis which can interfere with diagnostic tests. A second sample of blood should be obtained 2 to 3 weeks later. Both serums should be sent simultaneously to the virus diagnostic laboratory. Changes in antibody titers are most meaningful when paired serums are tested concomitantly.

Neutralization, complement fixation, hemagglutination inhibition, indirect hemagglutination, immunofluorescence, immune adherence hemagglutination, radioimmunoassay, and ELISA are procedures used to measure viral antibodies. After systemic viral infections neutralizing antibodies confer long-lasting immunity. Complement-fixing antibodies, on the other hand, often fall (or disappear) with convalescence. Particular tests are most appropriate for certain viruses (Table 176-4).

Isolation of virus coupled with a fourfold or greater rise in antibody titers between acute and convalescent-phase specimens is diagnostic of recent infection but is not necessarily diagnostic of the clinical syndrome in question. The most striking example of the possible disparity in isolation of virus and its etiologic relationship is herpes simplex virus (HSV), type 2, the cause of herpes labialis and HSV encephalitis. Biopsy of the brain is required for definitive diagnosis of HSV encephalitis. Rises in complement-fixing antibodies to HSV occur with herpes labialis which may accompany pneumococcal meningitis. Nevertheless, in most virus infections fourfold rises in specific antibodies strongly suggest the proper diagnosis. Cross-reactive antibodies among enteroviruses and among herpesviruses are possible and can be confusing. Isolation of virus from diseased tissues is definitive.

Group-specific antibody tests (e.g., group B arboviruses, influenza A, influenza B) often employ the complement-fixation method and are helpful, lessening the number of diagnostic antigens which must be available. If an initial serum is taken later in the illness, a high single titer or high constant titers in both acute and convalescent serums may be found. Single high titers are probably diagnostic if the disease is rare in the area, if the antibody is short-lived (e.g., complement fixing), or if the

TABLE 176-3
Appropriate specimens for virus isolation (or recognition)

Clinical syndrome	Viruses	Throat/ sputum*	Stool/ rectal swab*	CSF*	Urine*	Vesicular fluid*	Other
Meningitis-encephalitis	Mumps	+	−	+	+	None	Usually none
	Enteroviruses:						
	Coxsackieviruses, group A or B	+	+	+	−‡	+†	Blood, brain, skeletal muscle, heart, pericardial fluid, testicle
	Echoviruses	+	+	+	−‡	+†	
	Polioviruses	+	+	−	−	None	Brain, spinal cord
	Herpes simplex:						
	Type 1	+	−	−	−‡	+	Brain, buffy coat of blood
	Type 2	+	−	+	−	+	
	Arboviruses	−	−	+	−	None	Brain
Respiratory diseases	Influenza/parainfluenza viruses	+§	−	−	−	None	Lung, blood, heart
	Rhinoviruses	+	−	−	−	None	Usually none
	Adenoviruses	+	+	−	+	None	Conjunctiva
	Enteroviruses (see above)						
Exanthems	Rubeola (measles)	+	−	−	+	None	Brain
	Rubella	+	−	−	+	None	Brain
	Variola	+	−	−	−	+	
	Vaccinia	−	−	−	−	+	
	Varicella-zoster	−	−	−	−	+	Lung, heart
	Herpes simplex (see above)						
	Enteroviruses (see above)						
Myopericarditis	Enteroviruses (see above)						
Hepatitis	Hepatitis A and non-A, non-B	−	¶	−	−	None	
	Hepatitis B	−	−	−	−	None	Blood ¶
Virus diarrheas	Rotaviruses	−	¶			None	
	Parvoviruses	−	¶			None	
Other	Cytomegalovirus	−	−	−	+	None	Buffy coat of blood
	Progressive multifocal leukoencephalopathy	−	−	−	+	None	Brain
	Jakob-Creutzfeldt disease	−	−	?	−	None	Brain, eye

* +, present; −, absent.

† Vesicles are only occasionally present during coxsackievirus or echovirus infections.

‡ These viruses have occasionally been isolated from urine.

§ These viral antigens can also be promptly recognized in these specimens by immunofluorescent methods.

¶ Hepatitis A and non-A, non-B have been recognized by immune electron microscopy in feces. These viruses "appear" similar to enteroviruses. They have not yet been isolated in tissue cultures. Hepatitis B has been recognized by electron microscopy in blood and liver but has not yet been grown in tissue cultures. Diagnosis is usually made by immunochemical studies of blood (see Table 176-4). HBs, HBe, and DNA polymerase also identify this virus infection. Rotaviruses and parvoviruses have been recognized in feces of patients by immune electron microscopy, radioimmunoassay for virus antigen, and enzyme-linked immunoassay (ELISA) for virus antigen.

antibody is IgM. A fourfold fall in antibody titers is also suggestive. Similar paired serums may be tested from other members of the patient's family for they may be in different stages of apparent or inapparent infection with the same virus.

Nucleic acid hybridization using tumors may recognize viral nucleic acids implicating these viruses in the case of cancers. Herpes simplex virus, type 2, has been linked to cervical cancer and Epstein-Barr virus with Burkitt's lymphoma.

PREVENTION OF VIRUS DISEASES Prevention of virus disease has been achieved largely through the development of viral vaccines, either live attenuated and "killed" or inactivated. Inactivated vaccines are generally available for influenza A, influenza B, rabies, and polioviruses, and on a limited and/or experimental basis inactivated viral vaccines have been developed for adenovirus, Japanese-B, equine, and Russian spring-summer encephalitis. Vaccines derived from attenuated tissue cultures are available for rubella, mumps, measles, poliomyelitis, and yellow fever. Indications for use of these vaccines are discussed in Chap. 114.

Passive immunization with pooled human immune serum globulins or globulins with high titers to specific agents such as rabies, hepatitis B, or varicella has also been used in the prophylaxis of virus infections. These preparations generally are most useful when given early during the incubation period in order to prevent clinical illness. In selected instances, use of hyperimmune globulins may be useful in ameliorating illness once symptoms have developed. Lassa fever is an example. Specific indications for the use of passive immunization in the treatment and prevention of viral infections are discussed in Chap. 114.

Patients with slow virus infections of the central nervous

TABLE 176-4
Serologic tests employed in virus infections

Virus	Complement fixation	Neutralization	Hemagglutination inhibition	Indirect hemagglutination	Immunofluorescence	Immune adherence hemagglutination	Radioimmunoassay	ELISA	Immune electron microscopy
Mumps	+								
Enteroviruses		+							
Herpes simplex viruses	+			+	+	+		+	
Arboviruses	+		+						
Influenza/ parainfluenza	+		+		+				
Rhinoviruses	+	+							
Adenoviruses	+								
Rubeola (measles)	+				I				
Rubella			+						
Variola	+								
Vaccinia	+								
Varicella-zoster	+			+		+			
Hepatitis A	+					+			
Hepatitis B							+		
Cytomegalovirus	+			+					
Rotavirus	+				+				I
Parvovirus	+				+				+

system (Jakob-Creutzfeldt disease) undergoing neurosurgical or ophthalmologic procedures are contagious by means of contaminated surgical equipment. Prolonged autoclaving (121°C, 15 psi, 60 min) and 5% hypochlorite or iodine soaks for 60 min will inactivate large infective doses of this unusual virus. Chemoprophylaxis against smallpox with oral N-methylisatin β-thiosemicarbazone (Marboran) is effective as is amantadine hydrochloride (Symmetrel) taken by mouth throughout the period of exposure to influenza A. Amantadine is not effective against strains of influenza B.

TREATMENT OF VIRUS INFECTIONS Two topical preparations, idoxuridine and adenine arabinoside, are effective, approved, and available therapeutic agents for herpes simplex virus keratitis. Intravenous adenine arabinoside (ara-A) is also an effective therapeutic agent for the treatment of herpes simplex virus encephalitis occurring after the perinatal period. This agent has its maximal effect when it is begun before the onset of paralysis or coma. Ara-A (IV) is also effective in promoting healing and in limiting dissemination of herpes zoster in immunosuppressed patients. These drugs have minimal toxicity and are available for general use.

Experimental testing of ara-A in other herpesvirus infections as well as in chronic active hepatitis (HBs positive) is underway. Controlled clinical trials have also proved that pharmacological megaunits of leukocytic-derived human interferon are effective therapy for disseminated herpes zoster in immunocompromised patients. Exogenous megaunit human interferon (with or without ara-A) will also suppress HBs antigenemia in chronic active hepatitis. Currently, clinical trials of exogenous human interferon are limited by its small supply and great expense. However, no other antiviral agents have proved efficacy or can be recommended. Corticosteroids suppress leukocyte chemotaxis and T and B lymphocytes; they should not be given during the period of active virus multiplication.

REFERENCES

EVANS AS: *Viral Infections of Humans. Epidemiology and Control.* New York, Plenum, 1976

HORSFALL FL JR, TAMM I: *Viral and Rickettsial Infections of Man,* 4th ed. Philadelphia, Lippincott, 1965

JAWETZ E et al: *Review of Medical Microbiology,* 11th ed. Los Altos, Lange, 1974

NOTKINS AL: *Viral Immunology and Immunopathology.* New York, Academic, 1975

Respiratory viruses

177
GENERAL CONSIDERATIONS OF VIRAL RESPIRATORY DISEASES

VERNON KNIGHT

The viral respiratory diseases as a group are responsible for one-half or more of all acute illnesses, and although influenza virus is the only agent among them which causes significant mortality in adults, several different viruses contribute to the 20 percent of childhood mortality due to respiratory disease. Respiratory disease morbidity, due primarily to virus infections, causes 30 to 50 percent of time lost from work by adults, and from 60 to 80 percent of time lost from school by children. These diseases are worldwide, and although studies in many areas are scanty, reports from Great Britain, Western Europe, U.S.S.R., Czechoslovakia, Latin America, and the Orient indicate many common denominators in cause, prevalence, and severity.

Viral respiratory diseases are associated with a spectrum of host responses ranging from asymptomatic carrier states to severe and sometimes fatal pneumonias. There is a recurring pattern of severe illness in infants and young children and of milder disease with increasing age. A few clinical and epidemiologic entities can be recognized without laboratory aids, such as acute respiratory disease (ARD) in military recruits, caused by adenovirus type 4 and rhinovirus coryza in adults. The causative agent in a large proportion of cases, however, cannot be identified with virologic study.

EPIDEMIOLOGY More than 150 serotypes, representing 12 groups of viruses, have been or may be associated with the majority of acute respiratory illness in humans. With the capacity to isolate this large group of agents and with the recognition of the role of *Mycoplasma pneumoniae* (Chap. 172) it is possible to define the cause of many respiratory illnesses. The recent identification of coronaviruses as a cause of respiratory illness increases the potential for diagnosis. Though some of the inability to identify agents is caused by lack of efficient application of known diagnostic methods, it is probable that additional viral and possibly other causes of respiratory illness remain to be discovered.

FREQUENCY AND SEVERITY Since 1957 the National Health Survey has made annual estimates from selected population samples of the incidence of acute respiratory illness in the United States. Since these estimates are designed to measure the socioeconomic impact of illness, cases are reported only if they caused restriction of daily activity or required medical care. There are in excess of 250 million cases of acute respiratory illness in the United States annually, an average of 1.4 illnesses per person per year. Loss of time from work or school averaged 4.2 days for the 80 percent of cases in which some restriction of activity was reported, and about 50 percent of individuals with respiratory disease sought medical attention. Analysis of these data indicates that two-thirds to three-fourths of the cases are caused by viruses; the remaining are divided principally among infections with *M. pneumoniae,* streptococcal sore throat, bacterial pneumonia, and sinusitis.

In other studies, milder illness has been included, with a corresponding rise in annual frequency of reported cases. The Cleveland Family Study found an annual rate of illness of 6.2 per person per year, amounting to an estimated more than 1 billion cases annually in the United States. The greatest proportion of these illnesses were so mild that they constituted no hazard to health, but they are significant in the spread of infection. In addition, it is known that wholly asymptomatic virus infections occur.

Acute respiratory disease is a special problem in relation to older persons who have chronic bronchitis. It is a familiar finding that those with chronic pulmonary disease often undergo exacerbations of their disease as a consequence of acute respiratory infections. The question also arises whether individuals with chronic pulmonary disease experience more frequent acute respiratory illness than those without such involvement. Monto and Ross have shown that adults with mild or intermittent chronic cough and sputum production and diminished pulmonary function experience more frequent respiratory illness than those who are asymptomatic. The finding was present at different levels of smoking frequency, apparently excluding the role of smoking in the occurrences. There was no unusual concentration of cases among any of the several etiologic agents studied. The higher frequency of infection, the prolonged morbidity due to exacerbations of chronic bronchitis, and the large and increasing numbers of such patients in our aging population identify a major health problem for which there is no present solution.

Age, sex, and seasonal variation Infants and young children have the greatest number of viral respiratory infections; children under 6 may have twice as many illnesses per year as the average for the entire population. Females have more illness than males. This difference is most marked in adults, where the excess is 25 percent. In children respiratory viral infections appear to affect the sexes about equally, but boys have more lower respiratory tract disease with respiratory syncytial virus infection than girls.

There are prominent seasonal differences in the frequency of acute respiratory illnesses; the rates are highest in winter, with about 30 cases per 100 persons per quarter. Illness is least frequent during the summer—about one-third of the maximum. Epidemics of influenza cause pronounced increases in wintertime frequency of respiratory illness and are the most significant cause of mortality among the respiratory viruses. In pandemic years influenza may begin in summer or fall.

ETIOLOGY The known viral causes of acute respiratory disease and their estimated relative frequency in adults and older children in relation to their common patterns of illness are shown in Table 177-1. In younger or older persons the same agents may cause disease but the distribution of cases by etiology will vary.

Viruses, as a group, cause about three-fourths of acute respiratory illness, and nearly one-half of these illnesses are due to one of the rhinoviruses. The principal nonviral causes of respiratory illness are *M. pneumoniae* and hemolytic streptococci.

TABLE 177-1
Patterns of illness with respiratory viruses in older children and adults

Agent	Relative frequency per 100 cases	Manifestation				
		Rhinitis	Pharyngitis	Tracheo-bronchitis	Pneumonia	Constitutional
Rhinovirus*	40	+ +	±	+	Rare	± (usually afebrile)
Herpesvirus*	10	+	+ +	Rare	Rare	+
Influenza A and B viruses	10	+	+	+ +	Severe when present	+ + (high fever common)
Parainfluenza viruses†	8	+	+ +	+ +	Rare except in infants	+
Coronaviruses	8	+	±	+	In infants, also bronchiolitis	+
Respiratory syncytial virus	6	+ +	+	+	As above	+
Adenoviruses	1	+	+ +	+ +	Infants and recruits	+ + (high fever)
Coxsackievirus and echoviruses	<1	±	+	+	No	+ + (fever, visceral, and CNS complications)
Other	13 +	?	?	?	?	?

* *College students; lower socioeconomic groups have primary infection earlier.*
† *Laryngeal involvement common.*
NOTE: *+ + = severe; + = moderately severe; ± = mild; ? = unknown or uncommon.*

Table 176-1 shows a current classification of the respiratory viruses based on size, structure, and biochemical and other properties. Adenoviruses and herpesvirus are DNA viruses, while the remainder possess RNA cores. Respiratory tract disease is not known to be associated with particular properties of the viruses except that the long incubation period of adenovirus infection may be related to its longer cycle of replication. The relatively nonspecific response of the respiratory tract to virus infection probably indicates that the target cells of the respiratory tract (i.e., the respiratory epithelium), when damaged by infection, have a limited variability of pathologic response. Classification of viruses will certainly assume greater importance, however, as new chemotherapeutic agents are developed, since many of them will act on specialized viral functions unique to single or related groups of viruses.

CLINICAL MANIFESTATIONS The descriptive term "common cold" was coined to describe the coryzal syndrome before its diverse causes were known. It refers to illness characterized by nasal obstruction and discharge, sneezing, moderate sore throat, and mild constitutional reaction, usually without fever. Patterns of illness shown in Table 177-1 demonstrate that most respiratory viral infections may produce this picture. However, in adults and older children, syndromes more or less restricted to these manifestations are caused by infection with rhinoviruses, respiratory syncytial virus, and coronaviruses. These three groups of viruses may account for as much as two-thirds of cases of acute respiratory viral disease. Herpesvirus causes disease usually localized to the pharynx and tonsils in this age group. The other agents listed, while causing coryzal syndrome, also cause varying degrees of involvement of the lower part of the respiratory tract, with additional symptoms.

The following chapter (Chap. 178) considers six of the seven groups of viruses chiefly responsible for respiratory disease, i.e., rhinoviruses, herpesviruses, parainfluenza viruses, coronaviruses, respiratory syncytial virus, and adenoviruses. Included also is a description of the small contribution to respiratory illness of the enteroviruses, coxsackieviruses A and B, and echoviruses, which are discussed in detail in Chap. 187. Influenza is described in Chap. 179. Respiratory diseases cased by *M. pneumoniae* and the psittacosis agent, both of which resemble viral respiratory diseases, are considered in Chaps. 172 and 175.

REFERENCES

KNIGHT V (ed): *Viral and Mycoplasmal Infections of the Respiratory Tract.* Philadelphia, Lea & Febiger, 1973

MONTO AS, ROSS HW: The Tecumseh study of respiratory illness: X. Relation of acute infections to smoking, lung function and chronic symptoms. Am J Epidemiol 107:47, 1978

178
COMMON VIRAL RESPIRATORY ILLNESSES
Rhinoviruses, herpesviruses, parainfluenza viruses, coronaviruses, respiratory syncytial virus, adenoviruses, coxsackieviruses, and echoviruses

VERNON KNIGHT

RHINOVIRUS INFECTIONS

ETIOLOGY More than 100 types of rhinovirus are known, and others are certain to be found. Some of the clinical properties of rhinoviruses are shown in Table 178-1. They resemble the other picornaviruses in being small (15 to 30 nm), non-lipid-enveloped, relatively stable agents. Rhinoviruses can be distinguished from enteroviruses, the other subgroup of picornaviruses, by their loss of infectivity when exposed to an acid medium for 1 to 3 h.

EPIDEMIOLOGY Rhinovirus infection is the cause of approximately 40 percent of respiratory illness in children and adults. While it occurs throughout the year, there are peaks of high incidence in spring and fall. Infection with rhinoviruses, as with other respiratory viruses, is much more frequent in infants and children than was previously thought. Children may develop second episodes of rhinovirus infection and illness with different serotypes within a few weeks. The disease is also more severe in children, especially those under two years of age. In the young, fever, cough, croup, and occasionally pneumonia occur.

Family infections are most often initiated by children, and up to three-fourths of family outbreaks may be introduced by children of preschool age; however, at all ages spread is much greater from ill than from well primary cases. Large families have more episodes of infection than small families. Family secondary attack rates are high at all ages, but highest in infants, of whom almost two-thirds of susceptibles may become infected. Infection occurs in about two-thirds or more of exposed persons without antibody, and about 60 percent of these develop illness. In persons with preexisting homotypic anti-

TABLE 178-1
Illness associated with rhinovirus infection

Diagnosis	Adults (n = 61)	Children (n = 32)	Adult volunteers with nasopharyngeal inoculation (n = 31)
Common cold	58 (92)*	14 (44)	26 (84)
Croup		1 (3)	
Bronchitis	1 (2)	7 (23)	2 (6)
Bronchiolitis		3 (9)	
Bronchopneumonia		3 (9)	
No disease	2 (3)	4 (12)	3 (10)

* Values in parentheses are given as percentages.
SOURCES: *Hamparian et al, Proc Soc Exp Biol Med 117:469, 1964; and Cate et al, J Clin Invest 43:56, 1964.*

body, rates of infection and illness are about half that of those without antibody. However, studies in volunteers indicate that high titers of homotypic antibody are uniformly protective. Before 1970 a majority of infections were caused by lower-numbered serotypes; more recently the proportion of infections caused by higher-numbered (and also more recently identified) serotypes has increased. Virus is shed in a high percentage of patients from the day before to 6 days after onset of illness. In general, about one-half of individuals whose infection is associated with virus shedding develop a significant serologic response.

CLINICAL MANIFESTATIONS The incubation period for rhinovirus infections is 1 to 2 days. The first signs of disease are scratchy throat, nasal congestion and discharge, malaise, and mild headache. There is usually no fever. Nasal secretions increase sharply between days 1 and 2 and then as promptly return to pre-illness values. Recovery is rapid and complete. Virus shedding begins a few hours after inoculation and continues for a week or more.

Table 178-2 summarizes clinical experience with naturally occurring rhinovirus infections in adults and children and artificial infection in volunteers. Most adults have only a common cold syndrome, with a rare case of bronchitis the only other form of illness. In contrast, more than one-half of children develop bronchitis, bronchiolitis, or bronchopneumonia. Although these findings resemble those of respiratory syncytial (RS) virus infection, rhinovirus disease is generally milder than that due to RS virus.

LABORATORY FINDINGS In illness with rhinovirus there is usually slight neutrophilia. About one-third of volunteers develop moderate elevations in sedimentation rate.

COMPLICATIONS No serious complications have been reported with rhinovirus infections.

DIFFERENTIAL DIAGNOSIS Among the respiratory viruses, rhinovirus infection most consistently causes coryzal illness. In

TABLE 178-2
Illness associated with adenovirus infection

Disease	Occurrence	Order of association (serotypes) Common	Less common	Respiratory tract involvement Common cold	Pharyngitis	Bronchitis	Pneumonia
Acute respiratory disease (ARD)	Epidemic in winter and spring in military recruits	4, 7	3, 14, 21	Often present	Most frequent, usually with fever, often with laryngitis	Frequent, usually with fever and laryngitis	Infrequent complication of ARD, but adenovirus pneumonia is an important type of pneumonia in recruits
Pharyngoconjunctival fever	Summer epidemics in civilians, often in school-age children, related to swimming pools. Sporadic cases of conjunctivitis may occur without pharyngitis	3, 7	4, 14	Often present	Most frequent, usually with fever and cervical lymphadenopathy, hoarseness	Uncommon	Rare
Febrile pharyngitis	Sporadic or epidemic, resembles ARD, often in children	3, 7	1, 2, 5	Often present	Most frequent, usually with fever	Frequent, especially in older children	Infrequent but severe complication
Pneumonia in children	Highly fatal illness in infants, sporadic or epidemic	3, 7		Sometimes present	Very frequent	Very frequent	Primary, with acidophilic necrosis of tracheal and bronchial mucosa resembling tissue culture cytopathogenic effect
Keratoconjunctivitis (EKC)	Epidemic disease in shipyard workers; also spread from infected eye solutions	8	11	Unusual	Uncommon	Not reported	Not reported
Acute hemorrhagic cystitis	Year-round sporadic disease	11	21	No respiratory disease syndrome; acute hematuria with dysuria, frequency, bladder pain, more common in boys			
Pertussis syndrome	Infrequent sporadic disease	1, 2, 3, 5		Often inconspicuous		Tracheobronchitis common	Bronchiolitis and bronchopneumonia described

any one case, however, the illness cannot be distinguished from coryza due to other agents. Except for rare confusion with an atypical case of streptococcal sore throat, only respiratory viral diseases and *Mycoplasma pneumoniae* infection need be considered in differential diagnosis.

TREATMENT AND PREVENTION There is no specific treatment, and no vaccines are currently available for rhinovirus infections. Analgesics, antihistamines, and nose drops may be beneficial.

HERPESVIRUS INFECTIONS

The purpose of this section is to consider the role of herpesviruses in acute respiratory disease. Other aspects of herpesvirus infection are discussed in Chap. 193.

EPIDEMIOLOGY Several studies have shown that about 10 percent of acute respiratory illness in college populations is due to herpesvirus hominis infection. The disease consists almost uniformly of acute ulcerative pharyngitis and tonsillitis, and illness is associated with a significant rise in herpesvirus-neutralizing and complement-fixing antibody, usually from initially immeasurable levels. In one study the early antibody response was predominantly in the IgM fraction, supporting the concept that the disease resulted from a primary infection. Moreover, lesions in the anterior mouth or on the lips were uncommon, suggesting that a superficial recurrent herpetic infection (fever blisters) did not mask disease of another etiology in the pharynx.

The high prevalence of primary disease does not occur at college age in low socioeconomic groups, probably because members of this group experience their primary herpesvirus infections at a much younger age.

The disease occurs predominantly in the fall and winter. The route of transmission is not known, but virus can be readily isolated from respiratory secretions of patients with pharyngitis, or from vesicle fluid of fever blisters and is occasionally present in the saliva of asymptomatic persons.

CLINICAL MANIFESTATIONS Herpesvirus infections are characterized by pharyngitis similar to that caused by beta-hemolytic streptococci. There are shallow ulcers on the tonsils and posterior pharynx, and in about one-half of patients there is a grayish pharyngeal exudate. Streptococcal infections produce a creamy exudate. Anterior cervical or submandibular glands are enlarged, and tender lymph nodes occur in about one-half of cases. Fever rarely exceeds 102°F and disappears in a day or so. Recovery is rapid without complications.

LABORATORY FINDINGS Leukocyte counts are normal. Herpesvirus can usually be isolated from throat swabs taken early in infection, and neutralizing-antibody titers rise from unmeasurable levels to 1:16 to 1:64 in convalescence. Complement-fixing antibody also shows significant rises in titer.

COMPLICATIONS No significant sequelae have been observed.

DIFFERENTIAL DIAGNOSIS The disease most resembles acute β-hemolytic streptococcal pharyngitis. However, the systemic response is less severe and acute. Adenovirus pharyngitis is similar to herpesvirus pharyngitis. Pharyngitis that accompanies other respiratory viral and *Mycoplasma pneumoniae* infections is usually less severe and does not show ulcerations.

PREVENTION AND TREATMENT The disease does not appear to be highly contagious, but isolation of patients acutely ill with pharyngitis and tonsillitis is probably indicated.

No specific treatment is recommended for this relatively benign, self-limited disease, although potent chemotherapeutic agents are used for other forms of herpesvirus infection. Analgesics are recommended for pain and discomfort, and hot saline gargles may decrease throat symptoms.

PARAINFLUENZA VIRUS INFECTIONS

ETIOLOGY On the basis of antigenic differences, parainfluenza viruses are divided into four types, of which type 4 is divided into two subtypes. They agglutinate avian and mammalian erythrocytes and grow slowly in tissue culture; only type 2 produces readily visible cytopathic effects. Growth of these agents in tissue cultures is detected by addition of guinea pig erythrocytes, which absorb on the surface of infected cells to form rosettes, a process known as hemadsorption. Parainfluenza viruses have antigens common to Newcastle disease and mumps viruses, but influenza virus does not share these. Parainfluenza serotypes are distinguished in complement fixation, hemagglutination inhibition, or tissue culture neutralization tests. The serotypes can also be identified and differentiated from one another by immunofluorescence.

Constitutional reaction	Other
Headache, malaise, often high fever for several days	Usually no other involvement
Headache, malaise, high fever for several days	Acute follicular conjunctivitis, usually unilateral, occurs with varying frequency. Preauricular lymphadenopathy common with conjunctivitis
High fever, malaise, headache	Nausea, vomiting and diarrhea may occur, especially in infants
High fever, prostration	Conjunctivitis, skin rash, diarrhea, intussusception, and CNS invasion in some cases
Usually afebrile	Usually unilateral severe, acute conjunctivitis followed by corneal subepithelial keratosis; preauricular lymphadenopathy common
Slight	Causes 19 to 91% of cases of hemorrhagic cystitis in children
Prostration, vomiting with coughing spells	Usually no other involvement

Parainfluenza virus can be isolated in primary monkey or primary embryonic kidney cell cultures, but grows slowly or not at all in embryonated eggs.

EPIDEMIOLOGY The first three types of parainfluenza viruses have been found in many parts of the world; type 4 has so far been isolated only in the United States. Infection with parainfluenza viruses occurs early in life. By the age of 8 years, a majority of children show antibody to types 1 to 3, and it appears that most adults have antibody to all four types.

In children, illness with parainfluenza viruses occurs throughout the year, with seasonal increases in different years in the fall, winter, or spring. Type 3 virus spreads more rapidly than types 1 and 2 and may occur endemically throughout the year. Heterotypic antibody rises are frequent, with antibody to type 3 developing in half the cases with type 1 infection. In both children and adults, reinfection is frequent. In one outbreak, 96 percent of children without antibody, 67 percent with low levels, and 33 percent with high levels of antibody became infected. In adults, the disease is almost invariably a reinfection and is much milder than in children.

The total contribution of parainfluenza infections to respiratory illness is variable; its frequency is increasing in institutions in which general health status is lower than average and levels of sanitation and personal hygiene are less than optimum. In studies in the United States parainfluenza infections accounted for 4.3 to 17 percent of respiratory illness in children. The milder illness of adults constituted less than 5 percent of respiratory illnesses.

CLINICAL MANIFESTATIONS In all age groups, the incubation period appears to be 5 to 6 days. The disease is most serious in infants and children, and fever is a constant feature of the disease. The characteristic syndrome with type 1 parainfluenza is laryngotracheobronchitis or croup. Type 2 disease is less frequent but resembles that caused by type 1. Type 3 parainfluenza infections are about equally distributed as causes of croup, tracheobronchitis, bronchiolitis, and bronchopneumonia in infants and children. In older children, the disease is less serious, usually without evidence of pulmonary involvement, and in adults the virus produces a common cold syndrome with hoarseness and cough. Occasionally, adults may experience severe tracheobronchitis with fever with parainfluenza infection.

Physical findings are not distinctive. The throat is reddened, with little or no exudate. There may be tender submandibular lymphadenopathy.

LABORATORY FINDINGS In adult volunteers given type 2 virus, leukocyte counts were not abnormal. In children there is a considerable variation in leukocyte counts early in illness, making it difficult to distinguish this disease from pneumococcal and other bacterial infections. No characteristic alterations have been reported in other laboratory indexes such as liver or renal function tests, electrocardiograms, and urinalyses.

COURSE AND COMPLICATIONS In children, *otitis media* has occurred as a complication more often with parainfluenza than with the other respiratory viral infections. It is more often caused by pneumococci, streptococci, or *Hemophilus influenzae.*

Parainfluenza virus infection is characterized by slow resolution of pulmonary involvement and long persistence of cough and other symptoms. In very young or debilitated children, the outcome can be fatal. In adults, bacterial sinusitis may occur, and in persons with chronic bronchitis, emphysema, or bronchiectasis, the possibility of pulmonary bacterial superinfections should be considered.

TREATMENT There is no specific treatment. Therapy is limited to symptomatic measures and efforts aimed at early detection and treatment of bacterial complications such as otitis media or pneumonia. Nursing care is important in pediatric cases, especially children with croup. In adults, analgesics, antihistamines, and small doses of codeine for cough are generally sufficient.

PREVENTION Vaccines against parainfluenza virus infections are not available. In hospitals, respiratory precautions should be carried out. At home, bed rest or room isolation during acute illness is advised, with special effort to avoid contact with very young or aged persons.

CORONAVIRUS INFECTIONS

ETIOLOGY The disease in humans is caused by an antigenically heterogeneous group of lipid-enveloped RNA viruses sharing morphologic and other properties with mouse hepatitis virus (MHV) and avian infectious bronchitis virus (IBV). A few serotypes of human coronaviruses recovered in tracheal organ culture share antigens with the murine agent.

EPIDEMIOLOGY The disease, characteristically a common cold syndrome, occurs in winter and spring outbreaks that vary from year to year, with greatest incidence in the 15- to 19-year-old age group, but it may involve adults of 40 years of age and older. The incubation period is 3 to 5 days. One study showed lower respiratory tract disease in young children probably caused by coronaviruses ranking in frequency only behind respiratory syncytial virus and parainfluenza 3 infection.

CLINICAL FEATURES The disease resembles rhinovirus common cold with profuse watery and later mucopurulent nasal discharge, sore throat, moderate cough, and mild constitutional symptoms. It is of short duration. In young children, pneumonia and bronchiolitis with coronavirus infection is clinically like that with other respiratory viruses. About one-half of infants may require oxygen because of respiratory distress. Diagnosis is based on isolation of the agent in organ culture or human embryo kidney culture or by antibody rise. The neutralizing antibody test is more sensitive than the complement fixation test, and rises in titer persist for a longer time. Both tests, however, will provide adequate diagnostic information.

TREATMENT AND PREVENTION Treatment is symptomatic; no preventive measures are available.

RESPIRATORY SYNCYTIAL VIRUS INFECTION

ETIOLOGY Respiratory syncytial virus (RS) is classified as a subgroup of the myxoviruses. In tissue culture, it causes formation of giant cells, or syncytia, from which its name was derived. It grows well in several human primary and continuous cell lines and in primary rhesus monkey kidney culture. There is a soluble complement-fixing antigen which, with the neutralization test, permits virus identification and serologic studies. Viral antigen can also be detected by immunofluorescence of exudates from infected patients or in infected cell cultures. Respiratory syncytial virus contrasts with other myxoviruses because it does not grow in mice, guinea pigs, rabbits, or chick embryos and does not cause hemagglutination or hemadsorption.

EPIDEMIOLOGY Epidemiologic studies have delineated a very substantial role of this agent in acute respiratory disease in children. Illness in young children occurs most commonly in epidemics in the late winter and early spring. Attack rates are nearly 100 percent among susceptibles, who are mostly children under 4 years of age, but the peak occurrence of bronchiolitis and bronchopneumonia is observed at 2 to 3 months of age. In older children and adults, the disease appears in non-epidemic patterns. The limitation of epidemic disease to the younger age group is also evidence for unchanging antigenicity of the agent, in contrast to the situation with influenza virus, in which antigenic shifts are associated with recurrent epidemics in persons of all ages. In serologic surveys of volunteers, all were found to possess a measurable titer of neutralizing antibody to RS virus. Despite this finding, a report described the occurrence of febrile tracheobronchitis with increased airway resistance lasting several weeks among medical personnel caring for children with RS disease. Mild upper respiratory illness appears to be the usual form of the disease in adults, but the virus has been isolated from cases of acute tracheobronchitis in older persons with chronic pulmonary disease.

It is probable that RS virus is transmitted by means of infected respiratory secretions. The incubation period of naturally occurring disease in children is about 4 days, and in adult volunteers approximately 5 days. Virus was generally recovered from volunteers a day or so before the onset of illness, and throat swabs yielded a higher proportion of positive cultures than nasal swabs. Virus shedding continues for 3 to 4 days after onset of illness.

CLINICAL MANIFESTATIONS Somewhat less than one-half of infected children have symptoms defined as a common cold; the remainder have bronchiolitis or bronchopneumonia. Fever occurs in about 90 percent of ill children, with an average elevation to 102°F. Cough is almost invariably present, and severe malaise is frequent. Pharyngitis is not usually severe. Fatalities have been reported in infants.

LABORATORY FINDINGS In children, leukocytosis occurs with some frequency, but no significant hematologic changes were observed in adult volunteers. Bacterial flora of the nasopharynx and other laboratory indexes show no significant alterations in either age group.

COMPLICATIONS Except for progression to overwhelming lower respiratory tract disease in a few young children, no special complications are known. There is no evidence of secondary bacterial infection or systemic invasion by the virus in children. In adults, bacterial sinusitis occasionally complicates the virus infection.

DIFFERENTIAL DIAGNOSIS The resemblance of this disease in children to influenza has been suggested. In adults, the differential diagnosis should include rhinovirus and parainfluenza infection and, less often, other respiratory viral disease and *M. pneumoniae* infection.

TREATMENT As with other respiratory viral diseases, treatment should include rest and palliative medications such as aspirin, nose drops, and medication for sleep when restlessness occurs. The possibility of bacterial sinusitis in adults should be kept in mind and antimicrobial treatment, drainage procedures, or other therapy instituted when necessary.

PREVENTION A Formalin-inactivated RS vaccine elicited a high frequency of antibody, but a few months later vaccinated children experienced more severe illness than nonvaccinated children in the same population. This paradoxical effect of vaccination is a major contraindication to further attempts to develop a vaccine. The infection spreads rapidly among children in institutions and poses a threat to debilitated or very young children.

ADENOVIRUS INFECTIONS

ETIOLOGY The adenovirus group contains 31 human and 17 animal serotypes. Strains of types 3, 7, 11, 12, 14, 16, 18, 21, and 31 have been shown to cause sarcomas when injected into newborn hamsters.

Adenoviruses share a common antigenic determinant on a surface structure of the virus called a hexon, designated α. This antigen is the basis for an adenovirus group-diagnostic complement fixation test. It is not exposed on the intact virus and is not associated with immunity. A type-specific antigen ε, exposed on the hexon of the intact virus, gives rise to neutralizing antibody and is associated with immunity. An antigen γ, exposed on the fiber portion of a surface structure called the penton, is type-specific and elicits neutralizing and hemagglutination inhibiting antibody. Serotypes 12 and 18 do not hemagglutinate. An immunofluorescent test is also available that uses antihexon antibody to detect adenoviral group antigen present in exudates from patients or in infected cell cultures. Human adenoviruses grow well in continuous cell lines of epithelial origin.

EPIDEMIOLOGY Adenoviruses are most prevalent in infants and children; they are found in the throat and rectum of both sick and well children. Adenovirus-associated illness occurs throughout the year and accounts for about 2 to 10 percent of all respiratory illness in infants and children, but the highest frequency is in the period from the fall through the spring. Isolations of virus from well children show a similar pattern of seasonal prevalence but a lower frequency of occurrence. Adenovirus types most commonly associated with illness in children are 1, 2, 3, and 5.

The second most frequent occurrence of adenovirus disease is among military recruits. In the general adult population the disease is sporadic. An appreciable prevalence of infection with many adenovirus serotypes is suggested by serologic surveys, but definite virus-associated illness is limited to about 10. These serotypes produce five major patterns of illness, all of which occur in epidemics. A summary of these is presented in Table 178-2.

Acute respiratory disease (ARD) is a respiratory illness of military recruits caused principally by adenoviruses types 4 and 7 that occur in winter and spring outbreaks. Adenoviruses account for 15 to 50 percent of ARD in military groups, but only for about 2 percent of respiratory illness in civilian adults.

Febrile pharyngitis due to adenoviruses usually occurs sporadically or in small outbreaks in children. Its manifestations are summarized in Table 178-2. *Pharyngoconjunctival fever* is febrile pharyngitis associated with acute follicular conjunctivitis. This disease occurs as summer epidemics, frequently among children in relation to exposure in swimming pools. Although it is not limited to swimming pool exposure, it is believed that eye irritation from water, sun, or chlorine may be a factor in its initiation. Conjunctivitis may occur without pharyngitis.

Pneumonia due to adenovirus infection is rare in civilian adults, but occurs in military recruits, usually as an extension of ARD. In infants and children, sporadic and epidemic occurrence of highly fatal adenoviral pneumonia has been described in several parts of the world. Such outbreaks have been principally caused by types 3 and 7. The severity of disease in this

TABLE 178-3

Respiratory illness associated with coxsackieviruses A and B and echoviruses

Diagnosis	Description	Associated viruses
Herpangina	Febrile pharyngitis, anorexia, and discrete vesicular eruption on anterior faucial pillars. Occurs chiefly in children in summer and early fall outbreaks. Similar illnesses without eruption caused by the same viruses probably occur. An illness with nonulcerating nodules on anterior pillars caused by coxsackievirus A10 has also been described	Coxsackieviruses A1 through A6, A8, A10, and A12
Febrile respiratory illness ("summer grippe")	Undifferentiated febrile illness marked by headache, sore throat, and anorexia occurring in summer or early fall. Includes epidemics in recruits with coxsackievirus A21 infection, in which illness patterns have been confirmed by experimental inoculation of volunteers	Coxsackieviruses A21, A24, B2, B3, B5, (?), and echoviruses 1, 3, 6, 19, 20
Upper respiratory illness associated with gastroenteritis	Cases occurring largely in infants and exposed mothers	Echoviruses 1, 11, 19, 20
Acute laryngotracheobronchitis (croup)	Winter outbreaks in nurseries and institutions. Association less definite than with other syndromes	Coxsackieviruses A9, B5, and echoviruses 11
Pneumonitis and pleuritis	Largely confined to young infants and children; uncommon	Coxsackieviruses A9, B4, B5, and echoviruses 9, 19, 20

young age group may reflect the lack of prior experience with these agents, but other factors such as size and route of inoculation, general health, or greater susceptibility due to immaturity may be important.

Acute hemorrhagic cystitis and *pertussis syndrome* are summarized in Table 178-2.

Incubation period The period of incubation for pharyngoconjunctival fever and ARD is 5 to 10 days, and is probably similar for other syndromes, since induced disease in volunteers has a similar period of incubation.

PATHOGENESIS When the conjunctival sac is swabbed with suspensions of adenovirus, conjunctivitis occurs and there is sometimes respiratory involvement. The initiation of illness appears to require a significant degree of conjunctival irritation. Administration of virus aerosol by inhalation also produces illness. Volunteers inoculated in this way have developed ARD and mild pneumonia.

These observations suggest the existence of at least two routes of inoculation for naturally occurring respiratory illness with adenoviruses: (1) ocular inoculation associated with eye irritation such as may occur in outbreaks around swimming pools, with the development of *pharyngoconjunctival fever*; (2) inoculation through inhalation of infectious aerosol generated by sneezing and coughing of ill recruits under the crowded circumstances incidental to recruit training. The route of inoculation of infants is less likely to be limited to aerosolized virus, and whatever the route of inoculation, the occurrence of pneumonia may represent primarily a lack of resistance in this young age group.

Nasopharyngeal inoculation in volunteers often produces virus infection without illness, suggesting that the high frequency of antibody to many serotypes in the population may result from asymptomatic infections. Antibody may also result from intragroup cross reactions among serotypes in the three broad immunologic groups of adenovirus.

CLINICAL MANIFESTATIONS *Acute respiratory disease* is an acute febrile illness lasting about 1 week and characterized by fever, cough, hoarseness, and sore throat. Fever has gradual onset and reaches a maximum of 103 to 104°F on the second or third day. There are associated malaise and often headache. Pharyngitis, the most prominent localized manifestation of the disease, reaches maximum severity after about 3 days. There may also be regional lymphadenopathy, pharyngeal injection, some edema, frequent lymphoid follicular hyperplasia, but little or no faucial exudate. Nasal obstruction and discharge occur in almost one-half of cases, but these abnormalities are not usually conspicuous. Cough is almost always present, and hoarseness is frequent.

Pharyngoconjunctival fever is usually a milder respiratory illness than ARD, although fever may be high for 5 or 6 days. Nontender submandibular lymphadenopathy is common even in the absence of sore throat. Lower respiratory tract involvement has not been described. Conjunctivitis is mild to moderate but may last longer than respiratory symptoms. It is an acute, nonpurulent, follicular conjunctivitis. In some cases, unilateral preauricular lymphadenopathy occurs. There is usually no involvement of the cornea or uveal tract.

Febrile pharyngitis without conjunctivitis resembles the foregoing illness, except for the absence of conjunctivitis.

Adenoviral pneumonia in children occurs as a primary illness and is associated with as much as 15 percent mortality. Pediatric texts should be consulted for further details.

For further details about *hemorrhagic cystitis* and *pertussis-like syndrome*, pediatric texts should be consulted.

DIFFERENTIAL DIAGNOSIS The differential diagnosis of ARD should include the respiratory viral diseases described in the present chapter and influenza (Chap. 179), nonpneumonic forms of *M. pneumoniae* infection (Chap. 172), streptococcal sore throat, and purulent sinusitis. Pharyngitis and upper respiratory illness may also accompany the onset of infectious hepatitis and infectious mononucleosis.

Differential diagnosis of *pharyngoconjunctival fever,* when conjunctivitis is prominent, includes leptospirosis, influenza, measles, herpangina, and the nonpurulent conjunctivitides, such as inclusion conjunctivitis and physical or chemical trauma to the eye.

TREATMENT There is no specific treatment for adenovirus infection. Treatment is limited to alleviation of general discomfort, headache, and coughing, with analgesics, cough syrup containing terpin hydrate, codeine, antihistamines, or other antitussives.

PREVENTION The communicability of adenovirus infection probably extends from a day or so before onset of illness to recovery, and conventional precautions against respiratory spread should be employed during acute illness for patients in the hospital and to the extent reasonably possible in care of patients at home. Avoidance of swimming pools during outbreaks of pharyngoconjunctival fever is recommended.

Formalin-treated vaccines against types 3, 4, and 7 afford significant protection against infection and illness, but these vaccines were withdrawn from civilian use when it was discovered that some serotypes of adenoviruses produced tumors in hamsters. A live adenovirus vaccine given orally in enteric-coated capsules is highly effective in preventing infection with adenovirus types 3, 4, and 7 in military recruits. More recently, a vaccine prepared from hexons and the fiber portion of penton demonstrated a high degree of protection against experimental infections in volunteers. No vaccine is now marketed for civilian use.

COXSACKIEVIRUS AND ECHOVIRUS INFECTIONS

Diseases produced by these agents are described in Chap. 187. Table 178-3 summarizes the respiratory illnesses sometimes seen with infections caused by these viruses.

REFERENCES

Adenoviruses

BRANDT CD et al: Infections in 18,000 infants and children in a study of respiratory disease: II. Variation in adenovirus infections by year and seasons. Am J Epidemiol 95:218, 1972

KASEL JA: Adenoviruses, in *Diagnostic Procedures for Viral, Rickettsiae and Chlamydiae Infections*, 5th ed, FH Lennette, NJ Schmidt (eds). New York, American Public Health Association, 1978

KNIGHT V, KASEL JA: Adenoviruses, in *Viral and Mycoplasmal Infections of the Respiratory Tract*, V Knight (ed). Philadelphia, Lea & Febiger, 1973

MUFSON MB, BELSHO RB: A review of adenoviruses in the etiology of acute hemorrhagic cystitis. J Urol 115:191, 1976

Coronaviruses

CAVALLARO JJ, MONTO AS: Community-wide outbreak of infection with 229E-like coronavirus in Tecumseh, Michigan. J Infect Dis 122:27, 1970

KNIGHT V, MAYOR HD: Coronaviruses, in *Viral and Mycoplasmal Infections of the Respiratory Tract*, V Knight (ed). Philadelphia, Lea & Febiger, 1973

McINTOSH K et al: Coronavirus infection in lower respiratory tract disease of infants. J Infect Dis 130:502, 1974

WENZEL RP et al: Coronavirus infections in military recruits. Am Rev Resp Dis 109:621, 1974

Herpesviruses

EVANS AS, DICK FC: Acute pharyngitis and tonsillitis in University of Wisconsin students. JAMA 190:699, 1964

GLEZEN WP et al: Acute respiratory disease of university students with special reference to the etiologic role of *Herpesvirus hominis*. Am J Epidemiol 101:111, 1975

MOGABGAB WJ: Acute respiratory illness in university (1962–1966) military and industrial (1962–1963) populations. Am Rev Respir Dis 98:359, 1968

Parainfluenza virus

GLEZEN WP et al: The parainfluenza viruses, in *Viral Infections of Humans*, AS Evans (ed). New York, Plenum, 1976, chap 15

MONTO AS: The Tecumseh study: V. Patterns of infection with respiratory disease, N Engl J Med 258:207, 1978

Respiratory syncytial virus

HALL WJ et al: Respiratory syncytial virus infection in adults. Clinical, virologic, and serial pulmonary function studies. Ann Intern Med 88:203, 1978

KNIGHT V: Respiratory syncytial viruses, in *Viral and Mycoplasmal Infections of the Respiratory Tract*, V Knight (ed). Philadelphia, Lea & Febiger, 1973

PARROT RH et al: Epidemiology of respiratory syncytial virus infection in Washington D.C.: II. Infection and disease with respect to age, immunologic status, race and sex. Am J Epidemiol 98:289, 1973

Rhinoviruses

CATE TR: Rhinoviruses, in *Viral and Mycoplasmal Infections of the Respiratory Tract*, V Knight (ed). Philadelphia, Lea & Febiger, 1973

FOX JP et al: The Seattle virus watch: V. Epidemiologic observations of rhinovirus infections, 1965–1969, in families with young children. Am J Epidemiol 101:122, 1975

179
INFLUENZA

VERNON KNIGHT

DEFINITION Influenza is an acute respiratory infection of specific viral etiology characterized by sudden onset of headache, myalgia, fever, and prostration. The terms *influenza* and "flu" should be restricted to those cases with clear-cut epidemiologic or laboratory evidence of infection with influenza viruses.

HISTORY According to the best available records, influenza was uncommon in Europe during the nineteenth century until the pandemic of 1889. Subsequently, the frequency and severity of epidemics increased, culminating in the disastrous pandemic of 1918, which caused an estimated 20 to 40 million deaths. The mortality rate from the disease has decreased progressively since 1918 owing in part to the introduction of antibiotics and also to such factors as possible change in virulence of the virus and improved living standards.

ETIOLOGY There are three distinct antigenic types of influenza virus, designated A, B, and C. Infection with one type confers no immunity to the other two. On the basis of intrinsic properties, the three types are grouped in a virus family named Orthomyxoviridae. The influenza viruses contain a single, segmented, negative strand RNA genome. They are spherical or filamentous enveloped particles, 80 to 120 nm in diameter, with glycoprotein structures termed *hemagglutinin (H)* and *neuraminidase (N)*, which protrude from the envelope. The former are responsible for attachment of virus to cell receptors; the latter enzymatically degrades the active receptor substance, frees virus from attachment sites if cell penetration is unsuccessful, and functions in the release of infectious virus from cells during the replication cycle. The H and N are antigenic and elicit antibodies which correlate with the prevention of infection and disease. Antihemagglutinin antibodies are more potent than those elicited by the N antigen.

The three types of influenza viruses are biologically related by their infectivity for chick embryos, capacity to agglutinate erythrocytes in vitro, and affinity for respiratory epithelium of various mammals.

EPIDEMIOLOGY Influenza A Influenza A viruses are the cause of epidemics that occur every 2 to 4 years and of pandemics that occur every decade or so. Recent studies have also revealed milder annual interepidemic occurrences of influenza A.

Influenza, especially type A infection, is a recurring disease, because the virus undergoes continuous antigenic variation with time, involving the surface antigens H and N. This progressive, but not necessarily regular, change produces viruses to which segments of the population become susceptible in numbers somewhat in proportion to the extent of antigenic variation. Thus the annual interepidemic outbreaks are not as severe nor as extensive as the less frequent epidemics. The origin of pandemic viruses is unknown, but they appear to arise by a different mechanism. The segmented genome of type A influenza virus exhibits a high recombination frequency. Consequently, a recombinational event between human and nonhuman type A influenza viruses could possibly give rise to antigenically different subtypes. Table 179-1 shows subtypes of influenza that have appeared in this century.

The characteristics of the 1918 virus are inferred from retrospective serologic analyses. The H antigen is the most important, and each new subtype has had a different H antigen (Hsw, H0, H1, H2, H3). The less mobile N antigen has changed only once, N1 to N2 in 1957.

Pandemics accompanied the introduction of three new subtypes, and the absence of pandemics in 1933 and 1947 is probably due to a limited antigenic relationship that existed among the 1918, 1933, and 1947 subtypes, so that individuals who were ill with swine virus influenza in 1918 had some resistance to the 1933 subtype, and similarly, individuals ill in 1933 had some resistance to the 1947 agent.

It was also noted that many older people did not become ill during the 1968 epidemic, and it was found that many of them possessed antibody to this subtype that was probably acquired in the period 1889 to 1890, when the subtype then prevalent shared antigenic properties with the 1968 subtype. There is also evidence that the 1957 virus shared antigens with the subtype that was prevalent before 1890, although due to the time lapse there were too few older people with antibody to have a measurable effect on the pandemic.

Variants within subtypes are identified by the site of first isolation of the new strain and the year of its isolation. The four most recent variants that caused epidemic disease in the United States and elsewhere are A/England/72 (H3N2), A/Port Chalmers/73 (H3N2), A/Victoria/1975 (H3N2), and A/Texas/1976 (H3N2). Differentiation among variants is important because vaccines to one variant show a progressive loss of protective effect against later emerging variants, so that after about 3 years the vaccine will have little effect.

In 1976 what was first thought to be a new pandemic strain, a virus resembling the 1918 swine virus, was isolated from recruits at Fort Dix, New Jersey. In preparation for a possible pandemic, millions of doses of vaccine against the new virus were prepared and given in the United States. The swine agent did not, however, spread to the general population, but an unexpected occurrence of a syndrome of peripheral neuritis (Guillain-Barré syndrome) was observed in association with persons immunized in a ratio of 1 case per 100,000 immunized. About 1 in 1 million had some degree of residual neurologic damage, and 1 in 2 million died.

These rates are eight- to tenfold greater than in an age-matched, unvaccinated control population. Such an observation would probably not have been possible if a swine virus influenza epidemic or pandemic had occurred. Whether or not this low-frequency occurrence has accompanied the use of other influenza vaccines is not known.

TABLE 179-1
Subtypes of influenza A and associated disease occurrences in the twentieth century

Pandemic 1918	A/Swine/1931 (HswN1)-like
Epidemic 1933	A/Puerto Rico/1934 (H0N1)
Epidemic 1947	A/FM1/1947 (H1N1)
Pandemic 1957	A/Japan/1957 (H2N2)
Pandemic 1968	A/Hong Kong/1968 (H3N2)

In 1978 a strain of influenza A of the H1N1 subtype similar to strains that prevailed in the period 1947 to 1957, but mostly resembling the variant of 1951, caused epidemics in China and Russia. Persons born after 1957, having never been exposed, will be susceptible to infection with this agent. Since limited outbreaks of disease were caused by the new H1N1 variant in 1977 to 1978, preparations have been made to include it in the vaccine to be distributed in 1978 and 1979.

Influenza A viruses infect pigs, horses, and fowl, especially ducks and turkeys. H and N antigens of some of these viruses are related to H and N antigens of human influenza A viruses. Recently, it was shown that the internal matrix protein of the virus is an antigen common to all influenza A viruses. The name *swine influenza* was given to the agent that caused the 1918 pandemic because an epidemic of influenza that occurred among swine at that time was thought possibly to have spread to swine from infected people. The swine agent has continued to infect swine populations since that time. The outbreak of "swine virus influenza" among military recruits at Fort Dix in 1976 was presumably an example of swine-to-human transmission. The pandemic A(H3N2) strain of 1968 shared antigens with an agent isolated from horses in 1963. Despite these findings and considerable experimentation with induction of infection across species lines, there is no solid evidence that lower animals are involved in the natural history of human influenza.

Influenza A epidemics start abruptly, reach a peak in 2 to 3 months, and subside almost as rapidly. The attack rate is variable but was noted in 1957 to exceed 50 percent in urban populations. An additional 25 percent of individuals may show serologic evidence of infection without clinical manifestations. Experiences in 1957 proved conclusively that crowding, even in summer months or in tropical countries, is a major factor predisposing to epidemics. School children, in particular, appear to be the primary focus and disseminators of infection in the United States. If the general immunity of a population is at low levels, community-wide epidemics may occur within a short period after the introduction of new strains of virus. If, however, immune individuals predominate, the case rate will rise slowly and may not reach epidemic proportions.

The mortality rate from all causes always increases markedly during epidemics of influenza. In the fall and winter of 1957 to 1958 it was estimated that 40 million persons in the United States became ill with influenza and the total number of influenza-associated deaths was reported to be in excess of 8000. In addition, approximately 60,000 more deaths from various causes occurred during this period than would be expected under normal conditions. The greatest incidence of excessive mortality occurred among infants under 1 year of age and adults over 60 years of age. Data from a small series of cases clearly indicate that influenza is frequently fatal in individuals with preexisting pulmonary or cardiac disease, regardless of age. Chronic rheumatic heart disease with mitral stenosis, in particular, appears to predispose to fatal influenzal pneumonia.

Influenza B and C Influenza B virus infection occurs sporadically or in localized outbreaks, particularly in schools and military camps and every 4 to 6 years causes more discrete epidemics than influenza A. Although influenza B virus possesses H and N coat proteins, it undergoes less variation than influenza A viruses, and it is not now the practice to designate the virus by these antigens. Illness with influenza B infection is less serious than that caused by influenza A viruses. The most serious problem with influenza B infections is a complication, Reye's syndrome, characterized by encephalopathy and fatty changes in the liver and other organs (see "Complications"). Illness with influenza C is rarely detected, although antibody surveys indicate a wide prevalence of the infection.

PATHOGENESIS Influenza is primarily an infection of the respiratory epithelium that is produced by inoculation with virus from respiratory secretions of infected persons. Experimental studies show that a small number of virus particles inhaled in a small-particle aerosol or severalfold larger doses in liquid suspension dropped in the nose will produce the disease. Infection thus could result from transfer of infected secretions by personal contact or fomites or, probably much more frequently, by inhalation of aerosols generated by sneezes, coughs, and other expiratory discharges of infected individuals.

After inoculation, the virus multiplies to maximum titers in a few days. In studies in volunteers the incubation period was prolonged up to 7 days with small inocula but was only a day or so with large inocula. Cells lining the respiratory tract, including ciliated epithelium, alveolar cells, mucous gland cells, and macrophages may become infected. Neutrophil leukocytes and endothelial cells do not appear to become infected. Evidence of virus infection by specific immunofluorescence is most conspicuous in cells that show fewest morphologic changes. Infected ciliated cells undergo degeneration after a day or so and are characterized by swelling of nuclei with shift from a longitudinal to a transverse position in the cell. Cytoplasmic changes are granulation, vacuolation, and swelling. Ultimately cells become necrotic and slough, in some areas to be replaced by flattened and metaplastic epithelial regrowth.

Based on the finding of high titers of virus in nasal washes and from throat swabs and a generalized inflammatory reaction in the nasopharynx, the nasopharynx must usually be widely involved with viral infection. Since tracheobronchitis is regularly a part of uncomplicated influenza, it seems probable that viral lesions also occur in this area. The finding of abnormal pulmonary function in apparently uncomplicated cases suggests that viral infection may ordinarily penetrate more deeply into the lung than earlier supposed. When pulmonary involvement is clinically detectable, high titers of virus are recoverable from sputum and tracheal aspirates and autopsy studies show large areas of pulmonary virus infection.

Despite often severe systemic symptoms, direct evidence of influenza infection beyond the respiratory tract is limited to the isolation of virus in fatal cases from lung, spleen, lymph nodes, liver, kidney, and heart. It is also possible that rare cases of encephalitis with influenza may be associated with viral infection of the central nervous system. Finally, one report describes the isolation of influenza virus A from the feces of children ill with the disease.

MANIFESTATIONS The disease assumes its typical form during major epidemics of influenza A, but clinical differentiation between influenza A and B is not possible in localized outbreaks. Sporadic infections with either influenza A or B are likely to result in relatively minor illnesses, with predominantly respiratory symptoms, similar to those of common respiratory disease. Influenza C is particularly difficult to recognize because of its mildness. Although the manifestations and severity of influenza A vary from year to year, cases in a single epidemic often follow a remarkably similar pattern. The clinical description that follows is a composite picture of epidemic influenza A of the past three decades.

The *incubation period* is usually 18 to 36 h but may be as long as 3 days. Mild prodromal symptoms of cough, malaise, and chilliness are sometimes present, but extremely sudden onset is often such a characteristic feature that many patients can recall its exact time. The most common initial symptom is severe generalized or frontal *headache*, frequently accompanied by stabbing retroorbital pain that is accentuated by lateral or upward gaze. Diffuse *myalgia*, particularly marked in the legs and over the lumbosacral area, occurs in more than half the cases. Pain and spasm of the abdominal muscles may simulate

acute peritonitis, and incapacitating periarticular pains are sometimes confused with acute arthritis. *Feverishness* and *chilliness,* or occasionally true rigors, may be the first manifestations, but more often they are preceded by headache and myalgia. The temperature rises abruptly to a maximum of 100 to 103°F several hours after onset; rarely it may reach 106°F. Thereafter, the fever and pain usually subside over a 2- to 3-day period but may persist for as long as a week. A common variant in the temperature course is rapid defervescence after the initial peak, with a secondary rise to the original level on the following day. In general, severity of illness parallels the height and duration of the fever. The pulse rate is usually slow in relation to the fever, but marked tachycardia may occur in severely ill patients.

Respiratory symptoms may be present at the onset but become most prominent when the systemic manifestations and fever begin to subside. They are frequently less pronounced than in common respiratory disease and may be entirely absent. Sneezing, watery nasal discharge, and stuffy nose occur in most cases; hoarseness and epistaxis are less frequent. Conjunctival suffusion and burning, itching, watery eyes are often noted. The throat may feel dry, and the pharynx often appears slightly injected. *Cough* develops during the course of the illness in more than three-fourths of the cases, and in about a third of these it is productive of small amounts of tenacious, mucoid sputum. *Chest pain,* usually substernal in location and accentuated by coughing but not by breathing, is present in almost half the patients. Pleurisy and pleural effusion are uncommon. Slight hyperpnea is often noted, but the most ominous, although infrequent, signs are dyspnea and cyanosis, which signal bronchiolar or pneumonic involvement. Findings on physical examination of the lungs are often negative in uncomplicated influenza, but scattered rhonchi, wheezes, and showers of moist rales have been reported in 5 to 40 percent of cases in different epidemics. These changes may persist for several days after apparent recovery. Patients with uncomplicated influenza may have restrictive ventilatory defects and increased alveolar-capillary oxygen tension gradients, suggesting the regular occurrence of lower pulmonary tract involvement in the disease. Influenzal bronchiolitis should be suspected if rales persist in the absence of x-ray evidence of pneumonitis and if the patient raises mucopurulent or blood-tinged sputum.

Prostration of some degree is almost invariable and is often the most prominent and alarming manifestation. The face is flushed, and the skin is hot and dry; however, profuse sweating and cold, mottled extremities are sometimes noted. Anorexia, nausea, and constipation are frequent secondary symptoms, but vomiting is rare. Diarrhea occurs with some frequency in children but is rare in adults. Meningoencephalitis, polyneuritis, cranial nerve palsies, transient nerve deafness, aphasia, hemiplegia, psychoses, and other neurologic disorders have been described in association with influenza but are very unusual. Hypotension, heart block, peripheral vasoconstriction, and fatal myocarditis have also been reported in a few cases.

COMPLICATIONS The chief complication of influenza is pneumonia, which occurs as a primary infection with influenza virus or as influenza virus pneumonia with superimposed bacterial pneumonia. In recent years, about 20 percent of pneumonic complications have resulted from primary viral infection. In patients whose pneumonia is complicated by bacterial infection, *Staphylococcus aureus* and pneumococci are the most frequent etiologic agents. Less frequent bacterial etiologies are *Hemophilus influenzae,* hemolytic streptococcus, and various gram-negative bacilli. Staphylococci and gram-negative bacilli are often resistant to some antibiotics and these resistant strains may have been selected by prior treatment with these drugs. In addition, the incidence of bacterial pneumonias without an apparent viral concomitant is greatly increased during influenza epidemics.

Primary influenza virus pneumonia typically has its onset about 1 week after the onset of influenza, often following a period of apparent improvement. The disease is characterized by severe dyspnea and cyanosis, scanty sputum containing gross blood, leukopenia, few physical signs, and perihilar infiltrates by x-ray. The disease has a rapid course and fatality, when it occurs, results from acute respiratory failure.

Pathologic findings in fatal cases of primary viral pneumonia consist of large areas of inflammatory reaction within alveolar septa, with little exudate in alveolar spaces. Involved septa are edematous and infiltrated with lymphocytes, macrophages, and occasionally plasma cells. Some neutrophils may be present. In severe cases, fibrin thrombi may obstruct alveolar capillaries and cause necrosis and hemorrhage. An eosinophilic hyaline membrane may be found lining alveoli and alveolar ducts, presumably resulting from transudation of fibrin through affected alveolar septa. The pleura are not usually involved. This picture is not specific for influenza virus infection and must be differentiated from *Mycoplasma pneumoniae* pneumonia and from the common respiratory viruses that cause pneumonia, predominantly in children.

Secondary bacterial pneumonia is usually detected by onset of production of purulent sputum, fever, and other signs of bacterial pneumonia after the initial episode of influenzal illness. It may occur at variable intervals in relation to the associated viral pneumonia. The pathologic findings vary with the bacterial etiology. In general, the changes associated with pyogenic infection will obscure the less conspicuous viral lesions.

Staphylococcus aureus causes a necrotizing tracheobronchobronchiolitis associated with a neutrophil leukocytosis, tissue necrosis, masses of staphylococci in necrotic areas, thromboses of small blood vessels, and hemorrhage. Purulent exudate plugs the respiratory passages. This process may extend into the lung parenchyma and cause bronchopneumonia associated with large and small abscesses surrounded by areas of hemorrhage, capillary thrombosis, edema, and fibrin deposition.

Pneumococcal pneumonia shows its characteristic fibrinous leukocytic exudate within alveolar air spaces. Necrotizing inflammation as with staphylococcal infection is rare, and the alveolar architecture is preserved. As with staphylococcal infection, the pneumococcal infection may obscure the lesions of viral infection. *Hemophilus influenzae* and gram-negative bacilli produce necrotizing tracheobronchobronchiolitis with lobular pneumonia and sometimes abscess formation. Bacterial pneumonia occurring during influenza epidemics that is not associated with influenza virus pneumonia is a more benign disease with pathologic findings typical of the particular infection.

Many studies have shown that pneumonic complications are most frequent and severe in the aged; in patients with rheumatic valvular or other heart disease, chronic lung disease, and serious systemic illness; and in pregnant women.

Sinusitis and otitis media caused by the usual common pathogens sometimes complicate influenza.

A complication of influenza B and, less frequently, of influenza A and other viral infections that has been identified increasingly is a syndrome of encephalopathy with acute cerebral edema and fatty infiltration of the liver called *Reye's syndrome*. Reduced activity of one or two mitochondrial hepatic enzymes of the urea cycle is noted in these patients. The mortality rate is high. Treatment has consisted of dexamethasone administration under continuous monitoring to maintain intracranial pressure at tolerable levels. Peritoneal dialysis is also used to remove excess blood ammonia commonly present in these patients.

Recovery from uncomplicated influenza is often complete in a week, but convalescence may be prolonged by "postinfectious asthenia" and depression particularly in elderly persons. Minor relapses with fever may occur but are uncommon.

LABORATORY FINDINGS Virus is isolated most readily during the acute phase of the disease by inoculation of throat swab or broth garglings into the amniotic cavity of chick embryos or into tissue cultures of monkey kidney cells. Influenza virus types A, B, and C may be identified in complement fixation tests. These tests depend on the nucleocapsid antigen found in the viral core and in soluble form in infected cells. Antiserum to whole virions readily detects the same or closely related strains by immunofluorescence in infected cell culture and, on occasion, directly in exudates from patients with infection. This methodology is useful in rapid diagnosis. Serologic diagnosis can be made most reliably by the hemagglutination inhibition test, using paired serum samples obtained in both the acute and convalescent phases. Type-specific antibody against soluble complement-fixing antigens of influenza A virus also appears in the circulation of patients during the acute illness.

In uncomplicated influenza the lungs usually appear normal by x-ray but pulmonary involvement with viral infection is often marked by increased vascular markings, basilar streaking, small areas of patchy infiltration, atelectasis or nodular densities. The blood leukocyte count may be low 2 to 4 days after onset of illness, but is often normal or slightly elevated. Leukocytosis with counts above 15,000 cells per cubic millimeter indicates secondary bacterial infection, but leukopenia may occur in severe pneumonia. Slight proteinuria is common during the height of the febrile illness.

DIFFERENTIAL DIAGNOSIS Many bacterial and viral infections simulate influenza at their onset, but few febrile diseases have such a self-limited course. Noninfluenzal respiratory diseases are generally characterized by more gradual onset; milder systemic manifestations; and predominant symptoms of coryza, rhinorrhea, pharyngitis, and conjunctivitis.

TREATMENT Antibiotics do not affect the course of uncomplicated influenza, nor is there any evidence that they prevent complications. Antibiotics should be reserved for secondary bacterial infections. Clinical trials have shown limited effectiveness of amantadine, a symmetric amine that inhibits an early step in replication of influenza virus, as a chemoprophylactic and therapeutic agent. Codeine affords relief from incapacitating cough and is more effective than salicylates for symptomatic treatment of headache and myalgia; salicylates often increase discomfort by causing drenching sweats and chills. Bed rest during illness and gradual return to full activities are advisable.

PROPHYLAXIS Formalinized egg vaccines purified by zonal ultracentrifugation or other methods and containing a mixture of influenza A (H3N2) and B viruses in whole or split forms are available commercially in the United States. Current vaccines can be expected to be effective when given in suitable dosage at an interval of several weeks to several months before exposure, and when the antigens of the vaccine are still closely related to the epidemic strain.

The U.S. Public Health Service strongly recommends routine yearly immunization with polyvalent influenza vaccine for high-risk groups, including persons of all ages who suffer from chronic rheumatic heart disease, other cardiovascular diseases, chronic bronchopulmonary diseases, diabetes mellitus, or

Addison's disease, and persons 65 years of age or older, regardless of their previous state of health. Pregnant women should be immunized only if they fall into one of the high-risk categories. For initial immunization of adults it is advisable to administer the vaccine subcutaneously in two doses of 0.5 ml each, the first injection in September and the second several weeks or months later. A single subcutaneous dose of 0.5 ml given each autumn is satisfactory as a yearly booster. Intradermal injection of vaccine is far less satisfactory because a sufficient antigenic mass cannot be administered.

Influenza vaccination is generally safe but not completely innocuous. The recent occurrence of the Guilliain-Barré syndrome as a complication of the use of inactivated swine influenza virus vaccine requires further evaluation. Fatal anaphylactic reactions and purpura have been reported in individuals sensitive to egg proteins, and inactivated virus itself is pyrogenic and can sometimes produce an illness similar to active influenza. Infants and children have experienced severe febrile convulsions following vaccination, and vaccine should be avoided in children with a history of this syndrome. A decision to vaccinate children, especially the very young, should be made on

an individual basis. The subject of influenza prevention is also discussed in Chap. 114.

REFERENCES

GLEZEN WP, COUCH RB: Interpandemic influenza in the Houston area, 1974–1976. N Engl J Med 298:587, 1978

HOCHBERG FH et al: Influenza type B-related encephalopathy, the 1971 outbreak of Reye's syndrome in Chicago. JAMA 231:817, 1975

MONTO AS, KIOUMEHR F: The Tecumseh study of respiratory illness: IX. Occurrence of influenza in the community, 1966–1971. Am J Epidemiol 102:553, 1975

MULDER J, HERS JFP: Influenza. Groningen, The Netherlands, Wolters-Noordhoff Publishing, 1972, pp 1–288

PRICE DA et al: Influenza virus A2 infections presenting with febrile convulsions and gastrointestinal symptoms in young children. Clin Pediatr 15:361, 1976

Exanthems and enanthems

180
APPROACH TO THE PATIENT WITH RASH AND FEVER

LAWRENCE COREY

Because many infectious and noninfectious diseases produce cutaneous lesions, specific diagnosis of an acutely ill febrile patient with a rash is a clinical skill with important therapeutic implications. The cutaneous manifestations of an infectious disease may result from direct innoculation of the organism into skin or indirectly from lymphogenous, hematogenous, or contiguous spread of the pathogen. Exanthems are cutaneous eruptions due to systemic or contiguous spread of an organism. These eruptions may be due to multiplication of the etiologic agent in the skin or dermal vasculature or to the host's immune responses to the organism. The cutaneous manifestations of infections may involve the epidermis or the vascular or extravascular structures of the dermis. Some exanthems are unique to a particular pathogen, others are common to numerous etiologic agents. Classification of exanthematous illness into (1) maculopapular, (2) vesicular, and (3) petechial eruptions is useful in determining the etiology and in understanding the pathogenesis of an exanthem.

PATHOGENESIS The pathogenesis of an exanthem may be caused by (1) multiplication of the pathogen in the skin, (2) carriage of the agent in plasma or in infected hematopoietic cells (leukocytes and/or lymphocytes) into integumentary blood vessels, and (3) antigen-antibody or delayed hypersensitivity reactions to antigens derived from the infecting microorganism. For example, in many viral diseases, such as rubella, rubeola, and the enterovirus infections, initial viral replication

occurs in the infected mucosal surface and regional lymphatic tissue. Primary viremia then ensues, and "seeding" of the virus into target organs, such as liver, muscle, central nervous system, or heart, may occur. Continued viral replication and a secondary viremia with hematogenous spread of the virus to the skin may then follow. In this model, regional multiplication of the virus, primary viremia, and visceral dissemination of virus occur prior to the development of the exanthem and explain why the initial clinical manifestations of many viral illnesses occur prior to the development of the rash. Humoral and cellular immune responses which prevent or ameliorate secondary viremia may prevent the development of a rash. This may explain why exanthems associated with enteroviruses occur more frequently in younger children than adolescents or adults: young children do not possess cross-reacting antibodies or cannot mount an anamnestic immune response to the infecting agent.

While some maculopapular exanthems appear to be related to direct viral or bacterial invasion of the skin, other exanthems result from local or systemic immune responses to the microorganism. Rubella virus can be recovered from rubella maculopapules as well as from areas of the body not involved by the exanthem. Administration of pooled immune serum globulin after exposure to rubella may not eliminate rubella viremia but does prevent rash. Similarly, the exanthem of rubeola may be a manifestation of an Arthus reaction produced by the deposition of viral antigen in the endothelium of dermal capillaries. Local factors such as exposure to light or local irritation of the skin have also been shown to modify the distribution of some exanthems.

Vesicular exanthems are usually associated with active viral invasion of the infected area. Characteristically, herpes simplex virus, varicella-zoster virus, or poxviruses can be demonstrated in vesicular fluid by viral culture or by immunologic techniques. Local host and immune responses are important in the progression of varicella lesions, and their duration has been correlated with both local and "immune" interferon production.

Petechial eruptions may arise from direct invasion of the cutaneous vasculature by a microorganism, as occurs with septic emboli, or may result from immunologic injury to the vascular endothelium. In Rocky Mountain spotted fever, *Rickettsia rickettsiae* can be demonstrated in the smooth-muscle wall of arterioles. Vascular damage, microinfarction, and extravasation of red blood cells produce the characteristic petechial exanthem. Occasionally, a petechial eruption may complicate previous maculopapular or vesicular exanthems, usually coinciding with the development of diffuse intravascular coagulation. This may be seen in hemorrhagic dengue, measles, or varicella. In some petechial eruptions, direct evidence of viral or bacterial invasion can be obtained by direct aspiration and culture of the lesion, by demonstration of the agent with Gram's stain, or by immunofluorescent stain to detect microbial agents.

CLINICAL DIAGNOSIS OF MACULOPAPULAR ERUPTIONS

Table 180-1 lists the numerous viral, bacterial, rickettsial, and noninfectious agents that may be associated with maculopapular exanthems. One helpful approach to the physical examination of viral maculopapular (*not* vesicular) rashes is that these eruptions *relatively* spare the palms and soles in contrast to eruptions associated with drug reactions, bacteria, mycoplasma, and rickettsial and/or immunologic diseases. In the latter entities, a prominent palmar or plantar distribution is often present.

While some exanthematous diseases produce characteristic cutaneous patterns, e.g., measles or erythema infectiosum, overlap in the cutaneous manifestations of viral induced maculopapular exanthems is the rule. Therefore, the presence of associated signs or symptoms as well as the epidemiologic characteristics of the disease such as the season of the year, the patient's age, and history of exposure and previous immunization are useful in formulating a diagnostic impression. Because viral maculopapular exanthems are manifestations of the agent's systemic spread, evidence of mucosal viral replication in the form of an enanthem is often a valuable aid in determining the etiology of a viral rash. Koplik spots in rubeola, ulcerative lesions on the hard and soft palate with herpangina due to coxsackievirus A, and palatal petechiae in early infectious mononucleosis are all helpful clinical signs. Associated clinical findings such as coryza, conjunctivitis, and cough with rubeola, mild fever and posterior auricular lymphadenopathy in rubella, or localized mastitis or furunculosis in staphylococcal scalded-skin syndrome should be looked for. Concomitant arthritis, renal disease, and/or heart disease generally suggests immunologically mediated entities such as acute rheumatic fever, subacute bacterial endocarditis, serum sickness, or collagen vascular disease.

The distribution of the rash provides important information. Erythema infectiosum presents with a diffuse erythema of the cheeks ("slapped cheeks"). In addition, central clearing of the eruption on the extremities results in a lace-like appearance of the exanthem. Erythema marginatum occurs in 10 percent of patients with acute rheumatic fever and is characterized by a ringed eruption which rapidly spreads to the trunk and extremities. Scarlet fever due to erythrogenic toxin elaborated by a group A streptococcus produces a rash that starts on the neck and spreads to the trunk and extremities within 36 h. The rash consists of numerous punctate papular lesions at the site of hair follicles and feels like rough sandpaper. Circumoral

TABLE 180-1
Differential diagnosis of patients with rash and fever

Macules or papules	Vesicles	Petechiae-purpura
VIRAL		
Rubeola	Herpes simplex	Enteroviruses (echovirus)
Rubella	Varicella-zoster	
Enteroviruses	Vaccinia	Viral hemorrhagic fevers
Cytomegalovirus	Enteroviruses (herpangina)	Dengue
Hepatitis B		Adenoviruses
Erythema infectiosum	Hand-foot-and-mouth disease (A16)	Yellow fever
Exanthem subitum	Orf	Atypical measles
Adenoviruses	Molluscum contagiosum	
Arboviruses		
Rhabdovirus group	Vesicular stomatitis virus	
Reoviruses		
Live virus vaccines (measles, rubella)		
BACTERIAL		
Group A streptococci:	Staphylococcal scalded-skin syndrome	Severe sepsis with diffuse intravascular coagulation
Scarlet fever	Bullous impetigo	Meningococcemia
Erysipelas		Gonococcemia
Erythema marginatum		Pseudomonas sepsis
Staphylococcal scalded-skin syndrome		Subacute bacterial endocarditis
Subacute bacterial endocarditis		*Listeria monocytogenes*
Secondary syphilis		
Typhoid fever		
Erysipelothrix		
Mycobacterium leprae		
Rat bite fever		
Leptospirosis		
Chronic meningococcemia		
Pseudomonas sepsis		
RICKETTSIAL		
Rocky Mountain spotted fever (early)	Rickettsialpox	Rocky Mountain spotted fever
Murine typhus		Epidemic (louse-borne) typhus
FUNGAL		
Candidiasis		
Sporotrichosis		
Cryptococcosis		
CHLAMYDIAL		
Psittacosis		
PROTOZOAL		
Toxoplasmosis		Trichinosis
Trichinosis		Plasmodia (blackwater fever)
UNKNOWN		
Mucocutaneous lymph node syndrome		
IMMUNOLOGIC		
Erythema multiforme	Stevens-Johnson syndrome	Henoch-Schönlein purpura
Erythema nodosum	Pemphigoid	
	Behçet's syndrome	
	Inflammatory bowel disease	
DRUGS		
Drug eruptions	Drug eruptions	Drug eruptions

pallor, large red fungiform papillae (strawberry tongue), extension of the rash into body folds including the antecubital fossae, concomitant tonsillitis and cervical lymphadenopathy, and the subsequent desquamation of the rash, especially on the palms and soles, confirm the clinical diagnosis. Erysipelas due to group A (uncommonly group G) streptococci and staphylococci is characterized by an edematous indurated superficial cellulitis. Characteristically, the rash is shiny with a sharply demarcated edge. Occasionally streptococci can be demonstrated on Gram's stain and culture of material aspirated from the advancing edge of the lesion.

Some strains of *Staphylococcus aureus* (phage group 2) can elaborate a toxin which produces a diffuse erythema of the skin (staphylococcal scalded-skin syndrome). The development of bullae resulting in the easy separation of the epidermis (Nikolsky's sign) may occur but is not specific for this entity.

The course of the eruption is also helpful in differentiating the etiology of viral exanthems. Rubeola usually starts in the hairline area and spreads downward until the involved areas coalesce into a diffuse morbilliform eruption. In contrast, the eruption of rubella tends to disappear from its original sites of involvement as it spreads.

The rash of Rocky Mountain spotted fever usually starts on the extremities and spreads centripetally to the trunk. In contrast, the rash of roseola subitum starts on the trunk and spreads centrifugally to the arms and legs. Pityriasis rosea is characterized by the development of papular lesions along the lines of cleavage of the trunk ("fir tree" effect). The development of the earlier appearing "herald patch" and the lack of fever characterize this exanthem.

While papular lesions may be a manifestation of viral disease, systemic bacterial and/or fungal disease may also produce these lesions. Chronic meningococcemia may be associated with pale rose colored maculopapular lesions that may be mistaken for erythema nodosum when located on the lower extremities. The cutaneous lesions tend to wax and wane with fever. Organisms usually are not demonstrated in Gram's stain or cultures of these lesions. However, blood cultures taken during febrile periods may be positive. The development of discrete papules on the trunk in a patient with a previous history of diarrhea should suggest the possibility of typhoid fever. These "rose spots" are 1- to 3-mm papules which disappear in 3 to 4 days. In the untreated patient new lesions will emerge over the next 2 to 3 weeks. Pseudomonas bacteremia can also produce small painless papules on the trunk. The papulosquamous lesions of secondary syphilis often involve the trunk, palms, soles, and mucous membranes and may be present for days to several weeks. The serology (VDRL) is invariably positive in secondary syphilis.

Papulonodular lesions can be identified in 10 to 15 percent of patients with disseminated candidiasis. The appearance of these lesions in febrile immunosuppressed patients who fail to respond to antimicrobials should suggest the possibility of disseminated candidiasis. Biopsy and culture of the lesions should demonstrate the blastospores and pseudohyphae of *Candida* species.

In all infectious diseases, knowledge of the epidemiologic milieu of the patient is of great aid in arriving at a presumptive diagnosis of a patient with fever and a maculopapular eruption. Erysipeloid should be considered in persons with exposure to swine or saltwater fish; rat bite fever in those with a history of rodent exposure; sporotrichosis in those with contact with roses or spaghnum; leptospirosis in those patients who have contact with potentially infected animals and who also have hepatitis, conjunctivitis, and/or meningitis; and Rocky Mountain spotted fever in individuals who live in areas endemic for tick bites.

Mucocutaneous lymph node syndrome Also termed *Kawasaki's disease* mucocutaneous lymph node syndrome is a multisystem disease that occurs in children and is being recognized more frequently in the United States.

This entity was first described in Japan in the 1960s. It affects children from 2 months to 9 years of age, with 50 percent of cases occurring in children under 2 years of age. Characteristically, the patient presents with a fever between 38.3 and 40°C (101 and 104°F) of 1 to 2 weeks' duration which is unresponsive to antimicrobials. Bilateral conjunctivitis; dryness, redness, and fissuring of the lips; diffuse erythema of the oral and pharyngeal mucosa; "strawberry tongue," and cervical adenopathy may be present. On the third to fifth day of illness, a macular erythematous eruption, usually starting on the extremities, appears. Pronounced reddening of the palms and soles is present, and the child's hands and feet may swell due to an indurative edema. Characteristically during the second week of the illness desquamation of the rash starts at the junction of the nails and skin of the fingers and toes. Myocardial involvement is common, with abnormal ECG findings in over 50 percent of patients. Coronary angiography may reveal aneurysms and pathological changes in the vessels similar to infantile periarteritis nodosa. In severe cases, myocardial infarction due to coronary thrombosis may occur. Arthritis, hepatitis, and "aseptic meningitis" may also be seen. Laboratory data include an abnormal sedimentation rate, normal antistreptolysin O (ASO) titers, presence of elevated C-reactive protein, and peripheral leukocytosis. The prognosis is usually good; death occurs in 1 to 2 percent of patients and is usually due to coronary thrombosis. In the United States, cases have been clustered geographically and temporally. The etiology of this entity is unknown.

CLINICAL DIAGNOSIS OF VESICULAR ERUPTIONS The distribution of the eruption is often helpful in determining a clinical and etiologic diagnosis of a vesicular exanthem. Varicella begins on the trunk, spreads centrifugally, and demonstrates lesions in all stages of healing, i.e., vesicles, ulcers, and crusts. Variola usually begins on the extremities, spreads centripetally, and is characterized by lesions in similar stages of development. The vesicular ulcerative pharyngeal lesions of herpangina are present only on the palate, whereas primary herpes simplex gingivostomatitis also involves the anterior gingival area and/or the lips. Hand, foot, and mouth disease due to coxsackievirus A16 presents as multiple linear vesicles or pustules on the palms and soles; this is an unusual distribution for either herpes simplex or varicella-zoster virus.

Primary herpes simplex virus (HSV) infection is clinically distinct from recrudescent disease. Initial oral or genital HSV infection is often accompanied by constitutional symptoms such as fever, malaise, and myalgias; numerous vesicles, bilateral, tender regional lymphadenopathy, and a 2- to 3-week course between the onset of lesions and their complete reepitheliazation are the rule. Contiguous spread of virus as evidenced by the appearance of new vesicles after onset of the initial lesions is common, and inoculation at distant sites such as the fingers, thighs, eyes, and buttocks may be seen in 10 to 20 percent of primary herpes simplex. In contrast, patients with recurrent HSV are usually afebrile and have only a few clustered unilateral lesions which last from 5 to 12 days. Patients will often complain of a "prodrome," a tingling sensation near or at the eventual site of lesion, from 2 to 48 h prior to the appearance of vesicles. Occasionally, HSV infection will present in a dermatomal distribution that is usually characteristic of herpes zoster. Because cytological techniques do not differentiate between these two agents, viral cultures or use of specific techniques such as immunofluorescence must be employed in order to differentiate these two viruses.

The appearance of the vesicles may be helpful. Herpes simplex and varicella lesions have a surrounding zone of erythema and a thin vesicular roof, and they are tender when irritated. The lesions of molluscum contagiosum are umbilicated, contain an expressible white core, and are usually not tender when scraped gently. The lack of surrounding erythema, the large size of the bullae, and the presence of Nikolsky's sign are helpful in differentiating pemphigus or toxic epidermal necrolysis from viral vesicular eruptions. The vesicular-ulcerative lesions associated with Behçet's syndrome or inflammatory bowel disease tend to be present for longer periods than those associated with herpes virus infection. The unremitting course, tendency of the lesions to produce a deep ulcer and the prevalence of associated clinical findings such as colitis, urethritis, arthritis, and neurological disease in Behçet's syndrome should suggest this entity.

PETECHIAL ERUPTIONS Many hematologic and immunologic entities produce thrombocytopenia as a result of defects in the production, maturation, sequestration, or destruction of platelets. A consequence is the development of petechiae. However, the physician who is presented with an acutely ill patient with a petechial exanthem must be concerned with systemic bacterial or rickettsial disease. The common microorganisms associated with petechial exanthems are listed in Table 180-1. However, any microorganism that is capable of initiating the cascade of hematologic events termed *disseminated intravascular coagulation* may produce a petechial exanthem.

Petechiae due to septic embolization are characteristic of subacute bacterial endocarditis. Lesions may occur anywhere on the skin and/or mucous membranes but are most common over the upper anterior trunk. Splinter hemorrhages under the nails are difficult to differentiate from traumatic lesions and may be seen in hematologic, malignant, and other infective disorders.

Petechial lesions associated with meningococcemia are small, irregularly shaped slightly raised pale grayish lesions with a vesicular-pustular center. The lesions are usually asymmetric and are seen most often on the trunk and extremities, although the conjunctivas and mucous membranes may also be affected. Fulminant meningococcal infection will produce coalescence of the petechiae into grossly ecchymotic areas (purpura fulminans).

Gonococcal infection usually produces lesions on the distal extremities, often over joints. The presence of these pustular, hemorrhagic skin lesions in a patient with asymmetric tenosynovitis or polyarthritis, involving the wrists, fingers, knees, or ankles, should suggest the gonococcal arthritis-dermatitis syndrome. The majority of patients with disseminated gonococcal infection do not have symptoms of urogenital, anorectal, or pharyngeal gonococcal disease.

The metastatic lesions of staphylococcal bacteremia include pustules, subcutaneous abscesses, and purulent petechiae. Aspiration of material from the purulent center of the lesion will often reveal gram-positive cocci in clumps. Pseudomonas septicemia may produce ecthyma gangrenosum, a round, indurated, painless, necrotic eschar usually located in the anogenital or axillary area. In addition, hemorrhagic lesions with surrounding erythema resembling erythema multiforme may be associated with pseudomonas sepsis.

Rickettsial disease may produce an arteriolar vasculitis that results in a petechial exanthem. The rash of Rocky Mountain spotted fever generally starts as a blanching maculopapular exanthem on the extremities, and after 2 to 4 days petechiae appear in the involved areas. The lesions no longer fade, and decreased capillary fragility, manifested by a positive Rumpel-Leede test, is often present. These cutaneous findings in a patient with the abrupt onset of fever, chills, headache, myalgias, and arthralgias should suggest this diagnosis. If the patient comes from an endemic area, and a tick bite or tick exposure is present, appropriate therapy should be instituted.

Summer febrile illness due to enteroviruses, especially the echovirus group, may occasionally produce a petechial eruption. While involvement of the face is common, the distribution of the exanthem is usually not distinctive, and because fever, headache, and meningismus may also be present, the clinical differentiation between *Neisseria meningitidis* infection and viral aseptic meningitis may be difficult.

Atypical measles is another viral exanthem that produces a petechial eruption. It begins on the arms and legs and spreads to the trunk and face. The rash differs from typical measles because it has features of raised papules, blisters, and pinpoint hemorrhages into the skin. Koplik's spots are not present, while high fever, cough, bilateral interstitial pulmonary infiltrates, and eosinophils usually are. Patients with this syndrome have a history of previous immunization with inactivated (killed) measles vaccine or of receiving live measles vaccine within 3 months after killed vaccine. The history of previous antigenic exposure to measles virus plus eosinophilia suggests a "hypersensitivity" reaction. A fourfold rise in measles complement fixation antibody titer between acute and convalescent specimens may be demonstrated.

Allergic vasculitis (Henoch-Schönlein purpura) is found most frequently in children less than 16 years of age. The presence of symmetrical red papules ("palpable purpura"), commonly occurring on the lower extremities, accompanied by abdominal pain, gastrointestinal bleeding and renal involvement (edema, hypoproteinemia, hematuria), and arthralgias characterizes this entity.

Petechial eruptions and profuse mucosal bleeding are often major manifestations of the viral hemorrhagic fevers. This syndrome is associated with a number of the arenaviruses (Lassa, Junin), arthropod-borne viruses (dengue), and rhabdoviruses (Ebolla, Marburg). Recent travel to endemic or epidemic areas, involvement of the liver, spleen, heart, kidneys, and lungs, and evidence of diffuse intravascular coagulation are usually present.

LABORATORY DIAGNOSIS The laboratory studies most useful in determining the etiology of an exanthem in an acutely febrile patient are directed at demonstrating the microorganism at the cutaneous site. Gram's stain and culture of the lesions, dark-field microscopy of putative spirochetal lesions, and the use of immunofluorescent miscroscopy of skin scrapings or skin biopsy specimens for the detection of microbial antigens should be employed. Because exanthems are generally manifestations of a systemic illness, blood cultures should be taken prior to antimicrobial therapy. The agent should also be isolated from other extravascular sites such as stool specimens in the case of *Salmonella* or enteroviruses or the throat or urethra in the case of gonococci. Histological identification of organism from skin biopsies of lesions may be of great help, especially with slowly growing agents such as fungi or mycobacteria.

Because local viral invasion is characteristic of vesicular exanthems, isolation of the agent from these lesions provides the diagnosis. The development of rapid viral diagnostic testing has been especially useful to the clinician in the differential diagnosis of vesicular lesions. Biopsies or scrapings of exfoliated cells from vesicular lesions of herpes group viruses (varicella-zoster, herpes simplex virus) contain multinucleated giant cells and/or intranuclear inclusions. However, because the Tzanck smear is only 40 to 70 percent as sensitive as viral isolation, the absence of giant cells does not rule out herpes infection. Herpes simplex and zoster can be differentiated by viral isolation as well as antigen detection techniques such as fluorescent microscopy or enzyme-linked immunoabsorbent assays (ELISA). Immunofluorescence may also be useful in confirming the diagnosis of immunologically related diseases such as pemphigus vulgaris.

Electron microscopy is useful in differentiating the distinct morphology of poxviruses, vaccinia, variola, and molluscum from herpes viruses. In addition, molluscum bodies can be demonstrated by light microscopy with use of a 10% KOH preparation.

In viral exanthems, demonstration of local viral replication in throat secretions or rectal swabs provides presumptive evidence of the etiology of the exanthem; an example is the demonstration of coxsackievirus A16 in throat secretions of patients with hand-foot-and-mouth syndrome. In Behçet's syndrome or in collagen vascular disease, the absence of viruses in an early vesicular or active ulcerative lesion is useful in relating these mucosal lesions to the underlying multisystem illness.

Serologic determinations of acute phase serums are helpful in the diagnosis of syphilis, leptospirosis, streptococcal disease, Epstein-Barr virus infection, hepatitis B, toxoplasmosis, typhoid fever, and occasionally rickettsial disease. Evidence of autoantibody fixation may be useful in diagnosing some collagen vascular diseases. Demonstration of a fourfold or greater rise in antibody titer between acute and convalescent serums will confirm the diagnosis in rubella, rubeola, cytomegalovirus, rickettsial, or chlamydial infection.

REFERENCES

FULGINITI VA et al: Altered reactivity to measles virus. JAMA 202:105, 1967

GILCHEST B, BARDEN HP: Photodistribution of viral exanthems. Pediatrics 54:136, 1974

HEGGIN AD: Pathogenesis of rubella exanthems. J Infect Dis 137:74, 1978

KAWASAKI T et al: A new infantile acute febrile mucocutaneous lymph node syndrome (MLNS) prevailing in Japan. Pediatrics 54:271, 1974

KIMURA A et al: Measles rash, light and electron microscopic study of measles skin eruptions. Arch Virol 47:295, 1975

MIMS CA: Pathogenesis of rashes in virus diseases. Bacteriol Rev 30:739, 1966

181
MEASLES (RUBEOLA)

C. GEORGE RAY

DEFINITION Measles, or rubeola, is an acute febrile eruption which has been one of the most common diseases of civilization. With the development of effective prophylactic measures it should become a rarity.

HISTORY Measles probably was not a significant problem before the building of large cities. Rhazes wrote about it in the tenth century, and Sydenham in the seventeenth century wrote a full account of the disease and differentiated it from other exanthems. In 1905 measles was transmitted by the blood of infected persons to human volunteers and in 1911 to monkeys by both blood and nasopharyngeal secretions that had previously been passed through bacteria-retaining filters. In 1954,

Enders and Peebles obtained an agent from patients with measles that produced cytopathic changes in cell cultures. This achievement allowed the investigation of the characteristics of the measles virus and of the pathogenesis of the disease, with subsequent development of diagnostic and prophylactic measures.

ETIOLOGY The measles virion is composed of a central core of ribonucleic acid with a helically arranged protein coat surrounded by a lipoprotein envelope with small, spike-like structures. The virion is 120 to 250 nm in diameter and is classified as a paramyxovirus.

The measles virus is isolated most easily from infected persons in the first 4 or 5 days of illness, by utilizing primary cell cultures of monkey or human kidney, although primary isolations have been accomplished by using cells from human amnion or chorion or dog kidney. After several passages, the virus can be propagated on a number of types of cell cultures, including chick embryo cells, upon which many of the vaccine strains are grown.

Measles virus infection of cells in culture results in the formation of multinucleated giant cells, many with eosinophilic intranuclear and intracytoplasmic inclusions.

EPIDEMIOLOGY Measles occurs naturally only in human beings, although infection with the virus can be demonstrated in laboratory colonies of monkeys exposed to infected individuals. Before active immunization was available, epidemics of measles occurred in 2- to 3-year cycles, usually during the spring months, and about 95 percent of town and city dwellers developed the disease before the age of 15 years. The virus is transmitted by transfer of nasopharyngeal secretions, either directly or in airborne droplets, to the respiratory mucous membranes or conjunctivas of susceptile individuals. Persons infected with the virus may transmit the disease during a period which extends from 5 days after exposure until 5 days after skin lesions have appeared. The virus is highly contagious, with secondary attack rates among susceptible household contacts usually exceeding 90 percent; asymptomatic primary infections are rare. Measles is typically a disease of childhood in populous areas, but may occur at any age in remote isolated communities if the disease is introduced. In recent years in the United States, there has been a distinct shift in age-specific attack rates, with outbreaks frequently occurring among teenagers and young adults. Infants are uncommonly affected under the age of 6 to 8 months, presumably because of the persistence of maternal antibody acquired by transplacental transmission.

PATHOGENESIS AND PATHOLOGY It is probable that, after infection, measles virus multiplies in the epithelium of the respiratory tract and is disseminated by way of the blood to distant sites. For a few days before the rash appears, and for 1 or 2 days after, the virus can be isolated from blood or washed white blood cells, conjunctiva, lymphoid tissue, and respiratory mucous membranes and secretions. The virus can be obtained from urine for as long as 4 days after the onset of the eruptions.

The mucous membrane lesions (Koplik's spots) consist of vesicle formation and epithelial necrosis. Histology of the Koplik's spots reveals cytoplasmic and intranuclear inclusions, giant cells, and intercellular edema. Electron microscopy of the Koplik's spots and skin lesions has demonstrated microtubular aggregates which are thought to be the measles virus, and suggests that both the exanthem and enanthem are associated with local viral replication. Large multinucleated epithelial giant cells can be found during the prodrome and acute stages of illness in the buccal mucosa, pharynx, tracheobronchial mucosa, and occasionally in the urine. In addition, reticuloendothelial giant cells (Warthin-Finkeldey cells) are found in hyperplastic lymphoid tissues, including lymph nodes, tonsils, spleen, and thymus. An unusually high number of white blood cells from patients with the disease contain broken chromosomes. The epithelium of the respiratory passages may become necrotic and slough, leading to secondary bacterial infection; in addition, interstitial pneumonia with giant-cell infiltration may be observed. Changes in the brain of patients with encephalitis resemble those seen in other postviral encephalitides and consist of focal hemorrhage, congestion, and perivenous demyelination.

MANIFESTATIONS The time from exposure to the development of the first symptoms of measles infection is usually 9 to 11 days, and from exposure to the appearance of rash is about 2 weeks. The initial manifestations of the disease are malaise, irritability, fever as high as 105°F, conjunctivitis with excessive lacrimation, edema of the eyelids and photophobia, moderately severe hacking cough, and nasal discharge. The prodromal period usually lasts 3 to 4 days, with a range of 1 to 8 days before the onset of a rash. Koplik's spots—small, red, irregular lesions with blue-white centers—appear 1 or 2 days before the onset of the rash on the mucous membranes of the mouth and occasionally on the conjunctiva or intestinal mucosa. The findings of the prodromal illness subside or disappear within 1 or 2 days after the appearance of skin lesions, although the cough may persist throughout the course of the disease.

The red maculopapular rash of measles breaks out first on the forehead, spreads downward over the face, neck, and trunk, and appears on the feet on the third day. The density of lesions is greatest on the forehead, face, and shoulders, where coalescence of individual spots usually occurs. The lesions in each area persist for about 3 days and disappear in the same order in which they appeared, resulting in total duration of rash of about 6 days. As the maculopapules fade, a brown discoloration of the skin may be noticed, and finely granular desquamation may occur. In adults the duration of fever may be longer, the rash more prominent, and the incidence of complications higher.

The course of measles can be altered by the administration of gamma globulin soon after exposure. The incubation period may be prolonged for as long as 20 days. The prodromal period of the modified disease may be shorter, the fever, respiratory symptoms, and conjunctivitis milder, and the rash less marked; Koplik's spots may not be present. An atypical, severe form of measles is seen in some persons who received inactivated measles vaccine several years before exposure. The prodromal period with prominent fever, headache, myalgias, and abdominal symptoms lasts for 2 or 3 days and is followed by an eruption of maculopapules, vesicles, and petechiae. In contrast to natural measles, the rash begins on the feet and progresses toward the head and is especially prominent on the legs and in the body creases. Peripheral edema and pneumonia have been prevalent in this form of atypical measles. The pneumonia is lobar or segmental; hilar lymphadenopathy and pleural effusion are frequent. Ill-defined nodular shadows may persist at the periphery of the lung for as long as 1 to 2 years.

COMPLICATIONS Measles, usually a benign self-limited disease, may be associated with a number of complicating illnesses. Viral involvement of the respiratory tract may lead to croup, bronchitis, bronchiolitis, or rarely to *interstitial giant-cell pneumonia*, which is seen most often in children suffering from severe systemic disease such as leukemia, congenital immunodeficiency, or severe malnutrition, and which is characterized by severe respiratory symptoms, pulmonary infiltrations, and the presence in the lungs of multinucleated giant cells. It may occur in the absence of the typical measles exanthem. *Conjunctivitis,* which is seen regularly in the course of uncomplicated measles, may occasionally progress to corneal ulceration, keratitis, and blindness. *Myocarditis,* characterized by transient changes in the electrocardiogram, occurs in about 20 percent of patients with measles, but clinical evidence of cardiac dysfunction is rare. Viral involvement of the mesenteric lymph nodes and appendix may result in abdominal pain and signs of peritoneal inflammation so severe that surgical exploration is considered. The situation is especially confusing if the evidence of appendiceal involvement becomes manifest during the preeruptive phase of the disease. Measles infection of pregnant women results in death of the fetus in about 20 percent of the cases; however, a teratogenic effect such as that observed in rubella has not been demonstrated.

Superimposed bacterial pneumonia caused by streptococci, pneumococci, staphylococci, or *Hemophilus influenzae* is considerably more common than giant-cell pneumonia and occasionally may progress to formation of empyema or lung abscess. Bacterial otitis media is a frequent sequel of measles infection in children. In tropical areas, stomatitis, probably of bacterial origin, progressing to cancrum oris may be encountered during the course of the disease.

In addition to conditions associated with the viral infection and the complications resulting from superimposed bacterial infection, several situations may arise after measles infection which are of uncertain pathogenesis. Clinically apparent *encephalomyelitis* occurs in 1 of 1000 patients with measles. It usually begins 4 to 7 days after the appearance of the eruption, but may precede the rash by 10 days or follow it by 24 days. It is characterized by high fever, headache, drowsiness, and coma, and in some patients by focal brain or spinal cord involvement. Death occurs in about 10 percent of affected individuals, and persistent signs of central nervous system damage, including mental changes, epilepsy, and paralysis, are encountered. Electroencephalographic abnormalities without other signs of central nervous system dysfunction may be demonstrated in 50 percent of patients with otherwise uncomplicated measles. Though it is generally postulated that the encephalomyelitis is "postinfectious" or allergic in origin, a report of isolation of the virus from the brain of a patient with a fatal case suggests direct viral invasion of the central nervous system. A progressive, fatal encephalitis has been described in children with lymphatic malignancies treated with immunosuppressive drugs, with onset 1 to 6 months after an episode of measles. Other, more unusual neurologic complications include transverse myelitis and ascending myelitis. An extremely rare condition, *subacute sclerosing panencephalitis* (Chap. 192), is now thought to be a late complication of measles. *Thrombocytopenia* may occur 3 to 15 days after the onset of symptoms and results in purpura as well as bleeding from mouth, intestine, and genitourinary tract. Measles is also associated with transient suppression of delayed hypersensitivity to tuberculin, exacerbation of existing tuberculosis, and an increased incidence of new tuberculous infections.

LABORATORY FINDINGS Leukopenia is frequent in the prodromal phase of measles, and the appearance of leukocytosis suggests bacterial superinfection or another complication. Extreme lymphopenia (less than 2000 lymphocytes per cubic millimeter) is considered to be a poor prognostic sign. During the prodrome and in the early eruptive phase, multinucleated giant cells can be identified in stained preparations of sputum, nasal secretions, or urine, and the measles virus can be isolated by inoculation of the same materials into appropriate cell cultures. Complement fixation, neutralization and hemagglutination inhibition tests are available for serologic confirmation of measles. Spinal fluid protein of patients with encephalomyelitis ranges from 48 to 240 mg/ml, and lymphocyte counts are usually in a range of 5 to 99 per cubic millimeter, although counts as high as 1000 per cubic millimeter have been reported. Bacterial infection can be identified by appropriate cultures.

DIFFERENTIAL DIAGNOSIS Measles, with its prodrome, Koplik's spots, and characteristic rash, is infrequently confused with other diseases. Rubella is a milder disease of shorter duration with mild respiratory complaints or none at all. Infectious mononucleosis and toxoplasmosis can be identified by the presence of atypical lymphocytes and by serologic tests. Secondary syphilis may display skin lesions similar to the measles rash. Other infections which can sometimes mimic measles include those caused by adenoviruses, enteroviruses, *Mycoplasma pneumoniae,* and *Streptococcus pyogenes,* e.g., scarlet fever. Drug reactions, particularly those associated with ampicillin and Dilantin, can also produce a morbilliform rash. The atypical form of measles in patients previously immunized with inactivated vaccine may suggest Rocky Mountain spotted fever.

PROPHYLAXIS Measles can be prevented by the administration of 0.25 ml/kg gamma globulin within 5 days of exposure. Passive immunization should be considered for any susceptible person exposed to the disease, but is especially important for children under 3 years of age, for pregnant women, for patients with tuberculosis, and for those patients in whom immune mechanisms are impaired. A modified, less severe form of the disease which results in some degree of active immunity may be observed if 0.04 ml/kg gamma globulin is given within 5 days of exposure (see "Manifestations," above). Prophylactic administration of antibiotics does not decrease the frequency or severity of bacterial superinfections.

Active immunity can be induced by the use of live, attenuated measles virus without spread to contacts of vaccinated individuals. Further attenuated vaccine strains (Schwarz, Attenuvax) derived from additional chick cell culture passages of the original Edmonston B strains are currently recommended and are associated with few local or systemic reactions. Vaccination with these preparations induces antibody formation in more than 95 percent of susceptible individuals. The vaccine can induce protection if given before, or within 2 days after, exposure. After this time, active immunization is less predictable in its ability to confer protection to the already exposed individual, although no ill effects have been noted when vaccination followed exposure by more than two days. Vaccination results in protection for at least 10 years, but the total duration of immunity is not known. Live measles vaccine should not be given to pregnant women, to patients with untreated tuberculosis, to patients with leukemia or lymphoma, or to those who are receiving therapy which depresses immune reponses. Hypersensitivity reactions have not been associated with the vaccine even among egg-sensitive individuals; however, the vaccine should not be given to persons known to be hypersensitive to vaccine components, such as trace amounts of antibiotics. Except in unusual circumstances, vaccination should not be given in the first 13 months of life. However, if epidemiologic circumstances suggest a risk to infants in the 6- to 13-month age group, the vaccine may be used, and a second dose administered at 15 to 18 months of age to ensure adequate seroconversion. The vaccine seems equally effective when administered alone or simultaneously in combination with rubella and mumps vaccines. Measles vaccination has been very effective in decreasing the incidence of measles in the United States without producing serious side effects. Measles occurs most commonly among the unvaccinated, who, for the most part, are members of low socioeconomic groups. The disease rarely occurs in those who have been vaccinated, although there have been vaccine failures. These failures are related, in part, to early vaccination of infants who still have maternal neutralizing antibody or to the use of improperly stored vaccine.

There is no indication for the use of *inactivated* vaccine because of severe atypical measles which has been observed in persons immunized with it (see "Manifestations," above).

TREATMENT No therapy is indicated for uncomplicated measles. Gamma globulin, although effective in prophylaxis, is of no value once symptoms are evident. Patients should be monitored for the development of bacterial superinfections, with specific antibiotic selection based on clinical and bacteriologic findings.

REFERENCES

AICARDI J et al: Acute measles encephalitis in children with immunosuppression. Pediatrics 59:232, 1977

COOVADIA HM et al: Immunoparesis and outcome in measles. Lancet 1:619, 1977

ENDERS JF, PEEBLES T: Propagation in tissue cultures of cytopathogenic agents from patients with measles. Proc Soc Exp Biol Med 86:277, 1954

HORSTMANN DM: Problems in measles and rubella. Dis Mon, vol 24, no 6, 1978

KRUGMAN S: Present status of measles and rubella immunization in the United States: A medical progress report. J Pediatr 90:1, 1977

Measles prevention. Morb Mort Week Rep, vol 27, no 44, November 3, 1978

MEULEN V et al: Isolation of infectious measles virus in measles encephalitis. Lancet 2:1172, 1972

RAND KH et al: Measles in adults: Unforeseen consequences of immunization? JAMA 236:1028, 1976

RUUSKANEN O et al: Measles vaccination after exposure to natural measles. J Pediatr 93:43, 1978

WITTE JJ: The epidemiology and control of measles. Am J Epidemiol 100:77, 1974

182
RUBELLA ("GERMAN MEASLES")

C. GEORGE RAY

DEFINITION Rubella ("German measles," "3-day measles") is usually a benign febrile exanthem, but when it occurs in pregnant women, it may lead to serious chronic fetal infection and malformations.

ETIOLOGY In the late 1930s and 1940s rubella was transmitted to humans and monkeys, and in 1962 a viral agent was recovered in cell cultures inoculated with nasopharyngeal secretions of infected persons. Human primary amnion cells infected with rubella virus display rounding, clumping of nuclear chromatin, and eosinophilic intranuclear inclusions. Rabbit kidney and some other cell lines also display cytopathic effects. Rubella virus can be detected indirectly in African green monkey kidney cells by the interference or exclusion method. In this system, cells infected with rubella appear normal but are resistant to superinfection with viruses such as echovirus 11 or coxsackievirus A9 that ordinarily produce a cytopathic effect in these cells. Complement-fixing antigen and a hemagglutinin have been identified.

The rubella virion, 50 to 85 nm in diameter, is a somewhat spheroidal RNA virus which has been tentatively classified in the togavirus family.

PATHOGENESIS AND PATHOLOGY Rubella can be induced in susceptible persons by the instillation of virus into the nasopharynx, and natural infection is probably induced in the same way. Virus is present in blood, throat washings, and occasionally feces for several days before the exanthem becomes apparent. It can be detected in blood for 1 to 2 days, and in throat washings for as long as 7 days before appearance of rash, to 2 weeks after onset. Lymph nodes show edema and hyperplasia.

Congenital rubella results from transplacental transmission of virus to the fetus from an infected mother, and may be associated with growth retardation, infiltration of liver and spleen by hematopoietic tissue, interstitial pneumonia, a decreased number of megakaryocytes in the bone marrow, and various structural malformations of the cardiovascular and central nervous systems. The virus can persist in the fetus during intrauterine life and may be excreted for 6 to 31 months after birth.

EPIDEMIOLOGY Rubella is not as contagious as measles, and immunity to the disease is not so widespread. Estimates of susceptibility to rubella among women of childbearing age range from 10 to 25 percent. Before the routine introduction of vaccine in 1969, epidemics occurred at 6- to 9-year intervals; however, it is not known whether this cyclical pattern will continue in the future. In 1964 more than 1.8 million cases of rubella were reported in the United States; in 1976, 12,491 cases were reported in this country. Rubella was once most frequent among children 5 to 9 years of age, but with the advent of immunization programs often directed primarily at this age group as well as at preschoolers, a greater proportion of cases is now being reported among older school children and young adults. Sixty percent of the reported cases in 1976 occurred in persons 15 years of age or older.

MANIFESTATIONS The time from exposure to the appearance of the rash of rubella is 14 to 21 days, usually about 18 days. In adults there may be a prodromal illness preceding the exanthem by 1 to 7 days, consisting of malaise, headache, fever, mild conjunctivitis, and lymphadenopathy. In children the rash may be the first manifestation of disease. It is apparent from serologic studies that rubella infection may be associated with no signs or symptoms, or may result in lymph node enlargement without skin lesions; however, rash without lymphadenopathy is uncommon. Respiratory symptoms are mild or absent. Small, red lesions (Forchheimer's spots) occasionally may be seen on the soft palate but are not pathognomonic of the disease.

The rash begins on the forehead and face and spreads downward to the trunk and extremities. The small maculopapular lesions, of lighter hue than those of measles, are usually discrete but may coalesce to form a diffuse erythema suggestive of scarlet fever. The rash may last from 1 to 5 days, but is most commonly present for 3 days. Enlarged, tender lymph nodes appear before the rash, are most impressive during the early eruptive phase, and may persist several days after the rash has disappeared. Splenomegaly or generalized lymphadenopathy may occur, but the postauricular and suboccipital nodes are most strikingly involved. Arthralgias and slight joint swellings may be a complication of rubella, especially in young women. The pain and swelling, involving wrists, fingers, and knees, are most marked during the period of rash and may persist for 1 to 14 days after other manifestations of rubella

have disappeared. Recurring joint symptoms for a year or more have also been reported. Purpura with or without thrombocytopenia may occur and may be associated with hemorrhage. Encephalomyelitis following rubella resembles other postinfectious encephalitides and is much less common than encephalitis following measles. Testicular pain is also occasionally reported in young adults.

Congenital rubella The syndrome of congenital rubella has conventionally been thought to consist of heart malformations—patent ductus arteriosus, interventricular septal defect, or pulmonic stenosis; eye lesions—corneal clouding, cataracts, chorioretinitis, and microphthalmia; microcephaly, mental retardation, and deafness. In the American epidemic of 1964, thrombocytopenic purpura, hepatosplenomegaly, intrauterine growth retardation, interstitial pneumonia, myocarditis or myocardial necrosis, and metaphyseal bone lesions were encountered frequently in association with the previously recognized manifestations, leading to the term *expanded rubella syndrome*. Some infants have also been found to have significant humoral and/or cellular immunodeficiency, which generally resolves as chronic viral excretion diminishes and eventually ceases. Any combination of lesions may be seen in an individual infant, and the severity is highly variable.

Later complications include an apparent higher risk of subsequent development of diabetes mellitus. In addition, there are reports of patients with congenital rubella who develop a progressive, subacute panencephalitis, with onset in the second decade of life. This is characterized by intellectual deterioration, ataxia, seizures, and spasticity.

Congenital rubella is usually the result of maternal infection during the first trimester of pregnancy, although well-documented cases have resulted from infection several days before conception; deafness may occur as a result of infection in the fourth month. In the 1964 epidemic, about 10 percent of women with clinically recognized rubella during the first trimester gave birth to infants with the rubella syndrome. Serologically identified, asymptomatic maternal rubella can also result in severe fetal disease. It is therefore desirable to ascertain the immune status of every woman, either before conception or as early in the pregnancy as possible, by history of previous immunization or by serologic testing. If rubella antibodies are present before or within 10 days after exposure, the patient is considered immune, and the risk of fetal damage is virtually nil. If antibodies are not detectable and exposure has occurred, acute and convalescent antibody titers should be determined simultaneously on sera obtained 2 to 4 weeks apart, depending upon the time after exposure when the acute sample was drawn.

DIAGNOSIS Rubella is frequently confused with other diseases associated with maculopapular exanthems such as those described in Chaps. 180 and 183, and with infectious mononucleosis (Chap. 195), as well as with drug eruptions and scarlet fever. *A certain diagnosis of rubella can be made only by virus isolation and identification, or by changes in antibody titers.* Rubella hemagglutination-inhibiting antibodies may be present by the second day of rash and increase in quantity over the next 10 to 21 days. Patients with the congenital rubella syndrome may lose hemagglutination-inhibiting antibodies at age 3 or 4 years. Therefore a negative serologic test in a child over 3 years does not exclude the possibility of congenital rubella. There are no other laboratory findings helpful in the diagnosis of rubella, although lymphocytosis with atypical lymphocytes may occur. Congenital rubella should be differentiated by appropriate serologic tests from congenital syphilis (Chap. 146), toxoplasmosis (Chap. 203), and cytomegalic inclusion virus disease (Chap. 194).

PREVENTION In adults and children rubella is usually a mild disease with infrequent complications. However, the severity of congenital infection has prompted efforts to prevent the disease. Administration of gamma globulin to exposed persons can abort the clinical disease, but seroconversion and transmission of the disease from mother to fetus may occur despite the administration of large amounts of gamma globulin soon after exposure.

Active immunization with live attenuated rubella vaccines prepared in duck, dog, rabbit, or human diploid fibroblast cells has been practiced in this country since 1969, especially among young children. The aim has been to decrease the frequency of the infection in the population, thus decreasing the chance that susceptible pregnant women will be exposed. Because of concern for a possibly enlarging pool of susceptible adolescents and adults, there has been increasing enthusiasm for serologic screening of pubertal females with no history of immunization, followed by selective immunization of those who are seronegative. Such immunization must of course be done with appropriate precautions, as noted below.

The attenuated virus can be detected in the respiratory secretions of vaccines for as long as 4 weeks after immunization, but transmission to other susceptible individuals rarely, if ever, occurs. This has not been shown to be a problem, even in households where susceptible pregnant women are in contact with children who are being vaccinated. The vaccine induces antibodies in about 95 percent of recipients, but the degree and duration of protection are still being evaluated. After heavy exposure in closed populations, vaccinated individuals sometimes develop subclinical infections (diagnosed by antibody rises and virus isolation). However, viremia has not been demonstrated in immunized persons, which suggests that previously vaccinated pregnant women will not infect their fetuses even if they acquire subclinical rubella.

Side effects of fever, rash, lymphadenopathy, polyneuropathy, or arthralgias occur very seldom in vaccinated children, but joint pain and swelling or paresthesias were seen in more than 25 percent of women who were immunized with the earlier vaccines. The risk has been reduced to 2 to 9 percent with the advent of vaccines prepared in rabbit or human embryonic fibroblast cell cultures. The joint symptoms usually begin 2 to 10 weeks after vaccination, and they may be confused with other forms of arthritis. *Rubella vaccine must never be given to pregnant women or to those who may be pregnant within 2 months of immunization.* This precaution is necessary because the vaccine virus has the theoretical potential to damage the fetus of susceptible women.

REFERENCES

Fox JP et al: Rubella vaccine in postpubertal women. JAMA 236:837, 1976

Horstmann D: Problems in measles and rubella. Dis Mon, vol 24, no 6, 1978

Krugman S: Present status of measles and rubella immunization in the United States: A medical progress report. J Pediatr 90:1, 1977

Modlin JF et al: Risk of congenital abnormality after inadvertent rubella vaccination of pregnant women. N Engl J Med 294:972, 1976

Plotkin SA et al: Immunologic properties of RA 27/3 rubella virus vaccine. JAMA 225:585, 1973

Schlossberg D, Topolosky MK: Military rubella. JAMA 238:1273, 1977

Sever JL et al: Rubella epidemic, 1964: Effect on 6,000 pregnancies. Am J Dis Child 110:395,1965

Townsend JJ et al: Progressive rubella panencephalitis: Late onset after congenital rubella. N Engl J Med 292:990, 1975

Weil ML et al: Chronic progressive panencephalitis due to rubella virus stimulating SSPE. N Engl J Med 292:994, 1975

183
OTHER VIRAL EXANTHEMATOUS DISEASES

C. GEORGE RAY

In addition to the diseases such as measles, rubella and chickenpox, which historically have been associated with prominent skin lesions, there are other virus infections in which skin manifestations may occur. Table 183-1 lists the other most commonly recognized causes of maculopapular eruptions. Some of them, particularly the enteroviruses, can also occasionally cause papulovesicular or petechial rashes; others are capable of provoking erythema multiforme-like eruptions. One helpful aspect of the physical examination is the observation that viral-caused maculopapular (not vesicular) exanthems usually *relatively* spare the palms and soles. This is in contrast to eruptions associated with drug reactions, bacteria, *Mycoplasma,* and *Rickettsia,* in which a prominent palmar or plantar eruption is often noted.

EXANTHEM SUBITUM (ROSEOLA INFANTUM) Exanthem subitum is a benign disease of infants 6 to 24 months of age that is characterized by a high fever and rash. The disease can be transmitted to humans and monkeys by the transfer of blood obtained from a patient during the first few days of illness. The infectious agent is probably a virus, although it has not been isolated. The first manifestations of disease, after an estimated incubation period of 5 to 15 days, are the abrupt onset of irritability and fever, which lasts for 3 to 5 days; the temperature may be as high as 105°F. There may be mild pharyngitis and slight lymph node enlargement; convulsions may occur during the height of the fever. On the fourth to fifth day of illness, there is a sudden drop in temperature to normal or below normal; several hours before or after defervescence the rash suddenly and surprisingly appears. It is characterized by faint 2- to 3-mm macules or maculopapules over the neck and trunk and may extend to the thighs and buttocks; it may last for only a few hours or may be present for a day or two. Leukopenia is frequently noted later in the febrile period. The disease is benign and not associated with complications, although rarely an infant may show sequelae as a result of febrile convulsions. In the early, preeruptive phase, the disease may be difficult to differentiate from an acute, occult bacteremia, particularly from one associated with *Streptococcus pneumoniae.* Though a leukocytosis with an increase in band forms is often seen in occult bacteremias presenting in this fashion, blood cultures are necessary to aid in precise diagnosis.

ERYTHEMA INFECTIOSUM (FIFTH DISEASE) Erythema infectiosum is a mild febrile exanthematous disease with little or no prodrome. The incubation period is probably 5 to 10 days. The first manifestations are low-grade fever and the appearance of indurated, confluent erythema over the cheeks, giving a

TABLE 183-1
Causes of maculopapular eruptions

Viral	Other
Measles	*Mycoplasma pneumoniae*
Rubella	Syphilis
Exanthem subitum	Typhoid fever
Erythema infectiosum	Bacterial toxins.
Enteroviruses: coxsackievirus, echovirus	streptococci and staphylococci
Infectious mononucleosis	Rat-bite fever
Adenoviruses	*Rickettsia*
Reoviruses	Live-virus vaccines
Arboviruses	Drug eruptions

"slapped face" appearance. A day or so later, a bilaterally symmetric eruption is seen on the arms, legs, and trunk, but rarely on the palms or soles. The lesions are maculopapular and tend to be confluent, forming slightly raised blotchy areas and reticular or lacy patterns. The rash usually lasts about a week, and during this time it may disappear, only to reappear in the same areas a few hours later. The waxing and waning eruption may occasionally persist for several weeks, and can be brought on by fever, heat, exercise, sunlight exposure, or emotional stress. Mild joint pain and swelling have been observed in a large proportion of adults with the disease. Erythema infectiosum affects all ages but is most common in children of school age and may occur in epidemic form. The mode of transmission of the disease is not known, and an infectious agent has not been recovered. A clinical diagnosis of this disease must sometimes be made with caution, since rubella and some enteroviruses have also been shown at times to cause a nearly identical syndrome.

ENTEROVIRAL EXANTHEMS Many individual enteroviruses have been associated with rash. Of these, polioviruses are rarely implicated. More commonly, echovirus serotypes 1 through 7, 9, 11, 12, 14, 16, 18, 19, 20, 25, and 30, coxsackievirus serotypes A4, A5, A6, A9, A10, A16, and B2, B3, and B5 have all been implicated. With the exception of hand-foot-and-mouth disease, usually associated with coxsackievirus A16 infection (Chap. 187), there is no set of clinical or epidemiologic features that aid in differentiating the specific enteroviral agent involved in a specific case. All are capable of producing maculopapular rashes which vary in intensity and duration, and can also occasionally produce petechial or papulovesicular exanthems and enanthems. In community and household outbreaks, younger children and infants are usually more likely to manifest exanthems, while other features of enteroviral infection, such as fever, myalgia, and aseptic meningitis, are more prominent among older children and young adults. Two enterovirus infections which have been frequently associated with rashes and have been studied extensively are described here as examples of epidemic enteroviral infections.

Boston exanthem (infections with echovirus 16) Echovirus 16 infection was described first and most extensively during an epidemic in Boston in 1951. Children who were infected usually had a disease characterized by exanthem and low-grade fever, while adult family contacts often developed high fever, prostration, and signs of aseptic meningitis with absent or fleeting rash. The first manifestation of the disease in children was fever of 101 to 102°F, lasting for a day or two, pharyngitis with small ulcerated lesions resembling herpangina, and slight enlargement of the cervical and postauricular lymph nodes. The rash appeared during fever or after defervescence and consisted of small pink maculopapules on the face, upper part of the chest, and occasionally on the whole body, including the palms and soles. The rash lasted for 1 to 5 days, and there were no important complications or sequelae. The disease resembled exanthem subitum but occurred in children of all ages and in adults.

Infection with echovirus 9 Infection with this virus in children and adults has been characterized by a febrile illness with a high incidence of aseptic meningitis. The incubation period is 5 to 8 days. About 30 percent of patients have a rash, which may occur with or without meningitis. It is usually maculopapular, developing at the onset of fever. The exanthem appears first on the face and neck, spreads to the trunk and extremities, may involve the palms and soles, although slightly, and persists for 3 to 5 days. Petechiae with or without maculopapules have

been recognized; when they are seen in association with meningitis, there may be confusion with meningococcal meningitis. This can be a point of some concern, since concurrent outbreaks of echovirus 9 and meningococcal disease have been observed. A vesicular eruption with crusting lesions has been seen occasionally. An exanthem on the buccal mucosa and soft palate occurs in about 30 percent of patients and consists of small red areas with white centers which resemble Koplik's spots. The disease is usually benign but rarely has been associated with permanent central nervous system damage.

REFERENCES

BALFOUR HH: Erythema infectiosum: Clinical description of 91 cases seen in an epidemic. Clin Pediatr 8:721, 1969

——— et al: Erythema infectiosum: Recovery of rubella virus and echovirus 12. Pediatrics 50:285, 1972

HALL CB et al: The return of Boston exanthem. Echovirus 16 infections in 1974. Am J Dis Child 131:323, 1977

LAUER BA et al: Erythema infectiosum. Am J Dis Child 130:252, 1976

LERNER AM et al: New viral exanthems. N Engl J Med 269:678, 1963

NEVA FA et al: Clinical epidemiological features of unusual epidemic exanthem. JAMA 155:544, 1954

WENNER HA: Virus diseases associated with cutaneous eruptions. Prog Med Virol 16:269, 1973

184
SMALLPOX, VACCINIA, AND COWPOX

C. GEORGE RAY

Poxviruses are a group of large (200 to 320 nm), brick-shaped DNA-containing viruses that possess a common antigen and have a predilection for skin. Many of the poxviruses, such as myxoma and fowl pox agents, cause disease mainly in lower animals. Smallpox (variola major), alastrim (variola minor), vaccinia, and cowpox agents are closely related members of the poxvirus group that cause human disease. All these viruses grow and produce pox on the chorioallantoic membrane of chick embryos and can be cultivated in cells from various mammalian tissues with formation of intracytoplasmic inclusions, rounding fusion and heaping up of cells, and eventual degeneration of the infected area. The poxviruses responsible for human disease may be distinguished from one another by minor antigenic differences and by the type and severity of lesions they induce in experimental animals and humans. Smallpox and alastrim viruses produce smaller pox on the chorioallantoic membrane than vaccinia, and there are differences in incubation temperatures at which poxviruses produce lesions.

SMALLPOX (VARIOLA)

DEFINITION Smallpox is a severe, contagious, febrile disease characterized by a vesicular and pustular eruption. Alastrim is a similar but milder illness, with a lower mortality rate. Though the difference in severity between these diseases is apparent, the agents of smallpox and alastrim are biologically and immunologically indistinguishable from each other in the laboratory.

PATHOGENESIS AND PATHOLOGY The virus gains access to the body by the respiratory tract and multiplies in unidentified sites, probably in lymph nodes or liver. After several days, during which there is no evidence of infection, viremia ensues, with swelling of the endothelium of blood vessels in the corium and perivascular inflammation. Loculated vesicles are the result of cellular destruction and exudation of serum. The infected epithelial cells are swollen and contain intracytoplasmic inclusions surrounded by a halo (Guarnieri bodies). The extent of skin involvement is greater in smallpox than in chickenpox and reaches into the corium. Pitting, most commonly seen on the face, is said to result from destruction of sebaceous glands, which are abundant in this area. The liver, spleen, and lymph nodes may be enlarged and may show focal accumulations of large mononuclear cells.

EPIDEMIOLOGY Smallpox is not as contagious as measles or influenza, and ordinarily face-to-face contact with an infected person is required to transmit the disease; however, airborne dissemination from contaminated fomites has also been shown to occur. A patient with smallpox is infectious from a day before the rash appears until all lesions have healed and the scabs have fallen off. During the early phase of the illness, the virus is transmitted in nasopharyngeal secretions; when the eruption is fully formed, the lesions themselves are a major source of infectious material. Variola virus may contaminate clothing, bedding, dust, or other inanimate objects and remain infectious for months, necessitating disinfection of articles in the patient's environment. The World Health Organization's program to eradicate smallpox has resulted in marked decrease in the incidence of the disease since 1966, and the prospects for ultimate eradication seem bright. Two important epidemiologic factors which would suggest that this is possible are the absence of nonhuman reservoir for the virus, and the apparent nonexistence of completely asymptomatic human carriers. Control and the ultimate eradication of the disease, therefore, rely on complete reporting of cases and identification of even very mild ones, as a prelude to specific quarantine and selective immunization.

By April 1978 no new cases of smallpox had been reported from anywhere in the world since a case with onset of rash in October 1977 was identified in Somalia. That country is considered to be the last remaining endemic area, and, if a total of 2 years of effective surveillance elapses without further cases, it will be declared smallpox-free.

In August 1978 a case of laboratory-associated smallpox was reported from the medical school in Birmingham, England. Presumably the patient was infected by airborne transmission from a smallpox laboratory to her office area one floor removed.

MANIFESTATIONS The incubation period of smallpox, from the time of exposure to the onset of the prodrome, is about 12 days, with extremes of 7 to 17 days. The disease can be divided into a prodrome, an early eruptive phase, and a period of vesiculation and pustule formation. The prodrome is characterized by a temperature of 102 to 106°F, headache, myalgia especially in the back, abdominal pain, vomiting, and in some patients by a transient, blotchy, erythematous eruption. After 3 or 4 days the fever subsides, the symptoms decrease, and the patient seems to recover. It is at this time, when the patient is afebrile, that the focal eruption begins. Early manifestations are painful ulcers on the buccal mucosa and macules which appear first on the face and forearms, and rapidly become firm, shotty papules. The papules increase in number and spread from the face and distal extremities to involve the trunk. The individual lesions may remain discrete and scattered, or they may become confluent and involve most of the body. They are most concentrated on the face and distal extremities, including the palms and soles, and are relatively sparse in the axilla. On the third or fourth day after the appearance of the focal rash, the papules progress to vesicles containing clear fluid, which, over the next few days, becomes cloudy because of infiltration

by pus cells and desquamated epithelial cells; hemorrhage into the vesicles and surrounding skin may also be seen. During the course of smallpox, the lesions at any one time, in one area, are all at the same stage of evolution. At the time the vesicles become pustular, there is recurrence of fever, which may persist until healing occurs. The pustules umbilicate and form crusts and scabs which usually fall off 3 weeks after the beginning of illness, leaving small scars or deep pits.

The above description applies to disease of moderate severity. A milder illness may occur in previously immunized persons or in some who have no history of vaccination. It is characterized by the usual incubation period and prodrome, but is followed either by focal eruption of fewer than 100 papules, or by a rash resembling chickenpox. Smallpox with prodrome but with no eruption of any kind has been recognized (variola sine eruptione). The disease may also occur in a rapidly fulminating form ("sledgehammer" smallpox). After the usual incubation period, the patient develops an initial illness characterized by severe prostration, fever, bone marrow depression, hemorrhagic skin lesions, and bleeding. The disease progresses from inception to death within 3 or 4 days without evidence of the typical focal skin lesions.

Alastrim is similar to mild and moderate forms of variola major in that it has the same incubation period and prodromal illness, but the skin eruption is less extensive, and fatalities are rare and usually related to secondary bacterial infections.

COMPLICATIONS Bacterial superinfections of the lesions usually with *Staphylococcus aureus*, may occur in the late pustular stage. Bacterial pneumonia and sepsis may be seen in severe forms of smallpox. Mild conjunctivitis is quite common, and iritis and keratitis have been recognized. Encephalomyelitis may occur in the late stage of the disease and is similar to other postinfectious encephalitides. Osteomyelitis and joint effusions may complicate the disease, and orchitis has also been reported.

LABORATORY FINDINGS Leukopenia is present during the prodromal illness, and there is usually leukocytosis during the pustular stage. Rapid diagnosis of poxvirus infection can be made by the finding of characteristic brick-shaped particles in preparations of vesicle fluid examined by electron microscopy. Specific precipitation in agar by use of antigen prepared from lesions and antivariola or antivaccinia immune serum may also allow detection of poxvirus within a few hours. These tests do not distinguish variola from vaccinia or other poxviruses but do allow rapid differentiation from herpes simplex and varicella-zoster viruses. For definitive identification the virus must be grown in cell culture or on the chorioallantoic membrane and neutralized with specific antiserum.

DIFFERENTIAL DIAGNOSIS The major problem in differential diagnosis is in distinguishing smallpox from chickenpox. Smallpox is preceded by a longer prodrome than chickenpox, and the eruption vesiculates over a period of days instead of hours. The smallpox lesions are all characteristically in the same stage of development, whereas those of chickenpox may, in one area, display all stages of evolution. Electron microscopy and agar precipitation techniques (see above) are especially useful in distinguishing between smallpox and chickenpox. Cytologic examination of scrapings of the base of a vesicle can also be helpful in the differential diagnosis. The presence of multinucleated giant cells and/or intranuclear inclusions strongly suggests a herpes group infection (varicella-zoster or herpes simplex); such findings are not seen with poxvirus infections.

Other conditions which are sometimes confused with smallpox include eczema vaccinatum, eczema herpeticum, rickettsialpox, drug eruptions, some cases of contact dermatitis, and Stevens-Johnson syndrome. The fulminant, hemorrhagic smallpox may closely resemble meningococcemia, typhus, and hemorrhagic fevers.

PREVENTION Smallpox may be prevented among the patient's contacts by vaccination. Because this procedure is most successful if carried out during the early part of the incubation period, all exposed persons, regardless of previous immunization, should be vaccinated immediately upon recognition of exposure. Large, controlled, clinical trials have demonstrated that oral administration of N-methylisatin 3-thiosemicarbazone (methisazone), a drug which interferes with poxvirus multiplication, can prevent smallpox and alastrim in patients exposed to the diseases. The use of a drug together with prompt vaccination results in greater chance of protection than either measure alone. A drawback to the use of methisazone is its tendency to induce vomiting. The combined use of vaccination and parenteral administration of vaccinia immune globulin early in the incubation period is also effective in the prevention of smallpox in exposed individuals. It is now usual to apply these control measures selectively to the primary and secondary contacts of a patient rather than to all the inhabitants of a community.

In order to avoid laboratory-acquired smallpox, storage of the virus should be restricted to the five World Health Organization reference centers.

TREATMENT There is no specific therapy for smallpox. Thiosemicarbazone, although effective in prophylaxis, has not been shown to be of value in the treatment of established cases. Fluid deficits should be replaced by the administration of appropriate solutions. During the vesicular and pustular phases of the disease, an attempt should be made to prevent bacterial infection by the use of sterile sheets and aseptic nursing procedures. Antihistamines may be helpful in decreasing pruritus. Application of lotions or ointment should be avoided. Later in the course of the illness, when desquamation has begun, showers or baths may be helpful in removing desquamating tissue. If bacterial infection develops, an antibiotic active against the infecting organism should be given by the parenteral route. Topical antibiotics should be avoided.

VACCINIA

Vaccinia is a virus disease of the skin which is induced by inoculation for the prevention of smallpox. The exact origin of the vaccinia virus is obscure. The material first used by Jenner in 1796 was derived from cowpox lesions, and the infectious agent was propagated for many years by successive passage from person to person through use of exudate from fresh skin lesions. The original agent possibly became contaminated with variola virus during the period when transfer was being carried out without strict controls. It has been suggested that vaccinia virus is a hybrid of cowpox and variola agents, a contention supported by the finding that laboratory-induced hybrids of variola and cowpox viruses have many of the characteristics associated with vaccinia.

VACCINATION Live, lyophilized vaccinia virus prepared from vesicle fluid of infected calves is commercially available and maintains potency for 18 months at 46°F. It is dissolved in a diluent solution just prior to use. The usual method for vaccination is to apply a small drop of vaccine to the skin over the deltoid muscle and to press a sterile needle through the vaccine several times in such a way that only the superficial layer of skin is entered, or by simultaneous puncture utilizing a plastic tine device. Vaccination should always induce some form of skin reaction; complete absence of any kind of lesion indicates that the vaccine was not viable or was not administered properly. The reaction which occurs in nonimmune individuals is characterized by a red papule at the site of inoculation 3 to 5 days after vaccination. The papule becomes vesicular on about the fifth or sixth day and pustular by the ninth or eleventh day after inoculation. The vesicle and pustule may be surrounded by a large area of erythema. About 2 weeks after vaccination, the pustule dries and develops a crust which falls off by the end of the third week, leaving a scar. Fever, malaise, and irritability are common in children during the vesicular and pustular phases, and axillary lymphadenopathy may develop and persist for several months. In the partially immune person, a modified reaction develops without fever or constitutional symptoms. A papule appears on the skin within 3 days, vesiculates in 5 to 7 days, and heals without much scarring. The so-called "immune" reaction described by some, where a papule and/or erythema appears in a few days, then recedes without vesiculation, is an "equivocal" reaction, and may simply represent allergy to the components of an inadvertently inactivated vaccine. A successful vaccination is defined as the presence of a Jennerian vesicle (vesicular, pustular, or crusted) 7 days after inoculation. If the criterion is not met, the patient should be revaccinated, preferably with vaccine from a different lot.

Revaccination every 3 years is required to ensure protection, *but vaccination is currently indicated only for a few laboratory workers who might have contact with variola virus and for travelers to countries which still require vaccination as a condition for entry. Absolute contraindications* to vaccination include individuals with congenital or acquired immune deficiencies, lymphoma, leukemia or other blood dyscrasias, patients being treated with steroids, antimetabolites, alkylating agents, or ionizing irradiation, and individuals with a history of vaccinia encephalitis. *Relative contraindications* include patients or household contacts with eczema or a history of eczema, severe acne, or other similar dermatologic problems, pregnancy, and infants under twelve months of age. If the necessity to vaccinate any individual in this latter group is great, simultaneous administration of vaccinia immune globulin (VIG), 0.3 ml/kg, is suggested, to be given at a separate site intramuscularly at the time of immunization.

COMPLICATIONS Healing of the primary vaccinal lesion may not occur, and some patients go on to develop slowly progressive necrosis with destruction of large areas of skin, subcutaneous tissue, and underlying structures *(vaccinia gangrenosum)*. In addition to the local destruction, there may be metastatic lesions on other parts of the skin surface and in bone and viscera. Vaccinia gangrenosum occurs most frequently in persons with disorders of immunity and, if untreated, is nearly always fatal. *Eczema vaccinatum* is a serious complication that is seen in persons with eczema or other types of chronic skin conditions. Widespread infection in the previously affected areas, as well as in normal skin, may result from direct vaccination of an eczematous patient or from exposure to a recently vaccinated individual. *Generalized vaccinia* in patients without preexisting skin disease is characterized by a few satellite lesions surrounding the inoculation site or by widely disseminated pox resembling the primary vaccination lesion. This condition is usually mild with generally complete recovery. Vaccinia virus may be transferred from the primary inoculation site to the eye or other sites by scratching. *Postvaccinal encephalomyelitis* appears from 2 to 25 days after vaccination. The patient suddenly becomes severely ill with nuchal rigidity, drowsiness, vomiting, convulsions, coma, and signs suggesting disease of the spinal cord. The period of coma lasts for a few days, and in those who recover there are usually no permanent sequelae. Death occurs in about 30 to 40 percent of the patients with encephalomyelitis. *Erythema multiforme bullosum, or diffuse blotchy erythema,* may occur in vaccinated patients 7 to 10 days after vaccination, and is thought to be an allergic reaction to the virus or other components of the vaccine.

The rates of adverse effects per million primarily vaccinated persons were vaccinia gangrenosum, 0.9; eczema vaccinatum, 10.4; generalized vaccinia, 23.4; vaccinal lesions resulting from accidental implantation of virus, 25.4; postvaccinal encephalitis, 2.9; other complications, 11.8; the death rate was 1 per million. In view of the current status of smallpox in the world, the risks of widespread routine immunization seem far greater than the risk of inadvertent introduction of disease in this country. Because of this, the sharp restriction of indications for vaccination appears to be justified.

Active treatment of vaccinia complications, aside from control of bacterial superinfection and treatment of any underlying defects, is limited. VIG is of possible value in accidental inoculation into secondary sites such as the eye, vaccinia gangrenosum, eczema vaccinatum, and generalized vaccinia. Dosage is usually 0.6 ml/kg intramuscularly, although much larger doses are sometimes used in severe cases. VIG is of no use in erythema multiforme or postvaccinal encephalitis. Thiosemicarbazone has apparently been of benefit in some cases of progressive vaccinia gangrenosum. 5-Iodo-2′-deoxyuridine, while not yet proved to be effective, is suggested for topical treatment of vaccinial keratitis and conjunctivitis.

COWPOX

Cowpox is primarily a disease of the teats and udders of cows. Humans are almost always infected by milking, but occasional spread to contacts may occur from an infected person. The human disease is characterized by low-grade fever and by small papules on the fingers and hand, which go through vesicular and pustular stages resembling the course of vaccinia infection. The lesions may be ruptured by trauma and spread to immediately adjacent areas on the hand and continue to ulcerate for several weeks. Edema, lymphangitis, and axillary lymph node enlargement are common. Very rare cases of postcowpox encephalitis and serious infections of eczematous persons have been reported. In general, the disease is benign, heals without scarring, and is usually uncomplicated.

PARAVACCINIA (MILKERS' NODULES)

Paravaccinia is a poxvirus which is antigenically unrelated to cowpox, but produces similar lesions in humans. It is primarily a disease of calves and milk cows, producing lesions on the teats of the cows and oral lesions in the suckling calf. Humans acquire infection through the skin by direct contact. The lesion is usually solitary, beginning as a macule on the finger, hand, or wrist, and progressing to a firm nodule, 1 to 2 cm in diameter, in 10 days. It then crusts and heals without scarring in 2 to 3 weeks. Occasionally, there is associated lymphadenitis. The lesion and its evolution are closely similar to ecthyma contagiosum (orf), a poxvirus of sheep, which can also infect humans by direct inoculation.

REFERENCES

BEDSON HS, DUMBELL K: Smallpox and vaccinia. Br Med Bull 23:119, 1967

BROWN GC (ed): Symposium: Is routine smallpox vaccination necessary in the United States? Am J Epidemiol 93:221, 1971

DIXON, CW: *Smallpox.* London, Churchill, 1962

DOUGLAS RG et al: Treatment of progressive vaccinia. Arch Intern Med 129:980, 1972

GOLDSTEIN JA et al: Smallpox vaccination reactions, prophylaxis, and therapy of complications. Pediatrics 55:342, 1975

JOKLIK WK: The poxviruses. Bacteriol Rev 30:33, 1966

Laboratory-associated smallpox—England. Morb Mort Week Rep, vol 27, no 35, September 1, 1978

LANE JM et al: Smallpox and smallpox vaccination policy. Annu Rev Med 22:251, 1971

RENNIE AGR et al: Ocular vaccinia. Lancet 2:273, 1974

WENNER HA: Virus diseases associated with cutaneous eruptions. Prog Med Virol 16:269, 1973

185
CHICKENPOX (VARICELLA) AND HERPES ZOSTER

C. GEORGE RAY

DEFINITION Chickenpox is a contagious disease characterized by fever and a disseminated vesicular eruption. Herpes zoster, or shingles, is characterized by segmental inflammation of the spinal or cranial nerves and their ganglions, and by a painful localized vesicular eruption of the skin along the distribution of the involved nerve. Chickenpox and herpes zoster are different manifestations of infection with the same viral agent.

ETIOLOGY In 1953 a virus was recovered from patients with chickenpox and herpes zoster that produced intranuclear, eosinophilic inclusions and multinucleated giant cells in lines of cells derived from various monkey and human tissues. The infectivity of varicella-zoster virus in culture is closely cell-associated, and ordinarily can be passed to other tissue cultures only by transfer of infected, intact cells. The structure of the varicella-zoster virion resembles that of herpes simplex and the other viruses of the herpes group.

PATHOGENESIS AND PATHOLOGY Varicella is presumably transmitted by the respiratory route, although the virus has only rarely been isolated from nasopharyngeal secretions of infected persons. Virus multiplication occurs at some unidentified site and probably results in intermittent viremia, as suggested by the successive crops of widely spaced lesions. Focal viral infection of blood vessels in the corium with intranuclear inclusions in endothelial cells, results in degeneration of the epidermis and formation of vesicles containing serum, polymorphonuclear leukocytes, and multinucleated giant cells. Virus can be isolated from vesicle fluid, but not usually from crusting lesions or scabs, for 3 to 4 days after eruption. In patients with varicella pneumonia, the tracheobronchial mucosa, the alveolar septa, and the interstitial areas of the lungs are edematous and contain monocytic inflammatory cells, cells with intranuclear inclusions and giant cells. The nodular areas of pneumonia may eventually become calcified. The changes in the central nervous system in patients with postinfectious varicella encephalomyelitis resemble those seen in measles. Rarely, encephalomyelitis with inclusion bodies resembling herpes simplex infection may occur, and varicella-zoster virus can be recovered from the central nervous system. In infants and children, acute encephalopathy with fatty infiltration of the viscera (Reye's syndrome) sometimes follows the acute phase of varicella; in this condition, only cerebral edema is found on pathologic examination of the brain.

The pathogenesis of herpes zoster is not clear (see "Epidemiology," below), but the tissue changes are well documented. The dorsal root ganglion of the affected nerve is swollen and hemorrhagic; the edema spreads along the peripheral nerve and may reach the spinal cord. The nerve tissue shows hemorrhagic infarction, inflammation, and necrosis of many of the ganglion cells, some of which contain intranuclear inclusions. The microscopic appearance of zoster skin lesions is almost identical with that described for chickenpox vesicles. Virus can be cultured from the lesions for as long as 8 days after onset.

EPIDEMIOLOGY Chickenpox is a highly contagious disease with attack rates of 80 percent or more among susceptible household contacts of an index case. The infectious period extends from a day or two before the rash until as long as 6 days after the appearance of new skin lesions, or until all vesicles have crusted over. Patients with herpes zoster may be the source of an outbreak of chickenpox among susceptible contacts. Children from 5 to 8 years of age are most commonly affected, but younger children, including newborn infants, and adults may develop chickenpox; an estimated 2 to 20 percent of cases occur in persons over the age of 15 years. Serologic surveys are limited, but indicate that as many as 9 percent of parturient women are susceptible to chickenpox. In the United States the disease is endemic, with superimposed epidemics every 2 to 5 years, usually in the winter or spring.

Herpes zoster is mainly a disease of adults who have previously had chickenpox. The epidemiologic evidence strongly suggests that herpes zoster results from reactivation of virus that has remained dormant in spinal ganglia since an episode of chickenpox. Exogenous acquisition of infection directly resulting in herpes zoster rarely, if ever, occurs. Most patients with zoster have had no recent exposure to patients with zoster or varicella, and the incidence of the disease does not increase during seasonal chickenpox epidemics.

Zoster occurs commonly in patients with neoplasms, most frequently in those with Hodgkin's disease, where the incidence may be as high as 25 percent. Advanced disease, cutaneous anergy, recent x-ray therapy to affected nodes, and possibly splenectomy predispose patients with Hodgkin's disease to zoster. The most significant common factor responsible for the development of zoster in these patients appears to be depressed cell-mediated immunity; there is no clear correlation with humoral immune status.

Recurrent herpes zoster is distinctly rare. If such a recurrence is documented, the likelihood of an underlying malignancy or immunodeficiency is great. When episodes of so-called recurrent zoster in healthy individuals have been carefully studied, herpes simplex virus has usually been found to be the causative agent. Like varicella-zoster virus, herpes simplex can cause zoster-like disease, but can also cause recurrent lesions.

MANIFESTATIONS Chickenpox The incubation period from the time of exposure to the appearance of varicella rash is 10 to 21 days, most often 14 to 17 days. There may be a 1- to 2-day prodrome with fever and malaise, but these symptoms usually begin when the rash appears. The first skin manifestations are pruritic maculopapules that evolve in a few hours to thin-walled vesicles which contain clear fluid and are surrounded by a red border. During the next day the erythema diminishes and the vesicles collapse in the center, forming annular or umbilicated lesions which dry further and form scabs that fall off, after several days, without scarring. New maculopapules continue to erupt during the first 3 or 4 days of illness and go through a similar evolution. The findings at one time, in one area, of skin lesions in all stages of development—maculopapules, vesicles, umbilicated lesions, and scabs—is characteristic of chickenpox. The rash is most concentrated on the trunk, but pox are frequently seen on the face and scalp, occasionally on the mucosal surface of the mouth or conjunctiva, and rarely on the palms and soles.

Chickenpox in adults is often more severe than in children, with more profuse rash, higher fever, and a greater incidence of pneumonia.

Herpes zoster Herpes zoster is a disease of nerves of the skin and other tissues that they supply. It most commonly affects the thoracic (55 percent of cases), cervical (20 percent), and lumbar and sacral nerves (15 percent), and the ophthalmic division of the trigeminal nerve.

Fever and pain that is localized to the areas served by the affected nerves may begin 4 or 5 days before or be concomitant with the appearance of the skin eruption. Rarely, characteristic pain and serologic evidence of zoster occur with no clinical involvement of the skin (zoster sine eruptione). The discomfort is mild to severe and can be sharp, burning, or dull. In addition to disorders of sensation, herpes zoster is occasionally associated with motor paralysis of arms, legs, intercostal muscles, or muscles innervated by cranial nerves. The skin lesion starts with local redness followed by red papules that progress over the next 2 weeks through vesicular, pustular, and crusting stages that resemble the evolution of individual pox of varicella. The lesions are arranged unilaterally in characteristic band-like clusters which follow radicular lines. They may run transversely along the hemithorax or vertically over the arm or leg.

Disease of the individual cranial nerves leads to characteristic groups of symptoms. If the trigeminal (Gasserian) ganglion is affected, there will usually be pain in the distribution of the nerve, headache, weakness of the eyelid muscles, and occasionally Argyll Robertson pupil. Lesions appear on the face, in the mouth, on the tongue, and frequently on the cornea. Iridocyclitis, anesthesia of the cornea, and scarring may result. If the geniculate ganglion is involved, there may be Bell's palsy, disorders of hearing, and vertigo, with unilateral herpetic lesions of the external ear and canal and of the anterior portion of the tongue. Central nervous system inflammation is prominent when herpes zoster attacks the cranial nerves, and meningeal signs and symptoms are frequent.

COMPLICATIONS Hemorrhage into vesicles and surrounding skin may be seen in adults with severe chickenpox or in children receiving adrenal steroids. Infection of the varicella lesions by bacteria, most commonly *Staphylococcus aureus*, results in delayed healing and scarring of skin, and occasionally in bacteremia.

Of adults with chickenpox, 15 percent develop primary *Varicella pneumonia*. Pneumonia is invariably associated with skin lesions and appears 1 to 6 days after onset of rash. The degree of pulmonary involvement correlates to some extent with the severity of the rash; patients may be virtually asymptomatic or may develop serious, life-threatening disease. Tachypnea, dyspnea, cough, and fever, with a temperature of 102°F or more, are present in most patients with symptomatic pneumonia; cyanosis, pleuritic chest pain, and hemoptysis each occur in 20 to 40 percent of the recorded cases. The physical examination may disclose no abnormalities, or there may be intercostal retractions, a few rhonchi, wheezes, scattered rales, and rarely, evidence of pleural effusion. In contrast to the paucity of physical signs, roentgenograms demonstrate widespread nodular infiltration of both lungs, most prominent at the hila and least evident at the apexes. Vital capacity is decreased, arterial oxygen saturation is diminished, and the airways may be blocked by tenacious bronchopulmonary secretions. Most patients with varicella pneumonia show symptomatic improvement when the rash begins to wane; however, seriously ill patients may remain febrile and dyspneic for as long as 2 weeks. Roentgenographic evidence of disease diminishes at the time of clinical improvement, but may persist for several weeks, followed in some cases by persistent miliary calcifications. Persistent abnormalities of pulmonary gas diffusion have been demonstrated several months after apparent recovery.

Central nervous system complications occur most frequently in children, with estimated rates as high as 1 in 200 cases. The most common manifestation is acute cerebellar ataxia, which usually begins 3 to 21 days after onset of rash and is usually benign. Other less common manifestations include acute encephalomyelitis, polyneuritis, ascending or transverse myelitis, optic neuritis, and Reye's syndrome.

Patients who contract *varicella while receiving steroids* may have recurrent crops of new skin lesions for as long as 3 weeks. They have a higher incidence of hemorrhagic and progressive gangrenous lesions and occasionally develop a fatal disseminated disease with viral infection in all the viscera. The fatal form of the disease has been encountered most frequently in children being treated with steroids for leukemia or other disease of the hematopoietic system, but it has also been seen in those receiving therapy for rheumatic fever and allergic disorders. Children with the rare syndrome of cartilage-hair hypoplasia may suffer from unusually severe and occasionally fatal chickenpox. *Other complications of chickenpox* such as myocarditis, corneal lesions, iritis, nephritis, nephrosis, monoarticular arthritis or polyarthritis, thrombocytopenic purpura, purpura fulminans, orchitis, and appendicitis have been recognized but are rare. Like measles, chickenpox can transiently produce anergy to tuberculin, and occasionally there may be reactivation of latent tuberculosis. Congenital infection with varicella can occur, and infants born of mothers with chickenpox may display the typical skin lesions. Congenital malformations as a result of infection in early pregnancy have been reported but are rare. The greatest mortality risk to the newborn infant appears to occur when onset of the maternal rash occurs in the 4-day period immediately before delivery or 48 h after delivery.

Postherpetic neuralgia may last for several months or years and become the most troublesome part of the disease. In nearly all patients with zoster, healing with loss of scab is complete within 2 to 3 weeks. In the young, pain persists for only a week or two after healing and then usually disappears, although hypo- or hyperesthesia may remain. However, in patients over 60 years of age, moderate to severe pain persists for more than 2 months in as many as 70 percent, even though the skin lesions have healed normally.

Zoster skin lesions do not always remain localized. *Generalized zoster* occurs in 5 percent of zoster patients with no underlying disease, and in as many as 70 percent of those with Hodgkin's disease, and is characterized by dissemination to all parts of the skin, producing a picture similar to that of chickenpox. The scattered lesions last 6 to 9 days in normal hosts, but they may persist for 3 to 4 weeks in those with serious underlying disease. In these patients dissemination may also involve the visceral organs (including the lungs) and occasionally results in death.

LABORATORY FINDINGS Multinucleated giant cells and epithelial cells with eosinophilic intranuclear inclusions can be identified in material scraped from the base of a vesicular lesion or in sputum from patients with varicella pneumonia. For specific diagnosis, virus can be isolated from vesicular fluid, and antigens can be demonstrated in vesicular fluid and in

crusts of lesions by the use of a simple gel-precipitin technique. Serologic confirmation is also possible, utilizing complement fixation or the more sensitive immune adherence hemagglutination or indirect immunofluorescent antibody tests. The white blood cell count in patients with uncomplicated chickenpox or zoster is normal. Mononuclear pleocytosis is present in the cerebrospinal fluid of patients with herpes zoster, especially those with involvement of the cranial nerves. The spinal fluid in varicella-zoster encephalomyelitis often contains increased protein, and cell counts may range from zero to 3000 lymphocytes per cubic millimeter.

DIFFERENTIAL DIAGNOSIS Chickenpox can usually be diagnosed by the history of recent exposure and the character of the rash. In situations where smallpox is a possibility, differentiation from chickenpox can be attempted by noting the distribution and evolution of the rash and by examining the cells from vesicles, but definitive diagnosis can be made only by identification of the virus or by serologic methods. Disseminated vaccinia lesions similar to chickenpox lesions may occur in patients, especially those with disorders of immunity or eczema, who have recently been vaccinated or exposed to a vaccinated person. Herpes simplex infection in patients with chronic eczema or neurodermatitis may present as a varicelliform eruption confined to previously involved areas of skin. The diagnosis can be confirmed by virus isolation. Rickettsialpox can be differentiated from chickenpox by the presence of an eschar in the area of mite bite, prominent headache, and specific complement-fixing antibodies to *Rickettsia akari*. Rarely, coxsackieviruses can produce a similar eruption in young children, although the lesions all tend to be in the same stage of development in one area. Stevens-Johnson syndrome has also been occasionally confused with chickenpox.

In the preeruptive stage, the diagnosis of herpes zoster is difficult, and the disease is usually confused with other causes of pain, such as pleurisy, appendicitis, pleurodynia, or collapsed intervertebral disk. After the unilateral eruption appears, the clinical features are so characteristic that the diagnosis is usually simple. Occasionally, localized herpes simplex along the distribution of a segmental nerve may simulate zoster, including the localized pain and tenderness. The diagnosis of herpes simplex infection can be confirmed in the laboratory by virus isolation.

PROPHYLAXIS Chickenpox can often be prevented or significantly modified by the administration of specific zoster immune globulin (ZIG) derived from the serum of patients recovering from herpes zoster, varicella-zoster immune globulin (VZIG) prepared from pooled plasma containing high titers of varicella antibody, or intravenous zoster immune plasma (ZIP). Both ZIG and VZIG should be given within 72 h of exposure to be effective, and limited data suggest some usefulness of ZIP if given within 6 days of exposure, in doses ranging from 3 to 14 ml/kg. Table 185-1 lists the current Center for Disease Control criteria which should be fulfilled before the use of VZIG in prophylaxis of chickenpox, and these also generally apply for ZIG and ZIP. Large doses of pooled human gamma globulin have also been shown to modify the disease if given shortly after exposure, but the quantity required to do so is so great (0.6 to 1.2 ml/kg) that this form of treatment is not generally recommended. There is no evidence that any of these preparations have any value in the prevention of herpes zoster, or the treatment of established infection of either type.

TABLE 185-1
Recommended criteria for the use of varicella-zoster immune globulin for prophylaxis of varicella

I One of the following underlying illnesses or conditions
  A Leukemia or lymphoma
  B Congenital or acquired immunodeficiency
  C Under immunosuppressive medication
  D Newly born of mother with varicella
II One of the following types of exposure to varicella or zoster patient
  A Household contact
  B Playmate contact (less than 1 h play indoors)
  C Hospital contact (in same two- to four-bed room or adjacent beds in a large ward)
  D Newborn contact (newborn whose mother contracted varicella within 4 days before delivery or within 48 h after delivery)
III Negative or unknown prior disease history
IV Age less than 15 years
V Request for treatment must be initiated within 72 h of exposure

Live, attenuated varicella-zoster virus vaccines have been tried as immunizing agents in high-risk children in Japan, but larger trials elsewhere have not yet been reported. Such vaccines are not available in the United States.

TREATMENT The patient with uncomplicated chickenpox seems to benefit most from cool, wet compresses or tepid water baths, rather than drying lotions, for the relief of itching. Secondary bacterial infections should be treated with appropriate antibacterial agents. Patients with varicella pneumonia require skillful nursing care, removal of excessive bronchial secretions, administration of oxygen, and on occasion assisted ventilation. Adrenal corticosteroids have been considered by some to be beneficial in the treatment of varicella pneumonia, but convincing evidence of their efficacy in this condition is not available. Patients suspected of having varicella-zoster infection of the eye should be promptly treated by an ophthalmologist. The therapy consists of analgesics for severe pain and the use of atropine to prevent synechiae. Some ophthalmologists recommend the use of steroids if uveitis is present. Topical 5-iodo-2′-deoxyuridine is of possible value for corneal or conjunctival ulcerative lesions.

Intravenous adenine arabinoside has been used in cases of severe zoster in patients on immunosuppressive therapy who are at high risk of dissemination, with encouraging results. Other studies, utilizing high doses of intramuscular human leukocyte interferon in similar patients, have also shown promise, but this form of treatment may be limited by the restricted availability of human interferon. However, further data are necessary before either mode of treatment can be more widely recommended. Moreover, there is no convincing evidence that such therapeutic modalities are effective in severe chickenpox or in herpes zoster after dissemination has already occurred.

It has been claimed that in older patients with herpes zoster and no underlying disease, the administration of a short course of adrenal steroids by mouth during the early eruptive phase of the disease reduces the incidence and duration of postherpetic neuralgia without inducing dissemination or other complications. Steroids should *not* be used for this purpose in patients with neoplasms or other underlying disease.

REFERENCES

ARVIN AM et al: Selective impairment of lymphocyte reactivity to varicella-zoster virus antigen among untreated patients with lymphoma. J Infect Dis 137:531, 1978

BABA K et al: Studies with live varicella vaccine and inactivated skin test antigen: Protective effect of the vaccine and clinical application of the skin test. Pediatrics 61:550, 1978

BALFOUR HH et al: Prevention or modification of varicella using zoster immune plasma. Am J Dis Child 131:693, 1977

BROOK I: Varicella arthritis in childhood. Clin Pediatr 16:1156, 1977

BRUNELL PA, GERSHON AA: Passive immunization against varicella-zoster infections and other modes of therapy. J Infect Dis 127:415, 1973

EAGLESTEIN WH et al: The effects of early corticosteroid therapy on the skin eruption and pain of herpes zoster. JAMA 211:1681, 1970

GERSHON AA et al: Antibody to varicella-zoster virus in parturient women and their offspring during the first year of life. Pediatrics 58:692, 1976

GROTH KE et al: Evaluation of zoster immune plasma. JAMA 239:1877, 1978

KREBS RA, BURVANT MU: Nephrotic syndrome in association with varicella. JAMA 222:325, 1972

MERIGAN RC et al: Interferon for the treatment of herpes zoster in patients with cancer. N Eng J Med 298:981, 1978

MINKOWITZ S et al: Acute glomerulonephritis associated with varicella infection. Am J Med 44:489, 1968

NORRIS FH et al: Herpes-zoster meningoencephalitis. J Infect Dis 122:335, 1970

RAIDER L: Calcification in chickenpox pneumonia. Chest 60:504, 1971

RUCKDESCHEL JC et al: Herpes zoster and impaired cell-associated immunity to the V-Z virus in patients with Hodgkin's disease. Am J Med 62:77, 1977

TRIEBWASSER JH et al: Varicella pneumonia in adults: Report of seven cases and a review of literature. Medicine 46:409, 1967

WEBSTER MH, SMITH CS: Congenital abnormalities and maternal herpes zoster. Br Med J 2:1193, 1977

WHITLEY RJ et al: Adenine arabinoside therapy of herpes zoster in the immunosuppressed. N Engl J Med 294:1193, 1976

Central nervous system viruses

186
APPROACH TO THE PATIENT WITH ASEPTIC MENINGITIS OR ENCEPHALITIS

LAWRENCE COREY

INTRODUCTION Viral infections of the central nervous system (CNS) can be classified into five clinical syndromes: (1) aseptic meningitis, (2) myelitis, (3) viral encephalitis, (4) postinfectious or "allergic" encephalitis, and (5) persistent or slow virus infections. While the predominant signs and symptoms of these syndromes differ, considerable overlap among them occurs. Aseptic meningitis, encephalitis, meningoencephalitis, encephalomyelitis, and myelitis are descriptive terms; the choice of term depends upon whether the major impact of infection is upon the meninges, the brain, the spinal cord, or combinations of the three. Many viruses are associated with inflammation and infection of one anatomic site; for example, enteroviruses cause predominantly aseptic meningitis, arthropod-borne viruses produce encephalitis, while varicella-zoster is associated with postinfectious encephalitis. However, meningoencephalitis due to coxsackievirus or lymphocytic choriomeningitis virus, or aseptic meningitis due to St. Louis encephalitis, may occur. In addition, many nonviral infectious agents, focal inflammatory processes, and neoplastic and immunologic diseases may mimic viral CNS syndromes. These entities are listed in Table 186-1 and are discussed in detail in the referenced chapters. Despite these overlaps, definition of a clinical viral syndrome helps the physician both prognostically and therapeutically. In the adult, aseptic meningitis due to herpes simplex virus (usually type 2) is a benign self-limited disease, not requiring antiviral chemotherapy. In contrast, encephalitis caused by herpes simplex virus is a disease with a 75 percent mortality if left untreated.

ASEPTIC MENINGITIS The clinical syndrome of aseptic meningitis is manifested by fever, signs of meningeal irritation (nuchal rigidity, Kernig's or Brudzinski's signs), and a lymphocyte pleocytosis of the cerebrospinal fluid (CSF). The differentiation of viral meningitis from early or partially treated bacterial meningitis is a common diagnostic problem. In aseptic meningitis the CSF demonstrates a lymphocytic cellular response which may vary from 10 to over 1000 cells per cubic millimeter. Generally, a pleocytosis of more than 2500 cells per cubic millimeter is associated with bacterial, rather than viral, infection. Occasional cases of lymphocytic choriomeningitis may demonstrate CSF cell counts in the thousands, almost all of which are mononuclear, distinctly different from the polymorphonuclear response that occurs in bacterial meningitis. While lymphocytes are the usual CSF cell type in viral CNS infections, early in viral disease many patients will demonstrate a polymorphonuclear response in the CSF. In addition, a slight decrease in spinal fluid glucose (between 25 and 50 mg/ml) can occur in aseptic meningitis. Because of these overlaps in the

TABLE 186-1
Etiology and differential diagnosis of viral CNS disease

I Acute encephalitis or aseptic meningitis
  A Enteroviruses (Chap. 187)
    1 Poliovirus types 1 to 3
    2 Coxsackieviruses A1, A2, A4 to A11, A16 to A18, A22 to A24
    3 Coxsackieviruses B1 to B6
    4 Echovirus types 1 to 11, 25, 30 to 33
    5 Enterovirus types 68 to 70
  B Herpes simplex virus (Chap. 193)
    1 Type 2: Adult, aseptic meningitis; neonate, meningoencephalitis
    2 Type 1: Child or adult, focal encephalitis; neonate, meningoencephalitis
  C Arboviruses (Chap. 190): In the United States: California, St. Louis, Western equine, and Eastern equine encephalitis
  D Mumps (Chap. 188)
  E Measles (Chap. 181)
  F Varicella-zoster (Chap. 185)
  G Rubella (Chap. 182)
  H Cytomegalovirus (Chap. 194)
  I Influenza (Chap. 179)
  J Adenovirus (Chap. 178)
  K Lymphocytic choriomeningitis (Chap. 191)
  L Epstein-Barr virus (Chap. 195)
  M Colorado tick fever (Chap. 190)
  N Encephalomyocarditis virus (Chap. 187)
  O Rhabdovirus (Chap. 189)
  P Cat-scratch disease (Chap. 197)
II Postinfectious agents
  A Measles (Chap. 181)
  B Varicella-zoster (Chap. 185)
  C Viral vaccines (rabies, vaccinia) (Chaps. 184, 189)
  D Mxyoviruses, including influenza (Chap. 179)
III Viral associated: Reye's syndrome (Chap. 369)
IV Nonviral infectious agents which may cause encephalitis-aseptic meningitis syndrome
  A Bacterial
    1 Bacterial meningitis (Chap. 368)
      a Early phase
      b Partially treated
    2 Mycobacteria (Chap. 143)
    3 Leptospirosis (Chap. 148)
    4 Syphilis (Chap. 113)
    5 Brain abscess (Chap. 368)
    6 Parameningeal focus (Chap. 368)
  B Mycotic: *Cryptococcus neoformans* (Chap. 153)
  C Rickettsial
    1 Rocky Mountain spotted fever (Chap. 164)
    2 Q fever (Chap. 170)
  D Chlamydial and mycoplasmal
    1 *Mycoplasma pneumoniae* (Chap. 172)
    2 Psittacosis (Chap. 175)
    3 Lymphogranuloma venereum (Chap. 174)
  E Parasitic
    1 Protozoa: Toxoplasmosis (Chap. 203), malaria (Chap. 200), trypanosomiasis (Chap. 202), *Naegleria* and other amoebas (Chap. 199)
    2 Nematodes (Chap. 207): *Toxocara, Trichinella* (Chap. 208), *Strongyloides stercoralis*, angiostrongyliasis cantonesis (eosinophilic meningitis) (Chap. 210), filariasis (Chap. 209)
  F Trematodes: Schistosomiasis (Chap. 211), cestodes, cysticercosis, echinococcosis (Chap. 213)
V Noninfectious causes of "encephalitis-like" syndromes
  A Toxic (lead, drug overdose, tick paralysis, botulism, tetanus)
  B Metabolic
  C Vascular (emboli, hemorrhagic)
  D Immune injury—"arteritis"
  E Carcinomatous
  F Mass lesions
  G Recurrent (Mollaret's) meningitis

CSF findings, the criteria which differentiate viral from bacterial infection cannot be interpreted too rigidly. Each patient must be evaluated both clinically and epidemiologically.

Aseptic meningitis occurs more frequently during the summer months and in patients under 40. In the summer, a child or young adult who presents with fever, headache, myalgias, a stiff neck, a mononuclear CSF pleocytosis, and a CSF Gram's stain lacking bacteria most likely has aseptic meningitis. Even if a polymorphonuclear pleocytosis is present, antibiotic therapy can be withheld and the lumbar puncture repeated in 8 to 12 h. A shift from a predominance of neutrophils to one of mononuclear cells, a stable or increasing CSF glucose, and the absence of organisms on a second CSF Gram's stain all suggest viral rather than bacterial infection. However, initial therapy with antimicrobial agents until bacterial culture results are complete is appropriate if the epidemiologic and clinical data do not suggest a viral etiology such as the occurrence of the illness in the winter months or in a patient over 40 years of age. If the patient has received antimicrobial therapy prior to CSF examination, the distinction between viral and bacterial infection may be very difficult. Laboratory techniques for the detection of viral or bacterial antigens or bacterial products may be helpful in this clinical situation.

Other causes of aseptic meningitis include leptospirosis, a nonviral pathogen which mimics aseptic meningitis. Exposure to animals (especially rodents), conjunctivitis, mild hepatitis, and/or renal abnormalities should suggest this diagnosis. Tuberculosis and cryptococcal meningitis may resemble aseptic meningitis. These infections are usually characterized by a more subacute course, a higher CSF protein concentration, and a lower CSF glucose concentration than are found in viral meningitis. In addition, evidence of cranial nerve palsies often occurs in tuberculous meningitis and is a helpful differential sign (Chap. 143).

Laboratory diagnosis Studies conducted in the 1950s and 1960s indicated that the enteroviruses, particularly poliomyelitis and mumps virus, were the most frequent cause of etiologically identified aseptic meningitis. Administration of mumps and poliomyelitis vaccines has decreased the incidence of these diseases and their neurological complications. In contrast, the sharp increase in genital herpes simplex virus infection has resulted in an increased recognition of the aseptic meningitis and sacral radiculitis syndromes associated with primary herpes virus infection. Echovirus and coxsackieviruses A and B account for the majority of cases of aseptic meningitis in the United States. However, the large number of serotypes of these agents (70 enteroviruses) preclude the use of routine "serologic batteries" for the evaluation of individual cases of aseptic meningitis. During localized outbreaks, consultation with regional viral diagnostic laboratories or public health officials may aid in the selection of appropriate serologic and/or culture techniques for isolating the virus.

In evaluating individual cases of sporadic viral CNS infection, viral isolation procedures are the most helpful laboratory tests in establishing an etiologic diagnosis. Isolation of a specific viral agent from the CSF or nervous tissue is diagnostic, while culture of an agent known to cause CNS disease from the throat, stool, or urine must be interpreted according to the patient's clinical syndrome and course. For example, isolation of mumps virus from saliva or urine in a young male with aseptic meningitis would be presumptive evidence of mumps meningoencephalitis. Similarly, the presence of clinical measles, the isolation of measles virus from nasopharyngeal secretions, or the demonstration of a fourfold or greater rise in anti-

body titer to measles virus in a patient with an acute encephalitis would also constitute presumptive evidence of CNS measles infection.

Nonpolio enteroviral excretion in feces occurs in up to 20 percent of the population, depending on the geography and season. Studies of coxsackie- or echovirus diseases indicate that the isolation of these agents from throat and rectal swabs occurs much more frequently in cases of aseptic meningitis and their household contacts than in well individuals.

Isolation of agents known to cause recurrent or persistent viral infection such as herpes simplex virus or adenovirus from throat washings, or cytomegalovirus from urine samples, should generally not be interpreted as having etiologic importance. On the other hand, many agents, including group A coxsackieviruses, flavovirus, many togaviruses, and lymphocytic choriomeningitis virus, will be detected only if specimens are inoculated into suckling or adult mice. Despite these shortcomings, the etiologic diagnosis of aseptic meningitis can be established with reasonable certainty in 60 to 75 percent of cases.

MYELITIS SYNDROMES Viral invasion of the CNS may also result in parenchymal spinal cord involvement. Poliomyelitis, with its devastating effect on motor neurons of the spinal cord and brainstem, was for many years one of the most feared of all infectious diseases. The advent of effective vaccines has markedly reduced but not eliminated this disease. To take its place, acute paralytic disease due to the nonpolio enteroviruses has become increasingly evident. Coxsackieviruses A4, A7, A9, A10, and B1 to B5 and echovirus types 1, 2, 4, 6, 9, 11, 16, and 30 have been associated with lower motor neuron involvement usually characterized by an asymmetric flaccid paralysis of the limbs. Generally, the illness associated with these agents is less severe and has a higher rate of recovery of neuromuscular function than poliomyelitis.

Acute transverse myelitis (Chap. 375) usually begins with the abrupt onset of bilateral weakness of the lower extremities with concomitant involvement of proprioceptive, pain, and touch pathways which may be due to noninfectious and infectious causes. Acute pyogenic spinal epidural abscess may present as an acute transverse myelopathy (Chap. 368). Similarly, transverse myelitis related to acute infection with mumps, measles, Epstein-Barr, herpes simplex, or varicella-zoster virus or echo-, polio-, or cytomegalovirus may occur. Occasionally, one of these agents may be isolated from the CSF or neural tissue. Because a slight lymphocytic pleocytosis may accompany the transverse myelopathy of noninfectious etiology, clinical differentiation may be difficult. In addition, antecedent viral infection or vaccination (smallpox, rabies, influenza) can initiate postinfectious transverse myelitis. The pathogenesis of the perivenous demyelination and perivascular cellular infiltration associated with postinfectious transverse myelitis is unknown but is thought to represent a form of "hypersensitivity." Corticosteroids have been used in the treatment of postinfectious myelitis, but their value in controlled studies has not been proved.

ENCEPHALITIS SYNDROMES When an acute febrile illness is associated with dysfunction of the cerebrum, brainstem, and/or cerebellum, then encephalitis must be considered. The distinction between viral encephalitis and an acute toxic (noninflammatory) encephalopathy may be difficult. Both entities present with the abrupt onset of disturbed consciousness. In addition, Reye's syndrome (acute encephalopathy with fatty degeneration of the viscera) usually is associated with a history of an antecedent febrile upper respiratory "viral" illness. An elevated blood ammonia level, a prolonged prothrombin time, and elevated serum aminotransferases in a patient with an acute encephalopathy are characteristic of Reye's syndrome. Cerebrospinal fluid examination is the best means of distinguishing between encephalopathy and an acute encephalitis. Cerebrospinal fluid pressures and protein concentrations may be increased in both entities; however, the presence of lymphocytic pleocytosis is characteristic of encephalitis.

Herpes simplex encephalitis (Chap. 193)   The advent of successful antiviral chemotherapy for herpes simplex virus encephalitis has altered the traditionally laissez-faire attitude toward the etiologic diagnosis of acute viral encephalitis. The ability of herpes simplex virus to cause rapid necrosis of neuronal tissue, combined with the fact that patients treated with intravenously administered adenine arabinoside early in the course of illness have a better survival rate and less neurological deficits than patients treated late in the course of the disease, makes prompt and accurate diagnosis of this entity necessary. Clinically, the most distinctive aspect of herpes simplex virus encephalitis is its tendency to cause focal, especially temporoparietal lobe, destruction. For this reason, patients who present with focal neurological signs and symptoms should undergo immediate evaluation with electroencephalograms and/or radionuclide scans, computerized axial tomography, or angiography to corroborate the presence of a focal or diffuse inflammatory process. If a focal defect is demonstrated, the diagnosis of herpes simplex encephalitis must be considered. Unfortunately, accurate, noninvasive techniques for differentiating herpes simplex virus (HSV) encephalitis from other focal encephalitides or focal pyogenic processes such as brain abscess are not available. Herpes simplex virus antigen in CSF by immunofluorescence is present in only 10 percent of confirmed cases. Moreover, HSV-specific CSF antibody usually cannot be detected early in the disease when accurate diagnosis and therapy are most needed. Brain biopsy remains the definitive procedure. This procedure is best performed in facilities that have the comprehensive virological support needed to diagnose HSV infections rapidly. The biopsy should be examined for HSV antigen by immunofluorescence or immunoperoxidase techniques, by electron microscopy for detection of herpes group virus in infected cells, and by histologic examination for evidence of intranuclear inclusions; then it should be submitted for viral isolation. Adenine arabinoside therapy may be initiated and, if no evidence of HSV infection is found, can be discontinued. Adenine arabinoside is not effective against RNA viruses and is not effective in suspected viral encephalitis. Moreover, its hepatic, hematopoietic, and neurological toxicity preclude its use in seriously ill patients with encephalitis who do not have HSV infection.

Diffuse encephalitis   An attempt to make an etiologic diagnosis of a patient with diffuse encephalitis is often unrewarding; more than 50 percent of the cases reported to the Center for Disease Control are of undetermined origin. The number of potential pathogens is large, and, more importantly, the prognosis varies among viral pathogens. Some agents, such as rabies and Eastern equine encephalitis, are associated with a high case fatality rate. California or measles encephalitis infrequently causes death but may result in a neurological residua in as many as one-third of cases. In contrast, in adults, Western equine encephalitis is associated with severe neurological deficits only rarely.

Knowledge of the patient's age, the season, and the history of exposure is helpful in determining an etiologic diagnosis. During the summer months, arthropod-borne encephalitis, leptospirosis, and enteroviral disease may prevail. St. Louis encephalitis is more frequent in adults than children, while the converse is true for California and Western equine encephalitis. In the winter months, encephalitis associated with measles,

mumps, rubella, varicella-zoster virus, or, rarely, influenza is most common. Regional variations in the incidence of rickettsial infections and brucellosis may also affect the incidence of encephalitis. Herpes simplex virus encephalitis is endemic, but as the incidence of all other types of encephalitis increases during the summer months, the proportion of cases of herpes virus encephalitis falls to levels that are lower than in the winter.

Comparing levels of antibody in acute and convalescent serums is the most frequently used method of obtaining an etiologic diagnosis in diffuse viral encephalitis. Viral isolation procedures may be helpful, particularly in childhood exanthems, mumps, and encephalitis related to the respiratory viruses. If neural tissue is obtained, cultures for viral isolation, including mouse inoculation, should be performed.

The clinical distinction between acute encephalitis due to direct viral invasion versus postinfectious or "allergic" encephalitis is difficult. A previous illness or vaccination 1 to 6 weeks prior to the onset of CNS dysfunction, and demonstration of a demyelinating process affecting primarily "white" matter, suggest a postinfectious etiology.

Supportive care is the mainstay of therapy for diffuse viral encephalitis. Control of intracranial pressure and correction of the metabolic problems, disseminated intravascular coagulation, bleeding, renal failure, and pulmonary emboli or pneumonia associated with the illnesses are required.

CHRONIC VIRAL INFECTION   Slow virus infections of the CNS can be divided into two categories: (1) diseases associated with persistent viral replication due to "conventional" viruses, and (2) the transmissible dementias or subacute spongiform encephalopathies associated with unconventional viruses (Table 186-2).

Chronic viral infection associated with persistent replication of measles, rubella or the papovavirus (Jakob-Creutzfeldt virus), involves both white and gray matter and shows histologic evidence of an inflammatory response. Isolation of virus from brain tissue, evidence of viral antigens in infected cells (immunofluorescence), or visualization of virions or viral byproducts by electron microscopy can be demonstrated. In subacute sclerosing panencephalitis associated with persistent measles virus and in progressive rubella panencephalitis, in-

TABLE 186-2
Chronic viral infections of the CNS (Chap. 192)

Disease	Agent
DUE TO CONVENTIONAL VIRUSES	
Subacute postmeasles leukoencephalitis	Measles
Subacute sclerosing panencephalitis	Measles
Subacute rubella panencephalitis	Rubella
Progressive rubella panencephalitis following congenital rubella	Rubella
Progressive multifocal leukoencephalopathy	Papovavirus Jakob-Creutzfeldt, SV40
DUE TO UNCONVENTIONAL VIRUSES	
In humans:	
Kuru	
Jakob-Creutzfeldt	
Familial Alzheimer's	
In animals:	
Scrapie	
Transmissible mink encephalopathy	

creased antibody titers to these respective agents are present in serum and CSF. The serum and CSF of these patients should be examined for an increased concentration of gamma globulin, particularly that of monoclonal origin (oligoclonal banding), CSF hemagglutination inhibition (HI) antibody titers to measles and/or rubella virus should also be determined. The definitive diagnosis is made by isolation of the viral agent from neuronal tissue. These procedures are employed only in research laboratories.

In contrast, the transmissible viral dementias such as Jakob-Creutzfeldt disease are not associated with a prominent inflammatory response, nor can evidence of the etiologic agent(s) be identified by immunofluorescence or electron microscopy. A clinical history compatible with spongiform degeneration on brain biopsy provides a presumptive diagnosis. Propagation of the agent by inoculating it into a susceptible host is available only in a limited number of laboratories.

REFERENCES

BELL WE, MCCORMICK WF: *Neurologic Infections in Children.* Philadelphia, Saunders, 1975

FEIGEN RD, SHAKELFORD PG: Value of repeat lumbar puncture in the differential diagnosis of meningitis. N Engl J Med 289:571, 1973

GAJDUSEK DC: Unconventional viruses and the origin and disappearance of Kuru. Science 197, 4307:943, 1977

WHITLEY RS et al: Adenine arabinoside therapy of biopsy-proved herpes simplex encephalitis. N Engl J Med 297:289, 1977

WILFERT CM: Mumps meningoencephalitis with low cerebrospinal fluid glucose, prolonged pleocytosis and elevation of protein. N Engl J Med 280:855, 1969

187
ENTERIC VIRUSES
Coxsackieviruses, echoviruses, polioviruses, reoviruses, parvoviruses, and rotaviruses

A. MARTIN LERNER

GENERAL CONSIDERATIONS

It has been over 35 years since Dalldorf and Sickles isolated the first coxsackieviruses by inoculating suspensions of feces from two children with signs of clinical paralytic poliomyelitis into suckling mice. Subsequently, some 71 enteroviruses, including polioviruses and coxsackieviruses, and echoviruses, have been shown to multiply at various times in the gastrointestinal tracts of human beings. These viruses include four newly recognized members of the group which have been termed enterovirus, types 68 to 71 (Table 187-1). Enteroviruses have been recovered wherever attempts have been made; their distribution appears global. With notable exceptions such as coxsackievirus, type A21, and echovirus 28, which are predominantly respiratory pathogens and are only incidentally isolated from feces, enteroviruses like *Salmonella* periodically multiply within the human alimentary canal and sometimes concomitantly produce disease. Available information suggests that there is no normal enteric virus flora. In addition to enteroviruses, adenoviruses, reoviruses, and hepatitis A, non-A, and non-B, parvoviruses and rotaviruses are commonly recovered from stools. The latter two agents recently have been recognized as the cause of viral gastroenteritis.

Coxsackieviruses are named for their site of origin, the village of Coxsackie on the banks of the Hudson River in the state of New York. Echoviruses were descriptively named: *E,*

TABLE 187-1
Classification of human enteroviruses

I Enteroviruses
   A Polioviruses (3 types)*
   B Coxsackievirus A (24 types)
   C Coxsackievirus B (6 types)
   D Echoviruses (34 types)†
II Newly recognized enterovirus types
   A Enterovirus, type 68
   B Enterovirus, type 69
   C Enterovirus, type 70
   D Enterovirus, type 71

* *Typing is by neutralization of infectivity with immune serums either in suitable tissue cultures or in suckling mice.*
† *Echovirus, type 10, has been reclassified as belonging to another taxonomic group, now known as reoviruses.*

for their *enteric* residence; *C,* the filtrable agents produce *cytopathic* effects in tissue cultures of rhesus kidney; *H, human; O, orphan,* indicating that their relationship to disease remained to be established. They were viruses "in search of a disease." It is increasingly evident that a wide but definite variety of illnesses may result from enterovirus infections. As observations accumulate, these illnesses (Table 187-2) are continually being defined.

Etiologic associations are difficult to establish and usually require virologic, serologic, epidemiologic, and, when ethically possible, volunteer studies. These are especially useful if viruses are isolated only from the pharynx or anus, where they often multiply without causing significant injury to tissues. More meaningful are isolations from blood, vesicular fluids of patients with rashes, urine, cerebrospinal fluid, or from tissues at biopsy or autopsy. Coxsackieviruses and echoviruses have been recovered from lung, heart, pericardial fluid, liver, spleen, testicle, kidney, muscle, and brain. Dual virus infections and possible bacterial-virus synergisms occur. Until enteroviruses had been repeatedly documented in infants by isolations from pneumonic lungs, the prevalent opinion was that they did not produce pneumonias. The same skepticism exists concerning etiologic associations of enterovirus infections and chronic myocardiopathies, nonrheumatic valvular deformities, subendocardial fibroelastosis, and other congenital malformations. Firm evidence for an enterovirus cause of a chronic myocardiopathy, at least in a murine model, has now been established.

CHARACTERISTICS OF THE VIRUSES The enterovirus group is icosahedral-shaped, with a particle diameter of 17 to 30 nm and a ribonucleic acid core surrounded by a capsid of protein. Enteroviruses share about 20 percent of their nucleotide sequences, while within a grouping such as coxsackievirus B, there is 30 to 50 percent homology among types. The subunit structure of the outer protein capsid (capsomere) determines species, tissue, and age specificities for infection, as well as antigenicity. The RNA of the virus within infected cells transcribes and translates its own genetic information independent of the DNA (deoxyribonucleic acid) of the host. Enteroviruses are quite stable in acid and lipid solvents. They can be protected from thermal inactivation by certain cations.

When inoculated into suckling mice, group A coxsackieviruses induce primarily inflammation and necrosis of skeletal muscle, whereas group B viruses cause lesions of the central nervous system and other viscera, but only focal muscular involvement. Coxsackieviruses B and echoviruses are cytopathogenic for cultures of monkey kidney cells, but this is not the case for coxsackieviruses of group A. These distinctions are not without exception. Some strains of echoviruses, types 6 and 9, have been adapted to produce lesions in baby mice, the former in viscera and the latter in skeletal muscles. Some strains agglutinate human erythrocytes obtained from adults or umbili-

TABLE 187-2
Illnesses (or syndromes) associated with coxsackievirus, echovirus, or enterovirus infections

	Coxsackievirus types		Echovirus types	New enterovirus types
	Group A	Group B		
I No illness (probably 75% of cases)	1–24	1–6	1–8,* 11–34	69
II Mild or moderate illness				
A Undifferentiated mild febrile illness (nonspecific)	1–24	1–6	1–8, 11–34	
B Upper respiratory syndromes (rhinitis, pharyngitis, including herpangina and lymphonodular pharyngitis, conjunctivitis)	1–10, 16, 21, 22, 24†	1–5	1, 3, 6, 9, 16, 19, 20, 28	70
C Laryngotracheitis	9	5	11	
D Exanthems (various)	5, 9, 16	3, 5	2, 4, 5, 9, 11, 16	
E Lymphadenitis, with or without splenomegaly	5, 6, 9	5	4, 9, 16, 20	
F Pleurodynia (sometimes with pleural effusion)	4, 6, 10	1–5	1, 6, 9	
G Orchitis		1–5	9	
H Gastroenteritis	9	3, 4	2, 3, 6–9, 11–14, 18, 19, 22–24	
I Chronic myopathy				
III Severe or life-threatening illness				
A Hepatitis	4, 9	5	4, 9	
B Hemolytic-uremic syndrome	4	4		
C Pneumonia	9	1, 4	3, 8, 9, 19, 20	68
D Diabetes mellitus‡		4		
E Cardiac				
1 Myocarditis/pericarditis	1, 2, 4, 5, 8, 9, 16	1–6	1, 4, 6, 7, 9, 11, 14, 16, 19, 22, 25, 30	
2 Chronic myocardiopathy		2, 4, 5		
3 Subendocardial fibroelastosis‡		3		
4 Endocardial deformities		4		
5 Constrictive pericarditis		1, 2		
6 Congenital malformations†	9	3, 4		
F Neurologic				
1 Aseptic meningitis/encephalitis including variants	7, 9, 16	1–5	1–9, 11–23, 25, 30–32	71
2 Acute cerebellar ataxia	3, 4			
3 Benign intracranial hypertension				
4 Transverse myelitis				
5 Postencephalitic parkinsonism				
6 Guillain-Barré syndrome‡				

* *Asymptomatic infection is common with echovirus, type 9. Variation in attack rates among types (and strains of a single type) occurs.*
† *Coxsackievirus A, type 21, is also known as Coe virus.*
‡ *Suggested (and probable), but cause not established.*

cal cords at the time of delivery. None of the coxsackieviruses or echoviruses has been adapted to grow in embryonated eggs.

EPIDEMIOLOGY Fecal-oral contact is the usual method of transmission. Personal hygiene (particularly hand washing) inhibits the infectious cycle. Toddlers often bring enteroviruses into a household. Insects, including flies and mosquitoes, may act as passive vectors. Echovirus, type 6, may multiply in the gastrointestinal tracts of dogs. This has not been noted with other coxsackieviruses or echoviruses, and with echovirus 6 canine-to-human transmission has not been demonstrated. Respiratory transmission by droplets or their nuclei also occurs.

The incubation period is 2 to 5 days. Multiple concurrent infections within a family are not unusual. Clinical manifestations of infection vary within the family and community. Thus a 2- to 3-year-old child may have a mild fever with rash, while an older sibling may have pleurodynia, myocarditis, or one of a number of syndromes heralding involvement of the central nervous system (Table 187-2). The mechanism of the varied expression of enterovirus disease is not well understood but may relate to developmental changes in the number or availability of specific receptors on the surfaces of susceptible cells.

Enterovirus infections are most common during the summer. Prevalence is mirrored by virus isolations from samples of sewage. Serotypes present in a community vary from year to year. The level of immunity of a population as reflected by the prevalence of type-specific neutralizing antibodies in serums apparently determines the likelihood of infection by a particular enterovirus. In an individual usually one enterovirus multiplies within the intestine at any one time. Vaccination with attenuated polioviruses has virtually eliminated these interfering agents, and there may be a real increase in infections due to coxsackieviruses or echoviruses. Improved hygiene and urbanization have led to an "epidemiologic shift" from infants to adults. On the basis of intrahousehold spread, infectivity of coxsackieviruses is fairly high (76 percent of exposed susceptibles and 25 percent of immunes). For echoviruses, apparent infectivity is substantially lower (43 percent of susceptibles) and immune contacts are rarely infected. At least 49 percent of coxsackievirus and 55 percent of echovirus infections are subclinical.

An interesting correlate has been a seasonal incidence of new cases of insulin-dependent diabetes mellitus in patients under 30 years old. This autumn peak has been correlated with an annual prevalence for coxsackievirus B4, but does not relate to other virus infections. Recent epidemiologic studies show that there is no family history of diabetes mellitus in cases of juvenile onset. These cases show a predilection for certain HLA types, and pathologically, lymphocytes are found in their destroyed pancreatic islets. These data are consistent with, but do not prove, an infectious cause for juvenile diabetes. Adult-onset diabetes mellitus has a strong familial clustering and appears to be inherited.

VIRUS ISOLATION Primary multiplication occurs in epithelial and paraepithelial lymphatic cells of the pharynx. During this early period of infection the patient may be asymptomatic or have mild malaise, sore throat, or low-grade fever. Slightly later virus multiplies in the intestine. If a critical virus concentration within the pharynx results, viremia follows. During the viremic phase the patient is asymptomatic. Secondary foci of virus multiplication may occur in various tissues (skin, muscle, heart, nervous system, etc.). Major illness of moderate to serious severity sometimes results (Table 187-2). Occasionally (especially during infancy) aspiration of pharyngeal virus leads to lower respiratory infection.

Virus may be isolated from the throat during the minor illness and for as long as a week thereafter. Virus shedding persists in feces for a longer interval. Viremia can be documented during the incubation period until type-specific neutralizing antibodies appear.

PROTECTIVE RESPONSES AND SEROLOGIC DIAGNOSIS Intracellular virus multiplication stimulates interferon production within the infected cell (Chap. 176). About 3 days after the onset of infection specific antibodies appear in saliva and serum. These immunoglobulins combine with extracellular virus to limit spread of virus. Virus-antibody complexes are eliminated by phagocytosis.

Secretory immunoglobulins in saliva and succus entericus are in the IgA class, while the earliest antibodies to appear in serum are IgM. Both species of macromolecules have complement-fixing and neutralizing qualities. Within 3 to 4 weeks complement-fixing antibodies reach their peak and decline. Neutralizing antibodies of higher avidity (IgG) replace the IgM molecule about 2 weeks after the onset of infection. IgG antibodies persist and provide permanent type-specific immunity.

This information is important in diagnosis, because IgM molecules are susceptible to reduction and resultant biologic inactivation with sulfhydryl active compounds such as 2-mercaptoethanol (2-ME). IgG immunoglobulins are resistant to 2-ME.

IgG antibodies to coxsackieviruses and echoviruses traverse the placenta freely. IgM immunoglobulins do not. IgA antibodies in colostrum and milk are not absorbed, but apparently provide some local protection in the intestines of nursing babies. Passively acquired antibodies in serums protect the newborn from viremia for 3 to 6 months. Since the half-life of IgG immunoglobulins is about 3 weeks, duration of firm neonatal immunity depends upon initial titers of the transferred antibodies. Passively acquired antibodies inhibit active synthesis of immunoglobulins, and also may not protect the respiratory tract. Active synthesis of secretory antibody in saliva and nasal secretions is required. The role of cellular immunity in enterovirus infections remains to be fully defined. However, in coxsackievirus B3 murine cardiomyopathy, antibodies inhibit virus replication. Cytotoxic T lymphocytes augment the pathologic changes.

A fourfold rise in neutralizing antibodies or a titer which is similarly diminished by 2-ME indicates recent infection. When applicable, hemagglutination inhibition tests are simpler, and the results parallel those obtained in more cumbersome neutralization tests. Complement-fixing antibodies to enteroviruses are not type-specific. Many cross reactions render these tests less useful.

The neutralizing antibody response is highly type-specific in primary or initial enterovirus infections. In subsequent infections heterotypic responses occur with increasing frequency; they presumably arise from a booster effect of the current infecting virus on the level of antibodies to other types with which the individual has previously been infected. Levels of heterotypic antibody frequently exceed the level of homotypic antibody. Neutralizing antibodies to group B coxsackievirus,

types 1 to 5, are frequently found in titers of 1:64 to 1:512 in patients without evidence of current coxsackievirus infections (Table 176-4).

OTHER LABORATORY FINDINGS Enterovirus infections are usually acute processes, and persistent or chronic infections are unusual [e.g., chronic myopathy (coxsackievirus A9) or chronic myocardiopathy (coxsackievirus B3)]. Hence, changes in concentrations of hemoglobin, albumin, or globulins are unusual. Occasionally hemolysis occurs (see "Group A Coxsackievirus Infections" and "Echovirus Infections," further on in this chapter). White blood cell counts and the erythrocyte sedimentation rates are only mildly elevated. If there is necrosis (e.g., liver, lung), a neutrophilic leukemoid reaction may be noted. Hyperbilirubinemia and elevated transaminase and alkaline phosphatase levels may be seen in cases of hepatitis. Albuminuria often occurs transiently, but hematuria is rare.

PROPHYLAXIS AND TREATMENT Antiviral chemotherapy is not available. The 71 antigenic varieties of coxsackieviruses and echoviruses make prophylaxis with a single vaccine impractical. Pooled human globulin contains enterovirus antibodies, but during serious infections administration is not helpful. Most human enterovirus infections are mild, and globulin prophylaxis is not often warranted. As with poliomyelitis, tonsillectomy and other inoculations are probably best delayed during an outbreak of enterovirus disease. In a murine model of coxsackievirus B3 myocarditis, virus was isolated in higher titer from hearts of mice vigorously exercised daily by swimming, and a benign myocarditis was transformed into a lethal infection. Rest is the cornerstone of symptomatic therapy.

It has been repeatedly shown in experimental animals that during the acute phase of infection administration of steroids appreciably increases the quantity of virus in tissues and the degree of ensuing injury. Corticosteroids also depress cell-mediated immune functions, interferon and antibody synthesis, and leukocyte migration to the area of injury. Therefore at least during the acute phase of enterovirus infections, steroids are contraindicated. Pregnancy may be associated with enhanced susceptiblity to these and other infections. Alcohol, cold temperature, and chronic undernutrition are also associated with an increased virulence of coxsackievirus and perhaps other virus infections. Alcohol depresses phagocytic function. Malnutrition suppresses T and B lymphocytes, early mononuclear cell migration, and interferon production. In the presence of agammaglobulinemia, persistent enterovirus infections have been observed.

GROUP A COXSACKIEVIRUS INFECTIONS

Group A coxsackieviruses cause herpangina, lymphonodular pharyngitis, upper and lower respiratory disease, cutaneous eruptions, hepatitis, aseptic meningitis, paralytic disease, including acute infantile hemiplegia and unilateral oculomotor palsy, myopericarditis, and some sudden unexpected deaths in infancy. A chronic myopathy in an eleven-year-old girl has been associated with coxsackievirus A9. Picornavirus-like particles were seen on electron microscopy, and virus was isolated from the diaphragm at autopsy. Pharyngeal multiplication may induce infection of superficial vessels or diffuse moderate erythema. Purulent exudate is not seen. More characteristic is *herpangina*, a common febrile illness characterized by small papular, vesicular, or ulcerative lesions on the anterior pillars, soft palate, tonsils, pharyngeal mucous membrane, and posterior part of the buccal mucosa. Herpangina has been seen during infections with coxsackieviruses, group A, types 1 to 10, 16, and 22. Vesicular lesions of herpangina have also been described in patients with illnesses due to coxsackieviruses, group B, types 1 to 5, and echoviruses, types 9 and 17. Coxsackievirus

A10 may induce *acute lymphonodular pharyngitis*. Lesions here are raised, discrete, white to yellow 3- to 6-mm papules surrounded by a zone of erythema. All the papules appear at the same time; they do not ulcerate, and they occur on the uvula, anterior pillars, and posterior pharynx. Large outbreaks of mild to severe conjunctivitis have been caused by coxsackievirus A24. Typically, rapid onset of swelling of the eyelids, lacrimation, preauricular adenopathy and, in some cases, a mucopurulent discharge occur.

Coxsackievirus A21 (Coe virus) is predominantly a respiratory pathogen, being regularly isolated from the throat and occasionally from feces. It has been associated with several outbreaks of an illness resembling the common cold in military recruits.

The first enterovirus etiologically implicated in pneumonia was coxsackievirus A9. Subsequently, a number of other enteroviruses have been implicated (Table 187-2). Fatal cases have occurred in infants or young children. Hyperpnea, cyanosis, hyperpyrexia, leukocytosis (or leukemoid reactions), and subsequently coma have been characteristic. Interstitial diffuse polylobed bronchopneumonia with alternate areas of atelectasis and emphysema have been found. Microscopically mixed alveolar septal infiltration without necrosis or formation of giant cells is seen.

A striking cutaneous vesicular eruption, *hand-foot-and-mouth disease* has repeatedly been associated with infections due to coxsackievirus, group A, type 16. Infants and children with coxsackievirus, group A, type 4 (also coxsackievirus B14) infections have been described with respiratory or gastrointestinal symptoms, acute renal disease, thrombocytopenia, and hemolytic anemia. Reticulocytosis, albuminuria, and hematuria accompany this constellation of findings, which has been described as the *hemolytic-uremic syndrome*. Aseptic meningitis with occasional paralytic disease (especially with A7) also occurs. Acute myopericarditis has been associated with infections with coxsackievirus A, types 1, 2, 5, 8, 9, and 16; there are firmer etiologic data for coxsackievirus, types 4 and 16. One estimate suggests that 23 percent of acute virus cardiomyopathies may be caused by coxsackievirus A. A significantly greater incidence of infection with coxsackievirus, group A, type 9, has been reported in mothers of infants with congenital heart disease.

GROUP B COXSACKIEVIRUS INFECTIONS

Infections with group B coxsackieviruses cause a number of upper respiratory syndromes, exanthems, diarrheas, pleurodynia, orchitis (with subsequent atrophy), pneumonia, hemolytic-uremic syndrome, and cardiac and central nervous system disease. Pleurodynia and cardiac disease due to enteroviruses were first associated with this group of enteroviruses (Table 187-2). In 1965 the Public Health Service (Britain) reported 1160 coxsackievirus B5 infections. Gastroenteritis (90 percent), aseptic meningitis (31 percent), myalgia and Bornholm's disease (23 percent), respiratory disorders (15 percent), and cardiomyopathies (5 percent) were included. There were 41 patients with pericarditis and 5 with myocarditis. Of 6 deaths, 2 each were due to neurologic, respiratory, or cardiac cause. During infancy, the mortality rate of patients with acute infectious myocarditis approaches 50 percent.

PLEURODYNIA (EPIDEMIC MYALGIA, BORNHOLM'S DISEASE, DEVIL'S GRIP)
Prodromal symptoms of malaise, sore throat, and anorexia are interrupted by increasing debility, fever, and sudden onset of muscle, pleuritic, and abdominal pain. Pain is sharp, severe, and paroxysmal over the lower ribs or substernal area. It is accentuated by moving, breathing, coughing, sneezing, and hiccuping, and may be referred to the shoulders, neck,

or scapulae. Pain and spasm of anterior abdominal muscles occur in about half the cases, often in combination with chest pain. Muscle tenderness is usually not prominent, but some patients complain of intense cutaneous hyperesthesia and paresthesia over the affected area. The illness usually lasts 3 to 7 days, but relapses may occur. Among differential diagnoses are myocardial infarction and acute surgical conditions of the abdomen. Coxsackieviruses B have been isolated from striated muscles of patients with pleurodynia during epidemics. Occasinally pleuritis is accompanied by effusion, and virus has been isolated from pleural fluid. Bornholm's disease may occur at any age but is most common in children and young adults.

Early in the course of illness meningitis, myocarditis, or hepatitis may ensue. Liver biopsy in patients with complicating jaundice shows subacute portal triaditis and intense cloudy swelling of central-zone hepatocytes. A late complication is orchitis, occurring in 3 to 5 percent of patients with pleurodynia during relapse.

CARDIAC DISEASE Acute myocarditis may be caused by coxsackieviruses of groups A and B as well as echoviruses. Infections with strains of coxsackievirus, group B, have been most frequent. When congenital or neonatal infection occurs, the course is often rapidly fatal, with concomitant myocarditis, encephalitis, hepatitis, and sometimes adrenal necrosis. Later in childhood or in adult life the heart and pericardium more frequently are involved as the single site of disease. Cardiac inflammation varies in intensity and degree of muscle necrosis. Pericarditis may dominate the clinical presentation, with myalgia, fever, precordial pain, friction rub, and even cardiac tamponade. There may be prominent signs of myocarditis, with myocardial failure or arrhythmias. Illnesses may be self-limited and recovery complete. However, of 22 episodes of acute virus cardiomyopathies associated with infections due to coxsackieviruses, group B, 12 patients developed chronic heart disease. Strict bed rest until all electrocardiographic changes have reverted to normal (or as stationary) is indicated. This may require 4 to 6 weeks. Since steroids increase virulence of coxsackievirus B myocarditis in mice, they are contraindicated. Some infections may heal with significant myocardial scarring.

Coxsackievirus particles have been localized along tubules of the sarcoplasmic reticulum in infected mice with myocarditis. There is epidemiologic evidence associating coxsackievirus B, types 3 and 4, with congenital heart disease. Most infections in pregnant mothers are subclinical and occur in the first trimester. Suggestive evidence indicates that the following conditions may be caused by infections with coxsackieviruses belonging to group B: chronic continuing cardiomyopathies (B2, B4, B5); congenital calcific pancarditis (B3); and constrictive pericarditis (B1 and B2), with or without superior or inferior vena caval obstruction.

The possible courses and pathogenesis of enterovirus cardiomyopathies have been extensively studied in mice. It is likely that the similarity to humans is great. Enteroviruses affect the myocardium and pericardium, but there is no conclusive evidence to support the occurrence of a murine virus valvulitis. Coxsackievirus A9 induces an interstitial myocarditis in adult mice healing without scar (Figure 187-1). On the other hand, coxsackievirus B4 produces a transmural necrotizing myocarditis in baby mice. Ventricular aneurysms, mural thrombi, and pulmonary emboli have followed. (There certainly is serologic evidence in humans that some "myocardial infarctions" may be, in reality, myocarditis.) In weanling mice

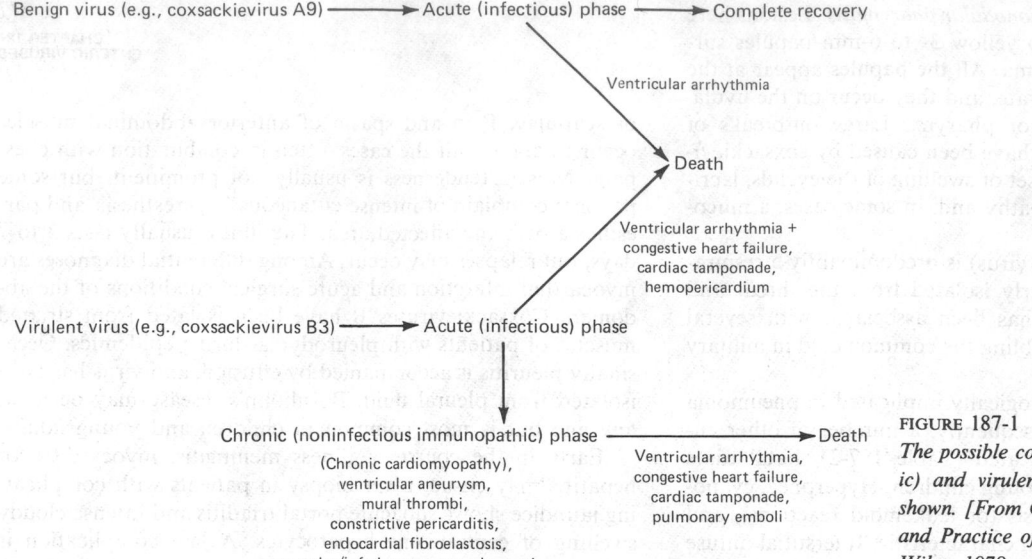

FIGURE 187-1

The possible courses of a benign (nonmyonecrotic) and virulent (myonecrotic) myocarditis are shown. [From GL Mandel et al (eds), Principles and Practice of Infectious Diseases, New York, Wiley, 1978, with permission.]

coxsackievirus B3 causes an immunopathic, cytolytic, T-lymphocyte–induced necrotizing myocarditis leading to a severe chronic cardiomyopathy. Constrictive pericarditis with or without superior or inferior vena caval obstruction, endocardial fibroelastosis, and congestive heart failure are other sequelae. The frequency of these illnesses in humans remains a major epidemiologic problem requiring resolution.

ECHOVIRUS INFECTIONS

Echovirus infections may be asymptomatic or mild, moderate, or life-threatening (Table 187-2). Mild to moderate are undifferentiated fevers, upper respiratory infections, various rashes, pleurodynia, and diarrheas. Pneumonia, myopericarditis, hemolytic-uremic syndromes, and neurologic involvement may be quite serious. They do not differ from similar illnesses caused by coxsackieviruses.

Enterovirus 70 is the most widespread of the new enterovirus types. It causes highly contagious infections which became pandemic in 1969 to 1971. After a 24-h incubation period, enterovirus 70 causes acute subconjunctional hemorrhagic conjunctivitis. The lesion may be discrete petechial to large and blotchy and covers the bulbar conjunctiva. Corneal involvement may occur but is transient.

ASEPTIC MENINGITIS (Chaps. 186 and 369) There may be a mild prodromal malaise, but major illness usually begins with fever, headache, and stiff neck. Papilledema and Kering's and Brudzinski's signs may be present. Localizing sensory or motor deficits are unusual. Confusion and delirium are common. These acute findings may persist for 4 to 7 days. Cerebrospinal pleocytosis is usually less than 500 cells per cubic millimeter. Early, there may be as many as 90 percent polymorphonùclear leukocytes, but within 48 h the cellular response becomes completely mononuclear. Persistence of polymorphonuclear leukocytes in the cerebrospinal fluid suggests pyogenic meningitis or intracerebral, subdural, or epidural abscess. Gram's stain and appropriate spinal fluid cultures must be done to exclude bacterial meningitis, tuberculosis, or mycotic meningitis. Protein concentration in the cerebrospinal fluid is moderately elevated, but glucose is normal. Early in the illness echoviruses may be isolated from spinal fluid. It usually takes several weeks before the cerebrospinal fluid reverts to normal.

For attempts at virus isolation, throat and rectal swabs, serum, and cerebrospinal fluid should be collected as early in the course as possible (Table 176-3). Acute and convalescent serums should be studied for rises in type-specific neutralizing antibodies.

It is not possible to distinguish clinically between aseptic meningitis due to various enteroviruses and mumps. Localizing findings, hemiplegia, prolonged fevers, oculogyric crises, coma, and bloody spinal fluid favor the diagnosis of herpes simplex virus encephalitis (Chap. 193). Although echovirus aseptic meningitis most often is self-limited and recovery in persons afflicted after the first year of life complete, about 10 percent of patients have more serious involvement of the central nervous system. Minor muscle weakness with reflex changes may persist for weeks to months, but over 90 percent of patients recover completely within a year. Occasionally, choreiform movements, ataxia, nystagmus, transverse myelitis, Guillain-Barré syndrome, coma, bulbar involvement, and death result.

As with coxsackieviruses, intact B lymphocytes are required for eradication of echovirus infections. Persistent echovirus infection of the central nervous system documented by the presence of echoviruses types 30, 19, 9, and 33 have been recovered for from 2 months to 3 years in five patients with congenital agammaglobulinemias. Additionally, three of the patients had a dermatitis-like syndrome.

POLIOVIRUS INFECTIONS

Enteric infection with the enteroviruses, poliovirus types 1, 2, or 3, is entirely analogous to other similar infections with coxsackieviruses or echoviruses. The unique aspect of poliomyelitis is the predilection of these three viruses for the anterior horn cells of the spinal cord and motor nuclei of the cranial nerves. Nervous tissues necessary for sensation are uninvolved.

ETIOLOGY Three distinct antigenic types have been defined: type 1 (Brunhilde), type 2 (Lansing), and type 3 (Leon). Natural infection leads to type-specific immunity with long-lasting neutralizing antibodies which can be measured in serum. The Nobel prize was awarded to Drs. John F. Enders, Thomas H. Weller, and Frederick C. Robbins in 1954 for their discovery that polioviruses multiply in nonneural tissue cultures producing easily recognizable cytopathic effects. It was this singular contribution which heralded the modern era of virology and allowed the preparation of effective vaccine prophylaxis.

EPIDEMIOLOGY AND PATHOGENESIS The occurrence, distribution, and pathogenesis (including incubation period) of polioviruses are similar to those of coxsackieviruses and echoviruses (see preceding portion of this chapter). Prior to vaccine prophylaxis with oral attenuated viruses, these were extraordinarily common agents with peaks in prevalence from July through September. Live attenuated vaccine eliminates polioviruses from feces and sewage, but the formalinized killed vaccine, which prevents viremia and neurologic illness, does not limit asymptomatic enteric infection. In countries with poor sanitation, infection and occasional disease occur early in life leading to the designation "infantile paralysis." Physical exertion increases the risk of clinically apparent or paralytic poliomyelitis.

VIRUS ISOLATION AND PROTECTIVE RESPONSES (See Chap. 176) Like coxsackieviruses and echoviruses, polioviruses can be recovered from the throat or feces during the first week of infection. In fatal cases polioviruses are easily recovered from affected brain or spinal cord. In aseptic meningitis (nonparalytic poliomyelitis) caused by polioviruses, virus is rarely recovered from cerebrospinal fluid (CSF). This is in contradistinction to the aseptic meningitis syndrome caused by coxsackieviruses or echoviruses in which these viruses are easily recovered from CSF. Long-lasting immunity is mirrored by the presence of serum-neutralizing antibody, which also follows natural infection with wild viruses.

CLINICAL MANIFESTATIONS Infections with polioviruses types 1, 2, or 3 may induce inapparent infection (95 percent of cases), undifferentiated febrile illness (minor illness), aseptic meningitis, or paralytic disease. Recovery is complete except in paralytic disease.

Necrosis and loss of motor nerve cells in any area of the spinal cord, brain, or cranial nerves causes various muscle paralyses. The precentral gyrus, reticular formation of the medulla, the cerebellum, Auerbach's and Meissner's plexuses, and sympathetic ganglia are frequently affected. Bulbospinal poliomyelitis is very serious.

Disease begins with fever and "minor illness." Classically, after several days, symptoms disappear. In 5 to 10 days fever recurs, and signs of meningeal irritation and paralysis ensue. Cramping muscle pain and spasm as well as coarse twitching in affected parts follows. In children younger than 5 years, paralysis of one leg is most common. In patients 5 to 15 years of age, weakness of one arm or paraplegia is most frequent, while in adults quadriplegia is common. Urinary bladder and respiratory muscle dysfunction are also frequent in adults. Inoculations of vaccines are associated with involvement of the muscles around the site of injection.

Tendon reflexes are diminished or absent. Sensation is intact, separating poliomyelitis from the Guillain-Barré syndrome. Paralysis due to heavy metal poisoning, on the other hand, may be more difficult to distinguish clinically from poliomyelitis.

Among paralytic cases, 6 to 25 percent may be bulbar. Tonsilloadenoidectomies should not be done during epidemics of poliomyelitis for 85 percent of patients under these circumstances develop bulbar disease. Myocarditis, hypertension, pulmonary edema, shock, nosocomial gram-negative or staphylococcal pneumonias, urinary tract infections, and emotional problems are among the complications of severe paralytic disease. Treatment is supportive. About 2 to 5 percent of children and 15 to 30 percent of adults with paralyzing infection die. Initially paralyzed muscles usually recover some function, gradually improving over 1 to 2 years.

PREVENTION Poliovirus vaccines, used widely since the introduction of inactivated poliovaccine (IPV) in 1955, have dramatically reduced the incidence of poliomyelitis in the United States. In 1954 there were more than 18,000 new cases, but

there were only 8 in 1976. The risk of poliomyelitis is generally very small in the United States today, but epidemics are certain to recur if the population's immunity is not sustained. Data from a national survey in 1976 indicated that 38 percent of 1- to 4-year-old children had not had primary vaccination against poliomyelitis! In disadvantaged urban and rural areas vaccination rates are even lower. It is essential to immunize all children beginning in infancy.

A Canadian product, inactivated poliovirus vaccine (IPV), is being marketed in the United States. It produces immunity in more than 90 percent of recipients. The vaccine is given by injection and can be administered simultaneously with diphtheria, tetanus, and pertussis antigens. Children or adults with immunodeficiency diseases or altered immune states who are at risk of exposure to poliomyelitis should receive IPV. An antibody response cannot be assured in these immunodepressed persons, but some protection probably results. Four doses are given, the first three at 1- to 2-month intervals and the fourth 6 to 12 months after the third injection. If adults are traveling to areas where poliomyelitis is present, or if they are exposed to vaccine virus following routine immunization of their children, IPV may be given. Except for the possibility of hypersensitivity reactions to the trace amounts of streptomycin and neomycin in IPV, there are no associated risks.

Trivalent oral poliovaccine (TOPV), licensed in 1963, combines all three strains of polioviruses. Full primary vaccination produces immunity in more than 90 percent of recipients. It is the preferred poliovirus vaccine in this country. In rare instances oral polio vaccine has been associated temporally with paralytic diseases in vaccine recipients or their close contacts. Of 193 million doses of TOPV, 55 "vaccine associated" cases have been reported. Primary immunization for infants (6 to 12 weeks old), children, and adolescents through age 18 is three doses, the first followed in 6 to 8 weeks by the second, and the third 8 to 12 months later. Routine polio vaccination for adults living in this country is not necessary. A susceptible adult at increased risk of exposure to infection because of travel to an area where poliomyelitis is common should receive complete primary immunization with IPV or TOPV. Supplementary single doses of TOPV should be given to children upon entering school and at the age of 11 or 12. There is no evidence that a pregnant woman or her fetus is at greater risk from TOPV than other persons. Persons with immunodeficiency or altered immune states should not receive TOPV because of the increased risk of vaccine-associated paralysis. These conditions include combined immunodeficiency, hypogammaglobulinemia, agammaglobulinemia, leukemia, lymphoma, generalized malignancy, or lowered resistance from therapy with corticosteroids, alkylating or antimetabolic drugs, or radiation.

REOVIRUS INFECTIONS

Reoviruses were discovered inadvertently in studies of the intestinal viral flora of healthy children and adults. They were initially classified as echovirus, type 10, but were later reclassified. They were named to emphasize their (1) *respiratory* or (2) *enteric* human origins, and their (3) *orphan* status.

Reoviruses are quite different from picornaviruses (Table 187-1). They are about 2½ times larger (70 nm in diameter) and show icosahedral symmetry. Their RNA is unique in that it consists of 10 discrete segments and is resistant to ribonuclease. The protein capsid consists of an inner core and 92 outer shell capsomeres. The capsid is composed of seven species of polypeptides. Unlike those of enteroviruses, reovirus cytopathic effects are nonlytic. Reoviruses multiply in primate and nonprimate tissue cultures. The particles hemagglutinate human or avian erythrocytes. On the basis of tests of hemagglutination inhibition antibodies (HIA) with type-specific serums, there are three serotypes.

Human infections with reoviruses are common, and their distribution is worldwide. Like coxsackieviruses and echoviruses, reoviruses spread by enteric and respiratory routes. Fifty to eighty percent of adults in the Western Hemisphere have had reovirus infections, as measured by the presence of persisting neutralizing or hemagglutinating antibodies. Infections are more frequent in winter but occur in every season. Reoviruses have been isolated from human nasal secretions, posterior pharyngeal and rectal swabs, spinal fluid, brain, and lung. In addition, reovirus isolations or serologic data indicate that natural infections occur in cattle, dogs, cats, mice, horses, swine, birds, and monkeys. Although animal-to-human transmission has never been demonstrated, its possibility is likely.

Widespread evidence of infection and few associations with disease indicate that most infections with reoviruses are asymptomatic. Isolations of virus and fourfold rises in HIA in individual patients with common colds, nonspecific febrile illness, exanthem, and diarrhea suggest an etiologic role in some instances. Provocative data came from three thoroughly studied fatal cases of encephalitis, myocarditis, hepatitis, or interstitial pneumonias. In these patients reoviruses and no other bacterial or viral pathogens have been isolated.

VIRAL GASTROENTERITIS

In 1929, Zahorsky first used the term *winter vomiting disease* to describe an epidemic gastrointestinal illness usually occurring in the winter and characterized by a short afebrile course, persistent vomiting, and the absence of an upper respiratory infection. Subsequently, a mild self-limited syndrome with more or less fever, nausea or vomiting, gripping abdominal pain, headache, malaise, and diarrhea or dysentery without identifiable bacterial or parasitic cause was repetitively described as "epidemic nonbacterial gastroenteritis," "epidemic diarrhea of the newborn," "winter-vomiting disease," or "viral dysentery." In 1947, this diarrheal disease was transmitted to human volunteers by the oral administration of fecal filtrates. However, it is only within the past 5 years with the use of electron microscopic examination of diarrheal specimens of feces that viral gastroenteritis in its epidemic and endemic forms could be effectively studied.

Viral gastroenteritis is the second leading cause of illness in the United States. In the chronically malnourished, the elderly, and in debilitated persons, death may result. Immune electron microscopic examination of virus particles isolated from fecal specimens has uncovered two major virus groups which cause viral gastroenteritis.

Parvoviruses are primarily responsible for disease in adults and older children, while reovirus-like agents cause diarrhea in infants and young children. The attack rates for both infections may reach 50 percent, and the incubation period is about 48 h, so that explosive outbreaks are common. Diarrhea may persist for 5 to 8 days and be followed by steatorrhea. A malabsorption syndrome with abnormal xylose and lactose absorption follows for another week. Other viruses (e.g., echoviruses, types 1 or 18, or coronaviruses) may from time to time be involved in sporadic outbreaks of gastroenteritis, but their overall importance seems minor.

The Norwalk, Hawaii, and Montgomery County agents are parvoviruses named after the sites of their original epidemics, and are distinctive in that immunity to one of the agents does not confer protection against the others. Parvoviruses contain

DNA genomes without lipid coats, have cubic symmetry with particle diameters of 27 nm, and are stable at pH 2.7 and 60°C (30 min.)

Human reovirus-like agents (HRLA) have also been described as *duoviruses, rotaviruses,* or *orbiviruses.* Their final nomenclature has not yet been decided. HRLA are responsible for worldwide sporadic and epidemic outbreaks of gastroenteritis, usually occurring in the winter or fall in infants and young children 6 to 24 months old. By the time children in the United States are 2 years old, 50 to 90 percent of them have antibodies to HRLA. Rotaviruses are easily recognized in duodenal biopsies by electron microscopy and are seen as 70-nm particles with double-shelled capsids completely similar to those of reoviruses. On biopsy, the proximal small intestine shows shortened villi, and crypts are hyperplastic. Polymorphonuclear leukocytes and mononuclear cells infiltrate the lamina propria. Normally, columnar surface cells are vacuolated and cuboidal. During acute illness, a transient peripheral lymphopenia involving all lymphocyte subpopulations ensues.

Parvoviruses and reovirus-like agents multiply in the small bowel to titers of 10^8 organisms per gram of feces. The viruses can be seen on electron microscopy or recognized for diagnosis by counterimmunoelectrophoresis of fecal filtrates. The Nebraska calf diarrhea virus can be used as antigen for HRLA (which has not yet been grown in tissue cultures) in complement fixation tests for antibody rises. Fluorescent antibody methods are also available. It is clear, however, that the presence of antibodies in serum does not confer absolute immunity for the bowel. The role of local coproantibodies needs to be explored.

REFERENCES

General

GELFAND HM: Occurrence in nature of coxsackie and ECHO viruses. Prog Med Virol 3:193, 1961

KOGON A et al: The virus watch program: A continuing surveillance of viral infections in metropolitan New York families. VII. Observations on viral excretion, seroimmunity, intrafamilial spread and illness association in Coxsackie and echovirus infections. Am J Epidemiol 89:51, 1969

MELNICK JL: Enterovirus, in *Viral Infections of Humans, Epidemiology and Control,* AS Evans (ed). New York, Plenum, 1976, p 163

PHILIPSON L et al: Structural model for picornaviruses as suggested from an analysis of urea-degraded virions and procapsids of coxsackie virus B-3. Virology 54:69, 1973

WOODRUFF JF, WOODRUFF JJ: Involvement of T-lymphocytes in the pathogenesis of coxsackie virus B-3 heart disease. J Immunol 113:1726, 1974

Coxsackievirus A infection

CHALHUB EG et al: Coxsackie A9 focal encephalitis associated with acute infantile hemiplegia and porencephaly. Neurology 27:574, 1977

HUEBNER RJ et al: Herpangina: Etiological studies of a specific infectious disease. JAMA 145:628, 1951

LERNER AM et al: Infections due to coxsackievirus, group A, type 9, in Boston, 1959, with special reference to exanthems and pneumonia. N Engl J Med 163:1265, 1960

TANG TT et al: Chronic myopathy associated with coxsackievirus A9. A combined electron microscopical and viral isolation study. N Engl J Med 292:608, 1975

Coxsackievirus B infection

BAIN HW et al: Epidemic pleurodynia (Bornholm's disease) due to coxsackie B 5 virus: The interrelationship of pleurodynia, benign pericarditis and aseptic meningitis. Pediatrics 27:889, 1961

BROWN GC, EVANS TN: Serologic evidence of coxsackievirus etiology of congenital heart disease. JAMA 199:151, 1967

EL-KHATIB MR et al: Coxsackievirus B4 myocarditis in mice: Valvular changes in virus infected and control animals. J Infect Dis 137:410, 1978

——— et al: Ventricular aneurysms complicating Coxsackievirus group B, types 1 and 4 murine myocarditis. Circulation, 1979 (in press)

JOHNSON RT et al: Acute benign pericarditis: Virologic study of 34 patients. Arch Intern Med 108:828, 1961

KIBRICK S: Viral infections of the fetus and newborn. Perspect Virol Symp NY 2:140, 1961

LERNER AM: Myocarditis and pericarditis, in *Principles and Practice of Infectious Diseases,* GL Mandel et al (eds). New York, Wiley, 1979, chaps 55, 56

———, WILSON FM: Virus myocardiopathy. Prog Med Virol 15:63, 1973

SAINANI GS et al: Adult heart disease due to Coxsackievirus B infection. Medicine 47:133, 1968

Echovirus infection

HORSTMANN DM, YAMADA N: Enterovirus infection of the central nervous system. Res Publ Assoc Res Nerv Ment Dis 44:236, 1968

WILFERT KM: Persistent and fatal central nervous system infections in patients with agammaglobulinemia. N Engl J Med 296:1485, 1977

Poliovirus infection

HENDERSON DA et al: Paralytic disease associated with oral polio vaccines. JAMA 190:41, 1964

Poliomyelitis prevention. Recommendation of the Public Health Service Advisory Committee on Immunization Practices. Morb Mort Week Rep 26:329, 335, 1977

WEINSTEIN L: Diagnosis and treatment of poliomyelitis. Med Clin North Am 32:1377, 1948

Reovirus infection

EL-EAI FM, EVANS AS: Reovirus infections in children and young adults. Arch Environ Health 7:700, 1963

JOKLIK WK: The molecular biology of reovirus. J Cell Physiol 76:289, 1970

ROSEN L: Serologic grouping of reoviruses by hemagglutination-inhibition. Am J Hyg 77:29, 1963

——— et al: Reovirus infections in human volunteers. Am J Hyg 77:29, 1963

TILLOTSON JR, LERNER AM: Reovirus, type 3, associated with fatal pneumonia. N Engl J Med 276:1060, 1967

Viral gastroenteritis

GORDON I et al: Transmission of epidemic gastroenteritis to human volunteers by oral administration of fecal filtrates. J Exp Med 86:409, 1947

SHREIBER DS et al: Recent advances in viral gastroenteritis. Gastroenterology 73:174, 1977

ZAHORSKY J: Hyperimmune hiemis or the winter vomiting disease. Arch Pediat 46:391, 1929

188
MUMPS

C. GEORGE RAY
ROBERT G. PETERSDORF

DEFINITION Mumps is an acute communicable disease of viral origin characterized by painful enlargement of the salivary glands and sometimes by involvement of the gonads, meninges, pancreas, and other organs.

ETIOLOGY The causative agent of mumps is a paramyxovirus of intermediate size (150 to 250 nm in diameter). It has a tight helical inner core (RNA) enclosed in an outer shell of lipid and protein. The virus of mumps causes in vitro agglutination of erythrocytes of fowl, human beings, and some other species, produces hemolysis, and has two components capable of fixing complement. These are the soluble, or S, antigens derived from the nucleocapsid, and the V antigen derived from the surface hemagglutinin. It elicits a delayed allergic reaction when used as an antigen in persons who have had mumps infection. The virus can be cultivated in chick embryos and in a variety of mammalian cell cultures, including HeLa, monkey kidney and human pancreatic beta cells.

EPIDEMIOLOGY Human beings are the only natural host for mumps. The disease is worldwide and is endemic in urban communities. Epidemics are relatively infrequent and are confined to closely associated groups who live in orphanages, army camps, or schools. The disease is most frequent in the spring, particularly during April and May. Although mumps is generally considered less "contagious" than measles and chickenpox, this difference may be more apparent than real because many mumps infections (at least 25 percent) tend to be inapparent clinically. In some surveys, 80 to 90 percent of an adult population had serologic evidence of previous infection with mumps. The incidence of mumps in the United States has reached its lowest point since reporting began in 1922; in 1977, there were 44.3 percent fewer cases than in 1976.

Infections are rare before the age of 2 years and then increase rapidly in frequency, reaching a peak at ages 6 to 10. Clinical mumps may be more common in males than in females. In North American cities, most infections are contracted from schoolmates and infected family members. The virus is transmitted in infected salivary secretions, although its isolation from urine suggests that the virus may also spread via this route. Mumps virus is rarely isolated from stools. The saliva is infectious for approximately 6 days prior to the onset of parotitis, and virus has been recovered from this site for as long as 2 weeks after onset of parotid swelling. Viruria also persists for 2 to 3 weeks in some patients. Despite this prolonged secretion of virus, the peak of infectivity occurs a day or two before onset of parotitis and subsides rapidly after the appearance of glandular enlargement.

One attack of clinical or subclinical mumps confers lasting immunity, and second attacks are most unusual. Unilateral parotitis affords protection just as effectively as does bilateral disease.

PATHOGENESIS The virus enters via the respiratory route; during the incubation period of 15 to 21 days it presumably replicates in the upper respiratory tract and cervical lymph nodes, from which it is disseminated via the bloodstream to other organs, including the meninges, gonads, pancreas, breasts, thyroid, heart, liver, kidneys, and cranial nerves. The salivary adenitis is thought by many to be secondary to viremia, but primary spread from the respiratory tract has not been ruled out as an alternative mechanism.

MANIFESTATIONS Salivary adenitis The onset of typical parotitis is usually sudden, although it may be preceded by a prodromal period of malaise, anorexia, chilly sensations, feverishness, sore throat, and tenderness at the angle of the jaw. In many cases, however, parotid swelling is the first indication of illness. The glands enlarge progressively over a period of 1 to 3 days, and the swelling resolves within a week after maximal enlargement. The swollen gland extends from the ear to the lower portion of the mandibular ramus and to the inferior portion of the zygomatic arch, often displacing the ear upward and outward. The skin over the gland is usually not warm or erythematous, in contrast to what happens in bacterial parotitis. There may be reddening and pouting of the orifice of Stensen's duct. Usually, pain and tenderness are marked, although at times they are absent. The edema of mumps has been described as "gelatinous," and when the involved gland is tweaked, it rolls like jelly. Swelling may involve only the submaxillary and sublingual glands and may extend over the anterior part of the chest, producing *presternal edema*. Involvement of submaxillary glands alone can cause difficulty in distinguishing mumps from acute cervical adenitis. Swelling of the glottis occurs rarely but may require tracheostomy. Parotitis is bilateral in two-thirds of cases and remains confined to one side in the remainder. The second gland tends to swell as the first is subsiding, usually 4 to 5 days after onset. In general, parotitis is accompanied by a temperature of 100 to 103°F, malaise, headache, and anorexia, but systemic symptoms may be virtually absent, particularly in children. In most patients, the chief complaints refer to difficulty in eating, swallowing, and talking.

Epididymoorchitis   Mumps is complicated by orchitis in 20 to 35 percent of postpubertal males. Testicular involvement usually appears 7 to 10 days after onset of parotitis, although it may precede it or appear simultaneously. Occasionally, orchitis occurs in the absence of parotitis. Gonadal involvement is bilateral in 3 to 17 percent of patients. Orchitis is heralded by recrudescence of malaise and appearance of chilly sensations, headache, nausea, and vomiting. Shaking chills and high fevers, with temperatures between 103 and 106°F, are frequent. The testicle becomes greatly swollen and acutely painful. The epididymis is often palpable as a swollen tender cord. Occasionally there may be epididymitis without orchitis. Swelling, pain, and tenderness persist for 3 to 7 days and gradually subside; lysis of fever usually parallels abatement of swelling. Occasionally, the temperature falls by crisis. Mumps orchitis is followed by progressive atrophy of the testicle in one-half the cases. Even after bilateral orchitis, sterility is unusual, provided no significant atrophy has taken place. However, if bilateral testicular atrophy occurs after mumps, sterility or subnormal sperm counts are quite common. Plasma testosterone levels are depressed during acute orchitis but return to normal with recovery. *Pulmonary infarction* has been noted to follow mumps orchitis. This may be the result of thrombosis of the veins in the prostatic and pelvic plexuses in association with the testicular inflammation. Priapism is a rare but painful complication of mumps orchitis.

Pancreatitis   Pancreatic involvement is a potentially serious manifestation of mumps, which may rarely be complicated by shock or pseudocyst formation. It should be suspected in patients with abdominal pain and tenderness together with clinical or epidemiologic evidence of mumps. It is difficult to document, since hyperamylasemia, the hallmark of pancreatitis, is also often present in parotitis. Many times the symptoms resemble those of gastroenteritis, and it is conceivable that the high incidence of gastrointestinal symptoms seen in association with the mumps epidemic in Great Britain in 1961 was due to involvement of the pancreas. Although diabetes or pancreatic insufficiency rarely follows mumps pancreatitis, several children have developed "brittle" diabetes a few weeks after mumps.

Central nervous system involvement   Nearly half the patients with mumps have an increased number of cells, usually lymphocytes, in the cerebrospinal fluid (CSF), although symptoms

of meningitis, stiff neck, headache, and drowsiness are less common. In typical cases, the onset of overt central nervous system signs and symptoms occurs 3 to 10 days after the onset of parotitis; however, the onset has also been noted to develop prior to the parotitis or 2 to 3 weeks later. In approximately 30 to 40 percent of laboratory-proved cases, there is *no* associated salivary gland involvement at any time in the course of illness. The CSF protein is moderately elevated, and CSF glucose tends to be normal, although in as many as 10 percent of patients low CSF glucose concentrations, in the range of 20 to 50 mg per 100 ml, may be seen. True encephalitis is unusual, although it is responsible for most of the central nervous system sequelae, including behavioral disturbances, headaches, seizures, deafness (usually unilateral), and visual disturbances. At least two cases of aqueductal stenosis and hydrocephalus have been reported as possible late sequelae to mumps encephalitis, but the association remains unproved. Mumps should also be recognized as capable of presenting a picture of mild paralytic poliomyelitis; definition of the cause depends on isolation of virus or serologic confirmation of mumps in the absence of changing antibody titers to poliomyelitis viruses. Rarely, mumps may produce a transverse myelitis, cerebellar ataxia, or the Guillain-Barré syndrome. Mumps meningitis, without clinical encephalitis, is generally thought to be benign.

Other manifestations   Mumps virus tends to involve glandular tissues; inflammation of the lacrimal glands, thymus, thyroid, breasts, and ovaries occurs occasionally. *Oophoritis* may be recognized by persistence of pain in the lower part of the abdomen and fever. It does not result in sterility. Mumps virus has been implicated in the causation of subacute thyroiditis; the diagnosis can be made serologically, and occasionally the virus can be isolated from the thyroid gland. A case of myxedema following mumps thyroiditis has been reported. Ocular manifestations of mumps include dacryadenitis, optic neuritis, keratitis, iritis, conjunctivitis, and episcleritis. Although these conditions may transiently interfere with vision, complete resolution is the rule. Mumps *myocarditis,* evidenced primarily by transient abnormalities in the electrocardiogram, is relatively common but does not usually produce symptomatic disease or impair cardiac function. Similarly, *hepatic* involvement may be manifested by mild abnormalities in liver function, but icterus and other clinical signs of hepatic damage are extremely rare. *Thrombocytopenic purpura* as a complication of mumps has been described, and an occasional patient has a leukemoid reaction involving predominantly lymphocytes. Tracheobronchitis and interstitial pneumonia have also been associated with mumps infection, particularly among young children.

A rare but interesting manifestation of mumps is *polyarthritis* which is often migratory. It is most common in males between the ages of 20 and 30. Joint symptoms begin 1 to 2 weeks after subsidence of parotitis; usually the large joints are involved. The illness lasts 1 to 6 weeks, and complete recovery is the rule. It is not clear whether arthritis is due to viremia or whether it is a "hypersensitivity reaction."

Acute hemorrhagic glomerulonephritis in the absence of streptococcosis has been reported after mumps. The relationship of these two diseases is not clear.

Late complications   With the exception of the rare central nervous system sequelae, the most serious of which is nerve deafness, which follow mumps encephalitis, and the occasional patient who is sterile following bilateral testicular involvement, mumps leaves no sequelae. There is no firm evidence that stillbirths and offspring with congenital defects are more common among mothers who have mumps during pregnancy. Likewise, the causal relationship between intrauterine mumps infection and endocardial fibroelastosis has not been clearly established.

LABORATORY FINDINGS In uncomplicated parotitis, the blood leukocyte count is normal, although there may be mild leukopenia with relative lymphocytosis. Patients with mumps orchitis, however, may have a marked leukocytosis with a shift to the left. In meningoencephalitis, the white blood cell count is usually within normal limits. The erythrocyte sedimentation rate is usually normal but may rise with testicular or pancreatic involvement. The serum amylase level is elevated both in pancreatitis and in salivary adenitis. It may also be elevated in some patients in whom the sole evidence of mumps is meningoencephalitis, and probably reflects subclinical involvement of the salivary glands. In contrast to the amylase, the serum lipase level is elevated only in pancreatitis, in which hyperglycemia and glucosuria also may occur. The cerebrospinal fluid contains 0 to 2000 cells per cubic millimeter, almost all mononuclear, although occasionally polymorphonuclear cells will predominate in the early stages. The pleocytosis in mumps meningitis tends to be greater than in aseptic meningitides caused by the poliomyelitis, coxsackie-, and echoviruses. There is no relationship between the cell count and the severity of central nervous system involvement. Transient hematuria and mild reversible abnormalities in renal function, including inability maximally to concentrate the urine and to clear creatinine, occur in association with the viruria of mumps.

DIAGNOSIS The definitive diagnosis of mumps depends on isolation of the virus from blood, throat swabs, secretions from Stensen's duct, cerebrospinal fluid, or urine. Immunofluorescence methods can detect positive cell cultures in 2 to 3 days rather than the 6 days required with standard methods. However, even with the simplification of viral isolation by means of tissue culture techniques, culture of the virus is rarely necessary in the typical case with associated parotitis. When an etiologic diagnosis is needed, as in aseptic meningitis or in atypical cases of parotitis, the complement fixation test is most commonly employed. Antibodies to the S antigen develop rather rapidly, often reaching a peak within 1 week after the onset of symptoms, and usually disappearing in 6 to 12 months. Complement-fixing antibodies to the V antigen follow a more typical pattern, reaching a peak titer within 2 to 3 weeks after onset, remaining elevated for at least 6 weeks, then persisting at lower levels for years afterward. Paired serums obtained 2 to 3 weeks apart are recommended. A fourfold increase in titer confirms recent infection. In cases where an acute serum is not obtained until later in the course of illness, an elevation of antibodies to the S antigen which exceeds the V antibody titer also suggests recent infection. The hemagglutination inhibition reaction is demonstrable somewhat later and persists for several months. The serum neutralization test is the most sensitive indicator of previous mumps infection, although it is more complicated to perform. However, it is a much better indicator of previous mumps infection than the skin test, and individuals with detectable specific neutralizing antibody are highly unlikely to contract mumps. The *skin test* consists of intradermal injection of killed mumps virus; previous exposure will result in a delayed reaction of the tuberculin type and an anamnestic antibody titer rise to mumps. The skin test is unreliable when used alone in determining the immune status of an individual, is useless in the diagnosis of acute mumps, and is no longer commercially available in the United States.

The diagnosis of mumps during an epidemic is usually obvious. Sporadic cases, however, must be distinguished from other causes of parotid enlargement. Parotitis may be caused by other viruses, notably parainfluenza, influenza, and coxsackieviruses. *Bacterial parotitis* usually occurs in debilitated patients with severe underlying diseases, such as uncontrolled diabetes mellitus, cerebrovascular accidents, or uremia. It may also follow surgical operations. The parotid glands are swollen, warm, and tender, and pus can be expressed from the orifices of Stensen's ducts. Marked polymorphonuclear leukocytosis is present. The disease is usually acquired in the hospital, and *Staphylococcus aureus* is the usual causative organism. Dehydration followed by inspissation of secretions in the salivary ducts is an important predisposing factor. *Calculus* in a salivary duct is usually detectable by palpation or by injection of radiopaque media into Stensen's duct. *Drug reactions* may produce tender swelling of the parotid and other salivary glands. "Iodine mumps" is the commonest type; it may follow such procedures as intravenous urography. Mercurialism and the antihypertensive agent guanethidine may also cause parotid enlargement and tenderness. A careful history usually serves to clarify the cause of these reactions. *Cervical adenitis* caused by streptococci, "bullneck" diphtheria, infectious mononucleosis, cat-scratch disease, sublingual cellulitis (Ludwig's angina), and cellulitis of the external auditory canal are usually easy to distinguish from mumps by careful examination. Parotid tumors and chronic infections such as actinomycosis tend to follow a more indolent course, with slowly progressive swelling. The common "mixed tumor" of the parotid is well circumscribed, nontender, and very firm, almost cartilaginous on palpation. Parotid swelling and fever, often accompanied by lacrimal adenitis and uveitis (Mikulicz's syndrome), may occur in tuberculosis, leukemia, Hodgkin's disease, and lupus erythematosus. The onset may be sudden, but the process is usually painless and of long duration. "Uveoparotid fever" of similar type may be the first manifestation of sarcoidosis; in this disease parotid swelling is frequently accompanied by single or multiple palsies of cranial nerves, particularly the facial nerve, and is referred to as Heerfordt's syndrome. Presternal edema may also be a manifestation of malignant lymphoma involving retrosternal lymph nodes. Bilateral painless parotid swelling unassociated with fever is found in patients with Laennec's cirrhosis, chronic alcoholism, malnutrition, diabetes mellitus, pregnancy and lactation, and hypertriglyceridemia.

Sjögren's syndrome (Chap. 363) is a chronic inflammation of the parotid and other salivary glands which is often associated with atrophy of the lacrimal glands and occurs most commonly in women past the menopause. With cessation of lacrimal and salivary function, there may be striking dryness of the conjunctiva and the cornea (keratoconjunctivitis sicca) and of the mouth (xerostomia). These patients may also have a variety of systemic manifestations, including arthritis of the rheumatoid type, splenomegaly, leukopenia, and hemolytic anemia. The chronicity of the process and its occurrence in elderly women make confusion with mumps unlikely. Finally, benign hypertrophy of both masseter muscles, presumably due to habitual clenching and grinding of teeth, may be confused with painless parotid swelling.

The causes of aseptic meningitis are discussed in Chaps. 186 and 369.

Orchitis occurring in the absence of parotitis is likely to remain undiagnosed. Serologic testing may later confirm the diagnosis of mumps. Orchitis may occur in association with acute bacterial prostatitis and seminal vesiculitis. It is a rare complication of gonorrhea. Occasionally testicular inflammation accompanies pleurodynia, leptospirosis, melioidosis, relapsing fever, chickenpox, brucellosis, and lymphocytic choriomeningitis.

TREATMENT There is no specific treatment for infections with the mumps virus. Patients with parotitis should receive mouth care, analgesics, and a bland diet. Bed rest is advisable only as long as the patient is febrile; contrary to popular belief, physical activity has no influence on the development of orchitis or other complications. Patients with epididymoorchitis may be acutely ill and in great pain. Many forms of treatment, including surgical decompression of the testicle, infiltration of the spermatic cord with local anesthetics, estrogens, convalescent serum, and broad-spectrum antibiotics, have not been regularly effective. Despite failure to document their effectiveness in controlled studies, adrenal steroids have been of considerable benefit in diminishing fever, as well as testicular pain and swelling, and in restoring the sense of well-being in a number of patients. It is important to give a single large dose corresponding to 300 mg cortisone or 60 mg prednisone, initially. During the ensuing 24 h the same quantity should be given in divided doses. Subsequently, administration of the hormone can be tapered off over 7 to 10 days. Adrenal steroids have not exerted an adverse effect on concomitant pancreatitis or meningitis, although they have not benefited patients with meningeal involvement, and their withdrawal has usually been accompanied by a recrudescence of symptoms. Adrenal steroids have not prevented the appearance of parotid involvement on the contralateral side. Mumps arthritis is usually mild and requires no treatment. Mumps thyroiditis may subside spontaneously, but excellent relief has been obtained with adrenal hormones.

PREVENTION A live attenuated mumps virus vaccine (Jeryl Lynn strain) has been highly effective in producing significant rises in mumps antibody in individuals who are seronegative prior to vaccination, and has afforded 95 percent protection to individuals subsequently exposed to mumps. The vaccine also has boosted antibody levels in vaccinated individuals who are seropositive. The vaccine produces an inapparent, noncommunicable infection which is not associated with fever or mumps-like symptoms. It has conferred excellent protection for at least 10 years and has not interfered with vaccines against measles, rubella, and poliomyelitis or with smallpox vaccination given simultaneously. Protection has been demonstrated in both children and adults.

Live mumps vaccine can be administered at any time after 1 year of age, and should be particularly considered for children approaching puberty, adolescents, and adult males who have not had clinical mumps or live mumps vaccine in the past. Individuals living in groups or in institutions should be vaccinated, particularly because it has been shown that physical isolation of mumps patients does not effectively prevent transmission of the infection.

Vaccination is contraindicated in babies under the age of 1 year because of the interfering effect of maternal antibody; in individuals with a history of hypersensitivity to vaccine components; in patients with febrile illnesses, leukemia, lymphoma, or generalized malignancies; in those receiving steroids, alkylating drugs, antimetabolites, or irradiation; and during pregnancy.

It is not known whether the vaccine will prevent infection when administered after exposure, but no contraindication to its use in this situation exists. Specific mumps-immune globulin in large quantity is of doubtful efficacy in aborting orchitis when given 1 to 2 days after exposure, and does not prevent parotitis. Ordinary gamma globulin is not at all effective.

REFERENCES

BEARD CM et al: The incidence and outcome of mumps orchitis in Rochester Minnesota 1935 to 1974. Mayo Clin Proc 52:3, 1977

BRAY PF: Mumps—a cause of hydrocephalus? Pediatrics 49:446, 1972

BRUNNELL PA et al: Ineffectiveness of isolation of patients as a method of preventing the spread of mumps. N Engl J Med 279:1357, 1968

CARANASOS GH, FELKER JR: Mumps arthritis. Arch Intern Med 119:394, 1967

KALTREIDER HA, TALAL N: Bilateral parotid gland enlargement and hyperlipoproteinemia. JAMA 210:2067, 1969

KARCHMER AW et al: Simultaneous administration to live virus vaccines. Am J Dis Child 121:382, 1971

KOCEN RS, CRITCHLEY E: Mumps epididymo-orchitis and its treatment with cortisone. Br Med J 2:20, 1961

LEVITT LP et al: Central nervous system mumps: A review of 64 cases. Neurology 20:829, 1970

MODLIN JF et al: Current status of mumps in the United States. J Infect Dis 132:106, 1975

Mumps vaccine. Morb Mort Week Rep 26:393, 1977

ST GEME JW JR et al: Immunologic significance of the mumps virus skin test in infants, children and adults. Am J Epidemiol 101:253, 1975

UTZ JP et al: Studies of mumps. IV. Viruria and abnormal renal function. N Engl J Med 270:1283, 1964

WILFERT CM: Mumps meningoencephalitis with low cerebrospinal fluid glucose, prolonged pleocytosis and elevation of protein. N Engl J Med 280:855, 1969

189
RABIES AND OTHER RHABDOVIRUSES

LAWRENCE COREY

RABIES

DEFINITION Rabies is an acute viral disease of the central nervous system that affects all mammals and that is transmitted by infected secretions, usually saliva. Most exposures to rabies are through the bite of an infected animal, but on occasion a virus aerosol or the ingestion or transplantation of infected tissues may initiate the disease process.

ETIOLOGY The rabies virus is a bullet-shaped ribonucleic acid (RNA) virus belonging to the rhabdovirus group. It has a diameter of 750 to 800 Å and varies in length. Excrescences, 60 to 70 Å long, each with a knob-like structure at the distal end, cover the surface of the virion. These surface structures elicit neutralizing and hemagglutination-inhibiting antibodies, while a nucleocapsid antigen induces a complement-fixing antibody. Following immunization or active infection, a third group of antibodies is elicited which, together with complement, reacts with surface membranes of infected cells to produce lysis and cell death. While the first two classes of antibody appear to correlate with protection against the disease, the third may have an important injurious effect. Isolates of rabies virus may exhibit different biologic properties, but little antigenic variation has been documented. Interferon is induced by rabies virus, particularly in those tissues with high virus concentrations, and may play some role in retarding progressive infection.

EPIDEMIOLOGY Rabies exists in two epidemiologic forms: *urban*, propagated chiefly by unimmunized domestic dogs and/or cats, and *sylvatic*, propagated by skunks, foxes, raccoons, mongooses, wolves, and bats. Infection in domestic animals usually represents a "spillover" from sylvatic reservoirs of infection, and human beings can be infected by either. Hence, human infection tends to occur in locales where rabies is enzootic or epizootic, where there is a large population of unimmunized domestic animals, and where human contact with the outdoors is common. While only about 800 rabies deaths are reported to the World Health Organization (WHO) each year, "guestimates" of the worldwide incidence of rabies is approximated at 15,000 cases per year. Southeast Asia, the Philippines, Africa, and the Indian subcontinent are areas where the disease is especially common. Imported rabies combined with the recent epizootic of fox rabies in Western Europe has increased the importance of this disease in Europe. In the United States human rabies is exceedingly rare.

In most areas of the world, the dog is the important vector of rabies virus, but the wolf (Eastern Europe, Arctic regions), the mongoose (South Africa, the Caribbean), the fox (Western Europe), and the vampire bat (Latin America) may also be prominent vectors of the disease. In the United States, the skunk and bat have been the most important recent sources of human disease, with raccoons, foxes, and unimmunized dogs and cats also playing a role. While in the United States rabies in wildlife accounts for over 75 percent of the reported animal rabies, over 50 percent of the reported cases of post-exposure prophylaxis are associated with dog bites.

PATHOGENESIS The first event is the introduction of live virus through the epidermis or onto a mucous membrane. Initial viral replication appears to occur within striated muscle cells at the site of inoculation. The peripheral nervous system is exposed at the neuromuscular and/or neurotendinal spindles. The virus then spreads centripetally up the nerve to the central nervous system, probably via peripheral nerve axoplasm. Experimentally, viremia has been shown to occur, but is not thought to play a role in naturally acquired disease. Once the virus reaches the central nervous system, it replicates almost exclusively within the gray matter and then passes centrifugally along autonomic nerves to reach other tissue—the salivary glands, adrenal medulla, kidney, lung, liver, skeletal muscle, skin, and heart. Passage into the salivary glands facilitates further transmission of the disease via infected saliva. The incubation period of rabies is exceedingly variable, ranging from 10 days to over 1 year (mean 1 to 2 months). The time period appears to depend upon the amount of virus introduced, the amount of tissue involved, host defense mechanisms, and the actual distance that the virus has to travel from the site of inoculation to the central nervous system.

The neuropathology of rabies resembles other viral diseases of the central nervous system: hyperemia, varying degrees of chromatolysis, nuclear pyknosis, and neuronophagia of the nerve cells; infiltration by lymphocytes and plasma cells of the Virchow-Robin space; microglial infiltration, and parenchymal areas of nerve cell destruction. The pathognomonic lesion of rabies is the Negri body. This eosinophilic mass, approximately 10 nm in size, is made up of a finely fibrillar matrix and rabies virus particles. Negri bodies are distributed throughout the brain, particularly in Ammon's horn, the cerebral cortex, the brainstem, the Purkinje cells of the cerebellum, and the dorsal spinal ganglia. Negri bodies are not demonstrated in at least 20 percent of rabies, and their absence in brain material does not rule out the diagnosis.

MANIFESTATIONS The clinical manifestations of rabies can be divided into four stages: (1) a nonspecific prodrome, (2) an acute encephalitis similar to other viral encephalitides, (3) a profound dysfunction of brainstem centers which produces the classic features of rabies encephalitis, and (4) rarely, recovery.

The prodromal period usually persists for 1 to 4 days and is marked by fever, headache, malaise, myalgias, increased fatigability, anorexia, nausea and vomiting, sore throat, and a nonproductive cough. The prodromal symptom suggestive of rabies is the complaint of parasthesias and/or fasciculations at or about the site of inoculation of virus. This symptom is present in 50 to 80 percent of patients.

The encephalitic phase is usually ushered in by periods of excessive motor activity, excitation, and agitation. Quickly, confusion, hallucinations, combativeness, bizarre aberrations

of thought, muscle spasms, meningismus, opisthotonic posturing, seizures, and focal paralysis appear. Characteristically, the periods of mental aberration are interspersed with completely lucid periods, but as the disease progresses, the lucid periods get shorter until the patient lapses into coma. Hyperesthesia, with excessive sensitivity to bright light, loud noise, touch, and even gentle breezes, is very common. On physical examination the temperature may be found to be as high as 40.6°C (105°F). Abnormalities of the autonomic nervous system include dilated, irregular pupils, increased lacrimation, salivation, perspiration, and postural hypotension. Evidence of upper motor neuron paralysis with weakness, increased deep tendon reflexes, and extensor plantar responses is the rule. Paralysis of the vocal cords is common.

The manifestations of brainstem dysfunction begin shortly after the onset of the encephalitic phase. Cranial nerve involvement causes diplopia, facial palsies, optic neuritis, and the characteristic difficulty with deglutition. The combination of excessive salivation and difficulty in swallowing produces the traditional picture of "foaming at the mouth." Hydrophobia, the painful, violent involuntary contraction of the diaphragm, accessory respiratory, pharyngeal and laryngeal muscles initiated by swallowing liquids, is seen in about 50 percent of cases. Involvement of the amygdaloid nucleus may result in priapism and spontaneous ejaculation. The patient lapses into coma, and involvement of the respiratory center produces an apneic death. The prominence of early brainstem dysfunction distinguishes rabies from other viral encephalitides and accounts for the rapid downhill course. The median survival after the onset of symptoms is 4 days, with a maximum of 20, unless artificial supporting measures are instituted.

If intensive respiratory support is used, a number of late complications may appear and include inappropriate secretion of antidiuretic hormone, diabetes insipidus, cardiac arrythmias, vascular instability, adult respiratory distress syndrome, gastrointestinal bleeding, thrombocytopenia, and paralytic ileus. Recovery is very rare and when it occurs has been gradual. There have been only three well-documented nonfatal cases of rabies in humans. Two of these survivors received partial postexposure prophylaxis and the third, a case of laboratory-associated rabies, probably from an aerosol exposure, had received preexposure prophylaxis.

Occasionally, rabies may present as an ascending paralysis resembling the Landry-Guillain-Barré syndrome (dumb rabies, *rage tranquile*). This clinical pattern occurs most frequently in those bitten by vampire bats or who have received postexposure rabies prophylaxis.

The difficulty of suspecting rabies when it is associated with ascending paralysis is illustrated by the documentation of person-to-person transmission of the virus by tissue transplantation. A corneal transplant from a donor who died of presumed Landry-Gullain-Barré syndrome resulted in death of the recipient 7 weeks later. Pathologic examination of the brain of both patients demonstrated Negri bodies, and rabies virus was subsequently isolated from the donor's frozen eye.

LABORATORY FINDINGS Early in the disease the hemoglobin and routine blood chemistries are normal, but abnormalities occur as hypothalamic dysfunction, gastrointestinal bleeding, and other complications ensue. The peripheral white blood cell count is usually slightly elevated (12,000 to 17,000 per cubic millimeter) but may be normal or as high as 30,000 per cubic millimeter.

As in any viral infection, the specific diagnosis of rabies depends upon (1) the isolation of virus from infected secretions [saliva, rarely cerebrospinal fluid (CSF), or tissue (brain)], (2) the serologic demonstration of acute infection, or (3) the demonstration of viral antigen in infected tissue, e.g., corneal impression smears, skin biopsies, or brain. Samples of brain obtained either on postmortem examination or from brain biopsy should be subjected to (1) mouse inoculation studies for virus isolation, (2) fluorescent-antibody (FA) staining for viral antigen, and (3) histologic and/or electron microscopic examination for Negri bodies. While the mouse inoculation studies for virus isolation and direct FA staining for viral antigen are quite reliable and sensitive, if the patient's life has been prolonged and high levels of neutralizing antibody are present in serum and CSF, "autosterilization" may occur, and these tests may be negative. The use of FA staining of skin biopsies, corneal impression smears, and saliva for evidence of rabies antigen has been helpful in diagnosing rabies during life. Confirmation of these findings either serologically or by demonstration of virus in brain should be sought.

If the patient has not received antirabies immunization, then a fourfold rise in neutralizing antibody to rabies virus in serial serum samples is diagnostic. If the patient has received rabies vaccination, then a clue to the diagnosis may be obtained from the absolute titers of serum-neutralizing antibody and the presence of neutralizing antibody to rabies in CSF. Postexposure rabies prophylaxis rarely produces CSF-neutralizing antibody to rabies. If present, it is usually in low titer, e.g., less than 1:64, whereas CSF titers in human rabies may vary from 1:200 to 1:160,000.

DIFFERENTIAL DIAGNOSIS There is little to distinguish rabies from other viral encephalitides, and the most helpful point in diagnosis is the history of exposure. Other problems to be considered include hysterical reactions to animal bites (pseudohydrophobia), Landry-Guillain-Barré syndrome, poliomyelitis, and allergic encephalomyelitis to rabies vaccine. The latter occurs most commonly after use of nerve tissue–derived vaccine and usually begins 1 to 4 weeks after vaccination.

PREVENTION AND TREATMENT Each year more than 1 million Americans are bitten by animals. In each instance, a decision must be made whether to initiate postexposure rabies prophylaxis. When deciding whether to institute rabies prophylaxis, the following considerations apply: (1) whether the individual came into physical contact with saliva or another substance likely to contain rabies virus; (2) whether rabies is known or suspected in the species and area associated with the exposure (e.g., all persons within the continental United States bitten by a bat that then escapes should receive postexposure prophylaxis); (3) the circumstances surrounding the exposure; and (4) the treatment alternative and complications. A guide for postexposure rabies prophylaxis is illustrated in Fig. 189-1.

If rabies is known to be present or suspected to be present in the animal species involved in a human exposure, the animal should be captured, if possible. Captured wild animals or any ill, unvaccinated, or stray domestic animal involved in a rabies exposure, particularly any animal involved in an unprovoked bite, exhibiting abnormal behavior, or suspected of being rabid, should be captured and killed, and the head should be sent immediately to an appropriate laboratory for rabies fluorescent antibody (FA) examination. If examination of the brain by the FA technique is negative for rabies, it can be assumed that the saliva contains no virus, and the exposed person need not be treated. Persons exposed to escaped wild animals capable of carrying rabies (bats, skunks, coyotes, foxes, raccoons, etc.) in an area where rabies is known or sus-

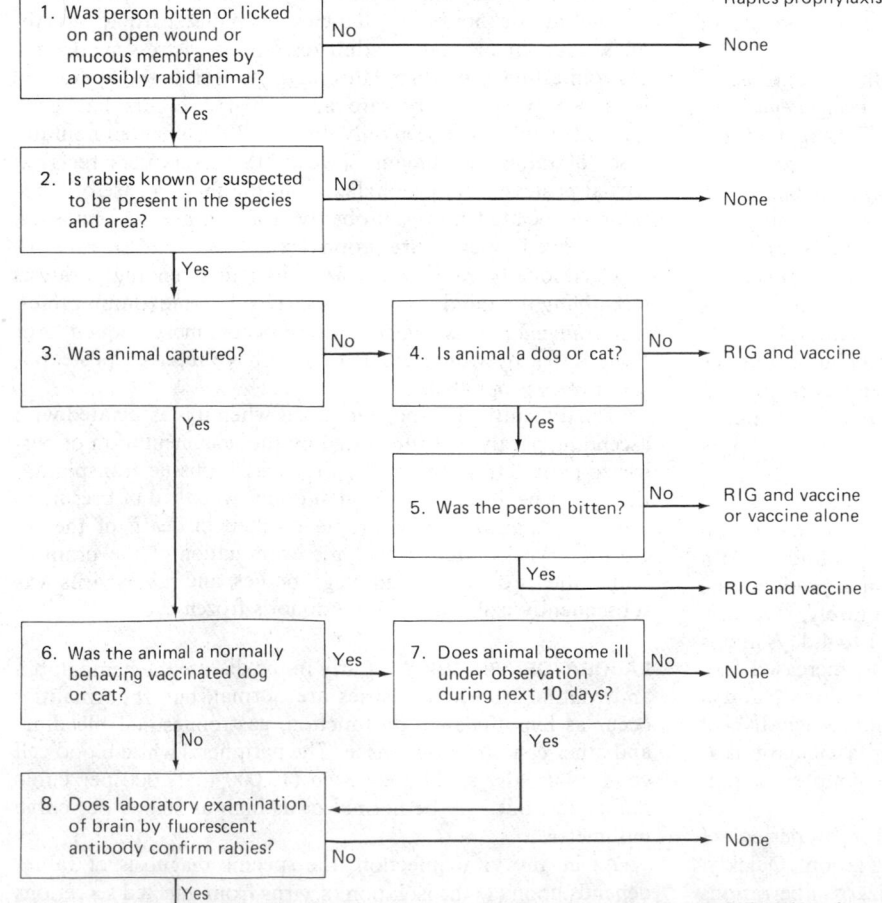

Rapies prophylaxis

FIGURE 189-1
Postexposure rabies prophylaxis algorithm. (Adapted from L Corey, MAW Hattwick, JAMA 232:272, 1975. Copyright 1975, American Medical Association.)

1. Was person bitten or licked on an open wound or mucous membranes by a possibly rabid animal? — No → None
   Yes ↓
2. Is rabies known or suspected to be present in the species and area? — No → None
   Yes ↓
3. Was animal captured? — No → 4. Is animal a dog or cat? — No → RIG and vaccine
   Yes ↓
4. (Yes) ↓
5. Was the person bitten? — No → RIG and vaccine or vaccine alone
   Yes → RIG and vaccine
6. Was the animal a normally behaving vaccinated dog or cat? — Yes → 7. Does animal become ill under observation during next 10 days? — No → None
   No ↓   Yes ↓
8. Does laboratory examination of brain by fluorescent antibody confirm rabies? — No → None
   Yes → RIG and vaccine

pected to be present should receive both passive and active immunization against rabies.

If a healthy vaccinated dog or cat bites a person, the animal should be captured, confined, and observed for 10 days. If any illness or abnormal behavior develops in the animal during the observation period, it should be killed for FA examination.

Postexposure prophylaxis Once a decision regarding the necessity to initiate postexposure rabies prophylaxis has been made, the general principle of postexposure therapy is to minimize the amount of virus at the site of inoculation with local treatment of the wound and to establish an early and long-lasting neutralizing antibody titer to rabies virus. The following therapeutic regimen is recommended:

1 *Local wound therapy* with generous scrubbing with soap and then flushing of the wound with water or ethyl alcohol, removing all vestiges of the soap. This is followed by a second scrubbing with a quaternary ammonium compound such as 1 to 2% benzalkonium chloride (Zephiran) or 1% cetrimonium bromide (Cetavlon). If indicated, tetanus toxoid and antibiotics (usually penicillin G) should be given.
2 *Active immunization* with antirabies vaccine. Duck embryo vaccine is the only currently licensed vaccine available in the United States. While major complications associated with duck embryo vaccine in postexposure prophylaxis are uncommon, local reactions, such as pain (100 percent), erythema (97 percent), and pruritus (13 percent) at the site of inoculation are common, and systemic symptoms, such as fever, malaise, or myalgia, occur in about 33 percent of postexposure recipients. Anaphylaxis is seen in less than 1 percent of recipients and usually occurs during administration of the first five doses. A history of hypersensitivity to avian products should be ruled out before initial therapy.

Central nervous system reactions to duck embryo vaccine are rare. Antihistamines will usually ameliorate local and systemic reactions to this vaccine. Corticosteroids interfere with the development of active immunity and may increase the likelihood of the development of clinical rabies; therefore use of these agents in treating adverse reactions is not recommended unless life-threatening complications to the vaccine occur.

A total of 23 doses of duck embryo vaccine should be given when it is used with hyperimmune serum. A primary series consisting of 21 doses of vaccine is given either as 21 daily doses or as two doses a day (separate injections or a double dose) for 7 days, followed by one dose daily for 7 days. This is followed by two booster doses on the tenth and twentieth days after completion of the primary series. Vaccine should be given subcutaneously in the abdomen or lateral aspect of the thigh, and rotation of injection sites is recommended. When vaccine is given alone, 14 daily doses are sufficient.
3 *Passive immunization* with antirabies antiserum of either equine or human origin. The latter is preferred when available, because of the high incidence of serum sickness (20 to 40 percent) with the equine product. Fifty percent of the total dose of 20 units/kg for human rabies immune globulin (RIG) and 40 units/kg for the equine antiserum is given by local infiltration of the wound, and the rest intramuscularly. Because many persons will not develop significant levels of neutralizing antibody [>1:5 by mouse inoculation or equivalent or 1:15 in the rapid fluorescent focus inhibition test (RFFIT)] after postexposure prophylaxis, a neutralizing antibody determination should be obtained after completion of therapy. "Nonresponders" may be candidates for the recently developed, more potent, tissue culture rabies vaccine.

An important development in rabies prophylaxis has been the development of several inactivated subunit human diploid cell strain rabies vaccines. These vaccines are licensed in Europe but are not yet available in the United States, except on a limited basis from the Viral Disease Division of the Center for Disease Control for those persons who (1) have a serious allergy to duck embryo vaccine, (2) do not show an adequate antibody response to duck embryo vaccine, or (3) have been bitten by an animal proved to be rabid. These tissue culture vaccines appear more immunogenic than duck embryo vaccine, and more than 95 percent of persons who received three doses of vaccines for preexposure immunization developed detectable antibody titers. While mild local reactions appear in 30 percent of recipients and febrile reactions in 5 to 10 percent, no serious neuroparalytic reactions have been identified. Data on the efficacy of these diploid vaccines in postexposure prophylaxis are still being accumulated, but published studies involving over 80 persons who have been bitten by animals proved to be rabid have indicated protection from clinical rabies. Treatment with a combination of human rabies immunoglobulin (20 ml/kg) on day 1 and six doses of tissue culture vaccine given on the first, third, seventh, fourteenth, thirtieth, and ninetieth days after exposure has been associated with an early, higher, and more sustained antibody response than that generally achieved with duck embryo vaccine. These vaccines require fewer doses, suggesting that morbidity associated with postexposure rabies prophylaxis will be diminished.

Preexposure prophylaxis The availability of the relatively safe duck embryo vaccine (DEV) has permitted the initiation of preexposure therapy for individuals with a high risk of contact with rabies virus: Veterinarians, spelunkers, laboratory workers, animal handlers, etc. Such preexposure therapy consists of two 1-ml subcutaneous injections of DEV given 1 month apart, followed by a 1-ml booster 7 months later. At the completion of the three-shot series, the neutralizing antibody titer should be checked.

Treatment While nonfatal human rabies has now been documented, once clinical symptoms develop, rabies is usually fatal. The basis for "therapy" of rabies must be prevention of acquisition of the disease through active domestic animal vaccination programs and postexposure prophylaxis. In the future, the availability of newly developed more immunogenic vaccines combined with the use of interferon or interferon-inducers may improve upon the efficacy and toxicity of the currently recommended regimens.

MARBURG VIRUS DISEASE

DEFINITION Marburg virus causes an acute systemic febrile illness characterized by the abrupt onset of headache, myalgias, pharyngitis, rash, and hemorrhagic manifestations. It was recognized first in 1967 when it caused simultaneous outbreaks in the Federal Republic of Germany and Yugoslavia among laboratory workers exposed to imported African green monkeys (*Cercopithecus aethiops*). The clinical manifestations are similar to other hemorrhagic fevers of the arenavirus class or flavovirus group (Argentina and Bolivian hemorrhagic fever, Chap. 191). The high case fatality rate and demonstrated ability for nosocomial spread has made recognition of this rare agent an important worldwide public health concern.

ETIOLOGY The Marburg virus has been isolated in guinea pig and various cell culture systems such as vervet monkey kidney. The virus particle contains lipid and RNA, and under the electron microscope the virus appears as an 80- to 100-nm elongated filamentous particle with occasional "blister-like excrescences." While the Marburg virus exhibits some morphologic relationship to other members of the rhabdoviruses (rabies, Ebola, and Mokola viruses), it appears antigenically distinct.

EPIDEMIOLOGY The initial outbreaks affected 31 patients in Marburg and Frankfurt, Germany, and Belgrade, Yugoslavia, and was epidemiologically linked to monkeys imported from the same source in Uganda. Virus was isolated from the blood and tissue of these monkeys. Of the 25 primary infections, there were seven deaths. Six secondary cases, involving two physicians, one nurse, a postmortem attendant, and the wife of a veterinarian occurred. Person-to-person transmission was felt to take place via accidental needle sticks or abrasions, although respiratory and conjunctival infection could not be ruled out. The wife of one patient developed Marburg virus disease at the onset of his illness; Marburg virus was demonstrated in semen of the original patient, despite the presence of circulating antibody, and this secondary case is believed to have been acquired through sexual intercourse. Subsequent investigations in the Lake Kyoga region of Uganda where the monkeys originated revealed no unusual illnesses or death among primates in the area. Complement fixation antibodies were demonstrated in 36 percent of *C. aethiops* trapped in the region, and antibody was detected in three monkey trappers.

PATHOLOGY Marburg virus appears "pantropic" and produces lesions in almost all organs including lymphoid tissue, liver, spleen, pancreas, adrenals, thyroid, kidney, testes, skin, and brain. In lymphoid tissue focal necrosis with degeneration of lymphoid tissue is apparent. In the liver, eosinophilic cytoplasmic bodies resembling the Councilman bodies of yellow fever have been noted. The lungs may show interstitial pneumonitis, as well as vascular lesions in small arterioles indicative of endarteritis. Neuropathologic changes consist of multiple small hemorrhagic infarcts with glial proliferation.

CLINICAL MANIFESTATIONS After an incubation period of 3 to 9 days, patients develop the abrupt onset of frontal and temporal headache, malaise, myalgias, especially in the lumbar area, nausea, and vomiting. Fever of 39.4 to 40°C (103 to 104°F) is characteristic, and about half the patients have conjunctivitis. Between 1 and 3 days after onset, watery diarrhea, which is often severe, lethargy, and a change in mentation are noted. An enanthem of the palate and tonsils, and cervical lymphadenopathy, may also be noted during the first week of illness. The most reliable clinical feature is the appearance of nonpruritic maculopapular rash which begins on the fifth to seventh day on the face and neck and spreads centrifugally to involve the extremities. A fine desquamation of the affected skin, especially the palms and soles, appears 4 to 5 days later. Hemorrhagic manifestations, including gastrointestinal, renal, vaginal, and/or conjunctival hemorrhages, generally develop between days 5 and 7 of disease.

During the first week, the temperature continues in the vicinity of 40°C (104°F), falling by lysis during the second week, to increase again between the twelfth and fourteenth days. Other clinical signs apparent in the second week of disease include splenomegaly, hepatomegaly, facial edema, and scrotal or labial reddening. Complications include orchitis, which may lead to testicular atrophy, myocarditis with irregular pulse and electrocardiographic abnormalities, and pancreatitis. The overall case fatality rate has been about 25 percent, with death usually occurring during the eighth to sixteenth days of illness. Recovery is often protracted over a 3- to 4-week period, and

during this period loss of hair, intermittent abdominal pain, poor appetite, and prolonged psychotic disturbances have been noted. Late sequelae including transverse myelitis and uveitis have been reported. Marburg virus has been isolated from the anterior eye chamber and semen nearly 3 months after onset of disease.

LABORATORY FINDINGS Abnormalities in granulocyte function are found, and leukopenia is detected as early as the first day, with leukocyte counts as low as 1000 per cubic millimeter and a neutrophilia by the fourth day. Subsequently, atypical lymphocytes, as well as neutrophils exhibiting the characteristic of the Pelger-Huet anomaly, may appear. Thrombocytopenia appears early and is most marked, often less than 10,000 cells per cubic millimeter, between the sixth and twelfth days. In fatal cases, evidence of disseminated intravascular coagulation can be demonstrated. Hypoproteinemia, proteinuria, and azotemia may occur. Elevations in serum glutamic oxaloacetic transaminase (SGOT) and alanine aminotransferase (SGPT) are usual. Lumbar puncture may be normal or reveal a minimal pleocytosis. The erythrocyte sedimentation rate is usually low.

DIAGNOSIS The characteristic clinical course and epidemiologic features are the basis of the diagnosis. Specific diagnosis requires isolation of the virus or serologic evidence of infection in paired serum samples. Viremia coincides with the febrile state of disease, and virus has been isolated from tissue as well as urine, semen, throat, and rectal swabs. Attempts to isolate virus must be carried out only in *specialized high-security laboratories*. All patients should be kept in strict isolation, and all specimens should be handled and shipped according to World Health Organization guidelines.

TREATMENT Patients have received a multiplicity of drugs without apparent influence on the course of the illness. Convalescent serum was administered to four patients, whose subsequent disease followed a mild course. However, similarly benign outcomes were observed in patients who did not receive serum.

EBOLA VIRUS

Between July and November 1976 simultaneous outbreaks of an acute febrile hemorrhagic disease occurred in Southern Sudan and Northern Zaire. "Secondary and tertiary" spread of infection, particularly among hospital staff, was noted. In the Sudan over 300 cases with 151 deaths and in Zaire 237 cases with 211 fatalities were reported. In one Sudanese hospital, 76 members of a staff of 230 were infected and 41 died. The virus isolated from patients in the Sudan and Zaire was morphologically similar to the Marburg agent but was antigenically distinct. The name Ebola virus, after the river in Zaire located near the epidemic, has been proposed.

Ebola virus has been propagated in tissue culture (Vero cells) and in suckling mice and guinea pigs. The source of the outbreak in both the Sudan and Zaire is unknown; however, as with other viral hemorrhagic fevers, peridomestic rodents are suspected as being a reservoir of the infection. Once established, nosocomial as well as community-acquired cases occur, especially among close and prolonged contact. Parenteral exposure to the virus through disinfected rather than sterilized needles may have played a role in transmission. Barrier nursing and strict isolation precautions using protective clothing appeared to decrease the number of nosocomial cases.

CLINICAL MANIFESTATIONS Clinically, the disease is similar to Marburg virus disease. The incubation period ranges from 4 to 6 days (mean is 7 days). Patients usually present on the fifth day of illness with a history of abrupt onset of headache, malaise, myalgias, high fever, diarrhea, abdominal pain, dehydration, and lethargy. Pleuritic chest pain, a dry hacking cough and a pronounced pharyngitis were also noted. A maculopapular eruption develops between days 5 to 7 of illness. On black skins the rash is often faint and not recognized until desquamation occurs. Hematemesis, melena, and bleeding from the nose, gums, and vagina are common. Abortion and massive metrorrhagia was a frequent complication among pregnant women. Death usually occurs in the second week of illness and is preceded by severe blood loss and shock.

TREATMENT Patients should be isolated until virological studies indicate they are free of virus, usually 21 days from onset of illness. Malaria parasites were frequently found in blood films of patients with Ebola virus infection in the Sudan indicating that the presence of parasitemia does not rule out concomitant viral illness. Treatment with plasma containing Ebola virus specific antibodies has resulted in diminished levels of viremia; however, further tests are required to establish the effectiveness of this form of therapy. Requests for viral isolation as well as convalescent plasma should be addressed to WHO Regional Centers in Atlanta or Geneva.

MOKOLA VIRUS

Mokola virus was first isolated from wild shrews captured in Nigeria and subsequently was shown to be related morphologically and serologically to rabies. However, neither of the two reported cases of human disease (both children) demonstrated classic clinical features of rabies. One patient had a nonfatal illness characterized by fever, pharyngitis, and convulsions. Mokola virus was recovered from her cerebrospinal fluid. The second patient initially had fever, cough, and vomiting, followed in several days by drowsiness, confusion, and generalized flaccid weakness. Her cerebrospinal fluid was normal. She progressed to deep coma and died within 10 days of onset. Mokola virus was isolated from her brain, and histopathologic sections revealed finely granular cytoplasmic inclusions that were distinguishable from Negri bodies in many neurons.

VESICULAR STOMATITIS VIRUS

Vesicular stomatitis is a viral illness of animals which can occasionally infect humans. It presents as an acute self-limited influenza-like disease. The disease in animals is found in the United States and South America and affects chiefly domestic cattle, horses, swine, and wild deer, raccoons, skunks, and bobcats.

In animals, vesicular stomatitis is characterized by the development of vesicles on the oral mucosa, particularly the tongue, udders, and heels. The mode of spread is probably by direct contact; however, epidemics tend to occur in warm weather, and the virus has been isolated from *Phlebotumus* sandflies in Panama and *Äedes* species in New Mexico, suggesting these as possible vectors. Two distinct serotypes, New Jersey and Indiana, have been recognized and most of the outbreaks in North America have been attributed to the New Jersey strain. The disease is most common in laboratory workers, and in one report three-fourths of laboratory personnel handling experimentally infected animals or manipulating the virus developed neutralizing antibodies. The disease is transmissible, however, under natural conditions among workers having direct contact with infected animals, especially cattle. The incubation period ranges from 1 to 6 days. This is followed by the sudden onset of fever, up to 40°C (104°F), chills, profuse sweating, myalgias, malaise, headache, and pain on ocular movement. One-third to one-half of patients have sore throat and cervical and/or submandibular adenopathy. Small

raised vesicular lesions may appear on the buccal mucosa. Conjunctivitis and coryza are present in about 20 percent of cases. Occasionally, small subcorneal, intraepithelial vesicles may appear on the fingers, usually associated with direct inoculation of the virus. Symptoms generally last 3 to 4 days, but occasionally a diphasic course may occur. Inapparent infection is common, and among laboratory workers with serologic evidence of infection, only about one-half reported clinical symptoms. In some areas of Panama, 17 to 35 percent of the population have neutralizing antibodies against vesicular stomatitis virus.

The differential diagnosis includes hand-foot-and-mouth disease, herpangina, primary herpetic pharyngitis and other mucocutaneous syndromes, and influenza. Viral isolation from patients is not common; however, a rise in complement fixation and/or neutralizing antibodies to vesicular stomatitis virus between acute and convalescent serums will help to confirm the diagnosis. Treatment is nonspecific.

REFERENCES

Marburg virus

GEAR JSS et al: Outbreak of Marburg virus disease in Johannesburg. Br Med J 4:489, 1975

MARTIN GA, SEIGERT R (eds): *Marburg Virus Disease.* New York, Springer-Verlag, 1971

SIMPSON DIH: Marburg and ebola virus infections: A guide for their diagnosis, management and control. WHO Offset Publication no 36, Geneva, 1977

Mokola virus

FAMILUSI JB: Fatal human infection with Mokola virus. Am J Trop Med Hyg. 21:959, 1972

Rabies

BAER GM: *The Natural History of Rabies.* New York, Academic, 1975

BAHMANYAR M: Successful protection of humans exposed to rabies. JAMA 236:2751, Dec. 13, 1976

COREY L, HATTWICK MA: Treatment of persons exposed to rabies. JAMA 232:272, 1975

HATTWICK MA et al: Recovery from rabies: A case report. Ann Intern Med 76:931, 1972

HOUGH SA et al: Human-to-human transmission of rabies virus by a corneal transplant. N Engl J Med 300:603, 1979

PLOTKIN SA, WIKTOR TJ: Rabies vaccination. Annu Rev Med 29:583, 1978

PUBLIC HEALTH SERVICE ADVISORY COMMITTEE ON IMMUNIZATION PRACTICES: Rabies prophylaxis. Morb Mort Week Rep 25(51):403, December 31, 1975

RUBIN RH et al: Adverse reactions to duck embryo vaccine. Ann Intern Med 78:643, 1973

190

ARBOVIRUS INFECTIONS

JAY P. SANFORD

Most viral infections in humans are either asymptomatic or present as undifferentiated illnesses characterized by fever, malaise, headache, and generalized myalgia. The similarities in clinical features between infections caused by viruses as dissimilar as the myxoviruses (e.g., influenza), the enteroviruses (e.g., poliovirus, coxsackievirus, echovirus), some of the herpesviruses (e.g., cytomegalovirus), and the arboviruses usually preclude an etiologic diagnosis based entirely on clinical manifestations without ancillary information regarding epidemiologic features and serologic findings. The purpose of this chapter is to direct attention to the ever-expanding list of viruses which produce febrile disease in humans. Because the number of agents is large, mention will be made of those which have been best documented, have demonstrated unusual features, or seem to be of greatest potential significance.

DEFINITION AND CLASSIFICATION It has not always been easy to determine that an agent is an arbovirus; hence with further characterization some agents which were initially registered as arboviruses have been reclassified, e.g., the zoonotic agents which have unique morphology on electron microscopy have been classified as arenaviruses (Chap. 191). Similarly, vesicular stomatitis virus, Mokola, and Lagos bat virus, provisionally registered as arboviruses, were found to be related to rabies virus and are now classified as rhabdoviruses (Chap. 189). The currently accepted definition of an arthropod-borne virus was published in 1967 by the World Health Organization:

Arboviruses are viruses which are maintained in nature principally, or to an important extent, through biological transmission between susceptible vertebrate hosts by hematophagous arthropods; they multiply and produce viremia in the vertebrates, multiply in the tissues of arthropods, and are passed on to new vertebrates by the bites of arthropods after a period of extrinsic incubation.

From this definition it can be appreciated that the term *arbovirus* is used in the ecological sense. Transmission by vectors is not correlated with virus architecture, which forms an important basis for current classification. Thus, the broad category arbovirus is being subdivided, and structurally related nonarthropod-borne agents may be classified with agents designated as arboviruses. Casal's serologic groups A and B arboviruses have been shown to be enveloped RNA agents with a spherical nucleocapsid forming the viral core, probably of icosohedral symmetry. Agents with these characteristics are now classified as togaviruses, with group A designated as alphaviruses and group B as flaviviruses. Other members of the togavirus group which are not transmitted by arthropods include rubella virus, equine arteritis virus, European swine fever/hog cholera virus, and viral disease of cattle agent.

There are more than 250 distinct arboviruses, which have been grouped into three families with some agents yet remaining unclassified. Within each family, the agents have been subdivided on the basis of antigenic differences (Table 190-1). The characteristics of individual members of this large group of viruses are not uniform; those in group A are 40 to 60 nm in diameter, and those in the Bunyamwera group are about 100 nm in diameter. The majority of agents contain single-stranded RNA, although some, such as Colorado tick fever, contain double-stranded RNA.

Arboviruses are of importance in both temperate and tropical zones. Representative viruses have been isolated in almost every geographic area outside the polar region.

Arbovirus infection of vertebrates is usually asymptomatic. The viremia stimulates an immune response which sharply limits the duration of the viremia. In arbovirus infections other than urban yellow fever, phlebotomus fever, chikungunya, o'nyong-nyong, mayaro, oropouche, and dengue, infection of humans represents an incidental occurrence which is tangential to the basic maintenance cycle of the virus. Hence, the isolation of virus from arthropod vectors or the detection of

infection in the natural vertebrate host may provide a means for early detection and enable control of epizootic infection before significant spread to humans occurs.

As determined by serologic evidence of host responses, at least 80 immunologically distinct arboviruses are capable of infecting humans, while somewhat fewer have been incriminated as causing clinical disease. The spectrum of clinical illness produced by the arboviruses is varied both in predominant features and in severity. Five broad, often overlapping, and somewhat arbitrary clinical syndromes may be delineated (Table 190-2).

TABLE 190-1
Classification of arboviruses

Family	Group	Specific agent	
Togaviruses	A (alpha-viruses)	Chikungunya*	Ross River*
		Eastern equine*	Sindbis*
			Venezuelan equine*
		Mayaro/ Semliki, Forest (Uruma)*	Western equine*
		Mucambo	
		O'nyong-nyong*	
	B (flavi-viruses)	Banzi	Nataya
		Bat salivary gland*	Negishi
		Bussuquara	Omsk hemor-rhagic*
		Central European encephalitis	Powassan
			Rocio
		Dengue 1–4*	Russian spring-summer
		Ilheus	
		Japanese (B)*	Spondwenii
		Kunjin	St. Louis*
		Kyasanur Forest*	Uganda S
			Usutu
		Louping ill	Wesselbron
		Murray Valley	West Nile*
			Yellow fever*
			Zika*
Bunyaviruses	C	Apeu*	Murutucui*
		Caraparu*	Oriboca*
		Itaqui*	Ossa*
		Madrid*	Restan*
		Marituba*	
	Bunyamwera	Bunyamwera	Ilesha
		Germiston	Wycomyia
		Guaroa	
	Bwamba	Bwamba	
	California	California LaCrosse*	Tahyna
	Ganjam	Dugbe	Ganjam
	Guama	Bimiti	Guama
		Catu	
	Quaranfil	Quaranfil	
	Sandfly fever (Phlebotomus)	Candiru*	Punta Toro*
		Chagres*	Sicilian type*
		Naples type*	
	Simbu	Shuni	Oropouche
	Thogoto	Thogoto	
	Ungrouped	Congo/ Crimean hemor-rhagic*	Tataguine
			Zinga
		Rift Valley fever*	
		Nairobi sheep disease	
Orbiviruses	Changuinola	Changuinola	Tribec
	Kemerovo	Kemerovo	Lipovnik
	Ungrouped	Colorado tick fever*	
Not classified		Nyando	

* *Discussed in the text.*

TABLE 190-2
Summary of clinical and epidemiologic features of arboviruses associated with infection in humans in the Western Hemisphere

Syndrome	Virus	Serologic group*	Vector	Known geographic range
Fever with malaise, *headaches,* and *myalgia*	Apeu	C	Mosquito	Brazil
	Anhembi	C	Mosquito	Brazil
	Candiru	Sandfly fever	Sandfly	Brazil
	Caraparu	C	Mosquito	Brazil, Panama, Trinidad
	Catu	Guama	Mosquito	Brazil, Trinidad
	Chagres	Sandfly fever	Sandfly	Panama
	Colorado tick fever	Ungrouped orbivirus	Tick	Western United States, Alberta, British Columbia
	Guama	Guama	Mosquito	Brazil, Trinidad
	Guaroa	Bunyamwera	Mosquito	Brazil, Colombia
	Itaqui	C	Mosquito	Brazil
	Madrid	C	?	Panama
	Marituba	C	Mosquito?	Brazil
	Mayaro	A	Mosquito	Brazil, Colombia, Central America, Trinidad
	Mucambo	A	Mosquito	Brazil
	Murutucui	C	Mosquito	Brazil
	Oropouche	Simbu	Mosquito	Brazil, Trinidad
	Ossa	C	?	Panama
	Punta Toro	Sandfly	Sandfly	Panama
	Quaranfil	Quaranfil	Tick	South America
	Restan	C	Mosquito	Trinidad
	Uruma	A	?	Bolivia
	U.S. Bat salivary gland	B	?	Southwestern United States
	Venezuelan equine encephalitis	A	Mosquito	Florida, Texas, Louisiana, Mexico, Central America, Ecuador, Peru, Colombia, Venezuela, Brazil, Trinidad, Surinam, Guyana
	Yellow fever	B	Mosquito	Central and South America
Fever with malaise, headaches, myalgia, *arthralgia,* and *rash*	Changuinola	Changuinola	*Phlebotomus*	Panama
	Mayaro	A	Mosquito	Brazil, Colombia, Central America, Trinidad
Fever with malaise, headaches, myalgia, rash, and *lymphadenopathy*	Dengue 1	B	Mosquito	Caribbean
	Dengue 2	B	Mosquito	Circumglobal
	Dengue 3	B	Mosquito	Caribbean
Fever with *central nervous system* involvement	California encephalitis	California	Mosquito	United States
	Eastern equine encephalitis	A	Mosquito	Eastern Canada, United States, Mexico, Dominican Republic, Jamaica, Panama, Trinidad, Brazil
	Ilheus	B	Mosquito	Northern South America, Trinidad, Central America, Florida
	Medoc		?	United States
	Powassan	B	Tick	Canada, New York
	Rocio	B	?	Brazil
	St. Louis encephalitis	B	Mosquito	Unites States, Caribbean, Panama, Brazil, Argentina
	Venezuelan equine encephalitis	A	Mosquito	Florida, Texas, Louisiana, Central America, Caribbean, Northern South America, Peru
	Western equine encephalitis	A	Mosquito	Canada, United States, Mexico, Brazil, Argentina
Fever with malaise, headaches, myalgia, and *hemorrhagic signs*	Dengue 1	B	Mosquito	Caribbean, including Puerto Rico
	Dengue 2	B	Mosquito	Caribbean, including Puerto Rico
	Dengue 3	B	Mosquito	Caribbean, including Puerto Rico
	Yellow fever	B	Mosquito	Central and South America

* Antibody responses to viruses in the same serologic group often show cross-reactions with other members of the group.

ARBOVIRUS INFECTIONS PRESENTING CHIEFLY WITH FEVER, MALAISE, HEADACHE, AND MYALGIA

PHLEBOTOMUS FEVER Phlebotomus (sandfly, pappataci, or 3-day) fever is an acute, relatively mild, self-limited infection caused by at least five immunologically distinct arboviruses (Naples, Sicilian, Punta Toro, Chagres, and Candiru). Serologic evidence of human infection has been demonstrated for four additional agents (Bujaru, Cacao, Karimabad, and Salehabad). Humans, the only known host, probably serve as a dead-end host. Voles are suspected of being an endemic host in the Middle East.

Prevalence The disease occurs throughout the Mediterranean Basin, the Balkans, the Near and Middle East, the eastern part of Africa, the Soviet republics of Central Asia, West Pakistan, and possibly certain parts of southern China. Recently, sandfly fever has been recognized in Panama and Brazil. In the Middle East and Central Asia native populations acquire the disease at an early age and develop and maintain high levels of immunity. Cases in Panama and Brazil are sporadic, occurring mainly in persons entering the forest. The apparent absence of phlebotomus fever in indigenous adult populations residing in areas where sandflies are abundant may present a deceptive picture of the actual risk to susceptible persons.

Epidemiology In the Middle East and Central Asia, the disease occurs during the hot, dry season (summer or autumn months) and is transmitted to human beings by the bite of infected sandflies (*Phlebotomus papatasi*). *Phlebotomus papatasi* is a small urban fly which can penetrate ordinary house screens. Only the female bites and usually does so during the night. In persons who are not sensitive, there is neither pain nor local irritation after the bite; hence only about 1 percent of patients will remember having been bitten. In contrast, most of the human-biting sandflies of tropical America are sylvan in their habits. Approximately 7 days after feeding on an infected individual, the fly acquires the capacity to transmit infection and remains infectious for its life span. Transovarial transmission of the virus to the next generation has been demonstrated and offers the best explanation for the mechanism of overwinter survival of the virus. In humans, the incubation period may be as short as 3 days. Viremia is present for at least 24 h before the onset of fever, but is not detectable for more than 2 days after the onset of illness.

Clinical manifestations   The onset of symptoms is abrupt in over 90 percent of patients, with the temperature rapidly rising to its highest point, which may vary from 37.8 to 40.1°C (100 to 105°F). Headache is nearly always present and often is accompanied by pain on moving the eyes and by retroorbital pain. Myalgia is common and may be localized to the chest, resembling pleurodynia, or to the abdomen. Other symptoms may include vomiting, photophobia, giddiness, neck stiffness, alteration or loss of taste, and arthralgia. Conjunctival injection is present in approximately one-third of patients. Small vesicles may be seen on the palate, and macular or urticarial rashes occur. The spleen is rarely palpable, and lymphadenopathy is absent. The pulse rate may be elevated in proportion to the temperature on the first day; thereafter bradycardia is often present. The fever persists 3 days in most patients, with gradual defervescence. Giddiness, weakness, and feelings of depression are frequently encountered during convalescence. Second attacks 2 to 12 weeks after the first occur in 15 percent of cases.

In common with other arbovirus infections, phlebotomus fever may be associated with *aseptic meningitis*. In one series, 12 percent of patients had symptoms and signs sufficient to warrant a lumbar puncture. Findings in these patients included pleocytosis, with an average cell count of 90 per cubic millimeter and a predominance of either polymorphonuclear or mononuclear leukocytes. Spinal fluid protein concentration ranged from 20 to 130 mg per 100 ml. In another series mild papilledema was observed in a few patients with severe illness.

Laboratory findings   The changes in leukocyte count constitute the only positive laboratory findings. Total leukocyte counts of less than 5000 per cubic millimeter are observed in 90 percent of patients if daily counts are done during the febrile period and convalescence. The leukopenia may not appear until the last day of fever or even after defervescence. The differential leukocyte count will reveal an absolute decrease in lymphocytes on the first day, accompanied by an increase in nonsegmented neutrophils. During the second or third day, the number of lymphocytes begins to return to normal and may constitute 40 to 65 percent of the total count. Concurrently, there is a reversal in proportion of segmented and band neutrophils. The differential count usually returns to normal within 5 to 8 days after defervescence. Erythrocyte values and urinalyses are usually normal.

Diagnosis   In the absence of a specific serologic test, the diagnosis must be made on clinical and epidemiologic grounds.

Treatment   The disease is self-limited, and no specific therapy is available. Symptomatic care, including bed rest, adequate fluid intake, and analgesia with aspirin, is recommended. Convalescence may require a week or longer.

Prognosis   No fatalities have been recorded among the tens of thousands of cases.

COLORADO TICK FEVER   Colorado tick fever is one of the two tick-transmitted virus diseases of human beings recognized in the United States and Canada, Powassan virus being the other. Though "mountain fever" had been described ever since the advent of immigrants to the Rocky Mountain region, Becker in 1930 differentiated it from mild Rocky Mountain spotted fever, established the clinical picture of disease, and renamed it Colorado tick fever.

Etiology   Colorado tick fever virus is classified as an arbovirus because it replicates in ticks, but is a reovirus (orbivirus) on the basis of both its structure and its content of double-stranded RNA.

Prevalence   The disease has been contracted in Colorado, Idaho, Nevada, Wyoming, Montana, Utah, the eastern portions of Oregon, Washington, California, and northern portions of Arizona and New Mexico, and Alberta and British Columbia. However, the virus of Colorado tick fever has been reported to have been isolated from the dog tick, *Dermacentor variabilis,* obtained from Long Island. This observation has not been confirmed, but suggests the possibility that Colorado tick fever may occur over a wider geographic area. The actual prevalence is difficult to assess, but the disease is relatively common. Mild and clinically inapparent forms of the disease occur, but its frequency has never been determined. The number of cases of Colorado tick fever reported in Colorado is 20 times greater than that of Rocky Mountain spotted fever. In fact, almost one-half of the patients diagnosed as having Rocky Mountain spotted fever in Utah were subsequently shown to have Colorado tick fever.

Epidemiology   Colorado tick fever is transmitted to humans by the adult hard-shelled wood tick, *Dermacentor andersoni.* The virus has been found in as many as 14 percent of this species of ticks collected in endemic areas. Transovarial transmission of the virus in the tick has been established. Illness occurs from late March through September, with most cases in May and June. Virus can be recovered from blood for 2 weeks in most patients, for at least 1 month in nearly one-half, and from spinal fluid during the acute illness. The virus persists within erythrocytes of convalescent patients for as long as 120 days. Virus can be readily isolated from washed erythrocytes 100 days following infection. Transfusion-associated Colorado tick fever has been reported.

Clinical manifestations   The incubation period is usually 3 to 6 days, and in 90 percent a history of tick contact within 10 days of onset of illness can be obtained. Failure to obtain such a history militates against the diagnosis. Persons affected usually are those whose occupational or recreational activities bring them in contact with ticks. The disease may occur at any age, although 40 percent in one series were 20 to 29 years of age. The clinical picture is characterized by the sudden onset of severe aching of the muscles of the back and legs, chilliness without true rigors, a rapid increase in temperature, which usually reaches 38.9 to 40°C (102 to 104°F), headache with pain on ocular movement, retroorbital pain, and photophobia. Abdominal pain and vomiting occur in one-fourth of patients; diarrhea is rare. The physical findings are not specific. Tachycardia in proportion to the temperature, flushed facies, and variable conjunctival injection may be present. Occasionally the spleen is palpable. Rash occurs in only 5 percent of patients, but on occasion a petechial rash involving primarily the arms and legs or a maculopapular rash over the entire body may occur. Rarely, punched-out ulcers may form at the site of tick bite. The fever with the associated symptoms lasts about 2 days, then abruptly lyses to normal or subnormal, leaving the patient very weak. After an afebrile period of about 2 days, the fever recurs, may be higher than in the first phase, and may last as long as 3 days. One-half of patients show this saddleback pattern of temperature. Rarely there may be three febrile phases. Convalescence of more than 3 weeks is reported in 70 percent of patients over age 30, while symptoms last less than 1 week in 60 percent of patients under 20. Prolonged convalescence has no relationship to persistent viremia.

Evidence of central nervous system involvement has been recorded in a few patients. The findings are those of either an aseptic meningitis with stiffness of the neck or encephalitis with clouding of the sensorium, delirium, and coma. Single instances of reported complications include epididymoorchitis and patchy pneumonitis.

Laboratory findings   The most important laboratory feature is moderate to marked leukopenia, although in one-third of confirmed cases leukocyte counts remain about 4500 per cubic millimeter. On the first day of illness, the total leukocyte count may be at normal levels, but usually by the fifth or sixth day there has been a decrease to 2000 to 3000 per cubic millimeter. Characteristically there is a proportionate decrease in lymphocytes and granulocytes. Toxic changes in neutrophils are often conspicuous, and "virocyte" types of lymphocytes are frequently observed. Bone marrow examination reveals "maturation arrest" in the granulocytic series. Erythrocyte values remain normal. Thrombocytopenia has been recorded in an isolated case report. The blood picture returns to normal within a week after the fever subsides.

Diagnosis   The diagnosis of Colorado tick fever is suspected on the basis of the epidemiologic history and clinical findings. Because of the infrequency of rash, patients who develop fever and rash after tick bites should be suspected of having Rocky Mountain spotted fever. The usual methods for confirming Colorado tick fever are mouse inoculation and fluorescent antibody (FA) staining of patients' erythrocyte; a combination of the two is best. Special handling of blood is not necessary for the FA test which remains positive during as well as several weeks after clinical illness.

Treatment   Treatment is entirely symptomatic.

Prognosis   The prognosis is excellent.

Prevention   Only one patient has been reported as having the disease twice. Active immunity with an attenuated virus has been produced, but the immunization itself frequently produced mild disease. Colorado tick fever is best prevented by avoiding contact with the wood tick. Convalescent individuals should be excluded as blood donors for at least 6 months.

VENEZUELAN EQUINE ENCEPHALITIS   Venezuelan equine encephalitis (VEE) was first noted in equines in Colombia in 1935.

Etiology   Like other alphaviruses, the causative agent of VEE is a relatively small, 40 to 45 nm, RNA virus. On the basis of serologic tests, differing serotypes have been identified, IA to IE, II, III, and IV. Strains ID, IE, II, III, and IV have remained sylvatic in distribution. IA was the original epidemic strain which occurred in Venezuela, and IB, which was recognized in Ecuador in 1963, spread through Central America into Mexico and was responsible for the epidemic in Mexico in

1971 which spread into southern Texas, with the occurrence of at least 76 laboratory-confirmed human cases. In early 1973, almost 4000 cases occurred in Peru.

Epidemiology   VEE has been primarily a disease of equines and other mammals, although occasionally the agent has infected humans. Evidence of human infection (virus isolation or specific neutralizing antibodies) has been found in Colombia, Ecuador, Panama, Surinam, Guyana, French Guiana, Mexico, Brazil, Curacao, Trinidad, Argentina, Peru, Florida, and Texas. The VEE virus complex in nature has been associated with numerous mosquitoes (at least 9 genera and 37 species), including *Aëdes, Mansonia, Psorophora,* and *Culex.* In this respect it differs markedly from other mosquito-borne encephalitogenic arboviruses, which usually are associated with only one to three vector species. VEE apparently has different vectors for its endemic-epizootic and its epidemic-epizootic cycles. The virus has a wide host range in wild mammals, with at least 20 genera, including capuchin monkeys, rats, mice, opossum, jack-rabbit, fox, and bats being naturally infected. Domestic animals other than equines which have been shown to be infected include cattle and pigs in Mexico and goats and sheep in Venezuela. VEE appears to multiply well in mammals with high titers of virus in the blood; e.g., infected horses may have titers of up to $10^{7.5}$ mouse intraperitoneal lethal doses per milliliter of blood. Though 29 species of wild birds have been shown to be naturally infected with VEE (20 percent of which are colonial nestling herons and related species), whether the VEE-viremia levels in birds are high enough to infect vector mosquitoes is not yet known. During the initial 3 days of illness, viremia has been detected in approximately two-thirds of patients. The levels of viremia are sufficiently high that humans could serve as a reservoir. VEE virus also has been isolated by pharyngeal swab in a few patients, suggesting the potential for person-to-person transmission. The available observations make it reasonable to consider that the natural vector is a mosquito, with the primary reservoir being either wild or domestic terrestrial mammals. However, natural infection can probably take place without an arthropod vector. Laboratory infections have occurred and are probably due to inhalation of aerosols.

Clinical manifestations   In humans, infection with VEE virus usually results in a mild acute febrile illness without neurological complications. No age is spared, and there is no sex preponderance. The incubation period is 2 to 5 days, followed by the abrupt onset of headache, fever often associated with rigors, malaise, and myalgia. Other common symptoms may include nausea, vomiting, diarrhea, and sore throat. Uncommon features include seizures, mental confusion, coma, tremors, and diplopia. On laboratory examination the cerebrospinal fluid may reveal pleocytosis with modest increases in protein concentration and normal glucose concentration. Virus may be isolated both from blood and from cerebrospinal fluid. The symptoms usually last 3 to 5 days in mild cases and up to 8 days in more severe cases, although one patient reported from Florida was febrile for 3 weeks. A biphasic course of illness may be encountered, with recrudescence of symptoms at the sixth to the ninth day. In one case report, palatine petechiae were noted and the patient vomited "coffee-grounds" material. In an epidemic in Venezuela in 1962, almost 16,000 cases of acute disease were evaluated; 38 percent were classified as encephalitis, but only 3 to 4 percent had severe neurological abnormalities: convulsions, nystagmus, drowsiness, delirium, or meningitis. The mortality rate was estimated to be less than 0.5 percent, and nearly all deaths occurred in young children.

RIFT VALLEY FEVER Rift Valley fever is an acute disease principally of sheep and cattle which is widespread throughout East and South Africa. It was first described in humans during an extensive epizootic of hepatitis in sheep in the Rift Valley in East Africa. A major outbreak occurred in Egypt, northeast of Cairo, including the province of Giza, and in Aswan in October to November 1977. An estimated 20,000 human cases occurred with several hundred deaths. Cases again occurred in the summer of 1978. Rift Valley fever had not occurred in Egypt previously. During an epizootic in South Africa in 1950–1951, an estimated 20,000 human beings became infected.

Virus has been found in several species of mosquitoes: *Eretmapodites chrysogaster, Aëdes caballus, Aëdes circumluteolus,* and *Culex theileri.* While antibodies to Rift Valley fever have been found in wild field rats in Uganda, the reservoir is unknown. Humans appear to be incidentally infected during the course of an epizootic. Although humans presumably can be infected by arthropods, many infections occur as a result of handling infected animal tissues. In addition, laboratory-acquired infections have been common, which suggests a respiratory route.

The incubation period is usually 3 to 6 days. The onset is abrupt, with malaise, chilly sensation or rigors, headache, retroorbital pain, and generalized aching and backache. The temperature rises rapidly to 38.3 to 40°C (101 to 104°F). Later complaints include anorexia, loss of taste, epigastric pain, and photophobia. Findings on examination are usually unremarkable except for flushing of the face and conjunctival injection. The temperature curve is often saddleback in type, with an initial elevation lasting 2 to 3 days, followed by a remission and second febrile period. Convalescence is typically rapid. Prior to the outbreak in Egypt, Rift Valley fever was a benign illness with almost no fatalities. In Egypt, approximately one percent of patients developed severe complications, such as encephalitis or hemorrhagic manifestations. Encephalitis appeared as the acute infection waned and was severe with serious residua in survivors. Hemorrhagic manifestations appeared as the disease evolved with generalized hemorrhages and icterus. Deaths from massive hepatic necrosis occurred at 7 to 10 days after onset of illness. Macular exudates, with decreased vision, occur. A characteristic finding is an initial normal total leukocyte count followed by leukopenia with a decrease in neutrophils associated with an increase in band forms. The diagnosis is made by isolating the virus from the blood by inoculation of mice. Three-fourths of patients are viremic (up to 10^8 mouse intraperitoneal lethal doses per milliliter blood) when first seen. Neutralizing antibodies have been demonstrated as early as 4 days after onset. There is no specific treatment. A killed vaccine which had been stockpiled in the United States is being utilized.

MAYARO-SEMLIKI FOREST VIRUS DISEASE Outbreaks involving a number of persons have occurred in Brazil and Bolivia. Survey for antibodies in serums obtained from residents in Rio de Janeiro showed that almost one-third were positive. Mayaro virus has been isolated from a wild mosquito, *Mansonia venezuelensis,* and can be maintained serially in *Aëdes aegypti* and *Anopheles quadrimaculatus.* Semliki Forest virus has been isolated from *Aëdes abnormalis* mosquitoes in Uganda and from various *Eretmapodites* mosquitoes in West Africa. Serologic surveys in humans document widespread virus activity. Antigenically these two alphaviruses are very closely related, suggesting that both may have been derived from one strain, with geographic separation having led to some antigenic variation. The mechanism of spread has not been determined, but the presence of viremia favors a biting arthropod vector. The predominance of illness and greater incidence of immunity in males suggest a forest infection.

Symptoms include fever of several days' duration, which may be marked during the first 1 to 2 days. Systemic complaints include severe frontal headache, epigastric pain, backache, nausea, photophobia, and vertigo. Signs have included conjunctival injection, mild icterus in a few patients, and arthritis in at least one patient. The leukocyte count is in the range of 5000 to 8000 per cubic millimeter. The fever lasts 3 to 5 days in most patients. Recovery is usually complete, although in Bolivia the illness was more severe, and several fatalities were reported.

BAT SALIVARY GLAND VIRUS During a survey of rabies infection in bats, a virus related to the St. Louis encephalitis complex was obtained from the salivary glands of Mexican free-tailed bats in Texas. It is not known how the virus is maintained in nature. Five laboratory-acquired infections have been recorded. The illnesses were characterized by fever associated with headache, myalgia, and a mild nonproductive cough. In two patients, there was evidence of central nervous system involvement with encephalitis and aseptic meningitis. One patient had oophoritis, and two developed orchitis. By the sixth to seventh day of illness, leukopenia in the range of 2000 to 3000 leukocytes per cubic millimeter was observed in two individuals.

ZIKA VIRUS Zika virus was first isolated from a captive rhesus monkey in Uganda and subsequently from wild mosquitoes. On the basis of serologic surveys, it is known to infect humans in Uganda and Nigeria. During investigation in eastern Nigeria of an outbreak of jaundice that was suspected of being yellow fever, physicians isolated Zika virus from one patient and noted that two others had a rise in neutralizing antibodies. The symptoms in these patients included fever, arthralgia, and headache with retroorbital pain. Jaundice was present in one, and bile was demonstrated in the urine of another. Albuminuria was noted in one patient. Prothrombin times were normal. The clinical syndrome appears to simulate mild yellow fever.

GROUP C ARBOVIRUSES Currently 11 viruses are classified as Bunyaviruses, group C, of which 9 have been isolated from blood obtained from humans. The geographic distribution includes Brazil (Apeu, Caraparu, Itaqui, Marituba, Murutucui, Oriboca), Trinidad (Caraparu, Restan), and Panama (Madrid, Ossa). Several of these viruses have been isolated from Culicine and Subethine mosquitoes, as well as from several species of rodents. Isolates have been obtained mostly from forest workers and laboratory technicians. Epidemics have not been recognized. The disease begins with headache, fever [with temperature up to 40.6°C (105°F)], and myalgia. Additional symptoms include malaise, photophobia, vertigo, and nausea. Illness is generally mild, lasting 2 to 4 days, and is occasionally followed by a relapse. No fatalities have been reported. Occasionally a prolonged period of convalescence ensues. Leukopenia, with total leukocyte counts as low as 2600 per cubic millimeter, is a common finding. Diagnosis has been established mainly by virus isolation.

BUNYAMWERA GROUP Representative viruses of this group are found in all inhabited continents except Australia. Only five viruses of the group—Bunyamwera itself, Germiston, Ilesha, Guaroa, and Wycomyia—have been associated with clinical disease. Serologic surveys give evidence of a high prevalence of inapparent infection in some areas. The clinical patterns of infection due to Germiston, Ilesha, and Guaroa viruses seem similar, while infection due to Bunyamwera virus is associated often with arthralgia and sometimes with a rash. The mild clinical illness is characterized by low grade fever, headache, and myalgia which last several days, and it may be followed by weakness during convalescence.

ARBOVIRUS INFECTIONS PRESENTING CHIEFLY WITH FEVER, MALAISE, ARTHRALGIA, AND RASH

CHIKUNGUNYA In 1952 an epidemic of a disease occurred in Tanzania, which was given the name *chikungunya* ("that which bends up") because of the sudden onset of joint pains. A group A arbovirus was isolated in 1956 both from serum of patients ill with the disease and from a pool of *A. aegypti* mosquitoes.

Chikungunya virus is responsible for a dengue-like illness in Africa, India, Southeast Asia, New Guinea, and Guam, as well as for a rather mild form of hemorrhagic fever in Asiatic children. Outbreaks have been associated with high attack rates, with as many as 80 percent of inhabitants in some settlements becoming ill. The only known host is the human being. *Aëdes aegypti* is a vector. Because virus has been isolated from *A. africanus* and because antibodies against the virus can be detected in chimpanzees, they may play a role in the natural cycle in Africa.

After an incubation estimated at no less than 9 days, the onset is typically abrupt, with a rapid rise in temperature to 38.9 to 40.6°C (102 to 105°F), often associated with a rigor and headache. Pain in large joints occurs early, incapacitating some individuals within a few minutes of onset. The arthralgia is often associated with objective arthritis. Sites of involvement include knees, ankles, shoulders, wrists, or proximal interphalangeal joints. Myalgia, especially backache, and malaise occur frequently. In 60 to 80 percent of patients a maculopapular eruption, which may appear at any time during the febrile course, is noted on the trunk or on the extensor surfaces of the extremities. Mild lymphadenopathy, predominantly in the axillary or inguinal areas, may be evident. Pharyngitis and conjunctival suffusion may be observed in a few patients. Fever continues for 1 to 6 days, and in some patients an afebrile interval of 1 to 3 days is followed by a secondary rise in temperature. The joint pains may continue after the temperature has returned to normal. In a few individuals joint pains have persisted for up to 4 months. Hematocrit values remain normal. Total leukocyte counts may be less than 5000 per cubic millimeter in some patients, while in others they remain normal. Urinalyses are normal. There is no specific antiviral treatment. Anti-inflammatory agents such as aspirin or indomethacin have been utilized. No second attacks have been recognized, and in the absence of the hemorrhagic fever syndrome, no deaths have been described.

O'NYONG-NYONG FEVER O'nyong-nyong fever was first noted as an epidemic illness characterized by joint pains, rash, and lymphadenopathy in the northern province of Uganda in 1959. The agent is a group A arbovirus which shows close antigenic relationships with chikungunya and Semliki Forest viruses. The original outbreak was associated with an explosive epidemic which spread to Tanzania and other areas in East Africa. By 1961, 2 million cases were recorded. In some areas, 91 percent of the population had either clinical disease or inapparent infection. Local outbreaks extended over the entire year. All age groups were affected. The most likely vector is *Anopheles funestus*. The clinical features are similar to those of chikungunya virus infection.

SINDBIS VIRUS Sindbis virus infection in humans rarely presents as a clinical disease. Of five cases from Uganda, one patient gave a history of joint pain. In the only well-studied clinical illness, a South African woman had arthritis as a prominent finding. Two days after a headache she noted swelling in her hands and feet. Soon thereafter she developed a confluent macular rash, followed by vesicle formation. The small joints of the hands and feet were swollen at the time of examination. Slight swelling of the fingers was present at 10 weeks, although she had otherwise recovered.

ROSS RIVER VIRUS Epidemics of polyarthritis associated with rashes have been observed in Australia since 1928. Outbreaks occur almost entirely in the period December to June. There is a predilection for women, and children are seldom involved (an obvious similarity with rubella, another Togavirus). The onset is characterized by headache, mild catarrh, and occasionally tenderness of the palms and soles. Initially fever may be absent or minimal [highest 38°C (100.4°F)]. In about one-half of patients, arthritis, involving mainly the small joints, wrists, and ankles and sometimes associated with swelling, and paresthesias precede a rash by 1 to 15 days. In the other half, the rash precedes the arthralgia. The rash, which lasts 2 to 10 days, is usually maculopapular, appears on the cheeks and forehead, occasionally spreads to the trunk, or may be restricted to the limbs. The rash may be pruritic. Vesicles occur rarely. Tender lymphadenopathy occurs in one-fifth of the patients. Joint symptoms persist for 3 weeks to 3 months. Patients with this syndrome have shown serologic evidence of infection with Ross River virus, although virus has not been isolated from synovial fluid. Serologic evidence of infection is common in New Guinea.

OTHER ARBOVIRUSES Mayaro and Bunyamwera viruses occasionally have been associated with the syndrome of rash and arthralgia.

ARBOVIRUS INFECTIONS PRESENTING CHIEFLY WITH FEVER, MALAISE, LYMPHADENOPATHY, AND RASH

DENGUE FEVER Dengue is endemic over large areas of the tropics and subtropics. Outbreaks of dengue have occurred in the Caribbean including Puerto Rico and the U.S. Virgin Islands since 1969. A number of travelers return to the mainland United States with clinical illness (52 confirmed cases in 1978). Cases were also imported from Tahiti. Despite intensive surveillance no secondary cases have been found in the continental United States. It is now recognized that the dengue syndrome can be caused by other arboviruses; hence the exact etiology of some of the earlier epidemics is uncertain.

Etiology There are four distinct serogroups of dengue viruses, types 1, 2, 3, and 4, all of which are group B arboviruses. In the Caribbean, type 1 was associated with the 1977-1978 outbreak, type 2 in 1968-1969, and type 3 in 1963-1964.

Epidemiology So far as is known, dengue infections in nature involve only human beings and *Aëdes* mosquitoes. Attempts have been made to implicate lower vertebrates, especially monkeys, as reservoir sylvatic hosts, but the data are inconclusive. *Aëdes aegypti* is the most important worldwide vector species. This species, as well as the less common vector species, is peridomestic, biting humans readily or even preferentially and breeding in small collections of water such as cisterns and backyard litter. They fly during the day. Humans appear to be uniformly susceptible, and susceptibility is not influenced by age, sex, or race. The disappearance of dengue from an area may be the result either of elimination of the vector or of exhaustion of the susceptible population. During outbreaks, attack rates may be very high; in Puerto Rico and the U.S. Virgin Islands, the overall rate of clinical illness was 20 percent, with infection rates as determined by serologic survey as high as 79 per 100. Over 10,000 cases of dengue-like illness were reported from Puerto Rico in 1978. For the first time in nearly 40 years, dengue was confirmed in Central America (Honduras and El Salvador).

Clinical manifestations   Dengue viruses frequently produce inapparent infections in humans. When symptoms develop, three broad clinical patterns may be encountered: classic dengue, hemorrhagic fever, and a mild atypical form. Classic dengue (breakbone fever) occurs primarily in nonimmune individuals, specifically nonindigenous adults and children. The usual incubation period is 5 to 8 days. Prodromal symptoms such as mild conjunctivitis or coryza may occur, followed in hours by the abrupt onset of a severe splitting headache, retroorbital pain, backache, especially in the lumbar area, and leg and joint pains. The headache is aggravated by movement. At least three-fourths of patients have ocular soreness, with pain on moving the eyes. A few have mild photophobia. Though true rigors are common during the course, they are usually not present at the onset. Additional symptoms include insomnia, anorexia with loss of taste or bitter taste, and weakness. Mild transient rhinopharyngitis occurs in as many as one-quarter of the individuals. Cough is almost never seen. Epistaxis has been observed. Examination reveals scleral injection (90 percent), tenderness upon pressure on the ocular globe, and nontender posterior cervical, epitrochlear, and inguinal lymphadenopathy. Over one-half of patients have an enanthem characterized initially by pinpoint-sized vesicles over the posterior half of the soft palate. The tongue is often coated. Skin rashes, varying from diffuse flushing to scarlatiniform and morbilliform, are frequently present over the thorax and inner aspects of the arms. These are transient and fade, only to be followed by a more definite maculopapular rash which appears on the trunk on the third to the fifth day and spreads peripherally. The rash may be pruritic and generally terminates with desquamation. Extreme bradycardia is not observed. Within 2 to 3 days after the onset, the temperature may decrease to nearly normal and other symptoms disappear. The remission typically lasts 2 days and is followed by return of fever and the other symptoms, although they are generally less severe than during the initial phase. This "saddleback" diphasic febrile course is considered characteristic, but often is not encountered. The febrile illness usually lasts 5 to 6 days and terminates abruptly. Complaints of fatigue for several weeks after infection are common.

In addition to this "classic" syndrome, an atypically mild illness may occur. Symptoms include fever, anorexia, headache, and myalgia. On examination, evanescent rashes may be seen, but lymphadenopathy is usually absent. The course is usually less than 72 h in duration.

At the onset both in classic and in mild dengue, the leukocyte counts may be low or normal; however, by the third to the fifth day, leukopenia, usually with counts of less than 5000 leukocytes per cubic millimeter, and neutropenia are usually seen. Occasionally albuminuria of moderate degree occurs.

Diagnosis   Virus isolation by tissue culture of serum obtained during the first days of illness is definitive. Diagnosis can be made by serologic tests employing paired serums for hemagglutination inhibition tests and complement fixation tests. Specific serologic diagnosis is complicated by cross reactions with other group B arbovirus antibodies such as those following immunization with yellow fever vaccine.

Treatment   Treatment is entirely symptomatic.

Prognosis   Mortality is nil.

Prevention   An attenuated vaccine for dengue type 2 is undergoing early experimental evaluation. Control depends upon mosquito abatement.

WEST NILE FEVER   West Nile virus is a group B arbovirus distributed from South Africa to southeastern India, but has been shown as a cause of significant disease only in the Near East, where it can produce a clinical picture closely resembling dengue. Outbreaks of disease involving several hundred patients occurred in Israel in 1950 to 1952. In one outbreak, over 60 percent of the population developed overt disease.

Epidemiology   The disease is highly endemic in Egypt but goes largely unrecognized. Presumably most of the adult population is immune, and the infection in childhood is an undifferentiated mild febrile illness, whereas in Israel it mainly affects adults. The infection occurs in the summer both in Israel and in Egypt. The transmission cycle in Egypt is believed to be bird-to-mosquito-to-bird, with *Culex univittatus* as the principal vector. Although humans and a variety of other vertebrates are infected by the virus, their involvement is believed to be tangential. In Israel, the most probable vectors are *Culex molestus* and *C. univittatus.*

Clinical manifestations   Most of the patients in Israel have been young adults, with neither sex predominating. The onset is usually abrupt and without prodromal symptoms. The temperature quickly rises to 38.3 to 40°C (101 to 104°F), with chills occurring in one-third of patients. Symptoms include drowsiness, severe frontal headache, ocular pain, and pain in the abdomen and back. A small number of patients have anorexia, nausea, and dryness of the throat. Cough is uncommon. Signs observed include flushing of the face, conjunctival injection, and coating of the tongue. The prominent finding is general enlargement of lymph nodes, which are of moderate size but are not hard and are only slightly tender. Occipital, axillary, and inguinal nodes are usually involved. The spleen and liver are slightly enlarged in a small proportion of patients. In one-half the patients a rash may appear from the second to the fifth day of illness and may persist for several hours or until defervescence. The rash occurs predominantly over the trunk and consists of pale roseolar maculopapular lesions. The illness is self-limited and lasts 3 to 5 days in 80 percent of patients.

In a few patients, transitory meningeal involvement may be encountered. Spinal fluid examinations may reveal a pleocytosis and some increase in protein concentration.

Leukopenia occurs in the majority of patients, and total leukocyte counts are lower than 4000 per cubic millimeter in one-third. Differential counts vary from a moderate shift to the left to a slight lymphocytosis.

Convalescence is often prolonged, lasting 1 to 2 weeks, with prominent symptoms of fatigue. Enlargement of lymph nodes subsides over several months. Only rarely have complications, sequelae, or fatalities been seen in natural infections, although in one outbreak in a group of elderly patients a high proportion of patients developed meningoencephalitis, and four fatalities ensued.

Accurate diagnosis rests on virus isolation, which can be accomplished because viremia persists for as long as 6 days, or the demonstration of a rising specific antibody titer.

The treatment is symptomatic.

ARBOVIRUS INFECTIONS PRESENTING CHIEFLY
WITH CENTRAL NERVOUS SYSTEM
INVOLVEMENT

831

CHAPTER 190
ARBOVIRUS INFECTIONS

Four arboviruses are presently recognized as numerically important causes of central nervous system disease in the United States: St. Louis encephalitis virus, Eastern equine encephalitis virus, Western equine encephalitis virus, and the California encephalitis group of viruses. The spectrum of infection caused by these agents includes inapparent infection, fever with headache, aseptic meningitis, and encephalitis. Of the 4308 patients reported with encephalitis during 1975, over 2000 cases (49 percent) were due to arboviruses. Widespread epidemics of St. Louis encephalitis were responsible for 86 percent of these cases. For 10 of the 21 years from 1955 through 1975, St. Louis encephalitis virus was the most common cause of arboviral encephalitis in the United States. In contrast, from 1967 through 1975, the California encephalitis group of viruses accounted for one-half or more of the reported cases of human arthropod-borne encephalitis in each year except 1971, 1974, and 1975.

Etiology Despite the diversity of specific viral etiologies (Table 190-2), in individual patients the clinical manifestations of aseptic meningitis and encephalitis are very similar, and preclude an etiologic diagnosis without ancillary information regarding epidemiologic and serologic features (Table 190-3). The clinical features of aseptic meningitis due to arboviruses are indistinguishable from those due to the more prevalent enteroviruses, which are discussed in Chap. 187. Since transmission to humans in the United States and Canada involves arthropods, specifically mosquitoes, except for Powassan and Colorado tick fever, indigenously acquired disease occurs at times when mosquitoes are prevalent, such as late spring through early fall. The broad clinical picture of arbovirus encephalitis will be discussed; then the specific epidemiologic and prognostic features which characterize the major types will be presented.

Clinical manifestations The clinical features of arbovirus encephalitis differ among age groups. In infants under 1 year of age, the only consistently noted symptoms are sudden onset of fever, which is often accompanied by convulsions. Convulsions may be either generalized or focal. Typically the fever ranges between 38.9 and 40°C (102 and 104°F). Other physical findings may include bulging of the fontanelle, rigidity of the extremities, and abnormalities in reflexes.

In children between 5 and 14 years of age, subjective symptoms are more easily elicited. Headache, fever, and drowsiness of 2 to 3 days' duration before medical attention is sought are common. The symptoms may then subside or become more

intense and may be associated with nausea, vomiting, muscular pain, photophobia, and, less frequently, convulsions (less than 10 percent except in California encephalitis). On examination, the child is found to be acutely ill, febrile, and lethargic. Nuchal rigidity and intention tremors are often present, and on occasion muscular weakness can be demonstrated.

In adults, the initial symptoms commonly include the fairly abrupt onset of fever, nausea with vomiting, and severe headache. The headache is most often frontal but may be occipital or diffuse in location. Mental aberrations, represented by confusion and disorientation, usually appear within the subsequent 24 h. Other symptoms may include diffuse myalgia and photophobia. The abnormalities found on physical examination predominantly relate to the neurological examination, although conjunctival suffusion is frequently seen and skin rashes may occur. Disturbances in mentation are among the most outstanding clinical features. These range from coma through severe disorientation to subtle abnormalities detected only by cerebral function tests such as the subtraction of serial 7s. A small proportion of patients show only lethargy, lying quietly, apparently asleep unless stimulated. Tremor is common and is observed more frequently in individuals over 40 years of age. The tremors vary in location and may be continuous or intention in type. Cranial nerve abnormalities resulting in oculomotor muscle paresis and nystagmus, facial weakness, and difficulty in deglutition may occur, and are usually present within the initial several days. Objective sensory changes are unusual. Hemiparesis or monoparesis may occur. Reflex abnormalities are also common; these include exaggerated palmomental reflexes, and suck and snout reflexes. Superficial abdominal and cremasteric reflexes are usually absent. Changes in the tendon reflexes are variable and inconstant. The plantar response may be extensor and fluctuates almost hourly. Dysdiadochokinesia often exists.

The duration of the fever and neurological symptoms and signs varies from several days to a month but usually ranges from 4 to 14 days. Clinical improvement generally follows the subsidence of the fever within several days unless irreversible anatomic changes have occurred.

Laboratory findings Erythrocyte values are usually normal. Total leukocyte counts often reveal both a slight to moderate leukocytosis (occasionally greater than 20,000 leukocytes per cubic millimeter) and neutrophilia. Examination of the cerebrospinal fluid usually reveals several hundred cells per cubic millimeter, but on occasion cloudy cerebrospinal fluid with cells in excess of 1000 per cubic millimeter may be seen.

TABLE 190-3
Features of arboviral encephalitides common in the United States

Etiology	Geographic predominance in the United States	Urban/ rural	Age, years	Sex	Unique clinical features	Mortality, %	Residua
California encephalitis	Midwest	Rural	5–10	M	Seizures	2	Seizures (one-fourth who had them in acute phase), behavioral problems (15%)
Eastern equine encephalitis	Eastern seaboard	Both	<5 >55	=	CSF may have >1000 WBC/mm³	50	Children < 10 years have emotional lability, retardation, convulsions
St. Louis encephalitis	Eastern and Midwest	Both	>35	=	Dysuria	2–12	Ataxia, speech difficulties (5%)
Western equine encephalitis	Entire	Both	<1 >55	=	None	3	Children <3 months have behavioral problems, convulsions

Within the first several days of illness, polymorphonuclear neutrophils may predominate. The initial cerebrospinal fluid protein is usually only slightly elevated but on occasion may exceed 100 mg per 100 ml. The level of spinal fluid sugar is normal; a significant decrease should raise serious consideration of an alternative diagnosis. As the illness progresses, mononuclear cells in the cerebrospinal fluid tend to increase so that they predominate and the protein concentration may increase. Other laboratory studies have been performed only sporadically, but abnormalities may include hyponatremia, often due to the inappropriate secretion of antidiuretic hormone, and elevations in serum creatine phosphokinase.

Diagnosis Specific diagnosis requires the isolation of the virus or detection of antibodies with a rising titer between the acute phase of disease and convalescence. Antibodies can be detected by hemagglutination inhibition, complement fixation, or virus neutralization techniques.

Treatment Treatment is entirely supportive and requires meticulous attention in the comatose patient.

CALIFORNIA (LACROSSE) ENCEPHALITIS A previously undescribed virus was isolated in 1943 from mosquitoes in Kern County, California. Since 1963, a large number of agents now designated as the California group of viruses have been isolated. Almost all the isolates have been LaCrosse virus.

Since 1966 in the Midwest United States, California (LaCrosse) encephalitis has been incriminated in 5 to 6 percent of cases of acute central nervous system disease, ranking above all agents except the enteroviruses.

Epidemiology Infection has been demonstrated to occur in the Midwest, especially in Ohio, Indiana, and Wisconsin, in wooded areas of eastern Texas and Louisiana, and along the Eastern Seaboard. The principal animal reservoir is the squirrel. The mosquito vectors are primarily woodland mosquitoes belonging to *Aëdes* species, principally *A. triseriatus*. The LaCrosse virus appears to overwinter in eggs of *A. triseriatus*. Transovarial transmission of California group viruses then occurs. California encephalitis occurs during the summer months (June to October), most often involving boys (60 percent) 5 to 10 years of age (60 percent) who live in rural areas.

Clinical manifestations Two clinical patterns have been defined. One is a mild form with a 2- to 3-day prodrome of fever, headache, malaise, and gastrointestinal symptoms. About the third day the temperature increases to 40°C (104°F), and the patient becomes lethargic and develops meningeal signs. These findings abate gradually over a 7- to 8-day period without overt sequelae. The second pattern, a severe form which occurs in at least one-half of the patients, begins abruptly with fever, headache, and vomiting, followed shortly by lethargy and disorientation. During the first 2 to 4 days the course is rapidly progressive with the occurrence of seizures (50 to 60 percent), focal neurological signs (20 percent), pathological reflexes (10 percent), and coma (10 percent). Focal neurological signs may include asymmetrical flaccid paralysis. Uncommon findings have included arthralgia and rash. Clinical laboratory features include peripheral leukocyte counts ranging from 7000 to 30,000 per cubic millimeter (median 16,000 per cubic millimeter) with neutrophilia. Cerebrospinal fluid examination reveals 10 to 500 cells per cubic millimeter, usually with a predominance of mononuclear cells, protein concentrations of less than 100 mg per 100 ml, and normal sugar concentrations. Electroencephalograms are abnormal in at least 80 percent of patients, revealing slow deltawave activity. In one-half of the patients the abnormality is asymmetrical, suggesting focal destructive lesions. Brain scans using [99Tc]pertechnetate also may be abnormal, and localized asymmetrical increased uptake has been observed. Beginning about the fourth day and proceeding over the next 3 to 7 days, there is progressive improvement, with almost all patients becoming afebrile, seizure-free, and ready for discharge from the hospital within 2 weeks after onset.

Diagnosis Neutralizing and hemagglutination-inhibition antibodies usually are present a few days after the onset. Complement-fixing antibodies become detectable 10 to 12 days after onset.

Treatment Initial seizure activity is frequently prolonged and difficult to control. The most effective anticonvulsant medication has been parenteral diazepam. Patients with the severe form of disease should be discharged on anticonvulsants such as phenobarbital for 6 to 12 months.

Prognosis The case fatality ratio is low (2 percent or less); however, one-third of patients may have abnormal neurological findings at the time of discharge. During the early convalescent period, emotional lability and irritability are common. In one series, recurrent seizures occurred in one-quarter of the patients who had seizures during the acute phase. In this same series EEGs were abnormal in one-third of patients evaluated 1 to 8 years after their acute illness. In another series, 15 percent had sequelae, predominantly personality or behavioral problems.

EASTERN EQUINE ENCEPHALITIS Eastern equine encephalitis, a group A arbovirus, was first isolated in 1933 from the brain tissue of horses during an outbreak of equine illness in New Jersey. The first recognized human outbreak occurred in Massachusetts in 1938.

Epidemiology The virus is distributed along the eastern coast of the Americas from Northeastern United States to Argentina. Viral isolations also have been reported in the Philippines, Thailand, Czechoslovakia, Poland, and the U.S.S.R., but the question of type specificity has not been resolved. In the Northeastern United States, epidemics occur in the late summer and early fall. Epizootics in horses precede the occurrence of human cases by 1 to 2 weeks. The disease affects mainly infants, children, and adults over 55 years of age. There is no sex preponderance. Inapparent infection occurs in all age groups, suggesting that the decreased likelihood of developing overt infection in the 15- to 54-year age group is not the result of decreased exposure. The ratio of inapparent infection to overt encephalitis approximates 25:1.

The natural reservoir is unknown. Isolations have been made from numerous species of wild birds and also from amphibians, reptiles, and mammals. The natural vector is the mosquito, including *A. sollicitans* and *Culiseta melanura*. *Aëdes sollicitans,* a salt-marsh mosquito which is an avid human feeder, has been postulated as the epidemic vector, while *C. melanura* is important in bird-to-bird transmission. Equine animals and human beings are probably "dead ends" in the transmission cycle, and infection in them is accidental.

Clinical manifestations Though human infections have been thought usually to result in serious, if not fatal, central nervous system involvement, the detection of inapparent infection as well as relatively mild disease establishes the occurrence of milder forms. In many patients, the cerebrospinal fluid is cloudy and contains in excess of 1000 cells per cubic millimeter.

Diagnosis The hemagglutination-inhibition or neutralization tests are the serologic methods of choice. The complement fixation test may be negative in patients with confirmed infections.

Prognosis The mortality rate in clinical infection exceeds 50 percent. In the most severe cases, death occurs between the third and fifth days. Children under 10 years of age have a greater likelihood of surviving the acute illness, but they also have a greater likelihood of developing severe disabling residuals: mental retardation, convulsions, emotional lability, blindness, deafness, speech disorders, and hemiplegia.

ST. LOUIS ENCEPHALITIS St. Louis encephalitis (SLE) was first recognized as an entity during a major outbreak in St. Louis, Missouri, and the surrounding area in 1933. Sporadic, unpredictable outbreaks occurred, for example, in Houston, 1974, Dallas, 1966, Memphis, 1974, Northern Mississippi and Illinois, 1975. The attack rate in Greenville, Mississippi, in 1975 was the highest which has been encountered, 10 per 10,000 population.

Epidemiology In the United States, epidemics of SLE fall into two epidemiologic patterns. One pattern is found in the West, where mixed outbreaks of Western equine encephalitis and SLE have occurred primarily in irrigated rural areas. The vector has been *Culex tarsalis*. The second pattern occurred in the original St. Louis outbreak and the numerous subsequent epidemics in the Midwest, Texas, New Jersey, and Florida. These outbreaks have been more urban in location and are characterized by a marked tendency for the development of encephalitis in older persons. In such urban-suburban epidemics, the epidemic vectors have been mosquitoes of the *Culex pipiens-quinquefasciatus* complex with the exception of the Florida epidemic, in which *Culex nigripalpus* was incriminated. The presence of SLE virus outside the United States has been proved by isolations in Trinidad, Panama, Jamaica, Brazil, and Argentina. However, except for Jamaica, SLE has not been reported outside the United States. The basic transmission cycle is that of wild bird-mosquito-wild bird. The virus survives the winter in female mosquitoes which ingested a blood meal from a viremic bird before overwintering. The disease in humans usually appears in midsummer to early fall. There is no sex preponderance. The human represents an accidental host and plays no role in the basic transmission cycle. Serologic studies following most urban epidemics indicate that infection rates are similar in all age groups, and that the increasing age-specific attack rate for clinical encephalitis which is typical of urban St. Louis encephalitis is probably due to age differences in host susceptibility to overt disease rather than to a higher rate of infection.

Clinical manifestations Infection with SLE virus most commonly results in an inapparent infection. Of the patients with confirmed disease, approximately three-fourths have clinical encephalitis; the remainder present with aseptic meningitis, febrile headaches, or nonspecific illness. Virtually all patients over 40 years of age have encephalitic manifestations. Urinary frequency and dysuria have been symptoms in approximately 20 percent of patients despite sterile routine aerobic urine cultures. SLE virus has been isolated from urine; this may account for the occurrence of urinary tract symptoms.

Diagnosis The occurrence of either encephalitis or aseptic meningitis as manifested by febrile illness with cerebrospinal fluid pleocytosis in the months of June through September in an adult, especially over 35 years of age, should raise the suspicion of St. Louis encephalitis. Because approximately 40 percent of patients with SLE have antibodies detectable by hem-

agglutination inhibition at the onset of illness, acute serum for serologic studies should be submitted promptly to a competent laboratory.

Prognosis The case fatality ratio in the original St. Louis epidemic was 20 percent. In most subsequent outbreaks the mortality rate has varied from 2 to 12 percent. Subjective nervous complaints, including nervousness, headaches, and easy fatigability and excitability, appear to be the most common residuals. Late organic defects such as speech defects, difficulty in walking, and disturbances in vision were demonstrated in approximately 5 percent of patients 3 years following infection.

WESTERN EQUINE ENCEPHALITIS Western equine encephalitis (WEE) virus is a group A arbovirus which was isolated in 1930 in California from horses with encephalitis. In 1938 it was recovered from a fatal human infection.

Epidemiology WEE virus has been isolated in the United States, Canada, Brazil, Guyana, and Argentina. Human disease has been diagnosed in the United States, Canada, and Brazil. In the United States, the virus is found in virtually all geographic areas. The central valley of California represents an important endemic area. The disease occurs mainly in early summer and midsummer. Wild birds, which develop viremia of sufficiently high titer to be able to infect mosquitoes that feed on them, are the basic reservoir, although nonavian vertebrate hosts may be important. *Culex tarsalis* is the principal vector in the Western United States. In areas east of the Appalachian Mountains, another vector must be operative. The virus has been repeatedly isolated from *Culiseta melanura;* however, the importance of this species has been questioned, since it is not primarily a human-biting mosquito. The ratio of inapparent infection to disease, as evidenced by serologic survey studies, varies from 58:1 in children to 1150:1 in adults. Approximately one-fourth of patients are less than 1 year of age. The highest attack rates occur in persons 50 years or older. In the summer of 1975, following the flooding of the Red River in North Dakota, an increase in equine and human cases of WEE occurred; 41 cases were reported from this region.

Prognosis The fatality rate approximates 3 percent in laboratory-confirmed cases. The incidence and severity of sequelae are related to age. Sequelae among very young infants are frequent (appearing in 61 percent of a group of patients less than 3 months old) and severe; they consist of upper motor neuron impairment, involving the pyramidal tracts, extrapyramidal structures, and cerebellum, and result in behavioral problems and convulsions. Both the incidence and severity of sequelae diminish rapidly after 1 year of age. Adults may complain of nervousness, irritability, easy fatigability, and tremulousness for 6 months or longer after the acute illness. Probably not more than 5 percent of adults have sequelae which are sufficiently severe to be of practical significance. Postencephalitic seizures are rare.

JAPANESE ENCEPHALITIS The name Japanese B encephalitis was employed during an epidemic which occurred in 1924 to distinguish it from von Economo's disease, which was designated as type A encephalitis. The designation as Japanese B no longer seems useful, and the term Japanese encephalitis will be employed.

Epidemiology Japanese encephalitis virus infection is known to occur in eastern Siberia, China, Korea, Taiwan, Japan, Malaya, Vietnam, Thailand, Singapore, Guam, and India. In temperate climates, the disease shows a late-summer early-fall seasonal incidence. In tropical climates there is no seasonal variation. The mosquito *C. tritaeniorhynchus* is the major vector species. It is a rural mosquito which breeds in rich fields and preferentially bites large domestic animals, such as pigs, but also feeds on birds and humans. The human is an accidental host in the transmission cycle. In several outbreaks, a higher incidence of cases has been reported in children than in adults. The ratio of inapparent infection, as evidenced by a serologic survey study of Australian troops in Vietnam, was 210:1.

Clinical manifestations   The occurrence of severe rigors at the onset has been noted in almost 90 percent of patients. On admission, most patients are alert, but deterioration of mental status occurs in about three-fourths of patients within 3 to 4 days. Localized paresis is found more often than with other arboviral encephalitides, e.g., in 31 percent of cases, with predominantly upper extremity involvement; however, it resolves rapidly with defervescence. Weight loss has been very striking. The failure of the temperature to lyse, appearance of diaphoresis, tachypnea, and the accumulation of bronchial secretions are grave prognostic signs.

Prognosis   The immediate mortality rate has varied from 7 to 33 percent or higher. The rate of occurrence of sequelae varies inversely with the fatality rate; in those series with high fatality rates (33 percent), sequelae occurred in 3 to 14 percent. In another series with a fatality rate of 7.4 percent, the sequelae rate was 32 percent. Individuals who had neurologic abnormalities during the acute phase but survived have no more than an 80 percent chance for complete recovery. Sequelae consist of seizures, persistent paralysis, ataxia, mental retardation, and behavioral disorders.

OTHER ARBOVIRUSES WITH CENTRAL NERVOUS SYSTEM INVOLVEMENT   A large group of additional arboviruses have been associated with encephalitis or aseptic meningitis. Some of these agents are listed in Table 190-2. Though the epidemiologic picture of each of these agents is unique, the general features are sufficiently similar to require laboratory support for their differentiation.

ARBOVIRUS DISEASES PRESENTING CHIEFLY WITH HEMORRHAGIC MANIFESTATIONS

For 300 years, yellow fever was the only epidemic viral disease known to be accompanied by grave hemorrhagic manifestations. Since the 1930s diverse viral etiologies of the hemorrhagic fever syndrome have been recognized and are now known to be responsible for the variety of epidemiologic situations in which this syndrome occurs (Table 190-2). Additional agents include: Central Asian hemorrhagic fever, Chikungunya, Congo-Crimean hemorrhagic fever, Kyasanur Forest disease, Omsk hemorrhagic fever, Rift Valley fever, and the arenaviruses (Chap. 191). Despite the diverse viral etiology, there are many similar clinical manifestations. The onset is usually sudden, with headache, backache, generalized myalgia, conjunctivitis, and prostration. From approximately the third day, the initial stage is followed by hypotension, and hemorrhagic manifestations may occur; these are characterized by bleeding gums, epistaxis, hemoptysis, hematemesis, melena, petechiae, ecchymoses, and hemorrhages into most visceral organs. Early mild leukopenia develops, but with the appearance of hemorrhagic manifestations, leukocytosis may occur. The pathophysiology of the cardinal signs is attributable to hematopoietic and capillary damage, with variable localization of lesions. On the basis of limited confirmatory observations, variable degrees of disseminated intravascular coagulation may be in part responsible for the pathophysiology of the hemorrhagic fever syndromes. Death usually occurs in the second week of disease, at which time a high titer of antibody has developed and the patient may have become afebrile. Death is usually associated with coma, which is due not to encephalitis but to an encephalopathy. The pathological changes may be similar despite diverse viral etiologies, with midzonal hepatic necrosis and acidophilic cytoplasmic inclusions similar to the Councilman bodies of yellow fever.

YELLOW FEVER   Yellow fever is an acute infectious disease of short duration and extremely variable severity; it is caused by a group B arbovirus and is followed by lifelong immunity. The classic triad of symptoms—jaundice, hemorrhages, and intense albuminuria—is present only in severe infections, which now compose only a small proportion of the total.

Prevalence   Yellow fever remains the most dramatically serious arbovirus disease of the tropics. For more than 200 years, after the first identifiable outbreak occurred in Yucatan in 1648, it was one of the great plagues of the world. As late as 1905, New Orleans and other Southern United States ports experienced at least 5000 cases and 1000 deaths. Because of the existence of the sylvatic form of the disease, protective measures must be maintained against human disease, as demonstrated by outbreaks in Central America in 1948 to 1957, the Congo in 1958, the Sudan and Ethiopia in 1959 to 1962, Senegal in 1965, central West Africa in 1969, Brazil in 1973, Panama and Colombia in 1974, and Ecuador in 1975.

Epidemiology   Human infection results from two basically different cycles of virus transmission, urban and sylvatic. The urban cycle is human-mosquito-human, i.e., *Aëdes aegypti*-transmitted yellow fever. After a 2-week extrinsic incubation period, mosquitoes can transmit infection. Sylvan yellow fever differs under various ecologic circumstances. In the rain forests of South and Central America, species of treetop *Haemagogus* or *Sabethes* mosquitoes maintain transmission in wild primates. Once infected, the mosquito vector remains infectious for life; hence it may serve as a reservoir as well as a vector. When humans come into proximity with the forest-canopy mosquitoes, sporadic cases or focal outbreaks may occur. With sylvan yellow fever, males predominate. Focal outbreaks may be quite extensive; in Brazil in 1973 at least 21,000 persons out of 1.5 million (1.4 percent) were infected. In East Africa, the mosquito-primate cycle is maintained by the forest-canopy mosquito, *A. africanus,* which seldom feeds on humans. The peridomestic mosquito *A. simpsoni* feeds upon primates entering the village gardens and can then in turn transmit the virus to humans. Once yellow fever is reintroduced into urban areas, the urban cycle can be reinitiated, with the potential for epidemic disease. Why yellow fever has never invaded Asia despite widespread distribution of human-biting *A. aegypti* mosquitoes has never been satisfactorily explained.

Pathology   The diagnosis of yellow fever may be suspected by the presence of necrobiosis and acidophilic necrosis of the parenchymal cells of the liver with the formation of Councilman bodies which occur in a characteristically discontinuous fashion in the midzones of the liver lobules. In the kidney, the virus produces necrosis of the tubular epithelium. Multiple minute hemorrhages occur in the gastrointestinal tract. In the brain, the chief lesion is perivascular hemorrhage, which is most frequently found in the subthalamic and periventricular regions at the level of the mammillary bodies.

Clinical manifestations The incubation period is usually 3 to 6 days. In accidental laboratory- or hospital-acquired infections longer incubation periods (10 to 13 days) have been reported. In considering the clinical features, it is advantageous to classify the illness as to severity: inapparent, mild, moderately severe, and malignant. In mild yellow fever the only symptoms may be the abrupt onset of fever and headache. Additional symptoms may include nausea, epistaxis, relative bradycardia known as Faget's sign [e.g., with a temperature of 38.9°C (102°F) the pulse may be only 48 to 52 beats per minute], and slight albuminuria. The mild illness lasts only 1 to 3 days and resembles influenza except that coryzal symptoms are lacking.

Moderately severe and malignant attacks of yellow fever are characterized by three distinct clinical periods: the period of infection, the period of remission, and the period of intoxication. Prodromal symptoms are usually absent. The onset is characteristically sudden, with headache, dizziness, and temperature elevations to 40°C (104°F) without a relative bradycardia. Young children may have febrile convulsions. The headache is followed quickly by pains in the neck, back, and legs. Often there is nausea with vomiting and retching. Examination reveals a flushed face and injection of the conjunctiva. The congestion of the eyes persists until the third day. The tongue characteristically shows bright red margins and tip and a white furred center. Faget's sign appears by the second day. Epistaxis and gingival bleeding are common. On the third day of illness, the fever may fall by crisis and the patient enters remission, or, in the malignant form, copious hemorrhages, anuria, or delirium may occur. The stage of remission lasts from several hours to several days. In the third stage, the "classic" symptoms develop; the fever returns but the pulse remains slow. Jaundice becomes detectable about the third day; however, jaundice often is not prominent even in fatal illnesses. Increased epistaxis, melena, and uterine hemorrhages are common, but gross hematuria is rare. Of the classic signs, "black vomit" is more characteristic than is jaundice. Hematemesis usually does not occur before the fourth day and is often associated with a fatal outcome. Albuminuria, which rarely develops before the third day, occurs in 90 percent of patients and may be quite marked (3 to 20 g albumin per liter). In spite of this massive albuminuria, edema or ascites has not been reported. In malignant infections, coma frequently occurs 2 to 3 days before death. Shortly before death, which usually occurs between the fourth and the sixth days, it is not uncommon for the patient to become delirious and wildly agitated. Though the duration of fever in the third stage is usually 5 to 7 days, the period of intoxication is the most variable of the stages and may last up to 2 weeks. Clinical yellow fever is relatively free from complications, suppurative parotitis being the most striking of those which do occur. Clinical relapses are not characteristic of yellow fever.

Laboratory findings Early in the disease, progressive leukopenia may occur. By the fifth day, total leukocyte counts of 1500 to 2500 per cubic millimeter often are found, the decrease being due mostly to a decrease in neutrophils. Total leukocyte counts return to normal by the tenth day, and in fatal cases there may be a marked terminal leukocytosis. Hemoglobin values remain normal except terminally, when hemoconcentration or bleeding may occur. Platelet counts are reported to be normal. Detailed coagulation studies have been performed only in rhesus monkeys experimentally infected with yellow fever. Within 72 h after viral inoculation and prior to apparent clinical illness, a coagulation defect was observed. This was characterized by a prolonged one-stage prothrombin time and a prolonged partial thromboplastin time, reflecting measured deficiencies in factors II, V, VII, VIII, IX, X, and XI. Both the euglobulin lysis time and the thrombin time were prolonged, suggesting a depression of plasminogen activation and accu-

mulation of fibrinogen degradation products. At this time platelet counts and chemical measurements of fibrinogen were normal. During the subsequent 48 h, these coagulation defects worsened as the monkeys developed clinical illness; terminally, depression of platelet counts and fibrinogen levels occasionally was observed. The disturbances in coagulation occurred during the stage of viremia and existed before the stage of hepatic necrosis in liver biopsy specimens. These data suggest that the *hemorrhagic manifestations are primarily caused by a disseminated intravascular coagulation rather than by hepatic failure.* Also, in experimental infections in primates, modest increases in total bilirubin and alkaline phosphatase levels and marked increases in serum glutamic oxalacetic transaminase occur. In Brazil in 1973, 7 of 29 patients with a clinical diagnosis of viral hepatitis had serologies compatible with recent yellow fever and lacked hepatitis B surface antigen. Electrocardiograms may show T-wave changes. Clinical examinations of cerebrospinal fluid have not revealed abnormalities.

Diagnosis There are three established procedures for the laboratory diagnosis of yellow fever:

1 Isolation of the virus from blood. This must be done early, preferably during the first 3 days. Caution must be exercised to avoid autoinoculation.
2 Demonstration of increase in neutralizing antibody.
3 Demonstration of the typical, although not completely specific, histopathologic lesions on liver biopsy.

Treatment The management has been symptomatic and supportive and should be based upon assessment and correction of the circulatory abnormalities. If evidence of disseminated intravascular coagulation is present, the administration of heparin should be considered. Close attention to fluids and electrolytes is essential.

Prognosis The overall fatality rate in yellow fever is between 5 and 10 percent of clinical cases; it may be even less since many infections are mild or inapparent.

Prevention Effective control measures are available. Immunization has been effective in the prevention of outbreaks. With the occurrence of sylvatic outbreaks, work in the area of epizootic activity should be discontinued and intensive mosquito abatement measures should be instituted. These measures may provide the time necessary for a mass immunization program.

MOSQUITO-BORNE HEMORRHAGIC FEVERS The term *hemorrhagic fever* was first applied to illness in Southeast Asia in the Philippines in 1953. Subsequently the hemorrhagic fevers have grown steadily as a disease problem. Initially they were classified on the basis of geography as Philippine, Thai, and Southeast Asian hemorrhagic fevers. With further study it appeared more rational to classify the syndromes as hemorrhagic dengue or chikungunya, depending upon the etiology. These diseases are caused by viruses transmitted by *A. aegypti.*

Etiology At least four (dengue types 1, 2, 3, 4) and possibly six types of dengue and chikungunya virus have been isolated from arthropods and humans during outbreaks of hemorrhagic fever.

Prevalence Once regarded as an inevitable but trivial infection, dengue is now both a feared killer and a pathogenetic enigma. The reasons for the apparent sudden "appearance" of the syndrome in the past 26 years are completely obscure. However, during the 1922 epidemic of dengue fever in Louisiana, hemorrhagic manifestations, including epistaxis, bleeding gums, melena, menorrhagia, and even "black vomit," were observed. Hemorrhagic disease with dengue also was seen in Durban in 1927, in Athens in 1928, and in Curacao in 1968. Yet no deaths were attributed directly to the dengue. During the past 15 years, dengue has resulted in 200,000 hospital admissions with 5 to 10 percent deaths, and involved every country in tropical Asia except Bangladesh. In Asia, hemorrhagic fever is a disease of children, with virtually all cases occurring in children under age 14 years. In 1962 in Bangkok and Thonburi, an estimated 10 to 20 percent of children under age 15 had illness due either to dengue or to chikungunya virus. Approximately 5 percent of children with dengue or chikungunya had hemorrhagic fever. Dengue hemorrhagic fever occurs almost exclusively in indigenous populations; it has been observed only rarely in Caucasians of European descent despite the frequent occurrence of classic dengue in this group. During the 1975 dengue-2 epidemic in Puerto Rico, three patients with hemorrhagic manifestations, but without shock, were reported. Elsewhere in the Western Hemisphere, since 1967, dengue hemorrhagic fever has occurred in Curacao and Jamaica.

Epidemiology *Aëdes aegypti* is the vector of both dengue and chikungunya viruses. It is an urban mosquito which breeds in artificial containers and receptacles. Outbreaks are confined to the rainy season, although in areas without marked seasonal rainfall cases may occur throughout the year. Human-mosquito-human transmission of dengue is responsible for urban epidemics. Recent isolates of chikungunya virus from *Culex tritaeniorhynchus* in Thailand where human population densities are low suggest a nonhuman reservoir for this virus.

Clinical manifestations The hemorrhagic dengue syndrome is almost exclusively a disease of children. There is no sex predominance. Illness begins abruptly with a minor stage characterized by fever, cough, pharyngitis, headache, anorexia, nausea, vomiting, and abdominal pain which is often severe. This continues for 2 to 4 days. In contrast to classic dengue, myalgia, arthralgia, and bone pain are unusual. Physical signs include fever varying from 38.3 to 40.6°C (101 to 105°F), injection of the tonsils and pharynx, and palpable lymph nodes and liver. The initial state is followed by abrupt deterioration, with the rapid onset of lassitude and weakness (Table 190-4). On examination the child is found to be restless and to have cold clammy extremities with a warm trunk and a pallid face with circumoral cyanosis. Petechiae, most frequently located on the forehead and distal extremities, are seen in half the cases. Occasionally there may be a macular or maculopapular rash. The extremities are frequently cyanotic. Hypotension, with narrowing of the pulse pressure, and tachycardia occur. Pathological reflexes may be observed. Most fatalities occur in the fourth or fifth day of illness, melena, hematemesis, coma, or unresponsive shock being poor prognostic signs. Cyanosis, dyspnea, and convulsions are terminal manifestations. Following this critical period, survivors show steady and quite rapid improvement.

Laboratory findings In one study, hemoconcentration was found in one-fifth of the children. The majority had leukocyte counts between 5000 and 10,000 per cubic millimeter, with one-third showing a leukocytosis. Only 10 percent of children had a true leukopenia. The most characteristic findings were thrombocytopenia, rarely with blood platelets under 75,000 per cubic millimeter, positive tourniquet test, and prolonged bleeding time. Prothrombin time and partial thromboplastin times were usually near normal values. Depression of clotting factors V, VII, IX, and X may be present. Bone marrow examination may reveal maturation arrest of megakaryocytes. In Manila or Bangkok, hematuria has been infrequent even with other serious bleeding manifestations; however, in Tahiti, gross hematuria was common. Cerebrospinal fluid examinations are usually normal. Other abnormal laboratory findings may include hyponatremia, acidosis, elevated blood urea nitrogen levels, elevation in serum glutamic oxalacetic transaminase levels, mild hyperbilirubinemia, and hypoproteinemia. Electrocardiograms may reveal diffuse myocardial abnormalities. Two-thirds of patients have radiological evidence of bronchopneumonia, with many showing pleural effusions.

Diagnosis Specific virological diagnosis of dengue virus infection by serologic means often is difficult because broad antibody responses to group B arboviruses occur. Virus isolation may provide the only means of identifying the specific agent. Chikungunya virus diagnosis poses less difficulty, since it can be isolated from acute serum in suckling mice or hamster kidney cells. Serologic responses can also be demonstrated.

Pathophysiology The pathophysiologic processes that occur in dengue hemorrhagic fever (DHF) and that distinguish it from unmodified dengue fever are increased vascular permeability in which an increased hematocrit is accompanied by a decrease in serum protein concentration due to selective extravasation of albumin, decreased plasma volume, hypotension, thrombocytopenia, and a hemorrhagic diathesis. The association of DHF with a secondary-type antibody response suggested that primary dengue infection "sensitizes" the host to a severe response accompanying infection with a second type. Anamnestic antibody responses with high titers of anti-dengue IgG antibody early in the course of DHF support this concept. Activation of both the classic and alternate complement pathways, with depression of C1q, C3, C4, C5 to C8, and C3 proactivator levels, has been shown in most patients. In dengue shock syndrome (DSS), the blood clotting and fibrinolytic systems are activated, and levels of factor XII (Hageman factor) are depressed. Presumably, dengue virus acting in the presence of complement-fixing IgG antibody is responsible for activation of this system. However, this does not explain the occasional cases of DSS which occur with initial infections. Moreover, there is a limit to the time period after primary infection in which a second infection can precipitate DSS. Halstead and associates have reported enhanced growth of dengue viruses in peripheral blood leukocytes obtained from immune, compared with nonimmune, donors. Circulating leukocytes capable of supporting replication of dengue virus in vitro disap-

TABLE 190-4
World Health Organization's clinical classification of dengue hemorrhagic fever

	Grade	Clinical features	Laboratory findings
DHF*	I	Fever, constitutional symptoms, positive tourniquet test	Hemoconcentration Thrombocytopenia
	II	Grade I plus spontaneous bleeding (e.g., skin, gums, gastrointestinal tract)	Hemoconcentration Thrombocytopenia
DSS*	III	Grade II plus circulatory failure, agitation	Hemoconcentration Thrombocytopenia
	IV	Grade II plus profound shock (blood pressure = 0)	Hemoconcentration Thrombocytopenia

* *DHF, dengue hemorrhagic fever; DSS, dengue shock syndrome.*

pear within months to a few years. These observations may relate the difference between benign and severe disease to the number of infected cells.

Treatment The mainstay is correction of circulatory collapse while avoiding fluid overload. Administration of 5% glucose in 0.5 *N* saline at a rate of 40 ml/kg restored blood pressure within 1 to 2 h in one-half of patients. When stable, the rate of administration of intravenous fluids was slowed to 10 (ml/kg)/h. If improvement did not occur, plasma or a plasma expander (20 ml/kg) was administered. Transfusion of whole blood is not recommended. Glucocorticosteroids have been used, but doses of 25 mg/kg have not resulted in significant improvement. Since the evidence for severe disseminated intravascular coagulation is questionable, use of heparin is not clear-cut, although in a group of Filipino children with type 3 dengue virus, administration of heparin (1 mg sodium heparin per kilogram) was associated with a dramatic rise in number of platelets and level of plasma fibrinogen. Antibiotics are not indicated, and sympathomimetic amines are contraindicated. Recovery from vascular collapse usually occurs within 24 to 48 h, at which time diuretics and digitalis may be necessary.

Prognosis Mortality has varied from 6 to 23 percent. Deaths have been most common in infants under 1 year of age.

Prevention At present, vector control is the only method available to prevent hemorrhagic fever.

TICK-BORNE HEMORRHAGIC FEVERS Crimean hemorrhagic fever At the close of World War II, a new disease entity was recognized in the Crimea region of the U.S.S.R. Retrospective studies demonstrated that an almost identical syndrome had been recognized in the south central Asian republics of the U.S.S.R. for many years. Soviet workers repeatedly isolated virus strains during 1967 to 1969.

ETIOLOGY The virus of Crimean hemorrhagic fever (CHF) has been shown to be antigenically identical with Congo virus, which has been isolated from patients, cattle, and ticks in Africa (Kenya, Uganda, Congo, and Nigeria). CHF-Congo isolates now have been made from an area extending from southwestern and central U.S.S.R. to Pakistan and across central Africa from Nigeria to Kenya.

EPIDEMIOLOGY Approximately 30 cases of CHF have been recorded annually in each of the known areas of occurrence in the U.S.S.R. The cases occur between April and September. The sex distribution of CHF is equal, and 80 percent of the cases occur in the 20- to 60-year age group, with the majority occurring in milkmaids and agricultural workers. The major arthropod vectors for transmission to humans are ticks which belong to the genus *Hyalomma*. Cattle and wild hares appear to be important reservoirs, and rooks and other birds have been implicated, although the detailed epidemiology has yet to be defined.

CLINICAL MANIFESTATIONS The onset is abrupt, with temperatures to 40°C (104°F), dizziness, headache, and diffuse myalgia. The course of fever is occasionally biphasic, with an average duration of 8 days. Physical signs include flushing of the face, conjunctival injection, vomiting, and, on occasion, epigastric pain. Hepatomegaly is found in half the patients. Splenomegaly has been reported in 2 to 25 percent of patients. Respiratory symptoms or signs are unusual. Hemorrhagic manifestations generally begin on the fourth day with petechiae on the oral mucosa and skin, epistaxis, gingival bleeding, hematemesis, and melena. Neurological abnormalities, seen in

10 to 25 percent of patients, include nuchal rigidity, excitation, and coma. Laboratory findings show leukopenia, with the number of white blood cells falling as low as 1000 per cubic millimeter, and thrombocytopenia, which is often severe. Proteinuria and microscopic hematuria are common, but azotemia and oliguria are not. Convalescence may be prolonged. Death is usually attributed to shock or intercurrent infection. Sequelae include transient alopecia and mononeuritis or polyneuritis. Although the clinical disease seen in Africa due to Congo virus generally has not been associated with hemorrhagic manifestations, one fatal case with gastrointestinal bleeding has been reported from Uganda.

TREATMENT The major approach to therapy has been transfusions of blood or plasma. The clinical similarities to other hemorrhagic fever syndromes in which the phenomenon of intravascular coagulation seems to occur are sufficient to suggest that appropriate studies should be done. If evidence of disseminated intravascular coagulation is demonstrated, treatment with heparin should be considered.

PROGNOSIS The reported mortality rate has shown variation between 9 and 50 percent.

Omsk hemorrhagic fever OHF is an acute febrile disease which occurs in the Omsk and Novosibirsk oblasts in the U.S.S.R. and is caused by a group B arbovirus of the Russian spring-summer complex.

EPIDEMIOLOGY The seasonal occurrence of OHF shows a biphasic pattern with peaks in May and August. OHF is transmitted to humans either by the bite of infected ticks of the genus *Dermacentor* or by the handling of infected muskrats. The natural reservoir includes muskrats, other rodents, and ticks. Epidemics occurred from 1945 to 1948, but recently the disease has been less prevalent.

CLINICAL MANIFESTATIONS Following an incubation interval of 3 to 8 days, illness begins abruptly with fever, headache, and hemorrhagic manifestations, which include epistaxis and gastrointestinal and uterine bleeding. Rarely, neurologic abnormalities may occur. Laboratory features include leukopenia. In contrast to many of the other hemorrhagic fevers, OHF has a low case fatality rate (0.5 to 3.0 percent).

Kyasanur Forest disease Kyasanur Forest disease was first recognized in south India in 1957 as a discrete clinical entity shown to be due to an arbovirus.

ETIOLOGY The virus is a group B arbovirus immunologically related to the Russian spring-summer complex.

EPIDEMIOLOGY Kyasanur Forest disease occurs following occupational exposure to *Haemaphysalis spinigera* ticks in the tropical forests of western Mysore in southern India. The silent reservoir cycle which infects the primate- and bird-feeding *Haemaphysalis* ticks is now believed to be *Ixodes* ticks transmitted among small forest mammals, especially the shrew. Laboratory-associated infections have been common.

CLINICAL MANIFESTATIONS The major symptoms include abrupt onset of fever, headache, fatigue, myalgia (especially of the lumbar area and calf muscles), and retroorbital pain. Cough and abdominal pain occur in half the patients. Additional symptoms may include photophobia and polyarthralgia. Epistaxis and hematemesis are observed in some patients. On examination, findings include relative bradycardia, conjunctival injection, and generalized lymphadenopathy. Fine and coarse rales are frequently heard. Hepatosplenomegaly has been encountered occasionally. During the initial phase, generalized hyperesthesia of the skin occurs occasionally. The fever usually lasts from 6 to 11 days. After an afebrile period of 9 to 21 days, approximately half the patients may develop a second phase, which lasts from 2 to 12 days. This is manifested by recurrence of fever, severe headache, neck stiffness, mental disturbance, coarse tremors, giddiness, and abnormalities in reflexes, as well as by recurrence of many of the initial symptoms. No sequelae have been observed, but convalescence is often prolonged.

Only limited laboratory studies have been performed. During the initial phase, leukopenia is a constant feature, with a total leukocyte count of fewer than 3000 per cubic millimeter by the fourth to sixth day. The leukopenia is associated with neutropenia. During the second phase there is a mild leukocytosis. Lumbar puncture during the second phase has shown a pattern of aseptic meningitis.

DIAGNOSIS Diagnosis is based upon virus isolation from blood; this is readily accomplished, since viremia is prolonged. Serologic tests of paired serums also can be performed.

TREATMENT The management is supportive.

PROGNOSIS The mortality rate is approximately 5 percent.

REFERENCES

Arboviruses: Definition and classification

HORZINCK MC: The structure of Togaviruses. Prog Med Virol 16:109, 1973

THE SUBCOMMITTEE ON INFORMATION EXCHANGE OF THE AMERICAN COMMITTEE ON ARTHROPOD-BORNE VIRUSES: Catalogue of arthropod-borne and selected vertebrate viruses of the world. Am J Trop Med 20:1018, 1971

WHO SCIENTIFIC GROUP: *Arbovirus and Human Disease,* WHO Tech Rept Ser 369. Geneva, 1967

WHO STUDY GROUP: *Arthropod-borne Viruses,* WHO Tech Rep Ser 219. Geneva, 1961

Arbovirus infections characterized by fever, malaise, headaches, and myalgia

BECKER FE: Tick-borne infections in Colorado. Col Med 27:36, 1930

BRICENO ROSSIE AL: Rural epidemic encephalitis in Venezuela caused by a group A arbovirus (VEE). Prog Med Virol 9:176, 1967

CENTER FOR DISEASE CONTROL: Rift Valley fever—Egypt. Morb Mort Week Rep 39:113, 1978

DAUBNEY R et al: Enzootic hepatitis or Rift Valley Fever. J Pathol Bacteriol 34:545, 1931

DIASIO JS, RICHARDSON, FM: Clinical observation on dengue fever. Milit Surg 94:365, 1944

FLEMING J et al: Sandfly fever. Review of 664 cases. Lancet 1:443, 1947

FLORIO L et al: The etiology of Colorado tick fever. J Exp Med 83:1, 1946

GOODPASTURE HC et al: Colorado tick fever: Clinical, epidemiologic and laboratory aspects of 228 cases in Colorado in 1973–1974. Ann Intern Med 88:303, 1978

HUGHES LE et al: Persistence of Colorado tick fever virus in red blood cells. Am J Trop Med Hyg 23:530, 1974

LENNETTE EH, KOPROWSKI H: Human infection with Venezuelan equine encephalomyelitis virus. JAMA 123:1088, 1943

SABIN AB: Research on dengue during World War II. Am J Trop Med 1:30, 1952

———— et al: Phlebotomus (Papataci or sandfly) fever; disease of military importance: Summary of existing knowledge and preliminary report of original observations. JAMA 125:603, 693, 1944

SCHERER WF et al: Ecologic studies of Venezuelan encephalitis virus in Southeastern Mexico: VII. Infection of man. Am J Trop Med 21:79, 1972

SIDWELL RW et al: Epidemiological aspects of Venezuelan equine encephalitis virus infections. Bacterial Rev 31:65, 1967

SMITHBURN KC et al: Rift Valley fever. J Immunol 62:213, 1949

SPRUANCE SL, BAILEY A: Colorado tick fever. A review of 115 laboratory confirmed cases. Arch Intern Med 131:288, 1973

SULKIN SE et al: Bat salivary gland virus: Infections of man and monkey. Tex Rep Biol Med 20:113, 1962

TESH RB et al: Antigenic relationships among Phlebotomus fever group arboviruses and their implications for the epidemiology of sandfly fever. Am J Trop Med Hyg 24:135, 1975

Arbovirus infections presenting chiefly with fever, malaise, arthralgia, and rash

CLARK JA et al: Annually recurrent epidemic polyarthritis and Ross River virus activity in a coastal area of New South Wales. I. Occurrence of the disease. Am J Trop Med Hyg 22:543, 1973

DELLER JJ JR, RUSSELL PK: Chikungunya disease. Am J Trop Med 17:107, 1968

DOHERTY RL et al: Studies of epidemic polyarthritis: The significance of three group A arboviruses, isolated from mosquitoes in Queensland. Aust Ann Med 13:322, 1964

MALHERBE H et al: Sindbis virus infection in man. Report of a case with recovery of virus from skin lesions. S Afr Med J 37:547, 1963

ROBINSON MC: An epidemic of virus disease in Southern Province, Tanganyika territory in 1952–53: I. Clinical features. Trans R Soc Trop Med Hyg 49:28, 1955

SHORE H: O'nyong-nyong fever: An epidemic virus disease in East Africa: III. Some clinical and epidemiological observations in the Northern Province of Uganda. Trans R Soc Trop Med Hyg 55:361, 1961

Arbovirus infections presenting chiefly with fever, malaise, lymphadenopathy, and rash

MARBERG K et al: The natural history of West Nile fever: I. Clinical observations during an epidemic in Israel. Am J Hyg 64:259, 1956

PERELMAN A, STERN J: Acute pancreatitis in West Nile fever. Am J Trop Med Hyg 23:1150, 1974

TAYLOR RM et al: A study of the ecology of West Nile virus in Egypt. Am J Trop Med 5:579, 1956

Arbovirus infections presenting chiefly with central nervous system involvement

ALTMAN R et al: The impact of vector-borne viral diseases in the middle Atlantic States. Med Clin North Am 51:661, 1967

BALFOUR HH JR et al: California arbovirus (LaCrosse) infections. Pediatrics 52:680, 1973

DICKERSON RB et al: Diagnosis and immediate prognosis of Japanese B encephalitis. Observations based on more than 200 patients with detailed analysis of 65 serologically confirmed cases. Am J Med 12:277, 1952

FEEMSTER RF, HAYMAKER W: Eastern equine encephalitis. Neurology 8:882, 1958

FINLEY KH et al: Western equine and St. Louis encephalitis. Preliminary report of a clinical follow-up study in California. Neurology 5:223, 1955

GRABOW JD et al: The electroencephalogram and clinical sequelae of California arbovirus encephalitis. Neurology 19:394, 1969

HILTY MD et al: California encephalitis in children. Am J Dis Child 124:530, 1972

KETEL WB, OGNIBENE AJ: Japanese B encephalitis in Vietnam. Am J Med Sci 261:271, 1971

LUBY JP et al: The epidemiology of St. Louis encephalitis (SLE): A review. Ann Rev Med 20:329, 1969

SCHNEIDER RJ et al: Clinical sequelae after Japanese encephalitis: One year followup study in Thailand. Southeast Asian J Trop Med Public Health 5:560, 1974

WEAVER OM et al: Japanese encephalitis: Sequelae. Neurology 8:887, 1958

Arbovirus diseases presenting primarily with hemorrhagic manifestations

BOKISCH VA et al: The potential pathogenic role of complement in dengue-hemorrhagic fever syndrome. N Engl J Med 289:996, 1973

CASALS J et al: A current appraisal of hemorrhagic fevers in the USSR. Am J Trop Med 15.751, 1966

Dengue. Lancet 2:239, 1976

DENNIS LH et al: The original hemorrhagic fever: Yellow fever. Blood 30:858, 1967

HALSTEAD SB: Mosquito-borne haemorrhagic fevers of South and Southeast Asia. Bull WHO 35:3, 1966

KERR JA: Clinical aspects and diagnosis of yellow fever, in *Yellow Fever*, GK Strode (ed). New York, McGraw-Hill, 1951, p 389

KIRK R: An epidemic of yellow fever in the Nuba Mountains, Anglo-Egyptian Sudan. Ann Trop Med Parasitol 35:67, 1941

LOPEZ-CORREA RH et al: Dengue fever with hemorrhagic manifestations: A report of three cases from Puerto Rico. Am J Trop Med Hyg 27:1216, 1978

LOW GC, FAIRLEY NH: Laboratory and hospital infections with yellow fever in England. Br Med J 1:125, 1931

NELSON ER: Hemorrhagic fever in children in Thailand: Report of 69 cases. J Pediatr 56:101, 1960

PINHEIRO FP et al: An epidemic of yellow fever in Central Brazil 1972–1973: I. Epidemiological studies. Am J Trop Med Hyg 27:125, 1978

PONGPANICH B et al: Management of shock associated with dengue hemorrhagic fever based on pathophysiological findings. Southeast Asian J Trop Med Public Health 6:115, 1975

Technical guides for diagnosis, treatment, surveillance, prevention and control of dengue hemorrhagic fever. World Health Organization, Geneva, 1975

191
ARENAVIRUS INFECTIONS

JAY P. SANFORD

DEFINITION AND CLASSIFICATION The term *arenavirus* is the proposed designation for a group of RNA viruses which have unique morphology (Table 191-1). The virions are round, oval, or pleomorphic, with diameters between 60 and 350 nm, and contain an electron-dense membrane with projections and 2 to 10 inclusion-like dense particles (resembling ribosomes) that give the virion an appearance of having been sprinkled with sand (Latin *arenaceus*, "sandy"). A special property of arenaviruses that causes disease in humans, especially Machupo and lymphocytic choriomeningitis, is their capacity to induce persistent infection in their reservoir hosts with no ill effects and in the absence of an immune response.

LYMPHOCYTIC CHORIOMENINGITIS The first-recognized arenavirus was lymphocytic choriomeningitis (LCM) virus, isolated in 1934 from a laboratory monkey in the course of studies of the 1933 St. Louis encephalitis outbreak. It was recognized early that LCM was carried by apparently healthy laboratory mice. Clinically LCM has been considered primarily in the context of aseptic meningitis; however, it is associated with at least two clinical syndromes in humans: central nervous system and influenza-like illness which may be associated with rash, arthritis, or orchitis. LCM virus has provided a valuable model for the study of chronic, persistent, and generally symptomless viral infections in laboratory animals.

Prevalence In the United States, at present, human infection with LCM virus is rare; however, seroepidemiologic studies on specimens obtained in 1935 to 1940 from persons with no history of central nervous system disease from all parts of the United States revealed neutralizing antibodies in 10 to 28 per cent. In a study of aseptic meningitis, Meyer and associates incriminated LCM in 8.1 percent. In recent years, the prevalence of infection seems to have decreased markedly.

Epidemiology The virus of LCM is worldwide in distribution. Although infection can be induced in a variety of animals, mice are the major natural reservoir as well as the primary host in which latent, asymptomatic infection occurs. The latency of infection in the mouse depends upon immunologic tolerance. Animals infected in utero or shortly after birth excrete LCM virus for life without overt disease. Human infections are secondary to contact with an infected rodent. The mode of transmission is thought to be via airborne spread or contact with excrement from infected animals. In the past, most cases have arisen in persons living in rodent-infested houses, but lately outbreaks of LCM virus disease in humans have been reported from Germany and from the United States in which the source of infection was traced to laboratory animals and household pets, specifically hamsters which, like mice, can shed LCM virus in urine and stool. LCM occurs throughout the year but has been more frequent in the colder months when "the mice come in from the fields." Person-to-person transmission has not been demonstrated.

Pathogenesis In natural infection, the portal of entry of the LCM virus is probably through the respiratory tract. Virus multiplication occurs initially in the respiratory epithelium, and an influenza-like illness develops. Dissemination of virus to extrapulmonary sites, presumably to reticuloendothelial cells, with multiplication and viremia occurs. LCM virus crosses the blood-brain barrier. In mice, the resulting meningi-

TABLE 191-1
Classification of arenaviruses

Virus	Clinical disease	Reservoir	Known geographic range
Lymphocytic choriomeningitis	Aseptic meningitis, meningoencephalitis, influenzal syndrome, orchitis, arthritis	Mice, hamsters	Worldwide except Australia
Tacaribe		Bats	Trinidad
Junin	Argentinian hemorrhagic fever	*Calomys musculinus*	Argentina
Machupo	Bolivian hemorrhagic fever	*Calomys callosus*	Northeast Bolivia
Amapari			Brazil
Latino			Bolivia
Parana			Paraguay
Pichinde			Colombia
Tamiami			Florida
Lassa	Lassa fever	*Mastomys natalensis*	Nigeria, Liberia, Sierra Leone, Republic of Guinea, Central African Republic
?	Far Eastern hemorrhagic fever (Korean, nephropathica epidemica)	*Apodemus agrarius*	U.S.S.R., Manchuria, China, Korea, Scandinavia

tis is attributed to a cell-mediated immune reaction. Support for this hypothesis derives from observations that disease but not infection can be prevented in experimental animals by neonatal thymectomy, irradiation, or immunodepressant drugs such as cyclophosphamide. Similar pathogenetic mechanisms may operate in humans, although isolation of LCM virus from the CSF of patients with aseptic meningitis is quite common.

Clinical manifestations The exact incubation period is not known. Following experimental inoculation of LCM virus into volunteers, fever occurred in 1½ to 3 days, while an influenza-like constellation of symptoms developed 5 to 10 days after exposure. An influenza-like illness with many features of other arenavirus and arbovirus infections is the commonest clinical pattern. In some patients, up to one-half in some series, the illness may be biphasic with subsequent aseptic meningitis or encephalomyelitis. Fever, usually from 38.3 to 40°C (101 to 104°F), associated with rigors, is uniformly noted. Other symptoms which are encountered in over one-half of patients include malaise, weakness, myalgia (especially lumbar aching), retroorbital headache, photophobia, anorexia, nausea, and light-headedness. Other prominent symptoms which occur in one-fourth to one-half of patients include sore throat, vomiting, and dysesthesias. Later arthralgias, especially in the hands, occur. Less common complaints (up to one-quarter of patients) include aching pain in the chest, associated with pneumonitis; increased hair loss progressing to generalized alopecia of the scalp, 2 or 3 weeks after the onset of illness; testicular pain or frank orchitis, usually unilateral, again 1 to 3 weeks after onset; and parotid pain, which may lead to a misdiagnosis of mumps. Physical findings in the first week of illness are few. Patients often have a relative bradycardia. Pharyngeal injection without exudate is commonly seen (60 percent). Mild nontender cervical or axillary lymphadenopathy may occur. The initial phase lasts from 5 days to 3 weeks followed by improvement. After a remission of 1 to 2 days many patients relapse with recurrent fever and more prominent headache. Physical signs may include skin rashes, swelling of metacarpophalangeal and proximal interphalangeal joints, meningeal signs, orchitis, parotitis, and alopecia of the scalp. Convalescence generally is of 1 to 4 weeks' duration, characterized by easy fatigability, an excessive need for sleep, dysesthesias, and occasional dizziness. Patients with aseptic meningitis almost always recover without sequelae. With encephalitis, 25 to 30 percent of patients have neurological residua.

Laboratory findings Leukopenia and thrombocytopenia are almost uniform during the first week of illness. Although leukocyte counts usually vary between 2000 and 3000 per cubic millimeter, counts as low as 600 per cubic millimeter have been recorded. Differential counts generally show slight relative lymphocytosis. Platelet counts are usually between 50,000 and 100,000 per cubic millimeter. Anemia is not encountered. The erythrocyte sedimentation rate often is normal. Mild elevations of the serum enzymes, serum glutamic oxaloacetic transaminase (SGOT) and lactic dehydrogenase (LDH), may occur. Chest radiographs may suggest basilar pneumonitis. In patients with meningeal signs examination of the cerebrospinal fluid usually reveals several hundred cells per cubic millimeter, although cell counts in excess of 1000 per cubic millimeter are reported in one-half patients in some series. Lymphocytes predominate (greater than 80 percent) even early. The initial cerebrospinal fluid protein is usually slightly elevated, but on occasion levels may exceed 150 mg per 100 ml. Although a normal cerebrospinal fluid glucose level is considered the hallmark of viral meningitides, hypoglycorrhachia has been observed in up to 27 percent of patients with LCM, glucose values as low as 15 mg per 100 ml with normal simultaneous blood sugar levels having been reported.

Diagnosis The diagnosis of LCM can be established with certainty by recovery of the virus from blood or spinal fluid. Complement-fixing antibodies are usually detectable 1 to 2 weeks after the onset of infection, peak at 5 to 8 weeks, and are gone by 6 months. Neutralizing antibodies appear after 6 to 8 weeks, increase in titer slowly, and remain high for years. Immunofluorescent studies have detected antibody to LCM virus earlier in the course of illness, and its appearance seems to parallel the development of the neurological phase. The clinical manifestations of LCM cannot be differentiated from those produced by numerous other viruses. A detailed discussion of aseptic meningitis appears in Chap. 186.

Treatment The management is supportive and symptomatic.

HEMORRHAGIC FEVER WITH RENAL SYNDROME Synonyms for this disease include Korean hemorrhagic fever, Far Eastern hemorrhagic fever, endemic or epidemic nephrosonephritis, Manchurian epidemic hemorrhagic fever, Songo fever, and Churilov's disease. The same disease in Scandinavia has been called *nephropathica epidemica.*

Epidemic hemorrhagic fever (EHF) is an acute febrile, often fatal, otherwise self-limited illness caused by an agent, most likely an arenavirus, which has been propagated in the rodent *Apodemus agrarius* and that is characterized by severe toxemia, widespread capillary damage, hemorrhagic phenomena, and renal insufficiency. In 1932, the Russians first observed the disease in southeastern Siberia along the Amur River. In April 1951, a previously unknown illness, subsequently recognized as EHF, broke out among the United Nations forces in Korea.

Etiology In 1978, Lee and associates reported a yet to be identified agent in the lungs of the rodent *A. agrarius* which reacted with serums from patients convalescing from Korean hemorrhagic fever. Diagnostic increases in immunofluorescent antibodies were demonstrated in 113 of 116 cases of severe EHF. The agent has not yet been cultivated in tissue culture or in laboratory animals, although it has been passed in *A. agrarius.*

Prevalence In Korea between April 1951 and January 1953, 2070 cases of EHF were reported among United Nations personnel. The disease usually occurs as an isolated event; hence, overall attack rates have relatively less meaning. With this reservation, attack rates in two United States Army divisions stationed in Korea varied between 1.9 and 2.9 cases per 1000 persons per epidemic season. Approximately 800 cases per year have continued to occur; however, most cases are now seen in Korean civilians and military with less than 10 cases per year in U.S. military personnel. The U.S.S.R. reports 500 to 2000 cases yearly.

Epidemiology In Korea the majority of cases occur in May to June and in October to November. These peaks coincide with the dry seasons. Geographically, EHF originally occurred among troops stationed in the vicinity of Seoul north of the 38th parallel. More recently cases have been encountered throughout the Korean peninsula. The epidemiology of EHF observed in Korea remains unknown. No vector is known or suspected although earlier, chiggers, especially *Trombicula pallida,* correlated closely with the epidemiology of EHF in Korea. Since World War II, rather remarkable outbreaks have occurred in northeast Asia between November and January.

In these outbreaks, the peak of the epidemic was preceded by a marked increase in forest rodent populations (usually the red-backed vole *Clethrionomys glariolus*), which migrated into the fields, barns, and even houses near the forest. Nephropathica epidemica, a disease encountered in Scandinavia and in Eastern Europe which is clinically similar to EHF, has been shown to be related to the agent causing Korean hemorrhagic fever. There may be a very narrow variety of rodent hosts which distribute virus in urine or by eating dead carcasses. Humans are probably an incidental host who may become infected by the aerosol route.

Clinical manifestations   The incubation period in EHF is usually 10 to 25 days, with possible extremes of 7 and 36 days. Individuals who contract the disease in an endemic area may easily not develop illness until their return to the United States. Inapparent or mild disease is less common than typical EHF.

The clinical course of EHF may be divided into phases on the basis of the underlying physiological aberrations: febrile, hypotensive, oliguric, diuretic, and convalescent. There is considerable variation among patients in the severity of the illness. In one study two-thirds of the 264 cases studied were classified as mild, while 14 percent were termed severe. The illness in most patients was of comparable severity in each phase.

FEBRILE (INVASIVE) PHASE   From 10 to 20 percent of patients describe vague prodromal symptoms resembling mild upper respiratory infections. The onset is then usually abrupt, often initiated by a chill and accompanied by fever, headache, backache, abdominal pain, and generalized myalgia. Anorexia and thirst are almost universal, while nausea and vomiting are common although not constant symptoms. The headache is most commonly frontal or retroorbital. Eye symptoms, especially mild photophobia and pain on movement of the eyes, are characteristic. Diarrhea is not a feature. Fever is present in almost all patients; the temperature ranges from 37.8 to 41.1°C (100 to 106°F), reaches a peak on the third or fourth day after onset, and falls by lysis on the fourth to seventh day. There is a relative bradycardia. Initially the blood pressure is normal. One of the most typical early findings is a diffuse reddening of the skin, most marked over the face and V area of the neck. It may resemble a severe sunburn. The erythema blanches on pressure. Dermographism can be demonstrated in over 90 percent of patients at the same time as the flush. Slight edema of the upper eyelids causes a bleary-eyed appearance. Bulbar and palpebral conjunctivas show injection. Conjunctival petechiae may develop by the third or fifth day of illness. Subconjunctival hemorrhages may be striking. Intense pharyngeal reddening without significant sore throat is typical. The first location for petechiae is usually the palate, where they occur in half the patients. Within 12 to 24 h, petechiae appear at pressure areas such as the axillary folds, lateral chest wall, belt line, hips, and thighs. Retinal hemorrhages occur rarely. Cervical, axillary, and inguinal nodes are moderately enlarged but nontender. Abdominal and costovertebral tenderness is almost a constant finding. Splenomegaly is unusual and in Korea was generally attributable to malaria with which EHF coexisted in about 1 percent of patients. The degree of flush, fever, and conjunctival injection and the number of petechiae correlate quite well with the overall severity of illness.

Laboratory studies during this phase are often not striking. Initial hemoglobin and hematocrit values are usually normal. Prior to the fourth day, leukocyte counts range from 3600 to 6000 per cubic millimeter but are associated with neutrophilia. Early in the course urine specific gravity may be high. Albuminuria, which is an almost universal finding, appears often abruptly, between the second and fifth days of illness. The urinary sediment reveals microscopic hematuria and hyaline, granular, red blood cell casts, and/or white blood cell casts. Erythrocyte sedimentation rates are normal during the first week. Capillary fragility tests are usually positive at the time of admission and become most abnormal by the ninth day. Electrocardiographic abnormalities may be seen in 15 to 30 percent of patients; these include sinus bradycardia and low or inverted T waves. Lumbar punctures may reveal gross blood in the spinal fluid.

HYPOTENSIVE PHASE   On about the fifth day of illness, during the last 24 to 48 h of the febrile phase, hypotension or shock may occur. In mild cases, only a transient fall in blood pressure occurs; among moderately and severely ill patients shock may persist for 1 to 3 days. In 828 patients, 16.5 percent had clinical shock, and another 14 percent had hypotension without shock. Headache often diminishes, but thirst persists. In the beginning of the hypotensive phase, most patients have warm, dry skin and extremities. As the hypotensive phase progresses and the systolic blood pressure decreases and pulse pressure narrows, the skin becomes cool and moist. Tachycardia replaces the relative bradycardia.

At this stage, an increase in hematocrit with no change in total serum protein level is found. This is thought to reflect a loss of plasma through damaged capillaries. On about the fifth day, all patients develop marked proteinuria. The previously normal urine specific gravity begins to fall and in 2 to 3 days is usually around 1.010. Blood urea nitrogen concentrations begin to increase. Other laboratory findings include leukocytosis with white blood cell counts of 10,000 to 56,000 per cubic millimeter with neutrophilia and toxic granulation. The number of platelets often decreases to less than 70,000 per cubic millimeter. In a single patient who became ill 30 days after leaving Korea and who was studied on the fourth day of illness (i.e., in the hypotensive phase), there was marked thrombocytopenia, hypofibrinogenemia, and hypoprothrombinemia with a prolonged thrombin time. The deficiency of multiple blood coagulation factors suggests that the bleeding defect was due to disseminated intravascular coagulation.

OLIGURIC PHASE (HEMORRHAGIC OR TOXIC PHASE)   About the eighth day of illness, blood pressure returns to the normal range and in some instances increases to hypertensive levels. While oliguria may have appeared during the shock phase, it now becomes a prominent feature. Oliguria develops even though hypotension was not recognized. Symptomatically patients continue to feel weak and thirsty and have more severe backache. Protracted vomiting and hiccups may ensue.

Blood urea nitrogen levels increase rapidly and are associated with hyperkalemia, hyperphosphatemia, and hypocalcemia. Metabolic acidosis is rarely severe. Although platelets begin to return to normal, hemorrhagic manifestations become more prominent and include petechiae, hematemesis (analogous to "black vomit" in yellow fever), melena, hemoptysis, gross hematuria, and hemorrhages into the central nervous system. The enlarged lymph nodes may now become tender.

With the onset of diuresis on about the seventh day in moderately ill patients and the ninth to eleventh day in severely ill patients, symptoms of fluid and electrolyte abnormalities and central nervous system or pulmonary complications may appear. Central nervous system symptoms include disorientation, extreme restlessness, lethargy, paranoid delusions, and hallucinations. Grand mal seizures, pulmonary edema, and pulmonary infection occur in some patients.

DIURETIC PHASE With the onset of diuresis, progressive improvement is the rule. Most patients begin to eat and regain their strength. In fatal cases the diuretic phase is associated with a daily urine output of less than 4 liters and often less than 2 liters, in contrast to larger volumes in surviving patients.

CONVALESCENT PHASE The convalescent phase lasts 3 to 6 weeks. Weight is regained slowly. Complaints include muscular weakness, intention tremor, and lack of stamina. Hyposthenuria and polyuria are present; however, within 2 months most patients are able to concentrate their urine to a specific gravity of 1.023 or greater after a 12-h period of water deprivation.

Diagnosis Serologic tests are not currently available; hence, diagnosis is based on clinical-epidemiologic features. The following criteria are necessary for diagnosis: the patient must have been in the endemic area within the limits of the incubation period, and there must be a characteristic history, hemorrhagic findings, and evidence of renal involvement. In addition, studies to exclude other forms of the hemorrhagic fever syndrome must be undertaken, particularly in the sporadic cases.

Pathology The most characteristic fundamental alteration is widespread capillary and endothelial damage, with all subsequent manifestations being the result of this damage. This is manifested by dilatation of all small vessels in tissues, congestion, plasma transudation, and multiple small hemorrhages. Three features are prominent and characteristic: hemorrhage, particularly in the renal medulla, right atrium, and gastrointestinal submucosa; a peculiar type of necrosis of the renal pyramids, anterior lobe of the pituitary body, and adrenal gland; and a mononuclear cellular infiltration of the myocardium, spleen, and liver. Moderate to severe retroperitoneal edema was present in three-fourths of patients who died in the hypotensive phase of EHF.

Pathophysiology The physiological changes correlate with the clinical features. During the early febrile phase, the cardiac index is normal. Late in the febrile phase widespread capillary dysfunction becomes evident. This is manifest by loss of protein-rich plasma through damaged capillaries and results in hemoconcentration and a progressive fall in cardiac output. Measured total peripheral resistance is low, a finding compatible with the observed capillary dilatation and refractoriness to l-norepinephrine. During the hypotensive phase, the increases in hematocrit values and decreases in plasma volume are accentuated. These findings have the pathological corollary of marked retroperitoneal edema. The hypotensive phase is associated with a reduction in cardiac output and an increase in peripheral vascular resistance. The reduced cardiac output is probably the result of reduction in circulating blood volume, inadequate vasoconstriction, and possibly myocardial damage. Although adrenal hemorrhages can be seen at necropsy, adrenal insufficiency does not seem to be a contributing cause of shock. The initial pathophysiologic changes may result in impairment of circulation through various organs, with the development of functional and morphologic changes secondary to inadequate perfusion with its attendant hypoxemia. The hemorrhagic manifestations appear to be the result of capillary damage, with diapedesis of erythrocytes and the development of disseminated intravascular coagulation.

The plasma loss and arteriolar dysfunction are limited in duration, and, for unknown reasons, the sequestered plasma rather abruptly returns to the vascular system at the time of oliguric phase. During this phase, examination of nail bed capillaries reveals increased vasomotor activity and vasoconstriction. When patients who became hypertensive were divided on the basis of the presence or absence of diuresis, the clinical and hemodynamic differences became more apparent. During the hypertensive phase in anuric or oliguric patients, some individuals presented with full veins, an exaggerated cardiac apical thrust, and wide pulse pressure. In this group the cardiac index was high, and the peripheral resistance and hematocrit were low. Hypertensive patients who had begun to have diuresis had normal cardiac outputs and significantly elevated values for peripheral vascular resistance.

Although diuresis is a harbinger of convalescence, a daily urine output of 3 to 8 liters contributes to further serious fluid and electrolyte imbalances. If fluid output exceeds intake, low cardiac indexes may be seen and shock may ensue. Conversely, if fluid intake exceeds output, hypertension and pulmonary edema may develop.

Treatment Clinical management primarily revolves around meticulous supportive care. Trials with a variety of agents including antibiotics, adrenocortical steroid hormones, antihistamines, and convalescent serum were without significant beneficial effect during the Korean epidemics. The treatment of shock is discussed in Chap. 109 and that of acute tubular necrosis in Chap. 275.

Prognosis The Soviet experience indicates a mortality rate of 3 to 32 percent; in other early reports the mortality has ranged from 10 to 15 percent. Between April 1951 and December 1976 the overall case fatality ratio in Korea was 6.6 percent.

Residua are uncommon. Of 783 surviving patients cared for at the Hemorrhagic Fever Center in Korea between April and December 1952, only 16 were unable to return to duty within a period of 4 months. Fifteen of these individuals still had hyposthenuria. Follow-up studies on former EHF patients 3 to 5 years later showed that they had many more subsequent hospital admissions for urologic problems than did a control group and that the relative frequency correlated with the severity of the acute episode of EHF. Asymptomatic residual renal tubular dysfunction may be more common than has been appreciated.

ARGENTINIAN AND BOLIVIAN HEMORRHAGIC FEVERS The first cases of a new American hemorrhagic disease were seen near the Argentinian town of Junin near Buenos Aires in 1953. A virus was isolated from patients' blood and from local rodents and their mites. In 1959, cases of a disease thought to resemble severe epidemic typhus were noted among rural workers in northeastern Bolivia. The similarity between these syndromes was recognized. In 1963, the causal virus was isolated from patients and rodents and named the Machupo virus. Machupo virus is serologically related to but distinct from Junin virus.

Prevalence Junin virus infections have occurred in epidemic form since 1958 with between 100 and 3500 cases reported annually. The hemorrhagic disease in Bolivia has been particularly severe. Of a total population of 4000 to 6000 in the endemic area, 750 persons were affected between 1959 and 1963.

Epidemiology Argentinian hemorrhagic fever occurs in sharply endemic seasonal form (February to August), mostly among male rural workers, especially those exposed to fields at the time of the maize harvest. Virus is transmitted in the urine of rodents with chronic infection and viruria. Humans acquire the virus through contact with items or foodstuffs which have been contaminated with infected rodent urine. The main reservoir is two species of cricetidae, *Calomys laucha* and *C. musculinus*.

Bolivian hemorrhagic fever is similarly transmitted by the urine of *C. callosus* (a mouse-like rodent) chronically infected with Machupo virus. Direct person-to-person transmission is possible and may have occurred in the outbreak in Cochabamba. Disease has not occurred in medical personnel attending infected patients.

Clinical features Argentinian hemorrhagic fever presents manifestations of renal, cardiovascular, and hematologic involvement. Inapparent infections are rare. The incubation period is estimated to be 7 to 16 days, followed by a gradual onset of chills, fever, headache, malaise, myalgia, anorexia, nausea, and vomiting. The temperature reaches 38.9 to 40°C (102 to 104°F), facial flushing may be prominent, and there is a painless enanthem of the pharynx. Lymphadenopathy and splenomegaly are not present. From 3 to 5 days after the onset, the signs and symptoms worsen, with the appearance of signs of dehydration, hypotension to 50 to 100 mmHg, oliguria, and relative bradycardia. In the more severe cases, hemorrhagic manifestations, including bleeding from the gums, hematemesis, hematuria, and melena, occur. Progressive oliguria and tremor of the tongue and extremities may develop. Some patients develop psychic manifestations, with agitation, delirium, or stupor. Progressive shock, hypothermia, gallop rhythm, or gastrointestinal bleeding may occur from the seventh to tenth days. In fatal cases, pulmonary edema usually is the cause of death. During convalescence a temporary alopecia has been noted. Erythrocyte counts are normal or elevated. The total leukocyte count drops to 1200 to 3400 blood cells per cubic millimeter. Thrombocytopenia may occur. Complement components C2, C3, and C5 are decreased. The urine is dark and may approach the color of mahogany, with intense albuminuria. Blood urea nitrogen levels rise rapidly.

The clinical picture of Bolivian hemorrhagic fever is similar to Argentinian, although epistaxis and hematemesis at the onset is more common.

Diagnosis Complement-fixing antibodies appear in 15 to 30 days in about 75 percent of the clinically diagnosed cases.

Treatment Available reports do not provide details as to therapy. Supportive measures, including peritoneal dialysis to correct both the azotemia and the pulmonary edema, would seem to offer the most reasonable approach.

Prognosis The mortality rate among patients with Argentinian hemorrhagic fever is usually 3 to 15 percent, while that in Bolivian hemorrhagic fever is 5 to 30 percent.

Prevention In Bolivia, rodent control measures directed primarily against *C. callosus* populations in the houses resulted in a prompt and dramatic cessation of human cases.

LASSA FEVER A new virus disease, which is both highly contagious and virulent, occurred in a missionary nurse in Lassa, a town in northeast Nigeria, in 1969.

Epidemiology Since the initial outbreak at Lassa in 1969, during which one of the patients was transferred to New York City, there have been other outbreaks near Jos in Northern Nigeria in 1970 (32 suspected cases with 10 deaths), in Zorzor, Liberia, in 1972 (11 cases with 4 deaths), and in the eastern province of Sierra Leone with 63 suspected cases admitted to two hospitals between 1970 and 1972. In Jos and Zorzor, outbreaks apparently resulted from person-to-person nosocomial spread from the index case to hospital workers or other patients. In Sierra Leone, the great majority of cases were acquired outside the hospital, although hospital workers were at high risk. *Mastomys natalensis*, a multimammate rat wide-

spread in Africa, is known to be an animal reservoir of the virus, and primary human cases probably result from contamination of foodstuffs with rodent urine. Human-to-human transmission may occur through contact with urine, feces, vomitus, or saliva through droplets and aerosols, and particularly through wounds contaminated with blood. Intrafamilial outbreaks have occurred around several cases. There are a number of cases which have been acquired through accidental autoinoculation with needles while starting intravenous fluids. At least one laboratory-acquired infection has occurred. In Sierra Leone 6 percent of the population surveyed had complement-fixing antibody against Lassa virus, while only 0.2 percent had recognized disease, suggesting mild disease or inapparent infection. In Liberia 10 percent of hospital personnel had antibodies. Positive serums were also obtained from individuals in Cameroon and Benin (formerly Dahomey).

Clinical features The incubation period is 1 to 24 days, being 10 days following accidental inoculation. Patients have ranged from 5 months to 46 years of age; approximately two-thirds are women. Three of eight women in one series were 22 to 28 weeks pregnant during their illness. The apparent predilection for women may relate to exposure to contaminated food or work in hospitals rather than to differences in susceptibility. The onset of illness was described by most patients as insidious. The most frequent initial symptoms are fever (100 percent), chilliness and true rigors, headache (50 percent), malaise (100 percent), and myalgia (50 percent). Most patients did not seek medical attention for 4 to 9 days after onset. Symptoms of a systemic viral illness then developed with anorexia, nausea, vomiting, myalgia, and pain in the chest, epigastrium, and lumbar area. Headache was usually present. Early examination reveals fever and flushing of the face and V area of the neck. Pharyngitis developed early and became progressively more severe during the first week; examination may reveal raised patches of whitish exudate occurring on the palatine arches which occasionally coalesce into a pseudomembrane. Oral ulcerations have been noted in up to one-half of cases. Generalized nontender lymphadenopathy occurred in one-half of patients. During the second week severe lower abdominal pain and intractable vomiting are common, and facial and neck swelling with conjunctival edema and infection frequently develop. Occasionally patients have tinnitus, epistaxis, bleeding from the gums and venapuncture sites, maculopapular rashes, cough, and dizziness. During the acute stage, systolic blood pressures of less than 90 mmHg with pulse pressures of less than 20 mmHg occurred in 60 to 80 percent of patients. Initially, relative bradycardia was common. During the second week, the patients who recovered defervesced, while the patients who died often developed signs of shock, clouding of the sensorium, rales, signs of pleural effusion, agitation and, on occasion, grand mal seizures. The duration of illness in surviving patients ranged from 7 to 31 days (average 15 days), while that in fatal cases was 7 to 26 days (average 12 days). The mortality rates in Jos and Zorzor were 52 percent and 36 percent, respectively, while in Sierra Leone the rate was 8 percent. During convalescence occasional flurries of rapid involuntary eye movements (oculogyric crises) occurred. Late sequelae include deafness in a number of patients (two of six in one series) and alopecia in one patient.

Laboratory features The hematologic findings include relatively normal hematocrit values and early leukopenia (less than 4000 cells per cubic millimeter in 36 percent) with a relative neutrophilia and immature forms of leukocytes. In two cases in which it was recorded, the erythrocyte sedimentation rate was normal. Urinalyses revealed proteinuria, which was often massive. Chest radiographs may suggest basilar pneumonitis and pleural effusions. Electrocardiographic abnormalities compatible with diffuse myocardial disease have been encountered. Levels of serum enzymes, serum glutamic oxaloacetic transaminase (SGOT), creatinine phosphokinase (CPK), and lactic dehydrogenase (LDH) have been elevated. Lassa virus has been recovered from cerebrospinal fluid in two patients.

Diagnosis Diagnosis may be made quickly by staining conjunctival scrapings with fluorescent labelled anti-Lassa antiserums. Confirmation involves growth of the virus in tissue culture and a complement fixation test; however, the latter is rarely positive before the fourteenth day of illness.

Treatment The management has been supportive. Infusion of immune plasma from convalescent patients resulted in a dramatic effect in three of four patients. Because of the self-limited nature of the disease, these results cannot be assessed easily. In view of the hospital association and the presence of virus in pharyngeal secretions and urine, strict isolation is required. Known contacts should be kept under medical surveillance for at least 3 weeks.

REFERENCES

BAUM SG et al: Epidemic non-meningitic lymphocytic-choriomeningitis virus infection. N Engl J Med 274:934, 1966

CASALS J: Arenaviruses. Yale J Biol Med 48:115, 1975

DENNIS LH, CONRAD ME: Accelerated intravascular coagulation in a patient with Korean hemorrhagic fever. Arch Intern Med 121:499, 1968

FARMER TW, JANEWAY CA: Infections with the virus of lymphocytic choriomeningitis. Medicine 21:1, 1942

FRAME JD et al: Lassa fever, a new virus disease of man from West Africa: I. Clinical description and pathological findings. Am J Trop Med Hyg 19:670, 1970

GREISMAN SE: Capillary observations in patients with hemorrhagic fever and other infectious illnesses. J Clin Invest 36:1688, 1957

HIRSCH MS et al: Lymphocytic choriomeningitis infection traced to a pet hamster. N Engl J Med 291:610, 1974

JOHNSON KM et al: Hemorrhagic fever of Southeast Asia and South America. A comparative approach. Prog Med Virol 9:105, 1967

LEE HW et al: Isolation of the etiologic agent of Korean Hemorrhagic Fever. J Infect Dis 137:298, 1978

MACKENZIE RB et al: Epidemic hemorrhagic fever in Bolivia: I. A preliminary report of the epidemiologic and clinical findings in a new epidemic area in South America. Am J Trop Med Hyg 13:620, 1964

MERTENS PE et al: Clinical presentation of Lassa fever cases during the hospital epidemic at Zorzor, Liberia, March–April 1972. Am J Trop Med Hyg 22:780, 1973

MEYER HM JR et al: Central nervous syndromes of "viral" etiology: Study of 713 cases. Am J Med 29:334, 1960

MONATH TP et al: Lassa fever in the Eastern Province of Sierra Leone, 1970–1972: II. Clinical observations and virological studies on selected hospital cases. Am J Trop Med Hyg 23:1140, 1974

POWELL GM: Hemorrhagic fever. A study of 300 cases. Medicine 33:97, 1954

RUBINI ME et al: Renal residuals of acute epidemic hemorrhagic fever. Arch Intern Med 106:378, 1960

SHEEDY JA et al: The clinical course of epidemic hemorrhagic fever. Am J Med 16:619, 1954

VANZEE BE et al: Lymphocytic choriomeningitis in University hospital personnel. Clinical features. Am J Med 58:803, 1975

ZWEIGHAFT RM et al: Lassa fever: Response to an imported case. N Engl J Med 297:803, 1977

192

DISEASES CAUSED BY SLOW VIRUSES

DONALD H. HARTER

Slow virus diseases are characterized by a long asymptomatic period, often on the order of months or years, between the introduction of the infectious agent and the appearance of clinical illness.

The factors responsible for this protracted incubation period have not been defined. Viruses causing slow infections do not appear to have any unique or common features, and the slowness of the disease may be due in large measure to the manner in which the host reacts or accommodates to the virus.

Some slow viruses provoke a conventional inflammatory response during the time they are clinically silent; others are able to reside within cells for long periods without causing detectable cytopathic changes. The role of immunity in slow virus infection is largely unknown. Some slow virus infections occur in the presence of elevated levels of circulating antibodies; in others, there may be no detectable immune response. Viruses such as poliovirus and echovirus, which ordinarily cause a rapidly evolving illness, cause persistent or chronic infections of the central nervous system in immunodeficient patients.

In animals, slow viruses are known to produce a variety of pulmonary, hepatic, renal, and neurologic disorders. In addition to viral hepatitis, there are five definitely identified slow virus infections of human beings. These are five infrequently encountered neurologic diseases: *kuru, Creutzfeldt-Jakob disease, progressive multifocal leukoencephalopathy, subacute sclerosing panencephalitis,* and *progressive rubella encephalitis.* Kuru and Creutzfeldt-Jakob disease share common neuropathologic features and are referred to as the *subacute spongiform virus encephalopathies.* Although these diseases have been shown to be of infectious etiology by the transmission of neurologic illness to higher primates, the causative agents are still incompletely characterized. Viruses have been recovered from the nervous system of patients with subacute sclerosing panencephalitis, progressive multifocal leukoencephalopathy, and progressive rubella encephalitis, but the pathogenesis of these disorders is still largely unknown. At present, there is no consistently effective therapy for any of the five diseases.

KURU Kuru, or "trembling with fear," is a progressive and fatal neurologic disorder which occurs exclusively among natives of the New Guinea Highland.

Difficulty in walking is usually the first sign of kuru. This usually progresses from a minor disturbance in gait rhythm to marked side-to-side lurching and staggering. Eventually, ambulation becomes incoordinated, and the patient is unable to use his or her limbs. As the disease progresses, cerebellar involvement (intention tremor, inability to perform rapid alternating movements, slurring of speech, hypotonia), abnormal involuntary movements resembling myoclonus, athetosis, or chorea, and convergent strabismus appear. There are no blood or cerebrospinal fluid abnormalities. Dementia develops in the later phases of the disease. The illness terminates fatally in 4 to 24 months, usually from decubitus ulcers or bronchopneumonia. Approximately 80 percent of adults afflicted with the disease are women. The incubation period may be more than 30 years in older patients.

Pathologic changes are limited to the central nervous system and include widespread neuronal loss, intense astrocytic and microglial proliferation, loss of myelinated fibers, and the presence of plaque-like bodies. Perivascular cuffing by lymphocytes and mononuclear cells has been observed occasionally.

It was the close similarity between the neuropathologic and clinical findings found in kuru and in scrapie, a slow infectious disease to sheep, that suggested the possibility that kuru was caused by a virus or other infectious agent. The infectious origin of kuru was confirmed subsequently by the appearance of a kuru-like syndrome in chimpanzees 10 to 82 months after intracerebral inoculation of suspensions of brain from human cases. Disease has also been produced in chimpanzees by inoculation of tissues other than brain. The clinical illness in chimpanzees lasts 3 to 11 months. The disease has also been successfully transmitted to a number of New World and Old World monkeys as well as to minks and ferrets. Although a number of known and novel viruses have been recovered from tissue explants prepared from chimpanzees with the kuru syndrome, the specific agent responsible for the disease has not been fully characterized.

Cannibalism has been considered as the probable mode of transmission of kuru. Native custom in New Guinea dictates that marrow, viscera, and brain be cooked and eaten. The agent may be introduced by conjunctival, nasal, or skin contamination during the practice of ritual cannibalism. The marked predilection of kuru for the adult female may be explained by the observation that cannibalism appears more prevalent among women and that males who practice cannibalism seldom eat the bodies of women. The recent influx of foreign settlers into the kuru area has led to increasing rejection of cannibalistic practices, and this, in turn, may be responsible for the progressive decline in the number of cases of kuru since 1960. Oral feeding of kuru brain to chimpanzees has not yet been reported to produce disease.

CREUTZFELDT-JAKOB DISEASE Creutzfeldt-Jakob disease is a fatal degenerative disease of the central nervous system which afflicts persons between 40 and 60 years of age and presents as a rapidly evolving dementia with myoclonic seizures. Unlike kuru, the disease is not geographically limited.

Although Creutzfeldt-Jakob disease may have a diverse clinical presentation, it is usually first manifested by organic mental changes similar to those seen in the presenile dementias. The earliest changes include impairment of reasoning and judgment, memory disturbances, and bizarre behavior. The patient may complain of headaches and distortions in the shape and appearance of objects. Hallucinations, delusional ideas, and confusion occur as the disease progresses, and myoclonic movements and convulsive episodes develop. Ataxia, dysarthria, muscular atrophy, and other signs of anterior horn cell damage may be noted in some cases. Spasticity and rigidity appear later. About 10 percent of cases show a familial pattern of inheritance. The disease progresses rapidly to death within 3 to 12 months, often from intercurrent infection. There are no abnormalities in the cerebrospinal fluid, but the electroencephalogram is usually abnormal.

The cerebrum and cerebellum are affected predominantly. Widespread status spongiosus in gray matter and intense gliosis are seen. Vacuoles are located within the neuropil, within and around neurons. There is a marked proliferation of astrocytes and disappearance of nerve cells. Inflammatory changes are absent. In the spinal cord, anterior horn cells may be damaged or lost, and there may be degeneration of the corticospinal tracts.

A neurologic disease with the clinical and pathologic features of Creutzfeldt-Jakob disease occurs in chimpanzees 11 to 71 months after inoculation with brain suspensions from patients with Creutzfeldt-Jakob disease. It is also possible to transmit the disease to monkeys, the domestic cat, and guinea pigs. The agent persists for many months in tissue cultures of human brain cells without loss of virulence. Neutralizing antibodies to the Creutzfeldt-Jakob agent have not yet been demonstrated in the serums of patients with the disease of primates with the experimental disease.

There is an unexpectedly high incidence of previous brain or eye operations among patients with Creutzfeldt-Jakob disease. Human-to-human transmission has occurred by corneal transplantation and by implantation of contaminated stereotactic electroencephalographic electrodes after an incubation period of 15 to 20 months.

The Creutzfeldt-Jakob agent has been found in lymph nodes, liver, kidney, spleen, lung, cornea, and cerebrospinal fluid of patients afflicted with the disorder. The agent is also present in leukocytes of infected guinea pigs.

Exposure to breath, saliva, nasopharyngeal secretions, urine, or feces of the Creutzfeldt-Jakob patient should not be of special concern, but the patient's blood or cerebrospinal fluid should be considered a potential source of infection. Maximum caution should be taken to avoid accidental percutaneous exposure to blood and cerebrospinal fluid or tissue. Guidelines for the handling of materials from patients with these disorders have been developed. These should be rigorously applied to all patients who have evidence of intellectual deterioration, particularly if it is associated with myoclonic activity, when no space-occupying lesion is demonstrated in the brain.

PROGRESSIVE MULTIFOCAL LEUKOENCEPHALOPATHY This rare neurologic condition, first described in 1958, usually occurs in patients who have leukemia, malignant lymphomas, carcinomatosis, immunosuppressive therapy, or a variety of other chronic disease processes. The disease is consistently associated with disorders of cell-mediated immunity in which deficits in humoral antibody response may or may not coexist.

The disease affects adults of both sexes, and its duration from onset of symptoms to death is 1 to 4 months. The neurologic signs and symptoms show diffuse, asymmetric involvement of the cerebral hemispheres. Hemiplegia, hemianopsia, aphasia or dysarthria, and organic mental changes are frequent; visual field abnormalities and complete or incomplete transverse myelitis may develop. Headache and convulsive seizures are rare, but electroencephalographic abnormalities consisting of diffuse or focal abnormalities are often present. White matter lesions may be recognized in computerized tomographic brain scans. Cerebrospinal fluid is normal in most cases.

The pathologic changes consist of multiple areas of demyelination with little or no perivascular infiltration. The presence of distinctive intranuclear inclusions in oligodendrocytes first suggested that the disease was of a viral etiology. Electron microscopic observations show the intranuclear inclusion bodies to be composed of closely packed spheres, which have the physical dimensions and properties of the polyomavirus genus of the papovaviruses.

By employing tissue cultures derived from human fetal brain it has been possible to recover a new human polyomavirus serotype (JC virus) from the brains of patients with progressive multifocal leukoencephalopathy. A variant of SV40 virus has been incriminated as the causative agent in a few cases. Abundant numbers of virus particles are present in brain. Rapid identification of the virus in brain is possible using fluorescence antibody staining or electron microscopic agglutination with monospecific hyperimmune rabbit serum. Serologic diagnosis using the patient's serum is unreliable.

The virus has not been demonstrated in tissues other than brain; the disease has not been transmitted to animals.

There are isolated reports of clinical remission with cytosine arabinoside, or adenine arabinoside, but viral infection may remain active despite clinical improvement.

Progressive multifocal leukoencephalopathy may result from the activation of a polyomavirus which has been latent in brain or other tissues since childhood infection. Alternatively, there may be certain individuals who fail to acquire immunity in childhood and have their first encounter with the virus when a disease which interferes with cell-mediated immunity develops. The demyelination which occurs may be related to virus-induced damage of oligodendroglia, cells which appear to be required for the normal maintenance of myelin.

SUBACUTE SCLEROSING PANENCEPHALITIS (INCLUSION-BODY ENCEPHALITIS)

This progressively fatal disease of children and adolescents has been suspected to be of viral origin since its initial description by Dawson in 1932. Measles virus or a virus very closely related to measles virus has been recovered from the brains of patients with the disease. The disorder may be considered to be a "slow" form of measles encephalitis.

Subacute sclerosing panencephalitis occurs between 4 and 20 years of age; 80 percent of patients are under 11. The disease affects boys three to ten times as frequently as girls. The incidence of the disease has fallen recently. Most patients are from rural areas or small towns. They are entirely well until the disease begins. Onset is usually insidious, and mental deterioration, often expressed by a decline in the patient's schoolwork, is the presenting symptom. Incoordination, ataxia, and myoclonic jerks develop along with abnormalities of the pyramidal and extrapyramidal motor systems. Cortical blindness, papilledema, and optic atrophy may be present, and focal chorioretinitis has been described. A few cases have occurred in association with infectious mononucleosis.

The patient becomes bedridden within 6 to 9 months. Death occurs from superimposed pulmonary or urinary tract infections or from decubiti. Signs of meningeal irritation do not occur.

The cerebrospinal fluid gamma-globulin level, as determined by electrophoresis, quantitative immunochemical assay, or colloidal gold curve, is elevated, but the fluid is otherwise normal. The electroencephalogram typically shows a "burst suppression" pattern characterized by synchronous and symmetric spike and high-voltage slow wave activity. Elevated levels of measles antibody are found in serum and cerebrospinal fluid. Brain biopsy may be required to make a definitive antemortem diagnosis.

Pathologic findings include round-cell infiltration about small cerebral arteries and veins, intranuclear and intracytoplasmic inclusions in neurons and glial cells, and varying degrees of demyelination.

Measles virus is now considered to be the etiologic agent. Electron microscopic studies show that the intranuclear inclusions in brain cells are composed of hollow tubular filaments resembling paramyxovirus internal nucleocapsid component. Staining of brain tissue from patients with the disease demonstrates measles virus antigen in the inclusions. An agent serologically identical with measles virus and having measles virus properties has been recovered from brain by cocultivating cell cultures originated from brain tissue with established laboratory cell lines.

Attempts to transmit the disease to animals have met with variable results. Ferrets inoculated with suspensions of brain from patients with the disease develop a nonfatal neurologic disorder with electroencephalographic changes.

Subacute sclerosing panencephalitis appears many years after the patient's initial experience with rubeola. There is evidence that subacute sclerosing panencephalitis patients have clinical measles at an unusually early age. A few reported cases may have been related to measles vaccination. The risk of subacute sclerosing panencephalitis following measles vaccination appears to be less, however, than the risk following natural measles. The disorder appears to represent an unusual response of the nervous system to measles infection. It is possible that the virus is present in a defective form or that a carrier state is produced wherein cells may continue to elaborate intracellular viral antigen without producing detectable amounts of mature infective virus. Similar virus-cell interactions may be important in the development of other diseases of the central nervous system such as parkinsonism and multiple sclerosis.

PROGRESSIVE RUBELLA ENCEPHALITIS

A chronic progressive encephalitis developing in the second decade of life and sharing some of the features of subacute sclerosing panencephalitis has been described in patients with congenital rubella.

Deterioration of mental and motor functions begins after a stable period of 10 or more years. The cerebrospinal fluid has an increased cell count and the protein and IgG levels are elevated. High titers of antibody to rubella virus can be detected in both serum and cerebrospinal fluid. Rubella virus has been recovered from the brain by use of the cocultivation technique.

Unlike subacute sclerosing panencephalitis, patients with rubella panencephalitis have the stigmata of congenital rubella before the onset of progressive disease. Myoclonus is less constant, and the electroencephalogram does not show the "burst suppression" observed in subacute sclerosing panencephalitis. Histologic examination of the brain shows mineralization, but not the inclusion bodies characteristically found in subacute sclerosing panencephalitis.

The progressive rubella encephalitis also resembles the rare cases of juvenile paresis which may occur in patients with congenital syphilis. The immune status of patients with this disorder has not been fully defined, and the pathogenesis of the disease remains obscure.

REFERENCES

AGNARSDÓTTIR G: Subacute sclerosing panencephalitis, in *Recent Advances in Clinical Virology*, AP Waterson (ed). Churchill Livingstone, Edinburgh, 1977, chap 2, p 21

FREEMAN JM: The clinical spectrum and early diagnosis of Dawson's encephalitis. J Pediatr 75:590, 1969

GAJDUSEK DC: Unconventional viruses and the origin and disappearance of Kuru. Science 197:943, 1977

———— et al: Precautions in medical care of, and in handling materials from, patients with transmissible virus dementia (Creutzfeldt-Jakob disease). N Engl J Med 297:1253, 1977

MEULEN V TER et al: Subacute sclerosing panencephalitis: A review. Curr Top Microbiol Immunol 57:1, 1972

MODLIN JF et al: Epidemiologic studies of measles, measles vaccine and subacute sclerosing panencephalitis. Pediatrics 59:505, 1977

PADGETT BL et al: JC papovavirus in progressive multifocal leukoencephalopathy. J Infect Dis 133:686, 1976

RICHARDSON EP: Progressive multifocal leukoencephalopathy. N Engl J Med 265:815, 1961

ROOS R et al: The clinical characteristic of transmissible Creutzfeldt-Jakob disease. Brain 96:1, 1973

WEIL ML et al: Chronic progressive panencephalitis due to rubella virus simulating subacute sclerosing panencephalitis. N Engl J Med 292:994, 1975

ZURHEIN GM: Association of papova-virions with a human demyelinating disease (progressive multifocal leukoencephalopathy). Prog Med Virol 11:185, 1969

Herpesviruses

193
INFECTIONS WITH HERPES SIMPLEX VIRUS

A. MARTIN LERNER

Herpes simplex virus types 1 and 2 (HSV1, HSV2), sometimes known as *herpesvirus hominis,* establishes diverse relations with humans. Acute disseminated primary infection (gingivostomatitis), chronic infection with continued or intermittent virus shedding (herpes keratitis and herpes labialis), and clinical reactivation occur. Virus multiplies in many tissues, including lymphocytes, and by its intracellular locus is able to escape anti-HSV antibodies. Herpes simplex virus antibody complexes may be infectious, and when this is the case, are called "sensitized virus." Interactions with the complement system are important in neutralizing sensitized virus. Since the decline of poliomyelitis with the development of an effective vaccine, herpes simplex virus encephalitis is the most frequent endemic encephalitis in this country. Type 2 herpes simplex virus is the second most frequent sexually transmitted disease (after gonorrhea). It has been associated with carcinoma of the cervix, but the etiologic association has not been proved.

ETIOLOGY The virus particle consists of DNA, protein, lipid, and carbohydrate. On an average there are 100 parts DNA, 25 parts carbohydrate, and 320 parts phospholipid to 1000 parts protein. Virus DNA is double-stranded with densities of 1.727 (type 1) and 1.729 (type 2). The molecular weight of the virion is about 100×10^6 daltons. By phosphotungstic acid staining on electron microscopy the virion is seen to consist of a roughly spheric central area or "core" of DNA which measures 75 nm in diameter, and a stable "capsid" which measures 100 nm in diameter; it appears to be an icosahedron with a 5:3:2 axial symmetry consisting of 162 capsomeres (9 to 10 nm by 12 to 13.5 nm) of which 150 are hexagonal and 12 pentagonal in cross section, and a surrounding envelope derived from host cell membranes, 145 to 200 nm. Particles appear with or without envelopes [enveloped and/or with or without cores ("full" or "empty")].

Although complete virions are more efficient, both "enveloped" and "naked" particles can infect cells. Phagocytosis of virions by susceptible cells, viropexis, precedes the digestion of virus envelopes and proteins. After initiation of infection, virus absorption is complete in 3 h. New virus infectivity rises sharply from the sixth to the ninth hour, when it levels off. Viral DNA enters the nucleus where new virus DNA is synthesized. Virus proteins are synthesized in the cytoplasm and migrate to the nucleus. The complete virion has a triple-layered envelope. The inner envelope is made within the nucleus, while the second and third are formed by evagination processes at the nuclear and cytoplasmic membranes, respectively. Host materials make up major portions of the envelope. An infected cell may produce about 1000 virus particles, but only 5 to 10 percent are infectious.

BIOLOGIC CHARACTERISTICS By means of neutralization kinetics, hyperimmune unitypic serums in conventional neutralization tests or direct immunofluorescent methods, strains of herpes simplex virus can be readily typed. Type 1 strains are recovered from the eye, nasopharynx, skin (other than thigh or buttocks), and brain in cases of postnatal encephalitis. Type 2 strains are usually related to the adult genital tract. Isolates have been recovered from the penis, cervix, endocervix, vagina, vulva, skin (usually, but not always below the waist), and spinal fluid. In infections of the newborn, HSV2 has been recovered from brain, liver, adrenal, and lung.

Optimal virus isolation occurs in rabbit or baby hamster kidney and human foreskin tissue cultures. Cytopathic effects are usually evident within 72 h after inoculation. However, when isolation of virus by brain biopsy is attempted, trypsinized suspensions of cells, rather than ground tissue suspensions, should be planted, both for primary growth and for cocultivation with HSV-susceptible tissue cultures. Typical of in vitro and in vivo cytopathic effects is the type A inclusion of Cowdry, an eosinophilic mass surrounded by a halo in a nucleus with marginated chromatin (Fig. 193-1).

In addition to site of recovery, a number of other properties separate type 1 from type 2 herpes simplex virus: HSV2 produces (1) larger pocks on the chorioallantoic membrane of embryonated eggs, (2) greater virulence in female mice which have been infected by the genital route, and (3) greater tendency toward formation of giant cells in tissue cultures. These strains also exhibit (4) difference in density and base composition of DNA and (5) antigenic distinctiveness. Likewise, (6) minimal inhibitory concentrations (MIC) of idoxuridine (IDU; 5-iodo-2′-deoxyuridine) for type 1 strains are 6.25 µg/ml, while similar values for type 2 herpesviruses are 62.5 µg/ml.

IMMUNOLOGY Following primary exposure to herpes simplex virus, humoral antibodies appear. Different polypeptides of the virus capsid probably stimulate distinct antibodies which rise and fall, describing separate kinetic curves. In contrast to other antibodies, such as conventional neutralizing, complement-fixing, and passive hemagglutination antibodies, complement-requiring neutralizing antibodies peak during the acute phase of primary infections with HSV1 and fall during convalescence.

After initial exposure IgM antibodies appear in serum within 1 week. In respiratory secretions IgA antibodies form. In cases of encephalitis, antibodies which are produced locally can be measured in cerebrospinal fluid. Seven days after infection IgG antibodies appear in serum, and antiherpesvirus IgM synthesis decreases. Complement-fixing antibodies appear in 14 days. After an initial exposure, complement-fixing antibodies fall to low levels within several months, while neutralizing antibodies persist for many years. Reactivations of infection evoke variable rises in serums of conventional neutralizing or complement-fixing IgG antibodies. There are some low-titered cross-reactions when anti-HSV antibodies are measured against varicella-zoster or cytomegalovirus.

Cellular immunity is also stimulated and may be the more important factor in inhibiting virus multiplication and relapse. Techniques for quantitating cell-mediated responses are being developed but are not yet routinely available.

CLINICAL FINDINGS: HSV1 Primary infection with HSV1 causes *acute gingivostomatitis, rhinitis, keratoconjunctivitis, me-*

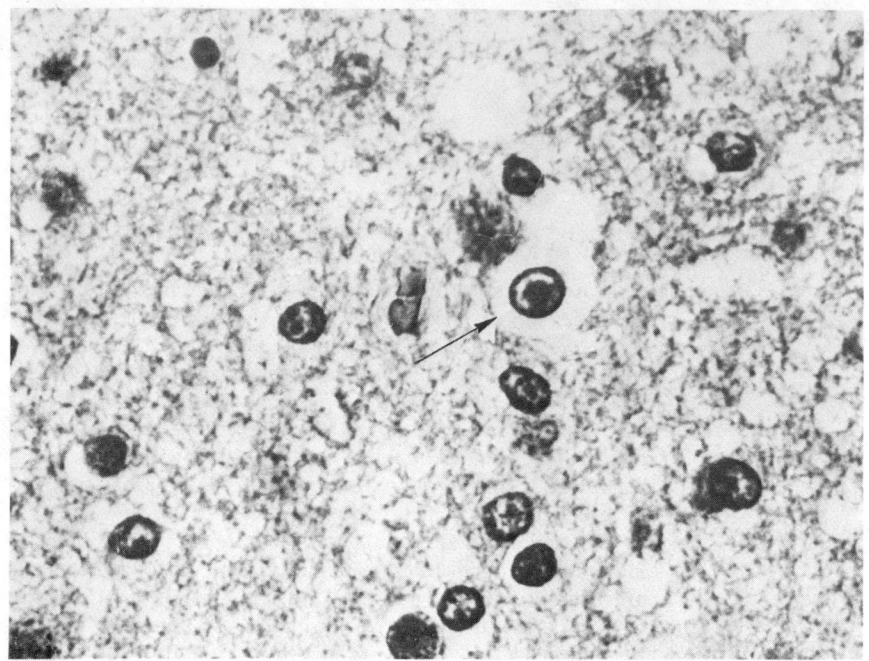

FIGURE 193-1

Cowdry type A ("owl-eye") intranuclear inclusions are seen in this hematoxylin-eosin section (600 ×) in the brain of a patient with encephalitis (arrow). [From ESE Hafez et al (eds), The Human Vagina in Health and Disease, Amsterdam, Elsevier/North-Holland, 1978, with permission.]

ningoencephalitis, *eczema herpeticum* (Kaposi's varicelliform eruption), and *traumatic herpes,* including *herpetic whitlow* and *generalized cutaneous herpes simplex* in burned patients or wrestlers (*herpes gladiatorum*). In immunosuppressed patients initial infection or clinical reactivation may induce esophageal ulceration or interstitial pneumonia.

The incubation period is 2 to 12 days, averaging 6 or 7 days. The route of infection is contact with infected skin or mucosal surfaces. There is little or no evidence to support respiratory contagion by droplets or their dehydrated nuclei. During acute herpetic gingivostomatitis there are fever, irritability, red swollen gums, a vesicular eruption on the mucous membranes of the mouth, oral fetor, and local submaxillary adenopathy. A visit to the dentist may precede an attack. Any portion of the oral mucosa may be affected. Viremia during which the virus is free in plasma or is limited to mononuclear cells may occur. A generalized vesicular eruption may follow and appear in crops. Lesions are generally smaller than those of varicella. In the eczematous infant or adult (Kaposi's varicelliform eruption), large quantities of fluid, electrolytes, and protein may be lost.

Within the tense vesicles is a clear fluid. An impression smear of an opened vesicle demonstrates syncytial giant cells undergoing ballooning degeneration (Fig. 193-2). Intranuclear inclusions are seen. Virus is readily isolated from the fluid; no bacteria are seen by Gram's stain, and none may be cultured. Later, vesicles collapse and ulcerate. Sometimes the nose is the site of primary infection. Tiny vesicles surrounding reddened areolae appear in the nostrils. Usually, there is fever and the anterior cervical lymph nodes enlarge.

Patients contaminate their fingers or those of hospital personnel by introducing infected secretions through unnoticed abrasions, producing *herpetic whitlow* in persons without previous experience with HSV. *Herpetic paronychia* may be caused by HSV1 or HSV2. Painful deep vesicles appear suddenly and spread locally for about a week. The nail may be separated from its matrix by a lesion at its base. Recrudescent relapses may occur at any time, but the initial infection seems to occur in immunologically "virgin" persons. The importance of wearing rubber gloves when working about the mouth and of handwashing in prevention of infection is obvious.

Follicular conjunctivitis (often unilateral) with chemosis, edema of the lids, and conjunctival ulcers may be seen. The cornea may be involved in primary or recurrent infections; most of these infections are due to HSV1. When the cornea is affected, a diffuse epitheliolitis develops with superficial punctate erosions which extend into small dendritic ulcers. If untreated, this ulcer increases in size to form a large, anesthetic "geographic" ulcer. Erosions of the cornea recur. *Deeper interstitial keratitis* with secondary bacterial invasion, hypopyon, iridocyclitis, synechia, and opacification of the lens follows.

Others with preexisting neutralizing antibodies in serums may suffer *recurrent attacks of herpes labialis* or trigeminal neuralgia. Pneumococcal and meningococcal, but not gram-negative infections; menstruation; emotional upset; and other little-understood events seem to trigger recurrent localized episodes. Quiescence and recurrences of herpes labialis may be associated with alternating low and higher titers of virus shedding, but reactivation of latent infection also occurs. In the prodromal and erythema stages of herpes labialis mean virus titers are $< 10^1$ PFU (plaque-forming unit), but when vesiculation occurs 24 h later, fluids contain $10^{4.7}$ PFU of HSV. Herpes simplex virus resides in a quiescent state within sacral or trigeminal ganglia for years, intermittently releasing virus along nerve fibers. After traversing the axon, HSV reaches the skin, and vesiculation occurs.

Encephalitis Occasionally, and for ill-defined reasons, HSV1 begins an ascent from the respiratory epithelium of the nose up the olfactory tract to reach the frontal and temporal areas of the brain. An often fatal or severely damaging necrotizing encephalitis results. The immediate mortality of patients with seizures and paralysis who are in coma is about 38 percent, but the majority of the survivors are severely impaired and unable to live productive lives.

Patients of any age, either sex, and of any socioeconomic status may be affected. About 15 percent of patients who develop herpes simplex virus encephalitis have histories of recurrent herpes labialis. Prodromal illnesses begin 3 to 4 days before admission to the hospital. Various combinations of headache, rhinorrhea, sore throat, fever, nausea, or vomiting are noted. Less frequently photophobia, vertigo, insomnia, or anorexia occurs. One-third of the patients develop concurrent fever blisters during the course of their illness. Personality changes, lethargy, or seizures necessitate hospitalization, but only a few (3 of 15 brain-biopsy-proved cases) have paralysis

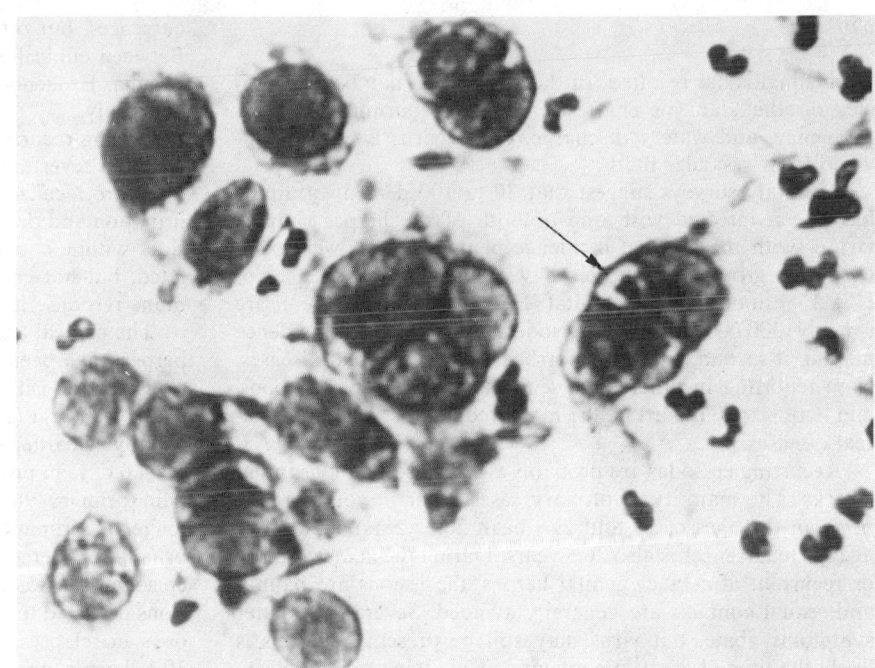

FIGURE 193-2

Characteristic intranuclear inclusion bodies of herpes simplex virus infection along with exfoliated multi- and single nucleated cells are shown (high power magnification). Note "ground glass" appearance of nuclear inclusion with peripheral rim of nuclear chromatin (arrow) or scattered polymorphonuclear leukocytes seen in the background. This is a Tzanck impression smear which may be obtained from an opened cutaneous vesicle or from the cervix. (From JW Regan, SF Patten, Cytology of the Female Reproductive Tract, Chicago, American Society of Clinical Pathologists, 1966, with permission.)

or coma at the time of hospitalization. The occurrence of paralysis and coma indicates that irreparable neurologic injury has occurred. In order of frequency, disorientation, personality change, hallucinations, photophobia, ataxia, facial weakness, incontinence of stool or urine, tremors, and amnesia appear. Patients with proved herpes simplex virus encephalitis have been mistaken for inebriates or psychotics. Neurologic signs include stupor, seizures (Jacksonian or generalized), coma, extensor plantar reflexes, nuchal rigidity, motor deficit, cranial nerve palsies, sensory deficit, decorticate and decerebrate posture, abnormal conjugate deviation of eyes, frontal lobe signs (glabella, snout, sucking), asymmetric deep tendon reflexes, and dysphasia. Coma (absence of response to all stimuli) indicates an ominous prognosis.

Leukocyte counts average 13,000 per cubic millimeter with a shift to the left. Cerebrospinal fluid samples are completely normal or contain only a few to several hundred leukocytes which may be predominantly mononuclear or polymorphonuclear. Grossly bloody spinal fluid is an ominous sign of far-advanced disease. Cerebrospinal fluid protein is normal or elevated as high as 250 mg per 100 ml. Glucose in cerebrospinal fluid is usually normal but may be low. In every case electroencephalograms are diffusely abnormal, or show focal lesions in the temporal or frontal regions. The abnormal electroencephalogram is an especially important finding, particularly in cases in which the cerebrospinal fluid is normal. Computerized tomography (CT scans) or carotid angiograms are indicated to rule out an epidural, subdural, or intracerebral hematoma, abscess, or tumor. In a few cases of HSV1 encephalitis, the focal hemorrhagic necrotic mass deviates carotid vessels, and craniotomy may be necessary for differentiation and diagnosis. Significant rises in HSV antibodies in serum do not determine the diagnosis of encephalitis caused by this virus because rises in these antibodies occur nonspecifically with bacterial pneumonias or bacterial meningitis and in uncomplicated herpes labialis and other conditions. Cowdry type A ("owl-eye") intranuclear inclusions may be demonstrated in the brain (Fig. 193-1). Attempts at isolation of other (e.g., enteroviruses) viruses from throat or rectal swabs, urine, and cerebrospinal fluid as well as, when possible, from brain, spinal cord, and vesicular fluid should be made. Paired serums should be tested for high titers of antibody against mumps virus or other agents known to be prevalent at the time of infection.

Isolation of HSV by brain biopsy is the only definitive means of diagnosing HSV encephalitis. Brain biopsy must be done as soon after admission to the hospital as possible before the onset of irreversible paralysis or coma, because if intravenous therapy with adenine arabinoside (ara-A) is begun before the onset of coma, full recovery may occur. Efforts toward earlier definitive nonsurgical diagnosis of HSV encephalitis continue. For example, serial concomitant paired serums (S) and cerebrospinal fluids (CSF) were taken from 8 patients with biopsy-proved HSV encephalitis. These specimen pairs were compared to 28 others from patients with various neurologic conditions. Both before and after reduction with 2-mercaptoethanol, a ratio of S to CSF antibody titers of ≤ 20 with either the passive hemagglutinating (PHA) or immune adherence hemagglutinating (IAHA) antibody tests occurred in three patients prior to biopsy of the brain, and in four patients by the tenth day of neurologic disease. Among controls, a ratio of S to CSF titers >20 was observed in all but four patients, each of whom had easily distinguishable neurologic diagnoses (e.g., HSV2 meningitis, active multiple sclerosis, varicella zoster encephalitis). This work is promising, but it would be better if HSV antigen could be detected in CSF earlier in the course of the disease. Another, perhaps more promising approach, is the early detection of virus-specific glycoproteins in the CSF.

CLINICAL FINDINGS: HSV2 Infection with HSV, type 2, is usually sexually transmitted. In one study seven of eight female contacts of men with penile herpetic infection showed evidence of current HSV genital infection. Similarly, 63 out of 64 HSV isolates from male genitalia and 155 of 162 from the female genital tract were HSV2. This infection is the most common cause of genital vesicles and/or ulcers found in women, and is second only to primary syphilis as the cause of such lesions in males. Teenagers make up one-fourth to one-half of patients with genital herpetic infections.

Neutralizing antibodies to HSV2 are reported to be present in 35.7 percent of patients who subsequently develop carcinoma in situ of the cervix, and are found in only 7.1 percent of matched controls. However, an etiologic relation between carcinoma of the cervix and infection with HSV2 is not established.

During primary infections fever, malaise, and inguinal adenopathy may be seen and viremia may follow. A benign aseptic meningitis has resulted. In the male there may be tiny vesicles on the glans or shaft of the penis, burning, urgency, frequency, and watery discharge. Herpesvirus is easily cultivated from vesicular fluids.

Antibody surveys suggest that 30 to 100 percent of adults have been infected with one or both of the herpes simplex viruses with the greatest incidence being among lower socioeconomic groups. Prostitutes have the highest frequency of HSV2 antibodies. For genital HSV2 infections, there are roughly 300,000 reported episodes each year, an incidence making it second only to gonorrhea among venereal diseases. Case reporting in other than venereal disease clinics is poor, and herpes may indeed be the most frequent of all of the venereal diseases.

Recurring episodes are probably twice as common as initial attacks. The majority of primary cases occur in young adults between the ages of 19 and 27 (mean 26.5 years). The mean age for recurrences is also 26.5 years. During the acute primary or recurrent attacks of genital herpes, the lesions are painful and sexual contacts are generally avoided. Several days later symptoms abate, but virus may still be present, and this is likely the time of greatest contagion. The attack rate with sexual contact is one in three.

Following recovery from an original episode, no further attacks may occur, or recurrences may vary from occasional to frequent. The reasons for the variability in the clinical course are unknown. Viremia probably occurs only during initial episodes when serum antibody is absent. Following primary HSV2 infections, virus follows a retrograde course along sensory nerves to reach spinal dorsal, lumbar, or sacral ganglia. Here the virus remains in a latent stage until lapses in cell-mediated immunity allow retrograde release of virus along nerves to the previously involved sites upon the skin or mucous membrane. Recurrences frequently involve the same locus on skin or mucous membrane.

In women, within several days after sexual relations with an infected partner, paresthesia and burning of the vulva begin and dyspareunia, dysuria, and tenesmus set in. There may be fever, malaise, headache, neuralgia, and tender inguinal nodes as well.

On examination, the skin and mucous membranes of the vulva, genitocrural folds, perianal region, and cervix show crops of 0.5- to 1.5-cm reddened papules which progress to vesicles and then ulcers. The vagina and urethra are affected infrequently. The vesicles on the vaginal vestibule ulcerate within several days, while those on less traumatized or cornified surfaces progress more slowly. Lesions within the vagina consist of mucous patches with collapsed gray, slightly elevated epithelium. The cervix is eroded and may appear as a necrotizing mass with a clear profuse or irritating discharge. Following viremia, similar skin lesions appear at distant sites. A tender enlarged liver and nuchal rigidity attest to the mild hepatitis and benign aseptic meningitis which may accompany primary HSV2 infection in the postnatal period.

Over several days systemic signs resolve, but lesions may persist for weeks. Unless secondary bacterial infection follows, ultimately healing is complete without scarring. The subsequent course is variable: (1) some patients remain well and culture negative indefinitely; (2) others have recurring episodes of differing severity at varying intervals; and (3) still others become symptomatic or asymptomatic HSV2 carriers in their cervical secretions. These patients have an increased incidence of cervical dysplasia.

Approximately two of every three women with primary HSV2 genital infection suffer relapses. Fever, menstruation, and physical or emotional trauma seem important in some recurrences, but often no obvious inciting cause is recognized. Between clinical episodes the virus remains latent in sensory ganglia. Exogenous reinfection has also been documented occasionally.

During recurrence, the clinical findings are usually milder. Malaise, fever, and adenopathy are often absent and the lesions are localized, less painful, and less numerous. Pain on urination and defecation is absent, and the entire episode subsides within 7 to 10 days. The milder course reflects a stimulated, but not completely effective, humoral and cellular immune response to latent HSV2.

The clinical and laboratory findings in initial and recurrent herpes have been studied carefully. The mean number of lesions at first visit for initial (primary) episodes is 6.3, while it is 4.7 in recurrent (secondary) attacks, but patients sought medical advice earlier in relapses (2.5 days in secondary cases versus 4.6 days in primary cases). All attacks were associated with pain (primary, 96 percent; secondary, 89 percent), which lasted longer in primary episodes (13.0 versus 8.6 days). Virus was usually (87 percent) present in cervical secretions in primary episodes but was found rarely during relapses (4 percent). Lesions persisted for 16.6 days in primary attacks opposed to 10.5 days in relapses. During episodes new vesicles appeared for 10.1 days in primary, but for only 4.7 days in secondary disease. Virus could be recovered from lesions for 8.0 days (primary) versus 4.5 days, (secondary) and from the cervix for 11.4 days (primary) versus 3 days (secondary).

Cytomegalovirus, varicella zoster virus, variola virus, Behçet's disease, drug or contact dermatitis, autoimmune disorders, or infections with herpes simplex viruses may cause clusters of vulvovaginal vesicles or ulcers on an erythematous base. Cytologic examinations from open vesicles, the bases of ulcers, or the cervix (Fig. 193-2) and appropriate attempts at isolation or recognition of virus are necessary for the diagnosis. Comparison of antibody titers in paired serums is also useful in establishing the presence of herpes infection.

Tzanck smears are positive in preparations from fresh lesions in two of three cases. Multinucleated giant cells with or without intranuclear inclusions, epithelial cells, and lymphocytes are present. These findings do not differentiate HSV from varicella zoster virus infection. To perform a Tzanck test, several fresh vesicles are cleansed with alcohol, opened with a no. 22 needle, and a sterile cotton swab or wooden applicator is pressed to the base of the lesion. The swab is smeared onto several clean glass slides. Slides are immersed in 95% alcohol fixed as in Papanicolaou staining. For immunofluorescent staining for HSV2 antigen, slides are dried in air and fixed with acetone. Hematoxylin-eosin, Giemsa's, Papanicolaou's, Wright's, or Leishman's stains (Tzanck test) may be used.

Herpes simplex virus may be transferred from the vagina or cervix by the hand of patient or attendant to other areas of the skin or to the cornea (herpetic keratitis). Patients must be instructed concerning the importance of hand washing; medical personnel must wear gloves and gowns.

When *venereus herpes* occurs in the pregnant mother before the thirty-second week of gestation, the risk of neonatal infection is 10 percent, but when HSV2 is present at the time of delivery, 40 to 80 percent of the offspring are affected. Pregnant women with cytologically proven genital herpes during the first 20 weeks of gestation have a threefold increase in abortions. After the 20th week there is a slight increase in prematurity. In every case, effects upon the woman and fetus are most severe when the infection is a primary exposure.

Within 2 to 12 days after delivery, affected newborns may show conjunctivitis, keratitis, papulovesicular rashes, jaundice, cyanosis, seizures, and gastrointestinal bleeding, reflecting disseminated infection to the skin, eye, liver, central nervous system, adrenal glands, lungs, spleen, and bone marrow. Mortality in disseminated infection approaches 67 percent, and another 18 percent of the neonates survive, albeit with significant morbidity. Only 15 percent survive to develop as healthy babies.

Intrauterine transplacental congenital infection has been proved occasionally. The usual outcome is fetal death. However, mental retardation, microcephaly, microphthalmia, intracranial calcification, retinal dysplasia, and vesicles on the skin have been observed at the time of delivery. If HSV2 infection at the time of delivery is suspected clinically by Papanicolaou smear from the cervix or by culture of HSV2, delivery by cesarean section prior to rupture of the fetal membranes is indicated.

TREATMENT Neither a killed nor attenuated vaccine has been shown to be effective. When there is a history of recurrent herpetic vulvovaginitis coupled with a clinical exacerbation at term, delivery by cesarean section must be considered. If primary herpetic vulvovaginitis is documented during gestation, the fetus may be infected during the mother's viremia, and the indication for cesarean section is less clear.

Idoxuridine (5-iodo-2'-deoxyuridine, IDU) and adenine arabinoside (9β-D-arabinofuranosyladenine, vidarabine, ara-A) are effective topically in herpes simplex virus keratitis. For herpetic keratitis topical IDU is applied in a 0.1% solution every hour during the day and every 2 h during the night. A simpler means of application is a 0.5% ointment four to five times a day. There are no controlled clinical trials to support the efficacy of any local preparation in the treatment of herpes labialis or genital herpes simplex virus infection.

Intravenous ara-A is being evaluated in disseminated perinatal infections and encephalitis. Therapy with intravenous ara-A (15 mg/kg per day for 7 days) should be instituted if a newborn has cutaneous evidence by positive Tzanck smear from a lesion of HSV infection, because such early treatment may prevent dissemination. Interferon, interferon inducers, transfer factor, and corticosteroids have not been shown to be useful in HSV infections. On account of the development of resistance of strains of herpes simplex virus to photoactive heterotricyclic dyes (proflavine, neutral red) and the possible induction of malignant transformation by these agents, this treatment is not recommended.

Adenine arabinoside is now an established antiherpesvirus agent. It has been effective in varicella zoster in immunosuppressed patients (Chap. 185), and when given before the onset of coma in biopsy-proved HSV1 encephalitis, has a good therapeutic index (efficacy/toxicity). Since 1971 it has been used extensively in several university centers. It is active in preventing cytopathic effects in tissue culture of HSV1, HSV2, varicella zoster (VZ) virus, cytomegalovirus, and herpes B and vaccinia viruses. It is much less depressive to the bone marrow than older and now obsolete systemic nucleoside antiviral agents such as idoxuridine or cytosine arabinoside. Ara-A is not an immunosuppressive agent; it is immediately converted within cells by the ubiquitous enzyme adenosine deaminase to hypoxanthine arabinoside (ara-Hx), which, in turn, also has antiviral activity, albeit less than the parent compound. Ara-A specifically inhibits HSV DNA polymerase without inhibiting similar normal enzymes. The mechanism of action of ara-Hx is unknown. Experience to date suggests, but does not prove, that ara-A is useful in disseminated cutaneous HSV1 but is of dubious value in recurrent cutaneous HSV2 or cytomegalovirus infections. Permission must be obtained prior to each experimental use of ara-A.

Ara-A is diluted in 5% dextrose solutions at a ratio of at least 2 ml for each milligram of antiviral compound. Adenine arabinoside is given by slow, continuous intravenous infusions in a dose of 15 mg/kg per day for 10 days. The National Institute of Allergy and Infectious Diseases Collaborative Antiviral Study Group suggests that in suspected cases of HSV encephalitis ara-A should not be given without a brain biopsy and that treatment should be discontinued after 5 days if brain biopsies are negative for HSV. With ara-A, slight depressions in hemoglobin have been noted, and megaloblasts have been seen in the bone marrow. When patients are receiving other immunosuppressive or cytotoxic treatments or have renal insufficiency, toxicity of ara-A may be greater. A transient reversible akinetic mutism has been observed in several patients. Approximately 40 percent of the daily dose of ara-A is excreted in the urine within 24 h.

Considerable effort is being expended in development of antiviral pharmacokinetics so that antiviral drugs may be used predictively. For instance, ara-A and ara-Hx singly exhibit in vitro anti-HSV inhibitory (MIC) and lethal (MLC) activity at concentrations of drug not inhibiting cellular DNA, RNA, or protein synthesis. This in vitro finding may account for the beneficial therapeutic index in humans. An assay for the combined antiviral activity (AVA) in micrograms per milliliter of ara-A equivalents in human body fluids has been developed which is unaffected by the concomitant presence of anti-HSV antibody or interferon. The combined AVA of ara-A plus ara-Hx (the antiviral drug in vivo) is greater than the predicted values of each drug measured individually by chemical methods. Moreover, sustained AVA in serums (approximately 10 μg/ml) persists throughout the period of treatment. It is clear that the true AVA of ara-A is expressed intracellularly, and concentrations of drug within cells have not yet been measured by microbiologic assay.

REFERENCES

BARINGER JR: Recovery of herpes simplex virus from human sacral ganglions. N Engl J Med 291:828, 1974

BRYSON T et al: Determination of plaque inhibitory activity of adenine arabinoside (9β D-arabinofuranosyladenine) for herpesvirus using an adenosine deaminase inhibitor. Antimicrob Agents Chemother 6:98, 1974

CHAMPNEY KJ et al: Anti-herpesvirus activity in human sera and urines after administration of adenine arabinoside (in vitro and in vivo synergy of adenine arabinoside and arabinosylhypoxanthine in combination). J Clin Invest 62:1142, 1978

CRANE LR, LERNER AM: Herpetic whitlow: A manifestation of primary infection with herpes simplex virus type 1 or type 2. J Infect Dis 137:856, 1978

LAUTER CB et al: Microbiological assays and neurological toxicity during use of adenine arabinoside in humans. J Infect Dis 134:75, 1976

LEVINE DP et al: Simultaneous serum and CSF antibodies in herpes simplex virus encephalitis. JAMA 240:356, 1978

MARKOWITZ A, LERNER AM: Virus infections of the vagina, in The Human Vagina: In Health and Disease, ESE Hafez, TN Evans (eds). Amsterdam, Elsevier/North-Holland, 1978 p 451

NAHMIAS AJ, JOSEY WE: Epidemiology of herpes simplex viruses 1 and 2, in Viral Infections of Humans: Epidemiology and Control, AS Evans (ed). New York, Plenum, 1976 p 253

SHIPMAN C JR et al: Antiviral activity of arabinosyladenine and arabinosylhypoxanthine in herpes simplex virus infected KB cells: Selective inhibition of viral deoxyribonucleic acid synthesis in synchronized suspension cultures. Antimicrob Agents Chemother 9:120, 1976

SPRUANCE SL et al: The natural history of recurrent herpes simplex labialis. N Engl J Med 297:69, 1977

TERNI M et al: Aseptic meningitis in association with herpes progenitalis. N Engl J Med 285:503, 1971

WHITLEY RJ et al: Adenine arabinoside therapy of biopsy-proved herpes simplex encephalitis. NIAID Collaborative Antiviral Study. N Engl J Med 294:289, 1976

—— et al: Adenine arabinoside therapy of herpes zoster in the immunosuppressed. NIAID Collaborative Antiviral Study. N Engl J Med 294:1193, 1976

WILLIAMS BB et al: Inhibitory and lethal concentrations of 9β-D-arabinofuranosyladenine and its hypoxanthine derivative versus herpes simplex virus, type 1. J Lab Clin Med 89:687, 1977

——, LERNER AM: Some previously unrecognized features of herpes simplex virus encephalitis. Neurology 28:1193, 1978

194
CYTOMEGALIC INCLUSION DISEASE (SALIVARY GLAND VIRUS DISEASE)

C. GEORGE RAY

DEFINITION Cytomegalic inclusion disease (CID) is a viral infection which can affect human beings at all ages beginning with conception. The agent was initially called *salivary gland virus* and was thought to be primarily responsible for occasional cases of disseminated, fatal illness in newborn infants, or subclinical salivary gland involvement only. Since its initial cultivation in 1956, the virus has been demonstrated to cause a broad spectrum of disease in humans. In adults the manifestations are frequently those of an illness like infectious mononucleosis, or may constitute a terminal complication of chronic debilitating disease.

ETIOLOGY Cytomegalovirus (CMV) belongs to the herpesvirus group and produces large, intranuclear (10 to 15 nm), and inconspicuous cytoplasmic (2 to 4 nm) inclusions which occur in all types of normal and neoplastic tissues. The agent is affected by temperature and other environmental factors. Low temperatures ($-80°C$) with added stabilizers are needed for shipment and storage. Several antigenically heterogeneous, but closely interrelated, strains have been isolated which are largely species-specific for man and grow in human fibroblast cultures. Of the various immunologic procedures available for diagnosis, the complement fixation test is most widely used, since the different human strains share a common complement-fixing antigen. Species-specific CMV occurs in many different animals and animal models. The mouse CMV systems are particularly important in the experimental study of the infection.

EPIDEMIOLOGY The infection is worldwide and, in this country, highest prevalence rates are found among young, preschool children of low socioeconomic background. CMV infection may be congenital but is more often acquired during the first year of life. At birth 0.5 to 2 percent of infants have been found to be excreting virus in the urine, and by 12 months of age, between 9 and 60 percent of infants in various population groups have acquired infection, with viruria. Among healthy adults, asymptomatic excretion rates are usually less than 1 percent; in late pregnancy, urine and/or uterine cervical virus excretion increases to between 2 to 13 percent. Complement-fixing antibody is relatively infrequent in infancy, increases during childhood, and is present in about 35 to 80 percent of adults. The virus persists in the host for a long time, perhaps indefinitely, and is excreted in saliva, urine, and semen even in the presence of antibody. Breast milk and feces may also transmit the infection. Close and prolonged contact appears necessary for efficient transmission of the infection. Venereal transmission appears to be common among young adults. Transplacental passage of the virus produces congenital infection, and perinatal infection may follow exposure to the virus in the infected cervix uteri during delivery. In adults CID may represent either activation of latent infection or may be newly acquired. It can also be transmitted by transfusion of whole blood; the risk of infection per unit of fresh blood tranfused has been estimated as between 5 to 7 percent. The majority of these infections, however, are subclinical, and only detectable by serologic conversion.

PATHOGENESIS Localized or systemic CID which may be latent or active occurs in hematopoietic and lymphocytic-reticular disorders (various anemias, leukemias, lymphomas), other chronic debilitating disease, and often during immunosuppression. It is a potential complication of any therapy which results in an impairment of humoral and/or cellular immunity. Physiologic factors related to age or late pregnancy favor viral proliferation and dissemination. CID may be associated with stillborn, premature, or low-birth-weight infants. Self-limited forms with generally mild clinical manifestations are being recognized more frequently in apparently normal persons.

PATHOLOGY Enlarged cells, 25 to 40 nm in diameter, with the distinctive nuclear inclusions, are the morphologic hallmark of the infection, and are similar in all forms and sites of infection. Infected cells elicit an inflammatory cell response only after cell death. In adults localized infection most commonly consists of interstitial pneumonitis and gastrointestinal ulcers. Less frequently affected are the nasal mucosa, salivary glands, liver, and adrenals. Hepatitis with the distinctive inclusions has been related to CID by serologic studies. In the disseminated form nearly every tissue may be affected, including the central nervous system. Involvement of the latter, however, has been noted most often in the immunosuppressed adult. In infancy the localized form is largely confined to the salivary glands, hence the original designation of salivary gland virus disease. In disseminated disease the more common sites are salivary glands, kidney, liver, lung, pancreas, gastrointestinal tract, thyroid, adrenal, and central nervous system. Multiple infections are frequently associated with CID. Bacterial, fungal, and various forms of other herpesvirus infections are common. Concomitant infection with pertussis, toxoplasmosis, and *Pneumocystis carinii* are frequent. Interesting interactions between CMV and toxoplasmosis and Newcastle disease virus have been noted experimentally.

CLINICAL MANIFESTATIONS While the majority of CMV infections are occult, there are a variety of manifestations of active disease which mimic other conditions. The categories of clinical infection can be grouped as follows: (1) congenital CMV, (2) perinatally or postnatally acquired CMV, (3) acquired CMV in healthy children and adults (including the CMV mononucleosis syndrome), (4) disseminated CMV in immunosuppressed patients, and (5) acquired or reactivated CMV infection in organ or bone-marrow transplant recipients.

Congenital CMV infection This disease can be detected virologically in 0.5 to 2 percent of all newborns. Of these, an estimated 10 to 15 percent will incur some tissue damage, with a risk of permanent sequelae or death. The greatest risk appears to be among infants born to women who experienced a primary infection during that pregnancy and are actively shedding virus at parturition. The clinical manifestations range from mild jaundice, respiratory distress, and failure to thrive to a variable constellation of signs including hepatosplenomegaly with hepatitis and cirrhosis, purpura, maculopapular exanthems, encephalitis, microcephaly with microgyria, growth retardation, chorioretinitis, acute or chronic pneumonitis, hemolytic anemia, and pathological fractures of long bones. It has been estimated that 10 percent of newborns with virologically proved congenital infection will develop significant neurological impairment, usually in the form of sensorineural hearing loss and variable degrees of mental retardation. This risk also extends to some infants with asymptomatic or mild congenital CMV. The differential diagnosis includes congenital rubella, enteroviruses, syphilis, and toxoplasmosis; bacterial sepsis must also be considered in some cases.

Perinatally or postnatally acquired CMV infection in infants This is usually a much more subtle disease, with little or no risk for neurological sequelae, and is usually asymptomatic. The signs may include poor weight gain, hepatomegaly with mild to moderate liver function abnormalities, atypical lymphocytosis, and anemia. Occasionally, chronic interstitial pneumonitis has been attributed to infantile-acquired CMV infection, but its primary role as a pathogen is not clear. Recent studies, for example, have shown that CMV may coexist in the pulmonary tissue with other candidate lung pathogens in infants, such as *Chlamydia* and *P. carinii*. Also, there have been rare cases of severe hepatitis and cirrhosis presumed to be related to infantile-acquired CMV infection.

Acquired CMV infection in otherwise healthy children and adults This disease has been associated with a myriad of disorders. The most common of these is the *CMV mononucleosis syndrome,* an acute febrile illness with relative or absolute lymphocytosis and many atypical lymphocytes. The patient often complains of headache, back and abdominal pain, and sore throat. Rubellalike rashes, usually lasting only 1 or 2 days, have also been noted. The appearance of extensive rash and prolongation of its duration can be aggravated by inadvertent treatment with ampicillin, an event similar to that seen in infectious mononucleosis treated with the same agent. Other findings have included hepatitis with icterus, hemolytic anemia, thrombocytopenia, purpura, pneumonitis, conjunctivitis, myocarditis, pericarditis, arthralgias, and occasional splenomegaly. The heterophile test and ox cell hemolysins are negative, and specific serologies will not confirm an Epstein-Barr virus infection. Liver function tests are frequently abnormal, and elevated cold agglutinin titers are found in severe cases. The disease occurs spontaneously or after perfusion with fresh whole blood (the postperfusion syndrome) and usually resolves without residua in 3 to 6 weeks; however, some patients will continue to experience recurrent fevers and malaise with atypical lymphocytosis for periods as long as 1 year. On the basis of observations of the postperfusion syndrome, the incubation period has been estimated to be 20 to 50 days.

The *differential diagnosis* of acquired CMV mononucleosis most commonly includes Epstein-Barr virus infection and toxoplasmosis. In some patients, particularly those with a protracted illness, autoimmune diseases and hematopoietic malignancies can become a concern. Unlike infectious mononucleosis, CMV does not evoke a heterophile antibody titer, and exudative pharyngitis and significant lymphadenopathy are unusual. CMV mononucleosis is more commonly seen among young adults, while infectious mononucleosis typically affects a slightly younger, although overlapping age group. Acquired toxoplasmosis can usually be differentiated by appropriate serologic testing.

There are other recognized manifestations of acquired CMV infections which may or may not be found in association with the CMV mononucleosis syndrome. These include the Guillain-Barré syndrome, in which it is estimated that as many as one-third of cases may be CMV-related. Occasional cases of acute encephalitis, thyroiditis, ulcerative gastrointestinal disease and protein-losing enteropathies, acute thrombocytopenic purpura, chorioretinitis, and granulomatous hepatitis have also been reported to be associated with CMV. Despite the common occurrence of viruria and inclusion-bearing cells in the kidney, progressive renal disease has not been a problem at any age.

Disseminated CMV in immunosuppressed patients This disease can be manifested as a severe, sometimes fatal form of the CMV mononucleosis syndrome, but atypical lymphocytosis is variable. Major organs involved include the lungs, liver, gastrointestinal tract, central nervous system, and eyes. Signs vary, but frequently include severe pneumonitis, jaundice, diarrhea, fever, and retinitis. The retinitis in such patients is often punctate, exudative, and hemorrhagic, and raises such differential diagnostic considerations as sarcoid, cryptococcosis, toxoplasmosis, and disseminated candidiasis. The interstitial pneumonitis may be difficult to distinguish from opportunistic bacterial, fungal, or protozoon infections, such as *P. carinii;* in fact, it is not uncommon for CMV to coexist with one or more of these pathogens, and a lung biopsy may be required to resolve the diagnosis.

CMV infection in transplant recipients This has become increasingly recognized as a serious problem. The situation is analogous to that of other immunosuppressed patients, but is also complicated by the fact that graft-versus-host reactions can reactivate latent infections and intensify both primary and reactivation disease. For kidney or heart transplant recipients, those who are seronegative before transplantation appear to be at greatest risk for active infection; in the case of renal transplantation there appears to be an even greater risk if the donor is seropositive and the recipient is seronegative for CMV, suggesting transmission of the primary infection via the transplanted organ. On the other hand, bone marrow recipients appear to have a higher risk of serious disease if they possess preexisting CMV antibodies, and no clear relation regarding risk could be correlated with the antibody status of the donor. While the spectrum of clinical disease is similar to that described for immunosuppressed patients, the major problems of CMV infection in transplantation are most often related to progressive, often fatal, interstitial pneumonia, a significant predisposition to pulmonary bacterial superinfection, and an increased incidence of graft rejection.

DIAGNOSIS Virus isolation from blood, body fluids, or tissues establishes the presence of active infection but cannot always be equated with disease, particularly in groups in which high asymptomatic infection rates are known to occur. Demonstration of significantly rising antibody titers are of some help, particularly in cases of acquired disease. However, spontaneous, wide fluctuations of complement-fixing antibody titers in healthy individuals have been demonstrated in one longitudinal study, and this rather unique lability of specific antibody tests should also be kept in mind when interpreting results. In congenital infections, the finding of elevated IgM-specific CMV antibody in the newborn generally correlates with active disease. However, false-positive results due to circulating rheumatoid factor have been found in some infants, and this possibility must be considered when interpreting the data. Morphologic demonstration of CMV inclusions is a relatively insensitive method of diagnosis, compared with cultures and serology. Roentgenographic and laboratory findings are nonspecific except for the lymphocytosis and atypical lymphocytes in CMV mononucleosis.

TREATMENT No specific therapy is available. Trials of interferon, interferon inducers, immunopotentiators such as levamisole, and viral antagonists such as adenine arabinoside have been limited, and without clearly beneficial results. A live, attenuated CMV vaccine is also under investigation, but is not available for routine use. The first use for such vaccine in the future, if it is at all effective, may be in the pretransplantation immunization of seronegative organ recipients.

REFERENCES

DOWLING P et al: Cytomegalovirus complement fixation antibody in Guillain-Barré syndrome. Neurology 27:1153, 1977

HANSHAW JB: Congenital cytomegalovirus infection: A fifteen year perspective. J Infect Dis 123:555, 1972

JORDAN MC et al: Spontaneous cytomegalovirus mononucleosis: Clinical and laboratory observations in nine cases. Ann Intern Med 79:153, 1973

MURRAY HW et al: Cytomegalovirus retinitis in adults. Am J Med 63:574, 1977

NEIMAN PE et al: A prospective analysis of interstitial pneumonia and opportunistic viral infection among recipients of allogeneic bone marrow grafts. J Infect Dis 136:754, 1977

PASS RF et al: Productive infection with cytomegalovirus and herpes simplex virus in renal transplant recipients: Role of source of kidney. J Infect Dis 137:556, 1978

PHILLIPS CA et al: Cytomegalovirus encephalitis in immunologically normal adults. JAMA 238:2299, 1977

PLOTKIN SA et al: Clinical trials of immunization with the Towne 125 strain of human cytomegalovirus. J Infect Dis 134:470, 1976

RAND KH et al: Increased pulmonary superinfections in cardiac-transplant patients undergoing primary cytomegalovirus infection. N Engl J Med 298:951, 1978

REYNOLDS DW et al: Congenital cytomegalovirus infection: Relation to auditory and mental deficiency. N Engl J Med 290:291, 1974

SUWANSIRIKUL S et al: Primary and secondary cytomegalovirus infection. Arch Intern Med 137:1026, 1977

WANER JL et al: Patterns of cytomegaloviral complement-fixing antibody activity: A longitudinal study of blood donors. J Infect Dis 127:538, 1973

WELLER TH: The cytomegaloviruses: Ubiquitous agents with protean clinical manifestations. N Engl J Med 285:203, 269, 1971

195
EPSTEIN-BARR VIRUS INFECTIONS, INCLUDING INFECTIOUS MONONUCLEOSIS

JAMES C. NIEDERMAN

DEFINITION Epstein-Barr virus (EBV), a lymphotropic herpes virus, infects all human populations. Primary infection in childhood is usually asymptomatic, but in adolescence or early adulthood, clinical manifestations of infectious mononucleosis (IM) develop in approximately 50 percent of infections. The characteristic clinical picture consists of fever, pharyngitis, lymphadenopathy, an increase of peripheral lymphocytes with a high proportion of atypical cells, and the development of transient heterophile and persistent EBV antibody responses.

ETIOLOGY EBV, which has the structural and immunologic characteristics of a member of the herpes group, was originally discovered by electron microscopic studies of tumor cells from biopsies of Burkitt's lymphoma grown in tissue culture. EBV antibodies measured by immunofluorescence techniques, complement fixation, immunodiffusion, enzyme-linked immunosorbent assay (ELISA), and virus neutralization are consistently absent before infectious mononucleosis, regularly develop during the course of the disease, and persist with little change for many years thereafter. In addition to IgG, EBV-specific IgM antibody is present during acute infectious mononucleosis in serums obtained 7 to 70 days after onset, and usually persists for several months.

Further evidence of a causative relationship is the presence of EBV in leukocytes cultured from serums of patients with acute mononucleosis as well as from subjects with a past history of the disease. The classical heterophil antibody of infectious mononucleosis has been produced experimentally in squirrel monkeys inoculated with EBV-transformed autologous leukocytes. In addition, inadvertent transmission of EBV by transfusion has been reported and in several instances was associated with the development of clinical infectious mononucleosis, including heterophil antibody.

EPIDEMIOLOGY Infectious mononucleosis has been recognized in all parts of the world. Although no yearly or seasonal trends are present in the general population, early fall and spring are periods of high frequency among college students. The most characteristic epidemiologic feature of the disease is its occurrence among young adults, especially in the 15- to 25-year age group.

Seroepidemiologic studies have demonstrated that the absence of EBV antibody correlates with susceptibility to infectious mononucleosis and its presence indicates immunity. The age at which infection is acquired is related to socioeconomic factors and hygienic environment. Among disadvantaged groups such as children living in certain tropical countries, antibody is acquired early. In contrast, in middle and upper socioeconomic groups, only 50 to 60 percent have detectable antibody during adolescent years and at the time of entry into college. Among these individuals, infectious mononucleosis is a well-recognized disorder. Studies measuring both apparent and inapparent infections suggest a clinical/subclinical ratio of 1:2 to 1:3 in young adults.

When EBV infection develops in early childhood, a mild and nonspecific or an inapparent illness occurs, both of which are associated with the appearance and persistence of specific antibody. If primary infection is delayed until adolescence or young adulthood, the clinical response is frequently typical infectious mononucleosis with the development of both heterophil and EBV antibodies.

Epidemiologic and laboratory evidence has suggested that transmission of EBV occurs through the oropharyngeal route

TABLE 195-1
Recovery of EBV in pharyngeal excretions from 25 cases of infectious mononucleosis

Time after onset of symptoms, days	No. specimens tested	No. specimens positive	Percent positive
0–14	16	13	81.3
15–28	12	10	83.3
29–150	11	11	100.0
>150	3	2	66.7
Total	42	36	85.7

SOURCE: *Miller et al.*

during close personal contact. Table 195-1 indicates that EBV is present in small amounts in throat washings from 1 week to many months after clinical illness.

This prolonged carrier state following clinical infectious mononucleosis, and perhaps also after inapparent EBV infection, may serve as a principal source of transmission. Investigations utilizing the presence of EBV antibody as an index of immunity have confirmed the low contagiousness of both the infection and the disease among susceptible college roommates; secondary attack rates for EBV infection within family units have also been low.

PATHOLOGY Generalized involvement of lymphoid tissue with lymphadenopathy, nasopharyngeal lymphoid hyperplasia, and splenomegaly is the outstanding pathologic feature. Widespread focal and perivascular aggregates of mononuclear cells, including atypical lymphocytes, are found throughout the body. Nonspecific hyperplastic changes in lymph nodes are present without infiltration of the capsule or surrounding tissues. Nonlymphoid organs and tissues, including liver, heart, kidneys, and central nervous system, are also infiltrated, and changes in these organs may be associated with functional disturbances. Bone marrow hyperplasia develops, and occasionally small granulomas are present.

MANIFESTATIONS In young adults an incubation period of 30 to 50 days has been suggested on the basis of contact infection studies. Infectious mononucleosis associated with the development of heterophil and EBV antibody has occurred in several patients 5 weeks following blood transfusion. Children appear to have shorter incubation periods, in the range of 10 to 14 days, but there is relatively little information on this point.

During a prodromal period of 3 to 5 days, mild symptoms, including headache, malaise, and fatigue, are common. Frank clinical features usually present over the next 7 to 20 days; they are variable in severity, but in over 80 percent of cases include fever, sore throat, and cervical adenopathy. In adults, temperature elevations which peak at 101 to 103°F may persist for 7 to 10 days. In severe cases, a daily rise in temperature to 105°F may continue even longer. On the other hand, children often have little or no fever accompanying the infection.

Sore throat occurs in the first week and is the most common feature of infectious mononucleosis. Hyperplasia of pharyngeal lymphoid tissue with inflammation and edema develops. A grayish white exudative tonsillitis persisting for 7 to 10 days is present in approximately 50 percent of cases. The uvula and palatal arch frequently have a gelatinous appearance. *Palatine petechiae*, located near the border of the hard and soft palate, are observed in about one-third of patients toward the end of the first week of illness. Although highly suggestive, their presence is not pathognomonic of the disease.

Lymph node enlargement is a hallmark of infectious mononucleosis. The onset is gradual, and anterior and posterior cervical chains are most commonly involved. Generalized adenopathy, including axillary, epitrochlear, and inguinal nodes, may also develop during the course of the disease. The nodes are affected singly or in groups and may be small or grape-sized; they are firm, discrete, and moderately tender on palpation.

Splenomegaly occurs in approximately one-half the patients, and enlargement is greatest during the second and third weeks of illness. Although extremely rare, splenic rupture is one of the few potentially fatal complications of the disease.

Percussion tenderness over the liver and hepatomegaly develop in only about 10 percent of patients, but the majority (90 percent) have abnormal liver function test results which persist for several weeks. Jaundice occurs in no more than 4 to 5 percent of cases and is usually mild and uncomplicated.

During early stages of the disease a transient faint erythematous maculopapular eruption on the trunk and extremities is present in about 10 percent of patients. The rash often resembles rubella, but may be urticarial, hemorrhagic, or scarlatiniform in nature. *Bilateral supraorbital edema* may also be a transient finding early in the course of disease.

A wide variety of neurologic manifestations has been described, but they occur only rarely. Aseptic meningitis, encephalitis, blurred vision, coma, acute cerebellar syndrome, and the Guillain-Barré syndrome may appear at any time during the illness. Most patients experience complete recovery from central nervous system involvement; however, severe paralysis and/or respiratory incapacity occur in rare instances and are potentially fatal complications.

LABORATORY FINDINGS **Blood picture** Essential to the diagnosis of infectious mononucleosis is an increase in relative and absolute numbers of lymphocytes and monocytes, including 10 to 20 percent atypical forms. Early in disease this is the result of increased numbers of both B and T cells, and later of a predominance of T lymphocytes. The atypical lymphocytes are large cells with oval, horseshoe-shaped, or indented nuclei and basophilic, vacuolated foamy cytoplasm. Nuclear chromatin is usually dense and irregular, and nucleoli are rarely seen. During the first week of illness, either the total leukocyte count is normal or there may be a leukopenia due to granulocytopenia. The total count then rises to between 10,000 and 20,000 leukocytes per cubic millimeter by the second or third week of illness; rarely, the number of leukocytes may range as high as 50,000 per cubic millimeter. Characteristic leukocyte changes often persist for 4 to 8 weeks or more. Anemia is rare in infectious mononucleosis, but hemolytic anemia has been reported as a complication. Slight to moderate thrombocytopenia, which is usually symptomless, has been recognized during the early weeks of disease. In a few reported cases, the clinical picture has suggested idiopathic thrombocytopenic purpura.

Serologic diagnosis The serum of IM patients characteristically contains heterophil antibodies, i.e., agglutinins against sheep red blood cells, in high titer. Heterophil antibody is associated with the IgM fraction of serum and usually declines over a period of 3 to 6 months. In general, the higher the titer developed during clinical illness, the longer the antibodies will remain detectable in convalescence. Though a nonspecific serologic response, the heterophil antibody of infectious mononucleosis differs from other antibodies in human serums that also agglutinate sheep red blood cells. The latter are found at low levels in normal human serums and in high titers in serum sickness. Differentiation is based on absorption techniques utilizing guinea pig kidney and beef erythrocytes. The sheep cell agglutinins of infectious mononucleosis are completely absorbed by beef red blood cells but not by guinea pig kidney. Serum sickness agglutinins are absorbed by both, whereas nonspecific Forssman agglutinins are absorbed only by guinea pig kidney. A high order of specificity has now been achieved with other qualitative heterophil antibody tests which utilize formalin-treated horse red blood cells, ox red blood cells, and enzyme-treated and -untreated sheep cells.

Usually sheep cell agglutinins are present in the first week of illness, but they may be delayed in appearance. During the first 2 weeks after onset of the illness, 60 percent of young adult patients develop a positive heterophil antibody test. This percentage increases to 80 to 90 percent by the end of 1 month.

The height of the titer is not related to severity of the disease or to the degree of lymphocytosis. In the presence of clinical and hematologic findings, a sheep cell agglutinin titer of 1:224 or higher before guinea pig kidney absorption and 1:28 after absorption has diagnostic significance. In the beef cell hemolysin test, a titer of 1:280 or higher may be considered significant. A rising titer in early stages of disease is the best criterion.

During acute infectious mononucleosis an increase in total serum IgM levels up to 100 percent over control values and a 50 percent increase in IgG levels has been observed. Other protein alterations associated with the IgM fraction which may be present in the disorder include cold agglutinating antibody and transiently positive serologic tests for syphilis and rheumatoid factor. In IM, the presence of EBV antibody is a regular feature. Prospective clinical studies have shown that the disease occurs only in individuals who lack antibodies to EBV; patients become seropositive in almost all cases by the time acute symptoms appear. As measured by immunofluorescence techniques, levels of 1:80 to 1:320 are often found during early illness, and in only 15 to 20 percent of cases are significant antibody rises demonstrable. Rarely, the development of both EBV and heterophil antibodies is delayed several weeks following onset of symptoms. The relationships between clinical features and antibody levels in typical heterophil positive cases are shown in Fig. 195-1. In addition to development of antibody to EB viral capsid antigen, which is the most widely used clinically, antibodies to early antigen and EBV-specific IgM occur in 75 to 90 percent of patients with acute mononucleosis. Antibodies to other EBV-associated antigen systems (membrane, nuclear, complement-fixing, neutralizing, and immunoprecipitating) are also absent before infection and appear during the course of disease.

No direct correlation has been found between the levels of EBV and heterophil antibodies, nor between the anti-EBV titer and severity of clinical symptoms or hematologic findings. Heterophil antibody levels are highest during the first 4 to 6 weeks after onset, and then decline or disappear after several months. EBV antibodies also reach peak titers within 3 to 4 weeks but persist at lower levels for many years thereafter, if not for life. Antibody titers of 1:20 to 1:40 have been demonstrated in serum collected 45 years after laboratory documentation of heterophil-positive IM.

The appearance of EBV antibody has also been demonstrated in cases which have the clinical and hematologic characteristics of IM but do not develop heterophil antibody. These EBV-positive, heterophil-negative cases are apparently frequent in infants and children but rare in adults.

Other laboratory abnormalities These consist primarily of abnormal liver function tests and may include an elevation in alkaline phosphatase level, retention of bromsulphalein, mild abnormalities in serum glutamic oxaloacetic transaminase and serum glutamic pyruvic transaminase, and mild icterus. With recovery, all these values return to normal.

Acute infectious mononucleosis is associated with depressed cell-mediated immunity manifested by loss of skin hypersensitivity and lymphocyte hyporesponsiveness to in vitro stimulation by a variety of mitogens and specific antigens.

DIAGNOSIS The main diagnostic features of infectious mononucleosis are (1) irregular fever, sore throat, and lymphadenopathy; (2) an absolute increase in lymphocytes and monocytes exceeding 50 percent and including more than 10 percent atypical lymphocytes in the peripheral blood; (3) the transient appearance of sheep cell agglutinins and beef cell hemolysins; (4) the development of persistent antibody against Epstein-Barr virus; and (5) abnormalities of liver function tests.

Since many of these features are also seen in other diseases, IM may resemble a number of febrile disorders, especially those associated with fever, sore throat, adenopathy, and leukocytosis. In early stages of the disease, it is often difficult to distinguish IM from other forms of febrile exudative pharyngotonsillitis such as *streptococcal infections, exudative tonsillitis of viral etiology, Vincent's angina,* and *diphtheria.* Differentia-

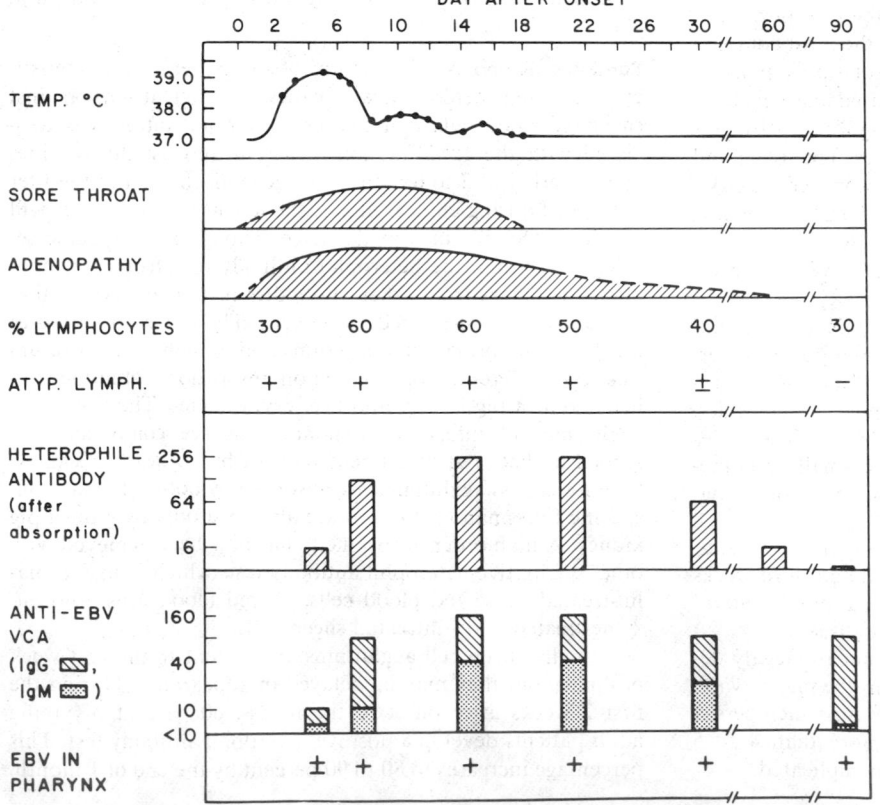

FIGURE 195-1

Scheme of symptoms, antibody responses, and EBV oropharyngeal shedding in typical cases of infectious mononucleosis.

tion depends on the results of throat cultures and the development of the hematologic and serologic features characteristic of infectious mononucleosis.

Diseases with some similarities in hematologic abnormalities such as *acute leukemia* and other lymphoproliferative disorders may be mistaken for IM. Demonstration of very immature leukocytes in blood or bone marrow and the presence of anemia, severe thrombocytopenia, and a negative heterophil antibody test distinguish these disorders from IM.

Cytomegalovirus (CMV) mononucleosis usually involves a slightly older age group, i.e., 20 to 30 years. Splenomegaly, hepatic involvement, and the presence of atypical lymphocytes in blood are common features of this disease, whereas sore throat and cervical adenopathy are usually absent. In transfusion-associated CMV infections, cytomegalovirus is excreted in the urine and a rise in complement-fixing antibody can be demonstrated.

Acute infectious lymphocytosis, a benign disorder of children, should be considered in the differential diagnosis among younger age groups. The majority of these cases are associated with signs of an upper respiratory tract infection; adenopathy is minimal, and splenomegaly is absent. The major feature is leukocytosis consisting of small mature lymphocytes; this abnormal blood picture may persist for 4 to 5 weeks, and occasionally for several months. The heterophil antibody test is negative, and no relationship to EBV antibody has been found.

The prodromal stage of *rubella,* associated with fever, malaise, postauricular and posterior cervical adenopathy, and lymphocytosis, may be indistinguishable from early infectious mononucleosis. A distinguishing feature of the rash of rubella is its invariable presence on the face, while that of IM is prominent on the trunk and usually spares the face; it is rarely as florid as in typical rubella. The appearance of large numbers of atypical lymphocytes in the blood and the development of heterophil and/or EB viral antibodies indicate infectious mononucleosis. Isolation of rubella virus from the throat and demonstration of a rising rubella antibody titer will confirm a diagnosis of rubella.

Acquired *toxoplasmosis* may be associated with fever, generalized adenopathy, splenomegaly, and lymphocytosis. A definitive diagnosis is based on direct isolation of *Toxoplasma gondii* and/or the demonstration of the development of specific serologic responses.

Infectious mononucleosis with jaundice can frequently be confused with *infectious hepatitis*. In hepatitis, fever is often lower and disappears when jaundice develops. Similarly, the presence of atypical lymphocytes is usually transitory during the preicteric phase of hepatitis, and the disease is less frequently associated with splenomegaly and leukocytosis.

TREATMENT Therapy is symptomatic. Antibiotics have no effect on uncomplicated cases of infectious mononucleosis. During the febrile period rest in bed is advisable. Salicylates or other analgesics are usually sufficient to control headache and discomfort from sore throat. Gargling and irrigation with saline solutions provide symptomatic relief of pharyngitis and stomatitis. As a rule, most patients recover uneventfully on this regimen in 2 to 4 weeks, with gradual return to normal activities. Patients with splenomegaly should be cautioned against heavy lifting and strenuous athletics until splenic enlargement has disappeared.

In patients with severe toxic exudative pharyngotonsillitis associated with extensive pharyngeal edema, corticosteroids are useful to induce a prompt anti-inflammatory effect. A short course of prednisone may be administered, starting with 40 to 60 mg the first day and decreasing this total dose 5 mg daily over 7 to 10 days. Steroids are not necessary in treatment of the usual patient with IM. However, full dosages of steroids should be employed in the management of severe complications, including (1) airway obstruction, in which a tracheostomy may also be required, (2) neurologic complications, (3) hemolytic anemia and thrombocytopenic purpura, and (4) myocarditis and pericarditis.

Approximately 20 percent of patients with infectious mononucleosis experience concurrent beta hemolytic streptococcal pharyngotonsillitis and should receive antibiotic treatment; a full 10-day course of penicillin V 250 mg four times daily, erythromycin 250 mg four times daily, or procaine penicillin G 600,000 units every 12 h, should be administered. Ampicillin should be avoided because of the high frequency of erythematous macular or maculopapular skin rashes associated with the use of this drug in patients with infectious mononucleosis.

Severe abdominal pain is rare in IM except in association with splenic rupture. This serious complication requires massive transfusions and immediate splenectomy.

REFERENCES

CARTER RL, PENMAN HG: *Infectious Mononucleosis.* Oxford, Blackwell, 1969

EPSTEIN MA, ACHONG BG: Pathogenesis of infectious mononucleosis. Lancet 2:1270, 1977

EVANS AS et al: Seroepidemiologic studies of infectious mononucleosis with EB virus. N Engl J Med 279:1121, 1968

HENLE G et al: Relation of Burkitt's tumor associated herpes-type virus in infectious mononucleosis. Proc Nat Acad Sci USA 59:94, 1968

———: Observations on childhood infections with Epstein-Barr virus. J Infect Dis 121:303, 1970

———: Antibodies to Epstein-Barr virus-associated nuclear antigen in infectious mononucleosis. J Infect Dis 130:231, 1974

MANGI RJ et al: Depression of cell-mediated immunity during acute infectious mononucleosis. N Engl J Med 291:1149, 1974

MILLER G et al: Prolonged oropharyngeal excretion of Epstein-Barr virus following infectious mononucleosis. N Engl J Med 288:299, 1973

NIEDERMAN JC et al: Infectious mononucleosis: Clinical manifestations in relation to EB virus antibodies. JAMA 203:205, 1968

———: Prevalence, incidence and persistence of EB virus antibody in young adults. N Engl J Med 282:361, 1970

———: Infectious mononucleosis: Epstein-Barr virus shedding in saliva and the oropharynx. N Engl J Med 294:1355, 1976

Miscellaneous and presumptive viral infections

196
WARTS AND MOLLUSCUM CONTAGIOSUM

LAWRENCE COREY

WARTS

DEFINITION Warts are benign neoplasms of the skin and contiguous mucous membranes caused by a member of the papovavirus group.

ETIOLOGY Warts or papillomata of several different clinical types are caused by the human papovavirus. Papovaviruses are spherical, small, double-stranded, DNA-containing viruses which replicate in the nucleus of the cells. Viruses composing the papovavirus group of agents include (1) the papilloma viruses (human wart virus, Schope papilloma virus of rabbits), (2) the polyoma viruses of mice, and (3) the vacuolating viruses of monkeys (SV40). These agents have been shown to induce the transformation of cells in tissue culture as well as to cause tumors in experimental animals. Human wart virus has been demonstrated by electron microscopy in extracts and thin sections of warts, and it has been propagated in a human epithelial cell line. Experimentally, cell-free filtrates of human warts will induce the formation of these lesions at the inoculated skin sites of human volunteers. The incubation period based upon these experimental inoculation studies varies from 1 to 20 months (mean 3 to 4 months).

EPIDEMIOLOGY Warts are found in approximately 7 to 10 percent of the population, with the highest frequency in the early teen-age years. They occur mainly on the skin areas unprotected by clothing except for the feet. Person-to-person transmission by direct contact with wart tissue and indirectly by virus contamination through contaminated secretions or instruments may occur. Autoinoculation of virus to contiguous or distant sites is frequent. Although warts of several animal species are caused by similar viruses, convincing evidence of interspecies transmission is lacking.

PATHOLOGY AND PATHOGENESIS The skin lesions induced by the wart virus are due to an abnormal proliferation of epidermal cells. In normal epidermis, cell division occurs mainly in the basal layer; however, in the wart, mitotic figures are seen in cells several layers higher. In addition, there is thickening of the cell layers, elongation and broadening of the interpapillary processes with the development of long, thin papilli containing blood vessels extending high into the wart. These vessels cause bleeding points when the wart is trimmed and, if thrombosed, may appear as small dark spots. Hematoxylin and eosin staining of warty lesions may reveal cells that contain both nuclear and cytoplasmic inclusions. The nuclear inclusions tend to be basophilic and represent aggregates of virus particles, while the cytoplasmic inclusions appear eosinophilic and are felt to represent deranged development of keratohyalin.

Warts are skin colored, can be single or occur in multiple clusters, and are often widely dispersed over the body. While warts may persist and spread within the same person for several years, or may recur in an individual several years after a total remission, most studies indicate that two-thirds of warts will resolve spontaneously within a 2-year period of time. Whether this is related to a limited life span of infected cells or is due to the host's defenses is unclear. The development of antiwart antibodies has been correlated with clinical regression of the lesions. In addition, warts have been known to increase in size during pregnancy and to reappear and disseminate during immunosuppressive therapy; hence cellular immunity has been implicated as an important aspect of the host's defenses to human wart virus.

CLINICAL MANIFESTATIONS Although many clinical types of warts exist, the same virus is thought to cause most varieties of warts. The clinical manifestations of the lesions are determined by the host response and the location of the lesions. For convenience, lesions are classified according to location and morphology.

Common warts (verrucae vulgaris) may occur anywhere on the skin but are most common on the hands or around the fingernails. Most lesions appear as solid, rounded tumors with rough, horny projections which may vary considerably in size (1 mm to 2 cm). Lesions occur in both children and adults, either singly or in clusters, may be localized along a scratch (Köbner phenomenon), and are usually asymptomatic.

Plantar warts occur beneath pressure points on the soles of the feet, particularly in children and young adults. The surfaces of the lesions are firm and flat and may occur individually or in mosaic-like clusters. These warts possess a conical shape, probably due to the pressure induced by walking. The lesions are covered by hyperkeratotic epithelial tissue which, upon removal, reveals the papillary structure of the soft whitish core containing thrombosed capillaries that appear as small dark specks. With further paring, capillary bleeding, which is diagnostic of warts rather than a callous corn or scar, can be induced. Local pressure upon the plantar wart usually induces pain which can be severe upon walking.

Flat warts (verrucae planae) present as skin-colored, smooth, flat, or slightly elevated, round or polygonal papules that vary between 1 and 5 mm in diameter. The common sites are the face, neck, chest, dorsum of the hands, and the flexor surfaces of the forearms and shins. The mucous membranes are involved rarely. The surfaces of these lesions show a stippled appearance when examined under a magnifying glass. Flat warts are most frequently confused with the lesions of lichen planus. Multiple lesions on the dorsum of the hands may be mistaken for one of the inherited disorders known as acrokeratosis verruciformis, epidermodysplasia verruciformis, or Darier's disease.

Warts which project finger-like structures are termed *filiform warts;* when present on the scalp, they are called *digitate warts.* Filiform warts are most frequent in adult males, usually on the bearded area of the face. The lips and eyelids may also be involved. The lesions are either single or multiple, and they grow to considerable size when left unattended. The differential diagnosis includes cutaneous horns and epidermal nevi.

Condylomata acuminata, or venereal warts, generally appear as multiple, polymorphic lesions which may coalesce to large masses in the genital and/or anal area. In men, they are found most frequently in the coronal or frenum area of the penis. Urethral warts usually affect the anterior urinary meatus. In women, warts may occur on the fourchette, on the adjacent labia and/or vulva, the cervix, and the lower and upper one-third of the vagina. In about 20 percent of patients, the lesions spread to the perineum and anal area. Anal warts may, however, appear without concomitant penile or vulvar disease and may extend into the anal canal.

The clinical and virological relationship between skin and genital warts has excited controversy. Even though the viruses from these lesions appear structurally identical, there is some evidence that there are antigenic and biochemical differences between the viruses extracted from skin and genital warts. Moreover, both the epidemiology and clinical manifestations of these two entities appear distinctive. While there are a small number of patients with skin warts who develop flat warts in the genital area due to autoinoculation, most studies indicate that genital warts is a disease of sexual maturity, and patients with genital warts do not have more skin warts than controls. The data suggest that genital warts are sexually transmitted. In one study, 60 percent of patients who had sexual contact with partners having active genital warts subsequently developed the disease, usually after an incubation period of 2 to 3 months.

The differential diagnosis of genital warts includes condylomata lata of secondary syphilis (darkfield microscopy for *Treponema pallidum* and serologic testing will differentiate between these two entities), granuloma inguinale in tropical countries, and carcinoma of the penis. Vulvar warts must be differentiated from fibroepitheliomas, molluscum contagiosum, and, in older women, seborrheic keratosis.

COMPLICATIONS Occasionally, a giant condyloma may cause destruction of the affected areas, e.g., the penis in Buschke-Lowenstein tumor. Despite its benign histology, this lesion may cause extensive perforation and destruction of tissue and may simulate a malignant growth. Biopsy is recommended. Vulvar warts may enlarge enough during pregnancy to cause problems in the management of labor and delivery.

Laryngeal papillomatosis of childhood appears related to condyloma acuminatum. These lesions, which are usually multiple, develop within the first 6 months of life, and most mothers of children who develop these multiple lesions have been noted to have genital warts at parturition. This condition appears to be etiologically distinct from the solitary laryngeal papilloma of elderly patients which tends to become malignant. Malignant transmission of warts is rare. An example is epidermodysplasia verruciformis, a condition with a familial predisposition that begins with multiple lesions similar to common warts on the dorsum of the hands and feet and soon spreads over the entire body surface.

TREATMENT There is no specific treatment for warts, although a variety of physical and chemical methods are used for their removal. These methods include electrodesiccation and curettage, surgical excision, x-ray, and cryosurgery by applying liquid nitrogen or dry ice. Repeated paring of warts

followed by the application of caustic agents, such as mono- or trichloracetic acid, calicylic acid, cantharidin, or silver nitrate, is helpful. Topical antimetabolites such as 5-fluorouracil have also been used.

Condylomata acuminata are treated effectively by repeated topical application of a 25% podophyllum resin and tincture of benzoin. This preparation is applied to the lesions, washed off after 3 to 4 h, and repeated once or twice a week, while the time of application is lengthened until the lesions have resolved. Large quantities of podophyllum are toxic, however, and may cause hypokalemia and neuropathy. It is also advisable to avoid podophyllum in pregnancy. Radical therapy of warts should be eschewed because most warts will disappear eventually spontaneously without leaving any scars.

MOLLUSCUM CONTAGIOSUM

Molluscum contagiosum is an infectious disease of the skin and mucous membranes caused by a member of the poxvirus group. The virus of molluscum contagiosum is the largest of the true viruses to cause human disease, and, because of its size, 240 to 320 nm in diameter, it can be demonstrated in direct touch preparations of lesions using oil immersion light microscopy. Molluscum contagiosum is a disease of worldwide distribution occurring in all races and is seen most frequently in children. Occasionally, epidemics of the disease are seen in closed populations as in boarding schools or among wrestlers. Infection can be transmitted experimentally by injecting material expressed from the lesions. Clinically, infection can be transmitted directly through sexual intercourse or, like other poxviruses, through fomites such as shared towels. The incubation period varies between 2 weeks and 2 months.

Proliferation, hyperplasia, thickening, and degeneration of the epidermis characterize the lesions. Infected epithelial cells become enlarged and develop large intracytoplasmic eosinophilic hyalin inclusion bodies which displace the nucleus to one side.

Molluscum contagiosum is characterized by single or multiple, rounded dome-shaped waxy, pearly white pustules with an umbilical central pore. A cheesy material that stains blue with Giemsa's stain can be expressed from the central core. Microscopically, the umbilicated central porous area is composed of horn lamellae, debris, dyskeratotic cells, and molluscum bodies.

These molluscum bodies appear as a mass of viral particles on electron microscopy. The lesions may vary in number and size and range from 1 mm up to 1 to 2 cm in diameter. The principal sites of involvement include the face, especially the eyelids, the trunk, and the anogenital areas. The conjunctiva, lips, and buccal mucosa are involved rarely. Molluscum lesions are frequently traumatized resulting in autoinoculation. Occasionally, secondary bacterial infection occurs. The lesions are usually present for 6 months to a year but may persist and spread for 3 to 4 years. Spontaneous regression without scarring occurs eventually. In contrast to warts, recurrences are rare. Patients with underlying immunologic defects may develop extensive involvement with an intractable course.

The diagnosis of molluscum contagiosum is easy, especially when multiple lesions are present. A single lesion may be confused with a keratoacanthoma, basal cell epithelioma, or pyogenic granuloma. The definitive diagnosis can be made histologically from smears of expressed material or by electron microscopy. Treatment by sharp curettage or by expression of the porous material with a curved forceps will help clear up the lesion with little if any scarring.

REFERENCES

EISINGER M et al: Propagation of human wart virus in tissue culture. Nature 256:432, 1975

ORIEL JD: Genital warts. Sexually Transmitted Dis 4:153, 1977

ROWSON KEK, MAHY BJW: Human papova virus. Bacteriol Rev 31:110, 1967

SANDERS BB, STRETCHER GS: Warts, diagnosis and treatment. JAMA 235:2859, 1976

197
CAT–SCRATCH DISEASE

ROBERT G. PETERSDORF

DEFINITION Cat-scratch disease is an infection characterized by indolent, occasionally suppurative, regional lymphadenitis, secondary to a primary cutaneous lesion at the site of inoculation, usually a cat scratch. Because more than 90 percent of the reported cases have originated from cat scratches and a history of close contact with cats is often elicited, the name *cat-scratch disease* has become popular. However, rarely a similar disorder has been acquired from injury due to splinters, thorns, beef-bone fragments, and dog and monkey scratches, and in some patients no inciting trauma is recalled.

ETIOLOGY A specific etiologic agent has not been identified. Among the agents that have been incriminated are atypical acid-fast bacteria, organisms of the psittacosis-lymphogranuloma group, herpes-like (EB) virus, and most recently chlamydia. The evidence for ascribing a definitive causative role to any of these is not convincing.

EPIDEMIOLOGY Cats act only as vectors for the diseases. They are not ill, and have negative skin tests. The disease occurs mostly in children (75 percent), and several cases have been described in siblings, because of contact with the same cat. The disease is most common in fall and winter. Cats may act as long-term carriers, a hypothesis supported by the familial occurrence of several infections interspersed by months or years.

PATHOLOGY The histopathologic appearance of lymph nodes is not specific. Three stages have been described: (1) early lesions show reticulum-cell hyperplasia; (2) intermediate lesions show granuloma formation; and (3) late lesions show microabscesses. These reactions are not readily distinguished from those induced by the tubercle bacillus. However, acid-fast bacilli are invariably absent.

MANIFESTATIONS The incubation period lasts a few days to several weeks, with an average of 3 to 10 days. In a typical case the primary lesion consists of a raised, slightly tender, nonpruritic papule crowned by a small vesicle or eschar; it often resembles an indolent furuncle or insect bite. Multiple primary lesions have been described. In some patients a primary lesion cannot be found.

Regional lymphadenopathy becomes evident in a few days or as long as 6 weeks after infection. Adenopathy is unilateral and asymmetric; in most instances only one node is involved. The axillary, cervical, preauricular, submandibular, epitrochlear, femoral, or inguinal nodes (in decreasing order of frequency) on one side become visibly swollen and tender, often with redness of the overlying skin. The nodes occasionally suppurate, soften, and drain spontaneously; fistulas heal completely with only slight scarring. Usually the tenderness subsides gradually, and nontender, firm, enlarged nodes remain palpable for some weeks or even months. With rare exceptions, there is no generalized glandular enlargement, and the spleen is not palpable.

Systemic symptoms are usually mild and consist of headache, fever, and malaise, which subside within a few days. Shaking chills and fever with temperatures as high as 104°F can occur but are unusual. Many patients are entirely symptom-free. A transient macular or vesicular rash which subsides within 48 h is rarely present during the early stages. Erythema nodosum and multiforme have been reported.

Clinical forms of this disease other than that described above may be delineated. These include (1) encephalitis characterized by fever, convulsions, alterations in consciousness, mild cerebrospinal fluid pleocytosis and elevation in protein, and complete recovery; (2) Parinaud's oculoglandular syndrome characterized by granulomatous conjunctivitis and enlargement of the homolateral preauricular node; (3) more rarely, mesenteric lymphadenitis; (4) osteolytic bone lesions, which subside spontaneously; and (5) thrombocytopenic as well as nonthrombocytopenic purpura. In all these syndromes the diagnostic criteria for cat-scratch disease must be present before the illness can be ascribed to cat-scratch disease.

DIAGNOSIS The following criteria should be fulfilled before a diagnosis of cat-scratch disease is established: (1) history of contact with cats, (2) finding of a primary lesion, (3) regional lymphadenopathy, (4) positive intradermal skin test, (5) biopsy of lymph node with demonstration of histopathologic changes consistent with cat-scratch disease (this may not be necessary if the skin test is positive), and (6) failure to demonstrate other causative agents.

The specific diagnosis is made by means of a skin test. Antigen for this is prepared by mixing one part pus aspirated from infected lymph nodes with three parts saline solution, and inactivating the mixture by heating or by irradiation. A positive reaction is of the delayed tuberculin type, consisting of 5-mm induration and 1-cm erythema, that appears in 24 to 48 h. Although batches of antigen vary in potency, in general, patients reacting to one batch react to another. Skin test material can be preserved by freezing. The test becomes positive within 30 days after infection and may persist for many years. Each batch of antigen must be tested against patients known to have had the disease. A well-standardized batch should provide highly reliable results. Approximately 10 percent of normal individuals have false positive reactions. The chance of carrying hepatitis virus in the antigen is remote.

Other laboratory abnormalities include mild leukocytosis (up to 15,000 cells per cubic millimeter), occasional mild eosinophilia, and an elevated sedimentation rate. The Frei test is negative.

Patients with cat-scratch disease show significantly depressed lymphocyte transformation responses to phytohemagglutinin and *Candida albicans*. These reactions revert to normal as the disease subsides.

Cat-scratch disease is a benign illness, and the prognosis is uniformly good. Its main clinical importance lies in its possible confusion with other more serious diseases of the lymphatics. Diseases to be considered are tularemia, lymphatic tuberculosis, sporotrichosis, histoplasmosis, coccidioidomycosis, toxoplasmosis, and bacterial adenitis. Because of the indolent character of the adenopathy, Hodgkin's disease or other lymphomas may be suspected. Neck masses may be confused with thyroglossal duct cysts, bronchial cleft cysts, dermoids, cystic hygromas, thyroid and parathyroid adenomas, salivary gland tumors, carotid body tumors, aneurysms, pharyngeal or esophageal diverticula, and mesodermal tumors, as well as lymphomas. Appropriate serologic and cultural tests serve to rule out other infections; biopsy may be needed to exclude tumor, but a positive skin test with cat-scratch antigen effectively rules out the necessity for biopsy. Cat-scratch disease must be differentiated from tularemia, which occasionally can be transmitted by cats.

TREATMENT In instances of node suppuration, aspiration of accumulated pus affords relief of pain (and incidentally, serves as a source of material for the preparation of skin-test antigen). Aspiration is required in only a few cases. Antibiotics and steroids are ineffective.

REFERENCES

CARITHERS HA et al: Cat-scratch disease: Its natural history. JAMA 207:312, 1969

EMMONS RW et al: Continuing search for the etiology of cat-scratch disease. J Clin Microbiol 4:112, 1976

FUTRELL JW et al: Unsuspected etiology of lateral neck masses. Arch Otolaryngol 95:277, 1972

LYON LW. Neurologic manifestations of cat-scratch disease. Arch Neurol 25:23, 1971

MARGILETH AM: Cat-scratch disease: Nonbacterial regional lymphadenitis. Study of 145 patients and a review of the literature. Pediatrics 42:803, 1968

SCHULKIND ML, AYOUB EM: Cell-mediated immunity in cat-scratch disease. J Pediatr 85:199, 1974

WARWICK WJ: The cat-scratch syndrome: Many diseases or one disease? Prog Med Virol 9:256, 1967

section 14 | Infections caused by protozoa

198
APPROACH TO THE PATIENT WITH PROTOZOAN INFECTION

JAMES J. PLORDE

Protozoan diseases such as *malaria, trypanosomiasis, leishmaniasis, amebiasis,* and *toxoplasmosis* remain among the major causes of human sickness and death in the world today. Over 500 million people still live in malarious areas, and it is estimated that 100 million of these are infected at any given time. Of those infected, 1 million die of the disease annually.

In Africa, from the Sahara in the North to the Kalahari Desert in the South, human strains of *Trypanosoma brucei* cause one of the most lethal of all human diseases, *sleeping sickness*. Animal strains of this species limit food supply in the same area through their impact on animal husbandry. In South America, a related organism, *T. cruzi*, infects several million people, leaving many with severe heart and gastrointestinal lesions (*Chagas' disease*).

Leishmaniasis is found in parts of Europe, Asia, Africa, and South and Central America where it may present as a chronic, highly lethal infection of the reticuloendothelial system (kala azar), a mutilating mucocutaneous infection (espundia), or a self-limiting skin ulcer (oriental sore).

Ten percent of the world population, including 2 to 5 percent in the United States, are infected with the intestinal protozoa *Entamoeba histolytica*. Invasive disease resulting in an ulcerative colitis and/or liver abscess is particularly common in Mexico, western South America, South Asia, and West and Southwest Africa.

Toxoplasmosis, giardiasis, and *trichomoniasis* are three cosmopolitan protozoan infections well known to American physicians. The first infects perhaps one-third of the world's population. Although it is usually asymptomatic, congenital toxoplasmosis may result in abortion, stillbirth, prematurity, or severe neurological defects. Even when there are no obvious signs at birth, chorioretinitis with visual impairment may occur years later. Asymptomatic infection may also result in fatal encephalitis during periods of immunosuppression later in life.

In contrast, giardiasis and trichomoniasis seldom result in severe disability; nevertheless their morbidity can be attested to by millions of otherwise healthy individuals.

The pathogens responsible for these diseases are unicellular and possess a true, or membrane-limited, nucleus. Morphological differences in the cytoplasmic organelles of locomotion are useful in separating the protozoa pathogenic for human beings into four major groups: *flagellates, ciliates, amebas,* and *sporozoa*. The structures concerned with the motility of the first two groups are self-evident. Amebas move by means of pseudopodia, while the sporozoa generally lack any specific locomotor structures. Nuclear morphology, particularly the distribution pattern of the chromatin and karyosome (nucleolus), is used in distinguishing the species of certain organisms in the above groups.

Characteristically, the flagellates, ciliates, and amebas reproduce by asexual binary fission, while the sporozoa have alternating cycles of asexual (*schizogony*) and sexual (*sporogony*) reproduction. In the process of asexual multiplication the nucleus of the intracellular trophozoite first divides into several portions to form a schizont. Cytoplasmic division then occurs, resulting in the formation of daughter cells, or *merozoites*. These invade new host cells in which they become trophozoites, thus completing the asexual cycle. After one or more such cycles some merozoites initiate the sexual phase of reproduction by differentiating into male and female gametocytes. These mature and effect fertilization; the fertilized zygote, upon encysting, becomes known as an *oocyst*. *Sporozoites* formed within the oocyst are released, penetrate tissue cells, and begin another asexual cycle as trophozoites. These alternating sexual and asexual cycles may occur within the same (*Toxoplasma* spp., *Isospora* spp.) or different hosts (*Plasmodium* spp.).

The mode of transmission of these protozoa depends upon whether they are luminal or tissue parasites. Those which inhabit human gastrointestinal or genitourinary tracts are passed from human to human either directly as in the case of *Trichomonas vaginalis* or indirectly by the ingestion of contaminated food or water (fecal-oral transmission), e.g., *E. histolytica* and *Giardia lamblia*. In the former situation the infecting agent is the vegetative form, or trophozoite; in the latter it is a cyst capable of survival in the external environment for prolonged periods. Blood and tissue parasites, on the other hand, are generally transmitted via an arthropod which functions as both a vector and a second host. In the case of *Plasmodium* spp. this alternation of human and arthropod host is associated with the alternation of asexual and sexual generations described above.

These differences in transmission have a profound effect on both the distribution and control of protozoan diseases. Those spread by the fecal-oral route are essentially diseases of poverty and are found throughout the world wherever there is inadequate hygiene and sanitation. Their control depends upon the improvements in these areas which invariably accompany economic development. In contrast, the geographic distribution of the blood and tissue parasites is determined by the ecologic factors, particularly climate, responsible for the persistence of the arthropod vector. Attempts at disease prevention are characteristically directed at the control or elimination of the specific vectors. However, malaria, trypanosomiasis, and leishmaniasis can also be passed from person to person via blood transfusion, and careful screening of donors from endemic areas is important.

Clinically, protozoa exert their effects in a number of ways. In diseases such as malaria, the primary pathogenic mechanism appears to be the invasion and subsequent alteration or destruction of erythrocytes by the parasite. *Entamoeba histolytica* destroys host cells via enzymes or toxins without actual cellular invasion. In still other diseases, clinical manifestations are the result of a host-mounted inflammatory reaction, and in several, immunologic mechanisms are responsible for clinical findings, e.g., nephrotic syndrome in quartan malaria. *Giardia lamblia*, on the other hand, is thought by some to produce

TABLE 198-1
Antiprotozoal agents available through the Parasitic Disease Drug Service*

Infection	Therapeutic agent
Amebiasis	Dehydroemetine Diloxanide furoate
Chagas' disease (*Trypanosoma cruzi*)	Bayer 2502 (Lampit)
Leishmaniasis	Sodium antimony gluconate (Pentostam)
Malaria	Parenteral chloroquine hydrochloride Parenteral quinine dehydrochloride
Pneumocystosis	Pentamidine isothionate
Sleeping sickness (*Trypanosoma brucei*)	Melarsoprol (Mel B) Pentamidine isothionate Suramin (Antrypol)

* *Parasitic Disease Branch, Bureau of Epidemiology, Center for Disease Control, Atlanta, Ga. 30333. Day telephone: (404) 633-3311, ext. 3496; nights, weekends, and holidays: (404) 633-2176.*

malabsorption by simply covering a significant proportion of the microvilli in the small bowel.

By themselves, the clinical manifestations of disease are not always specific enough to ensure prompt diagnosis. Furthermore, general laboratory findings are often of little diagnostic aid. Although eosinophilia has been recognized as an important clue to the diagnosis of parasitic diseases, this phenomenon is characteristic of helminthic, not protozoan, infections. A carefully elicited travel, transfusion, and socioeconomic history often first suggests to the physician the possibility of a protozoan infection.

Reliable serologic tests have become available in the United States for many of the protozoan infections including malaria, amebiasis, toxoplasmosis, leishmaniasis, and South American trypanosomiasis. Many of these tests are performed by local institutions. For the remainder, blood samples can be sent to the individual state health departments for forwarding to the Center for Disease Control in Atlanta, Georgia. However, the definitive diagnosis usually rests upon the recovery and morphologic identification of the parasite from the genitourinary tract, intestinal contents, tissue, or blood.

Most intestinal protozoan agents are passed in the feces intermittently or in fluctuating numbers, and the examination of a single normally passed stool will detect only one-third to one-half of involved patients. The testing of three such specimens collected at intervals of 2 or 3 days will improve this yield substantially. Alternatively, a saline cathartic is administered to evacuate the cecal area where many protozoa are concentrated, and the entire purge is then examined. The stool must be free of interfering substances such as antidiarrheal or contrast agents, antacids, and antibiotics. If the appropriate specimens can not be obtained prior to administration of such substances, testing should be delayed for 1 week or, in the case of antimicrobial agents, 3 weeks after their discontinuation. The results of antiprotozoal therapy should be monitored by checking specimens at 1, 3, and 6 months. Occasionally, specimens other than stool must be examined. In the case of small-bowel infections such as giardiasis and coccidiosis, the diagnosis at times can be established only by sampling the duodenal contents or by performing a jejunal biopsy. Similarly, the recovery of large-bowel pathogens such as *E. histolytica* may require sigmoidoscopic aspiration of colonic ulcers. Whenever intestinal aspirates or soft to watery fecal specimens are collected, they should be immediately placed in a preservative such as polyvinyl alcohol (PVA) to prevent rapid disintegration of fragile trophozoites and allow the preparation of permanently stained smears. Formed stools generally contain the most resistant cyst forms. These will survive for 1 to 2 days at room temperature and indefinitely if placed in 5% formaldehyde.

Direct examination of the blood is useful for the detection of malaria parasites, leishmania, and trypanosomes. Preferably, fresh capillary blood should be used to prepare thin and thick blood smears and, when appropriate, wet mounts. Only specially prepared glass slides should be used as traces of soda lime or potash on uncleaned slides may alter the pH of the stain, making recognition of parasites difficult. If an experienced technologist is not available to assist in the bedside preparation of smears, it is preferable to collect venous blood in an EDTA Vacutainer and send it to the laboratory. As the concentration of malaria parasites in the peripheral blood may fluctuate, specimens should be collected three to four times a day for 2 or 3 days.

Many of the drugs used to treat protozoan infection are either not generally available or have not yet been approved for use in the United States. Fortunately, many of these agents are available through the Parasitic Disease Drug Service of the Center for Disease Control, Atlanta, Georgia. These drugs are listed in Table 198-1.

REFERENCES

BROWN HW: *Basic Clinical Parasitology,* 4th ed. New York, Appleton-Century-Crofts, 1975

Drugs for parasitic infections. Med Lett 20(4):17, 1978

Health information for international travel 1978, US Department of Health, Education, and Welfare Publication (CDC) 78–82. Morb Mort Week Rep, vol. 27, suppl, September 1978

HUNTER GW III et al (eds): *Tropical Medicine,* 5th ed. Philadelphia, Saunders, 1976

199
AMEBIASIS

JAMES J. PLORDE

DEFINITION Amebiasis is an infection of the large intestine produced by *Entamoeba histolytica*. It is an asymptomatic carrier state in most individuals, but diseases ranging from chronic, mild diarrhea to fulminant dysentery may occur. Among extraintestinal complications, the commonest is hepatic abscess, which may rupture into peritoneum, pleura, lung, or pericardium.

ETIOLOGY There are seven species of ameba that naturally parasitize the human mouth and intestine, but of these only *E. histolytica* causes disease. *Entamoeba coli* and *E. hartmanni* are the two species with which it is most likely to be confused in examination of stools.

Entamoeba histolytica exists in two forms: the motile trophozoite and the cyst. The trophozoite is the parasitic form and dwells in the lumen and/or wall of the colon, divides by binary fission, grows best under anaerobic conditions, and requires the presence of either bacteria or tissue substrates to satisfy its nutritional requirements. When diarrhea occurs, the trophozoites are passed unchanged in the liquid stool, where they can be distinguished by their size (10 to 20 μm in diameter), directional motility, sharply demarcated clear ectoplasm with slender finger-like pseudopodia, and finely granular endoplasm. In dysentery, the trophozoites are larger (up to 50 μm in diameter), and often contain ingested erythrocytes. In the absence of diarrhea, the trophozoites usually encyst before leaving the gut. The cysts are highly resistant to environmental changes, chlorine concentrations found in water purification systems, and gastric acid. With rare exception they are responsible for transmission of disease. Young cysts have a single nucleus, a glycogen vacuole, and sausage-shaped chromatoid bodies. As the cyst matures, it absorbs its cytoplasmic vacuoles and becomes quadrinucleate. The cysts of *E. histolytica* can be distinguished from those of *Entamoeba coli* by the presence of one to four nuclei with small centric karyosomes and fine peripheral chromatin and by their thick chromatoid bodies with round ends.

Entamoeba histolytica had been classified into large and small races depending upon whether they form cysts measuring more or less than 10 μm in diameter. Strains of the small race, however, are not pathogenic for human beings and are now considered as a distinct species, *Entamoeba hartmanni.*

Entamoeba histolytica-like amebas are organisms isolated from humans that are morphologically indistinguishable from true *E. histolytica*. However, unlike *E. histolytica* they are nonpathogenic, grow best at 20°C, and can multiply indefinitely in hypotonic solutions.

Entamoeba histolytica can be cultivated in artificial media, a procedure that is useful in direct diagnosis and in the preparation of purified antigens for serologic testing.

EPIDEMIOLOGY Infection with *E. histolytica* is worldwide. Stool surveys indicate that the prevalence of infection in the United States is between 1 and 5 percent. Rates as high as 50 percent may occur in tropical areas where the level of sanitation is low. Symptomatic amebiasis is unusual below the age of 10 years in temperate climates, and both intestinal and hepatic lesions predominate in adult males to an extent that is not readily explainable on the basis of different rates of exposure to infection. Reports of amebic liver abscess suggest that invasive amebiasis is concentrated in comparatively few parts of the world, most notably Mexico, western South America, South Asia, and West and Southwestern Africa. In the United States, the incidence of amebiasis has decreased sharply in the past 20 years. Furthermore, an increasing proportion of reported cases are now acquired outside the United States. Cases of dysentery and liver abscess can still be found, however, in institutions for the mentally retarded, Indian reservations, and migrant labor camps.

Although the parasite can sometimes infect rats, cats, dogs, and primates, human beings are the principal host and reservoir. Because trophozoites die rapidly after leaving the intestine, asymptomatic cyst passers are the source of new infections. The cysts are usually spread through contaminated food or water. Direct fecal-oral spread occurs between sexual partners and in conditions of poor personal hygiene. Venereal transmission appears to be particularly common among male homosexuals. Cases of amebic dysentery are usually sporadic, but epidemics, which are sometimes waterborne, have occurred. Outbreaks of amebiasis are never explosive, as are those produced by pathogenic intestinal bacteria.

PATHOGENESIS AND ANATOMIC CHANGES After ingestion, cysts undergo further nuclear division. In the small intestine, the cyst wall disintegrates, and trophozoites are released. The immature amebas are carried to the large intestine, where they live in the lumen of the gut as commensals feeding on bacteria and debris. On occasion the amebas may invade the mucosa, causing ulcerations that are sufficiently extensive to produce symptoms. The factors responsible for this are not completely understood, but the state of the host and the virulence of the infecting organism both play roles. Epidemiologic evidence suggests that amebic strains indigenous to temperate climates are usually avirulent. It has also been shown, however, that invasiveness is not a stable strain characteristic. It can either be lost after continued cultivation in vitro or enhanced by rapid animal passage. The virulence of various strains of *E. histolytica* is dependent upon the association with living bacteria.

Amebic ulceration of the intestinal wall is characteristic. A small mucosal defect overlies a larger, burrowing area of necrosis in the submucosa and muscularis, producing a bottle-shaped lesion. There is little acute inflammatory response, and in contrast to the picture in bacillary dysentery, the mucosa between ulcers is normal. The sites of involvement in order of frequency are cecum and ascending colon, rectum, sigmoid, appendix, and terminal ileum. In the cecum and sigmoid, chronic infection may lead to the formation of large masses of granulation tissue or *amebomas*. Amebas can enter the portal circulation and lodge in venules; liquefaction necrosis of liver tissue leads to the formation of an abscess cavity. Rarely, embolization results in lung, brain, or splenic abscess.

CLINICAL MANIFESTATIONS Asymptomatic cyst passer In the majority of patients with this common form of amebiasis, *E. histolytica* probably lives as a commensal in the bowel lumen. Individuals infected in temperate climates are unlikely to develop significant tissue invasion. However, invasion does occur occasionally, and so treatment of cyst passers is warranted.

Symptomatic intestinal amebiasis In some patients there is intermittent diarrhea consisting of one to four foul-smelling loose or watery stools daily. The stools sometimes contain mucus and blood. Loose stools alternate with periods of relative normality and may persist for months or years. Flatulence and abnormal cramping are frequent. The only physical findings are occasional tender hepatomegaly and slight pain when the cecum and ascending colon are palpated. Sigmoidoscopy sometimes reveals typical ulcerations with areas of normal mucosa interspersed. The diagnosis depends upon finding the organism in the feces or in ulcers.

Fulminating attacks of amebic dysentery are less common. Waterborne outbreaks may occur, but fulminating dysentery is more likely to occur spontaneously in debilitated individuals. Attacks may be precipitated by pregnancy or corticosteroids. The onset in half the cases is abrupt with high fever, between 40 and 40.6°C (104 and 105°F), severe abdominal cramps, and profuse, bloody diarrhea with tenesmus. There is diffuse abdominal tenderness, often so severe that peritonitis is suspected. Hepatomegaly is very frequent, and sigmoidoscopy almost always demonstrates extensive rectosigmoid ulceration. Trophozoites are numerous in stools and in material obtained directly from the ulcers.

In some cases there may be extensive destruction of the colonic mucosa and submucosa, massive hemorrhage or perforation of the bowel wall, with resultant peritonitis. Repeated severe attacks of intestinal amebiasis can lead to an ulcerative postdysenteric colitis. Amebas can usually not be demonstrated in this condition, but serologic tests are strongly positive. Invasion of the appendix may lead to a clinical picture of *appendicitis*. Penetration of trophozoites through the muscle wall of the bowel may result in the development of large masses of granulation tissue. When the entire circumference of the intestine is involved, there may then be partial obstruction, and a movable, tender, sausage-shaped mass is often palpable. This lesion or ameboma is most frequently seen in the cecum where a palpable mass and radiologic demonstration of a ragged encroachment of the lumen may lead to a mistaken diagnosis of adenocarcinoma.

Hepatic amebiasis The parasites usually reach the liver through the portal vein; rarely, they may traverse the lymphatic vessels. It has been believed for a long time that amebas which lodged in the liver could produce a diffuse hepatitis. Careful postmortem and biopsy studies indicate that the syndrome of tender hepatomegaly, right upper quadrant pain, fever, and leukocytosis in patients with amebic colitis is not a result of amebas in hepatic tissues, is accompanied by nonspecific periportal inflammation, and is rarely, if ever, a prelude to hepatic abscess. It is evident, then, that these manifestations are best regarded as an accompaniment of colitis and do not merit a separate diagnosis of "diffuse amebic hepatitis."

Hepatic abscess may develop insidiously, with fever, sweats, weight loss, and no local signs other than painless or slightly tender hepatomegaly. In other patients, there is abrupt onset, with chills, fever to 40.6°C (105°F), nausea, vomiting, severe upper abdominal pain, and polymorphonuclear leukocytosis. Initially, cholecystitis, perforated ulcer, or acute pancreatitis may be suspected.

Most commonly, the abscess occurs singly and is localized in the posterior portion of the right lobe of the liver, because this lobe receives most of the blood draining the right colon through the "streaming" effect in portal vein flow. This loca-

tion is responsible for several features that aid in diagnosis. *Point tenderness* in the posterolateral portion of a lower right intercostal space is frequent even in the absence of diffuse liver pain. Most abscesses enlarge upward, producing a bulge in the diaphragmatic dome, obliteration of the costophrenic gutter, small hydrothorax, basilar atelectasis, and pain referred to the right shoulder. Liver function tests may be mildly to moderately disturbed but are of little diagnostic aid. Jaundice is uncommon. Radiologically, unruptured abscesses do not show a fluid level, and calcification of the liver parenchyma is very rare. Isotope liver scan utilizing two, or preferably three, projections is invaluable in confirming both the presence and location of a liver abscess. Ultrasonic scanning reveals a fluid-filled cavity often with scattered internal echoes. It has been reported that hepatic tomograms will visualize amebic abscesses following intravenous Hypaque infusion. Serologic tests are positive in over 90 percent of patients.

Needle puncture results in the withdrawal of "pus" which consists of liquefied, necrotic liver. Typically, it is thick and odorless, resembling "chocolate syrup" or "anchovy paste." It may, however, be thin in consistency and yellow or green in color. The pus contains no polymorphonuclear leukocytes (barring secondary bacterial infection) and, usually, no amebas. The parasites are localized in the cyst wall and may be demonstrated in the terminal portion of the aspirate or, at times, by a Vim-Silverman needle biopsy of the cyst wall following aspiration of the abscess.

Hepatic abscess complicates asymptomatic infection of the colon more often than symptomatic intestinal disease, another factor making recognition difficult. Trophozoites or cysts are demonstrable in the feces of only about one-third of patients with abscess, and fewer than one-half can recall significant diarrheal illness.

Pleuropulmonary amebiasis The right pleural cavity and lung are involved by direct extension from the liver in 10 to 20 percent of patients with liver abscess. Rarely, amebic lung abscess has resulted from embolization rather than direct extension.

Manifestations are those of a consolidating pneumonia or lung abscess. If perforation into a bronchus occurs, patients expectorate large amounts of the typical exudate, some patients even commenting that the sputum "tastes like liver." Cough, pleural pain, fever, and leukocytosis are the rule, and secondary bacterial infection is frequent. Rupture into the free pleural space results in a massive pleural effusion; aspiration of "chocolate" fluid is diagnostic.

Other extraintestinal lesions Extension of an abscess from the left lobe of the liver to the pericardium is the most dangerous complication of hepatic abscess. It may be mistaken for tuberculous pericarditis or congestive cardiomyopathy. Less frequently, rapid cardiac tamponade occurs with ensuing dyspnea, shock, and death. *Peritonitis* is a result of perforation of colonic ulcer or rupture of liver abscess. Painful ulcers or condylomata of the genitalia, perianal skin, or abdominal wall (draining sinuses) are unusual complications which may be mistaken for syphilitic, tuberculous, or neoplastic lesions. They usually result from direct extension of intestinal disease; some are thought to result from sexual transmission. Metastatic brain abscess is rare, and an etiologic diagnosis is seldom made clinically. Splenic abscess has been reported but is very unusual.

DIFFERENTIAL DIAGNOSIS **Intestinal amebiasis** Patients with nondysenteric amebiasis are often misdiagnosed as having irritable bowel syndrome, diverticulitis, or regional enteritis. Ameboma may mimic colonic carcinoma or granulomatous disease, while the clinical spectrum of amebic dysentery overlaps those of shigellosis, salmonellosis, ulcerative colitis, and, in endemic areas, schistosomiasis. The invasive bacterial infections are usually more acute, severe, and self-limited than amebiasis. Stools from patients with shigellosis, salmonellosis, and ulcerative colitis contain large numbers of polymorphonuclear leukocytes, while those in amebic infection do not. Nevertheless, amebiasis may closely resemble any of the above diseases both clinically and radiologically and must be considered in the differential diagnosis of any chronic diarrhea or dysentery.

The identification of *E. histolytica* in the stool, however, does not eliminate other diagnostic possibilities. Amebic infection is often superimposed on or exacerbated by other colonic disease including cecal carcinoma. For this reason, patients with intestinal amebiasis and abdominal complaints still require stool culture, sigmoidoscopy, and a barium enema.

Hepatic abscess Once a filling defect has been demonstrated by isotope liver scanning, the differential diagnosis includes hepatic neoplasm, hydatid cyst, and pyogenic abscess. Neoplasms can usually be differentiated on the basis of their ultrasonic scanning characteristics, while the lack of constitutional manifestations and presence of an appropriate epidemiologic history is helpful in recognizing echinococcosis. The most difficult problem lies in the exclusion of a pyogenic abscess. An insidious onset in an adult male, a history of chronic diarrhea, significant pleuritic chest pain, and a single right lobe lesion favors the diagnosis of amebiasis. High fever, hyperbilirubinemia, multiple hepatic filling defects, and foul-smelling hepatic aspirate are more suggestive of pyogenic disease. Ultimately, the separation of the two diseases rests upon laboratory procedures.

LABORATORY DIAGNOSIS The diagnosis of intestinal amebiasis depends upon *identification of the organism in the stool or tissues.* Formed stools are examined initially in saline and iodine mounts for amebic cysts; concentration methods such as the formalin-ether technique increase the yield two- to three-fold. Liquid or semiformed stools should be examined immediately in saline solution for the presence of motile hematophagous trophozoites. The addition of a supravital stain such as buffered methylene blue to the saline enhances nuclear detail and minimizes the possibility of confusing fecal leukocytes with amebic trophozoites, an error common to inexperienced parasitologists. If there is any delay in examination of the stool, a portion of the specimen may be refrigerated for a few hours at 4°C, or placed in polyvinyl alcohol and 10% formalin. Definitive identification of *E. histolytica* requires the examination of permanently stained slides prepared from the material preserved with polyvinyl alcohol. An ocular micrometer is necessary to separate *E. hartmanni* from its larger relative. Four to six stool specimens may be required for diagnosis. If possible, the stool should be examined before the administration of antimicrobial, antidiarrheal, or antacid preparations, because all these agents may interfere with the recovery of amebas. Likewise, enemas and radiographic procedures utilizing barium sulfate are best postponed until after a thorough search for *E. histolytica* has been made.

Sigmoidoscopy is of value in symptomatic cases. The mucosal lesions should be aspirated and the material examined for trophozoites as described above. Biopsy material obtained from such lesions and stained with periodic acid–Schiff solution also will frequently reveal trophozoites.

The diagnosis of extraintestinal amebiasis is difficult. The parasite usually cannot be recovered from stool or tissue. Cultivation of amebas from feces or pus is possible but is not practical in most laboratories. The most important diagnostic procedure in suspected liver abscess is a *therapeutic trial of antiamebic drugs.* The response is often dramatic within 3 days.

In the event that demonstrating parasites is difficult, the therapeutic trial should be instituted without hesitation.

Serologic tests employing purified antigens are positive in nearly all patients with proved amebic liver abscess and in a great majority of those with acute amebic dysentery. They are generally negative in asymptomatic cyst passers, suggesting that tissue invasion is required for antibody production. The persistence of significant antibody titers for months to years after complete cure makes serology, particularly in endemic areas, of more value in excluding the diagnosis than in confirming it. Some authors recommend the routine screening of all patients thought to have inflammatory bowel disease for serologic evidence of amebiasis. Steroid therapy could then be withheld in patients with positive tests pending the outcome of parasitological examination. Of the available tests, the indirect hemagglutination appears to be the most sensitive. Indirect immunofluorescence, countercurrent electrophoresis, and agar gel diffusion are also highly reliable. A number of rapid tests such as latex agglutination and cellulose acetate diffusion have made serologic testing available to most laboratories. Intradermal tests have been shown to be helpful in epidemiologic surveys, but their value in the diagnosis of amebiasis remains to be determined.

TREATMENT Treatment should be aimed at relief of symptoms, replacement of fluid, electrolyte, and blood losses, and eradication of the organism. Amebas may be found in the lumen of the bowel, in the intestinal wall, or extraintestinally. Most amebicides are not effective at all sites or when used alone, and a combination of drugs is often necessary to achieve cure. The available drugs based on their site of action fall into several different categories, as described below.

Luminal amebicides These oral agents act by direct contact with trophozoites dwelling in the bowel lumen but are ineffective against amebas in tissue. Of the large number of available drugs, diloxanide furoate (Furamide) is one of the most effective and well tolerated but is presently available in the United States only through the Center for Disease Control. A response rate of 80 to 85 percent has been noted; flatulence appears to be the only major side effect.

Diiodohydroxyquin has been effective in 60 to 70 percent of cases. As with its analogue iodochlorhydroxyquin (Entero-Vioform), myelooptic neuropathy has been reported after long-term use. However, no such case has been noted when the dosage was limited to that given in Table 199-1. The drug should not be used in patients with thyroid disease or preexisting optic neuropathy.

Tissue amebicides *Chloroquine diphosphate* (Aralen) is a systemic amebicide which is useful in hepatic disease because of its high concentration in the liver. It has little activity elsewhere.

Emetine is an alkaloid derivative of ipecac. When given intramuscularly, it is highly effective in destroying trophozoites in tissue including those in the wall of the intestine. It is ineffective against luminal amebas. Emetine is relatively toxic and may produce vomiting, diarrhea, abdominal cramping, weakness, muscle pain, tachycardia, hypotension, precordial pain, and electrocardiographic abnormalities. The common ECG changes include T-wave inversion and prolongation of the QTc interval. Rarely arrhythmias and prolongation of the QRS complex are seen. A synthetic derivative, dehydroemetine, is thought to be less toxic by virtue of its more rapid excretion and lower concentration in myocardial tissue. It is not free of toxicity, however, and patients treated with either drug should be at bed rest with ECG monitoring. Neither drug should be used in patients with renal, cardiac, or muscle disease, during pregnancy, or in children unless other drugs fail.

Metronidazole (Flagyl) is unique because it is both safe and effective against trophozoites at all sites, intestinally and extraintestinally. It is the drug of choice in most forms of amebiasis. For intestinal amebiasis it is given in dosage of 750 mg three times daily for 5 to 10 days. Smaller doses are effective in hepatic amebiasis. Metronidazole has an Antabuse-like action, and alcohol should be avoided during its administration. The recent evidence that this drug is carcinogenic and possibly teratogenic in animals when given in large doses is disturbing. The potential risk in human beings must be weighed against the severity of the disease, particularly in pregnant women.

Management (see Table 199-1) A course of diiodohydroxyquin or diloxanide furoate should be given in asymptomatic or mildly symptomatic patients. Stools should be examined monthly for 6 months to detect relapse. If it occurs, retreatment can be carried out with the alternate drug or metronidazole.

Treatment of acute dysentery involves control of symptoms as well as eradication of the organism. A number of regimens can be used:

For both mild and moderate dysentery, metronidazole given in a dose of 750 mg three times daily for 5 to 10 days is the simplest and least toxic regimen. This drug will cure about 90 percent of patients. The addition of one of the luminal amebicides will raise the cure rate close to 100 percent. Of some concern is the occurrence of amebic liver abscess in a few patients treated for dysentery with metronidazole. It is probable that this results from failure of metronidazole to eliminate luminal organisms in a small proportion of cases. For this reason, the routine addition of diiodohydroxyquin or diloxanide furoate seems indicated.

In severe dysentery, emetine or dehydroemetine should be

TABLE 199-1
Drug therapy of amebiasis

Clinical form and drug	Dosage
ASYMPTOMATIC INTESTINAL CARRIER	
Diiodohydroxyquin	600 mg tid for 20 days
or diloxanide furoate*	500 mg tid for 10 days
or metronidazole	750 mg tid for 5–10 days
MILD TO MODERATE INTESTINAL DISEASE	
Metronidazole	As above
plus diiodohydroxyquin	As above
or diloxanide furoate	As above
SEVERE INTESTINAL DISEASE	
Above regimen	
plus dehydroemetine*	1.0–1.5 mg/kg IM per day (maximum 90 mg per day) for up to 5 days
or emetine	1 mg/kg IM per day (maximum 60 mg per day) for up to 5 days
EXTRAINTESTINAL DISEASE	
Metronidazole	As above
or chloroquine phosphate	1 g per day for 2 days, then 500 mg per day for 4 weeks
plus dehydroemetine*	As above for 10 days
or emetine	As above for 10 days

* *Investigational drug available through the Parasitic Drug Service, Center for Disease Control, Atlanta, Ga., (404) 633-3311, nights and weekends 633-2176.*

added to the above regimen. These intramuscular agents rapidly control the acute attack, but because of their toxicity administration should be discontinued as soon as symptoms abate.

In extraintestinal amebiasis including hepatic abscess, metronidazole would appear to be the drug of choice; it is less toxic and probably just as effective as the chloroquine-emetine combination. In cases of relapse or in situations where the patient is unable to take oral medication, therapy with dehydroemetine or emetine should be instituted, and oral chloroquine added as soon as possible. Diagnostic trials should employ the chloroquine-emetine regimen because pyogenic liver abscesses may temporarily respond to metronidazole. Many authors prefer to add luminal amebicides to both the metronidazole and chloroquine-emetine programs. Treatment failures have been reported for both emetine-chloroquine and metronidazole. They appear to be unrelated to the organism's resistance.

There is debate over the value of routine aspiration of amebic liver abscesses. Certainly, if there is localized swelling over the liver, marked elevation of the diaphragm, severe localized liver tenderness, and failure to respond to systemic amebicides, it should be done. Adequate drainage can usually be accomplished by needle alone, and surgical drainage is rarely necessary. The greatest hazard in needling an abscess is secondary bacterial infection.

PROGNOSIS Intestinal amebiasis usually responds readily and completely to appropriate drugs. Parasitologic relapses sometimes occur, and posttreatment stools should be checked monthly for 6 months. Repeated relapses, however, are usually a manifestation of reinfection, complicating illness, inadequate therapy, or incorrect diagnosis. The fatality rate is less than 5 percent.

Hepatic and pulmonary amebiasis are still accompanied by an appreciable mortality, but no reliable figures are available.

PREVENTION For the individual, avoidance of contaminated food and water, scalding of vegetables, and the use of iodine-releasing tablets in drinking water (chlorine, in the form of halazone, is ineffective) are important measures. Globaline tablets, containing tetraglycine hydroperiodide, are convenient and effective.

Improvements in general sanitation and the detection of cyst passers and their removal from food-handling duties are general measures in prophylaxis, but such segregation of carriers is rarely practiced. Community control of amebic disease by periodic mass treatment with metronidazole and diloxanide furoate has been successful in some areas. At the present time, however, personal chemoprophylaxis for travelers is not recommended.

PRIMARY AMEBIC MENINGOENCEPHALITIS

Primary amebic meningoencephalitis is caused by free-living amebas, usually of the genus *Naegleria*. It most often affects children and young adults, appears to be acquired by swimming in fresh warm water, and is almost invariably fatal.

Free-living amebas are ubiquitous in nature where they are commonly found in soil and water. Although generally considered harmless, some varieties are clearly pathogenic for the central nervous system of mammals. In those instances of human meningoencephalitis where the responsible organism has been isolated and cultured, it has, with few exceptions, been identified as an amoeboflagellate, *Naegleria fowleri*.

Over 80 cases have been reported from different parts of the world including Australia, Czechoslovakia, Great Britain, New Zealand, and the United States. Serologic studies suggest that inapparent infections are much more common. Most of the 35 cases recognized in the United States have occurred in the Southeastern states, particularly Florida, Georgia, and Virginia. Characteristically the patients have fallen ill during the summer months approximately 1 week after swimming in fresh or brackish water. The 16 Czechoslovakian cases followed swimming in an indoor pool with chlorinated water maintained at 24°C, and 6 cases have been acquired apparently after bathing in hot mineral water. Histological evidence suggests that the amebas reach the central nervous system directly via the nasal mucosa at the level of the cribriform plate. Clinically, the illness is rapid in onset, brief in duration, and inexorable in course. The initial symptom is a severe, persistent, frontal headache followed by nausea, vomiting, fever, and nuchal rigidity. Unusual tastes or smells may be noted. Later, drowsiness, confusion, convulsions, and coma appear. Focal neurological findings may occur late in the course of the illness.

A more benign, chronic form of amebic meningoencephalitis has been linked to organisms of the genus *Acanthamoeba*. Patients with this clinical syndrome frequently lack a history of freshwater swimming and may recover spontaneously. Pathologically, the disease can be distinguished from *Naegleria* infections by the granulomatous nature of the inflammatory reaction and the presence of both trophozoites and cysts in the tissues. Unfortunately, the identification of the responsible organisms remains in some doubt as they have never been recovered by culture techniques. It is possible that the free-living ameba of several species are involved.

A careful examination of the cerebrospinal fluid is the single most helpful diagnostic procedure. The fluid is usually bloody or sanguinopurulent and demonstrates an intense neutrophilic response. The protein is elevated and the glucose diminished. No organisms are demonstrated on Gram's stain or routine culture. Early examination of a wet preparation of unspun spinal fluid will usually reveal viable trophozoites. They are 10 to 20 μm in diameter, possess a granular cytoplasm, a distinct ectoplasm, and bulbous pseudopodia. If the specimen is allowed to cool, the trophozoites may become immobile and more difficult to recognize. Although the amebas may be easily grown on ordinary culture media which have been seeded with coliform bacteria, this is not helpful in clinical management, so rapidly progressive is the disease. Treatment with standard antiprotozoal agents seems completely ineffective. *Naegleria*, however, is highly sensitive to amphotericin B, miconazole, tetracycline, and rifampin. To date only two patients have survived a *Naegleria* infection. Both were diagnosed early and treated, one with amphotericin B and the other with amphotericin B, miconazole, and rifampin. Intracisternal, as well as intravenous, administration of amphotericin is probably essential to rapidly obtain effective levels in the cerebrospinal fluid. The intraventricular dose is 0.5 to 1 mg for the first few days. The intravenous dose is similar to that for cryptococcal meningitis (Chap. 153).

If the source of the infection can be determined, further cases might be prevented by closing the area to bathing.

REFERENCES

Amebiasis

ADAMS EB, MACLEOD IN: Invasive amebiasis. Medicine 56:315, 1977

BARBOUR GL, JUNIPER K JR: A clinical comparison of amebic and pyogenic abscess of the liver in sixty-six patients. Am J Med 53:323, 1972

COHEN HG, REYNOLDS TB: Comparison of metronidazole and chloroquine for the treatment of amebic liver abscess. Gastroenterology 69:35, 1975

ELSDON-DEW R: The epidemiology of amebiasis. Adv Parasitol 6:1, 1968

GRIFFIN FH JR: Failure of metronidazole to cure hepatic amebic abscess. N Engl J Med 288:1397, 1973

JUNIPER K JR: Amebiasis. Clin Gastroenterol 7:3, 1978

KROGSTAD DJ et al: Amebiasis: Epidemiologic studies in the United States, 1971–1974. Ann Intern Med 88:89, 1978

——— et al: Current concepts in parasitology—amebiasis. N Engl J Med 298:262, 1978

The Medical Letter. 20(4):17, 1978

NEAL RA: Pathogenesis of amebiasis. Bull NY Acad Med 47:462, 1971

POWELL SJ et al: Metronidazole combined with diloxanide furoate in amebic liver abscess. Ann Trop Med Parasitol 67:367, 1973

SCHMERIN MJ et al: Amebiasis—an increasing problem among homosexuals in New York City. JAMA 238:1386, 1977

SODEMAN WA JR, DOWDA MC: Rapid serologic methods for the demonstration of *Entamoeba histolytica* activity. Gastroenterology 65:604, 1973

Primary amebic meningoencephalitis

CARTER RF: Primary amoebic meningoencephalitis: An appraisal of present knowledge. Trans R Soc Trop Med Hyg 67:193, 1972

DUMA RJ et al: Primary amebic meningoencephalitis caused by *Naegleria*. Ann Intern Med 74:861, 1971

———: Meningoencephalitis and brain abscess due to a free-living amoeba. Ann Intern Med 88:468, 1978

ROBERT VB, RORKE LB: Primary amebic encephalitis, probably from *Acanthamoeba*. Ann Intern Med 79:174, 1973

200
MALARIA

JAMES J. PLORDE

DEFINITION Malaria is a protozoan disease transmitted to humans by the bite of *Anopheles* mosquitoes. It is characterized by *rigors, fever, splenomegaly, anemia* and a *chronic relapsing course*. Despite the impressive results of the World Health Organization–sponsored malaria eradication program begun in the year 1956, technical and socioeconomic difficulties have led to a recent resurgence of the disease in many areas of the world. Consequently, malaria remains today, as it has been for centuries, one of the most serious infectious disease problems in the world. In the United States and Europe, several hundred imported cases are seen annually in travelers from endemic areas.

ETIOLOGY *The causative organisms are protozoa of the genus Plasmodium.* The four species known to infect human beings are *P. vivax, P. ovale, P. malariae,* and *P. falciparum.* Human infection begins when a female anopheline inoculates plasmodial *sporozoites* into the lymphohematogenous system while feeding. After a brief passage in the peripheral blood, these organisms invade hepatocytes where they initiate the preclinical hepatic (exoerythrocytic) phase of disease. By a process of asexual multiplication referred to as *schizogony,* a single sporozoite eventually produces 2000 to 40,000 hepatic *merozoites.* In 1 to 6 weeks, these daughter cells rupture back into the circulatory system. In *P. falciparum,* and presumably *P. malariae,* infections, the hepatic phase terminates at this point. In the other species, liver forms persist and produce new episodes of bloodstream invasion months to years later.

The erythrocytic or clinical phase of malaria starts with the attachment of a released merozoite to a specific receptor site on the red blood cell surface. This site appears to differ for each species of malaria; in the case of *P. vivax,* it is related in some way to the Duffy blood group antigens (Fy^a or Fy^b). Duffy-negative (FyFy) individuals, who include the majority of people of West African extraction, are resistant to vivax malaria, presumably for this reason. Following attachment, the merozoite invaginates the cell surface and is slowly interiorized. The intracellular parasite first appears as a ring-shaped trophozoite which later enlarges and assumes an irregular or ameboid shape. Its nucleus then divides into several portions to form a multinucleated *schizont*. Eventually, cytoplasm condenses around each daughter nucleus to form a new generation of merozoites. Forty-eight hours after its original invasion (72 h in the case of *P. malariae*) the erythrocyte ruptures, releasing 6 to 24 organisms, each of which is capable of initiating a new red blood cell cycle. With repetition of this cycle, some of the red blood cells become filled with *sexual forms* (gametocytes); these do not induce cell lysis and are unable to undergo further development unless ingested by an appropriate mosquito during a blood meal. In the stomach of the mosquito fertilization occurs, and the resulting *ookinete* encysts on the outer surface of the stomach and releases myriads of *sporozoites*. These migrate to the salivary glands and are inoculated into a human subject at the next feeding.

EPIDEMIOLOGY Malaria survives only in areas of the world where both the anopheline and infected human population remain above certain *critical densities* required for the sustained transmission of disease. Control measures are directed toward reducing both populations to levels that are too low for the infection to survive. Important procedures include drainage or filling of breeding areas, use of residual insecticide sprays, screening, use of skin repellents, effective treatment of cases, and large-scale suppressive drug programs in some human populations.

An active international cooperative program aimed at the eradication of malaria resulted in a significant decline in the incidence of the disease between 1956 and 1968. In over three-quarters of the original malarial areas of the world, the disease was eradicated, or active eradication programs were instituted. Presently, however, malaria still infects 125 million inhabitants of 104 countries throughout Africa, Latin America, South America, Asia, and Oceania (Fig. 200-1). Tropical Africa alone harbors 100 million of these afflicted individuals and contributes most of the 1 million deaths that occur annually from this terrible disease. The presence of mobile populations, outdoor-biting mosquitoes, and high levels of disease transmission make successful eradication in these remaining areas unlikely. Furthermore, the emergence of insecticide-resistant mosquitoes as well as a variety of administrative and socioeconomic problems has produced serious setbacks to several previously successful eradication programs, particularly those on the Indian subcontinent. Added to these difficulties has been the continuing spread of drug-resistant *P. falciparum* throughout Southern Asia, the Western Pacific, Central America, and South America. A limited number of resistant strains have now been discovered in Africa, an area previously free of this problem.

Endemic malaria did not disappear from the United States until the 1950s. Imported cases and occasional outbreaks of malaria acquired by mosquito transmission from imported infections (*introduced malaria*) have continued to occur, but until 1966 the total never exceeded 200 cases a year. This number rapidly increased with the return of infected military personnel from Southeast Asia, reaching a peak of over 4000 in 1970. Associated with this wave of imported malaria was a smaller increase in the number of infections induced by blood transfusion and intravenous heroin use. Although this epidemic has

FIGURE 200-1

Areas of risk for malaria transmission as of December 1974. (From WHO Weekly Epidemiologic Record no 45, 1975.)

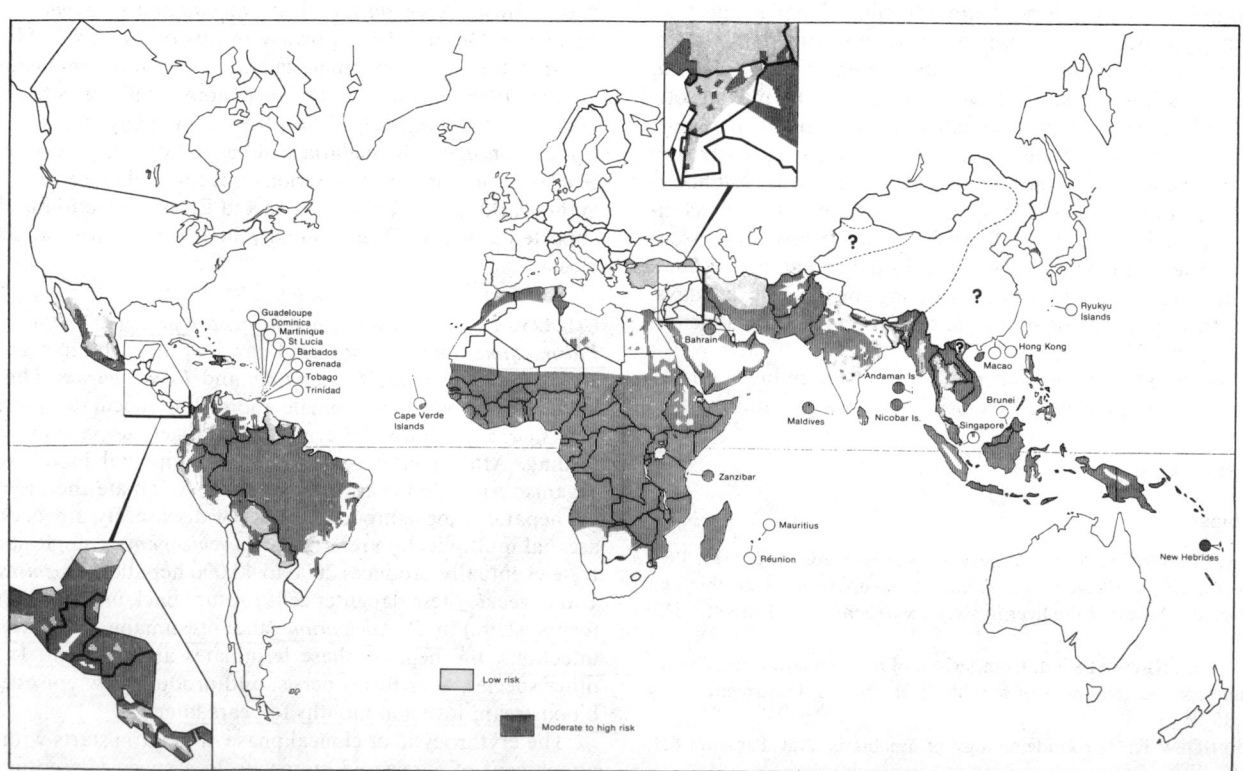

waned, the incidence of malaria in the civilian population has not (Fig. 200-2). From 1970 to 1977, the number of cases reported annually among tourists, businessmen, teachers, students, and other civilians rose from 151 to 466. With rare exceptions, malaria was acquired abroad: approximately 50 percent in Asia, 30 percent in Africa, and 10 percent in the Caribbean or Latin America. Clinical manifestations usually developed within 6 months of arrival in the United States, but in one-third of the vivax cases they were delayed beyond that point. In 1977, one-fifth of the cases and two out of the three deaths were caused by the virulent *P. falciparum*. Tragically, most of these cases could have been prevented with appropriate chemoprophylaxis. Until travelers are more fully informed of dangers inherent in traveling unprotected to malarious areas, the number of cases seen in this country each year will continue to increase.

PATHOGENESIS AND PATHOLOGY   The invasion, alteration, and destruction of red blood cells by malaria parasites, systemic and local circulatory changes, and immune phenomena are all important in the pathophysiology of malaria.

Red blood cell changes   Malaria species differ significantly in their ability to invade red blood cells. *Plasmodium vivax* and *P. ovale* attack only immature erythrocytes; *P. malariae*, only senescent ones. During infection with these species, therefore, no more than 1 or 2 percent of cells are involved at any one time. *Plasmodium falciparum* invades red blood cells regardless of age and may cause extremely high levels of parasitemia. Only the presence of certain abnormal hemoglobins, notably S, is capable of limiting parasitemia produced by the species. The same protective effect may be exerted in hemoglobin C, D, E thalassemia, and glucose 6-phosphate (G6PD) or pyridoxalkinase deficiency, since these abnormalities are found more commonly in malarious areas. In thalassemia and related hemoglobinopathies, the protection may be related in part to the persistent production of fetal hemoglobin since maturation of *P. falciparum* is retarded in cells containing hemoglobin F.

Once parasitized, the cells may be destroyed at the time of sporulation or in the presence of specific opsonizing antibody phagocytosed in the liver or spleen. In the spleen the parasites are also removed from some cells, and the intact erythrocytes are returned into the circulation. However, anemia usually develops and, in the case of falciparum malaria, may be severe. This species also induces physical changes in parasitized cells resulting in intravascular agglutination and sludging.

Although paroxysms of fever coincide with sporulation and the destruction of red blood cells, the cause of the fever remains obscure and may be related to release of an endogenous pyrogen from injured cells.

Circulatory changes   The circulatory changes in malaria are characterized by vasoconstriction during the "cold" stage followed by vasodilation during the "hot" stage. In falciparum malaria vasodilation in the skin is accompanied by hypotension, decreased central venous pressure, increased radioiodinated serum albumin space, and increased excretion of aldosterone, suggesting a decrease in effective circulating blood volume due to enhanced vascular permeability and/or capacitance. On the other hand, there may be localized vasospasm, kinin-induced capillary permeability with a resulting increase in blood viscosity, obstruction of capillaries with agglutinated red blood cells, and, occasionally, intravascular coagulation which may compromise perfusion to vital organs such as the kidney, brain, liver, and lung.

Immune phenomena   Normal as well as parasitized red blood cells are destroyed in malaria. The explanation for this phenomenon is unknown, although immunologic mechanisms including autoantibody production and adherence of antigen-antibody complexes to uninfected red blood cells have been suggested. The destruction is most profound in blackwater fever where there is massive intravascular hemolysis. More commonly, however, the red blood cells are sequestered and destroyed in the reticuloendothelial system of the liver and spleen. Thrombocytopenia is related to splenic pooling and shortened platelet life span. Both direct parasitic invasion and immune mechanisms may be operative in platelet destruction. Host γ and β-1C-globulin deposits have been noted along the glomerular capillary basement membrane of patients with the

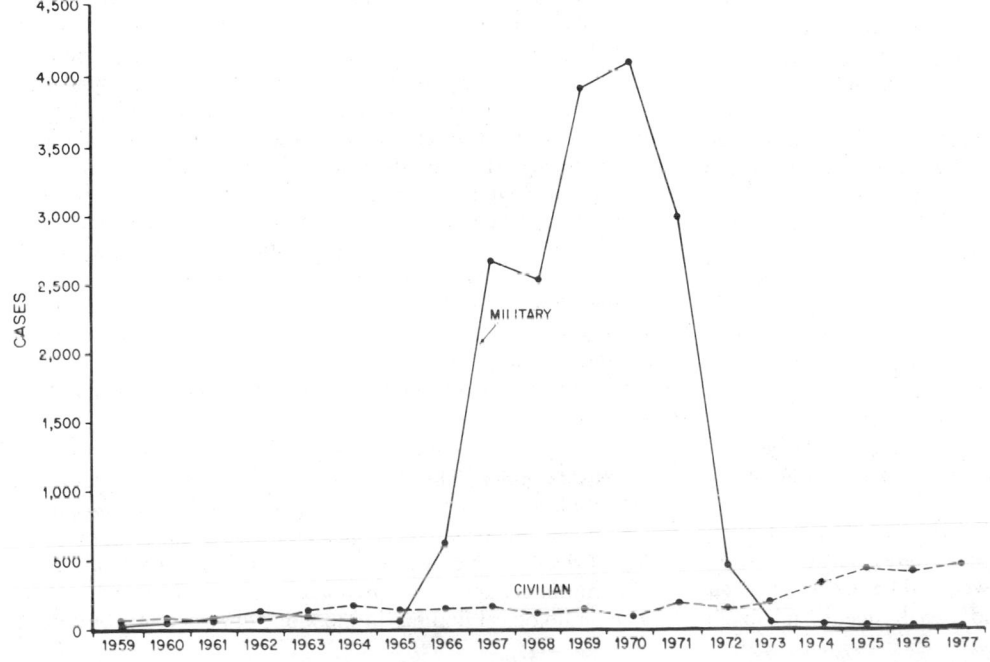

FIGURE 200-2
Military and civilian cases of malaria, United States, 1959–1977. (From Malaria Surveillance: Annual Summary 1977, Atlanta, Center for Disease Control, 1978.)

acute transient glomerulonephritis of falciparum malaria and the progressive nephrosis of chronic quartan malaria, establishing these as immune complex nephropathies.

IMMUNITY Recovery from malaria occurs slowly, apparently the function of acquired immunity. In simian malaria, this appears to require the presence of both T and B cell lymphocytes. Although the role of the T cell is known to be vital, its mechanism of action is uncertain. Some authors have suggested that it stimulates effector cells, perhaps macrophages, to release a nonspecific factor capable of inhibiting intraerythrocytic multiplication; others feel it may have a helper effect on antibody formation.

Strain-specific antiplasmodial antibodies do occur early in the course of parasitemia and reach high levels coincident with a fall in the number of circulating organisms. The relative rarity of malaria in young infants has been attributed to transplacental passage of IgG antibodies. It is uncertain whether these are directly lethal, act as opsonizing agents or block merozoitic invasion of erythrocytes. In simian malaria, antigenic change in the parasite results in cycles of recrudescent parasitemia and production of variant-specific antibodies. It seems probable that similar changes occur in humans, leading to the eventual disappearance of erythrocytic forms. In falciparum malaria, this results in cure. In vivax and ovale infections, the intracellular hepatic forms escape the humoral immune defenses and may later discharge fresh merozoites into the bloodstream to maintain the infection for a period of 3 to 5 years. *Plasmodium malariae* produces chronic disease of extremely long duration, up to 53 years in one case, despite the lack of a persistent exoerythrocytic focus. This effect is presumably due to long-term survival of circulating parasites in concentrations too low to be detected on routine blood films. How these parasites escape immunologic destruction is unknown. In a closely related simian malaria, however, splenectomy rapidly leads to termination of infection, suggesting that suppressor T cells in the spleen may play a protective role.

MANIFESTATIONS General The incubation period between the bite of the mosquito and onset of symptoms is usually 10 to 14 days in vivax and falciparum malaria and 18 days to 6 weeks in malariae infections. This period may be prolonged in persons who have taken antimalarial suppressants. In the United States, the interval between entry into the country and onset of disease exceeds 6 months in one-quarter of the patients developing vivax infections; it exceeds 1 month in a similar proportion of falciparum cases. There is some variation in clinical manifestations produced by the different plasmodia, but in all, chills, fever, headache, muscle pains, splenomegaly, and anemia are common. Herpes labialis is frequent and usually appears after the infection is well established. Hepatomegaly, mild icterus, and edema are often observed, especially in falciparum infections. Urticaria is common in patients with chronic malaria.

The hallmark of the disease is the malarial *paroxysm*, which recurs regularly in all but falciparum infections. The typical paroxysm begins with a rigor that lasts 20 to 60 min—the "cold stage"—followed by a "hot stage" of 3 to 8 h with temperature of 40 to 41.7°C (104 to 107°F). The "wet stage" consists of defervescence with profuse diaphoresis and leaves the patient exhausted.

First attacks are often severe, but repeated episodes become milder, although debilitation may be progressive. In untreated cases, the attacks may persist for weeks. The paroxysms eventually become more irregular and less frequent and finally cease, corresponding with the disappearance of parasites from the blood and marking the end of the primary attack. Relapses occur when exoerythrocytic parasites persisting in the liver reinvade the bloodstream.

Tertian malaria (*P. vivax* or *P. ovale*) This infection is rarely fatal, although relapses are common, and it is the most difficult to cure. A prodrome of myalgia, headache, chilliness, and low-grade fever for 48 to 72 h heralds the onset of the acute illness. Initially, the fever may be irregular because the maturation cycle of the parasite is not synchronized. Synchronization usually occurs toward the end of the first week, and typical paroxysms then occur on alternate days. The spleen becomes palpable at the end of the second week. Infections with *P. ovale* tend to be milder, and primary attacks shorter than those caused by *P. vivax.*

Quartan malaria (*P. malariae*) Paroxysms occur every third day and tend to be regular. The disease is usually more disabling than tertian but responds well to treatment. Edema, albuminuria, and hematuria (*not* hemoglobinuria), a clinical state similar to acute hemorrhagic nephritis, occasionally appear during the course. This complication should not be confused with *blackwater fever*. Chronic *P. malariae* infection may be associated with a clinically and histologically unique nephrosis. The prolonged duration of asymptomatic parasitemia characteristic of the species helps to explain the frequency with which it is implicated in transfusion-induced malaria.

Falciparum malaria (*P. falciparum*) Because of an asynchronous cycle of multiplication, onset may be insidious and fever continuous, remittent, or irregular. Typical paroxysms occur in a minority of patients. Splenomegaly occurs rapidly, and mental confusion, postural hypotension, edema, and gastrointestinal symptoms are common. If the acute attack is treated rapidly, the disease is usually mild and recovery uneventful. If left untreated, anemia becomes severe, and the decreased effective circulating blood volume results in capillary blockage that can give rise to serious complications. This feature of *P. falciparum* infections accounts for the protean manifestations of this form of malaria, and the high morbidity and mortality associated with it. Depending upon the organ system involved, several so-called *pernicious syndromes* are seen. *Cerebral malaria* can lead to hemiplegia, convulsions, delirium, hyperpyrexia, coma, and rapid death. When the *pulmonary* circulation is involved, there may be cough and blood-streaked sputum, leading to confusion with many other diseases of the lung. Severe pulmonary insufficiency closely resembling the "shock lung" syndrome frequently accompanies cerebral malaria. The splanchnic capillaries can be obstructed, with consequent vomiting, abdominal pain, diarrhea, or melena. Such patients are sometimes thought to have bacillary dysentery or cholera. Fever in these disorders may be low or absent. Indeed, in patients with predominantly gastrointestinal manifestations, there are usually cold, clammy skin, hypotension, profound weakness, and repeated syncopal attacks, so-called *algid malaria*. Tender hepatomegaly, with or without jaundice, and acute renal failure are common. The pernicious syndromes should be anticipated if the intensity of parasitemia exceeds 100,000 organisms per cubic millimeter.

Blackwater fever This is a disorder that occurs in association with malaria, particularly and perhaps only with *P. falciparum* infections. The usual attack begins with a rigor and fever followed by massive intravascular hemolysis, icterus, hemoglobinuria, collapse, and often acute renal failure and uremia. The pathological findings in the kidney are necrosis of tubules and occasionally hemoglobin casts. The mortality is 20 to 30 percent, and survivors are very likely to experience hemolytic episodes with subsequent malarial infections.

Although blackwater fever is often classified as one of the "pernicious" complications of falciparum malaria, its cause is obscure. In many patients, parasitemia is absent at the time hemolysis occurs. Because blackwater fever has usually occurred in patients with chronic falciparum infections who were treated with quinine, it was suggested that the hemolysis results from an autoimmune reaction to the red blood cells that have been altered by the drug, parasite, or both. However, blackwater fever can occur in patients not given drugs. The institution of an appropriate regimen for acute renal failure (Chap. 275) will reduce the fatality rate considerably.

Complications In addition to the several complications already mentioned, others deserve comment. Rupture of the spleen is relatively rare, but malaria is by far the commonest cause of spontaneous rupture and predisposes to traumatic rupture of this organ. It is most commonly seen in vivax infections.

Chronic malaria or repeated infection in an endemic area leads to anemia, debility, cachexia, and suppression of humoral antibody response to a variety of antigens. These manifestations are particularly severe in children under the age of 3 and in pregnant women. Infection in the latter population is associated with low birth weight of the resulting child and high neonatal mortality. Congenital malaria, although rare, does occur; it is probably most common in the offspring of nonimmune individuals. Secondary bacterial infection is frequent and is often the immediate cause of death. Bacillary dysentery, cholera, and pyogenic pneumonia are common. Tuberculous foci often extend in malarial patients, and miliary tuberculosis is occasionally observed.

Patients living in endemic malarious areas commonly present with chronic hepatosplenomegaly of unknown cause. In some of these, there is infiltration of hepatic sinusoids by lymphocytes, very high levels of serum IgM, and high malaria antibody titers. This condition, which is known as the *tropical splenomegaly syndrome,* is seldom seen before the age of 8. It differs from the ordinary hepatosplenomegaly of malaria in that parasitemia is rare. It has been suggested that the condition results from defective T-cell control of immunoglobulin production, leading to excessive macroglobulin production and immune complex formation. Long-term antimalarial therapy leads to a decrease in spleen size and a disappearance of hepatic sinusoidal lymphocytosis. The epidemiologic evidence implicating malaria as a contributory factor in the etiology of Burkitt's lymphoma has increased. It has been suggested that continuous stimulation of the lymphoid system in chronic malaria makes it more susceptible to neoplastic transformation in the presence of EB virus.

LABORATORY FINDINGS The blood leukocyte count is low or normal. The platelet count is often reduced, especially in falciparum malaria. The erythrocyte sedimentation rate is elevated. Plasmodia are demonstrable in smears of peripheral blood from the vast majority of patients with symptomatic malaria. When the disease is suspected, appropriately stained blood films should be examined diligently. For the inexperienced examiner, a thin smear of fingertip blood on a clean glass slide should be stained with Wright's or Giemsa's stain. Parasitized erythrocytes are most frequent at the edges of a smear; extracellular parasites are not found. Thick smears should be thoroughly dried and stained with diluted Giemsa's or Field stain. This method has the advantage of concentrating the parasites, but artifacts are numerous, and correct interpre-

tations of these preparations require much experience. The value of buffy coat smears in the detection of low-grade parasitemia remains to be determined.

The morphology of the four species of plasmodia that infect humans is specific enough to allow identification in blood smears. The parasitized red blood cells in *P. vivax* infections are enlarged and pale and may contain diffuse bright red dots (Schaffner's dots), and the parasite presents in a wide variety of shapes and sizes; in *P. ovale* infections, the red blood cells containing parasites are oval but otherwise resemble those in *P. vivax;* in *P. malariae* the red blood cells are of normal size and do not contain dots. The parasites often present in "band" forms, and the merozoites are arranged in a rosette around central pigment; in *P. falciparum* infections the rings are very small, may contain two rather than one chromatin dot, and often are found lying flat against the margin of the cell. Only the ring stages of the asexual forms are found in the peripheral smear, and there may be more than one ring in a single red blood cell. The gametocytes are distinctively large and banana-shaped.

There is no advantage of blood over material obtained by splenic or sternal puncture. The administration of epinephrine with the idea of dislodging parasites by producing contraction of the spleen has been advocated, but results are irregular. Serologic tests are used primarily for epidemiologic rather than diagnostic purposes but are also helpful in speciation of the infecting organism and in detection of occult malaria in the bloodstream. The indirect immunofluorescent test seems to be the most sensitive and specific.

DIAGNOSIS The most important diagnostic test is a careful medical history. The diagnosis must be considered in any febrile patient who has resided in or traveled to the Caribbean, Latin America, Asia, or Africa within the previous 12 months. History of previous attacks of malaria, typical malarial paroxysms, or some artificial exposure (blood transfusion, narcotic injections in an addict) should also suggest the disease. Splenomegaly is an almost invariable finding during the second week of illness. Leukocytosis is *not* a feature of malaria. The diagnosis is confirmed by demonstrating the parasites in the peripheral blood. Because the intensity of parasitemia varies greatly from hour to hour, particularly in *P. falciparum* infections, blood smears should be examined every 8 h for 2 or 3 days before the diagnosis is abandoned.

While final cure of malaria may be difficult, particularly in *P. vivax* infections, almost all cases will respond symptomatically to quinine or one of the newer antimalarial drugs, and failure of response to a therapeutic trial argues strongly against the diagnosis.

TREATMENT The use of appropriate chemotherapy can suppress symptoms in individuals exposed in endemic areas or cure malarial infection completely. However, the emergence of drug-resistant falciparum malaria in Southeast Asia, including Burma, Indonesia, and the Philippines, in South America, and in adjacent areas of Central America necessitates the use of drug combinations in the treatment of this infection.

Treatment of acute attack Treatment of an acute attack can be accomplished with chloroquine for all types of malaria except drug-resistant falciparum infection (Table 200-1). The drug usually produces complete subsidence of symptoms and destruction of the erythrocytic forms of the parasite. If vomiting is present, chloroquine hydrochloride should be given intramuscularly or, in the case of shock, intravenously. Oral therapy should be resumed as soon as possible. Although side effects are uncommon, this agent may produce epigastric distress, itching, and neurotoxicity, including involuntary movements and convulsions.

If patients have transfusion-induced malaria or have contracted the disease in an area known to harbor drug-resistant *P. falciparum*, they should be treated with a combination of quinine, pyrimethamine, and one of the sulfonamides or sulfones. *Quinine sulfate*, 0.6 g orally three times a day, should be given for 14 days. If nausea and vomiting preclude oral therapy, quinine dihydrochloride diluted in saline solution or glucose can be given very slowly intravenously. During infusion the pulse and blood pressure should be monitored constantly to detect arrhythmia or hypotension. Oral therapy should be instituted as soon as possible. In the presence of renal or hepatic failure, the dose of quinine should be limited to 0.6 g a day. An overdose of quinine produces cinchonism of which tinnitus is an early manifestation. The drug may also cause mild hemolysis, allergic purpura, and drug fever. The appearance of a Coombs-positive hemolytic anemia requires the immediate withdrawal of the drug. Pyrimethamine should be given orally in dosage of 25 mg two times daily for 3 days. This is an antifolate agent and may cause megaloblastic anemia. Sulfisoxazole or sulfadiazine, 2.0 g initially and then 0.5 g every 6 h for 5 days, should be given concurrently with the other two drugs. A variety of other combinations of antifolate agents with sulfonamides or sulfones have also been used with quinine to good effect. Fansidar, a fixed-drug combination containing 25 mg pyrimethamine and 500 mg sulfadoxine, has been particularly effective. However, it is presently not available in the United States. The combination of tetracycline 2.0 g per day for 7 days plus quinine has been suggested for the treatment of drug-resistant malaria.

Patients should be followed for 1 month to detect recrudescence of the infection. If there are circulating asexual erythrocytic forms, retreatment with pyrimethamine and a sulfonamide should be instituted. The presence of circulating gametocytes is not, however, an indication for retreatment.

Radical cure *Plasmodium vivax* and *P. ovale* persist in the liver in the exoerythrocytic stage and in this form are not affected by drugs used in the treatment of the acute attack. Unless destroyed, they will eventually reinvade the bloodstream. Primaquine base, 15 mg by mouth daily for 14 days, will effect a radical cure in most cases. If relapse occurs after primaquine therapy, a second course of the drug at twice the dosage should be given. Alternatively, 45 mg primaquine base can be given in combination with 300 mg chloroquine once weekly for 8 weeks. Primaquine may cause hemolysis in patients with G6PD deficiency, but in the dosage recommended this is rare and usually mild.

Treatment of complications This includes careful attention to fluid and electrolyte balance, prevention of fluid overload in patients with oliguria, and early diagnosis and treatment of renal failure. In severe hemolysis large doses of steroids may be helpful. Transfusions should be given in severe hemolysis, care being taken to match the donor's cells and plasma with those of the recipient. Intravenous low-molecular-weight dextran may be helpful in increasing capillary blood flow in cerebral malaria. Dexamethasone is used in management of cerebral edema. The value of heparin in this syndrome, even when evidence suggestive of intravascular coagulation is present, remains controversial.

PREVENTION General In areas of the world such as Africa where eradication is presently impractical, limited residual insecticides plus chemoprophylaxis for pregnant women and children are recommended. The long-term hope for eradication now depends on the development of new technologies. Two new areas of research hold some promise—biological control of mosquitoes and a malaria vaccine. The latter has been made more feasible by two recent achievements: the continuous culture of *P. falciparum* in red blood cells and the demonstration that merozoites can serve as effective immunogens. Although merozoite vaccines have already been used successfully in test animals, the adjuvants required preclude present use in humans. It is hoped that effective human vaccines can be developed within the next decade.

Personal protection In endemic areas, mosquito contact should be minimized through the use of house screens, mosquito netting around beds, insect repellants, and insecticides. In addition, patients traveling to endemic areas should receive chemoprophylaxis.

Chemoprophylaxis (see Table 200-2) Although it is not possible to prevent infection with chemotherapeutic agents, it is possible to suppress symptoms while the patient is residing in an endemic area by the administration of chloroquine base in dosage of 300 mg weekly (2 tablets Aralen). If the medication

TABLE 200-1
Malaria treatment

Purpose	Drug	Dosage
Cure chloroquine-resistant *P. falciparum* infection	Quinine sulfate* *or* quinine dihydrochloride*.†	650 mg PO tid for 10–14 days 600 mg in 300 ml normal saline IV over 1 h; repeat in 6–8 h; maximum 1800 mg per day
	plus pyrimethamine *plus* sulfadiazine	25 mg PO bid for 3 days 500 mg PO bid for 5 days
Cure *P. malariae* and chloroquine-sensitive *P. falciparum* infection	Chloroquine phosphate *or* chloroquine hydrochloride†	1 g (600 mg base) PO, then 500 mg in 6 h, then 500 mg per day for 2 days 250 mg (200 mg base) IM or IV every 6 h; administer IV dose as for quinine dihydrochloride above; maximum 900 mg per day
Cure *P. vivax* and *P. ovale* infection	Same as for *P. malariae* *plus* primaquine phosphate	26.3 mg (15 mg base) PO qd for 14 days

* If quinine is not immediately available, begin with chloroquine and switch when quinine arrives.
† For use when patient cannot take oral drug. Switch to oral therapy as soon as possible.

TABLE 200-2
Malaria chemoprophylaxis

Purpose	Drug	Dosage
To suppress clinical malaria in areas *without* chloroquine-resistant strains	Chloroquine phosphate	500 mg (300 mg base) PO once weekly, continued 6 weeks after leaving malarious area
	or amodiaquine dehydrochloride	520 mg (400 mg base) PO once weekly, continued 6 weeks after leaving malarious area
To suppress clinical malaria in areas *with* chloroquine-resistant strains	Same as above	
	plus pyrimethamine-sulfadoxine* (Fansidar, Hoffmann-LaRoche)	25 mg pyrimethamine and 500 mg sulfadoxine PO once weekly, continued 6 weeks after leaving malarious area
To prevent relapses of *P. vivax* and *P. ovale* infection	Primaquine phosphate†	26.3 mg (15 mg base) PO daily for 14 days or 79 mg (45 mg base) for 8 weeks; start during last 2 weeks of suppressive therapy or immediately upon its completion

* *Presently not available in the United States.*
† *Recommended only for travelers without G6PD deficiency who have had heavy exposure.*

is continued for 6 weeks after the patient has left the area, *P. malariae* and sensitive strains of *P. falciparum* will be eradicated. *Plasmodium ovale* and *P. vivax* will produce clinical manifestations some weeks or months after chloroquine is discontinued because of their persistence outside red blood cells. This can be circumvented by administration of primaquine after chloroquine is discontinued. Chloroquine is not effective in suppressing drug-resistant *P. falciparum*. In areas of the world where this is a problem pyrimethamine, 25 mg, plus sulfadoxine, 500 mg, can be taken orally once weekly. These drugs are available in combination form in most endemic areas. Leukopenia occurs in approximately 10 percent of patients using this regimen. Mefloquine, a highly effective prophylactic agent for chloroquine-resistant malaria, is currently undergoing clinical trials in several areas of the world.

Transfusions Transfusion malaria continues to occur in the United States; recently *P. falciparum* has been the most common cause. Adherence to recommendations of the American Association of Blood Banking will prevent most of these cases.

REFERENCES

Brown HW: *Basic Clinical Pathology,* 4th ed. New York, Appleton-Century-Crofts, 1975

Bruce-Chawatt LJ: Transfusion malaria. Bull WHO 50:337, 1974

Chemoprophylaxis of malaria. Morb Mort Week Rep Suppl 27(10):81, March 10, 1978

Drugs for parasitic infections. Med Lett 20(4):17, 1978

Heineman HS: The clinical syndrome of malaria in the United States. Arch Intern Med 129:607, 1972

Hendrickse RG et al: Quartan malarial nephrotic syndrome. Lancet 1:1143, 1972

Jeffery GM: Malaria control in the twentieth century. Am J Trop Med Hyg 25:361, 1976

Kean BH, Reilly PC Jr: Malaria—the mime. Recent lessons from a group of civilian travelers. Am J Med 61:159, 1976

Laderman C: Malaria and progress: Some historical and ecological considerations. Soc Sci Med 9:587, 1975

Miller LH: Current prospects and problems for a malaria vaccine. J Infect Dis 135:855, 1977

———: Hypothesis on the mechanism of erythrocyte invasion by malaria merozoites. Bull WHO 55:157, 1977

Trager W: Cultivation of *Plasmodium falciparum*. Arch Pathol Lab Med 101:277, 1977

Tropical splenomegaly syndrome. Lancet 1:1058, 1976

Wilson M et al: Comparison of the complement fixation, indirect immunofluorescence and indirect hemagglutination tests for malaria. Am J Trop Med Hyg 24:755, 1975

201
LEISHMANIASIS

JAMES J. PLORDE

DEFINITION Leishmaniasis designates a human disorder produced by flagellated tissue protozoa of the genus *Leishmania*. It is transmitted from animal to human being or sometimes from human to human by the bite of phlebotomine sandflies. The infection may be either visceral or cutaneous. The former, or kala azar, is characterized by chronic recurrent fever, splenomegaly, pancytopenia, weight loss, and high mortality. Cutaneous leishmaniasis may present as single or multiple chronic skin ulcers, destructive mucocutaneous lesions, or a disseminated infection resembling leprosy.

ETIOLOGY AND PATHOGENESIS There is confusion over speciation of *Leishmania*. These organisms appear morphologically identical and must be differentiated on serologic, biochemical, cultural, nosologic, and behavioral grounds which are not entirely satisfactory. Four main groups are generally recognized: *L. donovani, L. tropica, L. mexicana,* and *L. brasiliensis*. Each group contains a variety of strains which have been accorded separate species or subspecies status by some workers.

Leishmania donovani is the cause of kala azar, the visceral form of leishmaniasis.

Leishmania tropica causes Old World cutaneous leishmaniasis, or oriental sore, also known as Delhi boil, Bagdad boil, Aleppo button, and Salek and Pendeh sore. A variety of this organism, *L. tropica aethiopica,* causes both oriental sore and diffuse cutaneous leishmaniasis in Ethiopia.

Leishmania mexicana produces a cutaneous leishmaniasis known as bay sore and *chiclero ulcer* as well as the South American form of disseminated cutaneous disease. *Leishmania brasiliensis* is the cause of American mucocutaneous leishmaniasis also known as *espundia*. *Leishmania brasiliensis peruviana* produces *uta*, another type of cutaneous leishmaniasis.

In the sandfly, the parasites assume the flagellated leptomonas form, but in humans the organisms lose their flagella, enter mononuclear phagocytes, and multiply as small, rounded leishmanial forms 2 to 3 μm in diameter, containing a nucleus and kinetoplast, the pathognomonic Leishman-Donovan bodies.

In humans continued intracellular multiplication of the parasite leads to rupture of the affected phagocyte and invasion of other cells, resulting in extensive histiocytic proliferation. The course of the disease from this point is apparently determined by the host's cellular immunity as well as the species of the parasite. In cutaneous leishmaniasis, there is a marked lymphocytic infiltration associated with a reduction in the number of parasites, the development of a delayed skin (leishmanin) reaction, and spontaneous cure. In the mucocutaneous form, the spontaneous disappearance of the primary lesion may be followed by metastatic mucocutaneous lesions at some later date. The destructiveness of the cutaneous lesions is attributed to the development of hypersensitivity to parasitic antigens. An interesting exception to the general pattern in cutaneous disease is disseminated cutaneous leishmaniasis in which there is no infiltration of lymphocytes and plasma cells or reduction in the number of parasites, the leishmanin reaction is negative, and the skin lesions become chronic, progressive, and disseminated. In visceral leishmaniasis, the cellular changes are similar but the parasites spread to reticuloendothelial cells throughout the body. This spread is associated with development of marked hyperglobulinemia. As in the mucocutaneous form of the disease, circulating antibodies are detectable but do not seem to have a protective function. They may, in fact, be responsible for the pancytopenia and glomerulonephritis seen in visceral disease. A positive skin test develops in the visceral form after successful treatment.

KALA AZAR

DISTRIBUTION AND EPIDEMIOLOGY Kala azar occurs in China, Russia, India, the Middle East, Egypt, Sudan, East Africa, several Mediterranean countries, including Greece, Crete, and Malta, and a few areas of South and Central America. Although the manifestations of the disease throughout this area, which touches all continents but Australia, are basically similar, certain definite peculiarities in its behavior justify classification of visceral leishmaniasis into at least three main types. These differences are attributed to variations in the strains of *L. donovani* in a given area and, perhaps more important, to the length of time that the disease has been endemic in a population. It is believed that kala azar (and also infection by *L. tropica*) is introduced into a new area from animal reservoirs and that this "primitive" or zoonotic infection is likely to result in many cases of acute, rapidly fatal illness among the population coming into contact with the parasites for the first time. After generations, kala azar becomes endemic, the disease assumes a more chronic form, and the domestic dog becomes an important reservoir.

Mediterranean, or *infantile, kala azar* is seen primarily in the Mediterranean area, China, Russia, and Latin America. An outbreak in Kenya also appears to be of this type. It is a disease of children under the age of 4, but adults, particularly travelers to endemic areas, are not spared. Dogs, jackals, and foxes serve as reservoirs, and human-to-human transmission is thought to be rare. The strains responsible for the Eurasian and American diseases are sometimes referred to as *L. infantum* and *L. chagasi* respectively.

Indian kala azar affects older children and young adults, and males are involved more commonly than females. The human being is the only known reservoir, and transmission is carried out by anthropophilic species of sandflies. This form of disease has become uncommon as a result of antimalarial spraying.

African kala azar is found in the Eastern half of Africa from the Sahara in the North to the equator in the South. Its age and sex distribution is similar to that of Indian kala azar. It is endemic in gerbils and other rodents in many areas and is more resistant to therapy with antimony compounds than that found in the rest of the world.

MANIFESTATIONS The incubation period varies from 10 days to 1 year but is usually about 3 months. No lesion appears at the site of the infecting bite in most cases, but a primary "chancre" which heals with scarring before the onset of systemic symptoms is commonly noted in the African disease. The organisms multiply extensively in the macrophages of spleen, liver, bone marrow, lymph nodes, skin, and small intestine, accounting for many of the manifestations of the disease. Organisms may be found in the blood for several months before the onset of symptoms.

Fever, which is characterized at times by two daily spikes, may be abrupt or gradual in onset. It persists for 1 to 6 weeks and then disappears, only to reappear at irregular intervals during the course of the illness. Although prostration is absent even during periods of high fever, there is progressive weakness, pallor, weight loss, and tachycardia. Gastrointestinal disturbances are frequent in Indian cases. Physical findings include enormous splenomegaly, lymphadenopathy, hepatomegaly with signs of portal hypertension, and often edema, which tends to conceal the extent of the wasting. Hyperpigmentation is noted in light-skinned individuals, and mucocutaneous lesions similar to those seen in espundia occur in the African form of the disease. Anemia is the rule, and thrombocytopenia with gingival and other mucosal bleeding is common. The peripheral leukocyte count is low (usually less than 4000 per cubic millimeter); in children, agranulocytosis with cancrum oris (noma) and secondary pulmonary or intestinal infections contribute to the high mortality. The presence of a short erythrocyte life span, anti-red blood cell antibodies, positive Coombs' test, and antibody against white blood cells and platelets suggests an autoimmune basis for the pancytopenia.

Hypergammaglobulinemia is universally present. Proteinuria and hematuria are frequent in the course of kala azar and are thought to be related to the glomerular deposition of poorly soluble immune complexes. Uremia due to renal amyloidosis and symptoms of heart failure can occur.

Post-kala azar dermal leishmaniasis Patients treated successfully with antimony compounds for kala azar may develop cutaneous lesions called *leishmanoids,* in which *Leishmania* organisms are demonstrable. These are rare in Mediterranean or Chinese kala azar but develop in 3 percent of African cases almost immediately after systemic symptoms subside. They occur after a latent period of 1 to 2 years in as many as 10 percent of Indian cases. The lesions range from patchy areas of depigmentation to erythematous papules and confluent nodules which may involve the ears and mucous membranes and have been mistaken for leprosy. They are short-lived in African kala azar but may persist for years in the Indian variety, creating a persistent reservoir of infection.

DIAGNOSIS The diagnosis is made by finding *Leishmania* organisms in stained preparations of blood (often possible in Indian but rarely so in other forms), bone marrow, lymph nodes, or material obtained by splenic puncture. The last is the best source of organisms, but the spleen should be needled only when it is firm and enlarged well below the left costal margin. The organisms will grow out as flagellated forms in Nicolle-Novy-MacNeal (NNN) medium containing defibrinated rabbit blood incubated at 22°C.

Serologic tests are not totally satisfactory. The complement fixation test is sensitive and readily available but lacks specificity. Immunoelectrophoresis, by contrast, is highly specific but has a low sensitivity. The indirect immunofluorescence antibody test would appear to offer the advantages of both but is only group specific. A new enzyme-linked immunoabsorbent assay (ELISA) may be even more satisfactory.

The leishmanin skin test is negative during active kala azar but becomes positive several months after successful treatment of the disease.

TREATMENT   Rest, good diet, transfusions, and treatment of complicating infections, of which tuberculosis, bacterial pneumonia, amebiasis, and bacillary dysentery are more important, must supplement or precede specific therapy. Pentavalent antimony compounds are highly effective against the parasites. Owing to its lack of toxicity, Pentostam (sodium antimony gluconate) given intravenously or intramuscularly is the drug of choice. The adult dose is 0.6 g (6 ml) daily for 6 days in Indian kala azar and for 30 days is other forms.

More than 90 percent of cases respond promptly to antimony, except in Africa, where the cure rate is as low as 70 percent. Resistant cases can be treated with either one of the more toxic diamidines or with amphotericin B. Pentamidine is given intramuscularly in the dose of 4 mg base per kilogram of body weight dissolved in 3 to 4 ml water daily for 10 days. The course may be repeated twice after intervals of 10 days. Hypotension, renal damage, hypoglycemia, and diabetes mellitus can complicate therapy with this drug.

PROGNOSIS AND CONTROL   The mortality in untreated kala azar is 95 percent in adults and 80 percent in children. This has been greatly reduced by treatment with antimony and the aromatic diamidines. Relapses, occasionally several in number, occur in 5 to 15 percent of African and Mediterranean cases up to 2 years after treatment. Both relapses and post-kala azar dermal leishmaniasis should be re-treated in the same fashion as the initial illness.

The treatment of the disease in humans, the elimination of diseased dogs, and the use of DDT residual sprays against sandflies are the important preventive measures. Incidence of the disease has diminished greatly in many areas where DDT has been used to eradicate malaria—an unexpected added benefit of this program. When the vectors are exophilic, control is difficult. Attempts at vaccination with avirulent strains of *L. donovani* have been unsuccessful.

AMERICAN CUTANEOUS LEISHMANIASIS

These diseases occur in every country of Central and South America except Chile. In some areas, 10 to 20 percent of the population is infected. Three autochthonous infections have been reported from Texas. There are four varieties of American cutaneous leishmaniasis. All begin with a local lesion at the site of the infecting sandfly bite after an incubation period of from 10 days to 3 months.

Chiclero ulcer, which is found in Mexico, Guatemala, British Honduras, and possibly other parts of Central America, is a zoonosis caused by *L. mexicana.* The disease occurs naturally in several arboreal rodents. It is occasionally transmitted to persons entering forests to harvest chicle. In immunocompetent individuals, it is a relatively mild infection characterized by a single cutaneous lesion on the ear, face, or hand which is chronic and shows little tendency to ulceration. The leishmanin skin test is positive. Spontaneous healing usually occurs within 6 months. The parasites are never numerous in the lesions. Mucosal ulceration does not occur. Ear lesions cause extensive destruction of the pinna and should be treated with a single 350 mg intramuscular dose of cycloguanil pamoate. Immunization with live cultures of *L. mexicana* has been effective in forest workers.

Diffuse cutaneous leishmaniasis is found in Venezuela. It apparently results from a specific deficiency of cell-mediated immunity to leishmanial antigen. In South America, it is caused by members of the *L. mexicana* complex, usually *L. mexicana amazonensis.* This remarkable disease is characterized by massive dissemination of skin lesions without visceral involvement. The clinical picture often bears a striking resemblance to lepromatous leprosy. The diagnosis is not difficult, because the lesions contain a large number of organisms. In contrast to all other types of cutaneous leishmaniasis, the leishmanin skin test is negative. The disease is progressive and very refractory to treatment. Amphotericin B and pentamidine have been used to produce remissions, but cure is rare.

Uta, which occurs in cooler climates and at altitudes of more than 2000 ft, consists of single or multiple skin ulcers of the nose and lips in which parasites are readily demonstrable. Spontaneous healing within 3 months to a year is the rule, and mucosal spread is unusual. The etiologic agent is *L. peruviana,* a member of the *L. brasiliensis* group, and the reservoir is the domestic dog. With widespread use of insecticides in Peru, the disease has almost disappeared.

In tropical Latin America, *L. brasiliensis* causes the better-known and more serious *espundia.* The organism causes a natural infection in large forest rodents and is transmitted to human beings by sandflies when new settlements are made in jungle areas. The initial skin lesion enlarges progressively, and secondary bacterial infection is frequent. The disease may spread by direct extension or by lymphatics to the mucosal surfaces of the mouth and nose, where, after the primary lesion has healed, painful, destructive, and mutilating erosions scar and distort the involved structures. Fever, anemia, and weight loss accompany these mucosal complications. Destruction of the nasal septum produces a characteristic deformity called *tapir nose* or *camel nose.* The hard palate may be destroyed, and laryngeal erosion can lead to aphonia. In blacks, the lesion is often hypertrophic, and large polypoid masses deform the lips and cheeks, perhaps representing a type of keloid reaction. This can be mistaken for South American blastomycosis (Chap. 154). Secondary bacterial infection, inanition, and respiratory obstruction lead to death.

The diagnosis is made by finding the organisms in scrapings or by culture. The leishmanin skin test is specific and highly useful. Treatment consists of antibiotics for bacterial infections and pentavalent antimonials used as in kala azar. Cases that fail to respond to antimonials should be treated with amphotericin B, 0.25 to 1 mg/kg by slow infusion daily or every other day for up to 8 weeks.

The early lesions respond well, but even with repeated courses of antimony the mucosal complications of the espundia type heal slowly. In advanced cases, the prognosis is very poor.

OLD WORLD CUTANEOUS LEISHMANIASIS: ORIENTAL SORE

This, the least serious form of human leishmaniasis, consists of localized cutaneous ulceration which heals spontaneously and is endemic in the European countries bordering the eastern Mediterranean, in Africa, in Asia Minor, in Southwest Asia, and in India. Two major strains of the causative organism, *L. tropica,* produce similar but distinctive clinical syndromes. Homologous immunity after recovery from infection by either strain is solid and lifelong. Infection with *L. tropica major* protects against *L. tropica minor,* but the opposite is not the case. The rural type, caused by *L. tropica major,* has its reservoir in gerbils and other small rodents; the ulcers usually appear on the extremities 2 to 6 weeks after the bite of the sandfly and are accompanied by regional lymphadenopathy in a majority of cases. Spontaneous healing occurs within 3 to 6 months, leaving a depigmented, pitted scar.

The incubation period in the *urban,* or *dry,* type ranges

from 2 months to more than a year. The lesion is usually facial and begins as a pruritic, purplish nodule (the Aleppo button), which slowly enlarges and finally breaks down after 3 or 4 months. Lymphatic involvement is uncommon. Healing of the indolent, granulomatous ulcer may require a year or more. Occasionally, healing fails to occur, which results in lesions closely resembling lupus vulgaris. This condition, known as *leishmaniasis recidiva*, is thought to be the result of an exaggerated delayed hypersensitivity to leishmanial antigens. Humans and the domestic dog serve as the reservoirs of infection.

The typical oriental sore is a sharply punched-out, ragged ulcer about 1 in in diameter, surrounded by an erythematous rim. Satellite lesions which fuse with the original are not rare. The center of the granulating base of the ulcer frequently contains a hard excrescence called the *Montpellier sign* or the *rake* beneath which the parasites are most likely to be found when scrapings are examined.

The rural and urban types occur together in Asia Minor; indeed, it is not rare to find simultaneous infections in the same patient. In Southeastern Europe, India, and North Africa, the urban type is prevalent, while in the remainder of Africa the disease is predominantly rural.

A form of diffuse cutaneous leishmaniasis is seen in Ethiopia. It closely resembles the disease in Venezuela and appears to have a sylvatic reservoir.

Diagnosis is usually made on clinical grounds and is confirmed by finding the parasites, which occur both intra- and extracellularly. Pyogenic infection makes direct visualization difficult, but *L. tropica* can be cultured in NNN medium at room temperature, and a skin test using *L. tropica* antigen becomes positive in the vast majority of patients with the disease.

Treatment should include vigorous measures for bacterial infection, such as hot soaks and appropriate systemic antibiotics. Infrared heat treatment has also been suggested, as the leishmanial organisms are very heat-sensitive. Systemic antimonials may be required where ulceration is extensive or multiple. Pentostam is used as in kala azar in a course of 10 daily injections totaling 6 g. It may be injected locally in dosage of 0.6 g three to four times on alternate days. In endemic areas the custom is to withhold treatment directed against the parasite until the initial nodule ulcerates, to assure the development of immunity against reinfection.

Prevention consists of use of insect repellents on exposed parts of the body, residual DDT sprays, and fine-mesh screening for dwellings. The lesions should be covered to prevent infection of vectors and, of course, contact with the lesion or its discharges should be avoided.

REFERENCES

Bray RS: Leishmaniasis in the Old World. Br Med Bull 28:39, 1972
———: Leishmania. Ann Rev Microbiol 28:189, 1974
Brito T et al: Glomerular involvement in human kala azar. Am J Trop Med Hyg 24:9, 1975
Bryceson ADM: Diffuse cutaneous leishmaniasis in Ethiopia. Trans R Soc Trop Med Hyg 64:369, 1970
Hunter GW et al: *Tropical Medicine,* 5th ed. Philadelphia, Saunders, 1976
Kern F, Pedersen JK: Leishmaniasis in the United States: Report of ten cases in military personnel. JAMA 226:872, 1973
Laison R, Shaw JJ: Epidemiology and ecology of leishmaniasis in Latin America. Nature (Parasitol Suppl) 273:595, 1978
Marsden PD et al: Mucocutaneous leishmaniasis—an unsolved clinical problem. Trop Doctor 7:7, 1977
Shaw PH et al: Autochthonous cutaneous leishmaniasis in Texas. Am J Trop Med Hyg 25:788, 1976
Woodruff AW et al: The anemia of kala azar. Br J Haematol 22:319, 1972

202
TRYPANOSOMIASIS

JAMES J. PLORDE

SLEEPING SICKNESS

DEFINITION African trypanosomiasis, or sleeping sickness, is a disease caused by the hemoflagellate *Trypanosoma brucei*, which is transmitted to human beings by several species of tsetse fly belonging to the genus *Glossina*. Clinically, the untreated disease is characterized by an acute febrile lymphadenopathy followed, after a variable period, by a chronic lethal meningoencephalomyelitis. It occurs in two principal epidemiologic patterns: Gambian, or Mid- and West African, sleeping sickness, and Rhodesian, or East African, sleeping sickness.

ETIOLOGY Trypanosomes are fusiform protozoa recognized by an undulating membrane which extends along the length of the cell and terminates in an anterior flagellum. The morphological characteristics of many varieties are so nearly identical that they are distinguishable only by their pathogenicity for certain animals, differences in biochemical requirements, and ability to multiply in insects. *Trypanosoma brucei* strains are polymorphic organisms varying in shape from slender to stumpy and in length from 8 to 30 μm. The slender forms have a long flagellum that in the shorter types is rudimentary or absent. The Gambian and Rhodesian forms of sleeping sickness were previously thought to be caused by two distinct species of trypanosomes, *T. gambiense* and *T. rhodesiense*. It is felt now, however, that they, along with the animal trypanosome responsible for *nagana* in cattle, are all variants of a single species. The individual varieties are referred to as *T. brucei gambiense, T. brucei rhodesiense*, and *T. brucei brucei.*

Trypanosomiasis in animals is a great economic problem in many parts of the world. It is probable that an area of approximately 4 million square miles in Africa is not populated because of the impossibility of keeping animals in sites where tsetse flies are infected with trypanosomes.

EPIDEMIOLOGY Gambian sleeping sickness occurs in tropical, West, and Central Africa extending from the Sahara to the Kalahari Deserts and east to the Rift Valley. The incidence of disease is particularly high in Zaire. Rhodesian trypanosomiasis is found in tropical East Africa from Ethiopia in the north to Botswana in the south.

Transmission of the trypanosomes of sleeping sickness occurs by what is referred to as the "anterior station." After ingestion by a feeding tsetse, the parasites first develop in the intestine of the fly and then migrate to the salivary glands, where they are discharged when the host is bitten. In some situations it is possible that the trypanosomes can be mechanically transmitted from host to host by the tsetse and other hematophagous arthropods. This may be of importance during epidemics.

The Gambian strains of *T. brucei* are transmitted mainly by *G. palpalis* and *G. tachinoides*. These species live in shaded areas near water. Less than 5 percent of the flies are infected even in the most notorious endemic foci. Although *G. palpalis* and *G. tachinoides* are not exclusively anthropophilic, human beings are thought to be the only reservoir for Gambian sleeping sickness.

Rhodesian sleeping sickness, on the other hand, is primarily a zoonosis. It is transmitted to humans from the bushbuck, a small antelope, by the bite of *G. morsitans,* a savannah tsetse. It is seen typically in individuals who travel away from their villages to hunt or fish. Domestic cattle and sheep may also serve as reservoirs, and transmission from human to fly to human can occur.

PATHOLOGY AND PATHOGENESIS The tsetse fly inoculates the organism into the subcutaneous pool of blood that forms during its feeding. Some of the parasites may reach the bloodstream directly, but most remain at the site of inoculation, where they multiply to produce a local chancre. Following the appearance of this lesion, the trypanosomes spread through tissue spaces and lymphatics, eventually spilling over into the general circulation where they continue to multiply by longitudinal fission. The parasitemia is of low intensity and typically occurs in waves; each wave disappears coincidentally with the production of antibody to an exoantigen of the protozoan and reappears as a new antigenic variant arises. These waves of parasitemia, which are accompanied by fever and mononuclear leukocytosis, tend to become more infrequent and irregular in the later stages of the disease. At some time during this stage of dissemination, trypanosomes localize in the tissues of the central nervous system. This is first manifested as a diffuse leptomeningitis and later by a perivascular cerebritis. If untreated, this parenchymal inflammation gives rise to a demyelinating panencephalitis. Leishmanial or short forms have been demonstrated in experimental *T. brucei* infections, suggesting that this organism has an intracellular tissue phase in its developmental cycle. This could be of significance in occult infections.

The mechanism by which the trypanosome elicits tissue damage is unknown. It has been suggested that antigen-antibody reactions lead to the release of kinins. The release of proteolytic enzymes by degenerating phagocytes may be important. The parasitemia stimulates the production of large quantities of IgM immunoglobulin, perhaps in response to the rapid antigenic variation of the parasite. It is not known whether these antibodies are protective. They may, in fact, contribute to the pathogenesis of the anemia and thrombocytopenia sometimes seen in this disease. Cell-mediated immunity is probably important.

CLINICAL MANIFESTATIONS The Gambian and Rhodesian forms of sleeping sickness differ somewhat in symptoms, severity, and duration. Rhodesian trypanosomiasis is the more acute and severe of the two forms, usually terminating fatally within a year. Fever is higher, emaciation more rapid, and lymphatic involvement less evident. Death from intercurrent infections or myocarditis usually occurs before the typical sleeping sickness syndrome appears. In the Gambian variety there are often successive bouts of clinical activity with intervening latent periods that persist for a number of years. The early stages may be mild, and the disease may go unrecognized until the central nervous system is involved. In both forms of the disease, however, an entry lesion, a febrile period of dissemination, and a stage of central nervous system involvement are found to some degree. The *trypanosomal chancre* appears as an erythematous nodule at the site of inoculation 2 or 3 days after the bite of an infected fly. It may occur anywhere in the body but is most commonly seen on the head or limbs and is accompanied by regional lymphadenopathy. The lesion, which subsides spontaneously, is noted more frequently in Rhodesian sleeping sickness, perhaps because of the acute nature of the disease.

The incubation period is usually about 2 weeks, but in *T. brucei gambiense* infections may be several years. Systemic manifestations generally become apparent during the hematogenous dissemination of the trypanosomes. In the usual case the patient develops a high remittent fever, severe headache, insomnia, and inability to concentrate. In Caucasians a characteristic circinate erythema resembling erythema marginatum is frequent. Transient firm areas of painful subcutaneous edema localized to the hands, feet, and periorbital tissues may appear. All these signs and symptoms may disappear and reappear intermittently over a period of months to years. Tender lymphadenopathy with gradual induration of the nodes and splenomegaly are almost invariably present in Gambian sleeping sickness. The lymph nodes of the posterior cervical triangle are frequently prominent. This is referred to as *Winterbottom's sign*. Eventually the parasites enter the central nervous system. This may occur early in the course of the disease or may be delayed for as long as 8 years. Cerebral trypanosomiasis can be explosive, causing repeated convulsions or deep coma and death within a few days. Most patients show gradual progression to the classic picture of *sleeping sickness*. A vacant expression develops, the eyelids droop, the lower lip hangs loosely, and it becomes more and more difficult to gain the patient's attention or prod him or her to any activity. Patients will eat when offered food, but they never ask for it or engage in spontaneous conversation, and speech gradually becomes blurred and indistinct. Tremors of the hands and tongue, choreiform movements, seizures with transient paralysis, loss of sphincter control, ophthalmoplegia, extensor plantar responses, and finally death in coma, in status epilepticus, or from hyperpyrexia follows inexorably.

Death may also occur from intercurrent infection, of which bacillary and amebic dysentery, malaria, and bacterial (often pneumococcal) pneumonia are the most important.

DIAGNOSIS AND LABORATORY FINDINGS Anemia and *hypermacroglobulinemia* are invariably present, and spontaneous clumping of erythrocytes in blood specimens is grossly evident in many cases. The sedimentation rate is rapid, and peripheral monocytosis is frequent. When there has been invasion of the central nervous system, the *cerebrospinal fluid* shows mononuclear pleocytosis and increased protein concentration. The protein concentration is a better index of severity of disease and therapeutic response than the number of cells. The presence of IgM in the spinal fluid is almost pathognomonic of cerebral trypanosomiasis.

The definitive diagnosis depends upon finding the trypanosomes in the blood, aspirate of lymph node, or cerebrospinal fluid. These should be examined first in wet mounts; actively motile organisms are seen easily under high power. For final identification thin and thick blood films should be stained with Wright's or Giemsa's stain. If the blood smears are negative, citrated blood should be centrifuged at 1000 r/min for 10 min, the supernatant (including the leukocytes) recentrifuged at 2000 r/min for 15 min, and the sediment examined. Cerebrospinal fluid should be centrifuged at 2000 r/min for 15 min before examination. Alternatively the blood and spinal fluid may be centrifuged in a heparinized capillary tube at 12,000 r/min for 4 min and the tubes examined under a microscope using a 10-power objective. The trypanosomes are found at the junction of the plasma and buffy layer in centrifuged blood and near the sealed end of the tube in centrifuged spinal fluid. If these methods are negative, inoculation of rats or mice can be helpful in the diagnosis of Rhodesian disease. A severalfold increase in IgM globulins in the serum is of confirmatory value. Complement fixation and indirect fluorescent antibody tests utilizing stable antigens are useful in endemic areas.

TREATMENT Suramin (Bayer 205, Antrypol) is the most effective agent before central nervous system involvement has occurred. The initial dose should be limited to 0.2 g intravenously because of possible idiosyncrasy. If there is no evidence of sensitivity, a full course of therapy can be instituted the following day. One gram (10 ml fresh 10% solution) is given intravenously on the first, third, seventh, fourteenth, and twenty-first days for a total of 5 g. If red blood cells, casts, or significant amounts of protein occur in the urine, therapy should be discontinued. Pentamidine given in water intramuscularly each day for 10 injections is also effective in early disease. The dose is 3 to 4 mg pentamidine base per kilogram for each injection. When the agent is given too rapidly by the intravenous route, it may cause hypotension.

Lumbar puncture should always be performed in patients who are about to undergo therapy for trypanosomiasis. If the central nervous system is involved, agents that will penetrate the blood-brain barrier must be used; for this purpose the most effective agent is *melarsoprol* (Mel B). This drug, an arsenic derivative of British antilewisite (BAL), is effective at all stages of the disease but is more toxic than suramin. It is given intravenously in a 3.6% solution. The initial dose is 0.5 ml. Each subsequent dose is increased by 0.5 ml until the maximum single dose of 5 ml is reached. The first three doses are given at daily intervals followed by a 7-day rest. This schedule is repeated until a total of 37.5 ml has been given over a period of 1 month. If signs of arsenic toxicity occur, the drug should be discontinued. A reactive encephalopathy, probably due to the release of trypanosomal antigen, may occur early in the course of treatment. Pretreatment with suramin may help avert this complication. A hemorrhagic encephalopathy, a direct arsenic toxic reaction, may also occur and is usually fatal. BAL may be of some use in this situation.

Nitrofurazone can also be given for cerebral trypanosomiasis in an oral dose of 0.5 g three times a day for 7 days, but is more toxic than melarsoprol, and it should not be used unless the patients have failed to respond to this drug. The increasing incidence of drug-resistant parasites has limited the usefulness of *tryparsamide* in the treatment of certain *T. brucei gambiense* infections.

PROGNOSIS The disease is probably always fatal if untreated. If the infection is treated with suramin prior to central nervous system involvement, the cure rate is high and recovery is rapid and complete. When the nervous system becomes involved, the prognosis is less bright, and in far-advanced disease the survivors may suffer neurological damage. Relapses may occur, particularly following treatment with suramin, if the central nervous system was already involved at the time therapy was instituted. Less commonly they may be the result of drug resistance. Examination of the spinal fluid 6 and 12 months after therapy, or earlier if symptoms recur, is helpful in detecting relapse. Such patients must be re-treated with a second therapeutic agent.

PREVENTION Personal protection is best achieved by the use of repellents and protective clothing. A single intramuscular injection of pentamidine in dosage of 3 to 4 mg base per kilogram (maximum 300 mg) will protect against the Gambian form of disease for 6 months or more; its usefulness in Rhodesian trypanosomiasis is controversial. Because of the danger of cryptic infections occurring during chemoprophylaxis, it has been generally restricted to mass prophylactic campaigns. Other methods of disease control include clearing vegetation and the use of insecticides.

CHAGAS' DISEASE

DEFINITION American trypanosomiasis is an infection caused by *T. cruzi* that is characterized by an acute, often asymptomatic illness followed by chronic cardiac and gastrointestinal sequelae.

ETIOLOGY *Trypanosoma cruzi* circulates in the blood as a slender, fusiform hemoflagellate measuring 20 μm in length. In stained preparations, its narrow undulating membrane, large kinetoplast, and characteristic C shape are easily recognized. Unlike the trypanosomes of sleeping sickness, it does not multiply within the bloodstream. After invading tissue cells, it loses its undulating membrane and flagellum, assumes its leishmania form, and divides by binary fission. Eventually, new flagellated forms are produced which reenter the general circulation to initiate another cycle.

Strains of *T. cruzi* vary widely in both virulence and tissue tropism.

EPIDEMIOLOGY This infection is found from Chile and Argentina to Mexico, where it affects more than 7 million people. *Trypanosoma cruzi* has been found in insect vectors and wild animals in several areas of the Southern United States, and serologic studies have documented that acquisition of human infection occurs within this country. There are to date, however, only a handful of clinically apparent autochthonous cases reported from Texas.

The disease is transmitted to humans by reduviid ("assassin" or "kissing") bugs, primarily those of the genera *Triatoma, Panstrongylus,* and *Rhodnius.* These winged, hematophagous insects can be found in the burrows of animals and in the cracks and thatches of poorly constructed rural dwellings. The insect attacks human beings at night, usually biting the face at the mucocutaneous junction (most frequently the lip or outer canthus of the eye). The flagellated trypanosomes are ingested by the bug while feeding, and after multiplying and developing in the midgut of the insect for 8 to 10 days, are discharged in the feces; human infection occurs through contamination of the bite wound. This is referred to as transmission by the "posterior station." The reduviid may remain infected as long as 2 years.

Human beings, domestic animals (cats and dogs), and wild animals, especially the opossum and armadillo, may serve as reservoirs for the infection. The close association of human beings, domestic animals, and the vector within human dwellings is of prime epidemiologic importance, but the disease is occasionally transmitted by a blood transfusion and via the placenta to newborn infants.

PATHOGENESIS AND CLINICAL MANIFESTATIONS A local inflammatory reaction, manifested clinically as an erythematous nodule or *chagoma,* appears within 1 to 3 weeks at the site of inoculation of the protozoan. If, as is commonly the case, the portal of entry has been the conjunctiva, the presenting manifestations are a unilateral, painless conjunctivitis, palpebral edema, and preauricular lymphadenopathy (Romaña's sign). This primary complex may persist for 1 to 2 months during which parasites can be demonstrated in the lesion.

Following an incubation period of 2 weeks, trypanosomal forms reach the general circulation, producing a parasitemia and initiating the acute phase of the illness. After circulating in the blood for some time, the trypanosomes invade tissue cells, and, in the leishmanial form, multiply, producing intracellular pseudocysts. In 4 to 6 days these pseudocysts rupture, releasing both leishmanial and newly formed trypanosomal organisms. The leishmanial forms disintegrate, eliciting an intense inflammatory reaction, while the trypanosomal forms regain the bloodstream to maintain the infection and invade new tissues, particularly the heart, skeletal muscle, smooth muscle, and nervous system.

Clinically, the patient experiences a continuous or recurrent fever, generalized lymphadenopathy, hepatosplenomegaly, and in some cases extensive gelatinous edema of the face and trunk. A transient morbilliform or urticarial skin eruption may occur early in the acute phase. Although trypanosomes frequently can be demonstrated in the cerebrospinal fluid at this time, acute meningoencephalitis is relatively rare; newborn infants and young children are affected most commonly. Myocarditis characterized by tachycardia and electrocardiographic changes is very common. In severe cases, there may be conduction disturbances, cardiac dilatation, and heart failure. The duration of the acute illness is variable. In 5 to 10 percent of cases, meningoencephalitis or severe heart disease results in a fatal outcome within a few days or weeks. Most often it resolves slowly over a period of several weeks. Parasites become extremely scanty in both the tissues and blood, and the patient remains asymptomatic until the onset of the chronic phase 1 or 2 years later. Most patients presenting with late manifestations, however, deny a history of acute illness, suggesting that subclinical infections often result in chronic disease. It has been suggested that the basic pathogenetic mechanism is a hypersensitivity or autoimmune inflammatory reaction involving mesenchymal tissues, and recently antibodies reactive with endocardium, striated muscle, and vascular tissues have been described. On the other hand, lymphocyte-mediated destruction of myocardial tissue has been demonstrated in experimental animals, and lymphocytic infiltrates are commonly seen in patients dying of chagasic cardiopathy. Some authors have also suggested that the late manifestations of disease are primarily due to neuropathies caused by the destruction of ganglionic nerve cells during the acute phase of the disease and resulting in the dilatation and malfunction of the affected organs.

The most important late manifestation is heart disease which may affect as much as 10 percent of the rural population in endemic areas. Symptoms and signs range from arrhythmias and heart block to chronic congestive heart failure (predominantly right-sided). Thromboembolic phenomena and sudden cardiac arrest are relatively common. Echocardiography has been shown to be of value both in screening patients with infection for evidence of cardiac involvement and in following the progress of those with established cardiomyopathy. At autopsy the hearts of patients with Chagas' disease may show a peculiar herniation of the endocardium through the apical muscle bundles. Megacolon and megaesophagus are sequelae seen in southern South America, but they are less common in Central America and in northern South America. Neurological manifestations including mental deficiency and cerebellar symptoms also have been reported in the chronic state of disease.

DIAGNOSIS The diagnosis depends on the demonstration of *T. cruzi* in the patient or upon serologic tests. In the acute phase of the disease the parasite may be seen in the peripheral blood by means of the same direct methods described for African trypanosomiasis. If these are negative, blood may be cultured in Nicolle-Novy-MacNeal (NNN) or Warren's medium or inoculated into rats, mice, or guinea pigs.

Trypanosoma cruzi is easily grown in blood broth and incubated at 28°C; a more sensitive tissue culture method has been described recently. The technique of *xenodiagnosis* is often used in endemic areas; a laboratory-reared vector, known to be parasite-free, is allowed to feed on subjects with suspected cases, and 2 weeks later, the insect's intestinal contents are examined for parasites. Confusion sometimes arises from the finding of trypanosomes in blood. Many children in Venezuela and other South American countries are infected with a harmless species *T. rangeli,* which produces no symptoms but may be present in the blood for many months. By utilization of both culture and xenodiagnosis repeatedly, organisms can be recovered from most acute cases and from up to 40 percent of chronic ones. Biopsy of an involved lymph node or calf muscle may reveal the organism during the initial illness when the parasites cannot be recovered from the blood. The Machado-Guerreiro test (a complement fixation reaction) is most helpful in the diagnosis of chronic cases and in survey work. Fluorescent antibody and hemagglutination inhibition tests appear more sensitive and less specific. Rapid slide flocculation tests and enzyme-linked immunosorbent assay are currently being evaluated.

TREATMENT AND PREVENTION There is still no satisfactory treatment for Chagas' disease, although several drugs, including primaquine given in dosage suggested for malaria, will clear the blood of trypanosomes, but they do not affect the intracellular parasites. Bayer 2502 (Lampit), a nitrofurazone derivative given in dosage of 10 mg/kg per day for 3 or 4 months, shows promise as a curative agent. Chronic organ damage, however, is generally thought irreversible. Prevention consists of using residual insecticide sprays—of which benzene hexachloride (BHC) is the most effective—on the walls of houses, the main habitat of the vectors. Reinfestation, however, may occur within a year or two of spraying. Preliminary work on vaccine development is underway. Transfusion infections can be prevented by serologic screening of blood donors in endemic areas and by adding gentian violet to the blood. Immunosuppression may reactivate Chagas' disease, and patients from endemic areas should be serologically screened before such treatment is instituted.

REFERENCES

BARRETT-CONNOR E: Chemoprophylaxis of amebiasis and African trypanosomiasis. Ann Intern Med 77:797, 1972

BROWN HW: *Basic Clinical Parasitology,* 4th ed. New York, Appleton-Century-Crofts, 1975

COSSIO PM et al: Chagasic cardiomyopathy. Am J Pathol 86:533, 1977

GOODWIN LG: The pathology of African trypanosomiasis. Trans R Soc Trop Med Hyg 64:797, 1970

HOFF R et al: *Trypanosoma cruzi* in the cerebrospinal fluid during the acute stage of Chagas' disease. N Engl J Med 298:604, 1978

KABERLE F: Chagas' disease and Chagas' syndromes: The pathology of American trypanosomiasis. Adv Parasitol 6:63, 1968

LUMSDEN WHR: Trypanosomiasis. Br Med Bull 28:34, 1972

MAEGRATH BG, GILES HM: *Management and Treatment of Tropical Diseases.* Oxford, Blackwell Scientific Publications, 1971

MARTINI-CAMPOS JV, TAFURI WL: Chagas' enteropathy. Gut 14:910, 1973

PUIGBO JJ et al: Diagnosis of Chagas' cardiomyopathy by noninvasive techniques. Postgrad Med J 53:527, 1977

SPENCER HC JR et al: Imported African trypanosomiasis in the United States. Ann Intern Med 82:633, 1975

WHO MEMORANDA: Immunology of Chagas' disease. Bull WHO 50:549, 1974

203
TOXOPLASMOSIS

RIMA McLEOD
JACK S. REMINGTON

DEFINITION The term *toxoplasmosis* refers to disease caused by the obligate intracellular protozoan, *Toxoplasma gondii,* and must be differentiated from the more common asymptomatic infection caused by this organism. The infection and disease in older children and adults are discussed below. The reader is referred to the reference by Remington and Desmonts for information on congenital toxoplasmosis.

ETIOLOGY *Toxoplasma gondii* is classified among the coccidia and exists in three forms: trophozoite, cyst, and oocyst.

Trophozoites Also termed tachyzoites, trophozoites are crescent or oval, approximately 3 by 7 μm in size, and stain well with either Wright's stain or Giemsa's stain. Trophozoites invade all mammalian cells except nonnucleated erythrocytes and are found in tissues during the acute stage of infection.

Cysts Tissue cysts are formed within host cells and may contain thousands of organisms. They are 10 to 100 μm in size and stain well with periodic acid–Schiff stain; the cyst wall stains with silver stain. Cysts are important in transmission, as they may be present in animal tissues ingested by carnivores. They may persist in virtually every organ, but skeletal and heart muscle and the central nervous system appear to be the most common sites of chronic (latent) infection.

Oocysts Oocysts are oval and 10 to 12 μm in diameter. They are formed only in the mucosal cells of the intestines of members of the cat family and are subsequently excreted in the feces. The cat is the only animal in which the organism has a sexual cycle in the intestine, and cats have systemic infection with *T. gondii* as well. The time of appearance of oocysts in the feces depends on the form of the organism with which the cat becomes infected and varies from 3 to 24 days. Excretion continues for 7 to 20 days, and as many as 10 million oocysts are shed in the feces in a single day. Except under unusual conditions, once a cat has been infected and has excreted oocysts, it will not shed oocysts again. When a cat becomes infected with *Isospora felis,* renewed oocyst excretion has been reported to occur. Sporulation, which occurs from 2 to 3 days (at 24°C) after the oocysts are excreted, is required for the oocysts to become infectious and does not occur below 4°C or above 37°C. Oocysts may remain infectious for more than 1 year under favorable conditions (e.g., in warm, moist soil). This form presumably plays a major role in transmission by the oral route since ingestion of oocysts has been shown to transmit infection.

EPIDEMIOLOGY *Toxoplasma gondii* is ubiquitous and infects herbivorous, omnivorous, and carnivorous animals, including mammals, birds, and reptiles. Prevalence of infection varies with locale; prevalence of positive serologic reaction increases with age. In the United States, approximately 5 to 30 percent of individuals 10 to 19 years old and 10 to 67 percent of individuals over 50 years old have serologic evidence of infection. Generally, less infection occurs in cold regions, in hot and arid areas, and at high elevations. No particular genetic susceptibility has been documented for humans.

The natural mechanism of infection is by ingestion of cysts or oocysts or by transplacental transmission. Infection may also be acquired through blood transfusion, leukocyte transfusion, organ transplantation, and laboratory accident. Clinical illness due to reinfection from an exogenous source has not been reported.

Oral transmission Cysts are present in approximately 10 percent of lamb and 25 percent of pork used for human consumption; cysts have been isolated from beef, but their prevalence in beef has not been defined. Direct contact with any material contaminated by infected cat feces may result in ingestion of oocysts, and this form can be transmitted to food by insects. When humans or other animals (including cats) eat infected tissues (from any animal) or mature oocysts (excreted only by cats), the life cycle is completed. Approximately 1 percent of cats have been found to be excreting oocysts in their feces.

Transplacental transmission Accumulated data overwhelmingly support the concept that *Toxoplasma* is transmitted to the fetus in utero only if the pregnant woman is infected during the current pregnancy. Most often, when a mother is infected during pregnancy the outcome is a normal uninfected infant, but spontaneous abortion, stillbirth, or delivery of a premature or full-term infected infant may result. Congenital infection will occur in approximately one-third of infants born to mothers who acquire their infection during the current pregnancy. In infants born to mothers infected during the first trimester, congenital infection is least common (approximately 17 percent) but disease is most severe; in infants born to mothers infected during the third trimester, congenital infection is most common (approximately 65 percent) but is usually asymptomatic. The fetus is at risk whether or not the infection is symptomatic in the mother.

The following are general guidelines for ascertaining the risk of transmission of the organism to the fetus of a woman who is known to have been infected *prior to the pregnancy in question.* If a woman acquires *Toxoplasma* infection any time before gestation, she will not deliver an infected infant. If a woman had the acute infection during one pregnancy, whether or not she delivered an infected infant, she will not give birth to a child infected with *T. gondii* in a subsequent pregnancy. Studies in which data to the contrary have been presented lacked appropriate controls. Risk to the fetus in these settings, if present, must be exceedingly low. *Toxoplasma* has, however, been isolated on rare occasions from abortuses of women with chronic (latent) infection. At present, the frequency of chronic *Toxoplasma* infection as a cause of abortion has not been defined and is the subject of considerable controversy.

Transmission by blood or leukocyte transfusion *Toxoplasma* may be transmitted by blood or leukocyte transfusion. The organism has been isolated from leukocytes of individuals without recognized clinical evidence of *Toxoplasma* infection, and parasitemia has been reported to persist in otherwise normal individuals for as long as 1 year after acquisition of infection. The high incidence of isolation of the organism from the blood of patients who have chronic myelogenous leukemia and high antibody titers to *Toxoplasma* is particularly noteworthy. The organism has survived for 50 days in whole citrated blood stored at 4°C. Immunodeficient patients who require multiple blood transfusions may be particularly at risk for transmission of infection by this route.

PATHOGENESIS Organisms released from cysts or oocysts enter cells of the gastrointestinal tract, multiply, cause cell disruption, and then infect neighboring cells. Extracellular organisms or organisms within leukocytes are transported throughout the body via the lymphatic system and bloodstream and are capable of invading every organ and tissue. Proliferation of trophozoites usually leads to death of invaded cells, resulting in foci of necrosis, surrounded by an intense cellular reaction. The immune response of the host primarily governs the outcome of the acute process. Both humoral and cell-mediated immunity are important. In some apparently normal individuals and in immunodeficient patients, the acute infection may progress with acute necrotizing encephalitis, pneumonitis, or myocarditis which may be fatal. Trophozoites disappear from the tissues with development of the normal immune response.

A unique aspect of the infection is that organisms persist in cysts in many organs during the life span of the host. Either persistence of viable trophozoites within cells of the reticuloendothelial system or disruption of cysts may be the source of the recurrent parasitemias that occur in some asymptomatic individuals with chronic infection. Cysts are the probable origin of the organisms that cause recrudescent disease in immunocompromised patients or chorioretinitis in older children and adults with congenital toxoplasmosis.

PATHOLOGY The histopathologic changes in toxoplasmic lymphadenitis are characteristic and consist of reactive follicular hyperplasia with irregular clusters of epithelioid histiocytes that have vesicular nuclei and abundant eosinophilic cytoplasm and that encroach upon and blur the margins of germinal centers; numerous mitoses in the germinal centers; many necrotic cells and an associated focal distention of subcapsular and trabecular sinuses with monocytoid cells. Trophozoites or cysts are only rarely observed in conventionally stained sections.

Single or multiple foci of necrosis occur as the earliest manifestations of involvement of the eye. Infiltrates are composed largely of lymphocytes, plasma cells, and mononuclear phagocytic cells. There are intra- and extracellular trophozoites and cysts in the retinal lesions. Granulomatous inflammation of the choroid occurs secondary to necrotizing retinitis. Iridocyclitis, glaucoma, and cataracts may be complications of the chorioretinitis.

In cases of acute central nervous system infection, there is a focal or diffuse meningoencephalitis with necrosis and microglial nodules. Margins of areas of necrosis may be infiltrated with monocytes, lymphocytes, and plasma cells. Perivascular mononuclear inflammation frequently is present contiguous to areas of necrosis, and occasionally there is necrosis of vessel walls. Intra- and extracellular trophozoites are usually found at the periphery of areas of necrosis, and these areas of necrosis may mimic mass lesions. Cysts may be present after the first week of infection. The size of lesions and extent and location of central nervous system involvement vary considerably.

In cases of disseminated infection, pathologic changes occur in the heart, lungs, kidney, and multiple other organs. They consist of necrosis and the presence of trophozoites, cysts, and inflammatory cells alone or in combination. Glomerulonephritis with deposits of gamma-M globulin (IgM), fibrinogen, and *Toxoplasma* antigen and antibody has been reported. Involvement of the pancreas has been a prominent finding in infection in immunocompromised patients. Findings in skeletal muscle vary from parasitized fibers without pathologic changes to focal areas of infiltration to widespread myositis with necrosis.

CLINICAL MANIFESTATIONS Lymphadenopathy and other manifestations in the immunocompetent individual Lymphadenopathy is the most commonly recognized clinical manifestation of acute acquired toxoplasmosis. Cervical nodes are involved most frequently. Nodes may be single or multiple, and involvement may be symptomatic or asymptomatic. Asymptomatic lymphadenopathy may mimic lymphoma, and involvement of a pectoral node has been suspected to be carcinoma of the breast when detected on physical examination. Suboccipital, supraclavicular, axillary, inguinal, and mediastinal nodes may be involved. When mesenteric or retroperitoneal nodes are involved, abdominal pain and significant temperature elevation (e.g., up to 40°C) may occur. Involved lymph nodes vary in firmness, may be tender, do not suppurate, and are usually discrete. Malaise, fever, myalgias, headache, sore throat, maculopapular rash (which spares the palms and soles), hepatosplenomegaly, or reactive (atypical) lymphocytes may occur. Lymphadenopathic toxoplasmosis is self-limited, but malaise and/or lymphadenopathy may persist or recur for months.

Individuals who appear to be normal immunologically rarely may present with any of the following, alone or in combination: pneumonitis, myocarditis, pericarditis, hepatitis, polymyositis, encephalitis, or meningoencephalitis. Signs or

symptoms of involvement of these organs are nonspecific. Significant morbidity has occurred, and some of these patients have died of the infection.

Ocular involvement *Toxoplasma* has been estimated to be the cause of approximately 35 percent of cases of chorioretinitis in children and adults. Although chorioretinitis has been estimated to occur in approximately 1 percent of patients with the acute acquired infection, ocular disease is most often a consequence of congenital *Toxoplasma* infection. Blurred vision, scotomas, pain, photophobia, or epiphora may be due to active chorioretinitis. If the macula is involved, impairment or loss of central vision may occur. In children, strabismus may be an early sign of chorioretinitis. Associated signs of systemic infection occur only rarely. Vision improves, but frequently visual acuity recovers only partially as inflammation subsides. Commonly, episodic flares of chorioretinitis cause destruction of irreplaceable retinal tissue. These multiple recurrences may result in glaucoma or loss of vision and ultimately may necessitate enucleation. The acute lesions appear as yellowish white, cotton-like patches that have elevated, indistinct margins surrounded by a zone of hyperemia. Inflammatory exudate in the vitreous may obscure the fundus. Older lesions characteristically appear as atrophic, whitish gray plaques with distinct borders and black spots of choroidal pigment. Lesions usually are located near the posterior pole of the retina, although they may be peripheral. They may be single but are more commonly multiple, and lesions of varying age may be seen simultaneously. Panuveitis and papillitis with optic atrophy occur less commonly. Isolated anterior uveitis due to *Toxoplasma* infection has never been proved.

Toxoplasmosis in the immunocompromised patient All forms of toxoplasmosis that occur in normal individuals may also occur in immunocompromised individuals. Patients receiving immunosuppressive therapy for lymphoproliferative disorders (especially Hodgkin's disease), for hematologic malignancy, or for prevention of organ graft rejection have the greatest predilection for life-threatening toxoplasmosis. The untreated infection in these patients is frequently fulminant and rapidly fatal. Central nervous system involvement, present in greater than 50 percent of documented cases, is the most characteristic clinical feature of toxoplasmosis in immunocompromised patients. Therefore, the diagnosis of toxoplasmosis must be excluded in any immunosuppressed patient with symptoms or signs referable to the central nervous system. Symptoms and signs are manifestations of diffuse encephalopathy, meningoencephalitis, or cerebral mass lesions and include changes in mental status, headache, focal neurologic deficits, and seizures. Brain involvement has been established by demonstration of trophozoites in material from brain biopsy or in material aspirated from mass lesions that may have the characteristic appearance of a brain abscess on computerized tomography (CT) scan. Typically, the cerebrospinal fluid shows a mononuclear pleocytosis, a moderate elevation in protein, and a normal glucose. Immunocompromised patients also may have other nonspecific manifestations of the infection which are reflections of inflammation and necrosis of the organs involved, particularly heart and lungs.

Toxoplasmosis and *Toxoplasma* infection in the pregnant woman *Toxoplasma* infection acquired by the mother during pregnancy is symptomatic in only about 10 to 20 percent of cases. See also "Transplacental Transmission" above.

DIAGNOSIS Acute infection with *Toxoplasma* may be diagnosed by isolation of *T. gondii* from body fluids or blood (see qualification under "Isolation Procedures" below), demonstration of trophozoites in histologic sections or in impression smears of tissue or body fluids, demonstration of characteristic lymph node histology, and serologic tests.

Isolation procedures The organism can be isolated by inoculation of leukocytes, body fluids, or tissue specimens into tissue culture or by subcutaneous or intraperitoneal inoculation into mice. Body fluids should be processed and inoculated immediately, but blood and tissues may be stored at 4°C overnight. Freezing or treatment of specimens with Formalin kills the organism. Mice should be examined for the presence of organisms in their peritoneal fluid 6 to 10 days after inoculation, or earlier if they die. Mice that survive 6 weeks should be tested for *Toxoplasma* antibody in their serum. When antibody is present, visualization of *Toxoplasma* cysts in the mouse brain establishes the diagnosis. If cysts are not demonstrable in brains of mice with *Toxoplasma* antibody, portions of brain, liver, and spleen should be inoculated into other mice.

Isolation of *T. gondii* from body fluids reflects the acute stage of infection, as does isolation from blood in most patients. Although persistent parasitemia has been described in asymptomatic individuals with latent infection, this appears to be a rare occurrence, except, perhaps, in patients with chronic myelogenous leukemia. Isolation from tissues (e.g., skeletal muscle, lung, brain, or eye) obtained by biopsy or at autopsy may reflect the presence of tissue cysts and does not prove that infection is acute.

Histologic diagnosis Demonstration of trophozoites in tissue sections or smears (e.g., brain biopsy, bone marrow aspirate) or in body fluids (e.g., cerebrospinal fluid, amniotic fluid) establishes the diagnosis of the acute infection. It is difficult to identify trophozoites by ordinary staining methods; direct and indirect immunofluorescent antibody techniques have been used successfully for this purpose. Demonstration of tissue cysts does not differentiate between acute or chronic infection. When there are numerous cysts in any organ, infection is usually of recent onset. Characteristic histologic criteria establish toxoplasmic lymphadenitis (see "Pathology" above).

Serologic tests Methods most widely used to establish the diagnosis of acute *Toxoplasma* infection are the Sabin-Feldman dye test, indirect fluorescent antibody (IFA) test, and indirect hemagglutination (IHA) test. Methods that detect antigenemia, although presently experimental, are promising. Measurement of antibodies by enzyme-linked immunosorbent assay or radioimmunoassay is potentially valuable because these techniques may be automated.

The dye test, which measures primarily IgG antibodies, is sensitive and specific. The World Health Organization has recommended that dye test titers be expressed in international units (IU/ml) and will supply a standard reference serum.

The IFA test appears to measure the same antibodies as the dye test and is the most widely available procedure. In both tests, titers tend to be parallel. Dye test and IFA test antibodies usually appear 1 to 2 weeks after infection, reach high titers ($\geq$ 1:1000) in 6 to 8 weeks, and gradually decline over months to years; low titers (e.g., 1:4 to 1:64) commonly persist for life (Fig. 203-1). Magnitude of antibody titer does not correlate with severity of illness.

The IgM-fluorescent antibody (IgM-IFA) test is especially useful in establishing the diagnosis of acute infection with *T. gondii* because IgM antibodies appear early (as early as 5 days after infection) and disappear early as contrasted with gamma-G globulin (IgG) antibodies. In most cases, IgM-IFA test antibodies rise rapidly (to levels of 1:80 to $\geq$ 1:1000) and fall to low titers (1:10 or 1:20) or disappear within a few weeks or months (Fig. 203-1). However, in some patients they are present at low titer for as long as several years. Some immunodeficient patients with acute toxoplasmosis and most patients with only active ocular toxoplasmosis may not have IgM *Toxoplasma* antibodies. Rheumatoid factor may cause false-positive reactions in the IgM-IFA test. Removal of rheumatoid factor (e.g., by absorption) will eliminate false-positive test results in the IgM-IFA test. Antinuclear antibodies may cause false-positive reactions in both the IFA and IgM-IFA tests.

The antibodies measured in the IHA test may persist for years and are different than those measured in the IFA and dye tests. The IHA test may be helpful when titers in the IFA or dye test have stabilized since IHA test titers rise later. However, the rise in titer may occur so late that its demonstration is not helpful in diagnosis of the acute infection at a clinically pertinent time. Proper standardization of methodology for this and all other serologic tests is needed, as is quality control of commercial kits that are often employed by laboratories inexperienced in performing these serologic tests.

FIGURE 203-1

Antibody response in humans to Toxoplasma *infection. IgM antibodies (— —), detectable by the IgM-IFA test, reach maximum titer within the first few weeks after infection and may decline within a few weeks (----) or persist for months (——·——). IgG antibodies (——), detectable by ei-* *ther Sabin-Feldman dye test or conventional IFA test, reach maximum titer within 2 months, plateau for months or years, and then decline, but usually persist at a low titer for life. (After G Desmonts, Feuill Biol 16:61, 1975.)*

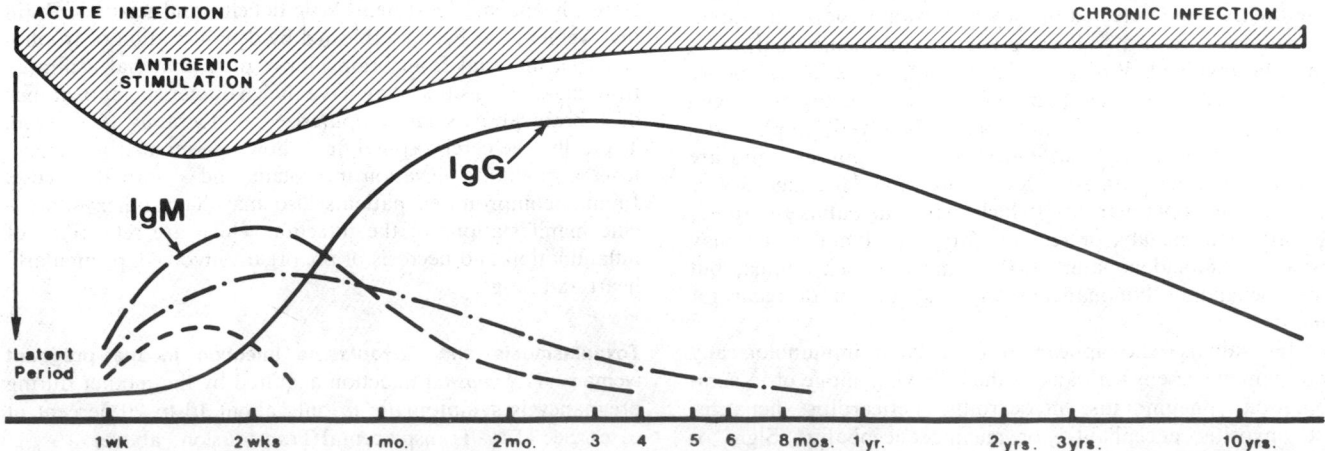

Titers in the complement fixation (CF) test also may appear several weeks later than those measured in the IFA and dye tests and also may persist for years. A negative CF test titer does not exclude acute or chronic infection, and a single positive CF test titer does not prove acute infection. A significant rise in CF test titer (i.e., of two serial dilutions performed at the same time on serums obtained several weeks apart) establishes recent infection.

Local production of antibody in active ocular or central nervous system toxoplasmosis may be demonstrated by comparison of level of *Toxoplasma* antibody in cerebrospinal fluid or aqueous humor. Application of the following equation may be used to assess local antibody production:

$$C = \frac{\text{antibody titer in body fluid}}{\text{antibody titer in serum}}$$
$$\times \frac{\text{concentration of gamma globulin in serum}}{\text{concentration of gamma globulin in body fluid}}$$

A significant correlation coefficient *(C)* is ≥ 8 and reflects local antibody production that signifies active central nervous system or ocular infection. It is usually not possible to demonstrate significant local antibody production by application of this formula if the dye test or IFA test serum titer is $\geq 1:1000$.

Acute acquired *Toxoplasma* infection in the immunocompetent individual In settings in which acute acquired infection is suspected in an immunocompetent individual, a negative dye test or IFA test virtually excludes the diagnosis. The diagnosis of recent acute acquired infection is confirmed if there is a serial two-tube rise in titer when serums drawn at 3-week intervals are run at the same time or if there is seroconversion from a negative to a positive titer (in the absence of transfer of antibody by transfusion). A single high titer in any test does not prove the presence of active infection.

Guidelines for interpretation of test results are presented below and in Table 203-1. Exceptions to these generalizations may occur.

A dye test or IFA test titer of $\geq 1:1000$ and a high IgM-IFA test titer ($\geq 1:80$) are probably diagnostic of recent acute infection whether or not symptoms are present. In an individual with a positive titer in the dye test or IFA test, absence of IgM-IFA test antibodies almost always excludes very recent acquisition of infection.

Ocular toxoplasmosis Diagnosis of ocular toxoplasmosis in older children and adults may be difficult because the level of antibody titer in serum does not necessarily correlate with presence of active lesions in the fundus. A patient with active *Toxoplasma* chorioretinitis usually has low serologic test titers (1:4 to 1:64). If a serologic test is negative when performed on undiluted serum, for practical purposes, toxoplasmic chorioretinitis is excluded. If retinal lesions are characteristic and serologic tests are positive (see also "Serologic Tests" above), the diagnosis can be made with a high degree of confidence. If retinal lesions are atypical and serologic tests are positive, diagnosis of toxoplasmosis is only presumptive; the high prevalence of *Toxoplasma* antibodies in the normal population precludes assumption of a causal relationship.

Active infection in the immunocompromised patient Because antibody formation may be deficient in immunocompromised patients, available serologic methods, including the IgM-IFA test, are at times insufficient for detection of active infection. Serologic tests to screen for *Toxoplasma* infection are useful in asymptomatic immunocompromised individuals in order to identify those patients who are at risk for primary infection or reactivation of latent infection (see also "Prevention" below).

Toxoplasmosis and *Toxoplasma* infection in the pregnant woman It seems advisable to perform serology in any woman considering becoming pregnant to determine whether she has *Toxoplasma* infection prior to pregnancy and to provide essential information when tests are performed during pregnancy (see "Transplacental Transmission" above).

In the absence of a routine screening program in which *Toxoplasma* serology is performed frequently during pregnancy, an IgM-IFA test should be performed if any other serologic test is found to be positive in any titer at any time during gestation. If the IgM-IFA test is not available, a repeat serologic test should be obtained in 3 weeks to determine if the

TABLE 203-1
Guidelines for interpretation of commonly employed serologic tests in the diagnosis of toxoplasmosis*

	Sabin-Feldman dye test	Indirect fluorescent antibody (IFA) test	Indirect fluorescent antibody test for IgM *Toxoplasma* antibodies (IgM-IFA)	Indirect hemagglutination (IHA) test	Complement fixation (CF) test
Positive titer	1:4, undiluted†	1:10‡	1:2 infants‡ 1:10 adults‡	1:16‡	1:4‡
Titer in acute infection	$\geq 1:1000$	$\geq 1:1000$	$\geq 1:80$	$\geq 1:1000$	Varies among laboratories
Titer in chronic (latent) infection	1:4–1:2000	1:8–1:2000	Negative to 1:20	1:16–1:256	Negative to 1:8
Duration of elevation of titer	Years	Years	Weeks to months; occasionally years	Years	Years
Special considerations	*1* No known cross reactions or false-positive results in humans.	*1* Antibody measured is same as that measured in dye test. *2* Antinuclear antibodies may cause false-positive results.	*1* Either antinuclear antibodies or rheumatoid factor (IgM) may cause false-positive results. Rheumatoid factor may be absorbed from serum.	*1* Not useful for diagnosis of congenital toxoplasmosis. *2* IHA antibodies rise later than in dye test and IFA. May be especially useful if rising IHA titer can be demonstrated.	*1* Antigen preparations have not been standardized. *2* CF antibodies also rise later than dye test and IFA; see special consideration 2 under IHA.

* *These guidelines are useful in the interpretation of test results, but exceptions to these generalizations may occur.*
† *In some cases of eye disease, the dye test may be positive only in undiluted serum.*
‡ *These values are representative, but normal values for each laboratory may differ significantly.*

titer is stable or rising. No further evaluation is necessary if the IgM-IFA test is negative and an IFA or dye test titer is stable and < 1:1000 (< 300 IU). If the dye test or IFA test is ≥ 1:1000 (≥ 300 IU) and stable (regardless of titer in the IgM-IFA test), the infection should be considered to have been acquired *at least* 4 weeks earlier and probably more than 8 weeks before the serum was obtained. Thus, for practical purposes, the fetus is not at risk if the dye test or IFA test titer is ≥ 1:1000 and stable in the first 2 months of pregnancy.

Whereas titers in the dye test or IFA test may have peaked and stabilized by 8 weeks after onset of infection, titers in the CF or IHA test may continue to rise for 4 to 6 months or longer after acquisition of infection. Therefore, rises in these latter two tests may not be helpful in defining when infection occurred relative to the time of conception and should not be used as the sole test for this purpose.

A common problem arises when an asymptomatic woman is tested for *Toxoplasma* antibody late in the first trimester or in the second trimester of pregnancy and her IFA or dye test titer is found to be in the vicinity of 1:2000, her IgM-IFA test titer is found to be negative, and no significant rise in titer in any test is demonstrable. It is not possible to establish whether infection occurred before, at, or after conception in this situation.

THERAPY Therapy in specific clinical settings The need for and duration of therapy are determined by the clinical severity of illness and by the underlying medical problem.

Most immunologically normal patients with lymphadenopathic toxoplasmosis do not require specific treatment. Indication for treatment in these cases is severe and persistent symptoms. Evidence of serious damage to vital organs is also an indication for therapy. Infections acquired via transfusions or in laboratory accidents may be more severe than naturally acquired infections and probably should be treated.

Patients with active chorioretinitis should be treated with specific therapy. When there is potential for serious visual impairment secondary to macular or optic nerve involvement, corticosteroids are added to the regimen.

Because of the high mortality rate associated with toxoplasmosis in patients whose resistance to infection is compromised by underlying disease or by therapy (e.g., corticosteroids or cytotoxic drugs), toxoplasmosis should be treated in all immunocompromised individuals. In immunocompromised patients, serologic evidence of acute infection (with or without signs and symptoms of infection) or demonstration of trophozoites in tissue (with or without serologic test titers or signs and symptoms) is an indication for therapy. Improvement has been reported to occur in the majority of patients to whom specific therapy was administered. Considering the diagnosis early enough to institute treatment is the major problem.

When a pregnant woman who acquired infection at any time during pregnancy is treated, the chance of congenital infection in her infant is decreased but not eliminated. In separate series reported from France and Germany, treatment decreased the incidence of infection significantly. The drugs employed were spiramycin in the study from France and pyrimethamine plus sulfonamide in the study from Germany. Spiramycin (not available in the United States) has been used safely for treatment in the first trimester. Pyrimethamine is a potential teratogen; therefore, sulfadiazine (which is highly effective in animal models when used alone) should be used alone if a decision is made to treat during the first trimester of pregnancy. When infection occurs during the first trimester, some authorities have recommended therapeutic abortion because of the high probability of severe damage when infection occurs early in fetal life. Other authorities recommend treatment rather than abortion because the risk of transmission of the infection to the fetus is low (approximately 15 percent) in the first trimester and because the incidence of congenital toxoplasmosis can be reduced significantly by intrapartum therapy. They reason that drug therapy would result in saving a significant number of healthy fetuses. Decision about mode of therapy ultimately must be made by both the well-informed physician and the well-informed patient who must be aware of the risks. Carefully controlled studies are needed to define whether a pregnant woman who has *Toxoplasma* antibody and a history of habitual abortion will benefit from treatment.

Pyrimethamine plus sulfadiazine or trisulfapyrimidines In vivo, pyrimethamine and sulfadiazine act synergistically against *Toxoplasma*. Clinical experience confirms efficacy of this combination. Comparative tests have shown that sulfapyrazine, sulfamethazine, and sulfamerazine are about as effective as sulfadiazine. In general, other sulfonamides are much less effective.

Pyrimethamine In adults, a loading dose of 100 to 200 mg pyrimethamine is given orally in two divided doses on the first day of treatment. In young children, a loading dose of 2 mg per kilogram of body weight (not to exceed adult loading dose) is given for the first 2 to 3 days of treatment. Maintenance dose is 1 mg per kilogram of body weight (with a maximum of 25 mg) in a single dose. In view of the drug's half-life of 4 to 5 days, administration of the maintenance dose at 3- to 4-day intervals has been suggested. Daily administration is recommended for the patient who is very ill, since there are no data concerning absorption of the drug in this situation. Daily therapy is also recommended for active ocular infection. Pyrimethamine is available only in tablet form.

Pyrimethamine is a folic acid antagonist and produces a dose-related, usually gradual, and reversible depression of the bone marrow. Anemia, leukopenia, and thrombocytopenia may occur. Platelet and peripheral blood cell counts should be evaluated twice weekly in any patient receiving pyrimethamine.

Folinic acid To prevent suppression of the bone marrow, folinic acid (calcium leucovorin) is administered in conjunction with pyrimethamine therapy. Optimal frequency for administration of folinic acid has not been established. A single oral dose of 5 to 10 mg daily is recommended. If folinic acid is not available, bakers' yeast (3 to 4 cakes daily) may be used to prevent toxicity due to pyrimethamine. Neither folinic acid nor bakers' yeast inhibits the action of pyrimethamine on *T. gondii*, whereas folic acid does.

Sulfadiazine and trisulfapyrimidines The loading dose is 50 to 75 mg per kilogram of body weight; thereafter, a total daily dose of 75 to 100 mg per kilogram of body weight is administered in four divided doses at intervals of approximately 6 h. Tablet and liquid oral forms as well as an intravenous form of sulfadiazine are available. The potential toxicities of sulfonamides (e.g., crystalluria, hematuria, and rash) must be carefully monitored.

Other drugs Trimethoprim alone or in combination with a sulfonamide has not been proved to be effective in treatment of toxoplasmosis in humans, but the activity of this combination in vitro and in vivo in animal models warrants carefully designed and controlled clinical trials. This combination is significantly less active than the combination of pyrimethamine with sulfadiazine.

Duration of therapy Optimal duration of specific therapy has not been defined for any form of toxoplasmosis. Specific therapy should be continued for 4 to 6 weeks in a patient who appears to be immunologically normal but who requires treatment for severe and persistent symptoms or evidence of damage to vital organs (e.g., chorioretinitis, myocarditis). Longer treatment may be necessary.

It seems advisable to treat an immunocompromised patient for at least 4 to 6 weeks *beyond* complete resolution of all signs and symptoms of active disease. Careful follow-up of these patients is imperative because relapse may occur and requires prompt reinstitution of therapy. Although therapy may be effective against *T. gondii* trophozoites and may induce a beneficial clinical response, it does not eradicate cysts from the central nervous system.

Desmonts and Couvreur suggest that an acutely infected pregnant woman be treated with spiramycin and use a total dose of 2 to 3 daily, administered orally in four divided doses. A 3-week course of treatment is alternated with 2 weeks without treatment from the time of diagnosis until term. Another treatment regimen was used in Germany and consisted of a course of sulfonamide and pyrimethamine followed by one or two courses of sulfonamide administered alone or in combination with pyrimethamine. Each course of therapy was given for approximately 2 weeks and was alternated with a 3- to 4-week interval without treatment. Pyrimethamine was not administered during the first trimester of pregnancy.

PREVENTION Measures for prevention of infection involve intervention in the cycle of transmission and are most important for immunodeficient patients and seronegative pregnant women. To kill cysts, meat should be heated to 60°C or frozen at −20°C. (Freezers available commercially do not reach or maintain this temperature reliably.) Hands should be washed after touching uncooked meat, and fruits and vegetables that may be contaminated with oocysts should be washed. Dry heat (66°C) or boiling water renders oocysts noninfectious. Contact with cat feces should be avoided.

There are no definitive data to allow for a firm recommendation regarding the use of whole blood, leukocyte transfusions, or organ transplants when a donor is seropositive for *Toxoplasma* antibodies. It seems reasonable, however, that whenever feasible, blood or blood products donated by an individual with *Toxoplasma* antibody should not be used in an immunosuppressed individual, and an organ transplanted to a seronegative recipient should be from an individual without serologic evidence of *Toxoplasma* infection.

A nontoxic drug that eliminates the organism in the cyst as well as the trophozoite form is needed for prophylaxis against the devastating complications of recrudescent infection in immunocompromised individuals.

See "Therapy in Specific Clinical Settings" above for guidelines concerning prevention of transmission to the fetus.

At present, no effective vaccine to prevent infection with *Toxoplasma* has been developed. Development of a vaccine for use in nonimmune women of childbearing age should be explored since maternal immunity appears to prevent congenital transmission of *T. gondii*. Vaccines that prevent oocyst development in cats could prove valuable by interrupting the life cycle of *T. gondii*.

REFERENCES

DORFMAN RF, REMINGTON JS: Value of lymph node biopsy in the diagnosis of acute acquired toxoplasmosis. N Engl J Med 289:878, 1973

DUBEY JP et al: Characterization of the new fecal form of *Toxoplasma gondii*. J Parasitol 56:447, 1970

FELDMAN HA: Toxoplasmosis. N Engl J Med 279:1370, 1431, 1968

JONES TC et al: Toxoplasmic lymphadenitis. JAMA 192:87, 1965

KIMBALL AC et al: Congenital toxoplasmosis: A prospective study of 4048 obstetric patients. Am J Obstet Gynecol 111:211, 1971

O'CONNOR GR: Manifestations and management of ocular toxoplasmosis. Bull NY Acad Med 50:192, 1974

REMINGTON JS, DESMONTE G: Toxoplasmosis, in *Infectious Diseases of the Fetus and Newborn Infant*, JS Remington, JO Klein (eds). Philadelphia, Saunders, 1976, p 191

RUSKIN J, REMINGTON JS: Toxoplasmosis in the compromised host. Ann Intern Med 84:193, 1976

SIIM JC: Acquired toxoplasmosis. JAMA 147:1641, 1951

TOWNSEND JJ et al: Acquired toxoplasmosis. Arch Neurol 32:335, 1975

204

PNEUMOCYSTIS CARINII PNEUMONIA (PNEUMOCYSTOSIS, INTERSTITIAL PLASMA CELL PNEUMONIA)

C. GEORGE RAY

DEFINITION *Pneumocystis carinii* pneumonia occurs in patients with impaired antibody and/or cellular immune responses, or severe debility with protein-calorie malnutrition. Progressive pulmonary insufficiency is the cardinal clinical manifestation

ETIOLOGY In vitro cultivation of *P. carinii* has only recently been accomplished, using primary embryonic chick epithelial lung cells. Its taxonomic position now appears to be that of a protozoan. Histologically, 1- to 2-μm oval or crescentic "merozoite" forms with a single nucleus-like, chromatoid body can be seen. These are usually arranged in groups of two to eight within cysts measuring 5 to 10 μm. Cyst rupture permits release of mature trophozoites, measuring 2 to 4 μm, into alveoli. The crescentic appearance of the cysts is thought to be due to partial collapse after encystment of trophozoites. Electron microscopic studies reveal a complex structure and suggest the capacity for protein synthesis and oxidative metabolism, while structures usually associated with phagocytosis are lacking. The agent can be best visualized with special stains, particularly methenamine silver, toluidine blue 0, Gram-Weigert, or Giemsa's stain (but not with hematoxylin-eosin), with phase microscopy, and with fluorescent antibody. The organism seen in human beings is morphologically similar to that in animals, but species-specific antigenic differences may exist.

EPIDEMIOLOGY The incidence of *P. carinii* infection is uncertain, and epidemiologic data are based on indirect evidence. It appears that latent infection is not rare in humans and is frequent in many wild, domestic, and laboratory animals. Indirect fluorescent antibody studies suggest that 75 percent or more of children develop antibodies to the agent by 2 to 4 years of age. In humans the disease is worldwide and occurs in all age groups either as epidemics in nurseries or as isolated cases. Clinical observations suggest that the disease can be contagious. This is based on evidence suggesting aerosol transmission in nurseries with debilitated and malnourished infants under 6 months of age, possible spread among patients in cancer hospitals, and isolated reports of intrafamilial spread. However, while it is possible that person-to-person or even animal-to-person spread of infection may occur, the presence of an underlying immunologic or nutritional deficiency is usually required for the development of overt disease. Intrauterine *P. carinii* pneumonia probably acquired by transplacental transmission has also been reported. The incubation period is estimated to be 1 to 2 months.

PATHOGENESIS The organism is of low virulence, proliferates slowly, and may require the presence of another microbial agent for multiplication. When affecting persons in the first year of life, the disease is usually associated with congenital immunodeficiency syndromes or severe protein-calorie malnutrition; in patients over 1 year of age, it is most commonly a complication of neoplasia, particularly of malignant lymphoreticular disorders, cyclic neutropenia, various anemias, collagen vascular and autoimmune diseases, renal failure, and in patients with transplants who are receiving immunosuppressive drugs and adrenal steroids. Surprisingly, among patients with acute lymphocytic leukemia, the clinical manifestations of infection are most frequently found during periods of remission. *Pneumocystis carinii* pneumonia has also been reported occasionally in the absence of demonstrated underlying disease. Progressive *P. carinii* infection has been produced in various laboratory animals by corticosteroid-induced immunosuppression or malnutrition, both of which apparently activated latent infection.

The largest group of patients with *P. carinii* pneumonia in the past were premature or debilitated newborns in whom the disease, first described as interstitial plasma-cell pneumonia, occurred at about the age of 3 to 4 months, often in nursery epidemics. These epidemics are virtually unheard of in this country, and are becoming increasingly rare in other areas, presumably as a result of improved infant nutrition and less crowding. However, cases continue to be reported and often involve young infants from orphanages in southeast Asia.

Many infections occur together with *P. carinii* pneumonia, and these are often multiple. Acute and chronic bacterial infections are common, and a wide range of concurrent viral, fungal, and some protozoan infections has been observed. Localized and disseminated cytomegalic inclusion disease is a particularly frequent concomitant infection.

PATHOLOGY In widespread disease the lungs are massively consolidated. The consolidation may be focal and confined to the central or dorsal lung areas. The alveoli are distended by a foamy material which suggests the diagnosis, and, when stained appropriately, the organisms can be seen. Hyaline membranes may be present. The sparse cellular response consists of mononuclear cells. Alveolar septal infiltration with plasma cells (interstitial plasma-cell pneumonia) is prominent in many cases and absent in others. Septal fibrosis is generally slight. The changes appear reversible. Granuloma formation, calcification, and focal and diffuse persistent fibrosis have also been noted. In latent infection the lesions are few and minute, organisms are scanty, the foamy intraalveolar material is lacking, and the cellular response is sparse. The infection is generally confined to the lung, but organisms have been seen in the regional lymph nodes. Pleuritis is characteristically absent, and systemic dissemination with focal lesions in distant sites is extremely rare.

CLINICAL MANIFESTATIONS Generally the onset is insidious. The fully developed clinical picture includes severe dyspnea and tachypnea. The patient displays all signs of extreme air hunger and is anxious and cyanotic. There may be a dry cough which, together with the cyanosis, is aggravated by any movement. Fever is absent or slight. Pulmonary physical findings are scanty in contrast to the grave clinical state and the extensive lung involvement seen roentgenologically. Roent-

genograms show hazy alveolar infiltrates spreading from the hilum and eventually affecting most of the lung. Some patients may develop peripheral, somewhat nodular infiltrates, which can be confused with other infections or malignant processes and usually require biopsy for confirmation of the diagnosis. Focal emphysema may be present, but pleural effusions are rare. Blood gas studies indicate impaired diffusion, with severe hypoxemia and normal or only slightly elevated P_{CO_2} values. Other laboratory studies are generally nonrevealing, except for a frequently observed lymphopenia. In young infants with combined immunodeficiency and *P. carinii* infection, significant eosinophilia has been observed. Complications include pneumothorax from a ruptured emphysematous bleb and rib fractures from forced respiratory movements. Death occurs by progressive asphyxia or cardiac failure within 1 to 10 weeks in untreated cases.

The differential diagnosis usually includes viral infection, particularly cytomegalovirus, disseminated pulmonary aspergillosis, and occasionally other bacterial and mycotic infections. In addition, pulmonary alveolar proteinosis, desquamative interstitial pneumonia, pulmonary hemorrhage, and pulmonary fibrosis, either idiopathic or secondary to irradiation or drugs, such as bleomycin, methotrexate, busulfan, cyclophosphamide, or nitrofurantoin, must be considered. The best way to resolve this differential is to do open lung biopsy, whenever possible.

DIAGNOSIS The diagnosis depends on the morphologic demonstration of the organism. Bronchial secretion, tracheal lavage, and gastric aspirate examinations have been variably successful. Needle or open lung biopsy is often diagnostic but entails some risk, particularly in far-advanced cases. Endobronchial brush biopsy has been reported as a simple, frequently successful procedure as has percutaneous needle aspiration of the lung in some series in children.

Serological testing, using indirect immunofluorescence or complement fixation is of limited value in diagnosis, and cannot be relied upon as an alternative to direct identification of the organism. Newer methods being developed for the detection of circulating antigen during acute disease may be useful in the future.

PROGNOSIS Morbidity and mortality figures are uncertain. *Pneumocystis carinii* infection is not rare at any age, and it seems likely that it will be recognized more frequently. The prognosis of *P. carinii* pneumonia is grave since it is generally a complication of a severe underlying disorder. A mortality of 40 to 50 percent has been suggested. However, remissions and spontaneous cures have been reported. The outcome is heavily dependent on the course of the underlying disease.

TREATMENT The current treatment of choice of *P. carinii* infection is a combination of trimethoprim and sulfamethoxazole in doses of 20 mg trimethoprim per kilogram of body weight and 100 mg/kg sulfamethoxazole per day, given orally or intravenously in four divided doses for 14 to 16 days. In high-risk groups of cancer patients, particularly children with acute lymphocytic leukemia, long-term prophylaxis with low-dose trimethoprim-sulfamethoxazole (5 mg/kg trimethoprim and 20 mg/kg sulfamethoxazole, divided into two doses daily) has significantly decreased the incidence of *P. carinii* pneumonia, without serious adverse reactions.

Pentamidine isethionate was the previous drug of choice, but it is now considered a secondary agent for patients unable to tolerate standard therapy. The recommended daily dose is 4 mg/kg given as a single intramuscular injection for 12 to 14 days. Approximately 40 percent of patients develop systemic side effects including azotemia, hypoglycemia, changes in liver function, and pulmonary fibrosis.

In patients with malnutrition and the histopathology of interstitial plasma-cell pneumonia, response to either form of therapy is often very slow. It has been suggested that concomitant corticosteroid therapy might benefit these patients by suppressing the alveolar inflammatory response until the organisms are eradicated. Treatment with oxygen is usually indicated, with the objective of trying to maintain Pa_{O_2} levels at 70 mmHg or above. The inspired oxygen concentration should be kept at less than 50 percent, if possible, to avoid oxygen toxicity. Careful monitoring and assisted ventilation are often required to achieve these goals. Antibiotics, convalescent serum, and commercial immunoglobulin have no effect.

REFERENCES

BURKE BA, GOOD RA: *Pneumocystis carinii* infection. Medicine, 57:23, 1973

CROSS AS, STEIGBIGEL RT: *Pneumocystis carinii* pneumonia presenting as localized nodular densities. N Engl J Med 291:831, 1974

DUTZ W: *Pneumocystis carinii* pneumonia. Pathol Annu 5:309, 1971

HUGHES WT et al: Successful chemoprophylaxis for *Pneumocystis carinii* pneumonitis. N Engl J Med 297:1419, 1977

——— et al: Comparison of pentamidine isethionate and trimethoprim sulfamethoxazole in the treatment of *Pneumocystis carinii* pneumonia. J Pediatr 92:285, 1978

———: *Pneumocystis carinii* pneumonia. N Engl J Med 297:1381, 1977

LAU WK, YOUNG LS: Trimethoprim-sulfamethoxazole treatment of *Pneumocystis carinii* pneumonia in adults. N Engl J Med 295:716, 1976

PIFER LL et al: *Pneumocystis carinii* infection: Evidence for high prevalence in normal and immunosuppressed children. Pediatrics 61:35, 1978

WEBER WR et al: Lung biopsy in *Pneumocystis carinii* pneumonia. Am J Clin Pathol 67:11, 1977

205
MINOR PROTOZOAN DISEASES

JAMES J. PLORDE

TRICHOMONIASIS Trichomoniasis is a venereal infection caused by the protozoan *Trichomonas vaginalis*. Of the many members of the genus *Trichomonas*, three are parasites of human beings: *T. hominis* in the intestine, *T. tenax* in the oral cavity, and *T. vaginalis*, the only one capable of producing disease, in the vagina, urethra, and prostate. All three exist only in the trophozoite stage and resemble one another morphologically. *Trichomonas vaginalis* is the largest, however, and confusion in diagnosis is rare because of the anatomic specificity of their habits.

Trichomonas vaginalis is transmitted by sexual intercourse. Although the organism may survive on moist washcloths for a few hours, transmission of fomites has not been convincingly demonstrated and is probably rare. Newborn children of infected mothers have, on occasion, acquired the infection. The parasite is cosmopolitan in its distribution, and estimates hold that up to 25 percent of the sexually active population may be infected.

In the female, trichomoniasis usually presents as a persistent vaginitis. Initial manifestations include itching, burning, and profuse, creamy yellow, frothy leukorrhea. This acute stage may persist for a week or months, often fluctuating in intensity; it may worsen following menstruation. Eventually the discharge and other symptoms subside and may actually disappear completely, even though the patient still harbors trichomonads. Examination shows inflammation ranging from

mild hyperemia of the vaginal vault to extensive erosion, petechial hemorrhages, and perianal intertrigo.

The prostate and urethra are the usual sites of infection in the male. It may present as persistent or recurring nonspecific urethritis, or, more commonly, it may be completely asymptomatic. Acute purulent urethritis occurs rarely.

The diagnosis is made by examining vaginal, prostatic, or urethral secretions for the presence of *Trichomonas*. The organism may also be found in the sedimented urine. A wet mount will usually reveal numerous motile organisms. A Giemsa-stained preparation is confirmatory. *Trichomonas vaginalis* may be grown in culture, but this technique is not generally available. A variety of serologic tests, including a complement fixation, an indirect hemagglutination, and an immunofluorescent reaction, have been described, but are not generally available or completely reliable.

Trichomonas is sometimes responsible for confusing changes in the cytologic pattern of exfoliated vaginal cells. Moreover, ordinary Papanicolaou preparations are not well suited to the diagnosis, and when trichomoniasis is suspected, fresh material should be looked at immediately.

Oral metronidazole (Flagyl), given either in dosage of 250 mg three times daily for 7 days or in a single 2-g dose, is an extremely effective therapeutic agent. Concurrent treatment of sexual partners will minimize recurrent infections.

The recent evidence that metronidazole is carcinogenic in rodents and mutagenic in bacteria has placed the role of this agent in trichomonas infections in doubt. The drug should not be used in pregnancy until further information on its teratogenicity is available. Some authorities suggest that the drug should not be used at all unless patients cannot be rendered asymptomatic by other means. Because of the agent's antabuse-like action, alcohol consumption is contraindicated during therapy and for 24 h following its completion.

GIARDIASIS *Giardia lamblia* is a pear-shaped multiflagellar protozoan that parasitizes the human duodenum and jejunum where it multiplies by longitudinal fission. Under a microscope, its two nuclei and central parabasal body give the organism the appearance of a face with two large eyes. It is actively motile but may attach itself to the intestinal mucosa by means of a large ventral sucker. Encystation occurs in transit through the colon. The resulting ovoid cysts are the infective form of the parasite and are transmitted by the fecal-oral route. Waterborne outbreaks involving well water, chlorinated community systems, and remote mountain streams have been reported. The latter episodes have been concentrated in the Rocky Mountains and suggest that wild animals may serve as alternate hosts. To date, only beavers have been implicated in an outbreak in Camas, Washington.

The infection is found worldwide and is particularly common in areas with poor sanitation and among populations unable to maintain adequate personal hygiene. In the United States, *G. lamblia* is isolated in 3.8 percent of examined stools, making it the single most frequently identified intestinal parasite. Children are three times more likely to be involved than adults and probably have more prominent clinical manifestations. Gastrectomy, decreased gastric acidity, and chronic pancreatitis in adults may increase their susceptibility. Giardiasis also has been reported frequently in patients with immunoglobulin deficiencies and may be a major cause of intestinal abnormalities in these patients. It has been suggested that this parasite is able to persist in such patients because of a relative deficiency in intestinal IgA. *Giardia lamblia* infections also appear to be a significant cause of travelers' diarrhea, particularly among visitors to the Caribbean, Latin America, India, Russia, and the Far East. Unlike the typical syndrome seen in travelers, however, the diarrhea usually begins late in the course of travels and may persist for several weeks. A study in New York demonstrated that all nontraveled immunocompetent males with giardiasis were homosexual. The actual prevalence of the disease in this population is unknown, but the opportunities for direct fecal-oral transmission suggest that it may be high.

Most often the infection is asymptomatic, but in some patients nausea, flatulence, epigastric pain, abdominal cramps, distention, and watery diarrhea occur. After a few days the stools may become semisolid, bulky, and malodorous. Symptoms and accompanying weight loss may persist for several weeks. These symptoms are more common in children and are usually self-limited. Rarely, fulminating and extensive duodenal ulceration has been described. Radiographically, asymptomatic carriers may show irritability of the duodenal bulb. Chronic giardiasis may lead to malabsorption of carbohydrate, fat, and vitamin B_{12}. Lactase intolerance and disaccharidase deficiencies have been described. The pathogenesis of these abnormalities is poorly understood. Mechanical blockage of microvilli or damage to their fuzzy coat by the parasite, organism-induced deconjugation of bile salts, altered motility, and mucosal invasion have been suggested as possible mechanisms. Patients with giardiasis and severe malabsorption had jejunal colonization with enterobacteria, suggesting that bacteria may potentiate the mucosal lesion and be responsible for the development of malabsorption. Jejunal biopsy of patients infested with *Giardia* sometimes shows flattening of the microvilli and an inflammatory infiltrate. Both malabsorption and the jejunal lesions have been reversed with specific treatment.

The diagnosis is made by identifying the cyst in formed feces or the trophozoite in diarrheal stools, duodenal secretions, or jejunal biopsies. In the majority of acute cases, the parasite can be easily demonstrated by the careful examination of one to three stool specimens. Excretion of the organism is often intermittent in chronic cases, however, making parasitological confirmation more difficult. Many of these patients can be diagnosed by examining specimens collected at weekly intervals for a period of 4 to 5 weeks. Alternatively, the duodenal contents can be sampled with a nylon string (Enterotest) or gastric tube and examined by direct wet-mount preparation. Occasionally, jejunal biopsy is required to establish the diagnosis in patients with typical clinical manifestations.

Treatment is usually carried out with quinacrine hydrochloride or metronidazole. Tinadazole, a third highly effective agent, is presently not available in the United States. Quinacrine, 0.1 g given three times daily for 5 days, eliminates the organisms in 70 to 95 percent of cases. Although the drug is usually well tolerated, it may produce gastrointestinal disturbances, exacerbate psoriasis, and, rarely, produce toxic psychosis. Metronidazole appears to be better tolerated and equally effective. However, it is not currently licensed for giardiasis, and there is concern over its mutagenicity. Household contacts and sexual partners of infected patients should be examined; individuals harboring the parasite should be treated even if asymptomatic to prevent the spread to others. Pregnant women, however, should receive therapy only if severely symptomatic.

COCCIDIOSIS This is an infrequently recognized disease characterized by fever, diarrhea, abdominal pain, and weight loss which results from ingestion of the oocysts of coccidia belonging to the genus *Isospora*. Coccidia are widespread in the animal kingdom; each vertebrate host harbors a specific species. *Isospora hominis* and *I. belli* are the two that most commonly infect human beings. Parasitization is much more common in children and is worldwide in distribution, particularly in tropical areas.

Like the related plasmodia, there is both an asexual and sexual stage of multiplication in *I. belli* infections. However, both occur within a single host. Following the ingestion of an oocyst, *sporozoites* are released which invade the epithelial cells of the intestine to become trophozoites. These multiply asexually producing a large number of *merozoites,* which in turn invade other epithelial cells to continue the cycle. In some cells sexual gametocytes are produced. With the fertilization of the female gametocyte, an oocyst is formed which is then passed in the stool. Transmission is by the fecal-oral route. Volunteers develop symptoms about 1 week after the ingestion of viable oocysts. The illness usually has an acute onset with fever, headache, abdominal cramps, and diarrhea. Stools are often fatty and weight loss is common. Coccidiosis may be associated with a malabsorption syndrome and abnormalities of the mucosa in the small bowel. Symptoms, which presumably continue as long as the asexual cycle of multiplication continues, usually subside spontaneously within a few weeks. In some cases, however, they may persist for months or even years, eventually resulting in death.

Isospora hominis is probably identical to *Sarcocystis fusiformis.* Its oocysts are believed to be infectious only for pigs and cattle in which it produces tissue sarcocysts. Humans become infected by eating undercooked pork or beef containing the cysts. These liberate trophozoites which invade intestinal epithelial cells to undergo gametogony with the formation of new oocysts. The disease in humans is usually asymptomatic, but mild self-limited gastrointestinal manifestations have been described.

A peripheral eosinophilia occurs in approximately half of the infected patients. The diagnosis can be made by examination of stool for oocysts. These are often scanty, and concentration techniques such as zinc sulfate flotation or the formol-ether method must usually be employed. Incubation of the stool for 2 days at room temperature improves the recovery rate. Duodenal aspiration and jejunal biopsy are less cumbersome and more reliable.

Isospora belli infections have been successfully treated with combinations of pyrimethamine-sulfonamide and trimethoprim-sulfamethoxazole. *Isospora hominis* infections do not require specific therapy.

BALANTIDIASIS *Balantidium coli,* the largest protozoon of human beings, inhabits the large intestine. In addition to producing an asymptomatic carrier state, it elicits disease ranging from mild recurrent diarrhea to fulminant ulceration with perforation and death. In many respects the disease is similar to amebiasis in its range of manifestations, exclusive of spread to the liver.

The illness has been reproduced by feeding the organism to volunteers. The diagnosis is made by finding the trophozoite or cyst in the stool, but repeated examinations may be required because shedding of *Balantidium* is intermittent. The disease is more likely to occur in tropical areas, but at least 60 cases have been reported in the United States. Swine and rats are frequent carriers of *B. coli* and may play an important role in the spread of the disease to humans. Outbreaks have been noted in mental institutions where coprophagy implicated direct person-to-person transmission.

The tetracyclines in ordinary doses are highly effective in treatment, as is diiodohydroxyquin given in the dosage of 650 mg three times daily for 20 days.

BABESIOSIS Known since biblical times, babesiosis is a cosmopolitan infection of domestic and wild animals caused by protozoan agents of the genus *Babesia.* These organisms are transmitted by ticks, multiply in red blood cells, and produce an acute febrile illness characterized by hemolytic anemia and hemoglobinuria. The parasite was first described by Babes in 1888 and demonstrated to be tick-borne by Theobald Smith in 1893. This marked the first time a blood-feeding arthropod was implicated in the transmission of a pathogen to a vertebrate host, antedating Ross's description of malaria transmission by 5 years.

The first human case was described in Yugoslavia by Skrabalo in 1957. This and four other European cases were particularly severe with high fever, hemoglobinuria, jaundice, and renal failure. In both their clinical presentation and in the presence of small intraerythrocytic parasites they closely resembled falciparum malaria with which they were originally confused. All five occurred in splenectomized patients, and three ended fatally. The causative agent was presumably a bovine parasite *B. divergens.* Some 20 cases have now been documented in the United States. The first occurred in California and closely resembled the European infections; it was thought to have been caused by an equine parasite. The remaining cases have been seen on a number of offshore islands between New York and Massachusetts, including Nantucket, Shelter Island, and Martha's Vineyard. These patients all had intact spleens and experienced a prolonged illness characterized by the insidious onset of fever, chills, sweating, myalgia, and mild to moderate hemolytic anemia. The physical examination was usually negative except for occasional splenomegaly. Most patients were over 50 years of age and all recovered. The carrier state persisted for weeks to months in some. Serologic studies suggest that mild or asymptomatic cases occur with some frequency.

The cases were apparently all caused by *B. microti,* a parasite of rodents. This organism has been found in field moles and deer mice in New York State and California in addition to the offshore islands of New England. Hard ticks of the genus *Ixodes* serve as vectors. This arthropod does not have specific host preferences and may transmit the disease to humans in both the immature and mature stages. Since the engorged nymph measures only 2 mm in diameter, infested patients may be oblivious to its presence. Transovarial transmission of other *Babesia sp.* has been demonstrated.

The diagnosis depends on the demonstration of the intraerythrocytic parasite in Giemsa-stained peripheral blood smears. Like malaria parasites, these organisms measure 2 to 3 μm in diameter and demonstrate red-staining nuclear material with blue cytoplasm. In some cases band forms resembling *Plasmodium malariae* may be seen. In contrast to malaria parasites, however, neither gametocytes nor pigment can be demonstrated. Unique basket shapes and tetrads produced by budding are also helpful distinguishing characteristics. In heavy infections organisms can be seen outside the red blood cell. Serodiagnosis is helpful in epidemiologic studies. Active infections have been demonstrated in smear-negative, serology-positive infections by inducing infection in experimental animals.

There are presently no satisfactory drugs available for the treatment of this infection. Although chloroquine has been recommended, it appears to have little activity against this parasite. Antitrypanosomal agents may be more effective. In life-threatening disease in patients without spleens, pentamidine or Berenil, both available from the Center for Disease Control, should be considered. Therapy with these toxic drugs does not seem warranted in self-limited *B. microti* infections.

REFERENCES

Babesiosis

DAMMIN GJ: Babesiosis, in *Seminars in Infectious Diseases,* L Weinstein, J Fields (eds). New York, Stratton Intercontinental Medical Book Corp, 1978, pp 169–199

MILLER LH et al: Failure of chloroquine in human babesiosis (*Babesia microti*). Ann Intern Med 88:200, 1978

RUEBUSH TK II et al: Human babesiosis on Nantucket Island. N Engl J Med 297:825, 1977

WOLF RE et al: Intraerythrocytic parasitosis in humans with *Entopolypoides* species (family Babesiide). Ann Intern Med 88:769, 1978

Balantidiasis

WALZER PD et al: Balantidiasis outbreak in Truk Islands. Am J Trop Med Hyg 22:33, 1973

Coccidiosis

BRANDBORG LL et al: Human coccidiosis: A possible cause of malabsorption. N Engl J Med 283:1306, 1970

SMITSKAMP H, OEY-MULLER E: Geographical distribution and clinical significance of human coccidiosis. Trop Geogr Med 18:133, 1966

TRIER JS: Chronic intestinal coccidiosis in man: Intestinal morphology and response to treatment. Gastroenterology 66:923, 1974

Giardiasis

AMENT ME, RUBIN CE: Relation of giardiasis to abnormal intestinal structure and function in gastrointestinal immunodeficiency syndromes. Gastroenterology 62:216, 1972

BRADY PG, WOLFE JC: Waterborne giardiasis. Ann Intern Med 81:498, 1974

JOKIPII L, JOKIPII AMM: Giardiasis in travelers: A prospective study. J Infect Dis 130:295, 1974

KAMATH KR, MURUGASU R: A comparative study of four methods for detecting *Giardia lamblia* in children with diarrheal disease and malabsorption. Gastroenterology 66:16, 1974

KNIGHT R: Giardiasis, isosporiasis and balantidiosis. Clin Gastroenterol 7:31, 1978

WOLFE MS: Current concepts in parasitology—giardiasis. N Engl J Med 298:319, 1978

Trichomoniasis

JIROVEC O, PETRU M: *Trichomonas vaginalis* and trichomonas, in *Advances in Clinical Parasitology,* vol 6, B Dawes (ed). London, Academic, 1968, p 117

KEIGHLEY EF: Trichomonas in a closed community: Efficacy of metronidazole. Br Med J 1:207, 1971

206

APPROACH TO THE PATIENT WITH HELMINTHIC DISEASE

JAMES J. PLORDE

Helminths that parasitize humans can be divided into three major groups: roundworms (nematodes), tapeworms (cestodes), and flukes (trematodes). In contrast to the protozoa, helminths are large, multicellular organisms which have excretory, nervous, and reproductive systems. Of these, trematodes are the most highly differentiated, possessing fully developed male and female sexual organs capable of producing enormous numbers of offspring in the form of eggs, or larvae. With few exceptions these offspring must pass out of the *definitive host* harboring the sexually active adults before they can mature into forms capable of infecting their next host. The eggs of *Enterobius vermicularis* require only a few hours of embryonation on the perianal skin before they become infective. The eggs and larvae of most of the intestinal nematodes, however, require a prolonged period of incubation in soil under appropriate conditions of temperature and humidity, while those of the cestodes and trematodes must undergo developmental changes in one or more *intermediate hosts* before they are capable of completing their life cycle.

These differences in life cycle have a determinative influence on the epidemiology of helminthic parasites. *Enterobius vermicularis,* which can be spread directly from host to host because of its brief embryonation time in the external environment, has a cosmopolitan distribution. The remainder of the intestinal nematodes are spread via contamination of soil by eggs or larvae-containing human excrement. They are thus found in all areas of the world with poor sanitation where the appropriate conditions of temperature and humidity pertain. Finally, the distribution of trematodes such as the various species of *Schistosoma* are limited by the ecologic niches of their intermediate hosts.

Human disease can result when humans serve as either the definitive host, harboring the mature adults (e.g., *Taenia saginata*), or the intermediate host to the larval stages of the worm (e.g., echinococcosis). Occasionally a person may function as both the definitive (*T. solium*) and intermediate host (cysticercosis) for the same helminth. Since most adult helminths are incapable of multiplying within their definitive host, the manifestations of illness are related to the total number of worms acquired by the host. Most small worm load infections are, in fact, asymptomatic, and many need not even be treated. As helminths are usually long-lived, however, repeated infections can result from very high worm loads with disability typical of infections, particularly in endemic areas.

The pathogenesis of helminthic disease is variable. *Diphyllobothrium latum* competes with the host for nutrients, *Strongyloides stercoralis* and *Capillaria philippinensis* interfere with the absorption of food across the intestinal mucosa, and hookworm causes loss of iron, an essential mineral. Other parasites such as *Clonorchis sinensis* and *Schistosoma haematobium* compromise the function of important organs by obstruction and secondary bacterial infections. Long-term infections with both of the organisms can also be carcinogenic. Disease can result from simple mass effect as in the case of echinococcosis. Actual tissue invasion and destruction by larval forms occur in many infections. Immunologic mechanisms are undoubtedly responsible for tissue damage and clinical manifestations in many helminthic diseases.

Once the clinician thinks of the possibility of a helminthic infection, the diagnosis is usually straightforward. Although these infections are not common in the United States, the continuous arrival of travelers and immigrants and the importation of food from endemic areas of the world make it necessary to consider them in the differential diagnosis. Patients should be carefully questioned about their travels and food intake. Many helminths can survive within the host for a decade or more after he or she leaves an endemic area.

Although eosinophilia has long been recognized as a clue to the presence of helminthic infections, the failure to detect it does not preclude this diagnosis. The eosinophilia presumably reflects an immunologic response to the complex foreign proteins of the worm and is most marked during the early stages of tissue migration and invasion. Once migration ceases and the worm matures to adulthood, the eosinophilia may diminish or disappear.

The definitive diagnosis usually rests upon the recovery and morphological identification of the parasite in stool, urine, sputum, blood, or tissues. This process is facilitated by the large and relatively constant numbers of morphologically distinct progeny discharged by gravid worms. A simple wet mount of fresh or concentrated stool suffices for detection of most significant gastrointestinal infections. In strongyloidiasis where larvae are released into the duodenum and jejunum, aspirates of the upper intestine may reveal parasites when stool examination has been negative. Similarly, eggs of *Enterobius* (pinworm) and *Taenia* (tapeworm) can frequently be found on the perianal skin when absent from the feces. Biopsy of the rectal valves is the most reliable diagnostic procedure for intestinal schistosomiasis. Helminths dwelling within the tissues of the host are more difficult to identify. Some discharge their offspring into the bloodstream (filaria) or sputum (lung flukes) where they can be found with appropriate concentration procedures. In others, larvae can be recovered with skin (*Onchocerca volvulus*) or muscle (*Trichinella spiralis*) biopsies. In diseases such as toxocaricosis, eosinophilic meningitis, and cysticercosis parasite recovery is uncommon. Immunodiagnostic tests, with the notable exceptions of those for trichinosis and ecchinococcosis, have been of limited help to date. However, introduction of purified homologous antigens and the adaption of the enzyme-linked immunosorbent and immunoelectrophoresis assays to helminthic infections are likely to improve this situation in the near future.

TABLE 206-1
Fecal egg counts associated with illness

Worm	Approximate egg output per female worm per day	Minimum egg output usually associated with illness
Necator americanus	25,000	>2000/ml
Trichuris trichiura	7500	>3000/g
Schistosoma mansoni	60–300	>200/g

SOURCE: After DP Stevens, Clin Gastroenterol 7:236, 1978.

TABLE 206-2
Antihelminthics available from the Parasitic Disease Drug Service*

Infection	Therapeutic agent
Dracunculosis	Niridazole (Ambilhar)
Fascioliasis	Bithionol
Onchocerciasis	Suramin (Antrypol)
Paragonimiasis	Bithionol
Schistosomiasis	Niridazole (Ambilhar) Sodium antimony dimercapto-succinate (Astiban)
Tapeworms (T. saginata, T. solium, Hymenolepsis nana, H. diminuta, Diphyllobothrium latum, Dipylidium caninum)	Niclosamide (Yomesan)

* Center for Disease Control, Atlanta, Ga. 30333.

The rational management of helminthic infections requires an estimation of the worm load. Since most worms do not multiply within the body and because disability is usually related to the intensity of infection, treatment is directed primarily at reducing the worm burden of moderately to heavily infected patients. Total eradication is often unnecessary and may be unwise considering the toxicity of many antihelminthics. Light infections should be treated only when (1) small numbers of worms may be dangerous as in the case of strongyloidiasis, (2) the chance of reinfection is slight, and/or (3) the antihelminthic agent in question is without serious side effects. The intensity of many intestinal infections can be determined by enumerating the eggs found in stool (Table 206-1). Multiplying the total seen on direct smear by 750 provides a rough estimate of the number present per gram of feces. The Stoll dilution and the various modifications of the Kato thick-smear technique provide more precise results.

Many antihelminthics are not generally available in the United States or have not yet been approved for use in that country. Fortunately, many of these are available through the Parasitic Disease Drug Service of the Center for Disease Control in Atlanta, Georgia (Table 206-2).

NEMATODE INFECTIONS

Nematodes are elongated, cylindrical, unsegmented organisms that vary in size from the tiny Trichinella spiralis and Strongyloides stercoralis, which are a few millimeters in length, to Dracunculus medinensis, which may measure more than a meter. They have a simple tubular digestive tract running from the mouth in the anterior end to the anus located ventrally near the tail. The sexes are separate, and the male, which is usually smaller than the female, generally has a curved posterior end. The life span varies from 1 to 2 months in the case of T. spiralis and Enterobius vermicularis to 10 years or more for hookworms. During this time the gravid female produces enormous numbers of progeny either as fertile eggs or larvae. With the sole exception of Trichinella, these offspring must undergo a period of development outside the definitive host.

Among the intestinal nematodes, this period of develop-

ment occurs without the benefit of intermediate hosts. The eggs of E. vermicularis, or pinworm, are fully embryonated when laid and become infective within hours of being deposited on the perianal skin. After being ingested, these eggs mature into adult worms within the alimentary tract of humans. The life cycle of the whipworm, Trichuris trichiura, is similar except that the eggs must pass in the stool and incubate several weeks in soil before becoming infective for humans on ingestion. The external development of Ascaris lumbricoides eggs is identical. However, following ingestion, the embryonated eggs hatch, releasing larvae which penetrate the intestinal wall and are carried to the pulmonary capillaries via the bloodstream. Here they penetrate the alveoli, ascend the respiratory tract, and reach the glottis. Then, after completing their pulmonary migration, the larvae are swallowed, regain the intestinal lumen, and develop into mature adults.

The eggs of Strongyloides and of hookworm, in contrast to those of the above three, hatch shortly before (Strongyloides) or after (hookworm) being passed in the stool, producing rhabditiform soil larvae. Following several molts, these larvae are transformed into infective or filariform larvae, penetrate human skin, and after migrating through the lung in the manner described above for Ascaris, reach the intestine.

The life cycle of Strongyloides differs from that of hookworm in two important respects. First, rhabditiform larvae may, under certain conditions, develop into free-living adult male and female worms which reproduce in the soil. Second, rhabditiform larvae may develop into the infective filariform larvae while still within the human intestine. These may then reinfect the original host directly (autoinfection) without first going through a period of incubation in the external environment (Table 206-3).

The offspring of the tissue nematodes such as Dracunculus and the filarial worms undergo their development in a second

TABLE 206-3
Life cycle of intestinal nematodes

Species	Route of infection	Migration in body	Diagnostic form	Site of larval development	Infective form	Free-living stage
Enterobius vermicularis	Mouth	Intestinal	Egg	Perineum	Egg	No
Trichuris trichiura	Mouth	Intestinal	Egg	Soil	Egg	No
Ascaris lumbricoides	Mouth	Pulmonary	Egg	Soil	Egg	No
Necator americanus*	Skin	Pulmonary	Egg	Soil	Filariform larvae	No
Strongyloides stercoralis	Skin	Pulmonary	Rhabditiform larvae	Soil, intestine†	Filariform larvae	Yes

* Also Ancylostoma duodenale.
† Intestine only in cases of autoinfection.

invertebrate host before they can complete their maturation in the human.

The nematodes infecting humans are usually divided into intestinal and tissue parasites. Those which produce clinical manifestations by virtue of the presence of the adult worm within the human alimentary tract are considered intestinal nematodes; they include *Enterobius, Trichuris, Ascaris,* the hookworms, and *Strongyloides.* A number of closely related nematodes infecting animals such as *Toxacara canis* and *Ancylostoma braziliense* which may infect, but usually fail to reach maturity within humans will also be included in this group in the following discussion. Listed among the tissue nematodes are those which produce disease by the migration of the adult and/or larval forms through tissues such as *Trichinella,* the filarial worms, and *Dracunculus.*

REFERENCES

Drugs for parasitic infections. Med Letter 20(4):17, 1978

Health information for international travel 1978, U.S. Department of Health, Education, and Welfare Publication (CDC) 78–82. Morb Mort Week Rep, vol 27, suppl, September 1978

HUNTER GW III et al (eds): *Tropical Medicine,* 5th ed. Philadelphia, Saunders, 1976

207
TISSUE NEMATODES

JAMES J. PLORDE

ANGIOSTRONGYLIASIS CANTONENSIS

DEFINITION *Angiostrongylus cantonensis,* the rat lungworm, is the etiologic agent of the common form of *eosinophilic meningitis* found in Southeast Asia in the tropical areas of the Pacific.

ETIOLOGY The delicate filariform adults (20 mm in length) reside and lay their eggs in the pulmonary arterioles of rats and certain other rodents. After hatching, the larvae break into the alveoli, migrate up the respiratory tract, are swallowed, and pass in the feces. They develop into infective third-stage larvae within snails and slugs, their natural intermediate host. Viable third-stage organisms may also be found in land planarians, crabs, and freshwater prawns. These carriers appear to acquire the larvae by feeding on the tissues of infected mollusks. Humans, like rodents, become parasitized when they ingest raw intermediate or carrier hosts containing the infective stage. In rodents the larvae migrate to the brain where they grow into young adults. After a period of further maturation, the worms travel to the lungs and begin to deposit eggs. The nematode does not complete its life cycle in humans and dies after reaching the central nervous system.

EPIDEMIOLOGY Human infections with *A. cantonensis* have been found in Thailand, Vietnam, Cambodia, Indonesia, the Philippines, Taiwan, Hawaii, and several smaller Pacific islands from Okinawa in the north to New Caledonia and Tahiti in the south. In addition, rodent infections have been found in the islands of East Africa, Sri Lanka, India, and China. The rat lungworm may have been spread from Madagascar to Asia and to the Pacific by the recent dispersal of the giant African land snail, *Achatina fulica.*

PATHOLOGY AND PATHOGENESIS The nematode can produce extensive tissue damage by moving through the brain when alive and provokes a marked inflammatory reaction when dead. The pathological lesions are characterized by (1) marked lymphocyte and eosinophilic infiltration of the meninges, (2) hemorrhagic and nonhemorrhagic worm tracts through the brainstem and spinal cord, (3) granuloma formation around dead parasites and necrotic debris which sheathes the worm, and (4) engorgement of almost all blood vessels, particularly the veins. Necrosis of vessel walls, aneurysmal dilatation of arteries, and perivascular hemorrhages have been noted. Living worms have been removed from the eyes of patients without central nervous system involvement.

CLINICAL MANIFESTATIONS The eosinophilic meningitis usually presents as an acute severe headache. Fever is usually mild or absent, and only 15 percent of patients show signs of meningeal irritation. Patients frequently complain of visual impairment and, in a majority of these, visual defects or blurring of the optic disk can be demonstrated. Paresthesias of the trunk and lower extremities are a common complaint, and paralysis of the sixth and seventh nerves is seen in 3 to 7 percent of cases. Paralysis of the limbs, convulsions, and loss of consciousness are rare. The disease usually ends in complete spontaneous recovery. The cerebrospinal fluid contains several hundred cells per cubic millimeter and many eosinophils, and the cerebrospinal fluid protein is elevated. There may or may not be an eosinophilia in the peripheral blood.

The second clinically distinct form of eosinophilic meningitis has been reported from Thailand. This presents as a radiculomyeloencephalitis with limb pain and paresis and is thought to be caused by the nematode *Gnathostoma spinigerum.* The cerebrospinal fluid eosinophilic leukocytosis is less marked than in *angiostrongylus* infections. The fluid is often xanthochromic. Death may occur from cerebral hemorrhage or destruction of vital centers.

DIAGNOSIS The diagnosis is made on the basis of the clinical manifestations in an endemic area. Angiostrongyliasis must be differentiated from other ectopic worm infections of the central nervous system including strongyloidiasis, filariasis, paragonimiasis, hydatid disease, schistosomiasis japonicum, trichinosis, cysticercosis, toxocariasis, and gnathostomiasis.

TREATMENT AND PREVENTION There is no known effective treatment. Anthelmintic therapy should not be given since the simultaneous death of many worms might produce a severe inflammatory reaction. Steroids may be beneficial in severe cases. Prevention depends upon avoidance or proper cooking of such foods as snails, prawns, and crabs. Raw vegetables should be carefully inspected for the presence of planarians and mollusks before they are eaten. Freezing of crustaceans and mollusks at −15°C for 12 h will destroy infective larvae of *A. cantonensis.*

ANGIOSTRONGYLIASIS COSTARICENSIS

Angiostrongylus costaricensis is a nematode that dwells in the mesenteric arteries of Central American rats. Larvae pass in the stool and develop in slugs, the intermediate hosts. Rats, and incidentally humans, are infected when they ingest slugs or vegetables contaminated with third-stage larvae. The larvae mature in the lymphatics and move to the mesenteric radicals of the cecum. Here they may cause arterial thrombosis, ischemic necrosis, ulceration, and eosinophilic granuloma formation. Infected patients present with fever, eosinophilic leukocytosis, abdominal pain, and a right lower quadrant mass.

Occasionally perforation of the bowel and generalized peritonitis occur. The fever may persist for up to 2 months. Children are more frequently involved than adults. Neither larvae nor eggs are seen in the stool of the human host. No specific therapy is available.

GNATHOSTOMIASIS

DEFINITION Gnathostomiasis is a tissue infection of humans caused by *Gnathostoma spinigerum,* an intestinal nematode of carnivores. Clinically it is manifest as migratory subcutaneous swellings, creeping eruption, or a lethal eosinophilic meningitis.

ETIOLOGY AND EPIDEMIOLOGY The parasite, which is found throughout the Far East, lives encysted in the gastric mucosa of dogs, cats, and wild felines. The ova are passed to the external environment via the feces, hatch in water, and are ingested by *Cyclops,* the first intermediate hosts. These in turn are eaten by freshwater fish, frogs, snakes, and eels in whose flesh the infective third-stage larvae develop. Ducks and chickens fed on these second intermediate hosts may also come to harbor infective larvae. Human infections, which are most commonly seen in Thailand and Japan, occur when humans ingest infected uncooked fish (somfak, sashimi), duck, or chicken.

PATHOGENESIS AND MANIFESTATIONS The parasite cannot complete its cycle in humans, and the immature worms migrate through the abdominal and thoracic organs producing localized areas of inflammation and hemorrhage. Clinically, this is manifest as fever, eosinophilic leukocytosis, urticaria, and pain. Typically, the systemic manifestations subside within a month as the worms make their way to the subcutaneous tissues. Here, their continued migration results in the production of transient serpiginous pruritic swellings, subcutaneous tunnels, and abscesses. If the worm invades the epidermis, the resulting lesions closely resemble those of cutanea larva migrans. Rarely the eye may be involved with orbital cellulitis, iritis, or uveitis. Migration into the central nervous system results in a lethal eosinophilic meningitis (see "Angiostrongyliasis cantonensis" above). This presents as a radiculomyeloencephalitis with limb pain and paresis. The cerebrospinal fluid eosinophilic leukocytosis is present but less marked than in *Angiostrongylus* infections. The fluid is often xanthochromic. Death may occur from cerebral hemorrhage or destruction of vital centers.

DIAGNOSIS AND TREATMENT Painless, recurrent migratory subcutaneous swellings and eosinophilic leukocytosis occurring in an endemic area make the diagnosis likely. It must be differentiated from cutanea larva migrans, however, and from angiostrongyliasis cantonensis when the central nervous system is involved. Definitive diagnosis depends upon the removal and identification of the worm. Other than excision, there is no specific therapy. The disease can be prevented by the adequate cooking of fish, chicken, and duck in endemic areas.

DRACUNCULIASIS

DEFINITION Dracunculiasis is an infection of human connective and subcutaneous tissues by the guinea worm, *Dracuncula medinensis.* The gravid female produces symptoms when she ruptures the skin to discharge her eggs.

ETIOLOGY AND EPIDEMIOLOGY Dracunculiasis affects about 50 million people in West, Central, and Northeast Africa, the Middle East, Iran, Pakistan, India, northeastern South America, and the Caribbean Islands. Humans acquire the parasite when they ingest raw drinking water containing infected copepods (*Cyclops* spp.) which serve as the intermediate host. Shallow ponds, cisterns, and wells are the usual habitat of these crustaceans. In the stomach the copepod is digested and the larvae are released. The larva penetrates the intestinal wall and matures in the connective tissue of the retroperitoneal space. The adult male is small, seldom seen, and presumably dies after mating. In contrast, the female *Dracunculus* is one of the largest nematodes known—1 to 2 mm in diameter and 300 to 800 mm in length. The female reaches gravidity in approximately one year and then migrates to the subcutaneous tissue of the lower extremities. When the anterior end of the worm approaches the skin, a blister forms. This breaks down in a few days, forming a superficial ulcer. When the protruding portion of the worm comes in contact with water, the uterus prolapses through the body and discharges large numbers of motile rhabditiform larvae. Following ingestion by one of several species of *Cyclops,* the larvae undergo further development, becoming infective in 10 to 12 days. Mammals other than humans may be infected, but their importance as a disease reservoir is uncertain.

PATHOGENESIS AND MANIFESTATIONS The infection is asymptomatic until the gravid female appears in the subcutaneous tissues where it may, on occasion, be palpable. A few days before the formation of the blister, the patient frequently has fever, generalized urticaria, periorbital edema, and wheezing. Blister formation is accompanied by intense local pain and pruritus; like the systemic manifestations, this is thought to represent an allergic reaction to prematurely liberated larvae. The local lesion is usually found over the feet and ankles but may occur on the trunk or the upper extremities. Multiple infections are common. With the rupture of the blister and the release of embryos, the systemic manifestations abate, and the worm is slowly extruded over a period of 4 to 5 weeks. Secondary infection and cellulitis are common, particularly if the worm is ruptured during the process of extraction. In Nigeria, guinea worm ulcers are a common portal of entry for the spores of *Clostridium tetani.* The female worm often fails to reach the surface and discharge her larvae. In most of these cases, it dies without producing symptoms. The calcified appearance on roentgenograms is characteristic. Occasionally the worm may invade the deep tissues, causing serious symptoms, and sterile abscesses may follow the release of embryos. Invasion of joint spaces by the adult worm or larvae results in arthritis.

DIAGNOSIS The clinical picture is characteristic. Placing a small amount of water on the worm results in discharge of larvae which can then be examined microscopically. A fluorescent antibody test may permit the diagnosis to be made prior to emergence of the gravid female.

TREATMENT AND PREVENTION If the outline of the worm can be clearly seen or palpated, it may sometimes be completely removed with a single incision. The gradual extraction of the worm can be accomplished by winding a few centimeters onto a stick each day. Administration of niridazole (Ambilhar) results in prompt remission of symptoms. The dose is 25 mg per kilogram of body weight given in three divided doses for 7 days. Thiabendazole in dosage of 25 mg/kg twice daily for 2 days or metronidazole 250 mg three times a day for

7 days is also effective in the relief of symptoms. At present, there is serious question whether any of the above agents hasten worm extrusion or death. Some authorities suggest the rapid symptomatic improvement induced by these agents is secondary to their antiinflammatory rather than anthelmintic properties. Dracunculiasis can be prevented by the chemical treatment of drinking water.

REFERENCES

ALICATA JE: Present status of *Angiostrongylus cantonensis* infection in man and animals in the tropics. J Trop Med Hyg 72:53, 1969

MORERA P, CESPEDES R: Abdominal angiostrongyliasis. A new human parasitic infection. Acta Med Costarric 14:159, 1971 (Spanish)

MULLER R: Dracunculus and dracunculiasis, in *Advances in Parasitology,* vol 9, B Dawes (ed). London, Academic, 1971, p 73

NYE SW et al: Lesions of the brain in eosinophilic meningitis. Arch Pathol 89:9, 1970

PUNYAGUPTA S et al: Eosinophilic meningitis in Thailand. Am J Trop Med 24:921, 1975

208
TRICHINOSIS

JAMES J. PLORDE

DEFINITION Trichinosis is an intestinal and tissue infection of humans and other mammals caused by the nematode *Trichinella spiralis.* The disease is characterized by diarrhea during the development of the adults in the intestine and by myositis, fever, prostration, periorbital edema, eosinophilic leukocytosis, and, occasionally, evidence of myocarditis or encephalitis during the stage of larval migration in tissue.

ETIOLOGY Trichinosis in humans is contracted by ingestion of meat containing the encysted larvae of *T. spiralis.* The meat has almost always been pork, but for the past several years about 10 percent of cases reported in this country have been attributed to bear meat. This has been particularly frequent in the Northern and Western states including Alaska, California, and Idaho. There are no intermediate hosts, and both the adult and larval stages develop in the same animal. Infection has been produced or observed in the bear, wild boar, wolf, coyote, fox, muskrat, horse, cow, dog, cat, rabbit, guinea pig, mouse, and marine mammals, in addition to the rat and the pig. Humans are particularly susceptible; most fowl are resistant. Among pigs, infection is contracted following feeding of the uncooked scraps, less often by eating infected rats. The incidence of infection in pigs has been reduced by laws requiring that garbage be cooked thoroughly before being fed. Rats also feed on uncooked pork scraps and, in addition, maintain a high incidence of infection by their cannibalism.

Soon after ingestion, the larvae are liberated from their cysts by gastric digestion and migrate into the intestinal mucosa, where copulation takes place. The male dies, and within a week, the viviparous female is discharging larvae (100 by 6 μm), which enter vascular channels and are distributed throughout the body. Larviposition continues for about 4 to 16 weeks, each female producing approximately 1500 offspring. The larvae enter skeletal muscle, grow, and begin encysting within 3 weeks; calcification of cysts begins in 6 to 18 months. The life span of the encysted organism has been estimated at 5 to 10 years. The muscles of the diaphragm, tongue, and eye, and the deltoid, pectoral, gastrocnemius, and intercostal muscles are most often affected. Larvae carried to sites other than skeletal muscles do not encyst but disintegrate. The life cycle can be carried further only if a new host ingests the encysted larvae.

The description of a fatal case of trichinosis in an immunosuppressed patient emphasizes the importance of the immune response in limiting the intensity of infection. Apparently, it does so by acting directly on circulating larvae, inhibiting the reproduction of the female worms, and accelerating the expulsion of the adult parasites from the intestine. Eosinophils as well as B and T cell lymphocytes are involved in the response. The T cells appear to have a "helper" function in promoting the production of antibodies which, in collaboration with eosinophils, mediate the protective response.

EPIDEMIOLOGY Trichinosis is particularly common in Europe and North America, but with the exception of Australia and Asia it is found world-wide. In the United States its prevalence as measured by finding cysts in human diaphragms at autopsy has declined from 16.1 to 4.2 percent over the past 20 years. This decline has been accompanied by a similar reduction of trichinosis in pigs. The prevalence appears highest in the New England, Mid-Atlantic, and Pacific states. Currently, it is estimated that 1.5 million Americans carry live trichinae in their musculature and that somewhere between 150,000 and 300,000 acquire new infections annually. The overwhelming majority of these infections are asymptomatic, and many of those that become clinically manifest are never correctly diagnosed. In 1977 only 142 cases and no deaths were officially reported in the United States. Large outbreaks are usually caused by consumption of ready-to-eat pork sausage prepared in noninspected facilities or at home. The incidence appears highest among Americans of Italian, German, Polish, or Portuguese descent, presumably because of their inclination to make and eat pork sausage. Notable epidemics have followed the ingestion of trichinae-infected wild pig in Hawaii and California and walrus in Alaska. The latter is the first reported outbreak caused by this host in North America. Each year, a few cases are acquired from ground beef, attesting to the frequency with which this meat is adulterated with pork.

PATHOLOGY The most striking lesions are in the skeletal muscles, where there is a severe myositis with basophilic granular degeneration of the invaded muscle fiber. Adjacent fibers exhibit hyalin or hydropic degeneration, and the focus becomes infiltrated with neutrophilic and eosinophilic leukocytes, some lymphocytes, and mononuclear macrophages. Hyperemia, edema, and hemorrhages are constant features.

Larvae do not encyst in cardiac muscle, but an intense myocarditis has been observed in fatal cases.

In cases of central nervous system involvement, there may be granulomatous nodules, and vasculitis involving small arterioles and capillaries of the brain and meninges. Encystment of larvae in the brain is unusual.

CLINICAL MANIFESTATIONS The severity of the clinical manifestations is generally related to the number of larvae disseminated to the tissues of the host; patients with severe disease usually harbor 50 to 100 larvae per gram of muscle, while those with 10 or less are often asymptomatic. The first symptoms usually appear within 1 to 2 days after ingestion of the uncooked or undercooked meat containing encysted larvae. At that time diarrhea, abdominal pain, nausea, and sometimes prostration and fever develop. The next stage, that of muscular invasion, begins about the end of the first week and may last as long as 6 weeks. During this period, patients have fever, edema of the eyelids, conjunctivitis and subconjunctival hemorrhages, muscle pain and tenderness, and often severe weakness. There may be a maculopapular rash which lasts for several days and subungual "splinter hemorrhages." Central nervous system involvement may be evident as polyneuritis, poliomyelitis, myasthenia, meningitis, encephalitis, focal or diffuse pareses, delirium, psychosis, and coma. Despite the severity of central nervous system involvement in some patients, the cerebrospinal fluid remains normal.

Myocarditis is characterized by persistent tachycardia or development of congestive heart failure. There are marked electrocardiographic alterations, including ST-T wave changes and conduction abnormalities in 20 percent of patients.

LABORATORY FINDINGS The most constant finding, and one of significance early in the course of the disease, is the eosinophilic leukocytosis (over 500 eosinophilic leukocytes per cubic millimeter) which generally appears before the end of the second week. In cases of moderate severity, the proportion of eosinophilic leukocytes ranges between 15 and 50 percent. In severe cases, particularly terminally, the eosinophilic leukocytosis may disappear entirely.

The skin test to larval antigen becomes positive early in the third week of infection and may remain so for up to 20 years. The usual positive response is a wheal of 5 mm or more appearing within 30 min. Unfortunately, the commercially available skin test preparations are not reliable and their use is currently discouraged.

There are a variety of serologic tests for trichinosis, including the precipitin reaction, the complement fixation test, the indirect fluorescent antibody test, and the bentonite flocculation test, which is probably the best. A commercially available latex agglutination test appears to give comparable results. These serologic tests all become positive by about the third week of the disease and may remain positive for a few years. Since each may occasionally be falsely negative, two or more tests should be used. The serologic tests are most valuable if they are negative initially and then in turn positive or if there is a change in titer.

Muscle biopsy when carried out during the third or fourth week of infection remains the most useful test for demonstration of larvae or cysts. The deltoid or gastrocnemius muscles are the most useful sites for biopsy. A small portion of the excised muscle should be compressed between glass slides and examined under a low-power microscope for the presence of larvae. Calcified cysts or larvae represent an old infection. The remainder of the biopsy should be submitted for routine processing because myositis is a significant finding even in the absence of larvae or cysts.

In severe trichinosis there may be marked hypoalbuminemia, probably because of protein leakage from damaged capillaries. During the fourth, fifth, and sixth weeks of the disease, concomitant with a rise in antibody, diffuse hypergammaglobulinemia occurs. Elevated levels of circulating IgE have been reported. There may be moderate rises in serum glutamic oxaloacetic transaminase, serum aldolase, and creatine-phosphokinase, probably related to myositis; the sedimentation rate is characteristically slow.

DIFFERENTIAL DIAGNOSIS Trichinosis must be differentiated from diseases which are characterized by eosinophilia (such as Hodgkin's disease, eosinophilic leukemia, and periarteritis nodosa) and from entities which are characterized by myopathy, such as dermatomyositis. When the central nervous system is involved, the diagnosis may be very difficult.

TREATMENT Thiabendazole, in dosage of 25 mg/kg bid for 5 to 7 days, has resulted in apparent improvement in a number of patients, with relief of muscle pain and tenderness and with

lysis of fever. The results have not been uniform, however, and the use of this drug in trichinosis has been associated with nausea, vomiting, abdominal discomfort, dermatitis, and drug fever.

Patients with "allergic" manifestations of trichinosis, including angioedema and urticaria as well as myocardial or central nervous system involvement, should be treated with prednisone in dosage of 20 to 60 mg per day. Response to steroids usually has been prompt, particularly in central nervous system trichinosis. Not all focal lesions have resolved, however.

Other measures should be directed at relief of pain and maintenance of adequate caloric and fluid intake.

PROGNOSIS The prognosis in trichinosis has improved markedly, and even when the central nervous system is involved, the mortality rate has fallen to under 10 percent. The overall mortality rate is probably less than 2 percent.

PREVENTION The responsibility for control rests with the consumer. Adequate cooking of pork involves heating all portions of the meat to 60°C. Freezing procedures to kill the larvae require a temperature of $-15°C$ for 20 days or $-18°C$ for 24 h. Proper smoking and pickling will also destroy the larvae. Important in control is the cooking of garbage fed to hogs. There is no practical method of inspection which will detect trichinous pork.

REFERENCES

BARRETT-CONNER E et al: An epidemic of trichinosis after ingestion of wild pig in Hawaii. J Infect Dis 133:473, 1976

BROWN HW: *Basic Clinical Parasitology*, 4th ed. New York, Appleton-Century-Crofts, 1975

DALESSIO DJ, WOLFF HG: *Trichinella spiralis* infection of the central nervous system. Arch Neurol 4:407, 1961

DESPOMMIER D: Immunity to *Trichinella spiralis*. Am J Trop Med Hyg 26:68, 1977

GRAY DF et al: Trichinosis with neurologic and cardiac involvement. Ann Intern Med 57:230, 1962

METZLER MH et al: Second-degree atrioventricular block in acute trichinosis. Am J Dis Child 124:598, 1972

MOST H: Current concepts in parasitology. Trichinosis— preventable yet still with us. N Engl J Med 298:1178, 1978

ROSENBERG EB et al: Increased circulating IgE in trichinosis. Ann Intern Med 75:575, 1971

SULZER AJ, CHISHOLM ES: Comparison of the IFA and other tests for *Trichinella spiralis* antibodies. Pub Health Rep 81:729, 1966

WAND M, LYMAN D: Trichinosis from bear meat. JAMA 220:245, 1972

ZIMMERMAN WJ: Prevalence of *Trichinella spiralis* in commercial pork sausage. Pub Health Rep 85:717, 1970

——— et al: Trichinosis in the U.S. population 1966-70. Pub Health Rep 88:606, 1973

209
FILARIASIS

JAMES J. PLORDE

DEFINITION Filariasis is a group of disorders produced by infection with the threadlike nematodes of the superfamily Filarioidea. These worms invade the lymphatics and subcutaneous and deep tissues of humans producing reactions ranging from acute inflammation to chronic scarring. The viviparous female discharges microfilariae into the blood or subcutaneous tissues where they live for weeks or months until taken up by hematophagous arthropods. Within these vectors they are transformed into filariform larvae which then infect a new host when the arthropod takes another blood meal. The clinical pictures produced by various species in this group are more or less specific. The term *lymphatic filariasis* is commonly used to designate the disease produced by *Wuchereria bancrofti* and *Brugia malayi,* the organisms responsible for lymphatic blockade and elephantiasis. *Loa loa* causes loiasis, a disease characterized by transient subcutaneous (Calabar) swellings, and *Onchocerca volvulus* produces the blindness and pruritic skin rash typical of onchocerciasis. *Mansonella ozzardi, Dipetalonema perstans,* and *D. streptocerca* cause infections of questionable clinical significance to humans.

These parasites are identified by the location, periodicity, and morphological characteristics of their microfilariae. Those of *W. bancrofti, B. malayi, L. loa, D. perstans,* and *M. ozzardi* are all found in the blood, and, with the exception of the last, all display nocturnal or diurnal periodicity. *Onchocerca volvulus* and *D. streptocerca* are found in the subcutaneous tissues and are nonperiodic. Morphologically, the microfilariae are distinguished by the presence or absence of a sheath and by the distribution of their deeply staining column of nuclei. The sheath, which is an elongation of the original eggshell, can be seen extending beyond the head and tail only in the microfilariae of *W. bancrofti, B. malayi,* and *L. loa.* The nuclear column extends to the very tip of the microfilariae of *B. malayi, L. loa,* and the two species of *Dipetalonema.*

Skin and serologic tests are group-specific, lack sensitivity, and may be falsely negative in other nematode infections. In the absence of microfilariae and other helminthic infections, however, they may be helpful in establishing a diagnosis in clinically suspect cases.

LYMPHATIC FILARIASIS (BANCROFTIAN AND MALAYAN)

ETIOLOGY AND EPIDEMIOLOGY   The threadlike adult worms live coiled together in human lymphatics. The male *W. bancrofti* measures 35 mm and the female 80 to 100 mm. The *B. malayi* adults are about one-half as long. Gravid females release microfilariae in large numbers into the lymphatics. These embryos, which are sheathed, measure approximately 200 to 300 μm. They eventually reach the peripheral blood, where further development depends on their ingestion by a proper mosquito vector. Species of *Culex, Aëdes,* and *Anopheles* transmit Bancroftian filariasis; *Mansonia* and *Anopheles* serve as vectors in Malayan disease. After further development in the vector, larvae migrate to the mouthparts. If the mosquito feeds on a human host, they penetrate the puncture site and reach maturity in about a year. In the absence of reinfection, humans harbor microfilariae for 5 to 10 years, the reproductive life of the adult worms. In most *W. bancrofti* and *B. malayi* infections, the microfilariae are found in the blood in greatest numbers between 9 P.M. and 2 A.M. During the day, apparently in response to changes in oxygen tension, they accumulate in the pulmonary vessels and disappear from the peripheral blood. However, in Polynesia and New Caledonia there is an *Aëdes*-transmitted variety of *W. bancrofti* (*W. pacifica*) that displays a diurnal periodicity in which the peak occurs in the early evenings (subperiodic form). Periodicity is of epidemiologic signif-

icance because it determines which species of mosquito serves as the vector. Furthermore, several subperiodic forms of *B. malayi* have been found in animals, suggesting the possibility that this disease has an animal reservoir. The human is the only known vertebrate host for *W. bancrofti.*

More than 250 million persons throughout the world are presently infected, and both the prevalence and distribution of the disease seem to be increasing in many parts of Africa and Asia.

Wuchereria bancrofti infection is endemic between latitudes 41°N and 30°S involving primarily Africa, the Pacific Islands, and Southeastern Asia from Korea on the north to India in the West. The West Indies, Central America, and the eastern coastal plains of South America are also involved. Distribution is irregular, and there are many peculiar "skip areas" in this geographic pattern, presumably because the endemic disease can be maintained only where human infection and mosquitoes are prevalent. *Brugia malayi* infection is much more restricted in its distribution and occurs in India, Burma, Thailand, Vietnam, China, South Korea, Japan, Malaysia, Indonesia, Borneo, New Guinea, and the Philippines. The parasite has recently disappeared from Sri Lanka.

Two new types of microfilaria have been described. One, found in Brazil, has been named *W. lewisi,* while the taxonomic status of the strain from Portuguese Timor has not been settled. It is provisionally called Brugia (Timor).

There were approximately 15,000 *W. bancrofti* infections among American military personnel in World War II. A small endemic focus of *W. bancrofti* once existed near Charleston, South Carolina, but no new cases have been observed since 1930.

PATHOGENESIS   Pathological changes are caused primarily by the presence of the adult worm in the lymphatics and may be divided into inflammatory and obstructive. The inflammatory response, most marked around molting larvae and dead or dying adult worms, consists of infiltration with lymphocytes, plasma cells, and eosinophils. This is followed by a granulomatous reaction which may lead to lymphatic obstruction. There are hyperplasia of lymphatic endothelium, acute lymphangitis, and thrombosis. Repetition of this process over a period of years leads to permanent lymphatic obstruction. The tissues become edematous, thickened, and fibrotic. Secondary streptococcal infections are common and may contribute to lymphatic blockade. Dilated lymphatics may rupture into surrounding tissue. Elephantiasis is actually a relatively unusual complication of filarial infections. If repeated reinfections do not occur, the disease is self-limited.

MANIFESTATIONS   The clinical manifestations vary with the geographic area, species of parasite, and intensity of infection. Light infections may be completely asymptomatic. Symptoms may occur within 3 months of infection, but ordinarily the incubation period is 8 to 12 months. The clinical findings closely reflect the pathological changes, with inflammation early in the disease followed by obstruction later. Inflammatory filariasis consists of a series of brief febrile attacks occurring over a period of weeks. Fever is usually low grade but may reach 40.6°C (105°F) and be accompanied by chills and sweats. Other symptoms include headache, nausea and vomiting, photophobia, and muscle pain. If the involved lymphatics lie close to the surface, the local symptoms dominate the clinical picture. Lymphangitis is very common, involving the legs more frequently than the arms. It often begins as a tender spot in the region of the malleoli or femoral area and spreads centrifugally. The involved vessels are palpably tender and painful. The overlying skin is red and swollen. When abdominal lymphatics are involved, the picture may simulate that of an acute abdomen. In Bancroftian filariasis the vessels of the spermatic cord and testes may be involved, resulting in painful orchitis, epididymitis, or funiculitis. Lymphadenitis almost always accompanies and may sometimes precede lymphangitis. The inguinal, femoral, and epitrochlear nodes are involved. Abscesses which may form about involved lymphatics and lymph nodes may discharge to the surface, resulting in persistently draining sinus tracts. The acute manifestations last only a few days and then subside spontaneously, only to recur at irregular intervals over a period of weeks or months. Recovery finally ensues. With repeated infections, slowly progressive lymphatic obstruction may develop in areas where the inflammatory reactions have occurred previously. Edema, ascites, lymph scrotum, hydrocele, pleural effusion, or joint effusion may appear as a result of interference with lymphatic drainage. Lymphadenopathy persists. The lymphatic vessels become palpably enlarged as tense elastic masses beneath the skin, especially in the femoral, inguinal, and scrotal areas. They may rupture and form draining sinuses. Internal rupture of lymphatics may give rise to chylous ascites or chyluria. In a small percentage of cases elephantiasis develops. This complication is rare below the age of 20 even in natives of heavily infested areas. The chronic obstructive phase of the disease often is punctuated by acute inflammatory episodes.

Tropical eosinophilia   Attention has been focused on an aberrant type of filariasis which is characterized by the presence of hypereosinophilia, circulating filarial antibodies, microfilariae in tissue but *not in the blood*, and a chronic, clinical course that can be terminated with specific antifilarial treatment. These amicrofilaremic forms were originally thought to be caused by zoonotic parasites, but it is more likely that they represent an atypical host response to various filariae including *W. bancrofti* and *B. malayi*. The syndrome is most commonly seen in India, Indonesia, Sri Lanka, Pakistan, and Southeast Asia, all areas of intense transmission for these organisms. Animal models suggest that hypersensitivity or immunity to microfilariae results in their being removed from the peripheral circulation and trapped in various tissue sites. Here, they incite an eosinophilic inflammatory reaction which, in time, progresses to granuloma formation and fibrosis. Clinically there may be marked enlargement of the lymph nodes and spleen (Meyers-Kouwenaar syndrome) and/or chronic cough, nocturnal bronchospasm, and miliary pulmonary infiltrates (Weingarten syndrome). The former syndrome is most frequently seen in children, and the latter in young male adults. Only one-quarter of the patients with pulmonary manifestations demonstrate obstructive defects on pulmonary function testing. All show restrictive disease, and irreversible pulmonary hypertension has been described in a few. A number of diseases characterized by pulmonary infiltration and eosinophilia (PIE) must be considered in the differential diagnosis of this disease. They include other helminthic infections, Loeffler's syndrome, chronic eosinophilic pneumonia, allergic aspergillosis, vasculitis, idiopathic hypereosinophilia, and drug allergies.

DIAGNOSIS   A history of exposure, the long incubation period, the occurrence of typical inflammatory episodes, and the finding of regional lymphadenopathy, thickening of the spermatic cord, or swelling of an extremity should suggest the diagnosis. There is usually eosinophilia during acute episodes. Lymphangiography may reveal dilated afferent and small efferent lymphatics. The definitive diagnosis depends on demonstration of the parasite. Although adult worms can be demonstrated in biopsied lymph nodes, biopsy is not recommended because it may interfere further with lymphatic drainage. Microfilariae are found in the blood during intermediate stages but not early or late in the disease. As they are motile, they can often be seen in a wet mount or counting chamber. Definite identification, however, requires staining with Giemsa. As in malaria, they are demonstrated best in thick smears. Either the Knott concentration or membrane filtration technique should be employed if the parasite is not found in thick smears. Because the appearance of microfilariae in peripheral blood is periodic, it is essential to obtain blood at appropriate times. When this proves difficult, the oral administration of 100 mg diethylcarbamazine usually produces positive blood specimens within 30 to 60 min. Microfilariae may also be found in lymphatic fluid, hydrocele fluid, ascites, and pleural fluid. Skin tests as well as complement fixation, indirect hemagglutination, bentonite flocculation, and soluble antigen fluorescent antibody tests are available and, although not completely reliable, are helpful when microfilariae cannot be demonstrated. An indirect immunofluorescent test utilizing adult *B. malayi* as the source of antigen appears to be both more sensitive and specific than previously developed procedures.

The diagnosis of *tropical eosinophilia* is confirmed by (1) a history of prolonged residence in an endemic area, (2) lack of microfilariae in the peripheral blood despite examination of both day and night specimens by concentration techniques, (3) peripheral eosinophilia in excess of 300 cells per milliliter, (4) high titers of filarial antibodies, (5) IgE levels of at least 1000 units per milliliter, and (6) response to diethylcarbamazine within 7 to 10 days of initiating therapy. Recovery of microfilariae from the tissues is uncommon, and biopsy is not warranted.

TREATMENT   Diethylcarbamazine (Hetrazan) rapidly eliminates microfilariae from the blood. It probably also kills or injures adult worms, impairing their ability to reproduce, and clears microfilariae permanently from the bloodstream of many patients. The drug is given in dosage of 2 mg/kg three times a day for 3 or 4 weeks. Treatment with this agent is often followed by allergic reactions to the dying parasite. These reactions may be quite severe, especially in Malayan filariasis. They can be controlled with aspirin, antihistamines, or steroid hormones. In heavy infections, it may be desirable to begin treatment with antihistamines before administration of Hetrazan.

Antimony compounds have no place in the treatment of filariasis.

Reassurance of the patient is very important in this disease. Vaccines and antiserums are valueless. Pressure bandages and surgery sometimes benefit elephantiasis. The prognosis for life is excellent, particularly if infected individuals leave endemic areas or otherwise avoid reinfections. Disease control is accomplished by combining mass treatment with mosquito control measures.

ONCHOCERCIASIS ("RIVER BLINDNESS")

DEFINITION   Onchocerciasis is a cutaneous filariasis caused by *Onchocerca volvulus*. It is characterized by subcutaneous nodules, a pruritic skin rash, and ocular lesions.

ETIOLOGY AND EPIDEMIOLOGY   The disease is found in focal areas within Mexico, Guatemala, Colombia, Venezuela,

Surinam, Brazil, and Yemen, and throughout tropical Africa. It is estimated that at least 40 million individuals are infected and that about 5 percent of these are blind as a result of the disease.

The infection is transmitted by black flies of the genus *Simulium,* which breed along fast-moving streams. An inoculated larva matures into a single male or female in approximately one year. Since larvae do not multiply within the human host, heavy parasite loads are the result of repeated infections. The adult worms are found coiled together in fibrous subcutaneous nodules. The gravid females, which may live as long as 15 years, release unsheathed microfilariae that are actively motile and migrate in the skin, subcutaneous tissue, and eye for up to 30 months or until they are ingested by a feeding *Simulium.*

PATHOGENESIS AND CLINICAL MANIFESTATIONS   The subcutaneous nodules which enclose the adult worms are usually 2 to 3 cm in diameter when fully developed. They are firm, nontender, and freely movable, although occasionally they may be adherent to underlying tissue. Their location on the body is related to the biting habits of the vector. In Central America, where the fly bites on the upper part of the body, the nodules are frequently over the head; in Africa they are primarily on the trunk and thighs. They usually number less than 10, but more than 100 have been reported in a single patient.

The important pathological changes occur as a result of a hypersensitivity reaction to the dead or dying microfilariae. Pruritus is often severe and constant. The skin lesion may appear as an erysipelas-like reaction over the face or a papular rash over one extremity. In chronic cases thickening, lichenification, and depigmentation may be present. In Africa gross skin lesions are common and may be associated with large folds of skin called *hanging groins.* Some authors believe elephantiasis may occur. Children living in endemic areas may not demonstrate these changes for decades even though microfilariae are present. The most serious complications of onchocerciasis are eye lesions which are usually found in patients repeatedly infected on the upper part of the body. A punctate keratitis, iridocyclitis, or less commonly a chorioretinitis may eventually lead to blindness.

DIAGNOSIS   The diagnosis is made by demonstrating microfilariae in a skin snip taken from an involved area. A thin sliver of superficial skin is removed with a razor or punch. Care must be taken to prevent bleeding and possible contamination with blood microfilariae. The skin is weighed and then is placed in saline, teased with a pair of sharp dissecting needles, and observed for emerging microfilariae over the next hour. The results should be expressed in microfilariae per milligram of tissue. Multiple skin snips may be necessary. In patients with eye lesions, microfilariae can sometimes be seen in the anterior chamber with a slit lamp. If organisms cannot be detected by the above methods, the patient may be given 50 mg diethylcarbamazine orally. The occurrence of a pruritic rash within 24 h strongly suggests the presence of cutaneous microfilariae (Mazzotti's test). One of the filarial serologic tests may also be helpful.

TREATMENT AND PREVENTION   Diethylcarbamazine is effective in destroying microfilariae but has little effect on the adult worm. The drug must be used with great care as rapid destruction of the parasites may cause a severe allergic reaction. If the eye is involved, this can result in further ocular damage. The initial adult dose is 50 mg orally. It is increased to 50 mg three times daily on the second day, 100 mg three times daily on the third day, and finally 200 mg three times a day for an additional 7 days. Antihistamines, or in rare cases steroids, can be used to control allergic reactions. In ocular reactions, the pupil should be dilated and topical steroids applied.

The adult worms may be eliminated by excision of nodules on the head and neck, a procedure which is useful in preventing ocular complications, or by chemotherapy with suramin. Details of the administration and toxicity of this drug are given in Chap. 202. The dosage is 0.1 g given intravenously to detect drug idiosyncrasy, followed by 1.0 g intravenously once weekly for five to six doses.

Chemoprophylaxis is not practical, and personal protection depends upon the use of protective clothing. Insecticides, mass therapy, and nodulectomies have been used but have not been very satisfactory.

LOIASIS

This form of filariasis is produced by *Loa loa* and is prevalent in West and Central Africa. The infection is transmitted by deer flies of the genus *Chrysops.* The adult worms, which like the other filariae may live for 10 to 15 years, migrate continuously through the subcutaneous tissue. The resulting localized areas of allergic inflammation, *Calabar swellings,* are the hallmark of the disease. Occasionally the adult worms may be seen crossing the eye subconjunctivally. This usually results in intense lacrimation, pain, and anxiety. Infestation may, however, be completely asymptomatic. An association between loiasis and endomyocardial fibrosis has been reported. The diagnosis can be made by finding the adult worm or by demonstrating the distinctive sheathed microfilariae in contents of the Calabar swellings or in the bloodstream during the daytime. Microfilariae are often not found. In these cases, there are usually marked eosinophilia and a positive filarial complement fixation test. Diethylcarbamazine, administered for 2 to 3 weeks in the manner described for onchocerciasis, will kill both adult worms and microfilariae. This drug must be used with great care as it may induce an encephalopathy in this disease. It is taken in a dose of 200 mg twice daily for 3 days each month and is also effective as a chemoprophylactic agent.

DIPETALONEMIASIS

Dipetalonema perstans (Acanthocheilonema perstans) is a filarial parasite of humans and other primates inhabiting the tropical areas of Africa and Latin America. The adult worm lives encysted in the subserosal tissues of the pericardium, pleura, and peritoneum, particularly the mesentery. The unsheathed microfilariae, which can be found in the peripheral blood throughout the day, have four to six nuclei in their tail. They are transmitted from host to host by blood-sucking gnats of the genus *Culicoides.* Most infections are asymptomatic, and their principal significance lies in the fact that they may be confused with other, more serious, forms of filariasis. Nevertheless, some patients complain of fever, pruritus, Calabar swellings, erysipelas-like rashes, and abdominal pain. Peripheral eosinophilia is common, but filarial complement fixation tests are generally negative. Diagnosis is made by finding the characteristic microfilariae in the peripheral blood. Treatment with diethylcarbamazine is of doubtful benefit.

Dipetalonema streptocera is found in Equatorial Africa where it inhabits the dermis and subcutaneous tissues of chimpanzees and humans. Like *D. perstans,* it is transmitted by *Culicoides.* The microfilariae inhabit the dermal collagen where they elicit a lymphocytic and eosinophilic inflammatory response, fibrosis, lymphatic dilatation, pruritus, hypopigmented macules, and a papular rash. The diagnosis is made by recovering the nonperiodic microfilariae from skin snips as described for Onchocerciasis above. They are unsheathed and possess a sharply crooked tail with nuclei. Diethylcarbamazine, as described for Bancroftian filariasis above, is effective.

MANSONELLIASIS OZZARDI

Mansonella ozzardi are found as adult worms in the mesentery and visceral fat of people living in the tropical areas of Latin America. This species is thought to be transmitted by flies of the genus *Simulium* and gnats of the genus *Culicoides*. The nonperiodic microfilariae are released into the peripheral blood where they can be identified by their lack of a sheath or caudal nuclei. This common infection is thought to be asymptomatic, but reports of patients presenting with fever, lymphadenopathy, and hydroceles have been published. Diethylcarbamazine is ineffective.

DIROFILARIASIS

Dirofilaria immitis (canine heartworm) is a large, cosmopolitan filaria of dogs which lives in their right ventricle and pulmonary arteries and releases its microfilariae into the peripheral blood. It is transmitted by several types of mosquitoes. Human infections are occasionally reported, particularly from the southern United States. The worm does not mature in humans, and hence microfilaremia is not present. Although cardiac infections have been noted at autopsy, most human infections present as well-defined pulmonary nodules. The patients may complain of cough and chest pain or, less commonly, of hemoptysis, fever, chills, and myalgia. The diagnosis is usually made by the microscopic examination of excised pulmonary nodules.

Other *Dirofilariae* may rarely invade humans producing subcutaneous eosinophilic granulomas of the eyelid, trunk, or extremities. The nodules, which measure 1 to 2 cm in diameter, may be painful or completely asymptomatic. In the southern United States, the filaria most frequently involved is *D. tenuis*, a parasite of raccoons. The nodules are removed by surgical excision.

REFERENCES

AKISADA M, TANI S: Lymphangioadenopathy of filariasis. Trans R Soc Trop Med Hyg 64:885, 1970

ANDERSON J, FUGLSANG H: Ocular onchocerciasis. Trop Dis Bull 74:257, 1972

CHRISTIE RW: *Dirofilaria tenuis* in Vermont. N Engl J Med 297:706, 1977

CONNOR DH et al: Onchocerciasis, onchocercal dermatitis, lymphadenitis and elephantiasis in the Ubangi territory. Hum Pathol 1:553, 1970

DAYAL Y, NEAFIE RC: Human pulmonary dirofilariasis. A case report and review of the literature. Am Rev Resp Dis 112:437, 1975

EDESON JFB: Filariasis. Br Med Bull 28:60, 1972

HAWKING F: The 24-hour periodicity of microfilariae: Biological mechanisms responsible for its production and control. Proc R Soc Lond B 169:59, 1967

IVE FA et al: Endomyocardial fibrosis and filariasis. Q J Med 36:495, 1967

MEYERS WM et al: Human streptocerciasis. A clinico-pathological study of 40 Africans (Zaireans) including identification of the adult filaria. Am J Trop Med Hyg 21:528, 1972

NEVA FA, OTTESEN EA: Current concepts in parasitology. Tropical (filarial) eosinophilia. N Engl J Med 298:1129, 1978

ONKEL TC: Infections with *Dipetalonema perstans* and *Mansonella ozzardi* in the aboriginal Indians of Guyana. Am J Trop Med Hyg 16:628, 1967

PAK SC: The course of lung function in treated tropical pulmonary eosinophilia. Thorax 29:710, 1974

WHO EXPERT COMMITTEE ON FILARIASIS: Third Report. Tech Rept Ser 542, 1974

210
INTESTINAL NEMATODES

JAMES J. PLORDE

ENTEROBIASIS

DEFINITION Enterobiasis (pinworm, seatworm, or threadworm infection, oxyuriasis) is an intestinal infection of humans caused by *Enterobius vermicularis* and characterized by perianal pruritus. Eggs of this parasite have been found in a 100,000-year-old coprolith, making it the oldest demonstrated infection of humans. It has been estimated that the worm infects 200 million people, 30 to 40 million of them in the United States and Canada.

ETIOLOGY The female averages 10 mm in length, the male 3 mm. They live with their heads attached to the mucosa of the cecum, appendix, and adjacent parts of the bowel. The gravid female migrates through the anal canal at night, deposits her 10,000 eggs on the perianal skin, and dies. In female patients the worm may enter the vagina and occasionally gain access to the peritoneal cavity through the fallopian tubes. Each egg contains an embryo which, within a few hours, develops into an infective larva. After the egg has been ingested, the larva is released in the small intestine and migrates down the bowel lumen to the cecum. In less than 1 month from the time of ingestion, newly developed gravid females are again discharging eggs. They are planoconvex and measure approximately 20 by 50 μm. The shell is clear and doubly contoured.

EPIDEMIOLOGY Humans are usually infected by the direct transfer of eggs from the anus to the mouth by way of contaminated fingers. Retroinfection, which is seen primarily in adults, may occasionally take place when eggs hatch in the perianal area and the larvae migrate back into the bowel to mature. The eggs, which are relatively resistant to desiccation, also contaminate nightclothes and bed linen, where they remain viable and infective for 2 to 3 weeks. Airborne transmission is possible, and spread within family and children's groups occurs readily. Enterobiasis is found in all climates and is probably the most common helminthic infection of humans. Its low incidence in some tropical areas, however, is not fully explained.

CLINICAL MANIFESTATIONS The most common symptom is pruritus ani, which is most troublesome at night, being related to the migration of the gravid female worms. Irritability, insomnia, enuresis, and other minor complaints are probably secondary to the pruritus. Scratching may lead to perianal eczema or pyogenic infection. Vaginal discharge has been reported, and rarely a chronic granulomatous salpingitis or endometritis results from the presence of ectopic adults. An association between enterobiasis and cystitis in young females has been reported. This, it is suggested, results from the transport of enteric bacteria into the bladder by the migrating worm. Other rare ectopic locations include the lung, liver, and peritoneum. Probably the worms can penetrate the bowel wall only if its continuity has been compromised by some other disease.

LABORATORY FINDINGS Examination for ova of material obtained from the perianal skin by means of a Scotch brand cellophane tape swab is the preferable method for the detection of enterobiasis. The tape is folded sticky-side out over the end of a tongue blade, pressed firmly against the perianal area, and then spread on a glass slide and examined under the lower power of a microscope. The swab should be taken at home by the patient on three to five consecutive mornings prior to bathing and brought to the laboratory for examination. Searching for ova in the feces is rarely helpful, but scrapings from under the nails may reveal ova. The diagnosis is sometimes made by finding adult worms in the perianal area or in the feces following a laxative or an enema. Eosinophilic leukocytosis may occur but is not a typical finding.

TREATMENT All infected individuals in a family or communal group should be treated simultaneously. The frequently recommended sanitary measures aside from daily bathing and hand washing before meals and after stools are of dubious benefit. It is relatively easy to eradicate the worms, but reinfection is frequent. Retreatment does not appear necessary unless symptoms recur.

Two highly satisfactory drugs are available. Pyrantel pamoate (Banminth) given in a single oral dose of 11 mg/kg (maximum 1.0 g) is probably the drug of choice. Alternatively, a single 100-mg oral dose of mebendazole (Vermox) can be used. This drug is not recommended for infants or pregnant women. Pyrvinium pamoate (Povan) and piperazine citrate are equally effective but less convenient. The former is given orally as a single dose of 5 mg/kg in tablet or liquid form. This compound turns the stool red and may stain bedclothes or undergarments. Piperazine citrate is given in dosage of 65 mg/kg (maximum 2.5 g) once daily for 8 days. When renal insufficiency is present, the dose should be reduced to avoid neurotoxicity. In heavily contaminated environments, treatment with the above drugs may be repeated after an interval of 2 weeks to eliminate any new infections.

PREVENTION Methods of preventing autoinfection and dissemination within a group involving children are extremely difficult to enforce. Personal environmental hygiene should be stressed, and anthelmintic and symptomatic treatment of pruritus ani should be instituted. To control infection within a group, simultaneous treatment of all cases is mandatory.

TRICHURIASIS

DEFINITION Trichuriasis (whipworm infection, trichocephaliasis) is an intestinal infection of humans caused by *Trichuris trichiura* and is characterized by invasion of the colonic mucosa by the adult trichuris. Five hundred million persons are thought to be infected with this parasite including 2 million in the United States. It may be the most commonly encountered helminthic infection in Americans returning from tropical areas.

ETIOLOGY The adult whipworms are found in the large intestine with their anterior ends deeply embedded in the mu-

cosa. They are 30 to 50 mm in length and possess a threadlike anterior two-thirds with a stouter posterior third, giving them a whiplike structure. The female produces about 5000 eggs each day. They are characteristically barrel-shaped (20 to 50 μm), brown, thick-walled, and translucent with knoblike ends. The eggs, like those of *Ascaris,* must incubate at least 3 weeks in soil before they become infective. After ingestion, the eggs hatch in the small intestine and the larvae become embedded in the intestinal villi. After several days they migrate to the large intestine where they mature in about 3 months. The adult worms may live for 4 to 8 years. Occasionally, *T. vulpis,* the whipworm of dogs, may infect humans. The eggs are larger (35 by 75 μm) but otherwise identical to those of the human parasite.

EPIDEMIOLOGY Whipworm is a cosmopolitan parasite but is most commonly found in the tropics where the level of sanitation is low and environmental conditions necessary for the incubation of the eggs are optimal. In the United States, it is found throughout the rural areas of the Southeast. Its distribution is similar to that of *Ascaris* and hookworm, but the eggs are less resistant than those of *Ascaris* to sunlight and drying. Because of their general lack of sanitary habits, children and the mentally retarded have the highest incidence of infection. For example, 13 percent of patients confined to hospitals for the mentally subnormal were found to harbor *Trichuris.*

PATHOGENESIS AND CLINICAL MANIFESTATIONS Symptomatic infection generally requires the presence of large numbers of adult whipworms and may be correlated in part with the degree of mucosal involvement. Heavy infections usually occur only in children and may be accompanied by nausea, abdominal pain, diarrhea, and dysentery. It has been estimated that infected patients lose 0.005 ml blood per worm per day. Infections with more than 800 worms often results in anemia. In heavier infections, the distribution of worms throughout the colon and rectum may result in rectal prolapse while straining at stool. Some investigators also feel that *Trichuris* infections predispose to amebic dysentery and bacterial gastroenteritis.

LABORATORY FINDINGS In symptomatic infection, large numbers of eggs are present in the feces, and there may be eosinophilic leukocytosis and anemia. In light infections, concentration techniques may be necessary to recover the eggs. Quantitation of egg output is helpful since only counts above 3000 eggs per gram of feces are likely to be associated with symptoms. Stools should be cultured for bacterial pathogens and examined for the presence of *E. histolytica.*

TREATMENT Treatment is unsatisfactory. Mebendazole in the oral dose of 100 mg twice daily for 3 days is the drug of choice. Its cure rate is 60 to 70 percent, and it achieves a 90 percent reduction in egg burden. The dose may have to be repeated in patients with heavy infections. It is not recommended for children under the age of 2 or pregnant women.

PROGNOSIS Whipworm infection, unless characterized by severe diarrhea, blood loss, and systemic reaction, usually responds well to treatment. Serious infections may require supportive treatment as well as chemotherapy.

PREVENTION Measures recommended for ascariasis apply also to trichuriasis.

ASCARIASIS

DEFINITION Ascariasis is an infection of humans caused by *Ascaris lumbricoides* and characterized by an early pulmonary phase related to larval migration and a later, prolonged intestinal phase. It is estimated that 25 percent of the world's population, including 4 million Americans, are infected with this nematode.

ETIOLOGY The adult ascarids are large (15 to 40 cm in length), cylindric worms with blunt ends which maintain themselves in the lumen of the jejunum by virtue of their muscular activity. Despite a life span of only 6 to 18 months, the female releases millions of eggs, both fertile and infertile, into the fecal stream; the daily output is estimated to be 200,000 per worm. Fertilized eggs are elliptic (30 to 40 μm by 50 to 60 μm) with an irregular, dense outer shell and a regular, translucent inner shell. They require a period of soil incubation before they become infective. Under optimum conditions of warmth and moisture this occurs in 2 to 3 weeks. The eggs may then remain viable for up to 6 years in temperate climates. When an infective egg is ingested, the larva is liberated in the small intestine. It migrates through the wall and is carried by the bloodstream or lymphatics to the lung. After about 10 days in the pulmonary capillaries and alveoli, the larvae pass in turn up the bronchioles, bronchi, trachea, and epiglottis, are swallowed, and return to the jejunum. There they develop into mature adult worms within 2 to 3 months of ingestion. *Ascaris suum,* a roundworm of pigs, may occasionally complete a similar life cycle in humans.

EPIDEMIOLOGY Infection follows the ingestion of the embryonated eggs contained in contaminated food, or, more commonly, the introduction of the eggs into the mouth by the hands after contact with contaminated soil. Geophagia may produce massive infections. In endemic areas, the infection is maintained primarily by small children who defecate indiscriminately in the area of the home. In dry, windy climates, eggs may become airborne, get into the mouth, and be swallowed. Since the eggs are relatively resistant to desiccation and wide variations in temperature, the disease is worldwide. In the developing areas of the world where the lack of sanitary facilities exposes populations to the greatest risk, the prevalence of infection may be as high as 80 to 90 percent; children are almost universally infected in these areas. In temperate areas, the infection occurs in family clusters.

PATHOGENESIS AND CLINICAL MANIFESTATIONS Because of the extensive migration of which both the larvae and adults are capable, the manifestations may be diverse. Bronchopneumonia characterized by fever, cough, dyspnea, wheeze, eosinophilic leukocytosis, and migratory pulmonary infiltrates may occur during the passage of the larvae through the lung. This is most commonly seen in communities where *Ascaris* transmission is seasonal. The severity of symptoms is apparently related to both intensity of infection and the degree of sensitization resulting from previous exposures. Significant arterial oxygen desaturation and, rarely, death may occur. Adult worms may produce no symptoms if the infection is light and may be detected accidentally when the adult worm is vomited or passed in the stool. Heavier infections may cause abdominal pain, and occasionally a bolus of worms may result in volvulus, intussusception, or intestinal obstruction in the iliocecal area. Children are most likely to have these complications because of their anatomically smaller intestine and larger worm loads. Up to 2000 worms have been found in children, although the usual load is less than 50. In the United States where worm loads are usually modest, the incidence of obstruction is 2 per 1000 infected children per year. It often follows a febrile illness or drug therapy which stimulates the worms to increase motility. Rarely, an adult worm will migrate into the appendix, bile ducts, or pancreatic ducts, causing obstruction and inflammation of these organs. Biliary tract obstruction may be associated with bacterial cholangitis and liver abscess. Worms may also penetrate the intestinal wall, particularly at a site of surgical anastomosis, and patients should be dewormed prior to elective surgery. Migration of the worms into the oral pharynx and mouth may lead to acute respiratory distress.

Ascariasis has been associated with mild to moderate malabsorption of fat, protein, carbohydrate, and vitamins. It seems likely that large worm loads may interfere with the growth of marginally nourished children.

LABORATORY FINDINGS The diagnosis is usually made by finding the ova in the feces. The fertilized eggs are usually numerous, characteristic, and not easily confused with those of other helminths. The occasional unisexual infection may pose diagnostic problems. The male produces no eggs, and the unfertilized ova produced by a single female may be atypical and difficult to recognize. Occasionally the worms may be seen after a barium meal, either as negative images or after ingesting barium themselves. In biliary ascariasis an intravenous cholangiogram will often demonstrate dilatation of the common duct and/or the negative image of the parasite. Ascaris pneumonia may be diagnosed by finding larvae and eosinophils in the sputum or gastric aspirate. Eggs will usually not be found until after the larvae have matured in the intestine. Eosinophilic leukocytosis is usually noted during larval migration, but diminishes and often disappears during the chronic intestinal phase of infection.

TREATMENT Only symptomatic treatment can be used during the period of pulmonary involvement by the migrating larvae. For removal of the adult worms from the intestines, either pyrantel pamoate or mebendazole should be used. Pyrantel is given as a single oral dose of 11 mg/kg (maximum 1.0 g). Mebendazole is given as described for trichuriasis and is the preferred agent if both *Ascaris* and *Trichuris* are present. An older agent, piperazine citrate, is highly effective, less expensive, but slightly more toxic than the above two agents. It is given as a flavored syrup administered in a single dose after breakfast on two successive days and will cure the majority of cases. The drug acts by paralyzing the ascarids, which are then passed in the stool. The dose of piperazine is 75 mg/kg with a maximum of 4 g. No particular dietary regulation is necessary. The drug must be administered with caution to patients with renal insufficiency, because impaired elimination may produce neurotoxic signs. In intestinal obstruction, nasogastric suction should be initiated. After vomiting is controlled, piperazine should be given through the nasogastric tube every 12 to 24 h in dosage of 65 mg/kg (maximum 1.0 g) for six doses. Surgery usually is not required.

PROGNOSIS The prognosis in intestinal infection is generally good. When acute or chronic obstruction of ducts of hollow viscera has occurred, the immediate prognosis is determined by the promptness of diagnosis and treatment. The case fatality rate of intestinal obstruction in the United States is 3 percent.

PREVENTION Ascariasis is primarily a household infection of rural areas. All infections should be treated, personal hygiene stressed, and adequate toilet facilities provided.

TOXOCARIASIS (VISCERAL LARVA MIGRANS)

DEFINITION This is a human infection with *Toxocara canis* or *T. cati.* The animal ascarids are usually unable to complete their life cycle in humans, but they may be widely disseminated in the body, producing a variety of clinical manifestations, collectively referred to as *visceral larva migrans.*

ETIOLOGY AND EPIDEMIOLOGY The large adult toxocaral worms live in the intestine of cats and dogs. Their eggs must be passed in the stool and incubate in soil for 2 to 3 weeks before they become infective. If the ova are then ingested by a human, larvae are liberated in the intestine, penetrate the wall, and are carried in the blood to the liver, where most remain, and lung. At the time the larvae reach the pulmonary capillaries, they are still very small (approximately one-half the size of *A. lumbricoides*) and many pass through the lungs to reach the systemic circulation. Larvae penetrate the tissues where their gradually increasing size approaches the diameter of the vessel through which they are traveling. Rarely the organisms break into the alveoli, ascend the respiratory tract, and are swallowed to reach the small intestine where they mature into adult worms. *Toxocara* infections of cats and dogs are common and widespread. Transplacental transmission occurs in canines and accounts for infection rates of 80 percent or more in young puppies; they can shed a large number of ova within 4 weeks of birth. Viable ova were found in 25 percent of soil samples taken from public parks in Great Britain. Although most human infections have been reported from the United States and Europe, it seems likely that the disease is present in other areas of the world as well. Children from the age of 2 to 5 years, because of their sanitary habits and intimate association with domestic pets, are most frequently involved. In Great Britain, 4 percent of children who play in public parks have positive skin tests to *Toxocara* antigens.

PATHOGENESIS AND CLINICAL MANIFESTATIONS The larvae migrate freely in tissues, causing hemorrhage, necrosis, eosinophilic inflammatory reaction, and eventually granuloma formation. The most frequently involved organs are the liver, lungs, brain, eye, heart, and skeletal muscles. Symptoms and signs are related to the number and location of the granulomas as well as sensitization to the parasite antigen. Commonly, only asymptomatic eosinophilia marks the presence of infection. Symptomatic patients most frequently present with fever and tender hepatomegaly. Splenomegaly, skin rash, and recurrent pneumonitis with wheezing respirations may occur in more severe infections. Respiratory failure with death has been reported. Most fatalities, however, result from involvement of the myocardium or central nervous system; the latter may result in convulsions, behavior disorders, or focal neurological defects. There is often a history of dirt eating and contact with cats and dogs. Leukocytosis with eosinophilia to high levels (over 60 percent) and hypergammaglobulinemia with raised levels of IgG, IgM, and IgE are common. These manifestations may persist for months or years. At surgery or autopsy the liver may be studded with small granulomas. A granulomatous endophthalmitis, which may be mistaken for retinoblastoma, may be observed in older children and adults. Typically, this is unilateral and occurs in the absence of other clinical manifestations of visceral larva migrans.

DIAGNOSIS The diagnosis can usually be made on the basis of clinical findings. Infections with *A. lumbricoides,* hookworm, and *Strongyloides stercoralis,* as well as other nonhuman nematodes, may also on occasion present as visceral larva migrans, making the etiologic diagnosis difficult. Eosinophilic leukemia, trichinosis, trematode infections, and periarteritis nodosa must be ruled out. Isoagglutinin titers of 1:1024 or greater are often present. Antibodies to *Toxocara* and *Ascaris* antigens may be found, but, as with the isoagglutinins, these tests are neither very sensitive nor specific. The adaption of larval antigens to the enzyme-linked immunoabsorbent assay has, for the first time, provided clinicians with a serologic test of diagnostic value. In one study, the sensitivity and specificity were 78 and 92 percent, respectively. A definitive diagnosis depends on the identification of the larvae in sputum or tissue granuloma. Biopsy of the liver with serial sections of the specimen may reveal eosinophilic granulomas or a *Toxocara* larva.

TREATMENT No uniformly effective therapy is available. Diethylcarbamazine as used in bancroftian filariasis (Chap. 209) is probably the drug of choice. Thiabendazole in dosage of 25 to 50 mg/kg for 7 to 10 days may be helpful. Adrenocortical steroids may be beneficial when respiratory difficulty is pronounced. Control measures are directed toward preventing ingestion of eggs. Removal and repeated worming of infected cats and dogs must be considered. Animals less than 6 months of age should be wormed monthly; older ones every 2 or 3 months.

ANISAKIASIS

Ascarids belonging to family Anisakidae infect seals, dolphins, porpoises, whales, and other large sea mammals. Their larval stages are found in the flesh of squid and several marine fish including cod, salmon, and herring. Humans are infected by eating raw, pickled, or slightly salted fish delicacies such as "green herring," sashimi, sunomono, creviche, and gravlax which contain the third-stage larvae. The infection may be asymptomatic and noted only when the worm is coughed or vomited up. More characteristically, the larvae burrow into the mucosa of the stomach, small intestine, or more rarely the colon. Here they produce eosinophilic granulomatous tumors with edema, thickening, and .induration of the bowel wall which may be mistaken for gastric carcinoma or regional enteritis. Occasionally, larvae may penetrate the intestinal wall to involve other abdominal organs. Perforations of the bowel with peritonitis have also been described. The pathological changes are thought to be the result of a hypersensitivity reaction. In the acute gastric syndrome common in Japan, the patient may develop epigastric pain, nausea, and vomiting within a few hours of ingesting infected fish. With a gastroscope 2- to 4-cm larvae can be seen penetrating the mucosa and can sometimes be removed. In Europeans, the small intestine has been the site most frequently involved. The clinical picture may be severe enough to simulate an acute surgical abdomen. More commonly, colicky pain, diffuse abdominal tenderness, fever, and leukocytosis develop a week or more after the ingestion of fish. Peripheral eosinophilia is not always present, and a definitive diagnosis can be made only by the identification of larvae in tissue. Serologic tests are being developed, but are neither highly reliable nor generally available. The disease usually subsides spontaneously with conservative therapy. Occasionally, a chronic illness develops which requires surgical resection of the lesion.

Hundreds of cases have been recognized in the Netherlands and Japan, and several cases have been reported from North America. The disease can be prevented by storing marine fish at −20°C for a single day or by cooking it at normal cooking temperatures.

HOOKWORM DISEASE

DEFINITION Hookworm disease is a symptomatic infection caused by *Ancylostoma duodenale* or *Necator americanus.* Asymptomatic infection may be termed simply *hookworm infection,* and the individual with such infection is called a *carrier.*

ETIOLOGY *Ancylostoma duodenale,* also known as the "Old World" hookworm, possesses four prominent hooklike teeth in its adult stage. The adults are about 1 cm long and inhabit the upper part of the human small intestine, where they attach to the mucosa by means of the mouth parts and suck blood. Each adult extracts approximately 0.20 ml blood daily. The adults migrate within the small intestine, and each site of attachment persists temporarily as a bleeding point. Following fertilization, the female liberates approximately 20,000 eggs per day. They measure about 40 to 60 μm and are usually in the two-to-four-celled stage when discharged in the feces.

Necator americanus, the "New World" hookworm, has a buccal capsule containing dorsal and ventral plates rather than teeth. It is slightly smaller, deposits fewer eggs, and causes much less blood loss than *A. duodenale* (0.03 ml per worm daily). *Ancylostoma cylonicum,* a hookworm of cats found in the Far East, may occasionally reach maturity in humans.

The life cycles of both hookworms are similar. Under appropriate conditions, the eggs hatch in 24 to 48 h, releasing free-living or rhabditiform larvae. Within a few days, these develop into infective or filariform larvae which may remain viable in the soil for several weeks. These, in turn, penetrate the skin to enter vessels which carry them to the lungs. The larvae leave the alveolar capillaries, enter the alveoli, ascend the respiratory tree, enter the pharynx, and are swallowed. They reach the intestine about 1 week after penetration of the skin and mature within 5 weeks. Larval development of *Ancylostoma* may be arrested or retarded in the human host. This may result in a prolonged latent period between the onset of infection and the appearance of gravid females in the intestine. Adults have been known to survive in the human intestine for as long as 14 years, but *A. duodenale* seldom persists beyond 6 to 8 years, and most *N. americanus* infections are eliminated within 2 to 4 years.

EPIDEMIOLOGY It has been estimated that hookworms infect 700 million people and cause the loss of 7 million liters of blood daily throughout the world from 45°N to 30°S latitude. *Necator americanus* is found predominantly in the tropical areas of Africa, Asia, and the Americas, while *A. duodenale* occurs in the Mediterranean Basin, the Middle East, northern India, China, and Japan. In many areas both species are found. In general, *Ancylostoma* presents a greater public health hazard than *N. americanus,* the species which is most prevalent in the southern United States, because it is more persistent in the environment, more harmful to the host, and less amenable to treatment. Conditions conducive to the development of the hookworm egg into infective filariform larvae are a mean temperature between 23 and 33°C, abundant rainfall, shade, and well-drained sandy soil. Hookworm infection occurs where there is opportunity for disease contact of the skin with soil contaminated by promiscuous defecation. The disease may also be acquired by oral ingestion of infective larvae, particularly those of *A. duodenale.* Lactogenic transmission may also occur with this species; presumably this results from the activation of larvae whose development within the tissues of the host has been arrested or retarded. Probably because of greater exposure, males show a higher incidence of infection than females. Infections are particularly common in closed, heavily populated communities such as coffee or tea plantations.

Repeated infections of hookworm in dogs result in immunity and elimination of the parasite. It seems probable that a similar phenomenon occurs in human infections. When the possibility of reinfection is eliminated, the majority of worms is eliminated spontaneously within 1 or 2 years.

PATHOGENESIS AND CLINICAL MANIFESTATIONS During the invasion of the exposed skin by the larvae, there may be an erythematous maculopapular skin rash and edema with severe pruritus. These manifestations, which may persist for several days, are more marked in *N. americanus* infection. The lesions are most common about the feet, particularly between the toes, and have been termed "ground itch."

During migration through the lungs, cough, pneumonia, and, in severe infections, fever may occur. Usually, however, pulmonary involvement does not give rise to clinical symptoms.

Various gastrointestinal symptoms, ranging from vague epigastric distress and pica to typical ulcer pain, have been reported in association with hookworm infection. Roentgenographic studies may reveal nonspecific changes such as excessive peristalsis and "puddling," particularly in the proximal jejunum. However, gross and microscopic examination of the bowel itself reveals conspicuously little damage. Previous reports of absorptive abnormalities in hookworm infection have not been supported.

The major clinical manifestations of hookworm disease clearly are those of iron-deficiency anemia and hypoalbuminemia consequent to chronic intestinal blood loss. Whether anemia develops and how severe it becomes depends on the balance between iron lost in the gut and iron absorbed from the diet. In many endemic areas, dietary iron is largely of vegetable origin and is absorbed poorly. General dietary deficiency also may lower resistance to parasitic infections. The severity of the disease and the prognosis depend on such factors as the age of the patient, the magnitude of the worm burden, the duration of the disease, and diet. Young children often have extreme anemia, with cardiac insufficiency and anasarca. These conditions may precipitate kwashiorkor. Those who survive to puberty show retarded physical, mental, and sexual development. Milder degrees of the disease, as seen in older children and adults, are characterized by lassitude, dyspnea, palpitation, tachycardia, constipation, and pallor of the skin and mucous membranes.

Asymptomatic infections outnumber symptomatic infections, considering all age groups, 20 to 40 times in endemic areas. The worm burden is small in asymptomatic infections, and the carrier state may be indicative of some degree of acquired host resistance.

LABORATORY FINDINGS In symptomatic infection, hookworm eggs are usually numerous enough to be detected by microscopic examination of a direct or concentrated fecal smear. A quantitative egg count, using the Stoll or Beaver technique, allows an estimation of the intensity of infection. If a stool specimen is allowed to stand for several hours before examination, the eggs may hatch, releasing larvae which are easily confused with those of *Strongyloides.* The eggs must be differentiated from those of *Trichostrongylus* and *Ternidens diminutus,* which are larger and in a later stage of maturation when observed in a fresh fecal specimen than are those of *Necator* or *Ancylostoma.* Abdominal and pulmonary symptoms appear before the eggs are discharged, although a presumptive diagnosis may be made on the basis of the clinical history and the eosinophilic leukocytosis. The feces seldom contain gross blood in hookworm disease, although tests for occult blood are usually positive.

Generally, the leukocyte count is normal. However, in some early cases, leukocytosis may be marked, with an eosinophilia as high as 70 or 80 percent. The anemia is characteristically hypochromic and microcytic.

The species of hookworm may be determined by the identification of the adult worm passed in the stool following treatment or by culturing the feces and identifying the third-stage larvae. This is seldom important in clinical practice.

DIFFERENTIAL DIAGNOSIS Since hookworm disease occurs in areas in which beriberi and malaria are also common, these diseases must be differentiated from hookworm disease, or their coexistence must be established.

TREATMENT Therapy specific for the infection and directed toward the improvement of nutrition and the anemia should be considered simultaneously. In areas where reinfection is likely, administration of anthelmintics to patients with light infections (less than 2000 eggs per milliliter of feces) is probably not beneficial. In most cases requiring specific therapy, anthelmintics may be administered immediately, followed by iron and a high-protein diet. A number of satisfactory anthelmintic agents are available, but two, pyrantel pamoate (see "Ascariasis" above) and mebendazole (see "Trichuriasis" above) are currently favored. Where expense remains a major consideration, the drug of choice is tetrachloroethylene (TCE). It is highly effective, nontoxic, inexpensive, and ideal for mass treatment. (The USP tetrachloroethylene available to veterinarians may be used.) In most instances a single dose of this agent will decrease the worm load substantially. Complete cure may require several courses of treatment but is not necessary in endemic areas; the aim of therapy is reduction of the worm load to an asymptomatic level. Tetrachloroethylene is administered as a single 5-ml oral dose. Children should receive 0.12 ml/kg (to a maximum of 5 ml) by the same route. The night before treatment, the patient is permitted a light fat-free meal. The following morning, breakfast is omitted and the drug is administered. No food is permitted for 4 h and no alcohol for 24 h. Treatment can be repeated in a week if complete cure is desired and has not been accomplished. If ascariasis is also present, it should be treated first with piperazine citrate (see "Ascariasis" above). Bitoscanate (Jonit) in oral dosage of 100 mg every 12 h for three doses is equally effective against *N. americanus* and *A. duodenale*. It is not available in the United States.

The anemia requires iron replacement. When anemia is severe and there is malnutrition with anasarca, blood transfusions and a high-protein diet should be given before drug treatment is begun. Blood should be given in an amount sufficient to raise the hemoglobin level to 10 g per 100 ml. In advanced cases it may be necessary to delay drug treatment for 2 to 3 weeks.

PROGNOSIS The immediate prognosis is good. When opportunity for reinfection persists and nutrition cannot be maintained, a state of chronic debility develops. Maturation of children is impaired, and intercurrent disease is a serious problem in adults.

PREVENTION Many of the measures required are obvious but difficult to apply on a large scale. Even if facilities for proper disposal of feces are provided, it is no simple matter to educate the population in their use. Soil pollution must be eliminated. Avoidance of direct skin contact with the soil (by wearing shoes) is often not practical in endemic areas. Periodic mass treatment of the population has been used in some hookworm control programs.

CUTANEOUS LARVA MIGRANS (CREEPING ERUPTION)

DEFINITION Creeping eruption is an infection of human skin caused by the larvae of the dog and cat hookworm, *A. brasil-*

iense. The other dog hookworms, *A. caninum* and *Uncinaria stenocephala,* as well as the human parasites, *Strongyloides stercoralis* and *Necator americanus,* may also produce the disease. The larvae of *Gnathostoma spinigerum,* a nematode found in the Orient, and *Gasterophilus,* the horse bat fly, may produce a similar cutaneous infection.

ETIOLOGY *Ancylostoma brasiliense* reaches adulthood regularly only in the dog and cat. The larvae emerging from eggs discharged in the feces develop to the filariform stage and then are capable of penetrating the skin. In humans, the larvae usually remain in the skin and migrate, producing an irregular erythematous tunnel visible on the skin surface.

EPIDEMIOLOGY AND DISTRIBUTION Transmission to humans requires environmental temperature and humidity appropriate for development of the egg to the infective filariform larva stage. Beaches and other moist, sandy areas are hazardous, because animals choose such areas for defecation, and the *A. brasiliense* eggs develop well in such soil. In the United States infection is found in the southern Atlantic and Gulf states.

PATHOGENESIS AND CLINICAL MANIFESTATIONS The site of penetration of the skin by the larvae becomes apparent in a few hours. The migration of the larvae in the skin is accompanied by severe itching. Scratching may lead to bacterial infection. In the course of 1 week, the initial red papule develops into an irregular, erythematous, linear lesion which may attain a length of 15 to 20 cm. The larvae may persist for weeks to months without treatment.

Loeffler's syndrome has been observed in 26 of 52 cases of creeping eruption. Transient, migratory pulmonary infiltrations associated with an increased number of eosinophils in the blood and sputum were interpreted as an allergic reaction to the helminthic infection.

LABORATORY FINDINGS Eosinophils occur in the lesion, but eosinophilic leukocytosis is slight, except when Loeffler's syndrome appears. The percentage of eosinophils in the blood may then rise to 50 percent and in the sputum to 90 percent. Only rarely are larvae found on skin biopsy.

TREATMENT Thiabendazole is the drug of choice; it should be given orally in the dosage suggested for hookworm. It may be repeated if necessary. Alternatively, it may be applied topically as a 10% aqueous suspension. Topical administration avoids systemic toxicity. Superficial bacterial infections are improved by the application of wet dressing and elevation of the extremity. For intense itching, oral antihistaminics may be of aid.

PROGNOSIS Untreated infections last several months. Treatment, which is usually sought because of severe pruritus, is usually successful.

PREVENTION Dogs and cats should be prevented from contaminating recreation areas and children's sandboxes.

TRICHOSTRONGYLIASIS

DEFINITION Trichostrongyliasis is an intestinal infection of herbivorous animals throughout the world. Humans are an intermediate host.

ETIOLOGY Almost a dozen species of *Trichostrongylus* are known to have infected humans. The disease is common in Asia, the Middle East, and South America, but few human infections have been reported in the United States. In view of the high frequency of animal infections here, the low incidence of human infections is difficult to understand. The possibility exists that some such infections are mistaken for hookworm infections.

The ova resemble those of the hookworm but are larger, have more pointed ends, and, when observed in a fresh fecal specimen, show a more advanced stage of segmentation (16- to 32-cell stage).

PATHOGENESIS Infection is acquired by ingestion of green leafy plants contaminated with third-stage larvae. On reaching the small intestine, they attach themselves to the mucosa and develop into adult worms within 4 weeks. The adult at that time sucks blood and maintains residence in the intestine for long periods. Sandground, who infected himself, observed infection to last more than 8 years.

MANIFESTATIONS Most infections are asymptomatic, but massive infections may result in epigastric distress and anemia. The parasite owes its importance primarily to the resemblance of its ova to those of the hookworms. Moreover, because the trichostrongylidae do not respond to anthelmintics effective in hookworm infection, it may be assumed incorrectly that refractory hookworm infection is present.

LABORATORY DIAGNOSIS The diagnosis depends on the finding of the ova in the feces. Since they are few, they are usually found only when a concentration method is used. In symptomatic infections, there may be leukocytosis with marked eosinophilia (for example, 80 percent).

TREATMENT These infections do not respond to tetrachloroethylene. Thiabendazole 25 mg/kg twice daily for 2 or 3 days, or pyrantel pamoate as used in hookworm infections, is effective in symptomatic infections. Both are considered investigational drugs for this condition by the U.S. Food and Drug Administration.

PREVENTION Leafy vegetables should be cooked before ingestion in endemic areas.

STRONGYLOIDIASIS

DEFINITION Strongyloidiasis is an intestinal infection of humans caused by *Strongyloides stercoralis*. Extraintestinal involvement may occur in severe cases.

ETIOLOGY The tiny (2 mm in length) adult female resides and lays her eggs in the mucosa of the upper part of the jejunum. In heavy infections, the biliary and pancreatic ducts, the entire small bowel, and the colon may be parasitized. The eggs quickly hatch, releasing rhabditiform larvae which enter the lumen of the bowel and are passed in the feces. On reaching the soil, the larvae develop into the infective filariform stage. There, as in the case of the filariform larvae of hookworm, they penetrate the skin and small blood vessels of humans. They are then carried to the lungs where they leave the alveolar capillaries, ascend the respiratory tree, enter the pharynx, and are swallowed. On reaching the small intestine, they mature and copulate. The fertilized female burrows into the jejunal mucosa, while the male is excreted in the stool. Oviposition begins 17 to 28 days after the initial infection. It is likely that the females also reproduce parthenogenetically. In addition to the *direct* host-soil-host cycle, *Strongyloides* has two alternative cycles. In the first, or *indirect,* cycle, the rhabditiform larvae, after passing from the host, develop into free-living adults which reside and reproduce in the soil, thus creating a reservoir of infection independent of the human host. Under certain environmental conditions, the free-living larvae are capable of

transforming back into filariform larvae which initiate a new cycle in humans. In the second, or *autoinfection,* cycle, the rhabditiform larvae develop into filariform larvae before they are passed in the stool. They may then invade the intestinal mucosa or perianal skin of the same host without first going through a soil phase. This may explain the long persistence (20 to 30 years) of strongyloidiasis in patients who have left endemic areas and may also account for the extremely heavy worm loads in some individuals. The early transformation of the filariform larvae is probably also responsible for the frequency with which strongyloidiasis is seen in crowded, unsanitary institutions for the mentally retarded. It appears to occur frequently in patients with achlorhydria, delayed intestinal transit time, and blind loops or diverticula.

EPIDEMIOLOGY The usual mode of infection is the penetration of the skin by larvae. Some infections may result from ingestion of contaminated food and drink, and some are believed to be transmitted by contact. This disease is endemic in the tropics, where the warmth, moisture, and lack of sanitation favor its spread. Sporadic cases appear among Puerto Ricans and throughout the rural south of the continental United States.

PATHOGENESIS AND CLINICAL MANIFESTATIONS The initial cutaneous penetration of the filariform larvae usually produces no symptoms. However, transitory skin eruptions characterized by blotchy erythema, serpiginous lesions, and urticaria may be seen. These may recur at irregular intervals thereafter and are particularly common following recovery from an acute febrile illness. In these situations the lesions are generally found over the lower back and buttocks and are related to episodes of autoinfection. Cough, dyspnea, gross hemoptysis, and bronchospasm may accompany migration through the lungs. Chest x-rays may show pulmonary infiltration at this time. The intestinal infestation is usually asymptomatic or productive only of vague abdominal complaints. In heavier infections, epigastric pain and tenderness, nausea, flatulence, vomiting, and diarrhea alternating with constipation may be observed. Peptic ulcer may be simulated, but food often aggravates the pain. The mucosal inflammation may be severe enough to produce subacute obstruction, segmental ileus, and impaired absorption. A severe form of ulcerative colitis, accompanied by intestinal perforation and peritonitis, has been encountered. In debilitated, immunodepressed, or steroid-treated patients massive autoinfection with widespread dissemination of larvae to the extraintestinal organs including the central nervous system may occur. This hyperinfection is often associated with severe enterocolitis, persistent gram-negative bacteremia, and occasionally gram-negative meningitis. Unrecognized, it usually leads to death. Disseminated strongyloidiasis should be considered in any compromised host with unexplained gram-negative bacteremia, abdominal complaints, and pulmonary infiltrates with or without eosinophilia.

LABORATORY FINDINGS Although clinical findings may be suggestive, the definitive diagnosis can be made only in the laboratory. Fresh fecal specimens should be examined to avoid confusion with hookworm infection; generally, fresh specimens contain *larvae* in strongyloidiasis infections, while in hookworm infection they contain *eggs*. Since the number of larvae in the stool is small and varies from day to day, several samples should be checked, using concentration and culture techniques. If pulmonary involvement is present, the sputum should be examined for larvae. Microscopic examination of the duodenal washings and jejunal biopsies may also establish the diagnosis. Alternatively, a weighted string can be passed into the duodenum, allowed to remain for a short time, and then withdrawn. The bile-stained section of the string is stripped of fluid which is then examined for the presence of larvae. The filarial complement fixation test is positive in approximately 75 percent of patients and may be helpful in the diagnosis of light infections.

Eosinophilic leukocytosis is common, except in very severe cases. When eosinophilia occurs in association with peptic ulcer symptoms, strongyloidiasis should be suspected.

TREATMENT All infected patients should be treated to prevent the occurrence of severe invasive disease. The drug of choice is thiabendazole, which should be given orally in dosage of 25 mg/kg twice a day for 2 or 3 days. In disseminated strongyloidiasis, treatment should be continued for 7 days or more. Lightheadedness, nausea, and vomiting are common accompaniments of therapy with this agent. Hypersensitivity reactions may occur but usually respond to treatment with antihistamines. The stools should be rechecked at intervals of 3 months because the parasite is not easily eradicated and retreatment may be necessary.

PROGNOSIS In the usual case, the prognosis is good. Since the occurrence of hyperinfection is unpredictable, every effort should be made to eradicate the infection in each case. In severe cases with hyperinfection, the prognosis is poor.

PREVENTION In general, the measures are those for the control of hookworm infection. In addition, it is well to remember that infection may be contracted by ingestion of contaminated food (especially uncooked vegetables) or of contaminated drinking water and by contact. Patients who have a history of residence in an endemic area should be carefully checked for the presence of the parasite prior to the initiation of steroid or immunosuppressive therapy. Because the larvae may not appear in the stool for several weeks after the initiation of such therapy, repeated examinations of stool and upper intestinal aspirates are indicated. Since sputum, vomitus, stool, and body fluids of patients with disseminated disease may contain infective filariform larvae, gloves and gowns should be worn by hospital personnel caring for such patients.

INTESTINAL CAPILLARIASIS

DEFINITION Intestinal capillariasis is an infection of humans caused by the roundworm *Capillaria philippinensis*. This species of *Capillaria* was first discovered in 1963 from a fatal human infection occurring in the Philippines. The infection results in intractable diarrhea with a high mortality rate. Clinical studies have shown a severe protein-losing enteropathy and malabsorption of fats and sugars.

ETIOLOGY *Capillaria* are nematodes of the family Trichuroidea and are closely related to comembers *Trichuris* and *Trichinella*. Adult *C. philippinensis* are small, measuring 2 to 4 mm in length. The peanut-shaped eggs have flattened bipolar plugs and an average size of 42 by 20 μm. The adults inhabit the mucosa of the small intestine, especially the jejunum. Adults, larval forms, and eggs are found in the stool.

EPIDEMIOLOGY The infection has been found almost exclusively in persons residing in the Ilocano ethnic region in Northwest Luzon, Philippines. Two cases from Thailand have also been reported. Since 1966 the disease has occurred in epidemic form, and more than 1000 cases and 100 deaths have been reported. Males are infected more frequently than females, perhaps because of occupational exposure. Prior to the discovery of an effective chemotherapeutic agent, the mortality rate in untreated cases was about 30 percent. With chemotherapy, the case fatality rate has been reduced to 6 percent.

The mode of transmission and life cycle of the parasite are not established. The presence of many adult worms, larviparous females, embryonated eggs, and all larval stages in human intestinal contents suggests that autoinfection may be part of the life cycle. In addition, indirect evidence indicates that person-to-person transmission occurs. The mechanism by which humans originally became infected remains obscure. Because the Ilocano people of the region eat many animal foods raw or semicooked, numerous species of local fauna have been examined for *Capillaria*, and developing larvae have been recovered from three species of fish.

PATHOGENESIS AND MANIFESTATIONS Adult worms in large numbers invade the small-intestinal mucosa and cause a severe protein-losing enteropathy and malabsorption. Hypokalemia, hypocalcemia, and hypoproteinemia are the rule. Autopsy studies have failed to show extraintestinal spread of the parasite. Initial symptoms of intestinal "gurgling" (borborygmi) and recurrent vague abdominal pain are followed, usually within 2 to 3 weeks, by a voluminous watery diarrhea. Other findings, consistent with the basic pathophysiologic process, are anorexia, vomiting, weight loss, muscle wasting and weakness, hyporeflexia, and edema. Abdominal tenderness and distention may occur. The period between onset of symptoms and death is usually 2 to 3 months. Subclinical infection has not been noted.

DIAGNOSIS The diagnosis is made by finding ova in the stool. The ova of *C. philippinensis* must be differentiated from those of *T. trichiura*, which are similar. Care must be taken that capillaria are not overlooked in patients with *Trichuris* infections because in the endemic area most patients with capillariasis have coexistent *Trichuris* infection.

TREATMENT Administration of mebendazole combined with fluid and electrolyte replacement leads to dramatic improvement; 400 mg per day in divided dosage should be given for 20 days to prevent relapse.

REFERENCES

AUR RJA et al: Thiabendazole in visceral larva migrans. Am J Dis Child 121:226, 1971

AZIZ MA, SEDDIQUI AR: Morphological and absorption studies of small intestine hookworm disease (ancyclostomiasis) in West Pakistan. Gastroenterology 55:242, 1968

BANWELL JG, SCHAD GA: Hookworm. Clin Gastroenterol 7:129, 1978

BLUMENTHAL DS: Current concepts—intestinal nematodes in the United States. N Engl J Med 297:1437, 1977

BROWN HW: *Basic Clinical Parasitology*, 4th ed. New York, Appleton-Century-Crofts, 1975

CROSS JH et al: Studies on the experimental transmission of *Capillaria philippinensis* in monkeys. Trans R Soc Trop Med Hyg 66:819, 1972

DAVIS CM, ISRAEL RM: Treatment of creeping eruption with topical thiabendazole. Arch Dermatol 97:325, 1968

KAMATH KR: Severe infection with *Trichuris trichuria* in Malaysian children. Am J Trop Med Hyg 22:600, 1973

LAYRISSE M et al: Blood loss due to infection with *Trichuris trichuria*. Am J Trop Med Hyg 16:613, 1967

MARKETT EK: Pseudohookworm infection—trichostrongyliasis: Treatment with thiabendazole. N Engl J Med 278:831, 1968

MARSEN JM, TURNER JA: Reinfection of enterobiasis (pinworm infection): Simultaneous treatment of family members. Am J Dis Child 118:576, 1969

MILLER MJ et al: Mebendazole. An effective anthelmintic for trichuriasis and enterobiasis. JAMA 230:1412, 1974

PAWLOWSKI Z: Ascariasis. Clin Gastroenterol 7:157, 1978

PHILLS JA et al: Pulmonary abnormalities and eosinophilia due to
Ascaris suum. N Engl J Med 286:965, 1972

PINKUS GS et al: Intestinal anisakiasis. First case report from North
America. Am J Med 59:114, 1975

SCHANTZ PM, GLICKMAN LT: Current concepts in parasitology—toxocaral visceral larva migrans. N Engl J Med 298:436, 1978

SCOWDEN EB et al: Overwhelming strongyloidiasis—an unappreciated
opportunistic infection. Medicine 57:527, 1978

WOLFF MS: Oxyuris, trichostrongylus and trichiuris. Clin Gastroenterol 7:201, 1978

ZINKHAM WH: Visceral larva migrans—a review and reassessment indicating two forms of clinical expression: visceral and ocular. Am J
Dis Child 132:627, 1978

211
SCHISTOSOMIASIS (BILHARZIASIS)

JAMES J. PLORDE

DEFINITION Schistosomiasis (biharziasis) designates a group
of diseases caused by three closely related species of digenetic
trematodes, or blood flukes, belonging to the family Schistoso-
matidae—*Schistosoma mansoni, S. haematobium,* and *S. japonicum.* These blood flukes inhabit the circulatory system of humans and animals living in tropical and subtropical countries.
Here they deposit large numbers of eggs, many of which are
retained within the body of the host with the production of
inflammatory lesions. The organs and tissues most frequently
affected are the colon, urinary bladder, liver, lungs, and central
nervous system.

ETIOLOGY AND LIFE CYCLE The adult worms, which grow
and mature within the portal venous system of the liver, measure 1 to 2 cm in length. The male has a central trough, the
gynecophoral canal, that enfolds the longer, more slender female during most of their 4- to 30-year life span. After copulation the male carries the female against the flow of portal
blood to the small mesenteric vessels. *Schistosoma japonicum*
ascends the superior and *S. mansoni,* the inferior mesenteric
vein. Both eventually reach the submucosal vessels of the intestine; *S. japonicum* settles in the small intestine and ascending
colon and *S. mansoni,* in the descending colon and rectum.
Schistosoma haematobium finds its way through the hemorrhoidal anastomoses to the systemic capillaries of the bladder and
other pelvic organs. When they can travel no further, the female deposits her eggs in clusters (or one by one in the case of
S. mansoni), slowly retreating down the vessel in front of them.
The daily egg output of each worm pair varies from 300 for *S.
mansoni* to over 3000 in *S. japonicum* infections. The eggs,
which remain viable for 3 weeks, secrete an enzymatic substance which destroys the surrounding tissue. If the eggs lie
close to the mucosal surface, they rupture into the lumen of the
gut (or bladder in the case of *S. haematobium*) and are carried
to the outside in the urine or feces. On reaching fresh water,
the embryonated eggs quickly hatch, liberating ciliated *miracidia.* These miracidia have a life span of 6 to 8 h in which to
search out and penetrate the specific snail host appropriate to
the species. Within the snail the miracidia are transformed by
a two-generation process of asexual reproduction into thousands of infective larvae called *cercariae.* When cercariae are
released 1 to 2 months after the original penetration of the
snail, they swim around vigorously, and if they contact human
skin within 2 days, they penetrate it and become *schistosomula.*
Within 24 h the schistosomula work their way into the periph-

eral venules and are carried to the right side of the heart and
then to the pulmonary capillaries. After some delay, they enter
the systemic circulation. Those parasites that survive the passage through the mesenteric capillary bed finally reach the portal venous system, where they mature into adult flukes in 5 to
12 weeks.

EPIDEMIOLOGY AND CONTROL Schistosomiasis is possibly
the most important of the helminthic diseases because of its
worldwide distribution and the extensive pathological changes
produced by the parasites. It is believed that over 200 million
people in 71 countries are affected by this condition, and it is
likely that increasing use of land irrigation in endemic areas
will increase this number substantially. Owing to the lack of
appropriate snail hosts, schistosomiasis is not transmitted in
the continental United States. Approximately 400,000 imported cases occur, however, particularly among the Puerto
Rican, Filipino, and Yemenite populations.

Within endemic areas, there are wide variations in both the
intensity and prevalence of infection. In most patients the
worm load is small, probably less than 10 worm pairs, and
disease manifestations are absent. Because adult worms do not
multiply within the body of their human host, heavy infections
are the result of repeated reinfections occurring over a period
of years. It is among this population that serious morbidity
and mortality occurs.

The continuing presence of schistosomiasis depends on the
disposal of infected human excrement into fresh water, the
presence of suitable snail hosts, and the exposure of persons to
water infested with cercarias. Promiscuous defecation, latrine
drainage, and unsanitary sewage disposal are the more important sources of pollution of streams and rivers. The disease is
contracted by persons washing clothes, bathing, wading, or
working in contaminated water. There is a close correlation
between the degree of water contact and infection rates in endemic areas. The infection rates and intensity of infection both
peak in the second decade of life and then decrease with advancing age. This might be explained in part by reduced exposure to contaminated water but also may reflect slowly developing immunity. In animal models, immunity arises in
response to the presence of viable adults, depends upon the
presence of antibody, and is mediated by eosinophils. It is directed only at newly invading immature parasites; the adults
appear to protect themselves by incorporating host antigen
into their tegument.

Of these three disease-producing blood flukes in humans, *S.
mansoni* is the most widespread and the only one present in the
Western Hemisphere. It was brought to the Caribbean area
and South America by African slaves. It is present in Venezuela, Surinam, Brazil, Puerto Rico, Dominican Republic, St.
Lucia, and several other islands in the Caribbean. In Africa, it
occurs in the Nile Delta, limited areas of East and South Africa, tropical Africa, and the Middle East including Yemen,
Saudi Arabia, and Israel.

Schistosoma japonicum affects the agricultural population in
Japan, China, the Philippines, the Celebes, Thailand, and
Laos. Men are more frequently infected than women. An important source of infection in the Orient is the use of human
excreta as a fertilizer in vegetable gardens.

Schistosoma haematobium is distributed widely throughout
the African continent and is found in several countries of the
Middle East. In Africa, it is highly prevalent among the agricultural population of the Nile Valley.

The best attack on schistosomiasis is prevention. Public
health measures, including proper disposal of human excre-

ment, provision of pure water supplies for domestic and recreational purposes, and mass anthelmintic therapy, should be carried out in endemic areas. The effectiveness of these measures is diminished if there are significant animal reservoirs of the disease, as in *S. japonicum* and possibly in *S. mansoni* infections. Extermination of the mollusk intermediate host by chemical agents has been used in areas where infestation rates are high. Available molluscicides include *N*-tritylmorpholine, yurimin, and niclosamide (Bayluscid). This drug appears to be the most effective, but the selection of an agent is determined in large part by the nature of the habitat. Biologic snail control methods, although showing promise, have not yet been demonstrated to be effective in the field. Careful attention to the design of irrigation systems in endemic areas is important. The use of concrete-lined ditches and intermittent or fluctuant application of water can be very effective in control of the snail population. The most successful control programs have combined mass therapy with mollusciciding and/or environmental control. Unfortunately, this approach is extremely costly and beyond the means of many countries.

SCHISTOSOMIASIS MANSONI (INTESTINAL BILHARZIASIS, SCHISTOSOMAL DYSENTERY)

ETIOLOGY *Schistosoma mansoni* is distinguished from the two other major species by the structure of its eggs and the adult flukes. The eggs are bluntly oval, have a lateral spine, and measure about 140 by about 60 μm. They are passed in feces and, rarely, in the urine. The intermediate snail hosts belong to the genera *Biomphalaria* and *Tropicorbis*. Humans are thought to be the principal host, but baboons in Kenya have been found to be infected naturally. It is not known as yet whether they constitute an important reservoir of the disease independent of humans.

PATHOGENESIS AND CLINICAL MANIFESTATIONS Schistosomiasis *mansoni* infections are usually asymptomatic. Serious disease occurs only in those who, by virtue of repeated exposures, develop and maintain heavy worm loads over prolonged periods. Clinical manifestations can be divided into three phases: (1) an early stage in which cercariae penetrate the skin and the resulting schistosomula are carried by the blood to the liver and mature into adult parasites within the intrahepatic portal veins, (2) an intermediate stage which begins with and continues through the duration of oviposition and egg extrusion, and (3) a late stage characterized by tissue proliferation and fibrosis in response to eggs that have been retained in tissue. Within a few hours of penetrating the skin, most cercariae die, producing a dermatitis characterized by round-cell infiltration, pruritus, and papular eruption. This is the result of both an immediate and delayed type of sensitivity reaction to cercarial antigen and rarely occurs in primary infection. The rash is commonly followed by headache, myalgia, abdominal pain, and diarrhea, manifestations presumably related to the migration of the schistosomula. These symptoms may persist for 1 or 2 weeks, terminating with a modest fever.

An acute, febrile illness, resembling serum sickness and beginning 1 to 2 months after exposure, marks the onset of oviposition and the beginning of the intermediate stage of illness. This so-called *Katayama syndrome* apparently represents an allergic response to the growing antigenic mass of ova and parasites. The illness is characterized by high spiking fever, chills, cough, urticaria, abdominal pain, diarrhea, and occasionally melena. Physical examination shows lymphadenopathy, enlarged tender liver, and fine scattered rales. Sigmoidoscopy reveals an inflamed, engorged mucosa with small areas of ulceration and hemorrhage. Laboratory tests demonstrate the presence of circulating immune complexes, nonspecific liver function abnormalities, and a marked eosinophilic leukocytosis. Eggs may not be present in the stool initially, and the clinical manifestations, with the exception of the eosinophilia, can be mistaken for typhoid. The acute illness may last as long as 3 months and on rare occasions may result in death. The syndrome is seen in its full intensity only in previously unexposed individuals who suffer a massive cercarial exposure. In endemic areas, it is most commonly brief and mild.

The late stage of illness is caused by the reaction of local tissue to the deposited eggs. Those which are extruded into the bowel lumen elicit little damage. The 50 percent or more that are retained, however, stimulate an eosinophilic and mononuclear-cell infiltration followed by edema, granuloma formation, and vascular obstruction. This has been demonstrated to be a delayed hypersensitivity reaction to a soluble antigen secreted by the egg. Early in infection the host response is vigorous, producing lesions which exceed the volume of the inciting egg by a hundredfold. In the chronic phase, however, this response appears to be moderated, and the pathological consequences are proportionately less severe. Healing occurs by fibrosis, calcification, and resorption.

In the bowel, these changes produce congestion, thickening, and, in severe infections, ulcerations and sessile or pedunculated polyps. Clinically, abdominal pain, diarrhea with or without blood, and a mild protein-losing enteropathy may be seen. Intestinal obstruction and rectal prolapse are rare complications. These changes often regress with treatment.

Of more severe consequence is the passage of eggs back into the venous system. These are carried to portal radicles of the liver where they produce an endophlebitis, pseudotubercle formation, acute vascular obstruction, and hepatic enlargement. With time, collars of fibrosis develop around the larger portal veins resulting in shrinkage of the liver and severe presinusoidal portal hypertension. The patient presents with hepatosplenomegaly and esophageal varices. Occasionally the enlarged spleen becomes enormous, producing a visible abdominal mass and the anemia, leukopenia, and thrombocytopenia of hypersplenism. Neovascularization and arterialization maintain hepatic blood flow at normal levels. As a result, hepatocellular function is usually well preserved, and spider nevi, gynecomastia, jaundice, and ascites are uncommon. Repeated bouts of esophageal bleeding may occur. Hepatic encephalopathy rarely results, however, and the outcome is usually favorable. When death does occur, it is the result of exsanguination.

With the development of portacaval anastomoses, some eggs are carried past the liver to the vessels of the lung where they may produce a similar histopathological reaction in the pulmonary arterioles. Interstitial fibrosis, destruction of pulmonary capillaries, and eventually pulmonary hypertension with cor pulmonale and aneurysms of the pulmonary artery may occur. On roentgenogram the granulomas may resemble miliary tuberculosis.

Occasionally ova are carried to the spinal cord through anastomotic venous channels or are deposited there by ectopic adults resulting in a transverse myelitis.

There is impressive evidence that circulating antigen antibody complexes may produce an immune-complex nephropathy in schistosomiasis *mansoni*. This has been observed primarily in patients with the chronic hepatosplenic form of the disease and may present as asymptomatic albuminuria, the nephrotic syndrome, or progressive renal failure. There is little information on its incidence or public health significance.

Chronic *Salmonella* and *Escherichia coli* bacteremias have been noted in patients suffering from hepatosplenic schistosomiasis. The chronicity of these infections may be related to the ability of adult parasites to harbor bacteria in their tegument. Antibiotic therapy is unsatisfactory unless the parasites are first eradicated with appropriate antischistosomal treatment.

DIAGNOSIS AND LABORATORY FINDINGS Diagnosis depends on finding the ova in the stools or the rectal mucosa. Stool concentration techniques such as gravity sedimentation or formol-ether centrifugation are often required for the detection of ova. Quantitation of the egg output by the Kato thick smear or similar methods is useful in estimating the severity of infection and in following response to therapy.

Rectal biopsy is probably the single most reliable method of diagnosis and it is often positive when repeated stool examinations are negative. By means of biopsy forceps and a proctoscope, mucosal snips are obtained from the valves of Houston, compressed between two glass slides, and examined under the low-power lens of a microscope. Eggs, often numbering in the hundreds, are clearly visible. Because dead eggs may persist in tissue for a long time after the death of the adult worms, active infection is confirmed only if the eggs can be shown to be viable. This may be done by observing the eggs for movement under the high-power lens or by hatching them in water.

Eosinophilia is usually present in schistosomiasis. An intradermal test of the immediate type becomes positive within 1 to 2 months of exposure and remains so for years despite parasitological cure. Since it is neither highly sensitive nor specific, it is of value chiefly as an epidemiologic tool. Twenty-five percent of patients with a history of swimmer's itch give a positive test.

Complement fixation, precipitin, counterimmunoelectrophoresis, and indirect fluorescent antibody tests can be done, but like the intradermal test most lack sensitivity and specificity.

Two tests show demonstrable improvement in both areas. One is an indirect fluorescent antibody procedure that utilizes frozen-sectioned adult antigens; the other a radioimmunoassay using purified egg antigen. Serologic tests become positive early in the course of infection, often before eggs can be recovered. A positive result should lead to a vigorous search for eggs by concentration methods or rectal biopsy, but by itself is not an indication for treatment.

TREATMENT No specific therapy is available for the treatment of schistosomal dermatitis or the acute illness resembling serum sickness seen in the early months of infection. Antihistamines and steroids have been used to control the manifestations of these two symptoms. Because late schistosomiasis is caused by the continued deposition of eggs by the mature worm pairs, the aim of therapy in this stage of the disease is the sterilization and destruction of these parasites. Adult schistosomicides are available for the purpose, but in light of their considerable toxicity, therapy should not be initiated unless the presence of an active infection is first proved by the recovery of *viable eggs* from the stool or rectal mucosa. Moreover, since the severity of disease is related to the intensity of infection, some authorities believe light infections (fewer than 50 eggs per gram of stool) do not require therapy. In heavier infections therapy will usually reduce egg output by 90 percent or more, and attempts to achieve cure by repeated use of toxic agents are unwise.

Trivalent antimony compounds, including tartar emetic (antimony potassium tartrate), stibophen (Fuadin), and stibocaptate (Astiban), have been the traditional agents for this disease. Only stibocaptate is still widely used and is probably the preferred agent. It is given by intramuscular injection as a 10% solution for five doses for a total of 35 to 50 mg/kg (maximum 2.0 g). Toxic side effects are mitigated if injections are given at weekly intervals.

Temporary ECG changes are common during therapy; they consist primarily of repolarization abnormalities which disappear a few days after the drug is discontinued. However, arrhythmias, collapse, and sudden death have been reported. Antimonials also may cause hepatitis, acute nephritis, hemolytic anemia, and thrombocytopenic purpura. Any of these complications calls for immediate discontinuation of therapy. Nausea and joint pains can usually be controlled by decreasing the individual dose or increasing the intervals between doses. Heart, renal, or liver disease constitutes a contraindication to therapy with this group of agents.

Ambilhar (niridazole) can be taken orally, 25 mg/kg every day in divided doses for 7 days. Since it is less toxic than the antimonials and probably just as effective, this agent has become the drug of choice in *S. mansoni* infections. Although ECG changes occur with this drug also, they are less common than with antimonial therapy. However, there has been a high incidence of neurological abnormalities, and as many as 80 percent of patients receiving the drug show electroencephalographic changes. Psychotic episodes or convulsions, which disappear when the drug is discontinued, have also been reported, particularly in adults. The incidence of neurological reactions seems to increase if there is serious liver disease with portacaval shunting. Niridazole should not be used in patients with a prior history of seizures.

Hycanthone is a new thioxanthone preparation that can be administered in a single intramuscular injection. Its hepatotoxicity and mutagenic properties may limit its usefulness. It is not available in the United States.

Success of treatment is judged by the disappearance of eggs from the stool, reduction in eosinophils, and alleviation of symptoms. Patients should be examined monthly for 6 to 12 months to detect relapses. The decision to retreat is based on factors such as intensity of egg output, presence of potentially reversible clinical manifestations, and the likelihood of reinfection.

Treatment of the patient with severe hepatic or pulmonary disease is largely symptomatic. There is little enthusiasm for portacaval shunting in the presence of esophageal varices. These patients usually have good hepatocellular function and, if treated carefully, will probably survive longer with repeated bleeding episodes than with surgery. Additionally, splenectomy makes these patients more susceptible to the recrudescence of chronic malaria.

PROGNOSIS The prognosis is good. Many patients never develop symptoms, and early states of colonic, hepatic, pulmonary, and central nervous system disease are completely reversible with adequate therapy. In the late fibrotic stage, the prognosis is worse.

SCHISTOSOMIASIS JAPONICA (KATAYAMA DISEASE)

ETIOLOGY The oval eggs are shorter, wider, and smaller than those of the other two species, measuring about 90 by 70 μm. Mature eggs have a minute hook, or spine, laterally situated and smaller than that of *S. mansoni*. The ova are passed in the feces only. The life cycle is similar to that of *S. mansoni*, except that amphibious snails of the genus *Oncomelania*, which are capable of prolonged existence away from water, are utilized as intermediate hosts, and water buffalo, horses, cattle, pigs, dogs, and cats as well as humans may harbor the adult worms.

Both factors add to the difficulty in disease control. *Schistosoma japonicum* lives in the superior mesenteric venules and frequently migrates to those of the colon for oviposition.

PATHOGENESIS AND CLINICAL MANIFESTATIONS The early manifestations of infection such as the pruritic dermatitis, cough, angioneurotic edema, diarrhea, and fever produced by the penetration and migration of the schistosomula are seen less commonly than in schistosomiasis *mansoni*. However, because *S. japonicum* eggs are deposited in greater number and in closer proximity to the liver than are those of *S. mansoni*, the intermediate and late manifestations of disease are usually both more frequent and more severe.

The allergic manifestations accompanying oviposition are particularly impressive in japonicum infections. Four to six weeks after exposure the patient notes the onset of a high spiking fever, chills, cough, urticaria, generalized lymphadenopathy, tender hepatosplenomegaly, and eosinophilic leukocytosis. The deposition of large numbers of eggs in the intestinal wall results in ulcerations, bloody mucoid stools, and abdominal pain. The acute illness may persist for 1 to 2 months but usually subsides leaving the patient relatively well. Death may occur in severe cases.

With continued oviposition fibrosis of the small bowel and liver develops. These changes are seen earlier than in *mansoni* infections, and as a result the entire disease may run its course in 2 to 5 years, ending in death.

In advanced cases the gross postmortem findings are emaciation and pallor; a large or contracted liver with periportal fibrosis; splenomegaly, with fibrosis of pulp; ascites; fibrotic nodules over the colonic peritoneum; fibrous thickening and rigidity of the colon, with small polyps projecting from the mucosa; and thickening and fibrosis of the omentum.

Clinically, signs of portal obstruction such as engorgement of superficial abdominal veins and ascites appear. Some individuals present marked splenomegaly, a small contracted liver, profound anemia, leukopenia, and thrombocytopenia associated with severe malnutrition and hypoproteinemia. The majority of individuals suffering from schistosomiasis japonica die of cirrhosis and cachexia, massive hemorrhage from rupture of esophageal varices, or intercurrent infections.

Central nervous system lesions occur more frequently in the brain than in the spinal cord, appear clinically as epilepsy in an expanding tumor, and usually result from the presence of ectopic adults.

DIAGNOSIS AND LABORATORY FINDINGS The characteristic ova must be found in the stools in order to establish the diagnosis. In established cases, ova are more difficult to demonstrate in the stools or in rectal biopsy; positive intradermal and serologic tests in suspected cases should lead to an intensive search for the egg.

TREATMENT In general, *S. japonicum* infections are more difficult to treat, and relapses are more frequent. There is debate over the preferred method of therapy. Some authorities recommend niridazole because of its limited toxicity and ability to substantially reduce worm load in most patients. Others, bothered by the relatively poor cure rate seen with this agent, prefer the more toxic and effective potassium antimony tartrate. It is administered as a freshly prepared 0.5% solution. The drug must be given slowly. Extravasation into surrounding tissue leads to painful necrosis. The initial dose is 0.04 g; subsequent doses are given on alternate days and gradually increased to a maximum of 0.12 g by the fifth dose. A total of 2.2 g should be given. The patient should be hospitalized during treatment and remain at bed rest for a few hours after each injection. If a lesion is present in the brain, prompt treatment may forestall the need for surgical intervention.

PROGNOSIS If the condition is not treated early, prognosis is poor in the majority of cases encountered in endemic communities.

SCHISTOSOMIASIS HAEMATOBIA (GENITOURINARY SCHISTOSOMIASIS, ENDEMIC HEMATURIA)

ETIOLOGY AND LIFE CYCLE The eggs are compact, elongated spindles, dilated in the middle and measuring about 140 by 50 μm. At one pole they present a short terminal spine. The ova are passed in the urine, and occasionally in the feces. The life cycle is similar to that of *S. mansoni*. The adult worms live in the hemorrhoidal plexus of veins, some going to the rectum for oviposition but most of them passing on to the vesical plexus. The intermediate hosts are snails of the genera *Bulinus, Physopsis,* and *Biomphalaria*.

PATHOGENESIS AND CLINICAL MANIFESTATIONS Large numbers of ova are deposited in the submucosa of the bladder where they incite an eosinophilic granulomatous reaction. The trigone is involved at first, but soon the entire mucosa is thickened and ulcerated. In chronic infections, the other coats become scarred and the muscularis hypertrophies. Pedunculated papillomas often develop at the trigone and about the urethral orifices. The bladder capacity becomes greatly reduced as the organ loses its contractility. Lesions occur in the distal third of the ureters in many cases, causing vesicoureteral reflux, obstruction, and hydronephrosis. Bacterial pyelonephritis may occur. In about 10 percent of cases, calculi develop in the bladder, renal pelvis, or ureters, and occasionally the entire calcified bladder can be visualized on roentgenograms. Fistulas between the urogenital tract and intestines may develop. The prostate and seminal vesicles in men and the cervix and vagina in women may be affected; lymphatic blockade with elephantiasis of the genitalia occurs rarely. Carcinoma of the bladder is a frequent late complication in Egypt but not in other areas. Because the ova are deposited in the vesical plexus, ectopic eggs are carried to the lungs where they produce miliary granulomas. Although in endemic areas the egg output usually decreases in adolescence, the pathological changes continue to progress in untreated infection.

MANIFESTATIONS Painful micturition, frequency, and terminal hematuria are the leading symptoms. Secondary bacterial infection of the urinary tract is frequent, and repeated hemorrhages from the bladder produce severe anemia. Chronic *Salmonella* bacteriuria with recurrent bouts of bacteremia have been reported from Egypt. An associated nephrotic syndrome which responds to antibiotic and anthelmintic therapy also occurred. With progressive obstruction, renal failure and uremia ensue.

DIAGNOSIS AND LABORATORY FINDINGS As in the other types of schistosomiasis, diagnosis is made by finding the characteristic ova in the urinary sediment, in tissues obtained from vesical mucosa, or, less frequently, in the stools. Egg output is highest in midmorning. Cystoscopy and biopsy of the bladder are usually diagnostic. In long-standing infections, urine cultures and intravenous urograms should be obtained.

TREATMENT Chemotherapy is very effective early in the disease and often results in dramatic reversal of symptoms and obstructive phenomena. The drugs are the same as those recommended for *S. mansoni*. Niridazole (Ambilhar) is the drug of choice. Surgery may be required for abscesses, fistulas, strictures, papillomas, and various other complications involving the bladder, but it should not be undertaken until the extent to which the lesions will resolve with medical treatment is known. Chemotherapy is indicated for secondary bacterial infections of the urinary tract, especially those caused by *Salmonella*. The criteria for cure are the absence of ova in the urine and bladder wall and the disappearance of ulcerative granulomatous lesions, as revealed by cystoscopic examination.

PROGNOSIS Provided treatment is started without delay, prognosis is good in recent infection, and fair when damage to the bladder and urinary infection have already occurred. Prognosis is very poor in chronic, late infections. After age 45, the mortality rate increases fourfold. The frequent coexistence of infection with *S. mansoni* aggravates prognosis and the clinical picture.

SCHISTOSOME DERMATITIS

DEFINITION AND GEOGRAPHIC DISTRIBUTION Certain nonhuman schistosome cercariae are capable of penetrating human skin but are unable to develop further. This results in a schistosome dermatitis similar to that seen with the species pathogenic for humans. This condition is also known as "swimmer's itch" and is common in many parts of the world. It apparently does not develop after a single contact with cercariae, but it ensues following multiple exposures. Definitive hosts of some of the schistosomes producing dermatitis are the muskrat and migratory birds. Both fresh- and saltwater mollusks serve as intermediate hosts.

Schistosome dermatitis has been reported from the freshwater areas of North Central and Western United States, Alaska, Canada, Central and South America, Western Europe (particularly Switzerland), and the Far East.

A seawater dermatitis believed to be produced by nonhuman schistosome cercariae has been reported in clam diggers and bathers along the coasts of New York, Rhode Island, California, Hawaii, and Florida.

PATHOGENESIS AND CLINICAL MANIFESTATIONS Because the dermatitis develops only after multiple exposures, it is believed to represent an allergic reaction, the nonhuman cercariae being the sensitizing agents. Exposed individuals show a positive intradermal reaction when tested with cercarial antigen. The initial symptom is usually a prickling sensation; occasionally urticaria is noted as the water evaporates from the skin. These manifestations disappear within an hour, leaving only a few macules to mark the site of cercarial penetration. Several hours later an intense itching accompanied by a papular and occasionally a vesicular rash begins. This is most intense on the second or third day and gradually subsides.

TREATMENT Local application of antipruritic lotions such as calamine with menthol or phenol is used to allay itching and thereby reduce the likelihood of secondary infection. Treatment with antihistaminic drugs will relieve the pruritus.

PREVENTION Immediate drying of the skin after swimming has been recommended as a prophylactic measure. This will not completely prevent lesions, since some penetration occurs during immersion. Dimethylphthalate cream has been reported as an effective cercarial repellent.

In some areas, control has been effected by destruction of snails. Copper sulfate and copper carbonate have been used for this purpose. Treatment of shallow waters where snails are abundant has been moderately effective.

REFERENCES

CHEEVER AW: A quantitative post-mortem study of schistosomiasis mansoni in man. Am J Trop Med 17:38, 1968

CLARK WD et al: Acute schistosomiasis mansoni in 10 boys—an outbreak in Caguas, Puerto Rico. Ann Intern Med 73:379, 1970

FALCAO HA, GOULD DB: Immune complex nephropathy in schistosomiasis. Ann Intern Med 83:148, 1975

JORDAN P: Epidemiology and control of schistosomiasis. Br Med Bull 28:55, 1972

LEHMAN JS JR et al: Urinary schistosomiasis in Egypt: Clinical, radiological, bacteriological, and parasitological correlations. Trans R Soc Trop Med Hyg 67:384, 1973

MAHMOUD AA: Current concepts—schistosomiasis. N Engl J Med 297:1329, 1977

MARCIAL-ROJAS RA, FIAL RE: Neurologic complications of schistosomiasis: Review of the literature and report of two cases of transverse myelitis due to *S. mansoni*. Ann Intern Med 59:215, 1963

ORRIS L, COMBES FC: Clam digger's dermatitis: Schistosome dermatitis from sea water. AMA Arch Dermatol Syphilol 66:367, 1952

PRATA A: Schistosomiasis mansonii. Clin Gastroenterol 7:49, 1978

SMITHERS SR: Recent advances in the immunology of schistosomiasis. Br Med Bull 28:49, 1972

WARREN KS: The pathology, pathobiology and pathogenesis of schistosomiasis. Nature (Parasitol Suppl) 273:609, 1978

———: Schistosomiasis japonicum. Clin Gastroenterol 7:77, 1978

212
OTHER TREMATODES OR FLUKES

JAMES J. PLORDE

The trematodes of humans are long-lived parasites which produce progressive damage to the tissues of their hosts. With the exception of schistosomes, they are similar in morphology and life cycle. The adult flukes are flat, leaflike hermaphrodites that vary in length from a few millimeters to several centimeters. Their digestive tract, unlike that of the nematodes, ends blindly. As their name indicates, they have two "holes" in the form of oral and ventral suckers which are used as organs of attachment and locomotion. The operculated eggs, which are passed in the feces or sputum, hatch in the water to produce a ciliated, free-swimming *miracidium*. The miracidium reaches and penetrates the tissue of an intermediate snail host to undergo a period of development, eventuating in the release of thousands of swarms of free-living *cercariae* from the snail. These thousands of tail-bearing larvae must, in turn, reach a second intermediate host, usually an aquatic animal or vegetation, where they encyst forming *metacercariae*. The definitive host is infected when he or she ingests the parasitized second intermediate host. The distribution of flukes is usually limited by the location of their molluscan intermediate host. With the exception of *Opisthorchis* and *Fasciola*, most hermaphroditic flukes are found only in tropical or subtropical areas.

PARAGONIMIASIS

DEFINITION Paragonimiasis (endemic hemoptysis) is a chronic infection of the lung caused by trematodes of the genus *Paragonimus*. Clinically, the disease is characterized by cough and hemoptysis. Ectopic worms may cause a variety of other manifestations. Geographically, it is probably the most widely distributed disease caused by hermaphroditic flukes.

ETIOLOGY AND EPIDEMIOLOGY Although *P. westermani*, which is widely distributed in the Far East, is the most common cause of human paragonimiasis, a number of other species, including *P. skrjabini, P. heterotremus* (China), *P. africanus, P. uterobilateralis* (Cameroons, Nigeria, and Zaire), *P. mexicanus, P. peruvianus,* and *P. caliensis* (Central and South America), may cause the disease. The short, plump adults (7 to 12 mm in length, 4 to 6 mm in width) have a life span of 4 to 5 years which they typically spend encysted in the lung parenchyma of the host. Their golden-brown operculated eggs (50 by 90 µm) reach the bronchioles from where they are coughed up and excreted in the sputum or swallowed and passed in the feces. They must embryonate several weeks in fresh water before hatching to release the miracidia.

The infection is acquired by ingestion of cysts in the second intermediate host, a crab or crayfish. The metacercariae excyst in the duodenum, burrow through the intestinal wall into the peritoneal cavity, and then usually migrate through the diaphragm and into the lung. The worms also may be found in the intestinal wall, liver, pancreas, kidney, mesentery, skeletal muscle, subcutaneous tissues, and central nervous system, particularly the brain. The dog, cat, pig, rat, and wild carnivores are definitive hosts for the parasite in addition to humans. In some of these, very young adults can be found in their striated muscles. Human infection has been reported following the ingestion of this undercooked flesh.

The incidence of paragonimiasis is often affected by food shortages or local customs. The metacercariae survive in vinegar, and lightly pickled or inadequately cooked food usually serves as the source of infection in the Far East. Fresh crab juice used for the treatment of measles in Korea and for infertility in the Cameroons may also transmit the parasite. Children may acquire the disease in endemic areas while handling or eating raw crabs during play.

PATHOGENESIS AND CLINICAL MANIFESTATIONS An eosinophilic granuloma forms about the adult worm, eventually leading to the formation of a fibrous cyst. The pulmonary lesions which measure up to 1 cm in diameter frequently communicate with a bronchiole, resulting in secondary bacterial infection. Small, fibrous nodules representing reaction around deposited eggs also occur. Clinically the picture is one of chronic bronchitis and bronchiectasis with production of brownish sputum and hemoptysis. A poorly resolving pulmonary infiltrate, lung abscess, or pleural effusion may be present in heavy infections. The roentgenographic findings vary with the stage of infection. Initially one or more soft infiltrates may be seen anywhere in the lungs excepting the apexes. These are then gradually replaced by round nodules which not infrequently cavitate. Eventually, fibrosis and calcification occur, presenting a picture closely resembling tuberculosis, a disease which often coexists with paragonimiasis.

An abdominal mass, pain, and dysentery characterize intestinal or peritoneal infections. Various types of paralysis and epilepsy occur in cerebral involvement. Homonymous hemianopsia, optic atrophy, and papilledema are common. The cerebrospinal fluid usually shows an eosinophilic leukocytosis and elevated protein. Cerebral calcifications are seen on x-ray in 50 percent of cases. *Paragonimus skrjabini* infections are characterized by migratory subcutaneous nodules that contain adult flukes.

LABORATORY FINDINGS Eosinophilia is a constant finding. Definitive diagnosis depends upon finding the characteristic operculated ova in the sputum, stool, pleural fluid, or tissue. Eggs may be rare or totally absent from the sputum during the first 3 months of infection but are eventually found in 75 to 85 percent of infected patients. Even later, however, repeated examinations using concentration techniques may be required for their recovery. Ziehl-Neelsen staining, often carried out for suspected tuberculosis, usually will not demonstrate the eggs. In fact, the sputum concentration techniques for tuberculosis may destroy the eggs that are present. Stool examination is frequently helpful in children. A complement fixation test is available, and the results correlate well with active infection. It usually becomes negative within 6 months of successful therapy. The skin test does not distinguish present and past infections and is used primarily for epidemiologic purposes.

TREATMENT AND PREVENTION Bithionol is the drug of choice. From 30 to 40 mg/kg in divided doses should be given every other day for a total of 10 to 15 treatment days. The symptoms disappear rapidly, and most infiltrates resolve within 3 months. Side effects are minor and consist of nausea, vomiting, and urticaria. Concomitant bacterial infection must be treated. Prevention of superinfection by the same parasite is important, because the disease is self-limiting.

The most practical control measure is the adequate cooking of all shellfish before they are eaten.

CLONORCHIASIS

DEFINITION Clonorchiasis is an infection of the biliary passages caused by *Clonorchis sinensis,* the most important liver fluke of humans. Although the infection is usually asymptomatic, heavy worm loads may produce manifestations of biliary obstruction.

ETIOLOGY AND EPIDEMIOLOGY *Clonorchis sinensis* is a small fluke (5 by 15 mm) that lives as long as 50 years in the biliary tree of its host. Here the flukes feed on mucosal secretions and pass operculated eggs into the feces. On reaching fresh water, the eggs are ingested by the intermediate snail host. After multiplication and development within the snail, the cercariae are released and penetrate freshwater fish. Infections result from ingestion of the raw, dried, salted, or pickled flesh of freshwater fish containing encysted metacercariae. The larva is released in the duodenum. It enters the common bile duct and migrates to the second-order bile ducts, where it develops into the adult form in about 1 month. In addition to humans, dogs, cats, pigs, and rats serve as disease reservoirs. The main endemic areas are Korea, Japan, Taiwan, Hong Kong, Southern China, and Vietnam where clonorchiasis may be perpetuated by the practice of fertilizing fish ponds with manure and human feces. Twenty-five percent of the population of Hong Kong and a small proportion of Chinese immigrants to this country have been shown to be infected. The disease may also be acquired in the United States by the ingestion of infected, dried, frozen, or pickled fish imported from the Far East. Clinically, apparent cases are restricted to the adult population in whom the accumulated worm load eventually produces pathological effects.

PATHOGENESIS AND CLINICAL MANIFESTATIONS Light infections are usually asymptomatic, but worm loads of 500 to 1000 flukes often result in clinical manifestations. During the migration of the larvae, the patient may have fever, chills, tender hepatomegaly, mild jaundice, and eosinophilia. The mature worm causes proliferation of the biliary epithelium, increased mucin production, adenoma formation, chronic pericholangitis, and periductal fibrosis. Hepatic parenchymal damage and portal hypertension are not seen in uncomplicated infections. Recurrent attacks of suppurative cholangitis with or without intrahepatic choledocholithiasis may follow biliary obstruction with dead flukes. These occasionally present as hypoglycemic coma. The occurrence of biliary stones in clonorchiasis is associated with an increased incidence of chronic *Salmonella typhi* carriage. Cholangiocarcinoma may occur in patients with severe, long-standing infections. The adult worms may infest the pancreatic ducts, where they can cause squamous metaplasia, periductal fibrosis, and acute pancreatitis.

LABORATORY DIAGNOSIS Clinical and epidemiologic findings often suggest the diagnosis. There may be elevation of the alkaline phosphatase and hyperbilirubinemia. Eosinophilia is variable. Occasionally, a plain film of the abdomen will demonstrate intrahepatic calcification. Liver scan is usually negative in asymptomatic infections but may show multiple areas of diminished uptake in acute symptomatic disease. Percutaneous transhepatic cholangiography in such patients often reveals dilatation of the peripheral intrahepatic bile ducts. The adult worms appear as round filling defects several millimeters in diameter. Definitive diagnosis depends on the demonstration of the eggs in the feces or the duodenal contents. They measure 29 by 16 μm, possess a conspicuous opercular rim as well as a posterior knob, and can be distinguished from the eggs of *Metagonimus, Heterophyes*, and *Opisthorchis* only with difficulty. An antigen extracted from adult worms can be used in a complement fixation test for the detection of the host's antibody response. Skin tests are also useful.

TREATMENT AND PREVENTION No consistently effective treatment is known, but some success has been noted with chloroquine diphosphate. Chloroquine is prescribed in a dose of 0.25 g three times daily for 6 weeks. Disturbances of mentation, vision, and gastrointestinal function are common during such prolonged therapy and may require a decrease in the daily dosage of chloroquine. In the majority of cases, egg output returns to pretreatment levels within 6 months, suggesting that the treatment of asymptomatic infections is not warranted. A number of experimental drugs have shown more satisfactory results in both experimental animal infection and humans; none are presently available in the United States. Thorough cooking of freshwater fish will prevent infection.

OPISTHORCHIASIS

Opisthorchiasis is caused by *Opisthorchis felineus* or *O. viverrini* and is characterized by hepatic lesions produced by adult worms in the larger bile ducts. The life cycle resembles that of *C. sinensis*. The geographic distribution differs in that *O. felineus* is endemic in Eastern and Central Europe and in Siberia and occurs in some parts of Asia, while *O. viverrini* is found in Thailand and Laos. Cats and wild carnivores act as the principal reservoir hosts, and the infection is found most commonly along rivers and lakes which harbor an abundant fish life. Up to 25 percent of inhabitants of northeastern Thailand are purported to carry the parasite. The clinical lesions are similar to those seen in clonorchiasis except that gallstones are rare. The diagnosis usually is based on the finding of the eggs in the feces

or duodenal contents. Treatment as recommended for clonorchiasis may be used. Infection can be prevented by eating only well-cooked fish.

FASCIOLIASIS

Fascioliasis is caused by *Fasciola hepatica*, which like *Clonorchis*, inhabits the bile ducts of the definitive host. When fully matured, the adult measures about 3 by 1 cm and discharges large operculate eggs 140 by 70 μm which must embryonate in fresh water before hatching.

Fascioliasis produces so-called "liver rot" in sheep, the principal definitive host. The disease is most common in sheep and cattle-raising countries but has been reported from many parts of the world. In North America it occurs in the Southern and Western United States, Central America, and in the Caribbean Islands.

Infection is contracted by ingestion of the encysted forms of the fluke attached to edible aquatic plants such as watercress. The larvae excyst in the duodenum, migrate through the intestinal wall, pass into the peritoneal cavity, penetrate the liver capsule, and finally reach the bile ducts, where they mature. Occasionally larvae may migrate to and mature in ectopic locations including subcutaneous tissue, chest cavity, or brain.

Early clinical manifestations are related to the migration of the larval form to and within the liver. Epigastric pain, fever, diarrhea, jaundice, urticaria, pruritus, arthralgia, and eosinophilia may be observed during this stage. Fibrosis of the liver similar to that found in clonorchiasis appears only after prolonged residence of many adult worms in the bile ducts. Obstruction of the bile duct occurs frequently and may be the presenting manifestation of disease. A pharyngeal form of the disease, called *halzoun*, can result from eating infected raw liver, the young adults attaching themselves to the pharyngeal mucosa, occasionally interfering with respiration.

The diagnosis usually is based on the finding of the eggs in the feces or in the duodenal contents. It is difficult to distinguish the eggs from those of *Fasciolopsis buski*. Complement fixation, hemagglutination, and precipitin tests have been reported to be helpful. A skin test is also available.

Treatment is unsatisfactory. Dehydroemetine dehydrochloride, 1 mg/kg per day intramuscularly for 10 days, may be helpful and at times curative. The drug should not be given to patients with chronic cardiac or renal disease or to children. Bithionol in an oral dose of 50 mg/kg every other day for 10 to 15 doses has also been effective and may be less toxic.

To prevent infection, aquatic plants such as watercress should not be eaten, vegetables grown in fields irrigated with polluted water should be boiled, and safe drinking water should be provided.

FASCIOLOPSIASIS

Fasciolopsiasis is caused by the large intestinal fluke *F. buski*, which inhabits the upper part of the intestine of its definitive host. The principal definitive host is the pig. In parts of China, India, and other areas in the Far East, infection of humans occurs following ingestion, or peeling with the teeth, of water chestnuts and other edible aquatic plants. The large adults attach themselves to the intestinal mucosa, and these sites may later ulcerate. The infection is usually asymptomatic. In heavy infections, diarrhea, abdominal pain, gastrointestinal hemorrhage, and intestinal obstruction may appear early. Later, asthenia with ascites and anasarca occurs. Diagnosis is based upon the history and the finding of eggs in the feces. The eggs resemble those of *Fasciola hepatica*. The prognosis in untreated heavy infections, especially in children, is poor. Tetrachloroethylene as given for hookworm infections is effective. Hexylresorcinol can also be expected to cure or markedly reduce the worm burden in the majority of cases.

HETEROPHYIASIS AND METAGONIMIASIS

Heterophyes heterophyes and *Metagonimus yakagawa* are small intestinal flukes of humans and other fish-eating mammals. They are found in the Far East and, in the case of *Heterophyes,* in India, Egypt, and Tunisia. Both are acquired by ingesting the raw or undercooked flesh of metacercarial-infected freshwater fish. The 2- to 3-mm adults attach themselves to the mucosa of the small intestine. If present in sufficient numbers, they may cause abdominal pain and/or diarrhea. Rarely the eggs have been found in sites such as the brain, spinal cord, or heart where they produce granulomatous lesions. Most commonly, they are passed in the stool where they very closely resemble those of *Clonorchis*. Both species can be treated with tetrachloroethylene as outlined in Chap. 210 for hookworm. As the life span of these trematodes is limited to a year or less, treatment is not indicated unless the patient is symptomatic.

REFERENCES

CHAN PH, TEOH TB: The pathology of *Clonorchis sinensis* infestation of the pancreas. J Pathol Bacteriol 93:185, 1967

JONES EA et al: Massive infection with *Fasciola hepatica* in man. Am J Med 63:842, 1977

KOENIGSTEIN RP: Observations on the epidemiology of infections with *Clonorchis sinensis.* Trans R Soc Trop Med Hyg 42:503, 1949

McFADZEAN AJS, YEUNG RTT: Hypoglycemia in suppurative pancholangitis due to Clonorchis sinensis. Trans R Soc Trop Med Hyg 59:179, 1965

OKUNDA K et al: Clonorchiasis studied by percutaneous cholangiogram and a therapeutic trial of 2,4-diisothiocyanate. Gastroenterology 65:457, 1973

PLANT AG et al: A clinical study of *Fasciolopsis buski* in Thailand. Trans R Soc Trop Med Hyg 63:470, 1969

SADUN EH, BUCK AA: Paragonimiasis in South Korea—Immunodiagnostic, epidemiologic, clinical, roentgenologic and therapeutic studies. Am J Trop Med 9:562, 1960

SEAH SKK: Digenetic trematodes. Clin Gastroenterol 7:87, 1978

YOKOGAWA M: *Paragonimus* and paragonimiasis. Exp Parasitol 10:81, 139, 1960

———: *Paragonimus* and paragonimiasis, in *Advances in Parasitology,* vol 7, B Dawes (ed). London, Academic, 1969, p 375

213
CESTODE (TAPEWORM) INFECTIONS

JAMES J. PLORDE

The tapeworms, or cestodes, are segmented ribbon-shaped hermaphroditic worms which inhabit the intestinal tract of many vertebrates. Unlike other helminths, these parasites lack a digestive tract, and they absorb food through their entire surface. Attachment to the host's intestinal mucosa is effected by means of sucking cups or grooves located on the head, or *scolex*. In some species, the head is also armed with hooklets which aid in attachment. Behind the globular scolex lies a short, narrow neck from which segments or *proglottides* de-

velop one at a time to form the chainlike *strobila* of the worm. These proglottides progressively mature as they are displaced further and further from the neck by the formation of newer segments. As each section reaches gravidity, it releases its mass of eggs by passing them through a uterine pore, by splitting open, or by simply disintegrating. Because the eggs of many tapeworms appear identical, species identification depends on the morphological characteristics of the scolex or gravid proglottides.

Except for *Hymenolepis nana* the tapeworm parasites of humans require one or more intermediate hosts for larval development. Among the *Taenia* group, there is a single intermediate. The eggs or *onchospheres* are passed onto the soil and ingested by the intermediate host in whose tissues they develop into cystlike structures. If the cyst contains a single scolex, it is referred to as a *cysticercus,* or *cysticercoid* in the case of *H. nana.* If several scolices develop within the cyst, it is called a *coenurus* (see "Coenurosis" below). However, if daughter cysts, each containing several scolices are formed, the structure is referred to as a hydatid (see "Echinococciasis" below).

Organisms belonging to the *Diphyllobothrium* genus require two intermediate hosts. The eggs, unlike those of the *Taenia* group, are operculated and must be deposited in fresh water. Here they hatch, releasing a free-swimming larva or *coracidium*. This is ingested by a suitable crustacean, the first intermediate host, and is transformed into a procercoid larva. If the infected crustacean is then swallowed by a freshwater fish, the larva invades the tissues of this second intermediate and develops into a plerocercoid larvae or sparganum (see "Sparganosis" below). In both the *Taenia* and *Diphyllobothrium* groups the definitive host is infected after ingesting the flesh of an intermediate host containing the infective larval form.

Human tapeworm infections fall into one of two major clinical groups. In the first, represented by taeniasis *saginata,* humans act as the definitive host, harboring the adult tapeworm in their intestine. In the second, humans are an intermediate host, and harbor the larval forms in their tissues. This is exemplified by sparganosis, coenurosis, and echinococcosis. Taeniasis *solium* is unique because the human may act both as the definitive and intermediate host.

TAENIASIS SAGINATA

DEFINITION Taeniasis saginata is an intestinal infection of humans caused by the beef tapeworm.

ETIOLOGY AND PATHOGENESIS In its adult stage, *Taenia saginata* inhabits the upper jejunum where it may survive for as long as 25 years. The cestode is 5 to 10 m in length and possesses a small, unarmed scolex with four prominent suckers and between 1000 and 2000 proglottides. The gravid segments are longer than they are wide (5 by 20 mm) and have 15 to 30 lateral uterine branches, thus distinguishing it from *T. solium,* which has 8 to 12. The eggs, which are passed within the intact proglottid, measure 30 by 40 μm, have a thick brown radially striated shell, and contain a fully developed embryo with three pairs of hooklets. They are indistinguishable from those of *T. solium.* After the eggs are deposited on soil or vegetation, they are ingested by cattle or other herbivores. The embryo is released in the intestine, invades the intestinal wall, and is carried by vascular channels to striated muscle in the hind limbs, diaphragm, and tongue. Here it is filtered out and is transformed over a period of 3 or 4 months into an ovoid bladder worm, or cysticercus. This form, which may remain viable for 1 to 3 years, measures about 5 by 10 mm and consists of a scolex held in a cystlike structure. After ingestion of the cyst in raw or undercooked beef by humans, about 2 months is required for the adult worm to develop in the intestine.

EPIDEMIOLOGY Taeniasis saginata occurs in all countries in which it is the custom to eat raw or undercooked beef. It is particularly prevalent in Ethiopia, Kenya, the Middle East, Yugoslavia, Mexico, and parts of South America and the U.S.S.R. Beef tapeworm transmission, although uncommon, continues to occur in the United States, particularly in the Northeastern and Western parts of the country.

CLINICAL MANIFESTATIONS In probably the majority of cases the disease is asymptomatic. Epigastric discomfort, diarrhea, hunger sensations, weight loss, irritability, nausea, and rarely an increase in appetite have been reported in association with *T. saginata* infections.

Movements of the worm are sometimes apparent, and occasionally proglottides may crawl through the anus, appearing in the bed linen or underclothing of the distraught host. Rarely, segments become impacted in the appendix or cystic or pancreatic duct producing obstruction and inflammation of these organs.

LABORATORY FINDINGS The diagnosis is usually made by the finding of proglottides in the feces. Several proglottides are shed daily, making their recovery relatively easy. Eggs may be distributed on the stool or perianal area if a proglottid ruptures during defecation, and should be looked for in the absence of segments. The perianal region may be examined as for pinworm infection, using the Scotch-brand tape swab. By this method 85 to 95 percent of infections may be detected, whereas by stool examination only 50 to 75 percent can be recognized. Since the eggs cannot be distinguished from those of *T. solium*, it is necessary to examine carefully either the proglottides or the scolex to identify the tapeworm species correctly.

TREATMENT Niclosamide (Yomesan) is a highly effective taenicide which kills the scolex and immature segments of the worm on contact. This drug may be given without preparation or purge in a single 2-g dose. Four 0.5-g tablets are thoroughly chewed at one time and swallowed with a small amount of water. Few side effects have been reported. As the worm is digested before it is passed in the stool, no attempt should be made to recover the scolex. The stool should be checked at 3 and 6 months to be certain a cure has been obtained. Alternatively, paromomycin, 1.0 g orally every 15 min for four doses, may be given. Quinacrine hydrochloride (Atabrine), for many years the standard medication for tapeworm, has been largely supplanted by the above medications because of its inconvenience and side effects. The agent does possess the advantage that the entire worm including the scolex is excreted intact, allowing morphological identification.

PREVENTION The only practical means of preventing infection is the thorough cooking of beef. Temperatures as low as 56°C for as little as 5 min will destroy cysticerci. Refrigeration and salting for prolonged periods or freezing at −10°C for 5 days also destroys the cysticercus. Adequate meat inspection and proper disposal of human excreta also aid in control.

TAENIASIS SOLIUM AND CYSTICERCOSIS

DEFINITION *Taenia solium,* the pork tapeworm, inhabits the intestinal lumen of humans, its only definitive host. The usual intermediate host is the hog, but in some circumstances, the larval or intermediate stages may also develop in humans, resulting in a condition referred to as *cysticercosis.*

EPIDEMIOLOGY Taeniasis solium is worldwide but is most common in the U.S.S.R., Eastern Europe, Asia, Africa, Mexico, and South America. At the present time the disease is practically nonexistent in the United States.

ETIOLOGY AND PATHOGENESIS The hermaphroditic adult resides in the upper jejunum and like *T. saginata* may live for decades. It is about 3 m in length and possesses a globular scolex containing a rostellum with two rows of hooklets. There are seldom more than 1000 proglottides. The gravid proglottid measures about 6 by 12 mm and contains a uterus with 8 to 12 lateral branchings. The eggs resemble those of *T. saginata* but are infective for both human and hog. Although humans may be autoinfected when gravid segments are returned to the stomach by reverse peristalsis, the eggs are more commonly transmitted by the fecal-oral route. When ova are ingested by the intermediate host, the embryo is released from the egg, penetrates the intestinal wall, and is carried by vascular channels to all parts of the body. Localization with development over a period of 2 to 3 months to the encysted larval stage ("bladder worm") occurs predominantly in striated muscle of the tongue, neck, and trunk. The cysticerci are ovoid, gray-white opalescent structures about 1 cm in diameter. They may survive for up to 5 years. Humans become infected with the adult stage following ingestion of undercooked pork containing cysticerci. The scolex is freed and attaches itself to the intestinal mucosa; development to the adult stage begins at this time.

CLINICAL MANIFESTATIONS Clinical manifestations of adult worm infestation resemble those associated with *T. saginata*. The clinical picture is entirely different when humans serve as the intermediate host. Cysticerci develop in the subcutaneous tissues, in muscles, in viscera, and—of most significance—in the eye and brain. Only a moderate tissue reaction occurs while the scolex is viable, but symptoms occur only in heavy infections. The dead larva, however, behaves as a foreign body and provokes a marked tissue response with muscular pains, weakness, fever, and eosinophilia. The involvement in the brain may be in the form of a meningoencephalitis when the cysticerci are widely distributed. However, epilepsy, brain tumor, encephalitis, and other types of neurological or psychiatric disorders may be simulated. Degenerated cysticerci ultimately calcify.

Infection with the adult worm can be detected by finding eggs in perianal scrapings or in the feces. However, to differentiate *T. solium* from *T. saginata* infection, proglottides or the scolex must be examined. Cysticercosis should be suspected in an individual who has lived in a hyperendemic area and who develops neurological findings. Biopsy of subcutaneous nodules may lead to the identification of typical encysted larvae. Roentgenograms of the soft tissues also often reveal calcified cysticerci. Cerebral arteriography, EEG, or computerized tomography (CT) or radioisotope scan will demonstrate the presence of several small space-occupying lesions. The cysticercosis hemagglutination or complement fixation test may be of help in the diagnosis. The prognosis is in large part determined by the stage and location of the parasite. Surgery may be necessary in cerebral and ocular cysticercosis.

TREATMENT For removal of the worm in the adult, Niclosamide or paromomycin is given as for taeniasis saginata above. However, because these drugs result in the maceration of worms with release of ova, cysticercosis could theoretically occur. To prevent this, a saline purge should be administered 1 h after completion of therapy.

COENUROSIS

This is a rare infection of humans by the larval stage, or *coenurus,* of the dog tapeworm *Multiceps multiceps.* As in cysticercosis, the subcutaneous tissue, eye, and central nervous system may be involved. Over 60 cases have been reported from around the world. In tropical areas the brain has usually been involved and the cases have ended fatally. Clinically, the presentation is one of a slowly growing tumor. Diagnosis and treatment both rely on surgical excision of the lesion.

HYMENOLEPIASIS NANA

DEFINITION Hymenolepiasis nana is an intestinal infection of humans, mice, and rats by *Hymenolepis nana,* the dwarf tapeworm. The infection is particularly common in children in whom it is usually asymptomatic.

ETIOLOGY The life cycle is unique in that both the larval and adult phases occur in the same host. The small, 2-cm adult lives only a few weeks, during which time it can be found in the proximal ileum. Its proglottides are wider than they are long and may number 100 to 200. The gravid segments break apart in the fecal stream releasing their spherical eggs. These measure 30 by 44 μm in diameter and have a double membrane enclosing the embryo with six hooklets. The inner vitelline membrane has four to eight slender filaments arising from each pole. The eggs are immediately infective and when ingested by a new host, the freed oncospheres penetrate the intestinal villi, becoming cysticercoids. Approximately 2 weeks later, the larvae migrate back to the intestinal lumen, attach themselves to the mucosa, and mature into adult worms. In some situations, the eggs hatch before passing in the stool, causing internal autoinfection.

DISTRIBUTION Dwarf tapeworm infection has been reported in temperate and tropical regions around the globe. It is the most common tapeworm found in the United States, most of the infections occurring in the Southern states. The infection is spread by the direct fecal-oral route and is most common in children and institutional populations.

CLINICAL MANIFESTATIONS This tapeworm infection is characterized by the presence of many adult worms in the host's intestine. When infection is massive, diarrhea and abdominal pain occur.

TREATMENT Niclosamide, as prescribed for taeniasis saginata above, is given each day for five consecutive doses. Children under 8 should receive one-half the adult daily dose and infants one-fourth the adult dose. Cure is obtained in 90 percent of patients. Paromomycin, 45 mg/kg daily for 5 to 7 days, may also be effective.

PREVENTION This is a difficult problem, similar to that encountered in enterobiasis. Only a single host is involved, and the eggs are immediately infective. Personal hygiene should be stressed. The contamination of food by rats and mice should be prevented.

HYMENOLEPIASIS DIMINUTA

Hymenolepis diminuta is a short-lived cestode of rats and mice that occasionally infects small children. Larval development

occurs in a wide variety of insect hosts including fleas and mealworms. Humans become infected with the adult tapeworm when they ingest uncooked cereal foods contaminated with these insects. Infection is usually asymptomatic, and the diagnosis is made only when the characteristic eggs are found in the stool. They resemble those of *H. nana,* but are longer (58 by 86 μm) and lack polar filaments. Niclosamide as prescribed for hymenolepiasis nana is the treatment of choice.

DIPYLIDIASIS

Dipylidium caninum is the common tapeworm of cats and dogs. The orange-brown proglottid, which resembles a pumpkin seed, is often passed intact in the stool or migrates through the anal canal. This may cause animals harboring this parasite to drag their buttocks across the floor. The characteristic egg packets are then expelled by the proglottides and ingested by fleas to develop into infective larval forms. The definitive host becomes infected by swallowing involved fleas. Human infections occur primarily in small children who ingest fleas in the process of playing with their pets. The diagnosis is made by recovering the characteristic proglottid or egg packet. Treatment is the same as for *T. saginata* above. Prevention consists of periodic deworming of pets.

DIPHYLLOBOTHRIASIS LATUM

DEFINITION *Diphyllobothrium latum,* the fish tapeworm or broad tapeworm, produces a disease in its definitive host, including humans, characterized by the presence of the adult worm in the intestinal lumen.

ETIOLOGY AND PATHOGENESIS The adult *Diphyllobothrium* lies attached to the mucosa of the ileum and occasionally jejunum by a pair of sucking grooves located on the scolex. It may live up to 20 years and achieve a length of 10 to 30 ft. The 3000 to 4000 proglottides are wider than they are long. Unlike *Taenia,* the gravid segments are retained by the worm, and each day a million operculated ova are passed directly in the stool. On reaching water, the egg hatches, releasing a free-swimming embryo. This is eaten by small freshwater crustaceans belonging to the species *Cyclops* or *Diaptomus,* in which it develops into a *procercoid.* When the infected crustacean is swallowed by a fish, the larva migrates into the flesh and grows into a *plerocercoid,* or *sparganum,* larva. Humans are infected by ingesting raw infected fish. The tapeworm matures in the intestine and after 3 weeks is an adult capable of discharging eggs.

EPIDEMIOLOGY The infection is common in the Baltic and Scandinavian countries, Switzerland, Italy, Russia, Japan, Chile, and Central Africa. It also occurs in the north central United States, south central Canada, and Florida. The maintenance of infection in these areas depends upon the continued disposal of raw sewage into freshwater lakes and the ingestion of improperly prepared fish. Women who sample lutefish or gefilte fish as they prepare these dishes often become infected. Among Ontario Indians, the infection is acquired by the ingestion of salted fresh fish.

CLINICAL MANIFESTATIONS Most infections are asymptomatic or produce slight, transient abdominal discomfort. Rarely, there may be severe cramping abdominal pain, vomiting, weakness, and loss of weight. Intestinal obstruction has been reported in multiple infections. In a small percentage of infected patients, a tapeworm anemia develops which has many features in common with Addisonian pernicious anemia including central nervous system involvement. The anemia appears to be related to the ability of the tapeworm to compete successfully with its host for vitamin B_{12}. A worm located high in the jejunum may take up 80 to 100 percent of labeled vitamin B_{12} ingested by a patient with anemia. Approximately forty percent of fish tapeworm carriers have low serum vitamin B_{12} levels, but only 0.1 to 2 percent develop anemia. These patients tend to be elderly, have diminished production of intrinsic factor, and have worms located in the proximal small bowel. Folate absorption may also be diminished and contribute to the anemia. It has been suggested that lysolecithin, a product of the tapeworm, contributes to the severity of the disease. Neurological manifestations of vitamin B_{12} deficiency are more common than in pernicious anemia and may occur in the absence of hematologic findings. Typically, they include paresthesias, impaired vibration sense, numbness, weakness, and, less commonly, central scotomas secondary to optic atrophy. These findings are reversible with expulsion of the worm.

DIAGNOSIS The characteristic eggs are discharged into the stools in large numbers, making the diagnosis quite easy. They measure 55 to 76 by 41 to 56 μm and possess a single shell with an operculum at one end and a knob on the other. Eosinophilia is often present.

TREATMENT Treatment as prescribed for taeniasis saginata will cure most infections. In the presence of severe macrocytic anemia, parenteral vitamin B_{12} should be given.

PREVENTION The most practical control measure is prohibiting the disposal of untreated sewage into freshwater lakes. Personal protection consists of thorough cooking of all freshwater fish. Freezing of fish at $-10°C$ for 24 to 48 h will also prevent transmission.

SPARGANOSIS

The *sparganum*, or plerocercoid larva, of *Diphyllobothrium*-related tapeworms belonging to the genus *Spirometra* will develop in humans following ingestion (usually in drinking water) of a *Cyclops* bearing the procercoid larva. Sparganosis also follows ingestion of infected frogs or application of infected fresh frog flesh as a poultice. The frog tissues contain the sparganum, which is capable of invading human tissues. The dog and cat are definitive hosts for *Spirometra*. The infection often presents as a painful subcutaneous swelling. The periorbital tissues may be involved with marked palpebral edema and destruction of the globe. A marked eosinophilia is usually present. The location of the larvae determines the prognosis of the infection in humans. Surgery and injection of ethyl alcohol with epinephrine-free procaine to kill the worms is the preferred method of treatment.

ECHINOCOCCIASIS

DEFINITION Echinococciasis is a tissue infection of humans caused by the larval stage of *Echinococcus granulosus* or *E. multilocularis*. These species of echinococcus are distinct morphologically and biologically. In humans, *E. granulosus* produces cystic, expanding lesions, involving the liver and lungs primarily, whereas the lesions of *E. multilocularis* are destructive because of their invasive character.

ETIOLOGY The adult *E. granulosus* is found in the jejunum of dogs, wolves, and other canines, where it may live for 5 to 20 months. It is a small worm measuring 5 mm in length. In addition to the scolex and neck, it has three proglottides, one immature, one mature, and one gravid. The gravid segment

splits, either before or after passage in the stool, to release eggs, which appear identical to those of *T. saginata*. When ingested by an appropriate intermediate host such as sheep, cattle, hogs, deer, camels, or humans, the embryos escape from the eggs, penetrate the intestinal mucosa, and enter the portal circulation. Approximately 60 percent are filtered out by the liver; 25 percent lodge in the lung, and the rest are carried into the general circulation to involve the brain, kidney, bones, and other tissues. The larvae that are not phagocytosed and destroyed develop into hydatid cysts, reaching the diameter of 1 cm within 5 months. Most cysts are unilocular and consist of an external laminated cuticula and an inner germinal layer. Fluid fills and distends the cyst. Brood capsules and second- or third-generation daughter cysts develop from the germinal layer. "Hydatid sand" found in the cyst consists of scolices liberated from ruptured brood capsules. Occasionally, evagination of the cyst wall occurs, with the development of a multilocular or alveolar type of lesion. In bone, the cysts are semisolid, invade the medullary cavity and slowly erode bone, producing pathological fractures. The cycle is completed when the hydatid cyst is ingested by a carnivore. The enormous number of scolices are released in the intestine and develop into adult worms. The life cycle of *E. multilocularis* is similar except that small rodents serve as the natural intermediate hosts, and the hydatid cyst is always of the multilocular or alveolar type. Most of the cysts develop in the liver, and progressive invasion of that organ usually occurs. The lesions may metastasize when growth extends into blood vessels.

EPIDEMIOLOGY The dog is the principal definitive host of *E. granulosa*. Sheep, cattle, and, in the Middle East, camels are common intermediates. Human echinococciasis, which is often acquired in childhood, has its highest incidence in countries where sheep and cattle raising is carried out with the help of dogs, particularly in East and South Africa, the Middle East, Central Europe, South America, Australia, and New Zealand. It has been reported from 15 states in this country, but most of these infections were probably contracted outside the United States. Only about 7 percent of cases diagnosed in this country are thought to be autochthonus. Most of these involve well-defined population groups, including the Southwestern Indians, Basque sheep farmers in California, and sheep raisers in Utah. A "sylvatic" focus of *E. granulosa* (var. *canadensis*) exists in Alaska and western Canada, where wolves act as the definitive host and caribou and moose as the intermediate host. A second sylvatic cycle involving deer and coyotes has been reported from California. When humans kill these herbivores and feed their viscera to dogs, a domestic cycle is initiated.

In *E. multilocularis* infection, rodents and deer mice are the natural intermediate hosts, while wolves, foxes, and coyotes serve as definitive hosts. A domestic dog and cat may also harbor the adult worms, and an urban cycle involving the cat and common house mouse has been described. Human infections have been reported from Russia, Central Europe, Canada, and Alaska. An extensive sylvatic focus has been described in the north central United States.

CLINICAL MANIFESTATIONS Enlarging hydatid cysts usually produce tissue damage by mechanical means. The resulting symptoms depend upon the site, type, and rate of growth of the cystic lesions. Approximately one-third of infected patients are asymptomatic when the diagnosis is made by routine medical examination. Of the remainder, most present with the complaint of local discomfort or pain of insidious onset. In 15 percent, however, hydatid rupture initiates an acute emergent illness. Most patients harbor a single hydatid, but as many as 40 percent may have multiple cysts involving more than a single site. The hydatids of *E. granulosa* var. *canadensis,* which occur principally in the lung, are small, grow very slowly, seldom cause symptoms, and are usually discovered on routine chest x-ray. The unilocular hydatids produced by other strains of *E. granulosa* grow somewhat more rapidly (0.25 to 1 cm per year) and eventually may reach enormous size. One-fifth rupture to produce cough, chest pain, and hemoptysis. Hepatic lesions may remain asymptomatic for 5 to 20 years, finally presenting as a palpable abdominal mass or abdominal pain. Rupture through the diaphragm, into the peritoneal cavity, or, most commonly, into the biliary tree occurs in 7 percent of patients. Intrabiliary extrusion often mimics acute recurrent cholecystitis. Obstruction of the bile duct may result in jaundice. Bone lesions with pathological fractures occur, and central nervous system involvement may be manifested by epilepsy or blindness. Cardiac cysts may produce embolic metastases. Unilocular lesions may be secondarily infected, resulting in abscess formation and sterilization of the cyst. Rupture of a hydatid into the bile duct, peritoneal cavity, lung, pleura, or bronchus may produce fever, pruritus, urticarial rash, or an anaphylactoid reaction which is occasionally fatal. Release of the numerous scolices leads to dissemination of echinococcal infection. The multilocular or alveolar cyst of *E. multilocularis* usually presents as a slowly growing hepatic tumor, with jaundice and portal hypertension.

DIAGNOSIS AND TREATMENT The clinical picture is seldom sufficiently characteristic to suggest the diagnosis. When eosinophilia is present, it is helpful. Pulmonary lesions usually present as round, somewhat irregular, masses of uniform density. A smooth rim of calcification is seen on plane x-rays of the abdomen in half of those with hepatic involvement. A liver scan with radioactive isotopes is extremely helpful in detecting the presence of hepatic lesions and should always be done in suspected cases. Ultrasonic scanning will detect small lesions missed with radioisotopic scanning and will reveal the lesion to be fluid-filled. Liver hydatids often show a characteristic rim of opacification on celiac arteriography. The skin test (Casoni's test) is usually positive, but lack of a standard antigen and testing technique limits its usefulness. Moreover, patients with other helminthic diseases, particularly schistosomiasis, may give false positive results. Until a single highly sensitive and specific test is available, immunodiagnosis should be carried out using a battery of tests. The indirect hemagglutination and latex agglutination are most frequently used for screening; they are positive in 90 percent of patients with hepatic and 60 percent of those with pulmonary hydatids. The complement fixation test, although less sensitive, rapidly returns to normal after surgical extirpation of cysts, making it a valuable screening test for residual or recurrent disease. Currently, indirect fluorescent antibody, enzyme-linked immunoabsorbent assay, and counterimmunoelectrophoresis techniques are being evaluated. It appears that the presence of "arc 5" in the recently described immunoelectrophoresis test allows the specific diagnosis of *E. granulosus* infections; technical considerations limit its wide-scale use at this time. Occasionally scolices may be demonstrated in the sputum with the Ziehl-Neelsen stain. Because of serious reactions to the leakage of cyst fluid into the tissues and body cavities, diagnostic aspiration should not be attempted.

There is no established medical therapy. Experimentally, prolonged administration of mebendazole has been shown to be larvicidal, but this treatment cannot be recommended until more information has become available. BCG administration is effective in suppressing the growth and metastasis of experimental *E. multilocularis* infections raising the possibility that effective immunotherapeutic modalities may be available in the future. At the present time, surgical treatment offers the only hope of cure. Patients with small calcified hepatic cysts and pulmonary hydatids of the "canadensis" variety need to be operated on only if they are symptomatic or the lesion continues to enlarge over time. All others should have their cysts excised or sterilized and drained. The cyst should be widely exposed and the contents sterilized with 10 ml 10% Formalin, 1% iodine, or 30% sodium chloride before an attempt is made to open it. The entire endocyst should then be removed if possible, and all biliary or bronchial fistulas carefully closed. The residual space must be obliterated to prevent postoperative infection or prolonged drainage. Omentoplasty is the procedure of choice in abdominal cases.

PREVENTION In prevention, (1) contact with infected dogs should be avoided, particularly fecal contamination of the hands and food; (2) infected carcasses and offal should be burned or buried, in order to prevent access of dogs to material containing scolices; and (3) dogs should be treated if found to be infected. The reduction of the incidence of echinococciasis in Iceland is an example of the efficacy of control measures.

REFERENCES

BARBOUR AG et al: Hydatid disease screening. Sanpete County, Utah 1971–1976. Am J Trop Med Hyg 27:94, 1978

CALAMAI G et al: Hydatid disease of the heart: Report of 5 cases and review of the literature. Thorax 29:451, 1974

GELFAND M, JEFFREY C: Cerebral cysticercosis in Rhodesia. J Trop Med Hyg 76:87, 1973

HERMOS JA et al: Fatal human cerebral coenurosis. JAMA 213:1461, 1970

JONES TC: Cestodes. Clin Gastroenterol 7:105, 1978

LITTLE JM: Hydatid disease at Royal Prince Alfred Hospital, 1964 to 1974. Med J Aust 1:903, 1974

MATOSSIAN RM: The immunologic diagnosis of human hydatid disease. Trans Roy Soc Trop Med Hyg 71:101, 1977

MOST H: Drug therapy: Common parasitic infections of man. N Engl J Med 287:495, 1972

NEWMAN CM, ARON BS: Roentgen diagnosis of tapeworm infestation. J Mt Sinai Hosp NY 28:91, 1961

PAWLOWSKI Z, SCHULTZ MG: Taeniasis and cysticercosis *Taenia (Taenia saginata)*. Adv Parasitol 10:269, 1972

PERERA DR et al: Niclosamide treatment of cestodiasis: Clinical trials in the United States. Am J Trop Med 19:610, 1970

PORAT S, JOSEPH KN: Hydatid disease of bone. Israel J Med Sci 14:223, 1978

SCHULTZ MG et al: Epidemiology of beef tapeworm infection in the United States. Public Health Rep 85:169, 1970

TAYLOR RL: Sparganosis in the United States. Report of a case. Am J Clin Pathol 66:560, 1976

VICARY FR et al: Ultrasound and abdominal hydatid disease. Trans Roy Soc Trop Med Hyg 71:29, 1977

VON BONSDORFF B et al: Vitamin B$_{12}$ deficiency in carriers of the fish tapeworm, *Diphyllobothrium latum.* Acta Haematol 24:15, 1960

WILLIAMS JF et al: Current prevalence and distribution of hydatidosis with special reference to the Americas. Am J Trop Med 20:224, 1971

WILSON JF et al: Cystic hydatid disease in Alaska. Am Rev Resp Dis 98:1, 1968

XANTHAKIS D et al: Hydatid disease of the chest. Report of 91 cases surgically treated. Thorax 27:517, 1972

214
SCABIES, CHIGGERS, AND OTHER ECTOPARASITES

JAMES J. PLORDE

SCABIES Scabies is a cosmopolitan skin infection commonly referred to as the "seven-year itch." It is caused by a burrowing mite, *Sarcoptes scabiei*, and is transmitted from person to person by close bodily contact, particularly among bed partners. Although the disease is more common in the poor and unclean, sporadic cases involve individuals of all socioeconomic groups. There has been a worldwide resurgence of this infection over the past 20 years, and in the United States it currently involves 2 to 4 percent of patients seen in dermatologists' offices.

The turtle-shaped female measures 0.4 mm in length and possesses four pairs of legs. With the help of the two anterior pair and her mouth, she burrows into the superficial layer of the epidermis. Here she deposits two or three enormous eggs daily until she dies 30 to 60 days later. The newly hatched larvae mature to adulthood within 2 weeks to continue the cycle of infection. Although an involved person may harbour thousands or occasionally millions of adult mites, the average number of adult females per infection is 11.

Two-thirds of the burrows are found in the upper extremities, particularly on the interdigital spaces of the hands and the flexor surface of the wrists. In heavy infections, other sites are typically involved. These include the dorsal surfaces of the elbows, anterior axillary folds, female breasts, periumbilical area, penis, and buttocks. In bedridden patients, lesions are often concentrated over pressure points. The face, head, palms, and soles are seldom involved in adults. Characteristically, a burrow appears as a short dark wavy line which may end in a small vesicle, the site of the adult female.

Sensitization to the mites and their products begins approximately one month after infection and results in a papular or eczematous reaction at the sites of involvement. Itching is often severe and tends to be more marked at night or after a hot bath. Scratching frequently leads to secondary infection with pustulation; acute glomerulonephritis has followed infection with nephrogenic strains of streptococci. Occasionally, reddish pruritic nodules are seen in the groin and axillary regions. Infected individuals with good personal hygiene usually have few lesions, and burrows may be difficult to identify. In mentally retarded, debilitated, or immunosuppressed patients, a particularly virulent infection known as *Norwegian scabies* is sometimes seen. Millions of mites may be present, producing a highly infectious exfoliative dermatitis; itching is often mild or absent. Scabies usually terminates spontaneously in a few months, but chronic cases do occur.

The diagnosis should be considered in any patient presenting with a pruritic eruption, particularly if it involves several members of a living group. The occurrence of symmetric lesions at the sites of predilection should initiate a search for the characteristic burrows. These should be vigorously scraped with a sterile needle or scalpel blade, and the scrapings transferred to a drop of 10% potassium hydroxide on a glass slide. A cover slip is placed over the top, and the preparation examined for adults, larvae, and eggs. The diagnosis can also be made on histological sections prepared from a punch biopsy. Considering the mode of disease transmission, individuals shown to have scabies should also be checked for venereal disease.

All sexual contacts and household members should be treated simultaneously with the patient to prevent the occurrence of "ping-pong infections." The therapeutic agents are applied topically, covering the skin thinly but completely from the neck down. Although the patient is rendered noninfectious within 24 h, up to 2 months may be required for the clinical manifestations of the disease to disappear completely. Needless retreatment during this period can lead to contact dermatitis.

A number of effective agents are available for use. Gamma benzene hexachloride (Gamene, Kwell) is left on for 12 h and then thoroughly washed off. Care must be taken to keep it away from eyes and mucous membranes. It should not be used in infants or pregnant adults. Benzyl benzoate (25%) is administered in a similar fashion. Crotamiton (Eurax) is massaged into the skin, and a second dose applied 24 h later. Antihistamines or salicylates are helpful in counteracting pruritus. Topical steroids may potentiate the infection and should not be used. Antibiotics are required occasionally when there is a significant bacterial superinfection.

CHIGGER MITES The term *chigger* is used to refer to larvae of harvest mites belonging to the family Trombiculidae. The cosmopolitan adults feed on vegetable matter and deposit their eggs upon the ground. The tiny (0.4 mm) emergent larvae crawl along the ground and upward onto vegetation. Here, they await the passage of a vertebrate host, upon which they must feed before again dropping to the ground and molting. In humans, the chigger usually attaches about the ankles, but some advance along the skin until they are stopped by tight-fitting clothing. It then pierces the skin, releases a digestant to liquefy tissue cells, and feeds for 3 or 4 days. Within a few hours, the chigger's secretions have produced an intensely pruritic papule 0.5 to 2 cm in diameter. This usually vesiculates, resulting in a chickenpox-like lesion. Occasionally, subcutaneous bleeding results in a surrounding area of ecchymosis. The lesion and itching may persist for several weeks. In the United States, most clinical cases are seen during the summer months; in warm climates, the seasonal pattern is missing. Treatment is directed at the relief of itching and the prevention of secondary infections. Insect repellants are highly effective prophylactic agents.

FLEAS Fleas are small wingless laterally compressed ectoparasites of humans and other warm-blooded animals. They tend to be found on the hairy portions of the host where they feed and deposit their eggs. The active larvae which hatch in 3 days can be found on the host, in its nest, or in dust. They eventually pupate and may remain dormant for weeks or months before completing their development to adults.

Medically, fleas serve as both vectors and agents of disease. Rodent fleas of the genus *Xenopsylla* are the most important. They are responsible for the transmission of both plague (*Pasteurella pestis*) and murine typhus (*Rickettsia mooseri*) from animal reservoirs to humans. Humans may also acquire the rat tapeworm *Hymenolepis diminuta* by swallowing fleas containing the cysticeroid. The dog tapeworm *Dipylidium caninum* may be transmitted in a similar fashion. The bites of these and other species of fleas belonging to the family Pulicidae can induce an irritating dermatitis. In addition, the tungidae (*Tunga penetrans*) may burrow into the subcutaneous tissues, producing a painful and debilitating disease.

Flea dermatitis The fleas of humans (*Pulex irritans*), cats and dogs (*Cetenocephalides*), and rodents (*Xenopsylla*) may all induce dermatitis. In many individuals, the bites seem completely innocuous, but in sensitive persons, the saliva induces an erythematous raised pruritic papule. Repeated scratching may result in secondary infection with pustulation or ulceration. The intense pruritus, the ability of the flea to escape capture by virtue of its prodigious jumping ability, and the difficulty involved in crushing their hard chitinous bodies has led to many a frustrating noctural safari dedicated to the destruction of this unwanted bed partner. Control is effected by the use of frequent vacuuming to remove eggs, larvae, pupae, and adults from the environment. Insecticide sprays are also of help, but fleas have developed resistance to many of these. Dogs and cats should be washed, flea collars should be applied, and kennels should be dusted or sprayed with DDT or Malathion. If rat runs can be located, they should also be dusted.

Tunga penetrans, sometimes referred to as a *jigger* or *chigoe flea*, is a burrowing flea found in the tropical areas of South America and Africa. These small (1 mm) free-living insects reside in sandy soil. The fertilized female burrows into the skin of the first warm-blooded animal encountered. In humans, they usually embed on the sole of the foot or under a toenail with only their anal pore exposed to the outside. Multiple infections are common. As the female becomes engorged with blood and eggs, a painful and pruritic pea-sized swelling is produced. Eventually, the overlying skin ulcerates, the flea dies, and the eggs are extruded. Secondary bacterial infections including tetanus and gas gangrene occur commonly. Autoamputation of the toes has been reported from Africa. The intact flea can usually be extracted by gently enlarging the entrance hole with a sterile needle and then applying pressure from the side. Alternatively, the lesion can be soaked in Lysol, the flea penetrated with a needle, and the lesion resoaked to kill the eggs and sterilize the wound. Antibiotics may be required to treat secondary bacterial infections.

PEDICULOSIS Lice are obligate human ectoparasites that complete their entire 30- to 40-day life cycle on the body of the host. *Pediculus humanis* var. *capitis* infests the head, *P. humanis* var. *corporis* the body and clothing, and *Phthirius pubis* (crab lice) the genital and occasionally other hairy areas of the body. All three are flattened dorsoventrally and measure 2 to 3 mm in length. The crab louse is broader and flatter than *Pediculus* and possesses powerful claws on its second and third legs with which it clings to the pubic hair. The females lay five or six eggs daily which they firmly attach to the hairs or, in the case of the body louse, the clothing of the host. These clearly visible tiny white nits hatch in 8 to 10 days. The resulting nymph

matures to adulthood in an additional 2 weeks. Both the larvae and adults take two blood meals daily, leaving behind a small purpuric puncture site. With repeated exposure, the host develops an inflammatory hypersensitivity reaction manifested as a small red papule at each new feeding site. Pruritus results in scratching, a weeping dermatitis, and secondary infection. Chronic infections of the scalp may result in a fetid mass of matted hair and exudate. On the body and genital areas, the lesions may become pigmented—so-called "vagabond disease." Heavy infections with *P. pubis* may involve the eyebrows and eyelids leading to blepharitis.

Lice can be transferred from person to person by direct contact or via discarded clothing in which the body louse can survive for up to a week. Migration is stimulated by fever, making *P. humanis* var. *corporis* an efficient vector of relapsing fever (*Borrelia recurrentis*), typhus (*R. prowazeki*), and trench fever (*R. quintana*). *Phthirius pubis* is not known to be a vector of human disease.

The diagnosis is suggested by the typical dermatitis and confirmed by finding the adults or nits on the hair or clothing of the patient. The treatment of choice is 1% gamma benzene hexachloride (lindane, Kwell). In head infections, the hair should first be shampooed with ordinary soap. Kwell shampoo is then rubbed in at least 4 min, the hair rinsed, dried, and combed with a fine-tooth comb to remove the nits. The process should be repeated in 7 days. The clothing and bedding of the patient with body lice are heat-sterilized. The patient's body should be lathered for 4 min with Kwell shampoo and then rinsed thoroughly. The therapy may be repeated in 7 days. In crab louse infestations, Kwell cream or lotion should be used on the involved areas and left for 24 h. In hirsute individuals, the treatment can be repeated in 1 week. If the eyelashes are involved, 0.25% physostigmine ophthalmic ointment is applied twice daily for 10 days. Lice and nits are carefully removed with a cotton-tipped applicator. Narrow-angle glaucoma should be ruled out before the physostigmine is used.

MYIASIS Infections with maggots or fly larvae are seen worldwide in a variety of animals. Human involvement occurs most frequently where people live in close contact with domestic animals. Many different species of flies are involved. In some, an animal host is required for larval development; in these, the larvae are capable of invading normal tissue or enter the body through the nose, mouth, or ears. Others are opportunists, depositing their eggs or larvae in the open wounds of debilitated patients. The clinical manifestations vary with the species of fly and site of involvement. Four of the more common clinical syndromes are described below.

Localized cutaneous myiasis In tropical America the lesions are produced by *Dermatobia hominis*, the human bot fly. This remarkable forest-dwelling diptera captures a mosquito or other blood-feeding insect on which to deposit its packet of eggs. When this unwilling vector then lands on a warm-blooded animal to feed, the eggs hatch and penetrate the feeding site. Within the skin of the host, the larva develops for 2 or 3 months. Finally, it emerges, drops to the ground, and pupates. The lesions are most frequently seen on unprotected areas of the body including the hands, feet, head, and neck. During the first week of infection, the pruritic lesion closely resembles a mosquito bite. As the larva grows and begins to move, it produces severe pain and itching. Tissue destruction and inflammation results in the development of a furuncle-like lesion. Generally, a central opening is present through which the posterior end of the larva protrudes. A dark serosanguinous discharge containing the feces of the insect may be noted.

In Africa, a similar lesion is produced by *Cordylobia anthropophaga* (Tumbu fly). These flies deposit their eggs on sandy soil or laundry laid out to dry. The larvae hatch and invade the unbroken skin of humans or wild rodents, where they mature in 8 or 9 days. In either case, the larvae can be surgically extracted without difficulty. In Tumbu fly infections, letting the larvae mature and drop off spontaneously may be appropriate. This process can occasionally be hastened by applying mineral oil to the central opening. This results in the suffocation of the larva and stimulates its early exodus.

Cutanea larva migrans This is usually caused by the large (1 to 2 cm) horse bot flies belonging to the genus *Gasterophilus*. When the larvae hatch on the skin, they penetrate to the lower epidermis. Because they do not mature in humans, they may migrate in the skin for several months. Clinically, the infection presents as a pruritic serpiginous band of erythema closely resembling cutanea larva migrans produced by *Ancylostoma braziliense*. The diagnosis can be made by placing a small drop of mineral oil on the skin just in advance of the worm tract. This allows visualization of black backward-directed spines on its body segments. The parasite can be easily removed with a sharp needle. Occasionally, the larvae may penetrate the eye. A similar clinical picture is sometimes produced by the larvae of *Hypoderma* spp. (cattle bot fly). These, however, often penetrate deeply into the subcutaneous tissue and produce more pain and less pruritus than *Gasterophilus* larvae.

Deep-tissue myiasis Screw flies of several genera can deposit large batches of eggs on unbroken skin or in wounds, ears, or the nose. After hatching, the larvae burrow into the tissues and develop for 2 or 3 weeks. The mature 1- to 2-cm larvae then drop to the ground and pupate. At times, they penetrate deep tissues, including the eye, nasal sinuses, and cranium, where they produce destructive foul-smelling lesions. Bacterial superinfection is common. In India and Africa, the flies are usually of genus *Chrysomyia* In the Western Hemisphere, *Callitroga* spp. are involved. The occurrence of human cases in the United States often accompanies epizootics of screw worm activity. Flesh flies of the family Sarcophagidae have also been implicated in deep-tissue myiasis both in the United States and elsewhere. In all the above infections, the lesions should be surgically incised and debrided, the larvae removed, and secondary infections treated.

Intestinal myiasis When humans ingest food contaminated with the eggs or larvae of several genera of flies, some survive passage through the stomach and later mature in the intestine before they are extruded in the stool. In the United States, *Tubifera tenax* is the most frequently implicated species. Invasions of the intestinal mucosa may occur with *Sarcophaga* infections.

REFERENCES

ACKERMAN AB: Crabs—the resurgence of *Phthirius pubis*. N Engl J Med 278:950, 1968

FAUST EC et al: *Craig and Faust's Clinical Parasitology*, 8th ed. Philadelphia, Lea & Febiger, 1970

HUNTER GW et al: *Tropical Medicine*, 5th ed. Philadelphia, Saunders, 1976

MACIAS EG et al: Cutaneous myiasis in South Texas. N Engl J Med 289:1239, 1973

MAEGRAITH BC (ed): *Adams and Maegraith Clinical Tropical Diseases*, 5th ed. Oxford, Blackwell Scientific Publications, 1971

ORKIN M, MAIBACH MI: Current concepts in parasitology. The scabies pandemic. N Engl J Med 298:496, 1978

215

DISORDERS CAUSED BY VENOMS, BITES, AND STINGS

JAMES F. WALLACE

INTRODUCTION Humans have the propensity to come into contact with a great variety of venomous animals. These contacts occur with many zoologic classes including snakes, lizards, sea animals, spiders, scorpions, and numerous species of insects. In general two types of injuries result: those due to the direct effect of venom on the victim, as exemplified in snakebite, and those due to indirect effects of the poison, of which hypersensitivity reaction to bee stings is an example. Each year in the United States at least 50 persons die as the result of venomous injuries. Three groups of animals—hymenopterous insects, snakes, and spiders—account for over 90 percent of the fatalities. Of even greater public health significance is the loss in economic productivity and human potential resulting from the many serious, nonfatal envenomations which occur annually in otherwise healthy children or working adults.

SNAKE BITE Epidemiology Fewer than one-tenth of the nearly 3500 known species of snakes are venomous. These poisonous varieties belong to five families or subfamilies: Elapidae (cobras, kraits, mambas, and coral snakes) found in all parts of the world except Europe; Viperidae (true vipers) found in all parts of the world except the Americas; Hydrophidae (sea snakes); Crotalidae (pit vipers) found in Asia and the Americas; and Colubridae (boomslangs, bird snakes) of the African continent. The poisonous varieties of the United States, with the single exception of the coral snake, are pit vipers and include rattlesnakes, the water moccasin, and the copperhead. Although this discussion centers around these species, the therapeutic measures outlined are applicable to snakes in all parts of the world.

The number of individuals bitten by poisonous snakes in the United States is estimated to be about 8000 per year, with a relatively large number occurring in the Southeastern and Gulf states, particularly Texas. Deaths are not reported separately but are undoubtedly rare, numbering fewer than 20 per year, and most are due to bites of various species of rattlesnake. In many European countries deaths from snakebite have averaged only one every 3 to 5 years for the last half-century. In contrast, the estimate of annual deaths from snakebite throughout the world is between 30,000 and 40,000 with the largest number occurring in the countries of Burma and Brazil, where 2000 deaths are estimated to occur each year.

Etiology The *coral snake* is found in the Southern states from Florida to Arizona. It is usually marked by alternating red and black bands separated by yellow rings; however, black and albino forms exist. Coral snakes are generally nocturnal in their activities, shy and elusive, and rarely bite humans. Their fangs are short and permanently erect; the highly toxic venom is injected into multiple puncture wounds produced by a series of chewing movements.

The *pit vipers* are so named because of a small pit between the eye and the nostril. Large venom glands in the temporal regions give the head a triangular appearance. They are generally aggressive and likely to strike if disturbed. The fangs are long and hinged, folding posteriorly when the mouth is closed. Pit vipers strike suddenly with a forward thrust of the head. The instant that the erect fangs make contact, venom is expressed by sudden muscular contraction.

The *rattlesnakes,* recognized by the horny rattle on the tail, which buzzes when the snake is disturbed, are widely distributed. The diamondbacks (*Crotalus adamanteus* in the Southeast and *C. atrox* in the Southwest) are the largest and most dangerous snakes in this country. Others include the prairie rattler (*C. confluentus*), the timber rattler (*C. horridus*), and the pigmy rattlers.

The *water moccasin,* or cottonmouth (*Agkistrodon piscivorus*), is found in swampy areas or along the banks of streams. It is a strong swimmer and can bite under water. This snake is notorious for inflicting severe facial bites when disturbed in the branches of small trees. The copperhead, or highland moccasin (*A. mokasen*), is a closely related species. Its bite is painful but rarely fatal.

Pathogenesis SNAKE VENOMS The venoms of most species which have been analyzed have been found to be mixtures of several toxic proteins and enzymes with diversified and complicated pharmacological effects. An an example, the venom of the Indian cobra (*Naja naja*) contains these distinct and separate substances: a neurotoxin, a hemolysin, a cardiotoxin, a cholinesterase, at least three phosphatases, a nucleotidase, and a potent inhibitor of cytochrome oxidase. Several venoms, including those of the pit vipers, contain hyaluronidase and numerous proteolytic enzymes. Although the exact roles of these components in toxicity are incompletely understood, the venom of a given species is usually predominantly neurotoxic or necrotizing, and frequently associated with hemolysis, abnormalities of blood coagulation, changes in cardiac dynamics, and alterations in vascular resistance. The venom of elapids, including the coral snake, is neurotoxic, with death resulting from respiratory paralysis probably caused by damage to brain centers and a curariform interference with transmission at the neuromuscular junction. The venom of crotalid snakes produces local tissue injury, hemorrhage, and hemolysis; death is often preceded by circulatory collapse associated with a marked fall in circulating blood volume resulting from pooling of blood in the microcirculation, and loss of plasma due to increased capillary permeability. Systemic absorption of venom occurs through the lymphatics, and therapeutic measures designed to reduce lymphatic function are helpful in controlling symptoms.

FACTORS AFFECTING SEVERITY OF SNAKE BITE Several factors affect the outcome of snake bite:

1 The age, size, and health of the patient. Envenomation in children is usually serious, and a fatal outcome more likely, since a relatively large dose of poison is injected into a small victim.

2 Location of bite. Bites on extremities or into adipose tissue are less dangerous than those on the trunk, face, or directly into a blood vessel. A direct strike of the fangs is more dangerous than a scratch, a glancing blow, or one hitting a bone. The discharge orifice of a fang is well above its tip so that the point of the fang can penetrate the skin without envenomation; even a thin layer of clothing may afford great protection. Because of the superficial nature of the wound as many as one-fifth of patients bitten by venomous snakes will have no evidence of envenomation, even though the fangs have penetrated the skin.

3 The size of the snake (a large pit viper can inject over 1000 mg venom, six times a lethal dose for an adult), the extent of its anger or fear (if hurt it may inject a larger amount of venom), the condition of the fangs (broken or recently renewed), and the condition of the venom glands (recently discharged or full). All these factors are important. Contrary to popular belief, the bite of a snake which has recently killed and fed is not necessarily less venomous for humans; the snake usually does not exhaust its venom in a single bite.

4 The presence of various bacteria, particularly clostridia and other anaerobic organisms, in the mouth of the snake or on the skin of the victim. This may lead to serious infection in the necrotic tissues at the local site.

5 Exercise or exertion, such as running, immediately after the bite. This speeds systemic absorption of toxin.

Manifestations Following the bite of a pit viper, severe burning pain develops within a few minutes at the site of the wound. Local swelling rapidly develops and spreads in all directions, accompanied by the appearance of ecchymoses and bullae over the involved area. As the edema spreads, serosanguinous fluid oozes from the puncture wounds. Later gangrene of the skin and subcutaneous tissues may develop. Systemic effects resulting from the absorption of venom and local tissue destruction may include fever, nausea and vomiting, circulatory collapse, bleeding into the skin and from all body orifices, low-grade jaundice, neuropathic muscle cramping, pupillary constriction, disorientation, delirium, and convulsions. Death may occur after 6 to 48 h. Survival may be attended by massive local tissue loss from gangrene or secondary infection, or may be complicated by acute renal failure, secondary to disseminated intravascular clotting and cortical necrosis, or by tubular necrosis following circulatory collapse.

The bite of the coral snake causes little pain and local swelling. There are usually multiple fang marks. Within 10 to 15 min numbness and weakness begin in the region of the bite followed by ataxia, ptosis, pupillary dilatation, palatal and pharyngeal paralysis, slurring of speech, salivation, and occasionally nausea and vomiting. The patient becomes comatose, develops respiratory paralysis and seizures, and dies within 8 to 72 h.

Cobra bites are painful and are often accompanied by severe hemolysis, local necrosis, and sloughing in addition to their neurotoxic effects. There is little pain and no edema at the site of a sea snake bite. Symptoms of systemic envenomation follow a latent period which may vary from 15 min to 8 h. Although the venom is both myotoxic and neurotoxic, the injury to skeletal muscle is most prominent and is characterized by generalized muscle pain, weakness, and myoglobinuria. Hemorrhagic manifestations predominate following envenomation by colubrids (boomslangs and bird snakes) and many pit vipers including certain species of rattlesnake.

Laboratory abnormalities In severe cases, laboratory abnormalities may include progressive anemia, polymorphonuclear leukocytosis of 20,000 to 30,000 cells per cubic millimeter, thrombocytopenia, hypofibrinogenemia, disordered tests of coagulation, proteinuria, and azotemia.

Treatment An attempt should be made to determine with certainty that the patient has been bitten by a poisonous snake. Absence of distinct fang punctures and failure of local pain, edema, numbness, or weakness to appear within 20 min are strong evidence against snake venom poisoning. If the species of snake is not known, the offending reptile should be killed for the purpose of identification.

FIRST AID This consists of reassuring and calming the victim and instituting measures to retard the absorption of venom and to remove it from the tissues as quickly as possible after the bite. The patient should be promptly placed at rest and the bitten extremity immobilized to reduce the rate of spread of the venom. If anatomically feasible, a wide tourniquet should be placed a few centimeters above the bite and made tight enough to allow one finger to pass beneath with difficulty. The purpose is to impede lymph flow; it is not necessary to obstruct venous return. The tourniquet should be loosened and moved proximally at hourly intervals when local swelling causes it to tighten. Unless the victim can be transported to a hospital within less than 15 min, incision and suction of the wound should be started prior to evacuation. By use of whatever antisepsis is available, 1.0 cm *linear* (not cruciate) incisions about 0.5 cm deep should be carefully made through each fang mark and suction applied. A rubber bulb, breast pump, or heated jar are all preferable to mouth suction, but if other means are not available and no oral lesions are present, this method may be employed. Suction should be continued for at least 1 h following the bite, or until antivenin has been administered. The practice of making multiple incisions along the advancing edge of edema as swelling progresses has not been found to be beneficial and is no longer advised. *Incision and suction are extremely important and should be diligently carried out in every poisonous snake bite.* When begun promptly, they may result in the removal of up to 50 percent of subcutaneously injected venom.

As soon as possible, the patient should be transferred to a hospital. Immobilization of the affected part during transportation is important in controlling lymph flow and is best achieved by splinting. Although ice packs relieve pain and slow lymphatic drainage, they do not neutralize venom, and even a small amount of cooling may result in irreparable damage to already injured tissues by causing ischemia. For this reason, it is recommended that no form of cryotherapy be used.

IMMEDIATE HOSPITAL CARE This should include appropriate treatment for shock and respiratory difficulty, antivenin, measures to combat infection, and general supportive care.

Antivenin is the only specific treatment of snake venom poisoning, and its use in severe bites is vital. In the United States polyvalent crotaline antivenin effective against all American pit vipers and antivenin for North American coral snake poisoning are commercially available. Both products are a lyophylized powder of refined horse serum. Kits are available containing antivenin powder (reconstituted by diluting with water to 10 ml per ampul), syringe, normal horse serum for prior sensitivity testing of the patient, and detailed instructions. Intravenously administered antivenin leads to the most rapid and effective response. It is not advisable to infiltrate antivenin at the local site. The initial dose should depend upon the amount of envenomation; for bites accompanied by local swelling but no systemic symptoms, 2 to 5 vials (20 to 50 ml) is usually sufficient. When swelling has progressed beyond the site of the bite, and mild systemic symptoms and/or hematologic abnormalities are present, moderate envenomation has occurred, and initial treatment should be 5 to 9 vials (50 to 90 ml). For severe bites, associated with marked local as well as systemic effects and evidence of hemolysis or coagulation abnormalities, 10 to 15 vials (100 to 150 ml) or more should be administered. Larger doses of antivenin should be given to children or small adults to neutralize the relatively higher venom concentrations. When progressive swelling in the bitten part ceases, an adequate dose has generally been achieved; improvement in the victim's clinical signs is often extremely rapid.

In the patient with severe envenomation who is allergic to horse serum, the relative risks of death from anaphylaxis rather than from venom poisoning should be carefully weighed before undertaking desensitization with small doses of diluted horse serum.

No antivenin for other snakes is manufactured in the United States, but antiserum for various types is usually kept on hand at large zoos all over the world. A national antivenin index is maintained by the Oklahoma City Zoo [(405) 271-5454], and telephone consultation service for physicians is also available at the Venom Poisoning Unit of the Los Angeles County/University of Southern California Medical Center.

Maintaining *respiration* by mechanical or other means is important. In patients bitten by elapid snakes, respiratory failure is usually reversible. *Tetanus toxoid* or *tetanus immune globulin* of human origin should be given. If wound infections appear, antibiotics should be used with the knowledge that the predominant microorganisms in the mouths of snakes are gram-negative pathogens. Treatment should be preceded by appropriate aerobic and anaerobic cultures. *Fasciotomy* may be necessary to prevent further ischemic injury to a massively swollen limb. *Surgical debridement* of vesicles and superficial necrotic tissue should be done near the end of the first week following the bite. *Relief of pain* with salicylates or meperidine, moderate sedation, maintenance of fluid balance, measures to combat shock and hemorrhagic diathesis, and appropriate management of coma or convulsions are all important.

The usefulness of corticosteroids to prevent tissue damage or systemic intoxication has not been convincingly demonstrated. However, these drugs may be of value in the management of severe shock associated with envenomation and for allergic reactions following the administration of antivenin.

Prevention In snake-infested regions long trousers, high shoes, boots or leggings, and gloves should be worn. Most important of all is to look where one steps or reaches. A sharp knife or lancet, tourniquet, suction bulb, and antiseptic suffice for an emergency kit, and in inaccessible areas, antivenin should also be carried.

POISONOUS LIZARD BITE Of the nearly 3000 species of lizard in the world, only two are venomous: the Gila monster (*Heloderma suspectum*) of the arid southwestern United States and the closely related Mexican beaded lizard (*H. horridum*) which inhabits the lowland forests of Western Mexico. These reptiles are not aggressive, and virtually every instance of their attacking a human has involved teasing or handling the animals in captivity. The venom is elaborated in eight glands in the floor of the mouth and secreted directly into the oral cavity, where it bathes the teeth, which are grooved posteriorly. The lizard clings tenaciously and is often dislodged only after considerable effort; envenomation occurs by contamination of the wound. The venom contains a potent neurotoxin which is undoubtedly responsible for its lethal effect on experimental animals. Death in humans following a bite is extremely rare. Most often, human envenomation results in tissue injury, excruciating pain, massive edema, and patchy erythema. Acute systemic symptoms may last for 3 to 4 days and include nausea, vomiting, hematemesis, blurred vision, dyspnea, dysphonia, and profound weakness. Intense hyperesthesia of the bitten extremity may persist for several weeks. There is no antivenin available. Treatment should consist of tourniquet, incision, suction, cooling of the bitten area, measures to prevent or combat infection, including tetanus, and supportive measures. Parenteral meperidine (Demerol) or infiltration of local anesthetic around the bite should be used to relieve pain.

SPIDER BITES The bite of many spiders is locally irritating, and several species can cause severe, even fatal systemic poisoning in man. The most numerous and important of the venomous spiders are members of the genus *Latrodectus,* widely distributed throughout the world. In the United States and Canada, *Latrodectus mactans,* the black widow or show-button spider, causes a majority of clinically significant arachnidism. In Florida, *Latrodectus bishopi,* the red-legged widow spider, has been reported to produce human poisoning resembling mild black widow bite. From the Southern and Midwestern states, there are increasing numbers of reports of poisoning from the bite of common brown spiders, including *Loxosceles reclusa* and *Loxosceles unicolor.* These bites are characterized by intense local pain and ischemic necrosis at the site, often followed by deep ulceration. Hemolysis occasionally is seen, and in severe cases hemoglobinuria and acute renal failure may occur.

The symptoms and mortality from bites of large, hairy spiders, the tarantulas, such as *Lycosa raptoria* and *Phoneutria fera* in Brazil or *Glyptocranium gastereanthoides* in Peru, and of such spiders as *Loxosceles laeta* in Chile are similar, with severe ulceration, necrosis, and hemolysis. Neurotoxic manifestations of the type produced by *Latrodectus* are sometimes admixed with local necrosis and hemolysis.

It is the female *L. mactans,* the black widow, that bites humans. She is glossy black with a body 1 cm in diameter, a leg span of 5 cm, and a characteristic red hourglass mark on her abdomen. She spins her web in woodpiles, sheds, basements, or outdoor privies, is very aggressive, and will bite on slight provocation. The venom produces diffuse central and peripheral nervous excitement, autonomic activity, muscle spasm, hypertension, and vasoconstriction.

In the United States, most black widow bites occur between April and October, and many patients are males bitten on the genitalia or buttocks while using a privy. After a momentary sharp pain at the site, there is cramping pain that begins locally within 15 to 60 min and gradually spreads. It may involve all extremities and the trunk. The abdomen is boardlike, and the waves of pain become excruciating, causing the patient to turn, toss, and cry out. Respirations are often labored and grunting. There are also nausea, vomiting, headache, sweating, salivation, hyperactive reflexes, twitching, tremor, paresthesias of hands and feet, and occasionally, systolic hypertension. A mild polymorphonuclear leukocytosis is usual, and many patients have slight fever. After several hours, the pains subside, although mild recurrences for 2 or 3 days are common. It may be a week before well-being is restored. Deaths due to cardiac or respiratory failure have occurred, mostly in children and the aged.

Because the bite itself is not prominent, patients are often thought to have some abdominal catastrophe such as perforated ulcer, pancreatitis, or volvulus. Renal colic, coronary occlusion, tetanus, strychnine poisoning, tabetic crisis, lead colic, and porphyria are other conditions to be ruled out. The abdomen is not tender to palpation in arachnidism, and pains in the extremities are not typical of most of these other disorders.

Treatment For *Latrodectus* poisoning, treatment consists of measures to relieve pain and administration of antiserum. Initial treatment should include a hot tub bath which affords prompt, although temporary, relief. An intravenous injection of calcium gluconate or magnesium sulfate usually produces dramatic, but transient, cessation of cramps. Opiates are sometimes necessary. When available, a single intramuscular injection of 1 ampul (2.5 ml) reconstituted antiserum usually is quite effective within a few hours. If the cramps return, administration of antiserum can be repeated.

Treatment of *Loxosceles* bites consists mainly of local wound management and treatment of secondary infection if it occurs. The parenteral use of corticosteroids within the first 24 h following a bite has been advocated in order to prevent progression of the lesion, but convincing evidence that this is efficacious is lacking. The ulcer usually heals spontaneously, although skin grafting may be required on occasion. Renal failure should be treated as advised in Chap. 275.

SCORPION STING Scorpions are eight-legged arthropods. Glands in the terminal segment produce venom, which is injected into the victim by a stinger located on the tip of the tail. Scorpions often enter dwellings. During the day they retreat into crevices; emerging at night, they often get into shoes and clothing and even into bedding. They do not deliberately attack humans, but accidental contact results in a sting.

Of about 650 species, roughly 40 occur in the United States, distributed over three-fourths of the nation. They are most numerous in the South from Florida to California, but the only two lethal species, *Centruroides sculpturatus* and *C. gertschi,* are limited to Arizona and portions of neighboring states. These two species reach a maximal length of about 7 cm. Their sting may be fatal to young children or old people, but seldom to a healthy adult.

Most of the nonlethal species of scorpions in the United States cause only minor reactions, like a bee sting. Some in the Southwest, however, produce local edema and ecchymosis, with burning pain. In contrast, many species whose venom has potentially dangerous systemic effects, including the Arizona *Centruroides,* evoke little or no visible reaction at the site of the sting. There is an immediate burning sensation followed by local paresthesia ("pins and needles"), hyperesthesia, or numbness. These sensations spread to involve the whole extremity, and within an hour or two, malaise, restlessness, lacrimation, rhinorrhea, salivation, perspiration, nausea, and vomiting appear.

The patient passes from an agitated state with hyperactive reflexes into coma; convulsions follow. In addition to these neurotoxic symptoms, cardiovascular effects due to myocarditis may be seen and include various arrhythmias and intractable heart failure. Death usually occurs within 12 h, but sometimes as late as 2 days after the sting.

Treatment This consists of immediately placing a tourniquet on the extremity just proximal to the sting in order to delay the absorption of venom. If available, ice packs may be applied to the wound and to the affected limb, with care not to create additional tissue injury through freezing. The tourniquet must be removed in 5 to 10 min, but the limb is kept cool for at least 2 h. After this time, if treatment has been applied promptly, no serious effects are experienced following the sting of *C. sculpturatus* or *C. gertschi.* If the sting is on the head, trunk, or genitalia, of course, a tourniquet cannot be used, but the area may be cooled.

Although tourniquet, incision, and suction as in the treatment of snake bite have been recommended, the amount of venom is minute; it produces no local necrotizing effect and is absorbed very rapidly.

Specific antivenin, reconstituted from lyophilized cat serum, is available in some areas and should be employed if the victim develops signs of central nervous system or cardiac involvement. Supportive therapy is directed at combating shock and dehydration. Barbiturates in large doses are useful in reducing restlessness.

Prevention This depends upon alertness in avoiding contact with scorpions in infested areas. Clothing and shoes should be well shaken before being put on in the morning. Towels and bedclothes should be inspected. A house infested with scorpions can in time be rid of them by closing all obvious ways of ingress; picking up debris in the environment, such as piles of brush, logs, stones; introducing a mixture of fuel oil or kerosene, containing a small amount of creosote, between the earth and the house foundation; and spraying with a mixture of 2% chlordane, 10% DDT, and 0.2% pyrethrins in an oil base.

HYMENOPTERA STINGS Each year in the United States, nearly twice as many people die as a result of bites by hymenopterous insects (including bees, wasps, hornets, yellow jackets and fire ants) as from poisonous snake bites. Occasionally, multiple stings in enormous numbers (500 to 1000) are the cause of death. However, the majority of systemic reactions and deaths are due to allergic reactions to the venoms of these insects.

Hymenopteran venoms contain histamine, various kinins, and other vasoactive substances, phospholipases, and hyaluronidase. They are hemolytic and neurotoxic in addition to being effective hypersensitizing agents. The usual reaction to a single wasp sting or bee sting is sharp pain, local wheal and erythema, intense itching, and in loose tissues, such as the eyelid or genitalia, considerable edema which subsides in a few hours. Only in the rare case when a bee is swallowed or inhaled and edema of the laryngopharynx or glottis develops is there danger. A sting directly into a peripheral nerve can destroy its function for a time, much as does an injection of alcohol. Bell's palsy has followed a sting into the trunk of the facial nerve. Unusual reactions such as optic neuritis, generalized polyneuropathy, and myasthenia gravis may follow a sting. The etiology of these reactions is unknown.

In hypersensitive individuals, a single sting may produce serious anaphylaxis with urticaria, nausea, abdominal or uterine cramps, bronchospasm, massive edema of the face and glottis, dyspnea, cyanosis, hypotension, coma, and death. Sensitization is usually the result of previous stings although most fatalities have occurred in individuals who experienced no apparent allergic reaction to the earlier envenomation. Beekeepers who develop allergic rhinitis followed by asthma when near bees or objects that have been in contact with bees are likely to have serious reactions to stings. It has been estimated that nearly 1 percent of the general population in this country has hymenoptera allergy.

Many species of ant can produce stinging bites with local redness and swelling. The most notorious of these is the fire ant (*Solenopsis saevissima*), whose bite may result in extensive vesiculation and skin necrosis similar to that caused by the brown recluse spider.

Treatment The wound site should be examined for a stinger which, if present, should be carefully removed in order to prevent further envenomation from the attached gland. The local reaction to the usual sting is treated by local cool application and antipruritic lotions or oral antihistamines. Epinephrine, 0.3 to 0.5 ml of a 1:1000 aqueous solution subcutaneously repeated every 20 to 30 min, may be lifesaving in patients with an anaphylactic reaction to a bee sting or wasp sting. A tourniquet to slow the absorption of venom and ice packs to relieve pain may be used. Oxygen, endotracheal intubation, vasopressors, and other supportive measures should be used as needed. In addition, corticosteroids should be employed in severe cases, although their maximum effect is not achieved until several hours after administration.

Prevention Allergic persons should make every effort to avoid contact with these insects, including wearing shoes when outside and not wearing perfumes or bright colors which may attract them. In addition, they should keep epinephrine readily

available for immediate use in case of a sting, without waiting for symptoms to develop. Sting kits containing premeasured doses of 1:1000 epinephrine in disposable syringes, tourniquets, and antihistamine tablets are commercially available. Careful instruction in their use should be provided by the person's physician.

Immunotherapy Desensitization by injection of extracts of crushed whole bodies of bees, wasps, hornets, and yellow jackets has been recommended for any patient who has had a systemic or generalized reaction to hymenopterous insect stings. This practice is based on retrospective studies suggesting benefit from this form of immunotherapy. However, skin testing with whole-body extracts has been found unreliable in identifying persons at risk for systemic reactions, and immunization with these extracts has been shown not to increase IgG-blocking antibodies to venom proteins, a response felt to be essential for protection in insect allergy. In contrast, purified hymenopteran venoms, currently available only for investigational use in the United States, have been found highly accurate in diagnosing insect sting allergy by skin testing and have provided much better protection than whole body extracts for immunotherapy of high risk patients. It is likely that purified venom antigens will soon be the preferred materials for diagnosis and desensitization.

TICK BITE The local reaction to the bite of a tick may be nothing more than an itching papule which subsides within a few days unless there is secondary bacterial infection. However, incomplete removal of a tick, with retention of the mouthparts, may result in the local formation of a nodule which continues to grow and is sometimes annoyingly pruritic. The definitive treatment is surgical excision of the nodule. Histologically, the nodule is a granuloma, but the inflammatory response is sometimes so bizarre and changes in the overlying epithelium are so striking that, in the absence of a history of tick bite, a mistaken diagnosis of malignant tumor may be made.

Removal of a tick by steady pulling is preferable to crushing. Touching with a hot object such as a glowing cigarette, freezing, or applying a drop of oil or nail polish facilitates removal without leaving embedded remnants.

Tick paralysis A progressive, ascending, flaccid paralysis which is reversible sometimes develops in humans and certain other mammals while a tick is engorging upon them. Human cases have most frequently been reported from the northwestern United States and Western Canada, where the wood tick, *Dermacentor andersoni* Stiles, is responsible. The dog tick, *D. variabilis* Say, has been identified in a number of cases occurring in the Southeastern states. *Amblyomma americanum*, the Lone Star tick, *A. maculatum*, the Gulf Coast tick, and *Ixodes scapularis*, the black-legged deer tick, have also been incriminated.

This disorder is caused by a neurotoxin apparently injected by the engorging tick. This toxin acts upon spinal and bulbar nuclei, slowing motor nerve conduction without affecting neuromuscular transmission. The toxin appears to be destroyed or excreted rapidly, for when the tick is removed the nerve cells soon regain normal function.

The tick must feed for several days before symptoms develop. Paralysis is seen in experimental animals after 5 to 6 days of engorgement. Male ticks feed for a shorter period than female ticks, a fact which may explain why they are less likely to cause paralysis.

Most human cases occur in children, generally in young girls. The tick is usually attached to the scalp and hidden by the hair, but may be found on any part of the body, especially the ear, axilla, groin, vulva, or popliteal region.

The patient may be irritable and have mild diarrhea for 24 h before frank motor involvement appears. There are weakness and poor control of the legs, the tendon reflexes in the legs are diminished or absent, and the Romberg sign is positive. Temporary improvement may occur, and if the tick is removed at this stage, true paralysis may never develop. Otherwise the symptoms recur within 24 h, with flaccid paralysis which extends in 24 to 48 h to involve the trunk, arms, neck, tongue, and pharynx. Sensory changes are usually absent, but there may be paresthesia and hyperesthesia in the affected extremities. Nystagmus, strabismus, truncal ataxia, and facial paralysis are sometimes noted. There is little or no fever unless a secondary infection is present. The leukocyte count is usually not elevated, but moderate leukocytosis may occur. The spinal fluid is almost always normal.

Tick paralysis is apt to be confused with poliomyelitis, the more so because ticks are active in warm weather when poliomyelitis is most prevalent. Among other diseases which might be considered in differential diagnosis are polyneuritis, transverse myelitis, the Guillain-Barré syndrome, myasthenia gravis, the Eaton-Lambert myasthenic syndrome, and botulism.

Definitive treatment is removal of the tick. Mouthparts retained in the skin should be promptly excised. The patient's body should be searched for other ticks. There is striking improvement within a few hours after removal of ticks.

If the tick is removed before bulbar involvement develops, the paralysis subsides and recovery is complete in a few days, sometimes within 24 h. The patient should be observed until the recovery trend is established, because if other ticks or retained mouthparts have been overlooked, the paralysis may progress. When bulbar or respiratory paralysis is present, death may occur if the tick is not removed in time. Other treatment is supportive.

OTHER ARTHROPOD BITES Flea bite There are many fleas that attack humans, including *Pulex irritans* and chicken fleas. In sensitive individuals, the salivary secretion of these bloodsuckers produces large, itching papules. It is thought that much of the papular urticaria of children is probably due to flea bites. Treatment is symptomatic only. Elimination of fleas from the environment may be very difficult, but persistent treatment of animals and of premises with appropriate insecticides is usually successful.

Centipede bite Local irritation is the usual reaction to centipede venom, although extensive necrosis and systemic illness have followed severe poisoning by tropical species. Treatment is purely symptomatic.

Caterpillar urticaria Contact with hairy caterpillars of many species produces irritation of skin or mucous membranes. The type of venom involved is not known, but severe pain, erythema, urticaria, and even blister formation may come on rapidly after direct contact with caterpillars, after handling cocoons, or on being exposed to windblown fuzz. There are often a regional lymphangitis and transient eosinophilic leukocytosis. The discomfort subsides within 24 h, but local soaks, oral antihistaminics, and, when pain is severe, oral codeine are often indicated.

Bedbug bite Members of the genus *Cimex* inflict bites that leave reactions varying from a simple puncture to large urticarial lesions, apparently depending on the sensitivity of the bitten individual. There is no specific treatment.

Chiggers or redbugs These are tiny mites which are commonly found in foliage, grass, etc., in many parts of the world. In the United States, the larval form of *Eutrobicula alfreddugesi* attacks the skin by secreting a substance which digests tissue, creating a red papule that itches intensely. The tiny reddish larva can be seen in the center of the lesion. Treatment is palliative and consists of antipruritic applications. The use of insect repellents, appropriate protective clothing, and prompt bathing after exposure reduce the risk of infestation considerably.

Bloodsucking-fly bite Many species of flies, particularly the horsefly and the deerfly, viciously attack and feed upon warmblooded animals, including humans. Occasionally, transmission of diseases such as anthrax, tularemia, loiasis, and trypanosomiasis has been attributed to horseflies and deerflies. More commonly in North America, however, their bites are responsible for painful, intensely pruritic cutaneous lesions which may be followed by delayed localized allergic reactions characterized by erythema, edema, and urticaria. Treatment should include thorough cleaning of the bite sites, topical corticosteroids, and oral antihistaminics for severe itching. Antibiotics may be necessary if the wounds become secondarily infected.

MARINE ANIMAL VENOM DISEASES The venoms of certain marine animals are known to cause illness in humans after injection or inoculation under naturally occurring conditions. Information concerning these toxins is limited; most appear to be composed of proteins and peptides as well as other substances that are pharmacologically active. Although probably less complex than the venoms of reptiles, many marine animal venoms are capable of causing several pathologic effects including neurotoxicity as well as local necrosis.

Portuguese man-of-war and jellyfish stings The burning discomfort induced by contact with sea nettles or jellyfish is familiar to most surf bathers. Contact with the tentacles of the colorful Portuguese man-of-war (*Physalia* species), which is found mainly in or near the Gulf of Mexico, or the more toxic jellyfish (*Chiropsalmus* of the Indian Ocean and *Rhizostoma* of the Atlantic) is followed by burning pain, swelling, and erythema. Severe, generalized muscular cramps, nausea, vomiting, and pulmonary edema may occur. Victims have died as a result of jellyfish stings, sometimes within minutes after contact. In nonfatal cases, systemic symptoms usually subside within several hours.

Treatment consists of removing any tentacles still clinging to the skin after first inactivating the toxins in their nematocysts with local application of alcohol, ammonia, or even dry sand. Analgesics should be used for pain control, and antihistaminics if there is an accompanying pruritic rash. Corticosteroids may be helpful in severe cases.

Sea anemone sting ("sponge diver's disease") Contact with certain sea anemones (especially *Sargatia elegans*) in Mediterranean and African waters produces extensive dermatitis with chronic ulceration. Occasionally, especially during August and September, systemic symptoms of headache, sneezing, nausea, chills, fever, and collapse are noted. Rare fatalities have occurred. No specific therapy is known; symptomatic treatment with topical steroids or oral antihistaminics may provide temporary relief.

Cone shell poisoning The colorful cone shells are highly prized by collectors. However, many species in the Pacific are venomous, a great danger to unwary hobbyists who pick them up. The poison, a neurotoxin, is delivered into a wound inflicted by pointed hollow teeth resembling darts in the long proboscis of the animal. Local manifestations include sudden intense pain, followed by swelling and numbness which may persist for several days. Symptoms of serious poisoning include muscular incoordination and weakness progressing to respiratory paralysis. Death may occur within 3 to 6 h, but recovery within 24 h is the rule. There is no specific therapy; recommended treatment is the use of tourniquet, incision, and suction (as for snake bite), and supportive measures which may include artificial respiration and administration of oxygen.

Sponge dermatitis Direct contact with several species of sponge results in a painful dermatitis, which may persist for several weeks. The lesions appear to be caused by mechanical irritation from the exoskeleton of the sponge as well as by toxins within its tissues. Delayed hypersensitivity reactions may also occur. Antihistaminics provide relief from the pruritus; dilute acetic acid ameliorates local pain strikingly, while alkali will intensify it. The lesions are self-limited.

Sea urchin sting Contact with the spines of some species of sea urchin results in painful erythema and ulceration, occasionally accompanied by neurotoxic symptoms of weakness and frank paralysis of lips, tongue, and face lasting for several hours. Treatment is purely symptomatic and supportive. The toxins isolated from sea urchins have produced paralysis in animals and are notably resistant to heat. Deaths from paralysis and drowning have been reported.

Paralytic and neurotoxic shellfish poisoning Certain dinoflagellates, which compose part of the marine phytoplankton, elaborate a potent neurotoxin. Occasionally, conditions in coastal waters become favorable for the growth of excessive numbers of these organisms, causing the water to develop an amber appearance termed the "red tide" and killing massive numbers of fish by exhausting their oxygen supply. When humans ingest shellfish which have themselves ingested toxic dinoflagellates, an illness occurs characterized by paresthesias of the face and extremities, dysphonia, and generalized muscular weakness, often accompanied by nausea, vomiting, and diarrhea and occasionally by paralysis and respiratory arrest. The more severe syndrome, known as paralytic shellfish poisoning, is encountered along the Pacific Northwest and New England coasts. A milder form, not associated with paralysis in humans, is seen along the Gulf and Atlantic coasts of Florida. Treatment should include induced emesis and purgation to remove unabsorbed toxin from the gastointestinal tract and whatever additional supportive measures are necessary. Spontaneous recovery usually takes place within 24 h. There is a standardized mouse bioassay procedure for demonstrating and quantitating toxin in shellfish but no diagnostic test for detecting toxin in clinical specimens.

Venomous fish stings The dorsal fins or spines of bullhead sharks, dogfish, and ratfish and the dorsal and other fins of the scorpion fish, weeverfish, toadfish, and catfish are grooved, and at their bases are found venom glands. Injury by these spines results in severe pain and swelling and, in some instances, neurotoxic manifestations. Local gangrene with extensive tissue loss is a complication of catfish stings that may prolong convalescence. Little or nothing is known of the venoms involved. Suction and hot application are advocated immediately after injury. Tetanus toxoid or antitoxin should be given also. Narcotics are often required to control the pain. Secondary pyogenic infection is a frequent complication.

Probably the most frequent type of venomous fish injury in the United States is that produced by the lashing tail of the stingray of the California coast (*Urobatis halleri*). The bony spine is encased in a sheath of epithelial cells containing venom which is expressed into the puncture wound. The wound may be several centimeters deep; portions of the bony spine may break off in it, or, more often, the integumentary sheath remains in the wound. The venom is a circulatory depressant in animals, but local injury predominates in humans. There are immediately severe pain and blanching followed by erythema and edema. Symptoms due to systemic absorption of venom are infrequent but may include salivation, muscle cramps and weakness, cardiac arrhythmias, seizures, and death. Treatment consists of application of a tourniquet (the vast majority of these injuries occur on the legs) and copious syringing of the wound with saltwater to remove fragments of sheath followed by immersion in water as hot as the patient can stand for 1 h. The venom is heat-labile, and extensive trials have indicated the usefulness of this last procedure. Tetanus toxoid or antiserum is indicated; as with other fish stings, pyogenic infection is a frequent complication.

REFERENCES

Hymenoptera stings

BARNARD JH: Studies of 400 hymenoptera sting deaths in the United States. J Allergy Clin Immunol 52:259, 1973
BROWN LL: Fire ant allergy. South Med J 65:273, 1972
BRUMLIK J: Myasthenia gravis associated with wasp sting. JAMA 235:2120, 1976
HUNT KJ et al: Diagnosis of allergy to stinging insects by skin testing with hymenoptera venoms. Ann Intern Med 85:56, 1976
——— et al: A controlled trial of immunotherapy in insect hypersensitivity. N Engl J Med 299:158, 1978
LIGHT WC, REISMAN RE: Stinging insect allergy: Changing concepts. Postgrad Med 59:153, 1976

Marine animal venoms

HALSTEAD BW: Poisonous and venomous marine animals of the world. Washington, DC, US Government Printing Office, 1965, vol I; 1970, vol III
HUGHES JM, MERSON MH: Fish and shellfish poisoning. N Engl J Med 295:1117, 1976
KEEGAN HL, MACFARLANE WV (eds): *Venomous and Poisonous Animals and Noxious Plants of the Pacific Region* Oxford, Pergamon, 1965
RUSSELL FE: Marine toxins and venomous and poisonous marine animals. Adv Marine Biol 3:255, 1965
SCOGGIN CH: Catfish stings. JAMA 231:176, 1975
SOUTHCOTT RV: Notes on stings of some venomous Australian fishes. Med J Aust 2:722, 1970

Other arthropod bites

FRAZIER CA: *Insect Allergy: Allergic and Toxic Reactions to Insects and Other Arthropods*. St Louis, Warren H Green, 1969
HANEVELD GT: Centipede bites. Br Med J 2:592, 1952
KINGERY FAJ: Sorting out bug bites. Med Times 105:102, 1977
MCMILLAN CW, PURCELL WR: Health hazard from caterpillars. N Engl J Med 271:147, 1964

Scorpion stings

BARTHOLOMEW C: Acute scorpion pancreatitis in Trinidad. Br Med J 1:666, 1970

Horen WP: Insect and scorpion sting. JAMA 221:894, 1972

Sita Devi S et al: Defibrination syndrome due to scorpion venom poisoning. Br Med J 1:345, 1970

Stahnke HL: Arizona's lethal scorpion. Ariz Med 29:490, 1972

Snake and lizard bites

Albritton DC et al: Venination by the Mexican beaded lizard (*Heloderma horridum*). Report of a case. S Dak J Med 23:9, 1970

Minton SA Jr: *Venom Diseases.* Springfield, Ill, Charles C Thomas, 1974

Russell FE: Pharmacology of animal venoms. Clin Pharmacol Ther 8:849, 1967

———— et al: Snake venom poisoning in the United States: Experience with 550 cases. JAMA 233:341, 1975

Stahnke HL et al: Bite of the Gila monster. Rocky Mt Med J 67:25, 1970

Watt CH Jr: Poisonous snakebite treatment in the United States. JAMA 240:654, 1978

Spider bites

Berger RS: A critical look at therapy for the brown recluse spider. Arch Dermatol 107:288, 1973

Gorham JR: The brown recluse spider, loxosceles reclusa and necrotic spider bite—a new public health problem in the United States. J Environ Health 31:138, 1968.

Horen WP: Arachnidism in the United States. JAMA 185:839, 1963

Spider bites. Lancet 2:509, 1969

Tick paralysis

Cherington M, Snyder RD: Tick paralysis: Neurophysiologic studies. N Engl J Med 278:95, 1968

Schmitt N et al: Tick paralysis in British Columbia. Can Med Assoc J 100:417, 1969

Tick paralysis. Br Med J 3:314, 1969

section 17 | Diseases of uncertain etiology

216
SARCOIDOSIS

CAROL J. JOHNS

INTRODUCTION At the 1975 Seventh International Conference on Sarcoidosis it was proposed that sarcoidosis be described as "a multisystem granulomatous disorder of unknown etiology most commonly affecting young adults and presenting most frequently with bilateral hilar lymphadenopathy, pulmonary infiltration, skin or eye lesions." Other organs commonly involved include peripheral lymph nodes, liver, spleen, mucous membranes, parotid glands, phalangeal bones, muscles, heart, and nervous system. The diagnosis is established most securely when there is involvement of more than one organ system with clinical and radiographic findings, supported by histological evidence of widespread noncaseating epithelioid-cell granulomas in one tissue, with the absence of known agents capable of inducing similar granulomatous lesions (beryllium, tubercle bacillus, fungi, etc.). The Kveim-Siltzbach reaction is frequently positive and lends support to the diagnosis. Impairment of cell-mediated immunity is manifest by depression of tuberculin-type delayed hypersensitivity but well-maintained or increased production of humoral antibodies (immunoglobulins). The clinical course varies from that of a self-limited one, with spontaneous resolution, to that of progressive widespread granulomatous inflammation and fibrosis. Corticosteroids produce clinical remissions and suppress inflammation and granuloma formation. Long-term treatment for many years may be required to prevent clinical relapse.

ETIOLOGY The cause of sarcoidosis remains unknown but most authorities agree it is a specific disease. Whether there is a single inciting infectious or other exogenous agent is unclear. The immunologic features and abnormalities have attracted increasing attention. Impaired regulation of the cell functions of thymus-derived lymphocytes (T cells) and bone-marrow-derived lymphocytes (B cells) is suspected. Such changes could be primary or secondary. A persistent antigen could stimulate release of an immunosuppressive lymphokine and the formation of epithelioid granulomas, probably derived from macrophages. Immune complexes may be implicated. There are other possible factors of genetic susceptibility, but no pattern of histocompatibility antigens has been identified in sarcoidosis. A possible role of the tubercle bacillus has been debated and may be significant in some cases. The disease may be a result of an interaction between an infective agent and a subject with unusual immunologic responses. It cannot be assumed that all cases of sarcoidosis are associated with the same inciting agent. Studies in mice suggest a transmissible agent from human sarcoid tissue, and the tubercle bacillus was identified in a few mice after serial passages through mice and a 0.2-μm filter.

EPIDEMIOLOGY Sarcoidosis has been observed in virtually every country in which it has been sought. Blacks are affected 10 times more frequently than Caucasians in the United States, and the incidence in females is usually double that in males. An increased incidence in relation to pregnancy and lactation has been noted, especially in patients with erythema nodosum. The disease is most frequent in the third and fourth decades of life, but the range begins in childhood, particularly around adolescence, and extends to the sixth and seventh decades. Familial associations are noted occasionally.

PATHOLOGY Granulomatous inflammatory changes of sarcoidosis may occur in almost any organ. Disseminated granulomas are probably often present even with clinically localized disease, i.e., hepatic granulomas with only asymptomatic hilar adenopathy. The hard tubercles are generally sharply demarcated from surrounding tissues but may coalesce. Some central fibrinoid or granular necrosis may occur, especially in association with systemic active febrile disease, but caseation is usually absent, and inflammatory reaction is minimal. Giant cells containing laminated calcific Schaumann bodies or stellate "asteroid" bodies are frequent, but neither of these inclusions is found solely in sarcoidosis.

Similar histological changes may be seen in tuberculosis, fungous infections, leprosy, tertiary syphilis, beryllium disease, "farmer's lung," foreign-body reactions, lymphomas, and lymph nodes draining malignant tumors. The histological picture in sarcoid is not specific for that disease alone, and the above-mentioned possibilities cannot be excluded in the absence of other data.

Adrenal corticosteroids cause a prompt reduction in the nonspecific cellular inflammatory reaction of an acute or subacute process and hasten involution and resorption of the "sarcoid" tubercles. It seems likely that these hormones prevent or lessen but do not erase progressive scarring.

Autopsy material on patients with long-standing sarcoidosis may reveal widespread tubercles in many organs, a few scattered tubercles or focal hyalin scarring, or, rarely, no residual changes.

MANIFESTATIONS Clinical manifestations of sarcoidosis generally depend on the activity, degree, and site of tissue involvement and vary from incidental radiographic findings without associated symptoms, to severe incapacity and death. Impaired function is caused both by active granulomatous disease and by secondary fibrosis. Symptoms are frequently mild or absent.

Constitutional symptoms Fever, weight loss, and fatigue are often nonspecific presenting complaints, occasionally without other localizing symptoms. Persistent daily spiking fever to 38.3°C (101°F) may be observed and necessitates careful exclusion of tuberculosis. This is most commonly observed in association with active granulomatous inflammation in the liver. Fever in association with erythema nodosum is another form in which sarcoidosis may become evident. This syndrome includes transient tender erythematous subcutaneous nodules over the pretibial areas, arthralgias, and pulmonary hilar adenopathy on x-ray. Hepatic tubercles and a positive Kveim reaction are frequent. This syndrome has been regarded as an early manifestation of sarcoidosis and noted frequently in young women in Scandinavia and Great Britain. It is also observed in the United States, may be overlooked easily, and has a favorable prognosis. Fever, hepatosplenomegaly, and hypercalcemia form another presenting syndrome, which is observed more commonly in Caucasian patients.

Lymph nodes Mediastinal and hilar nodes are most frequently involved. Vague substernal discomfort may be present. Readily palpable peripheral nodes which are discrete, firm, and nontender are often prominent. There may be generalized lymphadenopathy, or involvement may be localized to the cervical, axillary, and femoral nodes. Usually, the changes are symmetrical and the epitrochlear nodes are palpable.

Lungs Pulmonary involvement is the most common and, perhaps, the most important manifestation of sarcoidosis. Spontaneous permanent remissions are observed, but significant lung disease represents the most frequent indication for treatment. Serious parenchymal changes, with or without hilar adenopathy, are evident on x-ray in about 50 percent of all patients. Varying and impressive degrees of dyspnea and cough are noted. A discrepancy in which the radiographic changes exceed the symptoms and signs is a diagnostic clue in early sarcoidosis. In some patients, usually Caucasian, striking radiographic changes may be associated with no symptoms, and ventilatory and diffusion measurements are normal. In others, often blacks, pathological and physiological abnormalities may be present when the x-ray shows only hilar adenopathy. Dyspnea may be severe and is present in approximately half the patients with parenchymal disease. This results from extensive interstitial changes which impair oxygenation by disturbances of ventilation and perfusion ratios and loss of effective diffus-

ing surface. Compensatory hyperventilation is often noted. Large rounded intrapulmonary masses which may resemble metastatic tumor are probably a result of primary involvement of lymphoid tissue or localized infiltrates producing minimal physiological disturbance and minimal symptoms despite their dramatic x-ray appearance. Pleural effusions are unusual and should lead to the suspicion that other disease is present.

Cough may be severe and incapacitating and may occur in paroxysms which can even lead to vomiting. Sputum is scanty; occasional blood streaking results from the strain of coughing or endobronchial granulomas or in association with a picture that resembles bronchiectasis. Wheezing is occasionally produced by localized bronchial lesions with stenosis. Pulmonary obstruction is noted in late fibrotic chronic sarcoidosis. Physical findings are variable and nonspecific. Respiratory excursion may be restricted, crackling rales may be heard diffusely or at the lung bases, and the P_2 may be accentuated or split if pulmonary hypertension develops, or in the presence of bundle branch block.

Bronchoscopy generally reveals normal mucosa, although in a few cases it shows granulomatous inflammatory changes with endobronchial narrowing. Granulomas may be demonstrated occasionally in grossly normal-appearing mucosa.

In some patients sarcoidosis is a chronic progressive disease, and pulmonary insufficiency and cor pulmonale occur as late features. Bronchiolostenosis, resulting from peribronchial fibrosis and mucosal changes, may result in localized emphysema, giving rise to cystic changes, usually in the upper lung fields. With superimposed bacterial infection, a bronchiectasis-like picture results. Large cavitary or bullous lesions are rare but may lead to large and repeated hemoptyses, which are occasionally fatal. Such lesions may also form the locus for an aspergilloma, with recurrent hemoptyses. However, these "fungous balls" are usually saprophytic and often multiple. They may vary spontaneously in size and number over periods of 10 or more years, without invasive disease, even when steroid maintenance treatment is required. Surgical management is rarely feasible because of the diffuse and restrictive nature of the disease. Spontaneous pneumothorax is an occasional complication of lung involvement.

Eyes Acute granulomatous uveitis may be the initial manifestation of sarcoidosis. Ocular disease may progress to severe visual impairment and blindness with corneal and lenticular opacities and secondary glaucoma. A careful slit-lamp examination is worthwhile in all patients with sarcoid to detect early evidence of anterior uveitis. Lacrimal gland enlargement, conjunctival infiltrations, and keratoconjunctivitis sicca of the type seen in Sjögren's syndrome (Chap. 363) are common. Exophthalmos has been observed, as have retinal lesions with vasculitis producing papillitis and periphlebitis.

Skin Lesions occur in about 30 percent of patients, most dramatically around the nose, eyes, and mouth, and vary from extensive erythematous, infiltrated, and raised lesions to small nondescript plaques and papules. Mucosal lesions are often associated, extending into the nose, sinuses, and the hard palate. Increased or decreased pigmentation is frequently noted. Sarcoid changes often occur at sites of old scars or tattoos or recent injury. Subcutaneous nodular infiltrations occur, and in rare instances calcification of such lesions has been observed. Alopecia occurs if the scalp is affected. Skin lesions are associated with chronicity but often with otherwise mild disease. Erythema nodosum in early sarcoidosis usually presents a histologic picture of a nonspecific vasculitis.

Liver Clinical manifestations of hepatic sarcoidosis are present in only about 20 percent of cases. Nevertheless, hepatic tubercles can be found by biopsy in about 75 percent. Asymptomatic hepatomegaly is frequent. Severe jaundice is unusual, but mild increase in bilirubin and striking elevation of serum alkaline phosphatase level are observed. Intense pruritus may be the presenting manifestation. Intrahepatic cholestasis may occur with a picture resembling biliary cirrhosis. The spectrum of hepatic sarcoid includes the incidental tubercle, tubercles with surrounding nonspecific inflammatory reaction, chronic active granulomatous hepatitis, postnecrotic cirrhosis with or without portal hypertension, and portal hypertension without significant cirrhosis. Esophageal varices have been demonstrated in patients with portal hypertension, and shunt procedures occasionally have been required. Response to steroids has been disappointing in severe hepatic sarcoid, but steroids are indicated with a significant active inflammatory process. In some patients the granulomatous disease is limited to the liver, spleen, and abdominal nodes without other clinical or radiographic evidence of sarcoidosis.

Spleen Mild splenomegaly occurs in 20 to 30 percent of cases and often regresses promptly with administration of corticosteroids. Enlargement may be striking and associated with "hypersplenism," anemia, leukopenia, and thrombocytopenia. It may persist for 10 to 20 years without undue complications, although splenectomy will result in hematologic improvement.

Kidneys Impaired renal function may occur secondary to hypercalcemia and hypercalciuria, secondary to hyperuricemia, and, less commonly, because of direct granulomatous involvement. Nephrocalcinosis and renal calculi are observed.

Heart Effects are usually secondary to lung disease, with pulmonary hypertension and cor pulmonale. Primary myocardial sarcoidosis often is not recognized and is most commonly manifested by conduction disturbances, paroxysmal arrhythmias and infiltrative cardiomyopathy. Sudden death may result, and an artificial pacemaker may be required.

Salivary glands Asymptomatic enlargement of the parotid, sublingual, and submaxillary glands occurs in about 6 percent of cases. Spontaneous regression commonly occurs. A syndrome of fever, uveitis, and lacrimal and salivary gland enlargement is known as uveoparotid fever, or *Heerfordt's syndrome.* Facial nerve palsies may be associated with parotid disease.

Muscle Sarcoid granulomas occur in muscles far more frequently than is clinically indicated by pain and weakness. In a few cases symptoms may be severe and incapacitating. Muscle biopsy is likely to be positive in such patients and also in those with polyarthralgias.

Joints Arthralgias may occur independently as an early prominent feature and are common in association with erythema nodosum and fever. Sarcoid tubercles have been observed in biopsies of synovium. Transient knee effusions are occasionally noted. Chronic periarticular swelling and tenderness may be associated with bony changes in the fingers and toes and skin lesions. Monoarticular arthritis raises the suspicion of tuberculosis.

Bones Asymptomatic, punched-out lesions in the distal phalanges of the hands and feet are visible in roentgenograms in about 10 percent of cases. Associated overlying skin changes are common. Radiolucent skull lesions have been noted in a few patients. "Routine" hand x-rays are not likely to be abnormal in the absence of overlying skin changes.

Nervous system Neurological manifestations are variable. Cranial and peripheral nerves may be affected by direct involvement of the nerve sheaths or roots. Facial nerve palsies, which may be bilateral and sequential, are the commonest neurological finding and may undergo full remission. Swallowing disorders are observed. A granulomatous basilar meningitis can affect the cranial nerves and produce pleocytosis and elevation of the spinal fluid protein level. Pituitary involvement produces diabetes insipidus. Involvement of the choroid plexuses may obstruct the ventricles. Cortical changes may result in convulsive seizures.

Other tissues Involvement of the tonsils and laryngeal, buccal, and nasal mucosa (often with associated sinusitis) has been encountered. Bilateral nasal obstruction may be a presenting complaint. Submucous resections are contraindicated as they frequently result in septal perforations. Sarcoid lesions have been found in thyroid, parathyroid, and pancreatic tissues, and gastric granulomas have resulted in bleeding and perforation. Sarcoid involving the adrenal, cervix, uterus, epididymis, or testis is very unusual.

LABORATORY FINDINGS Mild anemia, leukopenia, eosinophilia, and elevated sedimentation rate are common in active disease. Thrombocytopenia is unusual but may be severe.

Delayed skin reactions Tuberculin anergy is noted in about two-thirds of patients, but a positive tuberculin reaction occurs if active tuberculosis supervenes. A previously known positive tuberculin reaction may become less reactive with active sarcoidosis. Associated generalized cutaneous anergy to other commonly occurring antigens such as *Candida albicans, Trichophyton,* and mumps virus has been noted. This depression of delayed skin reactivity is considered to be an important feature of sarcoidosis, but it varies with the duration and activity of the disease.

Chemical studies Hypergammaglobulinemia and reduction of serum albumin are common. Hypercalcemia and hypercalciuria are infrequent but apparently result from increased intestinal absorption of calcium, which is possibly related to increased sensitivity to vitamin D. Serum uric acid level may be elevated even in the absence of renal insufficiency. Elevation of serum alkaline phosphatase level is attributable to intrahepatic tubercles, rather than to bone lesions, and may reach very high levels.

Other studies Serum lysozyme levels are elevated in sarcoidosis (also tuberculosis) and are thought to reflect active granuloma formation. Levels seem to return to normal with corticosteroid therapy and inactivity of the disease. Elevated levels of serum angiotensin-converting enzyme (ACE) are similarly reported to correlate with the presence of active sarcoidosis. The specificity and sensitivity of ACE appears potentially useful. Elevated levels also have been observed in Gaucher's disease and occasionally in other diseases.

Roentgenographic studies Approximately 90 percent of patients show intrathoracic disease on chest x-ray. Bilateral hilar adenopathy, often with associated right paratracheal adenopathy, is a common feature. Unilateral hilar adenopathy is unusual and should initiate a search for other diseases. Patients may be grouped according to the apparent extent and chronicity of the radiographic picture as follows: group I, hilar adenopathy with no parenchymal changes; group II, hilar adenopathy and diffuse parenchymal changes; group III, diffuse parenchymal changes without hilar adenopathy; group IV, chronic parenchymal changes of more than 2 years' duration with pulmonary fibrosis. The pulmonary changes are generally symmetrical, and may present a diffuse ground-glass appearance, fine reticular or miliary lesions, large nodular lesions, or multiple large confluent infiltrates resembling metastatic tumors. Fine diffuse interstitial fibrosis may be present. Pulmonary fibrosis may produce contraction and distortion, and extensive cystic and bullous lesions are common in the late stages. Bony changes in the phalanges, skull, and vertebrae may occur.

Pulmonary function tests These tests commonly demonstrate restriction, decreased compliance, and loss of effective diffusing surface. Vital capacity is reduced. Measurements of carbon monoxide–diffusing capacity are frequently reduced even in the absence of demonstrable radiographic changes or clinical symptoms. Measurements of vital capacity and diffusing capacity may serve as indicators of progression of disease and response to treatment. In diffuse disease, arterial blood studies reveal with exercise a reduced P_{O_2} because of perfusion of poorly ventilated areas of the lung. The arterial P_{CO_2} is commonly below normal because of compensatory hyperventilation. Some abnormalities of airway function are frequently observed in severe, late stages of pulmonary fibrosis, but carbon dioxide retention with elevation of arterial P_{CO_2} is a late and unusual feature. Significant impairment of pulmonary function frequently remains even after radiographic clearing. Following steroid therapy or a spontaneous remission, the vital capacity tends to return toward normal, but may remain somewhat reduced. The diffusing capacity may improve significantly but usually stabilizes well below normal despite complete remission of all symptoms. Improvement in diffusing capacity is less frequent than is that of the vital capacity. Deterioration of pulmonary function may occur gradually and progressively.

DIAGNOSIS The diagnosis depends on the clinical features along with histological evidence of epithelioid tubercles from tissue biopsy or from a positive Kveim reaction. The amount of histological support required varies inversely with the certainty with which the pattern of clinical features is recognized. It is essential to exclude other recognized causes of granulomatous disease. To exclude local sarcoid tissue reaction, as in nodes draining a malignant tumor, clinical evidence of involvement of more than one site is desirable. Careful search for tubercle bacilli, fungi, and foreign bodies must be made in all histological sections. A positive Kveim reaction is a special feature and often helps to exclude other granulomatous processes, although the specificity and selectivity of this reaction are debated. Tissue biopsy for histological diagnosis is most readily and easily obtained from superficial or palpable lesions in skin, lymph nodes, conjunctiva, and nasal, buccal, and bronchial mucosa. Almost any palpable lymph node is likely to be positive. Liver biopsies reveal granulomas in 70 to 80 percent of cases even without clinical evidence of impaired hepatic function. Biopsy of the gastrocnemius muscle frequently reveals granulomatous changes in patients with arthralgias and erythema nodosum. In the absence of palpable peripheral lymph nodes or dermal or mucosal lesions, transbronchial lung biopsy or mediastinoscopy and node biopsy, or biopsy of liver or muscle is in order. Flexible fiberoptic bronchoscopy with transbronchial lung biopsy frequently provides a dependable histological diagnosis. Along with tissue showing granulomas provided by the biopsy, bronchoalveolar lavage reveals an increased number of lymphocytes but fewer than are seen in hypersensitivity pneumonitis. Open lung biopsy is generally reserved for patients in whom other diagnostic maneuvers have not been successful or in whom the exclusion of other diseases

is urgent. The indicated tissue biopsy is that which combines the least risk with the greatest likelihood of diagnostic yield. With typical clinical features with asymptomatic bilateral hilar adenopathy, a presumptive diagnosis may be justified, without histological verification. In mild or asymptomatic disease, when reliable Kveim material is available, this test is often useful in the diagnosis.

Kveim reaction In 50 to 80 percent of patients with sarcoidosis, the intracutaneous injection of a heat-sterilized suspension of human sarcoid tissues (spleen or lymph nodes) produces a papulonodular lesion with epithelioid tubercles. The nodule must be biopsied in 4 to 6 weeks for routine histological study. This reveals a spectrum from positive to negative, and includes a middle equivocal group. A positive reaction is limited to those with well-formed *epithelioid tubercles*. Test material must be assayed in patients of known reactivity, and experienced interpretation is essential. The Kveim reaction is very likely to be positive in the presence of sarcoid lymphadenopathy, in association with erythema nodosum, and when sarcoid skin lesions are present. The reaction is less likely to be positive in the absence of lymph node involvement and during steroid therapy. Tests in patients with a variety of granulomatous and collagen vascular diseases have revealed only 2 to 5 percent false-positive reactions, but many false-negative results are encountered in patients later shown to have sarcoidosis. The nature of the Kveim reaction is not understood, and its selectivity must be interpreted in concert with the clinical findings and the demonstrated performance of the particular Kveim preparation. This simple outpatient procedure is often useful.

COURSE Sarcoidosis is frequently no more than an incidental radiographic finding on routine chest x-ray. The course is often one of spontaneous remission over a period of 6 to 24 months, with little or no evidence of residual disease and with normal life expectancy. However, there may be persistent abnormalities with varying disability or progressive deterioration. Death related to sarcoidosis may ensue in 5 to 10 percent of cases and is most frequently related to advanced pulmonary disease. There may be impressive clearing of radiographic lesions, especially when the disease seems limited to the thorax. Following a spontaneous remission, recurrence is most unusual. Remissions are most frequent in the syndrome of erythema nodosum and hilar adenopathy. This "benign" form is more common in Caucasians than in blacks where chronic progressive diffuse systemic disease is more frequently encountered. Systemic manifestations in skin, bone, eyes, and salivary glands and hepatosplenomegaly herald a less favorable prognosis. Severe uveitis may progress to glaucoma, cataract formation, and blindness.

Steroids probably exert a favorable influence only when there is significant incapacitating disease and an active inflammatory process.

TREATMENT Relatively asymptomatic patients usually require no treatment. *Adrenal corticosteroids* dramatically suppress the active inflammatory reaction and provide important symptomatic improvement. Indications for treatment are (1) active ocular disease, (2) persistent or progressive pulmonary involvement, (3) persistent hypercalcemia or hypercalcinuria, (4) central nervous system involvement with significant functional impairment, (5) significant evidence of myocardial disease, (6) persistent systemic evidence of illness such as fever and weight loss, and (7) significant and progressive involvement of a vital organ. The disease remains in remission in some patients after administration of steroids, but it commonly recurs as the dose is reduced, even when therapy has been continued for 2 or more years. It is thought that steroids prevent the progression of disease, but healing may occur with hyalin scarring. Steroids clearly cannot reverse a fibrotic process. Early steroid therapy offers more hope than that initiated after 1 or 2 years of disease.

Steroids are most frequently required and beneficial for symptomatic lung disease. Uncertainty as to the value of steroids may stem from attempted evaluation of benefits in patients with asymptomatic minimal disease which probably required no treatment. Even relatively asymptomatic but significant lung disease should be treated if there is no evidence of spontaneous regression in 12 months, or if there is progression in 3 to 6 months. One should not wait for the appearance of symptoms when lung function is persistently and significantly reduced. Asymptomatic hilar adenopathy without clinical evidence of pulmonary parenchymal disease does not require therapy.

Prednisone is administered in initial divided daily doses of 40 mg, with 2-week periods on daily doses of 40, 30, and 25 mg, and then in single 8 A.M. daily maintenance doses of 20 to 10 mg. Symptomatic improvement occurs in 1 to 2 weeks, and the disease regresses over a period of several months. Therapy probably should be continued for a minimum of 6 to 8 months, with periodic attempts thereafter to reduce dosage or eliminate the drug. Objective criteria such as x-rays and measurements of pulmonary function are important. Maintenance therapy for many years has proved necessary in many patients in whom relapses recur at a dose below 10 to 15 mg. Dosage must be tapered slowly, with decrements of 2.5 mg no oftener than at 2- to 4-week intervals if long-term treatment has been used. Lifelong therapy may be required. Careful documentation and observation during tapering are essential in planning treatment. Alternate-day dosage may be used for maintenance therapy. It is probably not advisable for initial management. Endocrine side effects, with weight gain of 20 to 50 lb, have been observed in some women. Diabetes has appeared in some patients, particularly in association with significant hepatic involvement. Local steroid therapy has been effective in ocular sarcoid with anterior uveitis or iritis, although there is the risk of glaucoma. Intradermal steroids have been used with some success for disfiguring cutaneous lesions. Such lesions are not usually considered justification for systemic steroids.

Chloroquine (Aralen), in doses of 250 mg daily, after an initial period of 2 weeks with 500 mg daily, has been observed to induce dramatic improvement in skin and mucosal lesions over periods of several weeks, but relapse is common when the drug is withdrawn. With periodic ocular examinations and intermittent treatment periods of 6 months, no irreversible retinal damage has been encountered. Remission may be maintained with as little as 125 mg daily. Response to hydroxychloroquine (Plaquenil) has been slower and less satisfactory. Hypercalcemia has also appeared to respond to chloroquine.

Antituberculous therapy is ineffective in sarcoidosis. However, prophylactic isoniazid in association with corticosteroids is often recommended for black patients with extensive pulmonary disease, in areas with high risks of exposure to tuberculosis, and always for patients who are tuberculin-positive. If tuberculosis is really suspected, two drugs should be employed, e.g., isoniazid and ethambutol, especially if corticosteroids are to be administered.

COMPLICATIONS The complications are related to the effects of severe and progressive disease in various organs, the side effects of therapy, and superimposed infection. An increased incidence (2 to 5 percent) of tuberculosis in association with sarcoidosis has been recognized. Associated fungous infections seem to be increasing. Saprophytic *aspergillus* fungous balls (mycetomas) have been noted in pulmonary cysts. Candidiasis and cryptococcosis in association with sarcoidosis have also been noted. It is possible that long-term steroid and antimicrobial therapy predispose to these fungous infections, but the predisposing pulmonary anatomic changes represent the underlying problem.

REFERENCES

DELANEY P: Neurologic manifestations in sarcoidosis: Review of the literature, with a report of 23 cases. Ann Intern Med 87:366, 1977

DeREMEE RA: The present status of treatment of pulmonary sarcoidosis: A house divided. Chest 71:388, 1977

GUPTA RC et al: Pulmonary and extrapulmonary sarcoidosis in relation to circulatory immune complexes. Am Rev Resp Dis 166:261, 1977

JAMES DG et al: Immunology of sarcoidosis. Am J Med 59:388, 1975
——— et al: Sarcoidosis and respiratory disorders. Mt Sinai J Med 44:698, 1977

JOHNS CJ et al: Extended experience in the long-term corticosteroid treatment of pulmonary sarcoid. Ann NY Acad Sci 278:722, 1976

KOERNER SK et al: Transbronchial lung biopsy for the diagnosis of sarcoidosis. N Engl J Med 293:268, 1975

LEVINSON RS et al: Airway function in sarcoidosis. Am J Med 62:51, 1977

LIEBERMAN J: Elevation of serum angiotensin-converting-enzyme (ACE) level in sarcoidosis. Am J Med 59:365, 1975

LONGCOPE WT et al: A study of sarcoidosis: Based on a combined investigation of 160 cases including 30 autopsies from the Johns Hopkins Hospital and Massachusetts General Hospital. Medicine 31:1, 1952

MADDREY WC et al: Sarcoidosis and chronic hepatic disease: A clinical and pathologic study of 20 patients. Medicine 49:375, 1970

MAYOCK RL et al: Manifestations of sarcoidosis: Analysis of 145 patients with a review of 9 series selected from the literature. Am J Med 35:67, 1963

MITCHELL DN et al: Sarcoidosis. Am Rev Resp Dis 110:774, 1974
——— et al: Transmissible agents from human sarcoid and Crohn's disease tissues. Lancet 2:761, 1976

PROCEEDINGS OF THE EIGHTH INTERNATIONAL SARCOIDOSIS CONFERENCE, September 1978, Cardiff, Wales (in press)

ROBERTS WC et al: Sarcoidosis of the heart. A clinicopathologic study of 35 necropsy patients (group I) and review of 78 previously described necropsy patients (group II). Am J Med 63:86, 1977

SHARMA OP: *Sarcoidosis—A Clinical Approach.* Springfield, Ill, Charles C Thomas, 1975

SILVERMAN KJ et al: Cardiac sarcoid: A clinicopathologic study of 84 unselected patients with systemic sarcoidosis. Circulation 58:1204, 1978

Transactions of the New York Academy of Sciences: Seventh International Conference on Sarcoidosis and other Granulomatous Disorders. Ann NY Acad Sci 278:1, 1975

WEINBERGER SE et al: Bronchoalveolar lavage in interstitial lung disease. Ann Intern Med 89:459, 1978

217

FAMILIAL MEDITERRANEAN FEVER (FAMILIAL PAROXYSMAL POLYSEROSITIS)

SHELDON M. WOLFF

DEFINITION Familial Mediterranean fever (FMF) is an inherited disorder of unknown etiology, characterized by recurrent episodes of fever, peritonitis, and/or pleuritis. Arthritis, skin lesions, and amyloidosis are seen in some patients.

HISTORY Although the first report of FMF was by Janeway and Mosenthal in 1908, it was not until the report of five cases by Siegal in 1945 that attention was focused on FMF as a distinct entity. Subsequently, some authors have not applied strict clinical criteria, and many patients with other diseases have been reported as having FMF. The detailed and extensive descriptions by Heller and Sohar have clarified many of the clinical aspects of FMF.

TERMINOLOGY The variety of names given to FMF has led to confusion concerning its clinical features. None of the names, including FMF, is completely satisfactory, but FMF has received the widest acceptance. Such terms as *periodic disease, periodic peritonitis, la maladie periodique* are inaccurate because the disease often is not cyclical. *Benign paroxysmal peritonitis* is inappropriate because many of the patients have involvement of serosal surfaces other than the peritoneum, and some die of amyloidosis. *Familial paroxysmal polyserositis* is an acceptable alternative for the term *familial Mediterranean fever.*

ETHNOLOGY AND GENETICS FMF occurs predominantly in patients of non-Ashkenazic (Sephardic) Jewish, Armenian, and Arabic ancestry. However, the disease is not restricted to these groups, and has been seen in patients of Italian, Ashkenazic Jewish, and Anglo-Saxon descent as well as others.

The best studies of the genetics of FMF have been done in Israel, where relatively homogeneous population groups exist. In Israel, the disease appears to be inherited as an autosomal recessive. Nevertheless, approximately 50 percent of patients give no family history of the disease. Consanguinity among the parents of FMF patients is as high as 20 percent, a figure which may be an underestimate because most patients came from very inbred ethnic groups. Approximately 60 percent of patients are male.

ETIOLOGY Although numerous pathogenetic mechanisms have been suggested, the etiology of FMF is unknown. Fever and inflammation are such prominent signs that frequent attempts have been made to implicate infectious agents and/or their products. It has been suggested that FMF is a form of brucellosis or tuberculosis. Suffice it to say that extensive studies utilizing modern microbiological and serologic techniques have failed to implicate these or any other specific infectious agents.

It has been reported that FMF is due to an allergy or to hypersensitivity, but such hypersensitive states have not been substantiated. There is no firm evidence favoring an autoimmune etiology.

Reimann has suggested that FMF, like many other recurring illnesses (periodic disease), may be a pathological exaggeration of normal periodic temperature rhythmicity. However, extensive studies of temperature and other circadian rhythms in FMF patients have failed to demonstrate alterations from normal.

Because many FMF patients note that certain emotional or environmental changes may have profound effects on the frequency with which episodes of their disease occur, a psychosomatic basis has been suggested for the illness. There is no question that most patients eventually have transient or even permanent psychological alterations, which probably reflect their reaction to a chronic recurring illness that is forever threatening their social, economic, and personal well-being, but there is no evidence for a functional etiology for FMF.

The demonstration that FMF is inherited as an autosomal recessive disorder has led to the thesis that it is another inborn error of metabolism. Originally it was thought that the disorder might be one of altered lipid metabolism. Despite extensive studies, no such error has been found. Reported instances of

excessive urinary excretion of porphyrins in FMF are probably examples of true porphyria and not FMF.

It has been reported that blood levels of unconjugated etiocholanolone were elevated during fever in six patients with FMF. Subsequent studies, however, showed no correlation between levels of etiocholanolone and fever.

PATHOLOGY Despite the striking clinical manifestations during an acute attack of FMF, no specific pathological alterations have been found. Most FMF patients undergo at least one laparotomy, and only acute peritoneal inflammation in which the exudate contains a predominance of polymorphonuclear leukocytes is found to be present. A disproportionately large number of male patients develop gallbladder disease with and without cholelithiasis, but extensive histopathologic examination has failed to reveal any specific pathological changes. Pleural and joint inflammation are also nonspecific.

In the amyloidosis which accompanies FMF, amyloid is deposited in the intima and media of the arterioles, the subendothelial region of venules, the glomeruli, and the spleen. Aside from their vessels, the heart and liver are uninvolved.

MANIFESTATIONS In the majority of patients, the symptoms of FMF begin between the ages of 5 and 15, although attacks sometimes commence during infancy, and onset has occurred as late as age 52. The duration and frequency of attacks vary greatly in the same patient, and there is no set rhythm or periodicity to their occurrence. The usual acute episode lasts 24 to 48 h, but some may be prolonged for 7 to 10 days. The attacks range in frequency from twice weekly to once a year, but 2 to 4 weeks is the commonest interval. Spontaneous remissions lasting years have been seen. In the majority of cases, pregnancy is associated with an absence of acute episodes and many patients note less frequent attacks in the summer than in the winter. There may be a decrease in the severity and frequency of the attacks with age or with development of amyloidosis.

Fever Fever is a cardinal manifestation of FMF and is present during most but not all attacks. Rarely, fever may be present without serositis. The temperature may be preceded by a chill, and will peak in 12 to 24 h. Defervescence is often accompanied by diaphoresis. The fever ranges from 38.5 to 40°C but is quite variable.

Abdominal pain Abdominal pain occurs in more than 95 percent of patients, and may vary in severity in the same patient. Minor premonitory discomfort may precede an acute episode by 24 to 48 h. The pain usually starts in one quadrant and then spreads to involve the whole abdomen. The initial site is usually very tender. Tenderness may remain localized with referred pain in other areas, and there may be radiation to the back. There may be splinting of the chest and pain in one or both shoulders, typical of diaphragmatic irritation. Nausea and vomiting sometimes occur. The abdomen is usually distended, and may become rigid with decreased or absent bowel sounds. On x-ray, the wall of the small intestine may appear edematous, transit of barium is slowed, and fluid levels may be seen. Because the manifestations of an acute abdominal attack can simulate those of a perforated viscus so closely, patients should be advised to have an elective appendectomy between attacks so that acute appendicitis will not obfuscate the picture at a later date. An abdominal operation may precipitate an acute attack of FMF which may be confused with other postoperative complications.

Chest pain Most patients with abdominal attacks have referred chest pain at one time or another, and 75 percent also develop acute pleuritic pain with or without abdominal symptoms. In 30 percent, the attacks of pleuritis precede the onset of abdominal attacks by varying periods of time, and a small number of patients never develop abdominal attacks. Chest pain is usually unilateral and is associated with diminished breath sounds, a friction rub, or a transient pleural effusion.

Joint pain In Israel, 75 percent of patients report at least one episode of acute arthritis. Arthritis can be distinct from abdominal or pleural attacks, can be acute or, rarely, chronic, and may involve one or several joints. Effusions are common and the large joints are involved most frequently. Radiologic findings are nonspecific. Despite careful search, frank arthritis rarely has been seen in the United States. Some patients have a history of rheumatic fever-like illness in childhood, but in a large series of patients, including 30 from the Middle East, acute arthritis was not observed. Mild arthralgia is common during acute attacks but is nonspecific and can be seen in many febrile illnesses, including experimentally induced hyperthermia.

Skin manifestations Skin involvement is reported by 25 to 35 percent of patients. These lesions consist of painful, erythematous areas of swelling from 5 to 20 cm in diameter, usually located on the lower legs, the medial malleolus, or the dorsum of the foot. They may occur without abdominal or pleural pain and subside within 24 to 48 h.

Other signs and symptoms Involvement of other serosal membranes has been reported, but pericarditis is rare, and it is probable that descriptions of recurrent meningitis have been diseases other than FMF. Hematuria, splenomegaly, and small white dots called *colloid bodies* in the ocular fundus are among the findings of questionable significance. Rarely migraine-like headaches accompany acute abdominal attacks, and some patients have become somewhat irrational or show extreme emotional lability during attacks. Whether these are primary manifestations of FMF or secondary effects of pain and fever is not known.

Complications The most serious complication of FMF in the United States is drug addiction or habituation, and obviously efforts should be made to avoid use of narcotics. Depression and lack of motivation are common, and patients with FMF require considerable encouragement and support. A striking number of patients in one American series have developed gallbladder disease.

Another major complication of FMF is *amyloidosis*. Some investigators believe that few patients in Israel escape this complication and that it is an expression of the same gene that is responsible for the other manifestations of FMF. If the attacks occur first, as they do in over 90 percent of the patients, the patients are classified as being of phenotype I. Amyloidosis also occurs in siblings of FMF patients or precedes the abdominal attacks (phenotype II). The infiltration by amyloid involves the kidneys, and death is often attributable to renal failure.

Amyloidosis has been reported in Israel and North Africa, but there have been only three reported instances of amyloidosis complicating FMF in the United States. These findings are even more striking because there are probably as many known FMF patients in the United States as in Israel. These differences are unexplained and suggest that environmental or nutritional, as well as genetic, factors may play a role in the development of amyloidosis in FMF.

LABORATORY FINDINGS There is no specific diagnostic test. Polymorphonuclear leukocytosis ranging from 15,000 to 30,000 cells per cubic millimeter is almost invariable during acute attacks. The erythrocyte sedimentation rate is elevated during attacks but returns to normal between attacks. Plasma fibrinogen, serum haptoglobin, ceruloplasmin, and C-reactive protein increase during the episodes. Plasma lipids are normal, and there are no consistent abnormalities of hepatic or renal function. When amyloidosis is present, laboratory findings are typical of a nephrotic syndrome followed by renal insufficiency. Electrocardiographic and electroencephalographic changes are inconstant and nonspecific.

DIAGNOSIS When the typical acute attacks of FMF occur in an individual of appropriate ethnic background who has a family history of FMF, the diagnosis is easy. On the other hand, if the disease has not been present in the family and the patient resides in a community where FMF is rare, the diagnosis can be very difficult.

Most patients with undiagnosed FMF have had one or more abdominal operations with no relief of symptoms. When a patient is seen for the first time, a variety of other febrile illnesses must be excluded by appropriate study or observation. These include acute appendicitis, acute pancreatitis, porphyria, cholecystitis, intestinal obstruction, and other major abdominal catastrophes.

Some of the inherited forms of the hyperlipidemias may mimic the clinical picture of FMF, but measurement of serum cholesterol and triglycerides will eliminate them from consideration. The patient with FMF is not immune to the other diseases, and when an attack differs from the usual pattern or is more prolonged, consideration should be given to other diagnostic possibilities. The pleural form of the disease is sometimes difficult to differentiate from acute pulmonary infection or infarction, but the rapid disappearance of signs and symptoms resolves the problem. The joint manifestations may be more prolonged than other forms of FMF, and differentiation from septic arthritis, gout, and acute rheumatoid disease may be necessary. The erythema is sometimes difficult to differentiate from superficial thrombophlebitis or cellulitis.

Whether or not the patient is of the appropriate ethnic group, the most difficult diagnostic problem in FMF is the patient who presents with fever alone. In this situation, an extensive diagnostic work-up for fever of unknown origin may be required. Fortunately, such patients are rare, and all eventually develop serosal involvement. Until specific diagnostic tests for FMF are available, patients with recurrent fever but without signs of inflammation of one of the serosal membranes should not be categorized as having FMF.

PROGNOSIS The prognosis of patients with FMF varies greatly according to the country in which they live. In the United States, the prognosis for long life is excellent. Despite the severity of the symptoms during some acute attacks, most patients are remarkably free of any debilitation during the intervals between attacks. With encouragement and an understanding of their disease, most FMF patients lead fairly normal lives. The greatest hazard to patients is prolonged periods of hospitalization due to erroneous diagnoses or failure to understand the disease. The liberal and injudicious use of narcotics for analgesia in these patients can lead to major psychological and health problems. Establishment of a reasonable doctor-patient relationship and education of the patient avoids this hazard. In the United States, the prognosis of patients with FMF does not seem to be different from that of patients with other chronic nonfatal illnesses. Death usually results from causes unrelated to the underlying disease.

The complication of amyloidosis in Israel, parts of North Africa, Turkey, and other parts of the Middle East makes the prognosis quite different from that in America. Approximately 25 percent of FMF patients in Israel are known to have amyloidosis, and this complication usually leads to death. Because a majority of patients under observation in Israel are under 40 years of age, it has been suggested that fatal amyloidosis may eventually occur in nearly all patients. This would explain the rarity of older patients in that area.

TREATMENT Many forms of therapy had been tried in FMF, but until recently, nothing was effective. Among the therapies tried have been antibiotics, hormones (including estrogens and adrenal corticosteroids), antipyretic drugs, immunotherapy, psychotherapy, elimination and low-fat diets, chloroquine, and phenylbutazone. When carefully studied and followed up, none of these therapies proved effective.

During the past 10 years, the outlook of patients with FMF has been altered dramatically. Goldfinger reported in 1972 that the prophylactic use of colchicine in five patients dramatically reduced the number of attacks. Subsequently, controlled trials in the United States and Israel have shown that chronic administration of colchicine will greatly reduce the number of acute attacks of FMF. It is recommended that 0.6 mg colchicine be taken by mouth three times a day. Patients often develop gastrointestinal side effects with this dose, however, in which case the dose should be reduced to 0.6 mg taken twice a day. Although an occasional patient will respond to 0.6 mg taken only once a day, this amount is less likely to be beneficial. Most but not all FMF patients will respond favorably to colchicine prophylaxis.

Since colchicine is known to result in nondisjunction of chromosomes and in azospermia in some patients, it should not be given to any patient, especially a young one, unless the disease is severe enough to warrant taking the risk. In addition, everyone who requires therapy should first be tried on a course of intermittent colchicine. The patient should take 0.6 mg colchicine by mouth every hour for 4 h, then every 2 h for 4 h, and every 12 h thereafter for 48 h. The colchicine should be given at the first premonitory sign of an attack. When colchicine is taken on such a schedule, many patients will experience aborted attacks or no symptoms at all. If both acute and prophylactic colchicine therapy fail, supportive therapy is all that can be offered. Except for unusual circumstances, narcotics should not be given to FMF patients.

The mechanism of colchicine's action against acute attacks of FMF is unknown. It is postulated that it may work by preventing the normal cellular response to inflammation.

A few reports have appeared in which FMF patients with amyloidosis have had successful renal transplants.

REFERENCES

DINARELLO CA et al: Colchicine therapy for familial Mediterranean fever. A double-blind trial. N Engl J Med 291:934, 1974
—— et al: Effect of prophylactic colchicine therapy on leukocyte function in patients with Familial Mediterranean Fever. Arthritis Rheum 19:618, 1976
SCHWABE AD, PETERS RS: Familial Mediterranean fever in Armenians. Analysis of 100 cases. Medicine 53:453, 1974
SOHAR E et al: Familial Mediterranean fever. Am J Med 43:227, 1967
WRIGHT DG et al: Efficiency of intermittent colchicine therapy in Familial Mediterranean Fever. Ann Intern Med 86:162, 1977

218

WEGENER'S GRANULOMATOSIS AND MIDLINE GRANULOMA

SHELDON M. WOLFF

WEGENER'S GRANULOMATOSIS

DEFINITION Wegener's granulomatosis is characterized by necrotizing vasculitis and granulomatous inflammation which affects primarily the upper and/or lower respiratory tract and the kidneys. However, small vessels anywhere can be involved. Rarely is the disease restricted to the respiratory tract (localized Wegener's granulomatosis). In the vast majority of cases the kidneys are involved and such patients have generalized Wegener's granulomatosis.

ETIOLOGY The cause of Wegener's granulomatosis is unknown, but most studies suggest a hypersensitivity reaction. The vasculitis, glomerulonephritis, the occasional ultrastructural findings of subepithelial glomerular deposits which look like immune complex deposition, and the reported presence of immune complexes in the serums of a few patients strongly implicate immune complex formation as the basis for the pathogenesis of this disease. On the other hand, the granulomas seen in many tissues suggest that cellular immune responses may also be involved. The antigen initiating the response(s) is unknown but may be microbial or tissue in origin and probably has as its site of origin the respiratory tract.

PATHOLOGY In order to make the diagnosis of Wegener's granulomatosis both granulomas and necrotizing vasculitis must be demonstrated. These lesions can occur anywhere but are most commonly found in the sinus mucosa, lungs, and skin. The necrotizing vasculitis and granulomatous inflammation are in and of themselves not distinctive, but the demonstration of both is required. In the kidney the most common lesion is a focal and segmental glomerulonephritis, although on occasion frank vasculitis or even a granuloma may be observed.

CLINICAL FEATURES Wegener's granulomatosis has been reported as early as the first and as late as the eighth decade of life, but the mean age of onset is approximately 40 years. The disease occurs twice as often in males as in females. The initial signs or symptoms can occur anywhere but usually are seen in the upper or lower respiratory tract. For example, patients may have headache, sinusitis, rhinorrhea, and otitis media with or without hearing loss. Other prominent presenting symptoms can include fever, arthralgias, and anorexia. Cough, pain in the chest, and hemoptysis may predominate in some patients. Associated with the respiratory findings may be signs or symptoms of any of the organ systems involved, and these can include all organ systems. It is rare for a patient to present initially with signs or symptoms of renal failure, but this occurs in about ten percent of patients.

In most patients Wegener's granulomatosis is a generalized disease associated with involvement of multiple organ systems, often with manifestations of acute inflammation. The respiratory tract (upper, lower, or both) is involved in all patients. The sinuses are affected in over 90 percent of patients. Saddle-nose deformities are common, as is mucosal ulceration, but mutilation does not occur. Very often the sinuses become secondarily infected with bacteria, and such infections require aggressive antibiotic therapy and often surgical intervention. Radiographs demonstrate the sinus involvement in this disease. The pulmonary manifestations are varied. Signs and symptoms suggestive of a pneumonitis may occur. Similarly, pleuritic manifestations are sometimes seen. Occasionally massive hemoptysis or pneumothorax develops. The typical x-ray features are those of nodular and cavitary infiltrates. These lesions can be evanescent and spontaneously disappear even without therapy. Lung biopsy is commonly performed in these patients and often leads to the diagnosis.

Renal involvement is present in over 90 percent of patients with Wegener's granulomatosis and is a prerequisite for a diagnosis of the generalized form of the disease. Prior to the availability of effective therapy, the mean survival of patients with renal involvement was 5 months. The urinary findings are consistent with acute glomerulonephritis, and an active sediment is common. About one-half the patients have glomerulonephritis, and on biopsy a focal glomerulitis is seen. Others also have a picture compatible with the nephrotic syndrome. Approximately 10 percent of patients have rapidly progressive glomerulonephritis and on biopsy have necrotizing and proliferative glomerulonephritis and marked crescent formation. Such patients should be treated as medical emergencies. Deposition of immunoglobulins and possible immune complex deposits have been noted in some patients.

Approximately 50 percent of patients with Wegener's granulomatosis have involvement of the eyes. Iritis, scleritis, and conjunctivitis are common. Proptosis due to retrobulbar granulomatous inflammation is occasionally seen. About one-third of patients have cardiac involvement, ranging from coronary arteritis to pericarditis. In approximately one-quarter of the patients the nervous system is involved. Most commonly, patients have mononeuritis multiplex while others have cranial neuritis.

In addition to serous otitis media, hearing loss is common in Wegener's granulomatosis. Almost one-half of patients have dermatologic manifestations including petechiae, vesicles, and necrotic ulcerations. Although frank arthritis is uncommon, about two-thirds of Wegener's granulomatous patients have arthralgias.

LABORATORY FINDINGS   There are no specific laboratory abnormalities in Wegener's granulomatosis. A normochromic, normocytic anemia is sometimes present. Leukocytosis is present in some patients but is usually seen when a superimposed bacterial infection has occurred. Thrombocytosis is seen in approximately ten percent of patients with the generalized form of the disease. The sedimentation rate is increased in almost all patients with active disease and is the most useful parameter with which to follow therapeutic efficacy. About fifty percent of patients have a positive test for rheumatoid factor, and many patients have hyperglobulinemia, particularly IgA. When renal involvement occurs, there are changes in the urine consistent with an active glomerulonephritis, and as the disease progresses, renal insufficiency is reflected in the usual laboratory abnormalities of uremia.

DIFFERENTIAL DIAGNOSIS   The diagnosis of Wegener's granulomatosis is made when histological evidence of vasculitis and granulomatous inflammation is present. The purely vasculitic diseases such as polyarteritis nodosa and systemic lupus erythematosus do not have granulomatous inflammation as a histological hallmark. Conversely, granulomatous diseases such as tuberculosis, fungal disease, and sarcoidosis do not show histological evidence of vasculitis. Certain diseases do present problems in differentiation from Wegener's granulomatosis. Occasional patients with Wegener's granulomatosis will present with hemoptysis, pulmonary hemorrhage, and rap-

idly progressive renal failure, and a clinical diagnosis of Goodpasture's syndrome is suspected. However, appropriate biopsies and immunofluorescent studies should differentiate these two conditions. Midline granuloma is restricted to the head and neck and not associated with vasculitis. Lymphomatoid granulomatosis can present with a clinical picture indistinguishable from Wegener's granulomatosis. However, biopsy of involved organs (e.g., lung, skin) should demonstrate the characteristic cellular infiltrates. Occasional malignant tumors, particularly malignant lymphomas, will result in granulomatous inflammation and even vasculitis, but histological demonstration of the malignant cells leads to differentiation from Wegener's granulomatosis.

TREATMENT   The use of cytotoxic agents in Wegener's granulomatosis has resulted in one of the most striking examples of the way modern chemotherapeutic intervention can alter the course of a hitherto lethal illness. Properly treated, over 95 percent of patients will go into remission, and since some remissions have lasted up to 15 years, it is not inappropriate to talk of cures in this disease.

The treatment of choice is cyclophosphamide, although in many cases azathioprine is equally as effective. Other alkylating agents, such as chlorambucil, may be used. In those patients where the disease is progressing rapidly, intravenous cyclophosphamide therapy may be used, but in general the oral route is preferred. Therapy ordinarily begins at 2 mg/kg cyclophosphamide daily, and this dose is adjusted according to the peripheral white blood cell count. Generally, the dose will decrease with time owing to depression of the white blood cell count. Treatment should be carried on for 1 year after the patient goes into remission. In patients with irreversible renal failure, dialysis may have to be employed, but renal transplantation should be considered in such patients as well. Adrenal corticosteroids are often used as adjunctive therapy in patients whose disease shows active inflammation. The steroid regimen of these patients should be converted to an alternate-day schedule as early as possible.

MIDLINE GRANULOMA

DEFINITION   Midline granuloma is an uncommon disease characterized by localized inflammation, destruction, and often mutilation of the tissues of the upper respiratory tract and face. This condition has also been referred to as *lethal midline granuloma, malignant granuloma,* and *granuloma gangrenescens,* none of which is an appropriate term.

ETIOLOGY   The etiology of midline granuloma is unknown. In view of the intense granulomatous inflammation, the disease is thought to represent a localized hypersensitivity reaction which leads to tissue destruction and mutilation. However, the responsible antigen(s) is unknown, and there is no immunologic evidence supporting this hypothesis. A variety of microorganisms have been considered as possible causative agents, but detailed microbiologic investigations have failed to detect the consistent presence of pathogenic organisms. In view of the clinical and pathological features of the illness as well as the fact that some upper-airway tumors can elicit a similar intense inflammatory response, some authors have suggested a neoplastic basis for midline granuloma. However, when malignant tissue (usually of a lymphomatous nature) is found in the lesions, the diagnosis of midline granuloma is no longer tenable.

PATHOLOGY   The most characteristic pathological finding is acute or chronic inflammation with necrosis. Superimposed pyogenic infection of the involved tissues, including the sinuses, may contribute to nonspecific histological findings. The pathological hallmark, noncaseating granulomas, with or without giant cells, may be obscured by the inflammatory reaction, but when present are strong evidence in favor of the diagnosis. Primary vasculitis is seen rarely, and when it occurs, a search for other causes, most notably Wegener's granulomatosis, should be made. The presence of malignant cells makes the diagnosis of midline granuloma unacceptable. Until an etiology is established, the diagnosis of midline granuloma will rest on the characteristic clinical features outlined below.

CLINICAL FEATURES The disease may occur at any age, but the majority of patients are in the fifth and sixth decades. It is more common in women than men and has been reported in all races. Many patients report recurrent "sinus" problems, and some have histories of allergic rhinitis, although the significance of these features is unknown.

The major symptoms are usually related to the nose. Patients frequently complain of nasal stuffiness and occasionally of discharge. The first symptom in a smaller percentage of patients relates to ulceration of the mucosa of the nose, the buccal mucosa, or the gums. This has led to loosening of the teeth, and dentists are often first consulted by these patients. Rarely, patients will present first with eye findings related to conjunctival inflammation or even ulceration. Although the progression of symptoms in some patients may be slow, all too often the disease steadily, and sometimes rapidly, progresses. The characteristic symptoms of nasal discharge, difficulty in breathing through the nose, and pain over the sinuses, nose, or eye become more prominent with time. Once ulceration begins, the disease often progresses rapidly. The ulcers frequently involve the nasal septum and will lead to the characteristic septal perforation and a saddlenose deformity. The majority of patients develop ulceration and eventually perforations of the soft and hard palates. Untreated, the disease can lead to massive destruction and mutilation of the tissues involved, including the skin of the face and the eyes. Frequently, the necrotic tissue becomes infected, and systemic symptoms such as fever and anorexia appear. The destructive lesions can become very malodorous. The disease extends to involve local tissues and does not progress below the neck; if this happens, other diseases should be considered. As the necrotic process progresses and involves vital organs, patients may lose sight in the affected eye, experience dysphagia, and have difficulty in speech. Although spontaneous temporary remissions have been reported, untreated midline granuloma is fatal. The progression of the disease can be rapidly accelerated by surgical procedures in the affected areas. The patient usually dies from secondary infection, although erosion by the process into a major blood vessel or penetration into the central nervous system with superimposed meningitis can also cause death.

Aside from the granulomatous inflammation, necrosis, and destruction, no other specific clinical or pathological findings are associated with midline granuloma. Occasionally, with superimposed infection, local lymphadenopathy may be noted, but it is not characteristic of the disease per se.

LABORATORY FINDINGS With progression of the disease, a variety of nonspecific abnormalities may be noted. These changes are characteristic of inflammatory processes in general or of secondary infections. For example, mild anemia, leukocytosis, elevated sedimentation rate, and hyperglobulinemia are common in these patients. Radiographic examination reveals pansinusitis, and as the disease advances, destruction of bone in the involved areas is characteristic.

DIFFERENTIAL DIAGNOSIS The diagnosis of midline granuloma is made by finding the characteristic histological lesions in biopsies of the affected tissues. When the specimens show only inflammatory tissue, a presumptive diagnosis of midline granuloma can be made only when the characteristic clinical picture is present and other diseases with similar presentation have been excluded. The diagnosis of Wegener's granulomatosis is ruled out by the absence of vasculitis in the biopsy specimens and the localized nature of midline granuloma (i.e., no pulmonary or renal involvement). In addition, Wegener's granulomatosis rarely, if ever, causes erosion through facial tissues. It is often difficult to differentiate true midline granuloma from neoplasms of the upper airways such as malignant reticulosis and certain lymphomas. These may be clinically similar to midline granuloma and are often associated with granulomatous inflammation. Careful examination of generous biopsy material as well as concomitant work-up for disseminated neoplasm often provides the clinicopathological distinction. Other diseases to be excluded by appropriate laboratory techniques are histoplasmosis, blastomycosis, coccidioidomycosis, leprosy, tuberculosis, syphilis, mucocutaneous leishmaniasis, rhinoscleroma, and pseudotumor of the orbit.

TREATMENT The complications of midline granuloma such as superimposed infections can be treated specifically. Although adrenal corticosteroids are often used in the therapy of midline granuloma, they are of no value and probably are contraindicated if infection is present. Sporadic reports of therapy with cytotoxic agents are difficult to interpret, since some of the patients reported clearly had lymphoma or Wegener's granulomatosis, diseases where such agents are of definite value. Surgical removal of the involved tissue has been attempted but is useless and may, in fact, cause rapid progression of the disease.

The treatment of choice is radiotherapy to the local lesion. Although low dosages (1000 rads and below) have been reported to be effective, many patients relapse after such therapy. Radiotherapy should be given in a dose of 5000 rads to the involved areas. Where such a regimen is employed, long-lasting (more than 15 years) remissions and possible cures have been achieved. Following irradiation and after an appropriate period to allow for tissue healing (usually 1 year), reconstructive and plastic surgery, which may be of enormous cosmetic and functional value, can be undertaken.

REFERENCES

Midline granuloma

FAUCI AS et al: Radiation therapy of midline granuloma. Ann Intern Med 84:140, 1976

FECHNER RE, LAMPPIN DW: Midline malignant reticulosis. Arch Otolaryngol 95:467, 1972

WALTON EW: Reticuloendothelial sarcoma arising in the nose and palate (granuloma gangrenescens). J Clin Pathol 13:279, 1960

Wegener's granulomatosis

BLATT IM et al: Fatal granulomatosis of the respiratory tract (lethal midline granuloma—Wegener's granulomatosis) AMA Arch Otolaryngol 70:707, 1959

FAUCI AS et al: Wegener's granulomatosis: Studies in eight patients and a review of the literature. Medicine 52:535, 1973

—— et al: Wegener's granulomatosis and related diseases. Dis Mon 23:7, 1977

WOLFF SM et al: Wegener's granulomatosis. Ann Intern Med 81:513, 1974

219
TOBACCO SMOKING

JOHN H. HOLBROOK

Tobacco smoke is a ubiquitous personal and environmental pollutant. Although tobacco has been used in Western culture for more than 400 years, human inhalation of cigarette smoke is a twentieth century phenomenon with major medical and economic consequences. In industrialized nations cigarette smoking is a principal cause of preventable disease and premature death.

Important changes in smoking trends are occurring in the United States. In general, the trend is downward. For example, in 1977 per capita cigarette consumption for adults stabilized while consumption of cigar and pipe tobacco continued to decrease. More importantly, between 1965 and 1975 the proportion of adult cigarette smokers in the United States declined from 53 to 39 percent of men and 32 to 29 percent of women; this represented a decrease of 2.8 million adult cigarette smokers which occurred in the face of the population growth of more than 20 million adults (Table 219-1). The decline in smoking prevalence is due largely to men who have given up cigarette smoking. Unfortunately, an increasing number of teen-agers have taken up the smoking habit.

CIGARETTE SMOKE Large prospective epidemiologic studies have shown a strong association between cigarette smoking and several diseases (Fig. 219-1). Identification of more than 2000 substances in cigarette smoke provides a framework for understanding these diverse biologic effects.

Cigarette smoke is a heterogeneous aerosol produced by incomplete combustion of the tobacco leaf. It is composed of gases and vapors in which droplets are dispersed. Mainstream smoke emerges from the mouthpiece during puffing. Sidestream smoke is emitted between puffs at the burning cone and from the mouthpiece. The composition of the smoke is influenced by several factors including type of tobacco, temperature of combustion, length of the cigarette, porosity of the paper, additives, and filters. The major constituents of tobacco are carbohydrates, nonfatty organic acids, nitrogen-containing compounds, and resins. Cigarette temperatures vary greatly from 30°C at the mouthpiece to 900°C at the burning cone. In the presence of intense heat some tobacco constituents undergo thermic decomposition (pyrolysis). Volatile substances are distilled directly into the smoke. Unstable molecules recombine to generate new compounds (pyrosynthesis). Concentration of smoke constituents occurs as the smoke is filtered by unburnt tobacco and is redistilled by the burning cone. Some substances found in tobacco pass unchanged into cigarette smoke.

Each cigarette generates approximately 500 mg mainstream smoke of which 92 percent is present in a gas phase and 8 percent is present in a particulate phase. Mainstream smoke contains 2 to 5 billion particles per milliliter, with the particle size ranging from 0.1 to 1.0 μm. Nitrogen, oxygen, and carbon dioxide account for 85 percent of the smoke's weight. The remaining gases, vapors, and particulate matter are the substances of medical importance. (Selected constituents of cigarette smoke are listed in Table 219-2.) Some smoke constituents are absorbed directly through the mucosa of the mouth, nose, pharynx, and upper airways, while others are inhaled into the lungs where they are absorbed and retained. Concentrations of toxic constituents in smoke often far exceed threshold limits of industrial toxins.

PHARMACOLOGY Tissue and organ system responses to cigarette smoke inhalation are multiple and complex. Most studies in humans have dealt with exposure to whole smoke or selected constituents which are thought to pose the greatest risk to health, for example, nicotine and carbon monoxide. Relatively little is known about the individual effects and interactions of other potentially toxic smoke constituents that are often present in low concentrations.

Nicotine, the component most characteristic of tobacco, is a highly toxic alkaloid that is both a ganglionic stimulant and depressant. The average cigarette smoker who inhales absorbs about 2 mg nicotine per cigarette. The estimated acutely fatal oral dose for an adult is 1 mg/kg. Many of its complex effects are mediated by catecholamine release. Acute cardiovascular responses to nicotine observed in normal smokers include increases in systolic and diastolic blood pressure, heart rate, force of myocardial contraction, myocardial oxygen consumption, coronary artery flow, myocardial irritability, and peripheral vasoconstriction. Nicotine has also been shown to increase platelet aggregation and serum concentrations of free fatty acid and antidiuretic hormone. Nicotine plays an important but not exclusive role in maintaining the smoking habit.

Carbon monoxide is a toxic gas which interferes with oxygen transport and utilization. Because cigarette smoke contains 2 to 6 percent carbon monoxide, smokers inhale concentrations as high as 400 parts per million (ppm) and develop elevated carboxyhemoglobin (COHB) levels. While the range of COHB for smokers is 2 to 15 percent, levels for nonsmokers are near 1 percent. The average COHB level for moderate cigarette

TABLE 219-1
Estimated number of cigarette smokers in the United States, 1955, 1965, 1975

	Year	Total population, millions	Cigarette smokers, millions	% smokers
AGE GROUP, YEARS				
13–19	1955	16.0	2.2	14
	1965	24.4	3.5	14
	1975	29.5	6.0	20
20 and over	1955	104.8	39.6	38
	1965	118.0	49.7	42
	1975	138.8	46.9	34
SEX				
Adult male	1955	50.9	26.5	52
	1965	65.8	30.0	53
	1975	66.1	25.9	39
Adult female	1955	53.9	13.1	24
	1965	61.2	19.7	32
	1975	72.7	21.0	29

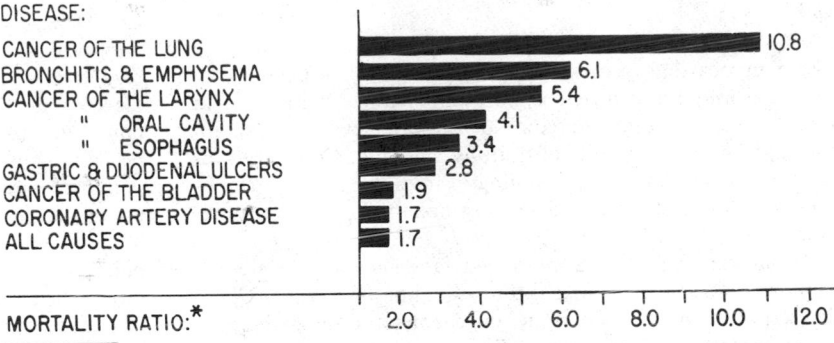

FIGURE 219-1
Mortality ratios for male cigarette smokers in seven prospective studies.

smokers is 5 percent. Carbon monoxide produces its adverse effects by reducing the amount of available oxyhemoglobin and myoglobin, and displacing the oxygen-hemoglobin dissociation curve to the left. Chronic, mild elevations of COHB due to smoking are a common cause of polycythemia and may produce subtle impairment of central nervous system function.

Cigarette smoke and its condensate are carcinogenic in several species of animals. The major carcinogens in cigarette smoke are polynuclear aromatic hydrocarbons (Table 219-2). Tumor promoters and tumor accelerators present in cigarette smoke greatly enhance its carcinogenicity. Cigarette smoke condensate is also mutagenic in a microbial test system.

Potent pulmonary irritants and ciliotoxins are found in cigarette smoke (Table 219-2). These substances cause increased bronchial mucus secretion, and they mediate acute and chronic decreases in pulmonary and mucociliary function.

EPIDEMIOLOGY Data from large prospective studies of populations in several countries show that cigarette-smoking men, taken as a whole, have 30 to 80 percent higher death rates than nonsmokers. This excess male mortality is present in all groups over the age of 35, but it is proportionately greatest in the age group 45 to 54. In a study of British physicians it was shown that 40 percent of 35-year-old men who smoked more than 25 cigarettes per day died before the age of 65, compared with 15 percent of nonsmokers in the same category. The excess mortality of smoking women has been somewhat less than that of men, but recent trends suggest it is increasing. Coronary heart disease is the chief contributor to smoking-related excess mortality in men, accounting for more than twice as many deaths as the second leading cause, lung cancer. In the United States cigarette smokers experience more disability due to chronic illness and report 45 percent more days absent from work than do nonsmokers.

A strong dose-response relationship exists between tobacco exposure and excess mortality, as measured by age at onset of smoking, cigarette consumption, and smoke inhalation. Cessation of smoking is associated with a decrease in the excess mortality. These observations together with clinical, experimental, and pathological studies suggest that smoking, per se, causes the excess mortality.

CHARACTERISTICS OF SMOKERS Demographic, anthropometric, physiological, and laboratory features distinguish cigarette smokers from nonsmokers. Smokers drink more alcohol, coffee, and tea than do nonsmokers. Their weight and blood pressure are slightly less and their heart rate is slightly faster than those of nonsmokers. In women the menopause comes earlier in smokers than in nonsmokers. Smokers have impaired maximum exercise performance. A markedly increased number of pulmonary alveolar macrophages is present in smokers, and these cells contain high levels of aryl hydrocarbon hydroxylase. Serum thiocyanate levels are much higher in smokers. When compared with nonsmokers, smokers show small

increases in total white blood cell count and serum cholesterol, as well as small decreases in serum high-density lipoprotein, vitamin C, uric acid, and albumin. Other laboratory findings observed more commonly in smokers than in nonsmokers include proteinuria, increased levels of carcinoembryonic antigen, and an increased frequency of antinuclear autoantibodies.

CLINICAL CORRELATIONS **Cardiovascular disease** Premature coronary heart disease (CHD) is one of the most important consequences of cigarette smoking (Chap. 244). The risk of fatal or nonfatal CHD is 60 to 70 percent greater in male smokers than nonsmokers. Sudden death may be the first manifestation of CHD, and it is two to three times more likely in 35- to 54-year-old smoking males than in nonsmokers. Women who smoke cigarettes and use oral contraceptives increase their risk of suffering an acute myocardial infarction more than fivefold. Cigarette smoking acts both independently and synergistically with other factors to increase the risk of developing CHD. Cessation of smoking is associated with decreased CHD mortality, an effect which is measurable within 1 year. Those who continue to smoke after an acute myocardial infarction are more likely to die from CHD than are those who quit smoking. Cigarette smoking produces an imbalance be-

TABLE 219-2
Selected cigarette smoke constituents

Substance	Effect
PARTICULATE PHASE	
"Tar"*	Carcinogen
Polynuclear aromatic hydrocarbons	Carcinogen
Nicotine	Ganglionic stimulator and depressor
Phenol	Cocarcinogen and irritant
Cresol	Cocarcinogen and irritant
β-Naphthylamine	Carcinogen
N-Nitrosonornicotine	Carcinogen
Benzo[a]pyrene	Carcinogen
Benz[α]anthracene	Carcinogen
Trace metals (e.g., nickel, polonium 210)	Carcinogen
Indole	Tumor accelerator
Carbazole	Tumor accelerator
GAS PHASE	
Carbon monoxide	Impairs oxygen transport and utilization
Hydrocyanic acid	Ciliotoxin and irritant
Acetaldehyde	Ciliotoxin and irritant
Acrolein	Ciliotoxin and irritant
Ammonia	Ciliotoxin and irritant
Formaldehyde	Ciliotoxin and irritant
Oxides of nitrogen	Ciliotoxin and irritant
Nitrosamines	Carcinogen
Hydrazine	Carcinogen

* The aggregate of particulate matter in cigarette smoke after subtracting nicotine and moisture.

tween myocardial oxygen supply and demand, a decrease in the threshold for ventricular fibrillation, and an increase in platelet aggregation; avoidance of these effects may explain the rapid cardiac benefits of quitting smoking. Coronary atherosclerosis and intimal thickening of intramyocardial arteries and arterioles are more frequent in smokers than in nonsmokers.

Cigarette smoking is a major risk factor for arteriosclerosis obliterans (Chap. 250) and thromboangiitis obliterans (Chap. 253). It also aggravates peripheral ischemia and may adversely affect peripheral bypass grafts. The mortality rate for atherosclerotic aortic aneurysm is greater in male smokers than nonsmokers. Cigarette smoking may also exacerbate proliferative diabetic retinopathy. Because of the association with chronic obstructive lung disease, cigarette smoking is an important factor leading to cor pulmonale.

Cancer Although the cause and effect relationship between cigarette smoking and lung cancer is one of the best documented in medicine, the current epidemic continues (Chap. 268). In 1978 more persons in the United States, an estimated 92,000, died from lung cancer than from any other tumor. The risk of developing lung cancer is quantitatively related to cigarette smoke exposure. Men who smoke one pack a day increase their risk tenfold compared with nonsmokers; men who smoke two packs a day may increase their risk more than 25-fold compared with nonsmokers. Workers in the asbestos and uranium mining industries who smoke cigarettes are at especially high risk for developing lung cancer. In the past 25 years cigarette consumption in the United States declined in men under the age of 60, and lung cancer mortality is beginning to plateau in this group. Cigarette consumption by women increased in the United States during this period, and lung cancer mortality is currently increasing at a faster rate in women than in men. Because 5-year survival rates for lung cancer are less than 10 percent, emphasis must be placed on prevention. An estimated 80 percent of lung cancer deaths are attributable to cigarette smoking and are preventable. Giving up cigarettes is associated with a gradual decline in the risk of developing lung cancer. After 15 years the ex-smoker's risk approximates that of the nonsmoker. Squamous-cell and oat-cell carcinoma are the histological types of lung cancer most closely associated with cigarette smoking.

Cigarette, cigar, and pipe usage in men is associated with a fivefold increased risk of developing cancer of the oral cavity, larynx, and esophagus; alcohol consumption contributes to the increased risk. Carcinoma of the bladder is also associated with cigarette smoking in men.

Respiratory disease Cigarette smoking is the most important factor contributing to the development of chronic obstructive pulmonary disease (COPD), that is, chronic bronchitis and emphysema (Chap. 263). Of the estimated 25,000 deaths from COPD that occurred in the United States in 1978, approximately 70 percent were attributable to smoking, and many of these deaths were preceded by prolonged respiratory disability. Depending upon the extent of smoke exposure, male cigarette smokers experience from 4 to 25 times higher mortality secondary to COPD than do nonsmokers. Chronic cough, sputum production, and breathlessness are much more common in smokers. Tests of pulmonary function including measurements of large and small airway obstruction, loss of elastic recoil, ventilation-perfusion mismatching, and defects in diffusing capacity are abnormal in smokers compared with nonsmokers. Subtle pulmonary function abnormalities may be present even in teen-age smokers. When compared with continuing smokers, ex-smokers experience a decrease in mortality from

COPD, a decrease in prevalence of pulmonary symptoms, and improved pulmonary function. British studies suggest that regular measurement of the forced expiratory volume in middle age may identify individuals who are at high risk for developing symptomatic COPD. Cessation of smoking would be especially valuable for these patients. Chronic inhalation of pulmonary irritants and ciliotoxins (Table 219-2) may contribute to the development of COPD. Studies of the pathogenesis of emphysema suggest that smoking may lead to an excess of pulmonary proteases. The major site of obstruction in chronic bronchitis is the bronchiole measuring less than 2 mm in diameter, and cigarette smoking is associated with bronchiolitis and increased stickiness of bronchiolar mucus. For most people in the United States cigarette smoking is a more important cause of COPD than are occupational or environmental factors; however, several factors may act conjointly to increase morbidity and mortality from COPD. In a rare disorder, homozygous α_1-antitrypsin deficiency, smoking accelerates the tendency to panacinar emphysema; smoking may play an additive role in individuals heterozygous for this state.

Cigarette smoking has been associated with an increased incidence of respiratory infections and deaths from pneumonia and influenza. Postoperative respiratory complications and spontaneous pneumothorax are also more common in smokers. Because tobacco smoke may increase airway obstruction, asthmatics should be urged not to smoke. Nicotinic stomatitis and chronic laryngitis occur more frequently in smokers than in nonsmokers.

Pregnancy Smoking during pregnancy may affect the fetus adversely. Infants whose mothers smoked during pregnancy weigh, on an average, 170 g less than infants whose mothers did not smoke. Maternal smoking during pregnancy is related to an increase in early fetal and neonatal deaths. This increased risk may be much greater in pregnancies already at high risk due to other factors.

Gastrointestinal disorders Gastric and duodenal ulcer disease is more prevalent and causes more deaths in male cigarette smokers than in nonsmokers. Smoking impairs healing of peptic ulcers, inhibits pancreatic bicarbonate secretion, and decreases the pressure of esophageal and pyloric sphincters.

Involuntary smoke inhalation Indoor atmospheres and other confined spaces are often contaminated by tobacco smoke which is inhaled involuntarily by both smokers and nonsmokers. Most of the atmospheric pollutants arise from sidestream smoke. It contains greater concentrations of many smoke constituents than does mainstream smoke, but since sidestream smoke is diluted in a large volume of air, the smoke exposure and health hazards of involuntary inhalation are much less than those associated with smoking.

The maximum acceptable ambient carbon monoxide level in the United States is 9 ppm, and in the setting of poor ventilation and heavy smoking this level may exceed 50 ppm. Breathing smoke-polluted air may exacerbate symptomatic CHD and COPD. Ocular and upper respiratory tract irritation is common in nonsmokers exposed to smoke-contaminated air.

Drug metabolism Tobacco smoke constituents induce hepatic microsomal enzyme systems which are important in the metabolism of many drugs. For example, cigarette smoking appears to increase the metabolism of phenacetin, propoxyphene, and antipyrine. The theophylline half-life is shorter in heavy smokers than in nonsmokers, and consequently smokers may require higher maintenance doses of this drug. With cessation of smoking, adjustment of the dose may be necessary.

TYPES OF SMOKING During the past 20 years the amount of tar and nicotine delivered by cigarettes made in the United

States decreased by more than 50 percent. Currently, the average United States cigarette delivers about 1.1 mg nicotine and 17 mg tar. Filter cigarettes now account for about 90 percent of sales. Death rates for CHD and lung cancer are somewhat lower for smokers of "low" tar and nicotine cigarettes than for smokers of "high" tar and nicotine cigarettes; nonetheless, death rates of nonsmokers are still much lower than those of smokers of "low" tar and nicotine cigarettes.

Cigar and pipe smokers usually inhale less smoke than cigarette smokers. This is presumably related to the alkaline pH of cigar and pipe tobacco, which is irritating to the respiratory tract. The smoke exposure and overall mortality rates of pipe and cigar smokers in the United States are substantially less than those of cigarette smokers. Death rates of cigarette, cigar, and pipe smokers are approximately equal for carcinoma of the oral cavity, larynx, and esophagus, sites where exposures to cigarette, cigar, and pipe smoke are similar. The mortality rates of most cigar and pipe smokers for cancer at other sites, CHD, and COPD are not greatly elevated above the rates of nonsmokers, but cigar and pipe smokers who inhale consistently may experience adverse health effects comparable with those of cigarette smokers.

CESSATION OF SMOKING Psychosocial forces lead to the onset of smoking, especially among teen-agers. Later, drug dependency and psychological factors maintain the smoking habit. It is estimated that more than 30 million people in the United States have stopped smoking. Many long-term smokers quit because of smoking-related health problems. This seems to explain Hammond's observation that the death rate of men smoking more than 20 cigarettes a day was somewhat higher in the months immediately after quitting than that of continuing smokers. Thereafter, a gradual decline in death rates was observed in ex-smokers. Ten or more years after quitting, the death rate of smokers of more than 20 cigarettes a day had dropped about two-thirds, and the death rate of individuals smoking 20 cigarettes a day or less was about the same as that of nonsmokers (Fig. 219-2). Ex-smokers usually experience prompt symptomatic improvement. On the average they also gain about five pounds.

In the United States more than 80 percent of cigarette smokers would like to stop smoking. Many self-care and organized programs are available to assist these individuals. Organized programs employ several techniques including instruction, counseling, withdrawal clinics, behavioral modification, hypnosis, aversive conditioning, self-monitoring, and drug therapy. Even though individual successes result from these programs, their value is uncertain. One-year abstinence rates of 20 to 30 percent are common. Relapse usually occurs during the 3-month interval after quitting. Successful programs emphasize maintenance of the nonsmoking state during this critical period.

All smokers should be encouraged to quit, especially those in high-risk groups with chronic pulmonary disease, coronary artery disease, and pregnancy. Physicians can help their smoking patients in the following manner:

1 Obtain a quantitative smoking history.
2 Explain the health risks in a personally relevant fashion.
3 Emphasize the benefits associated with cessation.
4 Advise and assist the patient to quit smoking.
5 Support the patient in a maintenance program.

Patients who are unable to stop cigarette smoking should be assisted to reduce their smoke exposure by smoking low-tar and low-nicotine cigarettes, smoking fewer cigarettes, inhaling less, taking fewer puffs, and leaving a longer stub.

Ultimately, primary smoking prevention in the pediatric and adolescent age groups may be the most effective program. Young people who understand the consequences of smoking to their health and who appreciate the difficulty of quitting are less likely to start smoking.

REFERENCES

AMERICAN HEART ASSOCIATION: Report of the ad hoc committee on cigarette smoking and cardiovascular diseases. Circulation 57:404A, 1978

HAMMOND EC: Smoking in relation to the death rates of one million men and women, in *Epidemiological Approaches to the Study of Cancer and Other Chronic Diseases,* W Haenszel (ed). National Cancer Institute Monograph no 19, 1966, pp 127–204

ROYAL COLLEGE OF PHYSICIANS: *Smoking or Health.* Tunbridge Wells, Kent, Pitman Medical, 1977

SCHMELTZ I, HOFFMANN D: Chemical studies on tobacco smoke. XXXVIII. The physicochemical nature of cigarette smoke, in *Proceedings of the 3rd World Conference on Smoking and Health.* DHEW Publication no (NIH) 76–1221, 1976, pp 13–34

SCHWARTZ JL: Smoking cures: Ways to kick an unhealthy habit, in *Research on Smoking Behavior.* NIDA Research Monograph 17, DHEW Publication no (ADM) 78–581, 1977, pp 308–336

U.S. DEPARTMENT OF HEALTH, EDUCATION, AND WELFARE: *Smoking and Health.* PHS Publication no 1103, 1964

———: *The Health Consequences of Smoking: A Reference Edition.* DHEW Publication no (CDC) 78–8357, 1976

———: The effects of smoking on health. Morb Mort Week Rep 26:145, 1977

WORLD HEALTH ORGANIZATION: *Smoking and Its Effects on Health.* WHO Technical Report Series no 568, 1975

FIGURE 219-2
Male mortality ratios for current and past cigarette smokers.

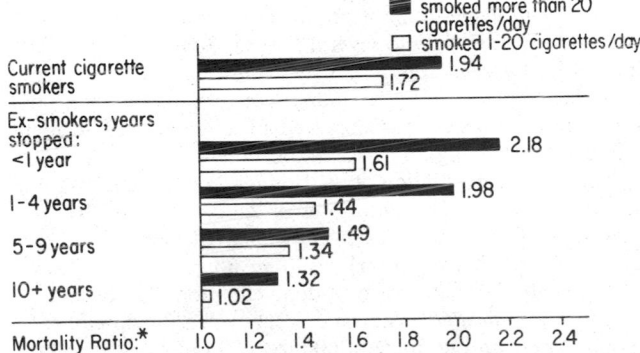

220
RADIATION INJURY

E. DONNALL THOMAS
EUGENE P. CRONKITE

TYPES OF RADIATION The types of ionizing radiation most often causing injury are x-rays, gamma rays, alpha rays, beta rays, protons, and neutrons. X-rays and gamma rays are photons. X-rays are produced by x-ray machines and as secondary emissions from particle accelerators or electron tubes. The energy spectrum of x-rays is continuous. Gamma rays are produced by radioactive decay. Beta rays are electrons. Alpha rays are composed of the nuclei of the helium atom with a mass of 4 and a charge of 2+. Protons are nuclei of hydrogen atoms with a mass of 1 and a charge of 1+. Protons are of interest because of their common use as primary particles in accelerators. They are also important because they are usually the secondary damaging particles produced by neutron interaction with tissue or other materials. Neutrons have a mass of 1 and a charge of 0. Biologic injury is produced primarily by ionization from secondary charged particles in diverse ways. Fast neutrons react principally with hydrogen atoms. As a result of collision, a portion of the energy is imparted to the hydrogen atom, and a proton is ejected causing the damage. With thermal or slow neutrons, damage is done by actual capture of the neutrons resulting in a secondary emission of ionizing radiation as the transmuted hydrogen, nitrogen, or other substance in tissue decays and emits radioactivity.

MECHANISM OF ACTION The major biologic effects of radiation occur in three interlinked steps. First, photons penetrate the protoplasm, interacting to produce ion pairs. This reaction takes on the order of 10^{-13} s. The second step is a radiochemical reaction of these ions primarily with water, producing free radicals such as H and OH. These reactions take about 10^{-9} s. These free radicals produce a further chain of reactions with themselves and tissue water to produce additional reactive forms such as H_2O_2 and HO_2. These products persist for microseconds or at most a few seconds. The last reaction takes place between these products and critical protoplasmic molecules. The nature of this last reaction is not known, but, because the actual amount of energy imparted to the system is small, the damage is generally thought to involve substances of low concentration but major importance to the living system such as nucleic acids or enzymes.

DOSE UNITS Two dose units are essential for the understanding of the quantitative effects of radiation. The *roentgen* (R), a measure of total exposure in air, is defined as the quantity of x-ray or gamma radiation such that the associated corpuscular emission per 0.001293 g air at standard conditions produces in air ions carrying one electrostatic unit of either sign. For energy to be deposited, there must be an interaction with matter. Hence, with x-rays passing through a vacuum, no radiation dose is delivered. In practice, the most important factor is the energy imparted to various tissues from a number of different types of radiation, and it is therefore essential to have a second unit of radiation which overcomes the limitation of the roentgen. This second unit, the *rad,* is a measure of absorbed dose equal to 100 ergs per gram of absorbed energy which applies to any type of radiation in any tissue. For small pieces of tissue in an x-ray beam of 1 R/min, the absorbed dose is very close to 1 rad/min. However, as irradiated objects become larger, the diminution in intensity due to the interaction of radiation and matter (buildup and then exponential attenuation) and the changing types of interaction (photoelectric effect, Compton effect, etc.) must be considered. In tissue of uniform density this leads to a decreasing absorbed dose in successive depth levels after equilibrium is attained. However, at interfaces such as soft tissue and bone, the absorbed dose may increase sharply. In addition to the exposure in roentgens and the absorbed dose in rads, attention must be given to the distribution of the absorbed dose in the anatomic area of interest.

The *density of ionization* in tissue varies with the energy and type of radiation as well as the composition of tissue. The density of ionization is referred to as *specific ionization* (ions per unit track length) or as *linear energy transfer* (LET) (kiloelectron volts deposited per unit track length). Among other factors, the density of ionization influences the biologic effect

for equivalent amount of energy deposited, with the effect being greater with more densely ionizing radiation. This leads to consideration of the relative biologic effectiveness (RBE), which is defined as the ratio of the dose in rads of standard radiation (usually x-ray or gamma radiation of 250 to 400 kV energy) to produce a given degree of biologic effect, to the dose in rads of an unknown radiation to produce the same degree of biologic effect. For example, if the median lethal dose (LD_{50}) of x-rays is 600 rads and for neutrons 300 rads, the RBE will be 2. The RBE may vary with the biologic response or the conditions of irradiation. For example, when the same radiations are used, a different value may be obtained for mortality, cataract, or tumor development. Another useful unit is the *rem,* which stands for *roentgen equivalent mammal.* Numerically, rem = rad × RBE.

Also of importance is the *dose rate.* In general, the lower the dose rate, the less will be the biologic effect. In a crude sense, dose rates in excess of approximately 5 rads/min give the same result. At lower dose rates the effect per unit of radiation becomes less as time becomes available for repair of radiation injury. In the past, genetic effects were believed to be independent of dose rate. This implies that all increments of radiation received by the gonads would add up directly as mutations. However, it is now known that there is a dose-rate dependence with respect to the production of mutations by irradiation of spermatogonia, and also for leukemogenesis in mice.

If the dose of radiation is sufficiently high, death of any living cell can be observed promptly as cell necrosis. However, after lower doses of radiation (precise values vary with the tissue) disturbances in cell proliferation are seen. These effects of radiation, other than the outright killing of cells, consist of interference with mitosis and DNA synthesis. DNA synthesis is impaired in two ways: (1) the rate of synthesis is slower, and (2) cells may continue DNA synthesis and become polyploid.

The diminution in the production of new cells in the tissues that are undergoing continual renewal (mucosa, bone marrow, gonads, etc.) results in a spectrum ranging from progressive hypoplasia to total atrophy, depending on the dose. Some cells still capable of mitosis that are not killed outright may be injured to such a degree that they will go through one or two generative cycles, producing abnormal progeny, such as giant metamyelocytes and hypersegmented neutrophils, before dying.

CLINICAL PHENOMENA IN RELATION TO DOSE AND TIME AFTER EXPOSURE Experience with radiation exposure of the entire human body is based on the effects of atomic bombs, laboratory and reactor accidents, and total-body radiotherapy. After any radiation accident close cooperation of the physician and health physicist is essential to obtain the best estimate of the radiation dose and to evaluate its probable effect in terms of the likely distribution of the absorbed dose.

The acute radiation syndromes may be classified generally as cerebral, gastrointestinal, and hematopoietic.

The *cerebral* syndrome is produced by acute uniform exposure of the whole brain to several thousand rads and is usually fatal. It is characterized by nausea, vomiting, listlessness, and drowsiness followed by tremors, convulsions, ataxia, and death. This sequence was observed in an industrial accident with death occurring 36 h after exposure.

Therapeutic irradiation of the brain is usually spaced over a period of 2 to 4 weeks, and doses of 2400 rads [used for prophylaxis of central nervous system (CNS) leukemia] to 6000 rads, (used for brain cancer) result in no recognizable acute CNS toxicity. Late effects from demyelination may occur.

The *gastrointestinal* syndrome occurs when the dose of radiation is lower, in the range of 600 to 2000 rads, and is usually maximal 3 to 5 days after exposure. At the higher doses it is characterized by intractable nausea, vomiting, and diarrhea leading to severe dehydration and vascular collapse. Severe injury to the gastrointestinal tract is caused by direct killing of a fraction of the crypt cells and by inhibition of mitosis. The mature epithelial cells continue to migrate out onto the villi in an orderly fashion, eventually being lost from the tip of the villi, producing a progressive diminution in the number of cells covering the villi. The epithelial cells become progressively cuboidal and then squamous in appearance, and ultimately the intestinal villi become denuded. Death from the gastrointestinal syndrome can be prevented by plasma, fluid, and electrolyte replacement. If the patient can be supported, regeneration of the gastrointestinal epithelium begins about the sixth day and is remarkably complete within 2 weeks.

The *hematopoietic* syndrome which occurs following whole-body exposure may be preceded by anorexia, nausea, and vomiting that is maximal between 6 and 12 h after exposure to doses of radiation between 200 and 1000 rads. Within 24 to 36 h after exposure the subject is usually asymptomatic, and a period of relative well-being is experienced until the onset of bleeding and/or infection secondary to bone marrow failure.

Lymphopenia begins immediately and becomes maximal within 24 to 36 h as a result of a direct killing of these extremely radiosensitive cells. Thereafter the lymphocytes remain at low levels for weeks and recover over several months.

A neutrophilic leukocytosis appears within a few hours after irradiation as a result of an inflammatory release of granulocytes from the bone marrow. The granulocytes are not directly damaged by the radiation, and therefore peripheral blood neutropenia does not begin until the bone marrow reserves are depleted of the more mature granulocytes. The primary damage is to the radiosensitive precursor cells so that the marrow becomes extremely hypoplastic after a few days. After sublethal and low lethal doses the minimum values of granulocytes occur in 4 to 6 weeks. After high lethal doses granulocytes diminish more rapidly, and values approaching 0 appear within 7 to 10 days. Reticulocyte production is halted within a few days, but anemia due to failure of red blood cell production is slow in onset because of the long life span of the red blood cell.

Thrombocytopenia develops slowly over a period of approximately 30 days after doses of 200 to 400 rads. After doses of 600 to 1000 rads, which effectively stop new platelet production, the decline in the platelet count reflects the life span of the platelet, and levels below 20,000 per cubic millimeter develop in approximately 9 days. The bleeding component of the hematopoietic syndrome is due to the lack of platelets and can be corrected by platelet transfusions.

Studies of decreased resistance to infection following total-body exposure have disclosed many contributing factors including granulocytopenia, lymphopenia, impaired antibody production, impaired granulocyte function, decreased cellular ability to kill phagocytosed bacteria, and damage to skin and bowel which provides portals of entry for infectious agents. However, in the acute hematopoietic syndrome, the greatest factor by far is the quantitative reduction in circulating granulocytes, and there is a high probability of bacterial infection when the granulocyte level falls below 200 cells per cubic millimeter.

INHOMOGENOUS EXPOSURE TO RADIATION The preceding description of radiation injury was based primarily on human clinical experience and animal experimentation in which the distribution of the dose absorbed by tissues was relatively uniform. However, conditions of exposure may be such that there are marked inhomogeneities in the absorbed dose. For example, an exposure may result in almost no irradiation to the lower part of the body and very heavy exposure to the abdomen and hands, resulting in extensive necrosis of the skin of these areas in addition to the fatal injury of deeper tissues. In evaluating radiation accident, the physical conditions and the probable distribution of absorbed dose within the body must be considered. What may initially appear as a fatal accident in terms of air exposure may be sublethal when effects of distribution of the absorbed dose are calculated.

MANAGEMENT OF ACUTE HUMAN RADIATION INJURY Presumptive evidence of exposure to radiation and the onset of nausea and vomiting indicate a possible medical emergency. Therapy is directed toward the management of both the gastrointestinal and hematopoietic syndromes and should be instituted as if the exposure were in the lethal range. If subsequent evaluation indicates less irradiation, therapeutic efforts can be reduced. The following is an outline of the therapeutic regimen assuming a lethal exposure:

1 If the exposure involves radioactive materials or neutrons, the patient must be monitored for radioactivity and decontaminated if necessary.
2 History, physical examination, and laboratory studies, including a complete hematologic evaluation, should be completed as quickly as possible. Cytogenetic preparations of direct bone marrow and phytohemagglutinin-stimulated peripheral blood lymphocytes should be set up for later analysis as biological dosimeters useful in estimating the level of radiation exposure. Lymphocytes should be obtained immediately, while still available, for human lymphocyte antigen (HLA) typing and storage for later mixed leukocyte cultures. The results of the typing will be useful for matching for granulocyte and platelet transfusions and for identification of a possible bone marrow donor.
3 Fluid and electrolyte balance should be monitored closely and restored with appropriate replacement solutions.
4 Ultraisolation techniques have been shown to be effective in preventing infection in patients undergoing treatment for leukemia or subjected to bone marrow transplantation. By analogy, the victim of a radiation accident should, if at all possible, be admitted to a laminar airflow room with a complete regimen of skin sterilization, a sterile diet, and oral nonabsorbable antibiotics for gut sterilization. If this is not feasible, measures should be initiated to prevent endogenous or exogenous infection. Reduction of the gastrointestinal flora is essential, and this is usually accomplished with oral nonabsorbable broad-spectrum antibiotics and an antifungal agent. Particular attention should be paid to oral hygiene and dental care. The patient should be nursed in a single-bed room, and reverse isolation precautions should be enforced vigorously.
5 Platelet transfusions should be given when the platelet count falls below 20,000 per cubic millimeter and continued until values above that level can be sustained. If the patient becomes refractory to random donor platelets, use of HLA-matched platelets from unrelated donors may become necessary. Family member transfusions should not be administered until the possibility of bone marrow transplantation has been excluded because such transfusions might sensitize the patient to the transplantation antigens of a potential marrow donor.
6 Granulocyte transfusions are indicated to prevent infection in patients who are not in ultraisolation when the granulocyte count falls below 200 per cubic millimeter. Granulocyte transfusions are indicated for therapy of any significant infection in a granulocytopenic patient. Once initiated, granulocyte transfusions should be continued on

a daily basis until the patient can sustain a granulocyte count above 200 per cubic millimeter.

7 Infection is an ever-present danger, and bacteriologic cultures should be obtained frequently. The onset of significant fever (38.5°C) should arouse a strong suspicion of infection in the granulocytopenic patient. Fever with clinical signs of bacteremia or fever sustained more than 24 h is an indication for initiating systemic antibacterial therapy even though cultures are negative. Since the most likely bacterial agent is a gram-negative organism from the normal bowel flora, initial therapy usually includes an aminoglycoside and carbenicillin with additional antibiotics added as indicated by culture results. Subsequently, if cultures are negative but fever persists, therapy with a combination of trimethoprim and sulfamethoxazole or, more rarely, with amphotericin may be considered. Once broad-spectrum antibiotic therapy has been initiated, it should be continued until the granulocyte count rises above 200 per cubic millimeter.

8 Packed red blood cells should be given as indicated to keep the hematocrit above 25.

9 All blood products should be given 1500 rads before infusion into the patient in order to inactivate lymphocytes that might subsequently proliferate and cause a graft-versus-host reaction in the immunosuppressed patient.

10 Bone marrow transplantation only rarely will be of value in an irradiation accident victim because of uncertainties about the magnitude of the radiation dose, inhomogeneity of the dose, and the requirement that the dose be within the limits of rescue by marrow transplantation, approximately 600 to 2000 rads. If marrow transplantation is indicated, immediate efforts should be made to locate a donor who is HLAA, HLAB, and HLAD identical with the patient. A genetically identical twin is an ideal donor, and one irradiation victim exposed to approximately 600 rads showed a rapid hematopoietic recovery following the infusion of marrow from his twin. The patient's family members should be typed in an effort to identify an HLA-matched sibling. By use of an HLA-identical sibling donor, marrow transplantation has resulted in a number of long-term survivors for patients with acute leukemia given 1000 rads total body irradiation. It is now possible to identify unrelated individuals who are HLA matched, but, owing to the heterogeneity of the HLA genetic region, the magnitude of such an undertaking is formidable.

PREVENTION AND ANTICIPATION Nothing can substitute for prevention. Shielding, distance, and limiting the exposure time are the only effective preventive measures against exposure from radiation sources, whether in industry, medical practice, military action, or civil defense. A series of drugs containing sulfhydryl groups will protect against radiation by effectively reducing the toxicity of the dose by approximately 50 percent if administered within minutes preceding exposure. However, the toxic effects of these drugs prevent continuous prophylactic administration. Another anticipatory maneuver is to store bone marrow in the frozen state for long periods which enables it to retain the viability necessary for successful engraftment. It would seem reasonable to store marrow of individuals at high risk against the eventuality of an accident that might produce marrow-lethal exposure. Such a program would be expensive and requires that individuals whose risk of accidental exposure is high enough to justify the expense be identified.

LONG-TERM EFFECTS Radiation alters the "information system" of proliferating somatic and germ cells. These dividing cells of the blood, gastrointestinal tract, skin, lens, gonads, and

other areas pass on either "bad" or "inadequate" information, presumably in the form of altered DNA, to their progeny, resulting in late somatic disease like cancer, cataracts, degenerative disorders, or nonspecific shortening of life. The survivors of the atomic bombs at Hiroshima and Nagasaki have been studied closely for 33 years. The most important finding has been an increased incidence of neoplasms in many organs, particularly leukemia and cancers of the thyroid, lung, and breast. The survivors continue to show increased posterior lenticular opacities and chromosome aberrations in peripheral blood lymphocytes. Impaired growth and development were observed following exposure during intrauterine life or childhood. To date no radiation-related genetic effects have been detected (see below).

In the course of radiation therapy of cancer, it is unavoidably necessary to expose normal tissues. Radiation injury results in a wide spectrum of tissue reaction depending upon injury to the tissue itself and to the small blood vessels supplying the tissue or organ. Rapidly dividing or growing tissues are most susceptible to injury, and the lag time for injury to appear is short. For example, irradiation of the scalp with 400 to 500 rads causes alopecia which is followed by prompt regrowth of hair, but irradiation of the testicle by 300 to 400 rads causes aspermia which persists for several years. Exposure of the kidney, liver, or lung results in injury that begins at about 1500 rads and increases progressively with increasing exposure. Radiation pneumonitis usually develops within 4 to 8 weeks after exposure, but fibrotic changes may occur over a period of months. Above 4000 rads, injury to the spinal cord is observed but may take 6 to 24 months to become apparent. Irradiation of muscle, bone, connective tissue, and the brain is usually well tolerated up to 6000 rads. Some late radiation effects, such as cancer of the skin, may take several decades to develop. Textbooks on radiation therapy should be consulted for details of these late effects of radiation injury.

Radiation can produce mutation of genes, the information and transmission centers for heredity. Not all mutations are harmful, but the chances are overwhelming that a change will be detrimental to the species. Not all mutations produce visible, immediately detectable effects. The concern is not only with an increase in the number of obvious malformations but with changes that will lead to such undesirable characteristics as lowered life expectancy, decreased fertility, a general increase in physical and mental disease, and an increase in fetal or neonatal death rates. The more obvious changes usually lead to early death of the individual and reduced fertility in those that survive. Therefore, the harmful mutant is relatively quickly deleted from the population. The more subtle changes, however, are propagated longer and may affect a larger number of individuals. The mutation may be dominant or recessive. Most dominant mutations are also lethal, and many such mutations may be missed because the fertilized egg never develops far enough to be recognized as a new individual. If the mutation is recessive, the mutant will not become evident unless both parents have the same mutant genes and transfer them to the child. If the mutation rate were increased by a single exposure of the population to radiation, the effects would be dispersed through many generations, and half the total damage produced would not be observed until some 30 to 50 generations had been born. For this reason, it is not possible to take negative evidence in populations that have been exposed to date as an indication that the genetic damage is small. If, for instance, an effect in the children born to individuals irradiated in Japan by the atom bombs were already obvious, it would mean that the total genetic effect would be great indeed. It has been hypothesized, but not proved, that radiation damage to the genetic material of the cell does not display a threshold effect. Therefore, the damage would be present, but not easily detected, even with very small doses, and would increase with increasing doses. Because exposure to irradiation cannot be avoided in modern industrial society and in the practice of modern medicine, and because of the uncertainty about its quantitative somatic or genetic effects, it is mandatory that exposure be minimal. Only by rigid control of radiation exposure can present generations be protected from its somatic effects, and future generations from its genetic consequences.

REFERENCES

ALAVI JB et al: A randomized clinical trial of granulocyte transfusions for infection in acute leukemia. N Engl J Med 296:706, 1977

BOND VP et al: *Mammalian Radiation Lethality*. New York, Academic, 1965

CASARETT AP: *Radiation Biology*. Englewood Cliffs, NJ, Prentice-Hall, 1968

CLIFT RA, BUCKNER CD: Supportive measures for patients with aplastic anaemia, in *Clinics in Haematology. Aplastic Anaemia*. Eastbourne, Saunders, 1978, chap 13.

——— et al: Granulocyte transfusions for the prevention of infection in patients receiving bone-marrow transplants. N Engl J Med 298:1052, 1978

CRONKITE EP, BOND VP: *Radiation Injury in Man*. Springfield, Ill, Charles C Thomas, 1960

HERZIG RH et al: Successful granulocyte transfusion therapy for gram-negative septicemia. A prospectively randomized controlled study. N Engl J Med 296:701, 1977

JABLON S, KATO H: Studies of the mortality of A-bomb survivors. 5. Radiation dose and mortality, 1950–1970. Radiat Res 50:649, 1972

LEVINE AS et al: Protected environments and prophylactic antibiotics. A prospective controlled study of their utility in the therapy of acute leukemia. N Engl J Med 228:477, 1973

RUBIN PR, CASARETT GW: *Clinical Radiation Pathology*. Philadelphia, Saunders, 1968

THOMAS ED et al: Bone-marrow transplantation. N Engl J Med 292:832, 895, 1975

221
ELECTRICAL INJURIES

JAMES F. WALLACE

EPIDEMIOLOGY Electrical injury has become progressively more common since the first human fatality from accidental electrocution was reported in 1879. In the United States, approximately 1000 deaths occur annually from electric current accidents, while another 200 persons die as a result of being struck by lightning. In addition, major electrical burns presently constitute nearly 5 percent of all admissions to burn centers in this country. Electrical injuries occur most commonly among utility pole linemen and construction workers who come into contact with high-tension current, but nearly a third result from accidents in the home or other settings including the hospital with its many electrically powered instruments and appliances.

PATHOGENESIS In understanding the fundamental aspects of electric current injury, it is helpful to consider some electrophysical principles. For an electric current to flow, there must be a closed pathway or circuit, and a difference in potential or voltage must exist between two points in this completed circuit. The flow of current is directly related to the voltage difference and inversely proportional to the electrical resistance between two points in the circuit (Ohm's law). High-resistance paths allow relatively small currents to flow, while low resistances permit large currents to flow. When the voltage is very high, the flow of current will likewise be relatively great, unless the resistance is increased proportionally to the voltage; however, if the potential difference between the two points can be minimized, the current flow can also be minimized regardless of resistance.

Although the end result of passage of an electric current through the human body is unpredictable in the individual case, many factors are known to influence the nature and severity of electrical injuries. Body tissues vary considerably in their *resistance* to the flow of current, with conductivity being roughly proportional to water content. Bone and skin offer relatively high resistance, while blood, muscle, and nerve are good conductors. The resistance of normal skin can be lowered by *moisture*, and this factor alone can convert what might ordinarily be a mild injury to a fatal shock. Of importance at the time of contact is *grounding* which, if effective, can minimize the voltage difference between two points in the electric circuit and lower the intensity of current passing through the body. The *pathway of the current through the body* is also crucial. An accident involving passage of a current between a point of contact on the leg and the ground is less likely to be injurious than one between the head and the foot, in which the heart lies between the two poles of the circuit. Similarly, a small current leak which would be innocuous when applied to the surface of the intact body may result in a fatal arrhythmia when conducted directly to the heart via a low-resistance intracardiac catheter. *Duration of contact* also influences the outcome of electrical injury. Alternating current is much more dangerous than direct current, partly because of its ability to produce tetanic muscular contractions which prevent the victim from being able to release contact with the circuit. This is usually accompanied by sweating, which lowers skin resistance, allowing current of still greater intensity to pass into the body until fatal cardiac arrhythmia results.

While the effects of electricity upon the body are incompletely understood, many pathophysiologic features of severe electrical injury have been described. In general, when sudden death occurs following low-voltage shock, it is due to the direct effect of relatively small amounts of current upon the myocardium resulting in ventricular fibrillation. With high-tension injury (greater than 1000 V) cardiac asystole and respiratory arrest occur probably as a result of injury to the medullary centers of the brain.

In addition, contact with high-intensity current may cause three types of thermal injuries. Current coursing externally to the body from the contact point to the ground may generate temperatures as high as 10,000°C and cause extensive carbonification of skin and immediately underlying tissues termed *arc* or *flash burns*. Such burns often ignite surrounding clothing or nearby objects which result in *flame burns*. Finally, there is injury due to the *direct heating* of tissues by electric current. As it traverses the skin, energy from current is converted into heat which produces coagulation necrosis at the points where it enters and exits from the skin as well as in striated muscle and blood vessels through which it passes. The associated vascular injury results in thromboses, often at sites distant from the body surface, and accounts for the observation that a greater amount of tissue destruction characteristically occurs in an electrical injury than is apparent on first inspection.

PATHOLOGY In patients who die immediately, autopsy findings are limited to burns and generalized petechial hemorrhages. If patients survive for a period of days or longer, postmortem examination reveals focal necrosis of bone, large blood vessels, muscle, peripheral nerves, spinal cord, or brain.

Renal tubular necrosis may also be seen when acute renal failure follows extensive tissue destruction.

CLINICAL MANIFESTATIONS Immediately after a severe electrical shock, patients are usually comatose, apneic, and in circulatory collapse from ventricular fibrillation or cardiac standstill. If they survive this stage, they often are disoriented, combative, and frequently may have seizures. Often they will be found to have fractures of bone caused either by convulsive muscular contractions accompanying the shock or from falls at the time of the accident. Hypovolemic shock often appears soon after high-tension electrical injury and is due to the rapid loss of fluid into areas of tissue damage, and from body surface burns. Hypotension, direct injury to the kidneys by the electric current, and renal tubular damage from myoglobin and hemoglobin pigments liberated during massive muscle necrosis and hemolysis may lead to acute renal failure.

Besides the extensive destruction of tissue occurring instantly in electrical burns, additional injury from ischemia produced by swelling of damaged tissues may appear later and is often accompanied by severe metabolic acidosis. Other serious complications which may be seen are gastrointestinal hemorrhage from preexisting or acute ulcers and both anaerobic and aerobic infections originating in inadequately debrided necrotic muscle masses.

Late effects include various neurological disabilities, visual disturbances, and the residual damage left by burns. Nervous system injuries are frequent and include peripheral neuropathies, incomplete transection of the spinal cord, and reflex sympathetic dystrophies, as well as late convulsive disorders and intractable headache. The development of cataracts of one or both eyes has been reported to occur up to 3 years following electrical injury.

LABORATORY FINDINGS Immediately following major electrical injury the hematocrit is elevated and the plasma volume reduced, reflecting sequestration of fluid in the wound. Unless extensive flame burns are also present, serial determinations of either of these parameters provide a good means of monitoring the adequacy of fluid replacement therapy. Myoglobinuria is seen frequently in association with severe shocks, and when it persists following establishment of urine flow, usually indicates massive muscle injury. In many patients arterial blood pH determinations will indicate the presence of metabolic acidosis. Lumbar puncture may show elevated pressure associated with cerebral edema or bloody spinal fluid as a result of intracerebral hemorrhage. The electrocardiogram not infrequently shows tachycardia and minor ST-segment alterations which can persist for several weeks following injury. Unexplained acute hypokalemia leading to respiratory arrest and cardiac arrhythmias has developed in some patients between the second and fourth weeks following injury.

TREATMENT Removal of victims from contact with the current should be accomplished immediately without touching them directly. Rescuers should use a rubber sheet, a leather belt applied as a sling, a wooden pole, or other nonconductive material to detach them, and this should be preceded by cutting off the source of current when possible. If the victim is not breathing, mouth-to-mouth ventilation should be instituted at once. Although most cases who survive develop spontaneous respiration within half an hour, complete recovery after longer periods occurs often enough so that respiratory support should be continued for at least 4 h. If there is no evidence of heartbeat, external cardiac massage should accompany ventilatory resuscitation. Persons struck by lightning frequently have cardiac asystole which responds to a manual blow to the chest, while victims of low-voltage shocks will usually require defibrillation to restore heart action. During cardiopulmonary resuscitation and evacuation to the hospital, attention should be paid to possible broken bones and spinal cord injuries incurred at the time of the accident.

Subsequent hospital management of patients with electrothermal injuries requires considerable specialized care; whenever feasible, they should be referred to an appropriate burn or trauma unit.

Rapid institution of fluid and electrolyte therapy for hypovolemic shock and acidosis is essential, with guidelines being the patient's urine output, hematocrit, osmolality, central venous pressure, and arterial blood gases. Standard burn formulas should not be used to estimate fluid therapy since these are based only upon extent of body surface area injury and do not take into account the extensive damage to muscle which is usually present. Instead, fluid replacement principles used in the treatment of crush injury, which electrical injury closely resembles, should be followed. Large volumes of fluid, preferably lactated Ringer's solution, should be administered in order to maintain urine output greater than 50 ml/h. If myoglobinuria persists after adequate urine flow has been established, the use of furosemide or an osmotic diuretic such as mannitol along with alkalinization of the urine is indicated. Management of the electrical wound should include adequate debridement of necrotic tissue and often will require fasciotomy to prevent further ischemic injury. Anticlostridial prophylaxis, including tetanus toxoid and high doses of penicillin, should be administered to all severely injured patients, while topical antimicrobial chemotherapy with mafenide (Sulfamylon) or silver sulfadiazine may be useful in preventing or delaying infections in extensive surface burns. Survivors of the acute episode often require extensive treatment for infection, cerebral edema, visceral injury, and delayed hemorrhage as devitalized tissues slough. If acute renal failure occurs, it should be managed as described in Chap. 275.

PREVENTION Proper installation of appliances, grounding of telephone lines and radio and television aerials, and the use of rubber gloves and dry shoes when working with electric circuits should be routine. Unused wall sockets should be kept plugged and live extension cords not left unattended, particularly in households where there are young children. During a severe thunderstorm, refuge near hilltops, riverbanks, hedges, telephone poles, and trees should be avoided. The safest shelter is the closed house, while a closed automobile, cave, ditch, or even lying on the ground curled up with hands close together is relatively secure. In hospitalized patients, the hazard of ventricular fibrillation precipitated by minute current leaks conducted directly to the myocardium from monitoring equipment via pacemakers or intravascular manometric catheters should be more widely appreciated. Hospital personnel should be aware that, in addition to medical instruments, patient contact with two or more other power line–operated devices such as television sets, radios, electric razors, lamps, and especially electric beds can also result in electrocution if the heart lies within the current path through the patient. These hazards can be minimized by proper grounding of equipment *before* a patient is connected to the instrument, periodic measurement for leakage of current supplied by each device, and by instruction in the principles of electrical safety for hospital personnel who use the complex and dangerous equipment that is so much a part of modern medical practice.

REFERENCES

APFELBERG DB et al: Pathophysiology and treatment of lightning injuries. J Trauma 14:453, 1974

ARTZ CP: Changing concepts of electrical injury. Am J Surg 128:600, 1974

BAXTER CR: Present concepts in the management of major electrical injury. Surg Clin North Am 50:1401, 1970

KAY NRM et al: The management of electrical injuries of the extremities. Surg Clin North Am 53:1459, 1973

KILPATRICK DG: The electrical environment. Med Clin North Am 55:1095, 1971

ROUSE RG, DIMICK AR: The treatment of electrical injury compared to burn injury. A review of pathophysiology and comparison of patient management protocols. J Trauma 18:43, 1978

TAUSSIG HB: Death from lightning—and the possibility of living again. Ann Intern Med 68:1345, 1968

222
DROWNING AND NEAR-DROWNING

JAMES F. WALLACE

EPIDEMIOLOGY   In the United States, drowning accounts for approximately 7000 fatalities per year and is one of the three leading causes of accidental death. In addition, although no national statistics are available, it has been estimated that as many as 48,000 persons annually are near-drowning victims: those who live at least temporarily following an immersion incident. Children and young adults are most often the victims, and nearly 80 percent are males. However, with the increasing popularity of boating and water sports in this country nearly half the population is at risk of drowning each year, especially during the summer months.

PATHOPHYSIOLOGY   Ten to twenty percent of drowning victims have no evidence of water aspiration in their lungs at autopsy ("dry drowning"). Death is due to asphyxia secondary to reflex laryngospasm and glottic closure. It is probable that a similar number of near-drowning victims also do not aspirate. If ventilation is reestablished before they sustain irreversible anoxic brain damage, prompt and complete recovery can be anticipated.

When aspiration accompanies drowning ("wet drowning"), the clinical situation is further complicated by the amount of surrounding water that is introduced into the respiratory tract as well as by the solutes and solids contained in it. A severe pulmonary injury often occurs, resulting in persistent arterial hypoxemia and metabolic acidosis even after ventilation has been restored.

In the past, an important distinction was made between the pathophysiology of saltwater and freshwater drowning with respect to changes in blood volume, serum electrolyte concentrations, and cardiovascular function. However, it has been established that the most important problem in human near-drowning is hypoxia and that the other disturbances are of considerably less significance in determining survival.

The mechanisms by which hypoxia develops in near-drowning with aspiration are often multiple: laryngospasm, bronchospasm, airway obstruction secondary to aspirated particulate matter, and pulmonary edema following prolonged hypoxia can take place regardless of the composition of the water aspirated, while other types of lung injury causing hypoxemia depend upon the osmolar and chemical characteristics of the immersion fluid. Aspiration of seawater, which is hypertonic compared with blood and chemically irritating to the pulmonary alveolocapillary membrane, causes a rapid shift of plasma proteins and water from the circulation into the alveolar lumen. Continued perfusion of these nonventilated, edema-filled alveoli results in an intrapulmonary right-to-left shunt and arterial hypoxemia. When hypotonic fresh water is aspirated, fluid is rapidly absorbed from the lung into the circulation.

Injury to alveolar lining cells takes place, altering or destroying the properties of pulmonary surfactant that maintains surface tension, and leading to alveolar collapse. Ventilation-perfusion ratios change in these atelectatic areas of lung, and hypoxemia is the result. Metabolic acidosis, which is present in as many as 70 percent of near-drowning victims, is a consequence of tissue hypoxia and may be severe.

Although changes in electrolyte concentrations occur, depending upon the type and volume of fluid aspirated, these disturbances are rarely life-threatening. Most persons who aspirate sufficient quantities to produce marked electrolyte abnormalities do not survive the immersion incident. Similarly, profound changes in circulating blood volume are unusual. However, hypovolemia requiring treatment may be seen in massive saltwater aspiration accompanied by shifts of fluid from the vascular space into the lung.

Although rarely of clinical significance, some hemolysis of red blood cells often takes place, especially with freshwater aspiration. Free hemoglobin may be found in the urine and blood, but the abnormality requires no specific therapy. Disseminated intravascular coagulation has been reported as a complication of freshwater near-drowning. It is thought that with extensive pulmonary injury "tissue factor" in lung parenchyma and plasminogen activator from pulmonary endothelium are released, triggering the extrinsic clotting and fibrinolytic systems. Other pathophysiologic events in near-drowning include the development of renal failure secondary to acute tubular necrosis, probably due to the combined effects of hypoxia and hypotension, and neurological deficits secondary to cerebral anoxia. Although the extent of the central nervous system injury tends to correlate with the duration of hypoxia, hypothermia accompanying the incident may be a moderating factor by reducing cerebral oxygen requirements. Complete neurological recovery has been reported in victims submerged as long as 40 min in water temperatures less than 20°C.

CLINICAL MANIFESTATIONS   The clinical features in near-drowning are variable and depend upon many factors including the amount and type of water aspirated and the promptness and effectiveness of treatment. Pulmonary and neurological abnormalities usually predominate. Patients may present with mild cough and tachypnea, or with fulminant pulmonary edema. At least a third will require endotracheal intubation and some type of ventilatory therapy for the management of pulmonary injury. Instead of gradual recovery during the first 48 to 72 h of treatment, some patients will develop the adult respiratory distress syndrome, associated with progressive respiratory failure and reduction in lung compliance (Chap. 271). Other pulmonary complications often include regional atelectasis due to aspirated particulate matter; secondary bacterial pneumonia; lung abscess; empyema; and injuries such as pneumothorax or pneumomediastinum sustained during resuscitation or related to ventilator therapy.

Early neurological manifestations include seizures, especially during resuscitative efforts, and altered mental status, ranging from normal alertness to agitation, combativeness, or coma. Patients may present with speech, motor, or visual abnormalities or with more diffuse organic brain syndromes. Some of these neurological deficits will improve gradually and resolve over several months. However, 5 to 20 percent of patients will have permanent sequelae, many of which prove ultimately fatal. Neurological status usually does not continue to worsen after a near-drowning victim is admitted to the hospital unless there has been a preceding deterioration in pulmonary status. The possibility of unrecognized head trauma coincident with the drowning episode or a subdural hematoma should be considered as well.

Near-drowning victims often require treatment for cardiac as well as respiratory arrest during resuscitation. If this is successfully accomplished, most patients experience few additional cardiovascular problems. Supraventricular arrhythmias are common but usually resolve promptly when acidosis and hypoxia are treated. Heart failure secondary to myocardial ischemia or acutely expanded blood volume is unusual. Instead, pulmonary edema and low cardiac output states are usually due to the pulmonary injury from water aspiration with extravasation of fluid into the lung, resulting in hypovolemia.

Fever, frequently greater than 38°C, is seen in most patients within the first 24 h following significant aspiration. Its appearance later in the hospital course usually indicates a complicating infection. Vomiting is common during and after resuscitation. This often is associated with gastric distention by large quantities of fluid and air swallowed during the near-drowning episode and may result in additional aspiration. Other rare, but clinically important, features which may be encountered include acute renal failure and a severe hemorrhagic diathesis.

LABORATORY FINDINGS Arterial blood gas and pH determinations on admission reveal varying degrees of hypoxia and acidosis; follow-up values are the most reliable indicators of the effectiveness of ventilatory therapy. In 25 percent of near-drowning victims the initial chest x-ray film may be normal; however, this finding does not exclude the possibility that the patient has significant hypoxemia. In the remainder of cases, radiologic findings range from fine, symmetric, perihilar infiltrates with relative sparing of apexes, bases, and lateral lung fields to massive bilateral pulmonary edema with little or no areas of sparing. Marked clearing of these abnormalities usually takes place within 72 to 96 h.

Alterations in serum sodium and potassium may be noted, but these are generally mild and require no corrective treatment. Although leukocytosis up to 40,000 white blood cells per cubic millimeter is common during the first 24 to 48 h following near-drowning, significant changes in hematocrit and hemoglobin are rare, irrespective of the type of fluid aspirated. A *falling* hematocrit should raise the possibility of bleeding, not hemolysis, which, if it has occurred, should be apparent at the time of initial evaluation. Thrombocytopenia, prolonged prothrombin and partial thromboplastin times, hypofibrinogenemia, and elevated fibrin degradation products may be seen if disseminated intravascular coagulation takes place (Chap. 318).

THERAPY The primary objective of therapy is to correct hypoxemia and acidosis as rapidly as possible. On-the-scene efforts should include immediate institution of mouth-to-mouth breathing and, if necessary, closed-chest cardiac massage. Time should not be wasted with attempts to drain water from the victim's lungs. However, it is important to establish and maintain a clear airway at the onset of resuscitation in order to avoid accidental overdistention of the stomach which might result in regurgitation and aspiration. One hundred percent oxygen should be administered by inhalation as soon as possible, and other necessary resuscitative efforts continued during evacuation to the hospital. Even if spontaneous ventilation returns and the patient seems coherent, high concentrations of oxygen should be continued, since severe hypoxemia and acidosis may be present even in persons who are alert and without cyanosis.

All near-drowning victims should be taken to a hospital for further evaluation. Initial diagnostic studies should include arterial blood gas and pH determinations, hemogram, serum electrolytes, and chest x-ray. Patients who are alert, have normal chest x-rays, and show no evidence of hypoxemia or acidosis usually require no further therapy. Nevertheless they should be observed over several hours for evidence of deterioration in blood gas and acid-base status prior to discharge. Metabolic acidosis should be treated by intravenous administration of sodium bicarbonate ($NaHCO_3$), and hypoxemia with supplemental oxygen. If bronchospasm is present, aerosol inhalation of a bronchodilator may be given. Patients with pulmonary edema or hypoxemia which fails to respond to increasing inspired oxygen tensions up to 40 percent should be intubated endotracheally and have positive end-expiratory pressure (PEEP) applied to the airways. When respiratory failure is present, lung compliance is markedly reduced, or the patient is unable to breathe spontaneously, mechanical ventilatory support should be used in addition to PEEP. Arterial blood gas tensions and pH should be determined frequently to assess the adequacy of respiratory therapy. Treatment with PEEP should be continued long enough for the lung injury to stabilize before it is withdrawn. This may take 48 to 72 h or even longer. Monitoring the magnitude of the intrapulmonary shunt, the pulmonary wedge pressure, and cardiac output by means of a Swan-Ganz intraarterial catheter is often very helpful in weaning patients from PEEP as well as in managing cases complicated by low cardiac output and hypotension.

Other therapeutic measures are largely supportive. Patients should be observed closely for evidence of pulmonary infection and treated with appropriate antibiotics on the basis of results of cultures of respiratory secretions. Prophylactic use of antibiotics and corticosteroids has been of no benefit in near-drowning victims. Fluid and electrolyte balance should be carefully maintained. If hypovolemia is associated with low urinary output or hypotension, plasma expanders may be required. Transfusion with packed red blood cells or whole blood, depending upon circulating blood volume status, may be used for significant anemia. Acute renal failure should be managed as described in Chap. 275.

PROGNOSIS The prognosis depends largely upon the extent and duration of the hypoxic episode. In addition, such factors as the temperature of the submersion medium, the availability and appropriate application of specific treatment, and coexisting medical illness or trauma are often important in determining the outcome. In general, patients who are alert and have normal chest x-rays upon arrival at the hospital can be expected to survive, while those who present in coma or cardiopulmonary arrest usually die or are left with significant neurological deficits. Prediction of outcome on the basis of other presenting neurological features or laboratory abnormalities is unreliable. The fact that nearly 90 percent of victims who live long enough to receive definitive hospital care will survive should serve to emphasize that extensive resuscitative efforts are advisable in all cases of near-drowning.

REFERENCES

FULLER RH: Drowning and the postimmersion syndrome: A clinicopathologic study. Milit Med 128:22, 1963

GIAMMONA ST, MODELL JH: Drowning by total immersion: Effects on pulmonary surfactant of distilled water, isotonic saline and seawater. Am J Dis Child 114:612, 1967

MODELL JH: Biology of drowning. Annu Rev Med 29:1, 1978

—— et al: Clinical course of 91 consecutive near-drowning victims. Chest 70(2):231, 1976

PETERSON B: Morbidity of childhood near-drowning. Pediatrics 59(3):364, 1977

PORTS TA, DEVEL TF: Intravascular coagulation in fresh water submersion: Report of 3 cases. Ann Intern Med 87:60, 1977

SIEBKE H et al: Survival after 40 minutes' submersion without cerebral sequelae. Lancet 1.1275, 1975

223
GENERAL CONSIDERATIONS AND PRINCIPLES OF MANAGEMENT

PAUL A. FRIEDMAN

Poisoning by chemical agents is a common and serious medical problem. In the United States accidental poisonings cause about 5000 deaths each year. Suicides by chemical agents annually number more than 6000. Malicious poisoning has become less common since the development of scientific toxicology, but toxic chemicals administered by homicides and abortionists are responsible for more deaths than is generally appreciated. In addition to fatal poisonings there is a much greater number of persons who are made seriously ill by chemical agents but recover after appropriate therapy. Unfortunately, some such victims are left with permanent sequelae of their intoxication. Finally, chemical agents impair the health of very many people by mechanisms not generally thought of as intoxications. Chemical carcinogenesis and mutagenesis, chronic alcoholic liver disease, allergic reactions, and chemical addiction and withdrawal syndromes are the most important examples.

Accidental poisonings may occur in the home or through industrial exposure. The former are far more frequent and usually acute; industrial intoxication is ordinarily the result of chronic exposure. Accidental poisoning is most commonly due to ingestion of toxic substances and involves children in the majority of cases. Each year 1 to 2 million American children accidentally swallow toxic materials, and approximately 1 ingestion in 1000 is fatal. Aspirin is involved in 25 percent of all ingestions, other medicines in another 25 percent. Cleaning and polishing agents are ingested by 15 percent, while cosmetics, pesticides, petroleum products, and turpentine paints account for 6 percent each. Younger children tend to ingest household products, older children are more likely to choose drugs.

The frequency of accidental poisonings reflects the enormous number of toxic substances found in the American home. Many such accidents could be avoided by simple preventive measures. Physicians can play an effective role in safety education. All toxic substances must be kept out of the reach of small children. Household chemicals and medicines should be kept in the original containers, and all such containers should be labeled. Before taking or administering any medicine, one should check the label carefully.

Despite all precautions, accidental, suicidal, and criminal poisonings will remain an important problem which every physician must be prepared to treat promptly and effectively. Besides their immediate therapeutic responsibilities, physicians have legal obligations in cases of attempted suicide, homicide, criminal abortion, and industrial exposure. The physician should also obtain psychiatric care for any patient who has attempted suicide by poison.

DIAGNOSIS OF CHEMICAL POISONING

Optimal management of the poisoned patient requires a correct diagnosis. Unfortunately, in many such patients poisoning is initially not even considered as a possible cause of the clinical picture. The patient may be unaware of exposure to poison or, as after attempted suicide or abortion, may be unwilling to admit it. Although the toxic effects of some chemical substances are quite characteristic, most poisoning syndromes can simulate other diseases.

Poisoning is usually included in the differential diagnosis of coma, convulsions, acute psychosis, acute hepatic or renal insufficiency, and bone marrow depression. It may not be considered when the major manifestation is a mild psychiatric disturbance or neurological disorder, abdominal pain, bleeding, fever, hypotension, pulmonary congestion, or skin eruption. Chronic, insidious intoxications are much more frequently missed than acute poisonings whose symptoms appear suddenly and may be immediately related to a specific event. Physicians should always remember the variegated manifestations of poisoning and maintain a high index of suspicion.

In every case of poisoning, identification of the toxic agent should be attempted. Specific antidotal therapy is obviously impossible without such identification. In cases of homicide, suicide, or criminal abortion the identity of the poison may be of legal importance. When poisoning results from industrial exposure or therapeutic mishap, accurate knowledge of the responsible agents is essential for future prevention.

In acute accidental poisoning the offending substance may be known to the patient. In many other cases information can be obtained from relatives or acquaintances, by a search for containers at the scene of the poisoning, or by questioning the patient's physician or pharmacist. Frequently such procedures yield only the trade name of a product, which gives no clue to its component chemicals. A number of books which identify the active ingredients of household products, agricultural compounds, proprietary medicines, and poisonous plants are listed in the references to this chapter. A small handbook of this type should be carried in every physician's bag. Poison control centers and manufacturers' representatives are other useful sources of such information. When poisoning is chronic, rapid identification of the toxic agent from the history is frequently impossible. It is therefore fortunate that the lesser therapeutic urgency of such cases usually permits the required painstaking exploration of the patient's habits and environment.

Some poisons can produce clinical features characteristic enough to strongly suggest the diagnosis. Careful examination of the patient may reveal the unmistakable odor of cyanide; the cherry-colored flush of carboxyhemoglobin in skin and mucous membranes; the pupillary constriction, salivation, and gastrointestinal hyperactivity produced by cholinesterase-inhibitor insecticides; or the lead line and extensor paralyses of chronic lead poisoning. Unfortunately, these features are not always present, and in any case telltales are the exception in chemical poisonings.

Chemical analysis of body fluids provides the most definite identification of the intoxicating agent. Some common poisons, such as aspirin, bromides, and barbiturates, can be identified and even quantitated by relatively simple laboratory procedures. Others require more complex toxicologic techniques, such as gas chromatography or bioassay, which are performed only in specialized laboratories. Furthermore, the results of toxicologic determinations are rarely available in time to guide the initial treatment of acute poisoning. Nevertheless, specimens of vomitus, gastric aspirate, blood, urine, and feces should always be saved for toxicologic study if diagnostic or legal questions are likely to arise. Chemical analyses of body fluids or tissues are of particular value in the diagnosis and evaluation of chronic intoxications. Finally, they are useful in following the success of some forms of therapy.

TREATMENT OF CHEMICAL POISONING

Although the physician should always try to identify the poison, such attempts must never delay vital therapeutic measures. Most poisons do not have specific antidotes. Essential supportive care must be given as indicated by the patient's clinical state and does not require knowledge of the toxic agent. Symptomatic treatment of circulatory, respiratory, neurological, and renal function should be immediately administered as to any other seriously ill patient.

Correct treatment of the poisoned patients thus requires knowledge of both the general principles of management and the details of therapy for specific poisons. Treatment involves four steps: (1) prevention of further absorption of the poison, (2) removal of absorbed poison from the body, (3) symptomatic or supportive therapy, and (4) administration of systemic antidotes (Table 223-1). The first three are applicable to most types of poisoning. The fourth is most often used only when the toxic agent is known and a specific antidote is available. However, sometimes naloxone is given if the index of suspicion is high that the patient has had an overdose of an opiate. Success often depends upon speed of treatment, and, when indicated by the clinical situation, several approaches should be used simultaneously.

PREVENTION OF ABSORPTION OF INGESTED POISONS If appreciable amounts of a poison have been ingested, one should always attempt to minimize its absorption from the gastrointestinal tract. The success of such endeavors depends upon the time elapsed since ingestion and upon the site and

TABLE 223-1
Treatment of acute chemical poisoning

I Prevention of further absorption of poison
  A Poisoning by ingestion
    1 Emptying the stomach
      a Induction of vomiting
      b Gastric lavage
    2 Minimizing gastrointestinal absorption
      a Neutralization and precipitation
      b Adsorption
      c Catharsis
  B Poisoning by other routes
II Removal of absorbed poisons from body
  A Detoxification—enzyme induction?
  B Biliary excretion—interruption of enterohepatic circulation
  C Urinary excretion
    1 Forced diuresis
    2 Alteration of urinary pH
  D Dialysis
    1 Peritoneal dialysis
    2 Hemodialysis
  E Charcoal or resin hemoperfusion
  F Exchange transfusion
  G Chelation and chemical binding
III Supportive therapy
IV Administration of systemic antidotes
  A Chemical agents
  B Pharmacological antagonists

speed of absorption of the poison. Prompt action is essential, and it is better to proceed with makeshifts than to waste time while waiting for special equipment or drugs. Conversely, it is unwise to temporize with unpredictable remedies when reliable and effective methods for removal of poison from the gastrointestinal tract are available. When skillfully applied, these methods do not lead to such complications as pulmonary aspiration, gastrointestinal perforation, or convulsions.

Evacuation of the stomach Attempts to empty the stomach are always worthwhile unless specifically contraindicated. They may be highly successful if made soon after ingestion. Significant amounts of poison may be recovered from the stomach hours after ingestion because gastric emptying may be delayed by gastric atony or pylorospasm.

Emesis occurs spontaneously after the ingestion of many poisons. In a minority of instances it may be induced in the home by mechanical stimulation of the posterior pharynx. The emetic action of syrup of ipecac (not the 14 times more concentrated fluid extract) in 15- to 30-ml dosage is more effective and is safe enough for home use. Its action has an average latent period of 20 min and depends in part on gastrointestinal absorption, so that it cannot be used in conjunction with other measures intended to minimize absorption of the poison. A second dose of ipecac should be given if the patient fails to vomit after 20 min (90 to 95 percent of patients will vomit after two doses). If not available at home, every effort should be made to locate a source of ipecac even if this requires taking the patient to the hospital. Apomorphine, 0.06 mg/kg intramuscularly, acts within 5 min but may cause prolonged vomiting. When given intravenously in doses of 0.01 mg/kg, apomorphine tends to produce almost immediate vomiting which is not followed by any other central nervous system effects. On occasion it is impossible to induce vomiting, and valuable time should not be lost with hopeful waiting. Induction of vomiting should not be attempted in severely depressed or convulsing patients, or (because of the danger of gastroesophageal perforation or tracheal aspiration of vomitus) in patients who have ingested strong caustics or liquid hydrocarbons which are potent lung irritants (e.g., kerosene, furniture polish).

In comparison with emesis, *gastric lavage* is more predictably and immediately active but usually no more effective in removing poison from the stomach. It can be employed in unconscious patients, and removal of gastric contents reduces the risk of aspiration of vomitus in such patients. It is, however, contraindicated after the ingestion of strong corrosives because of danger of perforating injured tissues. When properly performed, gastric lavage carries little risk of aspiration of gastric contents into the lungs. The patient should be prone, with head and shoulders lowered. A mouth gag is placed, and a gastric tube of sufficient diameter to permit withdrawal of particulate matter (size 30) is passed into the stomach. If central nervous system function is depressed and introduction of the tube produces retching, or if pulmonary irritants have been ingested, it is wise to place a *cuffed endotracheal tube* before lavaging. Gastric contents are withdrawn with a large syringe and usually contain most of the poison that will be removed. Thereafter 200 ml (less in children) of warm water or other lavaging solution is alternately instilled and withdrawn until the aspirate becomes clear.

Interference with gastrointestinal absorption Since neither emesis nor gastric lavage empties the stomach completely, one should also minimize absorption by administering substances which trap ingested poisons. Some toxic alkaloids can be precipitated and rendered insoluble by the administration of sulfate. Many other poisons are effectively adsorbed by powdered, activated charcoal. A good grade of activated charcoal can rapidly adsorb as much as half its weight of many common poisons. It is more effective than the so-called "universal antidote," which should be relegated to oblivion. A slurry of activated charcoal (20 to 50 g in 100 to 200 ml) should be administered after evacuation of the stomach.

Adsorption by charcoal is reversible, and the effectiveness of adsorption of many poisons varies with the pH. Acidic substances are adsorbed better in acid solutions and may therefore be released in the small intestine. It is desirable to speed the charcoal with its adsorbed poison through the intestine as quickly as possible. This will also decrease intestinal absorption of any unabsorbed poison which has passed beyond the pylorus. In patients with good renal and cardiac function this is best accomplished by oral or gastric administration of an osmotic cathartic such as magnesium or sodium sulfate (10 to 30 g given in solution at a concentration of 10% or less).

PREVENTION OF ABSORPTION OF POISON FROM OTHER SITES Most topically applied poisons can be removed by copious flushing with water. In certain instances weak acids or bases or appropriate organic solvents are more effective, but rapid and voluminous washing with water should always proceed while they are being obtained. Chemical antidotes can be hazardous because tissue injury may result from the heat of the chemical reaction.

The systemic distribution of injected poisons can be slowed by the application of cold to the injection site or by the proximal application of a tourniquet. Cruciate incision and suction is generally ineffective except after poisonous bites.

Following inhalation of toxic gases, vapors, or dusts, the victim should be removed into clean air and adequate ventilation maintained. If the patient cannot be moved, a protective mask should be applied.

REMOVAL OF ABSORBED POISON FROM THE BODY Unlike prevention or retardation of absorption, measures to speed removal of the toxic agent from the body rarely have much influence on the peak poison concentration. However, they can significantly abbreviate the time during which the concentration of many poisons remains above any given level and may thereby reduce morbidity, avoid complications, and save lives. In judging the need for such measures one must consider the patient's clinical state, the properties and metabolic fate of the poison, and the amount absorbed as judged by the history and the blood level. Removal of some poisons can be accelerated by several methods; selection depends on the clinical urgency, the amount in the body, and the skills and equipment available.

Biliary excretion Certain organic acids and active drugs are secreted into the bile against large concentration gradients. However, this process takes time and cannot be accelerated. The intestinal resorption of substances already secreted into the bile, such as glutethimide, can be decreased by the administration of charcoal every 6 h. The organochlorine pesticide, chlordecone, is slowly eliminated from the body (blood half-time 165 days). Cholestyramine (16 g per day) significantly accelerates elimination (blood half-time 80 days).

Urinary excretion Acceleration of renal excretion is applicable to a much larger number of poisons. Renal excretion of toxic substances depends on glomerular filtration, active tubular secretion, and passive tubular resorption. The first two processes should be protected by maintenance of adequate circulation and renal function, but for practical purposes they cannot be accelerated. On the other hand, passive tubular resorption of many poisons plays an important role in the prolongation of their action and can frequently be decreased by readily available methods.

The effectiveness of forced diuresis by administration of

large volumes of electrolyte solutions together with intravenous furosemide in increasing renal excretion has been demonstrated for many drugs such as salicylates, barbiturates, meprobamate, and glutethimide and is potentially applicable to all ultrafiltered poisons which are passively reabsorbed.

Alteration of the urinary pH can also inhibit passive back-diffusion of some poisons and increase their renal clearance. The renal tubular epithelium is more permeable to uncharged molecules than to ionized solutes. Weak organic acids and bases readily diffuse out of the tubular fluid in their un-ionized form but are trapped in it when ionized. Acidic poisons are largely ionized only at pHs above their pK_a. Alkalinization of the urine greatly increases the ionization in the tubular fluid of such organic acids as phenobarbital and salicylate. In contrast, the pK_a of pentobarbital (8.1) and secobarbital (8.0) is so high that renal clearance is not greatly increased by raising the urinary pH into the physiological alkaline range. Alkalinization of the urine is achieved by the infusion of sodium bicarbonate, sodium lactate, or tromethamine (which also acts as an osmotic diuretic) at a rate determined by the urinary and blood pH. Excessive systemic alkalosis or electrolyte disturbances must be carefully prevented. A combination of forced diuresis and alkalinization of the urine can raise the renal clearance of some acidic poisons tenfold or more and has been found highly effective in poisoning by salicylate and phenobarbital. The full range of its clinical applicability is undoubtedly much wider but remains to be established. Conversely, depression of the urinary pH beyond its usual range has been shown to augment significantly the clearance of amphetamines and phencyclidines.

Finally, the renal excretion of certain poisons can be increased in a highly specific fashion. An example is the removal of bromide by administration of chloride and chloriuretics. Such methods are discussed with the individual poisons.

Dialysis and hemoperfusion Dialysis has been found effective in the removal of many drugs including barbiturates, borate, bromide, chlorate, dimercaprol, diphenylhydantoin, ethanol, ethchlorvynol, ethinamate, glutethimide, glycols, isoniazid, methanol, salicylate, sulfonamides, and thiocyanate. Theoretically, it should accelerate the removal from the body of any dialyzable toxin which is not irreversibly bound to tissues. Obviously, its effectiveness does not extend to large-molecule, nondialyzable poisons and is decreased by a high degree of protein binding or lipid solubility of the toxic substance.

Peritoneal dialysis can be easily performed in any hospital and may be continued for long periods. It is valuable for the removal of poisons only if renal function is impaired, hemodialysis or hemoperfusion is not possible, or forced diuresis cannot be carried out.

Hemodialysis is unquestionably a more effective procedure for removing large amounts of dialyzable poisons. For barbiturates dialysance rates of 50 to 100 ml/min have been achieved, a removal rate two to ten times faster than during peritoneal dialysis or forced diuresis. Dialysis against solutions containing albumin or lipids can further speed removal of certain poisons. Perfusion of blood through activated charcoal or exchange resin achieves even higher clearance rates than hemodialysis for most poisons. Extracorporeal dialysis and hemoperfusion are clearly the procedures of choice for the rapid removal of poisons from patients who have absorbed amounts which make survival unlikely even under the best supportive care. Since the required equipment and skilled personnel are available only in a few hospitals, the possibility of transfer of such patients to one of these institutions should be considered.

Chelation and chemical binding The removal of some poisons is accelerated by chemical interaction with other substances followed by renal excretion. These substances are usually considered specific antidotes and are discussed with the individual poisons.

SUPPORTIVE THERAPY Most chemical poisonings are reversible, self-limited disease states. Skillful supportive therapy can keep many seriously poisoned patients alive and their detoxifying and excretory mechanisms functioning until the concentration of poison in the body has fallen to safe levels. Symptomatic measures are especially important when the poison is one of the many compounds for which no specific antidote is known. Even when an antidote is available, disturbances of vital functions must be prevented or controlled by appropriate supportive care.

The poisoned patient may suffer a variety of physiological disturbances. Most of these are not peculiar to chemical intoxications, and their therapeutic management is described elsewhere in this text. Only those aspects of supportive therapy specially relevant to poisonings are briefly discussed here.

Central nervous system depression Specific therapy directed against the depressant effects of poisons on the central nervous system is usually both unnecessary and difficult. Most poisoned patients will emerge from coma as from a prolonged anesthesia. During the period of unconsciousness meticulous nursing care and close observation are essential. If depression of medullary centers results in circulatory or respiratory failure, these vital functions must be immediately and vigorously supported by chemical or mechanical means.

The use of analeptics in the treatment of poison-induced central nervous system depression has been largely abandoned, for the following reasons: (1) Their effect is unpredictable, and their use in intoxicated patients produces an abnormal pattern of nervous activity in which paroxysmal excitation and convulsions may be superimposed on depression. (2) The availability of artificial ventilation and of effective measures to support the circulation has lessened the need for rapid restoration of normal medullary function. (3) It is doubtful that analeptics shorten the duration of coma sufficiently to justify their risks, and they have not been shown to improve prognosis. Certainly these agents should never be employed to restore consciousness, and it is doubtful whether their use to hasten the restoration of spontaneous breathing and active reflexes is ever justified. Naloxone, 0.4 mg administered intravenously, will generally reverse central nervous system depression secondary to narcotic overdosage.

Convulsions Many poisons (e.g., chlorinated hydrocarbons, insecticides, strychnine) cause convulsions by their specific excitatory effects. Poisoned patients may also have convulsions because of hypoxia, hypoglycemia, cerebral edema, or metabolic disturbances. In such cases these abnormalities should be corrected as far as possible. Regardless of the cause of the convulsions, anticonvulsant drugs are often required. Intravenously administered phenobarbital or one of the benzodiazepines, such as diazepam, is usually effective.

Cerebral edema Intracranial hypertension due to cerebral edema is also a characteristic effect of some poisons and a nonspecific result of other chemical intoxications. Cerebral edema is characteristically seen in poisoning by lead, carbon monoxide, and methanol. Symptomatic treatment consists of use of adrenocortical steroids and, when necessary, the intravenous administration of hypertonic solutions of mannitol or urea.

Hypotension The causes of hypotension and shock in the poisoned patient are legion, and often several of them coexist. Poisons can depress the medullary vasomotor centers, block autonomic ganglia or adrenergic receptors, directly depress the tone of arterial or venous smooth muscle, reduce myocardial contractility, or induce cardiac arrhythmias. Less specifically, the poisoned patient may be in shock because of tissue hypoxia, extensive tissue destruction from corrosives, loss of blood or fluids, or metabolic disturbances. When possible, these abnormalities should be promptly corrected. If the central venous pressure is low, fluid replacement should be the first therapeutic approach. Vasoactive drugs are often helpful and sometimes essential in the hypotensive poisoned patient, particularly in shock resulting from central depression. As in shock from other causes, choice of the most appropriate agent requires an analysis of the hemodynamic disturbance which goes beyond determination of the arterial pressure.

Cardiac arrhythmias Disturbances of cardiac impulse generation or conduction in the poisoned patient arise from the effects of certain poisons on the electrical properties of cardiac fibers or from myocardial hypoxia or metabolic disturbances. The latter should be corrected, and antiarrhythmic agents administered as indicated by the nature of the arrhythmia (Chap. 237).

Pulmonary edema The poisoned patient may develop pulmonary edema because of depressed myocardial contractility or because of alveolar injury from irritant gases or aspirated fluids. The latter type of edema is less responsive to treatment and may be associated with laryngeal edema. Therapeutic measures include suctioning, administration of high concentrations of oxygen under positive pressure, aerosols of surface-active agents, bronchodilators, and adrenocortical steroids.

Hypoxia Poisoning may cause tissue hypoxia by various mechanisms, and several of these may operate in one patient. Inadequate ventilation can result from central respiratory depression, from muscular paralysis, or from airway obstruction by retained secretions, laryngeal edema, or bronchospasm. Alveolar-capillary diffusion may be impaired by pulmonary edema. Anemia, methemoglobinemia, carboxyhemoglobinemia, or shock can interfere with oxygen transport. Cellular oxidation may be inhibited by cyanide, fluoroacetate, or general protoplasmic poisons. The highest priority in treatment must be given to maintenance of an adequate airway. The clinical situation and the site of obstruction may indicate frequent suctioning, insertion of an oropharyngeal airway or of an endotracheal tube, or a tracheotomy. If despite a clear airway ventilation remains inadequate, as judged by clinical appearance or by measurement of minute volume or blood gases, artificial ventilation by appropriate mechanical means is imperative. Administration of high concentrations of oxygen is indicated whenever tissue hypoxia occurs. When the central nervous system is severely depressed, oxygen administration often results in apnea and must be combined with artificial ventilation. Hyperbaric oxygen may be helpful in some situations. The treatment of methemoglobinemia, carboxyhemoglobinemia, and inhibition of cellular oxidation is discussed under the specific poisons which produce these changes.

Acute renal insufficiency Renal failure with oliguria or anuria may occur in the poisoned patient because of shock, dehydration, or electrolyte disturbances. More specifically, it may be due to the nephrotoxic potential of some poisons (e.g., mercury, phosphorus, carbon tetrachloride, bromate), many of which are concentrated and excreted by the kidney. Renal damage due to poisons is usually reversible. The management of acute renal insufficiency is outlined in Chap. 275.

Electrolyte and water disturbances Imbalances of fluid and electrolytes are common features of chemical poisoning. They may result from vomiting, diarrhea, renal insufficiency, or therapeutic maneuvers such as catharsis, forced diuresis, or dialysis. These disturbances are corrected or, ideally, prevented by appropriate therapy. Certain poisons produce more specific defects, such as metabolic acidosis (e.g., methanol, phenol, salicylate) or hypocalcemia (e.g., fluoride, oxalate). These abnormalities and any specific treatment are described under the individual poisons.

Acute hepatic insufficiency The primary manifestation of some poisonings (e.g., chlorinated hydrocarbons, phosphorus, cinchophen, certain mushrooms) is acute hepatic failure. Its management is described in Chap. 302.

ADMINISTRATION OF SYSTEMIC ANTIDOTES Specific antidotal therapy is available for only a few poisons. Some systemic antidotes are chemicals which exert their therapeutic effect by reducing the concentration of the toxic substance. They may do this by combining with the poison (e.g., ethylene diaminetetraacetate with lead, dimercaprol with mercury, sulfhydryl-containing reagents such as Mucomyst with a toxic metabolite of acetaminophen) or by increasing its excretion (e.g., chloride or mercurial diuretics in bromide poisoning). Other systemic antidotes compete with the poison for its receptor site (e.g., atropine with muscarine, naloxone with morphine, vitamin K_1 with coumadin anticoagulants; physostigmine reverses the anticholinergic effects of the tricyclic antidepressants, the antihistamines, and belladonna). Specific antidotes are discussed with the individual poisons.

REFERENCES

ARENA JM: *Poisoning*, 3d ed. Springfield, Ill, Charles C Thomas, 1974

ARLEFF AI et al: Coma following nonnarcotic drug overdosage—management of 208 adult patients. Am J Med Sci 266:405, 1973

BOURNE PG: *Acute Drug Abuse Emergencies*. New York, Academic, 1976

CASARETT LJ, DOULL J: *Toxicology: The Basic Science of Poisons*. New York, Macmillan, 1975

DREISBACH RH: *Handbook of Poisoning: Diagnosis and Treatment*, 9th ed. Los Altos, Calif, Lange, 1978

HAYDEN JW, COMSTOCK EG: Use of activated charcoal in acute poisoning. Clin Toxicol 8(5):515, 1975

LOOMIS TA: *Essentials of Toxicology*, 2d ed. Philadelphia, Lea & Febiger, 1974

LOVEJOY FH JR, ALPERT JH: Acute poisoning, in *Current Pediatric Therapy*, 8th ed, SS Gellis, BM Kegan (eds). Philadelphia, Saunders, pp 709–734, 1978

MOFENSON HC, GREENSHER J: The unknown poison. Pediatrics 54:336, 1974

Seminar on childhood poisoning. Paediatrician 6:3, 1977

SMITH RP, GOSSELIN RE: Current concepts about the treatment of selected poisonings. Annu Rev Pharmacol Toxicol 16:189, 1976

WINCHESTER JF et al: Dialysis and hemoperfusion of poisons and drugs—update. Trans Am Soc Artif Intern Organs 23:762, 1977

ZENZ C: *Occupational Medicine*. Chicago, Year Book, 1975

Toxic product information

Drug Identification Guide. Oradell, NJ, Medical Economics, 1975

GLEASON MN et al: *Clinical Toxicology of Commercial Products*, 4th ed. Baltimore, Williams & Wilkins, 1976

GOODMAN LS, GILMAN A: *The Pharmacological Basis of Therapeutics*, 5th ed. New York, Macmillan, 1975

HAYES WJ: *Toxicology of Pesticides*. Baltimore, Williams & Wilkins, 1975

The Merck Index, 9th ed. Rahway, NJ, Merck and Co, 1976

Poisindex. Englewood, Colo, Micromedex, 1974

Poisonous Plants and Fungi. Philadelphia, Rittenhouse, 1976

SCHERZ RG: The history of poison control centers in the United States. Clin Toxicol 12:291, 1978

WILSON CO, JONES TE: *American Drug Index*. Philadelphia, Lippincott, 1975

224
COMMON POISONS

PAUL A. FRIEDMAN

The poisons discussed in this chapter are some of those encountered by the general population such as commonly used drugs, household products, solvents, pesticides, and poisonous plants. It has been necessary to disregard many uncommon toxic materials as well as products to which exposure occurs only in specialized industrial environments. Details concerning poisoning by such compounds may be found in some of the references following Chap. 223. Toxic effects of many drugs are considered throughout this text in conjunction with their therapeutic use. Manifestations of hypersensitivity to chemicals are described in Chap. 71. The following discussions of specific poisons stress those details of their action which are pertinent to the recognition or treatment of clinical poisoning.

ACETAMINOPHEN Termed *paracetamol* in the United Kingdom, acetaminophen has become a popular alternative to salicylates as an analgesic and antipyretic. It is a frequent cause of poisoning. While the toxic and lethal doses of acetaminophen may vary from patient to patient, hepatic damage may be expected if an adult has taken more than 8 g as a single dose. A plasma concentration of greater than 200 μg/ml at 4 h after ingestion is also cause for concern. Clinical manifestations of acetaminophen poisoning are nonspecific. In the first few hours after ingestion lethargy, pallor, nausea, vomiting, and diaphoresis may occur; there are no acid-base derangements which may accompany aspirin overdose. Hepatic damage, the most important manifestation of acetaminophen toxicity, becomes evident 1 to 2 days after ingestion. While some patients show only elevation of serum transaminase and others show hepatic enlargement, tenderness, and jaundice, more severe damage can lead to hyperammonemia, asterixis, mental confusion, coma, bleeding, and death from acute liver failure. Acute tubular necrosis, pancreatitis, hypoglycemia, cardiac damage, and hypersensitivity reactions are sometimes seen.

There is good evidence that damage to tissue (especially liver) is caused by metabolites of acetaminophen and not the drug itself. At therapeutic doses acetaminophen is eliminated mainly conjugated to sulfate or glucuronic acid. A small amount of acetaminophen is activated by the cytochrome P_{450} system and conjugated with the sulfhydryl group of glutathione to yield a nontoxic mercapturic acid. After an overdose, the pathways of conjugation to the sulfate and glucuronic acid become saturated, an increasing fraction of the drug is activated by the P_{450} system, glutathione stores are depleted, and the reactive intermediates then become free to bind covalently to liver macromolecules and cause necrosis.

Treatment of acetaminophen poisoning should begin with induction of emesis or gastric lavage followed by administration of activated charcoal. Since endogenous glutathione appears to have a protective effect, the administration of several other sulfhydryl compounds has been studied for protection against acetaminophen hepatotoxicity. When administered orally within 10 h of ingestion, either *N*-acetylcysteine (Mucomyst) or cysteamine is effective in decreasing hepatotoxicity. A potentially toxic dose ($>$7.5 g) ingested within the previous 24 h is an indication for *N*-acetylcysteine therapy. Since early treatment is paramount, a patient suspected of having ingested a potentially hepatotoxic dose should be started on sulfhydryl therapy while awaiting the plasma acetaminophen level. A 5% solution of Mucomyst in a cola beverage or fruit juice is given with a loading dose of 140 mg/kg and a maintenance dose of 70 mg/kg every 4 h for 3 days. If sulfhydryl therapy is to be instituted, charcoal and osmotic cathartic administration are contraindicated since both may reduce absorption of the antidote. In a mixed poisoning, charcoal may be removed by lavage prior to administration of the antidote. The increment of acetaminophen clearance from forced diuresis is small compared with liver metabolism; both hemodialysis and charcoal hemoperfusion result in a greater clearance of drug, but as yet the effectiveness of these methods in reducing hepatotoxicity and mortality has not been demonstrated. Inducers of the cytochrome P_{450} enzyme system such as barbiturates should be avoided.

ACIDS Corrosive acids are used widely in industry and laboratories. Ingestion is almost always with suicidal intent. Death has occurred after an oral dose of 1 ml of a corrosive acid.

Toxic effects of corrosive acids are due to their direct chemical action. Ingestion of acids may produce irritation, bleeding, and sloughing in the mouth and esophagus with more severe burns occurring in the stomach, particularly in the pylorus. Perforations with peritonitis, though uncommon, may occur. Mouth and pharynx may be brownish black and may have a charred appearance. Yellow staining is seen after ingestion of nitric and picric acids. Severe pain in mouth, pharynx, chest, and abdomen is the rule and is soon followed by hematemesis and bloody diarrhea. Frequently profound shock develops. About half of those who ingest significant amounts of acid die from its immediate effects. Survivors can develop mediastinitis or peritonitis from esophageal or gastric perforation, and delayed perforation of the esophagus or stomach can also occur. Recovery from acid ingestion can be associated with stricture formation which most commonly involves the pylorus.

Ingested acid must be immediately diluted a hundredfold by water or milk. The danger of perforation contraindicates the use of emesis or gastric lavage except during the first 30 min after ingestion. Diagnostic esophagoscopy, if performed, should be done in the first 48 h after ingestion. Following the emergency measures, appropriate supportive therapy is administered for the relief of pain and the treatment of shock, perforation, and infection.

Certain gases found in industry (e.g., chlorine, phosgene) may combine with water in the lungs to form corrosive acids. During rapid decomposition of plant material in silos, oxides of nitrogen are released which form nitric acid in the lungs. Inhalation of such gases causes coughing and choking sensations which are followed after a latent period of 6 to 8 h by pulmonary edema. Treatment is supportive. Symptoms of dyspnea and hemoptysis may be prolonged, and frequent relapses may occur.

ALKALIES Strong alkalies such as ammonium hydroxide, potassium hydroxide (potash), potassium carbonate, sodium hydroxide (lye, Clinitest tablets), and sodium carbonate (washing soda) are widely used in industry and in cleansers and drain cleaners. Sodium and potassium phosphates find use as water softeners. Strong alkalies form soaps with fats and proteinates with proteins, resulting in penetrating necrosis of tissues. Fa-

talities have occurred from the ingestion of 5 to 30 g of such compounds.

The toxic effects of alkalies are due to irritation and destruction of local tissues. Ingestion is followed by severe pain in mouth, pharynx, chest, and abdomen. Vomiting of blood and sloughed mucosa and diarrhea are common. Reflex loss of vascular tone frequently leads to profound shock. Perforation of the esophagus or stomach may be immediate or delayed for several days. Mouth and pharynx show erythema and gelatinous necrotic areas. After ingestion of water softeners profound reduction in serum calcium may be seen and lead to tetany and hypotension. Survivors usually suffer from esophageal strictures.

Treatment consists of immediate administration of large amounts of water or milk. The volume of liquids should exceed that of the ingested alkali a hundredfold. Vomiting should be allowed to occur, and gastric lavage may be performed during the first half-hour after ingestion. Because of the danger of perforation, both are contraindicated thereafter. Esophagoscopy should be done within the first 48 h. With evidence of significant esophageal or gastric burns steroids are usually administered for about 3 weeks to decrease the incidence of stricture formation, although definitive evidence of efficacy is lacking. If steroids are given, a broad-spectrum antibiotic such as ampicillin or a cephalosporin should also be administered for prophylaxis. After the ingestion of water softeners (phosphates), calcium gluconate should be administered intravenously as needed. Treatment is otherwise symptomatic and directed at the relief of pain, respiratory obstruction due to edema of the hypopharynx, fluid loss, and shock.

Inhalation of ammonia, which is used as a refrigerant, results in irritation of the upper and lower parts of the respiratory tract. Laryngeal and pulmonary edema may occur and must be treated symptomatically.

ANILINE This substance is used in printing and clothmarking inks, paints, and paint removers. Both aniline and its derivatives, such as toluidine, nitroaniline, and nitrobenzene, are widely used in industrial synthesis. Aniline is absorbed from the gastrointestinal tract and through the lungs or skin. Ingestion of 1 g aniline has been fatal. Methemoglobinemia is the most important manifestation. Headache, dizziness, hypotension, convulsions, and coma may occur. If the acute period is survived, jaundice and anemia may appear. Treatment consists of correction of methemoglobinemia (see Chap. 315) and supportive measures.

ANTIHISTAMINES The common and unprescribed use of antihistamines makes them readily available for accidental overdosage and suicidal attempts. There is wide variation from patient to patient in tolerance to these drugs and in the manifestations of poisoning. A dose of 200 mg diphenhydramine has been fatal in one adult, whereas another tolerated 2 g. Manifestations of poisoning are central nervous system excitement or depression. In children the usual toxic manifestations are excitement, hyperthermia, hyperreflexia, tremors, and convulsions, followed by central nervous system depression. In adults depressive manifestations with drowsiness, stupor, and coma predominate, but convulsions followed by further depression may occur.

Treatment is supportive and directed toward removal of the unabsorbed drug and maintenance of vital functions. Convulsions may be controlled with phenobarbital or diazepam. Some antihistamines have prominent atropine-like properties. Patients poisoned with these drugs may show manifestations of atropine poisoning and are treated correspondingly.

ANTIMUSCARINIC COMPOUNDS Atropine, related belladonna alkaloids (hyoscyamine and scopolamine), and synthetic substitutes (e.g., benztropine, cyclopentolate, homatropine, methantheline, propantheline) are widely prescribed drugs and occur in many proprietary mixtures used in the treatment of gastrointestinal and upper respiratory diseases, asthma, and parkinsonism. Poisoning, especially in children, may also occur from the excessive use of ophthalmic solutions containing such compounds. Finally, children may be intoxicated by eating plants containing up to 0.5 percent of atropine or related alkaloids. Such plants are *Atropa belladonna* (deadly nightshade), *Hyoscyamus niger* (henbane), and *Datura stramonium* (Jamestown or Jimson weed).

Individual sensitivity to the toxic effects of belladonna alkaloids varies widely; fatalities have occurred from as little as 10 mg atropine, but doses of 500 mg have been survived. Young children are particularly susceptible to poisoning with belladonna alkaloids. Older persons appear to be more sensitive to the central nervous system effects of these drugs. Since atropine is both hydrolyzed in the liver and excreted unchanged in the urine, insufficiency of hepatic or renal function may lead to poisoning on therapeutic dosage.

The most characteristic manifestations of atropine poisoning are those of parasympathetic blockade: dryness of mucous membranes, thirst, dysphagia, hoarseness, xerophthalmia, dilated pupils, blurring of vision, rise in intraocular tension, flushing, dryness and increased temperature of the skin, fever, tachycardia, hypertension, urinary retention, and abdominal distention. This widespread parasympatholysis is almost diagnostic of belladonna poisoning, but the diagnosis can be further confirmed by the reversal of blockade by physostigmine (2 mg administered intravenously over several minutes).

Central nervous system symptoms are also very common during belladonna intoxication. Atropine and scopolamine produce similar toxic psychoses. Restlessness, excitation, confusion, and incoordination precede mania, hallucinations, and delirium. Patients intoxicated by scopolamine not infrequently show lethargy and somnolence rather than excitement. In severe intoxication with belladonna alkaloids, central nervous system depression and coma are the rule. When death results it is because of circulatory collapse and respiratory failure.

In the treatment of belladonna poisoning, emesis or gastric lavage should be followed by the administration of activated charcoal. Symptomatic treatment is directed at the reduction of body temperature, the moistening of mucous membranes, and, when necessary, urethral catheterization. Excitement or convulsions may require appropriate pharmacotherapy. Patients with deep coma, life-threatening cardiac arrhythmias, severe hallucinations, or severe hypertension have been treated with physostigmine with reversal of the effects. It has not been established whether physostigmine reduces mortality.

Death occurs in fewer than 1 percent of cases of atropine or scopolamine poisoning. No permanent sequelae have been observed, but manifestations may persist for several days.

BARIUM Poisoning may be due to the ingestion of rodenticides which contain soluble barium salts or of depilatories that contain barium sulfide. A soluble barium salt may be present as a contaminant in the insoluble barium sulfate used as a radiopaque contrast medium. Barium is extremely toxic, producing intense stimulation of muscles of all types. Its action on the gastrointestinal musculature causes vomiting, colic, and diarrhea. Skeletal muscle tremors and spasm are commonly seen. Arteriolar spasm results in marked hypertension. Cardiac arrhythmias may proceed to ventricular fibrillation. Anxiety, weakness, and convulsions may occur. Death is usually due to cardiac arrhythmia or respiratory arrest.

Treatment consists of the oral administration of 250 ml 10% sodium sulfate or 5% magnesium sulfate. This will precipitate and remove any unabsorbed barium in the gastrointestinal tract. A dose of 10 ml of a 10% solution of sodium sulfate should be slowly administered intravenously every 15 min until symptoms subside. Procainamide may be used to reduce the danger of fatal cardiac arrhythmias. Serum potassium may be reduced, in which case oral or intravenous supplementation is indicated. If necessary, pain should be relieved and artificial ventilation with oxygen administered.

BENZENE, TOLUENE These solvents are used in paint removers, dry-cleaning solutions, and rubber or plastic cements. Benzene is also present, to some extent, in most gasolines. Poisoning may result from ingestion or from the breathing of concentrated vapors. Toluene is the major ingredient in the cement used by teen-age glue sniffers.

Acute poisoning by these compounds causes central nervous system manifestations. With sufficient exposure, symptoms progress from an initial period of restlessness, excitement, euphoria, and dizziness to coma, convulsions, and respiratory failure. Ventricular arrhythmias may occur.

Chronic poisoning by benzene or toluene results from repeated exposure to their vapors in low concentration. Central nervous system symptoms include irritability, insomnia, headache, tremors, and paresthesias. Anorexia and nausea are also common. Fatty degeneration of the heart, liver, and kidneys may occur. By far the most important manifestation of chronic exposure to benzene is bone marrow depression, which may progress to aplastic anemia and complete aplasia of the bone marrow. Individual susceptibility to this effect varies greatly and may not become apparent for months after the initial exposure to the poison.

Treatment of both acute and chronic poisoning is symptomatic. After ingestion, emesis must not be induced, and gastric lavage should await placement of an endotracheal tube with an inflatable cuff. Neurological, pulmonary, or cardiovascular problems are treated as in poisoning by petroleum distillates.

BLEACHES Clorox, Purex, Sanichlor, and other bleaching solutions contain 3 to 6% sodium hypochlorite. The solution used for chlorinating swimming pools is 20%. Their corrosive action in mouth, pharynx, and esophagus is similar to that of sodium hydroxide. Acid gastric juice releases hypochlorous acid from such solutions. This compound is very irritating to mucous membranes, and inhalation of its fumes causes severe pulmonary irritation and pulmonary edema. However, the systemic toxicity of hypochlorous acid is low. Perforation and stricture formation are rare after the ingestion of bleaching solutions. The fatal dose is approximately 30 ml.

Treatment consists of dilution of the ingested bleach with water or milk. The usual bleaching solutions do not cause enough corrosive injury to the esophagus to preclude the induction of emesis or gastric lavage, but one should be wary of this possibility if a 20% solution has been ingested. Although sodium thiosulfate (100 ml of a 1 to 2.5% solution by lavage), which will reduce hypochlorite to nontoxic products, has been routinely administered to these patients, there is great doubt that it is of any use except in very large overdoses, very early after ingestion.

BORIC ACID This compound is a very weak germicide and has been widely employed in powders, lotions, solutions, and ointments. Though not highly toxic, boric acid is not nearly as benign as widely assumed. The lethal dose is approximately 15 g in adults and 5 g in infants. Such amounts can be absorbed through abraded skin, from serous cavities, and after ingestion.

Regardless of the route of administration, the first symptoms of poisoning are nausea, vomiting, and diarrhea. These are followed by headache, weakness, restlessness, and erythroderma which may progress to desquamation of skin and mucous membranes. Renal toxicity and shock are common, and more than 100 fatalities have occurred. Renal excretion of boric acid is slow, and clearance can be increased markedly by dialysis. Boric acid should always be labeled as poison, and since this substance has no therapeutic function which cannot be served equally well by less toxic preparations, it should be removed from home and hospital.

BROMATES These compounds are used as neutralizers in cold wave preparations. They produce widespread tissue injury, particularly in central nervous system and kidneys. The fatal oral dose of bromates is approximately 5 g. On contact of bromate with gastric acid, hydrogen bromate, an irritating acid, is formed. Ingestion of bromates is followed by vomiting, diarrhea, abdominal pain, drowsiness, coma, convulsions, hypotension, hematuria, oliguria, anuria, and hemolysis.

Treatment consists of emesis or gastric lavage with sodium bicarbonate solution followed by catharsis. A dose of 250 ml of a 1% sodium thiosulfate solution should be administered intravenously. Peritoneal dialysis or hemodialysis effectively removes bromate from the body. Appropriate supportive therapy should be given.

CARBON MONOXIDE Carbon monoxide is a colorless, odorless, tasteless, and nonirritating gas produced by the incomplete combustion of carbonaceous materials. Almost any flame or combustion device emits carbon monoxide. The gas is present in the exhaust of internal combustion engines in a concentration of 3 to 7 percent. Much higher concentrations are present in most illuminating and heating gases, but not in natural gas. Carbon monoxide is annually responsible for about 3500 accidental and suicidal deaths in the United States alone.

The toxic effects of carbon monoxide are the result of tissue hypoxia. Carbon monoxide combines with hemoglobin to form carboxyhemoglobin. Since carbon monoxide and oxygen react with the same group in the hemoglobin molecule, carboxyhemoglobin is incapable of carrying oxygen. The affinity of hemoglobin for carbon monoxide is two hundred times greater than for oxygen, and at equilibrium 1 part of carbon monoxide in 1500 parts of air will result in 50 percent conversion of hemoglobin to carboxyhemoglobin. Carboxyhemoglobin also interferes with the release of oxygen from oxyhemoglobin. This further reduces the amount of oxygen available to the tissues and explains why tissue anoxia appears in the carbon monoxide-poisoned person at levels of arterial oxyhemoglobin concentration well tolerated by the anemic patient.

The extent of saturation of hemoglobin with carbon monoxide depends on the concentration of the gas in inspired air and on the time of exposure. The severity of hypoxic symptoms depends further on an individual's state of activity, tissue oxygen needs, and hemoglobin concentration. As a general rule, no symptoms will develop at a concentration of 0.01 percent carbon monoxide in inspired air, since this will not raise blood saturation above 10 percent. Exposure to 0.05 percent for 1 h during light activity will produce a blood concentration of 20 percent carboxyhemoglobin and result in a mild or throbbing headache. Greater activity or longer exposure to the same concentration causes a blood saturation of 30 to 50 percent. At this point headache, irritability, confusion, dizziness, visual disturbances, nausea, vomiting, and fainting on exertion may be observed. After exposure for 1 h to concentrations of 0.1 percent in inspired air, the blood will contain 50 to 80 percent carboxyhemoglobin, which results in coma, convul-

sions, respiratory failure, and death. On inhalation of high concentrations of carbon monoxide, saturation of the blood proceeds so rapidly that unconsciousness may occur suddenly and without warning. When poisoning is more gradual, the individual may notice decreased exercise tolerance and dyspnea on exertion or even at rest. Excessive sweating, fever, hepatomegaly, skin lesions, leukocytosis, bleeding diathesis, albuminuria, and glycosuria have also been described. Cerebral edema and intracranial hypertension may result from the increased permeability of hypoxic capillaries. Myocardial hypoxia is reflected by electrocardiographic abnormalities.

The most characteristic sign of carbon monoxide poisoning is the cherry color of skin and mucous membranes, which is due to the bright red carboxyhemoglobin. If the characteristic flush is not present and carbon monoxide poisoning is suspected, 1 ml of the patient's blood can be diluted with 10 ml water; when 1 ml of 5% sodium hydroxide is added to this dilution, an oxyhemoglobin solution will turn brown. If significant amounts of carboxyhemoglobin are present, the solution will turn straw yellow ($<20\%$ carboxyhemoglobin) or will remain pink ($>20\%$ carboxyhemoglobin).

Treatment of carbon monoxide poisoning requires effective ventilation in the presence of high oxygen tensions and in the absence of carbon monoxide. If necessary, ventilation should be supported artificially. Pure oxygen should be administered. This will result not only in the replacement of carbon monoxide by oxygen in the hemoglobin molecule but also in the partial relief of tissue hypoxia by oxygen dissolved in the plasma. For the same reasons hyperbaric oxygen is helpful in seriously poisoned patients. Transfusion of blood or packed cells is also of value. In order to reduce tissue needs for oxygen, the patient must be kept absolutely quiet. Induction of hypothermia is not indicated. Cerebral edema should be treated with diuretics and steroids.

During the recovery from carbon monoxide poisoning symptoms regress gradually. If severe tissue hypoxia has obtained too long, neurological symptoms such as tremors, mental deterioration, and psychotic behavior may persist. Histological changes characteristic of hypoxia may be observed in cerebral cortex, medulla, myocardium, and other organs.

CASTOR BEANS The castor bean plant (*Ricinus communis*) is grown for commercial and ornamental purposes. The beans contain the protein ricin which is extremely toxic to mammalian cells. Like abrin, another toxic plant protein, ricin inhibits protein synthesis in eukaryotic cells. Both ricin and abrin consist of two polypeptide chains—one chain functions to bind the toxin to the cell surface while the second chain can then enter the cell and, in a specific and irreversible reaction, enzymatically inactivate the 60S ribosomal subunit, thus inhibiting protein synthesis. After a delay of several hours to 2 days following ingestion, abdominal pain, vomiting, and profuse diarrhea appear and produce severe dehydration. Extreme weakness, drowsiness, disorientation, stupor, coma, convulsions, respiratory depression, and circulatory collapse may develop. Intravascular clotting and hemolysis have been observed. If the patient survives the acute symptoms, oliguria may progress to anuria and uremia, with death after several days. Treatment consists of fluid replacement, alkalinization of the urine with sodium bicarbonate to prevent precipitation of hemoglobin in the kidneys, and supportive measures.

CHLORATES Sodium and potassium chlorates are strong oxidizing agents and are found in gargles, mouthwashes, matches, and weed killers. After oral ingestion, 2 g has been fatal for children and 10 g for adults. Chlorate ion acts as a catalyst in the production of methemoglobinemia, and absorption of a small amount can result in a high methemoglobin concentration. The symptoms of chlorate ingestion are those of local mucosal irritation and of methemoglobinemia (see Chaps. 53 and 315). Renal toxicity is common. Treatment is directed primarily at the methemoglobinemia. Absorbed chlorate can be removed effectively by dialysis.

CHLORINATED INSECTICIDES These compounds are ingredients of dusts, sprays, and solutions used as insecticides. The great majority of these compounds are chlorinated diphenyls (e.g., DDT, TDE, DFDT, DMC, Neotran) or chlorinated polycyclic compounds (e.g., aldrin, chlordane, dieldrin, endrin, heptachlor). Lindane is a hexachlorobenzene. Their toxicity has led to their greatly diminished use in recent years, and many are banned in certain locales, including the United States. The chlorinated insecticides are soluble in lipid and organic solvents but not in water. They are poorly absorbed unless dissolved in a vehicle such as kerosene, petroleum distillates, or other organic solvents. Under these circumstances they readily enter the body through the skin, lungs, or gastrointestinal tract. These compounds vary considerably in toxicity, and the toxicity of the dissolving vehicle must also be considered. The effects of the solvent may overshadow or modify those of the insecticide.

The initial symptoms of acute poisoning are nausea, vomiting, headache, dizziness, apprehension, excitement, and muscular tremors and weakness. These symptoms progress to generalized central nervous system hyperexcitability and delirium and clonic or tonic convulsions. This stage is in turn followed by progressive depression with paralysis, coma, and death. Except for endrin, which is strongly hepatotoxic, liver toxicity occurs only at extreme dosage levels. Treatment consists of induction of emesis or gastric lavage, activated charcoal administration, catharsis, anticonvulsive therapy, artificial ventilation, and other supportive measures. Sympathomimetic compounds should be avoided, since chlorinated insecticides apparently increase susceptibility to ventricular fibrillation. Cholestyramine accelerates the excretion of the chlorinated hydrocarbon kepone, and it may well have a similar effect on the excretion of pesticides such as DTT, dieldrin, chlordane, and heptachlor which remain in the body for prolonged periods.

CHOLINESTERASE INHIBITOR INSECTICIDES Many substances used in agriculture for control of soft-bodied insects are potent inhibitors of cholinesterase. Most of these compounds are organic phosphates (e.g., Parathion, Malathion, Systox, TEPP, HETP, OMPA), others are carbamates (e.g., Dimetan, Mactacil). The toxicity of these compounds varies widely. They are usually prepared for use by dilution with powders, organic solvents, or water. Formulations containing 1 to 95 percent of the active ingredient are available. The cholinesterase inhibitor insecticides are rapidly absorbed through the intact skin and after inhalation or ingestion.

The toxicity of these agents results from inactivation of acetylcholinesterase which allows accumulation of excessive amounts of acetylcholine at a number of sites: central nervous system, autonomic ganglia, parasympathetic nerve endings, and motor nerve endings. In the central nervous system coma and respiratory depression and less commonly seizures can occur. Toxic muscarinic effects include nausea, vomiting, diarrhea, involuntary defecation and urination, blurring of vision due to miosis, sweating, lacrimation, and salivation. Nicotinic effects include muscle twitching, fasciculations, weakness, and flaccid paralysis. Cardiac arrhythmias and pulmonary edema, as well as EEG abnormalities, also occur.

Management consists of emesis or lavage, charcoal instillation, catharsis, and washing of contaminated skin with soap and water. Atropine should be given immediately to block the parasympathetic and central nervous system effects. A dose of 2 mg is injected intramuscularly and repeated every 10 min until parasympathetic manifestations are controlled and signs of atropinization appear. The same dosage must be repeated frequently to maintain xerostomia and mild tachycardia. Fatal respiratory failure or pulmonary edema may occur quickly upon cessation of atropine therapy, and the drug should be judiciously withdrawn. Atropine is virtually ineffective against the autonomic ganglionic actions of acetycholine and against the peripheral neuromuscular paralysis. Relief of muscle weakness, in particular respiratory paralysis, can be achieved with certain oximes which can reactivate cholinesterase by reversing the phosphate ester bond formed by the organic phosphate at the enzyme active site. Pralidoxime is useful in the treatment of organic phosphate cholinesterase inhibition but should not be used if the inhibition is due to a carbamate. A dose of 1 g pralidoxime in aqueous solution is administered intravenously over a 5-min period, and this dose is repeated up to four times every 8 to 12 h. Supportive therapy includes administration of oxygen with artificial ventilation if necessary, removal of pulmonary secretions by suction, and treatment of convulsions with diazepam and phenobarbital. Energetic therapy with artificial ventilation, atropine, and pralidoxime allows survival after doses of organic phosphate esters vastly exceeding the usual fatal dose. In addition, charcoal hemoperfusion significantly increases the clearance of organophosphates and, when available, is indicated after large overdoses in which the patient cannot be supported with atropine and pralidoxime.

CYANIDE The cyanide ion is an exceedingly potent and rapid-acting poison, but one for which specific and effective antidotal therapy is available. Cyanide poisoning may result from the inhalation of hydrocyanic acid or from the ingestion of soluble inorganic cyanide salts or cyanide-releasing substances such as cyanamide, cyanogen chloride, and nitroprusside. Parts of many plants also contain substances such as amygdalin which release cyanide on digestion. Among these are the seeds of certain stone fruits (chokecherry, pin cherry, wild black cherry, peach, apricot, bitter almond), cassava roots, the berries of the jet berry bush, the leaves and shoots of elderberry, and all parts of hydrangea. The controversial drug laetrile, composed in part of an extract of apricot kernels, has been responsible for fatal cyanide poisoning. Cyanides are widely used in industry and for fumigation and may reach the home in photographic chemicals or silver polishes. As little as 300 mg potassium cyanide may cause death.

The extreme toxicity of cyanide is due to its ready reaction with the trivalent iron of cytochrome oxidase. The role of the enzyme in cellular oxygen utilization is inhibited by the formation of the cytochrome oxidase-cyanide complex. The resultant cytotoxic hypoxia leads to cellular dysfunction and death.

Inhalation of hydrogen cyanide may cause death within a minute. Oral doses act more slowly, requiring several minutes for the appearance of symptoms and up to several hours for death. The first effect is an increase in ventilation because of the blockade of oxidative metabolism in the chemoreceptor cells. As more cyanide is absorbed, there are headache, dizziness, nausea, drowsiness, hypotension, profound dyspnea, characteristic electrocardiographic changes, coma, and convulsions.

Cyanide poisoning is a true medical emergency. Treatment is highly effective if given rapidly. The chemical antidotes should be immediately available wherever emergency medical care is dispensed. The diagnosis may be made by the characteristic "bitter almond" odor on the breath of the victim, and physicians should familiarize themselves with this smell. Since the saturation of hemoglobin is not disturbed by cyanide, cyanosis is not seen until respiratory depression supervenes. The objective of treatment is the production of methemoglobin by the administration of nitrite. The trivalent iron of methemoglobin competes with cytochrome oxidase for the cyanide ion. The cytochrome oxidase-cyanide complex dissociates, and enzymatic function and cell respiration are restored. Further detoxification is then achieved by the administration of thiosulfate. The enzyme rhodanese catalyzes the reaction of thiosulfate with cyanide liberated by the dissociation of cyanmethemoglobin; thiocyanate, which is relatively nontoxic, is formed and readily excreted in the urine.

Since speed is of the essence, nitrite should be immediately administered by inhalation of amyl nitrite perles, one every 2 min unless blood pressure is below 80 mmHg. This is followed as soon as possible by the intravenous injection of 10 ml of 3% sodium nitrite over a 3-min period. An intravenous infusion of norepinephrine may be necessary to maintain blood pressure during this injection period. After the administration of sodium nitrite, 50 ml of 25% sodium thiosulfate should be administered intravenously over a 10-min period. Supportive measures, especially artificial respiration with 100% oxygen, should be instituted as soon as possible, but, unless methemoglobinemia is produced promptly, other forms of treatment are of no value. Administration of sodium nitrite and sodium thiosulfate may have to be repeated. Ideally, dosage should be based on methemoglobin determinations, and the methemoglobin should not exceed 40%. If the patient survives 4 h, recovery is likely but residual cerebral symptoms may persist.

DETERGENTS AND SOAPS These substances fall into the three groups of anionic, nonionic, and cationic detergents. The first group contains common soaps and household detergents. They may cause vomiting and diarrhea but have no serious effects, and no treatment is required. However, some laundry compounds contain phosphate water softeners whose ingestion may cause hypocalcemia. The ingestion of nonionic detergents is harmless and requires no treatment.

Cationic detergents, such as benzalkonium chloride (Zephiran) and many others, are commonly used for bactericidal purposes in hospitals and homes. These compounds are well absorbed from the gastrointestinal tract and interfere with cellular functions. The fatal oral dose is approximately 3 g. Concentrated preparations (>20% detergent) are corrosive to mouth and esophagus. Ingestion produces nausea and vomiting, and shock, coma, convulsions, and death may occur in a few hours. Treatment after ingestion of dilute preparations consists of minimizing gastrointestinal absorption by emesis and gastric lavage with ordinary soap solution, which rapidly inactivates cationic detergents. Emesis and lavage are contraindicated in the presence of esophageal injury which is unlikely to occur except after ingestion of concentrated preparations. Activated charcoal and an osmotic cathartic should be administered. If significant absorption has occurred, intensive supportive therapy may be required.

ERGOT This fungus (*Claviceps purpurea*) grows on rye and contains a number of highly toxic alkaloids (e.g., ergotamine, ergonovine) which are used in the treatment of migraine or as uterine stimulants. Poisoning may be due to therapeutic overdosage, particularly in patients with severe infections or liver disease, but more commonly results from the use of ergot as an abortifacient. The epidemic form of chronic ergot poisoning due to the ingestion of contaminated grain is now rarely seen. Ingestion of 1 g ergot has been fatal; ergotamine has caused gangrene in doses of 10 mg per day. Symptoms of acute or chronic ergot poisoning are vomiting, diarrhea, burning abdominal pain, severe muscle pains, ischemic peripheral gangrene, headache, psychotic behavior, muscle tremors, convul-

sions, and coma. Circulatory disturbances are due both to prolonged vasoconstriction and to intimal hyperplasia and thrombosis. Treatment of ergot poisoning is symptomatic. Vigorous vasodilator and analgesic therapy should be employed.

FLUORIDES Fluoride salts are widely used in insecticides. The gases fluorine and hydrogen fluoride are used in industry. The latter is a strong corrosive. Fluorine and fluorides are cellular poisons which inhibit a number of enzymatic reactions, probably the most important of which is to block the glycolytic degradation of glucose. Fluorides also form an insoluble precipitate with calcium and cause hypocalcemia. Finally, in an acid medium fluorides form the corrosive hydrofluoric acid. Ingestion of 1 to 2 g sodium fluoride may be fatal.

Inhalation of fluorine or hydrogen fluoride produces coughing and choking. After an asymptomatic period of a day or two, fever, cough, cyanosis, and pulmonary edema may develop. Ingestion of fluoride salts is followed by nausea, vomiting productive of corroded tissues, diarrhea, and abdominal pain. Consequent to the decrease in serum calcium the victim develops muscular hyperirritability, fasciculations, tremors, spasms, and convulsions. Death is due to respiratory paralysis or circulatory collapse. If the patient survives the acute period, jaundice and oliguria may appear. Chronic fluoride poisoning (fluorosis) is characterized by weight loss, weakness, anemia, brittle bones, and stiff joints. Mottling of teeth is seen when exposure occurs during enamel formation.

Acute fluoride poisoning is treated by immediate administration of milk, lime water, calcium gluconate, or calcium lactate solution to precipitate calcium fluoride. After lavage or emesis and charcoal instillation, calcium (e.g., calcium gluconate, 10 g) can be given again followed by an osmotic cathartic. Then 10% calcium gluconate or 1% calcium chloride should be slowly injected intravenously and repeated as needed to prevent a positive Chvostek's sign. Symptomatic and supportive therapy is administered as indicated.

FORMALDEHYDE This gas is available as 40% solution (Formalin) which is used as a disinfectant, fumigant, or deodorant. Poisoning by Formalin may be diagnosed by the characteristic odor of formaldehyde. Formaldehyde reacts chemically with cellular constituents, depresses cellular functions, and causes cell death. The fatal dose of Formalin is about 60 ml.

Ingestion of Formalin immediately causes severe abdominal pain, nausea, vomiting, and diarrhea. This may be followed by collapse, coma, severe metabolic acidosis, and anuria. Death is usually due to circulatory failure.

Since any organic material can inactivate formaldehyde, milk, bread, soup, etc., should be administered immediately unless activated charcoal is available. Formaldehyde is a corrosive, and emesis and lavage are not recommended.

Parenteral administration of sodium bicarbonate is indicated to combat acidosis. The treatment is otherwise supportive.

GLYCOLS Ethylene glycol and diethylene glycol are commonly used in antifreeze solutions. The more than 50 annual deaths from these compounds usually result from intentional drinking of antifreeze by alcoholics. The fatal dose of ethylene glycol is about 100 g, that of diethylene glycol somewhat lower. Glycols are metabolized by alcohol dehydrogenase to the aldehyde which is ultimately converted to oxalate. It is the metabolites of the glycols (particularly the aldehyde and oxalate) which are most responsible for toxicity after glycol ingestion.

The initial symptoms of acute poisoning by these glycols resemble those of alcoholic intoxication. They may progress to vomiting, stupor, coma with absent reflexes and anisocoria, and convulsions. Tachypnea, bradycardia, and hypothermia are commonly seen, as are metabolic acidosis and hypocalcemia. After massive ingestion death may occur from respiratory failure within a few hours or from pulmonary edema within a day or two. If the patient survives this stage, acute tubular necrosis often develops.

Intravenous infusion of ethanol to maintain a blood level of 100 mg per 100 ml is effective in competing for alcohol dehydrogenase, thus slowing the conversion of glycol to the more toxic aldehyde. Pyridoxine (100 mg daily administered intravenously) and thiamine (1 mg daily administered intravenously) are given to stimulate conversion of glyoxalate, the immediate metabolic precursor of oxalate, to the nontoxic metabolites, glycine and α-hydroxy-β-ketoadipate, respectively. However, the effectiveness of these latter procedures has not been definitely established. Dialysis is highly effective in the removal of ethylene and diethylene glycol from the body. Acidosis and hypocalcemia must be treated vigorously.

HALOGENATED HYDROCARBONS Halogenated hydrocarbons (carbon tetrachloride, ethylene chlorohydrin, ethylene dichloride, methyl halides, trichloroethane, trichloroethylene) find wide industrial use as solvents, refrigerants, fumigants, and in chemical synthesis. They enter the home in household cleaners, floor waxes, fire extinguishers, and rubber or plastic cements. These compounds are highly fat-soluble and produce cell damage either directly or after conversion in the body to other compounds. Individual halogenated hydrocarbons differ considerably in the degree and the exact manifestations of their toxicity, but in sufficient concentration all these compounds are capable of inducing central nervous system depression and varying amounts of hepatic and renal toxicity. Myocardial depression, vascular damage, and pulmonary edema may also occur.

The most important halogenated hydrocarbon is carbon tetrachloride, which is still widely employed as a nonflammable solvent and fire extinguisher fluid but which has largely been replaced in products intended for household use by the less toxic trichloroethane. Poisoning may occur from inhalation of the vapor, ingestion, or, rarely, percutaneous absorption. An oral dose of as little as 4 ml may be fatal. Absorption from the gastrointestinal tract is slow and unpredictable but is increased by the presence of fats and alcohol. Abdominal pain, hematemesis, and hepatic damage are more common and severe after ingestion than when the poison is inhaled. Inhalation may lead to irritation of the upper part of the respiratory tract.

Acute systemic absorption of carbon tetrachloride results in nausea, dizziness, confusion, and headache within a few minutes. Depending upon the quantity absorbed, the symptoms may quickly progress to stupor, coma, convulsions, respiratory failure, hypotension, or ventricular fibrillation. The patient may recover from these immediate manifestations until evidence of hepatic or renal toxicity appears several hours to several days after the exposure. Liver and kidney damage may also occur in the absence of any severe early central nervous system effects. Initially tender hepatomegaly may be present, jaundice may be rapidly progressive, and death due to severe centrilobular necrosis may occur within days. The renal lesion has the characteristics of acute tubular necrosis, and manifests itself by proteinuria, hematuria, oliguria, or anuria. Uremia, acidosis, hypertension, and pulmonary edema may develop as complications of renal failure. Optic neuritis, pancreatitis, and adrenal cortical necrosis are less common manifestations of carbon tetrachloride intoxication.

Chronic poisoning may occur after repeated exposures to low concentrations of carbon tetrachloride and may also lead to liver or kidney damage. Usually it manifests itself by vague symptoms of fatigue, weakness, mental confusion, abdominal pain, anorexia, nausea, blurring of vision, and paresthesias.

Treatment of acute poisoning by halogenated hydrocarbons

includes vigorous effects at minimizing gastrointestinal absorption by lavage or emesis and catharsis. Treatment is otherwise symptomatic. Sympathomimetic drugs should be avoided because of the danger of inducing ventricular arrhythmias in the sensitized myocardium. Acute renal and hepatic failure must be carefully managed. Hemodialysis is often required and may be lifesaving until kidney function returns three or more weeks after poisoning. Both hemodialysis and hemoperfusion will effectively remove carbon tetrachloride and trichloroethane from the body but are potentially useful in preventing severe toxicity and death only when begun early in the postingestion period.

IODINE The traditional antiseptic iodine tincture is an alcoholic solution of 2% iodine and 2% sodium iodide. Strong iodine solution (Lugol's solution) is an aqueous solution of 5% iodine and 10% potassium iodide. The fatal dose of tincture of iodine is approximately 2 g. Iodides are very much less toxic, and no fatalities have been reported.

The diagnosis of iodine poisoning is suggested by the brown staining of the oral mucous membranes. The effects are largely due to the corrosive effects of the compound on the gastrointestinal tract. Burning abdominal pain, nausea, vomiting, and bloody diarrhea may occur soon after ingestion. If the stomach contained starch, the vomitus is blue or black. Tissue trauma from corrosive gastroenteritis and fluid loss by vomiting and diarrhea may result in shock. Severe edema of the glottis, fever, delirium, stupor, and anuria have also been observed.

Treatment consists of the immediate administration of milk, starch, bread, etc., or activated charcoal to provide a source other than human tissue with which the iodine can react. Catharsis should be induced. Sodium thiosulfate will reduce iodine to less toxic iodide; 100 ml of a 5% solution should be given orally and then an osmotic cathartic should be given. Ten milliliters of a 10% thiosulfate solution should also be given intravenously every 4 h. Induction of emesis and lavage should not be attempted if esophageal injury is suspected. With appropriate treatment most patients poisoned by iodine survive, but esophageal strictures may complicate their recovery.

IRON SALTS Ferrous or ferric salts produce gastrointestinal corrosive damage. Following mucosal damage, large amounts of iron may be absorbed, particularly in children. The fatal oral dose, calculated as elemental iron in the preparation, is about 300 mg/kg.

The potential toxic effects of iron ingestion can be divided conveniently into five phases: (1) within 30 min to 2 h there may be nausea, vomiting, abdominal pain, bloody diarrhea, lethargy, restlessness; (2) a period of apparent recovery may follow; (3) 2 to 12 h after ingestion the victim may develop shock, refractory acidosis, and fever; (4) 2 to 4 days after ingestion hepatic necrosis may occur; and (5) 2 to 4 weeks after ingestion gastrointestinal obstruction may develop—the end result of the initial corrosive effects of iron.

Treatment is initiated by emesis and lavage with a 5% sodium bicarbonate solution which will precipitate the ferrous ion. A dilution of Fleet's phosphate enema solution can also be used, but excessive lavage can cause hypernatremia, hyperphosphatemia, and hypocalcemia. When possible, at this point an abdominal roentgenogram should be obtained. If radiopaque tablets are still in the stomach, further lavage is indicated, and then an osmotic cathartic should be administered. Optimal management is aided by determination of the presence or absence of free serum iron. If free iron is present, if the total serum iron exceeds 350 meq per 100 ml, or if clinical symptoms are severe (coma, shock), the iron chelator deferoxamine methane sulfonate (Desferal) should be infused intravenously at no more than 10 (mg/kg)/h or given intramuscularly at a dose of 20 mg/kg every 4 to 6 h. The iron deferoxamine complex turns the urine pink to orange, and chelator therapy is continued until the urine loses this color. Treatment is otherwise supportive.

ISOPROPYL ALCOHOL This compound is used as a sterilizing agent or as rubbing alcohol. Ingestion produces gastric irritation and raises the danger of vomiting with aspiration. The systemic effects of isopropyl alcohol are similar to those of ethyl alcohol, but it is approximately twice as potent as the latter. Coma is readily produced but rarely lasts longer than 12 h. About 15% of an ingested dose of isopropanol is metabolized to acetone; transient acetonuria is common, but significant acidosis does not occur. Emesis should be induced, or gastric lavage should be performed. Supportive therapy is required only after ingestion of massive amounts, and there are no sequelae other than transient gastritis.

MAGNESIUM Magnesium sulfate is used intravenously as a hypotensive agent and orally as a cathartic. The magnesium ion is a profound depressant of the central nervous system and of neuromuscular transmission. Poisoning after oral or rectal administration is unlikely in the presence of normal renal function, because the kidney removes magnesium more rapidly than it is absorbed by the gastrointestinal tract. In the presence of impaired renal function an oral dose of 30 g may be fatal. Symptoms begin at a serum magnesium level of 4 meq per liter, and concentrations of over 12 meq per liter may be fatal. Oral ingestion of concentrated solutions may cause gastrointestinal irritation. Manifestations of systemic poisoning are depression of reflexes, flaccid paralysis, hypotension, hypothermia, coma, and respiratory failure. Respiratory death usually precedes significant myocardial depression. The actions of magnesium on neurological and neuromuscular function are antagonized by calcium. Treatment of magnesium poisoning therefore includes the intravenous administration of 10 ml of a 10% solution of calcium gluconate, which may be repeated as necessary.

METHYL ALCOHOL This simplest of alcohols, also called wood alcohol or methanol, is used as a solvent, antifreeze, paint remover, and as a denaturant in ethyl alcohol. Denatured ethyl alcohol preparations, such as Sterno or Solox, contain 5 to 15 percent methyl alcohol as well as other denaturants. Methyl alcohol poisoning is due almost entirely to its ingestion as a substitute for ethanol or to the drinking of denatured ethyl alcohol. The toxic dose is quite variable: death has occurred after a dose of 20 ml, but 250 ml has been ingested with survival. As little as 15 ml methanol has caused permanent blindness.

Methanol is less inebriating than ethyl alcohol, and inebriation is not a prominent symptom of methyl alcohol intoxication. Methanol is oxidized in the body by alcohol dehydrogenase first to formaldehyde and then to formic acid; these metabolites cause the toxic manifestations of methanol poisoning. The rate of its metabolism is only 15 percent that of ethanol for which alcohol dehydrogenase has a greater affinity and which can inhibit competitively the rate of metabolism of methanol. Formic acid and especially formaldehyde have toxic actions on many cells; the retina and optic nerve are specifically damaged. The toxic metabolites of methyl alcohol are also responsible for the severe acidosis, which is the most prominent feature of methyl alcohol poisoning. This acidosis is partly due to the accumulation of formic acid, but formate also appears to exert an inhibitory effect upon enzymes involved in the oxidation of carbohydrate with consequent accumulation of acid intermediates.

Symptoms of methanol poisoning usually do not appear until 12 to 24 h after ingestion, when sufficient toxic metabolites have acccumulated. Manifestations include headache, dizziness, nausea, vomiting, vasomotor disturbances, central nervous system depression, and respiratory failure. Visual disturbance is almost universal and ranges from mild blurring of vision to total blindness. Impairment of vision may be transient, but permanent blindness may follow survival of the acute intoxication. The pupils are dilated and nonreactive, and there is hyperemia of the optic disk and retinal edema. Acidosis is commonly severe (plasma carbon dioxide–combining power below 20 meq per liter).

In the treatment of methyl alcohol intoxication emesis and gastric lavage are of use only within the first 2 h after ingestion. Intravenous administration of large amounts of sodium bicarbonate combats acidosis. Return of acidosis is frequent after initial correction, and additional alkali must be administered as indicated by close observation of the patient and laboratory determinations. It is most useful to obtain a blood methanol level as soon as possible. At any time after ingestion, levels between 20 and 50 mg per 100 ml are associated with acidosis and significant symptomatology and are an indication for intravenous ethanol therapy (1 ml absolute ethanol per kilogram of body weight in 5% dextrose in water over 15 min to load, then 7 to 10 ml/h in adults to maintain the blood ethanol level at about 100 mg per 100 ml). Severely symptomatic patients should be treated even if a methanol level cannot be obtained. A methanol level exceeding 50 mg per 100 ml is indication for hemodialysis as well as ethanol therapy; dialysis is also indicated in the presence of severe acidosis with lower blood levels.

MUSHROOMS There are many species of poisonous mushrooms, but in the United States most poisoning is due to *Amanita muscaria* (fly agaric) or *Amanita phalloides* (destroying angel). More than 100 deaths result each year from consumption of wild poisonous mushrooms, 90 percent being due to *A. phalloides*. Fatalities have occurred after ingestion of only part of one mushroom.

Amanita muscaria contains the parasympathomimetic alkaloid muscarine, as well as variable amounts of a substance active on the central nervous system and a parasympatholytic alkaloid. Symptoms are largely those of parasympathetic stimulation: lacrimation, pupillary constriction, perspiration, salivation, nausea, vomiting, diarrhea, abdominal pain, bronchorrhea, wheezing, dyspnea, bradycardia, and hypotension. Muscular tremors, confusion, excitement, and delirium are common in severe poisoning. Very rarely symptoms of atropine poisoning have predominated. After ingestion of *A. muscaria* symptoms appear within minutes to 2 h. The patient may die within a few hours, but with appropriate therapy complete recovery in 24 h is the rule.

Amanita phalloides, some other *Amanita* species, and *Galerina venenata* contain heat-stable cyclopeptide cytotoxins which are rapidly bound to tissues. The principal toxin is α-amanitin which binds to and inhibits specifically the mammalian RNA polymerase responsible for messenger RNA synthesis. Severe cell damage and fatty degeneration may occur in liver, kidneys, striated muscle, and brain. Ingestion of these dangerous mushrooms is followed by a latent period of 6 to 20 h. Manifestations of cytotoxicity may then appear suddenly and consist of severe nausea, violent abdominal pain, bloody vomiting and diarrhea, and cardiovascular collapse. Headache, mental confusion, coma, or convulsions are common. Painful and tender hepatomegaly, jaundice, hypoglycemia, dehydration, and oliguria or anuria frequently appear on the first or second day after ingestion. The victim may die from acute hepatic necrosis (yellow atrophy) within 4 days. About one-half of all poisonings with *A. phalloides* have a fatal outcome in 5 to 8 days. Recovery tends to be slow.

Ingestion of other poisonous mushrooms may cause gastrointestinal symptoms, visual disturbances, ataxia, disorientation, convulsions, coma, fever, hemolysis, and methemoglobinemia.

Treatment of mushroom poisoning depends upon the species ingested. If parasympathomimetic manifestations are prominent, atropine in doses of 1 to 2 mg is given intramuscularly and repeated every 30 min until symptoms are controlled. Poisoning by cytotoxic mushrooms is treated mainly symptomatically. Fluid and electrolyte balance must be carefully maintained. Hypoglycemia should be avoided; large quantities of carbohydrate may exert some protective effect on the liver. Excitement, convulsions, pain, hypotension, and fever may need symptomatic therapy. Early intensive hemoperfusion can remove α-amanitin from the body and is probably indicated in *A. phalloides* poisoning. Both thioctic acid (α-lipoic acid) and cytochrome c have been advocated as antidotes for α-amanitin poisoning, but convincing data as to their efficacy are lacking.

NAPHTHALENE   Poisoning by this substance is almost always due to ingestion of moth repellents. An oral dose of 2 g has been fatal. Nausea, vomiting, and diarrhea are the initial symptoms. Larger doses may produce hepatic damage with jaundice and renal toxicity which may progress to hematuria, oliguria, or anuria. Depending upon the amount ingested, central nervous system manifestations may range from headache, mental confusion, and excitement to coma and convulsions. In persons with glucose 6-phosphate dehydrogenase–deficient red blood cells the ingestion of naphthalene will produce hemolysis. Treatment consists of emesis or gastric lavage, catharsis, and supportive measures.

NICOTINE   This alkaloid is an exceedingly potent and rapidly acting poison. It is a component of many insecticides. Nicotine is readily absorbed from the oral and gastrointestinal mucosa, from the respiratory tract, and through the skin. The lethal dose for an adult is approximately 50 mg, the quantity contained in two cigarettes. However, tobacco is much less toxic than would be anticipated on the basis of its nicotine content. Nicotine is poorly absorbed from ingested tobacco, and on smoking, most of the nicotine is burned. Nicotine acts on chemoreceptors, on synapses in the central nervous system and in autonomic ganglia, on the adrenal medulla, and on neuroeffector junctions. Furthermore, its transient initial stimulant effects are followed by a more persistent depressant phase of action. It is not surprising that the manifestations of nicotine poisoning are highly complex and somewhat unpredictable.

Small doses of nicotine produce nausea, vomiting, diarrhea, headache, dizziness, and neurological stimulation manifested by tachycardia, hypertension, hyperpnea, tachypnea, sweating, and salivation. Larger doses also cause cortical irritability, progressing to convulsions, and myocardial arrhythmias. Finally coma, respiratory depression and arrest, and cardiac arrest or fibrillation may supervene. Severe poisoning may cause death from respiratory failure within a few minutes.

Treatment consists of induction of emesis or gastric lavage, followed by the instillation of activated charcoal and the administration of an osmotic cathartic. Potassium permanganate will oxidize nicotine, and a 1:10,000 solution can be used for lavage. Atropine, 2 mg, and phentolamine, 5 mg, may be given intramuscularly or intravenously and repeated as often as required to control signs and symptoms of parasympathetic or sympathetic hyperactivity. These compounds are ineffective in preventing paralysis of the respiratory muscles and distur-

bances in cardiac rhythm. Careful attention must be given to artificial ventilation with oxygen and to therapy of catecholamine-induced cardiac tachyarrhythmias. Propranolol is the drug of choice for the latter purpose. Nicotine is rapidly detoxified in the liver, and recovery will be prompt if the patient can be tided over the initial period.

NITRITES   Poisoning by the nitrite ion may result from the ingestion of large amounts of drugs such as amyl nitrite or sodium nitrite. Nitrites are also used to preserve the color of meat, and amounts in excess of the allowable residue of 0.01 percent may appear in food. Ingested nitrates may be reduced to nitrite by intestinal bacteria, especially *Escherichia coli*. Except after the ingestion of very large amounts, adults usually absorb all nitrate before this reduction takes place. However, in children nitrite poisoning may result from the ingestion of nitrates or nitrate-containing well water. Fatalities have occurred from the oral ingestion of 2 to 4 g nitrites.

Acute nitrite poisoning may lead to severe headache, flushing, dizziness, hypotension, and syncope. Usually the patient need only be positioned to facilitate venous return to the heart. Pressor agents are seldom required. The most important toxic effect of the nitrite ion is its ability to oxidize hemoglobin to methemoglobin (Chaps. 53 and 315).

OXALIC ACID   This acid is found in ink eradictors and stain removers. Ingestion causes irritation and corrosion of mouth, esophagus, and stomach, followed by vomiting and abdominal pain. After absorption it precipitates serum calcium as insoluble calcium oxalate, and the resultant hypocalcemia leads to muscular tremors, tetany, convulsions, and cardiovascular collapse. Ingestion of 5 g may cause death within minutes. Following recovery from the acute episode there may be renal failure due to blockage of renal tubules by calcium oxalate crystals.

Treatment consists of precipitating oxalate in the gastrointestinal tract by giving calcium in any form orally such as milk, limewater, chalk, or calcium salts. If tissue corrosion is suspected, neither emesis nor gastric lavage is indicated. A dose of 10 ml of 10% calcium gluconate should be given intravenously and repeated as required to maintain normal serum calcium and prevent tetany. In supportive therapy the maintenance of a high urine output is essential.

PARAQUAT   Paraquat is a dipyridilium compound which is used in 5 to 20% aqueous solutions as a herbicide. An oral dose of 5 mg/kg may be fatal. Some victims die within 24 h in respiratory failure, often with refractive pulmonary edema. In others a serious toxic effect is the delayed (3 days to 2 weeks postingestion) development of progressive pulmonary fibrosis. The lungs selectively accumulate paraquat from the blood over several days until a critical concentration is reached, after which pulmonary edema and fibrosis ensue. Progressive respiratory failure is the usual cause of death. The metabolism of paraquat by lung tissue leads to the production of radical intermediates as well as the superoxide radical; the latter appears to be at least partly responsible for the toxicity of the compound.

Prolonged absorption (up to several days) of paraquat from the gastrointestinal tract is common. After gastric emptying, diluted bentonite (fuller's earth) or activated charcoal should be administered followed by an osmotic cathartic twice daily for 48 h. Forced diuresis, hemodialysis, and hemoperfusion significantly augment clearance of paraquat. Oxygen administration is associated with a higher mortality from paraquat poisoning in animals; it would seem prudent to avoid oxygen-enriched breathing mixtures in patients poisoned with paraquat if possible. Intravenous administration of superoxide dysmutase has been reported to decrease lung toxicity from paraquat in animals, but no beneficial effect has yet been demonstrated in humans.

PETROLEUM DISTILLATES Petroleum distillates (diesel oil, gasoline, kerosene, paint thinner, solvent distillate) are liquids with a boiling point between 50 and 325°C. They contain variable amounts of branched or straight-chain aliphatic and aromatic hydrocarbons. Kerosene is widely used as a fuel and as a vehicle for cleaning agents, furniture polishes, insecticides, and paint thinners. Not surprisingly, each year petroleum distillates cause about 100 accidental deaths in the United States, 90 percent of these in young children. Furthermore, these products are annually responsible for almost 20,000 hospitalizations. Ingestion of 10 ml kerosene has been fatal, but adults have recovered from as much as 250 ml. Petroleum distillates are central nervous system depressants; they damage cells by dissolving cellular lipids. Pulmonary damage manifested by pulmonary edema or pneumonitis is a common and serious complication.

Inhalation of gasoline or kerosene vapors induces a state resembling alcoholic intoxication. Headache, nausea, tinnitus, and a burning sensation in the chest may also be present. When aliphatic hydrocarbons are inhaled, these symptoms may progress to profound drowsiness or coma with absence of deep reflexes. If the distillate contains a high proportion of aromatic hydrocarbons, the coma is characterized by tremors, muscle jactitations, hyperactive reflexes, and convulsions. Death is usually due to respiratory depression, rarely to ventricular fibrillation.

The oral ingestion of petroleum distillates causes irritation of the mucous membranes of the upper part of the intestinal tract. When large amounts have been ingested, the same manifestations as after inhalation may appear. Frequently eructation or vomiting results in aspiration of petroleum distillates into the trachea. Because of their low surface tension, minute amounts of these substances may then spread widely throughout the lungs and produce pulmonary edema and pneumonitis. Pulmonary damage may also arise because of absorption of ingested petroleum distillates from the gastrointestinal tract. However, kerosene is at least one hundred times more toxic by the intratracheal route than when ingested.

In the treatment of poisoning by petroleum distillates extreme care must be used to prevent aspiration. If the patient is coughing when seen, aspiration is likely to have occurred already. When large amounts (>100 ml) have been ingested, gastric emptying is indicated. In the alert patient emesis may be induced; when vomiting occurs, the patient's head should be lower than his or her hips. Otherwise, gastric lavage should be performed but only after insertion of an endotracheal tube with an inflatable cuff. A saline cathartic may be administered. All victims of kerosene poisoning should be hospitalized for at least 24 h for observation. If signs or symptoms of pulmonary irritation appear, oxygen should be given. Steroids do not appear useful in treatment of this pulmonary lesion and may be detrimental. Prophylactic antibiotics are not indicated. Symptomatic therapy for central nervous system depression or treatment of convulsions may be necessary. Sympathomimetic amines should be avoided because of the danger of inducing ventricular fibrillation in the hydrocarbon-sensitized heart.

PHENCYCLIDINE Phencyclidine (PCP, "angel dust") has become a common and dangerous drug of abuse. It is structurally similar to ketamine hydrochloride and is used as a general anesthetic in veterinary medicine, but its powerful psychomimetic properties make it unsuitable for human use. The drug can be inhaled, smoked, swallowed, or injected; at doses as low as 1 to 5 mg euphoria, numbness, and emotional lability result. Higher doses cause disorientation, confusion, restlessness, and psychosis. Doses as high as 1 g have reportedly been taken and have resulted in prolonged comatose states, seizures, spasticity, opisthotonos, hypertension on occasion severe enough to cause intracranial hemorrhage, respiratory depression, and death.

Phencyclidine is metabolized by the liver, and the metabolites as well as some free drug are excreted in the urine. Treatment begins with emesis or lavage (even if the drug was not taken orally), charcoal instillation, and administration of an osmotic cathartic. The drug is a weak base, and its renal clearance can be increased as much as twentyfold by forced diuresis after acidification of the urine (pH<5). Oral ammonium chloride and intravenous ascorbic acid are used to achieve and maintain the urinary pH, and a diuretic is administered. In addition, a significant clearance of phencyclidine is obtained by a continuously draining nasogastric tube. Hypertension occasionally requires treatment, seizures should be controlled with diazepam, and psychosis is best treated with butyrophenones and not phenothiazines.

PHENOL Phenol and related compounds (creosote, cresols, hexachlorophene, hydroquinone, Lysol, resorcinol, tannic acid) are widely used as antiseptics, caustics, and preservatives. These substances poison all cells by denaturing and precipitating cellular proteins. The approximate fatal oral dose ranges from 2 ml for phenol and cresols to 20 ml for tannic acid.

Ingestion of phenolic compounds produces erosion of mucosa from mouth to stomach. The corroded areas may have a characteristic dead-white appearance. Hematemesis and bloody diarrhea may occur. After an initial phase of hyperpnea due to stimulation of the respiratory center, stupor, coma, convulsions, pulmonary edema, and shock are seen. The initial respiratory alkalosis is soon followed by a profound acidosis which results from the renal excretion of base during the alkalotic stage, from the acidic nature of phenol, and from disturbances in carbohydrate metabolism presumably due to defects in enzymatic function. If the patient survives the acute stage, acute tubular necrosis may lead to oliguria or anuria and hepatic toxicity to jaundice.

Poisoning by phenolic compounds may often be diagnosed by their characteristic odor. Development of a violet or blue color of the urine after addition of a few drops of ferric chloride indicates the presence of a phenolic compound.

Emesis and lavage are indicated for treatment in the absence of significant corrosive injury to the esophagus. Activated charcoal should be administered. Olive oil or castor oil, which dissolves phenol and retards its absorption, should be given, and followed with an osmotic cathartic. Supportive therapy consists of correction of the acidosis, the control of shock and convulsions, and the maintenance of a patent airway in the face of glottal edema by intubation or tracheotomy.

PHOSPHORUS Phosphorus occurs in two forms: a red, nonpoisonous form and a yellow, fat-soluble, highly toxic form. The latter is used in rodent and insect poisons and in fireworks. Yellow phosphorus and phosphides cause fatty degeneration and necrosis of tissues, particularly of the liver. The lethal ingested dose of yellow phosphorus is approximately 50 mg.

Ingestion of yellow phosphorus is followed within 1 h by burning pain in the upper part of the gastrointestinal tract, vomiting, diarrhea, and a garlic odor of the breath and excreta. The patient may die in coma during the first day or two, or symptoms may subside after a few hours. Then, 1 to 2 days later, the victim may develop tender hepatomegaly, jaundice, hypocalcemia, hypotension, and oliguria and may die following convulsions and coma. Death from acute hepatic necrosis may occur in a few days.

Treatment consists of induction of emesis or gastric lavage, instillation of activated charcoal, and administration of an osmotic cathartic. Calcium gluconate is given intravenously to maintain the serum calcium level. Treatment is otherwise supportive.

SALICYLATES Each year 30 million pounds of aspirin is consumed in the United States, and salicylates can probably be found in every American household. It is therefore not surprising that salicylates (aspirin, methyl salicylate, salicylic acid, sodium salicylate) are more commonly involved in poisonings than any other agent. Aspirin is found in almost all compound analgesic tablets. Methyl salicylate (oil of wintergreen) is present in most skin liniments, and salicylic acid is used in ointments and corn plasters. The ingestion of 10 to 30 g aspirin or sodium salicylate may be fatal to adults, but survival has been reported after an oral dose of 130 g aspirin. On the other hand 3 g salicylate in a teaspoon of methyl salicylate has been fatal in children.

Salicylate intoxication may result from the cumulative effect of therapeutic administration of high doses. There is considerable individual variation: toxic symptoms may begin at dosages of 3 g per day or may not appear when 10 g per day is given. Toxic symptoms are also poorly correlated with the serum salicylate concentration, but few patients become intoxicated at levels less than 15 mg per 100 ml and most at levels over 35 mg per 100 ml. Therapeutic salicylate intoxication is usually mild and is called "salicylism." The earliest symptoms are vertigo, tinnitus, and impairment of hearing. Further overdosage causes nausea, vomiting, sweating, diarrhea, fever, drowsiness, headache, dimness of vision, and mental aberrations. The latter may be characterized by confusion, excitement, restlessness, and talkativeness; this "salicylate jag" resembles alcoholic intoxication without the euphoria. The central nervous system effects may progress to hallucinations, convulsions, and coma. Toxic doses of salicylates also have a direct stimulant effect on the respiratory center, resulting in hyperventilation, loss of carbon dioxide, and respiratory alkalosis. Renal excretion of bicarbonate may partially compensate for this.

In acute salicylate poisoning due to accidental or suicidal ingestion of massive amounts, the same manifestations may be seen in more rapid succession. However, they are usually overshadowed by severe disturbances in the acid-base balance which follow a definite sequence. Early in the course of intoxication there may be only hyperpnea, and the seriousness of the poisoning may not be appreciated at that time. The hyperventilation causes a fall in blood P_{CO_2} and an increase in pH. Renal excretion of bicarbonate, sodium, and potassium will bring the pH back toward normal and produce a compensated respiratory alkalosis. At that point the buffering capacity of the extracellular fluid will have been significantly decreased. In young children and after large doses in adults further developments may then produce a combination of respiratory acidosis and metabolic acidosis which stems from a number of factors. High concentrations of salicylate depress the respiratory center and cause CO_2 retention. Renal function becomes impaired because of dehydration and hypotension, and inorganic, metabolic acids accumulate. Furthermore, salicylic acid derivatives may displace several milliequivalents of blood bicarbonate. Finally, salicylates impair carbohydrate metabolism and cause accumulation of acetoacetic, lactic, and pyruvic acids. Severe acidosis and disturbances in electrolyte balance are most commonly seen in febrile young children.

Blood salicylate levels are of value in the estimation of the severity of poisoning. Serious poisoning is rare at levels less than 50 mg per 100 ml but usual at levels between 50 and 100

mg per 100 ml. Levels above 100 mg per 100 ml during the first 6 h after poisoning signify severe intoxication and may be fatal. Excretion of salicylates is renal, and in the presence of normal renal function about 50 percent will be excreted in 24 h. Addition of a few drops of ferric chloride solution to 5 ml boiled acidified urine containing salicylate yields a violet color and may aid in diagnosis.

Treatment of salicylate poisoning consists of initially inducing emesis or of gastric lavage after which activated charcoal and then an osmotic cathartic are administered. Disturbances of acid-base or electrolyte balance and hypoglycemia are corrected by the intravenous administration of appropriate solutions. Respiratory depression may require artificial ventilation with oxygen. Convulsions may be treated with diazepam or phenobarbital. The renal clearance of salicylate is enhanced ten- to twentyfold if the pH of the urine can be kept between 7 and 8. In addition to intravenous bicarbonate and a diuretic it may be necessary to give potassium to prevent paradoxical aciduria to raise the urinary pH above 7. Peritoneal dialysis and hemodialysis are also highly effective in removing salicylate from seriously poisoned patients, but forced alkaline diuresis is so effective in clearing salicylate that these maneuvers are most often not required.

SMOKE Poisoning by smoke is usually due to carbon monoxide inhalation. However, burning material may also release irritant fumes. Many irritant gases combine with water to form corrosive acids or alkalies and cause chemical burns of exposed skin and of the upper part of the respiratory tract. Such gases (and the corrosives formed) are ammonia (ammonium hydroxide), nitrogen oxide (nitric acid), sulfur dioxide (sulfurous acid), and sulfur trioxide (sulfuric acid). These irritating gases as well as hydrogen sulfide may also be present in smog. Another highly toxic gas which may be inhaled by firefighters or victims is phosgene. This compound is formed by the high-temperature decomposition of chlorinated hydrocarbons and is released when carbon tetrachloride from fire extinguishers comes into contact with hot surfaces.

After inhalation of irritant gases the victim may notice burning pain in throat and chest and severe coughing. These symptoms may subside completely, but from several hours to a day after exposure dyspnea and cyanosis may appear and progress rapidly to severe pulmonary edema and death from respiratory and circulatory failure. Treatment consists of administration of oxygen and adrenal steroids and appropriate therapy of pulmonary edema, should that develop.

SULFIDES Hydrogen sulfide is a gas released by the decomposition of organic sulfur compounds and is widely used in industry. Carbon disulfide is an industrial solvent. Other sulfides have industrial uses and release hydrogen sulfide in contact with water or acids. Significant concentrations of hydrogen sulfide may be present in smoke or smog. Inhalation of hydrogen sulfide in concentrations above 50 ppm (50 times the minimum detectable by smell) causes conjunctivitis, headache, nausea, soreness of the upper respiratory passages, pulmonary edema, and drowsiness. Concentrations in excess of 300 ppm may cause coma, respiratory depression, and death. Ingestion of carbon disulfide or soluble sulfides is followed by vomiting, headache, hypotension, respiratory depression, tremors, coma, convulsions, and death. The fatal oral dose of carbon disulfide is approximately 1 g. Treatment of sulfide intoxication is supportive. Administration of sodium nitrite may promote the binding of sulfide in sulfmethemoglobin.

VOLATILE OILS The volatile or essential oils (citronella oil, eucalyptus oil, menthol, pine oil turpentine) are colorless liquids which irritate all tissues. Poisoning may result from occupational exposure (painters) and accidental or suicidal ingestion. Unfortunately, some volatile oils also have an undeserved reputation as abortifacients. Absorption occurs from skin, intestine, or lungs; the less volatile oils are more slowly absorbed. Ingestion of 15 g turpentine has been fatal.

Ingestion is rapidly followed by abdominal burning, nausea, vomiting, and diarrhea. Inhalation produces severe bronchial irritation and may be followed by delirium, coma, and convulsions. If the patient survives the acute stage of poisoning, evidence of renal damage may appear and progress to acute tubular necrosis with anuria.

Treatment is entirely supportive. When emesis is induced or gastric lavage is undertaken, aspiration must be prevented with extreme care. Hemodialysis may be required for renal failure.

REFERENCES

Acetaminophen

BARKER JD et al: Chronic excessive acetaminophen use and liver damage. Ann Intern Med 87:299, 1977

FARID NR et al: Hemodialysis in paracetamol self-poisoning. Lancet 2:396, 1972

GAZZARD BG et al: Charcoal hemoperfusion for paracetamol overdose. Br J Clin Pharmacol 1:271, 1974

LOVEJOY FJ, GOLDMAN P: Acetaminophen toxicity. J Pediatr 1979 (in press)

PETERSON RG, RUMACK BH: Toxicity of acetaminophen overdose. J Am Coll Emergency Physicians 7:202, 1978

PRESCOTT LF et al: Treatment of paracetamol poisoning with N-acetylcysteine. Lancet 2:432, 1977

Antimuscarinic compounds

GOWDY JM: Stromonium intoxication. JAMA 221:585, 1972

LEVY R: Jimson seed poisoning—a new hallucinogen on the horizon. J Am Coll Emergency Physicians 6:58, 1977

RUMACK BH: Anticholinergic poisoning: Treatment with physostigmine. Pediatrics 52:449, 1973

Barium

GOULD DB et al: Barium sulfide poisoning. Arch Intern Med 132:891, 1973

Benzene, toluene

BROWNING E: Toxic solvents: A review. Br J Ind Med 16:23, 1959

BROZOVSKY M, WINKLER EM: Glue sniffing in children and adolescents. NY State J Med 65:1984, 1965

GLASER HH, MASSENGALE ON: "Glue sniffing" in children. Deliberate inhalation of vaporized plastic cements. JAMA 181:300, 1962

HAYDEN JW: The clinical toxicology of solvent abuse. Clin Toxicol 9:169, 1976

Boric acid

VALDES-DAPENA MA, AREY JB: Boric acid poisoning. J Pediatr 61:531, 1962

WONG LC et al: Boric acid poisoning: Report of 11 cases. Can Med Assoc J 90:1018, 1964

Carbon monoxide

ANDERSON RF et al: Myocardial toxicity from carbon monoxide poisoning. Ann Intern Med 67:1172, 1967

COSBY RS, BERGERON M: Electrocardiographic changes in carbon monoxide poisoning. Am J Cardiol 11:93, 1963

MEIGS JW, HUGHES JPW: Acute carbon monoxide poisoning: An analysis of 105 cases. AMA Arch Ind Hyg 1:90, 1950

REMICK RA, MILES JE: Carbon monoxide poisoning: Neurologic and psychiatric sequelae. Can Med Assoc J 117:654, 1977

WINTER PM, MILLER JN: Carbon monoxide poisoning. JAMA 236:1502, 1976

Castor bean

BENSON S: On the mechanism of protein-synthesis inhibition by abrin and ricin. Eur J Biochem 59:573, 1975

BRUGHSCH HG: The castor bean. N Engl J Med 262:1039, 1960

Caustics

CAMPBELL GS et al: Treatment of corrosive burns of the esophagus. Arch Surg 112:495, 1977

RUMACK BH, BURLINGTON JD: Caustic ingestions: A rational look at diluents. Clin Toxicol 11(1):27, 1977

Chlorate

KNIGHT RK et al: Suicidal chlorate poisoning treated with peritoneal dialysis. Br Med J 3:601, 1967

Chlorinated insecticides

BOYLAN JJ et al: Cholestyramine: Use of a new therapeutic approach for chlordecone (Kepone) poisoning. Science 199:893, 1978

COBLE Y et al: Acute endrin poisoning. JAMA 202:489, 1967

ZAVON MR: Chlorinated hydrocarbon insecticides. JAMA 190:595, 1964

Cholinesterase inhibitor insecticides

LUZHNIKOR EA et al: Plasma perfusion through charcoal in methylparathion poisoning. Lancet 1:38, 1977

MANN JB: Diagnostic aids in organophosphate poisoning. Ann Intern Med 67:905, 1967

MILBY TH: Prevention and management of organophosphate poisoning. JAMA 216:2131, 1971

QUINBY GE: Further therapeutic experience with pralidoximes in organic phosphorus poisoning. JAMA 187:202, 1964

WYCKOFF W et al: Diagnostic and therapeutic problems of parathion poisonings. Ann Intern Med 68:875, 1968

Cyanide

BRAICO KT et al: Laetrile intoxication: Report of a fatal case. N Engl J Med 300:238, 1979

BURROWS GE et al: Effect of oxygen on cyanide intoxication. J Pharmacol Exp Ther 184:739, 1973

CHEN KK, ROSE CL: Treatment of acute cyanide poisoning. JAMA 162:1154, 1956

COPE C: The importance of oxygen in the treatment of cyanide poisoning. JAMA 175:1061, 1961

HUMBERT JR et al: Fatal cyanide poisoning: Accidental ingestion of amygdalin. JAMA 238:482, 1977

Detergents

ARENA JM: Poisonings and other health hazards associated with use of detergents. JAMA 190:56, 1964

WILSON, JT, BURR, IM: Benzalkonium chloride poisoning in infant twins. Am J Dis Child 129:1208, 1975

Fluorides

YOLKEN R et al: Acute fluoride poisoning. Pediatrics 58:90, 1976

Glycols

HAGSTAM KE et al: Ethylene glycol poisoning treated by haemodialysis. Acta Med Scand 178:599, 1965

MORIARTY RW, McDONALD RH: The spectrum of ethylene glycol poisoning. Clin Toxicol 7:583, 1974

PARRY MF, WALLACH R: Ethylene glycol poisoning. Am J Med 57:143, 1974

Halogenated hydrocarbons

BAERG RD, KIMBERG DV: Centrilobular hepatic necrosis and acute renal failure in "solvent sniffers." Ann Intern Med 73:713, 1970

OETTINGEN WF VON: *The Halogenated Hydrocarbons of Industrial and Toxicological Importance.* Amsterdam, Elsevier, 1964

RECHNAGEL RO: Carbon tetrachloride hepatotoxicity. Pharmacol Rev 19:145, 1967

SCHWARZBECK A, KOSTERS W: Extracorporeal hemoperfusion in acute carbon tetrachloride intoxication. Arch Toxicol 35:207, 1976

iron salts

FISCHER DS et al: Acute iron poisoning in children. JAMA 218:1179, 1971

JACOBS J et al: Acute iron intoxication. N Engl J Med 273:1124, 1965

LEIKIN S: Deferoxamine as a chelating agent. J Pediatr 72:148, 1968

Isopropyl alcohol

FREIREICH AW et al: Hemodialysis for isopropanol poisoning. N Engl J Med 277:699, 1967

Methyl alcohol

BENNET H JR et al: Acute methyl alcohol poisoning: A review based on experiences in an outbreak of 323 cases. Medicine 32:431, 1953

COOPER JR, KINI MM: Biochemical aspects of methanol poisoning. Biochem Pharmacol 11:405, 1962

KEYVAN-LARIJARNI H, TANNENBERG M: Methanol intoxication: Comparison of peritoneal and hemodialysis. Arch Intern Med 134:293, 1974

SMITH ME: Interrelations in ethanol and methanol metabolism. J Pharmacol 134:233, 1961

Mushrooms

LITTEN W: The most poisonous mushrooms. Sci Am 232(3):90, 1975

PAASO B, HARRISON DC: A new look at an old problem: Mushroom poisoning. Am J Med 58:505, 1975

Naphthalene

HAGGERTY RJ: Naphthalene poisoning. N Engl J Med 255:919, 1956

Nicotine

GEHLBACH SH et al: Nicotine absorption by workers harvesting green tobacco. Lancet 1:478, 1975

TAYLOR WJR et al: Pesticide poisoning in children. Drug Ther 1(11):15, 1971

Nitrites

KEATING JP et al: Infantile methemoglobinemia caused by carrot juice. N Engl J Med 288:824, 1973

Paraquat

FAIRSHTER RD, WILSON RF: Paraquat poisoning: Manifestations and therapy. Am J Med 59:751, 1975

OKONABE S, HOFMANN A: Efficacy of gut lavage, hemodialysis and hemoperfusion in the therapy of paraquat and diquat intoxication. Arch Toxikol 36:45, 1976

Petroleum distillates

BROWN J et al: Experimental kerosene pneumonia: Evaluation of some therapeutic regimens. J Pediatr 84:396, 1974

SHIRKEY H: Treatment of petroleum distillate ingestion. Mod Treat 8:580, 1971

TAUSSIG LN et al: Pulmonary function 8 to 10 years after hydrocarbon pneumonitis. Clin Pediatr 16:57, 1977

Phencyclidine

ARONOW R, DONE AK: Phencyclidine overdose: An emerging concept of managment. J Coll Emergency Physicians 7:56, 1978

COHEN S: Angel dust. JAMA 237:515, 1977

LIDEN CB et al: Phencyclidine: Nine cases of poisoning. JAMA 234:513, 1975

Phosphorus

SIMON FA, PICKERING LK: Acute yellow phosphorus poisoning. JAMA 235:1343, 1976

TALLEY RC et al: Acute elemental phosphorus poisoning in man: Cardiovascular toxicity. Am Heart J 84:139, 1972

WINEK CL et al: Yellow phosphorus ingestions: Three fatal poisonings. Clin Toxicol 6:541, 1973

Salicylates

ANDERSON RJ et al: Unrecognized adult salicylate intoxication. Ann Intern Med 85:745, 1976

BUSCHANUN N, RABINOWITZ L: Infantile salicylism: A reappraisal. J Pediatr 84:391, 1974

DONE AK: Salicylate intoxication; significance of measurements of salicylate in blood in cases of acute ingestions. Pediatrics 26:800, 1960

———: Salicylate poisoning. JAMA 192:770, 1965

———, TEMPLE AR: Treatment of salicylate poisoning. Mod Treat 8:528, 1971

HILL JB: Salicylate intoxication. N Engl J Med 288:1110, 1973

PROUDFOOT AT, BROWN SS: Acidaemia and salicylate poisoning in adults. Br Med J 2:537, 1969

SEGAR WE, HOLLIDAY MA: Physiologic abnormalities of salicylate intoxication. N Engl J Med 259:1191, 1958

225
HEAVY METALS

DAVID C. POSKANZER

Three highly effective chemicals, BAL, Versene, and penicillamine, are available for treatment of systemic poisoning with heavy metals by forming nontoxic, stable cyclic compounds with polyvalent metallic ions, thus permitting the offending material to be excreted safely in the urine.

The first to be developed was BAL (British antilewisite, 2,3-dimercaptopropanol, dimercaprol), which was originally intended as an antidote against the arsenical war gas, lewisite. Its tendency to combine with certain metallic ions such as arsenic, mercury, cobalt, nickel, antimony, and gold is so great that it can remove them from combination with the enzymes whose function they impair in the body. By itself BAL is not useful in treating lead poisoning. Because the effectiveness of BAL depends to some extent upon the speed with which its administration is begun, every attempt should be made to avoid delay in its use. For serious systemic intoxications, BAL should be given in doses of 5 mg per kilogram of body weight intramuscularly as a 10% solution in oil and 20% benzyl benzoate. No single dose should exceed 300 mg. This dose should be repeated every 4 h on the first day and every 6 h on the second day. Thereafter, it should be given three times daily for several days; doses should then be tapered and discontinued about 10 days after acute poisoning. When the dose of poison has been relatively small, the schedule of BAL administration may be reduced by one-third. Because BAL is excreted in part by the kidneys, it can accumulate to toxic concentrations in anuric patients. Overdosage results in nervousness, hyperactivity, muscle twitching, and hyperreflexia. Large doses may produce convulsions. The presence of the material in tears sometimes causes blepharospasm. In patients with anuria or oliguria, therefore, BAL should be administered with caution and at a lower dosage than outlined above. If symptoms of overdosage occur, sedatives should be administered.

The second antidote to metal poisons is the chelating agent Versene (ethylenediaminetetraacetate, EDTA), which forms cyclic, stable, soluble, nontoxic compounds with most metals.

Because Versene reacts with calcium in the same way as with other metals, it must be given as the calcium salt (Calcium Disodium Versenate, calcium disodium edetate) to avoid hypocalcemia. The material has been used with notable success in the treatment of lead poisoning. It is given in a dosage of 1.0 g in 250 ml of 5% glucose intravenously every 12 h for 5 days. After a pause to allow for further solution of metal from body stores, a second and even a third course may be given.

Penicillamine (Cuprimine, β,β-dimethylcysteine) is an excellent chelating agent for copper, mercury, and lead, promotes their excretion in the urine, and has the additional advantage of being well absorbed from the gastrointestinal tract. It may be given orally, while BAL and Versene require systemic injection. N-Acetyl-dl-penicillamine is even more effective than penicillamine in protecting against the effects of mercury, probably because it is more resistant to metabolic degradation, and it has the advantage of being less toxic. Penicillamine is administered orally in a dose of 1 to 4 g daily on an empty stomach to avoid chelation of dietary metals. It has much lower toxicity than BAL, the only other agent which is effective in the treatment of Wilson's disease (hepatolenticular degeneration), in which toxic amounts of copper are deposited in various tissues, but has the disadvantage of acute sensitivity reactions. It has also been shown to be useful in lead poisoning, but the excretion of urinary lead may not be as high after oral penicillamine as after intravenous Calcium Disodium Versenate.

N-Acetyl-dl-penicillamine, available as an investigational drug, has been demonstrated to be effective in mercury poisoning and has the advantage of allowing much higher doses with fewer toxic effects. It has less effect on copper levels than penicillamine and is, therefore, used in the treatment of mercury poisoning when one would wish to maintain copper levels. The administration of 1 to 2 g daily in divided doses for 10 days gives good results.

ANTIMONY Symptoms of poisoning after the ingestion of antimony may occur when an acid food is allowed to stand in cheap enamelware or "graniteware" for a sufficient time to allow solution of antimony, which is used in the manufacture of these products. Certain parasiticidal drugs also contain this metal. The symptoms are similar to those produced by arsenic, except that antimony causes a more rapid onset of gastrointestinal symptoms. Treatment is the same as for arsenic, including use of BAL. Circulatory collapse occurs early and requires vigorous supportive treatment.

ARSENIC Arsenic poisoning is usually the result of accidental or suicidal ingestion of insecticides or rodenticides containing paris green (copper acetoarsenate) or calcium or lead arsenate. Pesticides containing arsenic are a frequent source of poisoning in rural areas of the United States. Medications such as Fowler's solution (potassium arsenite) and the organic arsenicals (arsphenamines and arsenoxides) were once common causes of intoxication.

The toxic dose of inorganic arsenic varies considerably and seems to depend upon individual susceptibility. Orchardists have been found to ingest as much as 6.8 mg arsenic a day without any signs of intoxication. On the other hand, as little as 30 mg arsenic trioxide has been fatal. Arsenic has a predilection for keratin, and the concentration of arsenic in the hair and nails is higher than that in other tissues. Arsenic reacts with the —SH groups in certain tissue proteins and thus interferes with a number of enzyme systems essential to cellular metabolism. Pathological changes in fatal inorganic arsenical poisoning are fatty degeneration of the liver, hyperemia and hemorrhages of the intestine, and renal tubular necrosis. The peripheral nerves often show fragmentation and resorption of myelin, with disintegration of axis cylinders (*axonal neuropathy*).

The symptoms of acute poisoning by the oral route are nausea, vomiting, diarrhea, severe burning of the mouth and throat, and agonizing abdominal pains. The vomitus often contains blood. Circulatory collapse is frequent, and death may ensue within a few hours. With chronic exposure, the first signs of poisoning are usually weakness, prostration, muscular aching, or nervous system involvement; gastrointestinal symptoms are minimal. In patients exposed to arsine gas (hydrogen arsenide), the outstanding features are hemolysis, chills, fever, and hemoglobinuria.

Patients who recover from acute poisoning and those with chronic intoxication usually develop skin and mucosal changes, peripheral neuropathy, and linear pigmentations in the fingernails (see Chap. 377). The *cutaneous manifestations* appear within 1 to 4 weeks and consist of a diffuse, dry, scaly desquamation, occasionally with hyperpigmentation, over the trunk and extremities. Hyperkeratoses of the palms and soles and edema of the face and extremities may also occur. The mucous membranes also show evidence of irritation, with conjunctivitis, photophobia, pharyngitis, or irritating cough. About 5 weeks after exposure to arsenic, a transverse white stria, 1 to 2 mm in width, appears above the lunula of each fingernail (*Mees line*). Patients with more than one exposure to arsenic may show double lines several millimeters apart.

Symptoms of headache, drowsiness, confusion, and convulsions are seen in both acute and chronic intoxication. Evidence of peripheral neuropathy usually appears 1 to 3 weeks after exposure. There are numbness, tingling, and burning of the feet and hands, followed by muscular weakness. The extremities show a decrease in touch, pain, and temperature sensations, in a symmetrical "stocking-glove" distribution, and distal weakness with inability to walk or stand, weakness of grip, and wrist drop. Tendon reflexes are absent or diminished, and atrophy of the affected muscles develops rapidly.

The laboratory findings usually consist of moderate anemia and a leukopenia of 2000 to 5000 white blood cells per cubic millimeter with mild eosinophilia. There is slight proteinuria, and liver function tests show mild abnormalities. The spinal fluid is normal.

None of the clinical or laboratory manifestations of arsenic poisoning is specific, and the diagnosis depends upon analysis of the urine for arsenic. Because arsenic is found widely in nature, and hence in water and food, its discovery in hair and nails may not be diagnostic. Normal persons have an average concentration of 0.05 mg arsenic per 100 g hair. Concentrations of arsenic greater than 0.1 mg per 100 g hair are considered indicative of poisoning. The minimal level of arsenic in the urine indicating intoxication is difficult to establish. Normal persons have been found to excrete between 0.01 and 0.06 mg arsenic per liter, and a few individuals as much as 0.2 mg per liter. Although there is considerable overlap, most patients with evidence of arsenic intoxication will be found to excrete more than 0.1 mg per liter; soon after acute exposure, many will show levels greater than 1 mg per liter.

The treatment for acute ingestion is gastric lavage (see Chap. 223). Replacement of lost fluids and elevation of blood pressure by vasopressor agents is often indicated. Immediate treatment with BAL should be instituted. Patients with peripheral neuropathy rarely show significant improvement with BAL and continue to have sensory disturbances and weakness for many months. Dramatic responses, however, have been observed with the use of BAL in the treatment of exfoliative dermatitis, bone marrow depression, and encephalopathy caused by the arsphenamines and the organic arsenicals. BAL is of little value in the treatment of the hemolysis caused by inhalation of arsine.

BISMUTH Poisoning by bismuth was formerly almost entirely a complication of antisyphilitic therapy. Now it rarely complicates bismuth salts taken for intestinal disorder. Toxic manifestations may appear in the mouth (gingivitis, followed by stomatitis), the kidneys (albuminuria and nephrotic syndrome), the skin (exfoliative dermatitis), and an acute confusional psychosis, requiring immediate interruption of bismuth injections or of the ingestion. The development of a bluish stippled line of pigmentation just at the margin of the gums is not dangerous but suggests that oral hygiene should be improved. Bismuth subnitrate occasionally gives rise to methemoglobinemia (Chap. 315).

CADMIUM Poisoning is likely to occur after ingestion of an acid food prepared in a cadmium-lined vessel. The classic example is lemonade served from metal cans. Symptoms of nausea, vomiting, diarrhea, and prostration usually develop within 10 min after ingestion. Treatment is symptomatic, and symptoms ordinarily subside within 24 h. The short length of time after ingestion and the typical circumstances suggest the diagnosis. Inhalation of cadmium fumes in industry produces an acute, extremely severe pneumonitis. The use of BAL is not recommended for cadmium intoxication, as the BAL-cadmium complex dissociates in the kidneys and cadmium is nephrotoxic.

COPPER See Chap. 83 for discussion of disturbances in trace element metabolism, including copper, zinc, cobalt, nickel, silicon, and fluorine.

GOLD Because practically all cases of poisoning by gold are associated with its use in the treatment of arthritis, diagnosis is usually easy. Manifestations are skin rashes of various types, bone marrow depression, icterus, oliguria, nausea, vomiting, and gastrointestinal bleeding. Treatment consists of symptomatic relief of discomfort and the use of BAL, an effective antidote.

LEAD Poisoning results from inhalation of fumes as from burning storage batteries, from solder, paint spraying, or processes requiring the remelting of metallic lead. Ingestion of lead-containing materials such as paint, or water which has stood in lead pipes, is less important in adults. Illicit whiskey contaminated by lead solder in the pipes of stills has been responsible for cases of poisoning. Bullets or buckshot containing lead can cause poisoning years after becoming embedded in a serous cavity. The most common form of lead poisoning today is that encountered in children who ingest lead-containing outdoor paint, often used indoors in older houses. It has a sweetish, apparently attractive taste. Absorption is slow by any route, and prolonged exposure is required for the development of symptoms. Lead is a cumulative poison, excreted slowly. Acute poisoning is virtually nonexistent. Symptoms may develop suddenly after chronic exposure. Most of the absorbed lead is deposited in the bones; blood, urine, and feces contain only small amounts.

Manifestations of poisoning are colic, encephalopathy, peripheral neuritis, and anemia.

Lead colic, or painter's cramps, is characterized by agonizing, wandering, poorly localized abdominal pain, often with spasm and rigidity of the musculature of the abdominal wall.

There is no fever or leukocytosis. Needless surgery has been carried out in these patients for supposed perforation of peptic ulcer or other catastrophe. Morphine has surprisingly little effect upon the pain; intravenous injection of calcium salts affords relief within a short time, although pain may recur. Attacks of colic seem to be brought on by intercurrent infection or alcoholic overindulgence.

Encephalopathy occurs chiefly in children and is manifested by convulsions, somnolence, mania, confusion, or coma. The mortality rate is high when convulsive seizures and coma occur. In an unexplained acute encephalopathy of childhood, increased intracranial pressure associated with high protein and the absence of cells should suggest the possibility of lead poisoning.

Peripheral neuritis with paralysis, characteristically involving the muscles most used (e.g., wrist drop in painters, etc.), occurs in patients exposed to lead, often in the absence of other symptoms. It is rare in children. (See Chap. 375.)

Mild anemia, probably the result of increased brittleness of the erythrocytes as well as a defect in cell maturation, is common. Pallor is out of proportion to anemia in patients with chronic plumbism and is attributed to spasm of small vessels in the skin. Anemia is almost never severe and is characterized by the presence of large numbers of erythrocytes with basophilic stippling. This is seen in other hematologic disorders, but a smear showing stippling should arouse suspicion of lead poisoning. In patients with poor oral hygiene a "lead line" of black lead sulfide may develop along the gingival margins. This is not seen in edentulous persons and is rare in children.

Patients with lead poisoning excrete increased amounts of coproporphyrin III in the urine (see Chap. 96). This is so consistent that examination of a urine specimen for porphyrin is the best screening test in suspected cases. A few milliliters of urine should be acidified with acetic acid and shaken with an equal volume of ether. Exposure of a specimen prepared in this manner under a Wood's lamp will reveal reddish fluorescence of the ether layer if coproporphyrin is present. A positive test result is strongly in favor of lead intoxication. Urinary lead determinations are of aid in confirming the diagnosis; a level of 0.2 mg per liter or more is usually regarded as significant, although interpretations vary. Diagnosis can be confirmed by promoting lead excretion with three doses of Calcium Disodium Versenate (25 mg/kg) at 8-h intervals. Excretion of over 500 μg in 24 h is indicative of excessive lead burden. A single blood lead level is rarely of help in diagnosis in adults because blood is cleared promptly of circulating lead.

Lead encephalopathy occurs chiefly in children, has a significant mortality rate, and causes severe permanent brain damage in 25 percent of survivors. Encephalopathy in adults is rare and usually results from consumption of lead-contaminated illicit liquor. Once minor symptoms of poisoning are present, acute encephalopathy can develop with unpredictable rapidity. Any child with symptoms suggestive of lead poisoning should be considered to have a medical emergency and should be hospitalized immediately. The onset of encephalopathy is signaled by the development of gross ataxia, persistent vomiting, and intermittent lethargy and stupor. These symptoms are followed by convulsions, hyperactivity, and coma.

The most important single feature of treatment is removal of the patient from further exposure to lead. Once abnormal absorption is terminated, virtually all the lead in the body is shifted into bone. Chelating agents do not remove significant quantities of lead from bone. It takes approximately twice as long to excrete a given burden of lead as it does to accumulate it. As long as significant quantities of lead remain in bone, any intercurrent illness which causes demineralization can cause mobilization of toxic quantities of lead into soft tissues and exacerbate plumbism.

The treatment of lead encephalopathy is begun once adequate urine flow is established. A combination of BAL and Calcium Disodium Versenate is employed, and the Versene therapy continued for 5 to 7 days. If Calcium Disodium Versenate is given alone in the presence of very high tissue concentrations of lead, some of the toxic effects may be intensified. Acute symptoms usually subside within 48 to 72 h after Versene is begun. Within 2 weeks urinary excretion of coproporphyrin ceases, and there is sometimes a dramatic improvement in neuritis.

Symptoms of acute increased intracranial pressure are best treated with repeated doses of mannitol given intravenously. High-potency corticosteroids are also useful in relieving cerebral edema in patients with lead encephalopathy.

The problem of lead poisoning in children is so significant that many health departments are carrying out extensive programs for removal of lead-containing paints in old low-income housing areas.

In adults combined therapy with BAL and Calcium Disodium Versenate followed by oral penicillamine is probably indicated whenever blood levels exceed 100 mg lead per 100 g blood, even in the absence of symptoms. Evidence of lead toxicity is usually present at this level, and the risk of symptomatic episodes is considerable. The use of oral penicillamine alone in a dose of 1 to 1.5 g daily for 3 to 5 days in mildly symptomatic cases has been suggested and has the advantage of easy administration and the avoidance of painful injections.

MERCURY Poisoning occurs chiefly as a result of the acute ingestion of a soluble salt, usually mercuric chloride (bichloride of mercury). Toxic symptoms may occur with 0.1 g, and 0.5 g is almost always fatal unless immediate treatment is instituted. The mercuric ion is corrosive and produces severe local inflammation. Oral, pharyngeal, and laryngeal pain are severe; abdominal cramps with nausea and vomiting occur within 15 min. As mercury is absorbed, it is concentrated in the kidneys, where it poisons the tubular cells, producing a tendency to diuresis within the first 2 to 3 h. The combination of vomiting, dehydration, shock, and progressive tubular damage, however, soon leads to anuria and uremia. The poison is also excreted into the colon and produces severe enteritis, with bloody diarrhea and tenesmus. Death is usually from uremia. The chief objectives of treatment are to prevent the shock of dehydration and to remove mercury from the body. Early in treatment, copious quantities of fluid should be infused intravenously to prevent dehydration and to reduce the concentration of mercuric ion in the renal tubules. That the patient is anuric early is often simply the result of dehydration and shock. In such instances, forcing fluids is advisable. However, the gradual development of oliguria and anuria in a hydrated patient indicates renal damage by mercury, and at this stage a regimen for acute renal shutdown should be instituted (Chap. 275).

Chronic poisoning from metallic mercury vapor occurs in persons exposed to large amounts of the metal in laboratories or in industry and occasionally as a result of prolonged therapeutic use, as in vaginal douches. Manifestations may be those of subacute poisoning, with salivation, stomatitis, and diarrhea or primary neurological signs, including tremors of the extremities, tongue, and lips, ataxia and dysarthria, erethism, a state of easy embarrassment, irritability, apprehension, withdrawal, and depression.

Methylmercuric salts were discovered to have a special effect, mainly on the nervous system. First it was observed that workers exposed in the manufacture of an insecticide containing this compound developed an acute cerebellar ataxia. Later in Minimata, Japan, an effluent from a factory was noted to cause cerebellar ataxia and cortical blindness. In some cases there was involvement of peripheral nerves and impairment of neuromuscular transmission (Rustam et al.). The damage to the central nervous system usually is permanent. Public health measures have been taken to eliminate such compounds from the environment.

Some poison can be removed from the body by gastric lavage, but more important in treatment is the binding of the mercuric ion in a harmless compound by BAL. The therapeutic usefulness of BAL depends on its immediate administration. In chronic mercury poisoning, *N*-acetyl-*dl*-penicillamine may well be the drug of choice. It can be administered orally and appears to chelate mercury selectively, with considerably less effect on copper, which is essential to many metabolic processes.

SILVER Most poisoning by silver involves silver nitrate, a caustic salt. There are intense nausea, vomiting, and diarrhea after swallowing nitrate (lunar caustic), and death from shock may occur within a few hours. The mouth is usually deeply stained by silver nitrate. Treatment is entirely supportive, with fluid replacement and control of pain.

Chronic exposure (usually to nose drops) produces a peculiar bluish skin discoloration (argyria).

THALLIUM Thallium is a component of certain rodenticides and depilatories, and clinical poisoning is usually a result of accidental ingestion of these materials. The fatal dose is approximately 1.0 g. Manifestations are vomiting, diarrhea, and leg pains, followed by a severe and sometimes fatal sensorimotor polyneuropathy. About 3 weeks after poisoning, the patient's hair falls out, providing a strong diagnostic clue if the cause has not previously been determined. Treatment is symptomatic. The alopecia is temporary if the patient recovers.

REFERENCES

Arena JM: Treatment of mercury poisoning. Mod Treat 4:734, 1967

Aub JC et al: Lead poisoning. Medicine 4:1, 1925

Bank WJ et al: Thallium poisoning. Arch Neurol 26:456, 1974

Chisholm JJ Jr: Poisoning due to heavy metals. Pediatr Clin North Am 17:591, 1970

Doolan PD et al: Acute renal insufficiency due to dichloride of mercury: Observations of gastrointestinal hemorrhage and BAL therapy. N Engl J Med 249:273, 1953

Hamilton A, Hardy HL: *Industrial Toxicology,* 3d ed. Acton, Publishing Sciences Group, 1974

Heyman A: Systemic manifestations of bismuth toxicity: Observations on 4 patients with pre-existent kidney disease. Am J Syph Gonorrhea Vener Dis 28:721, 1944

Jenkins RB: Inorganic arsenic and the nervous system. Brain 89:479, 1966

Kark RAP et al: Mercury poisoning and its treatment with *N*-acetyl-*d,l*-penicillamine. N Engl J Med 285:10, 1971

Kendrey G, Roe FJC: Cadmium toxicology. Lancet 1:1206, 1969

Keusler CJ et al: Arsine poisoning, mode of action and treatment. J Pharmacol Exp Ther 88:99, 1946

Levine WG: Heavy-metal antagonists, in *The Pharmacological Basis of Therapeutics,* 5th ed, LS Goodman, A Gilman (eds). New York, Macmillan, 1975, p 912

Longcope WT, Luetscher JA: The use of BAL (British antilewisite) in the treatment of the injurious effects of arsenic, mercury, and other metallic poisons. Ann Intern Med 31:545, 1949

Rustam H et al: Evidence for neuromuscular disorder in methyl mercury poisoning. Arch Environ Health 30:190, 1975

226
ALCOHOL

MAURICE VICTOR
RAYMOND D. ADAMS

Intemperance in the use of alcohol creates many problems in modern society, the importance of which can be judged by the repeated emphasis they receive in contemporary writings, both literary and scientific. These problems may be divided into three categories—psychological, medical, and sociologic. The main psychological problem is why individuals drink excessively, often with full knowledge that such action will result in physical injury to themselves and irreparable harm to their families. The medical problem embraces all aspects of the diseases which result from the abuse of alcohol. The sociologic problem comprises the effects of sustained inebriety on the family and community.

The various problems raised by excessive drinking cannot be separated from one another, and physicians must, therefore, be conversant with all parts of the subject. They may be asked to help patients conquer their alcoholic tendencies or to diagnose and to treat the numerous diseases to which they are subject; often they must admit or commit patients to a general or mental hospital, according to the nature of the presenting clinical disorder; and lastly, they may be required to enlist the aid of available social agencies when such services are needed by either patients or their families.

Alcoholism has been defined as both a chronic disease and a disorder of behavior, characterized in either context by drinking of alcohol to an extent that surpasses the social drinking customs of the community and that interferes with the drinker's health, interpersonal relations, or means of earning a livelihood. Reduced to pharmacologic terms, it is addiction to alcohol. Alcoholics are individuals who satisfy these medical, social, and pharmacologic criteria. The precise number of such persons in the United States is not known. In 1971, the Department of Health, Education, and Welfare estimated that about 9 million men and women (7 percent of the adult population) "manifested the behavior of alcohol abuse and alcoholism." It requires little projection of the imagination to conceive of the havoc wrought by alcohol in terms of decreased productivity, accidents, crime, mental and physical disease, and disruption of family life.

PHARMACOLOGY AND METABOLIC EFFECTS OF ALCOHOL

Ethyl alcohol, or ethanol, is the active ingredient in beer, wine, whiskey, gin, brandy, and other less common alcoholic beverages. In addition, the stronger spirits contain enanthic ethers, which give the flavor but have no important pharmacologic properties, and small amounts of impurities such as amyl alcohol and acetaldehyde, which act like alcohol but are more toxic. Contrary to prevailing opinion, the content of B vitamins in American beer and other liquors is so low as to have little nutritional value.

Alcohol is absorbed unaltered from both the stomach and the small intestine. Its presence may be detected in the blood within 5 min after ingestion, and the maximum concentration is reached in 30 to 90 min. The ingestion of milk and fatty foods impedes the absorption of alcohol, and water facilitates it. The rate of absorption increases after Billroth I and II gastrectomies, and in these individuals maximum blood alcohol concentrations are higher and attained faster than in subjects with intact stomachs.

After entering the bloodstream, alcohol enters the various organs of the body, as well as the spinal fluid, urine, and pulmonary alveolar air, in concentrations which bear a constant relationship to that in the blood. It is eliminated chiefly by oxidation to carbon dioxide, less than 10 percent being excreted chemically unchanged in the urine, sweat, and breath. The energy liberated by the oxidation of alcohol is equivalent to 7 kcal/g.

Alcohol is metabolized primarily in the liver, via the cytoplasmic enzyme alcohol dehydrogenase, to acetaldehyde. It can also be oxidized by catalase and a microsomal oxidase, but the physiological and quantitative roles of these pathways are not entirely clear. Acetaldehyde is converted by acetaldehyde dehydrogenase of liver mitochondria to acetylcoenzyme A and acetate, and the latter are metabolized further through well-established normal pathways to yield carbon dioxide and water.

For all practical purposes it may be accepted that once absorption is ended and an equilibrium established with the tissues, ethyl alcohol is oxidized at a constant rate, independent of its concentration in the blood (about 150 mg alcohol per kilogram of body weight per hour, or about 1 oz 90-proof whiskey or 10 to 12 oz beer per hour). Actually, more alcohol is burned per hour when the initial concentrations are very high, but this increment is of little clinical significance. On the other hand, the rate of oxidation of acetaldehyde does depend on its concentration in the tissues. This fact is of importance in connection with the drug disulfiram (Antabuse), which raises the tissue concentration necessary for the metabolism of a certain amount of acetaldehyde per unit of time. Patients taking both Antabuse and alcohol will accumulate an inordinate amount of acetaldehyde, resulting in nausea, vomiting, and hypotension, sometimes pronounced and even fatal in degree. This pharmacologic principle underlies the treatment of alcoholism with Antabuse.

Only a few factors are capable of increasing the rate of alcohol metabolism. It seems well established that chronic alcoholics metabolize alcohol somewhat faster than normal individuals. Amino acids (especially alanine), insulin, and fructose also enhance ethanol metabolism, but the clinical usefulness of these agents in speeding the oxidation of alcohol is limited. Alcohol also reduces the intestinal absorption of nutrients such as glucose, amino acids, calcium, folate and vitamin B_{12}. This impairment of absorption may contribute to the malnutrition frequently found in alcoholic subjects. On the other hand starvation slows the rate of alcohol metabolism in the liver.

Alcohol has a number of other metabolic effects. In the area of *lipid metabolism* it can cause hypertriglyceridemia as well as lead to a fatty liver. It interferes with *carbohydrate metabolism* and can produce hypoglycemia by impairing gluconeogenesis; however, a significant degree of hypoglycemia will occur only if hepatic glycogen stores are depleted. Under certain conditions alcohol can also interfere with the peripheral utilization of glucose and produce hyperglycemia. When ethanol is oxidized, there is a simultaneous generation of reduced nicotinamide adenine dinucleotide (NAD); as a result pyruvate is converted to lactate. Thus alcoholism may result in increased levels of serum lactate, occasionally *lactic acidosis,* and also *hyperuricemia,* which is secondary to the inhibitory action of lactic acid on the renal excretion of uric acid.

Other renal effects of alcohol ingestion are an increased urinary excretion of *phosphate and magnesium,* resulting in low serum levels of these ions, and an *increased urinary excretion of ammonium.* In addition to lactic acidosis, alcoholics may have other types of metabolic and respiratory acidosis. The metabolic acidosis is presumably due to an accumulation of acid metabolites, especially β-hydroxybutyrate. The respiratory acidosis is attributed to a direct action of alcohol on the respiratory center.

There are also well-recognized effects of alcohol on water excretion; thus the ingestion of 4 oz 100-proof bourbon whiskey may result in a diuresis comparable with that which follows the drinking of large amounts of water. This diuresis is most likely due to the transient suppression of the release of antidiuretic hormone (ADH) from the supraopticohypophyseal system, since a relatively small amount of alcohol injected directly into a carotid artery evokes a prompt diuresis without a detectable rise in the concentration of alcohol in the systemic blood. Alcohol does not alter the sensitivity of the kidney tubules to endogenous or exogenous ADH (pitressin) and has no discernible effect on renal hemodynamic function in normal persons. The degree of diuresis seems to be more closely related to the duration of the rising blood alcohol level than to the rate of increase or the absolute level attained if the period of alcohol intoxication is sustained. Diuresis occurs only during the initial phase of alcohol administration and does not persist during prolonged drinking.

Alcohol also appears to inhibit the hypothalamic and neurohypophyseal release of vasopressin and oxytocin. It has been demonstrated that the administration of alcohol to normal young men for periods up to 4 weeks decreased the rate of production and the plasma concentration of testosterone. These abnormalities in testosterone metabolism were traced to both a central (hypothalamus-pituitary) and gonadal effect of alcohol and were independent of nutritional deficiency and liver disease.

Alcohol has a direct effect on the excitability and contractility of heart muscle. With intoxicating doses there is a rise in cardiac rate and output and in systolic and pulse pressures, and a cutaneous vasodilatation at the expense of splanchnic constriction. Some authors have stated that prolonged intoxication may have a damaging effect on cardiac and skeletal muscle, a degeneration of fibers supposedly due to suppression of myophosphorylase activity. Increased sweating and vasodilatation cause a loss of body heat and a fall in body temperature.

In low concentrations, by whatever route it is administered, alcohol stimulates the parietal cells of the stomach mucosa to produce acid, apparently by antral activation of gastrin release, and possibly by causing the tissues to form or release histamine. With the ingestion of alcohol in concentrations of over 10 to 15 percent, the secretion of mucus is increased, the stomach mucosa becomes congested and hyperemic, and the secretion of acid may then become depressed. This is a state of acute gastritis, from which recovery may be relatively rapid. The increase in appetite following ingestion of alcohol is due to the stimulation of the end organs of taste and to a general sense of well-being. Similarly, the reviving effect of alcohol in fatigue states is a cerebral one, not due to a direct stimulating effect on muscle or other organs.

PSYCHOLOGICAL (BEHAVIORAL) EFFECTS OF ALCOHOL AND THE PHENOMENON OF TOLERANCE The most obvious actions of acute, nonlethal doses of alcohol are those exerted on the nervous system, constituting the characteristic symptoms and signs of alcohol intoxication. It is now accepted that alcohol is not a stimulant of the central nervous system but a depressant. Some of the early effects of alcohol, manifested by garrulousness, aggressiveness, excessive activity, and increased electrical excitability of the cerebral cortex, all of which suggest stimulation, are due probably to the inhibition of certain subcortical structures (probably the high brainstem reticular formation) which ordinarily modulate cerebral cortical activity. Similarly, the initial hyperactivity of tendon reflexes may represent a transitory escape of spinal motor neurons from higher inhibitory centers. With increasing amounts of al-

cohol, however, the depressant action spreads to involve the cerebral cortical neurons as well as other brainstem and spinal neurons.

The behavioral effects of acute ingestion of alcohol (1 to 6 ozs) in the nonaddicted person have been the subject of many studies. They have shown that all manner of motor performance, whether the simple maintenance of a standing posture, the control of speech and eye movements, or highly organized and complex motor skills, is adversely affected by alcohol. The movements involved in these acts are not only made slower than normal but also more inaccurate and random in character and therefore less adapted to the accomplishment of specific ends.

Alcohol also impairs the efficiency of mental function by interfering with the learning process, which is slowed and rendered less effective. The facility of forming associations, whether of words or of figures, tends to be hampered, and the power of attention and concentration is reduced. The person is not as versatile as usual in directing thought along new lines appropriate to the problems at hand. Finally, alcohol impairs the faculties of judgment and discrimination and, all in all, the ability to think and reason clearly.

A scale relating the various degrees of clinical intoxication to the blood alcohol levels in nonhabituated persons has been constructed. At blood alcohol levels of 30 mg per 100 ml, a mild euphoria is detectable, and at 50 mg per 100 ml, a mild incoordination. At 100 mg per 100 ml, ataxia is obvious; at 200 mg per 100 ml, the patient is drowsy and confused; at 300 mg per 100 ml, the patient is stuporous; and a level of 400 mg per 100 ml is accompanied by deep anesthesia and may prove fatal. These figures are valid provided that the alcohol content rises steadily over a 2-h period.

It should be emphasized that such a scale has little or no value in the chronic alcoholic patient since it does not take into account the adaptive changes that the organism makes to alcohol, which are an increased rate of alcohol metabolism by the liver and particularly the development of tolerance. These phenomena account for the large amounts of alcohol that can be consumed by the chronic drinker without significant signs of drunkenness. In the chronic alcoholic the ingestion of a given amount of alcohol will result in a lower blood alcohol level than in a nonalcoholic individual; furthermore, for a given blood alcohol level one will observe lesser degrees of "drunkenness" or inebriation. The organism is capable of adapting to alcohol after a very short exposure. If the alcohol concentration in the blood is raised very slowly, no symptoms may appear, even at quite high levels. It would seem that the important factor in this rapid adaptability is not so much the rate of increment or the height of the blood alcohol level, but the length of time the alcohol had been present in the body. It has also been shown that if the dosage of alcohol which causes blood levels to reach a certain height is held constant, the blood alcohol concentration falls and clinical evidence of intoxication disappears. The cause of this fall in alcohol concentration is not clear. It appears that ethanol has an important effect upon the neuronal membrane, but the nature of this effect or how it contributes to central nervous system (CNS) depression or to the development of tolerance is still an enigma. Removal of alcohol from the habituated CNS results in another disturbance in neuronal function, presumably an overactivity.

CLINICAL EFFECTS OF ALCOHOLISM The possible damaging effects of chronic alcohol ingestion on cardiac and skeletal muscle have already been mentioned. These are considered further on and in Chaps. 247 and 383.

That alcoholics are often anemic and thrombocytopenic is common clinical experience. Until recently these abnormalities were attributed to the malnutrition, infection, and liver disease that complicate severe alcoholism, but increasingly it has become apparent that the chronic ingestion of alcohol has a direct damaging effect upon cells of the bone marrow.

The most frequent and important clinical effects of alcoholism are on the digestive organs and on the nervous system.

Effect on digestive organs Symptoms of disordered gastrointestinal function are particularly common in alcoholics; of these the most distinctive are *morning nausea and vomiting.* Characteristically, patients can suppress these symptoms by taking a drink or two, after which they are able to consume large quantities of alcohol without their recurrence until the following morning. Since sufficient alcohol actually relieves these symptoms, they are probably not due to the local effects of alcohol on the stomach, but have a "central" origin and represent the mildest manifestations of the withdrawal syndrome (see below).

Other complaints referable to the gastrointestinal system are abdominal distention, epigastric distress, belching, typical or atypical ulcer symptoms, and hematemesis. The most common pathological basis for these symptoms is a superficial *gastritis,* which is an almost invariable sequel to prolonged drinking. Most instances of gastritis are benign, and the symptoms subside after a few days of abstinence, but more severe forms are associated with mucosal erosions or ulcerations and may be the source of serious bleeding. The incidence of *peptic ulcer* is exceptionally high in alcoholics. A serious cause of hematemesis is the *Mallory-Weiss syndrome,* which is characterized by lacerations of the mucosa at or just below the gastroesophageal junction. In many of these cases bleeding is preceded by an episode of forceful vomiting or protracted retching. The typical lesions appear to depend upon raising the intragastric pressure to 100 to 150 mmHg, i.e., to the range of pressure attained by normal subjects during a period of induced straining and retching.

Patients admitted to the hospital following a period of prolonged drinking and severe dietary depletion almost invariably show enlargement of the liver because of infiltration of the parenchymal cells with fat (see Chap. 299). This fatty liver is essentially reversible provided that patients remain abstinent and receive a nutritious diet. A form of hepatocellular necrosis or *alcoholic hepatitis* is observed frequently in chronic alcoholics, especially following a severe drinking bout. About 8 percent of patients with severe alcoholism develop a permanent form of liver disease, i.e., *cirrhosis,* in which a diffuse proliferation of fibrous tissue replaces the normal lobular architecture of the organ. The alcoholic forms of liver disease are discussed in Chap. 304.

The excessive use of alcohol is also a significant factor in the causation of pancreatitis. The mildest form of this disorder may be attributed to gastritis or may go unnoticed, unless discovered by elevations of the serum amylase level. In more severe form pancreatitis presents as an acute abdominal catastrophe, i.e., with epigastric pain, vomiting, and rigidity of the upper abdominal muscles. In these circumstances the pancreas appears tense and edematous, often with a serosanguineous exudation of fluid on its surface. The most severe form is that of hemorrhagic pancreatitis (Chap. 309). Alcoholics may also develop a chronic relapsing form of pancreatitis. This type is often associated with irregular calcification of the pancreas. Steatorrhea is a not infrequent complication and is probably related to abnormalities of pancreatic exocrine function, malnutrition, and interference with intestinal absorption of fat.

[The *management* of the various gastrointestinal complications of alcoholism is considered in the section dealing with these diseases (Chaps. 287 and 291).]

Effect on nervous system A large number of neurological disorders are associated with alcoholism. The factor common to all of them is the abuse of alcohol, but the mechanism by which alcohol produces its effects varies from one group of disorders to another, a feature which serves as the basis for the following classification. For the most part, this classification is based on known mechanisms.

I Alcoholic intoxication—drunkenness, coma, excitement ("pathological intoxication," "blackouts")
II Abstinence or withdrawal syndrome—tremulousness, hallucinosis, "rum fits," delirium tremens
III Nutritional diseases of the nervous system secondary to alcoholism
  A Wernicke-Korsakoff syndrome
  B Polyneuropathy
  C Optic neuropathy ("tobacco-alcohol amblyopia")
  D Pellagra
IV Diseases of uncertain pathogenesis, associated with alcoholism
  A Cerebellar degeneration
  B Marchiafava-Bignami disease
  C Central pontine myelinolysis
  D Cerebral atrophy
  E "Alcoholic" cardiomyopathy and myopathy
  F Fetal alcohol syndrome
V Neurological disorders consequent upon Laennec's cirrhosis and portosystemic shunts
  A Hepatic stupor and coma
  B Chronic hepatocerebral degeneration

ALCOHOLIC INTOXICATION Drunkenness is such a common phenomenon that its clinical features require little elaboration. The signs consist of varying degrees of exhilaration and excitement, loss of restraint, irregularity of behavior, loquacity, slurred speech, incoordination of movement and gait, irritability, drowsiness, and, in advanced cases, stupor and coma. On rare occasions acute intoxication is characterized by an outburst of irrational, combative, and destructive behavior, which terminates when patients fall into a deep stupor and for which they may later have no memory. This state has been referred to as "pathological intoxication" or "acute alcoholic paranoid state." Allegedly this reaction may follow the ingestion of relatively small amounts of alcohol, and it has been variously ascribed to constitutional differences in susceptibility to alcohol, previous cerebral injury, and "an underlying epileptic predisposition." However, there are no critical data to support any of these contentions. An analogy may be drawn between this state of alcoholic excitement and a similar reaction which occasionally complicates the administration of barbiturates.

"Blackouts," in the language of alcoholics, refer to transient episodes of amnesia which accompany heavy intoxication. After patients become sober, they cannot recall events that had occurred over a period of several hours, even though the state of consciousness (as observed by others) was not importantly altered during this period. The significance of these episodes is not clear; they do not necessarily indicate progression of alcoholic addiction, as is generally assumed.

Alcohol acts on nerve cells in a manner akin to the general anesthetics. Unlike the latter, however, the margin between the dose of alcohol that produces surgical anesthesia and that which dangerously depresses respiration is a very narrow one, a fact which accounts for the occasional fatality in cases of alcoholic narcosis.

The signs of alcohol intoxication are distinctive, and most forms present no problem in diagnosis or management. On the other hand, coma due to alcohol may present difficulties in differential diagnosis. It should be stressed that the diagnosis of alcoholic coma is made not merely on the basis of a flushed face, stupor, and the odor of alcohol, but only after the careful exclusion of all other causes of coma (see Chap. 20).

Treatment of alcoholic intoxication Mild to moderate degrees of intoxication require no special treatment. Certain time-honored remedies such as a cold shower, strong coffee, forced activity, or induction of vomiting may be helpful, but there is no evidence that any of these methods influences the rate of disappearance of alcohol from the blood. *Alcoholic stupor* is also a short, self-limited state, and if the vital signs are normal no special therapeutic measures are necessary. *Pathological intoxication* may require the use of restraints and the parenteral administration of phenobarbital sodium (200 mg subcutaneously) or amobarbital sodium (500 mg intramuscularly), repeated once in 30 to 40 min if necessary.

Coma due to alcoholic intoxication is a medical emergency. The main object of treatment is to prevent respiratory suppression and the complications which it engenders. The management of the comatose patient is described in Chap. 20. One should like to be able to lower the blood alcohol level as rapidly as possible. The administration of insulin and glucose or fructose for this purpose is of little practical value. Analeptic drugs such as amphetamine, pentylenetetrazole (Metrazol), and various mixtures of caffeine and picrotoxin are antagonistic to alcohol only insofar as they are powerful cerebral cortical stimulants and overall nervous system excitants; they do not hasten the combustion of alcohol.

ABSTINENCE OR WITHDRAWAL SYNDROME A second category of alcoholic neurological disease comprises the tremulous, hallucinatory, epileptic, and delirious states. Although a sustained period of chronic intoxication is the underlying factor in each of these disorders, the symptoms become manifest only *after a period of relative or absolute abstinence* from alcohol—hence the designation *abstinence* or *withdrawal syndrome.* Each of the major manifestations of the withdrawal syndrome may occur distinct from the others and will be so described; more frequently, however, they occur in various combinations. The prototype of the patients afflicted with these symptoms is the spree or periodic drinker, although the steady drinker is not immune if, for some reason, he or she stops drinking.

Tremulousness By far the most common manifestation of the abstinence syndrome is a state of tremulousness, commonly referred to as "the shakes" or "the jitters," combined with general irritability and gastrointestinal symptoms, particularly nausea and vomiting. The symptoms first show themselves after several days of drinking, usually in the morning, after the short period of abstinence that occurs during sleep. Patients then need to "quiet their nerves" with a few drinks. Indeed the symptoms are relieved by alcohol, only to return on successive mornings with increasing severity. The usual spree lasts about 2 weeks, but the duration varies greatly. It is terminated not only because of recurrent tremor and vomiting, but for one or more other reasons such as lack of funds, weakness, self-disgust, injury, illness, or collapse. The symptoms then become greatly augmented, reaching their peak intensity 24 to 36 h after the complete cessation of drinking.

At this stage, patients present a distinctive clinical picture. They are alert and startle easily. Their faces are deeply flushed, the conjunctivas are injected, and there is usually tachycardia, anorexia, nausea, and retching. They may complain of insomnia and crave rest and sleep. Preoccupied with their misery, they are inattentive and disinclined to answer questions, and may respond in a rude or perfunctory manner. Patients may be mildly disoriented in time and have a poor memory for events of the last few days of the drinking spree but show no serious confusion, being generally aware of their surroundings and the nature of their illness.

Generalized tremor is an outstanding feature of this illness. It is of fast frequency (6 to 8 oscillations per second), slightly irregular, and variable in its severity, tending to diminish when patients are in quiet surroundings and to increase with motor activity or emotional stress. The tremors may be so violent that patients cannot stand without help, speak clearly, or feed themselves. Sometimes there is little objective evidence of tremor, and patients complain only of being "shaky inside."

Although the flushed facies, anorexia, tachycardia, and tremor subside to a large extent within a few days, patients do not regain their full composure for a much longer time. The overalertness, tendency to startle easily, and jerkiness of movement may persist for a week or longer; the feeling of uneasiness may not leave patients completely for 10 to 14 days, and only at the end of this time are they able to sleep undisturbed, without sedation. An attempt should be made to keep patients in the hospital for this length of time. To discharge them after a few days increases the likelihood that they will turn to alcohol to suppress their still-present tenseness and sleeplessness.

Hallucinosis Symptoms of disordered perception occur in about one-quarter of the tremulous patients. Patients may complain of "bad dreams"—nightmarish episodes associated with disturbed sleep, which are difficult to separate from real experience. Sounds and shadows may be misinterpreted, or familiar objects may appear distorted and assume unreal forms. Although these are not hallucinations in the strict sense of the term, they represent the most common forms of disordered sense perception in the alcoholic. Hallucinations may be purely visual or auditory in type, mixed visual and auditory, and occasionally tactile or olfactory. There is little evidence to support the popular belief that certain visual hallucinations are specific to alcoholism. They are more commonly animate than inanimate and may comprise various forms of human, animal, or insect life. They may occur singly or in panoramas; they may appear shrunken or enlarged; they may be natural in appearance or take distorted and hideous forms (see also Chap. 21).

ACUTE AND CHRONIC AUDITORY HALLUCINOSIS This form of alcoholic psychosis, in which vivid auditory hallucinations are the major abnormality, merits separate consideration. Kraepelin referred to it as the *hallucinatory insanity of drunkards or alcoholic mania.* The central feature of the illness, in the beginning, is the occurrence of auditory hallucinations despite an otherwise clear sensorium; i.e., confusion, disorientation, and obtundation are minimal or absent, and memory is not significantly impaired. The hallucinations may be musical in nature, like a low-pitched hum or chant, or they may take the form of unstructured sounds such as buzzing, ringing, shots, or clicking. Usually vocal hallucinations are associated. When the voices can be identified, they are attributed to the family, friends, or neighbors of patients, rarely to God, radio, or radar. The voices may be addressed directly to patients, but more frequently they discuss them in the third person. In the majority of cases the voices are maligning, reproachful, or threatening in nature and are disturbing to patients; a significant proportion, however, are not unpleasant and leave patients undisturbed. The voices are intensely real and vivid, and they tend to be exteriorized; i.e., they come from behind the door, from the corridor, or through the floor. Another quality of these formed auditory hallucinations (and of visual ones) is the appropriateness of the emotional responses of patients to them. They may call on the police for protection or barricade themselves against invaders; they may even attempt suicide to avoid what the voices threaten. The hallucinations are most prominent during the night, and their duration varies greatly—they may last for a few minutes to an hour or two or for days, and they may recur intermittently for days on end and, in exceptional instances, for weeks or months.

Most patients, while hallucinating, have no appreciation of the unreality of their hallucinations. As improvement occurs, patients begin to doubt their reality, are reluctant to talk about them, and may even question whether they had been sane during the episode. Full recovery is characterized by the realization that the voices were imaginary and by the ability to recall, sometimes with remarkable clarity, the abnormal thought content of parts of the psychotic episode.

A unique feature of this psychosis is the evolution of a chronic auditory hallucinosis in a small proportion of the patients. Such patients become quiet and resigned, even though the hallucinations remain threatening and derogatory. Ideas of reference and influence and other poorly systematized paranoid delusions become prominent. At this stage these patients show many of the symptoms of schizophrenia—illogical thinking, vagueness, tangential associations, and a dissociation of affect and of thought content. There is some evidence that repeated attacks of acute auditory hallucinosis render the patient more vulnerable to this chronic schizophrenia-like syndrome (see Chap. 25).

Withdrawal seizures ("rum fits")   In this particular setting (i.e., where relative or absolute abstinence follows a period of chronic inebriation) there is a marked tendency to develop convulsive seizures. Over 90 percent of seizures occur during the 7- to 48-h period following the cessation of drinking, with a peak incidence between 13 to 24 h. During the period of seizure activity electroencephalograms may be abnormal, but they revert to normal in a matter of days, even though patients may go on to develop delirium tremens. Also during the period of seizure activity patients are unusually sensitive to strobo-scopic stimulation. About half of these patients respond to this activating procedure with generalized myoclonus (photomyoclonus) or a convulsive seizure (photoconvulsion). In contrast, patients with idiopathic epilepsy rarely show this type of response to photic stimulation.

Seizures occurring in the abstinence period have a number of other distinctive features. There may be only a single seizure, but, more often, a flurry of two to six seizures occurs over a span of several hours, and an occasional patient develops status epilepticus. The seizures are grand mal in type, i.e., major generalized convulsions with loss of consciousness. A focal seizure or seizures should always suggest the presence of a focal lesion (usually traumatic) in addition to the effects of alcohol. Almost one-third of the patients with generalized seizure activity go on to develop delirium tremens, in which case the seizures invariably precede the delirium. The postictal confusional state may blend imperceptibly with the onset of the delirium, or there may be a clearing of the postictal state, over several hours or even a day or two, before the delirium sets in. Seizures of this type occur in patients who have been drinking for many years, so that they have to be distinguished from other forms of epilepsy beginning in adult life.

It is suggested that the term *rum fits* be reserved for seizures which possess the attributes described above. It is the term used frequently by the alcoholic and serves to distinguish seizures that occur only in the immediate abstinence period from those which occur in the interdrinking period, long after withdrawal has been accomplished. It is important to note that the "idiopathic" or posttraumatic forms of epilepsy may be influenced by alcohol. In patients with these types of epilepsy, seizures may be precipitated by only a short period of drinking (e.g., a weekend, or even one evening of heavy social drinking); interestingly, in these circumstances, the seizures occur not when patients are intoxicated, but usually the morning after, in the "sobering-up" period.

Electroencephalographic findings in patients with "rum fits" do not support the notion that the seizures merely represent latent epilepsy made manifest by alcohol. Instead, the electroencephalogram (EEG) reflects a sequence of changes induced by alcohol itself—a decrease in the frequency of brain waves during the period of chronic intoxication; a rapid return of the EEG to normal immediately after cessation of drinking; the occurrence of a brief period of dysrhythmia (sharp waves and paroxysmal changes) which coincides with the flurry of convulsive activity; and again, a rapid return of the EEG to normal. Except for the transient dysrhythmia in the withdrawal period, the incidence of EEG abnormalities in patients who have had "rum fits" is not greater than in the normal population, in sharp contrast to patients who are indeed subject to seizures (see Chap. 364).

Delirium tremens   This is the most dramatic and serious form of the alcohol withdrawal syndrome. It is characterized by profound confusion, delusions, vivid hallucinations, tremor, agitation, and sleeplessness, as well as by increased activity of the autonomic nervous system, i.e., dilated pupils, fever, tachycardia, and profuse perspiration. The clinical features of delirium have been presented in detail in Chap. 21.

Delirium tremens develops in one of several settings. The patients, excessive and steady drinkers of many years' duration, may have been admitted to the hospital for an unrelated illness, accident, or operation, and 2 to 4 days later become delirious. Or, following a prolonged spree, they may have already experienced several days of tremulousness and hallucinosis, or one or more seizures, and may even be recovering from these symptoms, when they suddenly develop delirium tremens.

In the majority of cases delirium tremens is benign and short-lived, ending as abruptly as it begins. Consumed by the relentless activity and wakefulness of several days' duration, patients fall into a deep sleep; they awaken lucid, quiet, and exhausted, with virtually no memory for the events of the delirious period. Less commonly, the delirious state subsides gradually; more rarely still, there may be one or more relapses, with several discrete episodes of delirium separated by lucidity and the entire process lasting for as little as several days or as long as 4 to 5 weeks. When the delirium occurs as a single episode, the duration is 72 h or less in over 80 percent of the cases.

Five to fifteen percent of cases of delirium tremens, as defined above, end fatally. In many of these there is an associated infectious illness or injury, but in a few no complicating illness is discernible. Patients frequently die in a state of hyperthermia or peripheral circulatory collapse; in some, death comes so suddenly that the nature of the terminal events cannot be determined.

Closely related to typical delirium tremens and about as common are the *atypical delirious-hallucinatory* or *confusional states,* in which one facet of the delirium tremens complex assumes prominence to the practical exclusion of the other symptoms. Patients may simply exhibit a transient state of quiet confusion, agitation, and peculiar behavior lasting several days or weeks. Other patients present a vivid hallucinatory-delusional state and abnormal behavior, consistent with their false beliefs. Unlike typical delirium tremens, the atypical states always present as a single circumscribed episode without recurrences, are only rarely preceded by epilepsy, and do not end fatally. This may be another way of saying that they are a partial or less severe form of the disease.

Pathological examination is singularly unrevealing in patients with delirium tremens. Edema and brain swelling have been absent in the authors' pathological material except when there was shock or hypoxia terminally, and there have not been any significant microscopic changes in the brain. Abnormalities of the spinal fluid, blood nonprotein nitrogen, serum sodium, chloride, sugar, potassium, calcium, and phosphorus occur unpredictably. The electroencephalographic findings have been discussed in relation to alcoholic epilepsy.

The *pathogenesis* of the tremulous-hallucinatory-delirious state has been a matter of considerable controversy. The idea that it simply represents the most severe form of alcohol intoxication is not tenable. The symptoms of toxicity, consisting of slurred speech, uninhibited behavior, staggering gait, stupor, and coma, are distinctive and different from the symptom complex of tremor, hallucinations, fits, and delirium. The former symptoms are associated with an elevated blood alcohol level, whereas the latter become evident only when the blood alcohol is reduced. Finally, the toxic symptoms increase in severity as more alcohol is consumed, whereas tremor and hallucinosis and even full-blown delirium tremens may be nullified by the administration of alcohol. Although much discussed in the past, there is no evidence that endocrine abnormality or nutritional deficiency plays a role in the genesis of delirium tremens and related symptoms.

It is evident, from observations in both humans and experimental animals, that the one indispensable factor in the genesis of delirium tremens and related disorders is the withdrawal of alcohol, following a period of chronic intoxication. The emergence of withdrawal symptoms depends upon a decline in the blood alcohol level from a previously higher level and not necessarily upon the complete disappearance of alcohol from the blood. The mechanism(s) by which the withdrawal of alcohol produces symptoms is only beginning to be understood. It has been shown that the early phase of alcohol withdrawal (beginning 7 to 8 h after cessation of drinking) is regularly attended by a drop in serum magnesium levels and a rise in arterial pH values, on the basis of respiratory alkalosis. Indeed it is possible that the compounded effect of these two factors, both of which are associated with hyperexcitability of the nervous system, might be responsible for seizures and perhaps for other symptoms which characterize the early phase of withdrawal. The elevation in pH and drop in P_{CO_2} are explained as withdrawal release of the neurons of the "respiratory center," which had been previously rendered insensitive to circulating CO_2. In the "rebound" phase these cells become more sensitive than normal to CO_2, with resultant hyperventilation and respiratory alkalosis. But as an explanation of delirium tremens, hypomagnesemia is probably not important, since the serum magnesium level has frequently been restored to normal before the onset of the delirium.

Treatment of alcoholic withdrawal syndrome   The general aspects of management of the delirious and confused patient have been described in Chap. 21.

More specifically the treatment of delirium tremens begins with a careful search, followed by appropriate treatment, for associated injuries (particularly head injury with cerebral lacerations or subdural hematoma), infections (pneumonia or meningitis), pancreatitis, and liver disease. Because of the frequency and seriousness of these complications, skull and chest roentgenograms should be obtained and lumbar puncture should be performed routinely. In severe forms of delirium tremens, the temperature, pulse, and blood pressure should be recorded at 30-min intervals in anticipation of peripheral circulatory collapse and hyperthermia, which, added to the effects of injury and infection, are the usual causes of death in this disease. In the case of shock, one must act quickly, utilizing whole-blood transfusions, fluids, and vasopressor drugs. The occurrence of hyperthermia demands the use of a cooling mattress in addition to specific treatment for any infection that may be present.

A very important element in treatment is the correction of fluid and electrolyte imbalance. Severe degrees of agitation and perspiration may require the administration of 6000 ml fluid daily, of which 1500 ml should be normal saline solution. The specific electrolytes and the amounts in which they are added are governed by the laboratory values for these electrolytes. Occasionally, the withdrawal syndrome is characterized by hypoglycemia, in which case the administration of glucose becomes of prime importance. Rarely, alcoholic patients present with severe ketoacidosis and normal or only slightly elevated blood glucose concentrations. Usually such patients recover promptly, without the use of insulin.

A special danger attends the use of glucose solutions in alcoholic patients. Usually these persons have subsisted on a diet disproportionately high in carbohydrate (alcohol is metabolized almost entirely as carbohydrate) and low in thiamine, and their reserves of B vitamins may have been further reduced by gastroenteritis and diarrhea. The administration of intravenous glucose may serve to consume the last available stores of thiamine and precipitate Wernicke's disease. For this reason it is good practice to add B vitamins in all cases requiring parenterally administered glucose, even though the alcoholic disorder under treatment, e.g., delirium tremens, is not primarily due to vitamin deficiency.

In respect to the use of drugs, it is important to distinguish between mild withdrawal symptoms, which are essentially benign and responsive to practically all sedative drugs, and delirium tremens, which has a serious mortality and is relatively unresponsive to drugs. In the case of minor withdrawal symptoms, the purpose of medication is to ensure rest and sleep. In delirium tremens, the object of drug therapy is to blunt agitation, prevent exhaustion, and facilitate the administration of parenteral fluid and nursing care; one does not attempt to suppress agitation at all costs, since to accomplish this requires an amount of drug that might seriously depress respiratory function.

A wide variety of drugs is effective in controlling withdrawal symptoms. Some of the more popular are prochlorperazine (Compazine), chlorpromazine (Thorazine), meprobamate, chlordiazepoxide (Librium), hydroxyzine (Vistaril), and diazepam (Valium). There is little difference in the therapeutic efficacy of these drugs, and it is not certain that any of them can prevent hallucinosis or delirium tremens or shorten the duration and decrease the mortality rate of the latter disorder. In general, phenothiazine drugs should be avoided because of their epileptogenic properties. Furthermore, the advantages of the oral administration of these drugs over paraldehyde have not been proved by controlled studies; in fact, there is some evidence that in the more severe forms of the withdrawal syndrome paraldehyde is superior to both chlorpromazine and promazine. Paraldehyde has the additional advantage of being extremely safe provided it is freshly prepared and kept in brown, tightly stoppered bottles to prevent deterioration and the accumulation of acetaldehyde. If the patient can take medication orally, doses of 8 to 12 ml in orange juice should be given. Paraldehyde may also be administered rectally, but the intramuscular route should be avoided if possible, since it may damage nerves, and it should be given intravenously only with great caution because of the danger of respiratory depression. If parenteral medication is necessary, sodium phenobarbital or sodium amytal in doses of 120 mg, repeated at 3- to 4-h intervals, may be given, provided there is no serious liver disease. Some physicians prefer to use intravenous diazepam, giving 10 mg initially and repeating this dose at 20- to 30-min intervals until the patient is calm but awake. Such treatment is effective but requires careful monitoring to avoid hypotension and hypoventilation. Adrenocorticotropic hormone and cortisone have no place in the treatment of the withdrawal syndrome.

Treatment of "rum fits"   In most cases the seizures that occur in the withdrawal period ("rum fits") do not require the use of anticonvulsant drugs. In this setting there may be only a single seizure or a brief flurry of seizures which usually have ceased by the time that certain medicines, such as phenytoin (Dilantin), become effective. The parenteral administration of sodium phenobarbital early in the withdrawal period could conceivably prevent "rum fits" in patients with a previous history of this disorder or in those who might be expected to develop seizures on withdrawal. Also, the long-term administration of anticonvulsants is not practical; if patients remain abstinent, they will be free of seizures, and if they resume drinking they usually abandon their medicines. Withdrawal seizures that take the form of status epilepticus should be managed like status of any other type (see Chap. 23). Alcoholics with a history of idiopathic or posttraumatic epilepsy should be urged to drink only in moderation or not at all, because of the deleterious effects of relatively short periods of drinking on their epilepsy, and they should be maintained on anticonvulsant drugs.

NUTRITIONAL DISEASES OF THE NERVOUS SYSTEM   These diseases compose a relatively small but serious group of illnesses in chronic alcoholics. In contrast to alcoholic intoxication and the abstinence syndromes, the role of alcohol in the genesis of nutritional diseases is secondary, serving mainly to displace food in the diet. These illnesses, the role of alcohol in their production, and their treatment, are discussed in Chap. 371, "Metabolic Diseases of the Nervous System," and Chap. 372, "Nutritional Diseases of the Nervous System."

ALCOHOLIC DISEASES OF UNCERTAIN PATHOGENESIS   Included under this heading is a group of diseases which have little in common except that they are either confined to or predominant in alcoholics. The relationship to alcohol is not understood in any one of these diseases and is probably not crucial, insofar as some of them also occur in nonalcoholics. There is indirect evidence that some of these disorders are nutritional in origin, but as yet this relationship must be regarded as unproved.

Alcoholic cerebellar degeneration   This term is applied to a nonfamilial type of cerebellar ataxia which occurs in adult life against a background of prolonged ingestion of alcohol. The symptoms may progress slowly over a long period, but more frequently they evolve in a subacute fashion (several weeks or months), after which they remain stationary for many years. Often they are present in mild form and worsen considerably after an attack of pneumonia or delirium tremens. The signs are those of cerebellar dysfunction, affecting stance and gait predominantly. The legs are involved more frequently and severely than the arms, and nystagmus and speech disturbances are rare. Once established, the signs change very little, although some improvement of gait (due mainly to recovery from complicating polyneuropathy) may follow cessation of drinking. The essential pathological changes consist of degeneration of varying severity of all the neurocellular elements of the cerebellar cortex, particularly of the Purkinje cells, with a striking topographic restriction to the anterior and superior aspects of the vermis and adjacent parts of the hemispheres.

The disorder of stance and gait seems to be related to the lesion in the vermis, and the ataxia of the limbs to involvement of the anterior lobe of the cerebellum. A similar clinical syndrome has been observed in a few nutritionally depleted nonalcoholic patients.

It is likely that the cerebellar lesions in this disorder and in Wernicke's disease represent the same disease process. The latter designation is used when the cerebellar abnormalities are associated with the characteristic ocular and mental disorders, and the term "alcoholic" cerebellar degeneration when only the cerebellar signs are clinically manifest.

Marchiafava-Bignami disease (primary degeneration of the corpus callosum)   This is a rare complication of alcoholism originally described in Italian men addicted to crude red wine. The symptoms are diverse and include psychic and emotional disorders, intellectual deterioration, convulsive seizures, and varying degrees of tremor, rigidity, paralysis, apraxia, aphasia, and sucking and grasping reflexes. The duration is variable, from several weeks to months, and recovery is possible. The pathological picture is more constant than the clinical one. It consists of symmetrical demyelination in the corpus callosum, particularly of the middle lamina, and less consistently of the anterior commissure and other parts of the white matter. Axis cylinders are better preserved than medullated fibers in these areas, and there are appropriate reactions in the macrophages and astrocytes. Various degrees of recovery may occur if abstinence from alcohol and good nutrition are established and maintained.

Central pontine myelinolysis (CPM)   This term refers to a unique pathological change affecting the center of the basis pontis, in which the medullated fibers are destroyed in a single symmetrical focus of varying size. In contrast, the axis cylinders, nerve cells, and blood vessels are relatively well preserved. Although the lesion is usually confined to the basis pontis, occasional cases also show symmetrically placed lesions of similar histological type in other parts of the brain. The disease may manifest itself clinically by pseudobulbar palsy, quadriplegia, and pseudocoma ("locked-in syndrome"), evolving over a period of several days, but usually the lesion is so small that it causes no symptoms and is found only at postmortem examination. Most cases of CPM have occurred in severely malnourished alcoholics, but the relationship of this condition to nutritional deficiency, alcohol, or other toxic factors is obscure. Recently, attention has been drawn to the frequent occurrence of *hyponatremia* in patients with CPM, but the significance of this finding is unclear also.

Cerebral atrophy   The pathological examination of relatively young alcoholic patients not infrequently discloses an unexpected degree of convolutional atrophy, most prominent in the frontal lobes, and a symmetrical enlargement of the lateral and third ventricles. In some of these cases the lesions of the Wernicke-Korsakoff syndrome, cerebral trauma, anoxic or hepatic encephalopathy, or communicating hydrocephalus are associated, but in others they are not. Ventricular enlargement and, less often, convolutional atrophy have also been found on pneumoencephalography, and more recently similar findings have been reported in chronic alcoholics examined by computerized tomography (CT) scan. The clinical correlates of these radiological findings have not been determined, however. Clinical examination may disclose various abnormalities of neurological and intellectual function, but many patients betray no symptoms or signs of neurological disease. Obviously, the nature of "alcoholic cerebral atrophy" remains to be defined, both clinically and pathologically.

"Alcoholic" myopathy Alcoholics as a group are particularly vulnerable to several disorders of cardiac and skeletal muscle, loosely referred to as alcoholic cardiomyopathy and alcoholic myopathy. Apart from their high incidence in alcoholics, these myopathies possess no unique features, and the same disorders may be observed in a variety of clinical settings in which alcohol plays no part.

One type of myopathic syndrome occurs acutely in the course of a prolonged bout of heavy drinking and is manifested by severe pain and tenderness and swelling of muscles, accompanied by cramps and muscle weakness. The muscular affection may be generalized or remarkably focal, and an affected limb may give the appearance of a deep phlebothrombosis or lymphatic obstruction. Some of the focal lesions are surely induced by trauma or pressure-ischemic injury during a period of alcoholic coma. Diffuse necrosis of muscle fibers, all in one stage of degeneration (rhabdomyolysis), is the underlying pathological change and is reflected by myoglobinuria (leading in some cases to fatal myoglobinuric nephrosis) and high serum levels of creatine phosphokinase (CPK). Some of these patients show a diminished rise in blood lactic acid in response to ischemic exercise, similar to that which occurs in McArdle's disease. In distinction to the latter, however, myophosphorylase levels are not consistently reduced in the alcoholic patients. How these biochemical abnormalities are related to muscle cramps and weakness is a matter of speculation. Most patients with this disorder recover, usually in a matter of weeks; in severe cases, complete restoration of motor power may take several months.

In other cases, a painless and predominantly proximal weakness develops over a period of several days or weeks in the course of a prolonged drinking bout and is associated with a severe degree of hypokalemia. The urinary excretion of potassium is not significantly increased. Usually the depletion of potassium is the result of vomiting and diarrhea, which precede the onset of muscular weakness, but sometimes the mechanism of depletion is unclear. In several reported cases with low serum phosphorus levels a bone tumor (e.g., an ossifying angioma) was found, and its removal restored muscle power to normal. The oral administration of phosphates has been beneficial in nontumorous cases. Some of the latter are accompanied by pain and stiffness.

From time to time, one observes in alcoholics the subacute or chronic evolution of painless weakness and atrophy of the proximal muscles of the limbs, especially of the legs, with only minimal signs of polyneuropathy in the distal segments of the legs and feet. Cases such as these have been referred to as *chronic alcoholic myopathy,* but the data are as yet insufficient to warrant this designation. Muscle biopsies that the authors have examined from such patients suggest that it may represent a proximal form of polyneuropathy. Treatment follows along the lines for alcoholic neuropathy, and complete recovery can be expected if the patient abstains from alcohol and improves his nutritional status.

Alcoholic cardiomyopathy is discussed in Chap. 247.

Fetal alcohol syndrome That maternal alcoholism may have an adverse effect on the offspring has been a recurrent theme in medical lore, but only in the past decade have the effects of alcohol abuse on the fetus been clearly documented. This congenital disorder has been termed the *fetal alcohol syndrome* (FAS). The affected infants are small in length in comparison with weight, and most of them fall below the third percentile for head circumference. They are distinguished also by the presence of short palpebral fissures (probably a reflection of microphthalmia) and epicanthal folds; maxillary hypoplasia, thin vermillion of upper lip, micrognathia, and cleft palate; dislocation of the hips, flexion deformities of the fingers, and limited range of motion of other joints; cardiac anomalies (usually spontaneously closing septal defects); anomalous external genitalia; and capillary hemangiomata. The newborn infants suck and sleep poorly, and many of them are irritable, hyperactive and tremulous; the latter symptoms resemble those of alcohol withdrawal, except that they persist. In one series of such infants there was a neonatal mortality of 17 percent. Seriously affected infants who survive the neonatal period fail to achieve normal weight, length, and head circumference and remain backward mentally to a varying degree, even under optimal environmental conditions.

The anatomic basis of this syndrome, and the mechanism by which alcohol produces its effects, are not known; the limited evidence to date favors a toxic effect of alcohol or perhaps one of its metabolites or contaminants, rather than a nutritional or genetic factor. The critical degree of maternal alcoholism that is necessary to produce the FAS and the critical stage in gestation during which it occurs also need to be determined. Cases of the FAS observed to date have occurred only in children born to severely alcoholic mothers who continued to drink heavily (80 ml absolute alcohol per day) throughout their pregnancy. Studies of the effects on the fetus of lesser degrees of maternal alcoholism are in progress.

NEUROLOGICAL DISORDERS CONSEQUENT UPON CIRRHOSIS AND PORTAL-SYSTEM SHUNTS *Hepatic coma* refers to an episodic disorder of consciousness which frequently complicates (or terminates) advanced liver disease and/or portal-systemic shunts. This condition and the more chronic type of acquired hepatocerebral degeneration are described in Chaps. 304 and 371.

TREATMENT OF ALCOHOL ADDICTION Following recovery from the acute medical and neurological complications of alcoholism, the underlying problem—that of alcohol dependence—remains. To treat only the medical complications and to leave the management of the drinking problem to patients themselves is indeed shortsighted. Almost always drinking is resumed, with a predictable recurrence of medical illness. For this reason the physician must be prepared to deal with the addiction or at least to initiate treatment.

The problem of excessive drinking is formidable but not necessarily as hopeless as it is made out to be. A common misconception among physicians is that specialized training in psychiatry and an inordinately large amount of time are required to deal with the addictive drinker. Actually, a successful program of treatment can be initiated by any interested physician, using the standard techniques of history taking, establishing rapport with patients, and seeing them frequently, though not necessarily for prolonged periods. A useful point at which to undertake this task is during convalescence from a serious medical or neurological complication of alcoholism or in relation to loss of employment, arrest, or threatened divorce. Such crises may help convince patients, better than any argument presented by families or physicians, that their drinking has reached serious proportions.

The requisite for successful treatment is total abstinence from alcohol, and for all practical purposes, this represents the only permanent solution. It is generally agreed that any attempt to curb the drinking habit will fail if patients continue to drink. There are said to be cases in which patients have been able to reduce their intake of alcohol and eventually to drink in moderation, but they must be extremely rare. Also, it is

frequently stated that patients must recognize that they are alcoholics, i.e., that their drinking is beyond their control, and they must express willingness to be helped. Undoubtedly there is truth in both these statements, but they should not be interpreted to mean that patients must gain this recognition and willingness entirely on their own initiative and that they will be helped only after they do so. Physicians can do a great deal to help patients understand the nature of their problem and thus to motivate them to accept treatment. Logic and reasoning must be used to convince them that abstinence is preferable to chronic inebriety. Patients must be made fully aware of the medical and social consequences of continued drinking and must also be made to understand that because of some constitutional peculiarity (like that of diabetics, who cannot handle sugar) they are incapable of drinking in moderation. These facts should be presented in much the same way as one would explain the essential features of any other disease. There is nothing to be gained from adopting a punitive or moralizing attitude; nor should patients be given the idea that they are in no way blameworthy for their illness. There appears to be an advantage in making patients feel that they are responsible for doing something about their drinking.

The prevalent belief that alcoholics will not stop drinking under duress also requires qualification. In fact, one of the few careful studies of this matter disclosed that relatively few patients would have sought help unless pressure had been exerted by family or employer; furthermore, patients who came to the clinic under duress of this sort did just as well as those who came voluntarily.

If earnest and sustained efforts by physicians fail to convince patients that alcohol offers a problem, it is usually impossible to modify their alcoholic tendencies. The only way to make such individuals discontinue drinking is to commit them to psychiatric hospitals or special institutions for the management of alcoholism in the hope that with forced abstinence and improvement in their physical state they will gain insight and later accept psychiatric or other forms of therapy.

On the other hand, if patients come to realize that their drinking is beyond their control and that they need to do something about it, their chances of being helped are raised considerably. Indeed, under these circumstances, many persons stop drinking of their own volition. Some of these patients, despite the best of intentions, will relapse. This should not serve as an excuse to abandon treatment; many patients have attained a state of prolonged sobriety after several false starts. A number of methods have proved valuable in the long-term management of patients. The most important of these are the use of Antabuse, psychotherapy, and the participation in social organizations for combating alcoholism.

Antabuse (tetraethylthiuram disulfide, disulfiram) interferes with the metabolism of alcohol, so that patients who take both alcohol and Antabuse accumulate an inordinate amount of acetaldehyde in the tissues, resulting in nausea, vomiting, and hypotension, sometimes pronounced in degree. It is no longer considered necessary to demonstrate these effects to patients; it is sufficient to warn them of the severe reactions that may result if they drink while they have the drug in their body. Treatment with Antabuse is instituted only after patients have been sober for several days, preferably longer. It should never be given to patients with cardiac or liver disease. The drug is taken each morning, or at another suitable time daily, in a dosage of 0.5 g, preferably under supervision. This form of treatment is of particular value in spree or periodic drinkers, in whom relapse from abstinence usually represents an impulsive rather than a carefully planned or premeditated act. Patients taking Antabuse, aware of the dangers of mixing liquor and the drug, are "protected" against the impulse to drink, and this protection may be renewed every 24 h by the simple expedient of taking a pill. The willingness with which patients accept this form of treatment also serves as a rough index of their motivation. Should patients drink when they are taking Antabuse, the ensuing reaction is usually severe enough to require medical attention, and a protracted spree can thus be prevented. Antabuse may in rare instances lead to a mild polyneuropathy if continued over a period of months or years. It must then be discontinued.

Alcoholics Anonymous (AA), an informal fellowship of former alcoholics, has proved to be the single most effective force in the rehabilitation of alcoholic patients. The philosophy of this organization is embodied in their so-called "twelve steps," a series of propositions about alcohol and alcoholism which guide the patient to recovery. The AA philosophy stresses in particular the practice of making restitution, the necessity to help other alcoholics, trust in God, the group confessional, and the belief that alcoholics are powerless over alcohol. AA philosophy also embodies the 24-h plan, in which alcoholics strive for just 24 h of abstinence (a concept inspired by the Sermon on the Mount) as a means of facilitating the maintenance of sobriety. Although accurate statistics are lacking, it is stated that about half the members who express more than a passing interest in the program have no relapses, and that a significant additional number relapse but eventually recover.

The methods used by AA are not suited to every patient; some prefer the more personalized approach offered by special clinics and centers for the treatment of alcoholism. The physician should, therefore, be fully aware of all the community resources which are available for the management of this problem and should be prepared to take advantage of them in appropriate cases.

Finally, it should be noted that alcoholism is frequently associated with psychiatric disease of some other type. There is among alcoholics an increased frequency of schizophrenia, psychoneurosis, sociopathy, and particularly manic-depressive disease. In the latter case, the prevailing mood is far more often one of depression than of mania, and is more often encountered in the female who is more apt to drink under these conditions than the male. The presence of concomitant psychiatric disease complicates the management of the alcoholism, and in these circumstances expert psychiatric help should be sought.

REFERENCES

Alcohol and Health. US Department of Health, Education, and Welfare Publication (HSM) 72-9099, 1971

CLARREN SK, SMITH DW: The fetal alcohol syndrome. N Engl J Med 298:1063, 1978

EPSTEIN PS et al: Alcoholism and cerebral atrophy. Alcoholism. Clin Exp Res 1:61, 1977

ISSELBACHER KJ: Metabolic and hepatic effects of alcohol. N Engl J Med 296:612, 1977

MENDELSON JH, MELLO NK: Behavioral and biochemical interrelationships in alcoholism. Annu Rev Med 27:321, 1976

THOMPSON WL et al: Diazepam and paraldehyde treatment of severe delirium tremens. A controlled trial. Ann Intern Med 82:175, 1975

VICTOR M: The pathophysiology of alcoholic epilepsy, in *The Addictive States.* Res Publ Assoc Res Nerv Ment Dis 46:431, 1968

————: Neurologic disorders due to alcoholism and malnutrition, in *Clinical Neurology,* AB Baker, LH Baker (eds). New York, Harper & Row, 1979

————, WOLFE SM: Causation and treatment of the alcohol withdrawal syndrome, in *Alcoholism: Progress in Research and Treatment,* PG Bourne, R Fox (eds). New York, Academic, 1973

227

OPIATES AND SYNTHETIC ANALGESICS

MAURICE VICTOR
RAYMOND D. ADAMS

The opiates, strictly speaking, include all the naturally occurring alkaloids in opium, which is prepared from the sap of the poppy *Papaver somniferum.* For clinical purposes, the term refers only to those alkaloids which have a high degree of analgesic activity, i.e., morphine and codeine (3-methoxymorphine). Thebaine, another opium alkaloid which, like morphine, possesses a phenanthrene nucleus, has few or no analgesic properties and is therefore not ordinarily considered an opiate. The terms *opioid* and *narcotic-analgesic* refer to any drug with actions similar to those of morphine. Compounds that are chemical modifications of morphine include heroin or diacetylmorphine (now the most commonly abused opioid), hydromorphone (Dilaudid), dihydrocodeinone (Hycodan), dihydroxycodeinone (Eucodal), oxymorphone (Numorphan), and oxycodone (Percodan). A second class of opioids comprises the *purely synthetic analgesics* pethidine or meperidine (Demerol), the merperidine derivatives anileridine and alphaprodine (Nisentil), methadone (Dolophine or amidone), metopon (6-methyldihydromorphinone), racemorphan (Dromoran), levorphan (*l*-Dromoran), *d*-propoxyphene (Darvon), diphenoxylate (the main component of Lomotil), and phenazocine (Prinadol). The latter drugs are similar to the opiates, both in their pharmacological effects and in the patterns of abuse, the differences being mainly quantitative. In fact, *d*-propoxyphene has such low addictive liabilities that it is not controlled by the federal narcotic laws. The same statement applies to the synthetic analgesic pentazocine (Talwin), and although its overall addictive quality is low, cases of physical dependency do occur.

As with alcohol and the barbiturates, the opioids will be considered from two points of view: (1) acute poisoning and (2) addiction.

OPIOID POISONING Because of the high incidence of addiction, which leads to irregular and nonmedical usage of opioids, poisoning is not an infrequent accident. This may happen as a result of ingestion with suicidal intent, errors in the calculation of dosage, variations in drug potency, or unusual sensitivity. Children may exhibit an increased susceptibility to opioids, so that relatively small doses prove toxic. This is true also in adults who have myxedema, Addison's disease, chronic liver disease, or pneumonia. Acute poisoning may also occur in addicts who are unaware that tolerance for opioids declines quickly after the withdrawal of the drug: upon resuming the habit a formerly well-tolerated dose can be fatal.

Varying degrees of unresponsiveness, shallow respirations, slow respiratory rate (e.g., two to four per minute), or periodic breathing, miosis, bradycardia, and hypothermia are the well-recognized clinical manifestations of acute poisoning. In the most advanced stage the pupils dilate, the skin and mucous membranes become cyanotic, and the circulation fails. The immediate cause of death is usually respiratory depression, with consequent asphyxia. Patients who have a cardiorespiratory arrest are sometimes left with a residuum of anoxic encephalopathy. Others who recover from coma may occasionally reveal a hemiplegia, presumably due to vascular occlusion. In the stage of mild intoxication, anorexia, nausea, vomiting, constipation, and loss of sexual interest are the only symptoms.

Treatment consists of gastric lavage (after oral ingestion), with a cuffed endotracheal tube in place should the patient be comatose. This procedure may be efficacious many hours after ingestion, since one of the toxic effects of opioids is severe pylorospasm, which may cause much of the drug to be retained in the stomach. Other measures must be directed toward the maintenance of an adequate airway and oxygenation, as described in Chap. 228, "Barbiturates," under "Management." If the patient does not respond rapidly to these measures, *naloxone* (Narcan) should be administered. This is a specific antidote to the opiates and also to the synthetic analgesics. It is now preferred to *N*-allylnormorphine (Nalline) because naloxone has no agonistic properties; hence, naloxone will not depress respiration further if the diagnosis of opioid poisoning is mistaken. For such poisoning, the dose of naloxone is 0.7 mg per 70 kg *intravenously,* repeated once or twice if necessary at 5-min intervals for an adequate respiratory response. The improvement in circulation and respiration is usually dramatic. In fact, failure of naloxone to produce such a response should cast doubt on the diagnosis of opioid intoxication. If an adequate respiratory response to naloxone is obtained, the patient should be observed carefully for 24 h, and further doses of naloxone (50 percent higher than previously found effective) may be given *intramuscularly* as often as necessary. Naloxone has little direct effect on the impaired consciousness, however, and the patient may remain drowsy for many hours. This is not harmful, provided respiration is well maintained.

A new oxymorphone-derived antagonist, *naltrexone,* promises to be even more effective than naloxone. Naltrexone is relatively free of agonistic activity and has the additional advantage of being effective orally. It is about twice as potent as naloxone in precipitating abstinence phenomena in patients dependent upon opiates, and its half-life of antagonistic actions is at least twice as long as that of naloxone.

Once the patient regains consciousness, usually in about 8 h, other complaints such as severe pruritus, sneezing, persistent obstipation, and urinary retention may necessitate symptomatic treatment. Nausea and severe abdominal pain, due presumably to pancreatitis (from spasm of the sphincter of Oddi), are other troublesome symptoms. The antidote must be used with great caution in an addict who has taken an overdose of opioid, because in this circumstance it may precipitate withdrawal phenomena.

In addition to the toxic effects of the opioid itself, the addict is exposed to a variety of neurological and infectious complications, resulting mainly from the injection of crude adulterants (quinine, lactose, powdered milk, fruit sugars) and various infectious agents (injections often administered by unsterile methods). Amblyopia, due probably to the toxic effects of quinine in the heroin mixtures, has been reported, as well as transverse myelopathy and several types of peripheral neuropathy. The spinal cord disorder expresses itself clinically by the abrupt onset of paraplegia with a sensory level on the trunk. Pathologically, there is an acute necrotizing lesion involving both grey and white matter over a considerable vertical extent of the thoracic and occasionally the cervical region. In some cases the myelopathy has followed the first intravenous injection of heroin after a prolonged period of abstinence. Involvement of single peripheral nerves, particularly of the radial nerve, and painful affection of the brachial plexus, independent of compression and remote from the site of injection, have been observed.

An acute generalized myopathy with myoglobinuria and renal failure has been ascribed to the intravenous injection of adulterated heroin. Brawny edema and fibrosing myopathy are the sequelae common to venous obliteration resulting from the administration of heroin and its adulterants by the intramuscular and subcutaneous routes. Occasionally there may be an inexplicable swelling of an extremity (sometimes massive) into which heroin had been injected subcutaneously or intramuscularly. Infection and venous thrombosis appear to be involved in its causation.

The diagnosis of drug addiction or the suspicion of this diagnosis should always encourage surveillance for infectious complications, particularly abscesses and cellulitis at injection, sites, septic thrombophlebitis, serum hepatitis, septic arthritis, and periarteritis. Tetanus, endocarditis (due mainly to *Staphylococcus aureus*), spinal epidural abscess, meningitis, brain abscess, and tuberculosis are found less frequently.

OPIOID ADDICTION Between 15 and 20 years ago there were about 60,000 persons addicted to narcotic drugs in the United States, not including those who were receiving drugs because of hopeless medical diseases. This represented a relatively small public health problem, in comparison with alcoholism and barbiturate addiction; and the addiction problem was of serious proportions in only a few cities—New York, Chicago, Los Angeles, Washington, and Detroit. In the past 15 years a remarkable increase in opioid (principally heroin) addiction has taken place. The precise number of opioid addicts is not known but was estimated by the Drug Enforcement Administration, in 1970, to be more than 600,000. The peak incidence of heroin dependence occurred in 1972. The incidence declined between 1972 and 1974, then increased again, and has fluctuated at near peak levels over the past 4 years.

Etiology and pathogenesis A number of factors, socioeconomic, psychological, and pharmacological, all contribute to the genesis of opioid addiction. In our culture, the most susceptible subjects are young men or delinquent youths living in the economically depressed areas of large cities, but a significant number are now found in the suburbs, in small cities, and in rural areas in Southern states. The onset of opioid use is usually in adolescence, with a peak at 17 to 18 years. Fully two-thirds of addicts start using the drug before the age of 21. A disproportionately large number are American Negroes and persons of Puerto Rican or Mexican descent. In the Southern states, addicts are predominantly white. Almost 90 percent of addicts engage in criminal activity, often necessary to obtain their daily ration of drug, but most of these have had arrests or convictions prior to addiction. Also, many of them show psychiatric disorders, psychopathy and psychoneurosis being the most common. Monroe et al. examined a group of 837 opioid addicts, using the Lexington Personality Inventory, and found evidence of characterologic disorder (psychopathy or sociopathy) in 42 percent, emotional disturbance in 29 percent, and thinking disorder in 22 percent; only 7 percent were asymptomatic. Nevertheless, the precise "personality" factor which renders certain individuals vulnerable to addiction has not been defined.

Association with addicts is the chief reason for beginning addiction. One addict recruits another person into addiction, and the new recruit does likewise. In this sense opioid addiction is contagious, and as a result of this pattern of opioid abuse, heroin addiction, since the late 1960s, has attained virtually epidemic proportions. A small, almost insignificant, proportion of addicts are introduced to drugs by physicians in the course of an illness.

Opioid addiction evolves in three successive phases: (1) episodic intoxication, (2) pharmacogenic or physical dependence, or addiction, and (3) the propensity to "relapse after cure."

Some of the symptoms of opiate intoxication have already been considered. In persons who are distressed by pain or pain-anticipatory anxiety, the administration of opioid produces a sense of unusual well-being, a state that has been referred to in medical writings as "morphine euphoria." It should be emphasized that only a negligible proportion of such persons continue to use opioids habitually after the pain has subsided. The vast majority of potential addicts are not suffer-

ing from painful illnesses at the time they initiate opioid use, and in them the initial effects of the drug are not aptly described as euphoric. The latter persons are mainly teenagers who self-administer opioids (mainly heroin) under the tutelage of their peers and who learn, after several repetitions, to recognize what they refer to as a heroin "high," despite the recurrence of unpleasant symptoms (nausea, vomiting, faintness). The repeated self-administration of drug ("reinforcement," in the language of operant psychology) is the most important factor in the genesis of addiction. Regardless of how one characterizes the state of mind that is produced by episodic reinitiation of the drug, the individual quickly discovers the need to increase the dose in order to obtain the original effect. Although the initial effects may not be fully recaptured, the progressively increasing dose of drug does abate the discomforts which arise as the effects of each injection wear off. In this way a new *pharmacogenically induced need* is developed and the use of opioids becomes self-perpetuating. At the same time a marked degree of tolerance is produced, so that enormous amounts of drugs, e.g., 5000 mg morphine daily, have been administered without the development of toxic symptoms. The mechanism of tolerance is still not understood fully, although it is a subject of much interest and speculation. The various theories related to physical dependence have been discussed fully by Wikler (see "References").

The altered physiological state that develops with continued use of the drug is manifested in another dramatic way at the time of withdrawal. This constitutes a specific illness, termed the *abstinence syndrome*. Strictly speaking, addiction is defined as physical or pharmacological dependence. This definition distinguishes between *addicting drugs* (opiates, alcohol, barbiturates) and *habit-forming drugs* (bromides, cocaine, and marihuana), since no consistent abstinence symptoms follow the discontinuation of the latter group, even after prolonged exposure. Stated in another way, all addicting drugs are habit-forming, but the opposite is not true. The place of amphetamines in this scheme is uncertain. Undoubtedly they are habit-forming drugs. Withdrawal of *d*-amphetamine, following prolonged oral or intravenous use, is regularly followed by prolonged sleep [of which a high percentage is rapid eye movement (REM) sleep], from which the patient awakens with a ravenous appetite. The deep sleep can be reversed by administration of *d*-amphetamine.

The intensity of the opioid abstinence syndrome depends mainly on the dose of the drug and duration of addiction, but also on individual factors. In respect to morphine it has been found that the majority of individuals receiving 240 mg daily for 30 days or more will show moderately severe abstinence symptoms following withdrawal, whereas mild abstinence signs can be precipitated by narcotic antagonists in persons who have taken as little as 15 mg morphine, or an equivalent dose of methadone or heroin, three times daily for 3 days.

The abstinence syndrome which occurs in the morphine addict may be taken as the prototype of the opioid group. The first 8 to 16 h of abstinence usually pass asymptomatically. At the end of this period yawning, rhinorrhea, sweating, and lacrimation become manifest. At first mild, these symptoms increase in severity over a period of several hours and then remain constant for several days. The patient may be able to sleep during the early period but is restless, and thereafter insomnia remains a prominent feature. Dilatation of the pupils, recurring waves of gooseflesh, and twitchings of the muscles appear. The patient complains of severe aches in the back, abdomen, and legs and of hot and cold "flashes" so that he covers himself with blankets. By the end of about 36 h the restlessness becomes more extreme, and nausea, vomiting, and diarrhea usually develop. The temperature, respiration, and blood pressure are slightly elevated. All these symptoms reach their peak intensity 48 to 72 h after withdrawal, and then gradually decline. The abstinence syndrome is rarely fatal. After 7 to 10 days, all clinical signs of abstinence have disappeared, although the patient may complain of insomnia, nervousness, weakness, and muscle aches for several more weeks, and a small deviation of a number of physiological variables can be detected with refined techniques for up to 10 months (protracted abstinence).

Two types of abstinence changes have been recognized: *nonpurposive* and *purposive.* The former comprises the various autonomic and neuromuscular signs and are relatively transient in nature. That these symptoms represent an altered physiological state and are not psychic in origin has been clearly demonstrated experimentally. Physical dependence on morphine and other opioids develops even in the lower limbs of dogs whose spinal cords have been transected; the flexor and crossed extensor spinal reflexes that are depressed or abolished by the opioid become remarkably exaggerated when the drug is withdrawn. The purposive changes refer to the patient's craving for the drug and the manipulative activity directed toward obtaining it. These symptoms may persist indefinitely and are important in relation to that characteristic of addiction referred to as *habituation, emotional dependence,* or *psychic dependence.* These terms are used interchangeably and refer to the substitution of drug-seeking activities for all other aims and objects in life.

Psychic dependence is regarded as the most important quality of addiction, since it is this feature which governs the initial use of the drug and relapse following apparent cure of addiction. Relapse to the use of the drug may occur long after the nonpurposive abstinence changes seem to have disappeared. The cause of relapse is imperfectly understood. It has been theorized that fragments of the abstinence syndrome may remain as a conditioned response, and that these abstinence signs may be evoked by the appropriate environmental stimuli. Thus, when a "cured" addict finds himself in a situation where narcotic drugs are readily available, or in circumstances that were responsible for the initial use of drugs, the incompletely extinguished drug-seeking behavior reasserts itself.

The characteristics of addiction and of abstinence are qualitatively similar with all the drugs of the opiate group as well as the related synthetic analgesics. The differences are mainly quantitative and are related to the differences in dosage, potency, and length of action. Heroin is two to three times more potent than morphine but otherwise the same; nevertheless, the heroin withdrawal syndrome encountered in hospital practice is usually mild in degree because of the low dosage of this drug in the street product. Dilaudid and metopon are more potent than morphine and have a shorter duration of action; hence the addict requires more doses per day, and the abstinence syndrome comes on and subsides more rapidly. The length of action of racemorphan is somewhat longer than that of morphine, but withdrawal phenomena are similar to those of morphine in temporal course and intensity. Abstinence symptoms from codeine, while very definite, are less than those from morphine. The addiction liabilities of *d*-propoxyphene are even less than those of codeine. Abstinence symptoms from methadone are less intense than those from morphine and do not become evident until 3 to 4 days after withdrawal; furthermore, autonomic signs are less severe in the abstinence period. For these reasons methadone is used in the treatment of morphine addiction. Meperidine addiction is of particular importance because of the high incidence among physicians and nurses and because there is still a widespread belief that this

drug is nonaddicting. Tolerance to the toxic effects of meperidine is not complete, so that the addict may show tremors, twitching of the muscles, confusion, hallucinations, and at times convulsions. Signs of abstinence appear 3 to 4 h after the last dose and reach maximum intensity between 8 and 12 h, at which time they may be worse than those of morphine abstinence.

Diagnosis of addiction This is usually made by the patient's statement that he is using and needs drugs. Should he decide to conceal this fact, one must rely on collateral evidence such as miosis, needle marks, emaciation, or abscess scars. Meperidine addicts are likely to have dilated pupils and twitching muscles. A method for the testing of the urine for opiates is now generally available. The finding of morphine or opiate derivatives (heroin is excreted as morphine) in the urine confirms the suspicion that the patient has taken or has been given a dose of such drugs within 24 h of the test.

Formerly it was necessary to isolate questionable cases and to observe the patient over a period of at least 2 days for signs of abstinence. Through use of the specific morphine antagonist *N*-allylnormorphine (nalorphine, Nalline) and naloxone (Narcan), a diagnosis of addiction to opiates and related analgesic drugs can be made within an hour. Naloxone, which is now preferred for this purpose, should be administered only in the presence of another physician or nurse, with the full understanding and permission of the patient. The drug is given intravenously, slowly, using a syringe containing 1 ampul (0.4 mg). The injection is stopped when pupillary dilatation, increased respiratory rate, lacrimation, rhinorrhea, sweating, and yawning appear. If, after 5 to 10 min, no such signs appear, a second injection may be given in the same way. If again the patient shows no abstinence signs, it may be assumed that he is not physically dependent upon opiates. Naloxone may be injected *subcutaneously,* in the same dosage as intravenously. Again, if the patient has taken more than occasional doses of the drug within a week of the test, the administration of naloxone will precipitate symptoms of abstinence. These become evident within 5 min of the first injection, reach their peak intensity in 20 min, begin to decline in 60 min, and disappear after 3 h. *N*-Allylnormorphine and naloxone do not precipitate abstinence symptoms in meperidine addiction, unless the patient has been taking more than 1600 mg daily.

Management and avoidance of addiction The ambulatory treatment of addiction never succeeds and should therefore not be undertaken, except in special settings, such as a carefully supervised methadone treatment program (see below). Addicts who are refused opiates may ask for methadone, meperidine, or racemorphine, on the ground that these drugs are synthetic and nonaddicting. These are addicting drugs and have been legally defined as such. Physicians should also be aware that they are breaking both the letter and the spirit of the regulations if they prescribe narcotics for an addict merely for the purpose of preventing abstinence changes. Occasional exceptions may be made in the case of seriously ill addicts who are awaiting treatment in a hospital or methadone program, or of patients who are suffering from incurable, painful disease.

An alternate method, and one that is used now almost exclusively, is to substitute methadone for opioid, in the ratio of 1 mg methadone for 3 mg morphine, 1 mg heroin, or 20 mg meperidine. Since methadone is long-acting and effective orally, it need be given only twice daily by mouth—10 to 20 mg per dose being sufficient to suppress abstinence symptoms. After a stabilization period of 3 to 5 days on this dosage of methadone alone, the drug may be reduced rapidly and withdrawn over a similar period of time. Regardless of the method of drug withdrawal employed, treatment is best carried out in an institution with proper facilities for postwithdrawal rehabilitation in a drug-free environment or where methadone or a morphine antagonist may be administered. Such institutions, private or municipal, are available in most large communities.

The physician must be constantly alert to the dangers of addiction, particularly in susceptible individuals, i.e., those with psychoneurosis, psychopathic personality, or alcoholism. The use of opioids should be limited to cases where pain is the chief problem; they should not be used primarily as sedatives, for the relief of asthma, or even in patients with chronic pain until all other measures have been exhausted. It follows that it is most important to make a precise diagnosis of the cause of pain, since in some cases measures other than opioids will suffice, while in others, such as hysteria and depression, narcotic analgesics are contraindicated.

If narcotics have to be used for the relief of pain, consideration should be given to the choice of the appropriate drug and to the mode of administration. Morphine is still the drug of choice for most patients requiring relief of severe pain for short periods. Demerol may be useful in patients who cannot tolerate morphine. Patients with chronic pain should be managed with the least potent and smallest dosage of drug that will relieve them; doses should be spaced as far apart as possible and discontinued as soon as the need for pain relief has passed. In general, the opioids should be administered orally whenever possible, and the intravenous route should be avoided, since this method produces maximum "euphoria" and, hence, the greatest danger of addiction. The oral administration of codeine and aspirin is a useful way to begin treatment of the patient with chronic pain. If these drugs fail to control the pain, the parenteral administration of codeine should be tried. If the more potent opioids are needed, methadone and levorphan should be used, because of their effectiveness by the oral route and the relatively slow development of tolerance. Should long-continued injections of morphine or meperidine become necessary, maximum analgesic effect is obtained with 10 mg morphine rather than with 15 mg, as is often prescribed, and with 60 to 70 mg rather than with 100 mg meperidine. In these cases, use of the narcotic antagonist pentazocine (Talwin) might be considered. It is claimed that this drug, administered parenterally in doses of 40 to 60 mg, has analgesic effects comparable with those of morphine and other opiates, but has less addicting properties. The respiratory depression produced by pentazocine, as by opiates, can be counteracted by naloxone.

Ambulatory treatment of opioid addiction   The most significant development in the treatment of opioid (almost exclusively heroin) addiction has been the establishment and growth of ambulatory methadone maintenance clinics. The scope of this activity, like the incidence of addiction, cannot be stated precisely, but can be judged by the fact that in 1974, 135,000 addicts were participating in such programs nationwide.

The method of treatment consists of the oral administration of methadone, once daily, in doses sufficient to suppress the craving for heroin and to abolish the euphoria-producing effects of that drug given intravenously (heroin blockade). The daily dosage of methadone required to achieve these effects varies between 60 and 100 mg; some patients can be maintained on as little as 40 mg per day, and with higher dosage they need take the drug only once in 48 h. Recently a longer-acting form of methadone—*l*-acetylmethadol—has become available, which can be taken thrice or even twice weekly. In principle, these effects could be achieved by multiple daily injections of heroin or morphine, but the effectiveness of methadone orally, its prolonged duration of action, and the fact that it precludes the desire and need for taking other opioids make methadone far more practical.

Methadone is no longer dispensed in tablet form but only as a liquid (dissolved in fruit juice), which is taken under supervision. The collection of urine samples is also supervised, and these are analyzed for opiates and other drugs, to monitor the patient's adherence to the program. Once this has been established, the patient is allowed to take home a 1- to 3-day supply. These measures are designed to prevent the diversion of methadone into illicit channels. Various forms of individual psychotherapy, group psychotherapy, social service counseling, and vocational guidance are included in most programs. The use of former heroin addicts (who are themselves on methadone treatment) as counselors is considered to be a particularly important adjunct to methadone treatment.

The results of methadone treatment are difficult to assess and vary considerably from one program to another. Even the best programs suffer an attrition rate of about 25 percent after several years. In the patients who remain, heroin use is markedly reduced, and between 75 and 85 percent achieve a high degree of social rehabilitation, i.e., they are gainfully employed and no longer engage in criminal behavior or prostitution. These have been the most notable achievements of the methadone maintenance programs.

Although the effectiveness of methadone treatment in the social rehabilitation of many addicts cannot be doubted, a number of questions about this method remain. The usual practice of methadone programs is to accept only adult addicts with a history of heroin addiction for several years. This leaves unanswered the problem of the adolescent addict. Although some individuals have been withdrawn from methadone, this has been accomplished so far in a relatively small number, and their capacity to maintain a drug-free existence appears doubtful. This means that the large majority of addicts now enrolled in methadone programs are committed to an indefinite period of methadone maintenance, and the effects of such a regimen are uncertain.

An alternate method of ambulatory treatment of the opioid addict involves the use of narcotic antagonists. Cyclazocine is the best known of these. After withdrawal of the opiate, cyclazocine is administered orally, in increasing amounts over a period of 2 to 6 weeks, until a dosage of 2 mg per 70 kg is being taken twice daily. The cyclazocine-stabilized individual is highly refractory to the euphoria-producing and pharmacological effects of opiates. The idea of treatment is to continue the administration of cyclazocine until all drug-seeking behavior is extinguished, after which it is withdrawn. Good results have been achieved with this drug, but only in small numbers of highly motivated patients who chose cyclazocine maintenance in preference to other forms of treatment. More recently, interest has centered about the opiate antagonist naltrexone which is virtually devoid of agonistic activity and twice as potent as naloxone; it has the added advantages of being effective orally and in much smaller doses than naloxone. The value of this kind of "extinction therapy" has not yet been determined, but the results in some patients have been encouraging, and the search for improved methods of using opioid antagonists continues. One such agent, buprenorphine, presently under investigation, shows promise both as an analgesic of low abuse potential and as a maintenance drug in narcotic addiction (Jasinski et al.).

Obviously none of these methods promise lasting success unless combined with reeducation, vocational habilitation, and social adjustment.

REFERENCES

HOLLISTER LE: Effective use of analgesic drugs. Annu Rev Med 27:431, 1976

JASINSKI DR et al: Human pharmacology and abuse potential of the analgesic buprenorphine. Arch Gen Psychiatry 35:501, 1978

MARTIN WR: Realistic goals for antagonist therapy. Am J Drug Alcohol Abuse 2:353, 1975

———— et al: Naltrexone, an antagonist for the treatment of heroin dependence: Effects in man. Arch Gen Psychiatry 28:782, 1973

MONROE JJ et al: The decline of the addict as "psychopath": Implications for community care. Int J Addictions 6:601, 1971

RICHTER RW et al: Neurological complications of heroin addiction. Bull NY Acad Med 49:3, 1972

WIKLER A.: Theories related to physical dependence, in *The Chemical and Biological Aspects of Drug Dependence,* SJ Mule, H Brill (eds). Cleveland, Chemical Rubber Press, 1972, p 359

————: Drug dependence, in *Clinical Neurology,* AB Baker, LH Baker (eds). Hagerstown, Md, Harper & Row, 1975

————: Characteristics of opioid addiction, in *Psychopharmacology in the Practice of Medicine,* ME Jarvik (ed). New York, Appleton-Century-Crofts, 1977, p 417

ZINBERG NE: The crisis in methadone maintenance. N Engl J Med 296:1000, 1977

228
BARBITURATES

MAURICE VICTOR
RAYMOND D. ADAMS

The high incidence of addiction, suicides, and accidental deaths attributable to the improper use of the barbiturate drugs is a matter of continuing concern to the medical profession. The production of barbiturates greatly exceeds the amount needed for therapeutic purposes. It is estimated that barbiturates account for 20 percent of acute poisonings admitted to general hospitals and that they are responsible for 6 percent of suicides and 18 percent of accidental deaths, figures exceeded by no other single poison. More than 15,000 deaths secondary to barbiturate poisoning are reported annually in the United States, and this figure is undoubtedly an underestimation. The Domestic Council Drug Abuse Task Force (1975) estimated the total number of regular users of barbiturates who were "in trouble" (suicidal and accidental overdoses as well as medical complications of barbiturate abuse) to be 300,000.

About 50 barbiturates have been marketed for clinical use, but only the following are encountered with any frequency: pentobarbital (Nembutal), secobarbital (Seconal), amobarbital (Amytal), aprobarbital (Alurate), thiopental (Pentothal), barbital (Veronal), and phenobarbital (Luminal). In the United States, pentobarbital, secobarbital, and amobarbital are the most commonly abused barbiturates. All the barbiturates are similar pharmacologically and differ only in their speed of onset and duration of action. The clinical problems posed by the barbiturates vary, however, according to whether the intoxication is acute or chronic, and these two types will be considered separately.

ACUTE BARBITURATE INTOXICATION Acute barbiturate intoxication results from the ingestion of large amounts of the drug either accidentally or with suicidal intent. Another form of accidental poisoning occurs in individuals who are intoxicated with barbiturates or with alcohol and who, being confused, ingest more of the drug than was intended. This type of poisoning has been termed *drug automatism.*

The ingestion of barbiturates with suicidal intent is most frequently the act of a depressed person. The hysteric or psychopath may take an overdose as a suicidal gesture and sometimes become seriously intoxicated because of a miscalculation or ignorance of the toxic dosage. At times, no psychiatric disease is present, the drug being taken impulsively or while the individual is inebriated. The combination of alcohol and barbiturate intoxication is frequent and particularly dangerous, since these drugs have an additive effect.

Site and mode of action of barbiturates Barbiturates decrease the excitability of nerve cells, although the mechanism is not fully understood. Attempts have been made to localize the action of barbiturates to certain anatomic regions, or even to specific nuclei within the nervous system, but it would appear that all parts are to some extent sensitive to the drug. Nevertheless, the reticular formation of the thalami and midbrain are particularly susceptible. There is little experimental evidence to support the notion that the administration of barbiturates first depresses cerebral cortical activity and then sequentially affects the anatomically lower centers. Reflex and other activities of the nervous system are probably depressed simultaneously, although in some cases the spinal reflexes appear to be accentuated in the early stages of poisoning.

Symptoms and signs The symptoms and signs of acute barbiturate intoxication vary with the type and the amount of drug, as well as with the length of time that has elapsed since it was ingested. Pentobarbital and secobarbital produce their effects after a short delay, and recovery is relatively rapid. Phenobarbital induces coma more slowly, and its effects tend to be prolonged. The duration of action of these drugs can be judged by the hypnotic effect of an average oral dose. In the case of the long-acting barbiturates, such as phenobarbital, barbital, and diallylbarbituric acid, it lasts 6 h or more; with the intermediate-acting drugs, amobarbital and aprobarbital, 3 to 6 h; with the short-acting drugs, secobarbital and pentobarbital, less than 3 h.

In general, much larger doses of long-acting barbiturates are required to produce a depth of unconsciousness comparable with that produced by the short-acting ones. The ingestion by adults of more than 3.0 g secobarbital, pentobarbital, amobarbital, or diallylbarbituric acid at one time may be fatal unless intensive and skillful treatment is applied promptly; it has been estimated that to produce a comparable effect, the following amounts of long-acting barbiturates would have to be ingested: 6.0 to 9.0 g phenobarbital, 5.0 to 20.0 g barbital, and 15.0 g aprobarbital. Because of the serious complications of prolonged coma, the fatalities are greater with the long-acting than with the short-acting drugs.

Clinically, it is useful to recognize three grades of severity of acute barbiturate intoxication, particularly in regard to prognosis and treatment. Mild intoxication follows the ingestion of approximately 0.6 g pentobarbital or its equivalent. Patients are drowsy or asleep, a state from which they are readily roused by calling their name loudly or by shaking them. The symptoms resemble those of alcohol intoxication, except that the face is not flushed, the conjunctivas are not suffused, and there is no odor of alcohol. Patients think slowly, and there may be mild disorientation, lability of mood, impairment of judgment, slurred speech, drunken gait, and nystagmus. Reflex activity and vital signs are not affected.

Moderate intoxication follows the ingestion of five to ten times the oral hypnotic dose. Here the state of consciousness is more severely depressed and is usually accompanied by depressed or absent deep reflexes and slow but not shallow respiration. Corneal reflexes are retained, with occasional exceptions. At times patients can be roused by vigorous manual stimulation; when awakened, they are confused and dysarthric and, after a few moments, drift back into coma. At other times they cannot be roused by any means. In the latter case the depth of coma and seriousness of the respiratory depression may be roughly judged by the response of respiration to the inhalation of 10% carbon dioxide or to painful stimulation such as the application of firm pressure to the sternum or supraorbital ridge. If these stimuli cause an increase in the depth and rate of respiration, the outlook for recovery is good, and only symptomatic treatment is indicated.

Severe intoxication occurs with the ingestion of fifteen to twenty times the oral hypnotic dose. Patients cannot be roused by any of the means indicated. Respiration is slow and shallow or irregular, and pulmonary edema and cyanosis may be present. The deep tendon reflexes are usually but not invariably absent. Most often, patients show no response to plantar stimulation, but in those who do the plantar responses are extensor. In the most advanced cases the corneal and gag reflexes may also be abolished. Ordinarily the pupillary light reflex is retained in severe intoxication and is lost only if the patient is asphyxiated. In the early hours of coma, there may be a phase of rigidity of the limbs, hyperactive reflexes, ankle clonus, extensor plantar signs, and decerebrate posturing; persistence of these signs indicates a severe degree of anoxia. The temperature may be subnormal, the pulse thready and rapid, and the blood pressure at shock levels.

Diagnosis The diagnosis of barbiturate intoxication is made from the history and physical findings. If a reasonable suspicion of the diagnosis exists, a careful search for drugs or their containers may be rewarding. One should also examine the mouth and gastric contents for any characteristically colored capsules. Acute barbiturate intoxication which presents as a state of coma must be distinguished from other forms of coma by the methods outlined in Chap. 20, "Coma and Related Disturbances of Consciousness." Actually there are few conditions other than barbiturate intoxication which cause a flaccid coma with reactive pupils, hypothermia, and hypotension. Glutethimide poisoning may produce an identical clinical picture, excepting that the pupils are always fixed (a parasympathomimetic action). Laryngeal spasm and sudden apnea also characterize glutethimide intoxication. In the differential diagnosis, hysteria presents the main problem.

The use of gas chromatography has provided a reliable means of identifying the type and amount of barbiturate in the blood. The major virtue of this method is in determining the precise cause of coma when this is in question. The blood level also helps to identify the drug as long- or short-acting, thus giving information as to whether the therapeutic problem will be short or prolonged. A blood barbiturate level of 2 mg per 100 ml in a *comatose* patient is usually due to poisoning with secobarbital or pentobarbital; although the immediate mortality is high in such instances, the therapeutic problem will be short. A level of 11.5 to 12.0 mg per 100 ml is usually due to poisoning with barbital or phenobarbital, and the comatose state will be prolonged. Because of the additive effects of alcohol, a patient who has ingested both drugs may be comatose with relatively low blood barbiturate levels. For this reason, and also because of differences in individual tolerance, the correlation between blood barbiturate levels and depth of coma is not entirely dependable.

The *electroencephalogram* may also be useful in diagnosis, since characteristic patterns accompany barbiturate intoxication (Chap. 364). In mild intoxication, the normal activity is replaced by fast activity, in the range of 20 to 30 Hz, appearing first in the frontal regions and spreading to the parietal and occipital regions as intoxication worsens. In more severe intoxication, the fast waves become less regular and interspersed with 3- to 4-Hz slow activity. In still more advanced cases, there are short periods of suppression of all activity, separated by bursts of slow (delta) waves of variable frequency. In extreme overdosage, all electrical activity ceases. This is one instance in which a "flat" EEG cannot be equated with brain death, and the effects are fully reversible, unless anoxic damage has supervened.

MANAGEMENT The management of acute barbiturate intoxication depends on its severity. In mild or moderate intoxication, recovery is the rule, and no vigorous treatment is required. If the type and amount of ingested drug cannot be ascertained, it is important to empty the stomach and analyze its contents. In the responsive patient, gastric lavage with a large tube is difficult, and a simpler procedure is to induce vomiting with syrup of ipecac. Once this has been accomplished, the patient should be checked at frequent intervals for signs of deepening stupor and coma. If the patient is unresponsive, special attention should be given to maintaining respiration and urinary excretion and to the prevention of infection. It is most important to establish a patent airway by the insertion of an endotracheal tube; suctioning should be used when necessary, and the patient should be turned frequently. Tracheotomy and bronchoscopic suctioning usually become necessary if atelectasis becomes manifest, or if intubation must be maintained for longer than 48 h. If there is any risk of respiratory depression or underventilation, it is advisable to support respiration, so as to provide adequate oxygenation and minimize the risk of atelectasis. Also, early on, an intravenous fluid system should be established to promote the renal clearance of drug and permit rapid administration of drugs and electrolytes. In the unresponsive, intubated patient gastric lavage may be a useful therapeutic as well as a diagnostic measure. It must be performed within several hours of ingestion of the drug, since barbiturates are absorbed rapidly and completely.

Cases of severe respiratory depression, with cyanosis and pupillary dilatation, represent a serious medical emergency. A clear airway should be secured immediately, and some form of assisted respiration begun with an automatic intermittent positive-pressure respirator. If the patient is in shock, the foot of the bed should be elevated, and norepinephrine and whole blood or plasma administered. Catheterization is required to determine the adequacy of urinary output, to obtain samples for laboratory examination, and to prevent distention of the bladder. Since the amount of barbiturate cleared by the kidney is directly proportional to the amount of urine formed, 8 to 10 liters of 5% glucose in saline solution should be given daily. Forced diuresis is also important because toxic amounts of barbiturate have an antidiuretic effect. Coma of any significant duration requires the administration of other electrolytes as well, the amounts being governed by their serum and urinary values. The occurrence of pulmonary and urinary infections calls for the use of appropriate antibiotic treatment.

Hemodialysis has proved to be an effective form of therapy and should be used in all patients with profound coma who fail to respond to the measures outlined above. It is particularly useful in cases of coma due to long-acting barbiturates and is mandatory if anuria or uremia has developed.

The treatment of severe barbiturate intoxication with analeptic drugs (Metrazol, picrotoxin, Megimide), which enjoyed a brief period of popularity, has been generally abandoned. These drugs are antagonistic to barbiturates only insofar as they are powerful cortical stimulants as well as overall nervous system excitants; they do not affect the rate of metabolism or excretion of barbiturate. Alkalinization of the blood by the use of large amounts of bicarbonate solution, as a means of mobilizing the barbiturate and increasing its rate of excretion, seems to be a useful measure, particularly where phenobarbital is the responsible agent.

Occasionally, in the case of a barbiturate addict who has taken an overdose of the drug, recovery from acute intoxication is followed by the development of abstinence symptoms, which have to be managed by the methods outlined below.

CHRONIC BARBITURATE INTOXICATION Barbiturate addiction The problem of chronic barbiturate intoxication is quite different from that of acute intoxication, because of the phenomena of tolerance and addiction as well as the effects of withdrawal of drugs. In these respects there is a close similarity to the problems of opioid and alcohol addiction.

Chronic barbiturate intoxication, like other addictions, tends to develop on a background of some psychiatric disorder, most commonly depression or psychoneurosis with symptoms of anxiety and insomnia, or so-called "character disorder." The drug is usually prescribed for nervousness and insomnia; as the desired effects are lost, the patient increases the dose gradually until he is taking an amount sufficient to produce symptoms when it is withdrawn. Individuals with character disorders are usually introduced to the drug by associates; since the drug is taken for its intoxicating effect, the dose tends to be increased rapidly. Addiction to alcohol or to opiates may predispose to barbiturate addiction. Alcoholics find that barbiturates effectively relieve their nervousness and tremor (cross tolerance); then they may continue to take both alcohol and barbiturates, or the barbiturates may replace the alcohol. Heroin and morphine addicts may turn to barbiturates when they are unable to obtain opiates. As with other addicting drugs, the incidence of barbiturism is particularly high in individuals with ready access to drugs, such as physicians, pharmacists, and nurses.

The symptoms and signs of chronic barbiturate intoxication may be described in relation to (1) the toxic effects of the drug, (2) the development of tolerance, and (3) the effects of sudden withdrawal of the drug after a period of prolonged intoxication.

The toxic manifestations of chronic barbiturism are much the same as those of mild acute barbiturate or alcohol intoxication. The barbiturate addict thinks slowly, shows an increased emotional lability, and becomes untidy in his dress and personal habits. The neurological signs are quite characteristic and include dysarthria, nystagmus, and cerebellar incoordination. Both the mental and neurological signs fluctuate greatly, being more severe if the drug is taken in the fasting state and tending to increase during the day as more of the drug is ingested. If the dosage is elevated rapidly, the signs of moderate or severe intoxication become manifest.

A characteristic feature of chronic barbiturate intoxication is the development of tolerance, sometimes striking in degree. The average addict will ingest about 1.5 g daily of a potent barbiturate and will not develop signs of severe intoxication unless this amount is exceeded. Tolerance to barbiturates does not develop as rapidly as to opiates. Daily doses of 2 g have been reached, but this takes many months. Individual variations in the degree of tolerance make it difficult to state precisely the minimal amount of drug which must be ingested before the resulting condition is designated as chronic barbiturate intoxication. Most persons can ingest 0.4 g daily for as long as 3 months without developing major withdrawal signs (seizures or delirium). With a dosage of 0.8 g daily, the efficiency at all tasks is greatly reduced, and after the daily ingestion of this amount for a period of 2 months, abrupt withdrawal will result in serious symptoms in the majority of patients. Even after 2 weeks at this dosage, some patients will show mild withdrawal symptoms and paroxysmal electroencephalographic changes with photic stimulation. Individuals

taking 0.4 to 0.7 g daily fall into an intermediate category; practically all show some mental dulling, and episodes of forgetfulness and occasionally severe withdrawal symptoms may occur.

Abstinence or withdrawal syndrome Following the withdrawal of barbiturates from chronically intoxicated individuals, a characteristic sequence of symptoms occurs. Immediately following withdrawal patients seemingly improve over a period of 8 to 12 h as they lose the symptoms of intoxication. After this short period a new group of symptoms appears, consisting of nervousness, tremor, postural hypotension, weakness, and generalized seizures. With phenobarbital or barbital, the onset of withdrawal symptoms may not occur until 48 to 72 h after the final dose. Seizures usually occur between the second and fourth days of abstinence, occasionally as long as 6 or 7 days after withdrawal. There may be a single seizure, several, or rarely status epilepticus. The convulsive phase may be followed directly by a delusional-hallucinatory state or a full-blown delirium, indistinguishable from delirium tremens, or a varying degree of improvement may follow the seizures, before the delirium becomes manifest. Death has been reported under these circumstances. The abstinence or withdrawal syndrome may occur in varying degrees of completeness; some patients have seizures and recover without developing delirium, and others have a delirium without preceding seizures. The abrupt onset of seizures or an acute psychosis in adult life should always raise the suspicion of addiction to barbiturates or other sedative-hypnotic drugs and withdrawal effects.

The electroencephalogram (EEG) shows a number of changes during chronic barbiturate intoxication and following withdrawal. During chronic intoxication, the predominant pattern is that of fast activity of moderate voltage, interspersed with some 6- to 8-Hz activity chiefly in the frontal and parietal regions. The EEG findings do not correlate closely with the degree of intoxication, but some subjects do develop "EEG tolerance," i.e., a disappearance of the fast activity while receiving moderate doses of barbiturate (400 mg daily for 90 days). On withdrawal of barbiturates the fast activity diminishes. Also in the first few days of abstinence, paroxysmal bursts of mixed spike and slow waves or 4-Hz "spike and dome" paroxysmal discharges may occur, not necessarily associated with seizures. Characteristically, in the withdrawal period, there is a greatly heightened sensitivity to photic stimulation, to which the patient responds with myoclonus or a seizure, accompanied by paroxysmal changes in the EEG. Most of these abnormalities disappear after 4 or 5 days, and the EEG pattern is usually completely normal in 2 weeks.

TREATMENT OF CHRONIC BARBITURATE INTOXICATION This should always be carried out in the hospital. If the diagnosis of addiction is made before signs of abstinence have appeared, the first step in treatment should be the determination of the "stabilization dosage." This is the amount of short-acting barbiturate required to produce mild symptoms of intoxication (nystagmus, slight ataxia, and dysarthria). Usually 0.2 g pentobarbital given orally every 6 h is sufficient for this purpose. The patient is examined 1 h after each dose. If the signs of intoxication are severe, the next scheduled dose is reduced or omitted. If, instead, tremulousness and postural tachycardia appear, an additional 0.1 g pentobarbital is given and the next scheduled dose is increased. This method is preferable to a blind reduction of dosage, since patients frequently underestimate the amount of drug taken. In such patients, establishment of the "stabilization dosage" may have diagnostic as well as therapeutic value. A patient who can take 0.8 g or more pentobarbital daily, without developing signs of intoxication, is probably physically dependent on drugs of this type. Then a gradual withdrawal of the drug is undertaken, 0.1 g daily. The reduction is stopped for several days if abstinence symptoms appear.

An alternate method of managing barbiturate addiction is to stabilize the patient with phenobarbital rather than pentobarbital. The longer-acting barbiturate is safer than the shorter-acting ones and permits a withdrawal characterized by fewer fluctuations in blood levels (Wesson and Smith). The initial dosage of phenobarbital is calculated by substituting one sedative dose (30 mg) of phenobarbital for each hypnotic dose (100 mg) of the short-acting barbiturate which the patient had been using.

With either of these methods a severely addicted person can achieve abstinence in 14 to 21 days. Patients undergoing withdrawal treatment require careful observation for symptoms of abstinence, and special precautions have to be taken to prevent the smuggling or concealment of drugs.

If the patient presents with severe withdrawal symptoms, such as seizures, he should be given 0.3 to 0.5 g Luminal sodium intramuscularly and then enough to maintain a state of mild intoxication. Most anticonvulsant medicines have been shown to be ineffective against barbiturate withdrawal convulsions. Withdrawal should then be carried out as indicated above. If the abstinence symptoms are not severe, it is not necessary to reintoxicate the patient, but treatment can proceed along the lines laid down for the delirious and confused patient (Chap. 21).

After recovery has taken place, whether from symptoms of chronic intoxication or withdrawal or from acute intoxication due to attempted suicide, the psychiatric problem requires evaluation and an appropriate plan of therapy. Many of the considerations in the management of alcoholism are equally applicable to the patient addicted to barbiturate or nonbarbiturate hypnotic drugs (Chap. 226, "Alcohol").

BARBITURATE PROVOCATION OF OTHER DISEASES At times the administration of one of the barbiturates may induce an attack of another disease. The most striking example of this is in hereditary porphyria where a severe and sometimes fatal outbreak of abdominal pain, psychosis, and polyneuropathy may follow the ingestion of a few capsules of Seconal (see Chap. 96). With severe liver disease, detoxification of barbiturates may be impaired, as is discussed in Chap. 299.

REFERENCES

BLOOMER HA, MADDOCK RK JR: An assessment of diuresis and dialysis for treating acute barbiturate poisoning, in *Acute Barbiturate Poisoning*, H Mathew (ed). Amsterdam, Excerpta Medica, 1971, chap 15

CLEMMESEN C, NILSSON E: Therapeutic trends in the treatment of barbiturate poisoning: The Scandinavian method. Clin Pharmacol Ther 2:220, 1961

DOMESTIC COUNCIL DRUG ABUSE TASK FORCE: *White Paper on Drug Abuse*. Washington, DC, US Government Printing Office, September 1975

ESSIG C: Chronic abuse of sedative-hypnotic drugs, in *Drug Abuse*, CJD Zarafonetis (ed). Philadelphia, Lea & Febiger, 1972, p 205

HARVEY SC: Hypnotics and sedatives. The barbiturates, in *The Pharmacological Basis of Therapeutics*, 5th ed, LS Goodman, A Gilman (eds). New York, Macmillan, 1975, chap 9

ISBELL H et al: Chronic barbiturate intoxication: An experimental study. Arch Neurol Psychiatry 64:1, 1950

PLUM F, SWANSON AC: Barbiturate poisoning treated by physiological methods. JAMA 163:827, 1957

WESSON DR, SMITH DE: *Barbiturates: Their Use, Misuse and Abuse*. New York, Human Sciences Press, 1977

229

NONBARBITURATE SEDATIVE-HYPNOTICS; PSYCHOTHERAPEUTIC, STIMULANT, AND PSYCHOTOGENIC DRUGS

MAURICE VICTOR
RAYMOND D. ADAMS

SEDATIVE-HYPNOTIC DRUGS

This class of drugs, also referred to as *depressants,* may be divided into two main groups. The first includes the barbiturates (Chap. 228), the bromides, chloral hydrate, and paraldehyde. In the past 15 years these drugs have been largely displaced by a second group of sedative-hypnotics, comprising meprobamate and other glycerol derivates, and the benzodiazepines, the most important of which are chlordiazepoxide (Librium) and diazepam (Valium). Indeed, the benzodiazepines are the most commonly prescribed drugs in the world today. Their advantages over the older sedatives and hypnotics are their *relatively* low toxicity and addictive potential and their minimal interactions with other drugs.

BROMIDES Bromides are now seldom prescribed by physicians but are contained in certain "nerve tonics" and proprietary remedies (Nervine, Neurosine), so that cases of bromide intoxication are encountered with some regularity. Acute poisoning with bromide is rare because large doses of the drug are irritating to the gastric mucosa, and vomiting prevents the attainment of significant blood levels. Taken in smaller doses, however, bromide tends to accumulate in the body because of its slow excretion by the kidneys, and toxic symptoms may appear in a matter of weeks. These symptoms are caused by the bromide ion itself and are not simply a reflection of a decrease in chloride due to the displacement of the chloride by the bromide ion.

The symptoms of chronic bromide intoxication are predominantly in the mental sphere and range from dizziness, drowsiness, irritability, and emotional lability to a quiet confusional state, with impairment of thinking and memory and, in severe cases, to delirium and mania or stupor and coma. Skin manifestations are associated in many cases, taking the form usually of acne-like eruption and less frequently of proliferative nodular lesions, resembling those of tertiary syphilis. Headache, mild conjunctivitis, gastric distress, anorexia, and constipation may be associated. The blood bromide levels and the severity of toxic symptoms do not necessarily correspond. As a general rule, levels of 75 mg per 100 ml (9 meq per liter) or more are considered abnormal and diagnostic of bromism, if the clinical picture suggests it. However, higher levels are sometimes well tolerated, and symptoms of bromism may persist for some days even after the blood levels have been reduced to normal or near-normal levels.

Treatment consists of removing the source of bromide and administering sodium chloride (at least 6 g daily, in divided doses). Ammonium chloride may be substituted if an accumulation of sodium is to be avoided and if there is no danger of an uncompensated acidosis or hepatic failure. Confused or delirious patients require sedation, and anorectic and emaciated patients need careful nursing care and special attention to diet. The administration of a mercurial or thiazide diuretic serves to promote a bromide diuresis. Hemodialysis is an effective means of removing bromide and should be utilized in the most severe cases of intoxication.

CHLORAL HYDRATE This is the oldest and at the same time one of the safest, most effective, and cheapest of the sedative-hypnotic drugs. After oral administration, chloral hydrate is reduced rapidly to trichloroethanol, which is the agent responsible for the depressant effects on the central nervous system. A significant portion of the trichloroethanol is excreted in the urine as the glucuronide, which may give a false positive test for glucose.

In large doses, chloral hydrate is toxic to the heart, kidneys, and liver, but only in the presence of preexisting disease in these organs. Chloral hydrate is a strong gastric irritant, so that it requires dilution and should not be taken on an empty stomach. Tolerance and addiction to chloral hydrate develop only rarely, and for these reasons it is an appropriate medication for the management of insomnia, particularly the type which is associated with depression. Poisoning with chloral hydrate is a rare occurrence and resembles acute barbiturate intoxication, except for the finding of miosis, which is said to characterize the former. In combination with alcohol, the well-known "Mickey Finn" or "knockout drops," its effects are additive, leading to a rapid onset of coma. Death from poisoning is due to respiratory depression and hypotension; patients who survive these events may show signs of liver and kidney disease.

PARALDEHYDE This hypnotic is also effective and safe, providing that certain precautions are taken in its preparation and administration. On exposure to light, paraldehyde decomposes to acetaldehyde, which is very toxic, and oxidizes to acetic acid. It must be freshly prepared, therefore, and stored in tightly stoppered, amber-colored bottles. Paraldehyde is unique in that a significant proportion is excreted unchanged through the lungs; the remainder is detoxified in the liver, so that it should be used cautiously in patients with liver disease.

Paraldehyde has a wide margin of safety when administered orally (or rectally), and even three or four times the usual dose of 8 to 10 ml causes no more than prolonged sleep or mild stupor. Intramuscular use of the drug should be avoided because of its propensity to produce sterile abscesses and to damage the sciatic nerve if injected too close to it. Intravenous injections should be made with caution and only in a hospital, because of their unpredictable effects on respiration. The main objections to this drug are its bitter taste (this can be obviated by diluting in fruit juice) and its lingering, unpleasant odor.

Paraldehyde is very effective in suppressing the tremulousness, restlessness, and insomnia that characterize the early phase (6 to 60 h) of the alcohol withdrawal period. Patients with these symptoms make repeated demands for paraldehyde, which is not surprising in view of the pharmacological similarities between this drug and alcohol and the effectiveness of both drugs in suppressing withdrawal symptoms. This should not present a problem in management, however, if the need for the drug is determined before each dose is given and the drug is withdrawn as soon as the agitation and tremor are under control. Should a relapse from abstinence then occur, substitution of paraldehyde for alcohol rarely if ever occurs.

BENZODIAZEPINE GROUP The foregoing drugs have been replaced to a large extent by two drugs, chlordiazepoxide (Librium) and diazepam (Valium). These latter drugs have been used extensively to control anxiety, and they are probably more effective than the barbiturates in this respect. They have also been used to control overactivity and destructive behavior in children and the symptoms of alcohol withdrawal. Diazepam is particularly useful in the treatment of delirious patients who require parenteral medication. The benzodiazepines possess anticonvulsant properties, and the intravenous use of diazepam is an effective means of controlling status epilepticus, as indicated in Chap. 23. In addition, diazepam has been used with moderate success in the treatment of certain extrapyramidal movement disorders and dystonic spasms.

Other widely used benzodiazepine drugs are flurazepam (Dalmane), which is useful in the treatment of insomnia (see Chap 22), and carbamazepine (Tegretol), which now has a definite place in the treatment of seizures, especially those of temporal-lobe origin with behavioral abnormalities, and tic douloureux (Chap. 376). Two newer members of this group, clonazepam and nitrazepam, have also proved to be useful in the management of seizure disorders.

The benzodiazepine drugs, while comparatively safe in the recommended dosages, are far from ideal. They frequently cause unsteadiness of gait and drowsiness and at times hypotension and syncope, particularly in the elderly. In severely disturbed schizophrenic patients, rage, hostility, uncontrollable excitement, confusion, and depersonalization may develop. Nausea, diminished libido, headache, skin rashes, leukopenia, eosinophilia, agranulocytosis, and enhancement of the effects of alcohol have all been reported but are rare. Additional central nervous effects are slurred speech, dysphagia, ataxia, confusion, and faulty memory.

CARBONIC ACID DERIVATIVES These drugs are capable of modest depressant action and are appropriate for relieving mild degrees of nervousness, anxiety, and muscle tension, although they have no advantage over the barbiturates. Maximal action occurs with relatively small doses. Meprobamate (Equanil, Miltown) is the best-known member of this group. With typical doses (400 mg, three or four times a day) the patient is able to function quite effectively; large doses cause ataxia, drowsiness, stupor, coma, and vasomotor collapse. Hypersensitivity reactions in the form of fever, pruritis, and erythematous, maculopapular, and occasionally urticarial or bullous eruptions have been reported. Cutaneous petechiae or ecchymoses may also occur, without thrombocytopenia. Diplopia, syncope, menstrual irregularities, angioneurotic edema, peripheral edema, leukopenia, thrombocytopenia, and pancytopenia are other rare complications.

It should be emphasized that addiction to meprobamate, though reported infrequently, does occur, and if four or more times the daily recommended dose is taken over a period of weeks to months, withdrawal symptoms (including convulsions) may appear, resembling those which follow withdrawal of barbiturate in chronically intoxicated patients. Several other nonbarbiturate sedative-hypnotic drugs, when taken in increasingly large doses, have the same liability. These drugs are glutethimide (Doriden), ethinamate (Valmid), ethchlorvynol (Placidyl), methyprylon (Noludar), chlordiazepoxide (Librium), diazepam (Valium), methaqualone (Quaalude), and perhaps oxazepam (Serax). As with the barbiturates, the toxic effects consist of slurred speech, nystagmus, ataxic gait, drowsiness, confusion, and coma. Also upon withdrawal of these drugs, hallucinations, seizures, and delirium, symptoms indistinguishable from those of the barbiturate and alcohol withdrawal syndrome, may appear. There have been occasional reports of death following the withdrawal of meprobamate, methyprylon, and diazepam in persons who had been taking large doses of these drugs for protracted periods. In view of these observations, physicians must exercise caution in prescribing new sedative drugs which are continually being introduced and which are said to possess no addicting or habit-forming properties.

The management of patients addicted to nonbarbiturate sedative-hypnotics follows the lines indicated in Chap. 228 under "Barbiturate Addiction." Thus, if the drug and its dosage can be determined, it should be withdrawn at the rate of one therapeutic dose per day. Should abstinence symptoms appear, the reduction in dosage is stopped for several days. If the offending drug cannot be identified, a barbiturate such as Seconal should be administered to the point of mild intoxication and then withdrawn, in the manner indicated in Chap. 228. It should be noted that phenytoin (Dilantin) and phenothiazine derivatives are not effective against abstinence convulsions.

ANTIPSYCHOTIC DRUGS

Since the mid-1950s, a large series of pharmacological agents, loosely referred to as *tranquilizers* (because of their sedative properties), has come into prominent use. They are also referred to as *neuroleptics* because of their ability to increase motor activity in some patients. Mainly these drugs are used for the control of schizophrenia and to a lesser extent for psychotic states associated with organic brain syndromes, and certain instances of manic-depressive disease. The mechanism by which these drugs ameliorate disturbances of thought and affect in these psychotic states is poorly understood but has been attributed to their ability to inhibit or partially block transmission in dopaminergic pathways in the brain. Probably their parkinsonian side effects are attributable to blockade of the dopaminergic striatonigral pathways.

A large number of antipsychotic drugs are on the market (almost two hundred have been given generic names), and no attempt will be made here to describe or even list all. Some have had only an evanescent popularity, and others have yet to prove their value. Chemically these compounds form a heterogeneous group, but six categories are of particular clinical importance: (1) the phenothiazines, (2) the thioxanthines, (3) the butyrophenones, and (4) the *Rauwolfia* alkaloids; (5) an indole derivative, molindone (Moban), and (6) a dibenzoxazepine derivative, loxapine (Loxitane), have been introduced only recently. Experience to date indicates that in the management of schizophrenia, molindone and loxapine are about as effective as the phenothiazines, and their side effects are also the same. The main use of the newer antipsychotic drugs is in patients who are not responsive to the older ones or who suffer intolerable side effects from them. A new antipsychotic agent, clozapine (a dibenzodiazepine derivative), is of great current interest since it appears to be uniquely free of extrapyramidal side effects. Clozapine, metiapine, and timozide (a diphenylbutylpiperidine) are presently under investigation in the United States.

PHENOTHIAZINES This group comprises some of the most widely used tranquilizers such as chlorpromazine (Thorazine, Largactil), promazine (Sparine), triflupromazine (Vesprin), prochlorperazine (Compazine), perphenazine (Trilafon), fluphenazine (Permitil, Prolixin), thioridazine (Mellaril), and trifluoperazine (Stelazine). In addition to their psychotherapeutic effects, these drugs have a number of other actions, so that certain members of this group are used as antiemetics (prochlorperazine) and antihistaminics (promethazine).

The phenothiazines have had their widest application in the treatment of the psychoses (schizophrenia and to a lesser extent manic-depressive psychosis). Their use outside psychiatry should be discouraged. Under the influence of these drugs, many patients who would otherwise be hospitalized are able to live at home and even work productively. And the use of these drugs has greatly facilitated the hospital care of hyperactive and combative patients.

Side effects of the phenothiazines are frequent and often serious. All of them may cause a cholestatic type of jaundice, agranulocytosis, convulsive seizures, orthostatic hypotension, skin sensitivity reactions, mental depression, disorientation and hallucinations, and disorders of the extrapyramidal motor system. Jaundice and blood dyscrasias have occurred less often with prochlorperazine, perphenazine, and fluphenazine than with other members of the group, but the extrapyramidal side effects have been relatively more pronounced. Several types of extrapyramidal symptoms have been noted.

1 A parkinsonian syndrome—masked facies, tremor, generalized rigidity, shuffling gait, and slowness of movement; these symptoms appear after several weeks of drug therapy.

2 Muscle spasms and dystonia, taking the form of involuntary movements of facial muscles and protrusion of the tongue (so-called buccolingual or oral masticatory syndrome), dysphagia, torticollis and retrocollis, oculogyric crises, and tonic spasms of a limb (dyskinesias); these complications usually occur early in the administration of the drug, sometimes after the initial dose, and often can be improved dramatically by the intravenous administration of diphenhydramine hydrochloride (Benadryl).

3 An inability to sit still and an inner restlessness, so that the patient paces the floor constantly (akathisia).

4 Lingual-facial-buccal dyskinesia, restlessness, and choreoathetotic movements of the trunk and limbs may occur as late and persistent complications (tardive dyskinesia) of long-term therapy with phenothiazines or haloperidol.

These extrapyramidal reactions must be recognized at once and the medication discontinued, but even then the disorder may persist for weeks or months, and often permanently. Administration of antiparkinsonian drugs of the anticholinergic type (trihexyphenidyl, procyclidine, benztropine) may hasten the recovery from some of the symptoms. Oral, lingual, and laryngeal dyskinesias are affected relatively little by any of the antiparkinsonian drugs. Sometimes, however, one such medication has a better effect than another. Amantadine (Symmetrel) in doses of 50 to 100 mg tid has been useful in some cases of postphenothiazine dyskinesia. Chlorprothixene (Taractan), a *thioxanthene* drug with effects similar to the phenothiazines, and thioridazine (Mellaril), although not the best tranquilizing agents, are favored by some because of their lesser tendency to produce symptoms of extrapyramidal motor disorder. The latter drug, however, if given in large doses over a period of time, may cause deposits in the macula of the retina with resulting visual impairment.

BUTYROPHENONES These drugs (haloperidol, trifluperidol) have much the same antipsychotic effects as the phenothiazines, as well as the same side effects. Unlike the phenothiazines, they have little or no adrenergic blocking action. The butyrophenones are effective substitutes for the phenothiazines in patients who are intolerant to the latter drugs, particularly to their autonomic effects.

RESERPINE This is the prototype of the *Rauwolfia* alkaloids. It was in relation to the sedative effects of these drugs that the term *tranquilization* was used for the first time. These drugs, so effective in controlling hypertension, are no longer recommended for the treatment of mental disorders, except perhaps in patients who cannot tolerate phenothiazines. When given in therapeutic doses, the *Rauwolfia* alkaloids often provoke a parkinsonian syndrome or a serious depression of mood, which may prove more troublesome than the disorder for which they were prescribed.

Meprobamate, chlordiazepoxide, and diazepam are often referred to as "minor tranquilizers," the implication being that these drugs share the properties of the "major tranquilizers" or antipsychotic drugs. This is not the case. The so-called "minor tranquilizers" differ from the antipsychotics in both their chemical structure and pharmacologic effects. In fact, the minor tranquilizers more closely resemble the barbiturates in their pharmacologic (depressant) effects (including the ability to produce tolerance and physical dependence) and are more appropriately referred to as *antianxiety* drugs.

It hardly need be pointed out that the tranquilizing drugs have been much abused. This would be suspected just from the frequency with which they are being prescribed. It is stated that in the decade 1955 to 1965, 50 million patients in the United States received chlorpromazine alone. These powerful medications have specific indications, noted above, and the physician should be certain of the diagnosis before using them. The fact that these drugs can produce tardive dyskinesia in nonpsychotic patients is reason enough not to use them for nervousness, apprehension, anxiety, mild depression, and the many normal psychological reactions to trying environmental circumstances. These drugs are not curative, but only suppress or partially alleviate symptoms, and they should not serve as a substitute for, or divert the physician from, the use of other measures for the relief of the abnormal mental state.

ANTIDEPRESSANT DRUGS

Two classes of drugs—the monoamine oxidase (MAO) inhibitors and dibenzazepine derivatives—are particularly useful in the treatment of depression. The adjective *antidepressant* refers to their therapeutic effect and is used here in deference to common clinical practice. *Antidepressive* or *antidepression* drugs would be preferable terms since *depressant* still has a pharmacological connotation which does not necessarily equate with the therapeutic effect. For example, barbiturates and chloral hydrate, which may ameliorate the symptoms of depression, are in fact depressants in the pharmacological sense but act as mood elevators or antidepressants. The meaning of these terms must not be confused, for reference is made on the one hand to a drug that reduces nervous system excitability and on the other to the capacity of the drug to ameliorate the symptoms of mental depression.

MONOAMINE OXIDASE INHIBITORS The observation that iproniazid, an inhibitor of MAO, had a mood-elevating effect in tuberculous patients initiated a great deal of interest in compounds of this type and led quickly to their exploitation in the treatment of depression. Iproniazid (Marsilid) proved exceedingly toxic and was soon taken off the market, as have several more recently developed MAO inhibitors; but other drugs, much better tolerated, have become available. These include isocarboxizid (Marplan), nialamide (Niamid), phenelzine (Nardil), and tranylcypromine (Parnate), the latter two being the most frequently used. Tranylcypromine has proved to be the most potent of these agents, but it has also produced the most serious toxic effects.

The exact mode of action of the MAO inhibitors has not been determined. They have in common the ability to block the oxidative deamination of naturally occurring amines (norepinephrine, epinephrine, and serotonin), and it has been suggested that the accumulation of these neurohormonal substances is responsible for the antidepressant effect. However, these drugs inhibit many enzymes other than monoamine oxidases and have numerous actions unrelated to enzyme inhibition. Furthermore, many agents with antidepressant effects like those of the monoamine oxidase inhibitors do not inhibit this enzyme. At the present time, one cannot assume that the therapeutic effect of these drugs has a direct relation to the property of MAO inhibition.

These drugs must be dispensed with great caution and a constant awareness of their potentially serious side effects. They may at times cause excitement, restlessness, agitation, insomnia, and anxiety; occasionally, with the usual dose and more often with an overdose, mania and convulsions may occur (especially in epileptic patients). Other side effects are increased neuromuscular activity in the form of muscle twitching and involuntary movement of an extremity, urinary retention, skin rashes, tachycardia, hepatic disturbance, jaundice, visual impairment, enhancement of glaucoma, impotence, sweating, muscle spasms, and a variety of paresthesias. Orthostatic hypotension of a serious degree may develop.

Patients taking MAO inhibitors must be warned against the use of dibenzazepine derivatives (Tofranil and Elavil) and also sympathomimetic amines and tyramine, for they may induce a severe hypertensive episode and cerebral vascular accident, headache, atrial and ventricular arrhythmia, pulmonary edema, and even death. Sympathomimetic amines are contained in some of the commonly used nasal sprays, nose drops, and so-called "coryza tablets," and in tyramine-containing foods (cheeses, yogurt, beer, and wine).

The MAO inhibitors have the ability to potentiate the effect of many other drugs. In particular, phenothiazines and other powerful central nervous system stimulants should not be given with the MAO inhibitors, since severe reactions and occasional fatalities have followed their concomitant use. Exaggerated responses to the usual dose of meperidine (Demerol) and other narcotic drugs have also been observed; respiratory function may be depressed to a serious degree, and hyperpyrexia, agitation, and pronounced hypotension may occur as well, sometimes with fatal issue. Unpredictable side effects may also accompany the simultaneous administration of barbiturates and MAO inhibitors.

DIBENZAZEPINE DERIVATIVES (TRICYCLIC ANTIDEPRESSANTS) Soon after the first convincing successes in the treatment of depression with MAO inhibitors, a new class of tricyclic compounds appeared. The first of this group was imipramine (Tofranil), which was soon followed by amitriptyline (Elavil), and then by desipramine (Norpramin), nortriptyline (Aventyl), protriptyline (Vivactil, Triptil), and doxepin (Sinequan). The first two members of this group have proved to be the most popular.

The exact mode of action of these agents is unknown, but there is evidence that these agents inhibit re-uptake of norepinephrine by adrenergic nerve terminals, and their antidepressant effect has been attributed to this action. In the absence of other considerations, they are presently the most effective drugs for the treatment of patients with depressive illnesses, particularly those with retarded depressions, that are associated with insomnia (early morning awakening), decreased appetite, weight loss and decreased libido. Persistence of their pharmacological effects after the drug is stopped is very short in comparison with the MAO inhibitors, and their side effects are far less frequent and serious.

The tricyclic or dibenzazepine compounds are potent anticholinergic agents, and their most prominent and serious side effects (orthostatic hypotension, urinary bladder weakness) are due to peripheral anticholinergic action. They may also produce central nervous system excitement, leading to insomnia, agitation, and restlessness, but usually these effects are controlled readily by the use of phenothiazines or chlordiazepoxide given concurrently or in the evenings. Occasionally they may cause ataxia and blood dyscrasias. The dibenzazepine drugs should never be given with an MAO inhibitor, since the reactions which may occur are frequently serious; hypertensive crises and lethal hyperpyrexia have been reported. These reactions have allegedly occurred when small doses of imipramine were given to patients who had discontinued the MAO inhibitor 1 week previously.

STIMULANTS

These drugs, which act primarily as stimulants of the central nervous system, have a relatively limited therapeutic use but assume clinical importance for other reasons. Some members of the group, e.g., the amphetamines, are much abused, and others are not infrequent causes of poisoning.

AMPHETAMINES Amphetamine (Benzedrine) and its *d*-isomer, dextroamphetamine, are powerful analeptics and in addition have significant hypertensive, respiratory-stimulant, and appetite-depressant effects. These drugs are useful in the management of narcolepsy, but they are much more widely and indiscriminately used for the control of obesity and the abolition of fatigue. Undoubtedly, the initial effect of a moderate oral dose of amphetamine is to reverse fatigue, postpone the need for sleep, and elevate mood, but these effects are not entirely predictable and certainly not indefinite, and the user must pay for the period of wakefulness with even greater fatigue and often with depression. The intravenous use of a high dose of amphetamine produces an immediate ecstasy, "the flash." Because of the popularity of the amphetamines and ease with which they can be procured, instances of acute and chronic intoxication are observed frequently. Nonetheless, dextroamphetamine in doses of 5 mg morning and noon is a useful agent in the treatment of certain reactive depressions, such as the ones which follow myocardial infarction or stroke, and in suppressing overactivity of children who are impulsive and inattentive. The toxic signs are essentially an exaggeration of the analeptic effects—restlessness, excessive speech and motor activity, tremor, and insomnia. Occasionally grimacing, tic-like, choreoathetotic, and dystonic movements, similar to those produced by the phenothiazines, may develop as an acute idiosyncratic reaction to amphetamine. The chronic administration of large doses of amphetamine may give rise to hallucinations, delusions, and changes in affect and thought processes, a state that may be indistinguishable from paranoid schizophrenia (See Chap. 25). Treatment consists of removal of the offending drug and the administration of antipsychotic drugs. Nitrites may be useful if the blood pressure is markedly elevated.

METHYLPHENIDATE Having much the same type of action as amphetamine, this drug (Ritalin) is useful in the treatment of narcolepsy and, paradoxically, like dextroamphetamine, in the management of overactive children.

PICROTOXIN A powerful nervous system excitant, this drug exerts its main effects by producing convulsive seizures and reversing respiratory depression induced by drugs, particularly by barbiturates. However, the modern treatment of barbiturate intoxication does not include the use of picrotoxin or other analeptics, because of their epileptogenic properties and because barbiturate intoxication can be managed successfully by other means (see Chap. 228). It has been shown by Eccles and his colleagues that picrotoxin increases neuronal activity by blocking presynaptic inhibition, i.e., blocking the action of inhibitory fibers that synapse with the presynaptic terminals of excitatory fibers.

STRYCHNINE The action of strychnine is to increase neuronal excitability by interfering with postsynaptic inhibition; the therapeutic value is negligible. In children accidental poisoning may occur from ingestion of AS&B cathartic pills or "rat biscuits." Very rarely, strychnine is taken with suicidal intent. After a period of heightened irritability and muscle twitching, tonic seizures occur, characterized by opisthotonus, rigid extension of the legs, facial tetanus, and apnea due to spasm of the muscles of respiration. Death from anoxia may follow several seizures. The immediate need, in the treatment of strychnine poisoning, is to control the convulsions. This calls for the intravenous administration of a short-acting barbiturate or the application of inhalation anesthesia, if the appropriate drug is not immediately available; endotracheal intubation is an important safeguard. The patient must then be observed carefully, and if any signs of irritability recur, more sedative should be given. During this period, supportive care is indicated, as for any comatose patient. Morphine, which is principally a medullary depressant, is contraindicated.

PENTYLENETETRAZOL This drug (Metrazol, Cardiazol) is a potent stimulant of all parts of the nervous system. For a number of years it served as the convulsive agent in shock treatment of depression and schizophrenia but was abandoned in favor of less dangerous and more effective forms of convulsive therapy. The use of this drug to activate latent epileptogenic foci or to reproduce convulsions, with the purpose of studying the underlying cerebral mechanisms, although once a common procedure, has been virtually discontinued.

BEMEGRIDE, NIKETHAMIDE These two drugs, the latter with the trade name Coramine, act much like pentylenetetrazol. For many years common clinical practice was to administer nikethamide as a final therapeutic gesture in patients dying of cardiac and respiratory failure, but there is little evidence that the drug has a significant stimulant effect on either heart or respiration. Poisoning with these drugs, which is usually due to parenteral overdosage, is best treated with barbiturates.

CAFFEINE The therapeutic value of caffeine and other xanthine derivatives stems from their diuretic effects and their ability to stimulate the heart and nervous system. The major use of these agents is to abolish fatigue and maintain wakefulness, and the usual mode of administration is in coffee, a cup of which contains 100 to 150 mg caffeine. Overdosage leads to insomnia, tremulousness, mild delirium, tinnitus, tachycardia, prominent diuresis, and cardiac arrhythmias. The excitatory effects are easily controlled with barbiturates, and fatalities due to caffeine poisoning are extremely rare.

CAMPHOR Formerly a popular stimulant, camphor is now rarely used therapeutically; however, occasional cases of poisoning are still seen as a result of ingestion of liniment (camphorated oil) or moth flakes. The manifestations of poisoning are headache, sensation of warmth, confusion, clonic convulsions, and terminal respiratory depression; the characteristic odor of camphor facilitates the diagnosis. Treatment consists of supportive care and the cautious use of barbiturates to combat convulsions.

PSYCHOTOGENIC DRUGS

Included in this category are a heterogeneous group of drugs, the primary effect of which is to alter perception, mood, and thinking out of proportion to other aspects of cognitive function and consciousness. This group of drugs comprises lysergic acid derivatives, e.g., lysergic acid diethylamide (LSD); phenylethylamine derivatives (mescaline and peyote); psilocybin; certain indolic derivatives, *Cannabis* (marijuana), and a number of less important compounds. They are also referred to as psychotomimetic drugs, hallucinogens, illusinogens, and psychedelics, but none of these names is entirely suitable.

Tolerance to LSD, mescaline, psilocybin, and other psychotogenic drugs develops rapidly, even on a once-daily dosage. Furthermore, subjects tolerant to any one of these three specific drugs are cross-tolerant to the other two. Tolerance is lost rapidly when these drugs are discontinued abruptly, but no abstinence syndromes ensue. In this sense, addiction does not develop, although users may become dependent upon them for emotional support. In the case of marijuana, reverse tolerance (i.e., increasing sensitization) may be observed initially, but on continued use, tolerance to the euphoriant effects of the drug has been observed in one of the few chronic experimental studies that have been made, and the subjects reported jitteriness during the first 24 h after abrupt cessation of marijuana smoking, although no objective withdrawal signs could be detected.

LSD, MESCALINE, PSILOCYBIN These drugs produce much the same clinical effects if given in comparable amounts. The perceptual changes are the most dramatic—the user describes vivid visual hallucinations, alterations in the shape and color of objects, unusual dreams, and feelings of depersonalization. An increase in auditory acuity has been described, but auditory hallucinations are rare. Cognitive functions are difficult to assess because of inattention, drowsiness, and inability to concentrate and to cooperate in mental testing. The somatic symptoms consist of dizziness, nausea, drowsiness, paresthesias, and blurring of vision. Sympathomimetic effects—pupillary dilatation, piloerection, hyperthermia, and tachycardia—are prominent, and the user may also show hyperreflexia, incoordination of the limbs, and ataxia.

MARIJUANA When taken by inhaling the smoke from cigarettes, marijuana produces effects which are prompt in onset and evanescent. In low doses the symptoms are like those of mild intoxication with alcohol. With increasing amounts of the drug, the effects are similar to those of LSD, mescaline, and psilocybin, and they may be quite disabling for many hours. Very large doses result in severe depression and stupor, but death is unusual.

The fact that small quantities of these drugs can produce gross mental aberrations has stimulated the search for similar but endogenous substances that may be responsible for schizophrenia and other psychoses. The mechanisms involved in producing and antagonizing the psychotomimetic effects are also being studied intensively, in the hope of elucidating the mechanisms of the psychoses and finding improved psychotherapeutic agents. Doubtless these studies are adding greatly to our knowledge of abnormal behavior, but the fundamental problems remain to be solved.

Numerous claims have been made that LSD and related drugs are effective in the treatment of mental disease and a wide variety of social ills and that they have the capacity to increase one's intellectual performance, creativity, and self-understanding. At this time, there are no acceptable studies that validate any of these claims.

LSD is not yet an approved drug, and use of marijuana is governed by the federal narcotic laws. Nevertheless, these drugs are very widely used. They are taken by narcotic addicts as a temporary substitute for more potent drugs, by "drug heads," i.e., individuals who use literally any agent that alters consciousness, and by many troubled, unhappy college and high-school students, often for reasons that they cannot ascertain. The unsupervised use of these drugs is attended by a number of serious adverse reactions, taking the form of acute panic attacks, long-lasting psychotic states resembling paranoid schizophrenia, "flashbacks" (spontaneous recurrences of the original LSD experience, often precipitated by smoking marijuana and accompanied by panic attacks), or by serious physical injury, consequent upon impairment of the user's critical faculties. Whether prolonged usage leads to permanent damage to the nervous system is not certain; there are some data suggesting that this may happen. The reports claiming that LSD may cause chromosomal damage remain to be validated. A discussion of the legal implications of the illicit use of these drugs and their social impact is beyond the scope of this chapter but can be found in the references cited below.

REFERENCES

BYCK R: Drugs and the treatment of psychiatric disorders, in *The Pharmacological Basis of Therapeutics,* 5th ed, LS Goodman, A Gilman (eds). New York, Macmillan, 1975

DiMASCIO A, SHADER RI (eds): *Clinical Handbook of Psychopharmacology.* New York, Science House, 1970

DiPALMA JR (ed): *Drill's Pharmacology in Medicine.* New York, McGraw-Hill, 1971

HOLLISTER LE: Mental disorders—antianxiety and antidepressant drugs. N Engl J Med 286:1195, 1972

———: *The Clinical Use of Psychotherapeutic Drugs.* Springfield, Ill, Charles C Thomas, 1973

———: Antipsychotic medications and the treatment of schizophrenia, in *Psychopharmacology: From Theory to Practice,* JD Barchas et al (eds). New York, Oxford University Press, 1975, p 121

IVERSEN SD, IVERSEN LL: *Behavioral Pharmacology.* New York, Oxford, 1975

MARKS J: *The Benzodiazepines: Use, Overuse, Misuse, Abuse.* Baltimore, University Park Press, 1978

WIKLER A: The marijuana controversy, in *Marijuana: Effects on Human Behavior.* New York, Academic, 1974, p 25

———: Drug dependence, in *Clinical Neurology,* AB Baker, LH Baker (eds). New York, Harper & Row, 1975

INTRODUCTORY COMMENTS

Since *Principles of Internal Medicine* is a textbook used internationally, in preparing the Appendix we have taken into account the fact that the system of international units (SI, Système international d'unités) is being adopted by many laboratories. To this end, where possible and appropriate, we have expressed common laboratory values in terms of both traditional units and SI units. *Values in SI units appear in brackets* after values in traditional units. The use of SI units in medicine was endorsed by the Thirtieth World Health Assembly (May 1977) with the purpose of implementing an international language of measurement.[1] The SI *base* units, SI *derived* units, and other units of measurement referred to in this Appendix are listed below.

Quantity	Name of unit	Symbol for unit	Derivation of units
SI BASE UNITS			
Length	meter	m	
Mass	kilogram	kg	
Time	second	s	
Thermodynamic temperature	Kelvin	K	
Amount of substance	mole	mol	
SI DERIVED UNITS			
Force	newton	N	$(m \cdot kg)/s^2$
Pressure	pascal	Pa	$N \cdot m^2$
Work, energy	joule	J	$N \cdot m$
Celsius temperature	degree Celsius	°C	K
OTHER UNITS RETAINED FOR USE			
Time	minute	min	
	hour	h	
	day	d	
Volume	liter	L	

[1] The SI for the Health Professions, *Geneva, World Health Organization, 1977.*

TABLE A-1
SI prefixes and their symbols

Factor	Prefix	Symbol for prefix
10^{-1}	deci	d
10^{-2}	centi	c
10^{-3}	milli	m
10^{-6}	micro	μ
10^{-9}	nano	n
10^{-12}	pico	p
10^{-15}	femto	f
10^{-18}	alto	a

ASCITIC FLUID

See Table 40-1, page 210.

BODY FLUIDS AND OTHER MASS DATA

Body fluid, total volume: 50 percent (in obese) to 70 percent (lean) of body weight
  Intracellular: 30 to 40 percent of body weight
  Extracellular: 20 to 30 percent of body weight
Blood:
  Total volume:
    Males: 69 ml per kilogram of body weight
    Females: 65 ml per kilogram of body weight
  Plasma volume:
    Males: 39 ml per kilogram of body weight
    Females: 40 ml per kilogram of body weight
  Red blood cell volume:
    Males: 30 ml per kilogram of body weight (1.15 to 1.21 liters per square meter of body surface area)
    Females: 25 ml per kilogram of body weight

$$meq/liter = \frac{mg/100 \ ml \times 10 \times valence}{atomic \ weight}$$

$$mg/100 \ ml = \frac{meq/liter \times atomic \ weight}{10 \times valence}$$

CEREBROSPINAL FLUID

Cells: < 5 per cubic millimeter, all lymphocytes
Pressure, initial (horizontal position): 7 to 20 cmH$_2$O [0.7 to 2.0 kPa]
Colloidal gold test: not more than 1 to 2 in first few tubes
Creatinine: 0.4 to 1.5 mg per 100 ml [35 to 133 μmol per liter]
Glucose:[2] 44 to 100 mg per 100 ml [2.4 to 5.6 mmol per liter]
pH:[2] 7.34 to 7.43
Protein:
  Lumbar: 14 to 45 mg per 100 ml; γ globulin <12 percent of total protein [0.14 to 0.45 g per liter]
  Cisternal: 10 to 20 mg per 100 ml [0.10 to 0.20 g per liter]
  Ventricular: 1 to 15 mg per 100 ml [0.01 to 0.15 g per liter]
γ globulin: <12 percent of total protein [<0.12]

CHEMICAL CONSTITUENTS OF BLOOD[3]

See also "Function Tests," especially "Metabolic and Endocrine."

Acetoacetate, plasma: <0.3 mmol per liter
Albumin, serum: 3.5 to 5.5 g per 100 ml [35 to 55 g per liter]

[2] *Since cerebrospinal fluid concentrations are equilibrium values, measurement of blood plasma obtained at the same time is recommended.*
[3] *IU = international units.*

Aldolase: 0 to 8 IU per liter [0 to 130 nmol/s per liter]

α-Amino nitrogen, plasma: 3.0 to 5.5 mg per 100 ml [2.1 to 3.9 mmol per liter]

Aminotransferases, serum:

Aspartate (AST): 10 to 40 Karmen units; 6 to 18 IU per liter [100 to 300 nmol/s per liter]

Alanine (ALT): 10 to 40 Karmen units; 3 to 26 IU per liter [50 to 430 nmol/s per liter]

Ammonia, whole blood, venous: 30 to 70 μg per 100 ml [17.6 to 41.2 μmol per liter]

Amylase, serum: 60 to 180 Somogyi units per 100 ml; 0.8 to 3.2 IU per liter [13 to 53 nmol/s per liter]

Arterial blood gases:

[HCO_3^-]: 21 to 28 meq per liter [21 to 28 mmol per liter]

P_{CO_2}: 35 to 45 mmHg [4.7 to 6.0 kPa]

pH: 7.38 to 7.44

P_{O_2}: 80 to 100 mmHg [11 to 13 kPa]

Ascorbic acid, serum: 0.4 to 1.0 mg per 100 ml [23 to 57 μmol per liter]

Leukocytes: 25 to 40 mg per 100 ml [1420 to 2270 μmol per liter]

Barbiturates, serum: nondetectable

Phenobarbital, "potentially fatal" level (Schreiner): approximately 9 mg per 100 ml [390 μmol per liter]

Most short-acting barbiturates: 3.5 mg per 100 ml [150 μmol per liter]

Base, total, serum: 145 to 155 meq per liter [145 to 155 mmol per liter]

β-Hydroxybutyrate, plasma: <0.5 mmol per liter

Bilirubin, total, serum (Malloy-Evelyn): 0.3 to 1.0 mg per 100 ml [5.1 to 17 μmol per liter]

Direct, serum: 0.1 to 0.3 mg per 100 ml [1.7 to 5.1 μmol per liter]

Indirect, serum: 0.2 to 0.7 mg per 100 ml [3.4 to 12 μmol per liter]

Bromides, serum: nondetectable

Toxic levels: >17 meq per liter; 150 mg per 100 ml [17 mmol per liter]

Bromsulphalein, BSP (5 mg per kilogram of body weight, intravenously): 5 percent or less retention after 45 min

Calcium, ionized: 2.3 to 2.8 meq per liter; 4.5 to 5.6 mg per 100 ml [1.1 to 1.4 μmol per liter]

Calcium, serum: 4.5 to 5.5 meq per liter; 9 to 11 mg per 100 ml [2.2 to 2.7 μmol per liter]

Carbon dioxide-combining power, serum (sea level): 21 to 28 meq per liter; 50 to 65 volume percent [21 to 28 mmol per liter]

Carbon dioxide content, plasma (sea level): 21 to 30 meq per liter; 50 to 70 volume percent [21 to 30 mmol per liter]

Carbon dioxide tension, arterial blood (sea level): 35 to 45 mmHg [4.7 to 6.0 kPa]

Carbon monoxide content, blood: symptoms with over 20 percent saturation of hemoglobin

Carcinoembryonic antigen (CEA): 0 to 2.5 ng/ml (in healthy nonsmokers) [0 to 2.5 μg per liter]

Carotenoids, serum: 50 to 300 μg per 100 ml [0.9 to 5.6 μmol per liter]

Ceruloplasmin, serum: 27 to 37 mg per 100 ml [1.8 to 2.5 μmol per liter]

Chlorides, serum (as Cl⁻): 98 to 106 meq per liter [98 to 106 mmol per liter]

Cholesterol: see Table A-2

Complement, serum:

Total hemolytic (CH_{50}): 150 to 250 units per milliliter

C3: 55 to 120 mg per 100 ml [0.55 to 1.20 g per liter]

C4: 20 to 50 mg per 100 ml [0.20 to 0.50 g per liter]

Copper, serum (mean ± 1 SD): 114 ± 14 μg per 100 ml [17.9 μmol per liter]

Cortisol (competitive protein binding): 5 to 20 μg per 100 ml at 8:00 A.M. [0.14 to 0.55 μmol per liter]

Creatine phosphokinase, serum:

Females: 5 to 25 units per milliliter [0.08 to 0.42 mmol/s per liter]

Males: 5 to 35 units per milliliter [0.08 to 0.58 mmol/s per liter]

Creatinine, serum: < 1.5 mg per 100 ml [< 133 μmol per liter]

Dilantin, plasma:

Therapeutic level: 10 to 20 μg/ml [40 to 79 μmol per liter]

Toxic level: >30 μg/ml [>119 μmol per liter]

Ethanol, blood:

Mild to moderate intoxication: 80 to 200 mg per 100 ml [17 to 43 mmol per liter]

Marked intoxication: 250 to 400 mg per 100 ml [54 to 87 mmol per liter]

Severe intoxication: >400 mg per 100 ml [>87 mmol per liter]

Fatty acids, free (nonesterified), plasma: <0.7 mmol per liter

Fibrinogen, plasma: 160 to 415 mg per 100 ml [0.5 to 1.4 μmol per liter]

Fibrinogen split products: titer 1:4 or less

Folic acid, serum: 6 to 15 ng/ml [14 to 34 nmol per liter]

γ-Glutamyl transferase (transpeptidase), serum: 4 to 60 IU per liter [0.07 to 1.00 μmol/s per liter]

Gastrin, serum: 40 to 150 pg/ml [40 to 150 ng per liter]

Globulins, serum: 2.0 to 3.0 g per 100 ml [20 to 30 g per liter]

Glucose (fasting), plasma:

Normal: 75 to 105 mg per 100 ml [4.2 to 5.8 mmol per liter]

Diabetes mellitus: >140 mg per 100 ml (on more than one occasion) [>7.8 mmol per liter]

Glucose, 2 h postprandial, plasma:

Normal: <140 mg per 100 ml [<7.8 mmol per liter]

Impaired glucose tolerance: 140 to 200 mg per 100 ml [7.8 to 11.1 mmol per liter]

Diabetes mellitus: >200 mg per 100 ml [>11.1 mmol per liter]

Hemoglobin, blood (sea level):

Males: 14 to 18 g per 100 ml [8.7 to 11.2 mmol per liter]

Females: 12 to 16 g per 100 ml [7.4 to 9.9 mmol per liter]

Immunoglobulins, serum:

IgA: 90 to 325 mg per 100 ml [0.9 to 3.2 g per liter]

TABLE A-2
Pressures: intracardiac and intraarterial

Site	Representative, mmHg	Range
Aorta:		
Systolic	120	100–140 mmHg [13.3–18.7 kPa]
Diastolic	70	60–90 mmHg [8.0–12.0 kPa]
Atrium:		
Left (mean)	8	2–12 mmHg [0.3–1.6 kPa]
Right (mean)	3	0–5 mmHg [0–0.07 kPa]
Pulmonary artery:		
Systolic	25	15–30 mmHg [2.0–4.0 kPa]
Diastolic	10	3–13 mmHg [0.4–1.7 kPa]
Wedge (mean)	9	5–13 mmHg [0.7–1.7 kPa]
Ventricle, left:		
Systolic	120	100–140 mmHg [13.3–18.7 kPa]
Diastolic	8	4–12 mmHg [0.5–1.6 kPa]
Ventricle, right:		
Systolic	25	15–30 mmHg [2.0–4.0 kPa]
Diastolic	3	0–5 mmHg [0–0.7 kPa]
Venous, antecubital	100	5–14 cmH2O [0.5–1.4 kPa]

SOURCE: *Based on data in Altman, Dittmer (eds.), Respiration and Circulation, Bethesda, Federation of American Societies for Experimental Biology, 1971.*

IgE: <0.025 mg per 100 ml [<0.00025 g per liter]
IgG: 800 to 1500 mg per 100 ml [8.0 to 15 g per liter]
IgM: 45 to 150 mg per 100 ml [0.45 to 1.5 g per liter]
Iron, serum:
  Males and females (mean ± 1 SD): 105 ± 35 μg per 100 ml [19 ± 6 μmol per liter]
Iron-binding capacity, serum (mean ± 1 SD): 305 ± 32 μg per 100 ml [55 ± 6 μmol per liter]
  Saturation: 20 to 45 percent
Ketones, total: 0.5 to 1.5 mg per 100 ml [5 to 15.0 mg per liter]
Lactate dehydrogenase, serum:
  200 to 450 units per milliliter (Wrobleski)
  60 to 100 units per milliliter (Wacker)
  25 to 100 IU per liter [0.4 to 1.7 μmol/s per liter]
Lactic acid, blood: <1.2 mmol per liter
Lead, serum: <20 μg per 100 ml [<1.0 μmol per liter]
Lipase, serum: 1.5 units (Cherry-Crandall)
Lipids: see Table A-2
Lipids, triglyceride, serum: 50 to 150 mg per 100 ml [0.5 to 1.5 g per liter]
Magnesium, serum: 1.5 to 2.5 meq per liter; 2 to 3 mg per 100 ml [0.8 to 1.3 mmol per liter]
Nitrogen, nonprotein, serum: 15 to 35 mg per 100 ml [0.15 to 0.35 g per liter]
5'-Nucleotidase, serum: 0.3 to 2.6 Bodansky units per 100 ml [27 to 233 nmol/s per liter]
Osmolality, serum: 280 to 300 mosmol per kilogram of serum water
Oxygen content:
  Arterial blood (sea level): 17 to 21 volume percent
  Venous blood, arm (sea level): 10 to 16 volume percent
Oxygen percent saturation (sea level):
  Arterial blood: 97 percent [0.97 mol/mol]
  Venous blood, arm: 60 to 85 percent [0.60 to 0.85 mol/mol]
Oxygen tension, blood: 80 to 100 mmHg [11 to 13 kPa]
pH, blood: 7.38 to 7.44
Phosphatase, acid, serum:
  Bessey-Lowry method: 0.10 to 0.63 unit [28 to 175 nmol/s per liter]
  Bodansky method: 0.5 to 2.0 units
  Fishman-Lerner (tartrate sensitive): <0.6 unit per 100 ml (up to 0.15 unit per 100 ml)
  Gutman method: 0.5 to 2.0 units
  International units: 0.2 to 1.8 [3 to 30 nmol/s per liter]
  King-Armstrong method: 1.0 to 5.0 units
  Shinowara method: 0.0 to 1.1 units
Phosphatase, alkaline, serum:
  Bessey-Lowry method: 0.8 to 2.3 units (3.4 to 9 units[4])
  Bodansky method: 2.0 to 4.5 units (3.0 to 13.0 units[4]) [0.18 to 0.40 nmol/s per liter]
  Gutman method: 2.0 to 4.5 units (3.0 to 13.0 units[4])
  International units: 21 to 91 per liter at 37°C [0.4 to 1.5 μmol/s per liter]

[4] *Values in parentheses are those found in children.*

King-Armstrong method: 4.0 to 13.0 units (10.0 to 20.0 units[4])
  Shinowara method: 2.2 to 8.6 units
Phospholipids, serum: 150 to 250 mg per 100 ml (as lecithin) [48 to 81 mmol per liter]
Phosphorus, inorganic, serum: 1 to 1.5 meq per liter; 3 to 4.5 mg per 100 ml [1.0 to 1.4 mmol per liter]
Potassium, serum: 3.5 to 5.0 meq per liter [3.5 to 5.0 mmol per liter]
Proteins, total, serum: 5.5 to 8.0 g per 100 ml [55 to 80 g per liter]
Protein fractions, serum:
  Albumin: 3.5 to 5.5 g per 100 ml (50 to 60 percent) [35 to 55 g per liter]
  Globulin: 2.0 to 3.5 g per 100 ml (40 to 50 percent) [20 to 35 g per liter]
    α_1: 0.2 to 0.4 g per 100 ml (4.2 to 7.2 percent) [2 to 4 g per liter]
    α_2: 0.5 to 0.9 g per 100 ml (6.8 to 12 percent) [5 to 9 g per liter]
    β: 0.6 to 1.1 g per 100 ml (9.3 to 15 percent) [6 to 11 g per liter]
    γ: 0.7 to 1.7 g per 100 ml (13 to 23 percent) [7 to 17 g per liter]
Pyruvic acid, blood: <0.15 mmol per liter [<150 μmol per liter]
Salicylate, plasma: 0 mmol per liter
  Therapeutic range: 20 to 25 mg per 100 ml [1.4 to 1.8 mmol per liter]
  Toxic range: >30 mg per 100 ml [2.2 mmol per liter]
Sodium, serum: 136 to 145 meq per liter [136 to 145 mmol per liter]
Steroids: see "Metabolic and Endocrine" under "Function Tests"
Transaminase, serum glutamic oxaloacetic (SGOT): 10 to 40 Karmen units per milliliter; 6 to 18 IU per liter [0.10 to 0.30 μmol/s per liter]
Transaminase, serum glutamic pyruvic (SGPT): 10 to 40 Karmen units per milliliter; 3 to 26 IU per liter [0.05 to 0.43 μmol/s per liter]
Transferase, γ-glutamyl, serum: 4 to 60 IU per liter [0.07 to 1.00 μmol/s per liter]
Triglycerides: see Table A-3
Urea nitrogen, whole blood: 10 to 20 mg per 100 ml [3.6 to 7.1 mmol per liter]
Uric acid, serum:
  Males: 2.5 to 8.0 mg per 100 ml [0.15 to 0.48 mmol per liter]
  Females: 1.5 to 6.0 mg per 100 ml [0.09 to 0.36 mmol per liter]

TABLE A-3
Plasma lipid concentrations in normal subjects*

Age, years	Total serum cholesterol (both sexes), mg/100 ml [mmol/liter]	LDL cholesterol (both sexes), mg/100 ml	HDL cholesterol, mg/100 ml		Triglyceride (both sexes), mg/100 ml [mmol/liter]
			Male	Female	
0–19	120–230 [3.1–5.9]	50–170	30–65	30–70	10–140 [0.1–1.6]
20–29	120–240 [3.1–6.2]	60–170	35–70	35–75	10–140 [0.1–1.6]
30–39	140–270 [3.6–7.0]	70–190	30–65	35–80	10–150 [0.1–1.7]
40–49	150–310 [3.9–8.0]	80–190	30–65	40–85	10–160 [0.1–1.8]
50–59	160–330 [4.1–8.5]	80–210	30–65	35–85	10–190 [0.1–2.1]

* *Statistical ranges, not ideal values.*
SOURCE: *After DS Frederickson et al, N Engl J Med 276:151, 1967.*

Vitamin A, serum: 20 to 100 μg per 100 ml [0.7 to 3.5 μmol per liter]

Vitamin B₁₂, serum: 200 to 600 pg per ml [148 to 443 pmol per liter]

Zinc, serum (mean ± 1 SD): 120 ± 20 μg per 100 ml [18 ± 3 μmol per liter]

FUNCTION TESTS

Circulation

Arteriovenous oxygen difference: 30 to 50 ml per liter

Cardiac output (Fick): 2.5 to 3.6 liters per square meter of body surface area per minute

Circulation time:
  Arm to lung, ether: 2 to 12 s
  Arm to tongue:
    Calcium gluconate: 12 to 18 s
    Decholin: 10 to 16 s
    Saccharin: 9 to 16 s

Ejection fraction, stroke volume/end-diastolic volume (SV/EDV):
  Normal range: 0.55 to 0.78
  A₁: 0.67

Left ventricular work:
  Stroke work index: 30 to 110 (g·m)/m²
  Left ventricular minute work index: 1.8 to 6.6 [(kg·m)/m²]/min
  Oxygen consumption index: 110 to 150 ml per liter

Pressures, intracardiac and intraarterial: see Table A-2

Pulmonary vascular resistance: 20 to 120 (dyn·s)/cm⁵ [2 to 12 kPa·s per liter]

Systemic vascular resistance: 770 to 1500 (dyn·s)/cm⁵ [77 to 150 kPa·s per liter]

Systolic time intervals: see Table A-4

Gastrointestinal   See also "Stool."

Absorption tests:
  D-Xylose absorption test: After an overnight fast, 25 g xylose is given in aqueous solution by mouth. Urine collected for the following 5 h should contain 5 to 8 g [33 to 53 mmol] (or >20 percent of ingested dose). Serum xylose should be 25 to 40 mg per 100 ml 1 h after the oral dose [1.7 to 2.7 mmol per liter].
  Vitamin A absorption test: A fasting blood specimen is obtained and 200,000 units of vitamin A in oil is given by mouth. Serum vitamin A levels should rise to twice fasting level in 3 to 5 h.

TABLE A-4
Systolic time intervals in normal individuals (in milliseconds)

Regression equation	SD of index
QS₂ (M) = −2.1 HR + 546	14
QS₂ (F) = −2.0 HR + 549	14
PEP (M) = −0.4 HR + 131	13
PEP (F) = −0.4 HR + 133	11
LVET (M) = −1.7 HR + 413	10
LVET (F) = −1.6 HR + 418	10

NOTE: *QS₂ = total electromechanical systole, PEP = preejection phase, LVET = left ventricular ejection time, HR = heart rate, M = male, F = female, SD = standard deviation of the systolic time interval index.*
SOURCE: *AM Weissler, CL Garrard, Mod Concepts Cardiovasc Dis 40:1, 1971.*

Gastric juice:
  Volume:
    24 h: 2 to 3 liters
    Nocturnal: 600 to 700 ml
    Basal, fasting: 30 to 70 ml/h
  Reaction:
    As pH: 1.6 to 1.8
    Titratable acidity of fasting juice: 15 to 35 meq/h [4 to 10 μmol/s]
  Acid output:
    Basal:
      Females (mean ± 1 SD): 2.0 ± 1.8 meq/h [0.6 ± 0.5 μmol/s]
      Males (mean ± 1 SD): 3.0 ± 2.0 meq/h [0.8 ± 0.6 μmol/s]
    Maximal [after subcutaneous histamine acid phosphate 0.004 mg/kg and preceded by 50 mg promethazine (Phenergan); or after betazole (Histalog) 1.7 mg/kg or pentagastrin 6 μg/mg]:
      Females (mean ± 1 SD): 16 ± 5 meq/h [4.4 ± 1.4 μmol/s]
      Males (mean ± 1 SD): 23 ± 5 meq/h [6.4 ± 1.4 μmol/s]
    Basal acid output/maximal acid output ratio: 0.6 or less

Gastrin, serum: 60 to 160 pg/ml [60 to 160 ng per liter]

Secretin test (pancreatic exocrine function): 1 unit per kilogram of body weight, intravenously
  Volume (pancreatic juice): >2.0 ml/kg in 80 min
  Bicarbonate concentration: >80 meq per liter [>80 mmol per liter]
  Bicarbonate output: >10 meq in 30 min [>10 mmol in 30 min]

Metabolic and endocrine

Adrenal function tests: see Chap. 336

Adrenal steroid values including cortisol, aldosterone, and adrenal androgens: see Table 336-1

Catecholamines, urinary excretion:
  Free catecholamines: <100 μg per day
  Metanephrine: <1.3 mg per day
  Vanyllylmandelic acid (VMA): <8 mg per day [<40 μmol per day]

Estradiol, plasma:
  Women: 20 to 60 pg/ml [0.07 to 0.22 nmol per liter], higher at ovulation
  Men: <50 pg/ml [<0.18 nmol per liter]

Gonadotropins:
  Women, mature, premenopausal, except at ovulation:
    FSH: 5 to 30 mIU/ml
    LH: 5 to 20 mIU/ml
  Ovulatory surge:
    FSH: 5 to 20 mIU/ml
    LH: 15 to 40 mIU/ml
  Postmenopausal:
    FSH: >30 mIU/ml
    LH: >30 mIU/ml
  Men, mature:
    FSH: 5 to 20 mIU/ml
    LH: 5 to 20 mIU/ml
  Children of both sexes, prepubertal:
    FSH: <5 mIU/ml
    LH: <5 mIU/ml

Gonadal function tests: see Chaps. 341 and 342

17-Hydroxyprogesterone: <2 ng/ml

Insulin, serum or plasma, fasting: 6 to 26 μIU/ml [43 to 186 pmol per liter]

Pancreatic islet function tests: see Chap. 331
Parathyroid function tests: see Chap. 350
Pituitary function tests: see Chap. 333
Progesterone:
  Men, preovulatory women, and postmenopausal women: <2 ng/ml [<6 nmol per liter]
  Women, postovulatory: >5 ng/ml [>16 nmol per liter]
Prolactin, serum: 2 to 15 ng/ml
Renin-angiotensin function tests: see Chap. 333
Thyroid function tests:
  Dynamic tests of thyroid function: see Chap. 335
  Radioactive iodine uptake, 24 h: 5 to 35 percent (range varies widely in specific geographic areas owing to variations in iodine intake)
  Resin T_3 uptake: 25 to 55 percent (varies among laboratories)
  Thyroxine (radioimmunoassay): 5 to 12 μg per 100 ml [64 to 154 nmol per liter]
  Triiodothyronine (radioimmunoassay): 80 to 160 ng per 100 ml [1.2 to 2.5 nmol per liter]
  TSH (radioimmunoassay): 0 to 6 μU/ml [0 to 6 × 10^{-3} IU per liter]

Pulmonary See Tables A-5 and A-6.

Arterial blood gas measurements in normal subjects (sea level):
  P_{CO_2}, seated (mean ± 1 SD): 38.0 ± 2.9 mmHg (no change with age) [5.0 kPa]
  P_{O_2}:
    Seated (mean ± 1 SD): (104.2 ± 0.27 mmHg) × age in years [13.8 kPa]
    Supine (mean ± 1 SD): (103.5 ± 0.42 mmHg) × age in years [13.8 kPa]

Renal

Clearances (corrected to 1.72 m² body surface area):
  Measures of glomerular filtration rate:
    Inulin clearance (Cl):
      Males (mean ± 1 SD): 124 ± 25.8 ml/min [2.1 ± 0.4 ml/s]
      Females (mean ± 1 SD): 119 ± 12.8 ml/min [2.0 ± 0.2 ml/s]
    Endogenous creatinine: 91 to 130 ml/min [1.5 to 2.2 ml/s]
    Urea: 60 to 100 ml/min [1.0 to 1.7 ml/s]
  Measures of effective renal plasma flow and tubular function:

TABLE A-5
Normal spirometric values for seated subjects

Age, years	Men	Women
FORCED EXPIRATORY VOLUME IN 1 s (FEV₁), LITERS		
20–39	3.11–4.64	2.16–3.65
40–59	2.45–3.98	1.60–3.09
60–70	2.09–3.32	1.30–2.53
FEV₁/VITAL CAPACITY (FEV%)		
20–39	77	82
40–59	70	77
60–70	66	74
MAXIMAL MIDEXPIRATORY FLOW (MMEF₂₅₋₇₅%), LITERS/s		
20–39	3.8	3.4
40–59	2.8	2.2
60–70	2.2	1.6

TABLE A-6
Prediction formulas* for lung volumes and spirometric tests in seated subjects

	Age (A), to nearest year	Height (H), m	Weight (W), kg	Constant (C)	Residual standard deviation (RSD)
MEN					
TLC, liters		+6.92	−0.017	− 4.30	0.67
VC, liters	−0.020	+4.81		− 2.81	0.50
FRC, liters	+0.015	+5.30	−0.037	− 3.89	0.56
FRC/TLC, %	+0.18		−0.12	+52.3	6.8
FEV₁, liters	−0.033	+3.44		− 1.00	0.50
FEV%	−0.37			+91.8	7.2
MMEF₂₅₋₇₅%	−0.0523			+ 5.85	1.00
WOMEN					
TLC, liters	−0.015	+6.71		− 5.77	0.48
VC, liters	−0.022	+4.04		− 2.35	0.40
FRC, liters		+5.13	−0.028	− 4.50	0.41
FRC/TLC, %	+0.16		−0.08	+45.2	4.7
FEV₁, liters	−0.028	+2.67		− 0.54	0.36
FEV%	−0.26			+92.1	5.4
MMEF₂₅₋₇₅%	−0.0579			+ 5.63	0.71

* Answer = (A × age) + (H × height) + (W × weight) + C ± 2 RSD. Example: The normal value and lower limit for the FEV₁ are sought in a man, age 40 years, height 1.77 m, and weight 76 kg. The following equation gives the normal value:

$$FEV_1 = (-0.033 \times 40) + (3.44 \times 1.77) + (-1.00) = 3.77 \text{ liters}$$

The lower limit of normal:

$$3.77 - 2 \times 0.50 = 2.77 \text{ liters}$$

Only 2.5% of a normal population will fall below this value (2 SD below the mean). NOTE: FRC = functional residual capacity; FEV₁ = forced expiratory volume in 1 s; FEV% = FEV₁ expressed as percent of nonforced expiratory VC; MMEF₂₅₋₇₅% = mean flow rate during the middle half of the forced expiratory vital capacity. SOURCE: G Birath et al, Acta Med Scand 173:193, 1963; G Grimby, B Söderholm, Acta Med Scand 173:199, 1963.

p-Aminohippuric acid (Cl_PAH):
  Males (mean ± 1 SD): 654 ± 163 ml/min
  Females (mean ± 1 SD): 594 ± 102 ml/min
Concentration and dilution test:
  Specific gravity of urine:
    After 12 h fluid restriction: 1.025 or more
    After 12 h deliberate water intake: 1.003 or less
Phenolsulfonphthalein:
  After intravenous injection:
    Excretion in urine in 15 min: 25 percent or more
    Excretion in urine in 2 h: 55 to 75 percent
Protein excretion, urine: <150 mg in 24 h [<0.15 g per day]
  Males: 0 to 60 mg in 24 h [0 to 0.06 g per day]
  Females: 0 to 90 mg in 24 h [0 to 0.09 g per day]
Specific gravity, maximal range: 1.002 to 1.028
Tubular reabsorption, phosphorus: 79 to 94 percent of filtered load

HEMATOLOGIC EXAMINATIONS

See also "Chemical Constituents of Blood."

Bone marrow See Table A-7.

Erythrocytes and hemoglobin See also Table A-8.

Carboxyhemoglobin:
  Nonsmoker: 0 to 2.3 percent
  Smoker: 2.1 to 4.2 percent
Fragility, osmotic:
  Slight hemolysis: 0.45 to 0.39 percent
  Complete hemolysis: 0.33 to 0.30 percent

TABLE A-7
Differential nucleated cell counts of bone marrow

	Normal,* mean %	Range†	AGL	CGL	CLL	Multiple myeloma	Hemolytic anemia
Myeloid:	56.7						
Neutrophilic series:	53.6						
Myeloblast	0.9	0.2–1.5	↑↑↑	↑			
Promyelocyte	3.3	2.1–4.1		↑			
Myelocyte	12.7	8.2–15.7		↑			
Metamyelocyte	15.9	9.6–24.6		↑			
Band	12.4	9.5–15.3		↑			
Segmented							
Eosinophilic series	3.1	1.2–5.3		↑			
Basophilic series	<0.1	0–0.2		↑			
Erythroid:	25.6						
Pronormoblasts	0.6	0.2–1.3					↑↑
Basophilic normoblasts	1.4	0.5–2.4					↑↑
Polychromatophilic normoblasts	21.6	17.9–29.2					↑↑
Orthochromatic normoblasts	2.0	0.4–4.6					↑↑
Megakaryocytes	<0.1						
Lymphoreticular:	17.8						
Lymphocytes	16.2	11.1–23.2			↑↑↑		
Plasma cells	1.3	0.4–3.9				↑↑↑	
Reticulum cells	0.3	0–0.9					

* From MM Wintrobe et al, Clinical Hematology, 7th ed, Philadelphia, Lea & Febiger, 1974.
†Range observed in 12 healthy men.
NOTE: AGL = acute granulocytic leukemia, CGL = chronic granulocytic leukemia, CLL = chronic lymphocytic leukemia.

TABLE A-8
Normal values at various ages

	Red blood cell count,* millions/mm³	Hemoglobin,* g/100 ml	Vol. packed RBCs,* ml/100 ml	Corpuscular values			
Age				MCV, fl	MCH, pg	MCHC, g/100 ml	MCD, µm
Days 1–13	5.1 ± 1.0†	19.5 ± 5.0†	54.0 ± 10.0†	106–98	38–33	36–34	8.6
Days 14–60	4.7 ± 0.9	14.0 ± 3.3	42.0 ± 7.0	90	30	33	8.1
3 months to 10 years	4.5 ± 0.7	12.2 ± 2.3	36.0 ± 5.0	80	27	34	7.7
11–15 years	4.8	13.4	39.0	82	28	34	
Adults:							
Females	4.8 ± 0.6	14.0 ± 2.0	42.0 ± 5.0	90 ± 7	29 ± 2	34 ± 2	7.5 ± 0.3
Males	5.4 ± 0.9	16.0 ± 2.0	47.0 ± 5.0	90 ± 7	29 ± 2	34 ± 2	7.5 ± 0.3

* The range of values represents almost the extremes of observed variations (93 percent or more) at sea level. The blood values of healthy persons should fall well within these figures.
NOTE: MCV = mean corpuscular volume, MCH = mean corpuscular hemoglobin, MCHC = mean corpuscular hemoglobin concentration, MCD = mean corpuscular diameter.
SOURCE: MM Wintrobe et al, Clinical Hematology, 7th ed, Philadelphia, Lea & Febiger, 1974.

Haptoglobin, serum (mean ± 1 SD): 128 ± 25 mg per 100 ml [1.3 ± 0.2 g per liter]

Hemochromogens, plasma: 3 to 5 mg per 100 ml [0.03 to 0.05 g per liter]

Hemoglobin, fetal: <2 percent of total

"Life span":
  Normal survival: 120 days
  Chromium, half-life ($T_{1/2}$): 28 days

Methemoglobin: up to 1.7 percent of total

Plasma iron turnover rate: 20 to 42 mg in 24 h (0.47 mg/kg)

Protoporphyrin, free erythrocyte (EP): 16 to 36 µg per 100 ml red blood cells [0.28 to 0.64 µmol per liter]

Reticulocytes: 0.5 to 2.0 percent of red blood cells

Sedimentation rate:
  Westergren: <15 mm in 1 h
  Wintrobe:
    Males: 0 to 9 mm in 1 h
    Females: 0 to 20 mm in 1 h

Leukocytes See Table A-9.

Platelets and coagulation

Bleeding time:
  Ivy method, 5-mm wound: 1 to 9 min
  Duke method: 1 to 4 min

Clot retraction, qualitative: apparent in 60 min, complete in <24 h, usually <6 h

Coagulation time (Lee-White):
  Majority and range (glass tubes): 9 to 15 min, 2 to 19 min
  Majority and range (siliconized tubes): both 20 to 60 min

TABLE A-9
Normal values

	Percent	Average	Minimum	Maximum
Total number, per mm³		7,000	4,300	10,000
Neutrophils:				
Juvenile and band	0–21	520	100	2,100
Segmented	25–62	3,000	1,100	6,050
Eosinophils	0.3–8	150	0	700
Basophils	0.6–1.8	30	0	150
Lymphocytes	20–53	2,500	1,500	4,000
Monocytes	2.4–11.8	430	200	950

Prothrombin time (Quick's one stage): comparable to normal control (with most thromboplastins, 11 to 16 s)

Partial thromboplastin time [PTT (Nye-Brinkhouse method)]: comparable to normal control (with standard technique, 68 to 82 s; activated, 32 to 46 s)

Plasma thrombin time: 13 to 17 s

Platelets (Brecher-Cronkite method): 290,000 (150,000 to 400,000) per cubic millimeter [2.9×10^{11} per liter]

Whole-clot lysis: >24 h

Schilling test

Excretion in urine of orally administered radioactive vitamin B_{12} following "flushing" parenteral injection of vitamin B_{12}: 7 to 40 percent

STOOL

Bulk:
  Wet weight: <197.5 (115 ± 41) g per day
  Dry weight: <66.4 (34 ± 16) g per day
Coproporphyrin: 400 to 1000 μg in 24 h [610 to 1500 nmol per day]
Fat (on diet containing at least 50 g fat): <7.0 (4.0 ± 1.5) g per day when measured on a 3-day (or longer) collection
  Percent of dry weight: <30.4 (13.3 ± 8.07)
  Coefficient of fat absorption: >93 percent
Fatty acid:
  Free: 1 to 10 percent of dry matter
  Combined as soap: 0.5 to 12 percent of dry matter
Nitrogen: <1.7 (1.4 ± 0.2) g per day
Protein content: minimal
Urobilinogen: 40 to 280 mg in 24 h [67 to 470 μmol per day]
Water: approximately 65 percent

URINE

See also "Metabolic and Endocrine" under "Function Tests."

Acidity, titratable: 20 to 40 meq in 24 h [20 to 40 mmol per day]

α-Amino nitrogen: 0.4 to 1.0 g in 24 h [28 to 71 mmol per day]

Ammonia: 30 to 50 meq in 24 h [30 to 50 mmol per day]

Amylase: 35 to 260 Somogyi units per hour

Amylase/creatinine clearance ratio [$(Cl_{am}/Cl_{cr}) \times 100$]: 1 to 5

Calcium (10 meq or 200 mg calcium diet): <7.5 meq in 24 h, <150 mg in 24 h [<3.8 mmol per day]

Catecholamines: <100 μg in 24 h

Copper: 0 to 25 μg in 24 h [0 to 0.4 μmol per day]

Coproporphyrins (types I and III): 100 to 300 μg in 24 h [150 to 460 nmol per day]

Creatine, as creatinine:
  Adult males: <50 mg in 24 h [<0.38 mmol per day]
  Adult females: <100 mg in 24 h [<0.76 mmol per day]

Creatinine: 1.0 to 1.6 g in 24 h [8.8 to 14 mmol per day]

Glucose, true (oxidase method): 50 to 300 mg in 24 h [0.3 to 1.7 mmol per day]

5-Hydroxyindoleacetic acid (5-HIAA): 2 to 9 mg in 24 h [10 to 47 μmol per day]

Ketones, total (mean ± 1 SD): 50.5 ± 30.7 mg in 24 h

Lactic dehydrogenase: 560 to 2050 units in 8 h urine

Lead: <0.08 μg/ml; <120 μg in 24 h [0.39 μmol per liter]

Protein: <50 mg in 24 h [<0.05 g per day]

Porphobilinogen: none

Potassium: 25 to 100 meq in 24 h (varies with intake) [25 to 100 mmol per day]

Sodium: 100 to 260 meq in 24 h (varies with intake) [100 to 260 mmol per day]

Urobilinogen: 1 to 3.5 mg in 24 h [1.7 to 5.9 μmol per day]

Vanillylmandelic acid (VMA): 0.7 to 6.8 mg in 24 h [3.5 to 34 μmol per day]

D-Xylose excretion: 5 to 8 g within 5 h after oral dose of 25 g [33 to 53 mmol in 5 h]

INDEX